# Medical-Surgical Nursing
## TOTAL PATIENT CARE

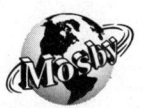

*Visit our website at* **www.mosby.com**

# NURSING CARE PLANS

# NURSING PROCESS BOXES

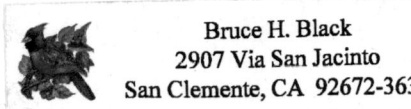

# Medical-Surgical Nursing
## TOTAL PATIENT CARE

**GAIL A. HARKNESS, DrPH, RN, FAAN**

Professor
University of Connecticut
School of Nursing
Storrs, Connecticut

**JUDITH R. DINCHER, RN, BSN, MSEd**

Professor Emeritus, Consultant
William Rainey Harper College
Department of Nursing
Palatine, Illinois

**TENTH EDITION**

*with 739 illustrations and 16 color plates*

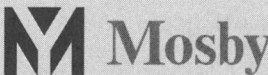
Mosby

*A Harcourt Health Sciences Company*

St. Louis   London   Philadelphia   Sydney   Toronto

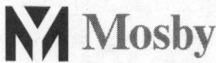

*A Harcourt Health Sciences Company*

Publisher: Sally Schrefer
Editor: Yvonne Alexopoulos
Associate Developmental Editor: Melissa K. Boyle
Project Manager: Patricia Tannian
Project Specialist: Suzanne C. Fannin
Design Manager: Gail Morey Hudson
Manufacturing Manager: Don Carlisle
Some illustrations drawn by Karen Merrill
Cover Design: Teresa Breckwoldt

**A Note to the Reader**

The author and publisher have made every attempt to check dosages and nursing content for accuracy. Because the science of pharmacology is continually advancing, our knowledge base continues to expand. Therefore we recommend that the reader always check product information for changes in dosage or administration before administering any medication. This is particularly important with new or rarely used drugs.

Mosby, Inc.
11830 Westline Industrial Drive
St. Louis, Missouri 63146

**Library of Congress Cataloging-in-Publication Data**

Medical-surgical nursing: total patient care/[edited by] Gail A.
Harkness, Judith R. Dincher. — 10th ed.
    p. cm.
  Includes bibliographical references and index.
  ISBN 0-323-00247-1 (alk. paper)
  1. Nursing.   I. Harkness, Gail A.   II. Dincher, Judith R.
RT41 .H65 1999
610.73—dc21                                                      98-46228

00  01  02  /  9  8  7  6  5  4  3  2

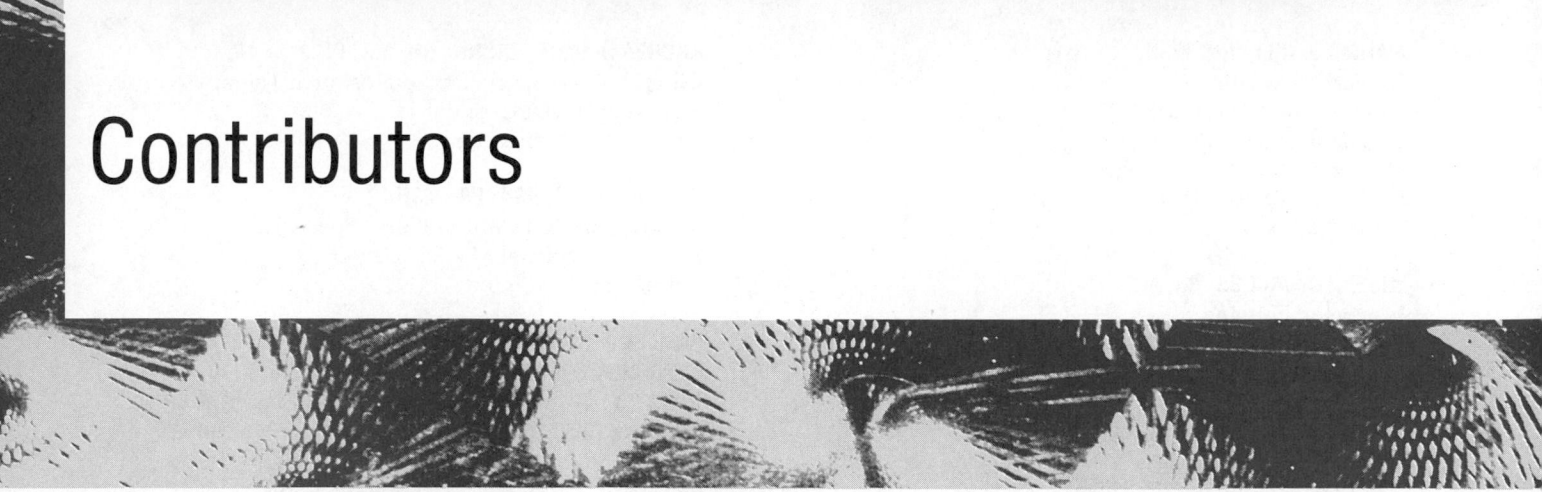

# Contributors

**LAURIE ANDREWS, RN, BSN, MPH**
HIV Clinical Trials Program Manager
AIDS Program, Yale University
New Haven, Connecticut

**JEAN K. BERRY, MS, PhD**
Clinical Assistant Professor
University of Illinois at Chicago
Chicago, Illinois

**SANDRA BLAKE, BSN, MS**
Infection Control Epidemiologist
Loyola University Medical Center
Maywood, Illinois

**JOYCE D. BLAU, RN, MS, ONC**
Clinical Nurse Specialist
Orthopaedics at Provena
St. Joseph Hospital
Lake Zurich, Illinois

**CATHERINE BENOIT, RNC, MSN**
Nurse Practitioner/Neurosurgery
Beth Israel-Deaconess Medical Center
Boston, Massachusetts

**CAROLE BOMBA, RN, MSN**
Adjunct Faculty, Nursing
William Rainey Harper College
Palatine, Illinois

**ANN CONNOR, RN, MS**
Stroke Nurse Specialist
Beth Israel-Deaconess Medical Center
Boston, Massachusetts

**CLAUDIA CONROY, RN, MS, AOCN**
Oncology Clinical Nurse Specialist
St. Alexius Medical Center
Hoffman Estates, Illinois

**JULIE A. D'AGOSTINO, RNC, BSN, MS, CEN, TNS**
Registered Nurse
Evanston Northwestern Healthcare
Evanston, Illinois

**CHERYL L. DURKEE, RN, BSN, MS**
Care Manager of Pulmonary Services
Lutheran General Hospital
Park Ridge, Illinois

**PATRICIA HENRY FOLCARELLI, BS, MA**
Clinical Nurse IV
Beth Israel-Deaconess Medical Center
Instructor of Surgery
Harvard Medical School
Boston, Massachusetts

**MARGARET M. GALLOWAY, RN, MSN**
Clinical Nurse Specialist
Allied Professional Staff
Alexian Brothers Medical Center
Elk Grove Village, Illinois

**ELAINE M. GEISSLER, RN, PhD, CTN**
Retired
School of Nursing, University of Connecticut
Storrs, Connecticut

**JEAN H. GENSTER, BSN**
Associate Professor of Nursing
William Rainey Harper College
Palatine, Illinois

**LISA L. HARRIS, RN, MS, CS**
Adult Nurse Practitioner
Hartford Hospital
Hartford, Connecticut

**MARCIA J. HILL, RN, MSN**
Clinical Associate
Office of Suzanne Bruce, MD, PA
Assistant Clinical Professor
Department of Dermatology
Baylor College of Medicine
Houston, Texas

**JOSEPH C. JACOBS, BA, MS**
Instructor, Nursing
William Rainey Harper College
Palatine, Illinois

**SANDRA KILGALLEN, ADN, BS, MEd**
Diabetes Nurse Educator
Team Leader, Nurse Educators
Joslin Diabetes Center
Boston, Massachusetts

**JEANNE LeVASSEUR, MS, RN, CS, FNP**
Assistant Professor
Quinnipiac College
Hamden, Connecticut

**KAREN S. MARTIN, RN, MSN, FAAN**
Health Care Consultant
Martin Associates
Omaha, Nebraska

**LORA McGUIRE, RN, MS**
Nursing Faculty and Pain Consultant
Joliet Junior College
Joliet, Illinois

**PATRICIA M. O'LEARY, MSN, RNCS**
Associate Professor/Clinical Specialist
William Rainey Harper College
Palatine, Illinois

**MILDRED OWINGS, RN, MSN, CS**
Professor
Patrick Henry Community College
Martinsville, Virginia

**MARION PHIPPS, MS, RN, CRRN, FAAN**
Rehabilitation Clinical Nurse Specialist
Beth Israel-Deaconess Medical Center
Boston, Massachusetts

**JOANNE M. PIER, RN, BSN, MA**
Consultant, Health Care Ethics
Menomonee Falls, Wisconsin

**E. CAROL POLIFRONI, BS, MA, EdD**
Associate Professor, School of Nursing
University of Connecticut
Storrs, Connecticut

**ANDREA D'AMATO QUINN, RN, MS, CS**
Clinical Nurse Specialist; Enterostomal Therapy Nurse
Yale New Haven Hospital
New Haven, Connecticut

**CLEO RICHARD, BSN, BA, MSN**
Medical-Surgical Clinical Nurse Specialist
St. Luke's Regional Medical Center
Boise, Idaho

**PAMELA J. SCHULTZ, RN, CRNO**
Clinical Nursing Coordinator: Ophthalmology
Rush Presbyterian St. Luke's Medical Center
Chicago, Illinois

**AMELIA K. SELPH, MN, RN, CS-ACNP, CCRN**
Nurse Practitioner
Columbia Nephrology Association
Columbia, South Carolina

**MARGARET HULL SPENCER, MS**
Family Nurse Practitioner
Trinity Hill Health Care Center
Hartford, Connecticut

**DONNA M. STARSIAK, RNC, MSN**
Assistant Professor, Medical-Surgical Nursing
Niehoff School of Nursing, Loyola University
Chicago, Illinois

**JEAN E. STEEL, RN, PhD, FAAN**
Professor and Chair
Advanced Practice Department
MGH Institute for Health Professionals
Boston, Massachusetts

**ELAINE SWEAT, MSN, APRN, CS**
Neuroscience Advanced Practice Nurse and Primary Care
    Nurse Practitioner
VA Healthcare System of Connecticut
West Haven/Newington, Connecticut

**PATRICIA TABLOSKI, PhD, RNCS, GNP**
Associate Professor
Boston College, School of Nursing
Chestnut Hill, Massachusetts

**PATRICIA TROTTA, RN, BSc, MSN, OCN**
Oncology Clinical Nurse Specialist
Veteran's Memorial Medical Center
Meriden, Connecticut

# Reviewers

**CARLA ABEL, MS, RNC**
Instructor
Iowa Western Community College
Council Bluffs, Iowa

**KATHY BLACK, MSN**
Assistant Professor
Iowa Western Community College
Council Bluffs, Iowa

**KATHLEEN M. BREWER, RN**
Chairman, Practical Nursing Programs
Delta Technical Institute
Jonesboro, Arkansas

**JEANNE COHEN, RN, EdD**
Nursing Instructor
Erwin Technical Center
Tampa, Florida

**SALLY FLESCH, RN, BSN, MA, EdS, PhD**
Chair, Allied Health Department
Black Hawk College
Moline, Illinois

**JOYCE HARRIS, RN, MAEd**
Director, Butler County Program-Practical Nurse Education
Butler County Joint Vocational School District
Hamilton, Ohio

**MARLENE MARTENSEN, BSN, RN**
Administrator, South Central Area Practical Nursing School
and School of Allied Health
South Central Area Practical Nursing School
West Plains, Missouri

**JOANN E. PEUTERBAUGH, MSN**
LPN Coordinator
Alton School District
Alton, Illinois

**ELAINE T. PRINCEVALLI, BSN, RN**
Instructor, Practical Nursing Education Program
State of Connecticut-Eli Whitney Regional Vocational
   Technical School
Hamden, Connecticut

**LYNN M. RIEBELING, RN, BSN**
LPN Instructor
Beck Area Vocational Center
Red Bud, Illinois

**SISTER BONAVENTURE SCHMEIDLER, RN, MSN**
Nursing Educator
Sisters of Charity
Mount St. Joseph, Ohio

**ALICE SKINNER, BSN, RN**
Clinical Nursing Instructor
Marion County School of Practical Nursing
Marion, South Carolina

**SHERRI L. SMITH, RN**
Practical Nursing Instructor
Delta Technical Institute
Jonesboro, Arkansas

**RUTH A. SPEAKMAN, BSN, MSEd**
Coordinator
Apollo School of Practical Nursing
Lima, Ohio

**SHIRLEY STAMFORD, BSN, RNC**
Practical Nursing Instructor
Hillsborough County School of Practical Nursing
Tampa, Florida

**KATHLEEN G. STILLING, RNC, MS**
Instructor
Johnston School of Practical Nursing
Baltimore, Maryland

**SHARON STINSON, RN, BSN, MA**
Clinical Nursing Instructor
The Health Institute of Louisville
Louisville, Kentucky

**FRANCES M. WARRICK, RN, BS, MS**
Program Coordinator, Vocational Nursing
El Centro College
Dallas, Texas

**KATHY WELLS, ADN, EMT-A**
Registered Nurse, EMT-A
HealthCare Plus
Pine Bluff, Arkansas

**KATHLEEN YOUNG, RN, BSN**
Practical Nursing Instructor
Greater Altoona Career Technology Center
Altoona, Pennsylvania

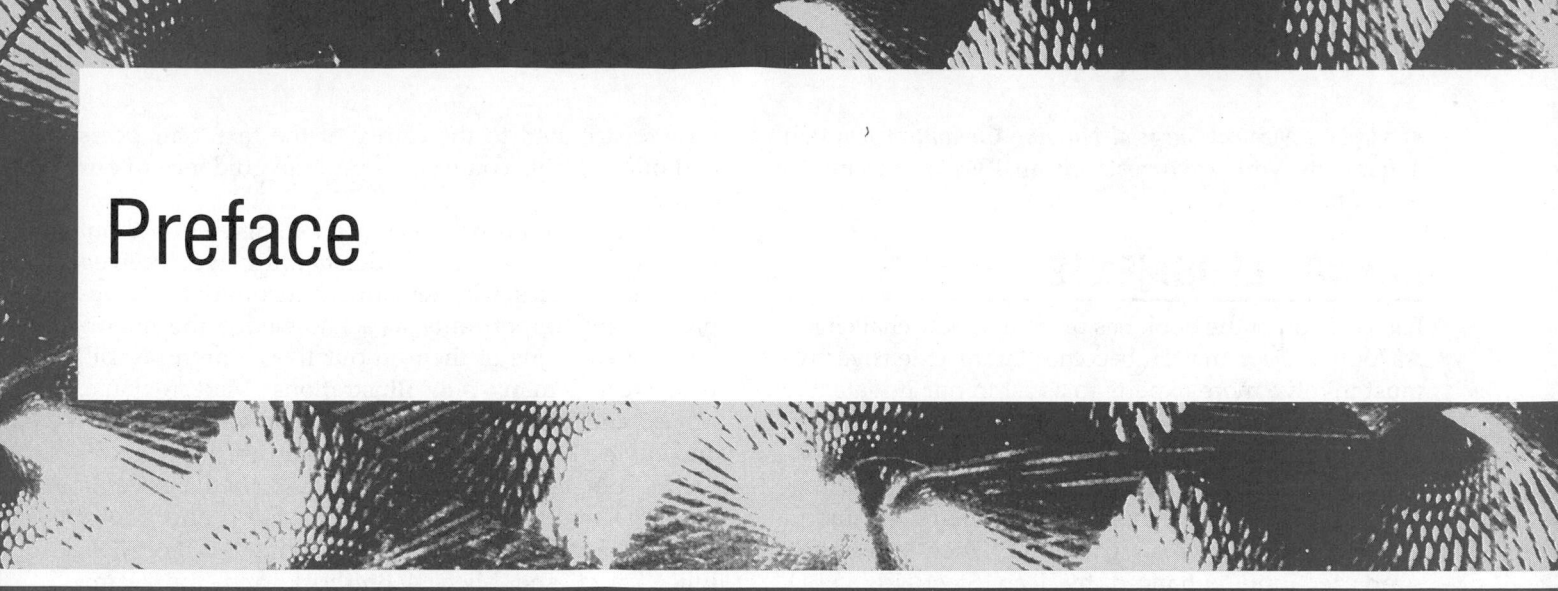

# Preface

*Medical-Surgical Nursing: Total Patient Care* has been a market favorite for 35 years and has served as a comprehensive text of adult health nursing for thousands of students embarking upon a technically focused nursing career. The tenth edition builds upon the strengths of this classic series of texts, addressing issues of contemporary nursing practice and providing the foundation to meet the needs of future health care demands.

This extensive revision features expanded content that includes new chapters on delegation and supervision of health assessment. Other chapters have been created to provide a clearer focus and increased content. These chapters include Cardiac Problems, Peripheral Vascular Problems, Hypertension, Arthritic and Rheumatic Problems, Neurologic Problems, Diabetes, Head and Spinal Cord Injuries, and Burns. The text continues to focus on the nursing process, with increased emphasis on patient teaching and older adult considerations. A contemporary look with many new illustrations provides visual appeal and enhances learning.

Boxes, tables, and numerous learning aids help students identify and retain important content. Each chapter contains critical thinking exercises, and most chapters also contain nurse alerts, older adult considerations, and ethical dilemma boxes to help prepare students for the realities of practice.

## LEARNING ENHANCEMENT FEATURES

- Completely revised and substantially expanded text.
- Chapter Objectives, Key Terms, and Key Concepts.
- Nursing Process boxes for key conditions that provide an increased focus on the nursing process.
- Medication tables for reference.
- Older Adult Considerations boxes with narrative discussions.
- Patient/Family teaching boxes and discussions.
- Ethical dilemma boxes based on realistic clinical scenarios.
- Nurse Alerts that emphasize critical responsibilities of the nurse and help with transition from theory to practice.
- Critical Thinking Exercises.
- Nursing Care Plans based on case studies that emphasize the nursing process.
- Consistent organization of disorder chapters, including a review of anatomy and physiology, diagnostic tests, and commonly occurring conditions.
- Inclusion of psychosocial factors that affect health and illness.
- Clear, readable writing style.

## TEACHING/LEARNING PACKAGE

- An accompanying workbook assists students to reinforce and evaluate their understanding of important concepts in the text. It includes a variety of learning activities such as key term exercises, clinical situations, matching exercises, crossword puzzles, and labeling and questions regarding text illustrations.
- The instructor's manual features a summary outline to aid faculty in class preparation. Critical thinking exercises for group discussion or written assignments are presented, along with guidelines for analysis of ethical dilemmas. Answers to workbook exercises are included. The revised test bank contains nearly 500 questions with answers.
- A CD-ROM Image Collection features key illustrations from the text.
- *Mosby's Instructor's Resource Kit* is a 3-ring binder that organizes all teaching materials in one handy location.

- *Mosby's Medical-Surgical Nursing Computest* lets you generate your own tests on an IBM or Macintosh computer.

## ACKNOWLEDGMENTS

Each edition of the book has presented new challenges. As our subject matter becomes more extensive, we must involve more experts to assist in our update. We have had the good fortune to work with many expert practitioners, and a special tribute belongs to our contributing authors. They accepted the challenge of presenting complicated technical information in an understandable and interesting format. Their work was supported and enhanced by Jean Steel, RN, PhD, FAAN, who served as editor during the majority of the manuscript development phase. We are grateful to all of our students, our fellow faculty members, our associates in clinical agencies, and the reviewers, whose efforts contributed to the clarity of the text. Our peers and our students continue to provide guidance to our efforts.

Our work could not have been completed without the love, patience, and understanding we received from our families, who remain our inspiration. We appreciate this opportunity to acknowledge the importance of each one of them in our lives: Karen Merrill, who created many new illustrations; Mike, Melanie, Mikey, and Maeanna Merrill, who provided support and advice; Doris and Ron Kerbs, who encouraged our work; Tom Dincher, husband, friend, and patriarch; John, Donna, Megan, Ryan, Bridget, and Colin Dincher; Todd, Liz, Zachary, and Samantha Bjur; Bob, Julie, Laura, and Michael Breshock; and Tom, Pam, Thomas, and John Kavanaugh.

**Gail A. Harkness**
**Judith R. Dincher**

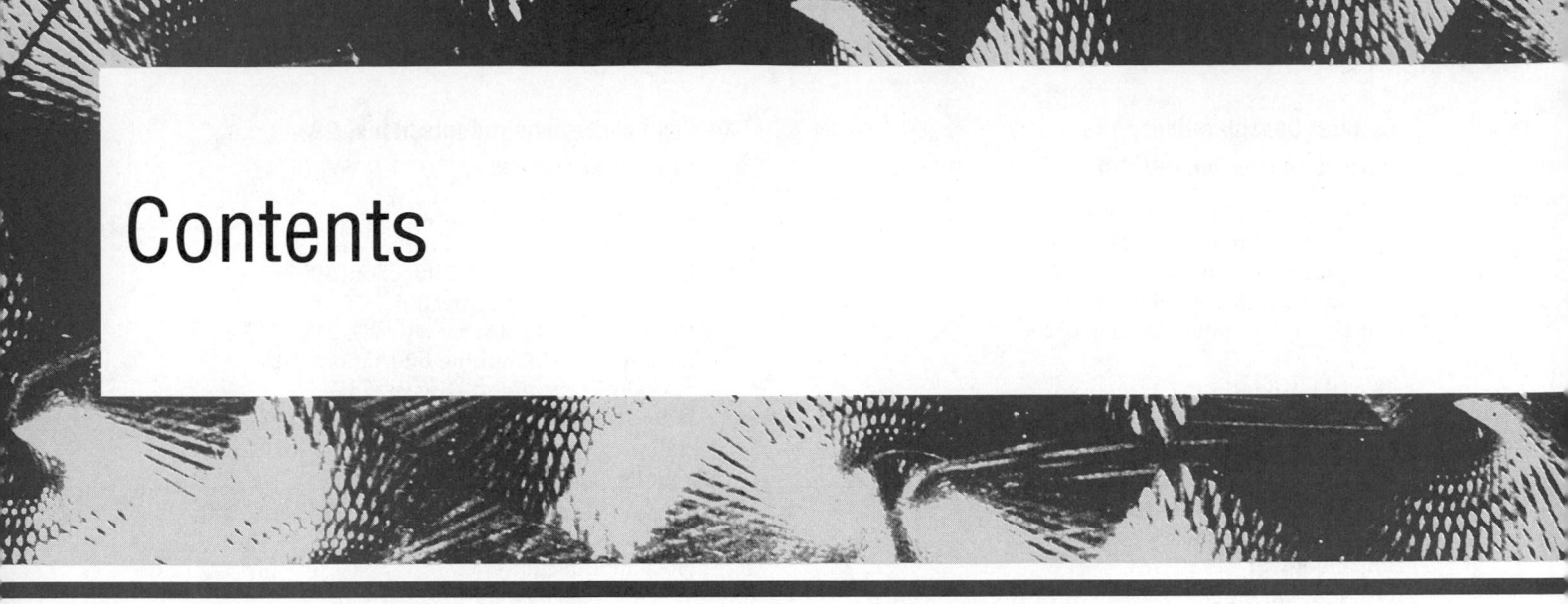

# Contents

# Nursing in the Health Care System

## KEY TERMS

acute care
ambulatory care
case management
diagnosis-related group (DRG)
extended care facility
functional nursing
health maintenance organization (HMO)
Healthy People 2000
holistic care
intermediate care facility (ICF)
long-term care
Medicaid
Medicare
multisystem
nonproprietary
preferred provider organization (PPO)
primary care
primary nursing
primary prevention
proprietary
prospective payment
quality assurance (QA) system
quality improvement (QI) system
retrospective payment
secondary prevention
skilled nursing facility (SNF)
standards
team nursing
tertiary prevention
total quality management (TQM) system

## TOTAL PATIENT CARE

Total patient care is a concept that serves as a basis for nursing practice. The word *total* means holistic, or whole, and it is used here to imply consideration of all human needs: physiologic, psychologic, sociocultural, developmental, and spiritual (Figure 1-1). Nurses

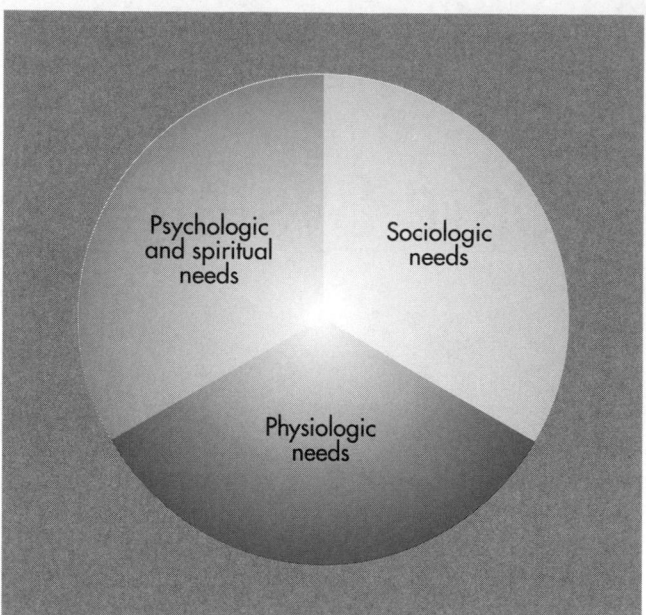

**Figure 1-1**   The total needs of the patient.

alone cannot meet all these needs, but they play a major role in identifying them and coordinating appropriate services and personnel. A patient is a person who is seeking health care. The word *patient* formerly implied a passive acceptance of services, but now the patient is viewed as an active participant in care and a thinking consumer of health services. Continued use of the term *patient* does not imply acceptance of a less active role for the health care consumer. The meaning of a word may change with time, and *patient* is used here to describe individuals who initiate, plan, and actively participate in their care. The word *care* refers to services that help patients maintain or regain optimum health. This text focuses on nursing care of medical and surgical patients who are hospitalized in an acute care or extended care facility to be cured, to improve after a specific illness or crisis, or to maintain optimum health.

## HEALTH

The World Health Organization (WHO, 1958), an agency of the United Nations that was established in 1948, defines health as "a state of complete physical, mental, and social well-being and not merely the absence of disease." Illness is an acute or chronic lack of adaptation to internal and environmental stressors. Implied in this concept is the belief that the body is constantly working to balance the internal environment (e.g., endocrine secretions, water, electrolytes, proteins, vitamins, minerals, and oxygen) as it re-

sponds to the stressors of the external environment. When the body is able to maintain this balance, or equilibrium, a state of homeostasis exists. Homeostasis is a dynamic process that requires constant bodily activity in response to change.

Because illness can arise from either deficiency or excess, the body must obtain needed materials and convert or eliminate excess materials. Stressors may be biologic (hemorrhage, bacterial toxins), psychologic (fear, worry), or sociologic (financial problems, marital difficulties), but all stressors produce a specific physiologic condition that requires adaptation. A person's ability to adapt to stressors varies; it depends on the individual's personal resources, the strength of the stressor, when the stressor appears, and whether its onset is gradual or sudden.

Society has begun to put greater emphasis on this complete state of well-being and on the values of preventive health care, health maintenance, physical fitness, and mental vigor. One national program launched to increase the healthy state of Americans is **Healthy People 2000**. This program addresses prevention of a wide range of disease conditions or reduction of serious complications. It also identifies the objectives of national health promotion and disease prevention that are to be incorporated into any national health program and is intended to serve as the foundation of any such plan (U.S. Department of Health and Human Services, 1990).

Efforts to prevent illness can be classified as primary, secondary, or tertiary. **Primary prevention** involves activities that promote general well-being and specific protection for selected diseases, such as immunizations for diphtheria, measles, and tetanus. **Secondary prevention** focuses on early diagnosis and implementation of measures that stop the progression of disease or handicapping disabilities. **Tertiary prevention** deals with rehabilitation of disabled patients to enable them to return to maximum usefulness (Stanhope, Lancaster, 1996).

## HEALTH CARE REFORM

The United States currently does not have a national health care system, but the government is developing new ways to provide universal care to all citizens. A variety of reform plans have been proposed, and each varies slightly in funding, implementation, and authority. President Bill Clinton's Health Security Act of 1993 called for universal access to affordable and appropriate health care. President Clinton believes that any system must incorporate "security, simplicity, savings, choice, quality, and responsibility" (Health Security Act of 1993, 1993).

In the early 1990s a group of 60 national nursing organizations developed and agreed to a "Nursing's Agenda for Health Care Reform" (American Nurses Association, 1991a). This agenda called on the public, legislators, and health care providers to reform their philosophy of care and to change their attitudes and systems to accommodate the public's demand for basic and equitable services. Universal access to quality care and affordable, appropriate services were key elements of the agenda.

Some type of health care reform will be initiated by the start of the twenty-first century. Nurse providers will be closely involved with and affected by the new direction of health care. A large number of nurses currently employed in hospitals will be relocated into community settings. It is estimated that by the year 2015, only one third of all nurses will work in a hospital setting; currently, two thirds of all nurses work in hospitals. Obviously this shift will affect the nursing profession, including where its members are educated and employed.

## Trends Affecting Health Care

The growing emphasis on preventing illness stems from the public's increasing awareness of health care. This awareness is only one of the trends affecting health care delivery in the United States. During the 1980s and 1990s many changes have occurred in society and health care, including demographic changes, scientific and technologic advances, and economic shifts.

The population of the United States is maturing. In 1900 the average life expectancy was 47 years, and only 4% of the population was 65 years of age or older. However, a baby boy born in 1992 can expect to live past age 73; a baby girl can expect to live past age 79. In 1994 the average life expectancy was 78 years for women and 72 years for men. The population of the United States was 260 million in 1994 and will exceed 275 million by the year 2000. In 1995 the majority of the population was female, and the median age was 34 years. Slightly more than 13% of the population was over 65 years of age, and that proportion is projected to increase to 14.9% by the year 2000. Scientific technology has advanced tremendously in the past 20 years, and these advances are reflected in modern health care. As death rates continue to decline, the number of frail elderly (generally considered to be those 85 years of age or older) will increase dramatically. Such increases in the older population will require more home care and long-term care facilities and more health care workers trained in geriatric care. The U.S. Bureau of the Census reports many statistics that

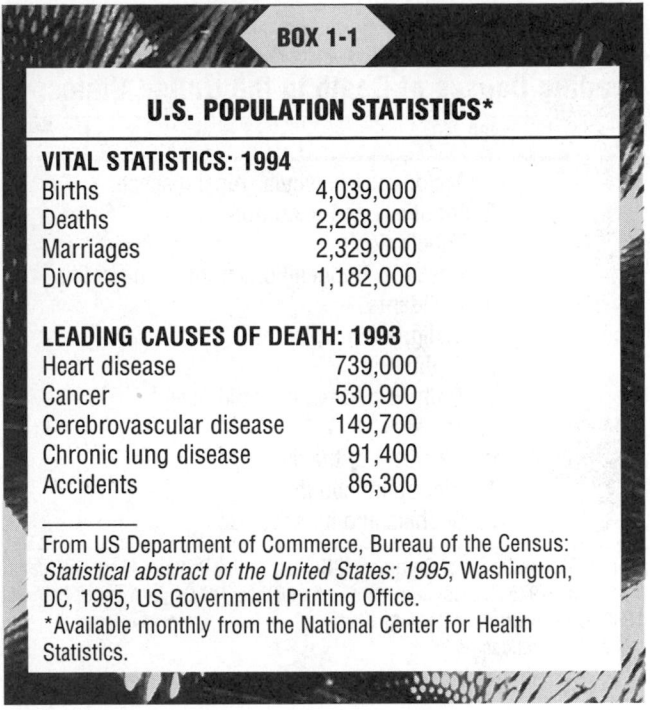

**BOX 1-1**

### U.S. POPULATION STATISTICS*

**VITAL STATISTICS: 1994**
| | |
|---|---|
| Births | 4,039,000 |
| Deaths | 2,268,000 |
| Marriages | 2,329,000 |
| Divorces | 1,182,000 |

**LEADING CAUSES OF DEATH: 1993**
| | |
|---|---|
| Heart disease | 739,000 |
| Cancer | 530,900 |
| Cerebrovascular disease | 149,700 |
| Chronic lung disease | 91,400 |
| Accidents | 86,300 |

From US Department of Commerce, Bureau of the Census: *Statistical abstract of the United States: 1995*, Washington, DC, 1995, US Government Printing Office.
*Available monthly from the National Center for Health Statistics.

are valuable in understanding the current demographics and that permit some latitude in projecting future changes (Box 1-1) (U.S. Department of Commerce, 1995).

Table 1-1 compares the leading causes of death in the United States in 1900 and 1990. A shift in causes of death from infectious diseases to noninfectious conditions is evident.

Emerging technologic advances in medicine are permitting an increasing number of outpatient diagnostic and therapeutic treatments. These advances are drastically reducing the inpatient stay for some procedures. A significant increase in same-day surgery has been noted. Also, many acute care requirements can be met in the home. New pharmaceuticals are developed almost weekly. Computerized information systems aid greatly in testing, interpretation, and diagnosis, bringing new dimensions to preventive health care. Computers are also used for scheduling, billing, payroll, budgeting, surveillance, ordering, documentation, and care plans; the list is endless.

Technologic advances have affected the economy of health care as well. Although many of these advances have reduced the cost of some services, the cost of research, development, and start-up for such technologies is high. The rising cost of health care and changes in reimbursement systems, discussed in more detail in the next section, have greatly affected health care delivery.

**TABLE 1-1**

## Leading Causes of Death in the United States: 1900 and 1990*

| 1900 | 1990 |
|------|------|
| 1. Major cardiovascular-renal diseases | 1. Diseases of the heart |
| 2. Influenza and pneumonia | 2. Malignant neoplasms |
| 3. Tuberculosis | 3. Cardiovascular accidents |
| 4. Gastritis, duodenitis, enteritis, and colitis | 4. Accidents |
| 5. Accidents | 5. Chronic obstructive pulmonary diseases |
| 6. Malignant neoplasms | 6. Pneumonia and influenza |
| 7. Diphtheria | 7. Diabetes mellitus |
| 8. Typhoid and paratyphoid fever | 8. Suicide |
| 9. Measles | 9. Chronic liver disease and cirrhosis |
| 10. Cirrhosis of the liver | 10. Human immunodeficiency virus |
| 11. Whooping cough | 11. Homicide and legal intervention |
| 12. Syphilis and its sequelae | 12. Nephritis, nephrotic syndrome, and nephrosis |

From US Department of Commerce, Bureau of the Census: *Historical statistics of the United States, colonial times to 1970, bicentennial edition,* part 2, Washington DC, 1975, US Government Printing Office; US Department of Commerce, Bureau of the Census: *Statistical abstracts of the United States,* Washington DC, 1995, US Government Printing Office.
*Excludes fetal deaths.

An increase in the "corporatization" of health care has brought a pervasive business orientation to the industry. The term *corporatization* refers to the development of the health care **multisystem**, an entity that manages a large network of health care facilities from a single corporate office. Such multisystems are believed to contain costs more efficiently than single institutions. Multisystem chains can include anything that concerns health care, such as hospitals, extended care facilities, health maintenance organizations (HMOs), clinics, outpatient facilities, pharmacies, medical supply distributors, and health insurance companies.

Multisystem chains include both national and regional systems that operate on a for-profit or a nonprofit basis. Managed care is a system instituted to control health care costs. Through the insurer, case managers review planned medical care, often prescribing the length of a hospital stay. Case managers often are nurses, who are employees of the insurance company.

The national economy also has also seen a steady increase in the standard of living and a concurrent rise in the demand for health care services. Inner cities and rural communities are particularly likely to have limited health care services and facilities, and both providers and residents are very concerned about access to affordable and appropriate care.

## Health Care Cost and Reimbursement

The gross national product (GNP) for health care was 10.7% in 1983; by 1996 it had exceeded 15% (Reddy, 1996). The United States currently spends more each year on health care than it does on national defense. Health expenditures totaled $247 billion in 1980, and 14 years later the amount had risen to $949 billion (The World Almanac and Book of Facts 1997, 1996) (Table 1-2). Enormous increases can be seen in hospital care, professional staff, drugs, nursing homes, and home care. Although people over 65 years of age make up only 12% of the population, they account for 29% of total health care expenditures (U.S. Department of Commerce, Bureau of the Census, 1995).

Since the inception of **Medicare** and **Medicaid,** the GNP for health care has more than tripled. Medicare and Medicaid are government programs that were created in 1965 through an amendment to the Social Security Act. These programs are funded by taxes on the earnings of those currently employed. Medicare is a federally administered health insurance program available to people over 65 years of age (regardless of income), to the disabled who have received Social Security benefits for more than 2 years, and to individuals with severe kidney disease. As with most private insurance plans, full Medicare coverage requires a monthly premium and involves a deductible charge for most services that must be paid by the individual or through supplemental private insurance. In 1996 this deductible was $42.50. The regulations for paid services change constantly and are difficult to interpret, both for the provider and the consumer (U.S. Department of Health and Human Services, 1996).

Medicaid is a cooperative federal and state medical assistance program for the poor. It is designed to cover areas that Medicare does not and to defray expenses

| TABLE 1-2 | | | | | |
|---|---|---|---|---|---|
| **Major Categories of U.S. Health Care Spending 1960-1994 (in Billions of Dollars)** | | | | | |
| CATEGORY | 1960 | 1970 | 1980 | 1990 | 1994 |
| Total national health care expenses | 26 | 73 | 247 | 697 | 949 |
| Hospital care | 9 | 28 | 102 | 256 | 338 |
| Professional services (other than physician or dentist) | 0.6 | 1.4 | 6.4 | 34.7 | 49.6 |
| Nursing home care | 0.8 | 4 | 18 | 51 | 72 |
| Home care | 0.1 | 0.2 | 2.4 | 13 | 26 |
| Drugs and nondurable equipment | 4 | 8 | 21 | 60 | 79 |
| Research and construction | 2 | 5 | 12 | 25 | 30 |
| Other | 9.5 | 26.4 | 85.2 | 257.3 | 354.4 |

From Famighetti R, editor: *The world almanac and book of facts 1997*, Mahwah, NJ, 1996, World Almanac Books.

for those who have exhausted their Medicare benefits or cannot meet the cost of Medicare contributions. The program is operated on a state level, but the federal government provides guidelines and a portion of the funds based on the per capita income of each state. A variety of benefits are available, and these differ from state to state. Medicare and Medicaid currently cover approximately 40% of health costs for the elderly and the poor. Many states have implemented major Medicaid reform, and other states will do so by the year 2000. The local state welfare office for Medicaid or the local Social Security office for Medicare can provide up-to-date information on the benefits available in a particular state.

Federal and state agencies, as well as private insurers, have implemented various regulations to curtail the upward spiral of health care costs through new incentive programs and payment systems. Until 1984 the traditional method of reimbursement for health care services was **retrospective payment** (i.e., all the costs of care were added up after they were incurred and eventually were paid by the government, private insurance companies, and the individual). In 1984 **prospective payment** was initiated in an attempt to curtail rising costs. This system, implemented by the Health Care Financing Agency (HCFA), requires hospitals to assign a **diagnosis-related group (DRG)** to all patients admitted as an incentive to reduce costs. The DRG system currently applies to acute care hospitals and long-term care institutions and covers any inpatient and outpatient health care service. The HCFA has established several hundred DRG codes, which are based on the physician's diagnosis, the patient's age and sex, and the required treatments. The DRG specifies the number of hospital days for which Medicare will pay. If a patient is discharged sooner than predicted for that DRG, the hospital profits. However, if a patient requires a longer stay, the hospital pays for the additional days. The DRG codes do not consider the

extensive nursing care some patients require. Managing patients who require intense nursing care has adversely affected institutional budgets.

Initially, implementation of DRGs affected only hospitalized Medicare patients. However, use of DRGs now has spread to the various prospective payment systems (PPSs) of many other government and private payors, including Medicaid, and is being extended to health care providers other than hospitals. Each type of PPS has a slightly different impact and its own advantages and disadvantages. DRGs have increased the emphasis on hospital discharge planning and hospital alternatives, such as skilled extended care, outpatient services, and home care. Although evidence shows that DRGs have helped cut some health care costs, critics find many shortcomings in the system. Their greatest concern is that DRGs put an emphasis on cost efficiency, perhaps at the expense of quality of care.

The new payment systems have vast implications for nursing because nurses constitute the major personnel expense in any hospital. The PPS provides an opportunity for nursing to demonstrate its value by clearly identifying nursing costs and by relating nursing care to positive patient outcomes. Nurses are in a position to maintain quality and cost-effective care as direct patient care providers and managers.

New methods of prepayment cannot provide all the answers to the problems of the troubled health care system. Designing systems that provide needed services to the uninsured is a major subject in state and federal legislatures and in health care reform. An estimated 39% of the total U.S. population has no health insurance and therefore has limited access to available services. Of those over 65 years of age, approximately 18% are not part of any health care insurance program. People significantly handicapped by the current health care payment system include single parents, the young, the homeless, individuals who have acquired immunodeficiency syndrome (AIDS), and the elderly.

# HEALTH CARE DELIVERY

Health care is provided in a variety of settings, such as hospitals, extended care facilities, HMOs, ambulatory care facilities, government and community health clinics, physicians' offices, nurses' offices, and patients' homes. More than 5 million people, including more than 2 million nurses, are involved in health care.

The health care system is divided into three areas of care: primary care (not to be confused with primary prevention), acute care, and long-term care. These terms also describe three areas of nursing practice and the three levels of care in the health care system.

**Primary care** is the first contact in a given episode of illness, and it leads to a decision on how to resolve the problem. This level of care is provided by the individual responsible for the continuum of care, which includes maintaining health, performing evaluations, managing symptoms, and making appropriate referrals. Primary care, then, is provided by physicians and advanced-practice nurses. The term *advanced-practice nurse* refers to the roles of nurse practitioner and clinical nurse specialist; it may also include the nurse midwife and nurse anesthetist. These primary care providers assume responsibility for the management of acute and chronic disease and for a variety of health promotion activities and services.

**Acute care** consists of services that treat the acute phase of illness or disability. In this type of care, the emphasis is on restoration of normal life processes and functions.

**Long-term care** consists of services that provide symptomatic treatment, maintenance, and rehabilitative services for patients of all ages in a variety of health care settings.

## Hospitals

Hospitals are the largest employers of nurses and other health care workers (Figure 1-2). They vary in size from fewer than 25 beds to more than 2000. A hospital may be governmental or nongovernmental, **proprietary** (for profit) or **nonproprietary** (nonprofit), and general or specialized (a children's hospital or cancer hospital). More than one third of all U.S. hospitals are owned, leased, managed, or sponsored by a health care multisystem.

A hospital has many departments, each of which is related to the total care of patients or to support services. Most hospitals have departments for nursing service; dietary and food service; laundry; business and finance; physical plant (maintenance, housekeeping); and other professional services such as radiology, a pharmacy, social service, speech therapy, respiratory therapy, a laboratory, and medical records. Many hospitals have education departments that oversee the orientation and continuing education of employees. Education may be undertaken within a specific department, such as nursing, or it may be central to the entire hospital. The volunteer department also is important. It includes auxiliary members, teenage volunteers, and friendly visitors. Volunteer workers provide support services and contribute to care without increasing costs.

Most hospitals provide both inpatient and outpatient services. Surgery, diagnostics, dialysis, and physical therapy are a few of the services that may be offered on an outpatient basis. Many hospitals also offer various wellness programs to the community.

## Extended Care Facilities

An **extended care facility**, also called a long-term care health center or nursing home, may be part of a hospital or may be a separate, freestanding institution. Most are proprietary organizations. These facilities provide nursing, medical, and rehabilitative care, as well as residential and personal services, to a wide range of patients. Residential care means providing a pleasant, healthy, and comfortable place to live, nutritious meals, clean laundry, barber and beautician services, and companionship. Personal care involves assistance with functional tasks such as dressing, bathing, toileting, eating, and walking. It also includes helping the resident to follow prescribed programs of medication, diet, and exercise and to attend scheduled activities. About 5% of those age 65 to 85 and 20% of those over age 85 make their homes in long-term care centers. The increase in the older population and the magnitude of

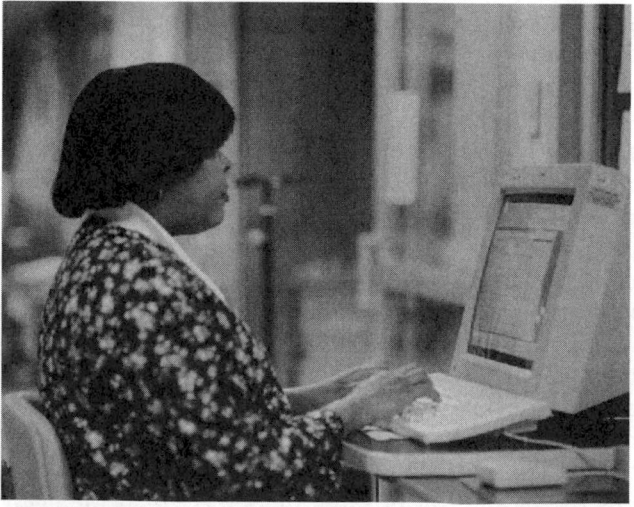

**Figure 1-2** Nurses and other health care workers manage patient information on a daily basis. (From Potter PA, Perry AG: *Fundamentals of nursing: concepts, process, and practice*, ed 4, St Louis, 1997, Mosby.)

their health needs have led to a proliferation of extended care facilities.

Long-term care centers can offer different levels of care. The Medicare and Medicaid programs have established two categories of extended care facilities. A **skilled nursing facility (SNF)** is a long-term facility that has been certified as being in compliance with federal standards. These facilities provide 24-hour nursing services, regular medical supervision, and rehabilitation therapy. An SNF cares for the recuperating patient who no longer needs acute nursing and medical attention but who still requires skilled nursing care. An **intermediate care facility (ICF)** is also certified as being in compliance with federal standards but provides less extensive health-related services and nursing supervision. These facilities primarily serve people who cannot live alone but who do not necessarily need 24-hour nursing care.

The terms *skilled nursing facility* and *intermediate care facility* describe the intensity of nursing care rather than the quality. Many extended care facilities are certified and licensed to provide their residents with both skilled nursing and intermediate care. Medicare and other third-party payors (insurance plans) do not pay to keep patients in a hospital beyond their need for hospital services. Therefore it is more cost-effective to move a patient to an extended care facility that provides skilled nursing care. Medicare covers at least part of a "period of illness," or up to 100 days of care in an SNF, but only after a hospital stay of at least 3 days. Medicaid also assists with the cost of care in an SNF and an ICF. For example, if care is needed beyond 100 days, the cost may be supplemented by Medicaid and private insurance programs.

Medicare and Medicaid programs are instituting a type of PPS for extended care facilities that is similar to the DRG categories currently used in hospitals. Local, federal, and state offices must be contacted for up-to-date information on these changes.

Care is also provided by continuing care retirement communities (CCRCs), which provide private housing to residents and access to an adjacent SNF. Preventing a temporary or permanent move away from one's home is viewed as a significant benefit for senior citizens and their families.

## Health Maintenance Organizations and Preferred Provider Organizations

A **health maintenance organization (HMO)** provides comprehensive health services to their members for a prepaid, fixed amount regardless of the extent of the services provided. The distinguishing feature of HMOs is prepayment, a type of annual prospective payment. Because the cost is fixed, the HMO profits more if the enrollee stays well or if unnecessary diagnostic tests and treatments are avoided. Health services, which may be provided directly or through arrangements with others, include the services of physicians, nurses, and other health care providers. HMOs also provide routine physical examinations, health maintenance programs (health education, fitness programs), and illness management.

HMOs have grown rapidly in some parts of the country, primarily in the urban areas of the West and Midwest. More than 425 HMOs serve approximately 11% of the U.S. population. Most HMOs are part of a proprietary multisystem. HMO members have 30% to 40% fewer inpatient days, which serves to reduce the overall cost of health care.

A **preferred provider organization (PPO)** offers a delivery system similar to that of the HMO. A PPO is made up of a number of physicians and nurses who have joined together to provide care as a group. Group members are not necessarily located in the same office, but they make referrals for each other. PPOs may or may not require a standard annual fee from each enrollee. Providers in the PPO furnish services on a discounted reimbursement basis in return for prompt payment and guaranteed volume. PPO enrollees are encouraged to use "preferred" providers through incentives such as lower insurance rates.

## Ambulatory Care and Home Health Agencies

The shift in emphasis away from overnight stays in the hospital has generated a proliferation of agencies offering **ambulatory care** and home health care. Many of these agencies are part of health care multisystems. A freestanding ambulatory care center may be associated with a hospital or may be operated by a group of physicians as an extended hours facility. These centers provide immediate and convenient access to episodic care at a relatively reasonable cost. There are more than 3000 ambulatory care centers in the United States, and some are open 24 hours a day.

Although most hospitals now have expanded outpatient surgery departments, freestanding outpatient surgery centers, or "surgicenters," have also grown in number. These facilities may or may not be hospital owned. The first surgicenter opened in Phoenix in 1975, and there are now well over 600 of them. The relatively low complication rates associated with procedures performed at surgicenters have been attributed both to the minor nature of the operations and to careful screening of patients before surgery.

Community nursing centers have been established throughout the country in recent years, their development often stimulated by a university school of nursing. The centers offer a variety of services needed by the community, and they are managed by professional nurses who work closely with community residents. Because of this close association, the center's services are directly related to the community's needs. Staff members in these centers have many collaborative relationships or contracts with other health care providers. More opportunities to fund the start-up of these systems are developing. It is anticipated that the community nursing center will be a major provider of primary care services, including management of acute and chronic disease and health promotion activities.

Home health care long has been provided by agencies such as the Visiting Nurse Association (VNA) and county health departments. This field has expanded greatly and now includes well over 6000 agencies in the country. The number of private proprietary and nonproprietary home health agencies has increased, but the number of government-based agencies has remained the same or declined. Hospitals are offering home health care more often than any other alternative service. Home health agencies provide services such as nursing, physical therapy, occupational therapy, social service, and home health aide or homemaker services in the patient's home. Because more complicated and invasive procedures are being performed in the home setting, the need for skilled nurses in these agencies has increased. The home health nurse may enjoy a greater sense of autonomy in this independent role.

In many communities hospice care is available to terminally ill patients who wish to remain at home. Hospice care addresses the physical, spiritual, emotional, psychologic, financial, and legal needs of dying patients and their families. The type of care is provided by an interdisciplinary team of professionals and volunteers and is available in many communities. These services frequently are part of the VNA.

## Government Health Departments

Health departments are found on the federal, state, and local levels. The federal system is widespread and offers many services, most notably through the Department of Veterans Affairs. State health departments have broad functions, usually in cooperation with federal agencies and local health departments. The average health care consumer deals most often with the local health department. Local boards of health vary in the services they provide. Their functions usually include control of communicable diseases, laboratory testing, environmental sanitation services, health screening, and health education. Public health nurses

may provide clinic services or care in the home or school.

## Other Health Care Facilities

Health care is provided in many settings beyond the walls of the hospital or nursing home. Physicians, dentists, and nurses in private practice and incorporated group practice centers offer a variety of services and expertise and play a major role in the health care system. Schools provide examinations and health teaching. Industries offer emergency services and physical examinations and are becoming more involved in programs that promote accident and illness prevention and health maintenance. Community health centers are playing a major role in bringing health care closer to people. The goal of the community health center is to provide needed services in an atmosphere of concern and understanding tailored to meet the needs of the community.

## HEALTH CARE TEAM

Regardless of the setting, comprehensive health care requires the efforts of a team that includes health professionals and paraprofessionals. The center of the team is the patient, to whom the team is ultimately responsible. Often the patient lacks the ability or resources to lead and coordinate the health team. It may be the nurse who spends the most time with the patient, providing continuity of care and assisting the patient with functional needs. Often the nurse represents the patient and coordinates the efforts of the physician, physical therapist, social worker, clergy, dietitian, respiratory therapist, psychologist, home care coordinator, occupational therapist, and others (Figure 1-3). The nurse assumes responsibility as a patient

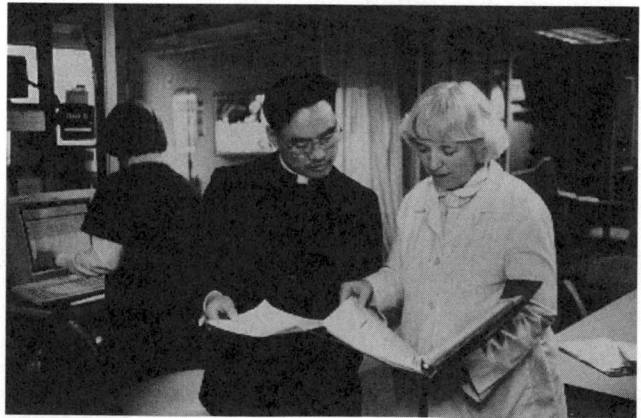

**Figure 1-3** The nurse serves as patient advocate and coordinates the work of others in meeting the varied needs of patients.

*advocate* and promotes the patient's needs, beliefs, and values for the development of a care plan. Each member of the health team is essential to the total care, or **holistic care**, of the patient (Figure 1-4).

## Collaboration Between Nurses and Physicians

The relationship between nurses and physicians has a significant impact on patient care outcomes (Steel, 1986). This relationship is receiving more and more attention as health care organizations look at systems and models for effective, efficient quality care. Health care organizations are realizing that the nurse-physician relationship significantly affects the provision of such care. The most desirable relationship between nurses and physicians is a collaborative one. Collaboration is defined as a relationship of interdependence and an understanding that joint planning of care improves its quality and quantity. Collaboration requires trust between the nurse and the physician and respect for the care each pro-

vides. Such a relationship improves patient outcomes and, in many situations, reduces patient cost. Collaboration is essential for evaluating patient care outcomes effectively, for analyzing variances in outcomes, and for modifying necessary practice patterns.

## NURSING PRACTICE

Nursing was once a simple function performed by an untrained individual. Until the Nightingale era, there was no organized system for preparation and quality management of patient care. Florence Nightingale opened the first formal nursing school, with a prescribed curriculum of study and practical experience. As nursing evolved as a profession, nursing leaders attempted to define it. Florence Nightingale wrote that the goal of nursing is "to put the patient in the best condition for nature to act upon him." Virginia Henderson (1966) developed a classic definition of nursing. She wrote that the nurse's purpose is "to assist the individual, sick or well, in the performance of

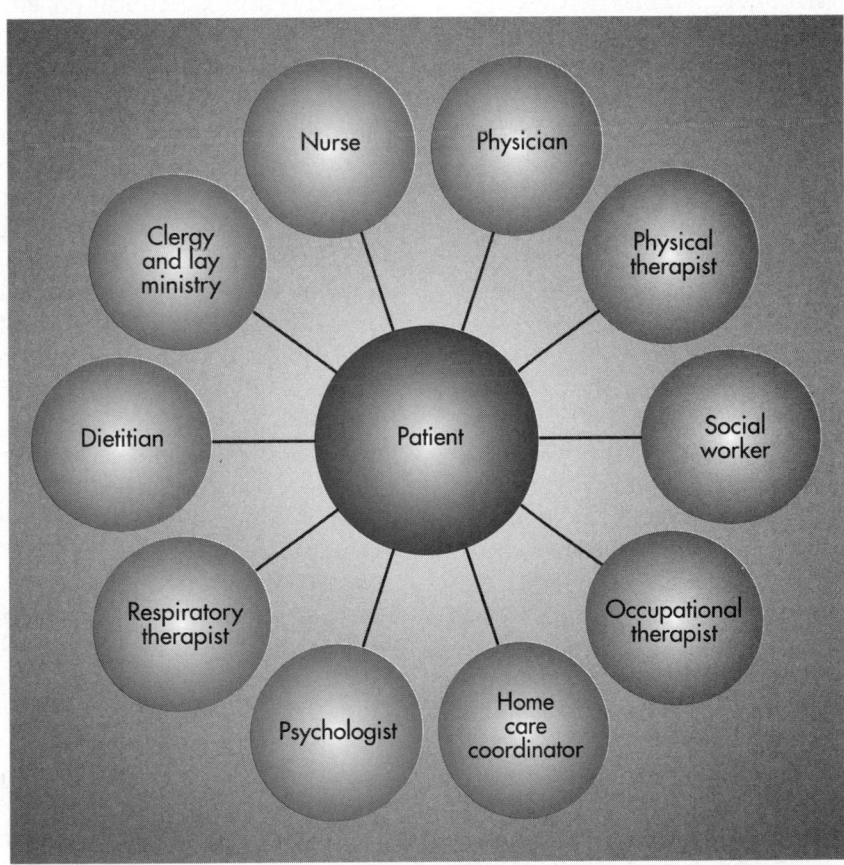

**Figure 1-4**   The health care team.

those activities contributing to health or its recovery (or to peaceful death) that he would perform unaided if he had the necessary strength, will, or knowledge. And to do this in such a way as to help him gain independence as rapidly as possible." The American Nurses Association (ANA) has defined nursing as "the diagnosis and treatment of human responses to actual or potential health problems" (American Nurses Association, 1980 and 1995). All these definitions illustrate the nurse's consistent orientation to providing nursing care that promotes the well-being of the people served.

Nursing long has been described as an art and a science. Early definitions emphasized the care of the sick, whereas more recent descriptions stress the role of the nurse in preventing disease and maintaining health. These modern definitions stress the need to view the patient as a whole person, encompassing physiologic, emotional, psychologic, intellectual, social, and spiritual factors, and acknowledging the interrelationship and interdependence of these factors as they affect health. Modern definitions also include references to the patient's family and significant others.

The functions of the nurse are likely to be categorized according to the degree of dependence or independence of the patient. Dorothy Orem goes beyond a definition to a theory of nursing when she describes the "locus of decision making" and places it with the nurse, with the patient, or with the nurse and patient together, depending on the patient's ability to make decisions or to perform health-related activities.

## Medical-Surgical Nursing

Medical-surgical nursing deals with any illness or disease that affects the physiology of adults. The illness may have begun in childhood, during or after pregnancy, or as a result of a psychiatric problem. Once the illness interferes with normal physiology, the patient is said to have a medical problem and is called a *medical patient*. When the problem is treated by surgical intervention, the individual becomes a *surgical patient*. Social and behavioral problems can affect or be affected by the physical illness and therefore are an important aspect of medical-surgical nursing. The knowledge required for medical-surgical nursing is complex and vast in scope.

A hospital medical service usually includes patients with serious conditions such as a myocardial infarction, terminal cancer, congestive heart failure, leukemia, and AIDS. The medical patient may have entered the hospital for a workup, which comprises diagnostic tests and examinations. After the examinations have been completed and a medical diagnosis has been established, the patient may be treated and discharged or prepared for surgery. Patients may have

medical and surgical conditions at the same time, such as a patient with diabetes who is admitted to the hospital for removal of the gallbladder.

The goal of medical-surgical nursing is to help patients help themselves. The degree of assistance each patient requires varies with the stage of illness. Nurses often are tempted to "do for" patients rather than encourage and assist with self-care. Sometimes it is faster to "do for" for the patient, and sometimes there is concern that the patient will not perform the activity well; most often, however, it is the need to help others that prompts the nurse to do what the patient should be doing independently or with assistance. Although most nurses cite the desire to help others as a reason for entering nursing, the role of the nurse is to promote independence while providing support and understanding. These two hallmarks of nursing are essential to maintaining and restoring optimum health (i.e., the patient's maximum possible level of health).

## Regulation of Nursing Practice

Nursing practice is regulated and controlled through credentialing of the individual nurse. Credentialing includes licensure, certification, and accreditation.

### Licensure

The state boards of nursing protect the public through approval of educational nursing programs and state licensure of individuals. In recent years the boards of nursing have achieved more extensive national standardization of requirements. This standardization provides nurses with more choices in the job market by giving them easier access across state boundaries. The development and implementation of the state board licensing examination (the National Council Licensure Examination, or NCLEX) assures the public that individuals are minimally safe to render nursing care. Each state has established broad definitions and standards for nursing care and monitors individuals through a renewal process. Some states require evidence of continuing education for license renewal. Many states also regulate advanced-practice nurses with a requirement for second licensure.

### Certification

Certification is the validation of a body of knowledge in a specialized or occupational field. The individual must pass an initial test and then maintains certification through a variety of mechanisms. This validation is based on professional standards of practice. Certification systems have been developed and implemented by national professional associations, including the ANA, and specialty nursing organizations, such as American Operating Room Nurses (AORN). Eligibility for certification varies among organizations. Although certification did not originate as a form of entry into practice, many state boards of nursing now require it for practice in advanced roles (e.g., nurse practitioners, clinical nurse specialists). Prescriptive authority and reimbursement may be granted to individuals who meet established criteria, including national certification.

## Accreditation

Accreditation is a system of review and approval of organized nursing education programs established to ensure that basic minimum expectations are included in the curriculum. Educational programs that provide continuing education credits may also be accredited. Programs are approved for a set period and are subject to reaccreditation. Individual nurses are not accredited.

## Nursing Education and Scope of Practice

Education within the nursing profession has evolved and changed since Florence Nightingale established the first school of nursing. Today, to become a licensed vocational nurse (LVN) or a licensed practical nurse (LPN), the student attends a 9- to 12-month program. To become a registered nurse (RN), an individual can attend a 2- to 3-year hospital diploma school, a 2-year associate's degree program at a community college, a 4-year baccalaureate program at a university, a generic master's program, or a generic doctoral program. Graduates of these programs complete their education with varying degrees of knowledge and differing skills and abilities.

The LVN and LPN are authorized to provide direct nursing care under the supervision and direction of an RN, a physician, a dentist, or a podiatrist. Supervision need not be direct and often is quite distant, but the supervisor is responsible for authorizing the LVN and LPN to provide care. The LVN and LPN are prepared to provide nursing care to patients with predictable nursing care problems in well-defined situations. LVN and LPN programs are offered by hospitals, community colleges, vocational centers, and some high schools. The program must be state approved for its graduates to be eligible to take the state board examination for practical nursing. All states except California use the National Council of State Boards of Nursing Licensure Examination for Vocational/Practical Nursing. California develops and administers its own examination.

Hospital-based diploma schools were the first educational programs offered in nursing. The functions and responsibilities of diploma school graduates involve direct patient care in hospitals, extended care facilities, and other health care agencies. However, the number of diploma schools in this country is declining. The high cost of maintaining such programs, using patient care dollars, and the moving of nursing education into the academic setting have contributed to this change.

A nursing graduate with an associate's degree (AD) is prepared to give direct care to patients with well-defined acute or chronic health problems or to those who need information or support to maintain health. This practice focuses on the individual patient in the context of that patient's relationships within a family, group, or community. The nurse with an AD can pursue study toward the baccalaureate degree. Some programs are designed to build directly on the AD program. Other baccalaureate programs admit AD graduates with advanced standing after evaluating transfer credits in the liberal arts and sciences. College credits can also be earned by passing standardized nursing examinations.

A nurse with a bachelor of science in nursing degree (BSN) is prepared to function in acute care and extended care facilities and in the community. The academic background provided in the baccalaureate program prepares the graduate to assume a greater share of responsibility for health care and for directing other members of the health care team. The curriculum emphasizes primary health care, preventive and rehabilitative services, acute and long-term services, health counseling, and education. Students have required studies in such areas as nursing leadership, community health nursing, and nursing theory and research.

Several schools have established a generic master's program for students who have earned a bachelor's degree in a field other than nursing. The 3-year curriculum includes nursing knowledge and skill, with a focus in an area of specialty. The student is eligible for the RN examination after 2 years of study and in the finishing year achieves the master's degree. These programs attract people who may have pursued another field before choosing nursing.

A generic doctoral program, which awards an ND degree, includes nursing sciences, clinical practice in a specialty, and research in clinical problems.

Graduate education in nursing is available to those who have earned a BSN degree and who meet the entrance requirements of a university graduate school. The master's degree allows a nurse to focus on an area of specialty and to become an advanced-practice nurse. Other programs prepare nurse administrators to manage health care delivery systems.

Several hundred doctoral programs in nursing are available in the United States. The primary focus of these programs is to prepare nurses to be scientists, engaged in research germane to the clinical field.

Although nursing has a variety of educational entry points, each type of graduate provides a unique service to patients and their families. The profession continues to differentiate the various types of practice according to education and experience.

## Collaboration Between Nursing Practice and Nursing Education

The many changes in the health care delivery system and pressures on educational institutions are forcing the issue of increased collaboration between education and practice. Some movement toward such collaboration has existed for the past 25 years, but today's pressures are causing practitioners and educators to examine the issues more seriously. Several good reasons support collaboration: (1) both educators and practitioners have the patient as their focus, (2) nursing education requires a practice laboratory for students, and (3) health care agencies must rely on nursing schools to produce practitioners to work in their agencies. Practicing nurses may not have the preparation or the time to do nursing research, but they can work closely with those already engaged in such research to identify phenomena encountered in practice.

## Standards of Nursing Practice

**Standards** are broad statements that encompass the full range of nursing's scope of practice. Standards reflect the values and priorities of the profession and provide a means of measuring the effectiveness of care. Clinical standards provide the public with a means to judge the quality of care provided. The ANA is responsible for establishing and maintaining the generic, or general, standards of nursing practice. Many nursing specialty organizations collaborate with the ANA to issue joint standards. Specialty organizations also develop standards related to each area of expertise. Nurses are responsible for incorporating these standards into their practice.

The ANA (1991b) has published the generic standards and organized them into Standards of Clinical Nursing Practice, which contain the standards of patient care and the standards of professional performance. These standards are used as the basis for quality assurance systems, databases, health care reimbursement policies, certification programs, and many other measurement systems. The standards are periodically modernized in an effort to keep current with contemporary practice (Box 1-2).

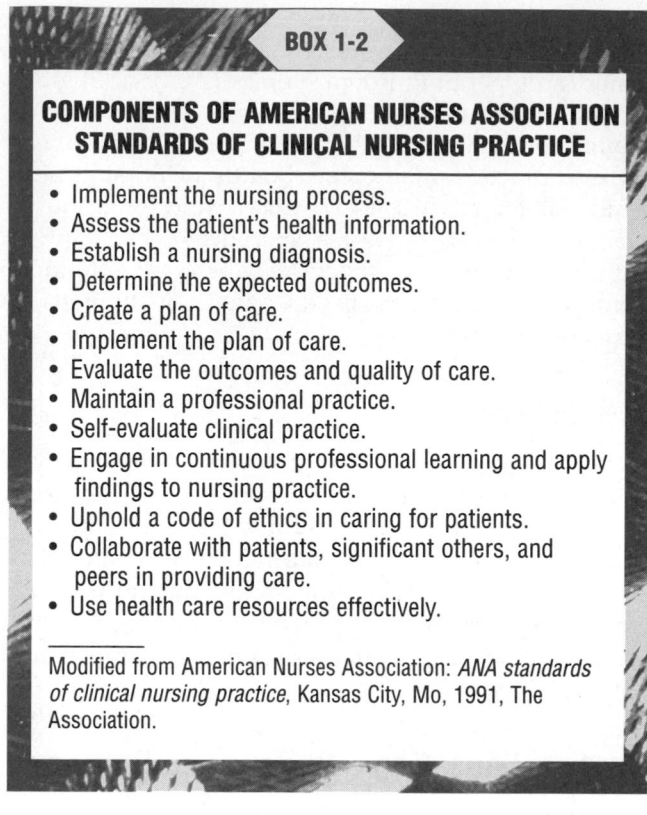

**BOX 1-2**

### COMPONENTS OF AMERICAN NURSES ASSOCIATION STANDARDS OF CLINICAL NURSING PRACTICE

- Implement the nursing process.
- Assess the patient's health information.
- Establish a nursing diagnosis.
- Determine the expected outcomes.
- Create a plan of care.
- Implement the plan of care.
- Evaluate the outcomes and quality of care.
- Maintain a professional practice.
- Self-evaluate clinical practice.
- Engage in continuous professional learning and apply findings to nursing practice.
- Uphold a code of ethics in caring for patients.
- Collaborate with patients, significant others, and peers in providing care.
- Use health care resources effectively.

Modified from American Nurses Association: *ANA standards of clinical nursing practice*, Kansas City, Mo, 1991, The Association.

## Quality Assurance and Quality Improvement

A significant component of nursing care is the measurement or evaluation of the outcome of that care. Although the phrase *quality of care* is difficult to define, it has been one of the hallmarks of professional nursing practice. Most formal nursing systems have developed some means of measuring the care provided. Nationally, **quality assurance (QA)** has been defined by the Joint Commission on Accreditation of Hospitals (JCAH) (1986) as a planned, systematic process for monitoring and evaluating the appropriateness of care, evaluating the quality of service, and resolving existing problems. Delivery systems appoint a QA committee with members from a clinical practice unit. In this way direct care providers are involved in QA measurement. Some systems incorporate a **quality improvement (QI) system** or a **total quality management (TQM) system.** In all these designs the major objective is to measure and evaluate the effectiveness and quality of care.

The characteristics of these evaluation systems are a focus on care, the involvement of a variety of professionals in the system of measurement, a focus on a particular problem and continuing problems, and the integration of quality and cost of care. In 1995 the Joint

**STANDARDS FOR QUALITY ASSESSMENT
AND IMPROVEMENT***

1. The health care organization must have a planned, systematic, organization-wide approach to designing, measuring, assessing, and improving its performance.
2. New processes must be well designed.
3. The organization must have a systematic process for collecting needed data.
4. Patient care services must be appropriately integrated throughout the organization.
5. The organization's leaders must establish expectations, develop plans, and manage processes to assess, improve, and maintain the quality of the organization's governance and management, as well as clinical and support activities.

Modified from Joint Commission on Accreditation of Healthcare Organizations: *Accreditation manual for hospitals: quality assessment and improvement,* Chicago, 1993, The Commission.
*Established by the Joint Commission on Accreditation of Healthcare Organizations.

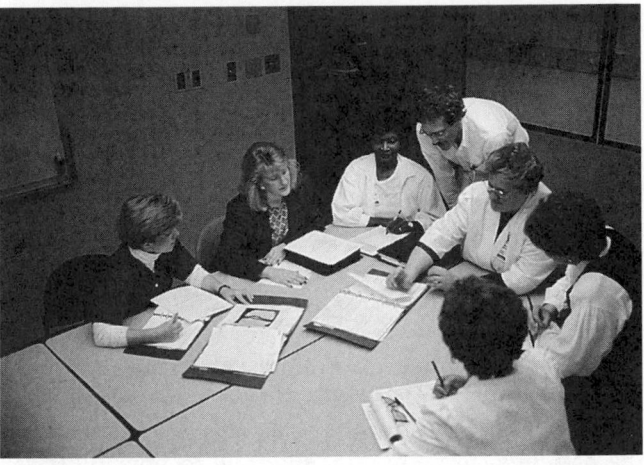

**Figure 1-5**   A variety of health care personnel work together to provide patient care. (From Potter PA, Perry AG: *Fundamentals of nursing: concepts, process and practice,* ed 4, St Louis, 1997, Mosby.)

Commission on Accreditation of Healthcare Organizations (JCAHO) recommended a systematic approach to identifying the ways care can be improved in the future (Box 1-3). The ultimate goals for quality assurance programs are to assure the public that the highest level of care is provided and that a system exists for constant monitoring of care. The professional provider and health care systems are involved in this monitoring. As a result of these measurement and evaluation efforts, health care systems redesign their policies or methods of providing service and individual care improves.

## Nursing Delivery Systems

In the early days of nursing, each nurse cared for and provided all necessary services to one patient, or "case," or a group of patients. This was known as the case method of patient assignment. As medicine and technology advanced, the nurse's responsibilities and duties became more complex. As a result of the nursing shortage during World War II, **functional nursing** was developed. This system uses auxiliary health workers trained in a variety of skills. Each person is assigned specific duties or functions, which are performed on all patients in a given unit. For example,

RNs give medications, LVNs and LPNs perform treatments, and aides and orderlies make beds and distribute meals. Functional nursing is still used in some institutions throughout the United States.

In the early 1950s **team nursing** was proposed as a way to take advantage of the skills of a variety of nursing personnel while providing more comprehensive care to the patient. The RN acts as the leader of a nursing team that is responsible for a predetermined group of patients. LPNs and LVNs, nursing assistants, and other nurses assist the RN in the care of those patients. The team leader knows and understands the condition of each patient and provides care by assigning team members according to their individual capabilities and personalities. The team leader also assimilates and dispenses knowledge and is the contact between the charge nurse and the physician.

The team leader also has certain responsibilities for promoting team morale, suggesting changes for team members, and evaluating individual work. Essential to the team nursing concept is the team conference, in which team members discuss a patient's needs and jointly establish a plan of care under the direction of the team leader. The team conference includes the patient whenever possible. The use of a variety of health care personnel, whose work is coordinated by the RN, is a modern version of team nursing (Figure 1-5).

**Primary nursing** is another type of nursing delivery system (not to be confused with the concepts of primary care or primary prevention, discussed earlier in this chapter). Under this system, each nurse is assigned a group of patients, preferably no more than five, and is responsible for their total care from admission to discharge. The initial assessment is performed by the primary nurse, who plans the care to be given. When the primary nurse is off duty, other nurses follow the directives of this care plan. The primary nurse involves the patients in their care, identification of goals, and discharge planning. This method provides continuity of care and enables the nurse to become better acquainted with and to provide specifically for the needs of patients and their families. As a result, patient-centered care becomes a reality. The primary nurse accepts responsibility for the care of the patient and establishes accountability.

Primary nursing requires all care to be delivered by nurses. Through delegation, the RN engages others in the patient's care while maintaining responsibility for the nursing care. Pairing an RN with a nursing assistant or technician (partners in practice) is a modification of primary nursing.

Other nursing delivery systems have evolved from the primary nursing concept. Among these are the collaborative practice model and its variations and the new **case management** model. Collaborative practice models encourage effective communication between the physician and primary nurse and emphasize their interdependent roles and the independent role of the professional nurse. The case management concept incorporates primary and team nursing and holds the RN, as case manager, accountable for specific clinical outcomes. Each agency must examine its resources, develop and state its philosophy of nursing care, and organize its approach to nursing accordingly. Because of the prospective reimbursement factor, the decision on which nursing delivery system to use may well rest on which approach is most cost-effective.

## Theory in Practice

Many theories or beliefs explain, predict, or describe the action of the nurse. Today, nursing practice is based on a wide range of theories developed by nurse scientists and others (Table 1-3) (Potter, 1997).

---

**TABLE 1-3**

### Summary of Nursing Theories

| THEORIST | GOAL OF NURSING | FRAMEWORK FOR PRACTICE |
|---|---|---|
| Nightingale (1860) | To facilitate "the body's reparative processes" by manipulating patient environment (Torres, 1986) | Patient environment is manipulated to include appropriate noise, nutrition, hygiene, light, comfort, socialization, and hope. |
| Peplau (1952) | To develop interactions between nurse and patient (Peplau, 1952) | Nursing is a significant, therapeutic, interpersonal press (Peplau, 1952). Nurses participate in structuring health care systems to facilitate natural ongoing tendency of humans to develop interpersonal relationships (Marriner-Tomey, 1989). |
| Henderson (1955) | To work interdependently with other health care workers (Marriner-Tomey, 1989); to assist patient in achieving independence as quickly as possible (Henderson, 1964); to help patient regain strength (Torres, 1986) | Nurses help patient meet Henderson's 14 basic needs (Henderson, 1966). |
| Abdellah (1960) | To provide service to individuals, families, and society; to be kind and caring but also intelligent, competent, and technically well prepared to provide this service (Marriner-Tomey, 1989) | This theory involves Abdellah's 21 nursing problems (Abdellah et al., 1960). |
| Orlando (1961) | To respond to patient's behavior in terms of immediate needs; to interact with patient to meet immediate needs by identifying patient behavior, reaction of nurse, and nursing action to be taken (Torres, 1986; Chinn, Jacobs, 1987) | Three elements (patient's behavior, nurse's reaction, and nurse's action) create the nursing situation (Orlando, 1961). |
| Hall (1962) | To provide care and comfort to patient during disease process (Torres, 1986) | Patient is composed of several overlapping parts: person (core), pathologic state and treatment (cure), and body (care). Nurse is caregiver (Chinn, Jacobs, 1987; Marriner-Tomey, 1989). |

Modified from Potter PA, Perry AG: *Fundamentals of nursing: concepts, process and practice,* ed 4, St Louis, 1997, Mosby.

TABLE 1-3

## Summary of Nursing Theories—cont'd

| THEORIST | GOAL OF NURSING | FRAMEWORK FOR PRACTICE |
| --- | --- | --- |
| Wiedenbach (1964) | To assist individuals in overcoming obstacles that interfere with the ability to meet demands or needs brought about by condition, environment, situation, or time (Torres, 1986) | Nursing as practice is related to individuals who need help because of behavioral stimulus. Clinical nursing has four components: philosophy, purpose, practice, and art (Chinn, Jacobs, 1987). |
| Levine (1966) | To use conservation activities aimed at optimal use of patient's resources | This adaptation model of individual as integral whole is based on "four conservation principles of nursing" (Levine, 1973). |
| Johnson (1968) | To reduce stress so that patient can move more easily through recovery process | This basic needs framework focuses on seven categories of behavior. Individual's goal is to achieve behavioral balance and steady state by adjustment and adaptation to certain forces (Johnson, 1980; Torres, 1986). |
| Rogers (1970) | To maintain and promote health, prevent illness, and care for and rehabilitate ill and disabled patient through "humanistic science of nursing" (Rogers, 1970) | "Unitary man" evolves along life process. Patient continuously changes and coexists with environment. |
| Orem (1971) | To care for and help patient attain total self-care | This is self-care deficit theory. Nursing care becomes necessary when patient is unable to fulfill biologic, psychologic, developmental, or social needs (Orem, 1985). |
| King (1971) | To use communication to help patient reestablish positive adaptation to environment | Nursing process is defined as dynamic interpersonal process involving nurse, patient, and health care system. |
| Travelbee (1971) | To help individual or family to prevent or cope with illness, regain health, find meaning in illness, or maintain maximal degree of health (Marriner-Tomey, 1989) | Interpersonal process is viewed as human-to-human relationship formed during illness and "experience of suffering." |
| Neuman (1972) | To assist individuals, families, and groups to attain and maintain maximum level of total wellness by purposeful interventions | Stress reduction is the goal of systems model nursing practice (Torres, 1986). Nursing actions are in primary, secondary, or tertiary level of prevention. |
| Patterson and Zderad (1976) | To respond to human needs and build humanistic nursing science (Patterson, Zderad, 1986; Chinn, Jacobs, 1987) | Humanistic nursing requires participants to be aware of their "uniqueness" and "commonality" with others (Chinn, Jacobs, 1987). |
| Leininger (1978) | To provide care consistent with nursing's emerging science and knowledge with caring as central focus (Chinn, Jacobs, 1987) | With this transcultural care theory, caring is the central and unifying domain for nursing knowledge and practice (Leininger, 1980). |
| Roy (1979) | To identify types of demands placed on patient, assess adaptation to demands, and help patient adapt | This adaptation model is based on physiologic, psychologic, sociologic, and dependence-independence adaptive modes (Roy, 1980). |
| Watson (1979) | To promote health, restore patient to health, and prevent illness (Marriner-Tomey, 1989) | This theory involves the philosophy and science of caring; caring is an interpersonal process comprising interventions that result in human needs being met (Torres, 1986). |
| Parse (1981) | To focus on individual as living unity and on individual's qualitative participation with health experience (Parse, 1990) (Nursing as science and art [Marriner-Tomey, 1989]) | Individual continually interacts with environment and participates in maintenance of health (Marriner-Tomey, 1989). Health is a continual, open process rather than a state of well-being or absence of disease (Parse, 1981; Marriner-Tomey, 1989; Chinn, Jacobs, 1987). |

BOX 1-4

## A PATIENT'S BILL OF RIGHTS

### INTRODUCTION

Effective health care requires collaboration between patients and physicians and other health care professionals. Open and honest communication, respect for personal and professional values, and sensitivity to differences are integral to optimal patient care. As the setting for the provision of health services, hospitals must provide a foundation for understanding and respecting the rights and responsibilities of patients, their families, physicians, and other caregivers. Hospitals must ensure a health care ethic that respects the role of patients in decision making about treatment choices and other aspects of their care. Hospitals must be sensitive to cultural, racial, linguistic, religious, age, gender, and other differences, as well as the needs of persons with disabilities.

The American Hospital Association (AHA) presents "A Patient's Bill of Rights" with the expectation that it will contribute to more effective patient care and be supported by the hospital on behalf of the institution, its medical staff, employees, and patients. The American Hospital Association encourages health care institutions to tailor this bill of rights to their patient community by translating and/or simplifying the language of this bill of rights as may be necessary to ensure that patients and their families understand their rights and responsibilities.

### BILL OF RIGHTS*

1. The patient has the right to considerate and respectful care.
2. The patient has the right to and is encouraged to obtain from physicians and other direct caregivers relevant, current, and understandable information concerning diagnosis, treatment, and prognosis.

    Except in emergencies when the patient lacks decision-making capacity and the need for treatment is urgent, the patient is entitled to the opportunity to discuss and request information related to the specific procedures and/or treatments, the risks involved, possible length of recuperation, and the medically reasonable alternatives and their accompanying risks and benefits.

    Patients have the right to know the identity of physicians, nurses, and others involved in their

care, as well as when those involved are students, residents, or other trainees. The patient also has the right to know the immediate and long-term financial implications of treatment choices, insofar as they are known.

3. The patient has the right to make decisions about the plan of care prior to and during the course of treatment and to refuse a recommended treatment or plan of care to the extent permitted by law and hospital policy and to be informed of the medical consequences of this action. In case of such refusal, the patient is entitled to other appropriate care and services that the hospital provides or transfer to another hospital. The hospital should notify patients of any policy that might affect patient choice within the institution.
4. The patient has the right to have an advance directive (such as a living will, health care proxy, or durable power of attorney for health care) concerning treatment or designating a surrogate decision maker with the expectation that the hospital will honor the intent of that directive to the extent permitted by law and hospital policy.

    Health care institutions must advise patients of their rights under state law and hospital policy to make informed medical choices, ask if the patient has an advance directive, and include that information in patient records. The patient has the right to timely information about hospital policy that may limit the hospital's ability to implement fully a legally valid advance directive.
5. The patient has the right to every consideration of privacy. Case discussion, consultation, examination, and treatment should be conducted so as to protect each patient's privacy.
6. The patient has the right to expect that all communications and records pertaining to his/her care will be treated as confidential by the hospital, except in cases such as suspected abuse and public health hazards when reporting is permitted or required by law. The patient has the right to expect that the hospital will emphasize the confidentiality of this information when it releases it to any other parties entitled to review information in these records.

From American Hospital Association: *Patient's bill of rights,* Chicago, 1992, The Association.
*These rights can be exercised on the patient's behalf by a designated surrogate or proxy decision maker if the patient lacks decision-making capacity, is legally incompetent, or is a minor. "A Patient's Bill of Rights" was first adopted by the American Hospital Association in 1973; this revision was approved by the AHA Board of Trustees on October 21, 1992.

BOX 1-4

## A PATIENT'S BILL OF RIGHTS—cont'd

7. The patient has the right to review the records pertaining to his/her medical care and to have the information explained or interpreted as necessary, except when restricted by law.

8. The patient has the right to expect that, within its capacity and policies, a hospital will make reasonable response to the request of a patient for appropriate and medically indicated care and services. The hospital must provide evaluation, service, and/or referral as indicated by the urgency of the case. When medically appropriate and legally permissible, or when a patient has so requested, a patient may be transferred to another facility. The institution to which the patient is to be transferred must first have accepted the patient for transfer. The patient must also have the benefit of complete information and explanation concerning the need for, risks, benefits, and alternatives to such a transfer.

9. The patient has the right to ask and be informed of the existence of business relationships among the hospital, educational institutions, other health care providers, or payers that may influence the patient's treatment and care.

10. The patient has the right to consent to or decline to participate in proposed research studies or human experimentation affecting care and, treatment or requiring direct patient involvement, and to have those studies fully explained prior to consent. A patient who declines to participate in research or experimentation is entitled to the most effective care that the hospital can otherwise provide.

11. The patient has the right to expect reasonable continuity of care when appropriate and to be informed by physicians and other caregivers of available and realistic patient care options when hospital care is no longer appropriate.

12. The patient has the right to be informed of hospital policies and practices that relate to patient care, treatment, and responsibilities. The patient has the right to be informed of available resources for resolving disputes, grievances, and conflicts, such as ethics committees, patient representatives, or other mechanisms available in the institution. The patient has the right to be informed of the hospital's charges for services and available payment methods.

The collaborative nature of health care requires that patients, or their families/surrogates, participate in their care. The effectiveness of care and patient satisfaction with the course of treatment depend, in part, on the patient fulfilling certain responsibilities. Patients are responsible for providing information about past illnesses, hospitalizations, medications, and other matters related to health status. To participate effectively in decision making, patients must be encouraged to take responsibility for requesting additional information or clarification about their health status or treatment when they do not fully understand information and instructions. Patients are also responsible for ensuring that the health care institution has a copy of their written advance directive if they have one. Patients are responsible for informing their physicians and other caregivers if they anticipate problems in following prescribed treatment.

Patients should also be aware of the hospital's obligation to be reasonably efficient and equitable in providing care to other patients and the community. The hospital's rules and regulations are designed to help the hospital meet this obligation. Patients and their families are responsible for making reasonable accommodations to the needs of the hospital, other patients, medical staff, and hospital employees. Patients are responsible for providing necessary information for insurance claims and for working with the hospital to make payment arrangements, when necessary.

A person's health depends on much more than health care services. Patients are responsible for recognizing the impact of their life-style on their personal health.

### CONCLUSION

Hospitals have many functions to perform, including the enhancement of health status, health promotion, and the prevention and treatment of injury and disease; the immediate and ongoing care and rehabilitation of patients; the education of health professionals, patients, and the community; and research. All these activities must be conducted with an overriding concern for the values and dignity of patients.

These theorists have made significant contributions to the nursing profession and society.

Other theories developed by those outside nursing have contributed to the understanding of behaviors and actions appropriate to the profession. For example, Abraham Maslow's work on understanding human needs has contributed to the field of nursing. Maslow identified five needs basic to all humans: physiologic needs, safety and security, love and belonging, esteem, and self-actualization. His work has helped give meaning to the concept of holism. Others also have contributed theories that help nurses understand and plan for change. Scientific theories offer guidelines for individual nurses and for nursing systems in making useful and timely changes and for explaining the reason for specific activities.

## PATIENTS' RIGHTS

Emphasis on the patient as an active participant in personal health care has prompted a variety of groups and individuals to make public statements about patients' rights. The House of Delegates of the American Hospital Association (AHA) adopted a "Patient's Bill of Rights" at its 1973 convention and revised it in 1992 (Box 1-4) (American Hospital Association, 1992). The AHA delegates believed that these rights would contribute to more effective patient care and to greater satisfaction for the patient, physician, and hospital.

## KEY CONCEPTS

➤ Total patient care involves consideration of physiologic, psychologic, sociocultural, developmental, and spiritual needs.

➤ The World Health Organization's definition of health is "a state of complete physical, mental, and social well-being and not merely the absence of disease."

➤ The "Nursing's Agenda for Health Care Reform" calls for universal access to affordable and appropriate quality care.

➤ Public politics, demographics, and economics affect the future of nursing as a profession and of nurses as providers of care.

➤ A wide variety of health care delivery systems are available and continue to be developed.

➤ Total patient care depends on collaboration among health care professionals and assistants.

➤ Entry into the practice of nursing is regulated by licensure and certification, which are organized by state boards of nursing and professional associations.

➤ Standards of care reflect the profession's values and priorities and provide a way to measure the care and competence of the nurse.

➤ Theories that explain, predict, and describe nursing actions are generated by nurse scientists and other theorists outside of nursing.

## CRITICAL THINKING EXERCISES

1. Select five key points from the chapter and write a paragraph that describes or explains each.
2. What examples can you give that demonstrate a violation of a patient's rights as identified by the American Hospital Association?
3. Discuss the factors that led to health care reform.

## REFERENCES AND ADDITIONAL READINGS

American Hospital Association: *Cost and compassion: recommendations for avoiding a crisis in care for the medically indigent*, Chicago, 1986, The Association.

American Hospital Association: *Patient's bill of rights*, Chicago, 1992, The Association.

American Nurses Association: *Nursing: a social policy statement*, Kansas City, Mo, 1980, The Association.

American Nurses Association: *Registered professional nurses and unlicensed assistive personnel*, Washington, DC, 1984, The Association.

American Nurses Association: *Environmental assessment: factors affecting long-range planning for nursing and health care*, Kansas City, Mo, 1985, The Association.

American Nurses Association: *Scope of nursing practice*, Kansas City, Mo, 1987, The Association.

American Nurses Association: *Classification systems for describing nursing practice: working papers*, Kansas City, Mo, 1989, The Association.

American Nurses Association: *Nursing's agenda for health care reform*, Kansas City, Mo, 1991a, The Association.

American Nurses Association: *ANA standards of clinical nursing practice*, Kansas City, Mo, 1991b, The Association.

American Nurses Association: *Directory of RN to BSN programs*, Kansas City, Mo, 1992a, The Association.

American Nurses Association: *Managed care and national health care reform*, Kansas City, Mo, 1992b, The Association.

American Nurses Association: *A social policy statement revised*, Kansas City, Mo, 1995, The Association.

Benner P: *From novice to expert*, Menlo Park, Calif, 1984, Addison-Wesley.

Benner P, Tanner C: Clinical judgment: how expert nurses use intuition, *Am J Nurs* 87(1):23-31, 1987.

Benner P, Wrubel J: *The primacy of caring*, Menlo Park, Calif, 1989, Addison-Wesley.

Bower K: *Case management by nurses*, Kansas City, Mo, 1992, American Nurses Association.

Dienemann J, editor: *Continuous quality improvement in nursing*, Kansas City, Mo, 1992, American Nurses Association.

Easterbrook G: The revolution in medicine, *Newsweek*, Jan 26, 40-74, 1987.

Ebersole P, Hess PL: *Toward healthy aging: human needs and nursing response*, ed 4, St Louis, 1994, Mosby.

Enthoven A, Kronick R: The consumer-choice health plan for the 1990's, *N Engl J Med* 320(1):29-37, 1989.

Famighetti R, editor: *The World Almanac and Book of Facts 1997*, Mahwah, NJ, 1996, World Almanac Books.

Farley E: How we survived a redesign, *Am J Nurs* 94(3):43-45, 1994.

Health Security Act of 1993, the White House, September 20, 1993.

Henderson V: *The nature of nursing*, New York, 1966, Macmillan.

Hickey J, Ouinette R, Venegoni S: *Advanced practice nursing: changing roles and clinical applications*, Philadelphia, 1996, Lippincott.

Ismeurt R et al: *Concepts fundamental to nursing*, Springhouse, Pa, 1990, Springhouse.

Joint Commission on Accreditation of Healthcare Organizations: *Accreditation manual for hospitals: quality assessment and improvement*, Chicago, 1993, The Commission.

Joint Commission on Accreditation of Hospitals: *Accreditation manual for hospitals*, Chicago, 1986, The Commission.

Kelley L: *The nursing experience: trends, challenges, and transitions*, New York, 1987, Macmillan.

Lindeman C, McAthie M: *Nursing trends and issues*, Springhouse, Pa, 1990, Springhouse.

Lynaugh J, Fagin C: Nursing comes of age, *Image J Nurs Sch* 20(4):184-189, 1988.

Lysought JP: *An abstract for action*, New York, 1970, McGraw-Hill.

Maglacas A: Health for all: nursing's role, *Nurs Outlook* 36(2):66-71, 1988.

McCloskey J, Grace H: *Current issues in nursing*, ed 5, St Louis, 1997, Mosby.

Mitty E: Prospective payment and long-term care: linking payments to resource use, *Nurs Health Care* 8(1):15-21, 1987.

Mullahy C: *The case manager's handbook*, Gaithersburg, Md, 1995, Aspen.

National Commission on Nursing: *Executive summary of final report*, Chicago, 1988, The Commission.

National Commission on Nursing, Implementation Project: *Characteristics of professional and technical nurses of the future and their educational programs*, Chicago, 1987, The Commission.

Phipps WJ et al: *Medical-surgical nursing: concepts and clinical practice*, ed 5, St Louis, 1995, Mosby.

Potter PA, Perry AG: *Fundamentals of nursing: concepts, process and practice*, ed 4, St Louis, 1997, Mosby.

Primm P: Differentiated practice for ADN and BSN prepared nurses, *J Prof Nurs* 3(4):218-225, 1987.

Reddy M, editor: *Statistical abstract of the world*, ed 2, Detroit, 1996, Gale Research.

Smith CE: DRGs: making them work for you, *Nursing* 15(1):34-41, 1985.

Stanhope M, Lancaster J: *Community health nursing*, ed 4, St Louis, 1996, Mosby.

Steel JE: *Issues in collaborative practice*, Philadelphia, 1986, Saunders.

Steel JE: Advanced nursing practice, *AACN Clin Issues* 5(1):71-76, 1994.

US Department of Commerce, Bureau of the Census: *Historical statistics of the United States: colonial times to 1970*, bicentennial ed, part 2, Washington DC, 1975, US Government Printing Office.

US Department of Commerce, Bureau of the Census: *Statistical abstract of the United States: 1995*, Washington DC, 1995, US Government Printing Office.

US Department of Health and Human Services: *Healthy People 2000: national health promotion and disease prevention objectives*, Washington DC, 1990, US Government Printing Office.

US Department of Health and Human Services: *The Medicare guide to health insurance for people with Medicare,* Washington, DC, 1996, US Government Printing Office.

US Department of Health and Human Services, Division of Nursing: *Report to the President and the Congress on the status of health personnel in the United States,* vol 1, part C: Nursing personnel, Washington, DC, 1984, US Government Printing Office

World Health Organization: *The first ten years of the World Health Organization,* New York, 1958, The Organization.

Zander K: Second generation primary nursing: a new agenda, *J Nurs Adm* 15(3):18-22, 1985.

# CHAPTER 2

# Nursing Process and Clinical Decision Making

## CHAPTER OBJECTIVES

1 Define critical thinking.
2 Identify characteristics and skills that demonstrate critical thinking.
3 Describe each phase of the nursing process: assessment, analysis, planning, implementation, and evaluation.
4 Distinguish between subjective and objective data.
5 List techniques for effective interviewing.
6 Define *nursing diagnosis* and explain how it differs from medical diagnosis.
7 Discuss the status of a universally accepted taxonomy of nursing diagnoses.
8 Identify the characteristics of an accurately written nursing diagnosis.
9 Describe the components of a nursing care plan.
10 Describe the essential characteristics of a well-stated expected outcome.
11 Identify the information that must be included in a written nursing action (order).
12 Discuss the importance of documentation.
13 Describe the problem-oriented record system and explain the activity called for by each letter of the acronym "SOAPIE."
14 Differentiate between standardized care plans, critical pathways (care maps), and individualized care plans.
15 Discuss the interrelationship of the phases of the nursing process.

## KEY TERMS

| | |
|---|---|
| assessment | nursing diagnosis |
| care map | nursing history |
| critical pathways | nursing process |
| critical thinking | objective data |
| documentation | planning |
| etiology | problem-oriented record |
| evaluation | SOAP |
| expected outcomes | standardized care plan |
| implementation | subjective data |
| nursing care plan | |

As the nursing profession has evolved, the process of nursing has been studied and documented. The practice of nursing requires the ability to think critically and to act on those decisions. It is generally accepted that critical thinking is used in an approach to problem solving known as the nursing process. This chapter examines critical thinking and the nursing process.

## CRITICAL THINKING AND DECISION MAKING

### Definition

There is no one right definition of **critical thinking**; it is a complex activity that can be described in more than one way. In her early work, Alfaro-LeFevre (1985) defined critical thinking as "purposeful, goal-directed thinking that aims to make judgments based on evidence (fact) rather than conjecture (guesswork)." She also gave a one-word definition: reasoning. In a more recent work, she added that "critical thinking requires you to 'personalize' information, to analyze it and draw conclusions about what it means to you rather than simply memorizing words"; she also described it as "a commitment to look for the best way, based on the most current research and practice findings" (Alfaro-LeFevre, 1998).

Richard Paul expanded on these concepts, describing critical thinking as "the art of constructive skepticism," which requires the thinker to challenge all information. It requires open mindedness and demands the absence of bias or prejudice. It is self-directed, in-depth, and rational learning that "certifies what we know and makes clear wherein we are ignorant" (Paul, 1990).

When we think critically, we evaluate information with an open mind, avoiding premature conclusions. A critical thinker is able to make a thorough and fair evaluation of his or her personal beliefs and viewpoints as well as those of others that are considered to be completely opposite (Paul, 1990). Assessing a patient, analyzing the data without bias or prejudice, and arriving at a decision about effective nursing actions require critical thinking.

## Elements of Critical Thinking

Nurses commonly use the elements of critical thinking as they provide care. Critical thinking is a process used to make sound, accurate, and reasonable decisions on the basis of thorough collection and analysis of data. This process includes elements of the scientific method, such as data collection, analysis, deductive reasoning (moving from a general premise to a specific conclusion) and inductive reasoning (from the particular to the general), as well as hypothesis testing and evaluation.

A person also uses critical thinking in everyday life. For example, someone who needs a new washing machine uses critical thinking in deciding what brand and model to buy. First, he or she gathers information about washing machines (data collection). The person then asks neighbors and relatives about their washing machines, goes to the library to check *Consumer Reports*, and reads the ads in newspapers and magazines. Keeping an open mind, the person gathers information from a variety of sources. Next, he or she uses critical thinking skills to analyze the data gathered. This information can be classified into categories; for example, features and facts that are important compared with those that are "nice" but not important. The cost and dependability of the various models also are analyzed. The person then makes a decision based on these facts.

The same critical thinking skills are used to make decisions in all areas of health care. Continuous development and improvement of critical thinking skills are essential at all levels of nursing practice.

## Characteristics and Skills that Demonstrate Critical Thinking

The American Philosophical Association (1990) has developed a statement that reflects the consensus of experts in the field. The statement describes a critical thinker as a person who is as follows:

... habitually inquisitive, self-informed, trustful of reason, open minded, flexible, fair minded in evaluation, honest in facing personal biases, prudent in making judgments, willing to reconsider, clear about issues, orderly in complex matters, diligent in seeking relevant information, reasonable in selection of criteria, focused on inquiry, and persistent in seeking results that are as precise as the subject and the circumstances of inquiry permit.

Richard Paul (1993) describes key traits of a critical thinker, which include a willingness to admit what one does not know; to evaluate one's own thinking and admit it when it may be flawed; to be able to face all ideas, beliefs, or viewpoints, including those about which one may have negative feelings; and to be able to see things from another's point of view, to be able to put oneself in another's place.

Researchers Noreen and Peter Facione have developed a test that measures seven habits of the mind demonstrated by critical thinkers. These habits are truth seeking, open mindedness, an analytic approach, systematicity (valuing organization, focus, and diligence in approaching problems of all levels of complexity), self-confidence, inquisitiveness, and maturity (Facione, Facione, Sanchez, 1994).

# NURSING PROCESS

Nursing is a dynamic and interpersonal problem-solving process. The process provides a framework for organizing both cognitive activities and the delivery of nursing care. Through the **nursing process,** the nurse helps the patient meet his or her health care needs. The skills and abilities a nurse must have to use the nursing process can be divided into three categories: cognitive (thinking, reasoning), psychomotor (doing), and affective (feelings, values). The five phases of the nursing process are (1) **assessment**, (2) analysis/**nursing diagnosis**, (3) **planning/expected outcome**s, (4) **implementation,** and (5) evaluation (Figure 2-1).

## Assessment
### Data Collection

Assessment is the process of collecting and recording objective and subjective data about the patient and grouping it into meaningful categories. Assessment begins when the patient enters the health care system and continues throughout the course of care. A complete assessment includes history taking and physical

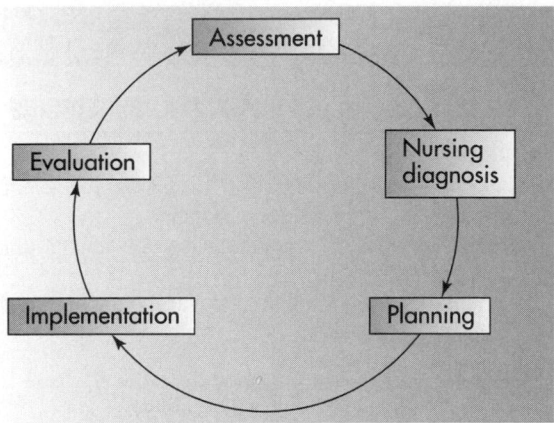

**Figure 2-1**　The nursing process.

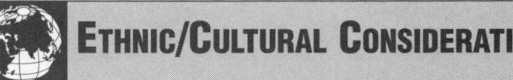

### ETHNIC/CULTURAL CONSIDERATIONS

In some cultures, as is common with people from India, a husband traditionally speaks for his wife. In these cases the husband would lose face in the eyes of his family if the nurse ignored him and sought information directly from his wife.

examination. Information about past and current health problems, subjective symptoms (those described by the patient), and psychosocial, sociocultural, spiritual, and developmental factors is obtained through an effective interview. Information also is obtained from the patient's chart, laboratory reports, family, and friends. Physical assessment requires a systematic examination of the patient. Both the history and the physical assessment are updated continually as the nurse provides care or obtains reports from other health care providers. Assessment continues throughout each phase of care.

### Subjective and Objective Data

Information the nurse receives from the patient or family, either spontaneously or in response to questions, is called subjective data. Subjective data is obtained from *statements* made by the patient or others. Data obtained directly through measurement, inspection, palpation, percussion, or auscultation is called objective data. Objective data is obtained through *observation*; it can be verified by others. Subjective data obtained from the chart or the patient's family should be validated with the patient when possible. Statements made by the patient that appear questionable should be verified with family members. For example, if a patient states that he just recently began to have trouble remembering things, the family should be asked when they first noticed a change in the patient's ability to remember recent events. The nurse should never convey disbelief to the patient or family. Most subjective data are obtained during the taking of the history, but information also may be contributed or elicited during the physical examination. It is the source of the information, not the time it is obtained, that differentiates subjective from objective data.

### Interviewing Techniques

The use of effective interviewing techniques enhances the quality of the **nursing history** (Box 2-1).

## Analysis/Nursing Diagnosis

After the assessment has been completed, the data obtained are analyzed, conclusions are drawn from the information, and the patient's health problem is described in a written nursing diagnosis. The nurse uses elements of critical thinking and the scientific method to analyze the assessment data so that valid conclusions about the patient are reached and accurate diagnoses are made.

### Definition

A nursing diagnosis describes a combination of signs and symptoms indicating an actual or potential health problem that nurses are licensed to treat and are capable of treating (Gordon, 1994). A nursing diagnosis describes human function or behavior. The term *behavior* is used here in its broadest sense, referring to an observable response that may be physiologic, psychologic, intellectual, emotional, or spiritual. Nursing diagnoses use a common language, which enables nurses to communicate the priority needs of the patient effectively and efficiently. The nursing diagnosis is the basis of the nursing care plan (Figure 2-2).

The nursing diagnosis differs from the medical diagnosis, which is concerned primarily with identifying an illness or injury (Box 2-2). The nursing diagnosis and related nursing care focus on the patient's *response* to an actual or potential health problem. For example, in caring for a patient with a medical diagnosis of stroke and left hemiplegia (paralysis), the nurse focuses on the self-care restrictions and the effects of immobility. The nursing diagnosis would describe the patient's problems related to function or behavior, rather than the disease itself. A patient with left hemiplegia is likely to have a nursing diagnosis of "impaired physical mobility related to paralysis, left leg and left arm."

---

<table>
<tr><td colspan="2">

**BOX 2-1**

## EFFECTIVE INTERVIEWING TECHNIQUES

- Introduce yourself to the patient.
- Approach the patient calmly and empathetically.
- Provide privacy and eliminate distractions.
- Explain that the purpose of the questions is to allow the nurse to provide better care by knowing more about the patient and family.
- Tell the patient approximately how long the interview will last.
- Use terminology familiar to the patient.
- Ask first about the patient's immediate concern or complaint; save delicate, personal questions until later.
- Consider the patient's condition when scheduling and conducting the interview. A weak patient will not have the energy to respond, and a patient in pain will not want to deal with questions.
- Call the patient by name.
- Speak clearly, slowly, and distinctly.
- Listen. Maintain the topic, but never interrupt.
- Show genuine concern.
- Ask open-ended questions that require more than a "yes" or "no" answer (e.g., "Tell me about your pain.").
- Use signals such as a nod, a comment such as "uh-huh," or a glance to encourage the patient to continue.
- Focus on what the patient is saying rather than anticipating answers or planning the next question.
- Even if the agency requires a checklist, do not sound as if you are using one.
- Relying on memory is dangerous; take brief notes but do not let it distract you from listening.
- Be aware of your own and the patient's nonverbal communication.
- Remain open, accepting, and objective even if the patient is hostile and uncooperative.
- Use good eye contact but never stare. Position yourself at the patient's eye level whenever possible.
- Select an appropriate time. Pain, fear, and anxiety are reasons to postpone the interview. In such cases obtain only the information needed to control the stressor and schedule the rest of the interview for another time.
- Be professional.

</td></tr>
</table>

**BOX 2-2**

## PRIMARY GOALS OF NURSING AND MEDICINE

**NURSING**
- Determine responses to health problems, the level of wellness, and the need for assistance.
- Provide physical care, emotional care, teaching, guidance, and counseling.
- Plan interventions aimed at helping the patient meet his or her own needs.

**MEDICINE**
- Determine the cause of illness or injury.
- Provide medical treatment and surgery.
- Plan interventions aimed at preventing and curing illness or injury.

From Lewis SM, Collier IC, Heitkemper MM: *Medical-surgical nursing: assessment and management of clinical problems*, ed 4, St Louis, 1996, Mosby.

to evolve as the common language of nursing. The National Conference Group on the Classification of Nursing Diagnosis began meeting in 1973. This group, now known as the North American Nursing Diagnosis Association (NANDA), meets annually to develop and validate nursing diagnoses. A list of accepted nursing diagnoses is published each year (see Appendix B).

## Characteristics of a Nursing Diagnosis

Despite different terms and philosophies, it generally is agreed that the nursing diagnosis must describe a behavior that is a problem for the patient and that requires nursing interventions. A NANDA diagnosis includes a problem statement, followed by a statement that describes the **etiology**, followed by the characteristic signs and symptoms. This format is referred to as the PES format: health problem (P), etiology (E), signs and symptoms (S).

The problem must be stated in terms that give the nurse direction in selecting nursing interventions and identifying desired expected outcomes. For example, "ineffective airway clearance" is an accepted NANDA nursing diagnosis, but it is not complete without a statement of etiology, a "related to" statement. To propose effective nursing interventions, the nurse must know why the airway clearance is ineffective (the etiology).

The nursing diagnosis statement can be modified to fit each patient. For example, "impaired physical mobility" is an accepted nursing diagnosis that becomes more meaningful when the impairment is further de-

## Classification of Nursing Diagnoses

To be useful, a nursing diagnosis must have universal meaning; therefore, it must be universally accepted. Nurses have been discussing the concept of the nursing diagnosis for more than 30 years, and it continues

| DATE INITIALS | NURSING DIAGNOSIS | INTERVENTION/PLAN | OUTCOME | EVALUATION |
|---|---|---|---|---|
| | Actual/potential impaired mobility due to: | 1. AROM/PROM q̄ _____ <br> 2. Reposition q̄ _____ <br> 3. Assist with ambulation as ordered <br> 4. Assistive devices—define: <br> 5. OOB _____ min. _____ times per day | 1. Mobility as defined: | 1. Date achieved: _____ <br> 2. Not achieved— define discharge plan/follow-up: <br><br> Initials |
| | Actual/potential alteration urinary elmination-incontinence/ retention due to: | 1. I & O <br> 2. Record time and amount of voiding <br> 3. Check for bladder distention <br> 4. Assess urine for character, frequency, dysuria <br> 5. Push fluids to ____ ml/day <br> 6. Maintain skin integrity <br> 7. Intermittent/indwelling cath. as ordered <br> 8. Establish toilet regimen— define: | 1. Bladder regimen established <br> 2. No urinary retention <br> 3. No skin breakdown <br> 4. Urine output appropriate to fluid intake | 1. Date achieved: _____ <br> 2. Not achieved – define discharge plan/follow-up: <br><br> Initials |
| | Actual/potential alteration bowel elimination— constipation due to: | 1. Push fluids to ____ ml/day <br> 2. Laxative/softeners as ordered <br> 3. Enemas as ordered <br> 4. Monitor frequency of stools <br> 5. Ambulate ___ times/day <br> 6. Instruct on fiber intake <br> 7. Check bowel sounds q̄ shift | 1. Soft formed stools within patient's established pattern <br> 2. | 1. Date achieved: _____ <br> 2. Not achieved— define discharge plan/follow-up: <br><br> Initials |
| | Actual/potential alteration bowel elimination— diarrhea due to: | 1. Assess frequency, appearance, volume of stools <br> 2. Stool chart <br> 3. Check for impaction <br> 4. Monitor lytes—report abnormals <br> 5. Maintain skin integrity <br> 6. Obtain stool specimens as ordered | 1. Soft formed stools within patient's established pattern <br> 2. No skin breakdown | 1. Date achieved: _____ <br> 2. Not achieved— define discharge plan/follow-up: <br><br> Initials |
| | Actual/potential ineffective coping due to: | 1. Allow to verbalize <br> 2. Offer support services <br>   A. Chaplain <br>   B. Reach for Recovery <br>   C. Stoma therapist <br>   D. Social service | 1. Coping evidenced by: | 1. Date achieved: _____ <br> 2. Not achieved— define discharge plan/follow-up: <br><br><br><br><br><br><br> Initials |

**Figure 2-2**  Sample of a nursing care plan. (Courtesy Central Healthcare and Affiliates, Arlington Heights, Ill.)

*Continued*

| DATE INITIALS | NURSING DIAGNOSIS | INTERVENTION/PLAN | OUTCOME | EVALUATION |
|---|---|---|---|---|
| | Actual/potential impaired gas exchange due to: | 1. Monitor ABG's–report abnormals<br>2. $O_2$ as ordered<br>3. H.O.B. up _____ °<br>4. Describe rate, depth, lung sounds, rhythm, color & sensorium q̄ _____<br>5. OOB ___ min. ___ times/day | 1. Tolerates activity<br>2. Achieves optimum sensorium<br>3. Independent of $O_2$ therapy<br>4. Stable on $O_2$ at ___ l/min. | 1. Date achieved:<br>_____<br>2. Not achieved– define discharge plan/follow-up:<br><br>Initials |
| | Actual/potential alteration in cardiac output due to: | 1. H.O.B. up _____ °<br>2. Assess lung sounds<br>3. $O_2$ as ordered<br>4. Monitor lytes & ABGs– report abnormals<br>5. I & O assess fluid balance<br>6. Auscultate apical pulse<br>7. Plan activity with rest periods–define: | 1. Tolerates activity<br>2. Independent of $O_2$ therapy<br>3. Stable on $O_2$ at ___ l/min. | 1. Date achieved:<br>_____<br>2. Not achieved– define discharge plan/follow-up:<br><br>Initials |
| | Actual/potential alteration in fluid volume–excess due to: | 1. I & O<br>2. Weights q̄ _____<br>3. VS q̄ _____<br>4. Lung sounds q̄ _____<br>5. Assess edema, L.O.C., orthopnea, neck vein distention<br>6. Monitor lytes & ABG's– report abnormals<br>7. Restrict fluids as ordered<br>8. Monitor reponse to diurectics | 1. Resolution of fluid imbalance as evidenced by: | 1. Date achieved:<br>_____<br>2. Not achieved– define discharge plan/follow-up:<br><br>Initials |
| | Actual/potential alteration in fluid volume–deficit due to: | 1. I & O<br>2. VS q̄ _____<br>3. Monitor tissue turgor & skin condition<br>4. Push fluids to ___ ml/day<br>5. Oral hygiene q̄ _____ | 1. Resolution of fluid imbalance as evidenced by: | 1. Date achieved:<br>_____<br>2. Not achieved– define discharge plan/follow-up:<br><br>Initials |
| | Actual/potential self-care deficit due to: | 1. Assist with feeding or feed<br>2. Assist/complete hygiene<br>3. Assist with self-care activities–define: | 1. Performs self-care activities within limitations– define:<br><br>2. | 1. Date achieved:<br>_____<br>2. Not achieved– define discharge plan/follow-up:<br><br>Initials |

NORTHWEST COMMUNITY HOSPITAL, Arlington Heights, Illinois

**PATIENT CARE PLAN**

Nurse-identify initials with signature

| Initials | Signatures | Initials | Signatures |
|---|---|---|---|
| | | | |
| | | | |
| | | | |
| | | | |

**Figure 2-2, cont'd**   For legend see page 25.

scribed as an "impaired physical mobility of right hand." The complete diagnostic statement could read "impaired physical mobility, right hand, related to joint inflammation." According to the NANDA format, the nursing diagnosis is followed by a description of the signs and symptoms that led to the diagnosis. Whether this grouping of significant signs and symptoms appears on the actual care plan depends on the format adopted by the particular health care agency.

Although much progress has been made, the goal of a universally accepted system, or taxonomy, of nursing diagnoses has not yet been reached. This period of development is particularly confusing to nursing students, who would like to be told precisely what is expected of them. While the nursing diagnosis continues to evolve, nurses will use diagnoses that have not been universally accepted, and they will not always agree on their appropriateness. Everyone in nursing must contribute ideas and become involved in testing the work of experts in the field. A universal taxonomy requires continual change to reflect current practice.

## Planning/Expected Outcomes
### Nursing Care Plan

In the planning phase of the nursing process, a concise, written design of action is developed on the basis of the nursing diagnosis. Priorities are set, specific expected behavioral outcomes are identified, and appropriate specific nursing actions or interventions are proposed. Expected outcomes are statements that describe specific, desired patient behaviors or results. An outcome is something that one hopes to achieve. The patient with immobility related to paralysis of the left leg and arm requires assistance with activities of daily living (ADL) and therapy to restore function. The care plan identifies the assistance required and activities aimed at improving strength and function. The expected outcomes identify goals that are realistic for the patient and measurable, such as "able to walk to the bathroom with the assistance of a walker."

Hospitals and other health care agencies require **nursing care plans** for all patients. These plans are used to communicate information among the staff, prevent complications, ensure continuity of care, identify and ensure patient teaching, and provide for discharge planning. The nursing care plan includes the nursing diagnosis or statements that identify the patient's problems and the proposed nursing interventions. Each diagnosis should have a statement of criteria for expected outcomes, given in specific and measurable behavioral terms. Each intervention may also have a statement of expected outcome criteria. Expected outcome criteria are the results anticipated from the interventions. For a hospitalized patient, the

nursing care plan focuses largely on the acute phase of care, but it should include a discharge plan as well. Ambulatory and home care services also use a formal plan of care to ensure that patients are given quality, comprehensive, and cost-effective care.

### Setting Priorities

After the nursing diagnoses have been identified, the nurse must determine the interventions needed and decide which problems need immediate attention. The life-threatening *a*irway, *b*reathing, and *c*irculation (ABC) problems always have top priority (see Chapter 21). Other theories, such as Maslow's hierarchy of needs (see Chapter 6) can guide nurses in setting other priorities. The patient's perception of what is most important should always be considered. If the patient does not agree with the priorities established by the nurse, the patient must be interviewed further to determine the basis for the disagreement. The patient's culture may be influencing his or her view of the situation and the choice of action to be taken. If cultural beliefs are not in opposition, instruction may be needed to help the patient understand. If the patient still disagrees after being fully informed on the situation, the nurse must respect the patient's wishes and make accommodations. Priorities change as the patient's condition changes.

### ETHNIC/CULTURAL CONSIDERATIONS

The nurse must be aware of cultural differences that might influence the patient's perception of priorities in a plan of care. If the patient believes that only natural substances should be used to treat illness, a belief common among the Amish, he or she may reject medication or technologically advanced treatments.

### Setting Goals and Outcome Criteria

After priorities have been established, long-term and short term goals are set and outcome criteria are established. Goals must be worded as expected outcomes, a statement that specifically describes the results or the patient's behavior when the goal is met, such as "ambulate length of hall independently by second day postoperative." The goals must be realistic and achievable. They must describe an expected behavior that can be measure or observed. Action verbs and specific numbers are critical elements of measurable outcome statements because they allow for precise measurement of outcome achievement. Goals should focus on the patient, describing the patient's condition or behavior, not the activity of the nurse. They should include a time frame and should be established mutually by nurse and patient. Short-term goals should be established for each long-term goal so that progress can be measured regularly. The expected outcome must be written so that it is clear to all caregivers when the outcome has been achieved.

## Planning Interventions

After the goals and outcome criteria have been established, the nursing actions to accomplish the desired behaviors should be planned. The nurse must use available resources and involve the patient and family in selecting effective measures. Other members of the health care team can be used as resources, and holding a patient-centered conference can help with planning. The nurse uses research findings and current literature in selecting interventions. The plan is then recorded on a chart or Kardex in specific terms. Anyone who reads the plan should have all the information needed to carry out the proposed intervention, including what should be done, how, when, for how long, how often, where, by whom, and with what. "Wet dressing qid" is not a clear nursing order; a specific, individualized nursing order would be "Apply two 4 × 4s soaked in Burow's solution to left leg wound @ 9-1-5-9. Leave open to air."

## Implementation

Implementation is the actual performance of the nursing interventions identified in the plan of care. The interventions may include direct care, observations or assessments, health teaching, or supervision of other actions beneficial to the patient. Nurses may perform the nursing interventions directly or, when safe and appropriate, they may be delegated to others. The nursing actions may be identified by the nurse in conjunction with the nursing diagnosis; they may be ordered by the physician as part of the medical treatment; or they may be essential ADL that the patient cannot perform independently.

 **ETHNIC/CULTURAL CONSIDERATIONS**

The Hmong place greater importance on the spoken word than on the written word; therefore health teaching will have a greater impact if given verbally rather than in written instructions.

## Documentation and Charting

**Documentation** is an important part of the implementation phase and the entire nursing process. It involves charting periodic patient assessments and all nursing interventions in the patient's record. Documentation is an important part of the patient's permanent record, which is considered a legal document. Under the auditing methods of diagnosis-related groups (DRGs), Medicare, Medicaid, and private managed care companies, inadequate nursing documentation can cause health care agencies to lose reimbursement through disallowance of services. Different agencies use different methods of documenting nursing interventions. Methods may vary from a narrative type to simplified flowsheets.

With the advent of standardized care plans and critical pathways, the use of flowsheets to document nursing interventions is increasing rapidly. Flowsheets usually involve "charting by exception," which means only observations other than those normally expected would be documented. The fact that the patient was observed would be indicated with a check mark in the appropriate place on a flowsheet. In FOCUS charting, the nurse's note is structured with a specific diagnosis or problem in mind. The diagnosis or problem is listed, and for each entry the assessment, activity, and

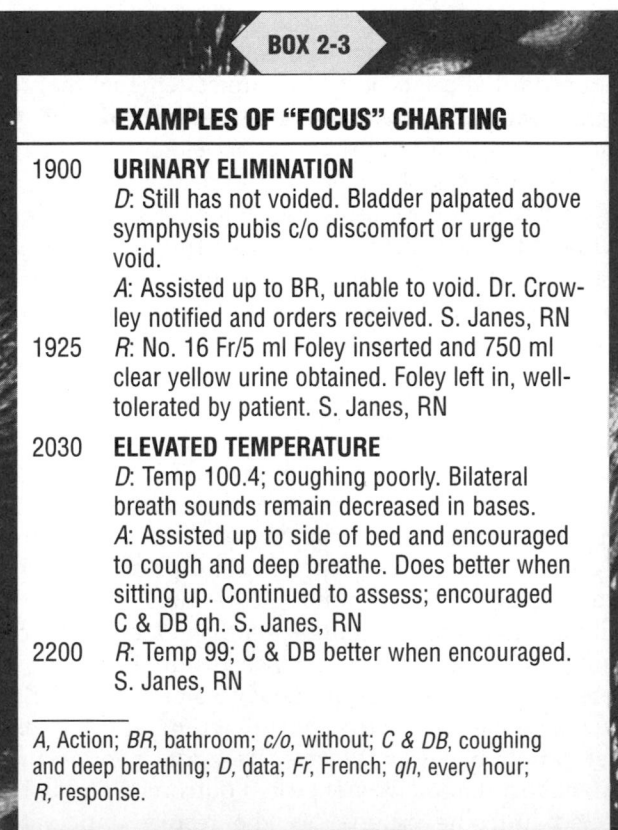

**BOX 2-3**

### EXAMPLES OF "FOCUS" CHARTING

1900 **URINARY ELIMINATION**
*D*: Still has not voided. Bladder palpated above symphysis pubis c/o discomfort or urge to void.
*A*: Assisted up to BR, unable to void. Dr. Crowley notified and orders received. S. Janes, RN
1925 *R*: No. 16 Fr/5 ml Foley inserted and 750 ml clear yellow urine obtained. Foley left in, well-tolerated by patient. S. Janes, RN

2030 **ELEVATED TEMPERATURE**
*D*: Temp 100.4; coughing poorly. Bilateral breath sounds remain decreased in bases.
*A*: Assisted up to side of bed and encouraged to cough and deep breathe. Does better when sitting up. Continued to assess; encouraged C & DB qh. S. Janes, RN
2200 *R*: Temp 99; C & DB better when encouraged. S. Janes, RN

*A*, Action; *BR*, bathroom; *c/o*, without; *C & DB*, coughing and deep breathing; *D*, data; *Fr*, French; *qh*, every hour; *R*, response.

response are recorded (Box 2-3). No matter what form is used, it is important that nursing documentation be complete and accurate.

## Problem-Oriented Record

One system of record keeping, the **problem-oriented record,** provides organization for the patient's chart. This system requires that all progress notes and orders be directly related to the patient's problems, which have been identified and assigned a number. All health care workers use the same progress notes and order sheets. Some institutions separate notes according to professional discipline and use a separate page for nurses, physicians, and other health care workers. The problem-oriented record consists of four parts: *s*ubjective data, *o*bjective data, *a*ssessment, and *p*lan; this often is referred to as the **SOAP** system (Box 2-4).

Others have expanded this system to SOAPIE by adding *i*ntervention and *e*valuation. The subjective data are the information the patient provides, whereas the objective data are the information the nurse obtains through observation and measurement. Assessment is based on *analysis* of subjective and objective data. The plan is the action to be taken as determined by the data and the diagnosis. The SOAPIE system is based on the nursing process but uses slightly different terminology in describing each step. The collection of subjective and objective data in SOAPIE are part of the assessment phase of the nursing process. Assessment in SOAPIE is comparable to the analysis phase of the nursing process. Planning, intervention or implementation, and evaluation are worded the same for both.

## PIE Charting

Another approach to charting follows the acronym PIE: the *p*roblem is stated and then followed by *i*ntervention, which is followed by *e*valuation. An example of PIE charting is presented in Box 2-5.

## Standardized Care Plans

Many health care institutions have developed standardized nursing care plans. **Standardized care plans** are adapted and individualized to the particular patient situation. The nurse selects from these plans only those elements that specifically apply to the patient (see Figure 2-2). In other health care settings, standardized care plans are used in conjunction with or are replaced by critical pathways.

## Critical Pathways (Care Maps)

A critical pathway is an interdisciplinary plan of care and method of documentation that indicates specific results and behaviors expected for a patient with a given medical diagnosis. **Critical pathways,** or **care maps,** are developed together and used by all disciplines: nursing, medicine, laboratory, dietary, physical and occupational therapy, and pharmacy (Figure 2-3).

Each agency designs or customizes critical pathways for conditions with highly predictable results that are commonly treated in that agency. The critical pathway identifies the responses expected in effective treatment and uncomplicated recovery for a given medical diagnosis, as well as the time and date by which the response should be expected. "Detours" from the normal pathways are documented. If the patient is progressing as expected, documentation

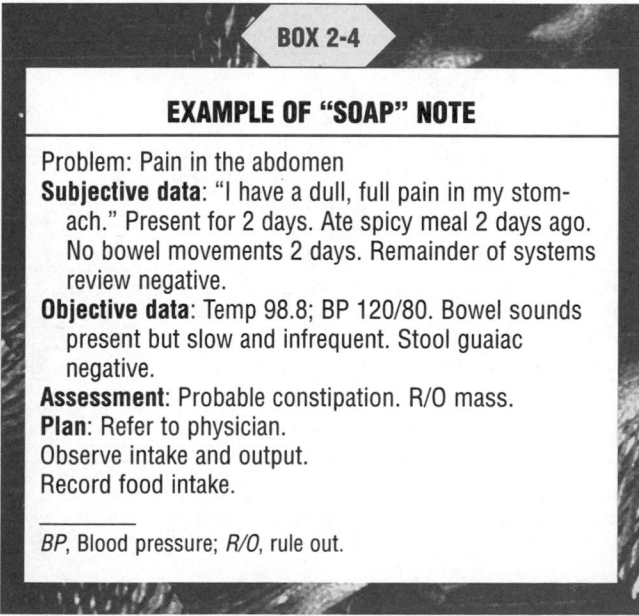

**BOX 2-4**

### EXAMPLE OF "SOAP" NOTE

Problem: Pain in the abdomen
**Subjective data**: "I have a dull, full pain in my stomach." Present for 2 days. Ate spicy meal 2 days ago. No bowel movements 2 days. Remainder of systems review negative.
**Objective data**: Temp 98.8; BP 120/80. Bowel sounds present but slow and infrequent. Stool guaiac negative.
**Assessment**: Probable constipation. R/O mass.
**Plan**: Refer to physician.
Observe intake and output.
Record food intake.

*BP*, Blood pressure; *R/O*, rule out.

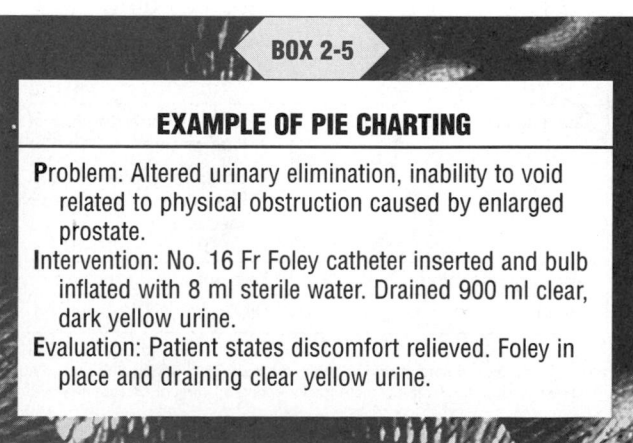

**BOX 2-5**

### EXAMPLE OF PIE CHARTING

**P**roblem: Altered urinary elimination, inability to void related to physical obstruction caused by enlarged prostate.
**I**ntervention: No. 16 Fr Foley catheter inserted and bulb inflated with 8 ml sterile water. Drained 900 ml clear, dark yellow urine.
**E**valuation: Patient states discomfort relieved. Foley in place and draining clear yellow urine.

**NORTHWEST COMMUNITY HEALTHCARE**
**Coordinated Care Map Summary**

☐ Lap Choley c̄ CC (DRG 493)
☐ Lap Choley s̄ CC (DRG 494)

Diagnosis: <u>Laparoscopic cholecystectomy</u>

National LOS: <u>493:4.3  494:1.7 (Geometric)</u>

NWCH: _____

Code Status: _____

Physician: _____

Demographics: <u>Adults with gallbladder dysfunction in need of surgery</u>

| Area of Treatment | Timeframe | Clinical Focus | Expected Outcomes |
|---|---|---|---|
| Physician's office | Preoperative 1-1½ hr | Gallbladder function/status Education • Procedure explanation/plan • Medication | Medical clearance addressed Understands teaching |
| PAT | 1-2 hr (1-6 days preoperative preferably 3 days) | PAT evaluation and testing Patient/SO teaching: • Preoperative/postoperative routines | Testing and evaluation completed Verbalizes understanding of teaching and surgical procedure |
| SDA | 2-3 hr | Preoperative assessment and preparation Anxiety | Secondary medical diagnoses addressed Assessment and preparation complete Verbalizes understanding of surgical plan |
| Operating room | 1-2 hr | Surgical procedure | Responsive with vital signs stable |
| PACU | 1-2 hr | Postanesthesia and postprocedure stabilization | Dressing and drain intact and evaluated Vital signs stable Pain managed |
| Surgical unit | 12-23 hr | Pain management Wound/skin integrity Activity progression Patient education | Pain managed Stable and tolerating diet Afebrile (99.6° F) before discharge |
| Physicians office | Postoperative within 7-10 days/1 hr | Postoperative evaluation | Independent activities of daily living— wound healed |

**Coordinated Care Map Timeframe (minutes, hours, days, weeks, visits)**

| Categories of Care | PAT          Preoperative (3-6 days) | Area:    SDA          DOS |
|---|---|---|
| Consults | Anesthesia Discharge planner as needed Other as needed | Anesthesia as needed Medical physician as needed Other as needed |
| Tests/specimens • Preoperative outpatient • USN of gallbladder • Biliary scan • Oral cholecystogram | Has acceptable test values for surgery  Date _____ Initials _____ • Routine preoperative testing • TXS if ordered, pancreatic function test/arterial blood gas | |
| Treatments/therapy | Completes early preoperative preparation  Assess  Date _____ Initials _____ • Per preoperative protocol • Verify routine medications | Ready for surgery as scheduled • Utilize preoperative protocol  Date _____ Initials _____ • Surgical preparation (if ordered) |
| Fluid balance | | • Start IV (#18) (Place PCA tubing, if ordered) |
| Medication | | • IV antibiotic order • Usual as ordered • Preoperative medication • Anticoagulant (if ordered) |
| Activity | Usual | Bedrest after preoperative medication |
| Miscellaneous | Secondary medical diagnosis addressed History and physical examination complete | • SCDs if ordered • TEDs if ordered • Secondary diagnosis addressed as needed |
| Teaching | Verbalizes understanding of surgical procedure • Plan of care   • What to expect postoperatively  • Scheduling/plan of care  Date _____ Initials _____ • Preoperative/postoperative course • Medication • Other _____ | Verbalizes understanding of plan of care/routines • Preparation • Pain management • IS if ordered) • Preoperative instructions verified  Date _____ Initials _____ • Preparation: review pain management • Postoperative care/routines |
| Discharge planning | Preassessment as needed | |
| Initials | D[  ]  E[  ]  N[  ] | D[  ]  E[  ]  N[  ] |

"The map is a suggested guide for all care providers involved in the patient's care, but it is not intended to establish the only appropriate care that a particular patient may need. Suggested treatments and interventions may be changed and individualized according to the patient's particular condition and assessment data. The map is not to be used as a substitute or replacement for independent clinical assessments and judgments."

**Figure 2-3**   Coordinated Care Map summary. (Care Map is a registered trademark of the Center for Case Management, Inc., South Natick, Mass.) (Courtesy Northwest Community Hospital, Arlington Heights, Ill.)

## Coordinated Care Map Timeframe (minutes, hours, days, weeks, visits)—cont'd

| Categories of Care | Area: Operating room 1-2° DOS Date: | Area: PACU 1° DOS Date: |
|---|---|---|
| Consults | Other (as needed) | |
| Tests/specimens | • Tissue/stone sample to laboratory | |
| Treatments/therapy • Vital signs/ abdominal status | Tolerates surgical procedure<br>• Stable vital signs and NS per anesthesia<br>• Cardiac monitor<br>• Pulse oximetry  Date ____ Initials ____<br>Anesthesia<br>• General<br>• IVA<br>• C-arm table for cholangiogram (if needed)<br>Assess<br>• Systems review in PSPA<br>• Procedure pre OR<br>Safe Environment Preserved<br>• Site/skin preparation  Date ____ Initials ____<br>• Routine surgical monitoring | Recovers from anesthesia with adequate RR/ volume and oxygen SAT per anesthesia<br>• Vital signs stable  Date ____ Initials ____<br>• Reflexes intact<br>• Routine PACU monitoring discontinued per protocol<br>• Extubate per protocol (if ordered)<br>• Oxygen as needed<br>• Vital signs per PACU protocol<br>• Follow postoperative protocol wound management<br>Assess<br>• Check if abdomen soft, check if distention |
| Fluid balance | • IVs<br>• Input and output | • IVs<br>• Input and output |
| Medication/ pain management | • Intravenous antibiotic in PSPA | Experiences pain relief with intravenous titration <5 on scale of 0-10<br>Pain management of<br>• Intravenous titration<br>• PCA (if ordered)<br>• Other _____ |
| Activity | Bedrest | Bedrest |
| Miscellaneous | • SCDs<br>• TEDs (if ordered)<br>• Preparation in PSPA per routine | • SCDs<br>• TEDs (if ordered) |
| Teaching | • Preparation for procedure and process | • Reinforce C & DB + leg exercises |
| Discharge planning | | |
| Initials | D[   ]   E[   ]   N[   ] | D[   ]   E[   ]   N[   ] |
| **Categories of Care** | **Area: Surgical Unit   DOS   Date:** | **Area: Surgical Unit   POD 1   Date:** |
| Consults | | Dietary PRN    Other PRN |
| Tests/specimens | | |
| Treatments/therapy • Vital signs/abdominal status | Recovery from anesthesia with vital signs stable<br>• Alert level of consciousness between pain meds  Date ____ Initials ____<br>• Respirations adequate volume/rate<br>• Vital signs per postoperative protocol<br>Incisions/sites clean and intact  Date ____ Initials ____<br>• Bandaids, steristrips, or dressings intact<br>• Utilize postoperative protocol wound management<br>Abdomen soft  Date ____ Initials ____<br>Assess<br>• Abdomen for distention<br>• Presence of shoulder pain<br>• Bowel function | Vital signs and respiratory status WNL for patient baseline  Date ____ Initials ____<br>• Clear lung sounds<br>• Afebrile<br>• Vital signs per postoperative protocol<br>Assess<br>• Temperature trends<br>Abdomen remains soft with steri strips/sites clean and intact  Date ____ Initials ____<br>Assess<br>• Follow postoperative protocol wound management<br>• Abdomen for distention<br>• Presence of shoulder pain<br>• Bowel function |
| Fluid balance/hydration | I&O balance  Date ____ Initials ____<br>• IVs<br>• I&O<br>• J-P PRN<br>• Clear liquids (as ordered)<br>Assess<br>• Voiding—urine output | I&O Balance  Date ____ Initials ____<br>• IVs<br>• I&O<br>• Discontinue IVs if patient tolerates diet<br>• Regular (low-fat) diet<br>Assess<br>• I&O |
| Medication | Acceptable comfort level <5 on scale 0-10 (with medication)  Date ____ Initials ____<br>Pain management<br>• PCA<br>• IM<br>• PO | Acceptable comfort level <3 on scale 0-10 (with medication)<br>Pain management<br>• PO pain medication<br>• Other _____ |

**Figure 2-3, cont'd**    For legend see opposite page.

Continued

## Coordinated Care Map Timeframe (minutes, hours, days, weeks, visits)—cont'd

| Categories of Care | Area: Surgical Unit    DOS    Date: | Area: Surgical Unit    POD 1    Date: |
|---|---|---|
| Medication—cont'd | Pain management—cont'd<br>• IV antibiotics<br>• IM nausea medication<br>• Other _____<br>Assess<br>• Comfort level | |
| Activity | Tolerates chair/OOB with moderate assistance<br>• Up to chair<br>• OOB with help<br>• BRP with help   Date _____ Initials _____ | • Up and about |
| Miscellaneous | • SCDs if ordered<br>• TEDs if ordered<br>• IS if ordered<br>• Medical service for orders | • IS if ordered |
| Teaching | • Start discharge teaching<br>• Reinforce C & DB and leg exercises | Performs self-care independently   Date _____ Initials _____<br>• Self care management<br>• Wound care<br>• Activity<br>• When to call for resource<br>• Diet instruction (PRN) |
| Discharge planning | | Preparations made for home   Date _____ Initials _____ |
| Initials | D[  ]    E[  ]    N[  ] | D[  ]    E[  ]    N[  ] |

## INDIVIDUALIZED CARE MAPPING PLAN

| Date | Patient Problem | Plan | Outcome | Date Met |
|---|---|---|---|---|
| | | | | |
| | | | | |
| | | | | |
| | | | | |
| | | | | |
| | | | | |
| | | | | |

## DETOURS

Admission Date: _____

Actual Discharge Date: _____

Case Type: Laparoscopic Cholecystectomy

Secondary Diagnosis: _____    DRG: 493/494

Surgical Procedures: _____    Expected LOS: __

Directions for use: Please code each entry with one of the listed codes below.

| Date | Time | Source no. | Description | Action Taken/Results | Int. |
|---|---|---|---|---|---|
| | | | | | |
| | | | | | |
| | | | | | |
| | | | | | |
| | | | | | |
| | | | | | |
| | | | | | |

### DETOUR SOURCE CODE

A. PATIENT/FAMILY
  1. Patient condition
  2. Pt/Family decision
  3. Pt/Family availability
  4. Pt/Family other

B. CAREGIVER/CLINICIAN
  5. Physician order
  6. Caregiver(s) decision
  7. Caregiver(s) response timelity
  8. Caregiver other

C. HOSPITAL/SYSTEM
  9. Bed/appt. time availability
  10. Information/data availability
  11. Supplies/equipment availability
  12. Department overbooked/closed
  13. Hospital other

D. COMMUNITY
  14. Placement/home care availability
  15. Ambulance delay
  16. Community other

Addressograph

**Figure 2-3, cont'd**    For legend see page 30.

involves a simple indicator, such as initialing, to convey that the patient's status is as expected. The nursing diagnoses commonly found for patients with a given medical diagnosis are identified to develop critical pathways. The common nursing interventions are specified, giving direction to appropriate nursing care.

As with standardized care plans, problems other than those expected can be added to a standard critical pathway or care map, allowing for individualized care for a specific patient. Because the nurse can compare the patient's progress to that normally expected, pathways can be used by administrators and accreditation committees to evaluate quality and productivity and by insurers as the basis for reimbursement. The nurse uses the nursing process and the nursing care plan in collaborating with other disciplines to develop critical pathways.

## Evaluation

Evaluation is the final stage of the nursing process. It requires a comparison of current results or patient behaviors to the expected outcome criteria or goals for each nursing diagnosis. The effectiveness of the plan of care is evaluated throughout the implementation phase, and the plan must be modified as necessary to achieve the desired or expected outcomes. The patient is assessed continually to determine progress toward goals and changes in condition. The nursing diagnoses are verified or modified as additional assessment data are obtained. Each intervention is evaluated in terms of its effectiveness in meeting expected outcomes. The outcome criteria are reviewed to determine if they are achievable and revised if they are not. The entire plan is maintained, modified, or completely revised in light of the patient's status and progress toward goals or outcomes.

## Interrelationship of Phases of Nursing Process

Although the nursing process has been described as comprising five phases, these phases do not occur in rigid progression. The process always begins with assessment, thus providing data required to develop a plan. The collection of data must be followed by a determination of what data are relevant. This analysis of relevant information guides identification of the nursing diagnosis. Once the nursing diagnosis has been identified, the plan can be developed. As part of the plan, expected outcomes are identified. As the nurse carries out the plan, the patient's responses are assessed during every intervention. The patient's response is compared to the expected outcome identified in the plan, which is a way of evaluating care. Evaluation requires further assessment. The results of the evaluation are used to make changes in the nursing diagnosis, to revise the goals or expected outcomes, and to modify the plan of care, including methods of intervention. The nursing process is a continuous cycle, and each step or phase does not always occur in isolation from the others.

## Roles in the Nursing Process

Critical thinking skills are used by all nurses as they engage in decision making and the nursing process. In a structured setting, where the licensed practical or vocational nurse (LPN or LVN) has an opportunity to consult with a registered nurse (RN), the LPN or LVN can determine the needs and provide care for patients with common, well-defined health problems. In this setting the LPN or LVN is able to contribute to the plan of care, perform identified nursing interventions, assess the patient's progress, and evaluate the effectiveness of care provided.

## KEY CONCEPTS

➤ Critical thinking is a process used to make sound, accurate, and reasonable decisions on the basis of thorough data collection and analysis.

➤ Critical thinking has five elements: (1) data collection, (2) analysis, (3) deductive and inductive reasoning, (4) hypothesis testing, and (5) evaluation.

➤ The nursing process is a dynamic, problem-solving process comprising five steps or phases: (1) assessment, (2) analysis/nursing diagnosis, (3) planning/expected outcomes, (4) implementation (performance and documentation), and (5) evaluation.

➤ Assessment requires the collection and recording of *objective data* obtained through observation and of *subjective data* obtained from statements made by the patient.

➤ Effective interviewing techniques are essential for obtaining a complete medical and family history.

➤ A nursing diagnosis describes a combination of signs and symptoms indicating actual or potential health problems that nurses are licensed to treat and are capable of treating.

➤ The nursing diagnosis focuses on the patient's response to an actual or potential health problem. It differs from the medical diagnosis, which is concerned primarily with identifying an illness or injury.

➤ A NANDA-approved nursing diagnosis includes a *p*roblem statement, followed by a statement that describes the *e*tiology, followed by the characteristic *s*igns and symptoms: the PES format.

➤ The use of nursing diagnoses provides a common language for nurses.

➤ In the planning phase of the nursing process, a concise, written design of action is developed on the basis of the nursing diagnosis. Expected outcomes are identified, priorities are set, and interventions are proposed.

➤ An expected outcome is a specific, objective, and desired result or patient behavior that will occur when the goal is met.

➤ Action verbs and specific numbers are critical elements of measurable outcome statements.

➤ Implementation involves the actual performance of the prescribed nursing interventions, including direct care, observations, and health teaching, supervision of others performing these activities, and documentation.

➤ Documentation of assessments and interventions is an important part of the patient's permanent record, which is considered a legal document.

➤ A problem-oriented record follows a format represented by the acronym SOAP: *s*ubjective data, *o*bjective data, *a*ssessment (or analysis of data), followed by the *p*lan.

➤ Standardized care plans are adapted and individualized to the particular patient situation.

➤ A critical pathway, or care map, is an interdisciplinary plan of care and method of documentation. It identifies the ideal responses expected in effective treatment and uncomplicated recovery for a given medical diagnosis.

➤ Evaluation is the final phase of the nursing process. The outcomes established in the planning phase are compared to patient behavior and symptoms.

## CRITICAL THINKING EXERCISES

1. Write a paragraph that explains what a nursing diagnosis is and how it differs from a medical diagnosis. Give an example of each.
2. Your hospitalized patient had surgery yesterday. The nurse in charge instructs you to ambulate your patient. What additional information do you need before carrying out the nurse's instructions?
3. Respond to the following statement: Assessment skills are more important than evaluation skills.

## REFERENCES AND ADDITIONAL READINGS

Alfaro-LeFevre R: *Critical thinking in nursing: a practical approach*, Philadelphia, 1985, Saunders.

Alfaro-LeFevre R: *Applying nursing process: a step-by-step guide*, New York, 1994, Lippincott.

Alfaro-LeFevre R: *Critical thinking in nursing: a practical approach*, Philadelphia, 1995, Saunders.

Alfaro-LeFevre R: Improving your ability to think critically, *Nursing Spectrum* 11(4):14-16, 1998.

Allen CV: *Nursing process in collaborative practice*, ed 2, Stanford, Conn, 1997, Appleton & Lange.

American Philosophical Association: Critical thinking: a statement of expert consensus for purposes of educational assessment and instruction. The Delphi Report: research findings and recommendations prepared for the Committee on Pre-College Philosophy, ERIC Document Reproductive Service 3:315-423, 1990.

Astedt-Kurki P, Hopia H: The family interview: exploring experiences of family health and well-being, *J Adv Nurs* 34(3):506-511, 1996.

Bandman B, Bandman E: *Critical thinking in nursing*, Norwalk, Conn, 1988, Appleton & Lange.

Doenges M, Moorhouse MF: *Guide: nursing diagnoses with interventions*, Philadelphia, 1996, Davis.

Facione N, Facione P, Sanchez P: Critical thinking disposition as a measure of competent clinical judgment: the development of the California Critical Thinking Disposition Inventory, *J Nurs Educ* 33(8):345-350, 1994.

Fry ST: The ethic of caring: can it survive in nursing? *Nurs Outlook* 36(1):48, 1988.

Gordon M: *Nursing diagnosis: process and application*, ed 3, St Louis, 1994, Mosby.

Greenwood D: Nursing care plans: issues and solutions, *Nurs Manage* 27(3):33, 37-40, 1996.

Hydo B: Designing an effective clinical pathway for stroke, *Am J Nurs* 95(3):44-51, 1995.

Leski J: Critical literacy: new ways to think and learn, *Nurs Spect* 6(6):9, 1993.

Miller M: *Critical thinking applied to nursing*, St Louis, 1996, Mosby.

North American Nursing Diagnosis Association: *Classification of nursing diagnosis: proceedings of the tenth conference*, New York, 1994, Lippincott.

Paul R: *Critical thinking*, Rohnert Park, Calif, 1990, Sonoma State University.

Paul R: *Critical thinking: how to prepare students for a rapidly changing world*, Santa Rosa, Calif, 1993, Foundation for Critical Thinking.

Snyder M, Egan ED, Nojima Y: Defining nursing interventions, *Image J Nurs Scholarsh* 28(2):137-141, 1996.

Varcoe E: Disparagement of the nursing process: the new dogma? *J Adv Nurs* 23(1):120-125, 1996.

Watson J: *Human science and human care*, New York, 1988, National League for Nursing.

Wilkinson JM: *Nursing process: a critical thinking approach*, Menlo Park, Calif, 1996, Addison-Wesley.

# CHAPTER 3

# Health Assessment

## CHAPTER OBJECTIVES

1 Define health assessment, its components, and its purpose.
2 Discuss the ways nurses use information obtained from the health assessment.
3 Explain the appropriate use of inspection, palpation, percussion, and auscultation in health assessment.
4 Identify and explain the equipment needed to perform a physical examination.
5 Demonstrate how to record information from a health assessment in an appropriate format.

## KEY TERMS

| | |
|---|---|
| auscultation | objective data |
| bruit | pallor |
| crepitus | palpation |
| cyanosis | percussion |
| edema | PERRLA |
| erythema | proprioception |
| inflammation | subjective data |
| inspection | turgor |
| jaundice | |

Health assessment is the process of obtaining subjective data and objective data from the patient. This assessment is the first step in the nursing process. Assessment of the patient includes a history of present illness, a past health history, and a family health history, as well as a physical examination. Nurses make their initial observations and determinations during the first contact with the patient, which may occur in the hospital, physician's office, outpatient department, or some other health care setting. The nurse repeats some parts of the assessment with each patient contact.

Whether assessing a patient for the first time or assessing a patient's health status during a lengthy hospital stay, nurses use the data collected in three ways: (1) to formulate nursing diagnoses and a plan of care, (2) to evaluate the effects of care, medications, and treatments, and (3) to determine health teaching and home care needs.

## GENERAL ASSESSMENT

### Baseline Assessment

The initial assessment of the patient may be very brief, such as an evaluation of the patient's status at the beginning of the shift. This assessment may be made while the report from the previous shift is being given, such as in walking rounds. It allows for introduction of the nurse to the patient, transference of care, and evaluation of assessment data that may point to a need for prompt action, such as the discovery of an infiltrated intravenous (IV) line.

The information obtained for a baseline assessment is determined by the type of unit to which the patient is admitted. On a telemetry unit, for example, this might involve reviewing the patient's cardiac rhythm; on a surgical unit, checking an abdominal dressing would be an appropriate assessment. Box 3-1 presents an example of a form that can be used to guide and record a baseline assessment. The form can be adapted to any specialty. It should be noted, however, that this abbreviated format should not take place of the thorough assessment that follows.

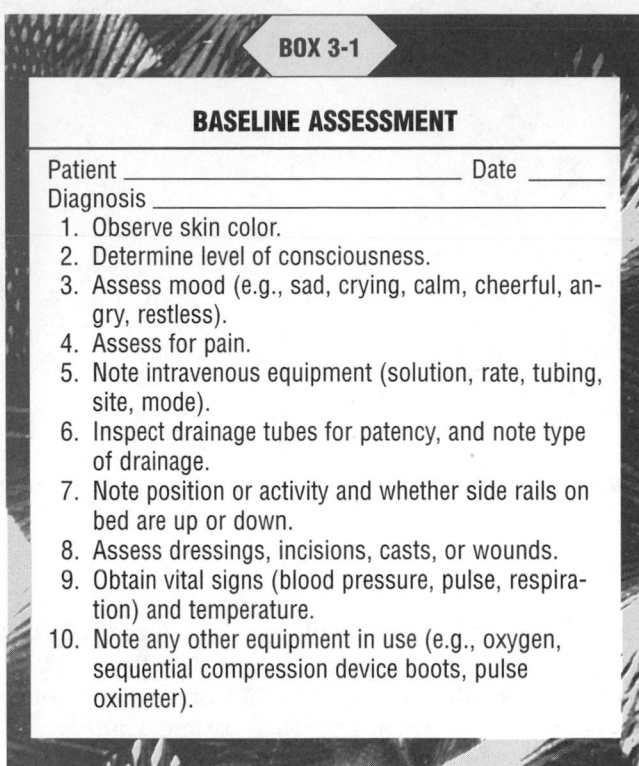

**BOX 3-1**

### BASELINE ASSESSMENT

Patient _____ Date _____
Diagnosis _____
1. Observe skin color.
2. Determine level of consciousness.
3. Assess mood (e.g., sad, crying, calm, cheerful, angry, restless).
4. Assess for pain.
5. Note intravenous equipment (solution, rate, tubing, site, mode).
6. Inspect drainage tubes for patency, and note type of drainage.
7. Note position or activity and whether side rails on bed are up or down.
8. Assess dressings, incisions, casts, or wounds.
9. Obtain vital signs (blood pressure, pulse, respiration) and temperature.
10. Note any other equipment in use (e.g., oxygen, sequential compression device boots, pulse oximeter).

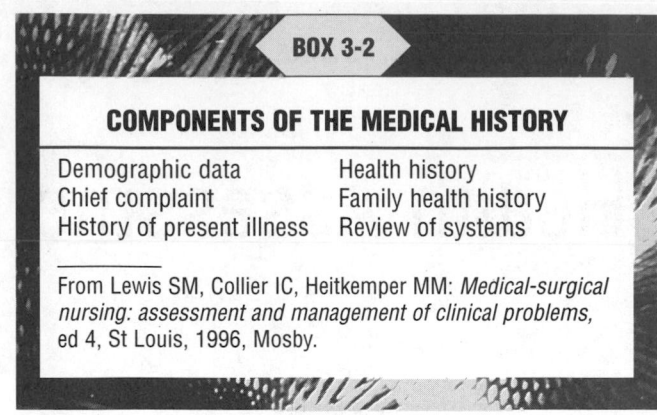

**BOX 3-2**

### COMPONENTS OF THE MEDICAL HISTORY

| | |
|---|---|
| Demographic data | Health history |
| Chief complaint | Family health history |
| History of present illness | Review of systems |

From Lewis SM, Collier IC, Heitkemper MM: *Medical-surgical nursing: assessment and management of clinical problems,* ed 4, St Louis, 1996, Mosby.

keep an open mind, and (3) avoid drawing rapid conclusions. Then the nurse should introduce himself or herself to the patient. The nurse should explain the purpose of the interview and the reason the information is needed. The patient should be reassured that the information obtained will be kept confidential. A nurse's skill in interviewing evolves over time. The nurse's experience, ability to accept the patient as an individual, ease in asking about sensitive topics, and ability to determine the patient's major concerns all affect the interviewing process.

A beginning nurse may obtain the patient's history during several sessions, gathering information from the patient or from a reliable family member. Information may need to be obtained from family members for patients with severe mental confusion, head and neck injuries, tracheostomies, stroke, or severe anxiety or withdrawal. Closed-ended questions, or questions that require a brief response (e.g., "Have you ever been hospitalized before?"), are used to collect some information. Sensitive topics may be addressed by asking open-ended questions, or questions that require more than a "yes" or "no" answer (e.g., "What type of recreational drugs do you use?"). Open-ended questions imply acceptance of the patient and a nonjudgmental attitude on the part of the nurse. (See Chapter 10 for a discussion of closed- and open-ended questions.)

# HISTORY

Physicians and nurses use the patient's medical history differently. Physicians use the medical history as a tool to make a medical diagnosis. (Box 3-2 presents the components of the medical history.) Nurses are concerned with "the diagnosis and treatment of human responses to actual or potential health problems" (American Nurses Association, 1980). Data gathered when the history is taken and during the physical examination allow the nurse to make nursing diagnoses. (See Chapter 2 for information on the nursing process.)

 ### ETHNIC/CULTURAL CONSIDERATIONS

A first-generation immigrant woman of East Indian, Hindu, culture is expected to sit passively by her husband, with all questions and inquiries directed to him. Seeking information directly from the wife may precipitate, on the part of the husband, feelings of personal humiliation and disrespect in the eyes of his family (Giger, Davidhizar, 1995).

The purpose of the history interview is to obtain information that will enable the nurse to provide the best care for the patient. Before beginning the interview, the nurse should resolve to (1) stay calm, (2)

 ### ETHNIC/CULTURAL CONSIDERATIONS

Navajo Native Americans believe that it is ethically wrong to speak for another individual. This belief makes it difficult to obtain a history from a relative or person other than the patient (Giger, Davidhizar, 1995).

When the patient's major concern differs from the nurse's priority, conflict can arise. It is important for the nurse to assess the patient's concerns and address them as soon as possible. Once that need has been met, the nurse's priorities can be met as well. For example, the nurse may want to explain a diagnostic test to the patient, but the patient may want relief from a headache. The nurse is wise to investigate the patient's concern before proceeding.

## Subjective Problem Assessment

A subjective complaint is a symptom the patient is experiencing but that is not observable by the nurse. For example, during the history interview, the patient may report pain, such as a headache. The nurse should further investigate this **subjective data**, or information reported by the patient, as to location, quality, intensity, chronology, setting, aggravating or alleviating factors, associated factors, and meaning for the patient. Box 3-3 presents a guideline for investigating a symptom. *It is important to allow patients to explain the problem in their own words.* (See Chapter 11 for a detailed explanation of pain assessment.)

## Obtaining the Health History

When interviewing a patient to obtain health information, it is important that the nurse ask questions about past and present medical problems, surgical procedures, and other treatments. Box 3-4 presents a format for recording a health history that is based on assessment of the patient's functional health patterns (Lewis, Collier, Heitkemper, 1996). The process of selecting nursing diagnoses becomes easier if these patterns are used to obtain information.

Questions about past health matters should cover childhood and adult illnesses, injuries, operations, and hospitalizations. The nurse also should ask the patient about the use of any prescription or over-the-counter (OTC) medications. It is important to ask about recreational drug use, including the consumption of alcohol, and about the patient's smoking history (see Chapter 10 for more information on substance abuse). The problem, when it occurred, its treatment, and the outcome are recorded.

## Assessing Health Patterns

The nurse is responsible for assessing both the patient's strengths and the areas in which a problem may exist or in which the patient may be at risk of developing a problem. This information is used in formulating nursing diagnoses (see Chapter 2 for detailed information on the nursing process). The patient should be asked about concepts of health and practices for staying healthy. The patient also should be asked about any allergies (to medications, food, or other substances, such as latex). Questions about a family history of major

---

**BOX 3-3**

### Guideline Questionnaire for Investigating a Symptom

**LOCATION**
Ask:      "Where do you feel it? Where is it located?"
Record:   Region of the body
          Local or radiating, superficial or deep

**QUALITY**
Ask:      "What does it (feel, look) like?"
Record:   The patient's analogy (e.g., "Like being burned")

**QUANTITY**
Ask:      "How often do you have this feeling? How bad is it? How much is it? How big is it?"
Record:   Frequency (mild, moderate, severe), volume, size, extent, number

**CHRONOLOGY**
Ask:      "When was the first time it occurred? Any particular time of day, week, month, or year?"
Record:   Time of onset, duration, periodicity and frequency, course of symptoms

**SETTING**
Ask:      "Where are you when this occurs? What are you doing?"
Record:   Where patient is when symptom occurs, what patient is doing, if symptom is related to anything

**AGGRAVATING OR ALLEVIATING FACTORS**
Ask:      "What makes it better? Worse? Is there any activity that seems to cause it? What have you done for it? Did it help? Was there some reason you didn't do anything about it?"
Record:   Influence of physical and emotional activities, patient's attempts to alleviate (or treat) the symptom

**ASSOCIATED MANIFESTATIONS**
Ask:      "What other things do you see or feel when it occurs? Has it affected your appetite? Elimination? Sleeping?"
Record:   Other symptoms

**MEANING OF THE SYMPTOM TO THE PATIENT**
Ask:      "How has it affected your life? Why have you sought care now? What do you think may be the cause?"
Record:   Patient's statements about the effect of the symptom and the cause of the symptom

From Lewis SM, Collier IC, Heitkemper MM: *Medical-surgical nursing: assessment and management of clinical problems,* ed 4, St Louis, 1996, Mosby.

BOX 3-4

## OBTAINING THE NURSING HISTORY (FUNCTIONAL HEALTH PATTERN FORMAT)

**DEMOGRAPHIC DATA**
Name, address, age, occupation

**IMPORTANT HEALTH INFORMATION**
Past health history
Medications
Surgery or other treatments

**FUNCTIONAL HEALTH PATTERNS**
**Health Perception–Health Management Pattern**
1. Reason for visit?
2. General state of health?
3. Any colds in past year?
4. Most important things done to keep healthy? Breast self-examination? Testicular self-examination? Other routine screening?
5. Health compliance problems?
6. Cause of illness? Action taken? Results?
7. Things important to you while here?
8. Family health history?
9. Illness and injury risk factors: use of cigarettes, alcohol, drugs?
10. Allergies? Immunizations?

**Nutritional-Metabolic Pattern**
1. Typical daily food intake (describe)? Supplements?
2. Typical daily fluid intake (describe)?
3. Weight loss or gain (amount, time span)?
4. Desired weight?
5. Appetite?
6. Food or eating: Discomfort? Diet restrictions?
7. Appetite?
8. Heal well or poorly?
9. Skin problems: Lesions? Dryness?
10. Dental problems?
11. Change in appetite with anxiety?
12. Food preferences?
13. Food allergies?

**Elimination Pattern**
1. Bowel elimination pattern (describe): Frequency? Character? Discomfort? Laxatives? Enemas?
2. Urinary elimination pattern (describe): Frequency? Problem in control? Diuretics?
3. Any external devices?
4. Excess perspiration? Odor problems? Itching?

**Activity-Exercise Pattern**
1. Sufficient energy for desired or required activities?
2. Exercise pattern? Type? Regularity?

3. Spare time (leisure) activities?
4. Dyspnea? Chest pain? Palpitations? Stiffness? Aching? Weakness?
5. Perceived ability for (code for level):
   Feeding _____ Cooking _____
   Grooming _____ Bed mobility _____
   Bathing _____ Home maintenance _____
   General mobility _____ Dressing _____
   Toileting _____ Shopping _____

**Sleep-Rest Pattern**
1. Generally rested and ready for daily activities after sleep?
2. Sleep onset problems? Aids? Dreams (nightmares)? Early awakening?
3. Usual sleep rituals?
4. Usual sleep pattern?

**Cognitive-Perceptual Pattern**
1. Hearing difficulty? Aid?
2. Vision? Wear glasses? Last checked?
3. Any change in taste? Any change in smell?
4. Any recent change in memory?
5. Easiest way to learn things?
6. Any discomfort? Pain? How managed?
7. Ability to communicate?
8. Understanding of illness?
9. Understanding of treatments?

**Self-Perception–Self-Concept Pattern**
1. Self-description? Self-perception?
2. Effect of illness on self-image?
3. Relieving factors?

**Role-Relationship Pattern**
1. Live alone? Family? Family structure diagram?
2. Difficult family problems?
3. Family problem solving?
4. Family dependence on you for things? How managing?
5. Family's and others' feelings about illness/hospitalization?*
6. Problems with children? Difficulty handling?*
7. Belong to social groups? Have close friends? Felt lonely (frequency)?
8. Work satisfaction (school)? Income sufficient for needs?*
9. Feel part of or isolated to neighborhood where living?

Modified from Fuller J, Schaller-Ayers J: *Health assessment: a nursing approach,* ed 2, Philadelphia, 1994, Lippincott.
*If appropriate.

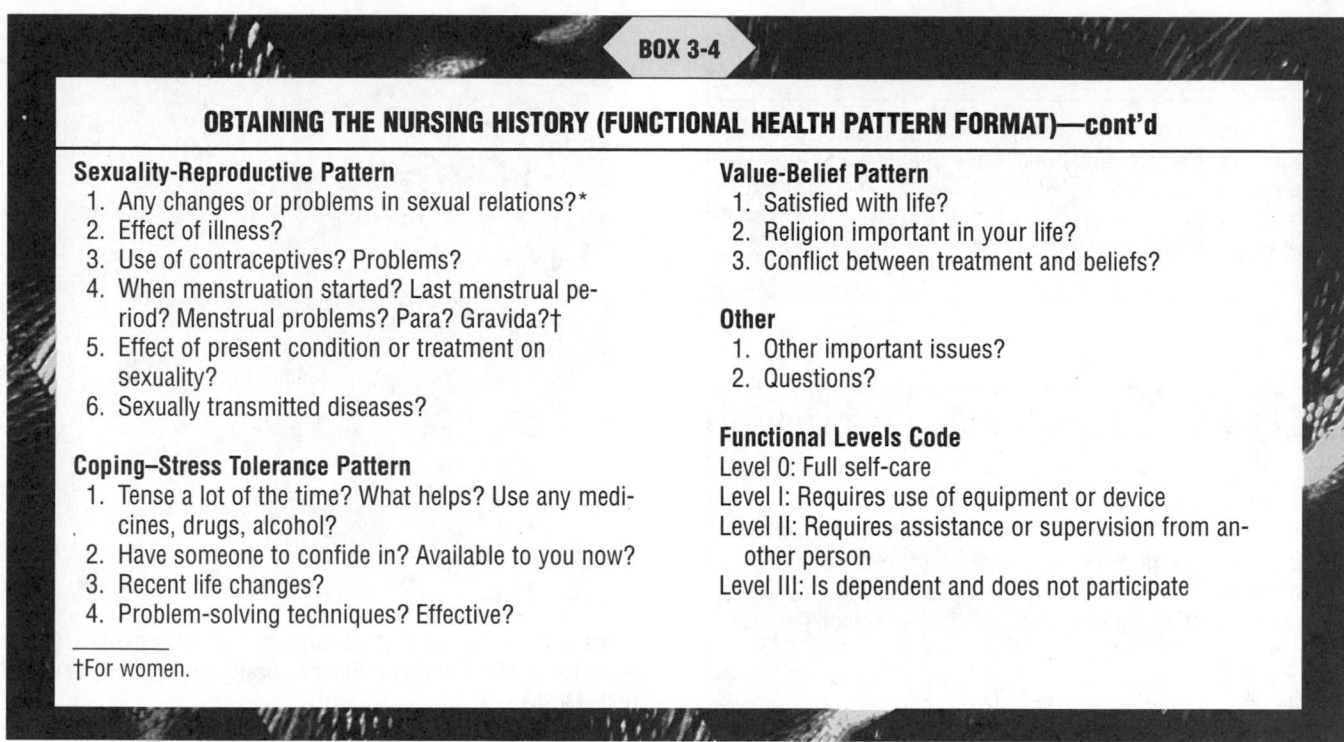

BOX 3-4

**OBTAINING THE NURSING HISTORY (FUNCTIONAL HEALTH PATTERN FORMAT)—cont'd**

**Sexuality-Reproductive Pattern**
1. Any changes or problems in sexual relations?*
2. Effect of illness?
3. Use of contraceptives? Problems?
4. When menstruation started? Last menstrual period? Menstrual problems? Para? Gravida?†
5. Effect of present condition or treatment on sexuality?
6. Sexually transmitted diseases?

**Coping–Stress Tolerance Pattern**
1. Tense a lot of the time? What helps? Use any medicines, drugs, alcohol?
2. Have someone to confide in? Available to you now?
3. Recent life changes?
4. Problem-solving techniques? Effective?

†For women.

**Value-Belief Pattern**
1. Satisfied with life?
2. Religion important in your life?
3. Conflict between treatment and beliefs?

**Other**
1. Other important issues?
2. Questions?

**Functional Levels Code**
Level 0: Full self-care
Level I: Requires use of equipment or device
Level II: Requires assistance or supervision from another person
Level III: Is dependent and does not participate

---

illnesses (e.g., diabetes mellitus, heart disease, cancer, hypertension, or psychiatric or behavioral disorders) or of drug or alcohol abuse or violence should be asked at this time. While obtaining this information from the patient, the nurse should assess the patient's knowledge of any problems, ability to manage problems, and developmental stage. All this information allows the nurse to develop a plan of care that addresses the patient's individual strengths and needs.

It is important that the nurse obtain the following information in assessing the patient's health patterns.
1. Question the patient about nutritional status. Ask the individual to recall the past 24-hour intake and to list foods liked and disliked. Ask about the number of servings, snacks, and times the patient eats. Does anxiety or depression play a part in how much or how little is eaten? Are budget constraints a factor?
2. Ask about bowel and urinary elimination patterns. Is pain associated with either? Does the patient use laxatives or enemas routinely? Does the patient have a catheter, colostomy, or other means of urinary or fecal diversion? Does he or she know how to care for it? Assess the skin surrounding any catheter or ostomy at this time.
3. Question the patient about exercise and activity. Assess the person's ability to perform activities of daily living (ADL). Box 3-4 includes a code for functional level that indicates the patient's ability to perform everyday activities.
4. Question the patient about ability to fall asleep, number of hours of sleep per night, and nightly routine. Does the patient take medication for sleep? If so, what kind, how much, and how often? What does the patient do to relax? Does he or she nap during the day?
5. Ask about any barriers to performing ADL. Does the patient have any problems affecting use of the senses (taste, touch, hearing, or vision)? When was the last eye examination? Ask questions to assess the patient's understanding of the illness and treatment. Any problems with memory? Assess pain at this time (review Box 3-3).
6. Determine how the patient perceives himself or herself. What concerns the patient? What feelings does the patient have about body image, abilities, and self-esteem?
7. Question the patient about relationships. Ask the patient to describe relationships at home and at work, as well as social relationships. Note the person's self-evaluation of these roles. Is the pattern stressful or satisfactory?
8. Ask the patient about any sexual or reproductive concerns. Formulate the questions so that they are age appropriate. For example, a 23-year-old, sexually active man should be questioned about his knowledge and use of condoms. A 70-year-old man might be asked about problems with urinary incontinence.

## ETHNIC/CULTURAL CONSIDERATIONS

Discussing topics concerning sex and reproduction may not always be appropriate in some cultures. For example, an Arabic woman traditionally would discuss these issues with women relatives but not with men or strangers (Giger, Davidhizar, 1995).

## ETHNIC/CULTURAL CONSIDERATIONS

Spanish-speaking and Native American patients speak more freely to a nurse of the same sex. When talking about sexual matters with a male child of Spanish-speaking, Pakistani, or Arabic parents, it is important to have the father present rather than the mother (Giger, Davidhizar, 1995).

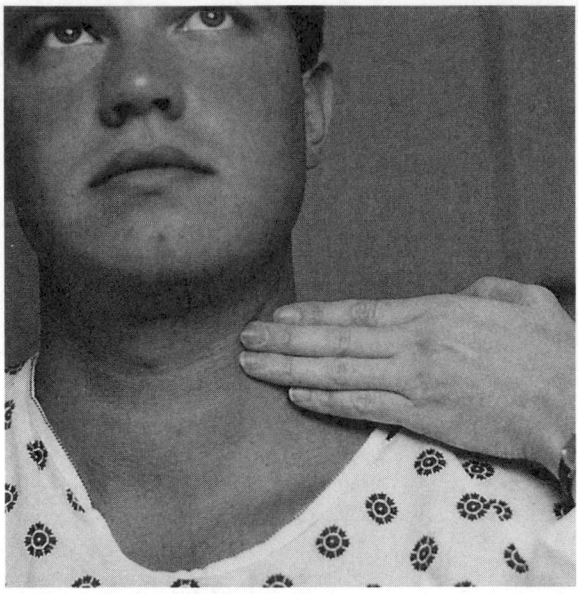

**Figure 3-1** Palpation is the examination of the body through the use of touch. (From Potter P, Perry A: *Basic nursing,* ed 3, St Louis, 1995, Mosby.)

9. To assess the patient's coping abilities and stress tolerance, ask him or her about any major stressors, either current or that occurred within the past year (e.g., loss of a job, divorce, or death of spouse). Ask the patient what measures are taken to help relieve stress or what has been done in the past that helped the patient cope with a stressful situation. Record the names of people the patient has found supportive. (See Chapter 6 for information on psychologic responses.)
10. Ask the patient about any spiritual, cultural, or ethnic practices that are important to the individual and to his or her care. Do any conflicts arise between these practices and the care provided? (Chapter 8 presents additional information on cultural considerations.)

## PHYSICAL ASSESSMENT TECHNIQUES

After completing the health history interview, the nurse is ready to begin the physical examination. This examination consists of a systematic review of the patient's physical and mental status. This information is considered **objective data**, or that observable by the nurse. As with the history, any positive finding is further evaluated using the criteria in Box 3-3. A negative finding, when a positive finding is expected, (e.g., *absent left pedal pulse*) is significant and is recorded.

Four examination techniques are used in performing a physical assessment: inspection, palpation, percussion, and auscultation. The proper equipment also is important.

## Inspection

**Inspection** is the direct observation of a part or area of the body to assess the condition of that area. The nurse uses focused observation to check over the area carefully. Comparisons are made between what is generally known and what is seen. For example, an observation of exophthalmos (bulging of the eyeballs) is an abnormal finding and indicates a need for investigation of thyroid function.

## Palpation

**Palpation** is the examination of a body area through the use of touch. Using palpation, the nurse can detect masses, tenderness, pain, swelling, and spasms. Pulses and lymph nodes can be felt more easily if the nurse palpates with the tips of the fingers. The dorsal part of the hand is best for assessing temperature. Figure 3-1 shows the use of palpation. (See the appropriate chapters for a detailed discussion of palpation for each area of the body.)

## Percussion

**Percussion** is a technique that involves placing the middle finger of the nondominant hand on the body's surface and striking the tip of the middle finger of the

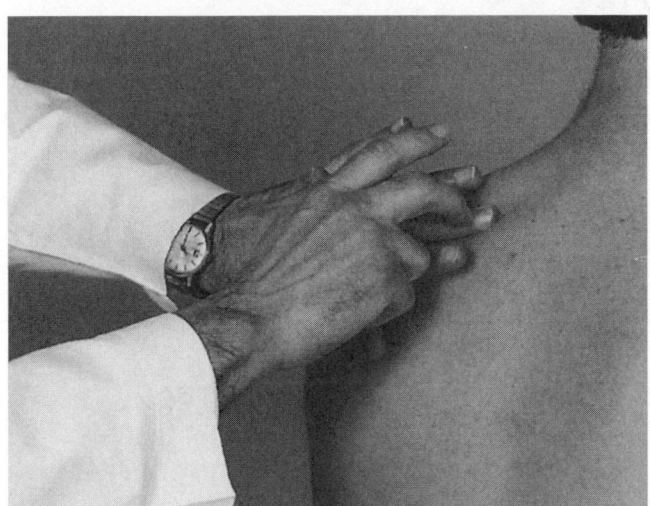

**Figure 3-2**   Percussion technique: tapping the interphalangeal joint. Only the middle finger of the nondominant hand should be in contact with the skin's surface, producing sound. (From Seidel H: *Mosby's guide to physical examinations*, ed 3, St Louis, 1995, Mosby.)

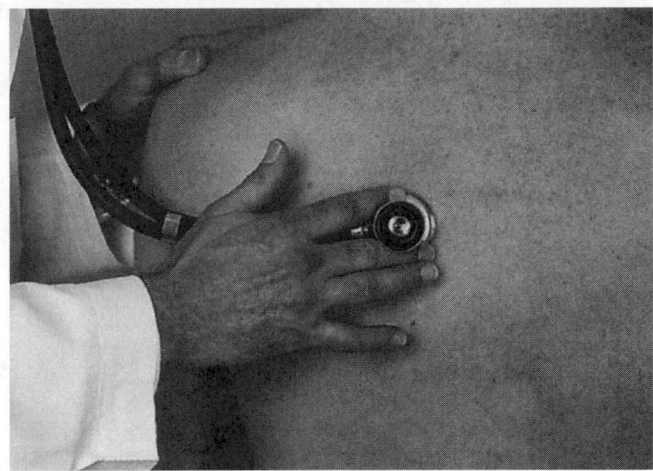

**Figure 3-3**   Auscultation is listening to sounds produced by the body to assess normal conditions and deviations from normal. (From Seidel H: *Mosby's guide to physical examinations*, ed 3, St Louis, 1995, Mosby.)

dominant hand against the finger of the nondominant hand (Figure 3-2). Percussion is performed to obtain information about an underlying area or organ. Using percussion, the examiner also can determine if fluid, air, or masses are present. (See the appropriate chapters for a detailed discussion of percussion sounds.)

## Auscultation

**Auscultation** involves the use of a stethoscope to amplify sounds (Figure 3-3). Low-pitched sounds are best heard with the bell of the stethoscope, whereas high-pitched sounds are best heard with the diaphragm. Auscultation is used to assess heart sounds, lung sounds, and sounds from the abdomen and vascular system. (See the appropriate chapters for a detailed discussion of auscultatory sounds.)

## Equipment

The use of specific equipment is discussed in the assessment section of the appropriate chapters. Box 3-5 presents a list of equipment that should be available for use during the physical examination.

## PHYSICAL EXAMINATION

### Approach

The physical examination should be performed systematically and efficiently, progressing in a logical manner. The patient's comfort, safety, and privacy must be en-

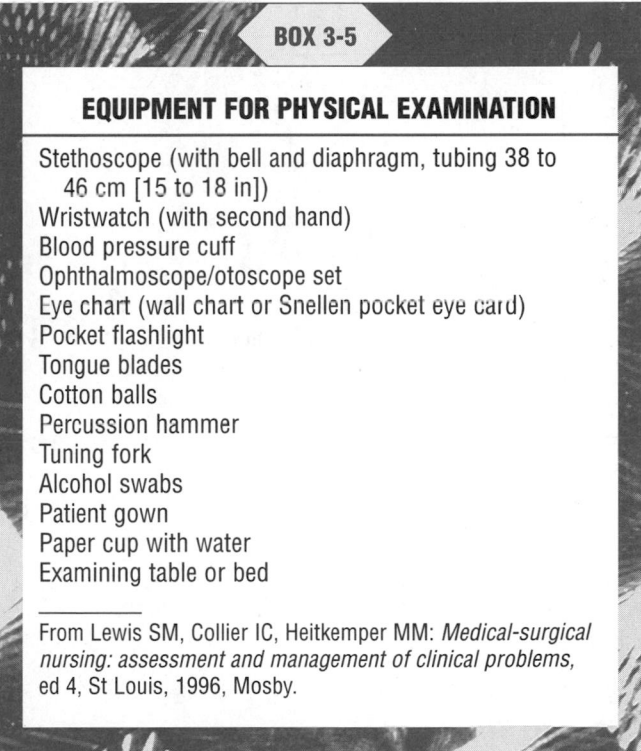

**BOX 3-5**

### EQUIPMENT FOR PHYSICAL EXAMINATION

Stethoscope (with bell and diaphragm, tubing 38 to 46 cm [15 to 18 in])
Wristwatch (with second hand)
Blood pressure cuff
Ophthalmoscope/otoscope set
Eye chart (wall chart or Snellen pocket eye card)
Pocket flashlight
Tongue blades
Cotton balls
Percussion hammer
Tuning fork
Alcohol swabs
Patient gown
Paper cup with water
Examining table or bed

From Lewis SM, Collier IC, Heitkemper MM: *Medical-surgical nursing: assessment and management of clinical problems*, ed 4, St Louis, 1996, Mosby.

sured. The nurse wears gloves when appropriate. Although there are various methods of performing a physical examination, this text reviews the outline presented in Box 3-6. Box 3-7 presents adaptations of the physical examination for the older adult. (See Chapter 9 for a complete discussion of the older adult.)

BOX 3-6

## PHYSICAL EXAMINATION OUTLINE

### 1. GENERAL SURVEY
**Observe General State of Health (Patient is Seated)**
Body features
State of consciousness and arousal
Speech
Body movements
Physical signs
Nutritional status
Stature

### 2. VITAL SIGNS
**Record Vital Signs:**
Blood pressure
Radial pulse
Respiration

**Record Height and Weight**

### 3. INTEGUMENTARY SYSTEM
**Inspect and Palpate Skin for the Following:**
Color
Lesions
Scars
Bruises
Edema
Moisture
Texture
Temperature
Turgor
Vascularity

**Inspect and Palpate Nails for the Following:**
Color
Lesions
Size
Flexibility
Shape
Angle

### 4. HEAD AND NECK
**Inspect and Palpate Head for the Following:**
Shape and symmetry of skull
Masses
Tenderness
Hair
Scalp
Skin
Temporal arteries
Temporomandibular joint

Sensory (CN V, light touch, pain)
Motor (CN VII, shows teeth, purses lips, raises eyebrows)
Looks up, wrinkles forehead (CN VII)
Raises shoulders against resistance (CN XI)

**Inspect and Palpate Eyes for the Following:**
Visual acuity
Eyebrows
Position and movement of eyelids
Visual fields
Extraocular movements (CN III, IV, VI)
Cornea, sclera, conjunctiva
Pupillary response
Red reflex
Eyeball tension

**Inspect and Palpate Each Ear for the Following:**
Placement
Pinna
Auditory acuity (Weber's or Rinne test, whispered voice, ticking watch)
Mastoid process
Auditory canal
Tympanic membrane

**Inspect and Palpate Nose and Sinuses for the Following:**
External nose
    Shape
    Blockage
Internal nose
    Patency of nasal passages
    Shape
    Turbinates or polyps
    Discharge
Discharge
Frontal and maxillary sinuses

**Inspect and Palpate Mouth for the Following:**
Lips (symmetry, lesions, color)
Buccal mucosa (Stensen's and Wharton's ducts)
Teeth (absence, state of repair, color)
Gums
Tongue for strength (asymmetry, ability to stick out tongue, side to side, fasciculations)
Palates
Tonsils and pillars
Uvular elevation (CN IX)

From Lewis SM, Collier IC, Heitkemper MM: *Medical-surgical nursing: assessment and management of clinical problems,* ed 4, St Louis, 1996, Mosby.
*AP,* Anteroposterior; *CN,* cranial nerve; *CVA,* costovertebral angle; *PMI,* point of maximal impulse; *RML,* right middle lobe.

BOX 3-6

## PHYSICAL EXAMINATION OUTLINE—cont'd

### 4. HEAD AND NECK—cont'd
Posterior pharynx
Gag reflex (CN X)
Jaw strength (CN XI)
Moisture
Color
Floor of mouth

### Inspect and Palpate (Occasionally Auscultate) Neck for the Following:
Skin (vascularity and visible pulsations)
Symmetry
Postural alignment
Range of motion
Pulses (carotid)
Midline structure (trachea, thyroid gland, cartilage)
Lymph nodes (preauricular, postauricular, occipital, mandibular, tonsillar, submental, anterior and posterior cervical, infraclavicular, supraclavicular)

### Inspect Neurologic Status:
Motor status observations
  Gait
  Toe walk
  Heel walk
  Drift
Coordination
  Finger to nose
  Romberg's sign
Spine (scoliosis)

### 5. EXTREMITIES
**Observe Size and Shape, Symmetry and Deformity, Involuntary Movements**
**Inspect and Palpate Arms, Fingers, Wrists, Elbows, Shoulders for the Following:**
Strength
Range of motion
Crepitus
Joint pain
Swelling
Fluid

### Test Reflexes:
Biceps
Triceps
Brachioradialis
Patellar
Achilles
Plantar

### Inspect and Palpate Legs for the Following:
Strength of hips
Edema
Hair distribution
Pulses (dorsalis pedis, posterior tibialis)

### 6. POSTERIOR THORAX
**Inspect for Muscular Development, Respiratory Movement, Approximation of AP Diameter**
Palpate for symmetry of respiratory movement, tenderness of CVA, spinous processes, tumors or swelling, tactile fremitus
Percuss for pulmonary resonance
Auscultate for breath sounds

### 7. ANTERIOR THORAX
Assess breasts for configuration, symmetry, dimpling of skin
Assess nipples for rash, direction, inversion, refraction
Initiate teaching or review of breast self-exmination
Perform upright examination
Inspect for PMI, other precordial pulsations
Palpate for thrills, lifts, heaves, tenderness over precordium
Inspect neck for venous distention, pulsations, waves
Palpate axillae
Inspect, palpate neck, check breasts for discharge (patient is supine)
Complete teaching of breast self-examination
Auscultate for rate and rhythm, character of $S_1$ and $S_2$; $S_1$ and $S_2$ in the aortic, pulmonic, Erb's point, tricuspid, mitral areas; bruits at carotid, epigastrium; breath sounds at RML

### 8. ABDOMEN
Inspect for scars, shape, symmetry, bulging, muscular development, position and condition of umbilicus, movements (respiratory, pulsations, presence of peristaltic waves)
Auscultate for peristalsis, femoral bruits
Percuss border of liver, all quadrants
Palpate to confirm positive findings; check liver (size, surface contour, tenderness); spleen; kidney (size, contour, consistency, tenderness, mobility); urinary bladder (distention); femoral pulses; inguinofemoral nodes

### 9. COMPLETION OF EXAMINATIONS OF EXTREMITIES
**Observe the Following:**
Range of motion of hips, ankles, feet
Crepitus

*Continued*

BOX 3-6

## PHYSICAL EXAMINATION OUTLINE—cont'd

**9. COMPLETION OF EXAMINATIONS OF EXTREMITIES—cont'd**
Joint pain
Swelling
Fluid
Muscle development
Coordination (heel to skin)
Homan's sign
Proprioception (position sense of great toe)

**10. GENITALIA***
**Male External Genitalia**
Inspect penis, noting hair distribution, prepuce, glans, urethral meatus, scars, ulcers, eruptions, structural alterations

Inspect epidermis of perineum, rectum
Inspect skin of scrotum; palpate for descended testes, masses, pain

**Female External Genitalia**
Inspect hair distribution; mons pubis, labia (minora and majora); urethral meatus; Bartholin's, urethral, Skene's glands (may also be palpated, if indicated); introitus
Assess for presence of cystocele, rectocele, prolapse (patient bears down)
Inspect perineum, rectum

*If the nurse has the appropriate training, the speculum and bimanual examination of women and the prostate gland examination of men should be performed after this inspection.

## Temperature

The nurse begins the physical examination by checking the patient's temperature. The route (e.g., oral, axillary, tympanic, or rectal) is specified on the data collection sheet. The normal range for an oral temperature is 36° to 37° C (96.8° to 98.6° F). A low body temperature (hypothermia) is indicated by a reading below 35° C (95° F); an elevated body temperature (pyrexia) is manifested by a reading of 38° to 40° C (100.4° to 104° F); a temperature above 41° C (105.8° F) is considered hyperpyrexia.

## Vital Signs
### Blood Pressure

The blood pressure should be checked at least once on both arms and recorded. Blood pressure readings vary with age. (See Chapter 25 for a discussion of hypertension.)

### Radial Pulse

Using the pads of the index and middle fingers, the nurse should palpate the radial pulse and count for 1 full minute. A heart rate of 60 to 100 beats per minute (bpm) is considered normal. Bradycardia is defined as a heart rate below 60 bpm, and tachycardia is a rate above 100 bpm. The nurse should note whether the rhythm is regular or irregular.

## Respirations

Respirations are counted for 1 full minute by observing the rise and fall of the chest as one cycle. A normal respiratory rate for an adult is 14 to 20 cycles per minute. The nurse should note whether the patient's breathing is regular or difficult (labored). (Chapter 22 discusses respiration in detail.)

## Height and Weight

The patient should be asked to stand, if possible, for height and weight measurements. If the patient cannot stand, a bed scale may be used. The nurse should note whether the patient is emaciated, slender, or obese. The patient's height and weight should be compared with the height and weight values shown in Table 3-1.

## Integumentary System
### Skin

The nurse should inspect and palpate the skin, noting color, moisture, texture, temperature, turgor, and vascularity, as well as any lesions, scars, bruises, edema, ulcerations, or excoriations. The nurse also should note the patient's hygiene. (Chapter 40 presents a detailed assessment of the skin.)

**Color.** The nurse should note whether the patient's skin is flushed, pink, pale, jaundiced, or cyanotic. The mouth also should be checked. With **cyanosis**, the mu-

## PHYSICAL ASSESSMENT TECHNIQUES FOR OLDER ADULTS

**GENERAL APPROACH**
Keep patient warm and comfortable because loss of subcutaneous fat decreases ability to stay warm. Adapt positioning to physical limitations. Avoid unnecessary changes in position. Perform as many activities as possible in the position of comfort for the patient.

**SKIN**
Handle with care because of fragility and loss of subcutaneous fat.

**HEAD AND NECK**
Provide a quiet environment free from distraction because of patient's sensory deficits (e.g., decreased vision, touch, hearing).

**EXTREMITIES**
Use nonvigorous movements and reinforcement techniques. Avoid having patient hop on one foot or perform deep knee bends because of patient's limited range of motion of the extremities, decreased reflexes, and diminished sense of balance.

**THORAX**
Adapt examination for changes due to decrease in force of expiration, weakened cough reflex, and shortness of breath.

**ABDOMEN**
Be cautious in palpating patient's liver because it is easily palpated with increased size. The older adult patient may have diminished pain perception in abdominal wall.

**GENITALIA**
Use a well-lubricated, smaller speculum for vaginal examination because dryness and atrophy of the female genitalia may cause discomfort.

From Lewis SM, Collier IC, Heitkemper MM: *Medical-surgical nursing: assessment and management of clinical problems,* ed 4, St Louis, 1996, Mosby.

**TABLE 3-1**

## Healthy Weight Ranges for Adults

| HEIGHT* | WEIGHT (IN POUNDS†) |
|---|---|
| 4'10" | 91-119 |
| 4'11" | 97-128 |
| 5'0" | 97-128 |
| 5'1" | 101-132 |
| 5'2" | 104-137 |
| 5'3" | 107-141 |
| 5'4" | 111-146 |
| 5'5" | 114-150 |
| 5'6" | 118-155 |
| 5'7" | 121-160 |
| 5'8" | 125-164 |
| 5'9" | 129-169 |
| 5'10" | 132-174 |
| 5'11" | 136-179 |
| 6'0" | 140-184 |
| 6'1" | 144-189 |
| 6'2" | 148-195 |
| 6'3" | 152-200 |
| 6'4" | 156-205 |
| 6'5" | 160-211 |
| 6'6" | 164-216 |

From *Report of the Dietary Guidelines Advisory Committee on the Dietary Guidelines for Americans,* 1995.
*Without shoes.
†Without clothes.
**Note:** The higher weights in each range apply to people with more muscle and bone, such as many men.

 **ETHNIC/CULTURAL CONSIDERATIONS**

1. When assessing patients with dark skin, changes in skin color are best observed in the conjunctivae, oral mucosa, tongue, lips, nail beds, palms, and soles.
2. **Pallor** may be seen as yellow-tinged or ashen gray skin.
3. Jaundice may best be seen in the sclerae, close to the center of the eye, or in the hard palate of the mouth.
4. The nail beds, conjunctivae, palms, and soles should be checked for evidence of cyanosis.
5. Petechiae are best seen in the conjunctivae and oral mucosa.
6. **Erythema** is best detected by palpating the skin for an increase in skin temperature.

cous membranes may look pale or bluish. If the patient has **jaundice,** the skin will appear yellow. To assess patients with dark skin for jaundice, the nurse should note the color of the sclerae. (Chapter 40 discusses assessment of individuals with dark skin.)

**Lesions, scars, and bruises.** The nurse should look for lesions, scars, or bruises, estimating the length and width of each and describing their locations. The color of bruised areas also should be noted.

**Moisture, texture, and temperature.** The skin's surface should be felt to determine the skin's moisture con-

tent. If the skin is extremely moist, the patient is said to be diaphoretic. Texture can be determined at the same time by noting whether the patient has rough or smooth skin. The dorsal aspect of the hand is used to assess skin temperature. The nurse should note whether the patient's skin is cool, warm, or hot. The skin normally feels slightly warm to the touch.

**Turgor.** **Turgor** refers to the skin's elasticity. The nurse should gently pinch the patient's skin and observe how quickly the fold returns to place. The speed of return determines the elasticity or the amount of moisture in the skin (see Chapter 28 for a detailed description).

### Nails

The nurse should note the color of the nails. The nails also should be checked for firmness, texture, flexibility, and thickness of the nail, and the nail bed should be assessed for shape and angle. Arterial flow to the extremities is assessed by checking capillary refill, which is done by pressing the fingernail firmly and then releasing it quickly. Normal color should return immediately or within 3 seconds. (Chapter 40 presents information pertaining to assessment of the nails.)

Box 3-8 presents normal physical assessment findings for the integumentary system.

## Head and Neck
### Head

The head and its structures should be inspected and palpated. The nurse should note the shape of the skull. The term *normocephaly* refers to a head that is normal in size in comparison with the body. The nurse should look and palpate for any depressed areas, masses, or tenderness. While inspecting the scalp, the examiner also should note the hair. It should be inspected for color, quantity (thick or thin), distribution (patchy or alopecic), and texture (fine or coarse). The hair should be parted in three places to allow inspection of the scalp for lesions or infestations. The temporal pulses

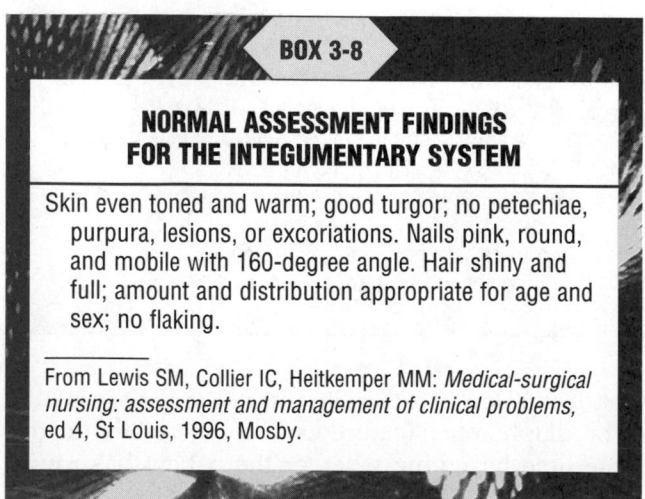

**BOX 3-8**

#### NORMAL ASSESSMENT FINDINGS FOR THE INTEGUMENTARY SYSTEM

Skin even toned and warm; good turgor; no petechiae, purpura, lesions, or excoriations. Nails pink, round, and mobile with 160-degree angle. Hair shiny and full; amount and distribution appropriate for age and sex; no flaking.

From Lewis SM, Collier IC, Heitkemper MM: *Medical-surgical nursing: assessment and management of clinical problems,* ed 4, St Louis, 1996, Mosby.

and the temporomandibular joint should be palpated. (Chapter 31 discusses cranial nerve assessment.)

### Eyes

The patient's visual acuity should be checked. (Chapter 38 provides assessment information for vision.)

**Eyelids, eyebrows, and eyelashes.** The eyebrows and eyelashes should be inspected for distribution of hair. Symmetry should be noted, and there should be no swelling or redness. The eyelids should be inspected for ptosis (drooping of the upper eyelid) and tremors (involuntary movement of eyelid).

**Movement.** Facing the patient, the nurse should assess the eyes for position and alignment. To assess extraocular movements of the eyes (the cardinal fields), the patient is asked to follow the examiner's finger or a pen as it makes a wide H in the air as follows: (1) beginning at the patient's extreme right (the nurse's left), (2) moving to the right and upward, (3) down on the right, (4) then without pausing in the middle, to the extreme left, (5) continue to the left and upward, (6) and finally down on the left. Any nystagmus (a fine rhythmic oscillation of the eyes) during the patient's upward lateral gaze should be noted.

**Cornea, sclera, and conjunctiva.** A flashlight should be shone into each of the patient's eyes to inspect the cornea for whitened areas (opacities). The corneas should appear clear. The color of the sclerae also should be noted; normally the sclerae are white. Normal conjunctivae appear pink. The lacrimal area should be inspected and assessed for excessive tearing or dryness. The nurse should observe for any swelling or discharge, and if drainage is present, the color should be noted.

**Pupillary reflex.** To check pupillary reflex, the nurse should darken the room and ask the patient to look into the distance. A flashlight is shone obliquely into each pupil, and the examiner notes the direct reaction (pupillary constriction in the same eye) and the consensual reaction (pupillary constriction in the opposite eye). The pupils' size, shape, symmetry, and reaction to light are assessed. Normal pupillary reaction is noted as **PERRLA** (pupils equally round and reactive to light accommodation). The size of the pupils is measured in millimeters (1 to 7 mm). The nurse must remember to compare the eyes.

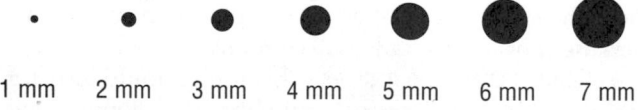

1 mm   2 mm   3 mm   4 mm   5 mm   6 mm   7 mm

**Red reflex.** The internal structures of the eye (iris, lens, vitreous, retina, and optic nerve) can be inspected directly with an ophthalmoscope. The structures can be seen through the clear cornea and the opening of the pupil. The examiner shines the light of the ophthalmoscope obliquely into the eye. When the posterior part of the eye is visualized, the color appears orange or red; the reflex results from the light reflecting off the retina, hence the name *red reflex.* Figure 3-4 compares a normal view with an abnormal view of the retina and optic area.

**NURSE ALERT**

**Always compare one side of the body with the other.**

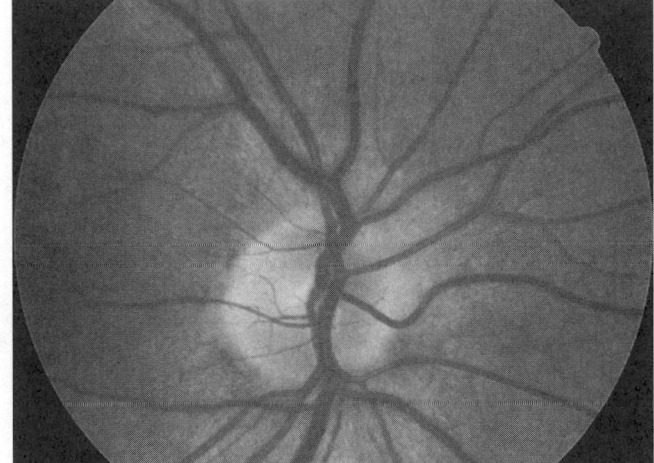

A

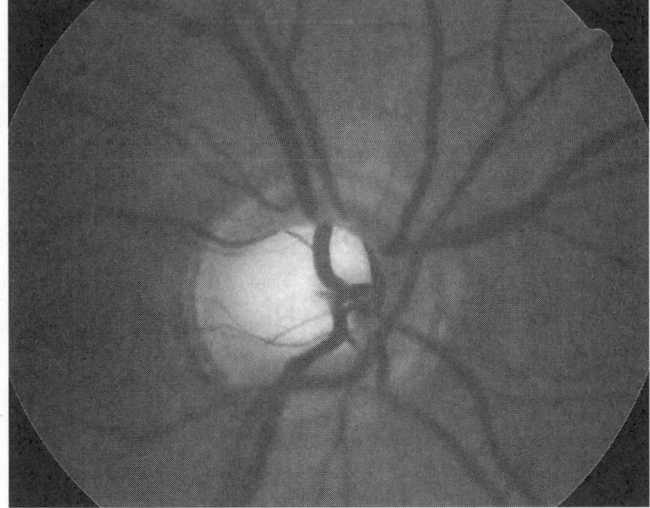

B

**Figure 3-4** **A,** In the normal eye, the optic cup is pink and shows little cupping. **B,** In a glaucomatous eye, the optic disk is bleached and optic cupping is present. (Note the appearance of the retinal vessels, which travel over the edge of the optic cup and appear to dip into it.) (From Lewis SM, Collier IC, Heitkemper MM: *Medical-surgical nursing: assessment and management of clinical problems,* ed 4, St Louis, 1996, Mosby.)

## Ears

The nurse should observe the ears for placement, size, symmetry, and skin integrity. The mastoid area is palpated for tenderness and nodules. (Chapter 39 presents specific information for assessing the ear and determining hearing acuity.)

**Auditory canal.** The external auditory canal is inspected before an otoscope is inserted. The nurse also should first ask the patient about any ear pain. The external canal should be inspected for cerumen, discharge, or edema. After this external inspection, the otoscope may be inserted (see Chapter 39 for proper technique). Using the otoscope, the examiner checks the internal ear canal for cerumen. Any discharge or lesions should be noted. Depending on the color and amount of cerumen, the tympanic membrane may or may not be visible. The tympanic membrane normally appears gray, white, or pink and is shiny and translucent.

## Nose and Sinuses

The external nose should be checked for shape and blockage. The nurse should press gently on the tip of the nose while looking into the nares, noting any masses or foreign bodies. The patency of the nasal passages can be determined by gently occluding one side and then the other while the patient exhales through the nose. Any discharge, and its color, should be noted. (Chapter 22 discusses problems associated with sinuses.)

The sinus areas can be palpated as follows:
- The *frontal sinus* is located above the eyebrows and middle of the forehead; palpate by pressing upward under the bony brows. Do not press on the eyes.
- The *maxillary sinus* is located behind the cheekbones; palpate by pressing upward on the cheekbone.
- The *mastoid sinus* is located behind the ear lobules; press behind the ear, assess for swelling or tenderness.

## Mouth

The mouth is inspected for symmetry of the lips, lesions, and color (the normal color is pink). The buccal mucosa and gums also are checked, and their normal color also is pink. The teeth are inspected for dental caries, abrasion, and state of repair. The nurse should note any partial or full dentures and how they fit. The color of the teeth and any absent teeth also are noted. The examiner should look at the hard and soft palates and the floor of the mouth, noting any lesions or masses. The patient should be asked if he or she has any difficulty swallowing. (Examination of the mouth includes further evaluation of the cranial nerves. A detailed assessment is found in Chapter 30.)

**Tongue.** The patient should be asked to stick out the tongue, and the nurse then checks its color (pink is normal), symmetry (equal), and position (midline). The patient then should be asked to move the tongue from side to side.

**Uvula and tonsils.** The examiner should ask the patient to open the mouth wide and say "Ahh." The normal position for uvular elevation is midline. The tonsils should be noted, if present, and the nurse should check for any masses, exudate, hyperplasia, or ulcerations.

## Neck

The skin of the neck is inspected and assessed for vascularity and visible pulsations. Symmetry is assessed by asking the patient to move the head from side to side and up and down. Normal findings would be equal with full range of motion (see Chapter 33).

The neck is inspected for venous distention and pulsations (see Chapter 24), and the carotid pulses are assessed. *Carotid pulses are assessed one at a time.* The midline structures are assessed next. The normal position of the trachea, thyroid gland, and cartilage is midline. The thyroid gland should be palpated.

**Lymph nodes.** The examiner should inspect and palpate for superficial lymph nodes, noting size, location, tenderness, temperature, erythema, and symmetry between sides. The nurse then has the patient sit up; standing in front of the patient, the nurse palpates the following areas (Figure 3-5):

1. Preauricular area (in front of the ear)
2. Postauricular area (behind the ear)
3. Occipital area (at the base of the skull posteriorly)
4. Mandibular area (halfway between the angle of the mandible and the jaw)
5. Tonsillar area (at the angle of the mandible, below the jaw)
6. Submental area (behind the tip of the mandible)
7. Anteroposterior cervical area (along the sternocleidomastoid muscle)
8. Infraclavicular area (below the clavicle)
9. Supraclavicular area (above the clavicle)

At this point in the assessment, some clinicians prefer to progress in a head to toe manner; others prefer to proceed with the examination of neurologic status. The order of progression is based on personal preference. Some might argue that this point is a logical break for the patient to be able to stand. As long as the progression is systematic and logical, the order is immaterial.

## Neurologic Status

Motor status is assessed by observing the patient's gait, toe walk, and heel walk (the patient is asked to walk normally, then to walk on the toes and on the heels). Cerebellar function is assessed by testing coordination. Coordination is assessed by asking the patient to stand with the feet together with no support from the arms. The nurse notes the patient's ability to stand upright, first with the eyes open and then with them closed. Minimal swaying should occur. The ability to perform this maneuver with minimal swaying is considered a negative *Romberg's sign.* (Chapter 30 presents information on neurologic problems.)

## Spine

While the patient is standing, the nurse should note the curves of the spine. The cervical and lumbar regions curve in a concave manner. The thoracic region is convex. Scoliosis is a lateral curvature of the spine. If seen on forward flexion, it is known as structural scoliosis. When an individual with structural scoliosis bends forward from the waist, this type of scoliosis is enhanced; the chest wall protrudes on one side, and the scapula is elevated. If the scoliosis does not involve vertebral rotation, the abnormal curvature disappears on forward flexion; this condition is known as functional scoliosis.

## Extremities

When assessing the extremities, the nurse should observe for size, shape, symmetry, deformity, and invol-

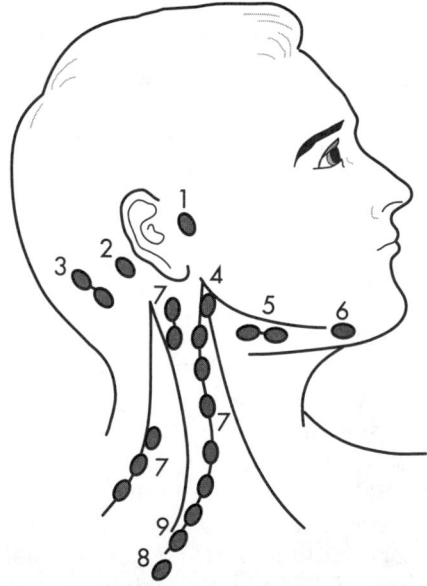

**Figure 3-5**   Locations of cervical lymph nodes. (See text for location of nine nodes.)

untary movements. (Chapter 33 discusses the musculoskeletal system.)

## Arms, Fingers, Wrists, Elbows, and Shoulders

**Strength.** The examiner should compare the size of the muscles, noting any atrophy. Flexion and extension are tested by asking the patient to move actively against the examiner or to resist the examiner's movement. The two sides are compared. The following methods can be used:

*Hand*: The patient squeezes two of the examiner's fingers as hard as possible. The finding is normal if the examiner has difficulty removing the two fingers from the patient's grip.

*Elbow*: The examiner has the patient push forward and pull back against the examiner's hand.

**Range of motion.** The patient's range of motion is checked (see Chapter 33). The nurse notes any abnormalities, such as **crepitus** (a crackling or grating sound between bones), joint pain, swelling, or fluid. The two sides are compared.

**Reflexes.** Deep tendon reflexes (Figure 3-6) are assessed by striking the tendon briskly using a rapid wrist movement (Figure 3-7); a reflex hammer may be used for this test. The examiner should use only the amount of force necessary to obtain a response. The speed and force of the reflex response are noted, and as always, the two sides are compared.

A scale of 0 to 4+ is used to grade reflexes:

| | |
|---|---|
| 4+ | Very brisk (hyperactive) |
| 3+ | Brisk (quicker than average) |
| 2+ | Average (normal) |
| 1+ | Diminished (low normal) |
| 0 | No response |

**Biceps.** With the patient's arms partially flexed at the elbow and the palms up, the examiner holds the patient's elbow with the examiner's thumb on the biceps

tendon. In the antecubital space the examiner then strikes the thumb with the reflex hammer, observing the patient for flexion of the elbow. The examiner also observes for and notes contraction of the biceps muscle.

***Triceps.*** The patient's elbow is flexed, the palm is turned toward the patient's abdomen, and the arm

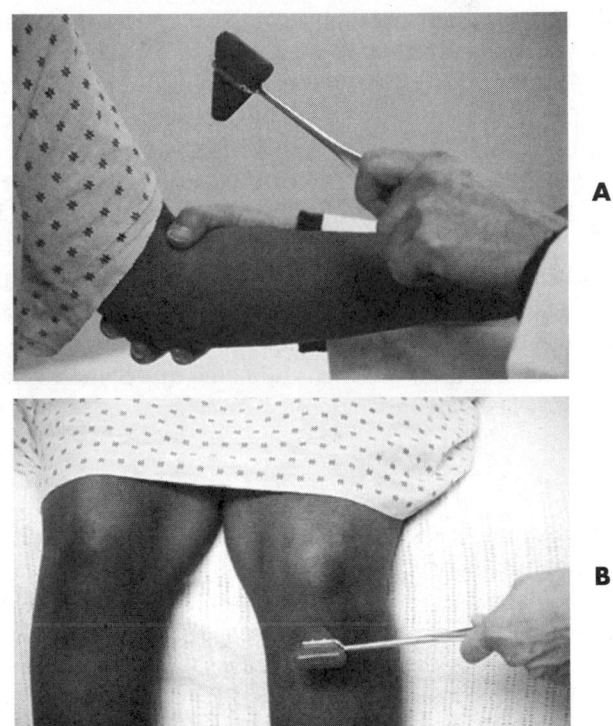

**Figure 3-7**    The examiner strikes a swift blow over a stretched tendon to elicit a stretch reflex and notes the response. (From Lewis SM, Collier IC, Heitkemper MM: *Medical-surgical nursing: assessment and management of clinical problems*, ed 4, St Louis, 1996, Mosby.)

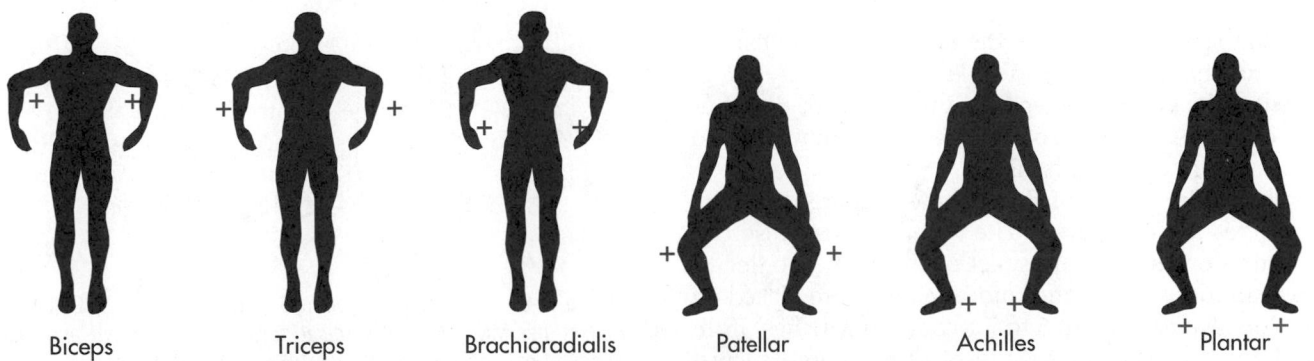

Biceps          Triceps          Brachioradialis          Patellar          Achilles          Plantar

**Figure 3-6**    Locations of deep tendon reflexes. Positions and methods to check reflexes.

is placed slightly across the chest. The examiner directly strikes the triceps tendon above the elbow and observes for contraction of the triceps muscle and extension of the forearm.

*Brachioradialis.* The patient rests the forearm on his or her lap or abdomen with the palm down. The examiner strikes the radial aspect of the forearm 2.5 to 5 cm (1 to 2 inches) above the wrist, watching for supination and flexion of the forearm.

*Patella.* The examiner directly taps the patellar tendon below the patella, observing for contraction of the quadriceps muscle with extension of the knee.

*Achilles.* The patient's foot is dorsiflexed. The nurse strikes the Achilles tendon and observes for plantar flexion.

*Plantar.* The nurse strokes the lateral aspect of the sole of the foot with a key, applicator stick, or pen. The motion should begin at the heel and curve toward the midline ball area of the foot. Normal movement results in flexion of the toes. A positive *Babinski's sign* is manifested by dorsiflexion of the great toe with fanning of the remaining toes, which indicates upper motor neuron disease.

### Legs

The examiner assesses the strength of the legs by having the patient push against the examiner's hands with his or her feet. Next, the examiner holds the patient's feet and has the patient pull against the hold while the examiner observes the patient's ability to perform this task.

**Edema.** The examiner should check for **edema**, or swelling, in the feet, ankles, legs, and coccyx area. The examiner presses a finger firmly but gently on the shin, ankle, and dorsal part of the foot for 5 seconds. The following grading scale can be used to assess edema:

    1+  Up to 0.59 cm (¼ inch) slight or mild
    2+  0.6 to 1.29 cm (¼ to ½ inch) moderate
    3+  1.3 to 2.5 cm (½ to 1 inch) moderately severe
    4+  over 2.5 cm (over 1 inch) very severe

If the rebound time for the skin is longer than 30 seconds, the edema is graded 4+.

**Hair distribution.** The legs are inspected for distribution of hair. An absence of leg hair on a man may be an indicator of vascular disease.

**Pulses.** The pulses of the feet are palpated, and the two sides are compared. The *dorsalis pedis* pulse can be found on the dorsal aspect of the foot. The tips of the examiner's index and middle fingers are placed on the dorsal aspect about 5 to 7.5 cm (2 to 3 inches) from the large toe. The *posterior tibial* pulse is located just

behind and slightly below the medial malleolus (Figure 3-8 shows the pulse points). Capillary refill is checked on the feet.

## Posterior Thorax

The posterior thorax is inspected for muscular development, respiratory movement, and assessment of the anteroposterior diameter. (Chapter 22 presents detailed assessments of respiratory function.)

### Respiratory Movement

The nurse assesses for symmetry of respiratory movement by placing both hands on the patient's back with

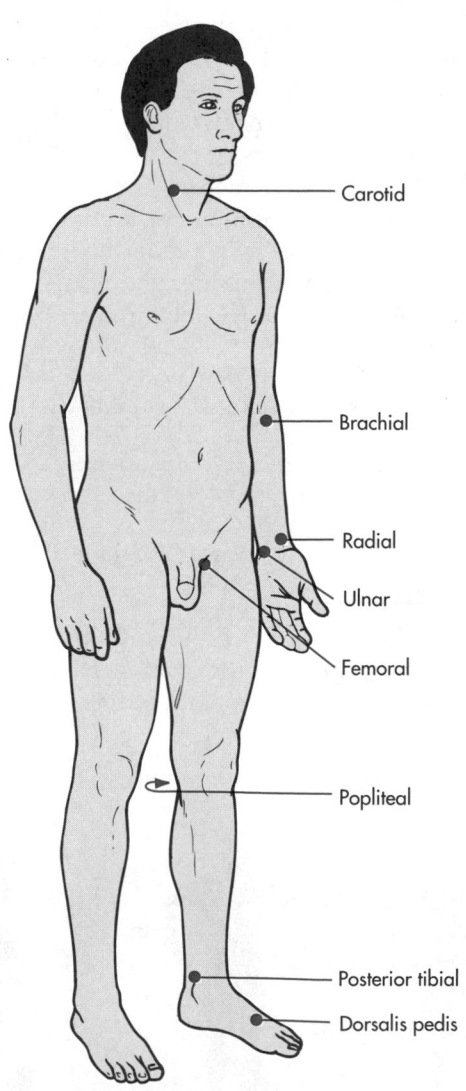

**Figure 3-8** Arterial pulse points. (From Lewis SM, Collier IC, Heitkemper MM: *Medical-surgical nursing: assessment and management of clinical problems*, ed 4, St Louis, 1996, Mosby.)

the thumbs together and the fingers spread. The patient takes several deep breaths while the nurse compares the two sides of the chest for movement. The nurse's thumbs should move apart equally on expiration. The chest area is palpated for tenderness. The spinous processes also are palpated. The nurse checks for tumors or swelling and palpates for tactile fremitus (see Chapter 22 for a detailed explanation). Auscultation of the breath sounds involves placing the diaphragm of the stethoscope on the patient's chest and listening to the respiratory cycle over all lung fields. Breath sounds are assessed both posteriorly and anteriorly. One side is always compared with the other. Chapter 22 provides information on percussion for pulmonary resonance and auscultation for breath sounds.

## Anterior Thorax
### Breasts

With the patient in a sitting position, the nurse inspects the breasts for configuration, symmetry, or dimpling of skin. The nipple area is inspected for direction, inversion, retraction, or rash. Normally the nipple projects outward and downward. Breast tissue is assessed by palpating for masses, and the breasts are inspected for discharge. At this point the nurse can begin instruction in or a review of breast self-examination. (Chapter 43 provides information on breast examination.) Male breast tissue should be inspected for nodules, swelling, or ulceration.

### Heart

The cardiac area is inspected for the point of maximum impulse and other pulsations. Normally none are visible unless the patient is very thin. The chest is palpated for thrills, lifts, heaves, and tenderness over the precordium. The heart is auscultated for rate and rhythm. The nurse listens to the heart with a stethoscope in the right second intercostal space close to the sternum; along the left sternal border in each intercostal space from the second through fifth spaces; and at the apex of the heart. The apical pulse is counted for 1 full minute. (Chapter 23 provides information on and techniques for cardiac assessment.) *Note: The neck can be assessed for venous distention at this time.*

### Abdomen

The patient is asked to empty the bladder. The abdomen then is assessed with the patient in a supine position. The order of assessment is *inspection, auscultation, percussion,* and *palpation.* Performing percussion and palpation before auscultating the abdomen may alter bowel sounds. The abdomen is inspected for scars, symmetry, muscular development, rashes, lesions, and dilated veins. The nurse also observes for pulsations and notes the contour of the abdomen, whether it is round, flat, hollowed, bulging, or symmetric. The umbilicus is inspected for contour, location, and signs of **inflammation** or herniation. The examiner also observes for peristalsis (normally seen only in very thin people). The examiner then auscultates for bowel sounds by placing the stethoscope on the abdomen and, beginning on the left, progressing to the right and down in a clockwise fashion (Figure 3-9). Normal bowel sounds are heard as clicks and gurgles at a rate of 5 to 30 per minute.

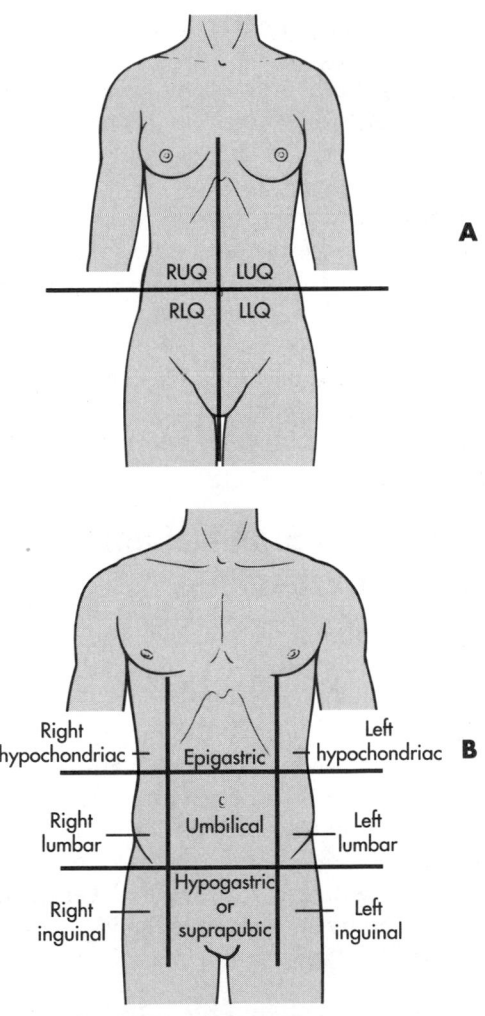

**Figure 3-9**   **A,** Abdominal quadrants. *RUQ,* Right upper quadrant; *LUQ,* left upper quadrant; *RLQ,* right lower quadrant; *LLQ,* left lower quadrant. **B,** Abdominal regions. (From Lewis SM, Collier IC, Heitkemper MM: *Medical-surgical nursing: assessment and management of clinical problems,* ed 4, St Louis, 1996, Mosby.)

The abdominal vessels also are auscultated. The examiner listens for an arterial **bruit** or venous hum over the aorta (7.5 cm [3 inches] above umbilicus), renal area (at the level of the aorta, 5 cm [2 inches] to the right or left), and at the iliac area (7.5 cm [3 inches] below the umbilicus, 5 to 7.5 cm [2 to 3 inches] to the right or left).

All quadrants are percussed. To do this, the examiner places his or her nondominant hand gently on the stomach. Using the dominant hand, the examiner taps the index and middle fingers over the joints of the nondominant hand and notes the sound produced. Tympany, a sound like a hollow drum, is heard over most of the abdomen. Next, the border of the liver is determined by percussing below the umbilicus (midsternal line) and progressing upward. The sound should change from tympany to dullness when the examiner reaches the border of the liver. The examiner percusses from the right lung, midclavicular area to the upper border of the liver.

The area of the liver is estimated in centimeters. A normal liver is 4 to 8 cm (about 1½ to 3 inches) at the midsternal line and 6 to 12 cm (about 2½ to 5 inches) at the right midclavicular line.

All quadrants of the abdomen are palpated by placing the fingers together and pressing with a slight downward motion. The examiner progresses slowly and notes any masses or areas of tenderness (Figure 3-10). The areas palpated should include the liver, spleen, kidneys, urinary bladder, femoral pulses, and inguinofemoral lymph nodes (see Figure 3-8 for pulse sites). Any bulges or tenderness in the groin should be noted.

## Completing the Examination of the Lower Extremities

The range of motion of the hips, knees, ankles, and feet should be assessed (see Chapter 33) and any crepitus, joint pain, or swelling noted. The examiner also should check muscle development. Coordination is assessed by having the patient place the heel on the opposite shin and move the heel downward. Normally, the motion is smooth, not jerky (see Chapter 30).

The nurse then assesses for deep vein thrombosis (Homans' sign) by sharply dorsiflexing each foot. The absence of calf pain with this maneuver is a negative response.

The nurse tests **proprioception** (position sense) by holding the patient's large toe between the thumb and finger. The toe is moved up and down, and the patient is asked to identify the direction. This test also can be performed on the thumb.

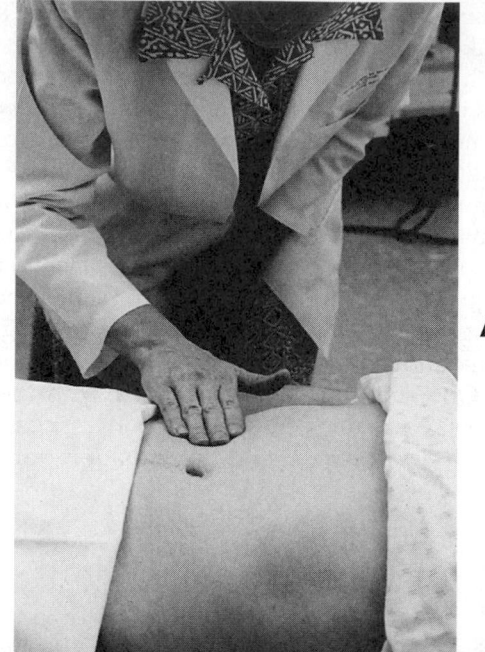

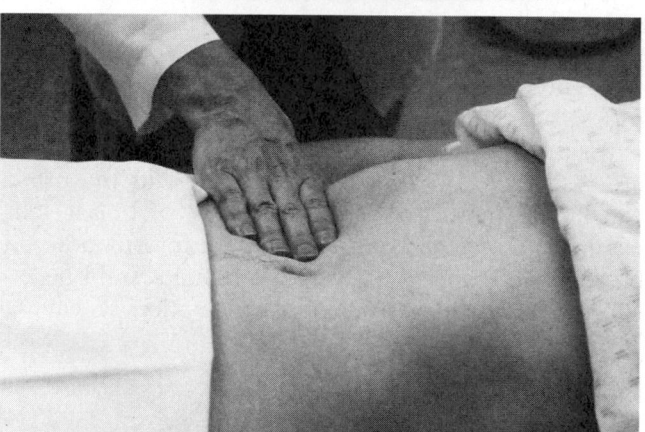

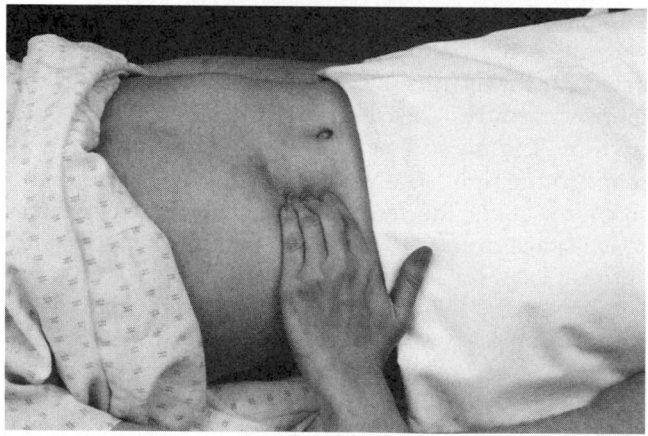

**Figure 3-10**   **A,** Technique for light palpation of the abdomen. **B,** Technique for moderate palpation using the side of the hand. **C,** Technique for deep palpation. (From Doughty DB, Jackson DB: *Mosby's clinical nursing series: gastrointestinal disorders*, St Louis, 1993, Mosby.)

## Genitalia

### Male External Genitalia

The nurse should drape the patient, ensure his privacy, and don gloves. The nurse then inspects the penis, noting hair distribution and the condition of the skin, and retracts the prepuce (if present) or asks the patient to do so. The glans and urethral meatus are checked. The examiner also looks for scars, ulcerations, inflammation, nodules, and discharge. The scrotum is inspected, and any swelling, lumps, or vein enlargement is noted. The nurse then palpates for nodules and undescended testes. At this point, the nurse can teach or reinforce testicular self-examination. (Male reproductive health is discussed in Chapter 42.)

### Female External Genitalia

The nurse assists the patient into the lithotomy position, drapes her, and ensures her privacy. The nurse then dons gloves and inspects the genital area for hair distribution. The labia (minora and majora), urethral meatus, and vaginal opening also are inspected, and any inflammation, discharge, or swelling is noted. The patient then is asked to bear down, and the nurse assesses for rectocele or cystocele. The nurse also palpates externally for nodules. With further education and training, the nurse can perform internal examinations. (Women's reproductive health is presented in Chapter 43.)

## Anus and Rectum

The patient is placed on his or her left side and draped, and privacy is ensured. The examiner dons gloves and inspects the perineum and rectum for excoriation, inflammation, or rashes. The anal area is checked for external hemorrhoids (a dilated vein seen as a swollen, reddish-blue mass). With further education and training, the nurse can perform an internal rectal examination.

## DOCUMENTATION OF THE EXAMINATION

Nurses can make notes about abnormal findings while performing the examination. However, they should not be continually writing down information because this disrupts the examination process. Box 3-9 presents

---

**BOX 3-9**

### SAMPLE RECORD OF A PHYSICAL EXAMINATION

Patient's Name _____
           Age _____

**GENERAL STATUS**
Well-nourished, well-hydrated, well-developed Caucasian woman or man in NAD, appears stated age, looks pleasant, smiles readily, speech clear and evenly paced; is alert and oriented × 3; cooperative, calm

**SKIN**
Clear $\bar{s}$ lesions, warm and dry, trunk warmer than extremities, turgor returns quickly, no ↑ vascularity, no varicose veins

**NAILS**
Well-groomed, round, 160-degree angle $\bar{s}$ lesions, nail beds pink, nails flexible

**HAIR**
Thick, brown, shiny, normal (male or female) distribution

**HEAD**
Normocephalic, sinuses nontender

---

From Lewis SM, Collier IC, Heitkemper MM: *Medical-surgical nursing: assessment and management of clinical problems*, ed 4, St Louis, 1996, Mosby.
↑, Increase in; *AC>BC*, air conduction greater than bone conduction; *AP*, anteroposterior; *bilat*, bilaterally; *BUS*, Bartholin's gland, urethral meatus, Skene's duct, *Coord*, coordination; *CVA*, costovertebral angle; *EOM*, extraocular movements; *FN*, finger to nose test; *ICS*, intercostal space; *LM*, landmarks; *LR*, light reflex; *MCL*, midclavicular line; *NAD*, no acute distress; *OD*, right eye (Lat. *oculus dexter*); *OS*, left eye (Lat. *oculus sinister*); *OU*, both eyes together (Lat. *oculi unitas*); *oriented* ×3, oriented to time, place, and person; *PER-RLA*, pupils equal, round, reactive to light and accommodation; *PMI*, point of maximal impulse; *prop*, proprioception, *reg*, regular; *resp*, respiratory; *ROM*, range of motion; $\bar{s}$, without; *TM*, tympanic membrane; *VA*, visual acuity; *WNL*, within normal limits.

*Continued*

BOX 3-9

# SAMPLE RECORD OF A PHYSICAL EXAMINATION—cont'd

## EYES

Visual fields intact on gross confrontation
VA: OD 20/20
    OS 20/20
    OU 20/20
    $\bar{s}$ glasses
EOM: Intact on all gazes $\bar{s}$ ptosis, nystagmus
Fundi: Red reflex present bilat no opacities, fundi WNL
Pupils: PERRLA, negative cover and uncover tests, negative Hirschberg's test

## EARS

Pinna intact, in proper alignment; external canal patent; small amount cerumen present; TMs intact; pearly gray LM, LR visible, not bulging; Rinne: AC>BC; Weber's: does not lateralize, whisper heard at 3 ft (about 1 m)

## NOSE

Patent bilaterally; turbinates pink, no swelling

## MOUTH

Moist and pink, soft and hard palates intact, uvula rises midline on "ahh," 24 teeth present and in good repair

## THROAT

Tonsils surgically removed, no redness

## TONGUE

Moist, pink, size appropriate for mouth

## NECK

Supple, $\bar{s}$ masses, $\bar{s}$ bruits, lymph nodes nonpalpable and nontender
Thyroid: Palpable, smooth, not enlarged
ROM: Full, intact, strong
Trachea: Midline, nontender

## BREASTS

Soft, nonpendulous, $\bar{s}$ venous pattern, $\bar{s}$ dimpling, puckering
Nipples: $\bar{s}$ inversion, point in same direction, areola dark and symmetric, no discharge, no masses, nontender

## AXILLAE

Hair present, shaved, no lesions, nontender

## LUNGS

No increase in AP diameter, resp rate 18, reg rhythm, no ↑ tactile fremitus, no tenderness, lungs resonant throughout, diaphragmatic excursion 4 cm (1.6 in) bilaterally, lung fields clear throughout

## HEART

Rate 82, reg rate and rhythm; no lifts, heaves
PMI: 5th ICS at MCL; nonpalpable thrills $S_1$, $S_2$ louder, softer in appropriate locations; no $S_3$, $S_4$; no murmurs, rubs, clicks
Carotid, femoral, pedal, and radial pulses present; equal, strong bilat

## ABDOMEN

No pulsations visible, rounded, active bowel sounds, no bruits or CVA tenderness, no palpable masses

## LIVER

Edge palpable, smooth, nontender; approximately 9 cm (3½ in) in size

## SPLEEN

Nonpalpable, nontender

## NEUROLOGIC SYSTEM

Cranial nerves I-XII intact
Motor (drift, toe stand) intact
Coord (FN, Romberg) intact
Reflexes: See diagram
Sensation (touch, vibration, prop) intact
  Grading Scale
  0   No response
  1+  Diminished
  2+  Normal
  3+  Increased
  4+  Hyperactive

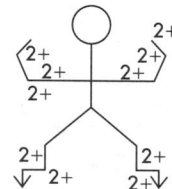

## MUSCULOSKELETAL SYSTEM

Well developed, no muscle wasting; $\bar{s}$ crepitus, nodules, swelling
ROM: Full, intact, and equal bilaterally; no scoliosis
Strength: Equal, strong bilat
Gait: Walks erect 2-ft steps, arms swinging at side $\bar{s}$ staggering

## FEMALE GENITALIA

External genitalia: No swelling, redness, tenderness in BUS; normal hair distribution, no cysts, rectocele
Vagina: No lesions, discharge; pink
Cervix: Os closed; no lesions, erosions, nontender
Uterus: Small, firm, nontender; pink
Adnexa: No enlargement; nontender
Rectovaginal: Sphincter intact; confirms above findings

## MALE GENITALIA

Normal male hair distribution
Penis: Urethral opening patent; no redness, swelling, discharge; no lesions, structural alterations
Scrotum: Testes descended; no redness, masses, tenderness
Rectal: No lesions, redness; sphincter intact; prostate small, nontender

## PSYCHOLOGIC STATUS

Affect appropriate; eye contact
Orientation: Oriented × 3
Mood: Pleasant, appropriate
Thought content: Intelligent, coherent
Memory: Remote and recent intact
Serial sevens test: Not done or intact

Signature _____

**TABLE 3-2**

## Physical Changes Caused by Aging

| SYSTEM | EXPECTED AGING CHANGES | CLINICAL MANIFESTATIONS |
|---|---|---|
| **Cardiovascular** | | |
| Cardiac output | Force of contraction decreased | Myocardial oxygen demand increased |
| | Fat and collagen increased | Stroke volume and CO decreased |
| | Heart muscle decreased | Fatigue, shortness of breath, tachycardia occur |
| | Ventricular wall thickened | Blood flow to vital organs and periphery decreased |
| Cardiac rate and rhythm | Dependence on atrial contraction increased | HR slow to increase with stress |
| | Loss of fibers from bundle of His | Decrease in maximum HR (e.g., 80-year-old person, 120 bpm; 20-year-old person, 200 bpm) |
| | Mitral valve stretching | Possible AV block |
| | Ventricles slow to relax | Resting HR constant |
| | Sinus node pacemaker cells decreased | Recovery time from tachycardia prolonged |
| | | Premature beats increased |
| Structural changes | Aortic valves sclerotic and calcified | Diastolic murmur present in 50% of older patients |
| | Baroreceptor sensitivity decreased | Heart position landmarks change |
| | Mild fibrosis and calcification of valves | |
| Arterial circulation | Elastin and smooth muscle reduced | Modest increase in systolic BP (160/90) |
| | Vessel rigidity increased | Rigid arteries contribute to coronary artery and peripheral vascular disease |
| | Vascular resistance increased | |
| | Aorta becomes dilated | |
| Venous circulation | Tortuosity increased | Inflamed, painful, or cordlike varicosities |
| Peripheral pulses | Arteries rigid | Pulses weaker but equal |
| | | Circulation slowed to periphery |
| | | Cold feet and hands |
| **Respiratory** | | |
| Structures | Cartilage degeneration | Kyphosis |
| | Vertebrae rigid | Anteroposterior diameter increased |
| | Strength of muscles decreased | Use of accessory muscles decreased |
| | Ciliary action decreased | Chest rigid and barrel shaped |
| | Respiratory muscles atrophy | Respiratory excursion decreased |
| | Thoracic wall more rigid | Cough and deep breathing diminished |
| Change in ventilation and perfusion | Pulmonary vascular bed decreased | Lung compliance decreased |
| | Alveoli decreased | Total lung volume unchanged |
| | Alveolar walls thickened | Vital capacity decreased |
| | Elastic recoil decreased | Residual volume increased |
| | Residual lung volume increased | Mucus thickened |
| | | $PaO_2$ and oxygen saturation decreased |
| | | Hyperresonance |
| Ventilation control | Response to hypoxia and hypercarbia decreased | Response to stress decreased |
| | | Ability to maintain acid-base balance decreased |
| | | Rate 12-24/min |

From Lewis SM, Collier IC, Heitkemper MM: *Medical-surgical nursing: assessment and management of clinical problems,* ed 4, St Louis, 1996, Mosby.
*AV,* Atrioventricular; *BP,* blood pressure; *bpm,* beats per minute; *BUN,* blood urea nitrogen; *CO,* cardiac output; *EEG,* electroencephalogram; *HR,* heart rate; *PaO₂,* partial pressure of arterial oxygen; *REM,* rapid eye movement; *ROM,* range of motion. *Continued*

an example of a written record of a physical examination performed on a healthy adult. Table 3-2 presents the changes caused by aging that may be seen in the physical examination of an older adult.

After completing the history and physical examination, the nurse evaluates the information obtained and selects appropriate nursing diagnoses. (See Chapter 2 for an explanation of the nursing process and its steps.)

**TABLE 3-2**

## Physical Changes Caused by Aging—cont'd

| SYSTEM | EXPECTED AGING CHANGES | CLINICAL MANIFESTATIONS |
|---|---|---|
| **Integumentary** | | |
| Skin | Collagen and subcutaneous fat decreased | Skin less elastic |
| | Sweat glands decreased | Wrinkles and folds increased |
| | Epidermal cell turnover slowed | Extremity fat lost; fat on trunk increased |
| | Skin tissue fluid decreased | Skin heals slowly |
| | Capillary fragility increased | Skin dry |
| | Pigment cells decreased | Skin tears and bruises easily |
| | Sebaceous gland activity decreased | Skin color uneven |
| | Sensory receptors decreased | Multiple senile lentigines |
| | Thresholds for touch, vibration, heat, pain increased | Normal skin lesions increased |
| | | Ability to respond to heat and cold decreased |
| | | Ability to feel light touch decreased |
| | | Cutaneous pain sensitivity decreased |
| Hair | Melanin decreased | Gray or white hair |
| | Germ center and hair follicle decreased | Hair quantity decreased and thinner |
| | | Scalp, pubic, axillary hair decreased |
| | | Facial hair on men decreased |
| | | Facial hair on women increased |
| Nails | Blood supply to nail bed decreased | Growth slowed |
| | Longitudinal striations increased | Nails thickened and brittle |
| | | Nails split easily |
| | | Potential for fungal infection increased |
| **Urinary** | | |
| Structural changes in kidney | Renal mass decreased | Protein in urine increased |
| | Number of functioning glomeruli decreased | Potential for dehydration |
| | Glomerular filtration rate decreased | Creatinine clearance decreased |
| | Renal plasma flow decreased | Serum creatinine and BUN increased |
| | | Excretion of toxins and drugs decreased |
| | | Nocturia increased |
| Bladder | Bladder smooth muscle and elastic tissue decreased | Capacity decreased |
| | | Less control: stress incontinence |
| Micturition | Sphincter control decreased | Frequency, urgency, nocturia increased |
| **Reproductive** | | |
| Male structures | Prostatic enlargement | Sexual response less intense |
| | Testicular volume decreased | Takes longer to achieve erection |
| | Sperm count decreased | Erection maintained without ejaculation |
| | Seminal vesicles atrophy | Force of ejaculation decreased |
| | Serum testosterone constant | |
| | Estrogen level increased | |
| Female structures | Estradiol, prolactin, progesterone diminished | Responses to changing hormone levels altered |
| | Size of ovaries, uterus, cervix, fallopian tubes, labia decreased | Cervical, vaginal secretions dry |
| | | Intensity of sexual response gradually decreased |
| | Associated glands and epithelium atrophied | Potential for vaginal infections increased |
| | Elasticity in pelvic area decreased | Potential for vaginal and uterine prolapse increased |
| | Breast tissue decreased | |
| | Vaginal pH becomes alkaline | |

| TABLE 3-2 |
|---|

## Physical Changes Caused by Aging—cont'd

| SYSTEM | EXPECTED AGING CHANGES | CLINICAL MANIFESTATIONS |
|---|---|---|
| **Gastrointestinal** | | |
| Oral cavity | Dentine decreased | Taste changes |
| | Gingival retraction | Potential loss of teeth |
| | Bone density lost | Gingivitis |
| | Papillae of tongue decreased | Bleeding gums and dry mouth |
| | Taste threshold for salt and sugar increased | Oral mucosa dry |
| | Salivary secretions decreased | |
| Esophagus | Lower esophageal sphincter relaxed | Epigastric distress |
| | Tone and motility decreased | Dysphagia |
| | | Potential for hiatal hernia and aspiration |
| Stomach | Gastric mucosa atrophy | Food intolerance |
| | Hydrochloric acid production decreased | |
| Small intestine | Intestinal villae decreased | Absorption of nutrients diminished |
| | Enzyme secretions decreased | Absorption of fat-soluble vitamins delayed |
| | Motility decreased | |
| Large intestine | Blood flow decreased | Potential for constipation and fecal impaction |
| | Motility decreased | |
| | Sensation to defecation decreased | Impaired fat absorption |
| Pancreas | Pancreatic ducts distend | Decreased glucose tolerance |
| | Lipase production decreased | |
| | Pancreatic reserve impaired | |
| | Number and size of cells decreased | Lower border extends past costal margin |
| | Hepatic protein synthesis impaired | |
| **Musculoskeletal** | | |
| Skeleton | Intervertebral discs narrowed | Height diminished 2.5 to 10 cm (1 to 4 in) |
| | Cartilage of nose and ears increased | Nose and ears lengthen |
| | | Kyphosis |
| | | Pelvis wider |
| Bone | Cortical and trabecular bone decreased | Bone resorption exceeds bone formation |
| | | Potential for osteoporotic falls and fractures |
| Muscles | Number of muscle fibers decreased | Strength decreased |
| | Muscle fibers atrophy | Agility decreased |
| | Muscle regeneration slowed | Rigidity in neck, shoulders, hips, knees increased |
| | Contraction time and latency period prolonged | Potential restless leg syndrome |
| | Flexion of joints increased | |
| | Ligaments stiffening | |
| | Sclerosis of tendons | |
| | Tendon flexor reflexes decreased | |
| Joints | Cartilage erosion | Mobility decreased |
| | Calcium deposits increased | ROM limited |
| | Water in cartilage decreased | Potential osteoarthritis |
| **Nervous** | | |
| Structure | Loss of neurons in brain and spinal cord | Conduction of nerve impulses slowed |
| | Brain size decreased | Peripheral nerve function lost |
| | Dendrites atrophy | Reaction time decreased |
| | Major neurotransmitters decreased | Response time precise and slowed |

*Continued*

| TABLE 3-2 |
| --- |

## Physical Changes Caused by Aging—cont'd

| SYSTEM | EXPECTED AGING CHANGES | CLINICAL MANIFESTATIONS |
| --- | --- | --- |
| **Nervous—*cont'd*** | | |
| Structure—*cont'd* | | Potential for altered balance, vertigo, syncope |
| | | Postural hypotension increased |
| | | Proprioception diminished |
| | | Sensory input decreased |
| | | EEG alpha waves decreased |
| Sleep | Deep sleep decreased | Difficulty remembering dreams |
| | REM sleep decreased | Difficulty falling asleep |
| | | Periods of wakefulness increased |
| | | Sleeptime averages 6 hours |
| **Visual** | | |
| Eye structure | Orbital fat lost | Eyes sunken |
| | Eyebrows and eyelashes gray | Eyes dry |
| | Elasticity of eyelid muscles decreased | Potential ectropion and entropion |
| | Tear production decreased | Potential conjunctivitis |
| Cornea | Corneal sensitivity decreased | Potential corneal abrasion |
| | Corneal reflex decreased | |
| | Arcus senilis | |
| Ciliary | Aqueous humor secretion decreased | Ability of lens to accommodate declines |
| | Ciliary muscle atrophy | Potential presbyopia |
| | | Peripheral vision decreased |
| Lens | Less elastic, more dense | Lens yellow and opaque |
| | Blue-green color discrimination decreased | Less ability to adapt to light and dark |
| | | Tolerance to glare decreased |
| | | Incidence of cataracts increased |
| | | Night vision impaired |
| Iris and pupil | Pigment lost | Visual acuity decreased |
| | Smaller | Pupils appear constricted |
| | Vitreous gel debris increased | Floaters |
| **Auditory** | | |
| Structure | Hairs in external auditory canals of males increased | Cerumen more dry |
| | | Potential conductive hearing loss |
| | Ceruminal glands decreased | |
| Middle ear | Middle ear long joints degenerate | Sound conduction decreased |
| | Ear drum thickens | |
| Inner ear | Vestibular structures decline | Sensitivity to high tones: "s," "t," "f," "g" decreased |
| | Hair cells lost | Understanding of speech decreased |
| | Cochlea atrophies | Discrimination of background voice decreased |
| | Organ of Corti atrophies | Equilibrium-balance deficits |
| | | Potential for tinnitus |
| Immune system | Secretory immunoglobulin (IgA) declines | Potential increase for infection on mucosal surfaces |
| | Thymus gland involved | Impaired cell-mediated immune response |
| | Thymopoietin decreased | Malignancy incidence increased |
| | Lymphoid tissue decreased | Response to acute infection reduced |
| | Stem cells impaired | Potential recurrence of latent herpes zoster and tuberculosis |
| | Antibody production impaired | Autoimmune disease increased |
| | T lymphocytes decreased | |
| | Autoantibodies increased | |

## KEY CONCEPTS

➤ Health assessment is the process of obtaining information from the patient to enable the nurse to provide care.

➤ The data collected during the health assessment are used to create a plan of care, to evaluate the effects of care, and to determine health teaching and home care needs.

➤ A subjective symptom, such as pain, is investigated promptly.

➤ The components of physical assessment include four examination techniques: inspection, palpation, percussion, and auscultation.

➤ The physical examination is performed systematically, and the patient's comfort, safety, and privacy are ensured.

➤ During the physical examination, the two sides of the body are always compared.

➤ The nurse must become proficient with various equipment before performing a physical assessment.

➤ Assessment information is recorded on appropriate forms, with significant data noted.

## CRITICAL THINKING EXERCISES

1. Discuss the process of health assessment. How is the information obtained in the assessment important to patient care?

2. Explain why it is important to compare the two sides of the body.

3. What examples can you give that demonstrate appropriate documentation of a normal health assessment?

## REFERENCES AND ADDITIONAL READINGS

American Nurses Association, Congress for Nursing Practice: *Nursing: a social policy statement,* Kansas City, Mo, 1980, The Association.

Darovic G: Assessing pupillary responses, *Nursing 97* 27(2): 49, 1997.

Fuller J, Schaller-Ayers J: *Health assessment: a nursing approach,* ed 2, Philadelphia, 1994, Lippincott.

Giger JN, Davidhizar RE: *Transcultural nursing: assessment and intervention,* St Louis, 1995, Mosby.

Gordon M: *Nursing diagnosis: process and application,* ed 3, St Louis, 1994, Mosby.

Heath H: Health assessment of people over 75 (continuing education credit), *Nurs Stand* 10(41):49-56, 1996.

Irwin MJ: Assessing color changes for dark skinned patients, *Adv Clin Care* 6(6):8-10, 1991.

Jarvis C: *Student laboratory manual for physical examination and health assessment,* ed 2, Philadelphia, 1996, Saunders.

Kirton CA: Assessing normal heart sounds, *Nursing 96* 26(2): 56-57, 1996a.

Kirton CA: Physical assessment: assessing for ascites, *Nursing 96* 26(4):53, 1996b.

Kirton CA: Physical assessment: assessing breath sounds, *Nursing 96* 26(6):50-51, 1996c.

Krenzer ME: Peripheral vascular assessment: finding your way through arteries and veins, *AACN Clin Issues* 6(4): 631-644, 1995.

Lewis SM, Collier IC, Heitkemper MM: *Medical-surgical nursing: assessment and management of clinical problems,* ed 4, St Louis, 1996, Mosby.

Nowazek V, Neeley MA: Health assessment of the older patient, *Crit Care Nurse Q* 19(2):1-6, 1996.

Poncar PJ: Who has time for a head to toe assessment? *Nursing 95* 25(3):59, 1995.

Scher HE: Chest pain: developing rapid assessment skills, *Orthop Nurs* 14(3):30-34, 1995.

Sneed NV, Hollerbach AD: Measurement error in counting heart rate: potential sources and solutions, *Crit Care Nurse* 15(1):36-40, 1995.

Thompson JM, Wilson SF: *Health assessment for nursing practice,* St Louis, 1996, Mosby.

Welsh JR, Arzouman J, Holm K: Nurses' assessment and documentation of peripheral edema, *Clin Nurse Spec* 10(1):7-10, 1996.

White JE: Using interactive video to add physical assessment data to computer-based patient simulations in nursing, *Comput Nurs* 13(5):233-235, 1995.

Wilson M, Lillibridge J: Health assessment: a study of registered nurses' knowledge and skill level, *Contemp Nurse* 4(3):116-122, 1995.

## CHAPTER 4

# Ethical Decision Making

## CHAPTER OBJECTIVES

1 Define ethics.
2 Define clinical ethics.
3 Discuss the principles that serve as a foundation for ethical decision making.
4 Discuss the concepts of respect and the nurse-patient relationship as a foundation for nursing ethics.
5 Use the nursing process as a framework for ethical analysis and decision making.
6 Discuss the purpose and importance of advance directives.
7 Apply the American Nurses Association Code of Ethics to the nursing experience.

## KEY TERMS

| | |
|---|---|
| advance directive | justice |
| autonomy | living will |
| beneficence | morals |
| bioethics | nonmaleficence |
| clinical ethics | power of attorney for |
| dilemma | health care |
| ethics | values |
| fidelity | veracity |

## ETHICAL ANALYSIS AND DECISION MAKING

### Introduction to Ethics

For thousands of years, people have raised questions about what it means to be good or excellent human beings. Basically, that is what ethics is all about: doing a good job of being a good person. In nursing, the fundamental question is this: How does ethics help us become good nurses as well as good people? An integral part of the profession of nursing and the administration of care is a concern for doing what is right for the patient. These issues touch on themes that run through all aspects of everyday life and work.

**Ethics** is a branch of philosophy that is the study of two facets of human existence: (1) how people should act and (2) what sort of character they should have. **Bioethics,** sometimes referred to as health care ethics, is the application of ethical principles and rules to biologic and medical issues. **Clinical ethics** refers to the application of bioethics to the identification, analysis, and resolution of moral problems that arise in the care of a particular patient. Box 4-1 presents a list of terms commonly used in discussions of ethics.

### Role of Ethical Theory

Interest in the ethical issues surrounding medicine and health care has been growing. The development of

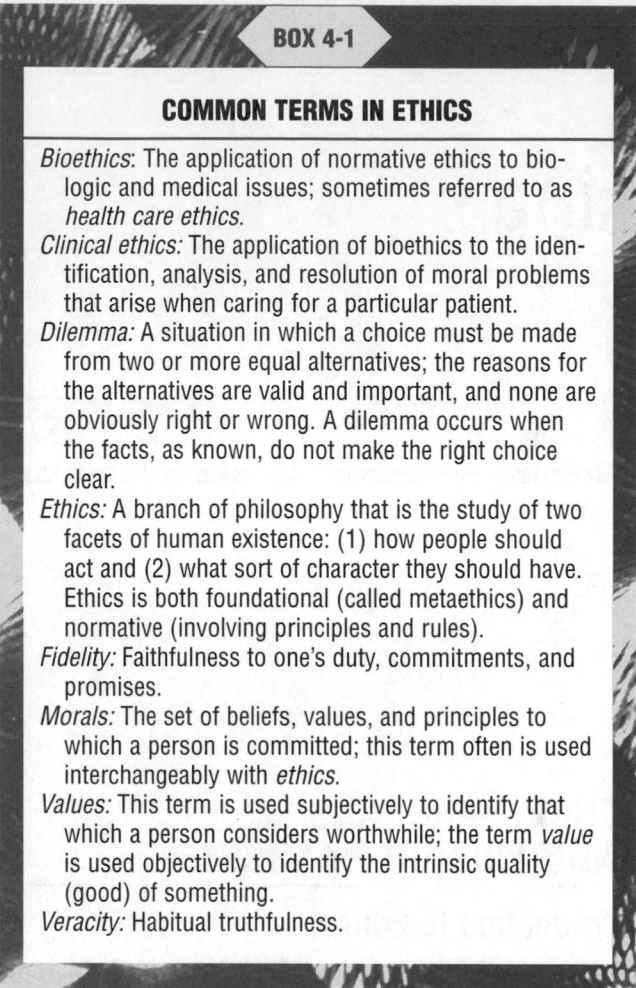

**BOX 4-1**

### COMMON TERMS IN ETHICS

*Bioethics*: The application of normative ethics to biologic and medical issues; sometimes referred to as *health care ethics*.

*Clinical ethics:* The application of bioethics to the identification, analysis, and resolution of moral problems that arise when caring for a particular patient.

*Dilemma:* A situation in which a choice must be made from two or more equal alternatives; the reasons for the alternatives are valid and important, and none are obviously right or wrong. A dilemma occurs when the facts, as known, do not make the right choice clear.

*Ethics:* A branch of philosophy that is the study of two facets of human existence: (1) how people should act and (2) what sort of character they should have. Ethics is both foundational (called metaethics) and normative (involving principles and rules).

*Fidelity:* Faithfulness to one's duty, commitments, and promises.

*Morals:* The set of beliefs, values, and principles to which a person is committed; this term often is used interchangeably with *ethics*.

*Values:* This term is used subjectively to identify that which a person considers worthwhile; the term *value* is used objectively to identify the intrinsic quality (good) of something.

*Veracity:* Habitual truthfulness.

new and sophisticated technology raises new possibilities for treating disease, increasing the life span, and caring for the disabled. However, the use of increasingly expensive technology also has a dark side. The conflict between the benefits and burdens of these developments leaves health care professionals and their patients with many difficult questions: Is it always appropriate to use this technology? Who makes this decision? What are the benefits? What are the costs, both in human suffering and in resources? The answers to these questions have significant consequences.

One problem in searching for these answers is that not all members of society come from the same cultural background, and they do not all hold the same moral values. Not everyone is committed to the same set of **values** or principles; such a society is known as a morally pluralistic society. Without a shared value system, how can people begin to discuss, let alone answer, these and other important questions?

A second problem is that in many situations, good reasons can be found for proceeding in different and sometimes conflicting ways. When conflicting choices arise, how does a nurse decide which is the ethical way to proceed? A normative ethical theory can provide the nurse with principles and rules to guide his or her actions.

## Basic Ethical Principles, Theories, and Rules

Philosophers Tom Beauchamp and James Childress (1989) have developed a normative ethical framework that uses four basic principles: nonmaleficence, beneficence, autonomy, and justice (Figure 4-1). **Nonmaleficence** means "to do no harm"; it also means preventing and removing harm. **Beneficence** directs the nurse to do good on the patient's behalf. The principle of **autonomy** affirms the right of people to govern their own lives, including the way they are treated as patients. This obligates a person to refrain from interfering with another person's autonomy without substantial reason.

The principle of **justice** is concerned with distribution of social benefits and burdens. It is a difficult principle to use in making decisions about individual patients because it requires consideration of society as a whole, such as who gets the benefits and who pays the burdens. Justice more often involves broad societal issues such as allocation of resources (e.g., who will pay for health care). The question of whether health care money should be spent on organ transplants while some children lack simple immunizations is a question of justice. A decision on which patient gets the only open bed in intensive care applies the principle of justice on a more individual level.

Beauchamp and Childress' four principles are supported by ethical theories that refer to the rightness or wrongness of an action in a more general way. These theories may help an individual think about the moral features of a situation in which he or she is trying to make an ethical decision. An ethical problem can arise in any of the three elements of a situation. Those elements are as follows:

- The actions being considered
- The consequences those actions probably will produce
- The people who would perform the actions

Three general orientations to ethics have evolved from emphasis on one of the three elements to the exclusion of the others (Fletcher et al, 1995). These orientations are the theories of deontology, utilitarianism, and virtue ethics.

Deontology theory focuses primarily on the action being considered in a situation. Deontologists believe that certain inherent features of an action determine the fundamental rightness or wrongness of that action. For example, lying is wrong because it is inherently

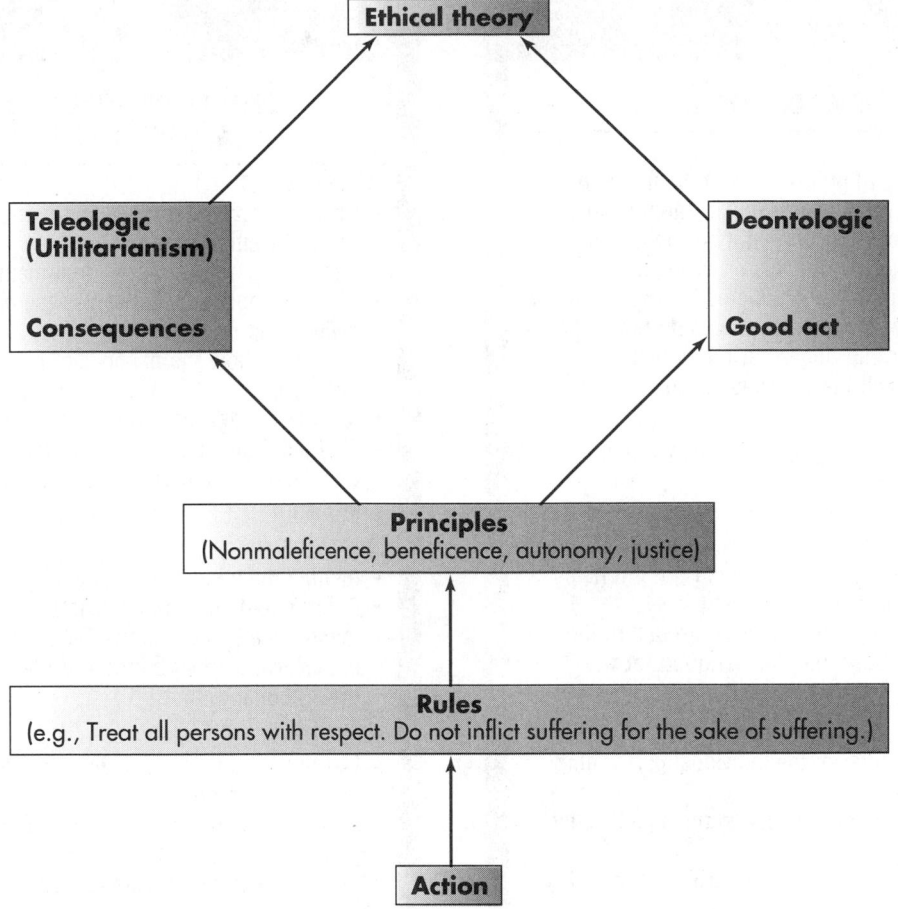

**Figure 4-1**   A framework for ethical decision making. The action in question is reviewed with rules in mind, which in turn are supported by the principles of nonmaleficence, beneficence, autonomy, and justice. Is the act good in itself (deontologic theory) or are the consequences good (teleologic theory/utilitarianism)? Answering these questions helps the nurse determine if the action is ethical. (Modified from Beauchamp T, Childress J: *Principles of biomedical ethics*, ed 3, New York, 1989, Oxford University Press.)

wrong, not because the consequences of lying may hurt people or deny them control over their lives.

Proponents of utilitarianism, in contrast, believe that one must look at the possible consequences of an action to decide if the action is right or wrong. Will lying bring about greater happiness than telling the truth? Will it help more people than it will harm?

Virtue ethics looks more closely at the people performing the action (the agents) and considers the actions they perform and how such actions reflect on their character. The main concern is how agents can develop good habits that contribute to a good character. Virtue ethics tries to cultivate good judgment by using those good characteristics in a complex situation (Fletcher et al, 1995).

Principles of justice also serve as supporting mechanisms for more specific rules and guidelines, such as

**veracity** (habitual truthfulness) and **fidelity** (faithfulness to one's duty, commitment, and promises). Beauchamp and Childress' principles and the theories of utilitarianism and deontology together serve as a framework to guide decision making in ethical issues and to justify ethical decisions (Figure 4-1 and Box 4-2).

## Nursing Ethics

A movement has arisen among health care ethicists to center ethical principles within the practice itself. In other words, the ethics of the practice would flow from the practice itself rather than from justification (Pelligrino, Thomasma, 1988). The current treatment of nursing ethics follows this initiative and is compatible with the belief that the nurse-patient relationship is the foundation of nursing practice (Watson, 1988; Fry,

BOX 4-2

## THEORIES OF ETHICS

### DEONTOLOGY
- Takes the position of philosopher Immanuel Kant
- Stems from the Greek word *deon,* meaning "duty"
- Involves the concept of moral duty or obligation
- Posits that the moral rightness or wrongness of a human action should be considered independently of its consequences; that consequences do not make an action right or wrong, but rather the principles or motivation on which the action is based

### UTILITARIANISM
- Found in the works of Jeremy Bentham and John Stuart Mill
- Referred to as *teleologic theory*, from the Greek word *telos*, meaning "end"
- Has the basic concept that an act is right if it helps bring about a good outcome, or end
- Involves weighing competing issues to determine which will bring about the greatest good for the greatest number

### VIRTUE ETHICS
- Looks at the character of the individual performing the act
- Emphasizes how actions reflect on the agent's character
- Focuses on cultivating habits that will be generally applied in guiding the agent's actions

BOX 4-3

## METHOD OF ETHICAL ANALYSIS AND DECISION MAKING

### ASSESSMENT
- Collect information and learn as much as possible about the situation.
- Identify the medical facts, treatment options, and nursing diagnoses, as well as the patient's values, beliefs, and religious preference.
- Determine how the patient's family is involved in the decision.
- Identify the decision maker or makers.
- Find out if any legal considerations are involved.
- Use these and any other pertinent data to define the problem.

### ANALYSIS
- Identify the ethical components.
- Determine if any conflict exists.
- Identify the source of any such conflict (e.g., conflicting values, conflict between professional duties, lying or withholding the truth).

### PLANNING
- List the options for resolving the conflict and their projected outcomes.
- Assess the benefit/burden ratio of the projected outcomes.
- Analyze each option with regard to the principle of respect for the patient.
- Determine which option can best fulfill that principle.

### IMPLEMENTATION
- Choose the option that best fulfills the principle of respect and begin justifying that option.
- Use the American Nurses Association Code of Ethics and the Beauchamp/Childress principles (nonmaleficence, beneficence, autonomy, and justice), which may be helpful for thinking through difficult issues.
- Apply each principle to the chosen alternative.
- Justify or list the ethical reasons for the decision.
- Formulate and consider the ethical reasons that would oppose the decision.
- Weigh the reasons that support and oppose the decision.
- Test other options in the same way if necessary.
- Make a decision.

### EVALUATION
- Determine if the patient's goals have been accomplished.
- Determine if the result is effective and realistic.
- Determine if the results are supported (justified) by ethical principles and theories.
- Determine what can be learned from this outcome for future situations.

1989; Catalano, 1992). Using this approach, the outcomes of ethical decision making remain compatible with Beauchamp and Childress' four principles, although a different framework is used for justification (Box 4-3).

## Nursing as an Inherently Moral Enterprise

The process of nursing involves the diagnosis and treatment of human responses to actual or potential health problems. The purpose of nursing is to enhance the well being of others. Because this is an inherently good human goal, nursing is an inherently moral enterprise (nursing is a science that is based on scientific knowledge and is directed by the need to help others). Applying this knowledge in a wise and humane manner is the art of nursing. The patient, as a unique person with individual needs, is the focus of nursing. Such a focus is based on the virtually universal moral obligation to respect all human beings. The belief underlying this obligation is that human beings possess dignity and an inherent worth on the basis of who they are as distinct human beings. The moral requirement to respect a person is not lessened for any reason, including socioeconomic status, personal attributes, or the nature of the health problem (American Nurses Association, 1985).

## Ethic of Care

The language of principles, as described previously, has been the dominant voice in biomedical ethics. However, recent work in moral psychology and ethics by Carol Gilligan (1984) has provided another way of looking at ethical issues in health care; Gilligan and subsequent proponents of this viewpoint refer to it as "ethics of care." Gilligan contrasts this way of thinking with the more abstract and logical forms of argument used in an ethical framework based on principles.

An "ethic of care" begins with relationships. It looks at the give and take of relationships; it includes empathy and concern in moral reasoning; and it emphasizes rules of responsiveness and responsibility in relationships with others. "Care" reasoning is contextual; that is, it involves all the details of the patient's situation. Its primary goal is to promote patients' dignity and respect for them as people. This means that nurses must pay attention to the particular details of individual patients, which counters all those forces that objectify and dehumanize people. It does not allow for just performing discrete tasks; rather, it requires knowing the patient as a person: as individual, as holistic, and as being in a situation (as a patient) that is only a part of a continuous life story. It requires prioritizing care according to the patient's values. It focuses not only on *what* nurses do, but also on *how* they do it.

In contrast, the principle or justice approach emphasizes autonomy and individuality and views ethical issues in the light of conflicting rules or abstract principles. Relationships are secondary, if taken into account at all. The issue of informed consent provides a good illustration. Traditionally, in obtaining informed consent, the emphasis has been on informing the patient about the benefits and risks of a treatment or procedure, pointing out what can go wrong, and then getting the patient's signature on the form giving consent for the procedure. More recently, the trend has been to pay more attention to the quality of patients' understanding of their situation. Ideally, more time is allowed for the communication process, which gives the patient the opportunity to comprehend the information and to ask questions.

This expansion of the informed consent process demonstrates that in a properly caring context, respect for autonomy, the principle that supports informed consent, involves not only prohibitions against coercion and manipulation, but also the responsibility to nurture and sustain the patient's capacity to exercise autonomous choices. This process requires more than the signing of forms; it requires sensitivity to the individual patient and to his or her fears, hopes, values, and capacities in the decision-making process.

Gilligan's ethics of care and Beauchamp and Childress' ethics of principles can work together to provide help in dealing with issues of clinical ethics. The principle approach helps identify the moral aspects of a given case and highlight the moral claims. The ethics of care approach helps fill out the picture and focus attention on the context of the case, especially the ethical aspects of communication, relationships, and nurse-patient interactions. Using the two approaches together allows the nurse to balance principles in a helpful way and to use the relationships that are part of an ethic of care to empower patients and families to make authentic autonomous choices.

## Personal and Professional Values

In addition to knowing the values of the nursing profession, found in the American Nurses Association (ANA) Code of Ethics (American Nurses Association, 1985), nurses need to identify their personal values. Such knowledge helps them respect the values of others and understand how they influence the nurse-patient relationship. It is important to try to prevent values and prejudices from affecting patient care. For example, a nurse who is opposed to elective abortions may want to avoid working in a setting that requires contact with those receiving abortions or that requires assisting with the abortion procedure.

## Ethics in Daily Practice

Understanding the nurse-patient relationship and its foundation of respect for human dignity is essential to the daily provision of compassionate nursing care. Too often life and death issues garner much attention, whereas ordinary but important issues receive little notice. Levine (1977) writes the following:

> There are overlooked ethical challenges in the mundane, everyday routine activities of professional practice, and these have largely gone unexamined. Ethical behavior is not the display of one's moral rectitude in times of crisis. It is the day-by-day commitment to other persons and the ways in which human beings relate to one another in their daily interactions.

This view of ethics encompasses a holistic framework that demands consideration of the patient's physical, psychologic, sociocultural, developmental, and spiritual dimensions.

# RESPECT FOR PATIENTS

## Impact of Illness on Respect

Any illness or injury breaks up the daily pattern of life, which often is taken for granted. The disruption affects jobs, daily activities, and family relationships. It can cause anxiety, frustration, suffering, and loss. Illness is marked by uncertainty. The patient asks, "What is wrong with me? Will I get better?" The forbidding and unfamiliar environment of the hospital or nursing home and the number of people involved in care add to the patient's uncertainty. The patient must also trust and rely on all these caregivers, who almost always are strangers. Hospital and nursing home care is intimate and personal, which places the patient in a very vulnerable position. Patients' needs are best served when they believe that the nurse and other caregivers respect them and address their legitimate needs, hopes, and fears.

## Demonstrating Respect

Showing respect requires serious consideration of the values and goals of others. It also demands that care not be limited by personal attitudes, beliefs, or values. The nurse shows respect for the patient by trying to provide freedom from anxiety and pain and to protect the patient's right to privacy and confidentiality. Respect is not a reward for good behavior; it is an inherent right of patients, coworkers, and oneself.

## Respect as the Application of Fidelity

The nurse's promise is a commitment to care that arises from respect for the patient. Nurses are morally committed to help care for patients in their living and dying. Doing this effectively requires knowledge and skills appropriate to the particular level of nursing. This commitment also requires honesty and integrity in accepting responsibility for providing the best possible patient care. Respecting a patient often is referred to as "following the principle of fidelity."

## Implication of Do Not Resuscitate Orders

Some patients and their families fear that if they choose not to be resuscitated (do not resuscitate [DNR] order), they will receive no further treatment and less intense nursing care. These patients often require significant medical and nursing care, and the principle of respect demands that they receive this care. It is important to provide essential nursing care and to assure the patient and family that they will not be abandoned because of a DNR order.

## Advance Directives

The principle of respect requires nurses to help a patient understand the concept of **advance directives,** which include the **living will** and the **power of attorney for health care** (Box 4-4). When appropriate, the nurse may also have a responsibility to speak with the patient or family, or both, to understand the patient's specific wishes pertaining to advance directives. Except in extremely rare situations and only with substantial overriding reasons, respect for patients demands that an advance directive be followed.

## Need for Patient Involvement in Decision Making

The nurse also is required to act in the patient's best interest, a concept identified as beneficence. Ethical **dilemmas,** or problems, may arise when the nurse tries to determine what is best for the patient without listening to the patient's views or obtaining the patient's agreement. The patient's best interest can be fully explored only by involving the patient. When patient involvement is not possible, the family or significant others must convey the patient's wishes.

## Respect for Privacy and Confidentiality

Respect for the patient demands respect for privacy and confidentiality. All information about a patient belongs to that patient. A nurse may not give out any information without the permission of the patient or legal guardian. Giving information without permission discounts the patient's unique dignity, infringes on the patient's autonomy, and may do significant harm. Breaches of confidentiality occur more often as a result of carelessness in elevators and cafeterias than as a purposeful and malicious violation of the patient's rights. As patient records become computerized, nurses need to be attentive to new possibilities for inadvertent violation of a patient's privacy. Students must be especially aware of these issues when submitting written or verbal assignments discussing the care of their patients.

## Pain Control

Pain control is an ethical issue because pain has a dehumanizing effect on patients and their families. Pain diminishes the quality of life. A major goal of nursing is to alleviate pain and provide comfort. This goal is supported by the ethical principles mentioned earlier in this chapter: *nonmaleficence,* not causing harm or re-

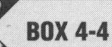

## BOX 4-4

### ADVANCE DIRECTIVES

**DEFINITION**

An advance directive is a written document that indicates your choices regarding the medical treatments you do or do not want and that names the person you want to act on your behalf as your health care agent. This document becomes effective if and when you become incapacitated and cannot express your wishes.

**TYPES OF ADVANCE DIRECTIVES**

The two types of advance directives are the living will and the power of attorney for health care.

**Living Will**

- Informs the doctor whether or not the patient wants life-sustaining procedures if he or she is terminally ill or injured and death is imminent or if the patient is in a persistent vegetative state
- Takes effect only if the patient is near death and unable to understand his or her health care options or express his or her wishes to others

**Power of Attorney for Health Care**

- Informs the health care provider that the patient has appointed another person (a *health care agent*) to make health care decisions for him or her if the patient is incapable of making them; the health care agent has authority to make a wide range of health care decisions for the patient, such as surgery, medications, or life support
- Takes effect only if two physicians or a physician and a psychologist agree in writing that the patient is no longer able to understand his or her treatment options or express his or her own wishes to others

**FACTS ABOUT ADVANCE DIRECTIVES**

- The patient must be 18 years old and of sound mind to make an advance directive.
- The patient can revoke or change his or her advance directive at any time.
- The patient's doctor or doctors and family members should have copies of the patient's advance directive. It should be kept where it can be easily found.
- The patient does not need a lawyer to complete the advance directive forms; however, two people must witness the patient's signature to these forms.
- Advance directives may vary from state to state; legal variations should be checked for the patient's particular state of residency.

moving harm that may cause pain; *beneficence*, providing good for the patient in the form of diminishing or eliminating pain; and *autonomy*, a consideration because a person is less capable of making authentic decisions when in pain.

It is a well-established fact that many patients in pain are still undermedicated despite the advances in research, medications, and knowledge that have occurred in the past 20 years. The reasons for undermedicating patients range from unfounded fear of addiction to fear of hastening death. Research has shown that the risk of addiction is extremely small and that good pain control, even with large doses of opioids, is unlikely to hasten death.

A great need exists to educate nurses about pain and about the uses of analgesics and opioids and the ways they can provide safe, effective pain relief for all patients, be they children, adults, or the elderly. Individual nurses must assume ethical responsibility for learning about pain management (see Chapter 11).

## ETHICAL DILEMMA

Mr. Stewart, who is 71 years old, has been admitted to a general medical-surgical floor in a small community hospital. He is diagnosed with metastatic cancer that has spread from his prostate to his spinal column and hip.

Mr. Stewart has been admitted to the hospital because he is too weak to walk, cannot care for himself, and can barely feed himself. With his physician's concurrence he has decided not to undergo chemotherapy. Because he is in the terminal stages of cancer, he is to be kept comfortable with a continuous intravenous infusion of narcotics.

Because of his emaciated condition, the skin over his coccyx has begun to break down. When nurses attempt to turn Mr. Stewart every 2 hours, he cries out in pain to such an extent that the nurse wonders if this nursing intervention is really helping him.

The staff decides to hold a care conference to discuss what they should do about Mr. Stewart's care. The head nurse insists that Mr. Stewart be turned at least every 2 hours because it is routine and minimal nursing care for bedridden patients. If he is not turned every 2 hours, his coccyx will become necrotic and an infection may result. Ms. Jones, his primary nurse, says she cannot stand to hear Mr. Stewart cry out in agony every time he is turned. Mr. Smith, another team member, suggests that Mr. Stewart have some say regarding his care. Mr. Smith says that turning or not turning will hardly make a difference in the overall outcome of his terminal illness. What should their decision be?

## ROLE OF THE ETHICS COMMITTEE

Sometimes an ethical dilemma is so difficult that consulting an institutional ethics committee may be helpful. Most hospitals and many long-term care institutions have an ethics committee. Such committees usually comprise many individuals with a variety of backgrounds and expertise (including ethics). These groups are skilled and experienced in assisting patients, families, and health care professionals in ethical decision making. More recently, a move has begun toward forming nursing ethics committees or nursing ethics forums in health care settings. The primary function of these groups is ethics education for nurses, but they also can provide help to nurses who may have a nursing ethics problem that would not require the attention of the hospital ethics committee.

## AMERICAN NURSES ASSOCIATION CODE OF ETHICS

Nursing is related to society. The state has given the profession the power to regulate and control its own practice. In return, the profession is obligated to see that acceptable standards are maintained. One important way to uphold this duty is provided by the ANA Code For Nurses (Box 4-5). This code, which consists of 11 statements, is a public expression of the values and goals of the nursing profession. Members of the nursing profession are required to follow this code, which is explicit about the importance of respect for patients (American Nurses Association, 1985).

## HEALTH CARE REFORM

### Managed Care

The focus in this chapter has been primarily on the individual patient and the nurse-patient relationship. However, health care has been undergoing significant changes, which will have an effect on the ethics of health care. The good of the individual is being balanced against the good of society. This change in focus puts health care professionals in a position of trying to promote common good while remaining responsive to the needs of unique individuals.

These changes fall under the heading "health care reform" in a general sense and under the heading of "managed care" in a more specific sense. The original intent of managed care was to achieve the best possible care for patients when resources are limited. It was to have been an integrated delivery system in which appropriate care would be provided in a variety of settings in a more cost-effective way. However, managed care, for the most part, has become a system that

---

**BOX 4-5**

### AMERICAN NURSES ASSOCIATION CODE FOR NURSES

1. The nurse provides services with respect for human dignity and the uniqueness of the patient, unrestricted by considerations of social or economic status, personal attributes, or the nature of health problems.
2. The nurse safeguards the patient's right to privacy by judiciously protecting information of a confidential nature.
3. The nurse acts to safeguard the patient and the public when health care and safety are affected by the incompetent, unethical, or illegal practice of any person.
4. The nurse assumes responsibility and accountability for individual nursing judgments and actions.
5. The nurse maintains competence in nursing.
6. The nurse exercises informed judgment and uses individual competence and qualifications as criteria in seeking consultation, accepting responsibilities, and delegating nursing activities to others.
7. The nurse participates in activities that contribute to continual development of the profession's body of knowledge.
8. The nurse participates in the profession's efforts to implement and improve standards of nursing.
9. The nurse participates in the profession's efforts to establish and maintain conditions of employment conducive to high-quality nursing care.
10. The nurse participates in the profession's efforts to protect the public from misinformation and misrepresentation and to maintain the integrity of nursing.
11. The nurse collaborates with members of the health professions and other citizens in promoting community and national efforts to meet the health needs of the public.

From American Nurses Association: *Code for nurses with interpretive statements*, Washington, DC, 1985, The Association.

---

stresses the administrative and financial aspects of health care delivery and places less emphasis on the traditional humane and caring values of medicine and nursing. Managed care is any system that provides health services thorough a network of parties who agree to abide by certain approaches established by a care management process. Generally, managed care providers receive a capitated payment (a specified amount per person) for providing all medically necessary services to its enrolled members. The goal of managed care is to change the behavior of providers and consumers of health care. It uses an economic model to improve efficiency and effectiveness and is viewed primarily as a business and as a commodity to be sold.

When it became apparent that the President and Congress would be unable to produce legislation for health care reform, the market stepped in and became the driving force behind health care reform, effecting a transition from fee for service to managed care, usually by the capitation process. These changes have raised concern that we have a system that emphasizes managed cost rather than managed care. Some are concerned that managed care organizations have few incentives to maintain standards of quality of care and safety when such standards may be expensive and costs are difficult to control. Presently, no regulations, standards, or guidelines have been developed to ensure quality and safety.

Managed care is seen as ethically problematic because of a fear of weakening professional commitment to beneficence and a concern for quality resulting from a cost reduction and a lack of regulations to ensure standards of quality.

What does this mean for nurses? How does managed care affect the nurse-patient relationship? With the emphasis changed from individual to common good, many managed care organizations have standardized treatments and created strict practice guidelines that limit the nurse's ability to meet the unique needs of the individual patients. These limitations may take the form of denying certain treatments, discharging patients earlier than in the past, and reducing staff. This situation creates a tension in nursing values. To accomplish humane and respectful nursing and health care, the nurse must be clear about the foundation of ethics and values that supports health care services in a pluralistic society. How can these values be balanced with economic and business values, which also are important?

Of special concern to nurses is the fact that some evidence indicates that the quality of patient care is being adversely affected by managed care. In a survey conducted by the ANA and the *American Journal of Nursing*, nurses reported that they were being assigned to care for an increasing number of patients. At the same time, those patients were more acutely ill. Other evidence shows that the quality of nursing care has deteriorated (Shindul-Rothschild, Berry, Long-Middleton, 1996), as seen in an increase in medication errors, skin breakdown, falls, and patient complaints and a decline in staff satisfaction.

The challenge for nurses who find themselves in settings that fit the previously mentioned descriptions is to remain faithful to the traditional values of nursing, which demand respectful and total care for the individual. Nurses need to be aware that the obligations and values in the ANA Code of Ethics to provide benefits for the sick and vulnerable within the general concerns of justice and fairness may be in conflict with the primary market values of efficiency and effectiveness of managed care.

Managed care, although neither new nor inherently evil, threatens to weaken professional commitments to beneficence and nonmaleficence, the foundations of the professional relationship, because of widespread demand that costs be reduced. How can nurses be assured that they will not be forced to compromise their professional principles by being compelled to participate in care they think is substandard? This is a significant concern, which has surfaced in studies by nurses associations, trade unions, and consumer groups; its twin is the concern that the goal of much of the restructuring is not to improve the quality of care, but rather to widen profit margins.

Although this simplified section on managed care has emphasized the downside of managed care, it is important to note that some managed care organizations do a good job of balancing the values of health care and business. It is in those organizations that do not do a good job of balancing these values that ethical concerns arise. It also is important to understand that cost effectiveness and efficiency can be important values. But values often are in conflict and cannot always be realized simultaneously. The economic value of controlling spiraling costs and the social and ethical value of providing adequate health care for all in need will remain in conflict for some time. To begin to reconcile this conflict, health care professionals must educate themselves on the issues and collaborate with all members of the health care team and with patients to realize the traditional values of health care and nursing in the most cost-effective way possible. For those who have the skill, getting involved in the legislative process, engaging in national debate on the rationing of health care, and helping to inform the local press on these issues are other ways of lessening the tension created by the conflict of values.

Meanwhile, all health care professionals must remain committed to the human values that are essential to the health professions and those who practice them. Nursing, especially, must take care to remain a caring profession rather than become a tool for the business of health care.

# KEY CONCEPTS

➤ Ethics is the branch of philosophy that is the study of how people should act and what sort of character they should have.

➤ The patient is the focus of nursing. This focus is based on the universal moral obligation to respect all people because, as human beings, they possess dignity and inherent worth.

➤ Ethics requires consideration of the whole patient in daily relationships.

➤ The nurse demonstrates respect by seriously considering others' values and goals and the ways these goals affect the nurse-patient relationship. Illness can threaten a patient's sense of respect.

➤ Nurses have a moral commitment to help care for patients, which arises from respect for all individuals.

➤ DNR orders do not justify abandonment; respect demands that care be given.

➤ An advance directive is a written document that indicates a patient's choices regarding medical treatment. Except in extremely rare situations with substantial overriding reasons, respect for the patient demands that an advance directive be followed.

➤ Patients must be involved in decision making.

➤ Respect for privacy and confidentiality grows out of respect for the patient.

➤ The ANA Code of Ethics describes a generally accepted set of nursing behaviors. Behavior that is inconsistent with these established guidelines may be deemed unethical.

# CRITICAL THINKING EXERCISES

1. Select an issue of biomedical ethics that has been in the news recently. Use the steps outlined in Box 4-3 to arrive at an ethical decision.

2. Mrs. Corona has been admitted from the emergency room with a diagnosis of congestive heart failure. In the emergency room she was asked if she had an advance directive. She does not, and she asks you to tell her what it is. Explain advance directives to Mrs. Corona. Describe the two kinds of advance directives and explain how they are different from one another.

3. After paying the rent and electric bills, Mary has no money to feed her two young children. She steals $50 from her employer. Apply the principles of utilitarianism and deontology to determine if this is an ethical action.

## REFERENCES AND ADDITIONAL READINGS

American Nurses Association: *Code for nurses with interpretive statements*, Kansas City, Mo, 1985, The Association.

Aroskar MA: Ethical decision-making in patient care, *Am Nurse* 26(3):10, 1994.

Aroskar MA: Managed care and nursing values: a reflection, *Trends Health Care Law Ethics* 10(1-2):83-86, 1995.

Bandman B, Bandman E: *Critical thinking in nursing,* Norwalk, Conn, 1988, Appleton & Lange.

Bandman E, Bandman B: *Nursing ethics in the life span*, Norwalk, Conn, 1985, Appleton, Century, Crofts.

Beauchamp T, Childress J: *Principles of biomedical ethics*, ed 3, New York, 1989, Oxford University Press.

Carse AL: The "voice of care": implications for bioethical education, *J Med Philos*, 16:5-8, 1991.

Catalano JT: Systems of ethics: a perspective, *Crit Care Nurse* 12(8):91-96, 1992.

Churchill LR: Trust, autonomy, and advance directives, *J Religion Health* 28(3):175-182, 1989.

Curtin L: The ethics of managed care, *Nurs Manage* 27(10):71-74, 1996.

Donley R: Ethics in the age of health care reform, *Nurs Econ* 11(1):19-24, 1993.

Fletcher J et al: *Introduction to clinical ethics,* Frederick, Md, 1995, University Publishing Group.

Fry ST: Toward a theory of nursing ethics, *ANS Adv Nurs Sci* 11(4):9-22, 1989.

Fry ST: The ethic of caring: can it survive nursing? *Nurs Outlook* 36(1):48, 1990.

Gilligan C: *In a different voice*, Cambridge, Mass, 1984, Harvard University Press.

Grant AB: Exploring an ethical dilemma, *Nurs 92* 22(12):52-54, 1992.

Husted GL, Husted JH: *Ethical dilemmas and nursing practice*, ed 2, St Louis, 1994, Mosby.

Levine M: Nursing ethics and the ethical nurse, *Am J Nurs* 77(5):845-849, 1977.

Miya PA, Megel ME: Confidentiality and electronic medical records, *Med Surg Nurs* 6(4):222-224, 1997.

Pelligrino E, Thomasma D: *For the patient's good: the restoration of beneficience in health care*, New York, 1998, Oxford University Press.

Shindul-Rothschild J, Berry D, Long-Middleton E: Where have all the nurses gone? Final results of our patient care survey, *Am J Nurs* 96(11):25-34, 1996.

Watson J: *Human science and human care,* New York, 1988, National League for Nursing.

## CHAPTER 5

# Delegation and Supervision

## CHAPTER OBJECTIVES

1 Define delegation.
2 Identify the "four rights" of delegation.
3 Compare and contrast the roles and responsibilities of the delegator and the delegatee.
4 Identify the characteristics of the delegatee.
5 Give examples of the relationship between the task and the situation in which the delegation will occur.
6 Compare and contrast responsibility, authority, and accountability.
7 Define supervision.
8 Explain the role of supervision in the delegation process.

## KEY TERMS

| | |
|---|---|
| accountability | health care delivery system |
| authority | responsibility |
| delegatee | roles and responsibilities |
| delegation | supervision |
| delegator | supervisory |
| desired objective | unlicensed workers |

Since the late 1980s, and with intense acceleration over the past 3 years, the **roles and responsibilities** of various employees in the **health care delivery system** have changed (Joel, 1994). New workers have been added, some job categories have been eliminated or markedly curtailed, and the roles of yet others have expanded. These changes were brought about by the rapidly rising cost of health care, and because of this crisis, cost has become a dominant concern in the health care delivery system.

Research data are replete with examples of **unlicensed workers** performing some aspects of patient care (Barter, Furmidge, 1994). The data also show that licensed caregivers (registered nurses [RNs]) have expanded their practice to areas previously reserved for other medical providers, and licensed practical nurses (LPNs) perform some activities that once were the province solely of RNs (Connecticut State Board of Nurse Examiners, 1995). In most of these instances the changes are driven by the twin factors of overall cost and the delivery of quality patient care within a specified dollar limit. Common sense shows that hiring an RN is less costly than hiring a physician and using an unlicensed worker is less expensive than using a licensed caregiver. For this reason the trend toward altering the characteristics of the work force is likely to continue throughout this decade and into the foreseeable future.

As roles have changed and job descriptions have been rewritten, a common theme has emerged: the act of **delegation.** This chapter defines delegation, addresses the purpose and expectations of delegation, explores the ways to accomplish effective and safe delegation, compares and contrasts the impact delegation has for the delegator and the delegatee, discusses problems in delegation, and concludes with some questions that are food for thought.

## DEFINITION OF DELEGATION

According to the American Nurses Association (ANA, 1993), delegation is "the transfer of **responsibility** for the performance of an activity from one individual to another while retaining **accountability** for the outcome." The National Council of State Boards of

Nursing (1990) defines delegation as "transferring the **authority** to a competent individual, authority to perform a selected nursing task in a selected situation." Delegation is defined as the assignment of personnel to achieve a **desired objective.**

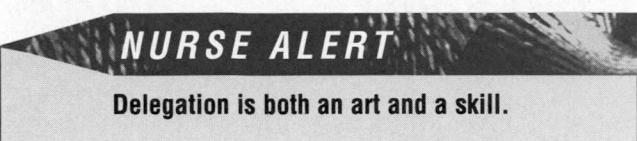

**NURSE ALERT**

**Delegation is both an art and a skill.**

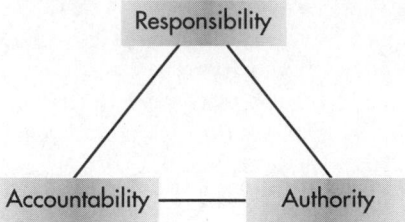

**Figure 5-1** Triad of responsibility, accountability, and authority.

These three definitions have many commonalities, but three points are of primary importance.

First, each definition limits what is being delegated. The ANA speaks of "an activity"; the National Council of State Boards of Nursing pinpoints "a selected task"; and Grohar-Murray and DiCroce use the phrase "a desired objective." Examples of activities that would satisfy all three definitions would be giving bed baths, ambulating a patient, feeding patients, delivering laboratory specimens, taking vital signs, changing dressings, or any of several hundred other activities.

Some institutions and state practice acts create lists of these activities; others address the issue in global rather than specific terms (Johnson, 1996). In each instance, however, delegation of the activity, task, or objective is accompanied by accountability. It must be stressed that, in most situations, the act of delegation in the context of nursing care involves a specific event, not an entire area of action. In other words, typically the act of changing a patient's dressing is delegated but not the entire care of a specific patient.

Second, each author addresses the notion of transferring performance of the action to someone else. The person delegating the activity is the **delegator**, and the recipient of the delegation, the person who performs the selected action, is the **delegatee.** Delegation, then, becomes the art of fulfilling one's own job description through the use of other personnel. More often than not the other personnel are less skilled or less experienced or have less expertise than the delegator. Appropriately, then, the overall cost of the delegatee (hourly wage or salary) is less than that of the delegator.

Third, the themes of authority, responsibility, and accountability are prevalent in each of the three references. Authority is the right and power to act. Responsibility is the condition of accepting important duties or obligations. Accountability means being answerable for something. The relationship between these three concepts should be envisioned as a triangle. Responsibility, accountability, and authority are the three corners of the triangle, equal in proportion (Figure 5-1). In other words, the three concepts are interre-

lated and interwoven. Every action, regardless of who starts or completes it, incorporates all three concepts. When one person delegates to another, the responsibility and authority for the activity go with the delegation. Accountability for the activity rests with both the delegator and the delegatee. Each individual is answerable for what has or has not been done. In the act of delegation, the delegator transfers the responsibility for the activity to another while retaining accountability for both the outcome and the act of transfer. The delegatee becomes responsible for the activity and is answerable for his or her actions.

Authority exists in the delegator-delegatee relationship in two ways. First, the delegator must have the authority to delegate (Davis, Farrell, 1995). Typically, the authority for delegation rests with the RN (Blegen, Gardner, McCloskey, 1992). A review of the literature and state practice acts reveals no evidence of an LPN or licensed vocational nurse (LVN) being given the authority to delegate to other parties (Johnson, 1996).

The second aspect of authority in the delegator-delegatee relationship, the authority to perform an activity, must be a component of the delegation process as well (Hansten, Washburn, 1995). Once the activity has been delegated to another individual, that individual must have the commensurate authority to perform the activity. If the delegatee does not have such authority, the act must not be delegated. For example, if an RN wants to delegate the administration of medications to the LPN but the LPN does not have the authority to administer medications, the activity cannot be delegated. On the other hand, if a dressing change is delegated and that activity is within the LPN's scope of practice and individual ability, the authority to change the dressing also exists.

Authority is an important element of the delegation process in another way as well. The person performing the delegated activity (i.e., the delegatee) must have the authority, the freedom, and the power to perform the activity in the manner he or she deems appropriate (Conger, 1994). If the delegator has a specific action in mind, that fact must be communicated to the delegatee before the action is performed (Ales, 1995). If no specifics are provided, the delegatee operates on the premise that full authority to fulfill the action is within his or her freedom and power. Certainly the delegatee must follow institutional protocol, policies, and procedures, but the exact and specific manner in which the activity is performed is left to the delegatee when authority is in proper perspective (Harrell, 1995).

> ## NURSE ALERT
> **Responsibility is accepting the consequences of one's own actions or inactions.**

Authority, responsibility, and accountability are often confused and misinterpreted. Everyone is accountable. No matter what one does or does not do, the individual remains answerable for the decision and subsequent action or inaction. Accountability is not eligible for delegation because everyone within the health care delivery system is already accountable. Responsibility also goes with the action, but the application may be different. In the case of RN delegators, their responsibility is limited to ensuring that the delegatee, the person receiving the delegation and performing the action, is capable of fulfilling that action. The delegatee is responsible for the action that actually is performed.

Consider this example: Mr. Jones has recently had an open reduction of his fractured hip. The RN (Betty) delegates to the staff LPN (Nancy) the act of assisting Mr. Jones to ambulate four times a day. During the afternoon session, Mr. Jones falls. Who is responsible for his fall? Both the LPN and the RN are accountable, and each is responsible for her own actions. The RN, Betty, is responsible for determining two key elements: (1) that it is safe, based on an assessment, for Mr. Jones to ambulate four times a day and (2) that the LPN, Nancy, has the both the ability and the experience to ambulate Mr. Jones. The LPN is responsible for the actual ambulation of the patient. Therefore one may question the RN (delegator) as to why the ambulation act was delegated to the LPN. If Betty explains that Nancy had ambulated patients successfully before and that Mr. Jones was stable in his ambulation and able to perform the expected activity, then Betty most likely acted appropriately. Her responsibility for appropriate delegation had been fulfilled.

The LPN, Nancy, is accountable for what happened to Mr. Jones and is responsible. However, it is important to assert that responsibility and harm are not synonymous, neither are fault and responsibility, nor negligence and responsibility. It is possible, and most probable, that Mr. Jones fell because of circumstances out of Nancy's control, and perhaps that of anyone else. Given that Mr. Jones had successfully ambulated in the past, Nancy was assisting him to do more of the same. Other circumstances may have caused the fall, such as a wet floor, a misstep, a sudden lack of balance, a trip over the belt on his bathrobe, or a physiologic reason that had not surfaced before this time. In other words, just because Nancy was assisting with ambulation does not mean that blame or fault is assigned. Responsibility means that Nancy is responsible for the act of ambulation, and she is answerable for the result of the ambulation activity. Without such an understanding, most people would fear doing anything in the health care arena. However, if one understands responsibility, authority, and accountability, there is little to fear.

Following through with this example, if Mr. Jones had told Nancy that he was dizzy, Nancy should have relayed that information to Betty so that another assessment could be made. If Nancy knew that Mr. Jones was dizzy and insisted that he ambulate without assessment by an RN, then Nancy is both responsible and accountable for that decision. If Mr. Jones did not say anything to either Nancy or Betty, both nurses remain accountable, but their knowledge base is necessarily limited.

> ## NURSE ALERT
> **Accountability means being answerable for all of one's actions and decisions.**

In summary, delegation requires an understanding of responsibility, accountability, and authority. The delegator is responsible for determining the act to be delegated (McCloskey et al, 1996) and selecting the appropriate delegatee (Juleff, 1995). When an act is delegated, the responsibility and authority for completion of the act also are delegated. The accountability for the delegation rests with the delegator, and the accountability of the delegatee is for the act as well.

## EFFECTIVE DELEGATION

From the above explanation, it is clear that both delegator and delegatee face certain expectations. The following information describes the reasonable expectations of both parties.

For the delegator, the person who is delegating an action to someone else, the expectations are many

(Parkman, 1996). First, and most important, the delegator must determine that the action is appropriate for delegation to someone else. In other words, the act being delegated does not require the expertise, experience, or skill of an experienced RN. For example, the act may be a simple dry dressing change, feeding a patient who has two fractured arms, or assisting a woman who had a stroke (cardiovascular accident) 5 days before to dress herself. In most instances an LPN or even an unlicensed worker may be both capable and skilled in simple dressing changes or clothing or feeding a patient.

However, the action must be examined in relation to the patient involved, the recipient of the action. In other words, a simple dry dressing may not be simple on a person experiencing clonic seizures. A depressed woman may not be the easiest to assist with clothing. The man with two fractured arms may have no desire to eat because he caused an accident in which someone died. These examples illustrate the relationship between the task and the patient, the person who requires the task itself. In each of the three examples, the task is simple but the situation is complex. Therefore the act may not be appropriate for delegation to someone who has not had experience with similar complex situations.

Thus the delegator must be certain that both the act and the situation are appropriate to delegate. Determining the appropriateness of delegating the act is the easiest of the two components. The situation determination is more complex. However, the approach to either determination is the same; it is based on an assessment. The delegator must assess both the patient within the situation and the act itself. Before making a delegation decision, the delegator must ascertain the complexity of the situation, the risk (likelihood or probability) of change in the complexity, the relationship between the complexity of the situation and the task, and the individuals available to be the delegatee. Several outcomes are possible once the assessment has been made. The delegator may decide not to delegate, may decide to delegate to a licensed individual, or may decide to delegate to an unlicensed individual.

The delegator's assessment activity forms the basis for the responsibility and accountability of the delegator. Without an assessment, the delegator is acting inappropriately and is both responsible and accountable for the potentially inappropriate delegation decision.

Once a decision to delegate has been made and the delegatee has been selected, the delegator transfers the responsibility and authority for the action to the delegatee. This transfer requires expert communication skills. The delegator must clearly explain what needs

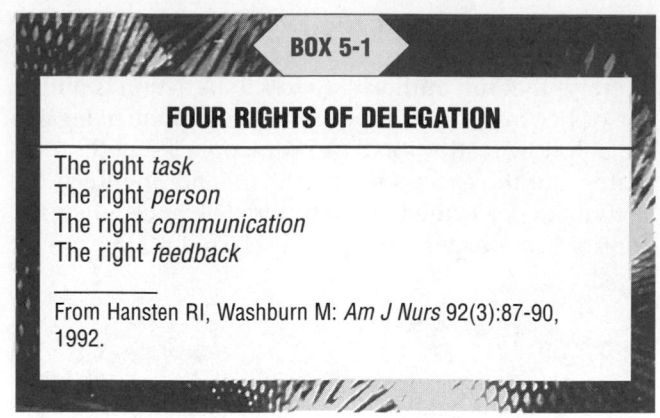

From Hansten RI, Washburn M: *Am J Nurs* 92(3):87-90, 1992.

to be done, to whom, when, under what conditions, and the expected outcome of the delegation.

Hansten and Washburn (1992) refer to these essential elements as the "four rights" of delegation (Box 5-1). The *right task* has been discussed previously. The delegator must make certain that the task is appropriate for delegation and within the legal and institutional authority of the delegatee. The *right person* refers to the delegatee, who must be competent, qualified, and capable of completing the task. The right person also needs to be interpreted to mean that the selected delegatee has the time within his or her overall assignment to complete the delegated activity. Last, the right person means that the delegator has the authority to delegate the task.

The *right communication* illustrates the need for a clear and cogent description of the task at hand, the specific objectives and outcomes the task is to accomplish, and the delegator's expectations of task accomplishment. The expectations of the delegator should include the time frame for the activity, the desired outcome of the activity, and the patient's status after the task has been completed. Finally, the *right feedback* is a determination of the result of the delegated activity and a sharing of information so that the staff may learn from the experience and patient care can improve continuously. Feedback is also known as evaluation and follow-up. Every delegated situation requires some type of follow-up and evaluation. Follow-up is simply the act of investigating and determining the outcome. Evaluation is the act of determining whether the outcome has had the positive desirable effect or some untoward result. The less-experienced delegator and delegatee necessarily require more follow-up. The evaluation component remains the same, regardless of experience. Follow-up may also be considered an element of **supervision.**

Supervision is the final component of effective delegation to be discussed. The delegator has the responsi-

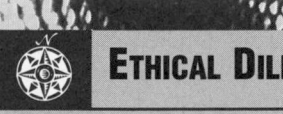

**ETHICAL DILEMMA**

**DELEGATION**

It is early morning in a subacute facility. There are 18 patients, and the staff consists of an experienced RN (yourself), an LPN who received her license 2 weeks ago, and a nurse's aide with 20 years of nursing home experience. Baths must be given, beds must be made, trays must be delivered, dressings need to be changed, medications must be administered, and patients want someone to talk with.

You have delegated all the dressing changes to the new LPN and assigned all the beds and baths to the nurse's aide. Knowing that all the patients are able to feed themselves, you have decided to deliver the food trays as you administer the medications to the patients.

All seems to be in order as the day progresses. During visiting hours that afternoon, Nancy, the daughter of a patient, Mr. Jones, asks you why the nurse's aide changed her father's dressing that morning. She knows that in the hospital, only RNs or LPNs changed the dressing. Knowing that you delegated the dressing change to the new LPN, you gather the details of what Nancy is telling you.

What information do you need? What do you say to the LPN to whom the dressing changes were delegated? What information do you gather from the aide and what do you do or say to the aide? Who is accountable and responsible? What happens next?

bility to supervise the act of delegation under the umbrella of responsibility. Once the delegator has delegated the activity, the delegator nonetheless retains the responsibility for continual assessment of the appropriateness of the delegation. In other words, the delegator should make additional assessments throughout the day if the act to be completed is not due till later in a worker's shift. A patient's condition changes quite regularly, and an assessment of such changes must be made before the delegated act is completed. Furthermore, the delegatee may require assistance with the task to ensure the desired patient outcomes. In this case the responsibility for assistance is the delegator's and is fulfilled through the act of supervision.

Both the delegator and the delegatee must be familiar with the "four rights" of delegation. The delegator has the responsibility to assess the rightness of the task, to determine the right person to do the task, to communicate the necessary information and to pro-

vide the feedback. The delegatee has the responsibility to receive the information *before* accepting the delegation. If complete information is not provided, the delegatee must not accept the delegation and the inherent responsibility.

Both the delegator and the delegatee need communication skills. Communication is built on respect and mutual understanding. If the patient remains the focus of the delegated activity and the subsequent communication, the result often is positive for all involved. If someone or something other than patients and their needs becomes the focus of the communication, the result usually is less than positive for everyone involved. Thus the heart of the delegation process is an orientation toward positive patient outcome.

## PROBLEMS IN DELEGATION

Although redesigned patient care is built around the premise that RNs will delegate those tasks that can be performed by others (Johnson, 1996; Parkman, 1996), the issue of delegation has given rise to significant resistance, reluctance, and a sense of the unknown. Lindstrom (1995) discusses the psychology of delegation in her classic article. She addresses the fact that delegation is neither a simple task nor necessarily a comfortable one. All too often, nurses are reluctant to delegate because they view delegation as an inability to do their job. Yet, administrators view delegation as an essential aspect of the RN job description, one that enables the work to be completed and patient outcomes assured. Thus a dichotomy potentially exists between a staff nurse's understanding and the expectations of an administrator. This is readily corrected and adjusted through open communication and dialogue about expectations, job descriptions, and evaluative criteria.

Additionally, some health care workers are reluctant to accept a delegated task for similar reasons. LPNs or LVNs and unlicensed workers often view delegation as add-on activities for them and as "doing someone else's work." Again, the reason for the delegation is not understood, and the patient is not at the center of the discussion and feelings. Solutions for this reluctance are similar to those already mentioned: communication and open dialogue.

Loss of control is another major reason nurses do not delegate freely. As discussed earlier in this chapter, responsibility, accountability, and authority are misunderstood. It is imperative that all parties involved understand the differences between these words and the expectations for both the delegator and the delegatee. Nurses may fear that if someone else performs the activity, they have lost control over the practice environment and patient care. Nurses must be assisted to see delegation as a means to accomplish better patient care, and they must learn to trust the other workers in the health care settings. Delegation does not mean loss of control, but rather greater control when it is the nurse who determines if an act is delegated or not. Additionally, the nurse decides to whom the act should be delegated. These two characteristics alone establish greater control rather than loss of control.

Research has shown that RNs are most concerned with the quality of the individuals (licensed and unlicensed) being hired to assist nurses in redesigned settings (Polifroni et al, 1996). No national standards have been set for unlicensed personnel (Connecticut State Board of Nurse Examiners, 1995). Each state and, in many situations, each institution determines how an unlicensed worker is trained and the minimal entry-level requirements. This has resulted in great confusion over the qualifications of the unlicensed worker. With a temporary or mobile work force, the uncertainty may also extend to licensed personnel, particularly the LPN/LVN. For this reason, greater collaboration is needed between administrators and all staff members in designing delivery systems to address these real issues. Without such collaboration, delegation remains a difficult task for most nurses.

Nurses generally have a desire to be liked by all in the health care environment. Telling someone what to do, a misperception of delegation, leads to dislike and negative work issues in regard to performance and willingness to cooperate. To avoid this difficulty, all members of the health team must have a full understanding of their roles in the health care environment. Ideally, this understanding is communicated on hiring and reinforced throughout the work years.

In most instances, both the delegator's and the delegatee's resistance to or dislike of delegation can be overcome through communication and attention to the patients' needs (Davis, Farrell, 1995). When the focus shifts away from the provider and to the needs of the patient and family, and when communication flows freely, resistance to and difficulty with delegation lessen significantly.

## SUPERVISORY ROLE

At some point in a nurse's career, he or she may be asked to assume a **supervisory** function in health care.

Labor laws generally define *supervisors* as individuals who have the authority to hire, fire, transfer, and promote employees (Yoder Wise, 1995). Supervisors are not eligible for membership in a collective bargaining unit by virtue of their role in personnel decisions.

Having defined the legal interpretation of *supervisors*, it is important to note that LPNs/LVNs generally do not function in this legal interpretation. Another word for directing, in this instance, is overseeing. When acting in a supervisory role within the directing capacity the LPN/LVN facilitates the delivery of patient care through others. In long-term care, in particular, the LPN/LVN may direct nurse's aides in providing aspects of direct nursing care. The LPN/LVN is responsible for making sure the aide or other LPN/LVN has the skills to provide the care. The LPN/LVN supervisor is determining that the aide has the ability, has had the appropriate orientation, and is capable of providing elements of direct nursing care such as giving bed baths, assisting with activities of daily living, assisting with ambulation, and perhaps ensuring that nonnursing functions of housecleaning and food preparation are accomplished.

Additionally, the LPN/LVN, as supervisor, is making sure that the performance of the nurse's aide or other LPN/LVN is consistent with the mission, policies, and procedures of the organization. If the work is not as it should be or is inconsistent, the supervisor must help the individual perform differently. The intensity of the supervision must be in line with the individual's abilities. Watching as the nurse's aide performs selected tasks and elements of care delivery is the best type of supervision; observing a process is more effective than hearing about it afterward.

The LPN/LVN supervisor also functions as coach for the employee (Gillies, 1994). In this role, the supervisor encourages, supports, motivates, and assists the individual to perform at a level consistent with both the individual's ability and the organization's need. The coach serves as cheerleader as well as evaluator.

The LPN/LVN, as supervisor, maintains accountability and responsibility for assigning a specific nurse's aide or other LPN/LVN to deliver the identified aspects of care. The aide or other LPN/LVN is responsible for the care that is delivered. This arrangement is consistent with the areas of accountability and responsibility discussed previously.

## KEY CONCEPTS

➤ Delegation is an element of practice in the health care delivery system.

➤ Delegation is complex and is based on the transfer of responsibility and authority to another individual.

➤ Delegation is framed and shaped by responsibility, accountability, and authority.

➤ Delegation requires assessment of the situation, the task to be delegated, and the appropriate person to whom the task should be delegated, all in the context of the desired outcome.

➤ The "four rights" of delegation demand determination of and provision for the right task, the right person, the right communication, and the right feedback.

➤ Patient care and the desired patient outcome form the heart of the delegation process.

## CRITICAL THINKING EXERCISES

1. What information must you have to accept an act of delegation?

2. On what grounds may you choose not to complete a delegated task?

3. If you are the delegator or the delegatee, what parameters assist you in the delegation process?

## REFERENCES AND ADDITIONAL READINGS

Ales BJ: Mastering the art of delegation, *Nurs Manage* 26(8):32A, 1995.

American Nurses Association: Position statement on registered nurse utilization of unlicensed personnel, *Am Nurse* 25(2):7-8, 1993.

Barter M, Furmidge ML: Unlicensed assistive personnel: issues relating to delegation and supervision, *J Nurs Adm* 24(4):36-40, 1994.

Blegen M, Gardner D, McCloskey JC: Survey results: who helps you with your work? *Am J Nurs* 92(1):26-31, 1992.

Conger MM: The nursing assessment decision grid: tool for delegation decisions, *J Contin Educ Nurs* 25(1):21-27, 1994.

Connecticut State Board of Nurse Examiners: *Memorandum of decision: declaratory ruling: delegation by licensed nurses to unlicensed assistive personnel*, Hartford, Conn, 1995, Connecticut State Board of Nurse Examiners.

Davis JM, Farrell M: Factors affecting the delegation of tasks by the registered nurse to patient care assistants in acute care settings, *J Nurs Staff Dev* 11(6):301-306, 1995.

Gillies D: *Nursing management: a systems approach*, Philadelphia, 1994, Saunders.

Hansten RI, Washburn M: Delegation: how to deliver care through others, *Am J Nurs* 92(3):87-90, 1992.

Hansten RI, Washburn M: Knowing how to delegate, *Am J Nurs* 95(7):16H, 16J, 16L, 1995.

Harrell MS: Practical strategies for delegation and team building in a redesigned environment, *Semin Nurse Manag* 3(4):180-184, 1995.

Joel LA: Restructuring: under what conditions? *Am J Nurs* 94(3):7, 1994.

Johnson SH: Teaching nursing delegation: analyzing nurse practice acts, *J Contin Educ Nurs* 27(2):52-58, 1996.

Juleff GL: Assessing competencies of the nursing assistant, *Nurs Manage* 26(8):77-80, 1995.

Lindstrom CC: The psychology of delegation, *Semin Nurse Manag* 3(4):175-179, 1995.

McCloskey JC et al: Nurses' use and delegation of indirect interventions, *Nurs Econ* 14(1):22-33, 1996.

National Council of State Boards of Nursing: *Concept paper on delegation*, Chicago, 1990, National Council of State Boards of Nursing.

Parkman C: Delegation: are you doing it right? *Am J Nurs* 96(9):43-48, 1996.

Polifroni EC et al: The how to's for effective performance in redesigned environments, University of Connecticut, Storrs, 1996 (unpublished manuscript).

Yoder Wise P: *Leading and managing in nursing*, St Louis, 1995, Mosby.

# CHAPTER 6

# Psychologic Responses

## CHAPTER OBJECTIVES

1 Discuss the stages of personality development.
2 Explain the normal use of defense mechanisms.
3 Define and differentiate between mood (affective) disorders, personality disorders, anxiety disorders, and psychosomatic disorders.
4 Identify three types of mood (affective) disorders, personality disorders, anxiety disorders, and psychosomatic disorders.
5 List five characteristics of schizophrenia.
6 Discuss the relationship between emotional and physical illness.
7 Describe regression and situational depression and the potential relationship of each to the ill or hospitalized nonpsychotic patient.
8 Identify four major sources of depression and list six symptoms.
9 List signals often given by individuals thinking about suicide.
10 List three behaviors that could signal emotional stress in a medically stressed patient.
11 List three common types of psychotropic drugs and one major side effect of each.
12 Describe, discuss, and demonstrate nursing techniques that are effective therapeutic tools in the care of both psychotic and nonpsychotic patients.

## KEY TERMS

Alzheimer's disease
anxiety
anxiety disorders
bipolar mood disorder
conscious
defense mechanisms
delusions
depression
ego
endogenous depression
hallucinations
Huntington's chorea
id
mental health
mental illness

mood (affective) disorders
organic brain syndromes
personality
personality disorders
posttraumatic stress disorders
psychoses
psychosomatic disorders
regression
schizophrenia
situational/reactive depression
subconscious
superego
unconscious

## RELATIONSHIP BETWEEN EMOTIONAL AND PHYSICAL WELL-BEING

Nurses may choose to practice in any of a variety of settings. Whatever the setting, however, the nurse must have a knowledge of **mental health** and **mental illness** and must understand the ways illness can affect a patient's emotional well-being. Emotional reactions occur in all patients with a physical illness, and these reactions increase the patient's need for emotional support. Mental health and mental illness are at opposite ends of an emotional spectrum. Without emotional support, the stress of a physical illness can move a patient toward mental illness.

Physical illness and mental illness are not clearly divided. Physical illness affects the patient's emotional well-being, and mental illness affects the body. A mentally ill person may have physical problems, and a physically ill patient may develop emotional problems. It is never safe to assume that a patient has only one or the other type of problem. Many patients currently seeking medical care have significant emotional problems that affect their physical states. Therefore almost all types of emotional problems can be seen in a general hospital, and many physical problems can be found in mentally ill patients. All people have similar needs that must be met to maintain their ability to function.

# NEEDS OF INDIVIDUALS AND MASLOW'S HIERARCHY

Each person is born with a definite set of basic needs, which are the same for everyone. These needs do not vary with age and are not changed by sex, color, race, religion, occupation, or marital status. They remain the same regardless of the individual's emotional or physical health. Maslow described these needs as having five levels. Starting with the most basic level, they are, in general: physiologic needs; a need for safety; a need for love; a need for esteem; and a need for self-actualization (Figure 6-1).

## Physiologic Needs

Maslow refrained from identifying the physiologic needs more specifically. The concept of homeostasis and recent studies of appetite that have linked homeostasis in an imperfect way to an actual chemical insufficiency in the body have led Maslow to believe it impossible and useless to list fundamental physiologic needs. He believes the list could become endless. In his study of Maslow, Goble (1970) identifies physiologic needs as food, liquid, shelter, sex, sleep, and oxygen. In nursing literature the physiologic needs commonly are identified as nutrition, elimination, oxygenation, activity, rest, sleep, and sexuality. If physiologic needs are not met, the individual focuses on obtaining them.

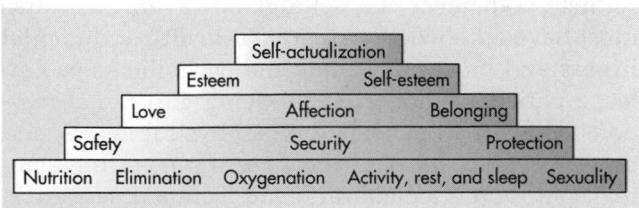

**Figure 6-1**   Maslow's hierarchy of human needs. (Modified from Goble FD: *The third force*, New York, 1970, Grossman.)

All other needs are ignored until the physiologic needs are adequately met.

## Safety

The needs that emerge on the next level are the safety needs. Maslow describes safety needs as security; stability; dependency; protection; freedom from fear, anxiety, and chaos; and the need for structure, order, law, limits, and strength in the protector. An organism can be dominated by the safety needs; they may serve as the almost exclusive organizers of behavior and may recruit all the organism's capacities. Such an organism may be fairly described as a safety-seeking mechanism.

In both children and adults, illness is a threat to safety and a disruption of order in the person's life. This disruption is particularly threatening to children, who need an organized and structured world. Children who frantically cling to their parents (which is often seen in hospitals and other health care agencies) are testimony to the parent's role as protector. The average child and the average adult generally prefer a safe, orderly, predictable, lawful, and organized world on which they can depend and in which unexpected, unmanageable, chaotic, or other dangerous things do not happen. In such cases the children have powerful parents or protectors who shield them from harm.

The healthy and fortunate adults in our society are largely satisfied in their safety needs and no longer have any safety needs as active motivators. The tendency to have some religion or world philosophy that organizes the universe into a satisfactorily coherent, meaningful whole is also partly motivated by safety seeking. Science and philosophy are partly motivated by safety needs. The need for safety is seen as an active and dominant mobilizer of the organism's resources only in real emergencies such as war, disease, crime waves, crisis, brain injury, and breakdown of authority.

## Love, Belonging, and Affection

If physiologic and safety needs are fairly well gratified, the need for love, affection, and belonging emerges. The individual is now keenly aware of the absence of friends, a sweetheart, a spouse, or children and hungers for a place in a group or family. The importance of a sense of belonging has been underrated. Belonging to a group, neighborhood, or culture now is recognized as a significant need. If society thwarts these needs, the unmet needs are most commonly at the core of maladjustment and more severe illnesses.

Maslow believed that love and affection needs and their possible expression in sexuality generally are viewed with ambivalence and customarily are hindered by many restrictions and inhibitions. Most theorists of psychopathology have stressed the thwarting of love needs as a basic factor in maladjustment. Maslow stresses that love is not synonymous with sex. Sex may be studied as a purely physiologic need. Sexual behavior usually is determined by a number of sexual and other needs, namely love and affection. Love needs involve both giving and receiving love.

## Esteem

At the next level are the needs related to esteem. All people in society (with a few pathologic exceptions) need or desire a stable, firmly based, and high evaluation of themselves, self-respect and self-esteem, and the esteem of others. These needs may be classified into two subsidiary sets. First is the desire for strength, achievement, adequacy, mastery and competency, confidence in the face of the world, and independence and freedom. Second is the desire for reputation or prestige (the respect or esteem of others), status, fame, glory, dominance, recognition, attention, importance, dignity, and appreciation. Satisfaction of esteem needs leads to feelings of self-confidence, worth, strength, capability, adequacy, usefulness, and importance. Thwarting these needs produces feelings of inferiority, weakness, and helplessness, and these feelings lead to basic discouragement or compensatory or neurotic trends. The most stable and healthy self-esteem is based on deserved respect from others rather than on external fame or celebrity and unwarranted adulation. Self-esteem must not be based solely on the opinions of others but must be perceived by the individual from within, based on real capacity, competence, and adequacy for the task.

## Self-Actualization

Even if all the previous needs are satisfied, discontent and restlessness soon develop unless the individual is acting according to personal capabilities. A musician must make music, and an artist must paint to be ultimately at peace. What a person *can* be, he or she *must* be; one must be true to one's nature. Maslow calls this need self-actualization. It refers to a person's desire for self-fulfillment, namely, the tendency for one to become actualized in what one potentially is and to become all that one can. Individual differences are greatest at this level. The clear emergence of this need usually rests on some prior satisfaction of the physiologic, safety, love, and esteem needs.

## Hierarchy of Needs

Maslow believes that the needs he described are satisfied to different degrees. Most members of society are both partly satisfied and partly unsatisfied with all their basic needs. A more realistic description of the hierarchy would be in terms of *decreasing* percentages of satisfaction at higher levels of the *hierarchy of prepotency* (superiority). The higher the level, the less often the need is satisfied by most members of society. Therefore emergence of a new need does not necessarily follow *total* satisfaction of the prepotent need. Instead, by slow degrees a gradual emergence from nothingness occurs. As the degree of satisfaction increases, emergence of the next need increases. For example, if only 10% of prepotent need "A" is satisfied, then need "B" may not be visible at all. As 25% of "A" becomes satisfied, 5% of "B" may emerge. If 75% of need "A" becomes satisfied, 50% of need "B" may emerge. At any given time, circumstances such as illness or personal catastrophe can necessitate that needs anywhere on the hierarchy take precedence. In other words, if we run a successful business and then suddenly lose all income, our priority needs may be reduced to the physiologic as we strive to feed ourselves and our families.

Maslow does not claim that these needs are to be understood as exclusive determinants of certain types of behavior. Any behavior tends to be determined by several or all of the basic needs simultaneously rather than by only one of them. For example, a person may eat partly to fill the stomach and partly for comfort and improvement of other needs.

Needs cease to play an active determining or organizing role as soon as they are gratified. Therefore a perfectly healthy, normal, and fortunate person has *none* of these needs. One who is thwarted in any of these basic needs may be seen as sick or at least as less than fully human. A healthy individual is primarily motivated by needs to develop and actualize his or her fullest potentialities and capacities.

Although health evolves from the gratification of basic needs, it does not produce selfishness. It is not ego centered. On the contrary, Maslow sees compassion and unselfishness in those who have had their basic needs gratified. Gratification assumes some positive growth tendency in the organism and drives it to fuller development.

If someone subscribes to Maslow's theory, self-actualization and health or wellness can be equated. Self-actualization is a goal and the ultimate need of all human beings, and it occurs when all other needs are gratified. Those involved with promoting wellness therefore can look to Maslow's theory of human motivation as a basis for their own theories. Maslow's theory treats the mind and body as a whole and has as its goal optimum wellness and self-actualization, which results in the most fully developed human individual.

# PERSONALITY

## Structure

Why do people appear to be so different? One person may be angry, aggressive, and ready to fight for the slightest reason, whereas another may be passive, submissive, and always ready to give in or compromise. An individual's response to a situation is based on **personality** structure, which is composed of a person's genetic makeup, life experiences, knowledge, and feelings.

Sigmund Freud is noted for deviating from the Viennese medical model by acknowledging the importance of emotions. He developed the concept of long-term psychotherapy called *psychoanalysis*. He referred to the awareness of the total environment as the **conscious** mind. He called the area just beneath consciousness where memories are stored the **subconscious** mind and named the reservoir of unremembered past experiences the **unconscious** mind. Because Freud was a scholar and a scientist, the goal he sought for his patients was not emotional happiness or mental health but self-knowledge and truth.

To describe and understand human behavior, Freud identified three parts of the personality: the id, the ego, and the superego. The **id** encompasses impulses and drives and operates at an unconscious level of thought. Id drives include hunger, sex, and warmth. Because the id operates on the pleasure principle, it demands almost immediate satisfaction. The **ego** deals with the way a person relates to the world. It is an awareness of the conscious self, or the "I." The ego sometimes has been called the executive of the personality because thoughts, feelings, compromises, and solutions are formed here. The ego attempts to satisfy the needs of the id while at the same time considering the pressures from the superego. The **superego** controls, inhibits, and regulates the impulses. It encompasses the notions of right and wrong as taught by parents and society. The superego operates at both the conscious and unconscious levels and aids in critical self-evaluation, self-punishment, and self-love.

## Development

The parts of the personality must achieve a balance before a person can function effectively and survive within a society. Like many theorists, Freud, Erikson, and Havighurst have attempted to explain how the personality develops.

Freud described stages of development from a psychosexual viewpoint. He identified three principal stages in the development of an individual: the *infantile stage,* which is divided into the *oral, anal,* and *phallic* stages; the *latent stage;* and the *genital stage.* Each of these stages has its own centers of importance and needs that must be met before the next stage can be entered successfully.

Erik Erikson's theory of personality development proposes that each stage of development involves a developmental task to be accomplished that not only contributes to some vital attribute of personality but also lays the groundwork for the next task. Erikson's first stages of emotional development are similar to those of Freud. Erikson described a sense of autonomy as the main emotional task of the early preschool years, a sense of initiative as the main task of the later preschool and early school years, and a sense of industry as the main task of the later childhood years. Havighurst also developed a specific set of tasks that must be accomplished in each developmental stage. Erikson's and Havighurst's theories together paint a mural of human development (Table 6-1).

# MENTAL HEALTH

There is no easy formula for judging normality. What is considered normal can and does vary from culture to culture, country to country, and town to town. From any point of view, the concept of normality and abnormality is a relative one.

A variety of writers have attempted to define mental health. Glasser (1970) states that a normal human being is one who can function effectively, obtain some degree of happiness, and achieve something of personal benefit within the rules of the society. Morgan and Johnston (1976) define mental heath as the ability to adjust to new situations, react to personal problems without marked distress, and productively contribute to society. An individual's degree of mental health may fluctuate from day to day and from situation to situation, but it maintains an overall consistency.

# ANXIETY

**Anxiety** is a major motivating factor in a person's emotional life. A person usually takes the course of action that reduces the apprehension, tension, and uneasiness that threaten the sense of self or the sense of control. These feelings stem from anticipated danger that may or may not be related to the reality of the situation. Some people are made anxious by love, some by hate, and some by the indifference of others.

## Sources of Anxiety

Anxiety is first experienced in infancy, when needs are not always met, and it continues to occur throughout the life cycle. All through life, an individual faces many conflicts that lead to anxiety. This anxiety can be

**TABLE 6-1**

## Comparison of Erikson's and Havighurst's Developmental Stages and Tasks

| DEVELOPMENTAL STAGE | ERIKSON | HAVIGHURST |
|---|---|---|
| Infancy | *Trust vs. mistrust*<br>1. Oral needs of primary importance<br>2. Adequate mothering necessary to meet infant's needs<br>3. Acquisition of hope | 1. Learning to walk<br>2. Learning to take solid foods<br>3. Learning to talk<br>4. Learning to control elimination of bodily wastes<br>5. Learning sex differences and sexual modesty<br>6. Achieving physiologic stability<br>7. Forming simple concepts of social and physical reality<br>8. Learning to relate oneself emotionally to parents, siblings, and other people<br>9. Learning to distinguish right and wrong and developing a conscience |
| Toddler years | *Autonomy vs. shame*<br>1. Anal needs of primary importance<br>2. Father emerges as important figure<br>3. Acquisition of will | |
| Early childhood | *Initiative vs. guilt*<br>1. Genital needs of primary importance<br>2. Family relationships contribute to early sense of responsibility and conscience<br>3. Acquisition of purpose | |
| Middle childhood | *Industry vs. inferiority*<br>1. Active period of socialization for child as he or she moves from family into society<br>2. Acquisition of competence | 1. Learning physical skills necessary for ordinary games<br>2. Building wholesome attitudes toward oneself as a growing organism<br>3. Learning to get along with age mates<br>4. Learning an appropriate sex role<br>5. Developing fundamental skills in reading, writing, and calculating<br>6. Developing concepts necessary for everyday living<br>7. Developing conscience, morality, and scale of values<br>8. Developing attitudes toward social groups and institutions |
| Adolescence | *Identity vs. identity diffusion*<br>1. Search for self in which peers play important part<br>2. Psychosocial moratorium provided by society<br>3. Acquisition of fidelity | 1. Accepting one's physique and accepting a masculine or feminine role<br>2. Developing new relations with age mates of both sexes<br>3. Achieving emotional independence of parents and other adults<br>4. Achieving assurance of economic independence<br>5. Selecting and preparing for an occupation<br>6. Developing intellectual skills and concepts necessary for civic competence<br>7. Desiring and achieving socially responsible behavior<br>8. Preparing for marriage and family life<br>9. Building conscious values in harmony with adequate scientific world picture |
| Adulthood | *Intimacy vs. isolation*<br>1. Characterized by increasing importance of human closeness and sexual fulfillment<br>2. Acquisition of love | 1. Selecting a mate<br>2. Learning to live with marriage partner<br>3. Starting family<br>4. Rearing children<br>5. Managing home<br>6. Getting started in occupation<br>7. Taking on civic responsibility<br>8. Finding congenial social group |

Modified from Sundeen SJ et al: *Nurse-client interaction: implementing the nursing process,* ed 6, St Louis, 1998, Mosby.

*Continued*

**TABLE 6-1**

**Comparison of Erikson's and Havighurst's Developmental Stages and Tasks—cont'd**

| DEVELOPMENTAL STAGE | ERIKSON | HAVIGHURST |
|---|---|---|
| Middle age | *Generativity vs. self-absorption*<br>1. Characterized by productivity, creativity, parental responsibility, and concern for new generation<br>2. Acquisition of care | 1. Achieving adult civic and social responsibility<br>2. Establishing and maintaining economic standard of living<br>3. Assisting teenage children to become responsible and happy adults<br>4. Developing adult leisure activities<br>5. Relating oneself to one's spouse as a person<br>6. Accepting and adjusting to physiologic changes of middle age<br>7. Adjusting to aging parents |
| Old age | *Integrity vs. despair*<br>1. Characterized by a unifying philosophy of life and a more profound love for mankind<br>2. Acquisition of wisdom | 1. Adjusting to decreasing physical strength and health<br>2. Adjusting to retirement and reduced income<br>3. Adjusting to death of spouse<br>4. Establishing explicit affiliation with age group<br>5. Meeting social and civic obligations<br>6. Establishing satisfactory physical living arrangements |

experienced in varying degrees, from mild anxiousness to a state of panic.

The sudden onset of an illness, a serious accident, or the death of a loved one may create anxiety and cause sleeplessness and other symptoms. An event that changes the family life-style or community status may produce a level of anxiety that makes a person feel helpless. A person in an acute state of panic who threatens to harm himself or herself or others may need the nurse to stay nearby until the panic has resolved.

## Effects of Anxiety

Anxiety is not always harmful, nor is it to be avoided at all costs. Mild anxiety actually can increase alertness and improve performance. Moderate anxiety, however, can diminish the ability to understand and make learning difficult. Panic results in complete incapacitation. Anxiety also has many physiologic effects that prepare the body for the "fight or flight" response.

## Symptoms of Anxiety

Anxiety can be recognized through many physical symptoms and communicative manifestations. A person may experience restlessness, fatigue, palpitations, increased perspiration, increased respiration and pulse rates, a loss of appetite, an inability to sleep, tremors, frequent urination, a "lump in the throat," vomiting, diarrhea, and a change in abdominal sensations ("butterflies" in the stomach). Anxiety also af-

fects communication. An anxious person may have a change in voice tone, speak at a higher pitch, or speak faster. He or she also may be preoccupied with personal thoughts and either avoid certain topics or continually discuss a particular subject.

## Defense Mechanisms

Because anxiety plays an essential role in influencing personality and behavior, it is helpful to explore the various mechanisms that people use to lower anxiety levels. **Defense mechanisms** are the attempts of the unconscious mind to protect the personality by controlling anxiety and reducing emotional pressures. Everyone uses defense mechanisms to reduce anxiety, and these mechanisms consequently affect behavioral responses. The use of defense mechanisms is not intrinsically unhealthy. Because illness, hospitalization, and incapacitation are anxiety-producing experiences, an understanding of defense mechanisms is essential to those caring for the ill.

Daily frustrations and conflicts usually can be resolved by using conscious coping mechanisms. More complex frustrations and conflicts are dealt with through unconscious defense mechanisms. The use of these defense mechanisms is not pathologic unless the individual's sense of reality is distorted. All defense mechanisms are automatic; they are not consciously planned by the individual. Their purpose is to reduce emotional pressures and prevent anxiety. Table 6-2 lists some of the more common defense mechanisms.

## TABLE 6-2

### Defense Mechanisms

| MECHANISM | DEFINITION | EXAMPLE |
|---|---|---|
| Compensation | The individual attempts to make up for real or imagined feelings of inadequacy. | The girl who has been made to feel unattractive works very hard to excel in school or other areas. |
| Conversion | Emotional conflicts that cannot be dealt with mentally are expressed through physical means. | A soldier on the front lines of battle is very fearful, but the thought of being a coward is unacceptable. Unable to resolve this conflict through thought processes, he becomes paralyzed, thus escaping the combat situation. He truly is unable to walk. |
| Denial | A person avoids painful or anxiety-producing reality by unconsciously denying that it exists. | A person denies unpleasant traits such as dishonesty or stubborness or refuses to believe that a loved one has died or has a terminal illness. |
| Displacement | Pent-up emotions are redirected toward objects or people other than the primary source of the emotion. | A nursing student is chastised by the instructor. After returning home, the student may kick the cat, slam the door, and argue with family. |
| Identification | A person unconsciously enhances self-esteem by patterning himself or herself after another person. | A hospitalized teenager so admires one of the nurses that she decides to choose nursing as a career. |
| Projection | A person protects himself or herself from being aware of his or her own undesirable traits or feelings by attributing them to others. | The nurse believes that a particular patient does not like him or her, when in reality, on an unconscious level, the nurse does not like the patient. The psychotic patient may state "He hates me" (I hate him) or "He thinks I am ugly" (I think I am ugly). |
| Rationalization | A person justifies inconsistent or undesirable behavior by giving acceptable explanations for them. (This has been called self-deception.) | A physician forgets to reorder medication for the patient and then criticizes the nurse for not giving a reminder. |
| Reaction formation | A person reverses unacceptable true feelings in exactly the opposite direction. | An overprotective and hovering mother actually resents and feels hostility toward her child. |
| Regression | A person returns to an earlier, less mature level of adaptation. Regression often results from lack of satisfaction or a threat to security. This behavior is seen to some extent in most hospitalized patients. | The 4-year-old boy suddenly starts to wet his pants and asks for a bottle after the arrival of a new baby at home. Some psychotic patients return to infantile behavior. |
| Repression | A person completely excludes from the conscious mind any impulses, experiences, and feelings that are psychologically disturbing because they arouse feelings of guilt or anxiety. Conflicts that remain repressed usually seek expression, as in dreams. | A daughter has very intense feelings of hatred for her father and wishes he would die. This thought is very unacceptable to the daughter and she excludes it from her conscious thought, yet she frequently has dreams of funerals and cemeteries. |
| Sublimation | Unconscious or unacceptable desires are channeled into socially acceptable activities. These desires are often sexual in nature. | A person may channel sexual drives into creating artwork or composing music. |
| Undoing | A person symbolically acts out in reverse something already done or thought that was unacceptable. The person attempts to erase the act or the guilt. | After slapping her child's hand, a mother keeps kissing her child's fingers. |

## Anxiety Disorders

**Anxiety disorders** are characterized by an anxious worrying that can result in a state of panic. Physical symptoms may include palpitations, shortness of breath, heavy perspiration, inability to concentrate, and sleeplessness, and these may be accompanied by unfocused feelings of dread. Anxiety disorders include panic disorders, phobic disorders, obsessive-compulsive disorders, conversion disorders, and **post-traumatic stress disorders** (Table 6-3).

**TABLE 6-3**

### Anxiety Disorders

| DISORDER | DESCRIPTION | EXAMPLE |
| --- | --- | --- |
| Panic disorder | General symptoms of anxiety | A person driving a car suddenly feels terrified and may have to stop driving. |
| Phobic disorder | Enormous fear of an object or situation, even though the person recognizes that it cannot really do any harm | A person may have a fear of open spaces (agoraphobia), closed spaces (claustrophobia), or heights (acrophobia). |
| Obsessive-compulsive disorder | Obsession: repetitive thoughts<br>Compulsion: repetitive acts that a person is unable to stop doing | A person constantly thinks about a love object, constantly drives by the love object's house, and makes him or her the total focus of all thoughts and activities. |
| Conversion disorder | Conversion type: blindness, deafness, paralysis<br>Dissociative type: split from the memory of the trauma and development of amnesia or multiple personalities | A person sees a shooting and suddenly goes blind.<br>A person is a victim of incest and remembers nothing of the incident. |
| Posttraumatic stress disorder | Numbness and decreased responses after the traumatic experience; flashbacks<br>Acute: within 6 months of the event<br>Delayed: more than 6 months after the event<br>Chronic: symptoms last longer than 6 months | A person experiences a traumatic event such as rape, earthquake, being held hostage, or war and demonstrates responses after the experience. |

# EMOTIONAL DISORDERS

Emotional disorders are difficult to define. They range from mild to severe, and definitions may vary according to the experiences of the person doing the defining and the cultural attributes and context of the patient in question. A person who is uncomfortable with the powerful expression of feelings may see a very angry person as being emotionally disturbed. A very emotionally expressive person may see a reserved person as being depressed. A nursing home patient who says, "I have stars on my ceiling and a monkey who eats orchids in my greenhouse," may be thought of by the nurse as senile or psychotic unless the nurse takes time to discover that the patient is recalling childhood memories, a time when the patient did indeed have a ceiling with stars and an orchid-eating monkey in the greenhouse.

A person who is emotionally distressed is less able to act and behave in a useful and productive way. He or she may be well oriented to persons, places, and things but may not know the reasons underlying a particular behavior and so cannot modify behavior merely by willing change.

## Pressures of Role Change

Whenever a person reaches a period of role change, new social and biologic pressures are brought to the surface. How well the transition occurs depends on the interpersonal resources and appropriate role models, as well as society's acceptance of the new role. The harder it is to make a smooth adjustment, the greater the conflict, the more intense the stress, and the more vulnerable the individual is to emotional and physical illness. Examples of difficult role changes are loss of a job, a death in the family, a career change, a divorce, an unwanted pregnancy, and school problems.

## Dealing with Hostility

Nurses may consider a patient with a physiologic illness to be a "difficult patient." Such patients' emotional response to illness and hospitalization makes them behave in ways that challenge the nurse to get past the negative emotional response and identify the

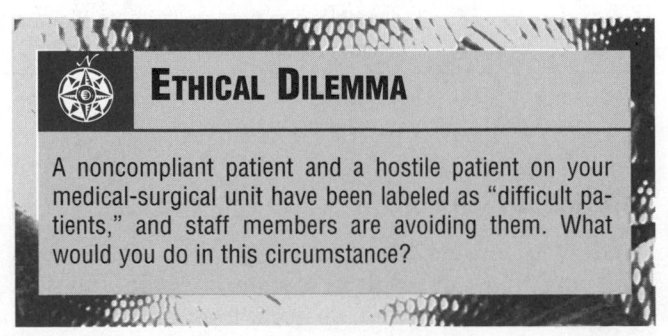

**ETHICAL DILEMMA**

A noncompliant patient and a hostile patient on your medical-surgical unit have been labeled as "difficult patients," and staff members are avoiding them. What would you do in this circumstance?

| | |
|---|---|
| **BOX 6-1** | **NURSING PROCESS** |

**MANIPULATIVE PATIENT**

**ASSESSMENT**

- Charming
- Intelligent
- Entertaining
- Too insistent
- Demanding/threatening

**NURSING DIAGNOSIS**

- Ineffective individual coping related to manipulation of others

**NURSING INTERVENTIONS**

- Identify the problem and the person who generated it.

- Provide a consistent environment.
- Point out manipulative behavior.
- Set clear, reasonable, firm limits.
- Reinforce positive regard for patient.

**EVALUATION OF EXPECTED OUTCOMES**

- Identifies own behavior
- States that anxiety has diminished
- Feels a trusting environment

behavioral needs. The emotional responses a patient can exhibit are hostility, manipulation, anxiety, and dependency.

A hostile patient exhibits anger and rage that usually masks feelings of fear and loss of control. In an effort to regain power or to control the situation, the patient resorts to a barrage of abusive language, threats, and constant complaints about the quality of care. Sometimes this behavior escalates to physical activity to relieve the pent-up anger. The nurse can detect the early warning signs of hostile behavior: a loud, menacing tone of voice, clenched hands, facial tautness, increased restlessness, pacing (if mobile), and listlessness (if in bed).

The nurse should not personalize the patient's expressions of anger, and the patient should be allowed to make choices and suggestions about his or her care. It is imperative that the nurse maintain open communication and avoid getting caught in a power struggle. The nurse also should ensure that the patient's environment is safe. Before the situation escalates and the patient loses control, the nurse should obtain help, and he or she should never try to manage a violent situation without adequate staff assistance. Quick tranquilization with chlorpromazine (Thorazine), lorazepam (Ativan), or haloperidol (Haldol) may be effective. Mechanical restraints may be needed to prevent the individual from doing personal harm or harm to others. Nurses need to know hospital protocols for initiating such an action. The nurse must also remember to maintain the patient's dignity and show respect even in the most chaotic time.

## Manipulative Behavior

Manipulative patients present an interesting dynamic. This type of patient may use charm, threats, flattery, or demands and may evoke feelings of guilt or pity. A manipulative patient is adept at splitting the staff by playing one staff member against another. The main purpose of this behavior is to gain control of the situation so as to have individual needs met. When dealing with a manipulative patient, the nurse should set realistic limits, be consistent, and be firm. This gives the patient set boundaries and diminishes the sense of loss of control (Box 6-1). The nurse must not get trapped into taking the patient's insults or threats personally. The nurse should explore the anger by accepting the patient but not the behavior. The nurse also should meet with other staff members to develop a consistent pattern of interaction. This strategy reduces the risk of the staff being split and provides a common basis for interaction.

## Anxious Patient

An anxious patient has an unpleasant feeling of apprehension and dread and may be unaware of the causes of these feelings. The nurse should help the patient explore his or her perception of harm and should use reality testing to assess the perceived danger. The nurse also should help the patient to verbalize his or her perceptions of events and their causes. The nurse should teach the patient the signs and symptoms of anxiety and should demonstrate ways to relieve anxiety, such as relaxation, meditation, exercise, and diversional activities. If antianxiety medications have been prescribed for the patient, the nurse should explain their use and intended effects.

## Dependent Patient

A dependent patient exhibits an inability to do things for himself or herself, may be demanding, and constantly rings for the nurse. Dependency may be exhibited during hospitalization because the patient loses confidence in his or her ability to function successfully. The nurse's first goal is to foster independence. This is done by ensuring that dependency needs are met and by gradually transferring daily care tasks to the patient. Setting a schedule with the patient and adhering to it enables the patient and the nurse to develop a trusting relationship and reassures the patient that his or her needs will be met. Praise and encouragement must be given after the patient performs even the most basic task.

## PSYCHOSES

It has been said that a neurotic person builds castles, whereas a psychotic person lives in them. **Psychoses** are a group of major emotional disorders characterized by bizarre behaviors and the inability to recognize reality and deal with life's demands (Fortinash, Holoday-Worret, 1996).

Psychoses resulting from or associated with organic brain syndromes are mental disorders caused by brain damage. These psychoses include those associated with chronic brain syndromes, alcoholic psychoses, intracranial infections, or endocrine problems.

Psychoses can also be caused by the stress of being in an intensive care unit (ICU). To diminish the potential for an ICU psychosis, the nurse should reduce the noise level, dim lights as necessary, and always explain what is being done. The patient should be kept oriented to time, place, and current events, and explanations should be kept simple. If hallucinations develop, the nurse should not repeat them but should continue to reorient the patient to reality. The nurse should assure the patient that this is a temporary state and that the hallucinations will go away as he or she gets better. Treatment varies according to the underlying physical situation (Box 6-2).

Psychoses that are not directly related to physical processes are called functional psychoses. These can be divided into three categories: schizophrenia, mood disorders, and personality disorders.

## Schizophrenia

**Schizophrenia** is the most prevalent form of psychosis. The term *schizophrenia* encompasses a large group of disorders involving disturbances in thinking, mood, and behavior. Schizophrenia comprises five major subdivisions, each with its unique characteristics, but the subgroups have several characteristics in common (Table 6-4).

The secondary symptoms of schizophrenia are those that characterize the major subdivisions of the disorder. These symptoms are a person's last desperate attempt to reduce enormous anxiety. Three of the major subdivisions of schizophrenia are disorganized, catatonic, and paranoid schizophrenia.

---

| BOX 6-2 | NURSING PROCESS |
| --- | --- |

### PSYCHOTIC PATIENT

**ASSESSMENT**

- Bizarre remarks
- Internal preoccupation
- Distractibility
- Mumbling to self
- Vacant look
- Tension
- Agitation

**NURSING DIAGNOSES**

- Anxiety related to mistrust
- Altered thought processes
- Sensory/perceptual alterations: visual, auditory
- Impaired verbal communication

**NURSING INTERVENTIONS**

- Provide a safe environment.
- Reduce stimulation.
- Make an effort to understand what patient means.
- Use physical contact sparingly.

**EVALUATION OF EXPECTED OUTCOMES**

- Protected from self-injury
- Feels decrease in stressors because of relaxed, restful environment
- Enters into trusting relationship
- Interprets physical contact appropriately

## Disorganized Schizophrenia

Disorganized schizophrenia often begins in adolescence. A patient with this disorder begins to demonstrate inappropriate emotions. The patient often withdraws from social contact and smiles and giggles in a silly manner. Severe **regression** occurs, until the patient's behavior becomes very childlike.

## Catatonic Schizophrenia

The catatonic type of schizophrenia has two forms. In one form the patient is completely inactive and mute and appears to be in a stupor. In the other form, the patient is in an agitated state, and his or her behavior often is impulsive and sometimes destructive.

## Paranoid Schizophrenia

In addition to displaying the other basic characteristics of schizophrenia, the paranoid schizophrenic is suspicious and aggressive and has **delusions** of persecution. The patient may hear voices that sometimes command action or may believe that the police are following his or her movements. This type of patient can be very convincing and often demonstrates manipulative behavior.

# Mood Disorders

Patients with a mood disorder show either extreme depression or extreme elation. **Mood (affective) disorders** include major depression, bipolar disorders, postpartum depression, and cyclothymic disorders.

## Major Depression

Major **depression** often occurs in middle age in people who have no history of depression. This condition also is called *involutional melancholia* and often is associated with menopause or with changes in a person's life situations. It is characterized by worry, agitation, guilt, and hopelessness.

## Bipolar Disorder

Bipolar disorder, formerly called manic-depressive illness, usually is characterized by wide mood swings that alternate between elation and depression. In the

---

**TABLE 6-4**

## Characteristics of Schizophrenia

| CHARACTERISTIC | DESCRIPTION | EXAMPLE |
|---|---|---|
| Thought and behavioral disturbances | The individual exhibits confused thought processes that are easily sidetracked or fragmented. The individual's speech lacks unity and clarity, and his or her behavior may be odd, sudden, and unreasonable. | Instead of thinking, "I'm cold. The window is open, and a breeze is blowing on me. I'll close the window," the schizophrenic person may think, "I'm hungry. Why is she staring at me? I see a red balloon." |
| Lack of affect | The individual does not display emotions, or displayed emotions are inappropriate. He or she fails to react to others in a meaningful way. | When informed of the death of a loved one, the individual may laugh. |
| Withdrawal | The individual becomes secluded from the rest of the world and exhibits decreased interest and initiative. He or she may have feelings of hopelessness, fear, and despair but remains acutely aware of the surroundings. | The individual may sit for hours staring into space without speaking to anyone. |
| Autism | The individual is detached from both reality and the world. | The individual is extremely withdrawn and involved with his or her inner thoughts. He or she ignores all that is occurring in the immediate area and fails to relate to others. |
| Regression | The individual retreats to past levels of behavior. | The individual's behavior becomes more infantile. |
| Delusions | An individual with delusional thoughts has false beliefs based on misconceptions. | The individual may refuse all food, fearing that it may be poisoned. |
| Hallucinations | The individual has sensory perceptions that cannot be explained by external stimuli. Any sense may be involved. | The individual may hear voices or exhibit unusual behavior such as talking to himself or herself, listening, or making unusual movements. |

manic phase the patient may make grandiose schemes and may not eat or sleep for days. The specific treatment of choice is lithium.

### Postpartum Depression

Postpartum depression can occur in the first 6 months of the postpartum period. It is characterized by weeping, lethargy, and feelings of being overwhelmed, incompetent, and helpless. Endocrine and hormonal changes, role changes, and stress, or a combination of these, have been proposed as causative factors.

### Cyclothymic Disorder

A cyclothymic disorder is characterized by mood swings between elation and depression. These mood swings are not as severe as those in a bipolar mood disorder.

## Personality Disorders

Personality disturbances fall somewhere in the middle range of emotional disorders. The behavior of people with **personality disorders** indicates serious inner problems. However, these people are in contact with reality, and most of them are able to adapt socially. People with personality disorders do not demonstrate the anxiety that is characteristic of other types of emotional problems. The more common personality disorders include the paranoid personality, the schizoid personality, the compulsive personality, the antisocial personality, and the passive-aggressive personality.

### Paranoid Personality Disorder

People with a paranoid personality tend to be overly sensitive, suspicious, rigid, jealous, and envious. They sometimes demonstrate an exaggerated sense of their own importance, and they tend to blame others. The paranoid patient has no **hallucinations** but has fixed delusions of grandeur or persecution that often center around religion. Other than these delusions, the personality is well balanced. There is some question as to whether paranoia is a separate disorder or simply a branch of schizophrenia.

### Schizoid Personality Disorder

People with a schizoid personality demonstrate emotional detachment, shyness, fearfulness, inability to socialize well with others, and a tendency to daydream and withdraw.

### Compulsive Personality Disorder

People classified as compulsive are rigid, neat, inhibited, conforming, and overly conscientious. They are excessively concerned with perfectionism and may show indecisiveness for fear of making a "wrong" decision.

### Antisocial Personality

People with an antisocial personality (sociopathic personality) are unable to form meaningful attachments to other people or groups or to society. They are selfish, irresponsible, impulsive, and unable to learn from punishment or past events. They feel no sense of guilt at causing harm or damage. Many prisoners are identified as having this personality type.

### Passive-Aggressive Personality

People with a passive-aggressive personality have considerable difficulty fulfilling dependent needs and responding to authority. Their behavior includes pouting, stubbornness, failure to keep appointments, procrastination, intentional inefficiency, and tardiness. The person may evoke feelings of anger in family members, friends, and coworkers.

## ORGANIC BRAIN SYNDROMES: DEMENTIA

Some forms of mental illness are caused by organic brain changes. These changes can be the result of a decrease in the blood supply to brain tissue, destruction of brain cells through trauma or disease, or age-related diminishment or destruction of brain tissue. Sometimes the symptoms of these **organic brain syndromes** can be slowed, but the symptoms are irreversible, and patients with these disorders progressively deteriorate. Senile dementia is the pronounced loss of mental, physical, or emotional control in the elderly, and it once was thought to be a normal result of aging. It is now known to have a variety of organic causes, including neuron degeneration in the cerebral cortex.

**Huntington's chorea** is a genetically transmitted disease. Everyone who has the gene develops a psychosis around midlife, and these individuals frequently require institutionalization. Parkinson's disease, which is caused by a lack of dopamine in the basal ganglia, is slowly progressive (see Chapter 30).

**Alzheimer's disease**, a more recently discovered chronic brain disorder, can manifest itself as early as the middle forties. This disease involves a progressive destruction of nervous system tissue and of brain cells, which come to have a twisted shape. The symptoms of Alzheimer's disease include involuntary muscle movements, slurred speech, memory lapses and loss, and gradual diminishment of thought processes and intellectual capabilities. Language disruption, emotional instability, inability to carry out daily tasks, and difficulty in following a set of instructions also may occur.

To give effective care to patients with dementia, the nurse should avoid overstimulating the patient and should ensure consistency in care. The nurse should use short, simple sentences when talking to the patient and should give him or her time to respond. Patients with organic brain syndromes are at high risk for injury when working around a stove or in other potentially dangerous areas. Such patients may wander away and may be unable to find their way back. These patients often cannot remember their name or address. The National Alzheimer's Association sponsors Safe Return, a program that provides identification bracelets and a national database for "wanderers."

## SOMATIC DISORDERS

In the psychoses and personality disorders, an individual's anxiety is expressed through behavior. In somatic reactions an individual's emotional conflict appears to be a major factor in the development of pathologic changes in a previously healthy organ of the body. The interaction between chronic anxiety and physical disease can be seen in a patient who develops essential hypertension as an adult. This person may have been raised in an environment that suppressed the expression of anger, and he or she may have lived for years with repressed hostility and underlying anxiety. Such a state can produce a slight but continual stimulation of the sympathetic nervous system and lead to a degree of arteriolar constriction in the kidneys, skin, and most visceral organs. A decrease in the blood supply to the kidneys can lead to the development of hypertension. Other conditions known to have a psychosomatic component are asthma, ulcerative colitis, hives, and migraine headaches. The specific causes of these disorders are unknown.

Not enough is known about these diseases yet to prove conclusively that they originate in the mind. The National Foundation of Ileitis and Colitis believes that ileitis and colitis have been incorrectly labeled as psychosomatic, and the foundation is involved in research to determine the cause of these diseases. A patient who has a disorder with a psychosomatic component may be angry that people think the illness is "all in your head."

Whatever the cause of the illness, it is the nurse's role to be supportive and caring. Those caring for patients with **psychosomatic disorders** may become impatient with or intolerant of a patient they think is "doing it to himself or herself." Consequently, an unsupportive and unsympathetic attitude may be conveyed to a patient who truly is suffering.

## DEPRESSION

Because of the high incidence of depression in the general population (the disorder is estimated to affect 1 in 12 individuals), a high incidence of depression among patients requiring nursing care can be assumed. The types of depression include grief, **situational/reactive depression, endogenous depression** (which occurs without an identified precipitating event), chronic depression, and bipolar mood disorder.

Depression has many signs and symptoms, some of which can actually mask the depression. All of the following symptoms should be considered when evaluating a patient for depression:

*Mood:* Sad, unhappy, blue, crying, appropriate to the situation

*Thoughts:* Helplessness, hopelessness, pessimism, guilt, low self-esteem, loss of interest and motivation, decrease in efficiency and concentration, inability to make decisions and choices

*Behavior and appearance:* Neglectful of personal appearance, angry/hostile, demanding, always smiling, seemingly the "good patient" (always compliant), perfectionistic, obsessive, anxious, hyperenergetic, withdrawn, dependent, indecisive, slowed in psychomotor capacities (speech and actions), agitated, apathetic

*Somatic or physical symptoms:* Loss or increase of appetite, loss or increase in weight, constipation, insomnia, fatigue or sleeping too much, chronic pain (especially backache, headache, and abdominal pains), menstrual changes, loss of interest in sex, sexual complaints or dysfunction, palpitations, hyperventilation, difficulty swallowing

### NURSE ALERT

A sudden elevation in a depressed patient's mood may indicate that he or she has developed a suicide plan and will act on it. A severely depressed person does not have the energy level or the ability to concentrate to carry out a plan effectively.

Many feelings underlie or contribute to depression, especially helplessness, hopelessness, and worthlessness. Other feelings that may cause depression include anger, despair, guilt, resentment, hostility, dependency, negativity, inferiority, low self-esteem, feelings of inadequacy, a poor self-image, a recent diagnosis of chronic or terminal disease, and loss. Loss can be defined in many ways and can include the loss of a significant other, a body part, a bodily function or mobility, a dependent state *(success depression)*, a symbolic object, self-esteem, or self-image.

Although feelings are significant factors in depression, depression also can be part of a symptom complex of certain diseases, including tapeworms, diabetes mellitus, thyroid disease, Addison's disease, Cushing's syndrome, systemic lupus erythematosus, uremia, hypoglycemia, gallbladder disease, stroke, cardiac disease, and Alzheimer's disease. Certain medications can induce depression, including reserpine, propranolol and other beta-blockers, methyldopa, diazepam, clonidine, corticosteroids, and oral contraceptives.

## Nursing Assessment of Depression

A nursing assessment and interview are useful not only for developing a nursing care plan but also to help the patient feel understood and cared for. A useful tool for evaluating a patient for depression is the phrase *in sad cages* (Box 6-3). In assessing a patient for depression, it is important to differentiate among the types and severity of depression and to recognize the following components of each:

*Grief:* Involves a real loss; lasts weeks to years; patient feels that everything has ended but knows better; reaction is proportionate to loss; no loss of self-esteem

*Reactive depression:* Related to loss in current life situation (either real or imagined; patient reacts to imagined losses as if they are real); comes and goes but can become chronic; reaction is disproportionate to loss; loss of self-esteem; patient manifests impaired

functioning, has distorted perceptions, and may be suicidal

*Endogenous depression:* Stems from a chemical imbalance and internal dynamics; same symptoms as reactive depression

*Psychotic depression:* Loss is not necessarily involved; patient has distorted thought processes and severely impaired functioning and suffers gross distortion of perceptions (hallucinations or delusions, or both); loss of self-esteem; patient reacts disproportionately and is suicidal

## Nursing Assessment of Suicide Risk

Suicide is one of the top five leading causes of death in the general population. It is the second most frequent cause of death for 15- to 24-year-olds and has a very high incidence among the elderly and the ill elderly. Therefore when a nurse assesses or suspects depression in a patient, it is extremely important to determine if the patient is suicidal. It is always appropriate to ask the patient very directly if he or she is suicidal or has ever thought about hurting or killing himself or herself. Directly asking patients if they are suicidal does not increase the risk of suicide. Patients often feel relieved at having the opportunity to talk about how terrible they feel. The nurse should always believe a patient if he or she expresses suicidal thoughts. Disbelieving a patient may lead to his or her death. The nurse might ask the following questions when assessing a patient's risk for suicide:

- Do you feel that life is worth living?
- Have you thought about hurting yourself or committing suicide?
- What do you think you might do?
- Do you have a plan to kill yourself?
- Have you ever tried to harm yourself before? What did you do?
- On a scale of 1 to 10, how suicidal are you?
- How do you see yourself in the future?
- Has any member of your family committed suicide?

Suicide is the ultimate expression of anger, hostility, hopelessness, and helplessness. Often the patient states the belief that "You have failed me." Many factors contribute to or increase the sense of hopelessness and helplessness and the risk of suicide in a patient, including the following:

- Previous suicide attempt
- Direct or disguised suicide threat, giving away belongings, or stating, "My family won't have to worry about me much longer."
- Chronic illness
- Isolation
- Bereavement or loss

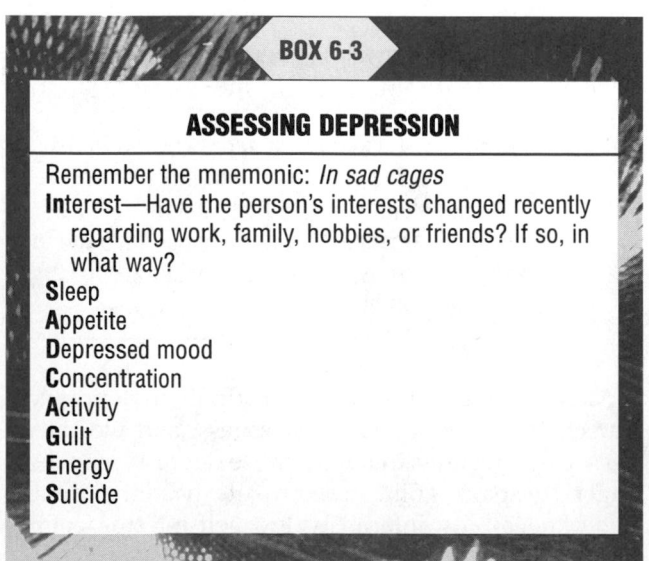

**BOX 6-3**

### ASSESSING DEPRESSION

Remember the mnemonic: *In sad cages*
**In**terest—Have the person's interests changed recently regarding work, family, hobbies, or friends? If so, in what way?
**S**leep
**A**ppetite
**D**epressed mood
**C**oncentration
**A**ctivity
**G**uilt
**E**nergy
**S**uicide

- Financial stress
- Severe depression or psychosis
- Alcoholism or drug abuse
- Chronic use of hypnotics or sedatives
- Family history of suicide
- Suicide of a close friend

Whatever the setting, it is important for the nurse to avoid trying to cheer up a depressed patient or to make statements such as "Things aren't that bad." The nurse should also avoid actions and attitudes that convey rejection, which can cause the patient to feel irritable and impatient and can lower self-esteem even more. Helpful actions include encouraging the patient to express anger and hostility; acknowledging the patient's statements about feeling depressed, sad, or worthless; and being nurturing, accepting, and respectful (Box 6-4). The nurse should think how he or she would want to be treated if the roles were reversed.

## NURSE ALERT

When dealing with a suicidal patient, ask specific questions about intent. Create a safe environment. Make a verbal contract with the patient that he or she will seek help from a staff member and will not harm himself or herself.

# THERAPEUTIC RELATIONSHIP IN NURSING

Psychologist Carl Rogers often is credited with refining the use of a therapeutic relationship in the treatment of the emotionally ill. In a psychotherapeutic relationship, therapists use interpersonal relationships with patients as a therapeutic tool. The therapists direct their own behavior in such a way as to treat the patient. The patient's behavior is analyzed as an expression of individual needs.

Nurses also need to establish therapeutic relationships with their nonpsychiatric patients. Whatever the setting, the nurse needs to use himself or herself as a therapeutic tool for patients and to develop a relationship that promotes healing. Nurses can develop meaningful and helpful relationships with their patients. Nurses have many opportunities to interact with them, observe their behavior, and react in a beneficial manner. Rogers has presented a variety of behaviors that are necessary for a helping relationship, including being genuine, offering warm acceptance of the person, and seeing the world as the patient sees it.

## Communication

To work effectively with a patient's psychologic needs, it is helpful to remember that the patient is attempting to communicate with the nurse verbally and behaviorally. The nurse is communicating with the patient in

---

| BOX 6-4 | NURSING PROCESS |
| --- | --- |

### DEPRESSED PATIENT

**ASSESSMENT**
- Anger
- Helplessness
- Hopelessness
- Apathy
- Crying
- Approval seeking
- Unkempt appearance
- Vague pain
- Fatigue
- Agitation/retardation
- Decreased social interest
- Focus on negative
- Appetite disturbance

**NURSING DIAGNOSES**
- Ineffective individual coping
- Altered thought processes

- Altered nutrition
- Potential for injury

**NURSING INTERVENTIONS**
- Accept patient.
- Be nonjudgmental.
- Encourage verbalization.
- Encourage patient to make his or her own choices.
- Help patient solve problems.
- Encourage participation in groups.
- Assess patient's ability to perform self-care tasks.

**EVALUATION OF EXPECTED OUTCOMES**
- Feels greater sense of self-worth
- Develops trust
- Gains self-control
- Receives positive feedback

the same way. The cornerstone in any relationship is communication. Communication implies a meaningful verbal and nonverbal exchange between people.

Verbal communication involves an exchange of words on a variety of levels. Each day one may greet a neighbor by saying, "Hi, how are you?" The neighbor may reply, "Fine, thank you, how are you?" This exchange is not meaningful communication. Neither person is really interested in how the other is feeling. Often a nurse cheerfully enters a patient's room with a bright "Good morning. Isn't it a beautiful day?" without observing that the patient is lying in bed quietly crying. The nurse is not in tune with the patient's nonverbal communication (crying). Successful communication involves four steps:

1. *Listen.* Often one is so involved with one's own thoughts or beliefs that the other person is not really heard. When a patient attempts to talk with the nurse, the nurse should really try to listen to what the patient is saying.

2. *Offer support.* A nurse can support what a patient is saying by not challenging or disagreeing with it. For example, a patient states, "I am really afraid to have surgery tomorrow. I wonder if my doctor knows what to do?" It would be easy to reply, "There is no reason to be afraid. The doctor knows what to do." This type of reply indicates that the nurse is not listening to the patient and supporting his or her feelings. Instead the nurse may say, "I can understand that the thought of surgery is scary. Let's talk about what worries you most." With this reply the nurse supports what the patient is saying and offers the patient the opportunity to discuss and perhaps resolve some of his or her fears.

3. *Empathize.* Empathy involves a sincere attempt by the nurse to understand situations as the patient perceives them. For example, it is easy for the nurse to become annoyed with a patient who refuses to learn to care for a colostomy. However, while talking with the patient, the nurse may learn that the patient's mother died shortly after having a colostomy. It is not always possible to determine why patients perceive things as they do. Situations have a variety of meanings for people, and nurses should be tuned in to what each patient is expressing.

4. *Use therapeutic responses.* Therapeutic responses are ways of communicating that encourage further discussion and indicate that the nurse is listening to what the patient is saying (Table 6-5). It is important that the nurse respond to the patient's feelings, not just to his or her words. It is also important that the nurse ask questions and not make assumptions about meaning. Fear and anxiety interfere with understanding. Therefore it is important for the nurse to realize that a patient who does not follow in-

structions is not attempting to "get the nurse" but may have difficulty understanding what the nurse wants. Because most patients want to please, the nurse's communications must be clear and easy to understand.

*Nonverbal communication* is also extremely important (Figure 6-2). It is "body language." Every move of the body and every gesture may convey a person's true feelings.

An incontinent patient in a nursing home who needs to have the bed changed for the third time in one evening may become only too aware of how loudly nonverbal communication speaks. The patient says to the nurse who is changing the bed, "I'm so sorry, my dear, I hope you don't mind." The nurse replies, "Oh, that's all right," while pulling and tugging at the sheets with an uncharacteristic roughness. The patient has "heard" the anger, although not a word of anger was actually spoken.

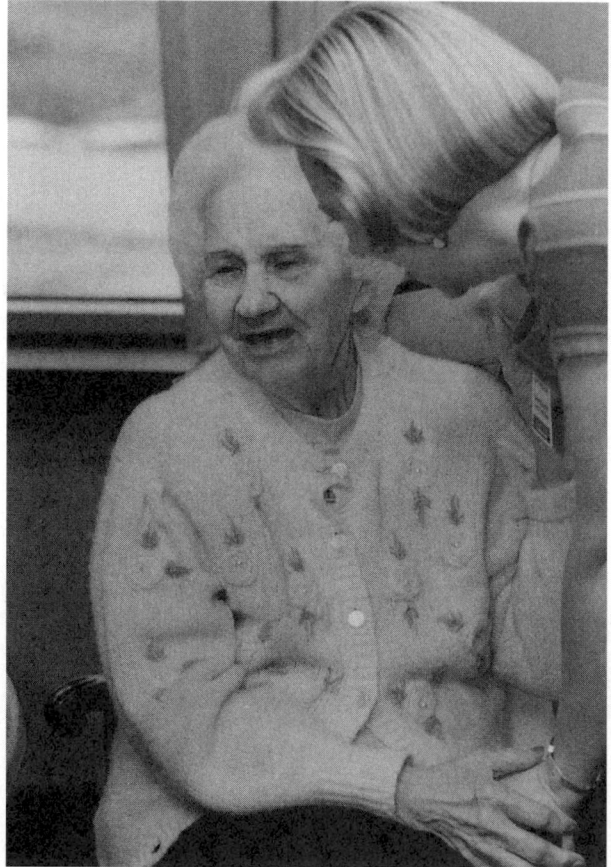

**Figure 6-2**   Touching a patient's shoulder and hand is an appropriate nonverbal gesture that expresses interest and support. (From Stuart GW, Sundeen SJ: *Principles and practice of psychiatric nursing*, ed 5, St Louis, 1995, Mosby.)

**TABLE 6-5**

## Techniques of Therapeutic Communication

**Technique: Listening**

*Definition:* An active process of receiving information and examining reaction to the messages received

*Example:* Maintaining eye contact and receptive nonverbal communication

*Therapeutic value:* Nonverbally communicates to the patient the nurse's interest and acceptance

*Nontherapeutic threat:* Failure to listen

**Technique: Broad Openings**

*Definition:* Encouraging the patient to select topics for discussion

*Example:* "What are you thinking about?"

*Therapeutic value:* Indicates acceptance by the nurse and the value of the patient's initiative

*Nontherapeutic threat:* Domination of the interaction by the nurse; rejecting responses

**Technique: Restating**

*Definition:* Repeating the main thought the patient expressed

*Example:* "You say that your mother left you when you were 5 years old."

*Therapeutic value:* Indicates that the nurse is listening and validates, reinforces, or calls attention to something important that has been said

*Nontherapeutic threat:* Lack of validation of the nurse's interpretation of the message; being judgmental; reassuring; defending

**Technique: Clarification**

*Definition:* Attempting to put into words vague ideas or unclear thoughts of the patient to enhance the nurse's understanding or asking the patient to explain what he or she means

*Example:* "I'm not sure what you mean. Could you tell me about that again?"

*Therapeutic value:* Helps to clarify the patient's feelings, ideas, and perceptions and to provide an explicit correlation between them and the patient's actions

*Nontherapeutic threat:* Failure to probe; assumed understanding

**Technique: Reflection**

*Definition:* Directing back the patient's ideas, feelings, questions, and content

*Example:* "You're feeling tense and anxious, and it's related to a conversation you had with your husband last night?"

*Therapeutic value:* Validates the nurse's understanding of what the patient is saying and signifies empathy, interest, and respect for the patient

*Nontherapeutic threat:* Stereotyping of the patient's responses; inappropriate timing of reflections; inappropriate depth of feeling of the reflections; inappropriate for the cultural experience and educational level of the patient

**Technique: Humor**

*Definition:* The discharge of energy through the comic enjoyment of the imperfect

*Example:* "That gives a whole new meaning to the word *nervous*," said with shared kidding between the nurse and the patient

*Therapeutic value:* Can promote insight by making conscious repressed material, resolving paradoxes, tempering aggression, and revealing new options; serves as a socially acceptable form of sublimation

*Nontherapeutic threat:* Indiscriminate use; belittling of the patient; screen to avoid therapeutic intimacy

**Technique: Informing**

*Definition:* The skill of information giving

*Example:* "I think you need to know more about how your medication works."

*Therapeutic value:* Helpful in health teaching or patient education about relevant aspects of the patient's well-being and self-care

*Nontherapeutic threat:* Giving advice

**Technique: Focusing**

*Definition:* Questions or statements that help the patient expand on a topic of importance

*Example:* "I think that we should talk more about your relationship with your father."

*Therapeutic value:* Allows the patient to discuss central issues and keeps the communication process goal directed

*Nontherapeutic threat:* Allowing abstractions and generalizations; changing topics

**Technique: Sharing Perceptions**

*Definition:* Asking the patient to verify the nurse's understanding of what the patient is thinking or feeling

*Example:* "You're smiling but I sense that you are really very angry with me."

*Therapeutic value:* Conveys the nurse's understanding to the patient and has the potential for clearing up confusing communication

*Nontherapeutic threat:* Challenging the patient; accepting literal responses; reassuring; testing; defending

**Technique: Theme Identification**

*Definition:* Underlying issues or problems experienced by the patient that emerge repeatedly during the course of the nurse-patient relationship

*Example:* "I've noticed that in all of the relationships that you have described, you've been hurt or rejected by the man. Do you think this is an underlying issue?"

From Stuart GW, Sundeen SJ: *Principles and practice of psychiatric nursing,* ed 5, St Louis, 1995, Mosby.

*Continued*

---

**TABLE 6-5**

## Techniques of Therapeutic Communication—cont'd

**Technique: Theme Identification—cont'd**
*Therapeutic value:* Allows the nurse to best promote the patient's exploration and understanding of important problems
*Nontherapeutic threat:* Giving advice; reassuring; disapproving

**Technique: Silence**
*Definition:* Lack of verbal communication for a therapeutic reason
*Example:* Sitting with a patient and nonverbally communicating interest and involvement
*Therapeutic value:* Allows the patient time to think and gain insights, slows the pace of the interaction, and encourages the patient to initiate conversation, while conveying the nurse's support, understanding, and acceptance

*Nontherapeutic threat:* Questioning the patient; asking for "why" responses; failure to break a nontherapeutic silence

**Technique: Suggesting**
*Definition:* Presentation of alternative ideas for the patient's consideration relative to problem solving
*Example:* "Have you thought about responding to your boss in a different way when he raises that issue with you? For example, you could ask him if a specific problem has occurred."
*Therapeutic value:* Increases the patient's perceived options or choices
*Nontherapeutic threat:* Giving advice; inappropriate timing; being judgmental

---

It is helpful for nurses to observe nonverbal communication carefully. Is the husband really listening to his wife when he is seated 2 feet from the television with his eyes glued to the screen? His body language says he is not. What is the mother conveying to her child when the child wraps his arms around her and she stiffens and draws away but says, "I love you"?

The use of verbal and nonverbal communication in nursing is as important as performing the proper techniques. Newcomers to the nursing field often are unsure of themselves when conversing with patients and are fearful of saying the wrong thing. However, patients can sense when nurses are sincere in their attempts to communicate. That attempt alone will be appreciated. Successful communication is worthwhile. It takes practice and effort, but its end results may be more important than any medication.

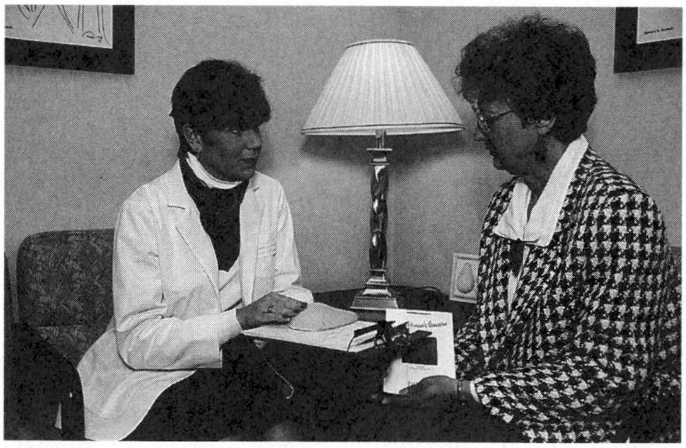

## Principles of the Therapeutic Relationship

Several general principles should be kept in mind when attempting to develop therapeutic relationships with patients. It is most important to accept the individual as he or she is. Patients should not be judged. Relationships are effective only if an individual perceives that the other party is interested in him or her as a human being worthy of dignity and respect.

The nurse should explain routines, procedures, and events according to the patient's level of understanding (Figure 6-3). Patients should be told that their feelings can be expressed and that they will be heard. Having patients participate in group sessions often is therapeutic. Mentally ill patients are usually anxious

**Figure 6-3** Explaining routines, procedures, and events helps maintain therapeutic communication with patients. (From Potter PA, Perry AG: *Fundamentals of nursing: concepts, process and practice,* ed 4, St Louis, 1997, Mosby.)

and should be treated with understanding and consistency. They should be offered reassurance for improvements in behavior, but false beliefs should not be supported. Any restrictions on behavior should be enforced consistently. Adhering to these principles can create a stable, supportive atmosphere that is conductive to mental health.

## PSYCHOPHARMACOLOGY

The use of medications to treat mental illness has revolutionized the field of psychiatry. Before the major tranquilizers were discovered in the 1950s, patients of-

**TABLE 6-6**

## Pharmacology of Drugs Used for Psychosocial Effects

| DRUG (GENERIC AND TRADE NAME); ROUTE AND DOSAGE | ACTION/INDICATION | COMMON SIDE EFFECTS AND NURSING CONSIDERATIONS |
|---|---|---|
| **Alprazolam** (Xanax) <br> **Route:** PO <br> **Dosage:** 0.25-0.5 mg 2-3 times daily as needed, not to exceed 4 mg/day; decrease dosage in debilitated or elderly patients | Benzodiazepine used in the treatment of anxiety, depression, and "panic attacks" | Dizziness, drowsiness, and lethargy |
| **Amitriptyline** (Elavil) <br> **Route:** PO, IM <br> **Dosage:** PO 30-100 mg/day in a single bedtime dose or in divided doses; dosage may be gradually increased to 150-300 mg/day; IM 20-30 mg 4 times daily | Antianxiety drug used in the treatment of depression | Drowsiness, sedation, lethargy, fatigue, dry mouth, dry eyes, blurred vision, hypotension, and constipation; potentially fatal reaction with MAO inhibitors; may interfere with antihypertensive drugs |
| **Chlordiazepoxide** (Librium) <br> **Route:** PO, IM, IV <br> **Dosage:** For alcohol withdrawal PO 50-100 mg, with repeated agitation, up to 400 mg/day; for anxiety PO 5-25 mg 3-4 times daily, IM, IV 50-100 mg initially then 25-50 mg 3-4 times daily as required | Benzodiazepine used in the treatment of anxiety and alcohol withdrawal; also used as a preoperative sedative | Dizziness and drowsiness; use with caution in patients with liver or kidney disease |
| **Chlorpromazine** (Thorazine) <br> **Route:** PO, IM, IV, Rectal <br> **Dosage:** For psychosis PO 10-25 mg 2-4 times daily, increase by 20-50 mg/day every 3-4 days (usual dosage is 200 mg/day); for nausea and vomiting PO 10-25 mg q 4-6 hr, IM 25-50 mg q 3-4 hr; rectal 50-100 mg q 6-8 hr; for intractable hiccups PO, IM 25-50 mg 3-4 times daily; IV up to 200 mg/day at rate of no more than 1 mg/min (usually given IV during surgery to prevent postoperative nausea and vomiting | Antipsychotic and antiemetic used in the treatment of acute and chronic psychoses, nausea and vomiting, and intractable hiccups; also used as a preoperative sedative | Sedation, extrapyramidal reactions, dry eyes, blurred vision, hypotension, constipation, dry mouth, and photosensitivity; use with caution in patients with liver and cardiac disease; may cause bone marrow suppression; may have adverse reactions with other CNS depressants |

*BP*, Blood pressure; *CNS*, central nervous system; *ECG*, electrocardiograph; *IM*, intramuscular; *IV*, intravenous; *MAO*, monoamine oxidase; *PO*, orally; *WBC*, white blood cell.

*Continued*

ten spent their entire lives in various institutions. Medications themselves do not necessarily cure the patient, but they often lessen symptoms sufficiently to allow the patient to participate more easily in other forms of treatment and to function more effectively in the community. As a result, the patient may be counseled in various community-based mental health centers rather than in an institutionalized setting.

Drugs that affect behavior are called *psychotropic drugs*. The major drug groups in this category are the antipsychotics, antianxiety drugs, and antidepressants. Antipsychotics and antianxiety drugs affect the individual's behavioral and emotional tone of feeling (affect). Antidepressants have a stimulating and energy-producing action that is particularly helpful in the treatment of depressive states (Table 6-6).

**TABLE 6-6**

## Pharmacology of Drugs Used for Psychosocial Effects—cont'd

| DRUG (GENERIC AND TRADE NAME); ROUTE AND DOSAGE | ACTION/INDICATION | COMMON SIDE EFFECTS AND NURSING CONSIDERATIONS |
|---|---|---|
| **Clorazepate** (Tranxene) Route: PO Dosage: 15-60 mg/day in divided doses | Benzodiazepine used in the treatment of anxiety and alcohol withdrawal and in the management of seizures | Dizziness, drowsiness, and lethargy; use with caution in previously suicidal or addicted patients |
| **Clozapine** (Clozaril) Route: PO Dosage: 300-600 mg/day; usual dosage is 12.5 mg 1-2 times daily, not to exceed 900 mg/day | Antipsychotic used in the treatment of schizophrenia that does not respond to other antipsychotic drugs | Sedation, fatigue, dizziness, tachycardia, hypertension, orthostatic hypotension, weight gain, seizure, and neutropenia; epinephrine may cause reverse (hypotensive) effects; requires weekly monitoring of WBC count; do not start or continue drug if WBC count is below 3500 mm² |
| **Diazepam** (Valium) Route: PO, IM, IV Dosage: For anxiety PO 2-10 mg 2-4 times daily or 14-30 mg extended release form once daily; for seizures and anxiety IM or IV 5-10 mg and may repeat q 10-15 min for a total of 30 mg; for alcohol withdrawal 10 mg 3-4 times daily in first 24 hr, decrease to 5 mg 3-4 times daily | Benaodiazepine used in the treatment of anxiety, seizures, and alcohol withdrawal; also used as a muscle relaxant, light anesthetic, and preoperative sedative | Dizziness, drowsiness, and lethargy; use with caution in debilitated individuals, in patients with renal or hepatic dysfunction, and in previously addicted or suicidal patients; drug has few compatibilities |
| **Fluoxetine** (Prozac) Route: PO Dosage: 20 mg/day in the morning; after several weeks may increase by 20 mg/day at weekly intervals (not to exceed 80 mg/day) | Antianxiety drug used in the treatment of depression | Anxiety, insomnia, headache, drowsiness, tremor, diarrhea, excessive sweating, and pruritus; may cause anorexia and weight loss; use with caution in the elderly and patients with renal or hepatic dysfunction |
| **Haloperidol** (Haldol) Route: PO, IM, IV Dosage: PO 0.5-5 mg 2-3 times daily; patients with severe symptoms may require up to 100 mg/day; IM 2-5 mg q 1-8 hr, not to exceed 100 mg/day; IV 0.5-50 mg, may be repeated in 30 min | Antipsychotic drug used in the treatment of acute and chronic psychoses | Extrapyramidal reactions, dry eyes, blurred vision, hypotension, constipation, dry mouth, and photosensitivity |
| **Lithium** (Lithium) Route: PO Dosage: 900-1200 mg/day in 3-4 divided doses; blood level monitoring is necessary to determine therapeutic dosage | Antimania drug used in the treatment of a variety of psychiatric disorders, especially bipolar affective disorders | Tremors, headache, impaired memory, lethargy, fatigue, ECG changes, nausea, anorexia, epigastric bloating, diarrhea, abdominal pain, polyuria dermatitis, hypothyroidism, leukocytosis, and muscle weakness; do not use in patients with severe cardiac or renal dysfunction or known alcohol intolerance; monitor drug levels closely |

TABLE 6-6

# Pharmacology of Drugs Used for Psychosocial Effects—cont'd

| DRUG (GENERIC AND TRADE NAME); ROUTE AND DOSAGE | ACTION/INDICATION | COMMON SIDE EFFECTS AND NURSING CONSIDERATIONS |
|---|---|---|
| **Lorazepam** (Ativan) **Route:** PO, IM, IV **Dosage:** PO 1-3 mg 2-3 times daily, up to 10 mg/day; decrease dosage in elderly; for insomnia PO 2-4 mg at bedtime; IM and IV routes used primarily as preoperative medication; IM 0.05 mg/kg for adults, up to 4 mg 2 hr before surgery; IV 0.44 mg/kg or a total of 2 mg, whichever is less, 15-20 minutes before surgery | Benzodiazepine used in the treatment of anxiety and insomnia; used preoperatively to induce sedation and anesthesia and for its amnesic effect; also used as antiemetic before chemotherapy | Dizziness, drowsiness, and lethargy; use with caution in debilitated individuals, in patients with renal or hepatic dysfunction, and in previously addicted or suicidal patients |
| **Olanzapine** (Zyprexa) **Route:** PO **Dosage:** 5-20 mg/day beginning with 5 mg/day and increasing to 10 mg/day within several days; target therapeutic dosage is 10 mg once a day | Antipsychotic drug used in the treatment of psychotic disorders | Orthostatic hypotension, drowsiness, headache, insomnia, and weight gain; instruct patient to avoid becoming overheated or dehydrated |
| **Oxazepam** (Serax) **Route:** PO **Dosage:** 10-30 mg 3-4 times daily; in older patients initial dosage should be 5 mg 1-2 times daily or 10 mg 3 times daily | Benzodiazepine used in the treatment of anxiety and alcohol withdrawal | Dizziness, drowsiness, and lethargy; use with caution in the elderly, in patients with hepatic dysfunction, and in previously addicted or suicidal patients |
| **Paroxetine** (Paxil) **Route:** PO **Dosage:** 20 mg as a single morning dose; may increase dosage by 10 mg/day at weekly intervals to a maximum dosage of 50 mg/day | Antianxiety drug used in the treatment of depression | Somnolence, dizziness, insomnia, tremor, nervousness, anxiety, headache, weakness, nausea, dry mouth, constipation, diarrhea, ejaculatory disturbance, male genital disorders, and sweating; potentially fatal reaction with MAO inhibitors; use with caution in the elderly and patients with renal or hepatic dysfunction |
| **Risperidone** (Risperdal) **Route:** PO **Dosage:** 4-8 mg/day; initial dosage is 1 mg 2 times a day; a total daily dosage as high as 16 mg/day may be required | Antipsychotic drug used in the treatment of chronic schizophrenia and other psychoses | Extrapyramidal reactions, insomnia, agitation, headache, anxiety, rhinitis, tachycardia, and weight gain; monitor for tardive dyskinesia (tongue thrusting, lip pursing and smacking, facial grimaces and chewing, muscle stiffness) |
| **Sertraline** (Zoloft) **Route:** PO **Dosage:** 50 mg/day as a single morning dose; may increase at weekly intervals to a maximum dosage of 200 mg/day | Antianxiety drug used in the treatment of depression | Headache, dizziness, tremor, insomnia, drowsiness, fatigue, dry mouth, nausea, diarrhea, male sexual dysfunction, and increased sweating; potentially fatal reaction with MAO inhibitors; use with caution in the elderly and patients with renal or hepatic dysfunction |

*Continued*

| TABLE 6-6 | | |
|---|---|---|
| **Pharmacology of Drugs Used for Psychosocial Effects—cont'd** | | |
| **DRUG (GENERIC AND TRADE NAME); ROUTE AND DOSAGE** | **ACTION/INDICATION** | **COMMON SIDE EFFECTS AND NURSING CONSIDERATIONS** |
| **Tranylcypromine** (Parnate) **Route:** PO **Dosage:** 30 mg/day, initially in a single dose or in divided doses; after 2 weeks may increase by 10 mg/day to a maximum dosage of 60 mg/day | MAO inhibitor used in the treatment of neurotic or atypical depression | Restlessness, insomnia, dizziness, headache, blurred vision, orthostatic hypotension, arrhythmias, constipation, anorexia, nausea, vomiting, diarrhea, abdominal pain, and dry mouth; watch for multiple drug reactions that could cause hypertensive crisis; foods containing tyramine (cheese, sour cream, beer, yogurt) can cause fatal hypertensive crisis; chocolate and caffeine can elevate BP |

It is important to note that neuroleptic malignant syndrome may develop suddenly in people receiving antipsychotic drugs. Patients with fluid and electrolyte imbalances, nutritional deficiencies, and organic brain disorders may be at risk. Because this is a life-threatening situation, early recognition of this syndrome is vital. A fever above 39.4° C (103° F), hypertension, tachycardia, diaphoresis, muscle rigidity, tremors, decreased consciousness, and incontinence may occur. Extrapyramidal symptoms and mental status changes also may be present. Neuroleptic malignant syndrome is a medical emergency, and the care delivered depends on the patient's symptoms. The neuroleptic drug should be discontinued immediately, and recovery may take 5 to 7 days. The patient should be told never to take the drug again.

General guidelines to give the patient for many, although not all, of these drugs include (1) do not get pregnant (use nonhormonal contraceptives) or use the drug if pregnant or lactating, (2) do not use over the counter (OTC) medications that have a sedative effect, and (3) do not stop taking the drug abruptly or without consulting a health care provider. The nurse should also be alert to the possibility of a patient "cheeking" or not swallowing a pill with the intent of hoarding it for a possible suicide attempt.

## ELECTROCONVULSIVE THERAPY

Electroconvulsive therapy (ECT) is an effective treatment for patients with severe depression. Muscle relaxants, general anesthesia, and proper education before the administration of ECT have reduced the fear of this treatment. The public's image of ECT as a mind-destroying, brutal, and indiscriminate therapy gradually is being replaced by the image of an effective therapy. Patients usually receive ECT three times a week for 4 to 6 weeks. They may experience temporary memory loss, learning loss, and confusion. Posttreatment nursing interventions help the patient perform routine and structured tasks and maintain adequate nutrition.

The goal of all treatments is to relieve symptoms and to help people learn new behaviors and different ways of relating to others. Some forms of psychotherapy can also help people to understand themselves better.

### NURSE ALERT

A sudden elevation in temperature, increased vital signs, diaphoresis, muscle rigidity, tremors, and an altered state of consciousness may herald neuroleptic malignant syndrome. This is a severe medical emergency that can occur in people taking antipsychotic drugs.

## NURSING CARE PLAN

## PATIENT WITH DEPRESSION

Marcus Overton is a 20-year-old college student who has been admitted to an acute inpatient psychiatric facility after an attempted suicide. He started to hang himself in his dormitory room but stopped because of severe neck pain and a change of intent. A college professor noticed the marks on his neck and referred him to Student Health Services, which recommended hospitalization.

| Medical History | Family History | Assessment Data |
| --- | --- | --- |
| Marcus witnessed the violent deaths of both parents at a very young age and has recurring bouts of depression and feelings of hopelessness and helplessness. He recently has been struggling with college academics, has difficulty maintaining social relationships, and has feelings of profound apathy. | Marcus currently lives in a dormitory on the campus of a large university. He is compatible with his roommate, but the two are not close friends. After his parents' death he went to live with his grandparents, with whom he still lives during the summer and between semesters. He has one older sister who also was severely traumatized by the loss of her parents. Marcus has a close relationship with family members but has few close friends. | Thin, quiet, and withdrawn male<br>Alert and oriented; responds appropriately to questions but gives short answers<br>Has flat affect and avoids eye contact<br>Reports feeling inadequate in college and feels helpless about what to do<br>Verbalizes difficulty concentrating because of sense of hopelessness and constant reminders of loss of parents<br>Acknowledges need for hospitalization and is interested in "getting better"<br>Denies suicidal tendencies at present<br>*Physical examination:* Within normal limits |

### NURSING DIAGNOSIS

Self-directed violence related to previous psychologic trauma, low self-esteem, depression, and hopelessness

| NURSING INTERVENTIONS | EVALUATION OF EXPECTED OUTCOMES |
| --- | --- |
| Explore suicidal thoughts and ideation.<br>Provide safe environment and close supervision at all times.<br>Develop contract in which patient states that he will not act on impulse and harm himself.<br>Encourage ventilation of feelings about previous loss and current difficulties.<br>Encourage participation in individual and group therapy.<br>Administer antidepressants as prescribed.<br>Spend extra time when available and convey care and concern. | Participates in program to full extent<br>Shows no evidence of behavior that could result in self-harm |

*Continued*

# NURSING CARE PLAN

## PATIENT WITH DEPRESSION—cont'd

### NURSING DIAGNOSIS

Hopelessness related to past trauma and current difficulties in college, as evidenced by verbal comments with such phrases as "giving up" and "nothing to live for"

| NURSING INTERVENTIONS | EVALUATION OF EXPECTED OUTCOMES |
|---|---|
| Assess for feelings such as hopelessness, lack of self-worth, and giving up. | Recognizes personal strengths and accomplishments |
| Assess for sources of hope, expectations for the future, and social support. | Expresses some optimism about the future |
| Encourage and assist with physical care that communicates care, concern, and respect. | |
| Encourage discussion of previous trauma and feelings of pessimism. | |
| Express hope for patient appropriately and realistically. | |
| Help him identify personal strengths, hopes, and future goals and to recognize accomplishments. | |
| Help him identify resources on campus that can help with academics. | |
| Encourage him and help him set realistic goals. | |

### NURSING DIAGNOSIS

Social isolation related to withdrawn behavior, low self-esteem, and fear of failure, as evidenced by lack of close friends, current hospitalization, and separation from environment

| NURSING INTERVENTIONS | EVALUATION OF EXPECTED OUTCOMES |
|---|---|
| Assess involvement with staff, other patients, and family. | Recognizes need to be involved with others |
| Encourage relationships as appropriate and participation in activities. | Works out plan to get involved with activities |
| Provide positive reinforcement when interacting with others and participating in groups. | |
| Educate regarding social skills if indicated. | |
| Help patient develop a plan to engage in social activities and pursue friendships with specific individuals after returning to school; this will enhance self-esteem. For example, encourage study groups, which will help academically and allow friendships to develop. | |

## KEY CONCEPTS

➤ Successful completion of developmental stages and tasks helps the patient respond to physiologic illness.

➤ Broken-down defense mechanisms create aberrant behavior.

➤ Patients who are extremely angry and out of control are at risk for becoming violent.

➤ The most serious risk of depression is suicide.

➤ Psychotic patients exhibit irrational behavior because their thinking pattern is irrational.

## CRITICAL THINKING EXERCISES

1. Mr. Rogers, who is 39 years old, has hypertension. He is supposed to take medication daily at bedtime. Recently he has been forgetting to take his medication. When his wife notices this, she reminds him. Mr. Rogers states that he does not need the medication because his headaches and dizziness have cleared up. He is feeling more relaxed, and the pressures at work have subsided. When Mrs. Rogers suggests he visit a physician just to make sure, he gets angry and says that he is fine and that she is the one who is sick and needs to see the doctor. He walks out of the room, slamming the door.
Identify the problem Mr. Rogers is having with the diagnosis of hypertension. What behaviors is he exhibiting (assessment)? What could be done to help him with the difficulties he is having relative to the diagnosis (nursing interventions)?

2. Mr. James is a patient in the medical unit where you are employed. You are assigned to care for the patient in the bed next to him. Your patient requires a lot of physical care, so you are in the room often and for extended periods. Your colleague is caring for Mr. James. You assess that Mr. James is trying to gain emotional support from his nurse. He communicates with his nurse and shares some of his concerns about his diagnosis, treatment, and prognosis. You hear your colleague making remarks such as, "How does your wife feel about it?" "Things will get better." "Don't worry about it; the physician has had a lot of experience."
What problems seem apparent in this situation? How might you handle the problems? Who might be able to assist you? What might happen if the situation is ignored? Consider the patient and your colleague; what might be the implications for future patient care?

3. Mrs. Frank, 72 years old, is admitted to the medical unit for regulation of her diabetes. It had been controlled by diet alone, but since the death of her husband 6 months ago, Mrs. Frank has been having difficulty. Her appetite is poor, and she has not felt like doing anything. She falls asleep at 9 PM but wakes up at 1 AM. She has refused recent social contacts with friends and has stopped going to church. Her son lives 300 miles away but is in weekly phone contact. She appears listless and cries easily when confronted about her feelings.
What are your perceptions of Mrs. Frank? What course of action can be taken to help her achieve control of her diabetes? How helpful can the son be in this situation? What are some of the precipitating factors of Mrs. Frank's depression?

4. Mr. Young, 25 years old, is admitted to the orthopedic unit for a fractured femur caused by an automobile accident. He also is diagnosed as having schizophrenia. After entering the room, you see him looking toward his left and mumbling to himself. You tell him that you are there to help set him up breakfast, and he asks you if you are with the FBI. How should you go about explaining to Mr. Young reality from your perception without agitating him? What drugs might he be taking for schizophrenia, and how might they interact with his medication for pain?

## REFERENCES AND ADDITIONAL READINGS

American Psychiatric Association: *Diagnostic and statistical manual of mental disorders,* ed 4, Washington, DC, 1994, The Association.

Breier A et al: Effects of clozapine on positive and negative symptoms in outpatient with schizophrenia, *Am J Psychiatry* 151:20-26, 1994.

Castner E: Dealing with the "difficult patient," *J Pract Nurs* 32:30, 1992.

Clayton B, Stock Y: *Basic pharmacology for nurses,* ed 11, St Louis, 1996, Mosby.

Collier S: Mrs. Hixon was more than "the CVA in 251," *Nursing* 22(5):62-64, 1992.

Daley DC, Bowler K, Cahalane H: Approaches to patient and family education with affective disorders, *Patient Educ Couns* 19(2):163-174, 1992.

Field WE Jr: Hearing voices, *J Psychosoc Nurs Ment Health Serv* 23(1):8-14, 1988.

Fortinash K, Holoday-Worret P: *Psychiatric mental health nursing,* St Louis, 1996, Mosby.

Glasser W: *Mental health or illness: psychiatry for practical action,* New York, 1970, Harper & Row.

Goble FD: *The third force,* New York, 1970, Grossman.

Hebert CP, Seifert MH Jr: When the patient is a problem: managing the difficult patient, *Patient Care* 24(1):59-62, 64-66, 69-71, 1990.

Jezierski M: Profile for depression, *J Emerg Nurs* 20(1):80-81, 1994.

Jones CP: Mr. Webb had a few reasonable requests, *Nursing* 22(1):60-62, 1992.

McDonald S: An ethical dilemma: risk versus responsibility, *J Psychosoc Nurs Ment Health Serv* 32(1):19-25; 40-41, 1994.

Messner RL, Lewis S: Double trouble: managing chronic illness and depression, *Nursing 95* 25(80):46-49, 1995.

Morgan AJ, Johnston MK: *Mental health and mental illness,* ed 2, New York, 1976, Lippincott.

Morrison M: *Foundations of mental health nursing,* St Louis, 1997, Mosby.

Paiva Z: Sundown syndrome: calming the agitated patient, *RN* 53(7):50-51, 1990.

Petersen S: Dealing with the difficult patient/family and remaining sane, *Caring* 9(11):23-25, 1990.

Piccinino S: The nursing care challenge: borderline patients, *J Psychosoc Nurs Ment Health Serv* 28(4):22-27, 40-41, 1990.

Stewart KB: What's wrong with this patient? *RN* 58(2):45-46, 1995.

Stolley MM: When your patient has Alzheimer's disease, *Am J Nurs* 94(8):34-41, 1994.

Stuart GW, Sundeen SJ: *Principles and practice of psychiatric nursing,* ed 5, St Louis, 1995, Mosby.

Wandal JC, Prince MR: Case studies: the care of patients with behavioral problems (including commentary by Mian P, Danis D), *J Prof Nurs* 7(2):126-135, 1991.

Whall AL: What is nursing treatment for depression? *J Gerontol Nurs* 20(1):42, 45, 1994.

# CHAPTER 7

# Physiologic Responses

## CHAPTER OBJECTIVES

1 Give an example of each of the major causes of illness and disease.
2 Describe the body's major physiologic defense mechanisms.
3 Identify the characteristics of the inflammatory process.
4 Describe nursing interventions for a patient with an inflammatory condition.
5 Explain the function of the immune system in combating and preventing disease.
6 Define the term *hypersensitivity*.
7 List the major assessment techniques used for allergic conditions.
8 Identify nursing interventions for people with allergies.
9 Discuss the nurse's responsibility in interventions for a patient in anaphylactic shock.
10 Identify diseases attributed to autoimmunity.

## KEY TERMS

allergen
antibodies
antihistamine
autoimmune
bacteriostatic
cell-mediated immunity
corticosteroids
desensitization
endotoxins
epinephrine
exotoxins
gram negative

gram positive
humoral immunity
hypersensitivity
immunity
immunoglobulins (Ig)
inflammation
leukocytes
normal flora
nosocomial infection
pathogenic
systemic infections
virulence

## CAUSES OF DISEASE

*Disease* is any condition in which the physiologic or psychologic functions of the body deviate significantly from that regarded as normal. Health and disease often are viewed as a spectrum, with excellent health on one end of the scale and disease, with permanent disability or death, on the other end (Figure 7-1). A person's state of health may vary periodically, and their position on the health-illness spectrum may change. In health a person successfully adapts to environmental stress, but in illness the capacity to adapt has been limited in some way. Homeostasis is the maintenance of a balance of physiologic processes in the body, and adaptation is the maintenance of a balance while interacting with the environment.

Most diseases are characterized by specific signs and symptoms. These signals arise from pathologic processes that interfere with normal body functioning. Because, in a state of health, the body functions as a

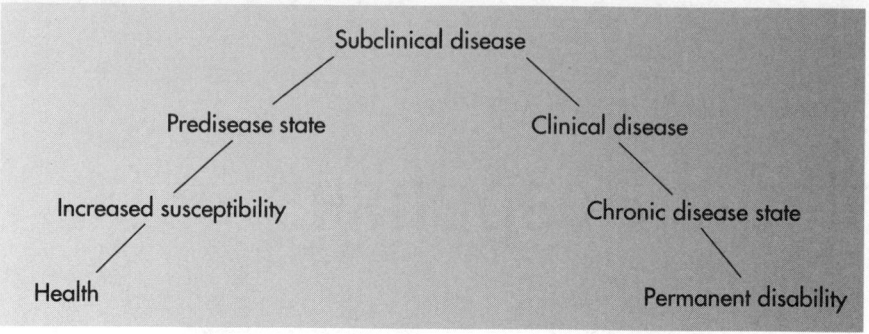

**Figure 7-1** Health-illness spectrum.

whole with all parts interdependent, a malfunctioning or abnormal condition of any part of the body may affect the entire body. Often more than one specific disease, each having a different cause, may be present in a person at the same time. The most common causes of disease are (1) microorganisms, (2) nutritional imbalances, (3) physical agents, (4) chemical agents, and (5) cellular abnormalities.

## Microorganisms

Microbiology is the study of microorganisms, or microbes. Microbes are living, minute organisms that usually have a one-celled structure. Many microbes live normally in the body without causing disease or illness; these are referred to as **normal flora,** which are found in places such as the gastrointestinal (GI) tract, the upper respiratory system, the genitourinary tract, and the skin. However, some microbes can become **pathogenic,** or disease producing; they invade the body, multiply, and cause disease. When this occurs, a person has an infection. Infections interfere with normal physiologic functioning and cause inflammation and possibly purulent discharge. The specific symptoms depend on the site of the infection. For example, an abscess in the brain tissue results in neurologic symptoms, whereas pneumonia results in respiratory distress. Microbes are classified as *bacteria, viruses, fungi,* or *protozoa.*

### Bacteria

Bacteria have many different characteristics. The three basic shapes are round, oblong, and spiral, but many variations of these shapes can be found. Some bacteria may be elongated or have pointed ends, and some may be flattened on one side. Some are shaped like a comma, and others appear square. Spirilla may be tightly coiled, like a corkscrew. During cell division some bacteria remain together to form pairs, whereas others form long chains. All these modifications are important in identifying specific types of bacteria.

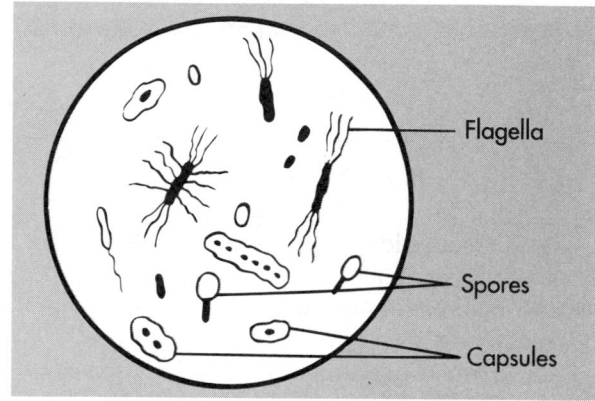

**Figure 7-2** Specialized structures of bacteria.

Bacteria may also have different chemical compositions, require different nutrients, and create different waste products. *Aerobic* bacteria grow only in the presence of oxygen, whereas *anaerobic* bacteria grow only in the absence of oxygen. Some bacteria are capable of movement; this motility is possible because of fine, hairlike projections called *flagella* that arise from the bacterial cell (Figure 7-2). These projections cause a wavelike motion that moves the cell. A bacterium may have only one flagellum attached to one end of the cell, or it may have many flagella surrounding the cell. Spirochetes, a type of spirilla, achieve locomotion by a wiggling motion that involves the entire cell body.

Some bacteria form a specialized structure called a *spore,* which is a round body formed by the bacterium in the presence or absence of oxygen (see Figure 7-2). Spores appear to form when conditions are unfavorable for growth of the bacterium. The spore enlarges until it is as large as the bacterial cell and is surrounded by a capsule. Eventually the portion of the cell that surrounds the spore disintegrates. The spore remains dormant until environmental conditions become favorable for growth. At that time the spore germinates and begins to reproduce in a normal manner. Spores are highly resistant to heat and disinfectants. In

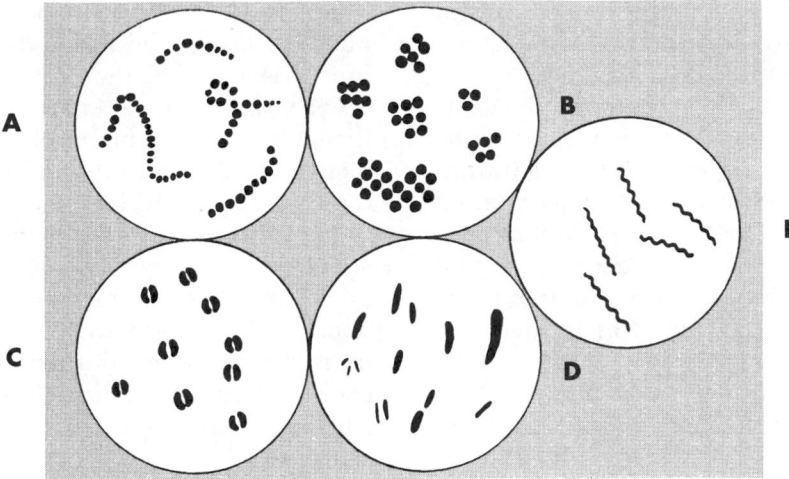

**Figure 7-3**   Common disease-causing bacteria. **A,** Streptococci. **B,** Staphylococci. **C,** Diplococci. **D,** Bacilli. **E,** Spirilla.

the laboratory they require special staining techniques because they cannot be stained by the usual methods.

Some bacteria have the ability to form *capsules* around the cell wall (see Figure 7-2). These mucilaginous envelopes seem to form when the bacterial environment is unfavorable. The formation may also protect the bacteria. The composition of the capsule varies with the species of bacteria, but it may include protein or fat substances or may contain nitrogen and phosphorus. As with spores, staining in the laboratory may require special procedures. When capsules are present, antibiotic therapy can be difficult because the capsule may prevent the drug from reaching the bacterium inside.

Many diseases cannot be diagnosed and properly treated until the specific microorganism causing the illness has been identified by specially trained laboratory personnel. Most bacteria cannot be seen until a special staining process has been done. Staining is accomplished by applying dye to a specially prepared glass slide that contains a small amount of the material to be examined. Most bacteria can be identified by this simple process, but some bacteria require additional staining. Depending on whether a color can or cannot be removed by a solvent, the organism is identified as being **gram positive** or **gram negative**. This simple laboratory test helps in the selection of effective antibiotics and is important in the treatment of the patient. Different antibiotics may be needed to destroy different bacteria. Some bacteria are known as acid-fast bacteria, depending on the staining process. As mentioned previously, special staining is required for bacteria that have flagella, spores, or capsules.

Body fluids and secretions suspected of containing pathogenic organisms can be collected in sterile containers and sent to the laboratory for culture and sensitivity tests. In the laboratory the collected specimens are transferred to a special culture medium that promotes growth. The culture is studied, and the pathogens are identified. Sensitivity tests are performed to determine which antibiotics effectively inhibit the growth of the pathogens. Appropriate antibiotics are ordered on the basis of these tests.

Bacterial infections are transmitted from person to person by direct contact, by inhalation of droplet nuclei, and by indirect contact with articles contaminated with the pathogen. Some infections are transmitted through ingestion of contaminated food and drink or through insect bites (see Chapters 14 and 15).

Bacteria are divided into four major groups: (1) cocci, (2) bacilli, (3) spirilla, and (4) rickettsiae.

**Streptococci, staphylococci, and diplococci.** The *Streptococcus* bacterium is responsible for more diseases than any other organism (Figure 7-3). Some strains produce serious or even fatal disease, others produce disease only under special conditions, and still others are nonpathogenic. Disease-producing strains include beta-hemolytic streptococci and the viridans group, also called *alpha-hemolytic streptococci.*

The beta-hemolytic group of streptococci causes about 90% of streptococcal infections. Some of the diseases caused by this group are extremely serious and may be fatal, including osteomyelitis, septicemia, scarlet fever, rheumatic fever, and pneumonia. This group also causes relatively common diseases such as tonsillitis and impetigo. The organisms also may invade surgical wounds or malignant lesions. Wound infection may occur as a result of improper hand washing before dressing changes. The organisms live in the upper respiratory tract and may be spread from one person to another by direct or indirect contact. Viridans streptococci may cause subacute bacterial endocarditis, which may affect the valves of the heart. Viridans streptococci also may be found in the nose and throat of healthy people. The two primary species of staphylococcal bacteria are *Staphylococcus aureus* and *Staphylococcus epidermidis*. *S. aureus* belongs to the pyogenic (pus-producing) group. Staphylococci, which can be found on the skin at all times, can cause boils (furuncles), abscesses, and carbuncles. They sometimes get into the bloodstream and cause serious complications. *S. epidermidis* is a nonpathogenic species of staphylococci that inhabits the human skin. Although this species may cause minor infections, the incidence of such infections is low.

There are several types of diplococcal bacteria. One type, which causes pneumonia, previously was called *pneumococcus* but now is known as *Streptococcus pneumoniae*. One characteristic of this organism is that it is encased in a capsule, or gelatinous envelope. Two other forms of diplococci cause gonorrhea (gonococcus) and meningitis (meningococcus). Further information about bacterial infections can be found in Chapter 14.

**Bacilli.** The term *bacillus* means "little rod." However, this rodlike shape can vary considerably (see Figure 7-3). Certain forms of bacilli produce spores, which are present in the intestinal tract of humans and animals and are discharged onto the soil. These spore-forming bacilli cause tetanus, gas gangrene, and anthrax (see Chapter 14). These organisms cause numerous other diseases as well, including tuberculosis, diphtheria, pertussis, typhoid fever, and bacillary dysentery.

**Spirilla.** Spirilla organisms have a corkscrew-like shape. Some forms of spirilla are rigid, whereas others (e.g., spirochetes) are flexible. One form, which resembles a comma, causes Asiatic cholera. Most diseases caused by the spirilla bacteria are uncommon. The spirochetes that cause syphilis are spiral shaped but have been separated and classified into a different order of bacteria. Lyme disease also is caused by a spirochete.

**Rickettsiae.** Rickettsiae are microorganisms that combine the characteristics of bacteria and viruses. They are parasites that flourish only within living susceptible cells, which provide a suitable environment and the nutrients needed for growth. The most serious disease caused by rickettsiae is Rocky Mountain spotted fever (see Chapter 14).

## Viruses

Before 1900, scientists discovered that certain agents, unlike bacteria, could pass through a laboratory filter. Scientists were unable to observe these tiny bodies with the ordinary microscope. In 1898 Martinus W. Beijerinck called these small bodies viruses, and they became known as filterable viruses. Viruses are the smallest known agents that cause disease. They are not complete cells but consist of a protein coat around a nucleic acid core, and they depend on the metabolic processes of the cell they enter to replicate.

For years scientists knew little about viruses even though they were able to observe their effect on humans and animals. In 1941 the electron microscope became available, which opened a new era in the study of human disease. With this technologic advance, the science of *virology* was born. In addition to the electron microscope, the use of certain dyes that become luminous when exposed to ultraviolet light (fluorescent microscopy), tissue culture methods, ultracentrifuges, cytochemistry, and the development of other technical laboratory aids have led to rapid advances in the study of viruses.

A virus may enter the body through the respiratory tract or the GI tract or through broken skin as the result of an animal bite. It also may be injected by a mosquito or hypodermic needle. Viruses are selective in the type of body cells they attack, but once they find cells that show affinity, they enter the cells and reproduce rapidly. As they multiply, they interrupt cell activities and use cell material to produce new virus material.

Viral infections usually are self-limiting. They run a given course, and the person recovers. One exception is rabies, which is almost always fatal. Other viral diseases may be fatal if complications occur or if they attack extremely weak, elderly, or debilitated individuals. The common cold is caused by a virus. The aches, fever, and chills may be relieved with rest and certain medicines, but colds cannot yet be cured. In nearly all viral diseases, antibiotics and sulfonamide agents do not alter the course of the disease. Some severe viral infections may be treated with an antiviral agent, such as interferon.

Certain diseases of human beings and animals appear to be caused by a protein that becomes an infective agent. These diseases, formerly called slow virus diseases, are neurologic infections; they include Creutzfeldt-Jakob disease and kuru in human beings, scrapie in sheep, and bovine spongiform encephalopathy in cattle. The exact cause is unknown, but the diseases have a long incubation period that ultimately results in severe microscopic degeneration of the brain.

Viruses can be classified according to the human diseases they cause (Table 7-1) or by the characteristics of a specific group. In the latter classification system, each subgroup may have many types of strains. The common viral infections are discussed in Chapter 14.

## Fungi

Fungal (mycotic) infections are among the most common diseases in human beings. Fungi belong to the

**TABLE 7-1**

## Major Groups of Viruses and Related Diseases

| VIRAL GROUP | DISEASE |
| --- | --- |
| Papovavirus | Papilloma (wart) |
| Adenovirus | Bronchitis, pneumonitis, pharyngitis |
| Herpesvirus | Herpes simplex (cold sore), herpes zoster (shingles) |
| Poxvirus | Rubella, rabies, smallpox |
| Picornavirus | Poliomyelitis, common cold |
| Reovirus | Believed to cause acute disease of the respiratory tract |

plant kingdom, and although many species are harmless, some cause infection. Fungi also are among the most plentiful forms of life; almost everyone is familiar with the fuzzy, black, green, or white growth on stale bread, rotten fruit, or damp clothing.

Mycotic infections are diseases caused by yeasts and molds. They often are superficial and involve the skin and mucous membranes. Scaling or cracking of the skin is characteristic, and blisters containing a watery fluid can develop. Most symptoms occur as a result of an allergic reaction to fungal products (Benenson, 1995). The areas most often affected are the external layers of the skin, hair, and nails. These infections are called *dermatomycosis* (ringworm). The most common site of ringworm in children is the scalp. The condition is considered infectious, and the child may not be permitted to attend school until the infection has been cured. Other sites include men's beards (barber's itch) and the feet (athlete's foot). The infection may occur on other parts of the body and often around the nails. Pets may have ringworm infection and often are the source of infection for human beings.

Fungi also invade the deeper tissues of the body. Most of these infections cause no symptoms, but some become serious and may be fatal. Those most common in the United States are coccidioidomycosis (valley fever) and histoplasmosis. Coccidioidomycosis was discovered in southern California, although it is found in other areas of the Southwest, where the climate is hot and dry. The disease affects the lungs and is believed to be contracted through inhalation of spores, which are present in the soil and are blown about by the wind. Histoplasmosis also affects the lungs. This disease is widespread throughout the world. In some areas 80% of the population may be infected, although overt clinical disease may not be present. The disease is contracted through inhalation of spores present in soil with high organic content and undisturbed bird droppings.

*Candida albicans* can cause either superficial infections or **systemic infections**. This fungus is a normal inhabitant of the GI tract, mouth, and vagina. An infection develops when something, such as a change in pH, interferes with the balance of the normal flora and allows the organism to grow. This change in balance can be caused by antibiotic therapy or immunosuppressive conditions.

## Protozoa

Protozoa are single-celled animals that exist in some form everywhere in nature. Some of the parasitic forms of protozoa are found in the intestinal tract, GI tract, and circulatory system of human beings and animals. The disease-producing protozoa are responsible for malaria, amebic dysentery, and African sleeping sickness. Another form of protozoa causes vaginal trichomoniasis in women, a condition often associated with pregnancy. It also may live in the male urethra and may be acquired or transmitted through coitus. Of the diseases caused by protozoa, the two of importance in the United States are malaria and amebic dysentery. The latter is more prevalent where sanitation is poor and personal hygiene is neglected. The source of infection can be the excreta of convalescent patients or carriers, and the disease is transmitted by food handlers or by contaminated food or water supplies. The common housefly may serve as an intermediary vector by transmitting the organism to food.

The malaria protozoan is transmitted to humans through the bite of the female *Anopheles* mosquito. Malaria is a worldwide health problem and is one of the most serious handicaps in the development of many countries (see Chapter 14).

## Nutritional Imbalance

Nutritional imbalance may be caused by (1) an insufficient or excessive diet, (2) an unbalanced diet, (3) increased use of a specific nutrient, and (4) failure of the body to use nutrients. Both nutritional excesses and deficiencies lead to an inadequate supply of nutrients to the cell. The general classes of nutrients that the body needs to perform vital functions are water, carbohydrates, proteins, lipids, vitamins, and minerals. The diet needs to include these essential nutrients for the body to be maintained, to grow, to repair, and to reproduce. The necessary amount of each nutrient varies from person to person and is influenced by factors such as age and level of activity.

Nutritional imbalance lowers the body's resistance to infection. Very young children, adolescents, pregnant women, the disabled, and the poor are especially vulnerable to malnutrition. There has never been greater emphasis on diet than now. For years it has been known that a deficiency of certain vitamins can cause scurvy, beriberi, and pellagra. Lack of adequate iron in the diet can lead to anemia. Minerals serve many functions in the body. Those present in large amounts are called *macrominerals* (Table 7-2). Of the minerals, 22 are known to be essential. Those present in small amounts are called trace minerals. These are arsenic, chromium, cobalt, copper, fluoride, iodine, iron, manganese, molybdenum, nickel, selenium, silicon, tin, vanadium, and zinc.

Obesity is a major health concern in affluent countries. Obesity, which is defined as an excessive amount of body fat, develops when the calories consumed exceed the calories used in the production of energy. Two types of obesity have been described: upper body (android, or male) and lower body (gynoid or female). Upper body obesity is characterized by larger fat cells and is more prevalent among men. The lower body type is more common among women. It is characterized by a greater number of fat cells, especially in the gluteal-femoral region. Obesity and diets high in saturated fats have been identified as risk factors in coronary artery disease. A high intake of dietary fat may also be associated with endometrial, breast, prostatic, ovarian, and rectal cancer. Obesity also can result in social isolation, glucose intolerance, hypertension, cholelithiasis, and menstrual irregularity.

Certain eating disorders have become significant health concerns. Anorexia nervosa is a psychologic and physiologic syndrome that involves the fear of becoming overweight. This fear results in fat and muscle depletion and produces severe symptoms and sometimes death. Bulimia is an eating disorder characterized by the consumption of food followed by vomiting or purging. Physical and psychologic problems can result.

Current research is concerned not only with the types of food necessary for health but also with how the body metabolizes and uses nutrients. A diet may be entirely adequate from a nutritional standpoint, but because of an organ or body part malfunction, the nutritional content of the food may not be used properly, and the person becomes ill. For example, in people with diabetes, the body cannot use carbohydrates despite an adequate intake.

In some countries the lack of food is so serious that people are predisposed to developing various diseases or dying from starvation. Protein-calorie malnutrition (marasmus, kwashiorkor) is of particular concern for children in developing countries. To help combat malnutrition, the United States has made millions of dollars' worth of surplus food and grains available to many of these countries. However, even in the United States, the problem of hunger and malnutrition is still of concern in some areas. Programs such as food stamps for low-income families have been created to increase the purchasing power of those who qualify.

## Physical Agents

Physical agents that can cause injury to the body include trauma, changes in external temperature, electric current, exposure to radiation, changes in atmospheric pressure, mechanical factors, and noise. Injuries from trauma can result in closed or open wounds, fractured bones, injured organs, and disruption of blood flow. Exposure to high environmental temperatures can lead to heat exhaustion or heatstroke. Severe environmental heat can cause life-threatening problems if not quickly recognized and treated appropriately. Overexposure to the sun's rays may result in severe burns and skin cancer. Fever is an example of internal heat production. A fever is a body temperature above 38° C (100° F) when the body is at rest. Heat also can be used therapeutically. For example, cautery is used to treat wounds, to stop bleeding, and even to cut tissue during surgery.

Exposure to extreme cold can cause frostbite or actual freezing of body parts and possibly death. Normally the body temperature never varies more than 1° from normal. The lethal limits for total body temperature range from approximately 22° to 42° C (71.6° to 107.6° F). Cold (*hypothermia*) generally is tolerated better than heat (*hyperthermia*). Controlled hypothermia is used in medicine as an anesthetic for minor pain; freezing techniques can be used for surgical purposes (*cryosurgery*); and profound hypothermia can be used for an extracorporeal bypass during cardiac surgery. General hypothermia may be used during surgery to decrease the activity of body tissues. This diminished activity results in a reduced need for oxygen and nour-

| TABLE 7-2 |
| --- |

## Macrominerals

| MINERAL | PHYSIOLOGIC FUNCTIONS |
| --- | --- |
| Calcium | Structural and maintenance role in bones and teeth |
| Chloride | Regulates stomach pH; major anion of extracellular fluid |
| Magnesium | Important intracellular cation; acts as activator for many enzymes |
| Phosphorus | Helps in bone formation and maintenance; important in enegy metabolism of adenosine triphosphate |
| Potassium | Major intracellular cation; necessary for transmission of nerve impulses, acid-base balance, and formation of protein and glycogen |
| Sodium | Major cation of extracellular fluid; regulates body fluid osmolarity and volume |

ishment circulated by the blood. An electric current may cause slight tingling, such as may be experienced in the home as a result of faulty wiring, or it can result in severe shock, burns, or death, as when a person is exposed to high voltage. Severe radiation injury can occur as a result of exposure to atomic radiation, and unless proper precautions are taken, injury also may result from x-ray or radium therapy.

Deviation from normal atmospheric pressure to increased or decreased pressure may cause illness or death. Persons traveling by air may experience extreme pain in the ears because of the rapid changes in atmospheric pressure. A condition known as the *bends* can occur in divers if water pressure declines too rapidly. The rapid decline causes the gases in the blood to come out of solution; the gases then can form emboli and obstruct blood vessels.

Mechanical injuries can be caused by physical impact or by irritation, and they often are related to occupational hazards. The field of occupational biomechanics deals with the prevention of overexertion disorders, which are caused by mechanical factors that affect the body (McCance, Huether, 1998). Noise is sound that can cause bodily injury. Noise-induced hearing loss can result from prolonged exposure to intense sound. However, a single, loud sound such as a gunshot also can cause acoustic trauma (McCance, Huether, 1998). Precautions must be taken in the workplace to prevent hearing loss.

## Chemical Agents

Studies indicate that poisoning is a major health problem. Substances known to be toxic in large doses, such as medicines, may be taken accidentally or intentionally. Many of the new drugs on the market may have no satisfactory antidote. Overdoses of some drugs cause respiratory and cardiovascular depression.

In contemporary society, the prevalence of chemical dependency is cause for great concern. The abuse of addictive and recreational substances, including drugs and alcohol, has long-term consequences that range from cardiac and liver disease to low birth weight and addicted newborns. Programs are available for helping people with a chemical dependence to gain access to treatment plans. These programs often can be found in hospitals and community agencies. Peer assistance programs also are available for health professionals to obtain treatment for their own chemical dependence. Substance abuse is discussed in Chapter 10.

Some chemical agents such as lye can be ingested, and others such as carbon monoxide are inhaled as gases. Carbon monoxide (CO) poisoning caused by faulty heating systems is becoming a major concern. CO is an odorless, colorless gas that can cause hypoxic

injury and death. Carbon monoxide detectors are recommended for home use to alert residents to dangerous levels of this gas.

Various industrial processes use chemicals that are injurious if inhaled or allowed to touch the skin. Caffeine and tobacco are two other commonly available chemical agents that have been shown to cause harm. Cigarette smoking has been closely linked with coronary artery disease and an increased incidence of lung cancer. A relatively new concern is the risk to nonsmokers who breathe secondhand smoke. Secondhand smoke has been linked to diminished pulmonary function, an increased number of respiratory infections, and exacerbations of asthma in children (Chilmonczyk et al, 1993).

Concern is increasing that the environment is becoming contaminated by insecticides and herbicides, lead from gasoline combustion, and industrial wastes. In certain high-risk occupations, such as mining, exposure to gases or dust may cause acute or chronic illness. In some older homes the potential for lead poisoning in children from lead-based paint is of particular concern. The sweet taste of the paint attracts youngsters to ingest it. In children, lead is readily absorbed from the intestine (McCance, Huether, 1998).

Hospitals, clinics, and other institutions have established poison control centers, where information about a drug is available usually on a 24-hour basis. Special educational displays, posters, and printed material have been placed in public buildings to inform people about the harmful effects of poisons. The U.S. government has curtailed the use of once-common food additives and some drugs because of possible harmful effects. State and local governments are becoming increasingly aware of the need for more public information and for legislation to control hazardous drugs, chemicals, insecticides, and sprays.

## Cellular Abnormalities

Cells are the smallest living structures capable of maintaining life functions and reproducing. Cells of varying structure and function form tissues, and tissues form organs, each of which contributes to the integrated, holistic function of the body. In all pathologic conditions, the cells that form tissues, organs, and other structures are affected.

Although the types of cells vary considerably, some structures are common to all. Figure 7-4 shows the structure of a typical body cell. The cell membrane forms the outer boundary, maintains the cell structure, and determines which substances may move into or out of the cell. Protoplasm, the internal substance of the cell, is composed primarily of the elements hydrogen, oxygen, carbon, and nitrogen. These elements are

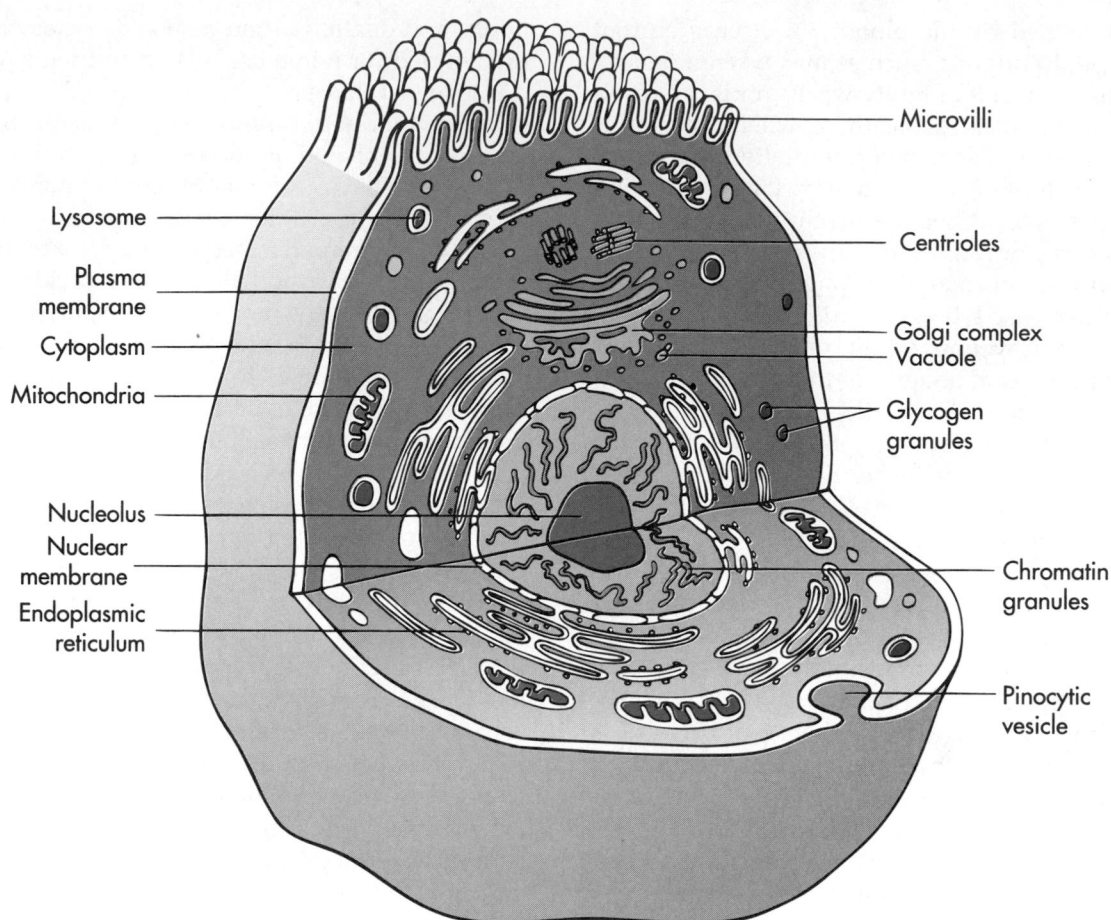

**Figure 7-4**    Structures of a typical body cell.

combined to form the major compounds: water, carbohydrates, proteins, lipids, and nucleic acids. Protoplasm minus nuclear material is called *cytoplasm.*

The specific internal structures of the cell are called *organelles* (Box 7-1). The number and types of organelles vary according to the type and specific function of each cell. For example, muscle cells have numerous mitochondria to provide energy for muscle contraction. Gland cells have large amounts of endoplasmic reticulum and Golgi complex to provide for secretion, and white blood cells (WBCs) have large numbers of lysosomes to destroy bacteria that invade the body.

Cells can be damaged in many ways. A lack of nutrients or oxygen may injure the cell membrane or other cell structures or cause cell death. An imbalance in the composition of the fluids surrounding the cells also can create cellular damage, and drugs or toxins can alter the functioning of the cell membrane (see Chapter 28). Tumors are caused by cells that have been altered in some way (see Chapter 12).

Defects in genes that carry inherited traits can result in abnormal metabolism that may or may not be compatible with life. Hereditary disorders such as phenyl-

ketonuria, hemophilia, and some neuromuscular disorders are examples of such disorders. Traits for these conditions are carried in the genes and passed from parents to offspring. Congenital defects also may be caused by environmental agents such as maternal disease and drugs. Many congenital defects are believed to occur during the first few weeks of embryonic life, even before the mother realizes she is pregnant. For example, if a mother contracts German measles during the first trimester, the baby may have a congenital defect. The evidence is increasing that other infectious diseases, including mumps, infectious hepatitis, and influenza, may play some part in spontaneous abortion, premature birth, stillbirth, and birth defects.

Congenital birth defects can affect any organ or system of the body, and several defects involving different organs or systems can occur in the same child. In recent years certain drugs have been shown to cause changes in fetal development. An excessive intake of caffeine during pregnancy has been associated with increased fetal loss. Alcohol ingestion and smoking also adversely affect fetal development (Clark, Queener, Karb, 1997).

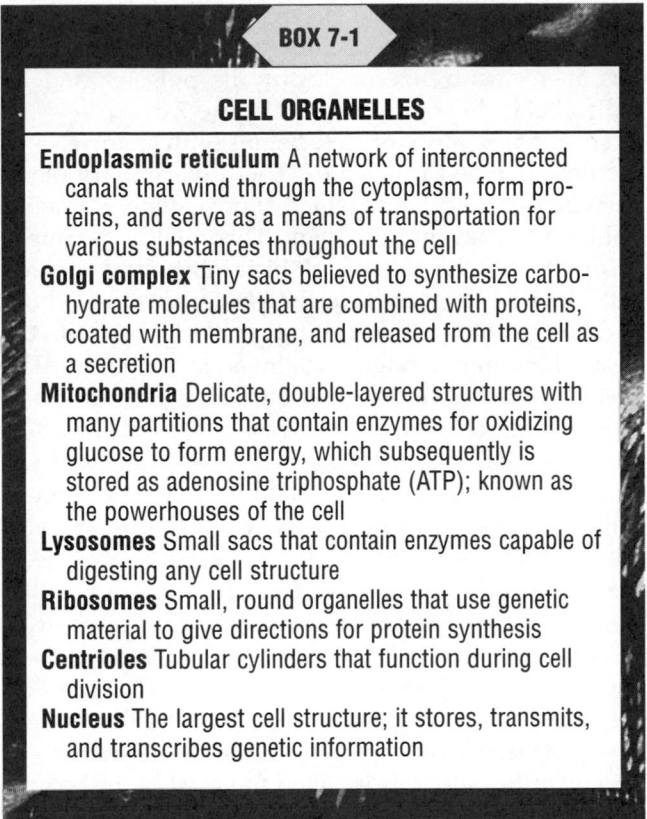

### CELL ORGANELLES

**Endoplasmic reticulum** A network of interconnected canals that wind through the cytoplasm, form proteins, and serve as a means of transportation for various substances throughout the cell

**Golgi complex** Tiny sacs believed to synthesize carbohydrate molecules that are combined with proteins, coated with membrane, and released from the cell as a secretion

**Mitochondria** Delicate, double-layered structures with many partitions that contain enzymes for oxidizing glucose to form energy, which subsequently is stored as adenosine triphosphate (ATP); known as the powerhouses of the cell

**Lysosomes** Small sacs that contain enzymes capable of digesting any cell structure

**Ribosomes** Small, round organelles that use genetic material to give directions for protein synthesis

**Centrioles** Tubular cylinders that function during cell division

**Nucleus** The largest cell structure; it stores, transmits, and transcribes genetic information

## PHYSIOLOGIC DEFENSE MECHANISMS

Nature has provided the body with various physiologic defense mechanisms that limit the ability of microorganisms and other substances to invade the body and cause disease. The first line of defense is the unbroken skin and the mucous membranes, which serve as mechanical barriers against invaders. Perspiration, the excretion of the sudoriferous (sweat) glands, has an average acid content of 5.65% on the skin, which is lethal to many bacteria. Lysozyme, an antibacterial enzyme present on the skin, dissolves some bacteria and is present in saliva and tears.

The mucous membranes lining the respiratory, GI, and urinary tracts secrete substances that are **bacteriostatic,** or able to inhibit the growth of bacteria. Lacrimal fluid (tears) can destroy some microorganisms, and it continuously bathes the eye, washing out foreign materials, including pathogens. The stomach's high acid content acts as a formidable barrier for swallowed pathogens. Any pathogens that enter the intestines may be destroyed by certain enzymes secreted by cells along the intestinal route. Vaginal secretions normally are acidic, and pathogens that enter the vagina usually are destroyed. Frequent vaginal irrigation, or douching, can reduce the pH (acid) concentra-

tion of the vagina, thereby diminishing the effectiveness of the natural barrier.

The nasal cavities, trachea, and bronchi contain fine, hairlike projections called *cilia,* which are in constant, wavelike motion. The cilia sweep pathogens toward the pharynx, where they may be swallowed or expectorated. If swallowed, they are destroyed by the stomach acids. The fine hairs around the external nares help prevent pathogens from entering; if they do get in, they are trapped by cavities.

The mouth has a high concentration of microorganisms. Many are swallowed and destroyed. Pathogens in the mouth usually do no harm as long as the mucous membrane remains intact. Involuntary acts also help the body rid itself of pathogens. Through acts or reflexes such as sneezing and coughing, pathogens may be eliminated from the respiratory tract. Vomiting and diarrhea eliminate bacteria and their toxins from the GI system.

Some cells constantly combat infectious agents and other substances that enter the body. Cells that line many of the vascular and lymph channels are capable of phagocytizing bacteria, viruses, and other foreign material. Lymph nodes are located intermittently along the course of the lymphatic vessels that drain the excess interstitial fluid surrounding the cells. These lymph nodes contain many cells that phagocytize foreign materials and prevent their general dissemination throughout the body. The spleen filters blood and removes not only old red blood cells from the circulation but also abnormal platelets, blood parasites, bacteria, and other substances. Kupffer's cells in the liver remove large numbers of bacteria that succeed in entering the body through the GI tract. The bone marrow has the ability to remove fine particles, such as protein toxins, from the bloodstream. Phagocytic cells in the tissues throughout the body also protect various organs against invading organisms or foreign material (Guyton, 1996).

The white blood cells **(leukocytes)** also combat invasion. Most of these cells are *polymorphonuclear leukocytes,* or granulocytes. The three types of polymorphonuclear leukocytes are the *neutrophils,* the *basophils,* and the *eosinophils.* The primary function of the neutrophils is phagocytosis, or ingestion and digestion of debris and foreign material throughout the body. Neutrophils are the first cells to arrive at the scene when an inflammatory reaction is stimulated. Basophils do not phagocytize, but they contain powerful chemicals, such as histamine, that can be released locally and assist in the inflammatory process. Eosinophils appear to play a role in allergic and foreign protein reactions. The mononuclear leukocytes, or monocytes, become large, phagocytic cells when stimulated and play an important role in inflammation. Lymphocytes are the cells primarily concerned with the development of immunity (Guyton, 1996).

## Inflammation

One of the more important defense mechanisms is the inflammatory response. **Inflammation** occurs when any agent (e.g., chemical substance, foreign body, severe blow, or bacteria) injures the tissue. The inflammatory process is characterized by five classic signs: redness (rubor), heat (calor), swelling (tumor), pain (dolor), and limitation of movement (Box 7-2). When

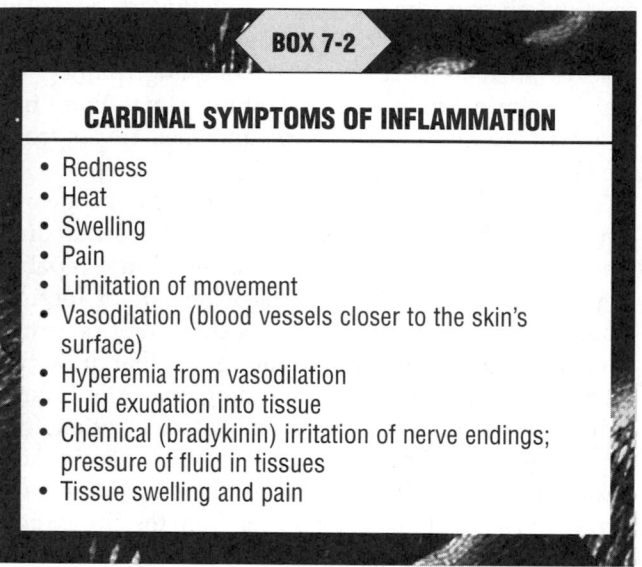

**BOX 7-2**

### CARDINAL SYMPTOMS OF INFLAMMATION

- Redness
- Heat
- Swelling
- Pain
- Limitation of movement
- Vasodilation (blood vessels closer to the skin's surface)
- Hyperemia from vasodilation
- Fluid exudation into tissue
- Chemical (bradykinin) irritation of nerve endings; pressure of fluid in tissues
- Tissue swelling and pain

tissue is traumatized, a defensive process begins in which the body tries to localize or eliminate the injurious agent, neutralize or destroy its poisons, and, finally, repair the injured tissue (Figure 7-5).

The inflammatory process begins with an increase in the flow of blood to the area. The tiny capillary blood vessels become dilated, which allows a larger amount of blood to pass through them. This dilation is caused primarily by the release of histamine from injured cells. The leukocytes have the power to move about and begin to migrate out of the capillaries and into the area where the pathogen has invaded the tissue. The first cells to arrive at the scene are the neutrophils, which begin to engulf and ingest any bacteria or foreign material. After several hours the monocytes follow; these cells are transformed into large, phagocytic cells called *macrophages.* It is believed that monocytes are stimulated by substances draining from the site. If the injurious agent is not removed from the site within 24 to 48 hours, lymphocytes begin to predominate at the site and the immune process is stimulated.

During the inflammatory process, some phagocytes are killed and some tissue is destroyed. The phagocytes, the destroyed cells, and some tissue fluid accumulate at the site; this is called the *exudate.* If the area has been invaded by microbes, or pathogens, an infection can occur and purulent drainage (pus) may be present. The characteristic heat and redness at the site are caused by the increased flow of blood to the area. Swelling results from the accumulation of exudate, and stimulation of the nerves in the area causes the

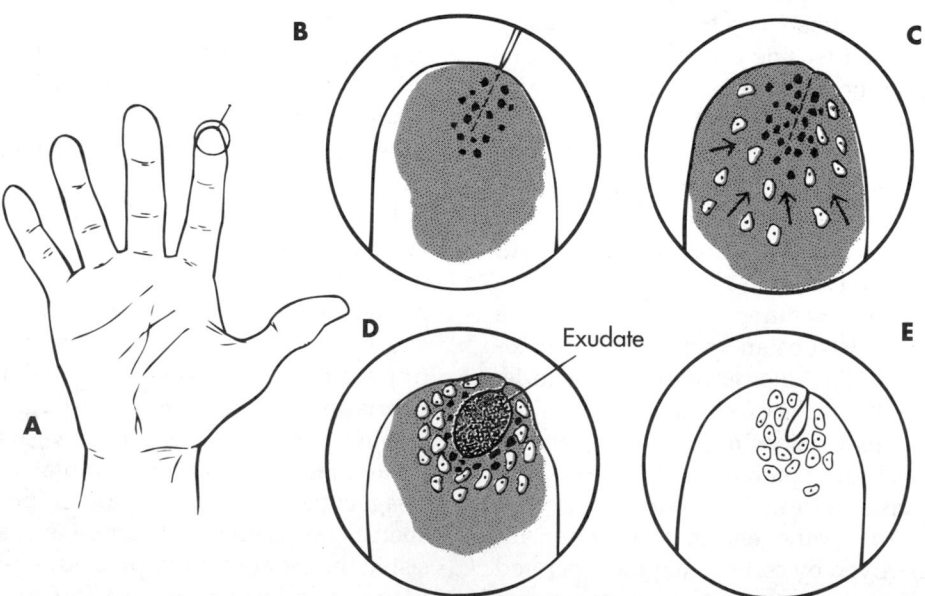

**Figure 7-5**  Inflammatory process. **A,** Pinprick introduces pathogenic bacteria into tissue. **B,** Blood supply to area increases. **C,** Leukocytes move out of blood capillaries. **D,** Phagocytes engulf and digest bacteria; dead phagocytes, cells, and tissue fluid escape as exudate. **E,** When phagocytosis is complete, wound begins to heal.

pain. Depending on the location, any effort to move the part may be painful, which may cause the individual to limit movement. When phagocytosis is complete, the inflammatory condition subsides and healing begins (see Figure 7-5).

Healing is the replacement of dead or damaged cells. Two overlapping stages occur in the process of healing: (1) the regeneration of lost cells with identical or similar tissue and (2) the formation of scar tissue. The body's ability to regenerate new tissue depends on the cells' ability to multiply and form units that can function physiologically like the original cell. Damaged brain, myocardium, and nerve tissue cannot regenerate. Scar tissue is formed by the proliferation of fibroblasts, which secrete collagen precursors. This preliminary stage is called *granulation* tissue. Collagen is a fibrous protein that is present in the connective tissues of the body. Layers of collagen are deposited at the site of injury, forming a dense area of scar tissue.

Wounds are repaired through a similar process. The three types of wound healing have been labeled primary, secondary, and tertiary intention. Healing by primary intention means that a wound heals with its edges close together or in close approximation and with a minimum of granulation tissue (Figure 7-6, *A*). Surgical wounds heal this way. Healing by secondary intention occurs when a greater amount of tissue is damaged and necrotic debris or inflammatory exudate is formed (Figure 7-6, *B*). These wounds take longer to heal and produce more scar tissue. Tertiary intention sometimes is called *delayed primary closure*. A wound that is closed surgically several days after the injury heals by tertiary intention. For example, a heavily contaminated wound may be left open intentionally to drain, after which it is closed.

## Infection

Pathogenic organisms may enter the body through the respiratory, digestive, reproductive, and urinary systems and through the skin. These organisms may leave the body through vomitus, feces, urine, draining wounds, drainage tubes, or discharge from the nose and throat. Pathogens also may enter via the urethral meatus in men or the vaginal canal in women. Certain pathogenic organisms, such as those causing malaria and hepatitis B, may be transferred through a blood transfusion. Infection with the human immunodefi-

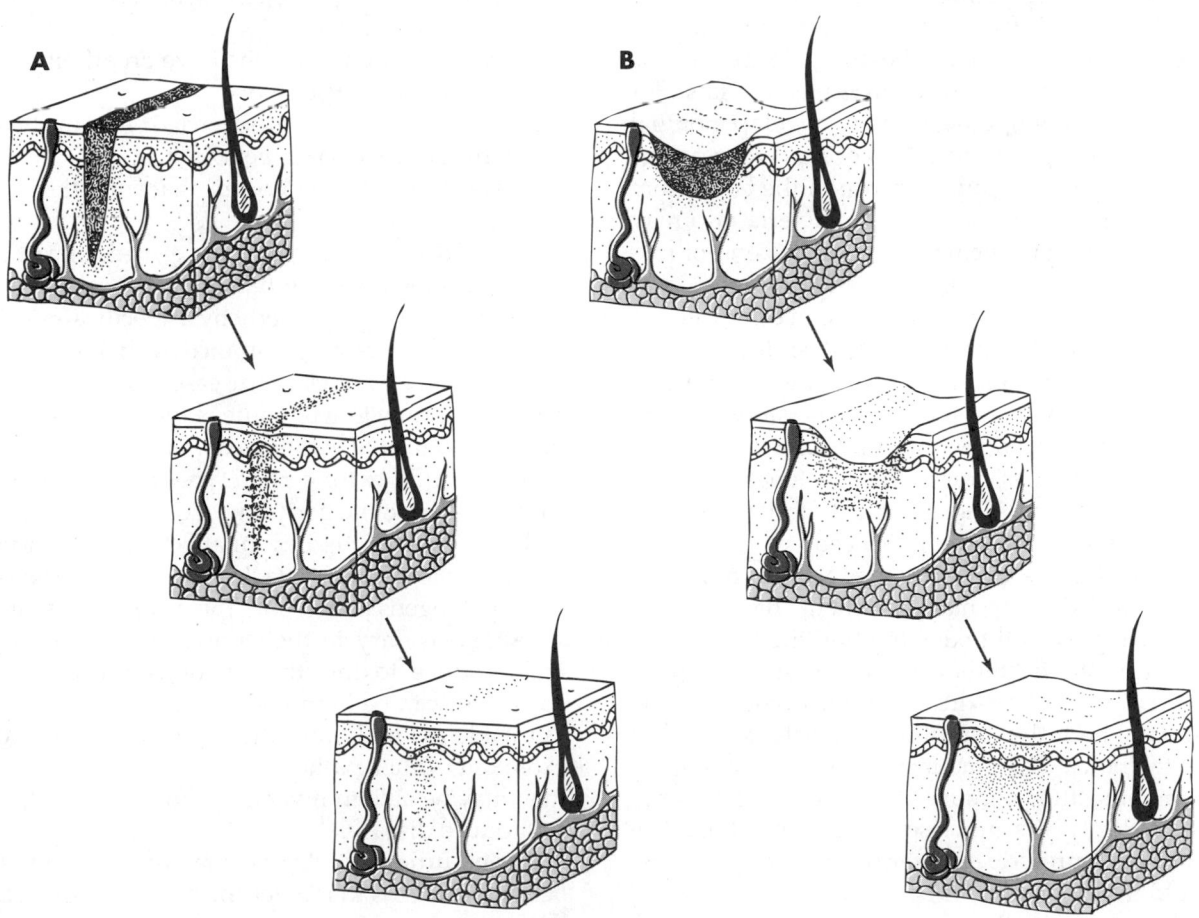

**Figure 7-6**    Types of wound healing. **A,** Primary. **B,** Secondary.

---

**TABLE 7-3**

## Classification of Infection

| CLASSIFICATION | DESCRIPTION |
| --- | --- |
| Primary infection | An acute infection that appears, runs its course, and resolves within a short time |
| Chronic infection | An infection in which the initial stages are the same as those for a primary infection, but in which symptoms persist and have a prolonged course |
| Secondary infection | Usually a complication of a primary infection; the bacteria that cause a secondary infection may not always be the same as those that caused the primary infection |
| Local infection | An infection confined to a single area |
| Generalized infection | An infection that spreads and involves the entire body |
| Focal infection | An infection in which bacteria have spread from the original site to other parts of the body |
| Latent infection | A condition in which bacteria are present in the body but are not active and do not cause symptoms |
| Specific infection | An infection caused by one type of microorganism |
| Mixed infection | An infection caused by more than one type of microorganism |

---

ciency virus (HIV) is transmitted by blood and some body fluids. Placental transfer of microorganisms to the fetus from the mother can occur in some cases, such as with syphilis. Individuals may enter a health care facility free of infection but may develop one during their stay; this is referred to as a **nosocomial infection**. An example of a nosocomial infection is oxacillin-resistant staphylococcal infection (see Chapter 15).

An endogenous infection can occur when microorganisms already present in the body cause disease as a result of compromised defense mechanisms. For example, patients with diabetes may develop monilial infections. An exogenous infection occurs when pathogenic microorganisms gain entrance to the body from the outside, such as in hepatitis B. Bacteria also may harm the body by producing powerful poisons, or toxins. These toxins are classified as **endotoxins** or **exotoxins**. Endotoxins are present in the cell walls of gram-negative rods and cocci. Most endotoxins are contained in organisms that cause enteric diseases, such as typhoid fever and bacillary dysentery. Exotoxins are produced by bacteria and released outside the cell. They are the most poisonous substances that can injure human beings. Cholera and botulism are diseases in which exotoxins are produced.

Some bacteria are powerful enough to resist the leukocytes and destroy many of them. Bacteria also may produce powerful toxins that kill the leukocytes. If this occurs, the bacteria causes disease, and either the bacteria or their toxins may be carried by the bloodstream and the lymphatic vessels to various parts of the body. The time factor is extremely important in an infection because the longer the bacteria have to multiply, the more severe the infection. The physician may prescribe bacteriostatic drugs to prevent rapid multiplication of bacteria.

Infection is classified in a number of different ways according to its location, extent, and severity (Table 7-3). When pathogenic microorganisms invade the body and cause inflammation or infection, they can cause different signs and symptoms, depending on the location of the infection (Table 7-4).

The following five factors influence the ability of invading pathogens to survive and cause disease (pathogenicity):

1. Whether the pathogens gain entrance by their characteristic route
2. Whether the pathogens have an affinity for only certain types of tissue
3. The ability of the pathogens to enter the body and produce toxins (virulence)
4. The number of pathogens that enter the body at a given time
5. The degree and character of resistance the host offers the invading pathogens

Most bacteria enter the body by a specific route. Unless they succeed in gaining entrance by their characteristic route, they may not cause disease. For example, bacteria whose characteristic route is the respiratory system may be harmless if swallowed. Some pathogens have a particular affinity for certain types of tissue. Once they gain entrance to the body, they go directly to that tissue and leave other tissues unaffected. The virus that causes poliomyelitis attacks only nerve tissue, and other pathogens attack only the respiratory system.

Pathogens vary in their power to invade the body and produce toxins; this factor is called **virulence.** Pathogens can be highly virulent, having great power to invade the body and the ability to produce deadly exotoxins. Other pathogens may be of low virulence; they may be able to invade the body but are too weak to produce disease.

The occurrence of disease may depend on the number of pathogens that enter the body at a given time. If a large number of pathogens enter the body, disease is more likely to occur than if only a few invade the host.

**TABLE 7-4**

## Signs of Infection

| SIGN | DESCRIPTION |
| --- | --- |
| Abscess | A walled-off area surrounded by inflamed tissue with a central, pus-filled cavity |
| Bacteremia | The presence of bacteria in the bloodstream |
| Carbuncle | An area of inflammation in the skin and deeper tissues that terminates with pus formation; constitutional symptoms sometimes accompany it |
| Cellulitis | A diffuse, poorly defined inflammatory process that usually involves the skin and subcutaneous tissues |
| Exudate | An accumulation of fluid within a cavity or area of inflammation that may contain cells, protein, and solid material |
| Furuncle | A boil or an inflamed, pus-filled swelling on the skin |
| Gangrene | Tissue death caused by poor arterial or venous circulation |
| Granulation | Budding projections formed on the surface of a wound that bring a rich blood supply to tissue |
| Necrosis | The death of tissue or small groups of cells |
| Purulent discharge | A discharge that contains pus |
| Pyemia | A condition in which purulent discharge in the bloodstream causes multiple abscesses to form in various parts of the body |
| Sanguineous discharge | A discharge that contains blood |
| Septicemia | The presence of pathogens or their toxins in the bloodstream |
| Serous discharge | A clear, watery, thin discharge |

However, invasion by a few highly virulent pathogens may result in disease, whereas a large number of pathogens of low virulence may be destroyed without having caused disease.

## Intervention

An inflammation can occur without infection, as is the case with sunburn. Infection, however, usually is accompanied by inflammation. Intervention depends on the type of injury, the extent of involvement, and the effectiveness of the body's defense mechanisms. An infection may be local (e.g., a boil); it may involve an entire body system (e.g., the respiratory system); or, if the infection is a bloodstream infection, it may affect the entire body (Box 7-3).

Local inflammatory conditions can be painful and can cause considerable discomfort. The goals of patient care are to relieve discomfort and to terminate the inflammatory condition before it can affect other parts of the body. To achieve these goals, it is necessary to monitor the injured or inflamed site, perform interventions that aid in the healing process and ensure adequate blood flow, and provide for adequate rest and nutrients. Treatment includes rest, elevation of the affected part, application of heat or cold, use of analgesics, and, occasionally, incision and drainage (I & D). Antibiotic therapy is required when an infection is present. Elevating the affected part above the level of the heart relieves pain and throbbing, which makes the patient more comfortable.

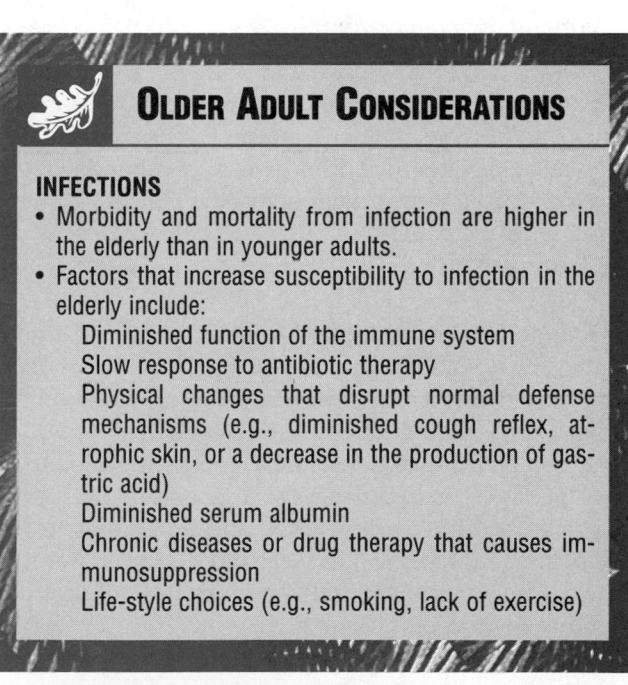

**OLDER ADULT CONSIDERATIONS**

**INFECTIONS**
- Morbidity and mortality from infection are higher in the elderly than in younger adults.
- Factors that increase susceptibility to infection in the elderly include:
    Diminished function of the immune system
    Slow response to antibiotic therapy
    Physical changes that disrupt normal defense mechanisms (e.g., diminished cough reflex, atrophic skin, or a decrease in the production of gastric acid)
    Diminished serum albumin
    Chronic diseases or drug therapy that causes immunosuppression
    Life-style choices (e.g., smoking, lack of exercise)

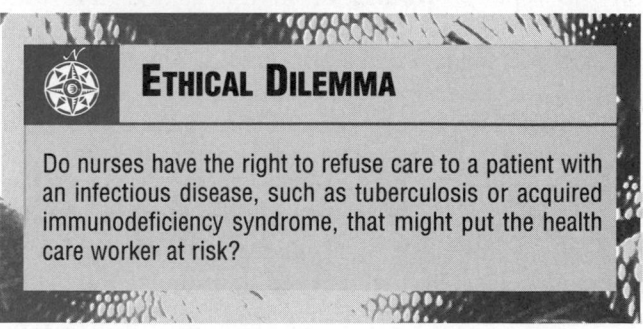

**ETHICAL DILEMMA**

Do nurses have the right to refuse care to a patient with an infectious disease, such as tuberculosis or acquired immunodeficiency syndrome, that might put the health care worker at risk?

---

BOX 7-3

## NURSING PROCESS

## RISK FOR INFECTION

### ASSESSMENT

- Vital signs q 4 hr
- Risk factors (e.g., inadequate bodily defenses, invasive devices or procedures, chronic disease)
- Laboratory values: whole blood cell count, culture, sensitivities
- Signs and symptoms of infection
- Respiratory status: adventitious sounds, sputum
- Urinary symptoms: urine color and consistency, burning with urination
- IV sites
- Wounds, skin condition (if applicable)
- Nutritional status
- Immunization status
- Recent exposure to individuals with acute infections
- Immunosuppression

### NURSING DIAGNOSIS

- Risk for infection

### NURSING INTERVENTIONS

- Wash hands carefully before and after contact.
- Maintain strict asepsis with required nursing care (e.g., IV therapy, Foley catheter care, suctioning).
- Change equipment, tubing, and solutions used for nursing care according to hospital policy.

- Maintain asepsis with invasive procedures.
- Screen visitors and staff for colds, nausea, vomiting, and fever.
- Keep patient in private room or protective isolation if required.
- Remove and prohibit fresh flowers, fresh vegetables, or water-filled vases if required.
- Keep skin clean, dry, and well lubricated with daily bathing.
- Encourage a high-protein, high-calorie diet if not contraindicated.
- Encourage liberal fluid intake if not contraindicated.
- Teach or provide perineal care.
- Teach or provide oral hygiene.
- Help patient to turn, cough, and deep breathe q 2 hr.
- Ambulate, if tolerated.
- Perform range-of-motion exercises if mobility is limited.
- Administer antimicrobials as ordered.

### EVALUATION OF EXPECTED OUTCOMES

- Absence of signs and symptoms of infection
- Patient and family demonstrate preventive measures

---

Heat and cold are applied to the body to aid in the healing process. Heat and cold cause different physiologic responses. The initial response to local application of heat is vasodilation of skin blood vessels, which increases blood flow to the area. Increasing the blood flow helps reduce pain and swelling and increases the movement of nutrients, WBCs, and antibiotics to the site. Application of cold reduces blood flow to the site, which prevents additional swelling and reduces inflammation and pain.

Whether dry or moist heat or cold is used depends on the type of wound or injury, its location, and whether drainage or inflammation is present. Compresses and packs can be hot or cold. A compress is a moist, gauze dressing that is applied to a specific area. If the skin is broken, a sterile technique is used. For a hot, moist compress the gauze is soaked in a solution with a temperature of 43° to 46° C (110° to 115° F). For a cold, moist compress the temperature is 15° C (59° F). Moist heat may also be applied with soaks or baths. For example, a sitz bath is used to immerse the pelvic

area in warm water. Soaks aid in the debridement, or cleaning, of wounds and are useful for applying medicated solutions.

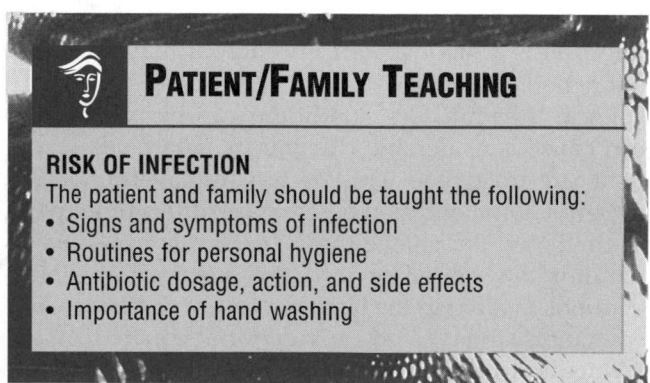

### PATIENT/FAMILY TEACHING

#### RISK OF INFECTION

The patient and family should be taught the following:
- Signs and symptoms of infection
- Routines for personal hygiene
- Antibiotic dosage, action, and side effects
- Importance of hand washing

Dry heat can be applied with an aquathermia pack, a hot water bottle, a heating pad, a heat lamp, or a paraffin bath. Aquathermia packs contain distilled water that circulates through tubes. The desired temperature is preset and is regulated by a temperature control unit. Hot water bottles rarely are used with hospitalized patients because they can injure the skin. Patients who use one at home should be instructed to fill it with warm tap water at a temperature of 43° to 46° C (110° to 115° F), cover it with a towel or pillow case, and apply it for 20 to 30 minutes. Before applying any type of heat, the nurse should consult the appropriate procedure manual and assess the patient's physical and mental status regarding his or her ability to tolerate heat. Because of the danger of burning the patient, the nurse should frequently assess the area receiving the heat treatment.

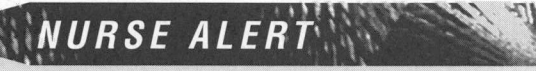

> **NURSE ALERT**
>
> When applying heat, assess the area often.

Moist cold is applied in the form of cold compresses, usually for short intervals and at specified periods. Dry cold is provided by an ice bag or ice collar. Because of the danger of injury to the tissues, an uncovered ice bag should never be applied directly to the skin and should not be used to cover wet dressings.

When local inflammation does not respond to treatment, a surgical incision may be required to allow the accumulated exudate to escape; this may be referred to as an I & D. Patients with generalized infections may be very ill, and they may have an extremely high temperature and a corresponding increase in the pulse and respiratory rates. The WBC count is elevated *(leukocytosis)*, and chills, loss of appetite, sweating, and delirium may occur. The patient usually is confined to bed.

Acetaminophen (Tylenol) or acetylsalicylic acid (aspirin) may be given to adults to lower their temperature. Aspirin is not recommended for children. In some cases a cooling blanket may be applied. A tepid or cool sponge bath may be given to remove waste products from the skin and provide comfort. Special mouth care should be given several times a day or as indicated. An emollient jelly may be used to lubricate the lips and nose to prevent dryness and crust formation. Accurate measurement of fluid intake and fluid loss from all sources is an important nursing intervention. Because the patient is losing greater amounts of fluid through the skin and respiratory system, adequate fluid intake should be encouraged. It is important that the patient continue to produce large amounts of urine to help eliminate toxins. Oral fluids should be high in nutrients, calories, and electrolytes. If sufficient fluids are not ingested, the physician may prescribe intravenous (IV) fluids. Weighing the patient

periodically yields information about loss of weight and body fluids. During the febrile period the diet should be liquid, followed by soft, easily digested foods and a gradual return to a general diet.

> **NURSE ALERT**
>
> Recording the fluid intake and output accurately is essential for patients with generalized infections.

Back rubs, a quiet, well-ventilated room, and freedom from annoying disturbances add to the patient's comfort. The nurse should ensure that patients who are young children, elderly, or delirious are protected from injury. Because most patients generally feel ill, the number of visitors should be kept to a minimum. The nurse should be careful to maintain medical asepsis, paying special attention to hand washing (see Chapter 15).

## Immunity

Immunology comprises the mechanisms by which the body's cellular and chemical systems recognize and react to foreign substances. This dynamic process occurs throughout life to counteract the effects of foreign materials, bacteria, viruses, foods, and chemicals that constantly enter the body. A person with an immune system that is functioning normally is immunocompetent.

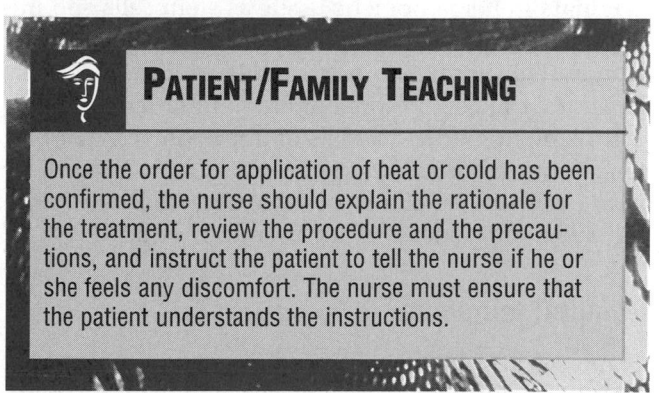

> **PATIENT/FAMILY TEACHING**
>
> Once the order for application of heat or cold has been confirmed, the nurse should explain the rationale for the treatment, review the procedure and the precautions, and instruct the patient to tell the nurse if he or she feels any discomfort. The nurse must ensure that the patient understands the instructions.

**Immunity** can be natural or acquired. Natural immunity is present at birth and depends on species, race, and heritage. For example, humans do not suffer from foot and mouth disease, which is found in cattle.

Acquired immunity is gained actively or passively by the individual. To develop active immunity, a person must contract the disease or be infected with an attenuated form of the disease-producing organism. This process does not provide immediate protection against the organism because the body requires time to develop a sufficient response. Passive immunity is gained from another source. A newborn acquires passive immunity from the mother through the placenta and breast milk. Others gain passive immunity by receiving disease-specific antiserum or pooled gamma-globulin that contains antibodies to a number of diseases. This is a temporary type of immunity and is used to protect an individual from disease immediately after exposure.

Any invading agent that can elicit an immune response is called an *antigen*. Antigens usually are large proteins or large polysaccharides, and many bacteria contain these substances. Some substances have a low molecular weight and cannot elicit a response by themselves. However, they do have antigenic sites and can combine with carrier substances. If these substances react with another material, they can stimulate an immune response. These substances, called *haptens*, include some drugs, chemicals in dust, and breakdown products from animal dander.

The immune system is comprised of specialized cells, central lymphoid tissue (bone marrow and thymus), and peripheral lymphoid tissue (lymph nodes, tonsils, spleen, and intestinal lymphoid tissue such as Peyer's patches and the appendix). The cells involved in the development of immunity are the lymphocytes and the macrophages. The lymphocytes are divided into two categories: (1) the B lymphocytes, which are responsible for antibody formation, or humoral immunity, and (2) the T lymphocytes, which are responsible for cellular, or **cell-mediated immunity**. Lymphocytes originate in hematopoietic tissue as stem cells and migrate to lymphoid tissue for maturation and expression of their immune functions (Figure 7-7).

Another major component of the immune system is complement, which consists of approximately 20 proteins found in normal human serum. The term *complement* refers to the ability of these proteins to enhance the other components of the immune system.

## Humoral Immunity

**Humoral immunity** results when an invading agent stimulates dormant B lymphocytes in the lymph nodes to produce **antibodies**. Antibodies are proteins that are developed to react with a specific *antigen*. The invading agent also stimulates the B lymphocytes to produce new lymphocytes that will continue to manufacture antibodies in the future. Therefore, immunity to the agent may continue over long periods. The antibodies are called **immunoglobulins (Ig)**, and they can react only with the antigen that first stimulated the B cell. Immunoglobulins are divided into five classes—

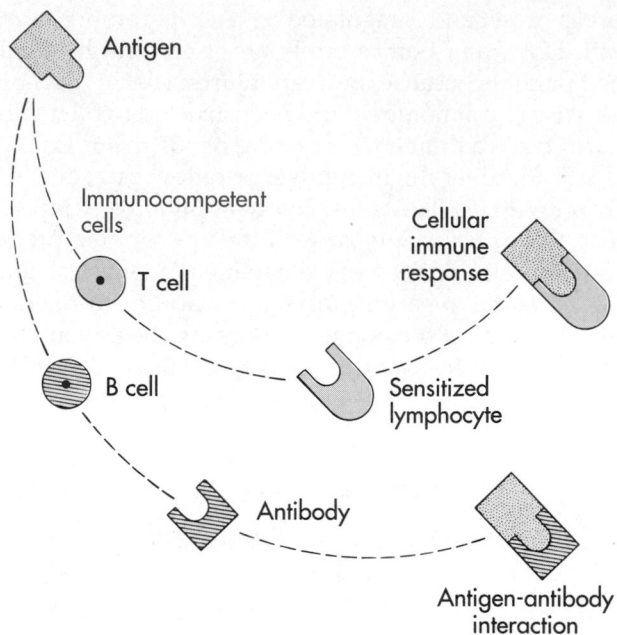

**Figure 7-7** Humoral (B-cell) immunity results in antibody formation. Cellular (T-cell) immunity results in production of a sensitized lymphocyte.

| TABLE 7-5 |
|-----------|

### Classes of Immunoglobulins

| NAME | CHARACTERISTICS |
|------|-----------------|
| IgG | Present in serum and amniotic fluid; activates complement; protects newborns |
| IgA | Present in serum, tears, saliva, gastrointestinal (GI) tract, secretions, colostrum; protects mucous membranes |
| IgM | Present in serum; activates complement; forms antibodies for ABO blood antigens |
| IgD | Present in serum and umbilical cord; action unknown |
| IgE | Present in serum and tissues; functions in allergic and hypersensitivity reactions |

IgA, IgG, IgD, IgM, and IgE—and each has its specific characteristics and functions. The IgE antibody, called the reaginic antibody, is primarily responsible for allergic reactions (Table 7-5).

The antigen-antibody reaction destroys or inactivates the invading agent through several processes. It can neutralize an antigen and diminish its toxic qualities; it can cause the agent to become insoluble in a solution or precipitate; it can cause agglutination, or clumping, of antigens; it can lyse cell membranes; or it can render the antigen susceptible to phagocytosis. Some antigen-antibody reactions can stimulate the activity of nine different enzymes that normally are inactive in plasma and body fluids; this is the complement system, which helps destroy and inactivate invading organisms.

## Cellular Immunity

The immune response referred to as *cell-mediated,* or *cellular,* is based on the function of T lymphocytes. The three major groups of T cells are the *helper, suppressor,* and *killer* cells. The helper T cells enhance the function of the B cells. The suppressor cells inhibit the activities of other lymphocytes and provide feedback to the system. The killer cells destroy targeted enemy cells by binding directly to their surface. Cellular immunity results when T cells are activated by an antigen. Whole cells become sensitized in a process similar to that which stimulates the B cells to form antibodies. Once sensitized, these T cells are released into the blood and body tissues, where they remain indefinitely.

The cellular type of immunity is stimulated by fungi, viruses, parasites, and some bacteria that live inside other cells. Tuberculosis stimulates cellular immunity. It is believed that an interaction occurs between humoral immune processes and cellular immune processes in which the helper T cells are used as a switch between the two processes.

No absolute immunity exists to any specific disease to which human beings are susceptible. The degree of resistance to a certain disease or agent may vary from person to person, and at different times in the same person.

# EXCESSIVE IMMUNE RESPONSES

## Allergy

The condition now known as **hypersensitivity,** or an *allergy,* first was observed in 1832 but was not seriously studied until 1890. Koch was the first to observe and describe the allergic reaction after he administered the tuberculosis test for a diagnosis of tuberculosis. The term *allergy* was not used until 1906, when von Pirquet used it to describe the changes associated with repeated contact with various antigenic substances. Since that time the term *allergy* has been accepted to designate hypersensitivity in certain individuals.

The terms *allergy* and *hypersensitivity* are used interchangeably. An allergy is an inappropriate and excessive response of the immune system to certain substances that are not harmful to most people. When an individual contacts the offending substance (antigen), the body is immediately stimulated to produce either antibodies or sensitized WBCs (T lymphocytes) to defend itself against the offending antigen. When the same antigen is contacted again, the antibodies or sensitized cells react with it and destroy or neutralize it, resulting in a group of symptoms referred to as manifestations of an allergy.

In some families, predisposition to an allergy is transmitted genetically. If a parent has an allergic disorder, the children may develop an allergic condition at some point in their life, but it may not necessarily be the same as the parent's allergy. The homeostasis of the body plays an important role when an individual has an inherited predisposition to allergy. Any episode that disturbs the homeostatic balance, such as a severe infection, a pregnancy, or an endocrine dysfunction, can cause or exacerbate an allergy.

An **allergen** can be transmitted directly from the mother to the fetus in utero by the placental blood supply. When an infant has been sensitized in utero to a specific allergen, contact with the allergen after birth may cause an allergic reaction.

Allergens can be classified as inhalants, ingestants, injectants, contactants, or infectants. The most common inhalants are pollens from grasses, weeds, trees, and grains, as well as dust. An allergy caused by inhaling pollens usually is seasonal and occurs when flowering and pollination occur. The most common type of allergy caused by pollens is hay fever. Ingestants usually are foods to which the individual may be hypersensitive. The most common offenders are the proteins of cow's milk, egg whites, chocolate, strawberries, shellfish, and nuts. Among the injectants are drugs such as antibiotics. Also, horse serum, which may be used in making antitoxins, can cause severe reactions. The venom from a snake bite or stings from some insects can cause a reaction in a hypersensitive person. Some individuals may be sensitive to contactants such as laundry powders, cosmetic preparations, nickel compounds used in costume jewelry, rubber compounds used in elastic, and the sap from plants such as poison ivy or poison oak (Figure 7-8). Factors related to infectants have been demonstrated in tuberculosis, typhoid fever, and anthrax.

Assessment for allergies includes an exposure history and recording of signs, symptoms, and other relevant information. A thorough physical examination is done, including a complete blood count (CBC) and differential count. Eosinophils are white blood cells that normally make up 1% to 3% of all leukocytes. During an allergic reaction the number of circulating eosinophils often increases. Eosinophils collect at sites of antigen-antibody reactions, such as in the nasal secretions. Another diagnostic blood study is the radioallergosorbent test (RAST), which uses a sample of the patient's blood to test for reaginic (IgE) antibodies.

## Pathophysiology

Most allergies are caused by an antigen-antibody reaction that damages some of the body's tissues; this type of response is called an *immediate* reaction. The body

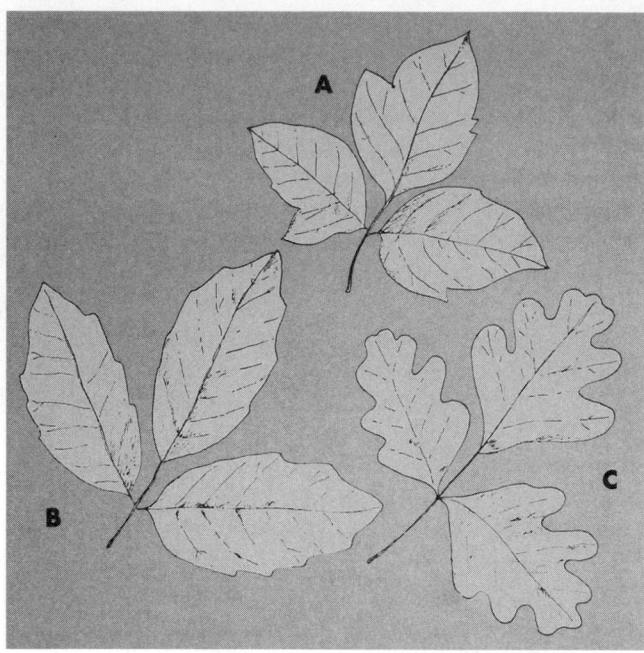

**Figure 7-8**   Plants and shrubs that commonly cause a severe skin reaction. **A,** Poison ivy. **B** and **C,** Types of poison oak. Note asymmetry in leaf formations.

| TABLE 7-6 | |
|---|---|
| **Hypersensitivity Reactions** | |
| **TYPE** | **REACTION** |
| Type I | Immediate reactions: IgE-mediated local or systemic anaphylaxis; atopic disorders |
| Type II | Cytotoxic reactions: IgG- and/or IgM-mediated destruction of cells; drug and transfusion reactions |
| Type III | Immune complex reactions: IgM- or IgG-mediated formation of antigen-antibody complexes; serum sickness; Arthus reactions |
| Type IV | Cell-mediated reactions: mediated by sensitized T cells; allergic contact dermatitis; delayed hypersensitivity reactions |

From Baere P, Myers J: *Principles and practice of adult health nursing*, ed 2, 1994, Mosby.

tissues commonly involved, called *target organs,* are the tissues that come in frequent contact with the external environment, such as the skin, mucous membranes, respiratory tract, and GI tract. A summary of hypersensitivity reactions is found in Table 7-6. Types I, II, and III reactions are related to humoral immunity and are the immediate result of interactions that involve circulating antibodies. Type IV reactions are delayed, are related to cell-mediated immunity, and are the direct result of interactions involving sensitized lymphocytes.

**Immediate hypersensitivity.** Individuals with a type I immediate hypersensitivity reaction must first come into contact with an allergen. The body may respond by forming specific antibodies that react with the allergen. Although this is essentially a normal mechanism, a hypersensitive individual produces an altered form of an antibody, called a *reaginic IgE antibody.* A nonallergic person would produce the IgG antibody. Subsequent contact with the allergen initiates an antigen-antibody reaction that damages tissues. Enzymes such as histamine and histamine-like substances are released from mast cells in the target organ to which the reaginic antibody and antigen have become attached. This process causes an increase in vascular permeability, constriction of smooth muscle, and increased secretion of mucus. A local inflammatory response is initiated.

The symptoms of this type of allergy depend on the chemicals and the lactation of the tissue in which the antigen-antibody reaction is occurring. If a sensitized

person inhales ragweed pollen, the antigen-antibody reaction occurs in the respiratory tract. Histamine causes vasodilation. Vessels become more permeable, allowing fluids to escape into the body tissues and cause edema. Constriction of the smooth muscle lining the airway and increased secretion of mucus all may lead to congestion, sneezing, coughing, and difficulty breathing (Figure 7-9).

Inhalants usually cause congestion of the nasal mucosa; sneezing; a thin, watery nasal discharge; red, itching conjunctivae; and increased lacrimation. Allergens that enter through the digestive tract may cause nausea, vomiting, and diarrhea. Various contact substances cause urticaria and dermatitis. Typical skin reactions, such as hives or wheals, are localized areas of swelling that are red, hot, and itchy. Hives also can develop in the GI tract, on the lining of the respiratory passageways, and along blood vessels. When histamine causes spasm and constriction of the bronchioles, bronchial asthma may occur.

Many local type I reactions are atopic or inherited. Usually the symptoms of atopic allergy are localized to the site of the antigen-antibody reaction. However, if large amounts of chemicals are released, they may enter the circulation and cause systemic effects. For example, drug allergies may cause a variety of reactions ranging from fever and skin rash to urticaria, anaphylactic shock, and death.

**Allergic reactions to insect bites or stings.** The bites or stings of various insects may cause local or systemic reactions. The local reaction at the site of the bite or sting is not considered an allergic reaction. However, the symptoms of systemic reactions are consistent with an allergy. Stings by bees, wasps, hornets, and yellow jackets may cause systemic reactions that vary from mild urticaria and itching to respiratory distress,

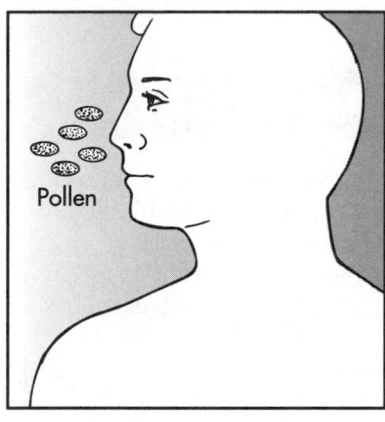

First exposure to pollen

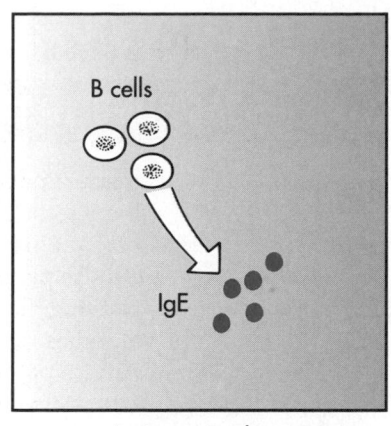

Antigen stimulates
B-lymphocyte to produce
IgE antibodies.

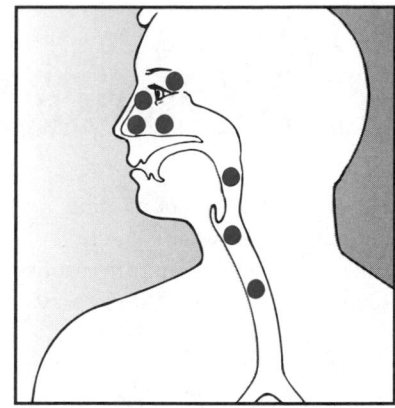

IgE lives on most cells
located in upper respiratory
tract, conjunctiva, and skin.

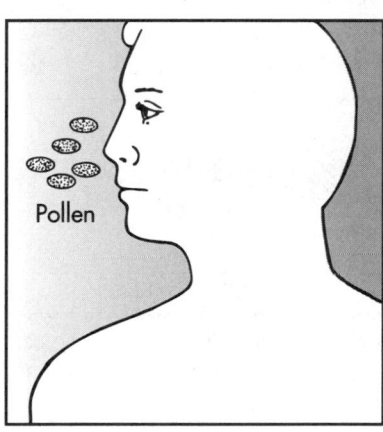

Second pollen exposure

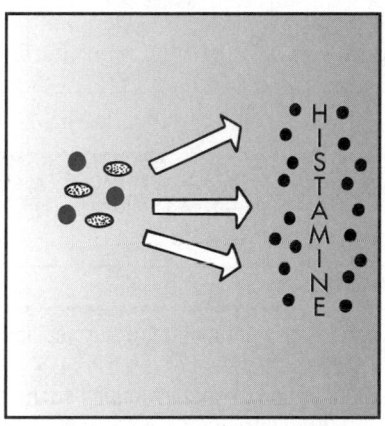

Antigen-antibody reaction occurs.
Histamine and other chemical
mediators are released.

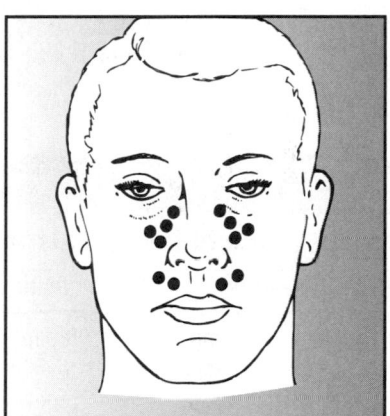

Symptoms of congestion,
sneezing, coughing, and difficulty
in breathing are exhibited.

**Figure 7-9**    Allergic response to ragweed pollen.

shock, loss of consciousness, and death. The antigen-antibody reaction may occur with all insects or with only a specific insect. The same process of antibody formation occurs as with other antigens. The first sting may cause no trouble, but a reaction may occur if the individual is stung again. The speed with which the reaction develops is in direct proportion to its severity. If a large number of stings occur at the same time, the reaction may be immediate and can be fatal as a result of the large amount of toxin injected. If the stinger is left in the skin, it should be scraped off. Squeezing should be avoided. The best treatment is prevention (Box 7-4). Patients with a known allergy to insect stings should carry an emergency medical information card or tag that explains the problem.

**Anaphylactic shock.** Anaphylactic shock is a systemic response to a type I hypersensitivity reaction. It follows exposure to a substance to which the individual is extremely sensitive. Anaphylactic shock is poten-

tially fatal and can appear within minutes in people who have been previously sensitized to the allergen. It is a sudden, severe, systemic reaction and is a true medical emergency. Although it is relatively rare, anaphylactic shock can occur after injection of vaccines, drugs, foreign sera, or allergenic extracts used in desensitization. Common causes of anaphylaxis are penicillin, bee or wasp venom, and substances containing iodine (which frequently are used as contrast media for x-ray examinations). Foods containing iodine often are implicated.

***Assessment.*** The initial symptoms of anaphylaxis are sneezing, apprehension, and edema and itching in the eyes and ears or at the site of injection. Edema of the face, hands, and other parts of the body can develop within seconds or minutes. Respiratory distress from bronchospasm, sneezing and coughing, wheezing, dyspnea, and cyanosis follow. Edema of the larynx and laryngospasm may lead to death. GI symptoms

---

> BOX 7-4

# NURSING PROCESS

## PREVENTING SEVERE REACTIONS TO INSECT STINGS

**ASSESSMENT**
- Local reaction at site of sting
- Evidence of systemic reaction
- History of severe allergic reaction
- Compliance with need to carry emergency kit

**NURSING DIAGNOSES**
- Knowledge deficit related to preventive measures
- Risk for injury related to severe allergic insect sting reaction

**NURSING INTERVENTIONS**
- Instruct patient to carry an emergency medical card or tag that identifies his or her condition.

- Instruct patient to carry an emergency kit containing injectable epinephrine (note expiration dates), oral antihistamines, and tourniquets.
- Advise patient to avoid perfumes, brightly colored clothing, flowers, and fields and to wear shoes at all times.
- Advise patient that he or she should always seek follow-up emergency treatment.

**EVALUATION OF EXPECTED OUTCOMES**
- Able to verbalize understanding of the need to avoid antigen in the future
- Demonstrates ability to initiate emergency treatment for anaphylactic shock

---

**TABLE 7-7**

## Emergency Care of Individuals in Anaphylactic Shock

| SIGNS AND SYMPTOMS | NURSING INTERVENTIONS | EXPECTED OUTCOMES |
|---|---|---|
| Rapid, shallow breathing; bronchospasms; dyspnea; cyanosis; restlessness; "sense of doom"; irritability; laryngeal edema | Prepare for oropharyngeal intubation or surgical insertion of tracheotomy; oxygen therapy per order. Prepare for administration of antihistamines such as diphenhydramine 25-50 mg intramuscularly, aminophylline IV drip; administer corticosteroids to reduce inflammation as ordered. | Maintains patent airway; demonstrates effective breathing pattern |
| Hypotension; rapid, thready pulse | Administer 0.1-0.5 ml 1:1000 epinephrine solution subcutaneously or intramuscularly into upper arm and massage site to hasten absorption; prepare to administer vasopressor drugs such as norepinephrine bitartrate (Levophed) and high-dose dopamine (Intropin); monitor pulse and blood pressure q 3-5 min until stable. | Maintains hemodynamic stability, as evidenced by blood pressure and pulse in normal range |
| Edema and itching at site of injection or insect bite | Place a tourniquet above the site of the antigen. Remove tourniquet q 10-15 min or until reaction is under control; apply ice. | Reduces systemic absorption of the antigen |

such as nausea and vomiting, abdominal pain, and diarrhea may be present. Cardiovascular signs such as dysrhythmia, tachycardia, or bradycardia may be followed by circulatory collapse, which is indicated by a falling blood pressure, pallor, and loss of consciousness. In extreme cases death may occur in 5 to 10 minutes after onset of the reaction (Table 7-7 and Box 7-5).

**Cytotoxic hypersensitivity.** Cytotoxic, or type II, hypersensitivity occurs when antibodies directed against antigens of the cell membrane stimulate complement (Levinson, Jawetz, 1994). A cytotoxic hypersensitivity reaction occurs when an incompatible blood product is

given to a patient. The antigen responsible for the antigen-antibody reaction is the donor red blood cell. This cell reacts with the recipient's antibody and complement to cause cell lysis. Some drug reactions are also cytotoxic reactions.

**Immune complex hypersensitivity.** Normally the products of the antigen-antibody reaction (immune complexes) are promptly removed, but sometimes they persist and are deposited in the tissues; this results in a type III hypersensitivity reaction (Levinson, Jawetz, 1994). Inflammation results, damaging the affected organ system. For example, a response to beta-hemolytic

| BOX 7-5 | NURSING PROCESS |
|---|---|

## ANAPHYLACTIC SHOCK

### ASSESSMENT

- Vital signs q 3-5 min until stable
- Respiratory status (dyspnea, tachypnea, wheezing, stridor, hoarseness)
- Breath sounds
- Arterial blood gases
- Level of consciousness, orientation
- Urine output
- Skin (temperature, flushing, urticaria, rash)
- Presence of facial edema
- Peripheral pulses
- Level of anxiety
- Coping mechanisms
- Knowledge of condition or allergies

### NURSING DIAGNOSES

- Decreased cardiac output related to severe allergic reaction
- Ineffective breathing pattern related to airway and facial edema, bronchospasm
- Impaired skin integrity related to urticaria, dermatitis
- Anxiety related to sudden, severe change in health status
- Knowledge deficit related to new medical condition, need for future prevention
- Ineffective individual coping related to variable nature of allergic reactions and necessity of altering life-style

### NURSING INTERVENTIONS

- If ingested food or drugs are the cause, help with forced emesis.
- If injected agents or insect bites are the cause, place tourniquet around site and apply ice directly to site. Remove tourniquet q 10-15 min and reapply.
- Administer medications as prescribed
    Epinephrine: 0.1-0.5 ml (1:1000 solution) subcutaneously or intramuscularly into upper arm; massage site to hasten absorption
    Diphenhydramine: 50-100 mg intramuscularly
    Aminophylline: IV infusion
    Corticosteroids
    Vasopressor drugs (norepinephrine bitartrate, dopamine)
- Place patient in position for shock, with head and trunk horizontal and lower extremities elevated 20 to 30 degrees, if indicated.
- Administer oxygen as prescribed.
- Stay with patient during acute distress; constantly assess and provide reassurance.
- Prepare for emergency intubation or tracheostomy if indicated.
- Administer IV fluids as ordered.
- Observe for development of rash.
- Explain all procedures and treatments.

### EVALUATION OF EXPECTED OUTCOMES

- Vital signs stable and within normal limits for patient
- Urine output >30 ml/hr
- Alert and oriented
- No evidence of respiratory distress
- Strong peripheral pulses
- Decrease in urticaria, rash
- Verbalizes anxiety and fear
- Verbalizes understanding of cause, prevention, and treatment of allergy

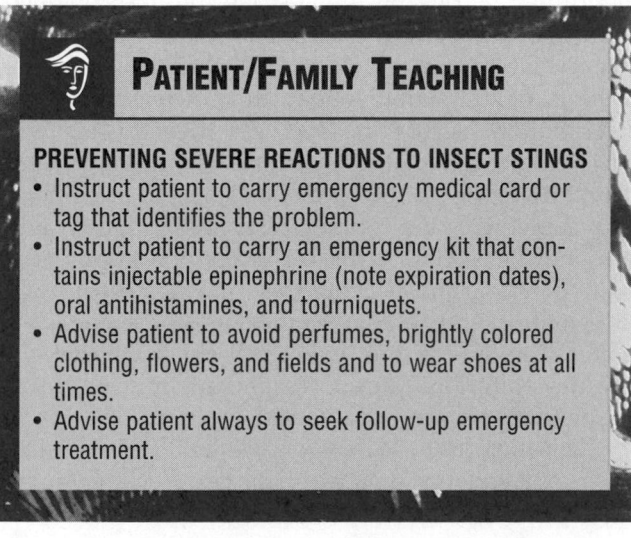

### PATIENT/FAMILY TEACHING

#### PREVENTING SEVERE REACTIONS TO INSECT STINGS
- Instruct patient to carry emergency medical card or tag that identifies the problem.
- Instruct patient to carry an emergency kit that contains injectable epinephrine (note expiration dates), oral antihistamines, and tourniquets.
- Advise patient to avoid perfumes, brightly colored clothing, flowers, and fields and to wear shoes at all times.
- Advise patient always to seek follow-up emergency treatment.

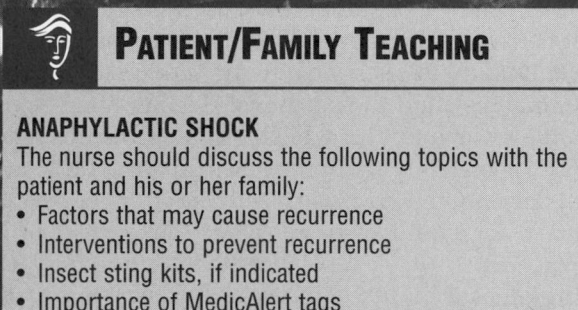

### PATIENT/FAMILY TEACHING

#### ANAPHYLACTIC SHOCK
The nurse should discuss the following topics with the patient and his or her family:
- Factors that may cause recurrence
- Interventions to prevent recurrence
- Insect sting kits, if indicated
- Importance of MedicAlert tags
- Importance of informing health care providers about the allergy or allergies

streptococci can result in acute poststreptococcal glomerulonephritis, which damages the nephrons of the kidney (see Chapter 38).

**Cell-mediated hypersensitivity.** Delayed reactions, or type IV hypersensitivity, may be local or systemic and may be delayed from hours to days. This type of hypersensitivity results from an alteration in the cell-mediated immune response in which entire lymphocytes (T cells) become sensitized to the antigen (see Table 7-6). Antibodies are not produced; rather, the whole cell attacks the antigen and destroys it. The most common example of a delayed reaction is the tuberculin skin test. Individuals who have been previously sensitized to the antigen respond to an intradermal injection of old tuberculin with erythema and induration after 24 to 48 hours.

Allergic contact dermatitis is the most common immunologic disorder treated by dermatologists. The most common sensitizing antigens are poison ivy, rubber compounds used in elastic, and nickel used in costume jewelry and buttons. These substances combine with skin proteins and create a non–self-antigen. A localized irritation of the skin (eczema) occurs, characterized by redness, edema, and scaling. Organ transplant rejection also is believed to be a type of delayed sensitivity. An individual's history of tension-producing situations, infection, endocrine disturbance, and work-related activities may be significant. Geographic movement may be important because of the change of climate or exposure to new types of allergens.

## Assessment of People with Atopic Allergies

Approximately 40 million Americans have some type of allergy. Because these hypersensitivity reactions occur so often, nurses in all fields must learn to assess the allergy patient appropriately. A careful, thorough allergy history is essential in identifying possible allergens (Figure 7-10). Genetic and congenital factors are extremely important in establishing a diagnosis. Patients should be asked about any family history of allergies and any previous allergic experiences. Past allergic reactions must be recorded and described in the assessment.

**Skin tests.** Skin tests include the scratch test, the intradermal test, and the patch test. Testing often begins with the scratch test, in which a small scratch is made through the skin with a blunt instrument. The scratch is not deep enough to cause bleeding. The allergen may be a powder, liquid, or paste. When the test is done on the forearm, an inert substance (the control) is placed on the other arm. If the individual is sensitive to the antigen, an area of redness and a wheal appears in 15 to 30 minutes; the control does not show any reaction.

The intradermal test may be used without previous use of the scratch test, or it may be used only for anti-

gens that failed to react to the scratch test. A minute amount of an antigen (0.01 to 0.02 ml) is injected into but not through the skin with a tuberculin syringe and a 26-gauge needle (Figure 7-11). The sensitivity reaction is similar to that of the scratch test and occurs in approximately 10 minutes. With the prick test a drop of allergen and a control substance are placed approximately 2 cm apart. A 26-gauge needle carefully pricks the skin through the drop and gently lifts it upward. Both the intradermal test and the prick test have grading systems for standardizing their interpretation.

Patch tests may be used when an allergy to specific substances is suspected for which commercial allergens are not available. The allergen is applied to the skin, covered, and secured with adhesive tape. The patch is removed in 2 to 3 days, and the skin is examined. The appearance of erythema or a wheal indicates sensitivity to the allergen. The nurse must be alert for any reaction that might indicate that the patient is developing a generalized allergic reaction. Sudden difficulty breathing, a change in vital signs, pallor, or dizziness should be reported to the physician immediately. A syringe of 1:1000 epinephrine (Adrenalin) should be available for immediate use. All patients undergoing testing should be kept under surveillance for at least 20 minutes after testing. If the patient has a reaction, the procedures outlined in Table 7-4 should be followed.

---

**NURSE ALERT**

When participating in skin testing, the nurse should be prepared for an anaphylactic emergency.

---

**Mucous membrane sensitivity tests.** Tests may also be performed by placing the allergen into the conjunctival sac of the eye. Nothing is placed in the opposite eye, which serves as a control. If the test is positive, itching of the conjunctiva and increased tearing (lacrimation) occur. The eyes are then flushed with physiologic saline solution to remove the allergen, and 1 or 2 drops of a 1:1000 aqueous solution of epinephrine is placed in the conjunctival sac. The nasal cavity also may be used for testing. The allergen is sprayed or sniffed into one nostril, and the opposite nostril serves as a control. A positive reaction causes sneezing, nasal congestion, and a thin, watery discharge. Because of the discomfort it causes the patient, mucous membrane testing is not widely used.

**Elimination tests.** When food is believed to be the cause of an allergy, a patient may be given an elimination diet to determine the specific food causing the

**ALLERGY SURVEY SHEET**

Name _John Richards_  Age _36_  Sex _m_  Date _Sept. 3, 1989_

**I. Chief complaint:** _stuffy nose & watery eyes_
**II. Present Illness:** _wheezing, clear nasal discharge, itchy eyes for 5 wks._
**III. Collateral allergic symptoms:** _same symptoms last fall._

| | | | | | |
|---|---|---|---|---|---|
| **Eyes:** | Pruritus ✓ | Burning — | Lacrimation ✓ | | |
| | Swelling ✓ | Infection — | Discharge — | | |
| **Ears:** | Pruritus — | Fullness — | Popping — | | |
| | Frequent infections — | | | | |
| **Nose:** | Sneezing ✓ | Rhinorrhea ✓ | Obstruction — | | |
| | Pruritus ✓ | Mouth breathing — | | | |
| | Purulent discharge — | | | | |
| **Throat:** | Soreness — | Post-nasal discharge ✓ | | | |
| | Palatal pruritus ✓ | Mucus in the morning — | | | |
| **Chest:** | Cough — | Pain — | Wheezing ✓ | | |
| | Sputum — | Dyspnea — | | | |
| | Color — | Rest — | | | |
| | Amount — | Exertion — | | | |
| **Skin:** | Dermatitis — | Eczema — | Urticaria — | | |

**IV. Family allergies:** _Father had eczemas. mother none._
**V. Previous allergic treatment or testing:** _no_
   **Prior skin testing:** _none_

| | | |
|---|---|---|
| **Drugs:** Antihistamines | Improved _yes_ | Unimproved |
| Bronchodilators | Improved _yes_ | Unimproved |
| Nose drops | Improved _yes_ | Unimproved |
| Hyposensitization | Improved _not done_ | Unimproved — |
|    Duration — | | |
|    Antigens — | | |
|    Reactions — | | |
| Antibiotics ⎫ _not_ | Improved — | Unimproved |
| Steroids ⎭ _used_ | Improved — | Unimproved |

**VI. Physical agents and habits:**

**Bothered by:**

| | | | |
|---|---|---|---|
| Tobbaco for — years | Alcohol — | Air cond. — | |
| Cigarettes — packs/day | Heat — | Muggy weath. — | |
| Cigars — per day | Cold — | Weath. chngs. — | |
| Pipe — per day | Perfumes — | Chemicals — | |
| Never smoked ✓ | Paints — | Hair spray — | |
| Bothered by smoke _yes_ | Insecticides — | Newspapers — | |
| | Cosmetics — | | |

**Figure 7-10**  Allergy survey sheet. (From Patterson R: *Allergic diseases,* ed 4, Philadelphia, 1993, Lippincott.)                    *Continued*

**VII. When symptoms occur:**

Time and circumstances of 1st episode:
Prior health:
Course of illness over decades: progressing _____✓_____ regressing _____
Time of year:
    Perennial ___✓___       Exact dates *Aug./Sept. 1988*
    Seasonal ___✓___                 *Aug. 1 – present 1989*
    Seasonally exacerbated ___✓___
Monthly variations (menses, occupation): *none*
Time of week (weekend vs weekdays): *no*
Time of day or night: *no*
After insect stings: *no*

**VIII. Where symptoms occur:**

Living where at onset: *Kansas City, Kansas*
Living where since onset: *Kansas City, Kansas*
Effect of vacation or major geographic change: *until June 1988 lived in N.W.*
Symptoms better indoors or outdoors: *indoors*           *Pennsylvania*
Effect of school or work: *better at work inside*
Effect of staying elsewhere nearby: *none*
Effect of hospitalization: —
Effect of specific environments: *went to park with increased severity of*
Do symptoms occur around:                         *symptoms*
old leaves ___✓___ hay ___✓___ lakeside ___—___ barns ___—___
summer homes ___—___ damp basement ___—___ dry attic ___—___
lawnmowing ___✓___ animals ___—___ other ___—___
Do symptoms occur after eating: *no*
cheese ___—___ mushrooms ___—___ beer ___—___ melons ___—___
bananas ___—___ fish ___—___ nuts ___—___ citrus fruits ___—___
other foods (list) *none* _____
Home: city ___—___ rural ___✓___
      house ___✓___ age *10 yrs*
      apartment ___—___ basement ___✓___ damp _____ dry ___✓___
      heating system *✓ Forced*
      pets (how long) *none* dog ___—___ cat ___—___ other ___—___

| Bedroom: | Type | Age | | Living room: | Type | Age |
|---|---|---|---|---|---|---|
| Pillow | *foam* | *3yrs.* | | Rug | *nylon* | *1yr.* |
| Mattress | *foam* | *5yrs.* | | Matting | *nylon* | *1yr.* |
| Blankets | *thermal* | *5yrs.* | | Furniture | *wood &* | *1yr.* |
| Quilts | *none* | *—* | | | *nylon fabric* | |
| Furniture | *wood* | *5yrs.* | | | | |

Anywhere in home symptoms are worse: *no* _____

**IX. What does patient think makes him worse:** *outside Aug./Sept.*

**X. Under what circumstances is he free of symptoms:** *in air conditioning*

**XI. Summary and additional comments:**

_____

**Figure 7-10, cont'd**   Allergy survey sheet.

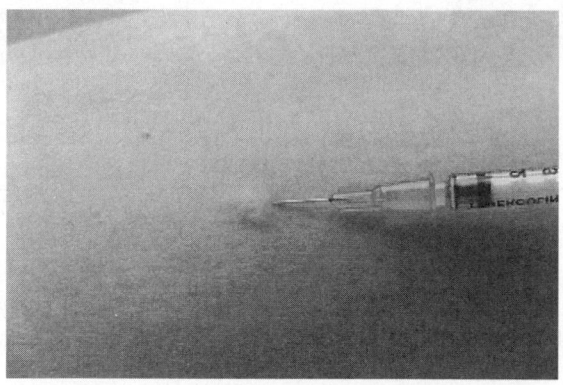

**Figure 7-11**    Intradermal skin testing for allergic response. (From Potter PA, Perry AG: *Fundamentals of nursing: concepts, process, and practice*, ed 4, St Louis, 1997, Mosby.)

trouble. One of two methods may be used. The patient may be asked to keep a record of all food eaten for a given period. After this period one food (e.g., milk, chocolate, or wheat products) is eliminated from the diet. Through gradual elimination of specific foods from the diet, the food causing the allergy may be identified.

Another method is to give the patient a diet consisting of foods that usually do not cause allergy. The diet is followed for a week. If allergic symptoms continue, changes are made in the diet. If the symptoms continue, it generally is considered that food is not the cause of the allergic reaction. However, if the symptoms disappear, other foods are added to the diet until the patient develops allergic symptoms. That food is then considered to be the probable cause and is eliminated from the diet. This type of testing may be used to identify the cause of urticaria, or hives.

Elimination testing also is used for patients with contact dermatitis. Offending agents such as cosmetics, hair spray, and certain types of clothing are eliminated until the dermatitis disappears. These agents then are reintroduced gradually to identify the causative agent.

## Nursing Interventions for People with Allergies

Nursing interventions for people with allergies include education in avoidance therapy, drug therapy, and immunotherapy **(desensitization)**. Patients should be taught the importance of maintaining optimum health, getting enough rest, and controlling stress. The patient's emotional status influences the severity of the allergic symptoms and the effectiveness of treatment.

**Avoidance of allergen.** The best treatment for an allergy is to prevent the person from coming in contact with the allergen. The specific allergen must be identified and necessary adaptations made. Adaptation may

change a person's way of life completely and also may affect family members. It may mean moving to another environment, changing employment, or changing the type of clothing worn. When animal dander is a factor, it may be necessary to remove pets or to avoid contact with farm animals. Picnicking or hiking into the woods may have to be eliminated. Air conditioning, damp mopping, dusting, and closed windows may help prevent allergic attacks caused by household dust or other allergens in the air. Rainy, damp, humid weather often is associated with asthma. Using a dehumidifier to remove moisture from the air may be beneficial in preventing asthma attacks. Individuals with allergies are advised to avoid exposure to infections. A common cold may precipitate an allergic reaction. A person may have to make many changes in environment and life-style.

**Drug therapy.** Antihistamines, epinephrine, topical decongestants, and corticosteroids commonly are used to treat allergies. Because of the antigen-antibody reaction, the cells release histamine, which is primarily responsible for allergic symptoms. Drug therapy is designed to counteract the effects of histamine.

An **antihistamine** is most useful in allergic conditions that affect the nasal mucosa (e.g., hay fever), rhinitis, itching, and acute urticaria. Antihistamines also are used for motion sickness, nausea and vomiting, vertigo, and sleeplessness. Antihistamines block the action of histamine on the bronchioles and blood vessels. The major side effect of these drugs is drowsiness; therefore people taking any of this group of drugs are advised not to drive motor vehicles. Other side effects include dizziness, dryness of mucous membranes, and weakness. Many antihistaminic preparations are available (Table 7-8). Antihistamines can be administered orally, and some are available for parenteral injection or rectal administration.

**Epinephrine** (Adrenalin) has several uses. It is used for serious hypersensitivity, such as anaphylactic shock. A 1:1000 aqueous solution is used for parenteral injection. Epinephrine counteracts the actions of histamine and helps reverse the pathologic condition that has occurred. It increases the strength and force of the heartbeat, increases blood pressure, and relaxes the smooth muscles of the respiratory tract.

Topical decongestants have an antiallergic effect and shrink congested nasal mucous membranes. Phenylephrine (NeoSynephrine) is one of the most widely prescribed topical nasal decongestants. It should be used at intervals of at least 4 hours to prevent rebound congestion. Rebound congestion can occur after prolonged and repeated vasoconstrictor stimulation initiates a compensatory vasodilation and subsequent increase in secretions. If this occurs, the drug treatment should be discontinued.

*Text continued on p. 136.*

## Pharmacology of Drugs Used for Physiologic Responses

| DRUG (GENERIC AND TRADE NAME); ROUTE AND DOSAGE | ACTION/INDICATION | COMMON SIDE EFFECTS AND NURSING CONSIDERATIONS |
|---|---|---|
| **ANTIBIOTICS** | | |
| **Amoxicillin** (Augmentin)<br>**Route:** PO<br>**Dosage:** 250-500 mg q 8 hr; gonorrhea, 3 g plus 1 g probenecid single dose | Antiinfective (extended spectrum penicillin) used for the treatment of skin and skin structure infections, otitis media, sinusitis, respiratory and genitourinary infections, meningitis, septicemia, endocarditis prophylaxis, and Lyme disease | Rashes and diarrhea; contraindicated in hypersensitivity to penicillins; use with caution in severe renal insufficiency and infectious mononucleosis |
| **Ampicillin** (Principen, Totacillin, Omnipen, Polycillin)<br>**Route:** IM, IV, PO<br>**Dosage:** All routes, 1-2 g/day in divided doses q 4-6 hr | Antiinfective (penicillin) used for all the above except Lyme disease | Rashes and diarrhea; contraindicated in hypersensitivity to penicillins; use with caution in severe renal insufficiency |
| **Cefazolin sodium** (Ancef, Kefzol)<br>**Route:** IM, IV<br>**Dosage:** Life-threatening infections, IM, IV, 1-1.5 g q 6 hr; mild/moderate infections, IM, IV, 250-500 mg q 8 hr | Antibiotic cephalosporin used to treat skin, skin structure, urinary tract, and bone and joint infections; also septicemia, intraabdominal and biliary tract infections, also used as a perioperative prophylactic antiinfective | Nausea, vomiting, diarrhea, rashes, phlebitis and pain at IV site; contraindicated in hypersensitivity to cephalosporins and serious hypersensitivity to penicillins; use with caution in renal impairment |
| **Cefoxitin** (Mefoxin)<br>**Route:** IM, IV<br>**Dosage:** IM, IV, 1-2 g q 6-8 hr (up to 12 g/day); uncomplicated gonorrhea, 2 g IM single dose with 1 g probenecid PO | Antiinfective (second-generation cephalosporin) used to treat respiratory tract, skin, skin structure, bone and joint, urinary tract, and gynecologic infections; also used in septicemia and for perioperative prophylaxis | Rashes, nausea, vomiting, diarrhea, phlebitis and pain at IV site, and anaphylaxis; contraindicated in hypersensitivity to cephalosporins and serious hypersensitivity to penicillins; use with caution in renal impairment |
| **Cephalexin** (Keflex)<br>**Route:** PO<br>**Dosage:** 250-500 mg q 6 hr (500 mg q 12 hr for cystitis) | Antiinfective (first-generation cephalosporin) used in the treatment of serious skin, skin structure, urinary tract, bone and joint, and respiratory tract infections; septicemia; and otitis media | Nausea, vomiting, diarrhea, rashes, phlebitis and pain at IV site, and anaphylaxis; contraindicated in hypersensitivity to cephalosporins and serious hypersensitivity to penicillins; use with caution in renal impairment |
| **Doxycycline** (Vibramycin)<br>**Route:** PO, IV<br>**Dosage:** PO, IV, 100-200 mg/day given once daily or in divided doses q 12 hr | Antiinfective (tetracycline) used most commonly to treat infections caused by unusual organisms, including *Mycoplasma, Chlamydia,* and *Rickettsia;* also useful in the treatment of gonorrhea and syphilis in patients allergic to penicillin; has been used for "traveler's diarrhea," exacerbations of chronic bronchitis, and Lyme disease | Nausea, vomiting, and diarrhea; can cause permanent straining of the teeth in children; use with caution in patients who are cachectic or debilitated or who have hepatic or renal disease |

*IM,* Intramuscular; *IV,* intravenous; *PO,* oral; *SC,* subcutaneous.

TABLE 7-8

# Pharmacology of Drugs Used for Physiologic Responses—cont'd

| DRUG (GENERIC AND TRADE NAME); ROUTE AND DOSAGE | ACTION/INDICATION | COMMON SIDE EFFECTS AND NURSING CONSIDERATIONS |
|---|---|---|
| **Erythromycin** (Erythromycin, Ilotycin) **Route:** PO, IV, topical, ophthalmic **Dosage:** PO, 250-500 mg q 6-12 hr, IV, 1-4 g/day in divided doses q 6 hr or as continuous infusion; topical, 2% ointment, gel, or solution bid; ophthalmic, 0.5% ointment to conjunctiva 1 or more times daily | Antiinfective (macrolide) used in the treatment of upper and lower respiratory tract infections, otitis media, skin and skin structure infections, pertussis, diphtheria, intestinal amebiasis, pelvic inflammatory disease, nongonococcal urethritis, syphilis, rheumatic fever, and Legionnaires' disease; used topically against acne and opthalmically against superficial ocular infections | Nausea, vomiting, and phlebitis at IV site; contraindicated in hepatic dysfunction; administer around the clock on an empty stomach, at least 1 hr before or 2 hr after meals; may be taken with food if GI irritation occurs; should not be taken with fruit juices |
| **Gentamicin sulfate** (Garamycin) **Route:** IM, IV, topical, ophthalmic **Dosage:** IM, IV, 3-5 mg/kg/day in divided doses q 8 hr; doses as low as 3 mg/kg/day given once daily or in divided doses q 12 hr have been used for uncomplicated urinary tract infection; topical, apply cream or ointment to cleansed area 3-4 times daily; ophthalmic, 1-2 drops of solution q 2-4 hr or ointment 2-3 times daily | Antiinfective (aminoglucoside) used in treatment of gram-negative bacillary infections and infections due to staphylococci when penicillins or other less toxic drugs are contraindicated; also used as part of a regimen for endocarditis prophylaxis | Ototoxicity and nephrotoxicity; use with caution in renal impairment; monitor serum electrolytes |
| **Nafcillin sodium** (Unipen) **Route:** IM, IV, PO **Dosage:** PO, 250-1000 mg q 4-6 hr; IM, 500 mg q 4-6 hr; IV, 500-1500 mg q 4 hr | Antiinfective (penicillinase-resistant penicillin) used in the treatment of infections caused by susceptible strains of penicillinase-producing staphylococci | Nausea, vomiting, diarrhea, rashes, and allergic reactions; contraindicated in hypersensitivity to penicillins; use with caution in renal impairment |
| **Neomycin sulfate** (Myciguent, Mycifradin) **Route:** PO, topical **Dosage:** Preparation for GI surgery, PO, 1 g q hr for 4 hr, then 1 g q 4 hr for 24 hr before surgery or 1 g given 19 hr, 18 hr, and 9 hr before surgery; minor skin infections, topical, 0.5% cream or ointment 1-3 times daily | Antiinfective (aminoglycoside) used to prepare the GI tract for surgery or to reduce the population of ammonia-producing bacteria in the management of hepatic encephalopathy; also used in the treatment of minor skin infections | Ototoxicity and nephrotoxicity; contraindicated in renal impairment; use with caution in neuromuscular diseases |
| **Penicillin G benzathine** (Bicillin) **Route:** IM **Dosage:** Streptococcal infections, 1.2 million U single dose; syphilis, 2.4 million U single dose (primary, secondary, or latent syphilis of <1 yr duration) repeated q wk for 3 wk; patients with neurosyphilis should be initially treated with aqueous penicillin G plus probenecid, then 2.4 million U penicillin G benzathine weekly for 3 wk; prevention of rheumatic fever, 1.2 million U q 4 wk | Antiinfective (penicillin) used in the treatment of a wide variety of infections, including pneumococcal pneumonia, streptococcal pharyngitis, and syphilis; also used to prevent rheumatic fever | Nausea, vomiting, diarrhea, epigastric distress, rashes, and pain at IV site; contraindicated in previous hypersensitivity to penicillins and benzathine; cross-sensitivity may exist with cephalosporins; use with caution in renal impairment |

*Continued*

TABLE 7-8

## Pharmacology of Drugs Used for Physiologic Responses—cont'd

| DRUG (GENERIC AND TRADE NAME); ROUTE AND DOSAGE | ACTION/INDICATION | COMMON SIDE EFFECTS AND NURSING CONSIDERATIONS |
|---|---|---|
| **Penicillin G potassium** (Pentids)<br>**Route:** PO<br>**Dosage:** Pneumococcal/streptococcal infections, 400,000-5 million U q 6-8 hr for 10 days (streptococcal) or afebrile for 2 days (pneumococcal infections); prevention of recurrence of rheumatic fever, 200,000-250,000 U bid continuously; gingivitis/pharyngitis, 400,000-500,000 U q 6-8 hr | Broad-spectrum antibiotic-natural penicillin used for emphysema, gangrene, anthrax, gonorrhea, mastoiditis, pneumonia, tetanus, osteomyelitis, meningitis, and urinary tract infections; used prophylactically in rheumatic fever, and effective for nonpenicillinase–producing gram-positive cocci | Coma, convulsions, increased bleeding time, bone marrow depression, granulocytopenia, hyperkalemia and hypokalemia, alkalosis, and hypernatremia; contraindicated in hypersensitivity to penicillin; use with caution with hypersensitivity to cephalosporins |
| **Penicillin G procaine** (Crysticillin, Wycillin)<br>**Route:** IM<br>**Dosage:** Moderate/severe infections, 600,000-1.2 million U/day, single dose or 2 divided doses; uncomplicated gonorrhea, 4.8 million U divided into 2 injection sites, preceded by 1 g probenecid PO | Antiinfective (penicillin) used to treat pneumococcal pneumonia, streptococcal pneumonia, streptococcal pharyngitis, syphilis, gonorrhea; used in enterococcal infections (requires the addition of an aminoglycoside) | Nausea, vomiting, diarrhea, epigastric distress, rashes, and pain at injection site; contraindicated in hypersensitivity to penicillin and procaine; use with caution with hypersensitivity to cephalosporins and in renal insufficiency |
| **Penicillin V** (Pen-Vee-K)<br>**Route:** PO<br>**Dosage:** 125-500 mg q 6 hr | Antiinfective (penicillin) used to treat infections such as pneumococcal pneumonia, skin and soft tissue infections, and streptococcal pharyngitis; used to prevent rheumatic fever | Nausea, vomiting, diarrhea, epigastric distress, rashes, and anaphylaxis; contraindicated in hypersensitivity to penicillin; use with caution with hypersensitivity to cephalosporins and in renal insufficiency; may be administered without regard to meals |
| **ANTIHISTAMINES** | | |
| **Chlorpheniramine** (Chlor-Trimeton, Tildrin)<br>**Route:** PO, SC, IM, IV<br>**Dosage:** PO, 4 mg q 4-6 hr or 8-12 mg of extended release formulation q 8-12 hr (not to exceed 24 mg/day); SC, IM, IV, 5-20 mg single dose (not to exceed 40 mg/day) | Antihistamine used for symptomatic relief of allergic symptoms caused by histamine release; most useful for nasal allergies and allergic dermatoses; also used for management of severe allergic or hypersensitivity reactions, including anaphylaxis and transfusion reactions | Drowsiness, sedation, hypertension, blurred vision, and dry mouth; contraindicated in acute attacks of asthma and alcohol intolerance; use with caution in glaucoma and liver disease and in the elderly |
| **Diphenhydramine** (Benadryl)<br>**Route:** PO, IM, IV, topical<br>**Dosage:** PO, 25-50 mg q 4-6 hr; IM, IV, 10-50 mg single dose (may need up to 100 mg dose, not to exceed 400 mg/day); topical, 1%-2% cream, lotion, or spray 3-4 times daily | Antihistamine and antitussive used for relief of allergic symptoms caused by histamine release, including anaphylaxis, nasal allergies, allergic dermatoses, Parkinson's disease; and dystonic reactions from medication; used to prevent motion sickness | Drowsiness, dry mouth, and anorexia; contraindicated in acute attacks of asthma and intolerance to alcohol; use with caution in the elderly and with severe liver disease, glaucoma, seizure disorders, and prostatic hypertrophy |

---

**TABLE 7-8**

## Pharmacology of Drugs Used for Physiologic Responses—cont'd

| DRUG (GENERIC AND TRADE NAME); ROUTE AND DOSAGE | ACTION/INDICATION | COMMON SIDE EFFECTS AND NURSING CONSIDERATIONS |
|---|---|---|
| **CORTICOSTEROIDS** | | |
| **Hydrocortisone** (Cortef, Hydrocortone, Solu-Cortef)<br>**Route:** PO, IM, IV<br>**Dosage:** PO, 10-320 mg/day in 1-4 divided doses; IM, IV, 100-500 mg q 2-6 hr (succinate, range 100-8000 mg/day); 15-240 mg (phosphate) q 12 hr | Short-acting glucocorticoid used in the management of adrenocortical insufficiency and short-term management of such inflammatory and allergic reactions as asthma and ulcerative colitis; chronic use is limited to mineralocorticoid activity; not suitable for alternate-day therapy | Depression, nausea, petechiae, decreased wound healing, adrenal suppression, decreased growth in children, hypokalemia, and sodium retention; contraindicated in serious infections; use with caution, chronic treatment with doses >20 mg/day may result in adrenal suppression; do not discontinue abruptly; during periods of stress, dose may need to be increased; use lowest possible dose for shortest period of time; may mask infection |
| **Prednisolone** (Delta-Cortef)<br>**Route:** PO, IM, IV, otic, ophthalmic<br>**Dosage:** PO, 5-60 mg/day single dose or divided doses (maintenance doses may be given as a single dose or every other day); multiple sclerosis, 200 mg/day for 7 days, then 80 mg every other day for 1 mo; IM, IV, 4-60 mg/day; ophthalmic, 1 drop q hr initially, then decrease to 2-4 times daily; otic, 3-4 drops 2-3 times daily | Glucocorticoid (intermediate acting) used systemically and locally for chronic illnesses such as inflammatory, allergic, hematologic, neoplastic, and autoimmune diseases; also used for replacement therapy in adrenal insufficiency | Depression, euphoria, hypertension, nausea, anorexia, decreased wound healing, petechiae, ecchymoses, fragility, hirsutism, acne, adrenal suppression, muscle wasting, osteoporosis, increased susceptibility to infections, and cushingoid appearance (moonface, buffalo hump); contraindicated in active, untreated infections and known alcohol intolerance; use with caution in children; chronic treatment with doses >20 mg/day may result in adrenal suppression; do not discontinue abruptly; during periods of stress dose may need to be increased; use lowest possible dose for shortest period of time; may mask infection |
| **Prednisone** (Deltasone)<br>**Route:** PO<br>**Dosage:** 5-60 mg/day single dose or divided doses; for multiple sclerosis, 200 mg/day for 1 wk, then 80 mg every other day for 1 mo | Glucocorticoid (intermediate acting) used systemically and locally in a wide variety of chronic diseases, including inflammatory, allergic, hematologic, neoplastic, and autoimmune diseases; suitable for alternate-day dosing in the management of chronic illness; also used for replacement therapy in adrenal insufficiency | Same as above |

*Continued*

---

**TABLE 7-8**

## Pharmacology of Drugs Used for Physiologic Responses—cont'd

| DRUG (GENERIC AND TRADE NAME); ROUTE AND DOSAGE | ACTION/INDICATION | COMMON SIDE EFFECTS AND NURSING CONSIDERATIONS |
|---|---|---|
| **Triamcinolone, acetonide** (Kenacort, Aristocort, Kenalog) **Route:** PO, IM, inhalation **Dosage:** PO, 4-48 mg/day in divided doses qd-qid; IM, 40 mg q wk (acetonide), 5-48 mg into neoplasms, 2-40 mg into joint or soft tissue; inhalation, 2 sprays 3-4 times daily (up to 12-16 sprays per day); nasal inhalation, 2 sprays each nostril once daily (up to 2 sprays in each nostril twice daily or 1 spray in each nostril 4 times daily) | Glucocorticoid (intermediate acting) antiinflammatory agent used systemically and locally to treat chronic inflammatory, allergic, hematologic, neoplastic, and autoimmune diseases; not suitable for alternate-day therapy | Same as above |
| **SULFONAMIDES** | | |
| **Sulfamethoxazole** (Gantanol, Azo Gantanol) **Route:** PO **Dosage:** 2 g initially, then 1 g q 8-12 hr | Antiinfective (sulfonamide) used in the treatment of urinary tract infections, nocardiosis, toxoplasmosis, and malaria | Nausea, vomiting, rashes, and fever; use with caution in severe renal or hepatic impairment |
| **Sulfisoxazole** (Gantrisin, Azo Gantrisin) **Route:** PO, ophthalmic **Dosage:** PO, 2-4 g initially, then 4-8 g/day in divided doses q 4-6 hr (not to exceed 12 g/day); ophthalmic, 1 drop 3 or more times daily, may increase interval as infection resolves | Antiinfective (sulfonamide) used in the treatment of urinary tract infections and nocardiosis, and in combination with other antiinfectives for malaria and pelvic inflammatory disease in prepubescent adolescents; ophthalmic uses for treatment of eye infections (e.g., *Chlamydia*) | Nausea, vomiting, rashes, aplastic anemia, agranulocytosis, and fever; contraindicated in hypersensitivity to sulfonamides; cross-sensitivity to Lasix, thiazides, sulfonylurea oral hypoglycemic agents, and carbonic anhydrase inhibitors may appear; use with caution in severe renal or hepatic impairment |

---

**Corticosteroids** are not used routinely for allergic disorders because of their serious side effects. However, steroid preparations are marketed as ointments, creams, and lotions for topical application. They are used in allergic dermatosis and applied two or three times a day. Systemic corticosteroids may be given to a patient with life-threatening asthma; in some cases of immediate allergic reactions, including anaphylactic shock; and for an allergic reaction to penicillin and other severe drug reactions. Corticosteroids help reduce the inflammatory reaction and help with recovery (see Table 7-8).

**Immunotherapy.** Immunotherapy, or desensitization, as it is sometimes called, is a form of immunization commonly referred to as *allergy shots*. Immunotherapy involves injecting an individual with increasing amounts of allergen to which the patient displays a type I hypersensitivity. The goal is to improve tolerance with fewer symptoms after exposure to the allergen. The precise mechanism of the improvement has not been definitively established.

The extract usually is given weekly, and the amount is increased gradually with each injection until the largest dose that causes no reaction has been given. This last dose is considered the maintenance dose. Desensitization has been most effective with hay fever. People who have a seasonal allergy are advised to begin injections early, before allergic symptoms appear. Immunotherapy is not a lifetime regimen. Most allergists consider a routine course to last 3 to 4 years.

## Autoimmune Disease

Normally the adult host shows tolerance to tissue antigens recognized as "self." However, sometimes this tolerance is lost, and immune reactions may develop against self-antigens, resulting in **autoimmune** diseases. These diseases tend to occur in genetically pre-

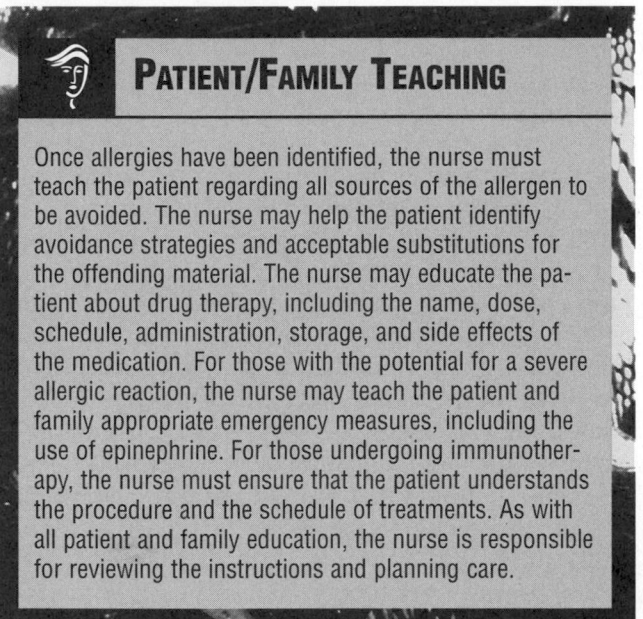

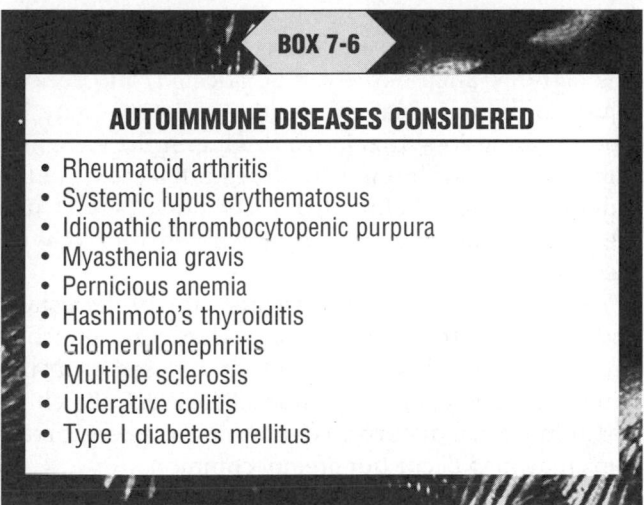

**BOX 7-6**

**AUTOIMMUNE DISEASES CONSIDERED**

- Rheumatoid arthritis
- Systemic lupus erythematosus
- Idiopathic thrombocytopenic purpura
- Myasthenia gravis
- Pernicious anemia
- Hashimoto's thyroiditis
- Glomerulonephritis
- Multiple sclerosis
- Ulcerative colitis
- Type I diabetes mellitus

disposed people who are exposed to an environmental agent that stimulates an immune response against normal tissue. Bacteria, viruses, and drugs may trigger the activation of T cells and B cells. Most reactions are mediated by antibodies. Diseases and disorders that result from this reaction may affect the eyes, skin, joints, thyroid gland, kidneys, brain, and vascular system (Levinson, Jawetz, 1994) (Box 7-6). Intensive study and research continue so that a better understanding of autoimmunity can be achieved.

Autoimmune diseases usually are treated with drug therapy aimed at interfering with the immune response. Immunosuppressants such as azathioprine (Imuran) and corticosteroids such as prednisone (Deltasone) may be administered.

# CHEMOTHERAPEUTIC AGENTS

Chemotherapy refers to the treatment of disease with chemical drugs. Some chemotherapeutic drugs are bacteriostatic, meaning that they arrest the multiplication of pathogenic bacteria; others are bactericidal, meaning that they kill bacteria. Still other drugs suppress the inflammatory response when pathogens are not involved (see Table 7-8).

## Sulfonamides

The sulfonamide drugs were the first chemotherapeutic agents to be discovered and were first used in the 1930s. They originally were used to treat both gram-negative and gram-positive infections. Thousands of sulfonamides have been developed, but only a few are in use today because of the development of bacterial resistance to sulfonamides and the discovery of newer, less toxic drugs. Many other antimicrobial agents have replaced or are used in combination with sulfonamides. The sulfonamides are primarily bacteriostatic and act by interfering with the metabolism of the invading microorganism to prevent further growth.

Some sulfonamide drugs are especially effective in treating uncomplicated infections of the urinary tract and preventing infection when long-term therapy is required. Sulfonamides are also common in the treatment of ulcerative colitis, chancroid, and burns (Clark, Queener, Karb, 1997). Patients receiving sulfonamide (sulfa) drugs should be encouraged to drink large amounts of fluid so as to provide 1200 to 2000 ml of urinary output over a 24-hour period; this prevents crystals in the urine. They also should be observed for side effects, the most common being anorexia and nausea and vomiting.

Sulfonamides also can cause a decrease in circulating red blood cells, white blood cells, and platelets, which can lead to the development of purpura, or bleeding into the skin. Any rash should be carefully observed. Signs of sensitivity such as sneezing or itching should be noted. Hematuria and the formation of crystals in the urine may be significant problems. A severe hypersensitivity reaction (Stevens-Johnson syndrome) is a rare reaction but has a mortality rate near 25% (Lehne, 1994).

## Antibiotics

The development of antibiotic drugs began in 1928, when Alexander Fleming, a British bacteriologist, discovered a substance he called *penicillin*. His findings were not immediately accepted, and it was not until about 1941 that intensive work began in the United States in the development of penicillin. In the early days only penicillin and streptomycin were available, but a large number of antibiotic agents are available today. Some antibiotic drugs are effective against only gram-positive or gram-negative bacteria; others, called broad-spectrum antibiotics, are effective against both gram-positive and gram-negative bacteria.

The penicillins are the most effective and widely used antibiotics. The penicillins and their semisynthetic derivatives prevent the development of the cell wall in bacteria and therefore are bactericidal. Penicillins are used to treat a variety of illnesses, including pneumococcal pneumonia, streptococcal infections, meningococcal meningitis, gonorrhea, syphilis, and *Salmonella* infections. However, some organisms, such as *S. aureus* and *Escherichia coli*, are capable of producing penicillinases, which are enzymes that destroy certain penicillins. Many new penicillins have been developed that are effective against these penicillinase-producing bacteria and against other virulent organisms. The penicillins are inexpensive and have a low incidence of toxicity. The development of "super" antibiotics has shortened infection times. They are expensive but have fewer side effects, and the patient feels better sooner.

Penicillin is available in different forms and under a variety of trade names. It is administered through intramuscular injection, intravenously, or orally. Under normal conditions penicillin is nontoxic, but allergic reactions can occur in some patients. These reactions vary from mild skin rashes to fatal anaphylactic shock. A nurse administering penicillin should first make sure that the patient has had no previous reaction to it and then should observe the patient carefully for several hours after administering the drug. Reactions do not always develop immediately, and fatal reactions have occurred several hours after the drug has been given.

No penicillin should be administered to anyone with a history of an allergic reaction to any member of the penicillin family. Oral preparations should not be taken for at least an hour before or after eating because they are poorly absorbed if acid is present in the stomach. Acidic fruit juices should not be used to administer the drugs.

The cephalosporin antimicrobial agents were first developed and used in the early 1960s. Cephalosporins are structurally similar to penicillin and have many of their physical characteristics. They are expensive, semisynthetic, and broad-spectrum antibiotics. Because they inhibit cell wall synthesis in microbes, they are bactericidal in action. Cephalosporins are classified into groups, called generations, that reflect their introduction and use. The difference between each generation stems from its effectiveness against gram-positive and gram-negative organisms. Cephalosporins should be avoided in patients who have severe or immediate reactions to penicillins. About 5% to 10%

of individuals allergic to penicillin show a cross-sensitivity to cephalosporins (Lehne, 1994). Caution is recommended when using cephalosporins for patients with preexisting renal conditions.

Tetracyclines were introduced in 1948 and were the first broad-spectrum antibiotics. They block the formation of proteins in microorganisms and are bacteriostatic. GI disturbances can occur with tetracyclines, but generally the drugs are nontoxic and allergic reactions are rare. The tetracyclines should not be administered with milk products, antacids, or iron preparations because the combination disturbs absorption of the drug. Tetracyclines are used in the treatment of adolescent acne, chlamydia, and other uncommon infections. They are the treatment of choice in rickettsial infections. Tetracyclines are not used in children and pregnant women because they bind to newly formed bones and teeth.

The group of antibiotics known as the *aminoglycosides* was in use as early as 1944 with streptomycin, but these drugs were further developed after 1952. Aminoglycosides also interfere with protein synthesis in invading microbes. They have widespread clinical use. However, toxic effects increase with increasing dosage. The eighth cranial nerve can be affected, and serious injury to the inner ear can result. Symptoms may include hearing loss, dizziness, ringing in the ears, and imbalance. In addition, these drugs can be toxic to the kidney nephrons (Lehne, 1994). The nurse is responsible for carefully monitoring intake and output with these drugs.

The macrolides (erythromycins) are bacteriostatic and inhibit protein synthesis. They are effective against gram-positive cocci and can be used as a substitute for penicillin in people allergic to penicillin. Gastrointestinal disturbances may occur. Allergic reactions may also occur but are not common.

Because a specific antibiotic may be ineffective against a particular organism, sensitivity tests should be done before any antibiotic is administered. Identifying the microorganisms causing the illness enables the physician to prescribe the most suitable antibiotic to cure the disease.

## Corticosteroids

The corticosteroids are used when inflammation is caused by some agent other than pathogens. These drugs, cortisone and hydrocortisone, are hormones produced by the adrenal cortex and are commonly referred to as adrenal steroids. One adrenal gland is located above each kidney and is comprised of two parts. The inner part is the medulla, and its primary secretion is epinephrine. The outer part is the cortex, which produces several substances, some of which are necessary for life. The cortex also produces cortisone and hydrocortisone. If the adrenal glands fail to function or have been removed surgically because of disease, hydrocortisone is administered to replace the normal secretion.

The first corticosteroids were prepared as glandular extracts around 1928. Today commercially available corticosteroids are of the same chemical composition but are made synthetically and have a higher potency. Chemical modification of the natural steroids has produced other, more selective synthetic steroids, which are used for replacement therapy and to suppress inflammatory and immune responses.

The beneficial effects of corticosteroid therapy are relief of inflammation, reduction of fever, and production of a feeling of well-being. The last effect probably is a result of symptom relief. For example, when cortisone is administered for an inflammatory condition, the classic signs of inflammation may be absent. Patients receiving cortisone feel encouraged because of the absence of symptoms. However, cortisone used therapeutically does not cure disease or alter its course and does not reverse any preexisting damage, such as crippling in arthritis. When used systemically the corticosteroids are powerful and dangerous drugs and can cause serious side effects that can affect every system of the body. Most physicians prescribe these drugs

extremely cautiously because of the toxic effects. Abrupt withdrawal and potentially life-threatening adrenal insufficiency is avoided by gradually decreasing the dosage. Corticosteroids can be administered orally, intravenously, or intramuscularly; they can be applied topically, such as in an ophthalmic preparation; or they can be injected directly into an inflamed joint or lesion.

Patients receiving any of the corticosteroid preparations must be carefully observed for undesirable or toxic effects. Clear instructions about the drug must be given when patients are transferred to other home health care facilities or discharged home. Other drugs used to relieve inflammatory conditions are the nonsteroidal antiinflammatory drugs (NSAIDs) and aspirin. Aspirin is used to diminish the joint inflammation associated with arthritis. NSAIDs and aspirin have a basic effect on the biochemistry of inflammation. However, both drugs can lead to serious bleeding complications and must be used cautiously; they should not be used in combination.

## NURSE ALERT

Check for allergies before giving any medication to a patient.

# KEY CONCEPTS

➤ Disease can be caused by microorganisms, nutritional imbalances, physical or chemical agents, or cellular abnormalities.

➤ Bacteria and viruses are examples of microorganisms. Nutritional imbalances include insufficient or excessive dietary intake, an unbalanced diet, excessive use of a specific nutrient, and failure of the body to use nutrients. Physical agents include trauma, changes in external temperature, electric current, radiation, atmospheric pressure, mechanical factors, and noise. Chemical agents include harmful substances and gases. Cellular abnormalities include cell damage from a lack of nutrients or oxygen, an altered environment, tumors, and defective genes.

➤ The major defense mechanisms of the body are the skin, mucous membranes, cilia, stomach acids, and reflexes, as well as the various cells and organs that participate in the inflammatory and immune responses.

➤ Characteristics of the inflammatory process include redness, heat, pain, swelling, and limitation of movement.

➤ Intervention for inflammation depends on the type of injury, the extent of involvement, and the effectiveness of the body's defense mechanisms. Heat and cold can be applied to affected areas to aid the healing process.

➤ The immune system works to counteract the effects of foreign materials, bacteria, viruses, food, and chemicals that constantly enter the body.

➤ Hypersensitivity is an inappropriate and excessive response of the immune system to certain substances that are not harmful to most people.

➤ Assessment techniques for allergic conditions include a detailed history, skin testing, mucous membrane tests, and elimination testing.

➤ Nursing interventions for people with allergies include administering drug therapy, assisting with immunotherapy, and teaching patients avoidance therapy.

➤ In an anaphylactic emergency the nurse is responsible for administering ordered medications, preparing for procedures such as oropharyngeal intubation, administering oxygen per order, and taking prescribed measures to prevent absorption of the antigen.

➤ Autoimmune diseases include rheumatoid arthritis, systemic lupus erythematosus, idiopathic thrombocytopenic purpura, myasthenia gravis, pernicious anemia, Hashimoto's thyroiditis, glomerulonephritis, multiple sclerosis, ulcerative colitis, and type I diabetes mellitus.

# CRITICAL THINKING EXERCISES

1. Relate the classic signs of infection to the underlying pathophysiologic changes.
2. What factors influence the pathogenicity of invading organisms?
3. Perform an allergy assessment on a friend or relative.
4. Design a plan for preventing insect stings for a small, rural community.

## REFERENCES AND ADDITIONAL READINGS

Beare P, Myers J: *Adult health nursing,* ed 3, St Louis, 1998, Mosby.

Benenson AS: *Control of communicable diseases manual,* ed 16, Washington, DC, 1995, American Public Health Association.

Chilmonczyk BA et al: Association between exposure to environmental tobacco smoke and exacerbation of asthma in children, *N Engl J Med* 328(23):1665-1669, 1993.

Clark SF, Queener SF, Karb VB: *Pharmacologic basis of nursing practice,* ed 5, St Louis, 1997, Mosby.

Guyton AC: *Textbook of medical physiology,* ed 9, Philadelphia, 1996, Saunders.

Howard BA: Guiding allergy sufferers through the medication maze, *RN* 57(4):26-31, 1994.

Huss K et al: Controlling allergies by assessing risks in the home, *Pediatr Nurs* 22(5):432-435, 1996.

Jacobs RL, Meltzer ED, Selner JC: Rhinitis: not just hay fever, *Patient Care* 23(6):168, 1989.

Lehne RA: *Pharmacology for nursing care,* ed 2, Philadelphia, 1994, Saunders.

Levinson WE, Jawetz E: *Medical microbiology and immunology examination and board review,* ed 3, Norwalk, Conn, 1994, Appleton & Lange.

Lewis SM, Collier IC, Heitkemper MM: *Medical-surgical nursing: assessment and management of clinical problems,* ed 4, St Louis, 1996, Mosby.

McCance KL, Huether SE: *Pathophysiology: the biologic basis for disease in adults and children,* ed 3, St Louis, 1998, Mosby.

Middleton E et al: *Allergy principles and practice,* ed 4, St Louis, 1993, Mosby.

Potter PA, Perry AG: *Fundamentals of nursing: concepts, process, and practice,* ed 4, St Louis, 1993, Mosby.

Thompson G, Ruane-Morris M, Lawton S: Lines of defence, *Nurs Times* 90(41):48-51, 1994.

Weigle WO: Immunologic tolerance: development or disruption, *Hosp Pract* 30(2):81-84, 1995.

Workman ML: Essential concepts of inflammation and immunity, *Crit Care Nurs Clin North Am* 7(4):601-615, 1995.

# CHAPTER 8

# Cultural Considerations

## CHAPTER OBJECTIVES

1 Gain beginning insight and skills into the delivery of culturally congruent nursing care.
2 Define culture.
3 Differentiate cultural customs, beliefs, and values.
4 Analyze one's own values and attitudes about common cultural concepts.
5 Explain the purpose of the field of transcultural nursing.
6 Name the three components of the transcultural triad.
7 Demonstrate the use of Leininger's three modes of nursing care decisions and actions.
8 Name two errors a nurse can make regarding patients who may be using alternative, nonconventional therapies.

## KEY TERMS

beliefs
cultural blindness
cultural conflict
cultural imposition
cultural relativity
culture
customs
ethnocentrism

monochronic time
polychronic time
stereotyping
subculture
sync time
transcultural nursing
values

It is hard to believe that for more than 100 years after the birth of modern nursing with Florence Nightingale in about 1860, the issue of a patient's culture was ignored. Dr. Madeleine Leininger, the first nurse to earn a doctorate in anthropology, began a lifelong crusade to change the status quo. Leininger's first book, *Nursing and Anthropology: Two Worlds to Blend*, published in 1970, awakened the profession of nursing to the relevance of culture in the causes and cures of illness and the cultural caring practices people expect when they are sick. It is now widely recognized that culture is a significant component of nursing care, but not all nurses know what *culturally congruent* nursing care is or how to provide it (Leininger, 1994). This chapter gives the nurse insight into the delivery of culturally congruent nursing care.

## PHENOMENON OF CULTURE

### What Culture Is. . .

When we hear the word *culture*, we often visualize only people who live in distant, exotic places and who behave in ways we may think are different and perhaps even strange or backward. However, culture is also the fabric of life. Every human being belongs to a culture.

**Culture** has been defined as values, beliefs, attitudes, and customs shared by a group of people that are passed from one generation to the next (Potter, 1997). Culture can be compared to an old pair of shoes; one does not think about them but just wears them comfortably day after day. Only when one puts on a brand new pair of shoes (i.e., is confronted with different cultural patterns) does one become uncomfortable.

Boyle and Andrews (1995) described the following four essential characteristics of culture.

First, as the definition clearly implies, culture is *learned* and transmitted. People begin learning their own culture from birth. Some who practice the Islamic faith whisper into the newborn's ear so that the first words he or she hears are from the Koran, the Holy Scriptures. Role relationships are part of a culture. One may believe that the term *brother* means a biologic sibling born of the same set of parents. However, African Americans may have a different meaning and define brother, or "bro," as any African American man. Other people may define a brother as any male first cousin on the maternal side of the family or even anyone who was breast-fed by the same woman. It soon becomes apparent that there are more cultural differences than similarities among the people of the world (Leininger, 1991). Thus a patient may completely misinterpret a nurse's very simple question about the patient's brothers. To avoid such misinterpretation, the nurse should be aware of these differences and clarify the meaning of the term with the patient.

> **NURSE ALERT**
>
> **Patients may misinterpret questions because of different cultural definitions of words or phrases. Be sure the meaning of a question is clear to the patient.**

Second, culture is *shared*. Members of the same group share culture both consciously and subconsciously. One may remember hearing, as a child, consciously shared rules such as, "Share your toys with your sister" or "You can't have dessert until you eat your vegetables." However, one probably does not remember learning that "baby boys don't wear the color pink." Such an idea probably was transmitted subconsciously. For most Americans it is culturally unacceptable for men to wear dresses. However, for people of Scottish heritage the skirt (kilt) is a symbol of pride and clan identity. In the Catholic religion priests wear cassocks that look like floor-length dresses. This sharing of common practices provides each group with part of its cultural identity. These exceptions to a so-called norm are culturally acceptable to most people, even if they do not belong to the group, often because these practices are widely recognized as a way of proclaiming who or what a person is.

Third, culture is an *adaptation* to one's environment that reflects the specific conditions, technical factors, and natural resources available to groups of people. For example, building homes with wide-open spaces in the outer walls instead of covered doors and windows would not be appropriate for the environmental conditions of cold northern climates. "Kangaroo care," a relatively new approach that began in Bogota, Colombia, is a means of survival for some low-birth-weight infants born into cultures in which "high-tech" equipment, such as an incubator, is unavailable. With kangaroo care the mother serves as a human incubator, like the kangaroo, which keeps its offspring warm in its pouch (Whitelaw et al, 1988). The mother holds the infant vertically between her breasts in skin-to-skin contact as much as possible. This cultural adaptation has been so successful that developed countries, including those with advanced technology, such as the United States, are adopting it as well (Miami Herald Medical Reports, 1995).

Fourth, culture is a *dynamic* and ever-changing process. Cultures change, but they change slowly in response to the conditions and needs of the group. Not too long ago the United States was known as a "throw away" society. Disposable needles and syringes replaced metal and glass ones, Styrofoam dishes and containers and plastic eating utensils replaced reusable ones, and disposable diapers replaced cloth ones. However, that "throw away" attitude is slowly changing as Americans become more aware of and responsive to the limited resources of the environment and the damage done by reckless use of these finite resources. In many cultures the roles of both men and women are changing. The idea of the man as the sole wage earner and the woman as the homemaker and child rearer is no longer the norm, and people are exploring alternative patterns of behavior that fit better with their needs and beliefs. The nursing profession in America is equally slow in changing and is still perceived as a female profession. Although every nurse belongs to a larger culture, nurses share many norms, values, and practices that make them a distinct group, known as a **subculture**. No culture can survive without being dynamic and adaptable to a changing world.

## . . . And What Culture Is Not

The characteristics a person acquires through genetics do not constitute culture. Racial and biologic characteristics and variations are part of the genetic legacy. When one member of a cultural group displays unique behaviors that are not common to the group, such behaviors are not a cultural characteristic. Just as there are more differences than similarities among cultures, so there are differences among individuals in a cultural group.

## Common Concepts

When a nurse cares for a patient of a particular culture and assumes that the patient will behave exactly as everyone else of that culture does, the nurse is **stereo-**

**typing.** Stereotyping prevents the nurse from performing an individualized assessment of the patient and his or her possible differences. In her research with Mexican American clinic patients, Shellenberger (1987) found that patients also stereotyped nurses. After interviewing her subjects about their health care practices, she noticed that no one had mentioned folk practices. She interviewed them again and was told that they had not talked about their cultural health practices because they thought an Anglo nurse would not be interested in hearing about them.

Unlike stereotyping, generalizing about the commonalities patients from a certain culture often hold increases a nurse's knowledge about that culture. Generalizing serves as a starting point for an individualized assessment of which cultural commonalities each individual patient believes and practices and which he or she does not (Geissler, 1994; Galanti, 1997).

Almost everyone has been guilty at some time of **ethnocentrism**, or harboring the attitude that one's own culture is the best one. Comparative judgments are made with other cultures that result in the conclusion that one's own culture is the only one that is normal and natural (Giger, Davidhizar, 1995). The opposite of ethnocentrism is **cultural relativity**. The nurse who approaches patients from the perspective of cultural relativity is open to the characteristics of culture and the wide variety of beliefs and practices that may result from being reared in different environments with different societal needs.

## Cultural Customs, Beliefs, and Values

Customs, beliefs, and values are the building blocks of all cultures. Although it is impossible for any nurse to be knowledgeable about every one of the thousands of cultures in the world, it is essential that nurses learn about a few of the cultures frequently encountered in their profession. Customs are the easiest to learn and recognize because they often are easy to see. **Customs** are habitual practices, or the usual way of acting under certain circumstances. When a patient wears a string of special blue beads around his or her wrist, when a patient does not look anyone directly in the eye when spoken to, when a woman cannot sign a consent form because she is a woman, when a man resists having his body hair shaved before a surgical procedure, or when a woman refuses to bathe after giving birth, deeply rooted cultural customs are being demonstrated.

**Beliefs,** or norms, are the rules that guide human behavior (Leininger, 1978). The rules tell a person what is appropriate or inappropriate behavior in a given situation or circumstance. Beliefs are more difficult to assess because they cannot be directly observed, but they can be learned by asking the right kind of questions,

such as, "What do *you* think caused this problem you're having now?" Some of the more common answers may include familiar Western biomedical explanations; or the problem may be explained as a punishment from God for a self-perceived transgression, as a loss of harmony or balance within the body, or as a hex cast on the patient either purposely or inadvertently by another person. Patients often believe that the cause of an illness dictates the type of treatment. Western biomedical caregivers cannot cure a magicoreligious type of problem. Special help is sought from a folk practitioner who is knowledgeable about the cause of and cure for these special problems.

**Values** are "goals to which behavior is directed" (Boyle, Andrews, 1995). Values are within the realm of the unconscious mind, and an individual may not even realize that he or she holds them. Therefore they are the most difficult to assess. Kluckholn (1953) conceptualized several options that different cultures commonly hold about the basic values of life. For example, one may be asked, "What is your basic value about the environment? Do you believe that the environment controls *you* or that you should live and coexist in harmony with the environment? Do you believe that human beings control the environment?" One may wonder, "Do I just think that's the way it should be, or do my behaviors demonstrate my belief?" One may also be asked, "What do you believe about your relationship to others? Do you believe that it is an ordered succession with a continuity that is based primarily on heredity and kinship, that the family as a group is more important than any individual within it, or that independence and autonomy of the individual are paramount?"

People differ in their views about health and illness. One person may believe that health is the result of choices and actions, another may believe that it is an inevitable balance of sickness and wellness throughout life, and another may believe that illness is sent by God or some supernatural force as punishment for wrongdoing. Such values have a subtle yet tremendous impact on patients' motivations and reactions to health care.

When a nurse and a patient and family believe and behave according to different values, beliefs, and customs, a **cultural conflict** can result. Figure 8-1 shows two icebergs. One iceberg represents the nurse and the other the patient. Customs reside near the tip of the icebergs, above the waterline, where they can be observed, acknowledged, and dealt with. Beliefs are close to the waterline and may or may not be observable. The greatest difficulty lies in the conflicting values, which are hidden well below the waterline. When these two icebergs collide, the collision is felt at this deepest level, where the impact actually occurs.

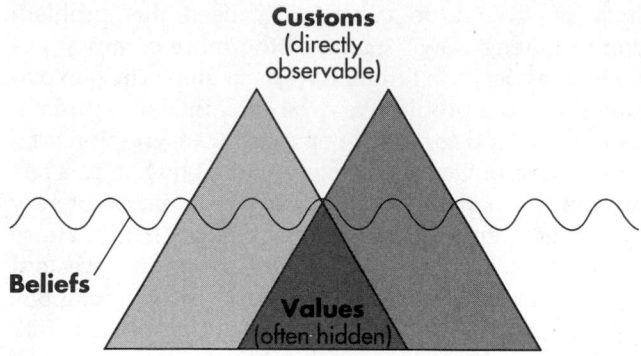

**Figure 8-1** One iceberg symbolizes the nurse's cultural customs, beliefs, and values, and the second iceberg symbolizes those of the patient and family. Cultural conflict may occur at any level but is most serious when deeply held and hidden values (i.e., those below the "waterline") clash and are not recognized by the participants.

## TRANSCULTURAL NURSING

The field of **transcultural nursing** is a formal area of study and practice conceived by Leininger in the mid-1950s. Leininger (1978) defined transcultural nursing as "the area of nursing which focuses upon the comparative study and analysis of different cultures and subcultures with respect to nursing and health-illness caring practices, beliefs, and values with the goal of generating scientific and humanistic knowledge, and of using this knowledge to provide culture-specific and culture-universal nursing care practices." Since the 1960s, courses and programs have been established by nursing leaders trained in anthropology and transcultural nursing. The Transcultural Nursing Society was founded in 1974 as a worldwide organization for nurses interested in and prepared to advance transcultural nursing. The society serves as a forum for bringing nurses with common and diverse interests together to improve care to culturally diverse people. The *Journal of Transcultural Nursing,* founded in 1989, focuses on transcultural nursing theory, research, and practice. Since 1989, nurses have been certified as transcultural nurses (CTNs) (Transcultural Nursing Society).

### Alternative Therapies

The *New England Journal of Medicine* reports that in 1990, one in three Americans, an estimated 61 million people, used alternative, nontraditional therapies for problems such as cancer, arthritis, chronic back pain, acquired immunodeficiency syndrome, gastrointestinal problems, chronic renal failure, and eating disorders (Eisenberg et al, 1993). Of the various therapies studied, relaxation techniques, chiropractic care, and massage were used most often. The estimated number

of visits to providers of these treatments was higher than the number of visits to traditional Western physicians in the same year. These data are even more significant because the study did not include visits to herbalists, curanderas, medicine men and women, or other important folk practitioners. The message is clear: Large numbers of Americans are consulting nontraditional health care practitioners.

Some people may use and combine nontraditional therapies with the biomedical regimens prescribed by their physicians. Others may decamp from the health care system because they are dissatisfied with the results obtained from Western medicine and want to seek help from folk practitioners. The nurse can make two serious errors with regard to patients who may be using alternative therapies. The first is failing to ask about alternative therapies that the patient may be using concurrently so that the effects of interaction between the two systems can be evaluated. The second is assuming that the patient who has not kept Western appointments or sought Western treatments has received no health care during this time. A nurse with an education in transcultural nursing can be a valuable resource when assessing, planning, and evaluating nursing care in situations involving culturally diverse patients.

### Transcultural Triad

The American Nurses Association's position statement on cultural diversity in nursing practice identifies three interacting systems in nurse-patient encounters: "the culture of the nurse, the culture of the patient, and the culture of the setting" (American Nurses Association, 1991). The patient is not the only person whose culture affects the nurse-patient relationship. Nurses bring their own customs, beliefs, and values into this *transcultural triadic relationship.* The nurse who understands the particular culture of a patient may still be missing part of the equation. Understanding oneself is the starting point for understanding the culturally diverse patient. When the two icebergs meet below the waterline, the nurse will be unable to understand fully why cultural conflict ensues unless the nurse recognizes his or her own subconscious cultural behaviors. Without cultural self-understanding, the nurse's negative reactions to cultural conflict may include ethnocentrism and stereotyping or cultural blindness and cultural imposition.

**Cultural blindness** occurs when the nurse ignores the patient's differences and proceeds to give care as if those differences do not exist. Cultural blindness is a sign of ignorance of the differences in cultural expression. **Cultural imposition** is closely tied to ethnocentrism. It occurs when the nurse expects the patient to conform to the cultural norms of the nurse and the hospital or health care agency. The nurse may be thinking, "You're here in my hospital, and you'll just have to do things our way." Such a negative reaction can cause a breakdown in nurse-patient communication, the nurse-patient relationship, and even in patient compliance because of the patient's feelings of loss of trust and security. Some hospitals ask patients who are about to be discharged to fill out a questionnaire rating their satisfaction with the care they received during their hospitalization. Although patients may have received very high quality nursing care, some may respond that they were dissatisfied with their care. One reason may be that their cultural needs were not recognized and met.

The third part of the triad is the often bureaucratic health care setting, with which the patient and family must interact and that often expects conformity with its norms. Some people believe that vigilance over a sick relative is a prescribed extended family role. Hospital rules that restrict visitors in an intensive care unit to two people for 15 minutes every hour are difficult to deal with. When a small waiting room becomes so full of this extended family that other patients' families complain about not having a place to sit, the nurse becomes involved.

## Nursing Care Decisions and Actions

Leininger's theory of cultural care diversity and universality offers three nursing strategies, called modes of action or decision, that guide nurses in providing culturally congruent care (Reynolds, 1993). These modes of action originate from the premise that "cultures have folk and professional care values, beliefs, and practices in Western and non-Western cultures" (Leininger, 1991). Elements of two different health systems may be in operation at one time. The nurse is operating under a professional system that influences the nurse's decisions and actions. At the same time, a culturally diverse patient may be operating, at least in part, under a folk system that guides his or her decisions and actions. The potential for conflict between the two systems exists. To avoid conflict and to make decisions that result in more culturally congruent care, the nurse gathers information from the patient and family about the customs, beliefs, and values relevant to promoting, maintaining, or restoring health within the patient's present circumstances. The nurse then chooses one of the following modes of action to minimize cultural conflict and meet the patient's needs.

1. "Cultural care preservation or maintenance refers to those assistive, supportive, or enabling professional actions and decisions that help patients of a particular culture to preserve or maintain a state of

health or to recover from illness and to face death" (Leininger, 1988).

For example, an East Asian woman who has no dietary restrictions wants her family to bring her an herbal tea that she always uses to calm her "nervous stomach." The nurse asks what is in the tea and learns that it contains nothing that would be contraindicated with her medications. Her family is encouraged to bring the tea. The decision and mode of action are not harmful to the patient and, in her opinion, may be beneficial. The worst that could happen would be that the tea would be medically neutral (i.e., neither harmful nor helpful). From the patient's point of view, however, it is important that her cultural belief has been preserved.

2. "Cultural care accommodation or negotiation refers to those assistive, supportive, or enabling professional actions and decisions that help patients of a particular culture to adapt to or negotiate for a beneficial or satisfying health status or to face death" (Leininger, 1988).

Either the patient or the hospital, or both, may need to accommodate in this mode. A classic example of unknown origin concerns a hospitalized, dying Gypsy king. According to the Gypsy culture, the king should die on the ground, but it was very cold outside and snow covered the ground. Two solutions were devised for resolving this dilemma: (1) When close to death, the king would be placed on the floor beside his hospital bed, or (2) a long rope would be brought in, one end placed in the king's hand, and the other end lowered through an open window until it touched the ground. Either of these creative solutions would meet the patient's needs in a culturally satisfying way.

3. "Cultural care repatterning or restructuring refers to those assistive, supportive, or enabling professional actions or decisions that help patients change their lifeways for new or different patterns that are culturally meaningful and satisfying or that support beneficial and healthy life patterns" (Leininger, 1988).

Nurses may be faced with situations in which they understand the patient's cultural belief but also believe that they could not professionally or ethically support or negotiate the practice because it would harm the patient. For example, some mothers believe that they should stop giving a baby fluids when the baby gets diarrhea. The nurse cannot respect this belief, nor can the nurse negotiate that the mother give the child only half the fluids it so desperately needs. Both are potentially life-threatening alternatives. In a respectful and nonthreatening way, the nurse tries to work with the mother to restructure this aspect of her belief system. For example, there may be one or two appropriate and cul-

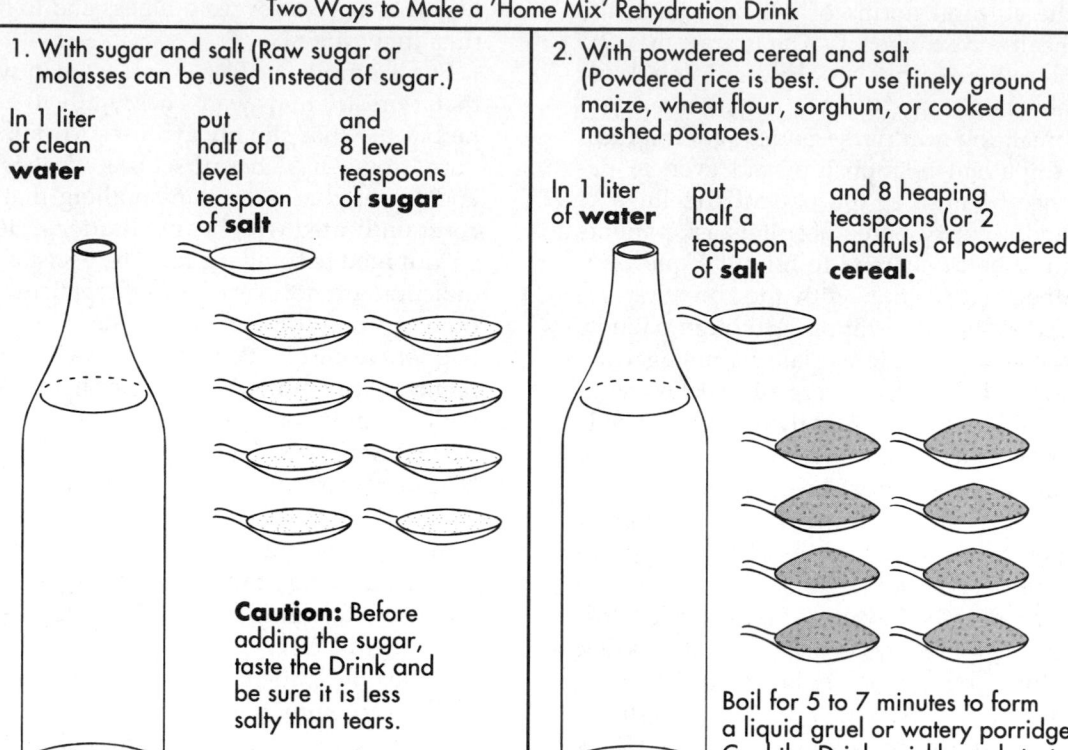

Two Ways to Make a 'Home Mix' Rehydration Drink

1. With sugar and salt (Raw sugar or molasses can be used instead of sugar.)

In 1 liter of clean **water** — put half of a level teaspoon of **salt** — and 8 level teaspoons of **sugar**

**Caution:** Before adding the sugar, taste the Drink and be sure it is less salty than tears.

2. With powdered cereal and salt (Powdered rice is best. Or use finely ground maize, wheat flour, sorghum, or cooked and mashed potatoes.)

In 1 liter of **water** — put half a teaspoon of **salt** — and 8 heaping teaspoons (or 2 handfuls) of powdered **cereal.**

Boil for 5 to 7 minutes to form a liquid gruel or watery porridge. Cool the Drink quickly and start giving it to the child.

To either Drink add half a cup of fruit juice, coconut water, or mashed ripe banana, if available. This provides potassium, which may help the child accept more food and drink.

**CAUTION:** Taste the Drink each time before you give it to be sure it is not spoiled. Cereal drinks can spoil in a few hours in hot weather.

**IMPORTANT:** Adapt the Drink to your area. If liter containers or teaspoons are not in most homes, adjust quantities to local forms of measurement. Where people traditionally give cereal gruels to young children, add enough water to make it liquid, and use that. Look for an easy and simple way.

Give the dehydrated person sips of this Drink every 5 minutes, day and night, until he or she begins to urinate normally. A large person needs 3 or more liters a day. A small child usually needs at least 1 liter a day, or 1 glass for each watery stool. Keep giving the Drink *often* in small sips, *even if the person vomits.* Not all of the Drink will be vomited.

**Figure 8-2**    A homemade or commercial oral rehydration mixture is an internationally recognized and potentially lifesaving method of treating dehydration. (From Werner D: *Where there is no doctor,* Palo Alto, Calif, 1992, Hesperian Foundation.)

turally preferred fluids that the mother would be willing to give the child, or the mother may be willing to be taught to make an oral rehydration mixture from home ingredients as a special "medicine" for her child (Figure 8-2) (Werner, 1992).

## CULTURAL VARIABILITY

In addition to cultural variations that involve health care beliefs and practices, there are variations in everyday behaviors to which little or no conscious thought is given (Figure 8-3). Awareness of such differences in

nurse-patient interactions is essential for effective interpersonal interactions, the development of respect and trust between individuals, and the patient's satisfaction with the self-perceived quality of nursing care.

## Perceptions of Time

Perception of time is one of the core values of a culture. People are controlled by time and usually believe that everyone else perceives time in exactly the same way. However, there are many different perceptions of time. Anthropologist Edward T. Hall (1983) has extensively

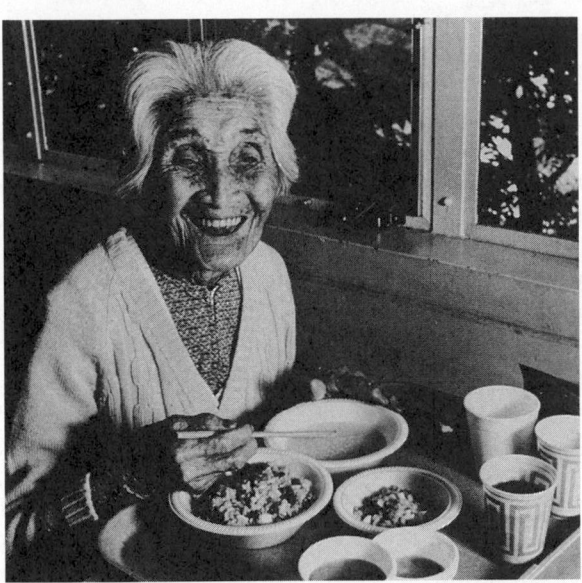

**Figure 8-3**    Oriental food and chopsticks make a meal enjoyable for this older Japanese woman. (Courtesy Ken Yamaguchi. From Castillo HM: *The nurse assistant in long-term care: a rehabilitative approach*, St Louis, 1992, Mosby.)

researched people's perceptions of time, and three forms of this perception are particularly relevant to nursing care.

**Monochronic time** is a form of time perception that is very familiar to many Americans (Hall, 1983). This form perceives time as linear and as clearly divided into yesterday, today, and tomorrow. People develop lists of priorities and concentrate on getting one thing done before moving on to the next. People often keep personal schedule books to organize their daily or weekly activities. Time is treated as a physical commodity that can be bought and sold. People who perceive time as monochronic speak about time that is spent, saved, killed, lost, wasted, or made up, and they use many other descriptive words usually used to refer to tangible objects. The primary goal for people with this perception of time is to get tasks done. As with all components of culture, this perception of time is arbitrary, learned, and transmitted from our early caregivers. It is neither correct nor incorrect but is just how some people view time. When the nurse says to a patient, "I'll be back in 15 minutes," the patient with a monochronic time view expects the nurse to reappear within approximately 15 minutes, not an hour later. The patient gets more annoyed as more and more time passes and the nurse does not return. Nurses react the same way when the situation is reversed.

People who share a **polychronic time** perception do not behave in a linear way. They prefer to be involved in and interacting with several people or things simultaneously. Schedules, if written at all, are not firm, and

plans may be changed at the last second. Rather than focusing on tasks and what should come next, those with polychronic perception focus on people and relationships. Caring about interruptions in human relationships has a much higher priority. For such people it is much more important to stop and chat than it is to break off a conversation just to be on time for an appointment. These people do not constantly look at the clock. Some Latin American, Middle Eastern, and Mediterranean cultures value this less rigid, nonlinear perception of time (Hall, 1983). Patients may miss or be late for clinic appointments for many reasons, including difficulties traveling to the clinic or in finding a responsible adult for child care, but another possibility is that the patient may be following a polychronic perception of time. The nurse may evaluate the late patient negatively, when in fact the patient is simply placing a higher value on people than on a bureaucratic and often rigid time schedule.

**Sync** (for synchrony) **time** is a form of time perception that has not been as widely researched but can be very significant in patient interactions. According to Hall (1983), greater awareness of sync time began when silent movies started to have soundtracks and it became necessary to synchronize the soundtrack with the moving pictures. Hall states that, "though it took the white man thousands of years to discover 'sync time,' the Mescalero Apaches have known its significance for centuries." Rhythm is the basic ingredient of synchrony and is an indispensable factor in nurse-patient relationships. Imagine a hospitalized patient who has been lying quietly in bed for several hours. Suddenly a nurse who has been busy running around the unit enters this patient's room and says, "I need to get you out of bed for a little walk once more before I go off duty in a few minutes. Are these your slippers? Where's your bathrobe? Do you want to use the bathroom while you're up?" At the same time the nurse is lowering the head of the bed and pulling down the patient's bedcovers. Nurse and patient are completely out of sync! To the patient, the nurse is trying to make him or her move at the speed of light, and to the nurse, the patient is not moving fast enough to accomplish this task in the time available. The entire mismatch can be avoided if the nurse lets the patient know in advance what is going to happen and gives the patient a chance to prepare mentally and physically. When the nurse recognizes the importance of being in sync with the patient on middle ground, the probable result is that the ambulation time will be more successful and satisfying for both.

Hall (1983) credits the Japanese with a much higher recognition of the impact of synchrony and gives the example of a sumo wrestling match in which the referee will not allow a match to start until the two wrestlers synchronize their breathing. Nurses need to learn to become referees during the many nursing care interactions and interventions affected by sync time.

For 15 years Levine (1990) researched people's attitudes toward time and the tempo of cultures, as well as the health consequences of both. The research was conducted in nine cities in each of the four regions of the United States. Results indicated that the pace of life is faster in the Northeast, followed by the Midwest, the South, and the West. A significant relationship existed between the pace of life, the rate of cigarette smoking, and death from ischemic heart disease.

The same study also was conducted in six countries with Eastern and Western cultures and varying degrees of economic development. The fastest pace was measured in Japan, followed by the United States, England, Taiwan, Italy, and Indonesia. Therefore self-selection of a fast track versus a slow track pace of life can be one indicator of the environmental dimension of culture.

## Use of Space

Hall (1966) coined the word *proxemics* to describe the study of people's use of social and personal space as a cultural phenomenon and nonverbal communication pattern. Within different cultures rather precise distances are considered appropriate or inappropriate, and these distances often depend on the roles of the individuals and the closeness of their social relationship. Breaking the unwritten and unspoken rules of culturally learned spatial distances can be stressful. A number of body organs and receptors are involved in the use of space. Seeing, hearing, smelling, heat gain and loss, and touch are important barometers that determine the range of space a person finds comfortable in a variety of situations. For example, being close enough to breathe on one another is a common behavior of many Arab cultures, whereas being close enough to detect body odor is avoided in other cultures (Hall, 1966). In some cultures being close enough to touch frequently is a vital component of communication, whereas in other cultures people stand in a crowded elevator with arms pressed in close to the body to avoid touching and feel relieved when some people exit the elevator and make more space available for their body.

Hall (1966) classifies the space envelopes, or protective personal invisible bubbles of space, into four general ranges. *Intimate space* is 15 to 45 cm (6 to 18 inches) and involves smell, heat, the feel of the other's breath, and distorted sight. In *personal space*, which is 45 cm to 1.2 m (18 inches to 4 feet), the visual distortion lessens, but one must still shift the gaze by looking into one eye

at a time. Body heat is not detectable, but even at its farthest distance people can still touch each other at arm's length. Personal discussions occur within this range, and individual cultures determine the degree of closeness needed for satisfying communication. *Social space,* which ranges from 1.2 to 3.6 m (4 to 12 feet), often is used for less personal business or social interactions. At its farther distances, the entire face can be taken in at a glance, and shifting from one eye to the other is not needed. Finally, *public space* is more than 3.6 m (12 feet), which causes significant changes in behaviors. At this distance people are more careful of their choice of words, and phrasing, grammar, and syntax are calculated to serve a more "speech-making" type of interaction.

A family member or professional colleague may approach a nurse at the nurse's station, and the nurse may take small backward steps because the person seems to be moving too closely into the protective space bubble. As the nurse moves backward, the person moves in to close the gap because he or she is becoming uncomfortable with the distance. Americans use the phrase, "Get out of my face," to express the discomfort experienced with this degree of closeness. The nurse may perceive this family member or colleague as pushy, aggressive, demanding, or intrusive. In contrast, the other person may be perceiving the nurse as uncaring, cold, aloof, or disinterested. Communication is breaking down on a subconscious, nonverbal level, regardless of how effectively the verbal words are being exchanged. Both parties come away dissatisfied and may not know why they feel as they do. However, the dissatisfaction may simply have been a result of the differences in cultural perceptions of space.

Each space category has both close and distant ranges that alter behavior, and these may overlap. For example, does the change of shift report occur in personal or social space? The size of the group, the size of the room, the presence of physical barriers such as a rectangular table around which everyone is seated, and how well the participants get along all dictate, or at least influence, the use of space. The rules may also be changed to accommodate the role of the individual. For example, a nurse must frequently enter a patient's intimate or personal space during nursing care activities. For some patients this may be acceptable, but for others the nurse should be aware that permission may be needed for such necessary closeness. For example, before urinary catheterization of a woman, a nurse might say to a patient, "I'm going to have to get really close to be able to see clearly the small hole into which I need to insert this catheter. The better I can see, the more comfortable I can make this for you." As with all cultural variations, the use of space varies both among and within different cultural groups (Dolphin, 1994).

## Use of Touch

As with space, the unspoken rules of and rather precise limits on the use of touch vary considerably. The appropriateness of touch is determined by several factors, including duration, location, intensity, frequency, action, and the sensation conveyed. Touch must also be situationally appropriate. In the United States touch is believed to be an important part of nursing care. Lack of knowledge about the reaction of a specific culture to touch may inhibit the nurse-patient interaction and even cause fear. In the Vietnamese culture the head is considered the seat of the soul. Touching and performing invasive procedures on the head or in the various openings of the head may be highly stressful because of the fear that the soul may be lost (Geissler, 1994). Even placing on a pillow a piece of clothing that is worn on the lower body may be objectionable to some Southeast Asian patients. People of English, German, or Japanese heritage may prefer minimal touching during interactions, whereas Hispanics and Arabs may prefer more touching.

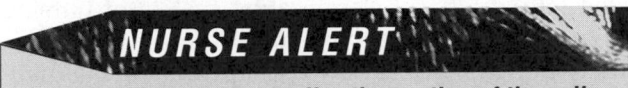

**NURSE ALERT**

Touch may neutralize the casting of the evil eye.

According to Spector (1991), the evil eye is one of the oldest and most common superstitions that exist in many cultures of the world. It is a common Hispanic and Mediterranean belief. The evil eye may be cast to project harm on an object or a person or when something, especially a child, is admired or criticized. There are many differing beliefs among people and cultures regarding who can cast the evil eye, the purpose for which it is cast, how it is cast, the effect it has on the person receiving it, and the cultural practices used to protect against it. Nurses may inadvertently cast the evil eye. Touch is one practice that may neutralize or undo the casting of the evil eye (Giger, 1991). For example, when telling a mother that her child is pretty or handsome, the nurse should simultaneously touch the child.

Nurses may or may not touch people frequently as a result of cultural values that guide their behaviors. Sensitivity to both the nurse's and the patient's desire for and reaction to touch should be assessed to deliver culturally congruent care. Touch should never be forced on or withheld from patients who have different perceptions of its meaning and importance.

## Eye Contact

People from some cultures, such as Arab ones, have such prolonged eye contact that they may seem confrontational to the uninitiated. Other cultural groups, particularly the Navajo people and Asians, use less eye contact or the "lighthouse sweep" during interactions (Geissler, 1994). Downcast eyes partly may reflect respect for authority figures. Some people are sensitive to the physiologic changes that occur in the pupil of the eye during interactions. Pupils tend to dilate slightly when one is interested and constrict slightly with disagreement or disinterest (Geissler, 1994). Cultures that prefer a narrower space between individuals may also be cultures that use more prolonged direct eye contact, with the ability to evaluate changes in pupil size.

**NURSE ALERT**

The nurse may be perceived as an authority figure. Patients may believe that looking the nurse directly in the eye for a sustained interval might challenge the nurse's authority and be considered unacceptable behavior.

Anglo-Americans use a moderate amount of direct eye contact during interactions. They are comfortable with some direct eye contact and may interpret a lack of eye contact as uncertainty, embarrassment, or even lying. These attitudes are reflected in the common phrase, "Now look me straight in the eye and tell me the truth." Yet Anglo-Americans are also comfortable with looking past the side of the face or away from the face. The former may be interpreted as "I'm thinking or considering what you are saying," and the latter, as long as it does not last very long, may be interpreted as a fleeting but acceptable momentary distraction. It is the total pattern that cultures find significant during an interaction rather than each discrete eye movement.

Time, space, touch, and eye contact are but a few examples of cultural variability. There are many other factors, including birth and death rites, reactions to pain, family dominance patterns, gender-specific roles, child-rearing beliefs and practices, communication patterns with authority figures such as health care professionals, and the family's role in hospital care. For example, some people from East Indian and Middle Eastern cultures insist on a professional caregiver of the same gender. Such restrictions should be honored whenever feasible by involving the family in care or by altering patient assignments. All these factors play simultaneous roles within some cultures and help determine when and when not to use a particular variable. The patient or family is the best data source for the assessment of cultural differences and similarities. The nurse must be aware of potential differences that could be critical to the patient's responses to nursing care, health restoration, and health maintenance.

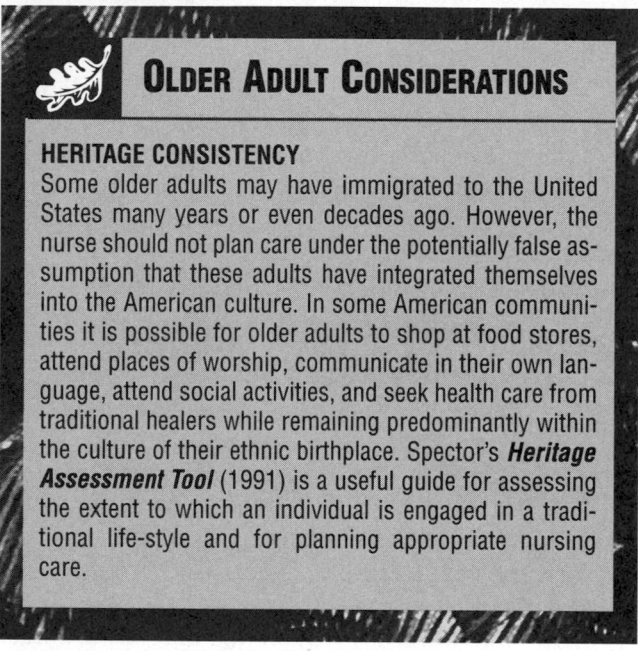

**OLDER ADULT CONSIDERATIONS**

**HERITAGE CONSISTENCY**
Some older adults may have immigrated to the United States many years or even decades ago. However, the nurse should not plan care under the potentially false assumption that these adults have integrated themselves into the American culture. In some American communities it is possible for older adults to shop at food stores, attend places of worship, communicate in their own language, attend social activities, and seek health care from traditional healers while remaining predominantly within the culture of their ethnic birthplace. Spector's *Heritage Assessment Tool* (1991) is a useful guide for assessing the extent to which an individual is engaged in a traditional life-style and for planning appropriate nursing care.

## NURSING DIAGNOSES

The use or misuse of nursing diagnoses with the culturally diverse patient has raised several questions in recent years (Leininger, 1990). Transcultural nursing recognizes that, regardless of a patient's medical diagnosis, it is important to plan nursing care that reflects the patient's unique health care beliefs and practices. The official list of nursing diagnoses of the North American Nursing Diagnosis Association (NANDA) does not adequately address the cultural needs of patients (Geissler, 1991, 1992). Nursing diagnoses that have been used with patients include actual, high risk, or potential for spiritual distress, impaired verbal communication, social isolation, noncompliance, and relocation stress syndrome.

A few examples illustrate the problem. When a patient does not speak English, who has the actual problem with verbal communication? Is the patient or the nurse to blame when both are adequately fluent in their own languages? The problem is one of mutual understanding or lack of it, not inability to communi-

cate verbally. Patients with limited English skills can experience extreme stress when trying to communicate in English. It can be frustrating and exhausting to express oneself in such a circumstance, and the patient may not be sure that the message was understood accurately.

The NANDA diagnosis is directed at verbal communication and does not address the critical role that nonverbal communication plays in human expression. Understanding nonverbal messages is important to mutual understanding. The diagnosis of noncompliance implies that a patient has made an informed decision to comply or not to comply, but for many the term *nonadherence* may be more acceptable. The term *compliance* implies that the patient must or should follow the medical and nursing regimens prescribed by the dominant health care system's practitioners. However, there are many valid ways of viewing health and illness. When a patient does not hold the same egocentric health care beliefs and values as the Western biomedical system, he or she may be falsely labeled as noncompliant. Therefore the nursing diagnosis of noncompliance can become a manifestation of the nurse's own culture, and a value conflict between the nurse and the patient may result.

Until transcultural nursing is adequately incorporated into an official classification system of nursing diagnoses, nurses may have to rely on their own creativity in writing culturally appropriate nursing diagnoses. Possible new nursing diagnoses have been suggested, including cultural distress, compromised health beliefs, broken beliefs, conflict in belief system, fear of witchcraft, biologic variations, alterations in caring patterns, and translocation syndrome.

## PATIENT AND FAMILY TEACHING

Patient and family teaching may present some unique challenges for the nurse because the patient may not speak or be sufficiently fluent in English to ensure understanding of the material being taught (Figure 8-4). A translator or interpreter may be used. However, there may be significant differences in the information communicated by translators and interpreters. Also, translators or interpreters may not be available, and too often the nurse resorts to using visitors or even other patients as interpreters. Languages cannot be translated word for word, and the risk of failing to communicate a message accurately is high. Sometimes a patient's young children who attend English language schools are used very inappropriately as interpreters, such as using a young boy to interpret a discussion about birth control to his mother. Despite how well the boy seems to speak English, he may not have the sex education background to interpret the words,

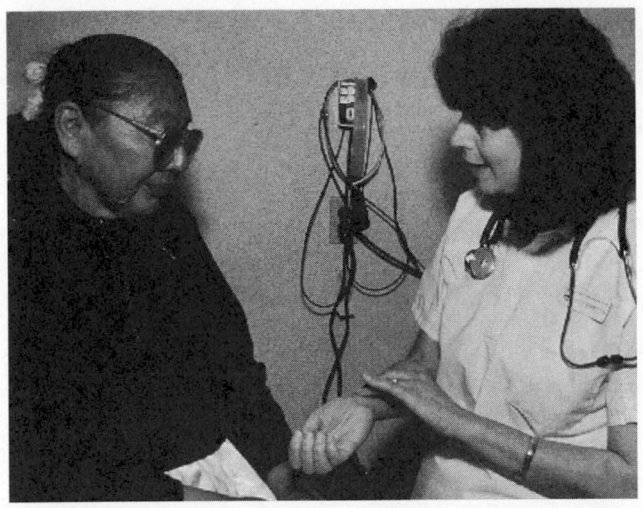

**Figure 8-4** A nurse shows a non-English-speaking patient how to take a pulse. (Courtesy Michael Clement, MD, Mesa, Ariz.)

**ETHICAL DILEMMA**

1 How should a nurse respond to a patient who confides that he or she is also currently under the care of a folk healer because the patient does not fully trust the physician's ability to heal?
2 How should a nurse respond when the same patient opens a bag in the bedside stand and displays the folk medicines that he or she is taking while in the hospital?
3 What should the nurse do if the same patient refuses to let the nurse tell anyone about the folk treatments?

or cultural taboos may be violated regarding what a child, especially a boy, can speak about with his mother.

The nurse may also need to include the husband or eldest member of the family in any discussions. Family dominance patterns may require these individuals to be involved in any decision-making or teaching-learning activities. The American culture tends to value the autonomy and independence of the individual patient in deciding what is best for him or her. However, this is not true in many other cultures in which family members, particularly the elders or males, play an integral role in deciding what is best for the patient. Therefore both the patient and significant family members must be well informed. In this situation teaching sessions become a dialogue among all participants rather than just a lecture given to the patient. The patient needs to be asked beforehand who should be included in the discussion, and a time for the teaching must be scheduled when the important individuals can be present. If relevant teaching materials are available in the patient's own language, they can be obtained in advance.

# KEY CONCEPTS

➤ Culture is defined as the homogeneous and learned patterns of behavior, values, and attitudes that are shared by a group of people and passed from one generation to the next.

➤ Culture is learned, shared, and dynamic behavior that represents an adaptation to the environment.

➤ Cultural definitions of words and phrases vary; therefore it is essential that the meaning of questions is clear to patients.

➤ Generalizing about the commonalities that patients from a specific culture often hold is a starting point for individualized assessment.

➤ Cultural relativity implies that a person is open to the wide variety of beliefs and practices that are characteristic of a specific culture.

➤ Cultural customs, beliefs, and values are the building blocks of all cultures.

➤ Transcultural nursing focuses on the comparative study and analysis of different cultures and subcultures as a way of providing universal and culture-specific nursing care practices.

➤ Common alternative therapies practiced by various cultures include relaxation techniques, chiropractic care, and massage.

➤ Nurse-patient relationships include three interacting systems that together are called the transcultural triad: the culture of the nurse, the culture of the patient, and the culture of the setting.

➤ Modes of action for nursing care decisions and actions include cultural care preservation or maintenance, cultural care accommodation or negotiation, and cultural care repatterning or restructuring.

➤ The nurse's understanding of cultural variability in the perception of time, the use of space, the use of touch, eye contact, and other factors is critical to the patient's response to nursing care, health restoration, and health maintenance.

➤ It is important to note that there may be significant differences in the communications that result from translators and interpreters.

# CRITICAL THINKING EXERCISES

1. An Asian American patient's family wants to prepare and bring all of her meals to the hospital. What must you consider and do to make this happen?

2. You are assigned to an alert patient who speaks no English. No family members are present when you give care, and no one on the unit speaks the patient's language. Although an interpreter is present in the hospital, she cannot be there when you are there. What creative ways might you devise to accomplish some very basic communication with your patient?

3. Your African American patient closely follows his Islamic faith. Friday is his day of worship, certain foods are forbidden, and he prays to Mecca five times a day. Describe how you would facilitate his culturally congruent religious care.

4. Choose a culturally diverse patient on your unit and examine the Kardex, nurses' notes, nursing diagnosis, and problem list. Are any cultural considerations noted in these records? If so, how are they actually carried over into the patient's nursing care? If not, should there be? What are your suggestions, and how would you put them into practice?

## REFERENCES AND ADDITIONAL READINGS

American Nurses Association: *Position statement on cultural diversity in nursing practice,* Kansas City, Mo, 1991, The Association.

Boyle JS, Andrews MM: *Transcultural concepts in nursing care,* Glenview, Ill, 1995, Scott, Foresman.

Dolphin CZ: Variables in the use of personal space in intercultural transactions. In Samovar LA, Porter RE, editors: *Intercultural communication,* ed 4, Belmont, Calif, 1994, Wadsworth.

Eisenberg DM et al: Unconventional medicine in the United States, *N Engl J Med* 328(4):246-283, 1993.

Galanti GA: *Caring for patients from different cultures: case studies for American hospitals,* ed 2, Philadelphia, 1997, University of Pennsylvania Press.

Geissler EM: Transcultural nursing and nursing diagnoses, *Nurs Health Care* 12(4):190-192, 203, 1991.

Geissler EM: Nursing diagnoses: a study of cultural relevance, *J Prof Nurs* 8(5):301-307, 1992.

Geissler EM: *Pocket guide to cultural assessment,* St Louis, 1994, Mosby.

Giger JN, Davidhizar RE: *Transcultural nursing: assessment and intervention,* St Louis, 1991, Mosby.

Giger JN, Davidhizar RE: *Transcultural nursing: assessment and intervention,* St Louis, 1995, Mosby.

Hall ET: *The hidden dimension,* Garden City, NY, 1966, Doubleday.

Hall ET: *The dance of life: the other dimension of time,* New York, 1983, Anchor Books.

Kluckholn FR: Dominant and variant value orientations. In Kluckholn C, Murray HA, editors: *Personality in nature: society and culture,* New York, 1953, Knopf.

Leininger MM: *Nursing and anthropology: two worlds to blend,* New York, 1970, John Wiley & Sons.

Leininger MM: *Transcultural nursing: concepts, theories, and practices,* New York, 1978, John Wiley & Sons.

Leininger MM: Leininger's theory of nursing: cultural care diversity and universality, *Nurs Sci Q* 1(4):152-156, 1988.

Leininger MM: Issues, questions, and concerns related to the nursing diagnosis cultural movement from a transcultural nursing perspective, *J Transcult Nurs* 2(1):23-31, 1990.

Leininger MM: Leininger's theory of cultural care diversity and universality, Livonia, Mich, 1991, Madonna University (videotape).

Leininger MM: Are nurses prepared to function worldwide? *J Transcult Nurs* 5(2):2-4, 1994.

Levine RV: The pace of life, *Am Scient* 78(5):450-459, 1990.

Miami Herald Medical Reports: *Mt. Sinai Medical Center: award-winning Kangaroo Care,* Miami, 1995, Miami Herald.

Potter PA, Perry AG: *Fundamentals of nursing: concepts, process and practice,* ed 4, St Louis, 1997, Mosby.

Reynolds CL, Leininger MM: *Cultural care diversity and universality theory,* Newbury Park, Calif, 1995, Sage Publications.

Shellenberger JM: A practice model for culturally appropriate nursing care in a primary healthcare setting for Mexican-American persons, Doctoral Dissertation, 1987, University of Texas at Austin.

Spector RE: *Heritage assessment tool: cultural diversity in health and illness,* ed 3, Norwalk, Conn, 1991, Appleton & Lange.

Transcultural Nursing Society: *Historical facts about the society,* Livonia, Mich, The Society (pamphlet).

Werner D: *Where there is no doctor,* Palo Alto, Calif, 1992, Hesperian Foundation.

Whitelaw A et al: Skin to skin contact for very low birth weight infants and their mothers, *Arch Dis Child* 63:1377-1381, 1988.

# CHAPTER 9

# The Older Adult

## CHAPTER OBJECTIVES

1 Discuss the effects on the health care system of the increasing number of people over age 65 in the United States.
2 Discuss socioeconomic and cultural factors that affect the older adult.
3 Identify biologic, psychologic, and social changes related to aging.
4 Identify the adjustments usually required of the aging individual.
5 Discuss the factors involved in maintaining mental health for a person over 65 years of age.
6 Discuss current theories of aging.
7 Discuss the effects of aging on intelligence and memory.
8 Identify the physiologic changes that occur with aging.
9 Identify assessment techniques used to evaluate the physiologic changes of aging.
10 Identify nursing interventions related to physiologic changes that occur with aging.
11 Discuss nursing measures that help prevent injury and promote function for the aged individual.
12 Describe the modifications in diet required by those over age 65.
13 Discuss the ways in which age-related pathophysiologic changes affect drug action and toxicity.
14 Identify alternatives to institutional care for the frail older adult.

## KEY TERMS

Alzheimer's disease
delirium
dementia
depression
diagnosis-related groups
drug interactions
geriatrics
gerontology
home care
Medicare

mini-mental status examination (MMSE)
nursing home
osteoporosis
quality of life
reality orientation
reminiscing
remotivation
retirement
senescence
sexuality

The term **geriatrics** is defined by *Webster's Medical Desk Dictionary* (1986) as the branch of medicine that deals with the diseases and problems of old age and aging people. The term is derived from the Greek word *geras*, meaning old age. **Gerontology** is defined as the scientific study of the process of aging and its effects (Webster's Medical Desk Dictionary, 1986). The science of gerontology is multidisciplinary, encompassing the social, biologic, spiritual, and psychologic aspects of aging. **Senescence** is the final stage in the life cycle. It denotes a time of gradual physical decline that is preceded by a period of attaining maturity. Senescence is not a pathologic condition but a normal biologic process (Figure 9-1). In American society the term *geriatrics* usually applies to individuals age 65 or over.

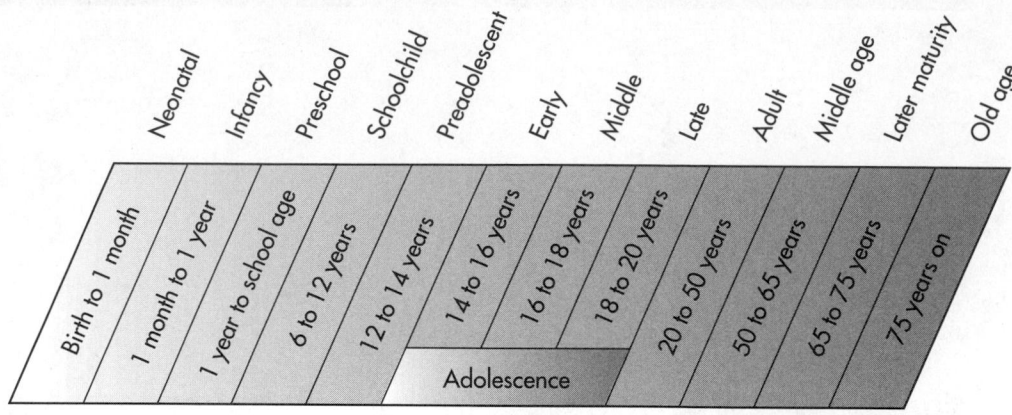

**Figure 9-1** The life span is continuous but has been divided into stages, each presenting different needs. Geriatric patients, who are near the end of the continuum, have their own special needs.

# DEMOGRAPHICS

Nurses must educate themselves about the health needs of older people. In the next several decades, the number of older people, especially those over age 85, will increase rapidly. Although the number of people over age 65 will more than double, from about 32 million today to more than 67 million by the year 2040 (U.S. Bureau of the Census, 1991), the number of people over age 85 is expected to quadruple. With this dramatic increase in the "old old" population will come an increase in the number of people with chronic health problems such as hypertension, chronic lung disease, sensory impairments, and memory deficits. In 1900 only 4% of the population was 65 years of age or older. In 1991 13.5% were age 65 or older. By the year 2030, 17% of the population, a predicted 50 million people, will be age 65 or older. There has been a corresponding increase in life expectancy. For example, a white woman at age 65 is expected to have another 20 years of life, and white men will have nearly 16 more years (Social Security Administration, 1994). Many older Americans continue to work full-time or part-time to supplement their retirement income and to remain active and engaged in life.

As the number and proportion of older adults increase, the proportion of working adults (ages 18 to 64) decreases. This means that fewer people will be contributing to the national economy and fewer family members will be providing support for the elderly, both financially and in times of crises. Adult daughters, who traditionally have been the caregivers of the older generation, now are more likely to be working in jobs outside the home. In view of such social and economic changes, the government may have to assume a greater role in providing these services to the older population (Burkhauser, Couch, Phillips, 1996).

Since the turn of the century, life expectancy has increased greatly from an average of 47.3 years in 1900 to 75 years for a person born in 1984. In general, women live longer than men. Among the more frequent causes of death for those who are age 75 or older, pneumonia and flu are the only infectious diseases remaining from the turn of the century (Table 9-1). To a large extent, the life expectancy has increased because deaths from infectious diseases and acute illnesses have been reduced. However, this has resulted in an increase in the death rate from chronic illnesses such as cancer and heart disease. People suffering from chronic illnesses require more health care and nursing services to remain functional. This may place additional demands on the health care system as the population continues to age and the number of older people continues to grow.

The social support system of the elderly person also is changing. Of those older than age 75, about 20% of men and 50% of women live alone. Of those who live alone, about 50% see their adult children at least once a week. The others either have no children or are separated geographically from their children and see them less often. Older individuals who require some form of care essential to their survival or to maintaining a high quality of life are a cause of concern. It can be predicted with reasonable accuracy that this trend will continue for many decades. The increase in life expectancy means that some older people will be healthier as they move into their later years. This group will need information and guidance for promoting and maintaining their health.

However, for the "old old" population (age 85 or older), the demand for long-term care will increase. The 7 million elderly people who currently need some long-term care assistance represent 24% of the elderly

**TABLE 9-1**

## Nine Most Frequent Causes of Death in Age Groups 75 to 84 Years and 85 or Older*

| | MEN | WOMEN | MEN | WOMEN |
|---|---|---|---|---|
| | 75-84 | | 85 OR OLDER | |
| Heart disease | 3239 | 2122 | 7830 | 6810 |
| Malignancies | 1861 | 982 | 2528 | 1292 |
| Cerebrovascular accident (CVA) | 603 | 523 | 1625 | 1738 |
| Chronic obstructive pulmonary disease (COPD) | 504 | 197 | 777 | 245 |
| Pneumonia and flu | 352 | 199 | 1428 | 1006 |
| Accidents | 143 | 84 | 375 | 225 |
| Diabetes | 127 | 123 | 229 | 219 |
| Suicide | 57 | 7 | 60 | 5 |
| Liver disease | 44 | 25 | 34 | 14 |

From US Bureau of the Census: *1991 Statistical abstract of the United States,* ed 111, Washington, DC, 1991, US Government Printing Office.
*By frequency of occurrence per 100,000 population of those age groups.

population. Most require assistance with activities of daily living (ADL) and personal care. About 78% of older people who receive long-term care live in the community, and the remaining 22% live in nursing homes. Nurses long have provided health care and illness care to the elderly, and such care will be needed far into the foreseeable future.

## PROGRESS AND RESEARCH

Since 1961, when the first White House Conference on Aging was held, there has been an awakening to the needs of the elderly. One of the most important recommendations submitted to this conference eventually led to enactment of legislation establishing **Medicare** and the Older Americans Act.

Benefits under Medicare became available July 1, 1966. Although changes have been made in the original act, millions of older Americans continue to receive hospital and medical care under its provisions. However beneficial it may be, Medicare does not cover all medical expenses for all elderly people. For example, it does not cover outpatient drug expenses, hospitalization carries a deductible charge, and only about 80% of outpatient services are reimbursed. The older person must pay these expenses out of pocket or buy additional insurance to close this gap. As the cost of prescription drugs continues to rise, unfortunately so does the cost of "medigap" insurance, which covers the cost of prescription drugs, putting this type of insurance beyond the reach of many older persons.

The Older Americans Act became law in 1965, and since then it, too, has undergone numerous changes. Parts of the act are administered by the federal government through the Department of Health and Hu-

man Services, and other parts are implemented by state and local agencies. The act covers a wide range of services to the elderly, with special emphasis on meeting the nutritional needs of older people. Programs funded under various parts of the Older Americans Act include homemaker services, home health aides, the foster grandparents program, employment referrals, housing, health screening, research and demonstration programs, and training programs in the field of aging.

The Social Security Act as revised in 1965 and its subsequent amendments provide monthly benefits for the elderly. Periodic increases in benefits have been granted to cover increased living costs. As the Social Security benefit has been increased, the ceiling on earned income has been raised without loss of the monthly benefit. This makes it possible for elderly people to continue working part-time.

Through Social Security, efforts also have been made to improve the aged person's quality of life through research. Many universities and medical centers have opened research centers to study the biologic and psychologic factors related to aging. Many health maintenance organizations (HMOs) now enroll older people, accepting the equivalent of the monthly premium as a capitation payment. Additional charges may apply for drugs, eyeglasses, hearing aids, and other services and equipment. Federal regulations to protect the rights of older people enrolled in HMOs and to ensure their right to appeal if they have been denied emergency services, referral to specialists, and the option of seeking second opinions are under consideration.

Although tremendous strides have been made in providing a better life for millions of elderly Americans, not all are receiving these benefits. Many communities have active programs, but others lag far behind and show little interest in improving the life of the elderly.

# FACTORS THAT AFFECT AGING

## Cultural and Ethnic Factors

The cultural patterns of different groups of people vary considerably. In early Oriental cultures the older members of society were revered and referred to as "the wise ones." In primitive cultures the elderly were the source of information and knowledge. They always knew where to find food and water, and they traveled with the tribe. When they became too feeble to travel and could not be cared for, they accepted death. In the early culture of the United States, the older citizens also were important sources of information. They were consulted about the political and educational affairs of the community. They were respected because of the knowledge they had acquired during their lives.

The current American culture is youth oriented, and the elderly occupy a lower position and endure less prestige. They may look back nostalgically to a time of solidarity of the family unit, a time when young people showed respect and devotion to the aged members of the family. The social system imposes retirement and forces the individual to find new roles at a time when it is more difficult to make decisions than it was at an earlier age. Limited financial resources come to affect many elderly people as inflation reduces the buying power of a fixed income from pensions or Social Security payments. (See Chapter 8 for a complete discussion of the importance of considering cultural factors when delivering nursing care.)

## Socioeconomic Factors

Housing is a pressing problem. Most elderly people wish to remain in their own homes, in familiar surroundings. However, this may be difficult or impossible with financial or health problems. Some older people have found themselves victims of urban renewal. They may have lived in areas in the city that recently became popular with the young urban working crowd and may have found their apartments being sold as condominiums or their rents raised drastically. This has resulted in an increase in the number of older people who are homeless. Other older people with health problems find they are no longer able to care for a large home and that rising taxes and maintenance costs have become a burden. When the adult children are all working outside the home or residing in other cities, it may be difficult for frail older people to care

for themselves, and they may be forced to leave their homes. Whether they move in with one of their children or enter an extended care facility, an adjustment is necessary and often difficult. Abrupt changes often are made without consideration for individual differences and needs. Lifetime patterns are not easily changed and must be evaluated in terms of what they mean to the individual.

Under the federal Housing Act, funds have been made available for construction of housing units for the aged. High-rise apartment complexes for the elderly are found in many urban and suburban areas. Although they may solve the problem of housing, many of these complexes provide no health services or cannot meet all the health care needs of the residents. For example, residents who are physically frail may need to have their vital signs monitored and their condition assessed regularly to prevent a health crisis and the resulting hospitalization. Support services such as visiting nurses, housekeeping, transportation, Meals on Wheels, and adult day care may supplement the services delivered in senior citizen housing and may allow some frail older people to remain independent in their own apartments.

---

### CASE STUDY

Mrs. Smith, an 83-year-old widow, lived in two small basement rooms of a house in a textile mill village. One day she fell and broke her wrist while carrying groceries down the stairs to her apartment. Mrs. Smith's daughter was afraid she would fall again and insisted that her mother give up her apartment and move in with her and her family on the other side of town. Mrs. Smith did not want to leave her neighbors and give up her independence, but she did not want to offend her daughter, so she sadly said "yes" and agreed to the move. Even after a 6-month adjustment period, Mrs. Smith seemed withdrawn and spent most of her time alone in her room.

---

Ambulatory services can be used to supplement housing and institutional services to keep older people from becoming permanent residents of long-term care facilities (Figure 9-2). Nurses play a pivotal role in this process by becoming involved in the linkage process and providing information, participating in discharge planning, working as case managers, and participating in multidisciplinary geriatric assessment teams.

Although many older people are forced to leave their homes because of urban renewal and must readjust their lifelong patterns of living, not all the elderly are confronted with this problem. Those with adequate health and financial resources are able to maintain their desired life-styles, but some of the elderly need assistance through community services. It is important to

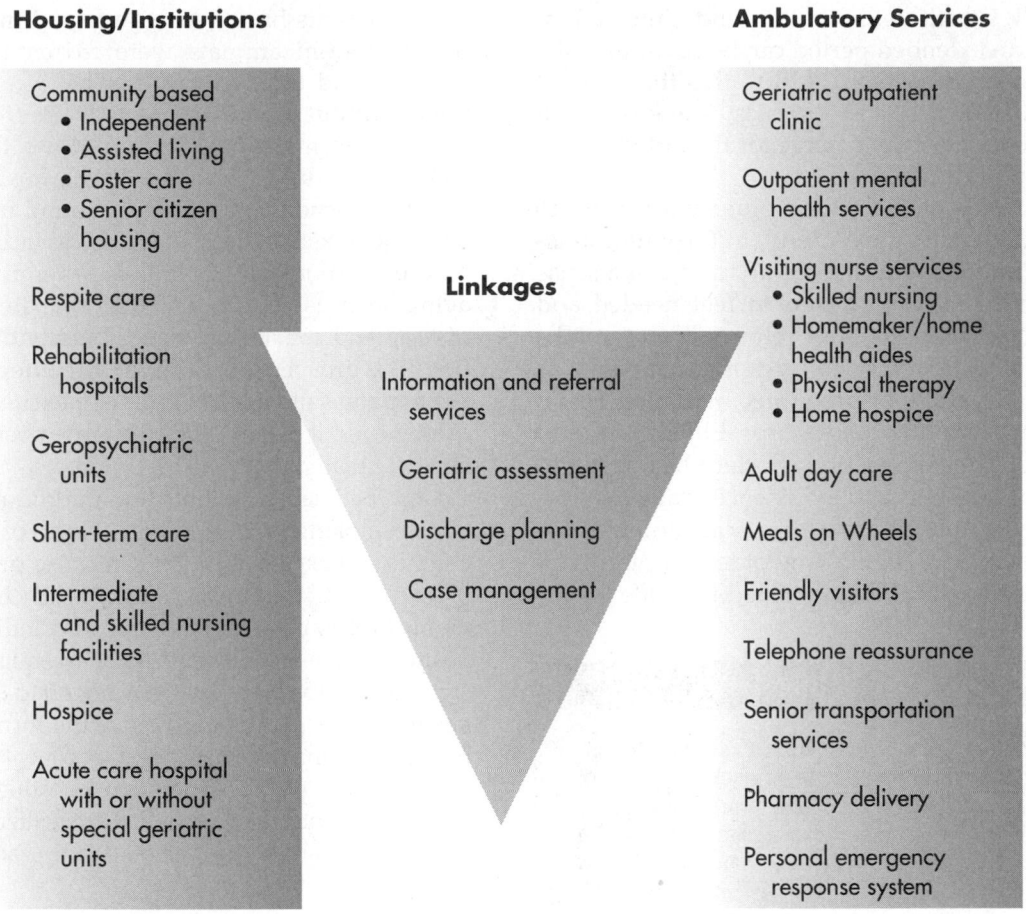

**Housing/Institutions**

Community based
• Independent
• Assisted living
• Foster care
• Senior citizen housing

Respite care

Rehabilitation hospitals

Geropsychiatric units

Short-term care

Intermediate and skilled nursing facilities

Hospice

Acute care hospital with or without special geriatric units

**Linkages**

Information and referral services

Geriatric assessment

Discharge planning

Case management

**Ambulatory Services**

Geriatric outpatient clinic

Outpatient mental health services

Visiting nurse services
• Skilled nursing
• Homemaker/home health aides
• Physical therapy
• Home hospice

Adult day care

Meals on Wheels

Friendly visitors

Telephone reassurance

Senior transportation services

Pharmacy delivery

Personal emergency response system

**Figure 9-2**    The long-term care continuum of services for older adults.

remember that most elderly people (95%) live independently in the community, with varying levels of assistance from family and friends. However, successful aging and retirement take planning and preparation, both of which should begin in middle age.

## Retirement and Aging

During the early history of the United States the economy was rural and agricultural, and there was little concern about retirement. Individuals worked well into their later years (after age 65), and when they were even more advanced in years, chores kept the elders occupied and provided an opportunity for them to make a contribution to society. Today's society remains essentially work oriented, but the older worker is pressured into retirement to provide jobs for younger workers.

Mandatory retirement was abolished for most people in the late 1970s, although many people continue to retire between ages 62 and 65. **Retirement** is thought of as a positive reward for labor, a special time free from worry, but many people facing retirement

have difficulty coping with this abrupt change in lifestyle. Many retired people become bored with their life-styles and inactivity after a brief "honeymoon" period. The increased number of women in today's labor force makes retirement a concern for men and women alike, but women usually adjust to retirement more easily than men do because they often have many social ties, continuing homemaker responsibilities, and ongoing family responsibilities.

In retirement, sustained activity is no longer required. The absence of social roles for the elderly

### CASE STUDY

Mrs. Clay had lived for 46 years in the home that had belonged to her parents. However, when urban renewal came, Mrs. Clay had to move. When asked about her new home, Mrs. Clay said, "I like it quite well, but it's very inconvenient. You see, I was right there in town. Out here I have to call a taxi every time I want to go to the store, and I don't always have the money."

makes a work substitute difficult to find. Enforced in-activity over an extended period can be harmful to the health of the retired person. Add to this the effect of bereavement over a spouse, friends, and even children, and a tendency may emerge for the individual to give up and withdraw.

The basic needs of the retired older worker are to feel financially secure, to be useful, to form new associations and interact with people, to maintain a sense of dignity and self-respect, and to feel needed and wanted in society. Many older retirees now can take free courses at community colleges and can serve as volunteers in a variety of programs, including Foster Grandparents, Vista, the Peace Corps, Elderhostel, and Retired Senior Executive Corps. Society has begun to recognize that the skills and experiences gained over a lifetime are valuable resources that can improve the situation of others while allowing older people an opportunity to feel helpful and involved with life.

### CASE STUDY

John, who had worked for 45 years in the electronics industry, was asked to take early retirement at the age of 62, when his company became less profitable. He was offered a financial retirement package that prompted him to accept the offer. However, John was bothered by the idea that people would think of him as "over the hill." After 3 months of retirement, he became bored with golf and television. His wife, who still worked part time in the town library, urged him to take up a new hobby or look for a part-time job. She was worried because John just did not seem like himself.

## Biopsychosocial Factors
### Biology of Aging

The biologic process of aging causes physiologic changes in the human organism. Changes usually develop slowly, and most older people consider themselves to be in good or excellent health. Scientists continue to investigate the cause of aging, not only to extend life but also to achieve a life free of degenerative disease. Some believe that the aging process is programmed by genes, whereas others theorize that it is related to a chemical blockage of thyroxine. The most recent evidence relates the aging process to the immune system. It has been found that a type of white blood cell, the T cell, provides resistance to cancer cells, viruses, bacteria, and fungi, but it loses its effectiveness with age, and the person therefore loses immunity to disease. It is believed that these cells become less effective because the thymus gland shrinks with age, and it is the thymus gland that secretes chemicals that stimulate the bone marrow cells to produce T cells.

Experiments have been conducted in which T cells removed from animals were frozen for as long as 15 years and then reinjected. The T cells maintained their youthful immune powers while frozen and were perfectly normal when thawed. When the frozen cells were reintroduced into the aging host, the immune system returned to the potency found in young adulthood. Scientists believe that this dwindling immunity may be responsible for the degenerative diseases of aging such as cancer, arthritis, diabetes, and kidney disease and for an increase in susceptibility to infection. The prospect of controlling the degeneration that accompanies old age is extremely exciting.

However, it is important to remember that life-style choices greatly affect the aging process and function in old age. Bad habits in youth and middle age, such as cigarette smoking, high-fat diets, lack of exercise, and chronic sun exposure, often can cause problems for the older person. Certainly genes influence aging, and a family history of certain diseases may indicate a threat to health, but life-style choices have an equal or even more significant impact on health (Schoenfeld et al, 1994). It is never too late to try to influence the formation of good habits, even in older patients. Good health is important to most older people. They fear becoming a burden to their spouse or children, and they realize that health is precious and should not be taken for granted.

### Mental Health

It is generally believed that individuals who are well adjusted and able to meet problems and make adaptations during their younger years are better prepared to face problems in advancing years. Erikson (1950) identified this stage of life as ego integrity versus despair. Erikson defines ego integrity as acceptance of one's own unique life cycle and the people who have become significant to it. He emphasizes that this life cycle and its significant people are something that must be and that, by necessity, allows no substitutions. Achieving integrity means that the individual accepts past events, experiences, and life-style, including the mistakes made along the way. The person who does not achieve ego integrity feels despair or disgust about the course of his or her life and may blame circumstances on someone or something else. Such a person feels regret that it is too late to start over or change that life.

An older person may be confronted with fears of illness, physical suffering, helplessness, and death. Chronic death or illness results in low morale, but when meaningful friendships exist, even when health is poor, the individual is less likely to suffer from low morale. At these times a caring nurse or a referral to a mental health clinic can provide emotional support and give the individual a feeling of friendship and warmth and a sense of personal worth.

Some elderly people depend on others for part or all of their care. Dependency can result in loss of dignity, diminished self-esteem, and low morale. When disease and illness are superimposed on the normal changes of aging, adaptation is difficult for the individual. The dependency that elderly people experience may give rise to feelings of resentment toward family, friends, or those trying to help. The dependent older person may become demanding, tend to magnify normal aches and pains, and complain of loss of sleep and various digestive disturbances. However, vague symptoms can be indications of underlying pathologic conditions. It must be remembered that older people have many adjustments to make during a period of their lives when they tolerate stressful situations poorly. Adjustments that older people may have to make include the death of a spouse or friends, retirement and reduced income, identification with an older age group, and adjustment to chronic illness and a gradually changing body.

**Depression** often goes unrecognized and untreated in the older population. Older people are less likely to complain of sadness or "feeling blue," but they may instead complain of weight loss, feelings of fatigue, memory loss and difficulty concentrating, anxiety, constipation, or other symptoms that are general in nature. Physical conditions associated with depression include cerebrovascular accident (CVA), thyroid disease, Parkinson's disease, and other chronic illnesses. Some of the medications known to cause depression in older people include beta-blockers taken for hypertension and some sleeping pills and tranquilizers. The Geriatric Depression Scale (GDS), which is used to assess depression, can be useful in the clinical setting (Brink, Yesavage, 1983). Van Marwijk and others (1995) have proposed using four questions from the GDS that can help identify depression in older individuals: (1) Are you satisfied with your life? (2) Have you dropped many of your activities and interests? (3) Do you feel happy most of the time? (4) Do you prefer to stay at home rather than going out and doing new things? Two or more positive answers are considered diagnostic of depression, and further investigation may be warranted.

Older people diagnosed with depression may be treated with counseling or antidepressant medications, or both. The success rate of treatment of depression in older people is equal to the success rate for treatment of middle-aged and young adults. Some of the newer antidepressant medications work well for elderly people and do not cause the harmful side effects associated with medications of the past. Some hospitals and long-term care facilities specialize in mental health problems of the elderly and accept patients for short-term stays (less than 2 weeks) to begin treatment and stabilize the patient on medications. These units are called geropsychiatric units.

Most elderly people become aware of the shortness of time. They become concerned about changes in their bodies and their loss of strength or the presence of disease. Grief after the loss of a spouse or close friend may cause the person to question his or her continued existence. The individual may progress to a state of depression and prefer self-destruction to continuation of life. With the increased incidence of geriatric suicide, the nurse caring for elderly patients should be alert to warning signs. The person who expresses a desire to die or makes threats of suicide should be taken seriously. The elderly are at the highest risk for successful suicides. It is during such periods of crisis that the individual needs emotional support. Each community has access to emergency mental health services, and the nurse should become familiar with the reporting process before a crisis occurs. An older person who speaks of death should be questioned carefully to see if he or she has a plan for dying and a means to carry it out. If so, emergency services must be mobilized immediately to prevent the person from harming himself or herself.

### CASE STUDY

Mr. Jones is a retired, 72-year-old man who has gradually lost the ability to walk because of Parkinson's disease. One day, while caring for Mr. Jones, the visiting nurse noticed a gun in the hall closet. When questioned about the gun, Mr. Jones said, "Yes, it's loaded, and I keep that gun close to me because one day I will use it to end it all." The nurse immediately called her supervisor and obtained emergency mental health services for Mr. Jones.

Many of the concepts concerning psychosocial factors in old age have never been proven and are now being questioned. It can no longer be assumed that all older people are lonely, depressed, uninterested in sex, fixated on their aches and pains, and happy to sit in a rocking chair all day. Only recently has research, although limited, enabled society to learn some of the factors that affect the social life and attitudes of elderly people. It has been stated that chronologic age may be unrelated to old age. Elderly people are individuals, and all 70-year-olds are not alike, just as all 20-year-olds are not alike. It has been suggested that older people represent a "subculture." Society has fostered such a culture through community programs that tend to segregate older people, such as senior citizen centers, golden age groups, and adult day care centers. These programs take older people out of the mainstream of society and provide little opportunity for interaction with younger people. New programs that encourage interaction and socialization with all age groups are needed.

The success of a mental health program for the elderly depends on a social consciousness within the community that is oriented toward mental health. The nurse can be a promoter of new ideas and a source of inspiration, not only to individuals but also to the community, in developing a mental health program for the elderly population.

Maintaining mental health does not mean doing *for* the older person; it means doing *with* the older person. A large number of elderly citizens want something to do and want to feel that they are useful. Many are ambulatory and able to remain in their own homes, where they are happier. For some, however, this is not possible. Older people face many social and economic problems in later life, and these problems can have a profound impact on their lives. A community counseling service should be available where the person can have privacy, quiet, and an unhurried atmosphere to talk over problems. Community groups of elderly people can be formed to develop social contacts. With the help of a group leader, the members of the group assist each other in devising methods to handle problems faced in the community.

## Aging and Intelligence

The belief that intelligence declines with age is a myth. Although the elderly achieve lower scores on intelligence tests, this usually is because their reaction times are slower and they need more time to complete the examination. The lower scores are not associated with a deficit in the ability to think. The elderly replace speed with accuracy, and research shows that they often do better than younger people when the time limit is removed. Leading an active life that includes mastery of new knowledge and skills is considered essential to maintaining intelligence in the elderly.

## Aging and Memory

It is common in our society to blame advancing age when a person experiences any lapse in memory. The basis for memory decline in old age is not well understood. Physical changes in the aging brain may be somewhat responsible, as well as other factors including lower educational levels among older people, changes in vision and hearing that may cause errors in encoding of information, lowered stress response, and the effects of physical illness (Nyberg et al, 1996).

The elderly sometimes are described as rigid in their approach to problem solving. The tendency to persist in a particular approach to a problem despite additional information suggesting a change is believed to be associated not with the age of the individual but with the level of education achieved. It has been demonstrated that the greater the number of years elapsed since the individual was involved in formal schooling, the more likely the individual is to solve problems by applying relevant knowledge from stored experience. Analyzing a problem and employing a new solution depend on recent exposure to this type of thinking, which commonly is found in the educational setting. All of these facts point to the importance of continuing lifelong learning in maintaining mental functioning.

Every older person who complains of memory loss should have a formal mental status assessment. A mental status assessment examines cognitive functions such as the ability to think and make decisions. In addition to establishing important baseline information about the older patient, the mental status assessment can be used to chart the progression of a cognitive deficit, if present, and document the effect of treatment and nursing interventions.

The **mini-mental status examination (MMSE)** is used widely in the clinical setting (Folstein et al, 1975). It assesses orientation, short-term memory, ability to attend to tasks (attention), calculation, recall (memory), and language. Each area provides neurologic information and may assist in identifying the cognition problem and its extent. With a possible score of 30, a score of 20 to 29 indicates a moderate cognitive deficit, and a score of 19 or below reflects a more serious deficit.

At first the nurse may be uncomfortable using the MMSE, but there are ways to become comfortable with this technique, such as trying out the MMSE on family and friends, watching geriatric nursing experts who use the examination often, and explaining to patients that the examination gives valuable information and helps ensure high-quality nursing care. If the patient misses answers, the nurse should move on to the next question and not dwell on failures. The nurse should be certain the older person is physically comfortable, can see the nurse, and can hear the instructions. When charting the results of the MMSE, the nurse should note the total score and where the patient had deficits (memory, orientation, or language). This information is vital to the nursing care plan.

## PHYSIOLOGY OF AGING

When a person has reached maturity, a gradual aging of all body tissues and organs begins. Loss of cells and loss of physiologic reserves may be the major way in which the body ages. By the time a person has reached 70 years of age, the aging process may be well advanced. The rate and extent of aging vary among individuals, and the rate at which various organs age may also vary. Among the various physiologic changes seen in the elderly, some begin when people are in their thirties (Table 9-2).

When normal aging progresses without the presence of disease, the end result is a loss of organ reserve. This means that normal function of the body continues as before, but the body is less likely to respond to stress in a positive manner. This may be why newspapers often carry a report of an older person suffering a heart attack while shoveling the driveway during the first snowstorm of winter. The older heart, which func-

**TABLE 9-2**

## Physiologic Changes of Aging

| BODY SYSTEM | PHYSIOLOGIC CHANGES | RESULTS |
|---|---|---|
| Cardiovascular | ↑ Number of heartbeat irregularities | ↓ Oxygenation |
| | ↓ Cardiac output | ↑ Chance of heart failure |
| | ↓ Heart rate | ↑ Blood pressure |
| | ↑ Atherosclerosis | ↓ Blood supply to peripheral areas |
| Sensory | ↓ Accommodation | ↓ Light to retina |
| | ↓ Diameter of pupil | ↓ Night vision |
| | ↑ Opacity of lens | ↑ Sensitivity to glare |
| | | ↓ Peripheral vision |
| | ↓ Sense of smell | ↓ Color vision |
| | ↓ Number of taste buds | ↓ High-frequency sounds |
| | ↓ Functioning of middle and inner ear | ↓ Balance |
| Integumentary | ↓ Sebaceous secretions | ↑ Dry skin |
| | ↓ Subcutaneous fat | ↑ Wrinkling |
| | ↓ Thickness of epidermis | ↑ Susceptibility to heat and cold |
| | | ↑ Thickness of nails |
| | | ↓ Hair color and distribution |
| Musculoskeletal | ↓ Bone calcium | ↑ Curvature of spine—osteoporosis |
| | ↓ Water of intervertebral disks | ↓ Height |
| | ↓ Blood supply | ↓ Mobility |
| | ↓ Elastic tissue | ↑ Risk of falls and fractures |
| | ↓ Muscle mass | |
| Nervous | ↓ Brain cells | ↓ Reflexes |
| | ↓ Nerve fibers | ↓ Short-term memory |
| | ↓ Touch receptors | ↓ Pain recognition |
| Digestive | ↓ Gastric secretions | ↑ Constipation |
| | ↓ Peristalsis | ↓ Appetite |
| | ↓ Sensory receptors | ↓ Ability to taste |
| | ↓ Number of teeth | ↓ Ability to chew |
| | | ↓ Nutritional status |
| Urinary | ↓ Blood supply | ↓ Urine concentration |
| | ↓ Nephrons | ↓ Bladder capacity |
| | ↓ Muscle tone | ↑ Residual urine |
| | ♂ ↑ Size of prostate | ↑ Chance of infection |
| | | ♂ ↓ Urinary stream |
| Respiratory | ↓ Elasticity | ↓ Gas exchange |
| | ↑ Thickness of capillaries | ↓ Vital capacity |
| | ↓ Number of capillaries | ↑ Risk of disease |
| | | ↓ Cough efficiency |
| Reproductive | ♀ ↓ Estrogen | ♀ ↓ Epithelial cells of vulva |
| | ♂ ↓ Testosterone | ♀ ↓ Vaginal secretions |
| | | ♀ ↓ Breast size |
| | | ♀ ↓ Ovary and uterus size |
| | | ♂ ↓ Ejaculation |
| | | ♂ ↑ Time to achieve erection |

↑, Increased; ↓, decreased; ♀, female; ♂, male.

tions well under normal conditions, may not be able to respond to the sudden demand for increased oxygen needed by the muscles during vigorous exercise. The zone of adaptation is smaller for an older person because of loss of organ reserve, presence of underlying chronic illnesses, and the effects of some drugs that many older people take to control symptoms of illness (Figure 9-3).

Although normal aging varies among individuals, some elderly people complain of physical symptoms that should be given medical attention. Many older people (and the physicians and nurses who care for them) think that fatigue, incontinence, falls, and confusion are normal parts of aging and therefore not worth mentioning to anyone. Because of negative stereotypes of aging, many older people suffer needlessly with conditions that can be treated. Older people who seek medical help and offer various complaints about their health deserve a complete investigation into the cause of the complaint.

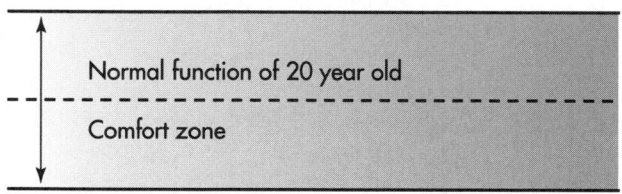

Wide adaptation range of young adult

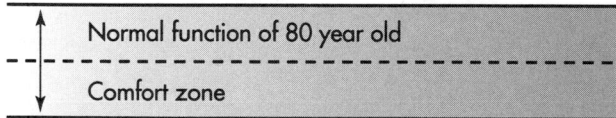

Adaptation range of older adult

Causes of narrowing of adaptation range

- Loss of organ reserve
- Underlying chronic illness
- Possible drug response

Threats to adaptation

- Illness (acute/chronic)
- Stress
- Social isolation
- Malnutrition/dehydration
- Depression/mental status change

**Figure 9-3** The physiology of aging and the narrowing of the adaptation range.

## Cardiovascular System

The size of the heart usually remains the same, but it may increase as a result of diminished activity or long-standing hypertension. With an enlarged heart the heart rate is slower in response to demand, and cardiac output is reduced. As a result, there is less rapid movement of blood carrying oxygen and nutrients to all the organs and tissues in the body. This in turn affects the function of these organs. In the presence of stress, either physical or psychologic, reduced cardiac output means that less oxygen is available to meet the greater need caused by the stress. Because the heart needs more rest between beats, tachycardia easily results in heart failure. Arteriosclerotic changes are common in the elderly, and these changes make the blood vessels less elastic and more resistant to blood flow, which results in elevated blood pressure. Exercise can increase cardiac output, and daily exercise, such as walking, is excellent for the elderly.

### Assessment

To begin assessment of the cardiovascular system, the nurse should note the rate, rhythm, and character of the pulse for 1 full minute with the patient in a resting state. Pulses are checked bilaterally for symmetry, because older people may have arterial insufficiency. Blood pressure is taken with the person first lying down and then standing. Orthostatic hypotension is common in the elderly. The medications the person is taking should be assessed for their effect on blood pressure. The presence or absence of pedal edema is evaluated when palpating pedal pulses. The temperature of the hands and feet is noted. Cool, dry extremities reflect a decrease in peripheral circulation. A family history of heart disease, if any, should be noted. The individual's life-style, including smoking, diet and obesity, exercise, and stress, should be assessed.

### Common Pathologic Conditions

Cardiovascular problems are among the most common diseases of the elderly. Some recent studies support the theory that life-style is the cause of many cardiovascular pathologic conditions. However, the effects of the aging process do contribute to the progress of pathologic conditions.

Hypertension is commonly found among the elderly and is defined as a blood pressure consistently above that considered normal. A person is considered hypertensive with a systolic blood pressure above 140 mm Hg or a diastolic pressure above 90 mm Hg. The diastolic reading is as important as the systolic pressure because the diastolic reading indicates the pressure in the cardiovascular system when the heart is at rest between beats, and the systolic reading indicates the maximum pressure on the system when the heart pumps. (See Chapter 25 for a complete discussion of the pathophysiology, assessment, and interventions for hypertension.)

**Arteriosclerosis and atherosclerosis.** The changes that occur in the heart and vascular system begin early in life and progress over the years. Arteriosclerosis, a condition in which the blood vessels lose their elasticity, is also known as hardening of the arteries. Atherosclerosis is a form of arteriosclerosis; it results from fatty deposits (plaque) that form in the intima of the blood vessels. These changes make it increasingly difficult for blood to flow through the vascular system. The flow of blood to the kidneys, brain, and lower extremities often is affected. The condition may become severe enough to cause serious heart disease, such as coronary artery disease, myocardial infarction, or congestive heart failure. Atherosclerosis has been directly linked to arterial occlusive disease. (See Chapter 25 for coverage of these conditions.)

CVA, or stroke, is one of the leading causes of death in the elderly and is the result of an interruption of circulation in the brain. Hypertension is a major factor in the occurrence of a stroke. (See Chapter 25 for pathophysiology and intervention for CVA.)

---

## CASE STUDY

Mary, an 82-year-old widow, always felt tired and slept most of the day. She had been told that at her age that was normal. However, Mary knew that until a few months ago, she had had plenty of energy, played bridge, and enjoyed brisk walks in good weather. Finally, Mary called her physician, who performed a physical examination and some blood tests. He found that Mary's thyroid gland was not producing enough of a hormone ($H_4$) needed for her normal function. A thyroid-replacement hormone was started (levothyroxine [Synthroid]), and now Mary is again enjoying a more active life.

---

## Nursing Interventions

The most important nursing interventions related to the cardiovascular system are prevention and management of cardiovascular disease. Promoting a healthy life-style in all individuals will reduce the incidence of cardiovascular pathologic conditions in the elderly. The importance of a good diet cannot be overemphasized. The nurse should encourage and help the elderly to reduce their intake of salt, saturated fats, and alcohol and to increase their intake of grains, fresh fruits, and vegetables. A regular program of exercise

tailored to the individual is very important. Smokers should be encouraged to quit.

Nursing interventions for individuals with cardiovascular problems include monitoring and evaluating the effects of the medical therapies. The nurse must teach the patient about the medications prescribed by the physician, their side effects, and the importance of continuing the medications. Careful monitoring of the patient for side effects is important because the patient who stops taking the medication because of fatigue, impotence, dizziness, or other complaints is at risk for increased blood pressure, cardiac enlargement, or possibly CVA. With the newer classes of antihypertension medication, most older people can attain adequate control of their blood pressure without suffering ill effects from their medication.

## Sensory System

The status of the individual's sensory system affects the way the individual reacts to the environment and the people in it. Deficits in hearing or vision have the effect of isolating an individual from what is going on around him or her.

### Vision

With aging, visual accommodation gradually declines. This means that the elderly require more time to focus when looking from one object to another. Night vision is reduced, and more time is needed for the eyes to adjust to the dark. Increased lens opacity causes light to scatter and makes the elderly person more sensitive to glare. These changes cause many older people to stop driving at night. Senile miosis, a condition that reduces the size of the pupils, results in a reduction in the amount of light reaching the retina, so that the elderly need more light to work, read, and walk safely. Peripheral vision, the ability to distinguish objects at the edges of the visual field, is reduced. Sometimes the elderly do not communicate with people sitting beside them simply because they do not see them. The lens yellows with age, causing the elderly difficulty in discriminating colors. Blues and greens tend to fade and are easily confused. Reds, oranges, and yellows can be seen best.

**Assessment.** The patient should be asked about visual problems such as double vision, blurring, tunnel vision, or any other visual disturbance. Headaches or pain in or around the eye should be noted. Vision can be assessed by using an eye chart or by determining if the person can recognize the number of fingers held up by the examiner standing a little more than 0.5 m (2 feet) and 3 m (10 feet) away. Newspaper headlines also can be used to check vision. Peripheral vision can be gauged by wiggling the fingers while slowly bringing them toward the patient's center of vision. Color discrimination can be checked by using a color chart, colored paper, or colors in the environment.

**Common pathologic conditions.** The most common visual problems of the elderly are cataracts, glaucoma, senile macular degeneration, and diabetic retinopathy. These problems are covered in Chapter 38.

**Nursing interventions.** Nurses should be aware of visual changes that occur with aging so that they can help elderly patients adapt to these changes. When moving back and forth between brightly lit and darker areas, such as coming indoors on a sunny day or coming out of a darkened theater into the daylight, elderly individuals should pause to allow the eyes to accommodate to the change. Sunglasses help reduce glare in bright daylight. Elderly people who drive at night can be advised to use lighted and divided highways to reduce the glare from oncoming cars. Indoors, lamps and windows should be shaded to allow adequate light but reduce glare. Supplemental light should be provided for tasks such as reading or sewing. Adequate lighting of stairs is essential. Stair edges should be marked with contrasting color. Night-lights will help the elderly when they need to get up during the night. Older patients who have diminished peripheral vision should be approached from the front, and objects should be placed directly in front of them.

## Hearing

Hearing impairment is common and is first demonstrated by an inability to hear the higher frequencies. This affects the individual's ability to discriminate words, and the individual will not hear certain words or will confuse them with other words. Peripheral conversation (background words) is not heard fully; this results in reduced sensory stimulation and may lead to withdrawal and social isolation. Changes in the middle ear and inner ear may result in some loss of balance. Ear wax becomes drier and may accumulate in the ear, causing further loss of hearing acuity.

**Assessment.** To assess hearing, the examiner should stand behind the individual and cover first one ear and then the other. Speaking in a normal voice, the examiner should ask the person to respond to questions or repeat a series of words. Both ears should be checked.

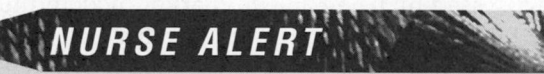

**NURSE ALERT**

**Shouting at the elderly may not help them to hear better.** ◆

**Nursing interventions.** When caring for the elderly, the nurse should stand face to face with the individual and speak clearly at a moderate rate. It is important not to overarticulate, shout, or mumble. Shouting may not help the person hear better. In fact, it may make hearing more difficult because when most people increase the volume of their voice, they also raise the pitch, and higher pitched sounds are more difficult for the elderly to hear. Hearing aids can help with some types of hearing loss. However, some individuals may refuse to wear a hearing aid because of vanity or because hearing aids often amplify background noise as well as conversation and can be difficult to adjust to.

## Taste and Smell

It generally has been thought that the senses of taste and smell decline with age. The sense of smell begins to decline in middle age and often continues to diminish during the later years (Knapp, 1989). The number of taste buds decreases with age, and as a result many older people choose salty and sugary foods in an attempt to enhance flavor (Pettigrew, 1989). Smoking and medications also can negatively affect taste and smell.

**Nursing interventions.** When caring for the elderly, the nurse should encourage them to use a variety of spices in cooking to increase taste. Dried or fresh herbs such as parsley, basil, or garlic can make a dish look attractive and taste better. Older people with deficits in smell should be medically evaluated for medication toxicity and for overall health status. Older people who lack a sense of smell should seek the help of others to make sure food has not spoiled in the refrigerator, and they should have smoke detectors to alert them in case of fire.

## Touch

Like the other senses, the sense of touch generally is thought to decline with age. Some evidence indicates that a person's ability to detect temperature extremes or pain is affected by age, but more and better research is needed in this area. Individuals with an impaired sense of touch may be unable to determine if a surface, such as a coffee pot, or water is hot enough to cause injury. With a diminished sense of pain, a person may not realize the extent of an injury such as a broken hip suffered in a fall. The nurse can assess the individual's sensitivity to temperature by using containers of hot and cold water. Pain sensitivity can be checked by using the ends of a cotton-tipped swab. Those whose sense of touch is diminished can be counseled to be particularly vigilant to prevent injury. Patients with diabetes may be at special risk because of diabetic neuropathies and slow healing time after injury occurs.

## Integumentary System

The signs of aging are perhaps most visible in the skin and hair. The epidermis and dermis become thinner, although there may be some thickening in areas exposed to sunlight. Decreased vascularity in the dermis leads to increased fragility of the skin. This results in easier bruising and greater susceptibility to skin problems such as decubiti. Secretion from the sebaceous glands declines, which causes the skin to become dry. Wrinkling of the skin is caused by loss of subcutaneous fat and by a decrease in the skin's water content. The nails become hard and brittle, leading to cracking and splitting. Hair becomes lighter and thinner. About half of the population over age 50 has at least 50% gray body hair. The elderly are more susceptible to heat and cold, so heat must be applied at a reduced temperature to avoid burns. Since reduced activity results in reduced heat production, elderly people often feel cold when others are comfortable.

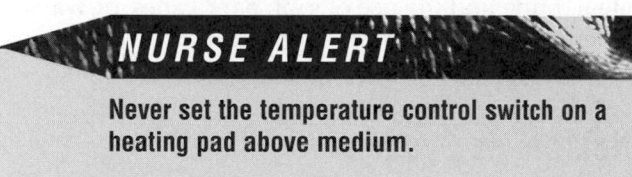

**NURSE ALERT**

**Never set the temperature control switch on a heating pad above medium.**

### Assessment

The skin should be examined by exposing all areas under good lighting. Pressure areas need to be checked for signs of redness or open lesions. Skin folds should be parted to check for irritation or signs of infection. The nurse should note the moisture of the skin and the size and location of any skin lesions. Older people bruise easily and may have reddened areas, called *senile purpurea*.

### Common Pathologic Conditions

The most common skin disorders among the elderly are skin cancers, keratoses, pigmentary disturbances, psoriasis, dermatitis, and urticaria (Ebersole, Hess, 1994). The immobile elderly are more likely to develop pressure sores. (See Chapter 40 for a discussion of these conditions.) Dryness and itching (pruritus) are common among the elderly. In most cases, dry skin is the cause of pruritus. However, if the patient has severe pruritus, other systemic problems should be ruled out. Conditions that may aggravate dry skin and itching include dry heat and air conditioning, daily hot baths or showers, and use of harsh or deodorant soaps.

### Nursing Interventions

The goal of nursing should be to maintain the integrity of the skin. Because the skin of the older person is more fragile, it should be given more gentle care. The use of very hot water, harsh or deodorant soaps, and rubbing alcohol should be avoided. A complete bath two or three times a week is sufficient when supplemented with partial baths. When bathing the elderly, the nurse should use gentle and superfatted soaps and should pat the skin dry rather than rub it. The nurse should use creams and lotions while the skin is still slightly damp. Bath oil must not be used in the water, because this makes the bathtub slippery and increases the likelihood of a fall. The nurse should use cornstarch rather than talcum powder in skin folds because talcum tends to cake and irritate when it becomes moist. The skin should be examined frequently for early signs of irritation or pathologic conditions. Proper humidity should be maintained in a heated or air-conditioned environment. Nutrition greatly influences the condition of the skin, and older people should be taught the importance of a sound, healthy diet.

## Musculoskeletal System

Aging of the musculoskeletal system affects bones, joints, muscles, and muscle attachments. Bone mass diminishes and the intervertebral disks of the spinal column thin, resulting in shortening of the trunk. This, along with a general flexion of the joints, results in a decrease in height, forward projection of the head and neck, and kyphosis (widow's hump). Loss of bone mass and postural changes increase the risk of fractures and falls. Fear of falling frequently leads to reduced mobilization, which decreases bone mass. Muscle fiber decreases, and muscle regeneration slows. Muscles atrophy and are replaced by fibrous tissue. These changes result in diminished muscle strength. Subcutaneous tissue is redistributed, with a decrease in the face and extremities and an increase around the abdomen and hips. Changes occur in the cartilage of the joints, especially the weight-bearing joints such as knees and hips, causing stiffness. These changes can be aggravated by joint stress, obesity, and a decrease in ambulation. Although the decrease in muscle strength and the increased joint stiffness cannot be halted, they can be significantly slowed with exercise.

### Assessment

The musculoskeletal system is assessed by first noting the curvature of the spine. The nurse should ask the individual to bend forward, sideways, and slightly backward to check the range of motion of the spine. The nurse should next ask the person to sit. This routine assesses the spinal muscles and hip muscles. The nurse should assess the upper extremities, symmetrically checking each joint in active and passive range of motion. The nurse should palpate the joints, noting deformities, tenderness, or areas of warmth. To check the lower extremities, the individual's gait should be observed. The nurse should examine the joints as with the upper extremities but should note carefully the internal and external rotation of the hips.

## Common Pathologic Conditions

The most common problems affecting the musculoskeletal system in the elderly include arthritis, osteoarthritis, gout, and fractures (see Chapter 33). **Osteoporosis** is a condition characterized by decreased bone density, resulting in weakness and brittleness of the bone. The bones become very fragile and fracture easily, often after only slight trauma. The sites most affected are the vertebrae, the hip, and the wrist. The kyphosis seen in many older women is caused by collapse fractures of the thoracic vertebrae. Osteoporosis results from the aging of the bone remodeling process. Before age 45 or so, bone formation, or absorption, is greater than bone loss, or resorption. After age 45 the process reverses, and bone mass is lost. Risk factors that appear to increase the occurrence of osteoporosis include cigarette smoking, high caffeine intake, excessive alcohol intake, a high-protein diet, a history of low dietary calcium, low vitamin D, a slender body build with little body fat, and a sedentary life-style. Bone loss increases significantly after menopause, which puts women at greater risk. Treatment of osteoporosis is aimed at prevention.

Ideally, prevention begins in the early years of life. Building up the bones throughout childhood and early adulthood by adequate calcium intake provides for greater bone mass. When bone loss begins later in life, a greater percentage of bone mass remains. Prevention of osteoporosis in mature people includes exercise, calcium, and estrogen replacement therapy.

Newer medications have been shown to increase spinal bone mass and reduce the rate of vertebral fractures. These medications include etidronate and intranasal calcitonin spray. However these medications are very expensive and may have significant side effects (Overgaard et al, 1992), and they do not negate the importance of preventive measures. Weight-bearing exercise such as walking, jogging, bicycling, and dancing stimulates bone formation and retards bone mass reduction (Goodman, 1987). Older adults without kidney disease should increase their intake of dietary calcium to the equivalent of three or four glasses of skim milk a day (1200 mg). Alternative sources of calcium include cheese, yogurt, canned salmon (with bones), and calcium supplements. Calcium carbonate is more easily absorbed from the gastrointestinal tract and is recommended. Estrogen replacement therapy after menopause may be recommended for those at high risk of osteoporosis.

## Nursing Interventions

A person's sense of self is directly affected by his or her ability to be independently mobile. Likewise, a healthy mental attitude will stimulate the individual to take measures to maintain motor function. Nurses can assist the older adult to assume a positive mental attitude and outlook on life. Exercise is extremely important in maintaining motor function. Every older adult can benefit from exercise, but it must be appropriate to the capabilities of the individual. Walking, swimming, dancing, jogging, stretching, and aerobics are all beneficial in maintaining muscle strength and joint movement. Pain management for elderly people who have muscle and joint pain is essential (Ebersole, Hess, 1994). Good nutrition is important in supplying the energy, vitamins, and minerals needed to maintain a healthy state.

Safety is of primary concern in preserving motor function. The nurse should assess the person's environment and recommend measures such as appropriate lighting and the use of grab bars, canes, or walkers when appropriate. Area rugs and other obstructions that could cause falls and injuries should be removed.

## Neurologic System

Changes in the nervous system of the aging adult include a decrease in the number of functioning neurons. This is a gradual change that becomes more pronounced over the age of 70. The loss of neurons means loss of neuronal interconnections, which results in slower conduction of nerve impulses. For this reason, it is more difficult for the elderly to maintain body homeostasis. Recovery from stress is slower and incomplete. The elderly are at risk for hypothermia and hyperthermia that may become life-threatening. Reaction time also is slowed among the elderly. Reflexes are diminished, and motor activity is slower. Tremors are common, especially in the head, face, and hands. The sense of pain also is diminished, and the elderly may be free of pain in such acute disorders as myocardial infarction or pneumonia. Older adults take longer to fall asleep, have shorter periods of deep sleep, and awaken more often during the night (Hamby et al, 1994).

## Assessment

Assessment of the nervous system is a complex process, but several simple techniques can provide valuable information. Careful observation of the person's gait will reveal the ability to coordinate muscle movements. The reflexes may be slowed but should be equal bilaterally. Sometimes severe arthritis can depress the knee-jerk reflex. Sensory testing can be done by using a cotton wisp for light touch and a cotton-tipped swab for deep touch. The nurse should touch the skin at different places bilaterally, from head to toe, while the person's eyes are closed. The person is asked to indicate when the wisp is felt. Deep touch is assessed in the same way, using a broken cotton-tipped swab, first the point, and then the head. The person is asked to identify "sharp" and "dull."

## Common Pathologic Conditions

The most common pathologic conditions of the neurologic system in older adults are **delirium** and **dementia**. Delirium (acute confusional states) is usually a temporary, reversible condition frequently associated with physical or mental illness in older adults (AHCPR Clinical Practice Guideline No. 19, 1996). Dementia (chronic brain syndrome) is a progressive decline in an individual's intellectual function.

Delirium is associated with metabolic changes and disruptions. It can be caused by cardiovascular changes such as CVA, decreased blood supply, congestive heart failure, or infection, as well as by metabolic disturbances such as hypokalemia, hyperkalemia, hypoglycemia, hyperglycemia, acidosis, or alkalosis.

Psychologic disturbances such as depression, grief, fatigue, or severe emotional stress, and environmental factors such as sensory deprivation or sensory overload also can be responsible for a state of delirium. Symptoms include sudden onset of confusion, disorientation, hallucinations, incoherent speech, anger, apathy, or changes in psychomotor activity. The delirium state usually is temporary and can be reversed by identifying and correcting the underlying condition causing it.

Dementia is a group of pathologic conditions characterized by a gradual decline in intellectual function, with symptoms such as loss of memory for recent and remote events, impaired ability to problem solve or to make judgments, and personality changes. The most common of the dementias is Alzheimer's disease.

## Alzheimer's Disease

**Alzheimer's disease** is a chronic, degenerative, irreversible disease. It is more common in women. No genetic links have been found, but it does have familial tendencies. The disease results in characteristic changes in the brain that can be identified only on autopsy: cerebral atrophy, senile plaques, and neurofibrillary tangles. The cause of Alzheimer's disease is unknown. A great deal of research is underway to isolate a cause, and many theories have been advanced, including environmental factors such as aluminum, head trauma, infection, immunologic factors, and genetic factors. Although aluminum is found in the damaged cells, some believe it enters the cell only as a result of the damage, not as the cause. There is no cure for Alzheimer's disease, and death usually occurs in an average of 5 to 8 years, although some victims have been known to live for 15 to 20 years after diagnosis.

Alzheimer's disease is classified into three stages. The *first stage*, the forgetful or mild stage, is characterized by short-term memory loss, mild disorientation for time and date, difficulty completing mathematical calculations, and subtle behavioral changes, such as a decreased interest in work, family, or recreation. The *second stage* is the confused stage, and symptoms include extreme confusion, suspiciousness and paranoia, and difficulty with ADL, such as driving, money management, and home maintenance. Patients are easily lost even in familiar places and will wander off, especially at night. They have difficulty functioning in environments other than home. During this stage patients neglect personal hygiene and withdraw from social groups, often becoming frustrated, and they may strike out at caregivers. Individuals may become extremely depressed if they are aware of what is happening. The *third stage* is the dementia or terminal stage, in which these patients have a flat affect and no longer ambulate. They do not recognize family or friends, are unable to communicate, and have no interaction with the environment. They become malnourished and emaciated and are incontinent. This last stage may progress to a condition known as "chronic vegetative state," in which the patient becomes unresponsive, even to pain, and lies in the fetal position. These patients are completely dependent on the nurse to maintain their skin integrity, nutritional status, and personal hygiene and to prevent injury.

## Assessment

No definitive tests are available to confirm a diagnosis of Alzheimer's disease. Only by examining the brain on autopsy can the diagnosis be confirmed. The diagnosis is made on the basis of cognitive and behavioral symptoms and by ruling out other physiologic and psychologic disorders. A complete history and physical examination are needed, and laboratory testing should include a complete blood count, blood chemistries, thyroid function tests, and folate and vitamin $B_{12}$ levels. A computed axial tomography scan of the head may also be needed. Careful review of all prescription and over-the-counter medications is imperative. A differential assessment for dementia, depression, and delirium should be performed, and experts in geriatric evaluation should be consulted to perform the examination and interpret the findings (Table 9-3). Since the goal of nursing care is to keep the individual

**TABLE 9-3**

## Differential Assessment of Dementia, Depression, and Delirium

| | NORMAL AGING | DEMENTIA | DEPRESSION | DELIRIUM |
|---|---|---|---|---|
| Onset | | Insidious | Acute | Rapid onset |
| Duration | | Months to years | Weeks to months | Hours to days |
| Behavior | Less physical; activity diminished and slower | Shuffling; restlessness; pacing | Slower; retarded movements | Increased or decreased activity level; change in level of consciousness |
| Mood | Appropriate to situation; normal, has energy | Normal; labile; sad | Sad; negative | Fear and suspicion may be prominent |
| Speech | Normal; may concentrate on past, separation, and death; speech is goal directed and has information | Confabulate; vague; focused on past | Negative; clear; repetitive; demanding | Slurred and incoherent |
| Thinking | Normal; intact | Illusions; old memories; suspicious | Distorted self-image and body image; distortion of others' motives; overpersonalized | Sensory misinterpretations; visual, auditory and tactile hallucinations may be florid |
| Memory | Slowing of memory storage, but easy access to information | Loss of recent memory; denies loss; conceals deficits | May be decreased by preoccupation; exaggerates loss; "I don't know" answers | Impaired by poor attention |
| Intelligence | Intact | Impaired; cannot recall previous learning | Intact; may be slow but will be accurate | Fluctuation of problem-solving ability |
| Orientation (time, place, person) | O.K. | First loses times, then place, and lastly orientation to person | Intact | Disoriented |
| Judgment (ability to evaluate a situation) | O.K.; perhaps better because of life experience | Impaired; decreased creativity; cannot use experience; cannot generalize | Intact except for evaluation of self | Fluctuation |

functioning at his or her highest possible level, the nurse must assess the patient's abilities on a continuing basis. Areas that should be assessed include level of consciousness, reality orientation, memory, ability to reason, ability to carry out ADL, interaction with others, and response to environmental stimuli.

### Nursing Interventions

Alzheimer's disease has no known cure. New drugs are being developed that may be effective for treating mild to moderate Alzheimer's disease, but research is still being done to evaluate the long-term effectiveness of the these medications. As with all new medications, these drugs are expensive and may have significant side effects. Medications may be used to reduce agitation or depression, but the use of these drugs is controversial. The focus of nursing care for Alzheimer's patients is to maintain the highest possible level of functioning for each person. Most Alzheimer's patients are cared for at home during the early stages of the disease and are institutionalized when the resources of the caregivers are exhausted. As the disease progresses, care becomes more and more difficult for family members. They need reassurance and help with developing and maintaining an ever-changing plan of care. Community resources for families of Alzheimer's patients often are lacking, but the nurse can assist by working through the political and social systems to provide this desperately needed support.

The Alzheimer's Association has many local chapters that conduct caregiver support groups and information sessions. Caregivers should be encouraged to attend these meetings. Care of the Alzheimer's patient at home or in an institution should establish effective verbal and nonverbal communication, provide a safe and structured environment, maintain normal daily living patterns, maintain mobility and exercise as much as possible, provide cognitive stimulation in the environment, maintain optimal nutritional status, and maintain bowel and bladder continence as long as possible (Box 9-1).

## Digestive System

Most of the problems associated with the gastrointestinal system of the elderly are the result of pathologic conditions and are not part of the normal aging process. The loss of teeth commonly attributed to aging is preventable if good dental hygiene has be followed earlier in life. Gastric secretion decreases slightly, and peristalsis in the bowel slows. This may lead to various complaints, one of the most frequent being constipation and its complications, colon flatus, and fecal impaction. Some older adults become lactose intolerant and find that eating or drinking milk products causes bloating and diarrhea. Avoiding foods high in lactose may alleviate this problem. Pathologic conditions in the older adult are the same as those seen in all adults. Chapter 35 provides a discussion of problems associated with the gastrointestinal system.

### Constipation

Constipation is a common complaint among the elderly. It is most important to determine the person's definition of constipation. Many people subscribe to the theory that daily bowel movements are necessary and that less frequent movements indicate constipation. They spend a great deal of time and money attempting to induce daily movements, and many become laxative dependent. The nurse can help to reeducate these elderly people about good bowel hygiene. Laxatives should be taken only under the direction of a physician.

### Assessment

Assessment of the elderly digestive tract includes a good oral examination. The condition of the mucous membrane should be noted. The nurse should examine the teeth for caries and evidence of good hygiene. If dentures are in place, the individual should remove them so that the nurse can inspect the gums. The nurse should question the older patient about fluid intake, because many older people restrict fluids or take dehydrating diuretics, both of which contribute to dry, hard stool and constipation. A stethoscope can be set lightly on the abdomen to listen for bowel sounds. It may take up to 1 minute to hear sounds in any one area. Increased sounds can mean a hyperactive intestine, as in diarrhea, and decreased sounds can be a sign of paralytic ileus or obstruction. A rectal examination provides information about anal sphincter tone. Fecal impaction may be present if large amounts of hard stool are in the rectum. The stool should be tested for signs of occult blood.

### Nursing Interventions

Nursing interventions for the gastrointestinal system focus on providing for and maintaining a healthy state of functioning in the patient. Good mouth care and attention to dental problems are essential. Teaching about and providing a healthy diet are important. It is not easy for older adults to change lifelong eating habits, so this may present a challenge to the nurse. Healthy bowel habits are necessary to prevent constipation. These include a sufficient intake of high-fiber foods and raw fruits and vegetables, six to eight

---

<table>
<tr><td colspan="2">BOX 9-1          NURSING PROCESS</td></tr>
<tr><td colspan="2">ALZHEIMER'S DISEASE</td></tr>
</table>

**ASSESSMENT**

- Mobility impairment
- Impulsive behavior
- Cognitive impairment
- Orientation to time, place, person
- Self-care ability and routine
- Patterns of elimination
- Coping mechanisms of patient and family
- Safety of environment

**NURSING DIAGNOSES**

- Risk for injury/trauma related to inability to recognize danger, deterioration, or weakness
- Altered thought processes related to loss of memory
- Self-care deficit related to impaired cognition, memory, or judgment
- Risk for total incontinence related to lack of sensation to void
- Risk for bowel incontinence related to impaired cognition
- Anticipatory grieving related to change in behavior
- Dysfunctional grieving related to perception in loss of loved one
- Caregiver role strain related to multiple demands, inadequate resources, or difficult situation

**NURSING INTERVENTIONS**

- Eliminate hazards in the environment.
- Redirect the patient's attention when he or she becomes agitated.
- Explore individual preferences.
- Provide the patient with an identification bracelet.
- Avoid use of restraints.
- Approach the patient in a calm manner.
- Speak in a low, slow voice.
- Use simple words and statements.
- Avoid criticism or confrontations.
- Provide a safe home environment.
- Explore the possibility of a home security device to reduce wandering.
- Make useful activities of repetitive activities (dusting, sweeping the floor, collecting junk mail).
- Administer medications as prescribed.
- Provide assistance with self-care activities, but encourage independence.
- Maintain a routine.
- Encourage regular intervals for toileting.
- Encourage adequate fluids but limit them after 6 pm.
- Use protective clothing or incontinence pads as needed.
- Identify support systems and support groups.
- Encourage the care provider to set aside time for himself or herself.

**EVALUATION OF EXPECTED OUTCOMES**

- Experiences no injury
- Participates in self-care activities
- Continent of bowel and bladder
- Caregiver competent and confident in care
- Caregiver knowledgeable about resources and support
- Family able to express concerns and discuss loss

---

glasses of water daily, a regular program of exercise, and a regular, unhurried time for bowel movements. Use of laxatives and enemas should be discouraged unless prescribed by a physician. Institutionalized elderly will need more assistance in assuming the above habits for healthy bowel management. Laxatives, cathartics, and enemas should not be used routinely in institutions that care for the elderly.

## Urinary System

With aging there is a decrease in the number of nephrons in the kidneys and a decrease in the blood supply that together adversely affect the functioning of the urinary system. The kidneys become less effi-cient in concentrating or diluting urine. The renal threshold for glucose is elevated, and individuals tested for high blood glucose will not show elevated levels in the urine. Excretion of drugs is altered, and the elderly must be closely observed for signs of drug toxicity. The smooth muscle and elastic tissue of the bladder are replaced with fibrous connective tissue. This results in decreased bladder capacity and increased frequency of urination. The elderly also experience more nocturia. The force of the stream diminishes, and some may experience stress incontinence. For these reasons many elderly people may avoid going out in public often or taking long trips. Some reduce their fluid intake to avoid embarrassment. Bladder outlet changes may cause obstruction in men and incontinence in women (Ebersole, Hess, 1994).

## Assessment

The urinary system is assessed indirectly by asking the elderly patient about his or her urinary habits. The kidneys themselves are rarely palpated. If a severe kidney infection is present, the individual may have flank tenderness. The amount, color, and odor of the urine can be a means of assessing the urinary system. The external meatus of both men and women should be inspected and kept clean to prevent infections. If the urinary bladder is overfilled with urine, it can be palpated above the pubic bone.

## Common Pathologic Conditions

Because of the age-related decrease in the function of the urinary system, certain pathologic conditions are seen regularly among the elderly. The diminished efficiency of the kidneys may result in acute and chronic renal failure (see Chapter 37). Bladder problems appear, such as urinary retention, urinary tract infections, and cancer of the bladder (see Chapter 37). Urinary incontinence is especially troublesome in women, whereas benign prostatic hypertrophy and prostate cancer are major problems for men (see Chapters 42 and 43).

## Nursing Interventions

The elderly may feel uncomfortable talking about a genitourinary problem and may live with the problem rather than face the embarrassment of mentioning it. The understanding nurse will appreciate these feelings and will provide a private, gentle, and sensitive environment for this discussion. Nursing interventions should focus on maintaining normal function of the urinary system. Mobility and activity promote normal urinary function, therefore the nurse should encourage the elderly to remain as active as possible. Older adults should be aware of their patterns of elimination and should plan their schedules accordingly. Medications that affect elimination, such as diuretics, should be taken in the morning so that they do not interfere with sleep.

When away from home the elderly should locate the washroom in any public place before it is needed. Clothing can be modified to permit ease and speed in removal. The environment also should be modified to accommodate individual needs, which might require providing unobstructed pathways to the bathroom, using a night-light, and having hand rails alongside the toilet to assist in getting up and down. Maintaining

adequate fluid intake is essential for bladder functioning, and good personal hygiene is important in preventing infection and controlling odor. The urine should be examined for indications of a urinary tract infection, and the patient should be treated if one is present. Women with dry, friable vaginal tissue benefit from topical estrogen cream. The patient can be taught Kegel exercises to reduce stress incontinence. These exercises involve tightening the muscles of the pelvic floor in a regular, scheduled pattern (see Chapter 17).

# Respiratory System

The function of the pulmonary system declines with age, and the loss reduces the reserve necessary during stress. These losses are not great enough, however, to interfere with ordinary activity (Matteson, McConnell, 1988). Skeletal changes reduce the flexibility of the rib cage, which tends to remain expanded. The respiratory muscles weaken, resulting in reduced ability of the thoracic cavity to enlarge with inspiration and to recoil with expiration. Smoking, immobility, and obesity can further compromise lung function. Because the lungs are less elastic, more air remains in the lungs, and less air is exchanged. Thickened and fewer capillaries reduce the exchange of oxygen and carbon dioxide in the lungs. The elderly become short of breath more readily and have greater difficulty recovering from respiratory diseases.

## Assessment

The respiratory system is assessed by first looking at the shape of the chest. The nurse should note the condition of the skin and whether the accessory muscles are used for breathing. Breathing should be unstrained and symmetric. The lungs are auscultated posteriorly first and then anteriorly, going side to side, top to bottom. The individual is asked to take a deep breath through the mouth while the stethoscope is placed on the chest. The nurse should observe the person carefully for signs of hyperventilation during this examination. Breath sounds may be distant but should be clear. Soft or loud crackles or wheezes are considered abnormal sounds.

## Common Pathologic Conditions

The most common respiratory diseases among the elderly include chronic obstructive pulmonary disease, emphysema, chronic bronchitis, asthma, tuberculosis, and lung cancer. These are not problems brought on by aging of the lungs but are the result of life-style and environmental factors, including smoking and air pollutants. Pneumonia also is common in older adults.

Several factors contribute to the increased incidence of pneumonia among the elderly, including a weakened immune system, immobility, chronic illness, and debility. Institutionalized elderly people are more vulnerable. These respiratory diseases are discussed in Chapter 22.

## Nursing Interventions

As with other systems, mobility and exercise play an important role in maintaining a healthy respiratory system. Exercise helps reduce the effects of aging on the lungs and increases the muscle tone of the chest and the individual's ability to fight off infection. The elderly who smoke should be encouraged and helped to quit. For older adults with lung problems, the nurse can assist in adapting the environment to reduce irritants. This might mean using filters, humidifiers or dehumidifiers, and air conditioning. Older people at risk for lung diseases should receive flu vaccines yearly in the fall. Pneumococcal vaccine should be administered once in a lifetime to prevent pneumonia. Colds and other respiratory infections should be attended to promptly (Matteson, McConnell, 1988).

## Reproductive System

After menopause women experience a decrease in estrogens, tissue changes in the vulva and vagina, thinning of the epithelial cells, and loss of normal vaginal acidity. The elderly woman is more susceptible to vaginitis because of these changes. The breasts, uterus, and ovaries begin to atrophy. Men experience a reduction in seminal fluid. The prostate may enlarge, and the testes may become smaller and less firm.

## Assessment

Assessment of the breast tissue in elderly women is important because cancer is a concern. The breasts are inspected for symmetry, nipple discharge, or dimpled skin. Circular palpation is done from the axilla, gradually working toward the nipple. A pelvic examination for the elderly woman can be helpful in determining pelvic muscle tone and in detecting a cystocele, rectocele, or uterine prolapse. All of these can contribute to incontinence. Some of these conditions can be noted with careful external inspection. A pelvic examination should be done by a physician or nurse practitioner. The elderly man is examined externally for signs of phimosis (tight foreskin), testicular swelling, hydrocele, or herniations. A physician or nurse practitioner should evaluate the status of the prostate gland by rectal examination.

## Common Pathologic Conditions

Problems of the reproductive system in elderly women include relaxation of the pelvic musculature (cystocele, rectocele, and uterine prolapse) and cancer of the reproductive organs. Breast cancer is the most common form. In elderly men benign prostatic hypertrophy and cancer of the prostate are often seen (see Chapter 42).

## Nursing Interventions

The focus of nursing interventions should be education. Many elderly people feel embarrassed about discussing problems related to their reproductive organs. The nurse needs to be sensitive to their embarrassment and provide an environment in which they can more easily discuss this subject. Adults should be taught breast self-examination or testicular self-examination and encouraged to practice it monthly. Annual mammograms are recommended for women over age 50. Regular physical examinations are recommended for both sexes, including Pap smears for women and digital rectal examinations for men.

# NURSING THE ELDERLY

The process of aging does not necessarily mean a process of decline. Although the elderly are more susceptible to illness, aging does not mean sickness. Physical changes do occur, but physical debility is not a normal part of the aging process. Nursing care of the aging requires the nurse to respect each individual as unique and valued. This includes the manner in which the person is addressed. Every adult should be asked how he or she would like to be addressed. Use of an elderly person's first name by a much younger person is considered by many as a breach of etiquette. To address an older adult as "Grandma" or "Gramps" or "dear" is inappropriate and demeaning. Care of the elderly includes procedures designed to maintain and improve functional ability, dignity, and quality of life, to protect against injury, to recognize individuality, to meet nutritional needs, to maintain personal hygiene, and to prevent complications from drug therapy.

## Maintaining and Improving Functional Ability

A functional assessment identifies the person's level of independence, focusing on abilities rather than disabilities. Each person's ability to perform ADL is assessed using a numeric scale.

Both physical activities of daily living (ADL) and instrumental ADL (IADL) need to be assessed. Physical

ADL include bathing, dressing, eating, ambulating, grooming, managing assistive devices, and using the toilet. IADL involve balancing a checkbook, housekeeping, going to the store, doing laundry, using the telephone, and managing medications.

---

### CASE STUDY

Mrs. Taylor is an 84-year-old woman who lives in a senior high-rise housing complex. She recently stopped bathing because she had difficulty getting out of the bathtub and was afraid of falling. However, she missed her baths very much and did not feel clean when just washing at the sink. Her nurse assessed her ability to rise from a sitting position and found her quadriceps muscles to be weak. She also noticed that the safety bath mat used by Mrs. Taylor in her tub was old and tended to slip. Mrs. Taylor and her nurse agreed to start a plan that eventually would allow her to bathe again. The plan was to strengthen her leg muscles by walking and exercising and to prevent injury by purchasing a new bath mat. In the meantime, Mrs. Taylor agreed not to bathe in the tub unless her daughter was present to help her should she have trouble getting out of the tub.

---

Assessment of functional ability allows the members of the health care team to design a care plan that considers the patient's ability to care for himself or herself independently. The assessment forms the basis from which goals and nursing interventions are developed. The patient should be involved in the plan of care and can assist in the goal-setting process. Each step can be discussed and a plan agreed upon.

The nurse may involve other members of the health care system who can assist in reaching functional goals. Physical therapy, occupational therapy, speech therapy, dietitians, social workers, and many others have skills that may improve the functional ability of the older person. The best care delivered to older people is multidisciplinary in nature. The nurse often plays the role of coordinator because nursing has a holistic focus.

The functional assessment also serves as a means of evaluation. Through periodic assessment, it can be determined whether abilities have improved or remained stable. In assessing functional status, each function may be evaluated numerically on a scale. As abilities change, the numbers change. The choice of a functional assessment instrument depends on the facility. Some instruments used in clinical practice include the Katz Index of ADL (Katz et al, 1963), the Barthel Index (Mahoney, Barthel, 1965), the PULSES Profile (Moskowitz, McCann, 1957), the Rapid Disability Scale (Linn, Linn, 1982), and the Scale for IADL (Lawton, Brody, 1969).

## Maintaining and Improving Quality of Life

Most older people want to live a life that involves autonomy, security, and the freedom to establish and maintain interpersonal relationships. Although defining **quality of life** is difficult, these concepts, among others, constitute what many older people would call a good life (Swan, Pickard, 1996). Gerontology focuses on improving the quality of life for older people because focusing only on length of life may not be adequate in many circumstances. Many older people prefer to live "a few good years" rather than many years of disability, pain, loneliness, and isolation.

Quality of life is of concern to nursing because the emphasis is on caring and on the well-being of the whole person. Nurses often intervene to improve the quality of life of an older person. Certainly, control of pain and improvement of function can improve the quality of a person's life, but this is just the beginning. Opportunities for growth and development, leisure activities, and privacy are necessary for most older people. Many of the concepts already discussed under the mental health section apply here.

---

### CASE STUDY

Mrs. Kline, age 84, recently returned home after hospitalization for a broken hip. Because she had to limit her activities until fully recuperated, Mrs. Kline could not go to the senior center. The home care nurse found her bored and angry. "I don't want to live like an invalid. I'm bored." The nurse realized that Mrs. Kline was fearful of isolation and that this negatively affected her quality of life. The nurse was able to arrange transportation so that Mrs. Carter, Mrs. Kline's best friend, could visit daily. The nurse also helped her contact the local library for home delivery of books. Although Mrs. Kline continued to be impatient for a full recovery, her feelings of boredom and isolation were lessened, and she greatly enjoyed Mrs. Carter's visits and reading her favorite library books.

---

Quality of life can be measured by asking older people to reflect on their day-to-day lives and to state their level of satisfaction with their life circumstances. Although the nurse may not be able to improve many things in an older person's life, many other areas may be addressed by the health care team.

Physical well-being, psychologic well-being, and quality of life are all closely correlated in the elderly patient. Nurses should make sure that the nursing care plan includes interventions designed to maintain and improve quality of life for the elderly.

## Group Work with the Elderly

Working with the aged in groups can be effective in meeting psychosocial needs. Group work of this nature is not to be confused with group psychotherapy, which deals with people who have psychiatric problems. Group work has been used to treat and prevent psychosocial problems in the elderly and to maintain mental health. Groups have been conducted for reality orientation, remotivation, reminiscing, and health teaching. In some instances the family also is involved with the group.

**Reality orientation** groups are used with regressed aged people, especially those with chronic brain syndrome. A small group of four or five meets daily with their leader, who emphasizes the time, day, month, weather conditions, and the like, which are then posted on a board for all to see throughout the day. **Remotivation** groups are the next step in progression after reality orientation. The leader must have specialized training to conduct these groups.

Reminiscing groups were pioneered by Ebersole, a psychiatric nurse (Ebersole, Hess, 1994). **Reminiscing** is an adaptive response to aging that can be used effectively to preserve and rebuild self-concept and maintain social integrity. It helps elderly individuals remember who they are and thus stimulates self-esteem.

Validation therapy is a technique used to validate the feelings of those with dementia, and reality is not emphasized. If an older person with dementia calls out for "mother," the feeling behind this call is explored. In other words, is the older person hungry, lost, in need of the special attention that mother can provide? Once the nurse identifies the feelings that underlie the request, appropriate reassurance and nursing care can be provided.

Nurses should be encouraged to investigate the possibility of working with groups, seek whatever training is required, and implement or assist in group work with the elderly when opportunities arise. Group work requires the support and cooperation of everyone in the agency if it is to be successful.

## Helping the Older Person Prepare for Death

Many older people wish to establish a living will, name a health care proxy or durable power of attorney, or leave advance directives regarding their health care with a close friend or relative. These concepts are fully discussed in Chapter 13. Although nurses may feel uncomfortable discussing these issues with essentially healthy older people, it should be remembered that preparation for death is one of the normal developmental tasks of aging. When and if a time comes when a person cannot make decisions for himself or herself,

it is important that someone be able to communicate the wishes of the patient. Although each individual is different, many older people have seen friends or loved ones die while on ventilators or in the critical care units of hospitals, and they may wish to die a "natural death." Natural death occurs when declining organ function becomes insufficient to sustain life (Fries, Crapo, 1981).

Individuals who have lived a long life and survived many threats of illness and accident may die in extreme old age without any obvious cause whatsoever. It is estimated that about one third of all deaths of elderly people are "natural deaths" that occur in the final stages of senescence.

### CASE STUDY

Mr. Watson, age 87, lives alone in his apartment near his son and daughter-in-law. His family notices that he is gradually failing, yet his doctor can find nothing wrong. For the next 6 months, he is just not himself and doesn't have his usual zest for life. One night he dies quietly in his sleep, and even after an autopsy no obvious cause of death can be found.

## Preventing Injury

Injuries resulting from accidents are a major and largely preventable cause of death and illness in the elderly. A great many accidental deaths are the result of complications that arise from falls.

Because most falls occur in the home, precautions should be taken to protect elderly people. Scatter rugs should not be used unless they are secured by rubber mats beneath them. Toys left on the floor and furniture moved to unfamiliar places may be responsible for a fall. Rubber mats should be placed in bathtubs, and support should be provided to assist those stepping from the tub (Figure 9-4). Bath oils should not be used because they may make the tub slippery.

Lights in bathrooms and on stairs should be left on at night, in addition to night-lights, and increased illumination should be provided in the evening. Elderly persons are susceptible to accidents on streets and highways at dusk or in the evening. To avoid such accidents, an elderly person should be accompanied, should carry a flashlight, and should have reflective material attached to his or her clothing.

## Recognizing Individuality

With aging comes increased diversity. Preferences and abilities become unique to each person with the aging

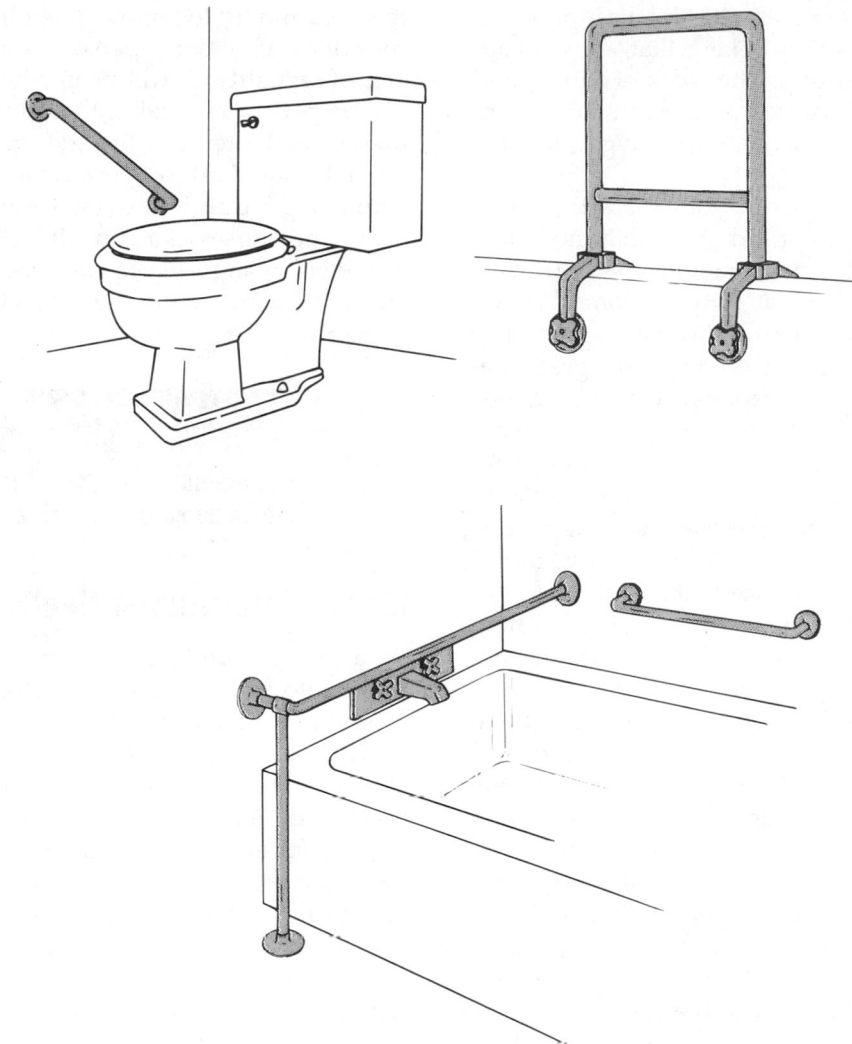

**Figure 9-4**    Hand bars placed on bathtubs and beside toilets provide support for the patient and prevent falls from loss of balance.

process. Society tends to stereotype the elderly as a group with members very like one another. In books, on television, and in most advertising, the elderly often are depicted as needing assistance, forgetful, and asexual. Sometimes nurses and physicians have the most negative stereotypes about aging because health care providers work mostly with sick older people, many of whom have cognitive deficits. However, there are great differences among older people. It is unfair for health care providers to limit an older person's choices and opportunities for rehabilitation because they assume that most older people are hard of hearing, dislike spicy food, care little about sexual relationships, and want a sedentary life-style without new experiences.

### NURSE ALERT

The individual preferences and abilities of each elderly patient must be carefully assessed and incorporated into the person's nursing care plan.

Society has held the stereotyped belief that sexual desire and activity begin to diminish in the mid forties and stop completely sometime in the later years and that this is appropriate. Sexually active elderly people are considered perverse or, at best, to be lying about their activities. Open expressions of sexuality between elderly partners are often met with the disapproval of grown children because they believe that sex is not appropriate for this age group. The work of Kinsey and Masters and Johnson, as well as recent studies conducted at Duke University, are proving quite the opposite.

Although Kinsey's work did not deal with a large sample of elderly people, it did show that most men over age 60 were capable of sexual intercourse (Kinsey et al, 1948) and that sexual activity in women varied more with marital status than it did with age (Kinsey et al, 1953). Masters and Johnson devoted a great deal of their study to the sexual responses of aged individuals. They found that physically, men over age 60 are slower to respond sexually and the physiologic response of women diminishes somewhat, but both are capable of orgasm, especially those often exposed to effective stimulation (Masters, Johnson, 1970). Studies continue to add to the evidence that sex plays an important role in the lives of many elderly people. These studies, along with the work of Masters and Johnson, lead to some overall conclusions that are different from the stereotype held by society, namely, that there is no specific age when sexual activity will and should cease. Frequency of sexual activity is related to the availability of a socially sanctioned partner rather than to age. An individual who has frequent sexual experiences earlier in life will continue to have more frequent sexual experiences later in life than will the person who is less active in early years. Good physical health affects sexual functioning and will affect the quality and quantity of sexual activity in the elderly.

---

### CASE STUDY

Mr. Jackson, age 69, recently had a stroke that left him paralyzed on his right side and unable to talk. He uses a wheelchair but is able to walk short distances with the assistance of a cane. Mrs. Jackson visits her husband each day in the rehabilitation unit of the hospital. Mrs. Jackson asked one of the evening nurses when she and Mr. Jackson could resume their sexual relationship, which she described as very intimate and satisfying to both of them. The nurse blushed with embarrassment and said, "I don't know. You'd better ask the doctor." Mrs. Jackson felt that she had said the wrong thing to the nurse and did not mention anything about sex again during the remainder of her husband's rehabilitation.

---

These current findings should be considered by the nurse working with the elderly. Nurses must become comfortable with the idea that the elderly have or desire to have an active sex life. The elderly do receive pleasure from sex, and sexual problems may, in turn, trouble older people. The nurse must educate others in this area and try to remove prejudices. The nurse must consider each elderly person as an individual in the area of **sexuality**, as well as in other human needs. The elderly person's sexual needs are affected by his or her present and previous life-style rather than by some concrete standard of performance. Again, the best gerontologic care is provided by a multidisciplinary team, and nurses can consult with other health care providers to set realistic goals for the older patient that are consistent with the individual's needs and strengths.

---

### NURSE ALERT

The prejudices of the nurse have no place in providing care to the elderly or anyone.

---

## Meeting Nutritional Needs

As a group, elderly people appear to be highly susceptible to malnutrition. In senescence, the metabolic processes decrease by 10% to 30%, physical activity decreases, and the individual needs fewer calories. However, if appetite fails, the individual becomes malnourished. Some elderly people are obese and continue to follow dietary patterns of overeating, particularly rich foods. They, too, may be undernourished, not in calories but in dietary essentials (Box 9-2).

The diet should include all the nutritional requirements, that is, carbohydrates, fats, proteins, vitamins, minerals, and water. Because of reduced physical activity and a decline in metabolic activity, elderly people need fewer calories than when they were younger. Caloric needs must be evaluated individually. Men may require more calories than women, and some people require more calories than others because they are more active and expend more energy. It has been suggested that calories should be reduced by 7% to 8% every 10 years after a person has reached age 25.

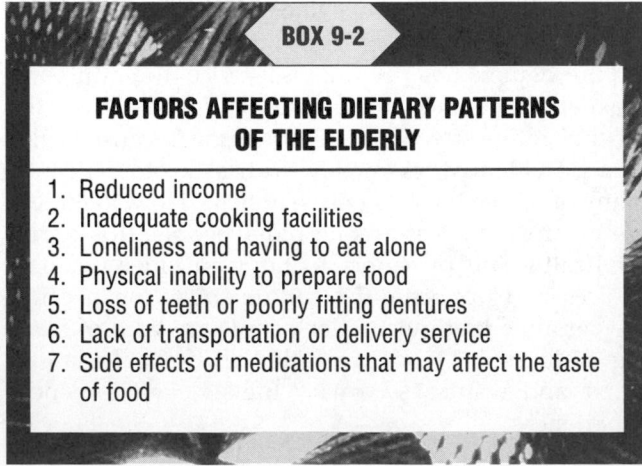

### BOX 9-2

#### FACTORS AFFECTING DIETARY PATTERNS OF THE ELDERLY

1. Reduced income
2. Inadequate cooking facilities
3. Loneliness and having to eat alone
4. Physical inability to prepare food
5. Loss of teeth or poorly fitting dentures
6. Lack of transportation or delivery service
7. Side effects of medications that may affect the taste of food

The diet should include the five basic food groups: (1) breads, cereals, pasta, and rice; (2) fruits; (3) vegetables; (4) milk and cheese; (5) meat, fish, poultry, eggs, dry beans, and nuts. The basic food groups apply to all people regardless of age, with the calories adjusted through smaller or larger servings. There is some evidence that proper use of food in the body requires that all nutrients be present at approximately the same time. Although the "basic five" diet provides a simple, systematic guide to food selection, it does not regulate intake of salt, cholesterol, and saturated fat. Additional information must be provided to guide the elderly in selecting a diet that is well balanced and at the same time low in salt, cholesterol, and saturated fat (Ebersole, Hess, 1994).

The frequency and amount of food served is also important, and it is recommended that the daily food requirement be divided into six small meals. Vitamin and mineral supplements should be used only on the advice of the physician. Whenever possible, the individual should eat with the family, and food should be prepared the way the person likes it and then served attractively. The elderly should be encouraged to participate in food selection and preparation if they are able, and guidance in including all essential foods in the diet should be provided as necessary. For those frail elderly who live at home and need assistance with meal preparation, home-delivered meals for the elderly (Meals on Wheels) may be appropriate. Many community senior citizen centers sponsor daily lunch programs at minimal cost for elderly people who attend activities at the center. In addition to a good meal, socialization and recreational activities may benefit the older person.

## Maintaining Personal Hygiene

Daily baths result in excessive dryness and scaling of the skin, often accompanied by itching. Inadequate rinsing may cause a dermatitis, causing a great deal of discomfort from burning and itching of the affected parts. Complete baths should be reduced to two or three a week, with careful rinsing and drying. However, attention should be given to the perineal area on a daily basis. Bath oils may be added to the water, but extra caution must be taken to prevent falls, since these oils may make the tub slippery. Showers, taken with a hand-held shower head in a stall that has a seat or is large enough for a bath chair, provide for thorough rinsing and are easier to maneuver in and out of than are bathtubs. An elderly person should not be alone in a locked bathroom. However, it is important to ensure privacy, which can be accomplished by a sign on the door or hanging from the doorknob to tell others than the room is occupied. Because of diminished activity of oil glands, the hair should be shampooed less often, and shampoos containing alcohol should be avoided because of their drying effect.

Cold weather and dry furnace heat can aggravate the problem of dry skin. Older people who spend the winter in cold climates should take extra precautions to prevent skin problems. Wearing soft clothing and using skin lotions can help prevent dryness. Care of the feet is also important. Warm soaks with thorough drying, particularly between the toes, followed by massage with baby oil or lanolin will prevent excessive drying. A member of the family or the nurse should trim the nails. If financial resources permit, the individual may be taken to a podiatrist for foot care. Visits may be scheduled at 4- to 6-week intervals. Corns, calluses, and infections require special care.

Many elderly people have partial or full dentures, and some have teeth missing. The loss of teeth, dental caries, and poorly fitting dentures can affect the person's general health by interfering with dietary needs. Normal shrinking of the gums exposes the soft parts of the tooth structure, which are more sensitive to injury. Improperly fitting dentures may cause the gums to become sore. Regular gum massage stimulates circulation and helps keep gums healthy. For those who have their own teeth, regular visits to the dentist are necessary. Teeth should be brushed after meals with a mild dentifrice and a soft-bristle brush; dentures also should be brushed after each meal.

Sluggishness of the bowel, which may accompany aging, is primarily the result of inactivity and faulty diet. When it occurs, it is not unusual for the person to resort to the use of a laxative that was seen advertised or that a well-meaning friend or neighbor has suggested. Laxatives, like any other medication, should be prescribed by the physician. Regular bowel habits should be encouraged and, when possible, the diet should include some soft bulk to facilitate bowel evacuation. Simple measures such as prune juice at night or a glass of warm water with a little lemon juice before breakfast may be all that is required.

Decreased muscle tone and reduced capacity of the bladder may cause urinary incontinence. This may result in embarrassment for the individual. A medical examination should be done to rule out infection or other pathologic condition. Clothing should be changed as often as necessary to prevent odor and skin excoriation. If no pathologic condition is found, incontinence can be prevented by planning frequent use of the bathroom, commode, or bed pan during the day and by limiting fluids after the evening meal.

The individual should be encouraged to maintain good personal hygiene and good personal appearance, particularly with reference to hair and clothing. For many elderly people some member of the family will have to help with or supervise daily care. The same principles of personal hygiene apply to the individual who may be hospitalized or in a nursing home.

## Preventing Complications from Drug Use

Twenty-five percent of all medications are taken by the 10% of the population who are over age 65. For this reason, and because of the physiologic effects of aging on drug action, drug use in the elderly must be carefully examined.

It is said that 85% of all prescriptions written by a physician are based on what the patient says. When an older patient complains of sleep problems, lack of energy, or feelings of sadness or chronic pain, a busy physician may be tempted to write a prescription for a medicine to solve the problem rather than get a full history relating to the problem. In other words, sometimes older people are treated for symptoms of physical problems without an adequate exploration of the cause of the problem. This approach sometimes makes the patient's problem worse because many medications may cause side effects and further reduce the patient's functional ability. These potential problems make it particularly important that older patients know about their drugs, understand their actions, and keep their physicians informed. It is equally important for the nurse to be aware of age-related factors that affect drug action and increase toxicity in this age group.

The age-related factors that account for changes in drug action and increased toxicity are numerous. Gastric emptying time is slowed in the older person, and the motility of the gastrointestinal tract is slower. Intestinal blood flow is reduced, and absorption by the cells also is reduced. For these reasons, drugs taken orally and absorbed in the gastrointestinal tract are absorbed more slowly than they would be in a younger person. Metabolism slows with age, and any drug that affects or is affected by metabolism will be needed in lower doses. For example, dosage of antibiotics should be reduced because an elderly person retains antibiotics in the body longer than a younger person. The absorption and distribution of a drug changes with age. Passage across the blood-brain barrier, however, is always good, which means that the drug will manage to get to the brain, even though it may not be supplied as well to other parts of the body. This accounts for the fact that confusion frequently is an early sign of drug toxicity in the elderly. Excretion is another factor affecting drug action. The nephrons in the kidney are reduced by 50% to 60% with aging, and liver function declines, both of which slow the rate at which drugs are excreted from the body. Cumulative actions can be a problem if doses are not reduced to account for the aging process.

When evaluating drug dosages ordered for the elderly, the nurse must remember that recommended drug dosages are tested on 25-year-old, healthy men weighing approximately 150 pounds. One commonly used drug, diazepam (Valium), has a recommended adult dosage of 15 to 50 mg per day, usually given in three or four doses. In the elderly it has been found that 5 to 15 mg of diazepam per day is the maximum that should be given and that 2 mg per dose or 6 mg per day is probably the most beneficial. Diazepam is commonly ordered for the elderly, but at 5 or 10 mg three times a day. Like diazepam, all tranquilizers and antidepressants should be administered in reduced dosages. Dosages ordered for elderly patients, as well as the symptoms they are exhibiting, should be examined. If a patient is showing confusion, it could be because these drugs are being excreted slowly by the body and are crossing the blood-brain barrier in toxic levels. Confusion may be one of the earliest signs of toxicity. When older people act confused, they are often labeled senile, but medications should be checked to see whether the confusion is, in fact, drug induced.

Sedatives and other nervous system depressants have an intensified effect on the elderly, therefore only small doses of the drugs should be given. Elderly people may exhibit bizarre behavior when given a sedative or hypnotic. Memory loss, disorientation, falls, and incontinence commonly occur.

Barbiturates include in their action an ability to slow the heart rate. For this reason, it is best to avoid the use of barbiturates for the elderly, and some authorities believe that they should not be used by anyone. Any elderly patient who is taking a barbiturate should be watched for signs of reduced heart action, and extreme care should be exercised if that patient has a heart problem. The nurse should be sure to report these symptoms to the main provider immediately so that the medication order might be reconsidered.

In drug idiosyncrasies, known to be common in the elderly, the action obtained from the drug is just the opposite of the intended action. For example, if a sleeping pill is given and the individual has an idiosyncrasy to that particular drug, sleeplessness rather than sleep will result.

**Drug interactions** are a problem not only for the elderly but for all individuals taking drugs. Drugs interact with foods and with other drugs in ways that may affect the action of the drug. The dangers of giving aspirin with anticoagulants and causing an increase in bleeding are well known. Antacids are not to be given with an antibiotic because they tie up the antibiotic and reduce its effectiveness. There are literally hundreds and hundreds of possible drug interactions; the nurse should consult drug references to identify the possible interactions for each drug the patient is taking.

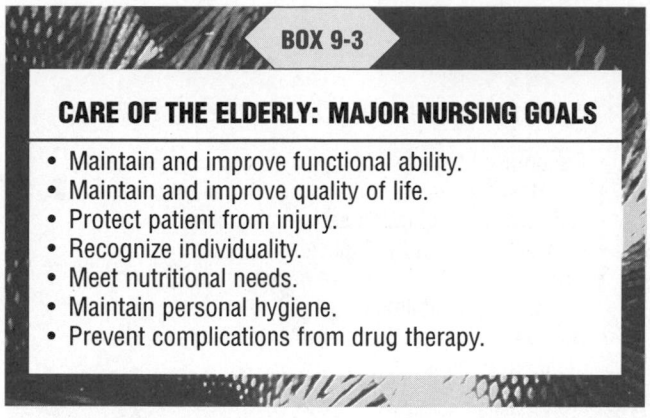

It is important that all drugs taken by the elderly be identified. This includes not only those prescribed by all providers but also the over-the-counter drugs that the elderly may not even consider as drugs or medications. A very careful history must be taken to identify every drug that the elderly person is taking to avoid interactions and possible toxic effects. The route and method of administration must be as clearly understood by elderly people as by younger persons. If the drug is to be taken under the tongue or taken without chewing, it is important that the person understand those directions to achieve the therapeutic effect.

An elderly person with dementia may resist taking medications. Some will very aggressively refuse. It is necessary to see the patient swallow the drug and to be sure that the patient has not hidden the drug under the tongue, in the buccal cavity, in the hand or bed linen, or in any number of other places. The nurse should stay with the patient while he or she takes the drug and ensure that it is gone from the mouth. It may even be necessary to check the mouth after the person supposedly has taken the drug to be sure that it has been swallowed and that he or she does not aspirate. Preventing complications from drug therapy is one of the major nursing goals in the care of the elderly (Box 9-3).

## CARE OF THE HOSPITALIZED ELDERLY PATIENT

Nursing elderly patients with acute mental or surgical conditions is different in many respects from nursing younger patients. The normal changes of aging produce physiologic and psychologic patterns that would not be observed in younger people. Nursing care of the elderly requires more time because these patients move and act more slowly. The time spent with the patient varies and is appropriate to the needs of each patient. More assistance may be required in performing ADL. A gentle touch is also important because the older person is susceptible to injury to skin, bones, and connective tissue. To avoid injury, assistance from other nursing personnel may be needed for turning, lifting, and ambulating the older patient.

## Mental Status and Vital Signs

The level of orientation, memory, and level of consciousness of older people may change when they are acutely ill. The acute confusional state is called delirium and was discussed previously. When delirium occurs, the nurse should conduct a careful search for the cause. This would include a complete examination of all medications, review of bowel function and vital signs, and inspection of the patient's physical environment. While protecting the patient from injury, the nurse and other members of the health care team can attempt to correct the cause of the delirium.

Elderly patients often do not tolerate sedative drugs as well as do younger patients, and after surgery they usually require smaller amounts of narcotics. Changing the patient's position, giving a warm drink, or sitting with an anxious patient often is of greater value than administering a drug. When a hypnotic is administered to an elderly person at bedtime, it is important for the nurse to check on the patient frequently. Often the patient may become confused, try to get out of bed, and fall, causing serious injury. When administering any medication to elderly people, it is advisable not to use the term "drug," since many of them associate drugs with addiction.

Blood pressure is influenced by age, but the range of systolic pressure may be rather wide; the diastolic range, however, is less wide. Any significant change in blood pressure should always be reported. The blood pressure of elderly people may be affected by chronic disease or the stress of illness. In the elderly person, a small change in blood pressure may be more important than it would be in a younger person, and the pulse's rate may be less significant than its volume and rhythm. The rate must be considered together with other symptoms and the patient's condition. It is not uncommon for the pulse in an elderly person to be intermittent, and patients who are receiving digitalis often exhibit changes in the normal rate and rhythm of the pulse. Most people over 70 years of age have premature beats, which occur sooner than expected in the rhythmic pattern. The nurse should develop a sensitivity to what is felt and be able to report it accurately.

## Intake and Output and Nutritional Needs

Total fluid intake, including that contained in foods, should be sufficient to produce 1500 ml of urine in 24 hours. Since many older people are dehydrated, fluids often are retained until a physiologic balance has been established. A severely dehydrated patient may retain and absorb solution administered as an enema. Persuading an individual to take oral fluids can be a frustrating experience, and small amounts at frequent intervals often are better accepted than a large amount at one time. When fluids are restricted because of a cardiac condition or other problem, the nurse should understand the amount permitted and calculate it carefully.

In some conditions and after surgery, the physician may order administration of solutions intravenously. An important factor in the administration of intravenous fluids to elderly people is the rate of flow. Severe cardiac disturbance may result if fluids are administered too rapidly. Unless ordered otherwise by the physician, 1000 ml of fluid should not be administered in less than 4 hours. Elderly people often do not tolerate blood transfusions well. The blood should be administered slowly, and the patient should be observed carefully during the procedure. Careful records of intake and output should be maintained, and accurate measurements should be made.

Nutrition for the hospitalized older person may be difficult because many older patients may not wish to eat on a hospital schedule or may dislike the quality and variety of foods served. If allowed, family members may wish to bring in favorite foods from home that the patient may enjoy. Food not eaten at mealtime can be labeled and stored in the refrigerator for a snack at bedtime. Liquid protein drinks can be given between meals to boost caloric intake and protein ingestion. Older patients who select their own daily menu should be urged to choose a wide variety of foods representing a balanced diet and extra protein choices to speed the healing process after surgery.

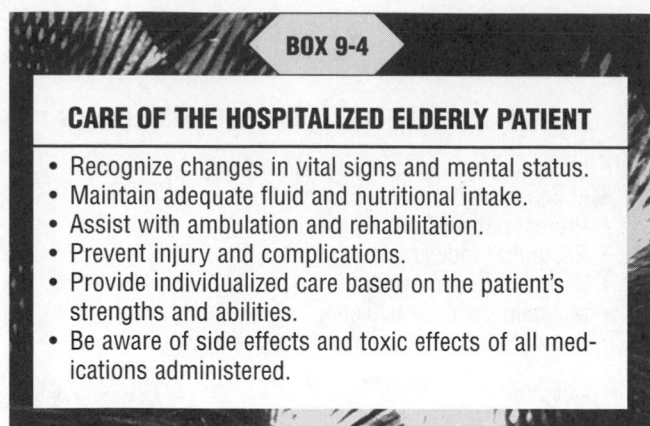

**BOX 9-4**

### CARE OF THE HOSPITALIZED ELDERLY PATIENT

- Recognize changes in vital signs and mental status.
- Maintain adequate fluid and nutritional intake.
- Assist with ambulation and rehabilitation.
- Prevent injury and complications.
- Provide individualized care based on the patient's strengths and abilities.
- Be aware of side effects and toxic effects of all medications administered.

---

> ### NURSE ALERT
>
> **Scheduling ambulation as soon as possible prevents possible side effects of hospitalization.**

## Ambulation and Rehabilitation

Recovery from acute illness often is accompanied by chronic disease, which may affect the rate of recovery. Older people require longer periods for recovery than do younger persons, and their progress is slower. The elderly should be out of bed as much as their condition permits to prevent complications of bed rest. The process of ambulation should be slow and progressive, beginning with elevating the patient in bed. The next steps are to have the patient sit on the side of the bed, then sit up in a chair for 15 to 20 minutes beside the bed, then take a few steps, then gradually lengthen the time up and the extent of walking. The patient should be observed for color, respiration, and pulse rate, and if faintness or dizziness occurs, the patient should be returned to bed. An elderly person out of bed for the first time should not be left alone.

The older patient recovering from surgery or serious illness may become anxious and frustrated because of the slow rate of recovery and long convalescence. The nurse should recognize that these emotions can affect the patient's desire to participate in care and continue with prescribed activities. A caring attitude, encouragement, and support are important aspects of care.

When caring for elderly patients in the hospital or in the home, the nurse should speak clearly and distinctly and be sure that the patient understands. This is especially important when giving medications or treatments, since the patient may respond to a name that is not his or her own. When working with elderly patients in the hospital or in the home, the nurse should not expect to make requests and secure a quick response. The patient may respond with "all right" or "in a minute." Directions should be given slowly, making certain that the patient understands. The patient may indicate that he or she understands, but action may be slow. The older person should not be hurried, since this may create confusion and render the patient unable to respond appropriately (Box 9-4).

## NURSING HOMES

Only 5% of the elderly population live in institutions, but of these, most are in **nursing homes.** Many of those residing in nursing homes could be cared for in their own homes. There is a move to provide additional services to families to make home care feasible, but nursing homes remain an important provider of health care. Nursing homes may provide sheltered care for the ambulatory patient, intermediate care, or skilled care for the patient requiring extensive nursing services. A home may provide only one or all three of these levels of care, and the home is chosen according to the nursing needs of the prospective resident.

Nursing homes approved for Medicare require that the personnel maintain nursing care plans for each patient. Plans should be based on the immediate and long-term needs of the patient. Like plans prepared in the general hospital, they should reflect the thinking of the entire nursing staff.

The average nursing home resident differs little from most other people of the same chronologic age. In addition to the normal degenerative changes, many nursing home residents have chronic diseases and may be malnourished and debilitated. The nursing care must be individualized according to the individual's particular needs. Some patients are ambulatory and can provide much of their own care, others need assistance with personal hygiene, and some must have total care. The patient's psychologic needs should be met. They should be reassured of their personal worth and should be helped to maintain a sense of dignity and self-respect. Chapter 18 discusses in more depth the problems related to caring for elderly residents in nursing homes.

# ALTERNATIVES TO INSTITUTIONAL CARE

## Home Care

If the patient is to be cared for in his or her own home, the family and the community must provide the necessary services. Most elderly people prefer to remain in their own homes and are happier when they can do so. Each person must be carefully evaluated medically and socially for **home care.** When the person's potential for self-care has been determined, an individualized program is planned. There may be a need for services available under the Older Americans Act, such as meals, transportation to physicians or clinics, home health aides, and homemaker service. Visits by the public health nurse or visiting nurse may also be needed. Home care can preserve the elderly person's independence, dignity, and identity (precious human qualities that are often lost when the elderly person is placed in an institution) (Hughes, 1996) (see Chapter 18). Medicare provides reimbursement for skilled nursing care in the home (see Chapter 19 for details).

With the introduction of the prospective payment system and **diagnosis-related groups**, the incentive to provide alternatives to hospitalization has become greater. Home care and preventive programs are expanding in an effort to keep elderly individuals from being hospitalized. HMOs have become more involved in providing Medicare benefits to the elderly. This involvement has created greater use of alternate care services such as home care, day care, and preventive programs.

## Day Hospital

Experimental programs for daytime care of the aged are being tried in both the United States and Canada. The objective is to prevent or delay admission to an institution and to promote independence. Individuals must be ambulatory, but they may be permitted to use a walker or cane. Emergency care is available if needed. A kitchen may be available for retraining and motivation. Transportation is provided, and a noon meal is provided in a cafeteria. Each person is encouraged to participate in group activities and in various crafts. A team approach is used, with the team usually consisting of a physician, nurse, dietitian, psychiatrist, and occupational therapist. The progress of each patient is evaluated, and some of those who become sufficiently independent to maintain themselves at home may leave the program as others are admitted.

## Foster Home

Care of the elderly in foster homes has had limited success. The concept that an elderly person will be happier in a home environment and be able to share in family relationships has been difficult to implement in many communities. Disadvantages have centered around the lack of medical care and the fact that the foster home is being operated for profit.

## Other Services

The extended care facility provides short-term, intermediate respite and convalescent care. It may be operated as part of a general hospital or as an independent institution. Its function is to provide care after an acute illness until the person is able to return home.

Many communities offer a variety of outpatient services, including mental health clinics, physical therapy, dental clinics, speech clinics, and numerous social services.

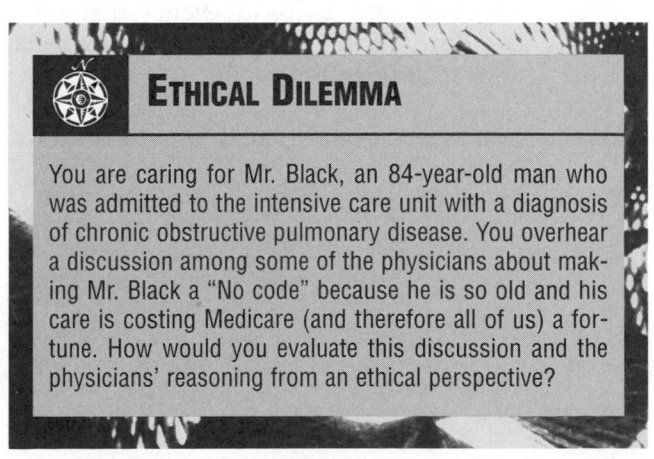

### ETHICAL DILEMMA

You are caring for Mr. Black, an 84-year-old man who was admitted to the intensive care unit with a diagnosis of chronic obstructive pulmonary disease. You overhear a discussion among some of the physicians about making Mr. Black a "No code" because he is so old and his care is costing Medicare (and therefore all of us) a fortune. How would you evaluate this discussion and the physicians' reasoning from an ethical perspective?

# KEY CONCEPTS

➤ Senescence, or biologic aging, is a normal process.

➤ The number of elderly people is increasing, and one result is the increasing demand on the health care system.

➤ Medicare benefits pay only part of the health care costs of the elderly.

➤ Cultural, ethnic, and socioeconomic factors affect the aging process.

➤ Retirement is a major transition in an older person's life, and it requires preparation and planning for success.

➤ Biologic aging is a slow, progressive process that affects all organ systems of the body.

➤ Mental health in old age involves coping with numerous losses, accepting changes in the body, and staying involved with society.

➤ Normal aging does not include senility or loss of intelligence.

➤ Cardiovascular problems are among the most common diseases of the elderly and are associated with the changes of aging and the effects of lifestyle.

➤ The senses of vision, hearing, touch, taste, and smell all tend to decline in old age.

➤ With aging, the skin becomes thinner, drier, and more prone to injury.

➤ Changes in the musculoskeletal system increase the older person's risk of falling and of injury from falls.

➤ Changes in the nervous system result in decreased reaction times, slowed reflexes, and diminished pain responses.

➤ Alzheimer's disease is a slow, progressive, irreversible dementia that requires careful evaluation by a multidisciplinary team of health care professionals.

➤ The changes in the aging digestive system require attention to oral hygiene, a balanced, high-fiber diet, and six to eight glasses of fluid per day.

➤ The kidneys become less efficient with aging. This may affect how older people metabolize drugs.

➤ Changes in the respiratory system may place the older person at risk for infection and pneumonia.

➤ The male and female reproductive systems change with aging, but satisfying sexual relationships are possible in the healthy older adult.

➤ Goals of nursing care for the elderly involve maintaining and improving functional ability, maintaining and improving quality of life, helping the older person prepare for death, preventing injury, recognizing individuality, meeting nutritional needs, maintaining personal hygiene, and preventing complications from drug use.

➤ Caring for the hospitalized elderly person requires careful monitoring of mental status and vital signs.

➤ Long-term care may be provided in nursing homes, patients' homes, day hospitals, foster homes, or a variety of community-based settings.

# CRITICAL THINKING EXERCISES

1. Today's elderly were born before 1925. Discuss the social, scientific, and political events that have taken place during their lifetime. How might these events affect their lives and health?

2. Discuss ways of increasing activity for the institutionalized elderly. Consider those who are ambulatory and those who are not.

3. Develop a nursing care plan for home care of a patient in the second stage of Alzheimer's disease.

## REFERENCES AND ADDITIONAL READINGS

Agency for Health Care Policy and Research (AHCPR): Pressure ulcers in adults: prediction and prevention, Clinical Practice Guideline No 3, AHCPR Pub No 92-0048, Rockville, Md, 1992, US Department of Health and Human Services.

Agency for Health Care Policy and Research (AHCPR): Urinary incontinence in adults, Clinical Practice Guideline, AHCPR Pub No 92-0038, Rockville, Md, 1992, US Department of Health and Human Services.

Agency for Health Care Policy and Research (AHCPR): Early identification of Alzheimer's Disease and related dementias, Clinical Practice Guideline No 19, AHCPR Pub No 97-0703, Rockville, Md, 1996, US Department of Health and Human Services.

Brink TL, Yesavage JA: Screening tests for geriatric depression, *Clin Gerontol* (1):37-43, 1983.

Burkhauser RV, Couch KA, Philips JW: Who takes early social security benefits? The economic and health characteristics of early beneficiaries, *Gerontologist* 36(6):789-799, 1996.

Ebersole P, Hess P: *Toward healthy aging: human needs and nursing response,* ed 4, St Louis, 1994, Mosby.

Erikson EH: *Identity and the life cycle: psychologic issues,* New York, 1950, International Universities Press.

Ferri R: *Care planning for the older adult,* Philadelphia, 1994, Saunders.

Folstein M, Folstein S, McHugh PR: "Mini-mental state": a practical method for grading the cognitive state of patients for the clinician, *J Psychiatr Res* 12(3):189-198, 1975.

Fries J, Crapo L: *Vitality and aging,* San Francisco, 1981, Freeman.

Goodman CE: Osteoporosis and physical activity, *AAOHN J* 35(12):539-542, 1987.

Hamby R et al: *Alzheimer's disease: a handbook for caretakers,* St Louis, 1994, Mosby.

Hughes S: Home health. In Evashwick CJ, editor: *The continuum of long term care: an integrated systems approach,* New York, 1996, Delmar Publishers.

Institute for Sex Research: *Sexual behavior in the human female,* Philadelphia, 1953, Saunders.

Kane RL, Ouslander JG, Abrass IB: *Essentials of clinical geriatrics,* New York, 1994, McGraw-Hill.

Katz S et al: Studies of illness in the aged: the index of ADL: a standardized measure of biological and psychosocial function, *JAMA* 185(21):914-919, 1963.

Kinsey AC: *Sexual behavior in the human male,* Philadelphia, 1948, Saunders.

Knapp M: A rose is still a rose, *Geriatr Nurs* 10(6):290-291, 1989.

Lawton HP, Brody EM: Assessment of older people: self-maintaining and instrumental activities of daily living, *Gerontologist* 9(3):179, 1969.

Linn MW, Linn BS: The rapid disability rating scale-2, *J Am Geriatr Soc* 30(6):378-382, 1982.

Mahoney F, Barthel D: Functional evaluation: the Barthel index, *Maryland State Med J* 14:61-65, 1965.

Masters WH, Johnson VE: *Human sexuality inadequacy,* Boston, 1970, Little, Brown.

Matteson MA, McConnell ES: *Gerontological nursing: concepts and practice,* Philadelphia, 1988, Saunders.

Miller C: *Nursing care of older adults: therapy and practice,* Philadelphia, 1995, Lippincott.

Moskowitz E, McCann C: Classification of disability in the chronically ill and aging, *J Chronic Dis* 5:342-346, 1957.

Nyberg L et al: Age differences in episodic memory, semantic memory, and priming: relationships to demographic, intellectual, and biological factors, *J Gerontol B Psychol Sci Soc Sci* 51(4):P234-P240, 1996.

Overgaard K et al: Effect of salcatonin given intranasally on bone mass and fracture rates in established osteoporosis: a dose-response study, *BMJ* 305(6853):556-561, 1992.

Pettigrew D: Investing in mouth care, *Geriatr Nurs* 10(1):22-24, 1989.

Roberts B, Dunkle R, Haug M: Physical, psychological, and social resources as moderators of the relationship of stress to mental health in the very old, *J Gerontol* 49(1):535-543, 1994.

Schoenfeld D et al: Self-rated health and mortality in the high-functioning elderly(a closer look at healthy individuals: MacArthur field study of successful aging, *J Gerontol* 49(3):109-115, 1994.

Social Security Administration: *Year 2000: a strategic plan.* Baltimore, 1994, Office of Strategic Planning, Social Security Administration.

Stolley J: When your patient has Alzheimer's disease, *Am J Nurs* 94(8):34-40, 1994.

Swan JH, Pickard RB: Mental health and mental retardation services. In Evashwick CJ, editor: *The continuum of long term care: an integrated systems approach,* New York, 1996, Delmar Publishers.

US Bureau of the Census: *Current population reports,* Washington, DC, 1991, US Government Printing Office.

US Department of Health and Human Services: Profile of older Americans: 1990, Program Resources Department, AARP, and Administration on Aging, Washington, DC, 1990, Department of Health and Human Services.

van Marwijk H et al: Evaluation of the feasibility, reliability, and diagnostic value of shortened versions of the geriatric depression scale, *Br J Gen Pract* 45(393):195-199, 1995.

Wallace M: Management of sexual relationships among elderly residents in long-term care facilities, *Geriatr Nurs* 13(6):308-314, 1992.

*Webster's medical desk dictionary,* Springfield, Mass, 1986, Merriam-Webster.

Yurick AG et al: *The aged person and the nursing process,* ed 3, Norwalk, Conn, 1989, Appleton & Lange.

# CHAPTER 10

# Substance Abuse

## KEY TERMS

| | |
|---|---|
| addiction | habituation |
| blackout | intervention |
| codependency | minimizing |
| cross-tolerance | relapse |
| delirium tremens (DTs) | substance abuse |
| denial | substance dependence |
| dry drunk | tolerance |
| flashbacks | withdrawal |

**Substance abuse** is the pathologic use of a mind-altering chemical that is accompanied by a loss of control over how much and how often the chemical is used. Substance abuse results in impaired thinking and functioning. The user may abuse the chemical occasionally or continuously over a period, or months may elapse between episodes of abuse. Substance abuse differs from **substance dependence (addiction)**, which describes the total psychophysical state of a person who must receive an increasing amount of the chemical to prevent the onset of withdrawal symptoms. The person's life is marked by an overwhelming involvement with getting and using the drug.

The abuse of legal and illegal substances is a major health and socioeconomic problem worldwide. In the United States the abuse of mind-altering substances affects millions of users, their families, their coworkers, and the population in general. Alcohol abuse, smoking, and illegal drug use cause illness and death and are related to domestic violence, child abuse, lost productivity, and crime. Substance abuse places a tremendous burden on the economy because it strains the health care system, social services, and the criminal justice system. The total cost of substance abuse is staggering. It is estimated that the health care costs of alcoholics are twice as high as for nonalcoholics. A considerable amount of money also is spent on health care and social services for close family members of addicted individuals because these family members often are at risk of developing physical and emotional illnesses. Money is spent, too, for services for the victims of crimes related to substance abuse.

Experts on substance abuse estimate that one out of every five people who seek medical treatment from a physician or clinic is a substance abuser. Between 20% and 35% of all admissions to hospital medical-surgical units are substance abusers and possible candidates

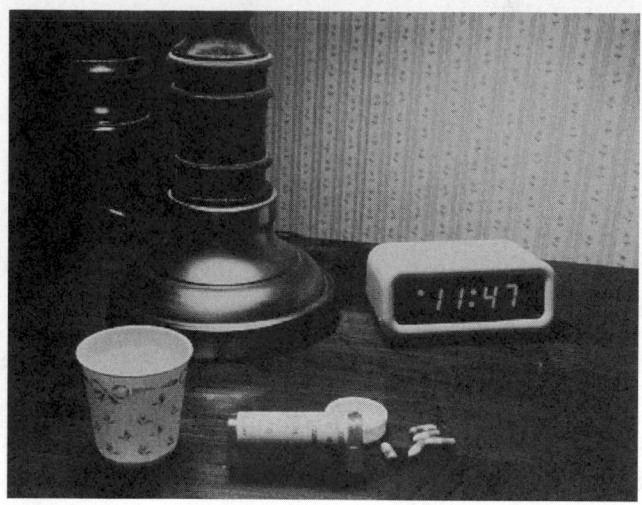

**Figure 10-1**   Abuse of prescription drugs is a major health problem. (Courtesy Michael Clement, MD, Mesa, Ariz.)

for withdrawal symptoms (Mendelson, Mello, 1992). The numbers are higher in critical care areas because of the link between alcohol and drug use and trauma (Sommers, 1994). Therefore it is wise to view every patient seen in a health care facility as a potential abuser. Mortality related to substance abuse remains high (Figure 10-1).

Fortunately, the general public is becoming more intolerant of substance abuse, possibly because of an increased awareness of its health risks and the cost of social programs that deal with its associated problems. Tobacco use and alcohol-related motor vehicle accidents are declining. As more people become aware of the incidence and impact of substance abuse, perhaps the nationwide educational and treatment activities will have a positive effect on the problem.

## TERMINOLOGY

To understand the problem of substance abuse, or chemical dependency, it is essential to become familiar with several terms. **Habituation** is an acquired tolerance that results from repeated exposure to a particular substance. Psychologic or emotional dependence may result from habituation, but there is little tendency to increase the dose, and withdrawal symptoms do not occur if the substance is discontinued. **Withdrawal** is a syndrome of potentially serious physical or psychologic symptoms that occurs when use of a drug is severely diminished or discontinued. Symptoms vary with the substance and occur until the substance is eliminated from the body. It is important to note that with heavy users, withdrawal symptoms may begin before all of the drug has been eliminated from the body. **Tolerance** describes the physiologic adaptation

to the effects of a chemical substance, which makes it necessary to increase the dose or frequency of use to obtain the original or desired effect. The ability of the human body to adjust to increasing doses of some chemicals is remarkable. Some heavy users ingest large amounts of drugs with seemingly few apparent effects, whereas the same dose may be life-threatening to an individual who has not developed a tolerance. It is unclear how long tolerance lasts in an individual. With some mind-altering substances, such as alcohol, tolerance may last for many years. **Cross-tolerance** occurs when a body that has developed a tolerance for one substance develops tolerance for substances in the same or similar categories. For example, a patient who is alcohol dependent can develop a tolerance for other central nervous system (CNS) depressants and may require larger doses of surgical anesthetics and pain medications to achieve the desired effects.

It is impossible to determine when a substance abuser becomes substance dependent. Estimates of the number of abusers who eventually become dependent vary, but some experts put the figure at approximately 50%. Substance abusers use mind-altering drugs for one reason: to change the way they feel. Initially substances are used to produce a feeling of well-being or pleasure. However, as dependence progresses the substance is used, in spite of the consequences, to function and to avoid withdrawal. Box 10-1 lists some alternate names for commonly abused substances.

## ETIOLOGY

Much research has been done to attempt to explain why some people are prone to substance abuse and others are not. Various theories focus on the biologic, psychologic, sociocultural, and behavioral-cognitive aspects of the problem.

The biologic theory states that substance abuse has a physiologic cause. For example, two distinct subtypes of alcoholism have been identified. Type A shows the features of sporadic, late-onset alcoholism, whereas type B shows the manifestations of familial, early-onset alcoholism during the teenage years. Type B is accompanied by a high incidence of violence during intoxication, increased impulsivity, and depression (Yoshino, 1996). A genetic predisposition to alcoholism is evidenced by studies that reveal a high incidence of alcoholism in families of alcoholics. Sons of alcoholic men appear to be particularly at risk; their chance of developing alcoholism ranges from 30% to 50%. Children of alcoholic birth parents who were adopted as infants and raised apart from their birth parents also have been found to have higher rates of alcoholism. Studies of adopted twins have shown that identical twins of an alcoholic parent have a 60% chance of becoming alco-

BOX 10-1

## "STREET" NAMES FOR COMMONLY ABUSED DRUGS

**MARIJUANA**
Acapulco gold
Blunt
Grass
Joint
Pot
Reefer
Roach
Tea
Weed

**PCP**
Angel dust
Cosmos
Jet
Mist
Peace pill
Rocket fuel
Superjoint
Tranq
Whack

**HASHISH**
Ganja
Hash
Rope
Sweet Lucy

**HALLUCINOGENS**
Acid (LSD)
Blue dots (LSD)
Cactus (mescaline)
Cube (LSD)
Love drug (MDA)
Magic mushroom (psilocybin)
Purple haze (LSD)

**COCAINE**
Blow
Coke

**COCAINE—cont'd**
Flake
Gold dust
Nose candy
Rock
Snow
Speedball (heroin and cocaine)
White girl

**HEROIN**
Brown
Horse
Junk
Shag
Smack

**STIMULANTS**
Bennies
Crystal
Dexies
Meth
Pep pills
Speed
Ups

**BARBITURATES**
Barbs
Blue devil (amobarbital)
Blues
Downer
Goof balls
Rainbows
Red devil (secobarbital)
Yellow jacket (pentobarbital)

**TRANQUILIZERS**
Blues (10 mg Valium)
Tranqs
Yellows (5 mg Valium)

holics. For fraternal adopted twins of an alcoholic parent, the risk of becoming alcoholics is only 30%.

Some evidence points to brain chemistry alterations among some substance abusers. Cocaine abusers show a deficiency in dopamine and norepinephrine. The enkephalins and endorphins are noted to be deficient in alcoholics and narcotic abusers. Many Japanese people may be protected from alcoholism by liver enzymes that allow high levels of acetaldehyde to accumulate in the blood, causing adverse reactions, such as a flushing response, after alcohol ingestion (Higuchi, 1995). Studies continue regarding evidence of metabolic defects and the possibility of abnormal enzyme levels in some chemically dependent individuals.

The psychologic theory proposes that substance abusers are responding to depression, low self-esteem, and other stressors and are self-medicating to deal with tension, anxiety, and various kinds of psychic pain. For example, chemical use initially may relieve the loneliness that results from a lack of meaningful relationships.

The sociocultural theory recognizes the importance of group values and attitudes. The group can be relatively permanent, such as a biologic family or ethnic group, or temporary, such as junior high school classmates. Social expectations and encouragement may promote irresponsible use of even legal substances. Many teenagers become chemically dependent because peer pressure is particularly strong (Figure 10-2). Cultural beliefs can encourage or discourage responsible use of substances (Mendelson, Mello, 1992). For example, people with an Irish, Scandinavian, or Native American heritage show a proclivity for substance abuse, whereas the rate of abuse among Jewish and Asian people is low. Low socioeconomic status and racial inequality are also precursors of chemical dependency, such as with Native Americans and poor, black men. It recently has become evident that older people, who long have been ignored in substance abuse studies, are at high risk of becoming chemically dependent.

The behavioral-cognitive theory assumes that using and abusing patterns are learned and continue because of positive reinforcement. When the use of mind-altering substances in the family or peer group is accepted as normal behavior and encouraged, it is viewed as a way to manage stress, deal with problems, or have fun or celebrate. Therefore consumption provides the individual with short-term rewards, which reinforces the consumption pattern. As an individual becomes substance dependent, certain cues are associated with consumption, including the end of the workday, a particular group of friends, or certain locations.

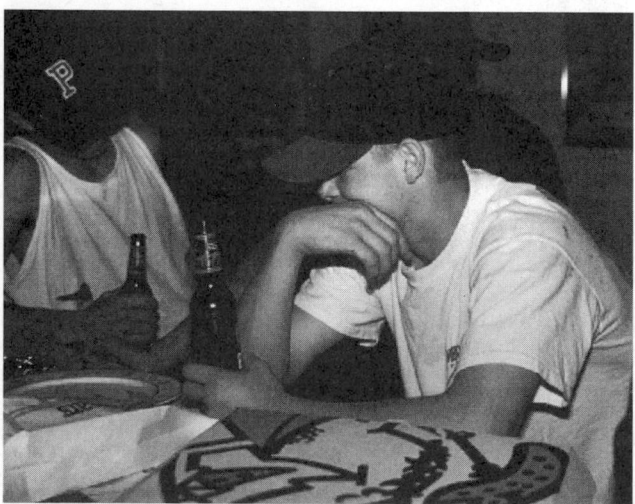

**Figure 10-2** Peer pressure leads many teens to experiment with drugs and run the risk of becoming chemically dependent. (Courtesy Michael Clement, MD, Mesa, Ariz.)

It is evident that substance abuse and dependence are the results of complex and incompletely understood processes. In some substance abusers no genetic link has been found. Many people believe that the interaction of genetic and environmental factors produces vulnerability to substance abuse. Therefore even though a genetic propensity may exist, substance abuse or dependency is not inevitable.

## SUBSTANCE ABUSE AS A DISEASE

In the United States Dr. Benjamin Rush recognized alcoholism as a disease as early as 1748. He described acute and chronic symptoms and observed hereditary and nongenetic influences. Beginning in the 1930s scientific studies of alcoholism were based on the understanding of alcoholism as a disease. In 1956 the American Medical Association officially accepted alcoholism as a disease (Report to Congress, 1990). The *Diagnostic and Statistical Manual of Mental Disorders IV* of the American Psychiatric Association (1994) identifies various forms of alcoholism and abuse of various substances, including not only illegal drugs but also nicotine and caffeine, as diseases.

The explanation of alcoholism and other substance abuses as diseases contrasts with historic moral explanations, in which any substance dependence is believed to come from a character defect that an individual can conquer by willpower. Even today some physicians and health care professionals only partly accept the idea that substance abuse is a disease. The reasons for this ambivalence are complex and may involve individual beliefs about moral judgment and free will and about the paradox of personal responsibility in the disease process. With some individuals this ambivalence may stem from having a substance abuser in the family (Miller, Toft, 1990).

## DYSFUNCTIONAL FAMILY

Health care professionals who treat substance abusers view substance abusers and dependence as a disease process that is a problem not only for the individual but also for the family or significant others. Much has been written about the dysfunctional family, which results when a substance abuse problem is present. In a dysfunctional family, family members assume clearly defined roles and interact and communicate in predictable patterns to maintain the relationship or family structure.

### Roles

As substance abuse progresses, one or more family members begin to act in ways that protect the abuser from the consequences of substance abuse. This behavior is known as enabling. The enabler begins to assume the roles or duties that the addicted person can no longer perform. A spouse may take a second job to ease the financial burden that occurs when the abusing spouse gets fired from a job. A significant other may lie to an employer or to school authorities about absenteeism or poor performance. Family members may make excuses when social events or family gatherings are missed. Such enabling behavior spares the abuser embarrassment, financial consequences, and other negative effects of alcohol or drug abuse.

Other roles assumed by family members include the scapegoat, mascot, hero, and lost child. The *scapegoat* is the child who may act out to divert attention away from the using family member and toward himself or herself. The scapegoat is blamed for the problems in the family. The *mascot* is the funny, playful, or especially loving child who diverts attention to himself or herself in an attempt to shift the focus from the family pain. The *hero* is the good child who gets excellent grades, always acts responsibly, and possibly helps the nonusing parent meet family responsibilities. The *lost* or *forgotten child* withdraws and tries to avoid attention. The lost child does not expect his or her needs to be met. All of these roles help family members cope with the dynamics of substance abuse in the family. These roles are considered adaptive, yet they become a dysfunctional way of coping to maintain homeostasis or equilibrium within the alcoholic family system.

## Codependency

Substance abuse affects all family members to some degree. As the substance abuser becomes more preoccupied with getting and using the chemical, family members become more focused on the abuser and his or her behavior and chemical use. They begin to change their own behavior in response to the abuser's life-style. For example, family members may try to control the drinking, activities, or friends of the alcoholic. They may attempt to keep peace within the family system and may begin to withdraw from activities outside the family. Their lives begin to focus entirely on the substance abuser and his or her problem, and the disease of **codependency** develops. Codependency itself has predictable traits that may parallel those of the chemically dependent person (Box 10-2). The concept of codependency began in relation to the treatment of alcoholism as a family disease and the awareness that the alcoholic was not the only person affected by the disease. During the past 10 years the concept of codependency has grown to include a broad range of definitions.

---

**BOX 10-2**

### SHARED TRAITS OF ALCOHOLISM AND CODEPENDENCY

**DENIAL** (Dishonesty)
*Alcoholic:* I can stop drinking any time I want.
*Codependent:* She doesn't get drunk every time she drinks.

**RATIONALIZATION** (Confused thinking)
*Alcoholic:* I only drink because the boss doesn't like me and has it in for me.
*Codependent:* If I could keep the house cleaner and the children quiet when he gets home, he wouldn't drink so much.

**MINIMIZING** (Denying the amount of alcohol consumed)
*Alcoholic:* I buy a lot of rounds at the bar, but I don't drink that much myself.
*Codependent:* She buys a lot of beer, but her friends drink most of it.

**FEAR**
*Alcoholic:* I'm afraid to stop drinking. I've been doing it so long, what would I do instead?
*Codependent:* I can't make it on my own if he leaves me.

**SELF-CENTEREDNESS**
*Alcoholic:* I don't care what he wants to do. I work hard all week and deserve to go out and have a few drinks if I want to.
*Codependent:* After all I've done for her, how could she do this to me?

**LOSS OF PERSONAL VALUES**
*Alcoholic:* I would never have taken that money from petty cash if I hadn't been buzzed from the drinks I had at lunch.
*Codependent:* I hate lying to his boss about him being sick, but if I don't he'll be fired because he's missed so many days.

**LOW SELF-ESTEEM**
*Alcoholic:* I'm really not as good as these other salesmen. I have to have a few drinks to loosen up before I can make my presentation.
*Codependent:* He's right. I can't do anything right.

**DEPRESSION**
*Alcoholic:* I'm sick and tired of feeling this way. My family would be better off if I just killed myself.
*Codependent:* I feel hopeless. Nothing is ever going to get better. No matter what I do, she still drinks.

# CENTRAL NERVOUS SYSTEM DEPRESSANTS

## Alcohol and Alcoholism

About two thirds of all adult Americans and a significant number of those under age 21 drink alcohol. Alcohol is rapidly absorbed from the gastrointestinal tract, beginning in the stomach and continuing in the small and large intestines. The rate of absorption is affected by the amount of food in the stomach and the concentration of alcohol in the drinks. Before reaching the bloodstream, some of the ethanol is metabolized in the stomach by gastric alcohol dehydrogenase. Men generally produce more of this protective stomach enzyme than women, which partly explains why women typically become intoxicated more quickly than men, even considering women's smaller size. All of the ethanol absorbed from the stomach is carried to the liver, which is the primary site of alcohol metabolism. Here the alcohol is converted to acetaldehyde and then acetate with the help of enzymes known as alcohol dehydrogenases. The rate of metabolism depends on the weight and tolerance of the drinker. The amount of ethanol excreted through the liver varies and depends on the amount ingested. Usually 5% to 10% of ethanol is excreted unchanged through the lungs and kidneys

---

**TABLE 10-1**

### Relationship Between Type and Amount of Alcoholic Beverages Consumed and Estimated Potential Blood Alcohol Concentration*

| | | | ESTIMATED POTENTIAL BLOOD ALCOHOL CONCENTRATION IN 1 HOUR† | | |
| | | | ONE DRINK | TWO DRINKS | THREE DRINKS |
| ALCOHOLIC BEVERAGE | ALCOHOL CONTENT (%) | NORMAL MEASURES DISPENSED | BODY WEIGHT 100 140 180 220 (% wt/vol) | BODY WEIGHT 100 140 180 220 (% wt/vol) | BODY WEIGHT 100 140 180 220 (% wt/vol) |
|---|---|---|---|---|---|
| **Beer** | | | | | |
| Ale | 5% | 12 oz bottle | 0.05 0.04 0.03 0.02 | 0.08 0.06 0.05 0.05 | 0.11 0.09 0.08 0.07 |
| Malt beverage | 7% | 12 oz bottle | 0.05 0.05 0.04 0.03 | 0.09 0.07 0.06 0.05 | 0.15 0.12 0.09 0.08 |
| Regular beer | 4% | 12 oz bottle | 0.04 0.03 0.02 0.02 | 0.07 0.05 0.04 0.03 | 0.10 0.08 0.06 0.05 |
| **Wines** | | | | | |
| Fortified (e.g., port, muscatel) | 18% | 3 oz glass | 0.04 0.03 0.02 0.02 | 0.07 0.05 0.04 0.03 | 0.10 0.08 0.06 0.05 |
| Natural (red, white) Champagne | 12% | 3 oz glass | 0.03 0.03 0.02 0.02 | 0.06 0.05 0.04 0.03 | 0.08 0.06 0.04 0.04 |
| **Cider (hard)** | 10% | 6 oz glass | 0.05 0.04 0.03 0.02 | 0.08 0.06 0.05 0.05 | 0.11 0.09 0.08 0.07 |
| **Liqueurs** | | | | | |
| Strong (sweet, syrupy) | 40% | 1 oz glass | 0.03 0.03 0.02 0.02 | 0.07 0.05 0.04 0.03 | 0.08 0.06 0.05 0.05 |
| Medium (fruit brandies) | 25% | 2 oz glass | 0.04 0.03 0.02 0.02 | 0.08 0.06 0.04 0.04 | 0.10 0.08 0.06 0.06 |
| **Distilled Spirits** | | | | | |
| Brandy, cognac, rum, scotch, vodka, whiskey | 45% | 1 oz glass | 0.04 0.03 0.02 0.02 | 0.07 0.05 0.04 0.03 | 0.09 0.07 0.06 0.05 |
| **Mixed Drinks and Cocktails** | | | | | |
| Strong (martini, Manhattan) | 30% | 3½ oz glass | 0.08 0.06 0.04 0.04 | 0.15 0.12 0.09 0.08 | 0.22 0.16 0.12 0.10 |
| Medium (Old Fashioned, daiquiri, Alexander) | 15% | 4 oz glass | 0.05 0.04 0.03 0.02 | 0.08 0.06 0.05 0.05 | 0.11 0.09 0.08 0.07 |
| Light (Highball, Sweet and sour mixed, tonics) | 7% | 8 oz glass | 0.05 0.04 0.03 0.02 | 0.08 0.06 0.05 0.04 | 0.12 0.09 0.07 0.06 |

Source data from US Department of Transportation, National Highway Traffic Safety Administration.
*The legal limit of intoxication is 0.08% in 15 states and 0.1% in 35 states at this time.
†For each hour additional subtract 0.015% wt/vol from the number shown.

without passing through the liver. If the blood alcohol level (BAL) is high, a relatively large amount of alcohol is excreted rather than metabolized (Mendelson, Mello, 1992).

The most serious effect of chronic excessive alcohol intake is alcoholism. Many terms have been used to describe alcoholism. It currently is defined as a chronic, progressive, and potentially fatal biogenic and psychosocial disease characterized by tolerance and physical dependence and manifested by a loss of control, diverse personality changes, and social consequences.

Alcoholism is found in all socioeconomic levels, all occupations, and all age groups from preteen through the end of the life span. The average alcoholic takes his or her first drink between 12 and 14 years of age, first becomes intoxicated between 14 and 18, and experiences the first alcohol-related problem between 18 and 25. The first major problems with alcohol occur between 23 and 33 years of age. A variety of drinking patterns may occur. Alcoholics may drink daily, two or three times a week, only on weekends, or in sporadic binges that occur every few weeks or months. According to Schuchit and Marc (1989), "The average alcoholic has spontaneous periods of abstinence and marked decreases in drinking, which appear to alternate with times of heavy drinking." It is easier for the alcoholic not to drink at all than to try to control the amount of alcohol that he or she ingests. Any alcoholic substance may be used by the alcoholic: beer, wine, or distilled spirits. It is a myth that a person must drink "hard liquor" to become an alcoholic.

The effects of alcohol are related to the level of alcohol in the blood and brain (Table 10-1). Symptoms of alcohol intoxication include impaired cognition (from drowsiness to stupor), ataxia, labile affect, slurred speech, diplopia, euphoria or violent, belligerent behavior, flushing, anorexia, and a depressed mood. An intoxicated individual may also experience **blackouts**. A blackout does not involve losing consciousness or passing out. It is a period of amnesia that occurs while a person seems to be functioning normally, and it is seen in someone who is or has been drinking heavily. The period of amnesia may range from a few minutes to several days. The blackout explains why a heavy drinker does not remember driving home, how a party ended, or what decisions were made at a business meeting.

If left untreated, alcoholism progresses through stages that Jellinek (1960) identified in his classic writings and studies (Box 10-3). Alcohol directly or indirectly affects every organ system in the body. Some people may be more predisposed than others to develop severe physical consequences from alcohol use (Box 10-4).

Because alcoholism involves a physical dependence, a significant decrease in the BAL or the sudden cessation of alcohol intake is likely to result in some withdrawal symptoms. Alcohol withdrawal is potentially life-threatening, although a large number of alcoholics do not experience severe signs of withdrawal. Withdrawal symptoms begin as the BAL declines (usually 4 to 12 hours after the last drink). Each alcoholic responds differently to withdrawal, and subsequent withdrawals in the same individual may progress differently. Mild physical symptoms are common, including an increase in pulse, blood pressure, respiratory rate, and temperature. Mild to moderate diaphoresis, anorexia, nausea and vomiting, diarrhea, irritability, anxiety, and insomnia also are common. More than half of those who experience mild to moderate withdrawal symptoms have tremors. The inexperienced observer may confuse the tremors commonly seen in withdrawal with **delirium tremens (DTs)**. Alcohol withdrawal syndrome, or delirium tremens, is the most serious stage of alcohol withdrawal; it is characterized by severe autonomic nervous system dysfunction, confusion, hallucinations, and grand mal

---

**BOX 10-3**

### JELLINEK'S STAGES OF ALCOHOLISM

**PHASE I: PREALCOHOLIC**
Uses alcohol to relax and deal with tension
Gradually increases tolerance

**PHASE II: EARLY ALCOHOLIC**
May begin experiencing blackouts
Sneaks drinks
Rationalizes drinking
Becomes defensive when someone mentions drinking
Has an increased preoccupation with drinking
Experiences guilt and denial

**PHASE III: CRUCIAL PHASE**
Has become fully addicted
Has lost control over drinking
Develops a physiologic dependence
Has severe problems with job, marriage, and interpersonal relationships

**PHASE IV: CHRONIC PHASE**
Experiences many physical and psychologic illnesses
Severe withdrawal results from abrupt cessation of drinking

---

Modified from Jellinek EM: *J Stud Alcohol* 13:673, 1952.

---

**BOX 10-4**

## PHYSIOLOGIC EFFECTS OF ALCOHOL ABUSE

**CARDIOVASCULAR**
Cardiomyopathy
Hypertension (systolic)
Beriberi
Heart disease

**GASTROINTESTINAL**
Cancer of the mouth, stomach, and pancreas
Gastritis
Peptic ulcer
Esophagitis
Esophageal varices
Hypoglycemia
Cirrhosis of the liver
Alcoholic hepatitis
Pancreatitis
Colitis
Malabsorption
Vitamin deficiencies
Malnutrition

**GENITOURINARY**
Impotence in males
Testicular atrophy
Gynecomastia in males
Menstrual irregularities in females

**HEMATOLOGIC**
Anemia
Hyperlipidemia
Lactic acidosis
Impaired immune response

**MUSCULOSKELETAL**
Reduced bone density
Increased risk of fracture
Skeletal myopathies

**NEUROLOGIC**
Cerebral atrophy
Impaired cognition and memory
Peripheral neuropathies
Wernicke-Korsakoff syndrome

**RESPIRATORY**
Diminished resistance to chronic infections (e.g., tuberculosis, pneumonia)
Chronic obstructive pulmonary disease (COPD)

**INTEGUMENTARY**
Spider angiomas
Palmar erythema
Bruising

---

seizures. Table 10-2 summarizes the stages of alcohol withdrawal.

Because alcoholics are more prone to developing medical problems than the general population, a physical examination and assessment are essential as the first step in the treatment of alcohol withdrawal. However, many people with alcoholism go through withdrawal at home and without any medical supervision (Mendelson, Mello, 1992). The goal of treatment during withdrawal is to provide a medically safe and reasonably comfortable period of detoxification (detox). Medications may be used to control the symptoms, make the patient more comfortable, and lessen the risk of seizures or DTs. Such treatment is especially important when the alcoholic has been diagnosed with hypertension or type I diabetes or has a history of seizure activity. Although there are indications that almost any CNS depressant can be used to detoxify a patient from alcohol, one or more of the benzodiazepines generally is used. Longer acting benzodiazepines, such as diazepam (Valium) or chlordiazepoxide (Lib-

rium), generally are given in decreasing doses and provide a safe detox or withdrawal. Shorter acting drugs from that class, such as oxazepam (Serax) or lorazepam (Ativan), are less likely to accumulate in someone with severe liver disease. However, if they are not given at least every 4 hours, they may add to the problem of alcohol withdrawal or precipitate seizures (Schuchit, Marc, 1989).

After alcohol withdrawal has been completed, most alcohol-dependent individuals require some form of ongoing treatment. During the first few weeks or months of recovery, disulfiram (Antabuse) may be prescribed to help prevent a relapse into drinking. Antabuse prevents the normal breakdown of alcohol in the liver. Disulfiram itself has few side effects. Drowsiness may occur for a few days, but taking the daily dose at bedtime may help alleviate the insomnia that many alcoholics experience for weeks after becoming sober. However, when Antabuse is in the body (up to 14 days after the last dose), as little as ½ ounce of alcohol in the bloodstream causes a physical reac-

| TABLE 10-2 | | |
|---|---|---|

## Alcohol Withdrawal Symptoms and Interventions

| STAGE | MEDICATIONS* | INTERVENTIONS |
|---|---|---|
| **Mild** | | |
| Tremors (begin 3-36 hr after last drink) | Librium | 1. Monitor vital signs (VS) q 1-3 hr. |
| Pulse < 92 | Valium | 2. Administer sedating medications as ordered, prn if needed. |
| BP < 140/90 | | 3. Offer small, high-cholesterol feedings q 2-3 hr. |
| Slight diaphoresis | | |
| Slight flushing | | 4. Offer clear or nourishing liquids as tolerated. |
| Anxiety | | |
| | | 5. Record intake and output (I&O). |
| **Moderate** | | 6. Administer vitamins as ordered. |
| Tremors | Librium | 7. Assist with activities of daily living (ADL) as needed. |
| Pulse 90 to 130 | Valium | |
| BP 140/90 to 160/110 | | 8. Allow and encourage ambulation if VS and gait are stable. |
| Moderate to profuse diaphoresis | | |
| Irritability; anxiety | | 9. Orient to time, place, and person if necessary. |
| Agitation; anxiety | | |
| Anorexia | | 10. Follow seizure precautions if any history of seizures. |
| Nausea and vomiting | | |
| | | 11. Spend time with patient and family. Be nonjudgmental and reassuring. |
| **Hallucinosis** | | |
| Moderate symptoms plus auditory or visual hallucinations | | |
| **Alcohol Withdrawal Syndrome (DTs)** | | |
| Begins 24-72 hr after last drink (mortality up to 35%) | Anticonvulsants intravenously (IV) per physician order | 1. Check patient q 15 min. |
| Pulse > 130 | | 2. Monitor VS q 1 hr. |
| BP > 160/110 | | 3. Assess neurologic status q 1 hr. |
| Confusion | | 4. Restrain if necessary to prevent injury. |
| Delirium | | 5. Monitor IV fluids and catheter. |
| Severe agitation | | 6. Administer medications as ordered. |
| Hallucinations | | 7. Assess for signs of trauma or skin breakdown. |
| Seizures | | 8. Provide calm, quiet atmosphere. |

*Each physician may have his or her own detoxification protocol. It is not uncommon to exceed usual medication parameters with a patient who is experiencing withdrawal from alcohol.

Maximum dosages:
Librium: 600 mg/24 hr ⎤
Valium: 120 mg/24 hr ⎦ administered by mouth (PO)

tion that begins with flushing, increased respirations, and an increased heart rate. This reaction begins within a few minutes and can progress to nausea and vomiting, aches, and weakness. Immediate medical help is needed if such symptoms occur.

Because of the potentially harmful effects of drinking or using alcohol-based products while taking Antabuse, a witnessed and signed consent form should be required of the patient. Teaching protocols are helpful for the nurse to use with a patient who is taking Antabuse because he or she needs to know the important contraindications while taking the medication. Some teaching issues include not giving blood while undergoing Antabuse therapy and avoiding products such as vinegar and alcohol-based shaving lotions and cough medications. It is very important to instruct the patient that after quitting the medication, the effects of the drug remain in the system up to 14 days, and therefore any use of alcohol or alcohol-based products will cause an adverse reaction.

## OLDER ADULT CONSIDERATIONS

Alcohol problems are much more common among older adults than professionals in health care and aging services generally recognize. Manifestations of alcohol abuse in older adults are more subtle, atypical, and non-specific than in younger people. Many older patients consume smaller quantities of alcohol than do younger patients and therefore may develop overt withdrawal states less often. Those who consume lesser quantities may not drink to the point of intoxication and therefore may appear to be more in control of their drinking. Because susceptibility to the toxic effects of alcohol increases with advancing age, a person can develop alcohol problems just by becoming older and without necessarily changing the amount of alcohol consumed. In such cases craving and compulsive use may not be apparent, but continued use in spite of negative consequences still defines problem drinking.

An alcohol intake that is considered moderate for a younger person may cause adverse consequences in an older adult, who has less physiologic reserve in meeting self-care needs such as grooming and housekeeping. A small, frail, older person who is barely functioning in terms of self-care capabilities and who consumes two or three drinks a day can tip the balance toward an inability to maintain himself or herself independently.

Approximately 80% of Americans over age 65 have at least one chronic disease. Many will have several chronic diseases, any or all of which may be complicated by even small amounts of alcohol. Unlike in younger adults, alcohol abuse in the older adult most likely manifests itself in the form of some combination of nonspecific, functional deficits, which makes it all the more difficult to diagnose.

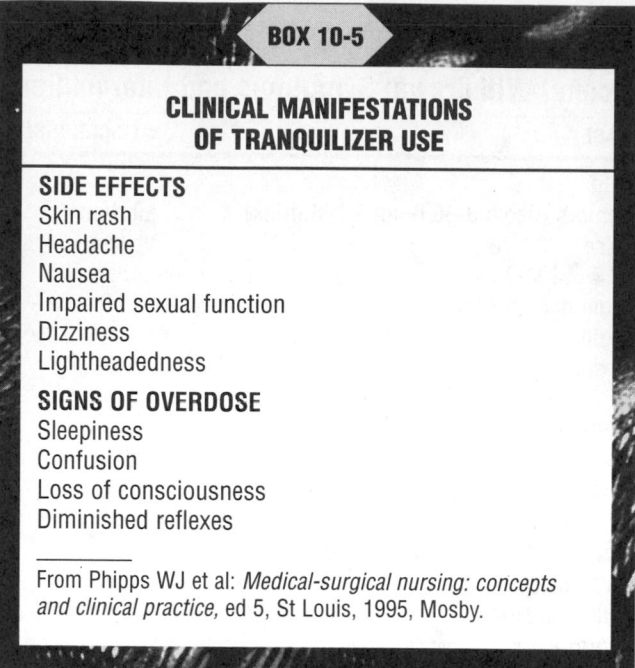

**BOX 10-5**

## CLINICAL MANIFESTATIONS OF TRANQUILIZER USE

**SIDE EFFECTS**
Skin rash
Headache
Nausea
Impaired sexual function
Dizziness
Lightheadedness

**SIGNS OF OVERDOSE**
Sleepiness
Confusion
Loss of consciousness
Diminished reflexes

From Phipps WJ et al: *Medical-surgical nursing: concepts and clinical practice*, ed 5, St Louis, 1995, Mosby.

## Tranquilizers

The most common type of tranquilizers are the benzodiazepines. These are psychoactive drugs used to lessen anxiety that also may be used as anticonvulsants and muscle relaxants. They include diazepam (Valium), alprazolam (Xanax), lorazepam (Ativan), chlordiazepoxide (Librium), oxazepam (Serax), clorazepate (Tranxene), and triazolam (Halcion) (Table 10-3). Benzodiazepines are available in tablet, capsule, and liquid form and are widely prescribed. Therefore they are often abused. The antianxiety effects of the minor tranquilizers are short-lived, and when the effects wear off, an individual may experience a greater level of anxiety (Box 10-5). Tolerance and physical and psychologic dependence can de-

velop. Withdrawal symptoms can develop within 12 to 24 hours. Many symptoms, including anxiety, insomnia, irritability, vomiting, diaphoresis, tremors, and seizures may occur during withdrawal, especially if use of the drug has been prolonged. Therefore the dosage is reduced gradually. Benzodiazepines have a synergistic effect with alcohol, and the combination may lead to an overdose (Table 10-4).

## Barbiturates

Barbiturates are synthetic drugs used to treat insomnia and epilepsy and to sedate surgical patients. Tolerance and physical and psychologic dependence can result from barbiturate use, regardless of whether it is a prescribed medication or a street drug. Barbiturates are available in oral form (capsules or elixirs) or suppository form or in a liquid form for injection. Taking another CNS depressant with a barbiturate may lead to an accidental overdose, with symptoms of slurred speech, disorientation, confusion, respiratory depression, cyanosis, hypotension, ataxia, a weak pulse, and death (Box 10-6). Withdrawal symptoms range from mild to life-threatening and can include irritability, insomnia, weakness, anxiety, nausea and vomiting, headache, mental confusion, hallucinations, convulsions, and delirium. The patient is best hospitalized for this withdrawal, which may involve substituting a long-acting barbiturate for the original abused substance. The dosage is slowly tapered over several weeks until the drug is discontinued.

**TABLE 10-3**

## Pharmacology of Drugs Used in Substance Abuse

| DRUG (GENERIC AND TRADE NAME); ROUTE AND DOSAGE | ACTION/INDICATION | COMMON SIDE EFFECTS AND NURSING CONSIDERATIONS |
|---|---|---|
| **Alprazolam** (Xanax)<br>**Route:** PO<br>**Dosage:** 0.25-0.5 mg 2-3 times daily as needed, not to exceed 4 mg/day; decrease dosage in debilitated or elderly patients | Benzodiazepine used in the treatment of anxiety, depression, and "panic attacks" | Dizziness, drowsiness, and lethargy |
| **Amitriptyline** (Elavil)<br>**Route:** PO, IM<br>**Dosage:** PO 30-100 mg/day in a single bedtime dose or in divided doses; dosage may be gradually increased to 150-300 mg/day; IM 20-30 mg 4 times daily | Antianxiety drug used in the treatment of depression | Drowsiness, sedation, lethargy, fatigue, dry mouth, dry eyes, blurred vision, hypotension, and constipation; potentially fatal reaction with MAO inhibitors; may interfere with antihypertensive drugs |
| **Chlordiazepoxide** (Librium)<br>**Route:** PO, IM, IV<br>**Dosage:** For alcohol withdrawal PO 50-100 mg, with repeated agitation, up to 400 mg/day; for anxiety PO 5-25 mg 3-4 times daily or IM, IV 50-100 mg initially, then 25-50 mg 3-4 times daily as required | Benzodiazepine used in the treatment of anxiety and alcohol withdrawal; also used as a preoperative sedative | Dizziness and drowsiness; use with caution in patients with liver or kidney disease |
| **Chlorpromazine** (Thorazine)<br>**Route:** PO, IM, IV, Rectal<br>**Dosage:** For psychosis PO 10-25 mg 2-4 times daily, increase by 20-50 mg/day every 3-4 days (usual dosage is 200 mg/day); for nausea and vomiting PO 10-25 mg q 4-6 hr, IM 25-50 mg q 3-4 hr; rectal 50-100 mg q 6-8 hr; for intractable hiccups PO, IM 25-50 mg 3-4 times daily; IV up to 200 mg/day at rate of no more than 1 mg/min, usually given IV during surgery to prevent postoperative nausea and vomiting | Antipsychotic and antiemetic used in the treatment of acute and chronic psychoses, nausea and vomiting, and intractable hiccups; also used as a preoperative sedative | Sedation, extrapyramidal reactions, dry eyes, blurred vision, hypotension, constipation, dry mouth, and photosensitivity; use with caution in patients with liver and cardiac disease; may cause bone marrow suppression; may have adverse reactions with other CNS depressants |
| **Clorazepate** (Tranxene)<br>**Route:** PO<br>**Dosage:** 15-60 mg/day in divided doses | Benzodiazepine used in the treatment of anxiety and alcohol withdrawal and in the management of seizures | Dizziness, drowsiness, and lethargy; use with caution in previously suicidal or addicted patients |

*CNS,* Central nervous system; *ECG,* electrocardiograph; *IM,* intramuscular; *IV,* intravenous; *MAO,* monoamine oxidase; *PO,* orally.

*Continued*

**TABLE 10-3**

## Pharmacology of Drugs Used in Substance Abuse—cont'd

| DRUG (GENERIC AND TRADE NAME); ROUTE AND DOSAGE | ACTION/INDICATION | COMMON SIDE EFFECTS AND NURSING CONSIDERATIONS |
|---|---|---|
| **Diazepam** (Valium) <br> **Route:** PO, IM, IV <br> **Dosage:** For anxiety PO 2-10 mg 2-4 times daily or 14-30 mg extended release form once daily; for seizures and anxiety IM or IV 5-10 mg and may repeat q 10-15 min for a total of 30 mg; for alcohol withdrawal 10 mg 3-4 times daily in first 24 hr, decrease to 5 mg 3-4 times daily | Benaodiazepine used in the treatment of anxiety, seizures, and alcohol withdrawal; also used as a muscle relaxant, preoperative sedative, and light anesthetic | Dizziness, drowsiness, and lethargy; use with caution in debilitated individuals, patients with renal or hepatic dysfunction, and previously addicted or suicidal patients; drug has few compatibilities |
| **Fluoxetine** (Prozac) <br> **Route:** PO <br> **Dosage:** 20 mg/day in the morning; after several weeks may increase by 20 mg/day at weekly intervals (not to exceed 80 mg/day) | Antianxiety drug used in the treatment of depression | Anxiety, insomnia, headache, drowsiness, tremor, diarrhea, excessive sweating, and pruritus; may cause anorexia and weight loss; use with caution in the elderly and patients with renal or hepatic dysfunction |
| **Haloperidol** (Haldol) <br> **Route:** PO, IM, IV <br> **Dosage:** PO 0.5-5 mg 2-3 times daily; patients with severe symptoms may require up to 100 mg/day; IM 2-5 mg q 1-8 hr, not to exceed 100 mg/day; IV 0.5-50 mg, may be repeated in 30 min | Antipsychotic drug used in the treatment of acute and chronic psychoses | Extrapyramidal reactions, dry eyes, blurred vision, hypotension, constipation, dry mouth, and photosensitivity |
| **Lithium** (Lithium) <br> **Route:** PO <br> **Dosage:** 900-1200 mg/day in 3-4 divided doses; blood level monitoring is necessary to determine therapeutic dosage | Antimania drug used in the treatment of a variety of psychiatric disorders, especially bipolar affective disorders | Tremors, headache, impaired memory, lethargy, fatigue, ECG changes, nausea, anorexia, epigastric bloating, diarrhea, abdominal pain, polyuria, dermatitis, hypothyroidism, leukocytosis, and muscle weakness; do not use in patients with severe cardiac or renal dysfunction or known alcohol intolerance; monitor drug levels closely |
| **Lorazepam** (Ativan) <br> **Route:** PO, IM, IV <br> **Dosage:** PO 1-3 mg 2-3 times daily, up to 10 mg/day; decrease dosage in elderly; for insomnia PO 2-4 mg at bedtime; IM, IV routes used primarily as preoperative medication; IM 0.05 mg/kg for adults, up to 4 mg 2 hr before surgery; IV 0.044 mg/kg or a total of 2 mg, whichever is less, 15-20 min before surgery | Benzodiazepine used in the treatment of anxiety and insomnia; used preoperatively to induce sedation and anesthesia; used as antiemetic before chemotherapy | Dizziness, drowsiness, and lethargy; use with caution in debilitated individuals, in patients with renal or hepatic dysfunction, and in previously addicted or suicidal patients |

**TABLE 10-3**

## Pharmacology of Drugs Used in Substance Abuse—cont'd

| DRUG (GENERIC AND TRADE NAME); ROUTE AND DOSAGE | ACTION/INDICATION | COMMON SIDE EFFECTS AND NURSING CONSIDERATIONS |
|---|---|---|
| **Methadone** (Dolophine)<br>Route: PO<br>Dosage: 15-20 mg orally (up to 40 mg orally) to suppress symptoms; maintenance dose of 20-120 mg daily to control abstinence | Narcotic analgesic that replaces heroin or other opioid analgesics in detoxification/maintenance programs | Sedation, confusion, hypotension, and constipation; euphoria is much less prominent, and the addict may eventually overcome compulsive need for "narcotic high" |
| **Oxazepam** (Serax)<br>Route: PO<br>Dosage: 10-30 mg 3-4 times daily; in older patients initial dosage should be 5 mg 1-2 times daily or 10 mg 3 times daily | Benzodiazepine used in the treatment of anxiety and alcohol withdrawal | Dizziness, drowsiness, and lethargy; use with caution in the elderly, in patients with hepatic dysfunction, and in previously addicted or suicidal patients |
| **Paroxetine** (Paxil)<br>Route: PO<br>Dosage: 20 mg as a single morning dose; may increase dosage by 10 mg/day at weekly intervals to a maximum dosage of 50 mg/day | Antianxiety drug used in the treatment of depression | Somnolence, dizziness, insomnia, tremor, nervousness, anxiety, headache, weakness, nausea, dry mouth, constipation, diarrhea, ejaculatory disturbance, male genital disorders, and sweating; potentially fatal reaction with MAO inhibitors; use with caution in the elderly and patients with renal or hepatic dysfunction |
| **Sertraline** (Zoloft)<br>Route: PO<br>Dosage: 50 mg/day as a single morning dose; may increase at weekly intervals to a maximum dosage of 200 mg/day | Antianxiety drug used in the treatment of depression | Headache, dizziness, tremor, insomnia, drowsiness, fatigue, dry mouth, nausea, diarrhea, male sexual dysfunction, and increased sweating; potentially fatal reaction with MAO inhibitors; use with caution in the elderly and patients with renal or hepatic dysfunction |
| **Tranylcypromine** (Parnate)<br>Route: PO<br>Dosage: 30 mg/day, initially in single or divided doses; after 2 wk may increase by 10 mg/day to a maximum dosage of 60 mg/day | MAO inhibitor used in the treatment of neurotic or atypical depression | Restlessness, insomnia, dizziness, headache, blurred vision, orthostatic hypotension, arrhythmias, constipation, anorexia, nausea, vomiting, diarrhea, abdominal pain, and dry mouth; watch for multiple drug reactions that could cause hypertensive crisis; foods containing tyramine (cheese, sour cream, beer, yogurt) can cause fatal hypertensive crisis; chocolate and caffeine can elevate blood pressure |

**TABLE 10-4**

## Serious Side Effects of Combining Some Substances with Alcohol

| SUBSTANCE | EFFECT OF COMBINING WITH ALCOHOL |
|---|---|
| Sedatives (anxiolytic) | Additive or synergistic increase occurs in sedative actions; psychosomatic impairment also occurs. |
| Tricyclic antidepressants | Both smoking and alcohol may accelerate the clearance of these antidepressants, therefore depressed alcoholics may not achieve the appropriate blood levels of antidepressants. |
| Monoamine oxidase (MAO) inhibitors | Some MAO inhibitors produce disulfiram-like (Antabuse) effects; dark beer and red wines contain tyramine and may cause episodes of hypertension. |
| Opioids | Respiratory depressant effects of both ethanol and opioids may be potentiated. |
| Cocaine | Cardiovascular effects may be potentiated. |
| Oral hypoglycemic agents | Blood sugar levels may decrease significantly if these drugs are ingested with alcohol. |
| Acetaminophen | Toxic metabolites may accumulate and increase susceptibility to acetaminophen-induced hepatotoxicity. |
| Salicylates and aspirin | Alcohol increases the tendency of salicylates to cause gastrointestinal bleeding. Aspirin increases alcohol absorption, which results in an elevated blood alcohol level. |
| Anticoagulants | Chronic drinkers metabolize warfarin more rapidly, necessitating close monitoring of anticoagulant effects, especially when the drinking pattern varies substantially. |
| $H_2$ antagonists | Cimetidine, ranitidine, and nizatidine (but not famotidine) may increase the blood alcohol level by reducing ethanol metabolism in the stomach. |
| Antimicrobials and antibiotics | With acute alcohol consumption, many antimicrobials (chloramphenicol, furazolidone, griseofulvin, metronidazole, and some cephalosporins) may produce a disulfiram-like (Antabuse) reaction. |

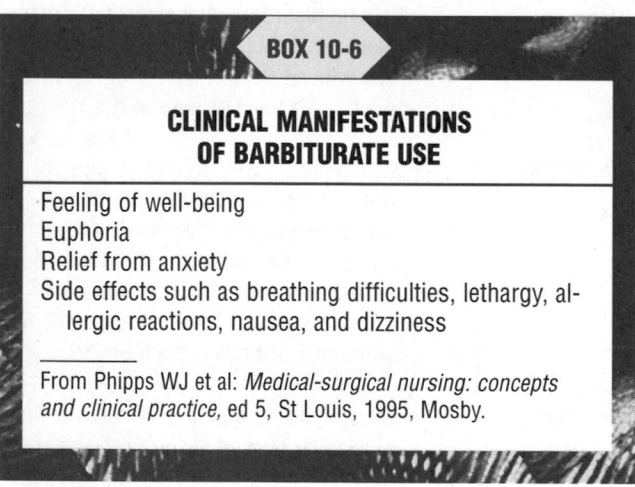

**BOX 10-6**

### CLINICAL MANIFESTATIONS OF BARBITURATE USE

Feeling of well-being
Euphoria
Relief from anxiety
Side effects such as breathing difficulties, lethargy, allergic reactions, nausea, and dizziness

From Phipps WJ et al: *Medical-surgical nursing: concepts and clinical practice*, ed 5, St Louis, 1995, Mosby.

**BOX 10-7**

### CLINICAL MANIFESTATIONS OF NARCOTIC USE

Relief of pain and feeling of well-being
Shallow breathing
Reduced hunger and thirst
Reduced sexual drive
Drowsiness
Euphoria
Lethargy
Heaviness of limbs
Apathy
Loss of ability to concentrate
Loss of judgment and self-control
*With overdose:* coma, convulsions, respiratory arrest, and death

From Phipps WJ et al: *Medical-surgical nursing: concepts and clinical practice*, ed 5, St Louis, 1995, Mosby.

## Narcotics

Narcotics include opium and its derivatives, heroin, codeine, morphine, hydromorphone, and synthetic opiates, including meperidine, methadone, propoxyphene (Darvon), and pentazocine (Talwin). Tolerance and physical and psychologic dependency can occur rapidly. Heroin is the most commonly abused of the opiate drugs, but dependency can occur with any of the narcotics. Heroin users report an initial euphoria followed by the "nod," which is a feeling of almost complete physical and mental relaxation that can last for several hours (Box 10-7). Once a drug used primarily by minorities in the lower socioeconomic class, heroin recently has been increasingly used by middle class whites. It may be inhaled through the nose (snorted) or injected. The use of contaminated needles creates a risk for human immunodeficiency virus (HIV), hepatitis, and septicemia.

Withdrawal symptoms may begin within 8 to 12 hours of the last dose. Heroin withdrawal is rarely life-threatening; it may produce mild, flulike symptoms such as diaphoresis, nausea, vomiting, a runny

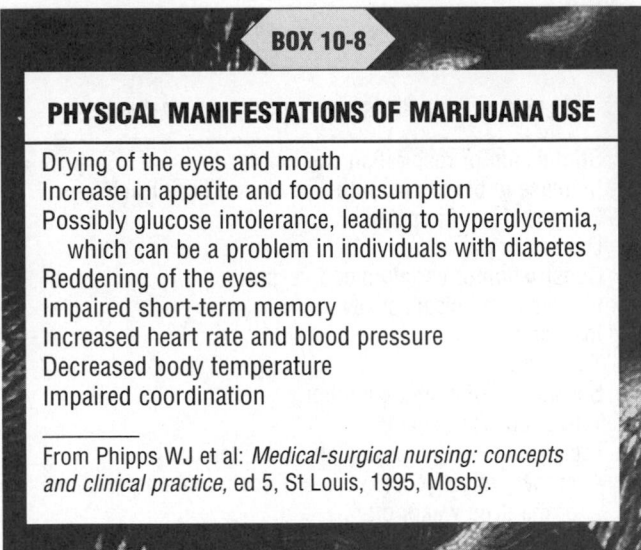

nose, increased lacrimation, yawning, and generalized musculoskeletal aches. More severe symptoms include anxiety, agitation, chills, fever, tremors, muscle spasms, and elevated blood pressure and pulse. Clonidine may be used to treat some of the withdrawal symptoms. Naltrexone (Trexan), a long-acting narcotic antagonist, may be used after the patient has been free of opiates for at least 5 days. Administering Trexan to a patient who is using opiates can precipitate a relatively severe withdrawal syndrome because Trexan negates the effects of the opiates. Therefore the patient must be properly screened to determine current opiate levels.

Methadone, a synthetic opiate, sometimes is used to diminish or eliminate the symptoms of heroin withdrawal. The patient may be enrolled in a methadone maintenance program in which he or she receives the drug over a period of weeks to years. Because methadone itself is addicting, its dosage must be tapered slowly. Not all professionals endorse the use of methadone, however; some recommend instead symptomatic treatment of withdrawal to reach complete abstinence.

## Marijuana

Marijuana, or cannabis, has been used as a mind-altering drug for thousands of years. It grows wild in many countries and is easily cultivated for street use. Marijuana comes from the dried leaves and flowers of the hemp plant, and it is smoked in a pipe or cigarette. "Bongs," or water-filled pipes, may also be used for smoking marijuana or hashish, which is a concentrated extract of the hemp plant. Marijuana is one of the most commonly abused illegal drugs in the United States, and it is particularly popular among young people. Cannabis is used in medicine to help control the side effects of chemotherapy, and occasionally it is used to reduce the eye pressure of glaucoma. Cannabis is a CNS depressant, and users may develop a psychologic dependence. The use of cannabis before or during activities that require concentration and motor coordination is dangerous. Driving a vehicle or operating machinery while under the influence increases the risk of injury or death, both to oneself and to others (Boxes 10-8 and 10-9).

# CENTRAL NERVOUS SYSTEM STIMULANTS

## Amphetamines

Amphetamines are synthetic psychoactive drugs used to increase a sense of alertness and wakefulness and to alter mood. They are legally available by prescription in tablet and capsule form. Methamphetamine is an illegal street drug produced in powdered form and mixed with a diluent for injection.

Amphetamines stimulate the brain and heart, resulting in an increase in blood pressure and pulse rate, dilated pupils, reduced fatigue, reduced appetite, and increased concentration. Large doses or prolonged use results in an unnatural wakefulness and euphoria, often followed by a "crash," or a period of physical and mental exhaustion and depression (Box 10-10). Amphetamines may produce tolerance and a psychologic dependence. It is unclear if physical dependence occurs.

Amphetamine withdrawal symptoms may include fatigue, lethargy, depression, muscle pain, and a toxic psychosis. Severe symptoms may require respiratory and cardiovascular support. Intravenous diazepam (Valium) for sedation and antihypertensives also may be ordered.

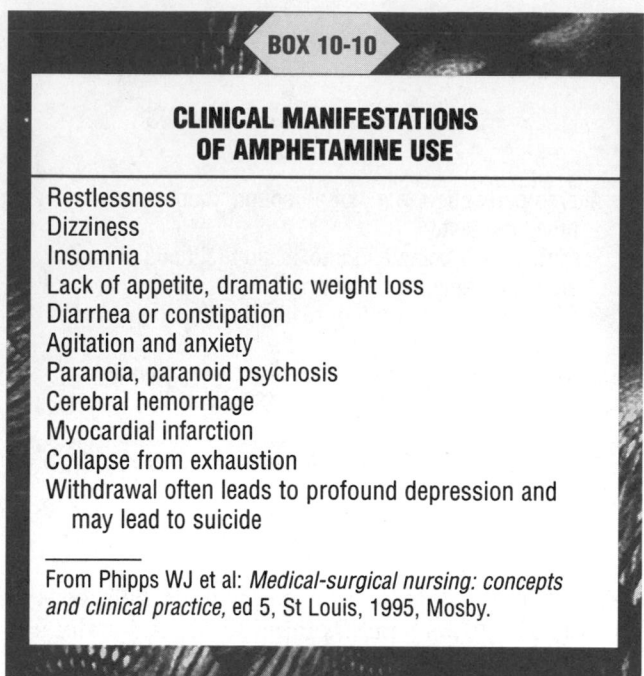

## Cocaine

Cocaine is a potent, highly addictive CNS stimulant, and its use has increased greatly in the United States during the past decade. Cocaine can be used in a variety of ways. A powdered form may be snorted or dissolved and injected intravenously. Crack cocaine is produced by heating cocaine with baking soda and water, which results in a purified substance that may contain as much as 90% pure cocaine. Crack is smoked in a pipe or mixed with tobacco and rolled and smoked as a cigarette. Freebasing involves heating the cocaine to separate it from the adulterants used to cut (or dilute) the drug. Free base cocaine may be smoked or injected intravenously. Cocaine is a rapidly acting but relatively short-acting drug. When it is snorted, the effects are felt within approximately 3 minutes and last 15 to 30 minutes. A more intense euphoria occurs when crack cocaine is smoked. The euphoria begins within 4 to 6 seconds but lasts only 6 to 7 minutes.

Tolerance and psychologic dependence can occur quickly with cocaine. The high usually is followed by a crash when the drug wears off. The feelings of well-being and confidence are replaced with fatigue and depression. The fast, intense effects of cocaine motivate an individual to use more of the drug, which leads to repeated abuse. To relieve the sometimes uncomfortable effects of CNS stimulation, users often also abuse a CNS depressant such as alcohol or heroin. Physical dependence may occur in some cocaine users. Cocaine acts on the neurotransmitters of the brain and prolongs the effects of norepinephrine and dopamine. Repeated or habitual use may break down the neurotransmitters and eventually deplete the supply of norepinephrine and dopamine to the brain and peripheral nerves.

Severe physical problems occur with cocaine use. Soon after taking cocaine, the user's blood pressure and pulse increase rapidly, and the user may report chest pain and a pounding heart. Death may be caused by a ventricular arrhythmia, seizures, a cocaine-induced stroke, or respiratory paralysis. Some users describe a cocaine psychosis, which includes hallucinations, insomnia and, in some individuals, an increased potential for violent behavior (Box 10-11). Withdrawal treatment depends on the patient's symptoms and may include the use of sedatives, tranquilizers, anticonvulsants, and antiarrhythmic drugs.

## Ritalin

Ritalin (methylphenidate), a CNS stimulant frequently prescribed for treatment of attention deficit disorder, is increasingly becoming a drug of abuse among young people. Available in tablets or sustained-release capsules, it is used to produce a high or to improve concentration and delay sleep while studying for examinations. Because it is prescribed often, young teenagers may obtain the drug from friends or brothers or sisters. Older students find it available as a street drug.

The effects of Ritalin include increased motor activity, mental alertness, a decreased sense of fatigue, and mild euphoria. Adverse reactions range from nervousness, insomnia, and anorexia to tachycardia, palpitations, chest pain, psychotic episodes, seizures, and coma. Deaths from cardiac collapse have been reported.

## Nicotine

Nicotine, which is found in tobacco, is used by 25% to 30% of all Americans. Tobacco may be smoked or chewed. Finely chopped tobacco in the form of snuff is placed between the gums and the cheek, and the nicotine is absorbed through the mucous membranes in the mouth. Nicotine is very addictive, perhaps more so than any other drug. It is both psychologically and physically addicting. The physically damaging effects of cigarette smoking are widely recognized (Figure 10-3). When tobacco smoke is inhaled, the effects are felt within seconds, and the nicotine is rapidly metabolized in the body. Because the effects of nicotine are brief, the user smokes anywhere from several times a day to several times an hour, depending on the tolerance that has developed and the opportunities for use.

Laws and policies are increasingly limiting the opportunities for smoking in public places. Although nicotine is a mild CNS stimulant, users report that smoking a cigarette may have an energizing or a calming effect, depending on the user's mood and the circumstances. Nicotine acts as a mild to moderate appetite suppressant and causes a temporary rise in blood pressure. In excessive doses it produces mild tremors and an increased respiratory rate. Withdrawal symptoms occur rapidly. Within 1 to 3 hours after smoking a cigarette, the craving for another may begin. Cravings may last for weeks or months after cessation but diminish in frequency and intensity over time. Other withdrawal symptoms include irritability, anxiety, poor concentration, headaches, fatigue, insomnia, and constipation or diarrhea.

Some nicotine addicts are resistant to treatment in spite of the well-known health risks, perhaps because, unlike other substances of abuse, nicotine does not produce substantial cognitive impairment. Nor does it produce pathologic alterations in mood. Some schizophrenics who smoke may be self-medicating aspects of their illness or some side effects of drugs (Docherty, 1996). Some evidence indicates that recent former smokers with a history of major depression or those with persistent withdrawal symptoms are at increased risk for posttreatment major depression, even weeks after smoking cessation treatment has ended (Covey, 1997).

A number of behavior modification programs that promote smoking cessation are available. Acupuncture and hypnosis have proven successful for some

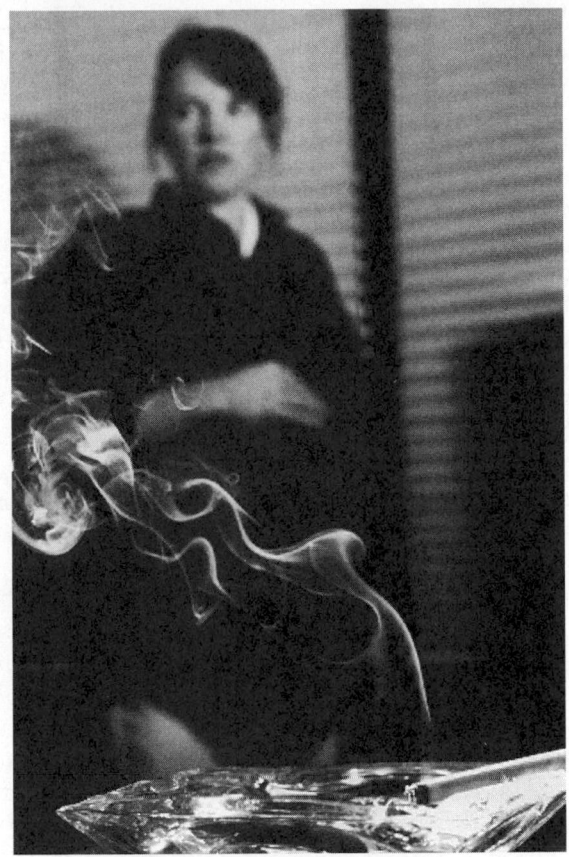

**Figure 10-3** The physically damaging effects of smoking are widely recognized. Women are advised not to smoke during pregnancy to prevent harm to the infant. (Courtesy Michael Clement, MD, Mesa, Ariz.)

smokers. Transdermal nicotine patches lessen physical withdrawal symptoms by providing small amounts of nicotine continuously through the skin. The patches are most effective when used in conjunction with a behavior modification program.

Zyban, a nicotine-free prescription medication supplied in sustained-release tablets, recently was approved by the U.S. Food and Drug Administration (FDA) as an aid to smoking cessation treatment. It appears to affect the nonadrenergic or dopaminergic mechanisms (or both) in the brain that have been identified as pathways of nicotine addiction. Patients treated with Zyban report reduced withdrawal symptoms and a lessening of the urge to smoke. The drug may be used in conjunction with a transdermal nicotine patch and is most effective when used as part of a comprehensive smoking cessation program. It is contraindicated in patients with a history of seizure disorders, bulimia, or anorexia nervosa and in those who have recently taken an MAO inhibitor.

# INHALANTS

Inhalants include a wide range of chemicals that emit vapors or fumes. Many household products such as glue, paint thinner, nail polish remover, spot remover, gasoline, kerosene, and cleaning products belong to this category. Aerosol products such as hair spray, antistain protectors, deodorants, and insecticides become drugs of abuse when the fumes are inhaled. Nitrous oxide and ether are anesthetics sometimes used recreationally. The user may sniff the vapors directly from an aerosol can or other container or may capture the fumes in a bag or balloon. Because these products are inexpensive, legal, easy to conceal and, except for the anesthetics, easily obtainable, most inhalant abusers are adolescents, and the incidence of inhalant abuse is rising rapidly in that age group (Lawson, 1992). Some inhalants cause tolerance and may cause physical dependency.

Most inhalants are CNS depressants. Box 10-12 lists the clinical manifestations of inhalant use. The solvents are fat-soluble organic substances that pass through the blood-brain barrier to produce a change in the level of consciousness similar to the more mild stage I or II level of anesthesia. The onset of mental change occurs rapidly, and the period of intoxication is relatively short, lasting 15 to 45 minutes (Robin, Michelson, 1988). Serious consequences may occur from excessive or repeated use of inhalants, including damage to the liver, kidneys, bone marrow, and brain. A life-threatening toxic event characterized by respiratory depression and cardiac arrhythmias can follow the use of inhalants, especially fluorinated hydrocarbons. Death may result from cardiac arrest or from suffocation as a result of displacement of oxygen in the lungs.

# HALLUCINOGENS

Hallucinogens are drugs that produce an acute change in thinking and in reality perception. Included in this group are lysergic acid diethylamide (LSD); mescaline; 2,5-dimethoxy-4-methamphetamine (STP); psilocybin; dimethyltryptamine (DMT); and methylenedioxyamphetamine (MDA). These street drugs became popular during the 1960s and 1970s. Hallucinogens are ingested orally and may be found in many forms, including tablets, capsules, powder, mushrooms, and peyote buttons. Sometimes they are mixed with food or put on sugar cubes. LSD is also found on blotter paper and on sheets of paper containing tattoos or pictures of cartoon characters.

Hallucinogens distort the user's perception of the environment and alter thought and emotional patterns (Box 10-13). Visual hallucinations and mood changes vary dramatically from person to person and also within the same person, depending on the circum-

---

**BOX 10-12**

## CLINICAL MANIFESTATIONS OF INHALANT USE

Slurred speech
Blurred vision, bloodshot eyes
Inflamed mucous membranes, episodes of nose
  bleeding
Bad breath/chemical odor
Lightheadedness
Ringing in the ears
Watery eyes
Loss of coordination/poor memory
Excessive nasal secretions
Loss of consciousness or seizures lasting 20 to
  45 minutes with large doses

Modified from Phipps WJ et al: *Medical-surgical nursing: concepts and clinical practice*, ed 5, St Louis, 1995, Mosby.

---

**BOX 10-13**

## CLINICAL MANIFESTATIONS OF HALLUCINOGEN USE

Initial stimulation followed by depression
Anxiety
Depressed appetite
Increased body temperature
Increased heart rate
Increased respiration
Dilated pupils (dizziness, facial numbness, and shivering also may occur with psilocybin use)
Altered sensory awareness (senses become more acute)
Sensation of "hearing" colors and "seeing" sounds
Fantasies and illusions
Hallucination-like happenings
Unawareness that hallucinations are not real
Melding of past and present experiences, leading to a feeling of oneness, compassion, and love for all things

Modified from Phipps WJ et al: *Medical-surgical nursing: concepts and clinical practice*, ed 5, St Louis, 1995, Mosby.

stances in which the drug is ingested. Hallucinogenic effects may last from 6 to 12 hours. A "bad trip" occurs when frightening images, panic, terror, or depression is experienced. Paranoid or violent behavior or psychotic episodes may occur.

Tolerance develops quickly and often after only a few days' use. Psychologic dependence may occur with frequent use, but no physical dependence occurs. Treatment aims at getting the patient into a quiet, nonstimulating environment and remaining with him or her until the effects of the drug wear off. Talking to the patient in a calm, reassuring way (i.e., talking him or her "down") may be helpful. **Flashbacks** occur when the user briefly experiences the original sensations experienced during use even when no drug has been ingested. Although the frequency of flashbacks varies, they may occur for many years after an individual's last use of hallucinogens.

## Phencyclidine

Phencyclidine, or PCP, is a psychoactive drug and is classified as an anesthetic-hallucinogen. It is available legally only as an animal anesthetic for use by veterinarians. It is available on the street in powder, capsule, or tablet form. It may be snorted, injected, or smoked with tobacco or marijuana.

PCP use results in symptoms that vary from person to person (Tables 10-5 and 10-6). It may act as a CNS stimulant, a CNS depressant, or a hallucinogen. PCP ingestion may be viewed as a psychiatric emergency because of its unpredictable and volatile effects. There is the potential for self-harm or harm to others. This drug is psychologically habit forming, but there is disagreement as to whether it is physically addicting.

## TREATMENT AND REHABILITATION

There is a difference between being sober and being a recovering alcoholic or substance abuser. To maintain sobriety and be in recovery, a person must make major changes in attitude, behavior, beliefs, and thinking. A **dry drunk** is one who abstains from alcohol completely but still exhibits the attitudes, impaired thinking, and behavior of an active alcoholic.

It often is difficult to convince an abuser (who

---

### TABLE 10-5

#### Dose-Related Physical Manifestations of Phencyclidine Use

| DOSE | EFFECTS |
| --- | --- |
| 5 mg (Low) | Physical sedation; numbness of the extremities; loss of muscle coordination; dizziness; constricted pupils, blurred or double vision, and involuntary eye movements; flushing and profuse sweating; nausea and vomiting; increase in blood pressure, heart rate and respiratory rate (breathing shallow) |
| 5 to 10 mg (Moderate) | Marked drop in blood pressure, breathing and heart rate; shivering, increased salivation, and watering of the eyes; loss of balance, dizziness, and rigidity of muscles; in some cases, repetitive movements, such as rocking; analgesic and anesthetic properties apparent |
| More than 10 mg (High) | Extreme agitation, followed by seizures or coma; symptoms similar to mental confusion and delusion of schizophrenia |

From Scott L: *PCP,* Charlotte, NC, 1981, Charlotte Drug Educational Center (pamphlet).

---

### TABLE 10-6

#### Dose-Related Psychologic Manifestations of Phencyclidine Use

| DOSE | EFFECTS |
| --- | --- |
| 5 mg (Low) | Euphoria; sense of intoxication; changes in body image; mood swings, from ecstasy to panic; hallucinations and confusion about time and space; in some cases, in the final stage, a sense of despair and emotional isolation, possibly leading to a feeling of paranoia and a sense of impeding death |
| 5 to 10 mg (Moderate) | Increase in effects felt at low dose; loss of sense of contact with environment |
| More than 10 mg (High) | Symptoms of mental and emotional confusion similar to schizophrenia |

From Scott L: *PCP,* Charlotte, NC, 1981, Charlotte Drug Educational Center (pamphlet).

frequently is still in **denial**) that treatment is needed. Vernon Johnson (1990) states in *I'll Quit Tomorrow*:

It is a myth that alcoholics (drug abusers) have some spontaneous insight and then seek treatment . . . typically, in our experience they come to their recognition scenes through a buildup of crises that crash through their almost impenetrable defense systems . . . they are forced to seek help . . . it was not only pointless but dangerous to wait until the (alcoholic/drug abuser) hit bottom . . . we came to understand that crises could be used creatively to bring about intervention . . . in all the lives we studied, it was only through crisis that intervention had occurred.

An **intervention** occurs when the patient's significant others, family, friends, and a professional who works with addicts unite with the goal of breaking through the patient's denial and getting him or her into appropriate treatment. The intensity level and type of treatment depend on a number of factors, including how long the dependence problem has existed, medical problems, family support relationships, available facilities, and financial resources.

Since 1990 many inpatient detoxification and treatment facilities have closed as a result of reduced reimbursement from insurers and changes in treatment methods. In view of this, detoxification may be done on an inpatient basis on a hospital medical-surgical unit or on an outpatient basis in which the patient makes a daily visit to a clinic to be monitored. Initial treatment after detox may also be done on either an inpatient or outpatient basis. Most alcohol and substance abuse rehabilitation programs last from 3 to 8 weeks and include education about the disease process, an orientation to Alcoholics Anonymous (AA), individual and group therapy, and the involvement of significant others.

**Relapse**, or the return of drinking or use of any mind-altering drugs, is common in recovering alcoholics. Follow-up treatment after the initial rehabilitation program significantly reduces the number of patients who relapse during their first year of recovery and for some time thereafter.

AA plays an important part in the recovery of many alcoholics. Founded in 1935 it is the original self-help group, with currently more than 1 million members in the United States. Members follow 12 steps and 12 traditions in an attempt to stay sober 1 day at a time (Box 10-14). AA is a spiritual program, but not a religious one, that promotes reliance on a higher power and the responsibility to help each other maintain recovery after admitting to powerlessness over alcohol. Subgroups of AA, such as Al-Anon, Alateen, Alatot, and Adult Children of Alcoholics, recognize the family disease of alcoholism and provide assistance to family members in their own recovery from codependency.

---

**BOX 10-14**

### TWELVE STEPS OF ALCOHOLICS ANONYMOUS

1. We admitted we were powerless over alcohol—that our lives had become unmanageable.
2. Came to believe that a Power greater than ourselves could restore us to sanity.
3. Made a decision to turn our will and our lives over to the care of God as we understood Him.
4. Made a searching and fearless moral inventory of ourselves.
5. Admitted to God, to ourselves, and to another human being the exact nature of our wrongs.
6. Were entirely ready to have God remove all these defects of character.
7. Humbly asked Him to remove our shortcomings.
8. Made a list of all persons we had harmed and became willing to make amends to them all.
9. Made direct amends to such people whenever possible, except when to do so would injure them or others.
10. Continued to take personal inventory and when we were wrong promptly admitted it.
11. Sought through prayer and meditation to improve our conscious contact with God, as we understood Him, praying only for knowledge of His will for us and the power to carry that out.
12. Having had a spiritual awakening as a result of these steps, we tried to carry this message to alcoholics and to practice these principles in all our affairs.

From *Alcoholics Anonymous*, New York, 1976, Alcoholics Anonymous World Sources.
The Twelve Steps of Alcoholics Anonymous have been reprinted with permission of Alcoholics Anonymous World Services. Permission to reprint them does not mean that AA is in any way affiliated with this publication or that it has read or endorses the contents thereof. AA is a program of recovery from alcoholism *only*—inclusion of these steps in this publication, or use in any other non-AA context, does not imply otherwise.

---

Some recovering addicts benefit from spending a few weeks or months in a halfway house, which provides a support system during early recovery. The emphasis is on assuming responsibility for one's own well-being and adjusting to living in a drug-free community. Residents are expected to find employment, help maintain the residence, and work toward continued recovery by attending the appropriate self-help meetings and counseling.

## NURSING MANAGEMENT

In the following sections, alcoholism is used as the model for all substance abuse and dependence disor-

---

**BOX 10-15**

### HELPFUL ATTITUDES IN TREATING ALCOHOLICS

1. Alcoholism is a chronic, relapsing illness.
2. Alcoholism is a treatable disease.
3. Alcoholism has definite signs and stages of progression.
4. Treatment of alcoholism often is successful.
5. Help is readily available in most communities.
6. Alcoholism could happen to anyone.
7. Recognizing the alcoholic's self-loathing, isolation, depression, and feelings of guilt while he or she is drinking is essential to successful treatment.
8. Alcoholics Anonymous and two subgroups of AA (Al-Anon and Alateen) can be effective self-help groups in treating alcoholism.
9. Standard psychiatric treatment methods generally are ineffective in treating alcoholism per se; in fact, the alcoholic can use them to avoid dealing with the alcoholism.
10. The alcoholic's spouse cannot cause the problem, although the spouse may aggravate it.
11. Members of the alcoholic's family need treatment as much as the alcoholic.
12. For all practical purposes, an alcoholic cannot return to normal, controlled drinking.
13. To the alcoholic, following through on a referral presents an extreme life crisis: a decision to not drink. This is akin to the heroin addict's giving up heroin. In the alcoholic's view, alcohol is the only means of survival.
14. The recovery process is a frightening, difficult, lifelong task. It requires a complete reordering of social aspects of the alcoholic's life; to accomplish this, the individual will need lifelong support.

Adapted from Norris JL: *Psychiatr Ann* 8(11):48-53, 1978.

---

**BOX 10-16**

### UNHELPFUL ATTITUDES IN TREATING ALCOHOLICS

1. Alcoholism is a self-inflicted illness.
2. Alcoholism is hopeless.
3. Recovering from alcoholism is simply a matter of will power.
4. Drinking in any amount is dangerous and can lead to alcoholism.
5. Let the poor, sick, unemployed, lonely, or old people with alcoholism continue to drink. They're better off that way.
6. Abstinence for an alcoholic is a primitive expectation. No one can live that way.
7. It is so hard for an alcoholic to abstain, one should merely expect the alcoholic to limit the amount.
8. Alcoholics are simply people who will not accept life's responsibilities as most people must do.

From Norris JL: *Psychiatr Ann* 8(11):48-53, 1978.

---

ders. The following information applies to the abuse of all mind-altering drugs.

Given the prevalence of alcoholism in the United States, all nurses may expect to encounter both diagnosed and undiagnosed alcoholics in any health care setting. It is important that the nurse recognize the signs and symptoms of alcoholism, its medical problems, and the physical symptoms of withdrawal and to identify the psychologic and social problems related to alcoholism.

The nurse may find it necessary to carefully examine his or her own views when dealing with alcoholics. As with any disease, not all alcoholics remain in recovery. Some relapse once or repeatedly, and many die as a result of the disease, which may cause feelings of anger or helplessness in the nurse. Without realizing it, nurses sometimes respond to the dysfunctional behavior of alcoholics and their family members in a rejecting, judgmental, or condescending way. Occasionally the nurse may become an enabler to the alcoholic or the family (Boxes 10-15 and 10-16).

## Assessment

Direct observation of the alcoholic patient and information gathered from a number of sources results in the most complete and accurate assessment possible. Because denial and impaired thinking are almost universally displayed in the untreated alcoholic, the information given by the patient may be inaccurate or incomplete. If possible, this information should be confirmed with a friend or family member.

Objective data helpful in assessing the alcoholic patient might include the following:
- General appearance (neat and clean or disheveled and dirty)
- General behavior (loud, aggressive, euphoric, combative, uncooperative, depressed)
- Speech (normal, slurred, incoherent)
- Memory (evidence of memory loss)
- Sensorium (clear, disoriented, hallucinations)
- Tremors (tremors, motor incoordination)
- Vital signs (depressed, elevated)
- Eyes (dilated or pinpoint pupils, normal or blurred vision)

- Skin color and integrity (well oxygenated, jaundiced, cuts, bruises, petechiae, needle marks)
- Gastrointestinal (nausea and vomiting, ascites, blood in stools)
- Breath (describe odor)
- Laboratory reports (note any abnormal results)

The following subjective data also should be gathered:

- Date and time of last drink or use
- Substances used, quantity used
- History of blackouts, tremors, seizures, hallucinations, delirium tremens
- Usual drinking or using pattern

Box 10-17 lists additional signs of substance abuse.

## Planning

The first priority in planning for the alcoholic patient is to ensure his or her medical safety if withdrawal symptoms are present or impending. Careful assessment may identify numerous problems that need attention. After withdrawal is complete, the nurse may help the patient accept his or her substance abuse problem and refer him or her to a substance abuse professional who can help clarify treatment options.

---

**BOX 10-17**

### SIGNS AND SYMPTOMS OF ALCOHOL OR SUBSTANCE ABUSE

1. Frequent illnesses and related illnesses
2. Undue preoccupation with the intake of drugs or alcohol
3. Mood swings
4. Violent or acting-out behavior
5. Denial about the use of substances
6. Financial difficulties
7. Loss of control over use
8. Use of alcohol or drugs in such a way as to endanger physical health, interpersonal relationships, or economic functioning
9. Use of substances as the universal answer to all problems
10. Loss of ability to express feelings
11. Use of defense mechanisms, including a strong denial of the problem that drugs or alcohol is causing

Data from Phipps WJ et al: *Medical-surgical nursing: concepts and clinical practice*, ed 5, St Louis, 1995, Mosby.

---

## Teaching

Health teaching is an essential part of the nursing care of alcoholic and other chemically dependent patients. Patients need to learn about the physiologic effects of mind-altering drugs, the disease concept of substance abuse, and the environmental factors that may contribute to the development of a full-blown dependence problem. Information about cross-tolerance to drugs in the same general category is important in preventing the patient from developing a polyabuse problem. Health teaching about HIV prevention is especially important in alcoholics. Alcoholics, especially women, are more likely to become sexually promiscuous while under the influence. They may deny that they are at high risk for exposure to HIV.

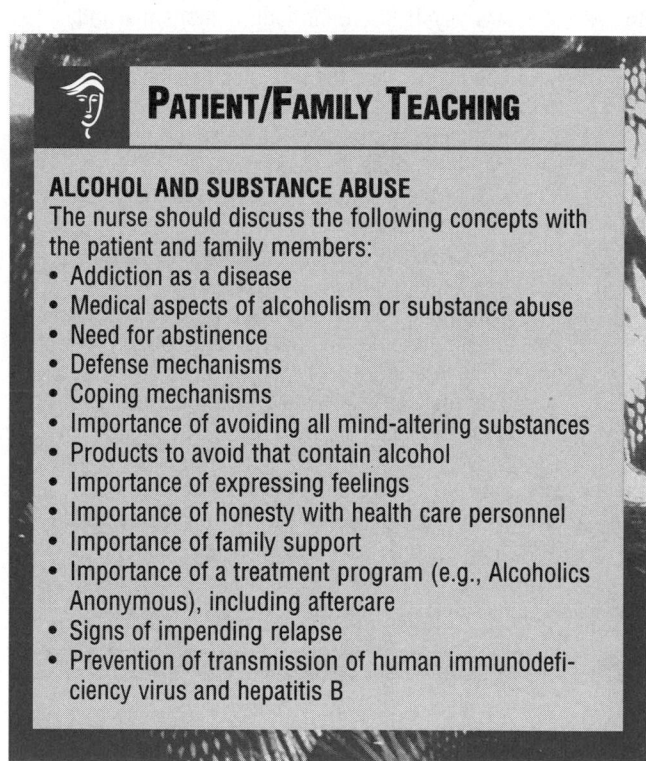

**PATIENT/FAMILY TEACHING**

**ALCOHOL AND SUBSTANCE ABUSE**
The nurse should discuss the following concepts with the patient and family members:

- Addiction as a disease
- Medical aspects of alcoholism or substance abuse
- Need for abstinence
- Defense mechanisms
- Coping mechanisms
- Importance of avoiding all mind-altering substances
- Products to avoid that contain alcohol
- Importance of expressing feelings
- Importance of honesty with health care personnel
- Importance of family support
- Importance of a treatment program (e.g., Alcoholics Anonymous), including aftercare
- Signs of impending relapse
- Prevention of transmission of human immunodeficiency virus and hepatitis B

## Pain Management

Another area of concern for the nurse and the patient is pain management. Even for a specific medical problem, patients committed to recovery often are hesitant to admit to the need for pain medication. However, some patients are drug seeking and demand more pain medication than they actually need so that they can get a mind-altering effect. The responsible nurse conducts a pain assessment and tries to determine the cause of pain. Even when the nurse has doubts about the credibility of the patient's record, it is wise to remember that the patient's report of pain must be considered the most reliable indicator of pain. Establishing a schedule for administering pain medication with input from the patient and physician may help resolve conflicts. Withholding pain medication as a result of distrust regarding the patient's report of pain usually serves no purpose.

Alcoholics and other chemically dependent patients have a higher tolerance for pain medication than do other patients. Therefore during periods of acute pain, such as the first 2 to 3 days after major surgery, the physician often orders larger than usual doses of pain medication to be given at more frequent intervals. The patient is then rapidly weaned from the pain medication and probably should not be discharged with a prescription for pain medication. Any questions about safe dosages should be discussed with the physician to clarify the parameters for administration of the medication.

## Evaluation

It is important to evaluate the patient's responses to medical and nursing interventions continually during hospitalization and also at the time of discharge (Box 10-18). If withdrawal symptoms are or were present, consider the following:
- Stability of vital signs
- Status of respiratory function
- Fluid volume status
- Nutritional intake
- Cognition
- Potential for harm to self or others

To evaluate the patient's understanding and acceptance of the substance abuse problem, consider the following:
- Absence of current substance abuse
- Verbalization of a willingness to obtain treatment
- Understanding of potential mental and physical problems caused by substance abuse
- Verbalization of a desire to cope with problems caused by substance abuse

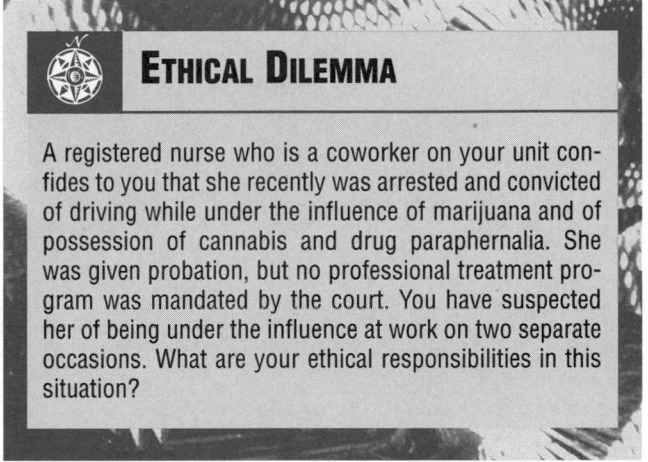

**ETHICAL DILEMMA**

A registered nurse who is a coworker on your unit confides to you that she recently was arrested and convicted of driving while under the influence of marijuana and of possession of cannabis and drug paraphernalia. She was given probation, but no professional treatment program was mandated by the court. You have suspected her of being under the influence at work on two separate occasions. What are your ethical responsibilities in this situation?

---

**BOX 10-18**    **NURSING PROCESS**

### ALCOHOL/SUBSTANCE ABUSE OR DEPENDENCY

**ASSESSMENT**

Assess often during acute phase of withdrawal
- Vital signs
- Fluid volume status
- Level of consciousness, mental status, and behavior
- Respiratory rate and depth and breath sounds as indicated
- Nutritional status and presence of nausea, vomiting, or anorexia
- Laboratory studies (electrolytes, liver function tests, ammonia, blood urea nitrogen [BUN], glucose, coagulation, arterial blood gases [ABGs])
- Effective coping mechanisms
- Family relationships

**NURSING DIAGNOSES**
- Risk for ineffective breathing pattern related to alcohol or drug toxicity and/or the sedative effect of drugs given to treat withdrawal
- Risk for injury related to seizures, cessation of alcohol or drug intake, and impaired cognitive and motor ability
- Risk for self-directed or other-directed violence related to altered thinking patterns, chemical alteration, and hostility
- Sleep pattern disturbance related to withdrawal, anxiety, and insomnia
- Altered nutrition: less than body requirements related to anorexia and inadequate intake
- Fluid volume deficit related to anorexia, nausea, vomiting, diarrhea, and impaired cognition

*Continued*

---

◄ BOX 10-18 ► NURSING PROCESS

## ALCOHOL/SUBSTANCE ABUSE OR DEPENDENCY—cont'd

- Sensory/perceptual alterations related to withdrawal, memory impairment, and impaired judgment
- Ineffective individual coping related to alcohol or drug dependence and loss of support system or employment
- Powerlessness related to inability to control alcohol or drug use
- Noncompliance related to alcoholic or drug-using life-style, denial, lack of resources, and physical or mental disability
- Altered family processes related to situational crisis of alcohol/substance abuse
- Knowledge deficit related to denial of the disease process, medical consequences of addiction, and treatment programs

**NURSING INTERVENTIONS**

- Maintain patent airway.
- Elevate head of bed.
- Encourage patient to turn, cough, and deep breathe q 2 hr.
- Have suction equipment and airways available.
- Maintain nothing by mouth (NPO) until alert.
- Avoid medications that cause respiratory depression.
- Administer supplemental oxygen as ordered.
- Institute seizure precautions.
- Assist with ambulation and self-care.
- Administer medications for withdrawal as ordered.
- Note onset of any hallucinations.
- Provide quiet environment with lights low.
- Restrict visitors.

- Reorient as needed.
- Restrain as necessary to prevent harm to self or others.
- Remove dangerous objects from environment.
- Approach patient nonthreateningly; take time to introduce self and describe procedures.
- Maintain IV fluids until patient tolerates oral (PO) intake.
- Encourage diet high in protein and carbohydrates.
- Provide small, frequent meals.
- Develop a trusting relationship.
- Project an accepting attitude toward patient.
- Help patient identify feelings and express thoughts.
- Confront patient with unacceptable behaviors.
- Reward positive behaviors.
- Involve patient and family in alcohol support groups.

**EVALUATION OF EXPECTED OUTCOMES**

- Respiratory status stable with clear lungs and no evidence of hypoxia
- Vital signs stable
- No physical injury to self or others
- Regains previous level of consciousness
- Reports absence of hallucinations
- Consumes adequate dietary intake
- Verbalizes understanding of effects of alcohol on nutrition
- Begins to recognize effect of self-destructive behaviors
- Refrains from alcohol and substance use
- Participates in a support group
- Identifies available resources

---

# CHEMICALLY IMPAIRED NURSES

The rate of chemical dependency in nurses and other health care professionals is greater than in the general public. The reasons may be complex, but the reality is that nurses generally have much greater access to mind-altering substances. Drug or alcohol abuse is a serious problem in any individual, but diminished judgment and performance in a caregiver threatens their patients' safety. Therefore if a nurse ever has reason to suspect that another nurse is chemically dependent, there is only one option for action: to document incidents and contact the state board of nursing or the state nurses association.

With the support of the American Nurses Association, many states within the last decade have developed peer assistance programs that assist impaired nurses with treatment and recovery. Other goals of peer assistance programs include protecting the public from the untreated nurse, helping the recovering nurse safely reenter nursing, and helping to monitor the recovering nurse for a period of time. Many states have laws that allow the impaired nurse to receive treatment without losing his or her professional license. Although practice may not be allowed for a period of time, the nurse is diverted from full disciplinary action.

## NURSING CARE PLAN
## PATIENT WITH ALCOHOL DEPENDENCE

Mr. DePaul is a 66-year-old man with carcinoma of the bladder who has been admitted to the hospital for cystectomy and urinary diversion via urostomy. His operation is uneventful and without complications. However, after surgery he is difficult to wean from the ventilator and requires 2 days in the critical care unit for respiratory management. It is now 2 days after surgery, and he has been transferred to the medical-surgical unit.

| Medical History | Psychosocial Data | Assessment Data |
|---|---|---|
| Emphysema (two packs a day for 45 yr) | Mother and father had a history of smoking and emphysema; both parents deceased | Barrel-chested, pale male, alert and oriented; irritable and angry at times |
| Reports drinking six beers a day for 8 yr | | Height 5' 10"; weight 91.8 kg (204 lb) |
| *Postoperative treatment:* | No siblings | *Skin:* Good condition; abdominal dressing dry and intact; staples intact; wound edges well approximated with no erythema or drainage at incision |
| D5 ½NS at 100 ml/hr | Wife in very good health | |
| Clear liquid diet | Married for 44 years, has two grown children who live out of state | *Chest:* Increased AP diameter; scattered crackles/rhonchi throughout; respiratory rate 24-32; shallow, symmetric respirations |
| Respiratory therapy with Alupent q 4 hr | | |
| Oxygen ($O_2$) at 2 L via nasal cannula | Limited contact with children and grandchildren | *Apical pulse:* 112 and regular, strong peripheral pulses; no peripheral edema; brisk capillary refill |
| Pulse oximetry q shift | Has few friends and describes himself as a "loner" | *Abdomen:* Obese; softly distended, positive bowel sounds |
| Urostomy to gravity drainage | | |
| Intake and output | Verbalizes difficulty adjusting to retirement | Urostomy patent and draining cloudy yellow urine >30 ml/hr |
| | *Hobbies:* Television and vegetable gardening | Full range of motion in all extremities; out of bed with assistance of one person; dyspneic with exertion; tremors of upper extremities |
| | | Further assessment of alcohol intake with wife reveals history of 24 beers a day, which has gradually increased since retirement |
| | | Physician informed and Ativan (1 mg q 8 hr) initiated |

### NURSING DIAGNOSIS
Risk for ineffective breathing pattern related to postoperative sedation, sedation from medication to prevent alcohol withdrawal, smoking history, and immobility

### NURSING INTERVENTIONS

Monitor respiratory status q 2 hr.
Auscultate breath sounds q 8 hr and prn.
Keep head of bed elevated 30 degrees at all times.
Encourage coughing and deep breathing.
Encourage change of position q 2 hr.
Encourage mobility.
Have suction equipment and airway available.
Administer and monitor $O_2$ at 2 L via nasal cannula.
Monitor pulse oximetry q 8 hr.
Educate patient and wife about importance of aggressive respiratory management and prevention of complications.

### EVALUATION OF EXPECTED OUTCOMES

No evidence of respiratory distress
Lungs clear
Oxygen saturation :>90% on room air
Coughs effectively and deep breathes with encouragement

*Continued*

# NURSING CARE PLAN

## PATIENT WITH ALCOHOL DEPENDENCE—cont'd

**NURSING DIAGNOSIS**

Risk for injury related to cessation of alcohol intake and effect of medications

| NURSING INTERVENTIONS | EVALUATION OF EXPECTED OUTCOMES |
|---|---|
| Monitor for evidence of alcohol withdrawal (e.g., tremors, tachycardia, diaphoresis, hypertension) q 8 hr. | No evidence of withdrawal symptoms |
| Monitor for loss of consciousness and orientation and orient prn. | No evidence of injury |
| Maintain bed in low position, side rails up, padded rails, call light within reach and observe often. | |
| Provide quiet environment. | |
| Restrain prn. | |
| Maintain seizure precautions. | |
| Include wife in treatment plan. | |
| Administer medications as prescribed. | |

**NURSING DIAGNOSIS**

Risk for impaired individual coping related to cessation of alcohol, denial of problem, withdrawal symptoms, and change in body image with urostomy

| NURSING INTERVENTIONS | EVALUATION OF EXPECTED OUTCOMES |
|---|---|
| Assess coping mechanisms and confer with wife if necessary. | Begins to recognize maladaptive behaviors |
| Have same staff care for patient to develop a trusting relationship. | Verbalizes feelings and concerns |
| Spend time with patient each day. | Patient and wife demonstrate effective coping mechanisms |
| Encourage patient to openly discuss alcohol use, feelings, fears, and concerns. | Patient and wife verbalize potential benefit of support groups |
| Encourage support and involvement of wife. | |
| Provide support and encouragement. | |
| Provide instructions for caring for ostomy. | |
| Refer to alcohol and ostomy support groups in the community. | |

## KEY CONCEPTS

➤ Substance abuse is a complex disease and is most likely precipitated by a combination of etiologic factors.

➤ Alcoholism is a progressive, chronic, and debilitating disease that significantly shortens life expectancy.

➤ Substance abuse is found in every age group from childhood through the life span and in all health care settings. It often goes undiagnosed.

➤ Substance abuse is a family disease. Family members and significant others usually react in predictable ways that become increasingly dysfunctional.

➤ Withdrawal from alcohol and other mind-altering substances is a complex nursing problem that may require medical supervision or hospitalization.

➤ Substance abuse is not curable, but continuous recovery is possible, especially with the assistance of professional help and self-help groups such as Alcoholics Anonymous and three subgroups of Alcoholics Anonymous (Cocaine Anonymous, Narcotics Anonymous, and Pills Anonymous).

➤ Recovery requires abstinence from all mind-altering chemicals.

➤ A variety of treatment options are available to help the patient and family with recovery.

➤ Drugs of abuse are categorized as depressants, stimulants, hallucinogens, and inhalants.

➤ Nurses are at greater risk than the general public of becoming chemically dependent.

## CRITICAL THINKING EXERCISES

1. During the second day of his hospitalization for detoxification, a patient complains to you that the nurse on the previous shift delayed each dose of his Valium, stating that, "The more uncomfortable you are, the less likely you will be to go out and drink again." One of your previous detox patients made a similar complaint about the same nurse. Is any action necessary on your part? Why or why not?

2. You are a nurse working in a clinic. One of your patients states that her family is in turmoil because her 10-year-old son will not behave in school. You see in her record that she has a history of alcohol abuse. Identify a possible reason for the son's behavior.

3. Give examples of the behaviors you would expect of a child who has an alcoholic parent and who is assuming the role of "hero."

## REFERENCES AND ADDITIONAL READINGS

Adams WL et al: Alcohol-related hospitalizations of elderly people: prevalence and geographic variation in the United States, *J Am Med Assoc* 270(10):1222-1225, 1993.

*Alcoholics Anonymous big book,* ed 3, New York, 1976, AA World Services.

American Psychiatric Association: *Diagnostic and statistical manual of mental disorders DSM-IV,* ed 4, Washington, DC, 1994, The Association.

Antai-Otong D: Helping the alcoholic patient recover, *Am J Nurs* 95(8):22-30, 1995.

Baberg HT, Nelesen RA, Dimsdale JE: Amphetamine use: return of an old scourge in a consultation psychiatry setting, *Am J Psychiatry* 153(6):789-793, 1996.

Boyle MH et al: Predicting substance abuse in late adolescence: results from the Ontario Child Health Study follow-up, *Am J Psychiatry* 149(6): 761-767, 1992.

Covey LS, Glassman AH, Stetner F: Major depression following smoking cessation, *Am J Psychiatry* 154(2):263-265, 1997.

Docherty JP: Nicotine dependence: perspectives on a new guideline from APA, *Am J Psychiatry* 153(10):1247-1248, 1996.

Higuchi S: Alcohol and aldehyde dehydrogenase polymorphisms and the risk for alcoholism, *Am J Psychiatry* 152(8):1219-1221, 1995.

Hughes JR et al: Practice guideline for the treatment of patients with nicotine dependence, *Am J Psychiatry* 153(10):1-31, 1996.

Huntington DD: Home care of the elderly alcoholic, *Home Health Nurse* 8(5):26-32, 1990.

Jellinek EM: *The disease concept of alcoholism,* New Brunswick, NY, 1960, Hillhouse.

Johnson V: *I'll quit tomorrow: a practical guide to alcohol treatment,* San Francisco, 1990, Harper & Row.

Lawson GW, Lawson AW, editors: *Adolescent substance abuse: etiology, treatment, and prevention,* Gaithersburg, Md, 1992, Aspen.

Lerner WD, Barr M, editors: *Hospital-based substance abuse treatment,* New York, 1990, Pergamon.

Mendelson JH, Mello N, editors: *Medical diagnosis and treatment of alcoholism,* New York, 1992, McGraw-Hill.

Miller N, Toft D: *The disease concept of alcoholism and other drug addiction,* Minneapolis, 1990, Hazelden Foundation.

Moss HB, Tarter RE: Substance abuse, aggression and violence: what are the connections? *Am J Addiction* 2(2):149-160, 1993.

Nicotine-free smoking cessation aid approved, *Pharmacol Ther* 22(8):375, 1997.

Phipps WJ et al: *Medical-surgical nursing: concepts and clinical practice,* ed 5, St Louis, 1994, Mosby.

Robin HS, Michelson JB: *Illustrated handbook of drug abuse recognition and diagnosis,* Chicago, 1988, Mosby.

Schuchit MD, Marc A: *Drug and alcohol abuse: a clinical guide to diagnosis and treatment,* ed 3, New York, 1989, Plenum.

Seventh special report to the US Congress on alcohol and health, Rockville, Md, Jan 1990, US Department of Health and Human Services.

Shaef AW: *Codependence: misunderstood—mistreated,* New York, 1966, Harper Collins.

Sommers M: Alcohol and trauma: the critical link, *Crit Care Nurse* 14(2):82-86, 1994.

Stimmel B: *The facts about drug use,* Binghamton, NY, 1993, Haworth.

Stuart G, Sundeen S: *Principles and practice of psychiatric nursing,* ed 4, St Louis, 1991, Mosby.

Sullivan EJ: *Nursing care of clients with substance abuse,* St Louis, 1995, Mosby.

Trimpey J: *The small book,* New York, 1992, Delacorte.

Twerski AJ: Avoiding relapse on medication, *Prof Couns* 6(2):10, 1991.

Volkow ND et al: Decreased brain metabolism in neurologically intact healthy alcoholics, *Am J Psychiatry* 149(8):1016-1022, 1992.

Wang MQ et al: Tobacco use among American adolescents: geographic and demographic variations, *South Med J* 87(6):607-610, 1994.

Wilson S: Can you spot an alcoholic parent? *RN* 57(1):46-50, 1994.

Yates WR, Meller WH: Comparative validity of five alcoholism topologies, *Am J Addiction* 2(2):99-108, 1993.

Yoshino A: Prediction of 3-year outcome of treated alcoholics by an empirically derived multivariate typology, *Am J Psychiatry* 153(6):829-830, 1996.

# CHAPTER 11

# The Patient with Pain

## CHAPTER OBJECTIVES

1 Discuss the nature of pain.
2 Identify applications of the gate control theory to pain management.
3 Discuss the role of the nurse in pain management.
4 Identify the components of a pain assessment.
5 Describe analgesics using the World Health Organization's Analgesic Ladder.
6 Discuss the nurse's role in administering analgesics.
7 Describe nonpharmacologic measures appropriate for the nurse to use in pain relief.
8 Identify neurosurgical interventions for pain relief.

## KEY TERMS

| | |
|---|---|
| acute pain | pain threshold |
| addiction | pain tolerance |
| chronic pain | patient-controlled analgesia |
| distraction | (PCA) |
| drug tolerance | phantom pain |
| endorphins | physical dependence |
| epidural analgesia | placebo |
| faces rating scale | referred pain |
| gate control theory | relaxation techniques |
| intrathecal analgesia | transcutaneous electrical |
| neurotransmitters | nerve stimulation (TENS) |
| opioids | visual analog scale |
| pain | |

The alleviation of **pain** is one of the most common problems faced by nurses when giving care to patients. Nurses have a well-established central role in the successful management of pain. Whether in a hospital, long-term care facility, physician's office, or patient's home, the nurse has numerous opportunities to work with patients who are anticipating or experiencing pain. The nurse's role includes assessing an individual who has pain, administering medications and other therapeutic modalities, teaching the patient and family about pain and its control, and monitoring the effectiveness of the interventions. The nurse can be the key link in facilitating communication between a patient who has pain and the health care team.

Pain is often the symptom that brings the patient to the physician. The physician assumes primary responsibility for diagnosing the cause of the pain and for treating the disease that is causing the symptom. However, the nurse has the most direct contact with the patient during the long hours that he or she is experiencing pain. Therefore the nurse is in a position to make a major contribution to any program of pain relief. Nurses are held accountable for managing the pain program for patients under their care.

> ### NURSE ALERT
>
> To be a true patient advocate, the nurse must make pain control a priority in patient care.

## NATURE OF PAIN

The nature of pain has been of considerable interest throughout history. Pain is a nebulous sensation.

Scientists cannot directly measure its intensity, nor can they see it in action. Patients often have trouble describing their pain and sometimes even have trouble pinpointing its location. Religion and culture may have a strong influence on an individual's experience of pain. Some people believe that they have pain because they have sinned and must suffer to make up for their wrongdoing. Others believe that they are suffering to improve or discipline themselves. The word *pain* is derived from the Latin word *poena*, which means punishment. Members of primitive cultures sometimes deliberately inflicted pain on themselves in an attempt to appease the gods and redeem their souls.

The beliefs, values, and customs that are passed from one generation to another (cultural factors) greatly influence how an individual reacts to pain. In some cultures and families it is important to be stoic and suffer in silence. In other cultures, outward displays of emotion are acceptable. It is important for the nurse not to stereotype individuals because they belong to a certain ethnic group and not to assume that the characteristics common to a particular sociocultural group occur in all members of that group.

In more recent years scientists have come to realize that pain is both a physical and a psychologic phenomenon. Pain can be viewed as having two components: (1) the sensation, or perception, of pain; and (2) the response, or reaction, to pain. The perception of pain depends on the intactness of the nerve pathways and brain and on the degree of physical damage. The pain reaction is a complex response and involves the highest cognitive (thinking) mechanisms. Many factors influence an individual's reaction to pain such as anxiety, previous pain experiences, age, culture, and the meaning of the pain-producing situation. Research has shown that the **pain threshold** (the point at which a sensation is perceived as pain) is essentially the same in all people under normal circumstances. However, **pain tolerance** (the point at which a pain sensation is no longer voluntarily endured) and the reaction to pain vary widely from one person to another and even in the same individual under different circumstances.

## Defining Pain

Pain is an intensely personal and complex biochemical event. The International Association for the Study of Pain (1986) defines pain as an unpleasant sensory and emotional experience that arises from actual or potential tissue damage. Much of the difficulty in precisely defining pain occurs because it is a personal, subjective phenomenon that can be interpreted only in terms of its meaning to the person experiencing it. To the patient, pain is simply "what hurts." Nurses can experience their own pain but can only make judgments about the pain of others. It is critical that health care providers believe the patient's report of pain and not depend on their own perceptions of how a person in pain should act. The definition of pain proposed by McCaffrey and Beebe (1989) best meets the needs of nurses caring for patients in pain: "Pain is whatever the experiencing person says it is, existing wherever he says it exists." Using this definition, the nurse accepts that the patient is in pain. The patient does not have to prove that pain exists.

> ### NURSE ALERT
> Believe the patient's report of pain. The patient does not need to act in any specific way to be experiencing pain. There is no test for pain.

## Function of Pain

Pain can serve as a protective mechanism for the body by signaling that tissues are damaged or threatened with damage. Pain is often the first symptom that tells an individual that something is wrong with the body or that urges a person to seek medical assistance. Pain can also protect the body from further injury. For example, the pain caused by contact with a hot object causes a person to withdraw from the object. However, the protective function of pain sometimes becomes lost or obscured, such as in long-term arthritis or chronic back pain. No longer is the pain a useful mechanism that warns of danger. In such individuals, reactions to pain and methods of adapting to and living with pain become of great significance to the health care team.

Individuals who cannot feel and respond to pain because of a loss of sensation (e.g., spinal cord injury) or because of an absence of pain receptors (genetic deficiency) are susceptible to injury. The nurse must be extremely vigilant when providing care to these patients. Whether a result of anesthesia, sedation, or neurologic damage, an unconscious patient is at great risk for skin integrity problems. The nurse is unaware of the pain that the unconscious patient is experiencing because the patient cannot communicate verbally or nonverbally.

## Pain Theories

Science does not yet have a satisfactory explanation for pain transmission and pain relief. Therefore it must resort to theory. In 1965 Melzack and Wall proposed the **gate control theory,** which has generated much research and has provided a partial explanation of how pain is transmitted and perceived (Figure 11-1). According to this theory, pain sensations travel along small-diameter C-delta fibers and enter the brain through a "gate" located in the spinal cord. Pain sensations can be blocked at this gate by stimulating the large-diameter A-delta fibers, which carry generalized sensations. The gate can also be closed by brain activity. Psychologic factors, memories of previous pain experiences, and many physical or mental activities can also influence the perception of pain. Applications of this theory include the use of transcutaneous electrical nerve stimulation (TENS), massage or back rubs, counterirritants such as Ben Gay and Deep Heat ointments, and heat or cold. In each case the fast-moving impulses coming from the peripheral nerve receptors reach the "gate" first and block the impulses traveling along the slower pain fibers. The brain receives and interprets the general sensation message and does not receive the pain message.

Current research on pain focuses on its neurochemical nature. It is now known that the body is capable of secreting narcotic-like substances called **endorphins** (West, 1981). Endorphins lock into narcotic receptors on nerve endings in the brain and spinal cord and block the transmission of pain sensations. Different individuals have different amounts of endorphins, which may help explain differences in pain perception. Research has shown that such things as prolonged pain or constant stress can decrease the amount of endorphins. Brief pain or brief stress increases the amount. It is interesting to note that intense physical exercise, such as jogging, can temporarily increase an individual's endorphin level.

> ## NURSE ALERT
>
> Different individuals have different amounts of endorphins, which may help explain differences in pain perception.

The body also produces a number of endogenous chemicals (e.g., histamine, substance P, serotonin, and prostaglandins) that act as **neurotransmitters** for the transmission of pain impulses (Paice, 1991). Much

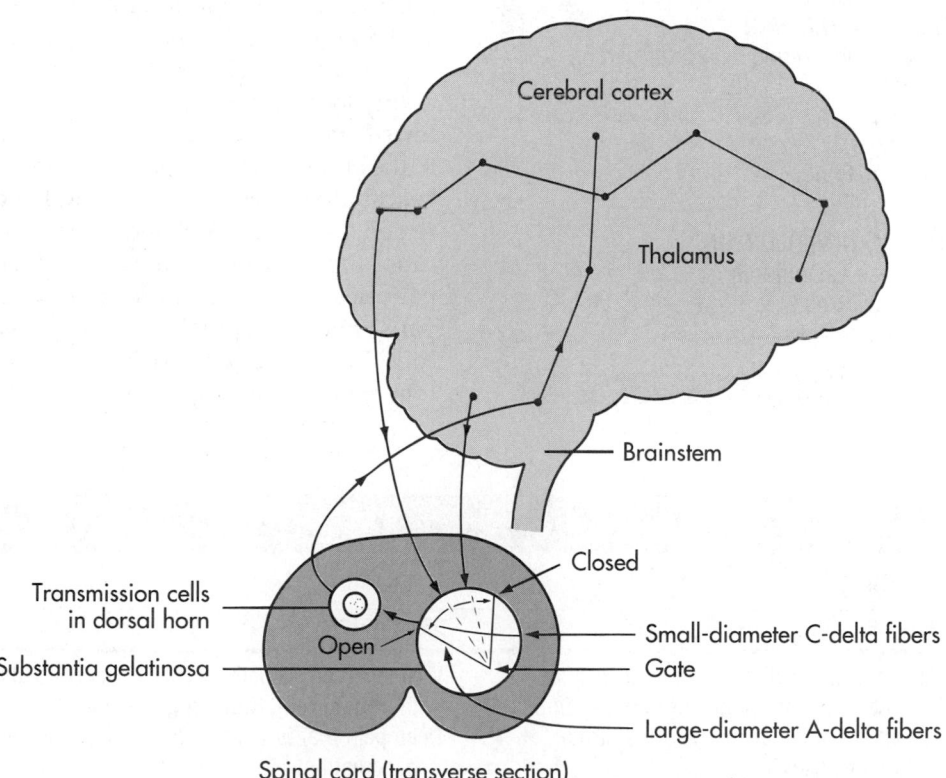

**Figure 11-1**   Gate control theory. Pain sensations, traveling along small-diameter C-delta fibers, pass through a "gate" in the substantia gelatinosa, through transmission cells, and into the brain. These sensations can be blocked at the gate by stimulating large-diameter A-delta fibers, which carry general sensations. The gate also can be closed by brain activity.

research is being done to discover medications that can block the actions of specific neurotransmitters. An example of such a drug are the nonsteroidal antiinflammatory drugs (NSAIDs), which inhibit the synthesis of prostaglandins. Further research on the roles of neurotransmitters will lead to better methods of inhibiting pain. Although much is known about the pain experience, more is yet to be discovered. For a person in pain, the answers cannot come quickly enough.

## Types of Pain
### Classified by Chronicity

Pain can be classified into two types: acute and chronic. The intensity can vary from mild to severe in

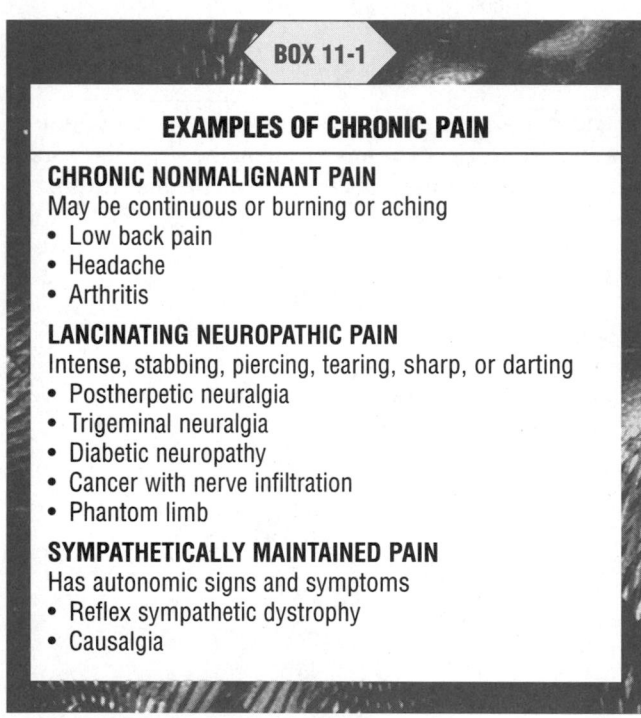

**BOX 11-1**

### EXAMPLES OF CHRONIC PAIN

**CHRONIC NONMALIGNANT PAIN**
May be continuous or burning or aching
- Low back pain
- Headache
- Arthritis

**LANCINATING NEUROPATHIC PAIN**
Intense, stabbing, piercing, tearing, sharp, or darting
- Postherpetic neuralgia
- Trigeminal neuralgia
- Diabetic neuropathy
- Cancer with nerve infiltration
- Phantom limb

**SYMPATHETICALLY MAINTAINED PAIN**
Has autonomic signs and symptoms
- Reflex sympathetic dystrophy
- Causalgia

either type. **Acute pain** usually has a short duration (less than 3 months), a sudden onset and, most often, an identifiable cause. Examples include pain after surgery, trauma, and burns and pain experienced in critical care. Acute pain usually is reversible because it seems to diminish with healing. Anxiety often accompanies acute pain, and measures to reduce anxiety are helpful in easing pain.

**Chronic pain** lasts longer than several months, and often the cause is not well defined. The pain usually begins gradually and persists. Because chronic pain is exhausting and unnecessary, patients may suffer from depression and fatigue. Examples of chronic pain include chronic cancer pain and chronic benign pain (low back pain, arthritis, headache) and lancinating neuropathic pain. Objective signs and symptoms are absent in chronic pain—there is no picture of a patient in pain. Box 11-1 lists examples of chronic pain.

### Classified by Source

Pain can also be classified by its location or source (Table 11-1). Superficial pain occurs when the skin or its surface structures are affected by a painful stimulus. The pain localizes to the site of the stimulation and usually is described as having a prickling or burning quality. Deep pain arises from deeper structures, such as the muscles and visceral tissue. Deep pain may be localized to the site of the stimulus but more likely is poorly localized and has a dull and aching quality. **Referred pain** is projected from various internal organs to the body surface, as in cardiac pain that arises in the heart but is projected to the jaw, left arm, or epigastric region (Figure 11-2). Referred pain probably occurs because the branches of the nerve fibers from the actual pain site and the fibers from the site of the perceived pain enter the spinal cord at the same place, which causes the brain to make a faulty interpretation. **Phantom pain,** an example of neuropathic pain, is com-

**TABLE 11-1**

## Types of Pain by Source

| TYPE OF PAIN | SOURCE | DESCRIPTION |
|---|---|---|
| Superficial | Arises from localized tissues, usually related to a disturbance of nerve endings | Well localized, usually described as constant, sharp, tingling or throbbing (e.g., bumping the elbow) |
| Visceral | Arises from somatic or visceral structures (muscles, organs) | Deep pain that is difficult to localize; may be dull or aching (e.g., pancreatitis) |
| Referred | Felt in an area away from the source of injury; usually originates in the viscera | A common example is pain in the shoulders when a patient experiences a myocardial infarction |
| Neuropathic | Arises from destruction or injury to a part of the central nervous system | Usually intense, severe, burning; may not always respond to narcotics (e.g., neuralgia, shingles, phantom limb) |

monly felt by an individual after amputation of a body part. The person feels as if the part is still there and may feel tingling, burning, itching, or other unpleasant sensations. Phantom pain is disturbing to the patient and may be difficult to treat. It is important for the nurse to assure the patient with phantom pain that there is a legitimate reason for the pain.

## Assessment of Pain

A detailed, accurate description of the patient's pain is essential for precise diagnosis and treatment of the underlying cause. Because pain is subjective, the patient should be encouraged to describe in detail the nature, intensity, and location of pain (Figure 11-3). Following a specific pattern for assessing each painful episode can be helpful (McCaffery et al, 1989).

### Pain Scales

Quantifying the degree of pain before and after administering medications or performing other interventions

is a useful way to monitor the effectiveness of the therapy. Two methods widely used to monitor treatment effectiveness are questionnaires and rating scales. The McGill-Melzack Pain Questionnaire measures both sensory and affective dimensions of pain (Melzack, Wall, 1988). Rating scales can be used in any patient care setting (McCaffery, Beebe, 1989). The patient is asked to rate his or her pain on a scale of 0 to 5, or 0 to 10, either verbally or on a **visual analog scale** (Figure 11-4). The visual analog scale is a 10-cm line that represents a continuum from no pain to the worst imaginable pain. The patient makes a pencil mark at the point on the line that describes the intensity of his or her pain at that time. A **faces rating scale** can be used for children or other people who cannot speak (Figure 11-5). The patient points to the face that best illustrates his or her pain. To maintain consistency with the 0 to 10 scale of the Agency for Health Care Policy and Research (AHCPR), shown in Figure 11-5, each number on the Wong-Baker faces scale is multiplied by 2.

Patients who are to undergo surgery must be taught the use of rating scales and must be told how their

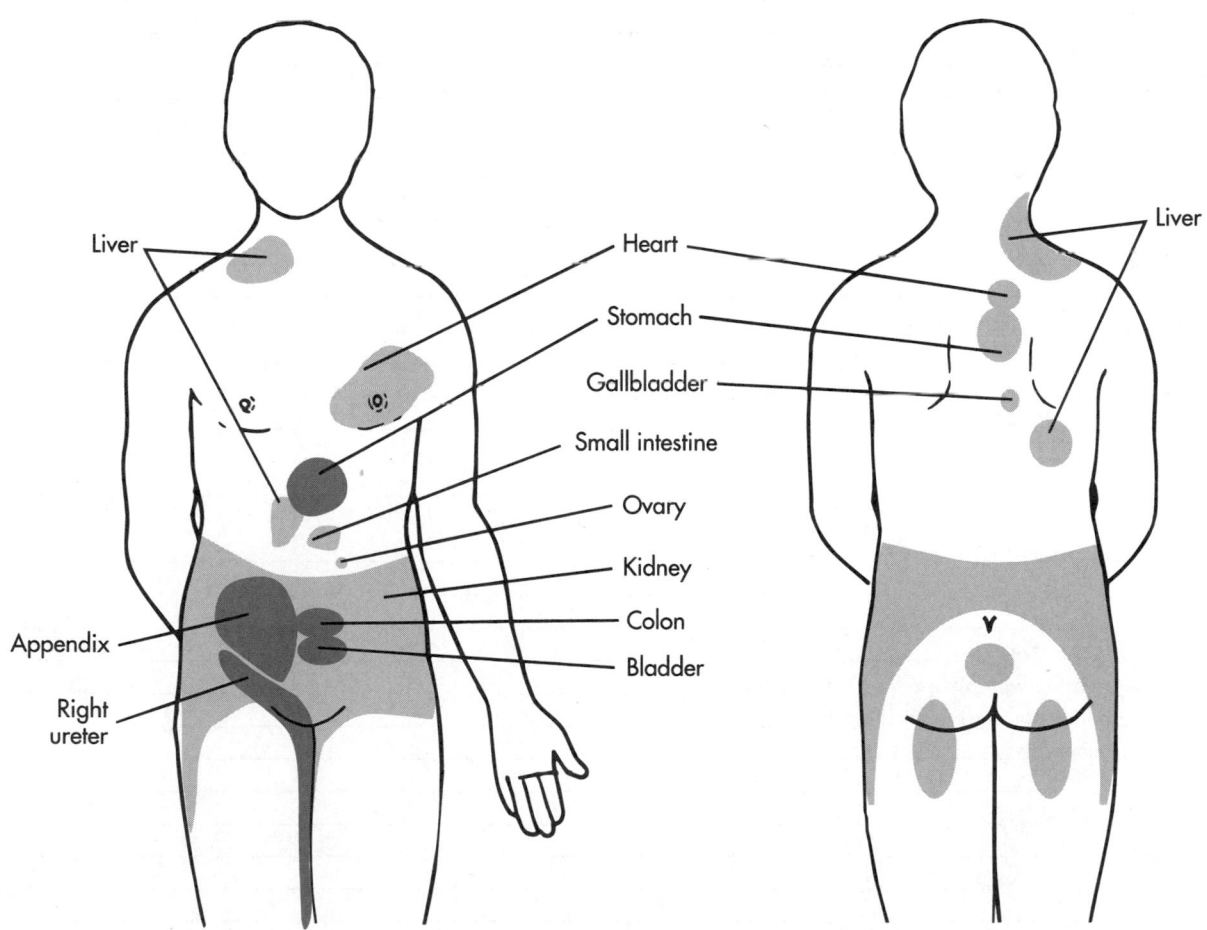

**Figure 11-2**    Areas of referred pain.

INITIAL PAIN ASSESSMENT TOOL                    Date_____

Patient's Name_____ Age_____ Room_____

Diagnosis_____ Physician_____

                                          Nurse_____

I. LOCATION: Patient or nurse mark drawing.

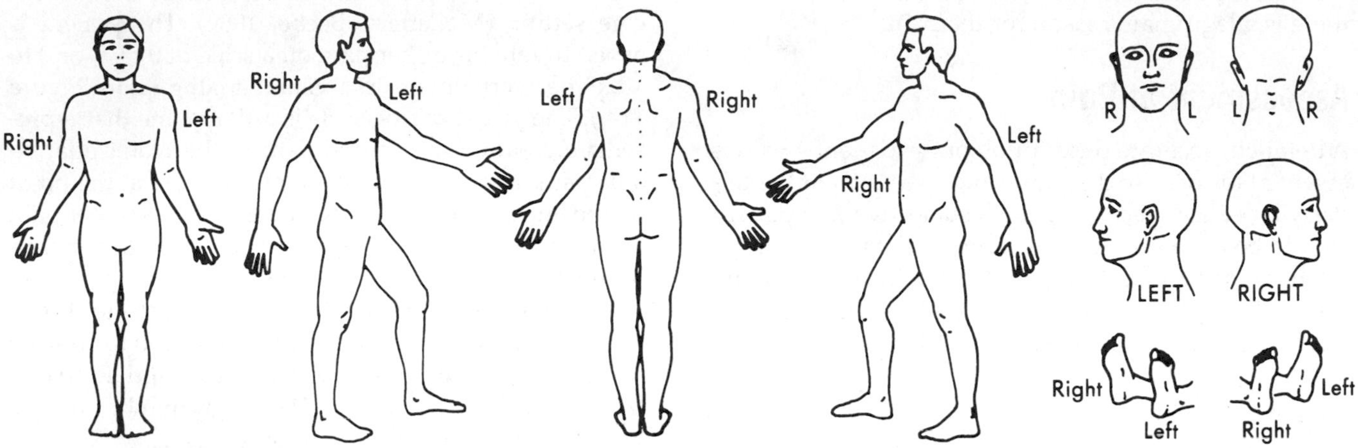

II. INTENSITY: Patient rates the pain. Scale used _____

    Present:_____
    Worst pain gets:_____
    Best pain gets:_____
    Acceptable level of pain:_____

III. QUALITY: Use patient's own words (e.g., prick, ache, burn, throb, pull, sharp)_____
_____

IV. ONSET, DURATION, VARIATIONS, RHYTHMS:_____
_____

V. MANNER OF EXPRESSING PAIN:_____
_____
_____

VI. WHAT RELIEVES THE PAIN?_____
_____
_____

VII. WHAT CAUSES OR INCREASES THE PAIN?_____
_____

VIII. EFFECTS OF PAIN: Note decreased function, decreased quality of life.
    Accompanying symptoms (e.g., nausea)_____
    Sleep_____
    Appetite_____
    Physical activity_____
    Relationship with others (e.g., irritability)_____
    Emotions (e.g. anger, suicidal, crying)_____
    Concentration_____
    Other_____

IX. OTHER COMMENTS:_____
_____

X. PLAN:_____
_____

**Figure 11-3**   Initial pain assessment tool. (From McCaffery M, Beebe A: *Pain: clinical manual for nursing practice,* St Louis, 1989, Mosby.)

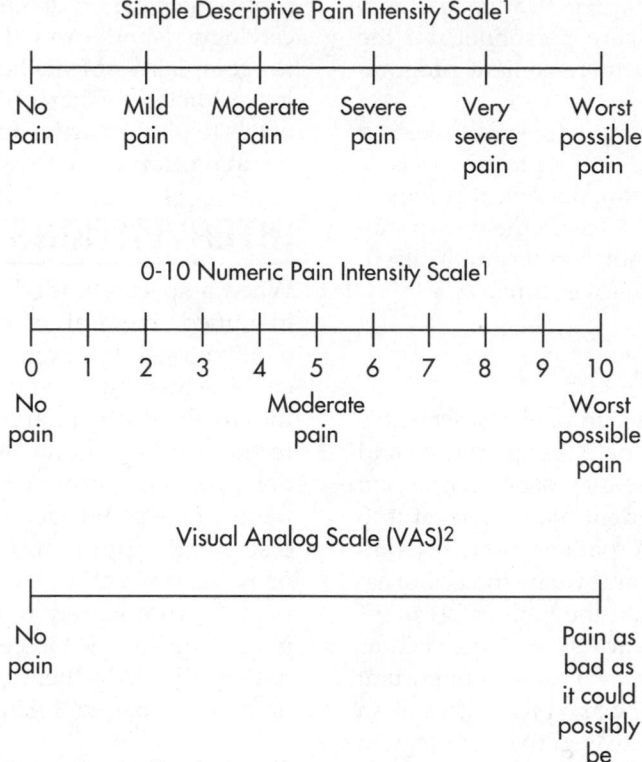

$^1$ If used as a graphic rating scale, a 10 cm baseline is recommended.
$^2$ A 10-cm baseline is recommended for VAS scales.

**Figure 11-4**    Pain intensity scales. (From Acute Pain Management Guideline Panel, Acute pain management: operative or medical procedures and trauma, Clinical practice guideline, Pub No 92-0032, Rockville, Md, 1992, Agency for Health Care Policy and Research, Public Health Service, US Department of Health and Human Services.)

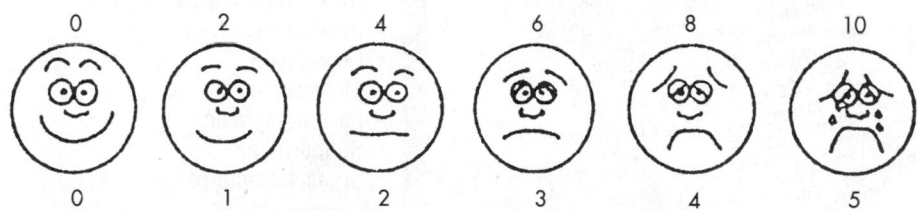

1) Explain to the child that each face is for a person who feels happy because he or she has no pain (hurt, or whatever word the child uses) or feels sad because he or she has some or a lot of pain.
2) Point to the appropriate face and state, "This face is . . .":
    0-0 —"very happy because he doesn't hurt at all."
    2 or 1 —"hurts just a little bit."
    4 or 2 —"hurts a little more."
    6 or 3 —"hurts even more."
    8 or 4 —"Hurts a whole lot."
    10 or 5 —"hurts as much as you can imagine, although you don't have to be crying to feel this bad."
3) Ask the child to choose the face that best describes how he or she feels. Be specific about which pain (e.g., "shot" or incision) and what time (e.g., now? earlier before lunch?).

**Figure 11-5**    Wong-Baker faces rating scale. (From Wong D: *Whaley and Wong's essentials of pediatric nursing,* ed 5, St Louis, 1997, Mosby.)

pain will be managed as part of preoperative teaching. It is essential that all health care personnel use the same scale and the same pain management program with each patient.

It is standard practice in many hospitals to keep a rating scale on the patient's bed or door to make it convenient for the nurse to check the patient. It is important to remember that all pain measurements are subjective. A single measure is not significant in itself. What is important is the change over time.

## Patient Descriptions of Pain

A problem that nurses often face in pain assessment is the wide variation in the ways pain is experienced and reported by patients. The nurse may use the term *pain* to mean one thing, but the patient may interpret it to mean something different. A patient may respond "No" to a question about pain and yet be in need of assistance. To determine just what the patient is experiencing, it is helpful to use a variety of terms such as *ache*, *pressure*, *hurt*, and *discomfort*. It is also important to use the phrase "patient reports" pain rather than "patient complains of" pain. The negative connotation of the word *complain* may influence the responses of the patient or significant others.

The young child and the elderly patient present special problems when the nurse is assessing pain (McGuire et al, 1982; McCaffery, Beebe, 1989; Ferrell, 1991; Herr, Mobily, 1991). The nurse needs to be especially alert to nonverbal cues. A child often cannot describe the pain or denies having pain for fear of receiving a "shot." An elderly patient often is reluctant to "complain" or fears being overmedicated or becoming addicted to narcotics. In either case, the nurse needs to play an active role to prevent undue suffering resulting from undertreatment of pain.

## INTERVENTIONS FOR PAIN RELIEF

When a specific underlying cause of the pain can be identified, medical management is directed toward eliminating it. For example, the pain of appendicitis or cholecystitis can be eliminated by surgically removing the involved organ, and the pain associated with infection can be relieved with antibiotics. When an underlying cause cannot be identified or eliminated, a patient may be referred to a pain clinic, where a multidisciplinary approach is used to diagnose and treat the pain. In such a clinic the major focus is on helping patients learn a variety of methods, such as distraction, guided imagery, biofeedback and relaxation techniques, that help them better manage their pain on a daily basis (Baque, 1989).

## Nurse's Role in Administration of Analgesics

Various medications are used to alleviate pain through their interaction with some aspect of the pain experi-

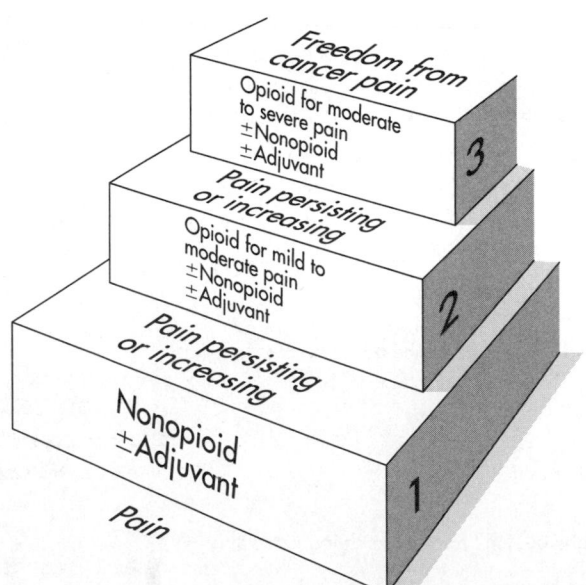

**Figure 11-6** World Health Organization analgesic ladder for cancer pain management. (From World Health Organization (WHO): *Cancer pain relief*, ed 2, Geneva, Switzerland, 1996 World Health Organization.)

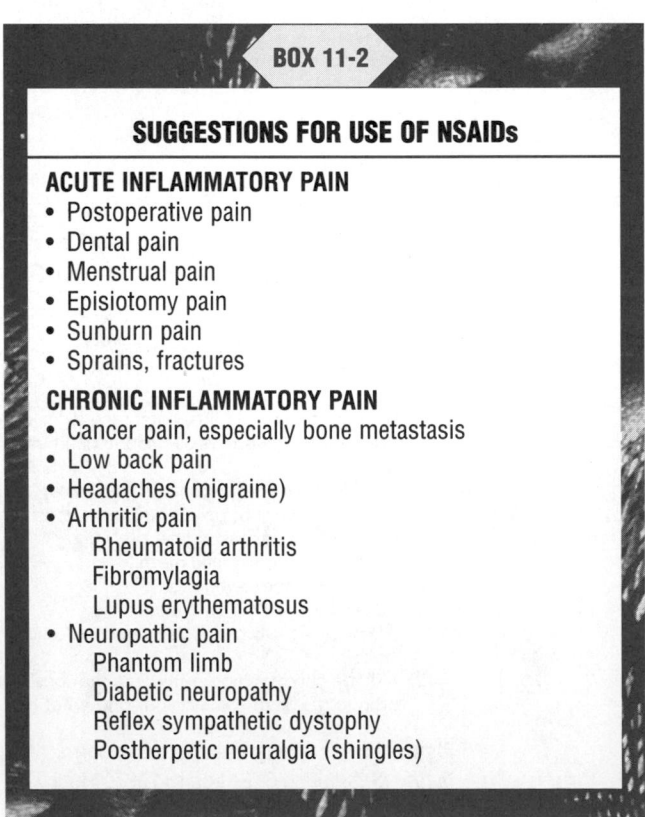

BOX 11-2

### SUGGESTIONS FOR USE OF NSAIDs

**ACUTE INFLAMMATORY PAIN**
- Postoperative pain
- Dental pain
- Menstrual pain
- Episiotomy pain
- Sunburn pain
- Sprains, fractures

**CHRONIC INFLAMMATORY PAIN**
- Cancer pain, especially bone metastasis
- Low back pain
- Headaches (migraine)
- Arthritic pain
    Rheumatoid arthritis
    Fibromylagia
    Lupus erythematosus
- Neuropathic pain
    Phantom limb
    Diabetic neuropathy
    Reflex sympathetic dystophy
    Postherpetic neuralgia (shingles)

ence. Three groups of medications are used to manage pain: nonnarcotics (nonopioids), narcotics **(opioids)**, and adjuvants (See WHO Analgesic Ladder, Figure 11-6). The first group is the nonopioid group, which includes aspirin and other NSAIDs commonly used for mild to moderate pain (0 to 5 on a 0 to 10 scale) (Acute Pain Management Guideline Panel, 1992, 1994). These drugs block the production of neurotransmitters near the injury that activate nerve endings and send pain signals to the brain. They reduce inflammation by inhibiting the synthesis of prosta-

glandins. Box 11-2 lists types of pain for which antiinflammatory drugs (NSAIDs) are useful.

Opioid drugs are used for moderate to severe pain (5 to 10 on a 0 to 10 scale) (Table 11-2). Morphine molecules fit into receptor sites on certain cells in the brain and central nervous system (CNS) and prevent the reception of pain messages. Combinations of drugs (e.g., aspirin and codeine) often are used to attack the pain problem from several approaches. Long-acting versions of morphine (e.g., MS Contin and Oramorph SR) and transdermal fentanyl patches

### TABLE 11-2

## Opioid Equianalgesic Chart (Doses Approximately Equal to 10 mg Morphine IM)

| DRUG | SQ/IM | PO | DURATION | COMMENTS |
|---|---|---|---|---|
| **Opioids for Mild to Moderate Pain** | | | | |
| Codeine | 130 mg | 200 mg | 3-6 hr | Schedule III opioid; short-acting, weak opioid; nausea, vomiting, and constipation occur with greater frequency and severity as dose increases<br>Tylenol #2 = Tylenol 325 mg + Codeine 15 mg<br>Tylenol #3 = Tylenol 325 mg + Codeine 30 mg<br>Tylenol #4 = Tylenol 325 mg + Codeine 60 mg<br>Aspirin (acetylsalicylic acid) 650 mg + Codeine 30 mg |
| Hydrocodone (Vicodin, Lortab, Vicodin ES) | NA | 50-100 mg | 3-4 hr | Schedule III opioid<br>Lortab, Vicodin = Hydrocodone 5 mg + Acetaminophen 500 mg<br>Vicodin ES = Hydrocodone 7.5 mg + Acetaminophen 750 mg |
| Meperidine (Demerol) | 75 mg | 300 mg | 2-3 hr | Schedule II opioid; poor oral bioavailability (50 mg PO = 650 mg aspirin); short acting, painful to administer, irritating to tissue; toxic metabolite, normeperidine, accumulates with repetitive dosing, causing CNS toxicities (numbness, tingling, twitching, confusion, seizure) especially in patients with decreased renal function; should *not* be used for more than 48 hr for acute pain and never for chronic pain, especially cancer pain |
| Oxycodone (Percodan, Percocet, Tylox) | NA | 30 mg | 3-6 hr | Schedule II, fast-acting oral opioid usually given in combination with nonopioid, which may limit ability to increase doses; plain oxycodone oral solution available in 5 mg/5 ml<br>Percodan = Oxycodone 5 mg + Aspirin 325 mg<br>Percocet = Oxycodone 5 mg + Acetaminophen 325 mg<br>Tylox = Oxycodone 5 mg + Acetaminophen 500 mg |
| Oxycontin 10 mg, 20 mg, 40 mg, and 80 mg sustained-release tablets | NA | 15-30 mg | 12 hr | Only long-acting form of plain oxycodone |

*CNS*, Central nervous system; *IM*, intramuscular; *IV*, intravenous; *PO*, oral; *SQ*, subcutaneous.

*Continued*

---

**TABLE 11-2**

## Opioid Equianalgesic Chart (Doses Approximately Equal to 10 mg Morphine IM)—cont'd

| DRUG | SQ/IM | PO | DURATION | COMMENTS |
|---|---|---|---|---|
| **Opioids for Moderate to Severe Pain** | | | | |
| Morphine and sustained-release morphine (15 mg, 30 mg, 60 mg, 100 mg, and 200 mg sustained-release tablets available) | 10 mg | 30-60 mg | 3-4 hr 8-12 hr | Schedule II opioid; standard narcotic to which all other analgesics are compared; drug of choice for severe pain; very versatile since it can be given by many routes (PO, SQ, IM, IV, rectal, intraspinal), available as concentrated oral solution 20 mg/ml; cancer pain experts recommend concentrated oral morphine solution or sustained-release tablets regularly around-the-clock; although no limit to the dosing of morphine, most patients can be controlled on 30-60 mg PO q 4hr; occasionally some patients require much higher doses |
| Diamorphine (Heroin) | 5 mg | NA | 4-5 hr | Schedule II opioid; not available in the United States but widely used in England for treatment of cancer pain; similar to morphine but shorter acting; no advantage over morphine for cancer pain |
| Hydromorphone (Dilaudid, Dilaudid HP) | 1.5 mg | 7.5 mg | 3-4 hr | Schedule II opioid; fast-acting, useful alternative to morphine; available orally in 2 mg, 4 mg, and 8 mg tablets, parenterally and by 3 mg suppository; high-potency parenteral strength available (10mg/1ml); shorter duration of action than morphine, may be more useful with the elderly |
| Fentanyl (Duragesic) 25 $\mu$g/hr, 50 $\mu$g/hr, 75 $\mu$g/hr, 100 $\mu$g/hr transdermal patches | 25-50 $\mu$g/hr patch | | 72 hr | Schedule II opioid; only transdermal opioid available, easy to use, noninvasive; because of skin reservoir, 12 hr delay in onset; monitor patient 24-36 hr after removal of patch |
| Methadone (Dolophine) | 10 mg | 20 mg | 4-8 hr | Schedule II opioid; long duration of action because of long half-life (24-36 hr); cumulative effect with repetitive dosing causes excessive sedation, thus careful observation of patient is needed; use with caution in elderly patients or patients with liver or renal dysfunction |
| Levorphanol (Levo-Dromoran) | 2 mg | 4 mg | 4-8 hr | Schedule II opioid; long duration of action (4-8 hr) because of long half-life (12-16 hr); careful monitoring and dosage adjustments needed to prevent excessive sedation; has accumulation problems similar to those with methadone |

---

(Duragesic) often are used for cancer pain and in the home setting. Meperidine is one opioid that is still commonly used and should be reconsidered because of its many disadvantages (Box 11-3 and see Table 11-2).

In addition to nonopioids and opioids, another group of medications, called adjuvants, is used for pain management. These medications are not true analgesics, but they can be helpful for certain types of pain, particularly chronic pain. Adjuvant analgesics have the ability to enhance the effects of analgesics or to counteract the side effects of analgesics. They may also have analgesic properties of their own.

Examples of adjuvants useful for chronic pain include tricyclic antidepressants (Elavil), anticonvulsants (Tegretol), and topical or local anesthetics (EMLA cream). Phenolthiazines, such as Phenergan, are not narcotic potentiators. In fact, these drugs may counteract the effect of the narcotic and increase the intensity of pain. They also lower seizure thresholds.

BOX 11-3

## DISADVANTAGES OF MEPERIDINE (DEMEROL)

- Irritating to tissues (causes lumps); if it must be administered, especially with Vistaril, Z-track method should be used
- Painful to administer
- Short acting; the younger the patient, the shorter the duration of action
- Oral dosages are rarely adequate; 300 mg Demerol PO = 75 mg Demerol IM, thus oral Demerol is ineffective and *not* recommended
- Active metabolite, normeperidine, accumulates with repetitive dosing and can cause central nervous system toxicities (twitching, numbness, seizures, hallucinations)
- Agency for Health Care Policy and Research (AHCPR) recommends using meperidine only for acute pain, and only for 48 hours; AHCPR recommends *against* the use of meperidine for cancer pain

*PO*, Orally; *IM*, intramuscularly.

## Timing Administration of Analgesics

Most analgesic drugs used to be administered on an "as needed" (prn) basis. The patient had to ask for pain relief. To manage any pain with analgesics, the preventive approach must be used; that is, the pain must be suppressed around-the-clock (ATC). Giving medications according to an ATC schedule enables the patient's body to maintain a sufficient level of drug to keep the pain under control; it also prevents anxiety from building and prevents the memory of suffering from becoming established.

Discomfort and anxiety increase if the patient must wait too long for relief and thus more medication is needed to achieve control. By careful assessment, the nurse detects indications for pain control and makes pain prevention possible.

### NURSE ALERT

Teach the patient to request pain medication as soon as pain occurs or before it increases.

It is critical that the nurse be aware of the significant variations in drugs, peak effects, duration of effects, and side effects. The nurse must also be alert to the differences that result from oral versus parenteral administration of a medication. The peak effect for most parenteral narcotics is 1 hour, whereas the peak effect of most oral forms of the same drug occurs 2 or more hours later. Oral analgesics usually have a longer duration of effect than parenteral drugs. A careful assessment of these factors must be made and incorporated into the plan of care for any patient receiving medications. If one analgesic is not providing satisfactory pain relief, another drug is likely to be substituted.

### NURSE ALERT

The onset, peak effects, and duration of analgesia differ from drug to drug and also may vary from individual to individual.

## Side Effects

Patients should be monitored for side effects with all medications. This is especially true of opioid (narcotic) drugs. All narcotics have the potential to cause respiratory depression as a result of the respiratory center's diminished sensitivity to carbon dioxide. The nurse must assess the patient carefully for respiratory changes. Respiratory depression is rare with oral opioids and rare with properly titrated doses. It is unfortunate that the concern over possible respiratory depression has become so exaggerated with health care professionals. A much more common problem is inadequate pain management. Treatments for respiratory depression include rousing the patient, establishing a patent airway, administering a narcotic antagonist such as naloxone, and providing artificial ventilation should it become necessary. Patients develop a tolerance to respiratory depression if the opioid continues to be used.

Constipation is the most common side effect of opioid administration. Opioids cause a decrease in peristaltic contractions in the gastrointestinal (GI) tract, which allows increased absorption of water from bowel contents. Tolerance to this side effect does not develop, nor does the side effect diminish over time. Because constipation can cause pain and discomfort, a program of constipation prevention must begin when opioids are started.

### NURSE ALERT

Constipation, drowsiness, and nausea are possible effects of narcotics; these side effects are time limited and easily managed.

## Risks for Older Adults

Older adults often suffer from several chronic and painful illnesses and often take many medications. Therefore they are at greater risk for drug-drug and drug-disease interactions. Aging may also alter the function of organs that are vital to the use and elimination of drugs, such as the liver and kidneys. Older patients may need to be given lower doses of certain drugs, and the interval between doses may need to be adjusted to compensate for the older patient's changed physiology (Ramsey, 1988; Ferrell, 1991; Acute Pain Management Guideline Panel, 1992).

## OLDER ADULT CONSIDERATIONS

Pain is not a normal part of aging. Older patients sometimes believe that pain cannot be relieved and are stoic in reporting their pain. The frail and those over age 85 are particularly at risk for undertreatment of pain. Aging need not alter pain thresholds or tolerance. The pain experiences of older and younger patients have far more similarities than differences.

Pain assessment can be difficult in the older adult. Cognitive impairment, delirium, dementia, and visual and hearing changes may interfere with the use of some pain assessment scales. When a verbal report is not possible, observe for behavioral clues to pain, such as restlessness or agitation. The absence of pain behaviors does not indicate the absence of pain. Older adults often suffer multiple, chronic, and painful illnesses and often take multiple medications. Therefore they are at risk for drug-drug and drug-disease interactions. Nonsteroidal antiinflammatory drugs (NSAIDs) can be used safely in older adults, but their use requires vigilance for side effects, especially gastric and renal toxicity. Opioids are safe and effective when used appropriately in older adults. However, older adults are more sensitive to the analgesic effects of opioid drugs and often experience higher peak effects and longer durations of pain relief.

### NURSE ALERT

A patient can be both sedated and in pain. Do not confuse sedation with analgesia.

## Addiction

Pain medications should not be withheld from patients for fear of tolerance or dependence. **Addiction** (psychologic dependence) must be distinguished from **physical dependence** or drug tolerance (Porter, Hick, 1980; McCaffery, Beebe, 1989; Ferrell, McCaffery, Rhiner, 1992).

With **drug tolerance,** increasingly larger doses are needed to provide the same effect as the original dose. The first sign of tolerance is a shortened duration of the drug's effect. The amount of pain relief obtained is then lessened. It is important to note that tolerance is rare. For example, with cancer pain, the need for increasing doses of opioids is because of the progression of the disease, *not* because of the tolerance to the drug.

If a patient receives narcotics continuously for several weeks, it is assumed that physical dependence will occur (McCaffery, Beebe, 1989). **Physical dependence** is an altered state produced by repeated administration of a drug. Withdrawal symptoms occur when the drug is stopped. In the clinical setting, pain seldom stops abruptly. Patients who become physically dependent can be weaned off the drug by gradually diminishing the doses as the pain subsides.

Addiction is a behavioral pattern rooted in a psychologic desire for the euphoric effects of narcotics. It is characterized by an overwhelming need to get and use the drug. Most patients do not request analgesics unless they have pain. In fact it is far more common for patients with pain to refuse analgesics unnecessarily because of a fear of addiction. Psychologic dependence (addiction) is rare when narcotics are administered to patients who experience pain.

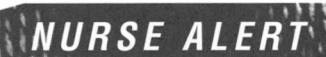

### NURSE ALERT

Focus on the patient's response to a medication rather than on the size of the dose.

## Placebos

Placebos have no role in clinical pain management. A **placebo** is an inactive substance or procedure that is prescribed by a physician for a patient as a supposedly effective treatment (Perry, Heidrich, 1981; McCaffery, Beebe, 1989). Placebos are commonly used as control measures in research. A placebo is documented on the patient's chart just like any other drug or therapy. Approximately one third of the population reacts to placebos and experiences effects of pain relief. However, on successive uses, patients report less or no pain relief.

Research has shown that the effects of placebos are physical as well as psychologic. The exact mechanisms by which placebos work are unknown, but research suggests that placebos stimulate the brain to produce endorphins and other chemicals, thus calling on "the doctor within." To a large extent the ability of a placebo to produce effects is a measure of the faith or confidence that the patient has in his or her physician or nurse. Administering placebos sometimes creates an ethical dilemma for the nurse. If a placebo is being given for an inappropriate purpose (e.g., to "prove" that the pain is not "real"), the nurse has the right to refuse to give it. In such a situation, the nurse should discuss the problem with the nursing supervisor so that the action has administrative support and the patient receives attention for his or her pain (McCaffery, Beebe, 1989). The obligation to manage pain and relieve the patient's suffering is at the core of a health care professional's commitment (Acute Pain Management Guideline Panel, 1992). The American Society of Pain Management Nurses (1997) has written a position paper adamantly opposing the use of placebos in the assessment and treatment of pain in all cases.

## Patient-Controlled Analgesia

**Patient-controlled analgesia (PCA)** is a method of delivering pain-killing drugs into an intravenous line (Figure 11-7) (Fitzgerald, Shamy, 1987; Jones, Brooks, 1990). A variety of intravenous infusion pumps are now used to allow patients to control pain by administering analgesic medications to themselves. The pumps are programmed to provide specific amounts of drugs at time intervals that are determined by the physician. The pumps are equipped with safety features that prevent overdoses. The patient should be told how often he or she can administer a dose and whether medications will be received after each attempt. It is important that the patient notify the nurse if pain relief is not satisfactory because a different order may need to be obtained from the physician. Research has shown that PCA can often provide better pain relief than periodic injections because patients can receive relief at the first sign of pain. Studies also show that patients like the idea of controlling their own pain. Anxiety and tension are decreased, and

---

## NURSE ALERT

The use of placebos can destroy a patient's trust in health care professionals; placebos are never to be administered for pain relief.

---

 ## ETHICAL DILEMMA

Mr. Jones, age 57, has come to the hospital with lung cancer that has spread to his bones and liver. Mr. Jones knows that he is dying and has signed an advance directive to prevent any "heroic measures." He has also made it clear that he does not want to die in pain. His medications include morphine every 3 hours.

One morning Miss Adams, his nurse, heard from the night nurse during report that Mr. Jones' respirations were only 8 per minute. Therefore the night nurse had withheld the last dose. Miss Adams discussed this situation with her fellow nurses, and they feared that another dose of morphine might kill him. Miss Adams talked to Mr. Jones and discovered that he was alert but fearful because his pain was getting worse.

1 Was it appropriate for the night nurse to withhold the medication?
2 How should Miss Adams follow up on this situation?

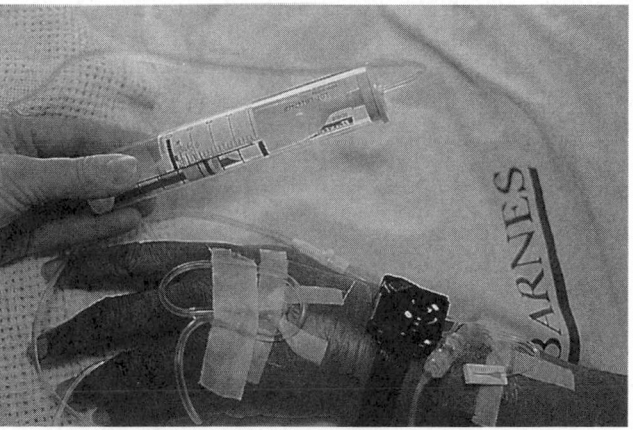
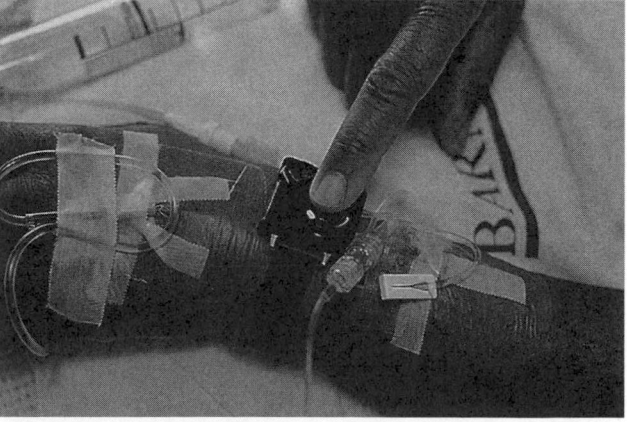

**Figure 11-7** Patient-controlled analgesia (PCA) devices. (From Perry AC, Potter PA: *Clinical nursing skills and techniques*, ed 4, St Louis, 1998, Mosby.)

often less narcotic is used. When using a PCA pump, it is important to assess the patient's pain at least every 4 hours and to maintain accurate records of the infusion on the flowsheet. The amount of medication used needs to be tailored to each patient's needs, regardless of how it is delivered.

## Intraspinal Analgesia

Opioids are sometimes administered via catheters into the epidural or subarachnoid space in the spinal cord (Haight, 1987; Wild, Coyne, 1992; Keeney, 1993). Analgesia results from the drug's direct effect on receptors in the spinal cord rather than in the brain. Fewer side effects (e.g., sedation and disorientation) are seen by this route than with systemic administration of narcotics. The spinal route can be used for both acute and chronic pain. Intraspinal analgesia is most commonly used for postoperative pain (e.g., cesarean section, orthopedic surgery) and for cancer pain that is poorly controlled by systemic medications. Nurses must have specific, additional inservice education in this method before being assigned to care for patients who have orders for **epidural** or **intrathecal analgesia.** Patients must be carefully monitored to be certain that the catheter remains in place and that no inflammation is present. The nurse must also monitor for side effects such as pruritus, urinary retention, nausea and vomiting, respiratory depres-

sion, and postural hypotension. Patients should be instructed to quickly report any side effects or lack of pain relief.

## Transcutaneous Electrical Nerve Stimulation

**Transcutaneous electrical nerve stimulation (TENS)** is most commonly used for pain that is fairly well localized (McCaffery, Beebe, 1989). TENS modulates pain by stimulating peripheral nerves with electrical current via electrodes that are applied to the skin and connected to a small battery-operated pulse generator (Figure 11-8). This stimulation enhances the production of endorphins and therefore mobilizes the pain defenses of the body. This method may be used alone or in conjunction with other modalities.

TENS is most often used to control chronic pain but may also be used for acute pain, especially postoperative pain, pain from orthopedic injuries, and pain from lacerations and sprains. Using TENS for a postoperative patient often diminishes (although does not eliminate) the patient's need for narcotic analgesics and therefore reduces unwanted side effects such as respiratory depression, nausea and vomiting, and slow bowel functioning.

In most clinical settings the physician or physical therapist introduces the patient to TENS. The treatment typically is administered by nurses who have

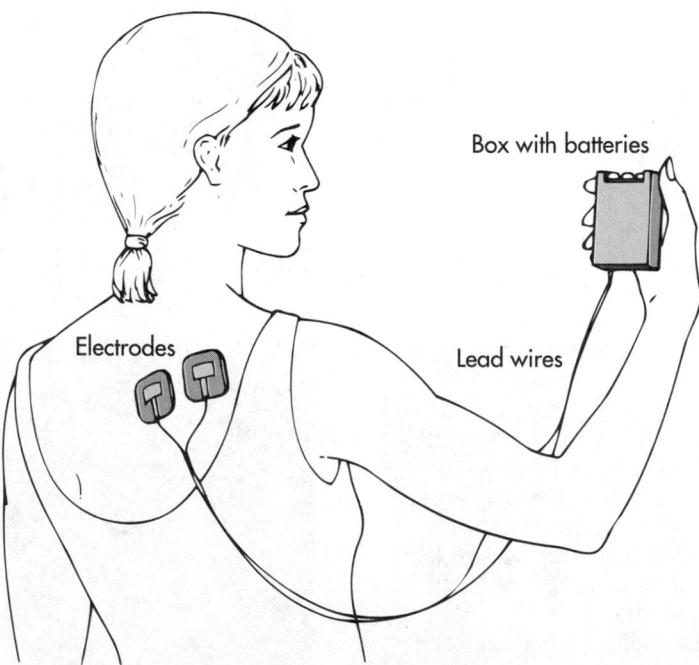

**Figure 11-8**   Three major components of a transcutaneous electrical nerve stimulation unit, with two electrodes placed on the patient's upper back to relieve shoulder pain. (From McCaffery M, Beebe A: *Pain: clinical manual for nursing practice,* St Louis, 1989, Mosby.)

had special education in the use of TENS. The patient is encouraged to handle the equipment and experiment with the settings to determine the best location for the electrodes and the most comfortable frequency and duration of current. Before the electrodes are attached to the skin, the nurse washes the area with soap and water (to reduce resistance), rinses the area, and dries it. The nurse applies enough electrode gel to ensure adequate conduction but not so much that the gel oozes from under the electrode. The nurse tapes the electrodes in place, turns on the stimulator, and slowly advances the output control until the patient feels stimulation. Most patients describe the stimulation as a buzzing or tingling sensation. The nurse helps the patient adjust the controls to provide the most comfortable sensation that gives the most pain relief.

Most patients obtain considerable relief from TENS. However, TENS does not work the same for everyone. Some patients experience great relief immediately. Others experience relief only after repeated applications. Some patients find that the analgesia may last for hours or even days after the current is turned off, whereas others experience relief only for a limited time. Nurses can provide support and encouragement to their patients while they experiment with this device.

## Noninvasive Interventions

A number of physical or mental activities can be used to help the patient focus his or her attention on sensations other than pain (Barbour, McGuire, Kirchhoff, 1986; Mast et al, 1987; McCaffery, Beebe, 1989; Acute Pain Management Guideline Panel, 1992; Watt-Watson, Donovan, 1992). **Distraction** is a useful technique if a patient is experiencing mild to moderate pain. With severe pain, distraction tends to increase anxiety and tension and thus increase pain. Examples of distraction include talking on the telephone, watching television, working on hobbies or crafts, and performing rhythmic breathing techniques. It is critical to remember that distraction does not make the pain go away but only makes it more bearable. Any procedure that helps the patient relax can help relieve emotional and muscular tension and lessen pain. A wide variety of **relaxation techniques** are available, such as progressive relaxation exercises, meditation, biofeedback, and self-hypnosis. The Lamaze method of childbirth is an example of a procedure that uses both distraction and relaxation procedures. Most relaxation techniques require time and effort to master but are useful, especially for a patient who has chronic pain. Nurses who have a knowledge of relaxation techniques can help their patients tolerate short-term painful procedures. They can also provide encouragement and support as their patients practice new methods.

> ### NURSE ALERT
>
> **Massage, heat, cold, ice, or menthol may be used to provide effective pain relief, and one may work as well as the other.**

Many patients have developed their own methods of coping with pain. The nurse should ask the patient to describe procedures that have helped in the past and should support and encourage the patient as he or she attempts to use them in the present pain situation. As with the use of analgesics, it is important to begin pain control methods before the pain becomes severe.

## Neurosurgical Interventions

A number of neurosurgical techniques for blocking pain transmission have been tried (McCaffery, Beebe, 1989; Acute Pain Management Guideline Panel, 1992; Miaskowski, 1993). Peripheral nerve blocks using local anesthetics such as lidocaine can temporarily relieve pain in some acute painful situations such as neuralgia, thrombophlebitis, or musculoskeletal conditions. If a local anesthetic is also needed, 0.06% bupivacaine is recommended. Preservative-free morphine or fentanyl are the opioids most commonly used for the intraspinal route. Surgical interruption of the pain pathways may be necessary if the pain becomes severe and cannot be controlled by any other means. A peripheral neurectomy (severing of a nerve) may be performed if the pain is localized to a specific area such as an arm or leg. When the pain is more diffuse (e.g., cancer pain), the pain pathways in the spinal cord may be interrupted. This procedure, known as a chordotomy, can be done at various levels depending on the location of the pain. The nurse must be aware that the body is no longer protected from injury as a result of the loss of sensation in the area affected by the surgery. Therefore such patients are particularly susceptible to pressure ulcers. Box 11-4 describes nursing care guidelines for patients who are in pain.

## PATIENT AND FAMILY TEACHING

It is important to work routinely with both the patient and the family. Patients who understand their pain and the possible ways to reduce it feel more in control of their life and are better able to actively participate in the available interventions. Nurses provide a vital service by teaching patients ways to manage the pain or discomfort they may face.

BOX 11-4

# NURSING PROCESS

## PATIENT IN PAIN

### ASSESSMENT

- History of pain: prior pain experiences, factors that precipitated the pain, activities that increase or decrease the pain, methods used to relieve the pain, usual time of occurrence of pain episodes
- Physiologic characteristics: increase in pulse and respiratory rates, increase in diastolic and systolic blood pressure, pallor, dilated pupils, diaphoresis, nausea; because of the body's ability to adapt to abnormal situations, these physiologic signs may be absent or decreased in prolonged acute pain or chronic pain
- Verbal statements: description of the quality or character of the pain (aching, burning, prickling), severity of pain using a scale (mild, moderate, severe), location of pain (precisely located or diffuse), frequency and duration of pain, meaning of pain to the individual

### NURSING DIAGNOSIS

- Pain, chronic pain (additional diagnoses may occur as a result of pain, such as anxiety, constipation, fatigue, or fear) related to pathophysiologic condition

### NURSING INTERVENTIONS

- Assure the patient that it is known that the pain is real and that he or she will have help in dealing with it.
- Provide general comfort measures such as turning, repositioning, providing back rubs, and changing damp dressings.

- Provide support for painful areas when moving the patient, such as placing a pillow to the abdominal incision area.
- Individualize pain control measures by considering a variety of approaches.
- Use pain control measures before pain becomes severe; get ahead of the pain. Include measures that the patient believes will help.
- Provide distraction and meaningful and interesting sensory stimulation such as radio, television, hobbies, and conversation.
- Provide cutaneous stimulation to block pain transmission, such as gentle massage, pressure, application of menthol rubbing agents to skin or around painful area, application of heat or cold as indicated, and TENS.
- Promote relaxation. Instruct the patient to breathe deeply and "let go" on expiration. Help patient to relax his or her body while contracting one muscle group (e.g., arm, leg).
- Help patient use guided imagery and imagine a pleasant event as a substitute for the pain experience.

### EVALUATION OF EXPECTED OUTCOMES

- Pain reduced or eliminated
- Understanding of the rationale for therapy
- Use of effective measures for relief of discomfort
- Anxiety and fear reduced or eliminated
- Side effects of medications controlled or minimized
- Demonstration of increased tolerance for pain by returning to work, using analgesics less often, or increasing daily activities

---

Every patient education plan must start with an assessment of what the patient needs to know and how much he or she already knows. The nurse must assess the patient's readiness and ability to learn. The severity and duration of the patient's pain often dictates what he or she is ready to learn. The nurse should then determine whether the patient has any barriers to learning, such as hearing or visual impairments, language difficulties, or a lack of reading skills. It is always wise to keep any instruction simple. Medical terminology may not be understood by patients or their families.

Prevention is a key concept that needs to be taught. Patients should ask for pain relief when the pain first begins. The nurse must make sure that patients (and their families) know how to use a pain rating scale and how to help with the pain relief by assessing and reporting their own pain. They should be assured that other measures of pain control are available and can be used if the current measures are not satisfactory.

Specific instructions for each pain relief measure are provided, and the procedures set forth by the physician or institution are followed. Nurses should learn and practice as many noninvasive measures as possible so as to be prepared to help a patient when the need and opportunity arise.

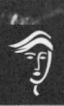 **PATIENT/FAMILY TEACHING**

- Explain what pain to expect and what will be done about it.
- Explain the concept of prevention; teach patient to take (or ask) for pain relief drugs when pain first begins.
- Explain how to use the pain rating scale and how it helps the staff to determine the best way to control pain.
- Provide instructions for whom to notify if pain relief is not satisfactory.
- Provide specific instructions for each pain relief measure (e.g., PCA, TENS, epidural, relaxation, distraction, medications).

## Pain Patient's Bill of Rights

The rights of the patient and family regarding pain management must be respected. These rights, identified by Cowles (1992), appear in Box 11-5.

## Pain Information Resources

The following are resources for information on pain:
American Pain Society
A National Chapter of the International Association for the Study of Pain
4700 W. Lake Avenue
Glenview, IL 60025-1485
1-847-375-4715
Agency for Health Care Policy and Research
(established by Congress to develop Clinical Practice Guidelines in several areas, including acute postoperative, and cancer pain)
AHCPR
Publications Clearinghouse
P.O. Box 547
Silver Springs, MD 20907
1-800-358-9295
American Society of Pain Management Nurses
(an organization of nurses specializing and interested in the management of pain)
1550 S. Coast Highway
Suite 201
Laguna Beach, CA 92651
1-888-34-ASPMN

**BOX 11-5**

### PAIN PATIENT'S BILL OF RIGHTS

**YOU HAVE A RIGHT TO:**
- Have your pain prevented or controlled adequately
- Have your pain and pain medication history taken
- Ask how much pain to expect and how long it might last
- Have your pain questions answered freely
- Develop a pain plan with your physician
- Know what medication, treatment, or anesthesia will be given
- Know the risks, benefits, and side effects of treatment
- Know what alternative pain treatments may be available
- Sign a statement of informed consent before any treatment
- Be believed when you say you have pain
- Have your pain assessed on an individual basis
- Have your pain assessed using the scale 0 = no pain to 10 = worst pain

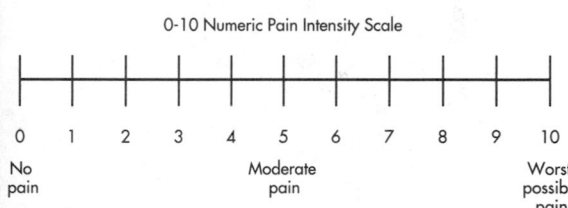

0-10 Numeric Pain Intensity Scale

0 No pain   1   2   3   4   5 Moderate pain   6   7   8   9   10 Worst possible pain

- Ask for changes in treatments if your pain persists
- Compassionate and sympathetic care
- Receive pain medication on a timely basis
- Refuse treatment without prejudice from your physician
- Seek a second opinion or request a pain care specialist
- Your records upon request
- Include your family in decision making
- Remind those who care for you that your pain management is part of your diagnostic, medical, or surgical care

From Cowles J: *Pain relief: how to say no to acute, chronic and cancer pain*, New York, 1992.

# NURSING CARE PLAN

## PATIENT WITH EPIDURAL ANALGESIA FOR PAIN MANAGEMENT

The patient is a 52-year-old woman who had an elective total knee replacement this morning. She is in good general health and has no known food or drug allergies. An epidural catheter is in place for pain management. The patient is a good candidate for epidural analgesia. Monitoring for actual or potential patient responses to epidural analgesia is an essential nursing responsibility.

| Medical History | Psychosocial Data | Assessment Data |
| --- | --- | --- |
| Good general health<br>Menopause at age 50<br>Discomfort from osteoarthritis for 6 yr | Both parents and husband in good health<br>Three grown children, living in vicinity<br>Married, lives with husband in own home<br>Employed as a teacher in local high school<br>Has good family support | Oriented to time, place, person<br>*Respiratory:* Lungs clear to percussion and auscultation; chest movements symmetric<br>*Cardiovascular:* Apical pulse strong and regular at 78; vital signs stable (T 99.6, P 76-84, R 18, BP 114/74)<br>*Epidural catheter:* Taped in place at L3; transparent dressing-surgical tape dry and intact; catheter connected to a continuous infusion with label on it stating "for epidural use"; catheter looped over left shoulder and secured on the back with tape; connected to infusion pump<br>*Pain:* States feeling no pain<br>**Medications**<br>Droperidol (Inapsine) 0.625-1.23 mg IV q 4 hr prn for nausea<br>IV fluids D5 with lactated Ringer's solution 1000 ml q 12 hr; may discontinue when PO intake is adequate<br>*Epidural infusion:* See epidural analgesia order form |

### NURSING DIAGNOSIS
Potential for knowledge deficit related to process of epidural analgesia

| NURSING INTERVENTIONS | EVALUATION OF EXPECTED OUTCOMES |
| --- | --- |
| Ask patient if clarification of terms or procedures is needed; review physician's explanation.<br>Remind patient to take a slow, gradual approach to changing position or ambulating.<br>Before ambulation, ensure that motor function (ability to bear weight) is present.<br>Encourage patient to report any numbness, tingling, or lack of sensation.<br>Observe for signs that patient may be more active than is safe. | Verbalizes an understanding of procedures and reports any side effects and/or lack of pain relief<br>After surgery, does not attempt activities beyond ability |

# NURSING CARE PLAN

## PATIENT WITH EPIDURAL ANALGESIA FOR PAIN MANAGEMENT—cont'd

**NURSING DIAGNOSIS**

Pain related to inadequate analgesia, catheter problems, pruritus, or nausea and vomiting

| NURSING INTERVENTIONS | EVALUATION OF EXPECTED OUTCOMES |
|---|---|
| Monitor and evaluate analgesic effect; ask patient about level of comfort; observe level of ease at which patient moves about.<br>Notify anesthesiologist if pain relief is inadequate with highest level of dosage range ordered.<br>Check catheter for breaks, knots, or leakage at dressing site or at catheter hub.<br>Observe for signs of scratching or rubbing, especially around the face or neck.<br>Promptly notify primary care nurse and physician of edema, urticaria, or respiratory difficulties.<br>Provide support measures such as lotions, cool/warm packs, or diversional activities as directed.<br>Observe for signs of nausea or vomiting. Notify primary care nurse and physician; administer droperidol (Inapsine) per physician's order.<br>Provide hygienic and emotional support; increase activities slowly. | Verbalizes pain relief<br>Verbalizes no pruritus or minimal pruritus that does not interfere with comfort<br>Verbalizes no nausea and experiences no vomiting |

**NURSING DIAGNOSIS**

Risk for ineffective breathing pattern related to side effects of spinal opioid

| NURSING INTERVENTIONS | EVALUATION OF EXPECTED OUTCOMES |
|---|---|
| Administer narcotics, sedatives, and other analgesics only as directed by physician.<br>Assess respiratory function q 1 hr for first 24 hr, then q 2-8 hr and as necessary; assess level of consciousness/sedation and color of mucous membranes.<br>Attach patient to apnea monitor if necessary.<br>Obtain and evaluate blood gases as ordered.<br>Notify physician if respiratory depression occurs; administer naloxone per physician's order. | Respiratory function maintained:<br>  Respiratory rate >12<br>  Respiratory depth adequate<br>Baseline level of consciousness maintained<br>Skin, nail beds, and mucous membranes pink<br>Arterial blood gases within normal limits |

**NURSING DIAGNOSIS**

Risk for altered urinary elimination/urinary retention related to side effects of spinal opioids

| NURSING INTERVENTIONS | EVALUATION OF EXPECTED OUTCOMES |
|---|---|
| Monitor intake and output q 8 hr, observe for symptoms of discomfort, urgency, or diminished output; gently palpate bladder for distention if no urinary catheter is in place.<br>Rule out other causes, such as fluid balance or positioning; assist patient with voiding.<br>Catheterize per physician's order. | Verbalizes no complaints of distention; bladder is not palpable; voids within 8 hr of surgery |

*Continued*

# NURSING CARE PLAN
## PATIENT WITH EPIDURAL ANALGESIA FOR PAIN MANAGEMENT—cont'd

**NURSING DIAGNOSIS**
Risk for injury related to postural hypotension

| NURSING INTERVENTIONS | EVALUATION OF EXPECTED OUTCOMES |
|---|---|
| Assess postural blood pressure and heart rate before ambulation. Assess fluid balance. Help patient sit up or ambulate the first time, then as needed. | Postural hypotension prevented or detected before ambulation Tolerates position changes without feeling dizzy or lightheaded |

# KEY CONCEPTS

➤ Pain is both a physical and a psychologic phenomenon.

➤ Pain is whatever a person says it is and exists wherever a person says it does.

➤ Nurses are held accountable for managing the pain program for patients under their care.

➤ The gate control theory at least partially explains how massage, heat and cold, counterirritants (e.g., Ben Gay), distraction, relaxation, and TENS affect the sensation of pain.

➤ A detailed and accurate description of the patient's pain is essential for accurately diagnosing and treating pain.

➤ Quantifying the amount of pain before and after administering medications or providing other interventions is a useful way to monitor the effectiveness of the therapy.

➤ Pain medications should be given on a set time schedule (ATC) to maintain a sufficient level of drug and to control the pain, prevent anxiety, and prevent the memory of suffering.

➤ Pain medications should be given before the pain becomes severe. Prevention of pain is the goal of satisfactory pain management.

➤ The peak effect of most parenteral drugs is 1 hour. For oral drugs the peak effect is 2 or more hours later.

➤ Addiction (psychologic dependence) is rare in people receiving narcotics for pain. Although physical dependence is to be expected if narcotics are used for several weeks, the patient can be "weaned" off the drug.

➤ The ability of a placebo to cause effects often is a measure of the faith or confidence that the patient has in his or her physician or nurse.

➤ Patient-controlled analgesia provides better pain relief than injections because patients can receive relief at the first sign of pain.

➤ Nurses must have special education to care for patients receiving intraspinal analgesia.

➤ Distractions such as watching television and visiting with friends are helpful if the pain is mild or moderate.

➤ Any activity that helps a patient relax can help relieve emotional and muscular tension and lessen pain.

# CRITICAL THINKING EXERCISES

1. How would you assess a non-English-speaking patient for pain after abdominal surgery?
2. Considering the current theories on the causes of pain, explain the advantages of patient-controlled analgesia.
3. The physician has ordered a placebo for your patient who has chronic pain because it is suspected that the patient is exaggerating the severity of the pain experienced. Would you administer a placebo when your patient requests pain medication? Explain your answer.
4. Discuss whether meperidine (Demerol) is appropriate for long-term use in a cancer patient.

## REFERENCES AND ADDITIONAL READINGS

Acute Pain Management Guideline Panel: Acute pain management: operative or medical procedures and trauma, Clinical practice guideline, AHCPR Pub No 92-0032. Rockville, Md, 1992, Agency for Health Care Policy and Research, Public Health Service, US Department of Health and Human Services.

Acute Pain Management Guideline Panel: Acute pain management in adults: operative procedures quick reference guide for clinicians, *MedSurg Nurs* 3(2):99-107, 1994.

American Society of Pain Management Nurses, Clinical Practice Committee, Position statement: Use of placebos for pain management, Laguna Beach, Calif, 1997, National Office of the Society.

Baque ML: What matters most in chronic pain management, *RN* 53(3):46-50, 1989.

Barbour LA, McGuire DB, Kirchoff KT: Nonanalgesic methods of pain control used by cancer patients, *Oncol Nurs Forum* 13(6):56-60, 1986.

Cowles J: *Pain patient's bill of rights,* New York, 1992.

DeWolf MS: The ethics of pain management, *MedSurg Nurs* 2(3):218-220, 1993.

Ferrell BA: Pain management in elderly people, *J Am Geriatr Soc* 39(1):64-73, 1991.

Ferrell BR, McCaffery M, Rhiner M: Pain and addiction: an urgent need for change in nursing education, *J Pain Symptom Manage* 7(2):117-124, 1992.

Fitzgerald J, Shamy P: Let your patient control his analgesia, *Nurs 87* 17(7):48-51, 1987.

Haight K: What you should know about epidural analgesia, *Nurs 87* 17(9):58-59, 1987.

Herr KA, Mobily PR: Complexities of pain assessment in the elderly: clinical considerations, *J Gerontol Nurs* 17(4):12-19, 1991.

International Association for the Study of Pain: Pain terms: a current list with definitions and notes on usage, *Pain* 3(27):S215-S221, 1986.

Jones J, Brooks J: The ABC's of PCA, *RN* 54(5):54-60, 1990.

Kaiko RF: Age and morphine analgesia in cancer patient's with postoperative pain, *Clin Pharmacol Ther* 28(6):823-826, 1980.

Kaiko RF et al: Central nervous system excitatory effects of meperidine in cancer patients, *Ann Neurol* 13(2):180-185, 1983.

Keeney SA: Nursing care of the postoperative patient receiving epidural analgesia, *MedSurg Nurs* 2(3):191-196, 1993.

Mast D et al: Relaxation techniques: a self-learning module for nurses, *Cancer Nurs* 10(6):141-147, 1987.

McCaffery M, Beebe A: *Pain: clinical manual for nursing practice,* St Louis, 1989, Mosby.

McCaffery M, Ferrell BR: How to use the new ACHPR cancer pain guidelines, *Am J Nurs* 94(7):42-47, 1994.

McCaffery M, Beebe A: Giving narcotics for pain: the secrets to giving equianalgesic doses, *Nurs 89* 19(10):161-165, 1989.

McGuire L: The nurse's role in pain relief, *MedSurg Nurs* 3(2):91-98, 1994.

McGuire L et al: Managing pain in the young patient . . . in the elderly patient, *Nurs 82* 12(8):52-57, 1982.

Melzack R, Wall P: Pain mechanisms: a new theory, *Science* 150(3699):971-978, 1965.

Melzack R, Wall P: *The challenge of pain,* ed 2, London, 1988, Penguin.

Miaskowski C: Current concepts in the assessment and management of cancer-related pain, *MedSurg Nurs* 2(2):113-118, 1993.

Paice JA: Unraveling the mystery of pain, *Oncol Nurs Forum,* 18(5):843-849, 1991.

Pasero CL: Pain control: are opioids right for chronic nonmalignant pain? *Am J Nurs* 97(6):20-22, 1997.

Pasero CL, McCaffery M: Managing postoperative pain in the elderly, *Am J Nurs* 96(10):38-45, 1996.

Perry S, Heidrich G: Placebo response: myth and matter, *Am J Nurs* 81(5):720-725, 1981.

Peterson AM: Pharmacology in practice: analgesics, *RN* 60(4):45-50, 1997.

Porter J, Hick H: Addiction rare in patients treated with narcotics, *N Engl J Med* 302(2):123, 1980.

Ramsey R: Adjusting drug dosages for critically ill elderly patients, *Nurs 88* 18(7):47-49, 1988.

Sherman R: A survey of current phantom limb pain treatment in the United States, *Pain* 8(28):285-295, 1987.

Szeto H et al: Accumulation of normeperidine, an active metabolite of meperidine, in patients with renal failure of cancer, *Ann Intern Med* 86(6):738-741, 1977.

Watt-Watson JH, Donovan MI: *Pain management: nursing perspective,* St Louis, 1992, Mosby.

West BA: Understanding endorphins: our natural pain relief system, *Nurs 81* 11(2):50-53, 1981.

Wild L, Coyne C: The basics and beyond: epidural analgesia, *Am J Nurs* 92(4):26-34, 1992.

Willens JS: Giving fentanyl for pain outside the OR, *Am J Nurs* 94(2):24-28, 1994.

# CHAPTER 12

# The Patient with Cancer

## CHAPTER OBJECTIVES

1. Discuss cancer as a health care problem.
2. Describe the predominant characteristics of cancer.
3. Identify the major causes of cancer.
4. List recommended methods of prevention and early detection.
5. Describe the common methods of diagnosis and treatment of cancer.
6. Discuss nursing care of the patient receiving radiation therapy.
7. Discuss nursing care of the patient receiving chemotherapy.
8. Discuss the emotional impact of cancer on the patient and family.

## KEY TERMS

| | |
|---|---|
| benign | malignant |
| biologic response modifier | metastasis |
| bone marrow transplantation | myelosuppression |
| carcinogens | neoplasms |
| carcinoma | oncogenes |
| chemotherapy | oncology |
| desquamation | radiation therapy |
| ionizing radiation | radioisotope |
| leukopenia | sarcoma |
| magnetic resonance imaging | thrombocytopenia |

Cancer is a group of diseases characterized by abnormal and unrestricted cell division and by the spread of these cells into healthy tissues of the body. Without appropriate medical intervention, this dissemination of cancer cells can become widespread and lead to tissue destruction, which ultimately may result in death. Cancer is one of the oldest diseases known to human beings. Its cause has been a puzzle for centuries and remains so. However, recent scientific breakthroughs have led to cautious optimism that the causes of most cancers can be identified and strategies for prevention, cure, or control can be developed.

In the United States the number of deaths caused by cancer each year is exceeded only by the number of deaths resulting from heart disease. In 1997 it was estimated that approximately 1,382,400 new cancer cases would be diagnosed and that approximately 560,000 Americans would die of cancer that year (American Cancer Society [ACS], 1997). According to current trends, 1 out of 4 individuals and 3 out of 4 families will be affected by cancer at some time. Cancer strikes rich and poor, young and old with equally devastating effects. The largest number of malignant tumors occurs in four areas of the body: the lungs, colon-rectum, breast, and prostate.

Lung cancer is the leading cause of death from cancer in both men and women. The incidence of lung cancer has been declining in men but continues to rise in women. Since 1987 more women have died each year from lung cancer than from breast cancer. In 1997 it was estimated that 160,400 people in the United States (94,400 men and 66,000 women) would die from lung cancer. The survival rate for lung cancer is extremely low—only about 14% of these individuals live as long as 5 years after the disease has been diagnosed. These statistics are unfortunate, because the disease is largely preventable. Cigarette smoking is directly related to at least 87% of the cases of lung cancer and accounts for approximately 29% of all cancer deaths (ACS, 1997).

According to 1997 estimates, colorectal cancer kills approximately 54,900 people each year. It ranks second as a cause of cancer deaths (ACS, 1997). The incidence of colorectal cancer has declined over the past two decades and the survival rate has risen, especially for women. However, the death rate for African-American men continues to rise. Approximately 2 out of 3 patients may be saved by early diagnosis and prompt treatment, the keys to survival. Digital rectal examination, stool blood tests, and sigmoidoscopy are the methods recommended for early detection.

Breast cancer is the most common cancer among women over 40 years of age. In 1997 it was expected that 180,200 new cases of breast cancer would be diagnosed

and that 43,900 women would die from the disease. When breast cancer is diagnosed early and at a localized stage, 97% of those affected survive 5 years or longer. When diagnosis and treatment are delayed and regional spread occurs, the 5-year survival rate drops to 76%. When distant metastases are present, the survival rate is 20% (ACS, 1997). The most recent data indicate that death rates are declining in white women and, for the first time, in younger African-American women. Earlier detection and improved treatment probably are contributing to this decline. Several prominent women have had breast surgery in recent years, which has resulted in better public awareness, and more women now perform breast self-examination (BSE), have screening mammograms, and seek health care early.

Prostate cancer, the second leading cause of death from cancer in men, was estimated to have caused 41,800 deaths in 1997. Between 1989 and 1993, the inci-

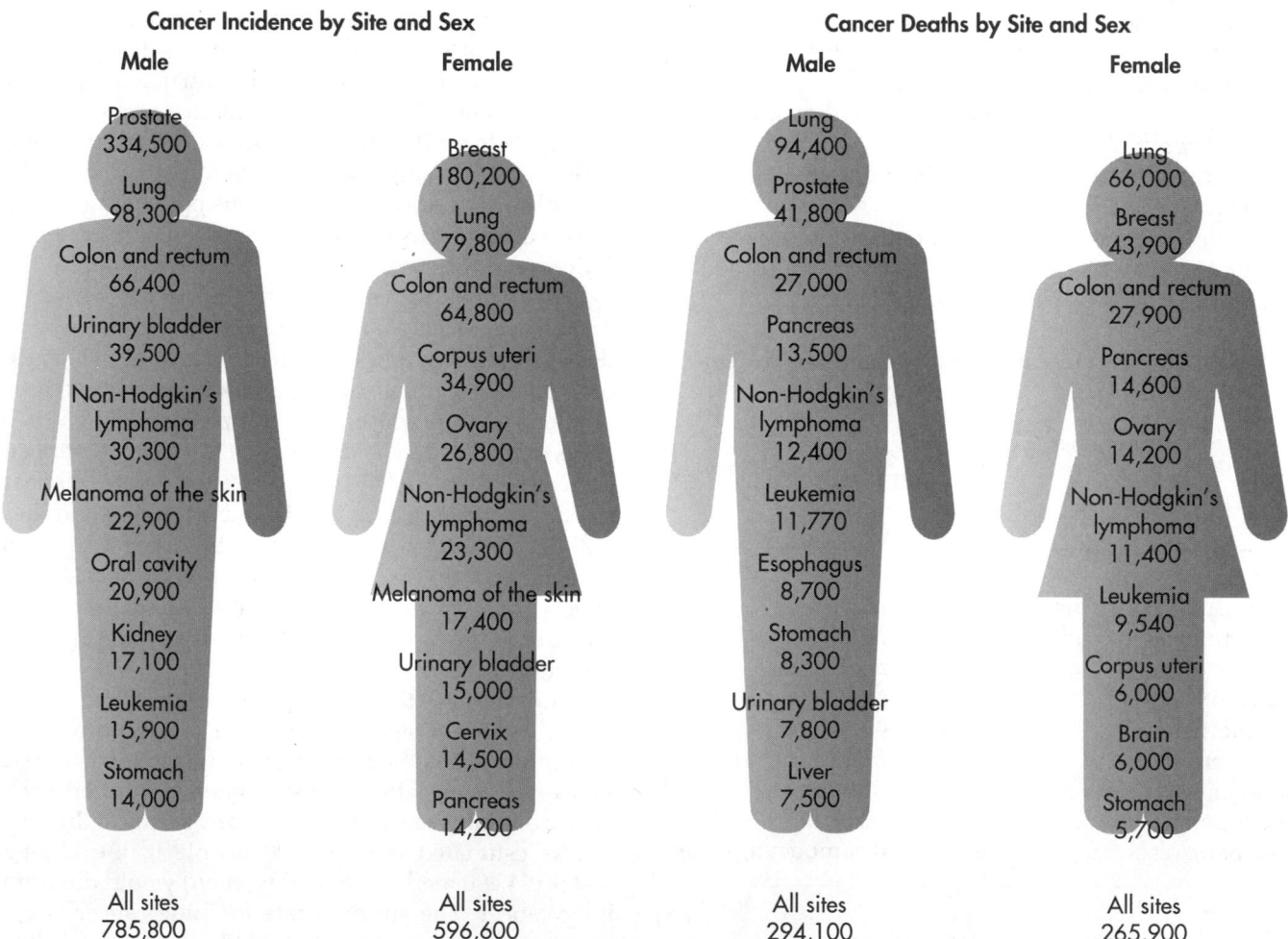

**Figure 12-1**  Leading sites of new cancer cases and deaths caused by cancer (1997 estimates; excludes basal and squamous cell skin cancer and in situ carcinoma except bladder cancer). (From American Cancer Society: *Cancer facts and figures—1997*, Atlanta, 1997, The Society.)

dence rate for prostate cancer increased 50%, largely as a result of improved detection. Black men have a 66% higher incidence than white men. Digital rectal examinations and prostate-specific antigen (PSA) serum screening tests are recommended for early detection. Prostatic ultrasound scans also are being used to improve early detection. The most common sites of malignant neoplasms and their mortality rates are presented in Figure 12-1.

Congress appropriates millions of dollars to the National Cancer Institute for research and training. It also provides grants and contracts to other organizations whose research activities may be applied to the prevention, detection, diagnosis, and treatment of malignant disease. The National Cancer Act of 1971 provided funds for establishing cancer research centers throughout the nation. These centers are carefully reviewed by the National Cancer Advisory Board and receive funding from the National Cancer Institute, the ACS, and many other sources. The ACS is one of the oldest and largest voluntary health agencies in the United States. It is dedicated to eliminating cancer through research, education, patient service, and rehabilitation. In 1995 the ACS invested over $92 million in cancer research (ACS, 1997).

The ultimate objective of all cancer research is to control cancer in human beings. Progress toward this goal is measured by (1) a greater knowledge of malignant disease, (2) identification and control of factors related to cause and prevention, and (3) improvement in detection, diagnosis, and treatment. Since 1990 small but measurable gains have been made in the fight against cancer. After several decades of a continuous rise, the overall, age-adjusted cancer mortality rates declined about 3.1% between 1990 and 1995 (Cole, Rodu, 1996). This favorable trend is the result of several different cancer control activities, including a reduction in smoking and improved medical care.

The financial costs of cancer are exceedingly high; they account for 10% of the total cost of disease in the United States. The National Cancer Institute estimates the overall annual cost of cancer to be $104 billion, a cost that certainly has a significant financial impact both on individuals and society as a whole. The current debate on health care reform has concentrated on ways to control the high cost of health care and ensure equal access for all Americans, including the more than 7 million people who are cancer survivors (ACS, 1997).

## PATHOPHYSIOLOGY

The basic structural unit of all forms of animal and plant life is the cell. Each organ of the body is composed of many different types of cells that are joined together to perform specific functions. It is the coordination of all cellular activities that allows the body to function as a whole organism. All cells have the genetic capability to divide and multiply, and they normally do so in response to a specific need of the body. However, a normal cell can undergo changes that transform it into a cancer cell. Cancer cells are able to divide and multiply, but not in a normal manner. Instead of limiting their growth to meet the specific needs of the body, cancer cells continue to reproduce in a disorderly and unrestricted manner. Whether benign or malignant, new growths of abnormal tissue are referred to as **neoplasms,** or tumors. **Benign** tumors normally do not progress or spread and are easily removed. Although benign tumors usually are harmless, they occasionally involve vital organs, such as the brain, with fatal results. **Malignant** tumors tend to become progressively worse, often resulting in the death of the individual.

Malignant tumors differ from benign tumors in several important aspects (Table 12-1). They are capable of continued growth that compresses, invades, and

---

### TABLE 12-1

#### General Characteristics of Neoplasms

| BENIGN TUMOR | MALIGNANT TUMOR |
|---|---|
| Slow, steady growth | Rate of growth varies, usually rapid |
| Remains localized | Metastasizes |
| Usually contained within a capsule | Rarely contained within a capsule |
| Smooth, well defined, movable when palpated | Irregular, more immobile when palpated |
| Resembles parent tissue | Little resemblance to parent tissue |
| Crowds normal tissue | Invades normal tissue |
| Rarely recurs after removal | May recur after removal |
| Rarely fatal | Fatal without treatment |

destroys normal tissue. Malignant cells break away from their original sites and are transported by the blood or lymph to new sites, where they begin to grow; this process is called **metastasis.** During metastasis malignant cells are stopped temporarily by the lymph nodes, but they may grow and multiply there. The immune system constantly tries to rid the body of these metastasizing cells, and generally it is successful, with only a fraction of 1% surviving. However, this small percentage may be sufficient to establish tumors in other parts of the body. Cancer spreads by the following processes (Figure 12-2):

1. Direct extension into adjacent tissue
2. Permeation along lymphatic vessels
3. Embolism through lymphatic or blood vessels
4. Diffusion or seeding within a body cavity

Malignant tumors are found in all types of tissue and in all parts of the body. **Carcinoma,** the most common form of cancer, arises from epithelial cells, the type of cells that form coverings, such as the skin, and that line cavities such as the mouth, stomach, and lungs. Other types of epithelial cells are found in glandular organs such as the breast. Another, less common form of cancer is a **sarcoma,** which arises from connective tissue such as bone, muscle, and cartilage. Carcinomas and sarcomas are called solid tumors. Cancer can also develop in the blood-forming and lymphoid organs. *Leukemia* is an abnormal, uncontrolled multiplication of white blood cells. *Lymphoma* arises in the lymph system, especially in the lymph nodes and spleen, and is characterized by overproduction of lymphocytes. Lymphoma has two main forms, Hodgkin's disease and non-Hodgkin's lymphoma. *Multiple myeloma* is caused by an overproduction of plasma cells in the blood and bone marrow.

## CAUSES OF CANCER

Cancer is a group of diseases that have many causes. Scientists now realize that healthy cells become malignant because of multiple mutations in the genes that control cell division. These mutations are caused by prolonged exposure to a variety of environmental agents, called **carcinogens.** Viruses, chemical agents, physical agents, hormones, and dietary factors all have been implicated as contributing to malignant changes in cells. Inherited genetic mutations that predispose an individual to some types of cancer also have been identified.

Although viruses are suspected of causing some forms of human cancer, it has been difficult to isolate specific types of such viruses. Cancer-causing viruses are able to enter a cell and alter the genetic material that controls the cell's growth. Burkitt's lymphoma and nasopharyngeal and cervical cancer are thought to be induced by viruses.

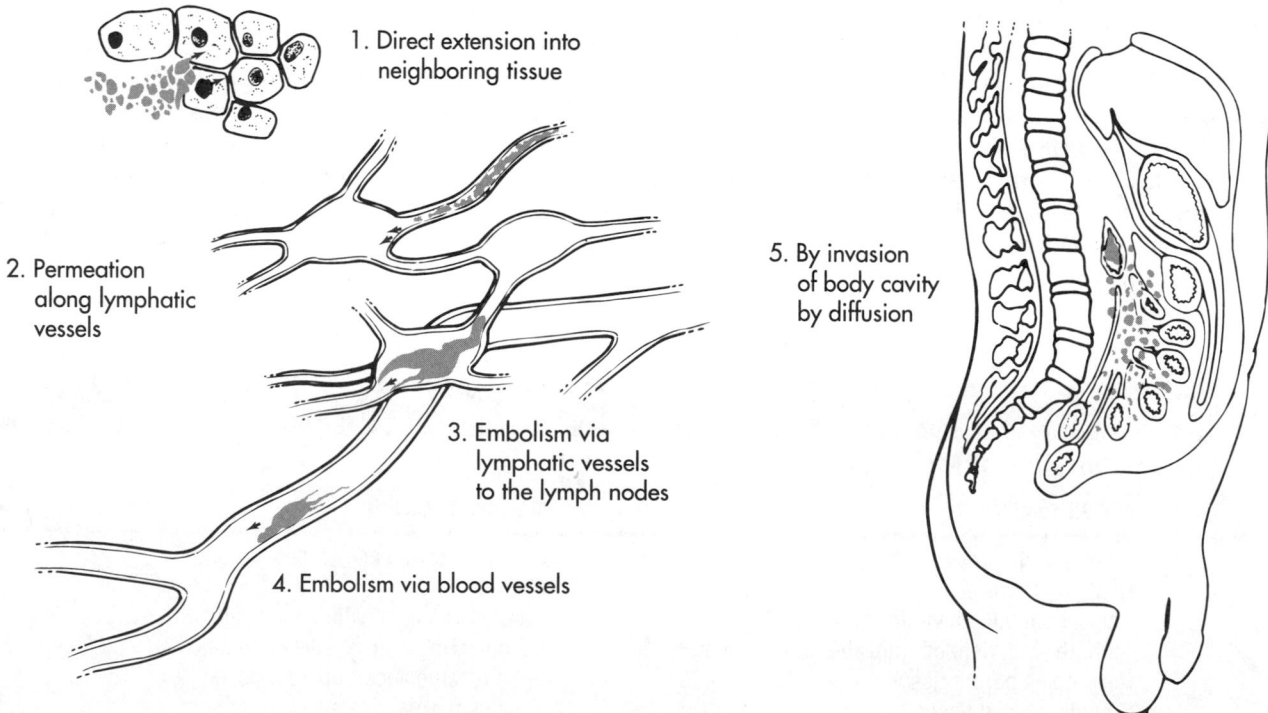

**Figure 12-2**   Modes of dissemination of cancer. (From Phipps WJ et al: *Medical-surgical nursing: concepts and clinical practice,* ed 5, St Louis, 1995, Mosby.)

Chemical agents include a wide variety of substances that often are found in greater amounts in certain occupations and in polluted environments. The most common chemical carcinogens are hydrocarbons found in cigarette smoke, air pollutants, tar, soot, aniline dyes, and benzene. Asbestos, vinyl chloride, cobalt, chromium, nickel, and arsenic compounds are other common chemical carcinogens. The relationship between cigarette smoke and lung cancer has been well established, and evidence is increasing that secondary smoke is a hazard. Snuff, a form of smokeless tobacco, has been implicated as a cause of mouth cancer and is a concern because of the increase in "dipping snuff" among young men (ACS, 1997). The recent popularity of cigar smoking among men and women also has raised concern about mouth and throat cancer.

Physical agents include ultraviolet radiation from sunlight and **ionizing radiation** from natural gamma-rays, x-rays, and radioactive isotopes. Skin cancer is found more often in people who have had prolonged exposure to sunlight, and it is more common in fair-skinned individuals. The greater pigmentation in dark skin appears to offer some protection against the effects of ultraviolet rays. People who have undergone short-term or chronic exposure to ionizing radiation have an increased incidence of cancer, especially leukemia. This phenomenon is seen in the survivors of the atom bomb attacks and in people cured of an earlier cancer by radiation therapy, and it also was seen in radiation workers before strict exposure precautions were enforced.

Hormones have been implicated in the development of some forms of cancer. Prolonged estrogen therapy has been linked to an increased incidence of endometrial cancer. Use of diethylstilbestrol (DES) during pregnancy has been related to the development of vaginal carcinoma in female children. In prostate cancer and in some breast cancers, tumor growth can be slowed by treatments that stop the natural production of sex hormones.

Dietary factors have been linked to the development of certain cancers. According to the ACS (1997), existing scientific evidence suggests that about one third of U.S. cancer deaths each year are due to dietary factors. It is thought that some diets may increase the risk of cancer, whereas other diets may offer some protection from cancer. High-fat diets have been associated with an increased risk of colon, breast, prostate, and endometrial cancer, whereas fiber is thought to have a protective role against colon cancer. Various vitamins, particularly vitamins A and C, may reduce the risk of cancer. A diet that includes many fruits, vegetables, and grains may protect against many cancers. Some food additives have been suspected of being carcinogenic, and excessive drinking of alcohol has been linked to an increased risk of cancer of the mouth, larynx, and esophagus.

In the past few years scientists have been able to identify specific genetic changes in some members of families with a strong history of cancer. Inherited cancer genes have been identified for breast, colon, and prostate cancer. Commercial testing for two breast cancer genes is now available.

Human cancer is thought to be caused by a combination of many environmental and genetic factors. Recent research suggests that each cell has certain genes that control cell growth. Some of these genes, called **oncogenes,** stimulate cell division whereas others, called tumor-suppressor genes, slow down cell division. In a normal cell the two types of genes work together to maintain healthy tissue growth and repair. However, mutations in either type can cause loss of control of cell division, and the cell begins to act like a car with a stuck accelerator pedal or no brakes (Nash, 1996). How these mutations occur is not yet known, but the effect of many of the carcinogens previously discussed are being studied. Some scientists believe that cancer cells form in the body throughout life and that the immune system is constantly detecting and eliminating the abnormal cells. This concept has stimulated research involving the immune system of the body. Some immunologists suggest that cancer may be caused by a failure of this system and that strengthening the body's natural immune defenses may help destroy malignant tissue.

## PREVENTION AND CONTROL

Cancer usually begins as an alteration in one microscopic cell of the body. The individual is asymptomatic and appears to be an active, healthy person. As the cancer cell begins to divide without restraint, symptoms eventually appear. The first symptoms are insidious and not readily apparent to the victim. A small, painless lump, a vague change in bowel habits, or a chronic cough may be the only warning sign of a devastating illness. Often these poorly defined symptoms are not considered valid reasons to seek health care. If left untreated, cancer cells continue to invade adjacent healthy tissue and eventually spread to other parts of the body, where new cancer growths are established.

Because of this characteristic pattern of development, cancer is difficult to detect in its earliest stages. However, if the disease is not readily diagnosed, the chances for cure are greatly reduced because the disease has already spread. The current survival rate is 4 in 10 patients, but early diagnosis and prompt treatment could save more than 50% of all cancer patients. It is clear that cancer must be prevented or controlled at an early stage. Future efforts must concentrate on promoting research, controlling environmental carcinogens, and educating health professionals and the public about prevention and early detection.

Nurses can play a particularly important role in these efforts by promoting primary and secondary prevention. Primary prevention refers to the steps that can be taken to avoid factors that might cause cancer (Box 12-1). Many of the risk factors are avoidable, and the risk declines as positive behavioral changes occur. Dietary guidelines and steps to reduce the risk of cancer recommended by the ACS are provided in Box 12-2.

Secondary prevention refers to the steps taken to diagnose cancer as soon as possible after it has developed and while it is still potentially curable. Early

detection of cancer in people without symptoms is a major goal of all cancer organizations. The ACS and other agencies recommend certain guidelines for cancer-related checkups (Table 12-2). Simple steps to early diagnosis include a monthly BSE (see Figure 43-7), testicular self-examination (TSE), and skin self-examination, as well as a regular mammogram, Papanicolaou (Pap) smear, digital rectal examination, stool-blood test, and sigmoidoscopy. All nurses should urge their patients to practice these preventive health behaviors and should teach them symptoms that possibly indicate cancer (Box 12-3).

Public awareness about the prevention and early detection of cancer is increasing. Cigarette advertise-

---

**BOX 12-1**

## RISK FACTORS FOR MAJOR CANCERS

**LUNG**
Cigarette smoking
Exposure to some industrial chemicals (e.g., arsenic, asbestos)
Radiation exposure, including radon
Secondhand smoke

**COLON-RECTUM**
Personal or family history of cancer or polyps of colon or rectum
Inflammatory bowel disease
High-fat and/or low-fiber diet

**BREAST**
Age over 40
Personal or family history of breast cancer
Early age at menarche
Late age at menopause
Never had children or late age at first birth
Higher education and socioeconomic status
High-fat diet

**PROSTATE**
Increasing age
Living in northwestern Europe or North America
African-American
Family history of prostate cancer
High-fat diet

**UTERUS (CERVIX)**
Early age at first intercourse
Multiple sex partners
Cigarette smoking
Infection with human papillomavirus (HPV)
Low socioeconomic status

**UTERUS (ENDOMETRIUM)**
Early menarche
Late menopause
History of infertility
Failure to ovulate
Unopposed estrogen therapy (without progesterone)
Obesity, diabetes, gallbladder disease, hypertension

**OVARY**
Increasing age
Never had children
Personal history of breast cancer
Family history of ovarian cancer

**MOUTH**
Cigarette, cigar, pipe smoking
Smokeless tobacco
Excessive drinking of alcohol

**SKIN**
Excessive exposure to ultraviolet radiation
Fair complexion
Occupational exposure to coal tar, pitch, creosote, arsenic, radium
Family history of skin cancer

**BLADDER**
Cigarette smoking
Urban living
Exposure to dye, rubber, or leather

**STOMACH**
Diet heavy in smoked, salted, or pickled foods
Family history of stomach cancer

> **BOX 12-2**
>
> ### DIETARY GUIDELINES AND STEPS TO REDUCE THE RISK OF CANCER
>
> 1. Choose most of the foods you eat from plant sources.
>    - Eat five or more servings of fruits and vegetables each day.
>    - Eat other foods from plant sources such as breads, cereals, grain products, rice, pasta, or beans several times each day.
> 2. Limit your intake of high-fat foods, particularly from animal sources.
>    - Choose foods low in fat.
>    - Limit consumption of meats, especially high-fat meats.
> 3. Be physically active: achieve and maintain a healthy weight.
>    - Be at least moderately active for 30 minutes or more on most days of the week.
>    - Stay within your healthy weight range.
> 4. Limit consumption of alcoholic beverages, if you drink at all.
>
> Reprinted by permission of the American Cancer Society, Inc.

**TABLE 12-2**

## American Cancer Society Guidelines for Cancer-Related Checkups in People Without Symptoms, According to Age

| SITE | INCREASING AGE → | | |
|---|---|---|---|
| Basic | All persons 20 to 39 years of age should have a cancer-related health checkup every 3 years. | All persons age 40 or over should have a cancer-related health checkup every year. | |
| Breast | Women age 20 or over should perform breast self-examination (BSE) monthly. Women 20 to 40 years of age should have a breast examination by a health care provider every 3 years. | All women should have a baseline mammogram by age 40. Women age 40 to 49 should have a mammogram every 1-2 years and a breast examination every year. | Women age 50 or over should have a mammogram and breast examination every year. |
| Colon-rectum | | Men and women over age 40 should have a digital rectal examination every year. | Men and women over age 50 should have a stool-blood test every year and a sigmoidoscopy every 3 to 5 years. |
| Cervix/uterus | Women age 18 or over and younger women who are sexually active should have an annual Pap smear and pelvic examination. After three or more consecutive normal annual examinations, a Pap smear may be done less frequently at the physician's discretion. | | High-risk women should have an endometrial tissue sample checked at menopause. |
| Lung | Primary prevention should focus on helping smokers to stop smoking and keeping nonsmokers from starting. | | |

Modified from American Cancer Society: *Cancer facts and figures,* Atlanta, 1997, The Society.

*Continued*

| TABLE 12-2 | | | |
| --- | --- | --- | --- |
| **American Cancer Society Guidelines for Cancer-Related Checkups in People Without Symptoms, According to Age—cont'd** | | | |
| SITE | INCREASING AGE | | |
| Prostate | | Men age 40 or older should have a digital rectal examination every year. If suspicious, a transrectal ulrasound examination is recommended. | Men age 50 or over should have an annual prostate-specific antigen (PSA) blood test every year. If suspicious, a transrectal ultrasound examination is recommended. |
| Skin | Primary prevention involves avoiding exposure to sunlight, using sunscreens, and protecting children from traumatic sunburns. Skin self-examination should be done every month. | | |

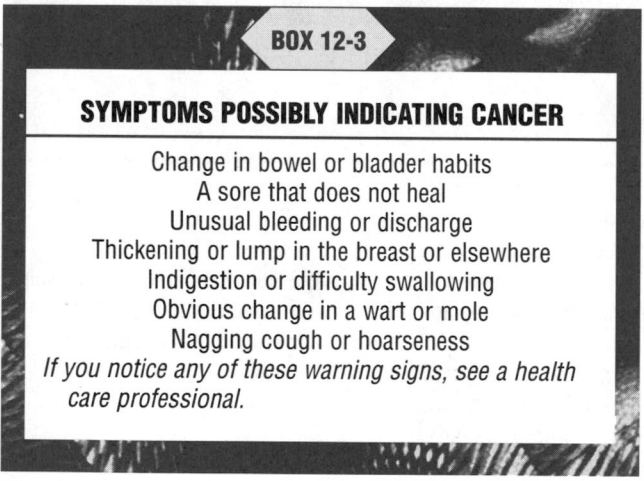

**BOX 12-3**

**SYMPTOMS POSSIBLY INDICATING CANCER**

Change in bowel or bladder habits
A sore that does not heal
Unusual bleeding or discharge
Thickening or lump in the breast or elsewhere
Indigestion or difficulty swallowing
Obvious change in a wart or mole
Nagging cough or hoarseness
*If you notice any of these warning signs, see a health care professional.*

ments have been banned on radio and television; airlines no longer allow smoking on flights; and many businesses, government agencies, and restaurants also have banned smoking. Educational programs in schools and short advertisements on television are designed to acquaint the public with the hazards of smoking and to encourage people who smoke to break the habit.

Smoking-cessation classes and support groups are now widely available and often are provided by companies for their employees. In the summer of 1996, President Bill Clinton announced new restrictions on the sale and advertising of cigarettes in an attempt to curb smoking among teenagers. Public education pro-

grams have alerted more women to the benefits of BSE, mammograms, and Pap smears. Since 1995 a federal grant has provided free mammograms and Pap smears to uninsured women over 50 years of age who cannot afford them. Colorectal, skin, and prostate screening programs often are run by cancer centers or community agencies.

The National Cancer Institute and the ACS spend a considerable amount of money on public and professional education. The Institute sponsors a toll-free information line, which is accessible in all parts of the country by dialing 1-800-4-CANCER. Trained counselors provide the most up-to-date answers about cancer prevention, detection, and treatment. The ACS has units in all states and provides free information about cancer, as well as services to people with cancer. The ACS unit phone numbers can be found in local phone directories or by calling 1-800-ACS-2345.

## DIAGNOSTIC TESTS AND PROCEDURES

Before a physician or pathologist can make a diagnosis of cancer, the patient must be examined carefully, a tissue sample must be obtained, and the primary location and anatomic spread (stage) of the cancer must be established. The degree of malignancy, or grade, is based on microscopic examination of the lesion. The higher the grade, the worse the prognosis. Staging is a classification that describes the extent of the spread of the tumor. Staging does not consider the microscopic characteristics of the lesion (Box 12-4).

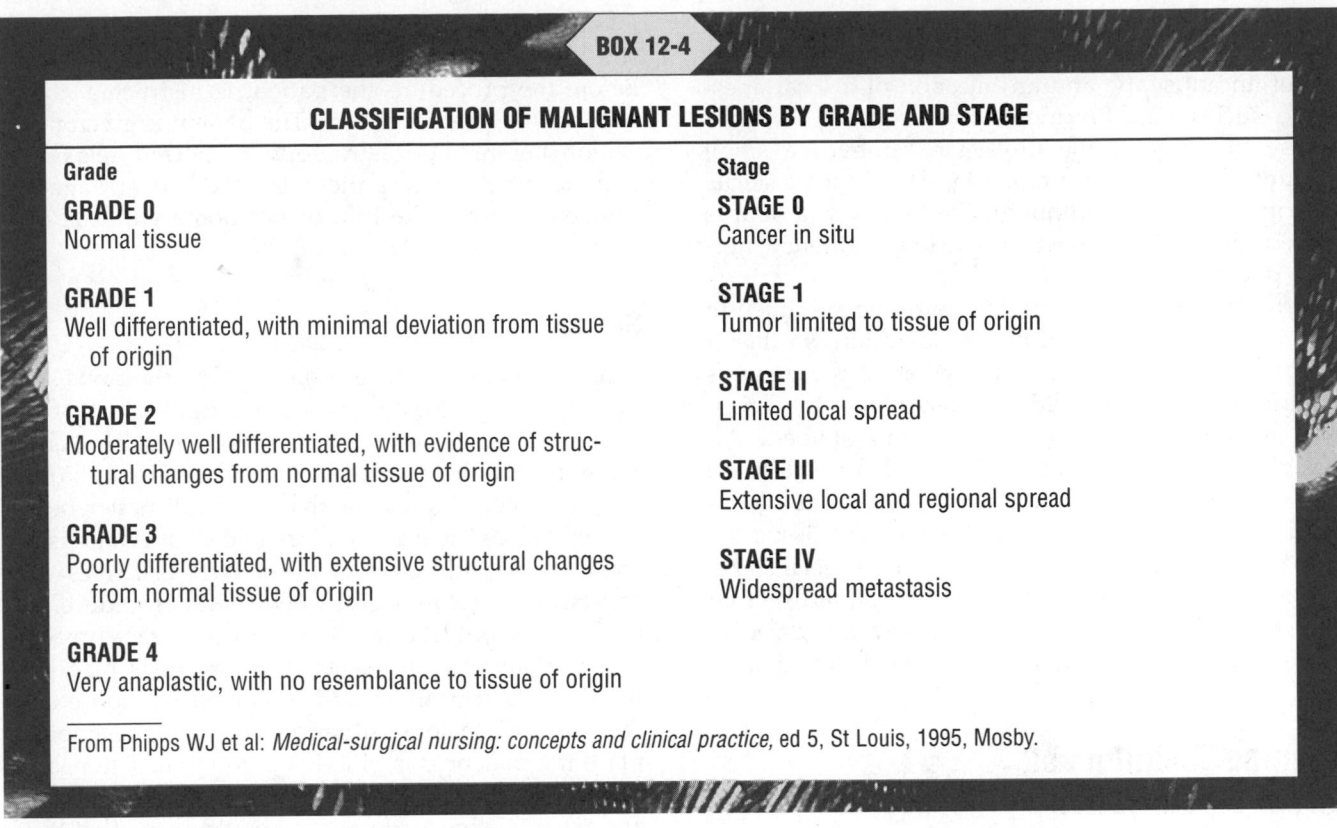

BOX 12-4

## CLASSIFICATION OF MALIGNANT LESIONS BY GRADE AND STAGE

| Grade | Stage |
|---|---|
| **GRADE 0**<br>Normal tissue | **STAGE 0**<br>Cancer in situ |
| **GRADE 1**<br>Well differentiated, with minimal deviation from tissue of origin | **STAGE 1**<br>Tumor limited to tissue of origin |
| **GRADE 2**<br>Moderately well differentiated, with evidence of structural changes from normal tissue of origin | **STAGE II**<br>Limited local spread |
| **GRADE 3**<br>Poorly differentiated, with extensive structural changes from normal tissue of origin | **STAGE III**<br>Extensive local and regional spread |
| **GRADE 4**<br>Very anaplastic, with no resemblance to tissue of origin | **STAGE IV**<br>Widespread metastasis |

From Phipps WJ et al: *Medical-surgical nursing: concepts and clinical practice,* ed 5, St Louis, 1995, Mosby.

## Tissue Sampling

A definitive diagnosis of cancer can be made only when a pathologist sees malignant cells in a tissue specimen that is viewed under a microscope. A number of techniques can be used to make a tissue diagnosis.

## Exfoliative Cytology

Exfoliative cytology, or the Pap smear test, is used to study cells that the body has shed during the normal sequence of body tissue growth and replacement. If cancer is present, cancer cells are also shed. By studying these cells under the microscope, malignant conditions can be diagnosed before the patient notices symptoms. The test originally was developed to diagnose early cancer of the cervix, but it now can be used effectively to study cells shed from the stomach, esophagus, lungs, colon, and bladder, as well as discharge from the breasts. If cancer cells are found, a biopsy is always done.

To detect cancer of the cervix, cervical secretions are obtained during a pelvic examination. The examination is a simple, painless procedure that should be performed annually in women age 18 or older. The nurse can help the patient by explaining how to prepare for the examination. The Pap smear is not done during the menstrual period. The patient should not douche for several hours before the test, and both coitus and tub bathing should be avoided for 24 hours before the test. A Pap smear is primarily a screening test, and further examination may be necessary to confirm a diagnosis. This simple test has resulted in a decrease in the death rate for cervical cancer.

## Biopsy

A biopsy is the surgical removal of a piece of tissue for microscopic examination. There are several biopsy techniques. An *incisional* biopsy involves taking a small sample out of a tissue mass, whereas an *excisional* biopsy involves removing all of the known tumor. An incisional needle biopsy can be performed when tumors are close to the skin, visible on x-ray films or scans, or seen during endoscopic procedures. Fine needle biopsies are easy to do but yield only a few cells. Larger bore needles give bigger tissue samples but are more difficult to perform.

Simple biopsies can be performed in a physician's office, but excisional biopsies that require sedation are performed in the hospital or an outpatient surgery center. Needle biopsies of internal organs often are done in the radiology department with the guidance of x-ray films or ultrasound scans. If the biopsy is taken from an external lesion, preparation includes use of an antiseptic and an injection of a local anesthetic, such as 2% Procaine solution. Using a special biopsy instrument, the physician removes a small amount of tissue for examination, after which a sterile dressing is applied. Although the biopsy is a simple procedure, it may not seem simple to a frightened, nervous patient.

A frozen-section biopsy allows a tissue specimen to be examined quickly during an operation, so that it can be determined immediately whether the tissue is benign or malignant. With this technique, the specimen is immediately frozen, cut, and stained. Although this method is not satisfactory for a detailed study of the cells, possible malignancies can be identified promptly. Permanent sections of the tissue are prepared so that the pathologist can use special stains to make a definite diagnosis. Patients should be told that these biopsies usually take several days to process and that a diagnosis may be delayed until then.

## Imaging Techniques: Direct Visualization

The primary location and anatomic spread of cancer can be determined by a number of imaging techniques that use direct or indirect visualization. Direct visualization techniques involve introducing fiberoptic endoscopy tubes into hollow organs to view internal surfaces. Fiberoptic tubes contain lighting, magnifying devices, and attachments that allow brushings or biopsies to be performed.

### Bronchoscopy

Bronchoscopy is the examination of the trachea and bronchi after local or general anesthesia has been induced. The bronchoscope is inserted through the nose and advanced into the upper airway. Biopsies or brushings of suspicious areas can be done through the tube. The patient's throat is numbed during this procedure to prevent discomfort and gagging. After the procedure, the patient is warned not to eat or drink until the gag reflex returns, which should occur within 2 hours. The nurse monitors the patient for signs of breathing difficulties or bleeding after the procedure.

### Esophagoscopy and Gastroscopy

Esophagoscopy and gastroscopy involve the visualization of the esophagus and stomach by using a flex-ible tube inserted through the patient's mouth. Biopsies or washings can be taken during the procedure. Before the procedure the patient is instructed not to eat or drink after midnight. The patient is given medication before the gastroscopy to permit relaxation and sleepiness. The patient is asked to arrange for someone else to take him or her home after the procedure.

### Sigmoidoscopy

Sigmoidoscopy is the examination of the anus, rectum, and sigmoid colon by use of a rigid tube that can be up to 25 cm (10 inches) long. Tumors, polyps, or ulcerations may be studied by examination and biopsy. It is extremely important that all fecal matter be removed before the examination, and this usually is accomplished with cleansing enemas. Laxatives and cathartics are seldom given before the procedure, but the nurse should be familiar with the exact preparation the physician requests. The patient is placed in the knee-chest position and is draped to expose only the anal area. In some situations it may be desirable to place the patient in a side-lying position. The patient should be given information about the examination and what to expect. He or she should know that there may be some discomfort but that the procedure usually is not painful. Because the examination often is fatiguing, especially for an elderly person, the nurse should arrange for the patient to rest after the procedure. Providing light nourishment may be appropriate.

### Colonoscopy

Colonoscopy involves the examination of the entire colon by means of a long, flexible tube. Preparation of the bowel for a colonoscopy is more extensive than for a sigmoidoscopy. The patient must be on a liquid diet and use laxatives and enemas before the examination.

## Imaging Techniques: Indirect Visualization

Indirect visualization techniques include radiographic tests such as chest x-ray examinations, mammograms, gastrointestinal series, barium enemas, computed axial tomography (CAT) scans, and **radioisotope** studies. They also include nonradiographic tests such as ultrasound scans and **magnetic resonance imaging** (MRI).

Radiographic studies can be done with or without contrast. Noncontrast x-ray examinations include chest x-ray examinations, mammograms, and abdomen and bone films. Contrast x-ray examinations use materials such as air, iodine-containing dyes, or barium to outline an organ. Contrast x-ray examinations include lymphangiograms, myelograms, and barium studies of the gastrointestinal tract.

X-rays, which are produced in a vacuum tube, are electromagnetic waves similar to light waves and heat waves. X-rays have the ability to penetrate most substances and alter a photographic plate, which produces an image of the substances through which the rays pass. The image reflects the varying densities of substances such as bone, soft tissue, fat, and air. Body cavities, organs, and bones can be visualized, which assists the physician in diagnosis and treatment. Fluoroscopy is an x-ray technique in which the radiologist views internal structures while they are functioning. For example, fluoroscopy of the chest enables the radiologist to view the expansion and contraction of the lungs. Nurses may be requested to assist while diagnostic x-ray films are being made. Precautions must be taken to avoid exposure to radiation. A nurse who remains in the room with the patient should wear a lead apron and possibly gloves.

## Mammography

Mammography is a safe, simple technique for detecting breast tumors. A low-energy beam is used to make films of the soft breast tissue without the use of a radiopaque medium. It often is possible to differentiate between a benign tumor and a malignant one. To obtain a good quality image, the breast must be compressed firmly, and women who have sensitive breasts may find this an uncomfortable procedure. A mammogram is recommended for women who have signs and symptoms of breast disease, a familial history of breast cancer, or large, pendulous breasts that make palpation difficult. A previous breast biopsy or breast surgery also is an indication for mammography. All women should have a baseline mammogram done at age 40 and then have one every 1 to 2 years until age 49. A yearly mammogram is now recommended as a screening test for all women age 50 or older.

## Barium Enema

A patient must be prepared carefully when the physician wants to visualize the colon above the sigmoid. It is important that all fecal matter be removed from the colon because any residue may interfere with a correct diagnosis. Usually the patient takes nothing by mouth after midnight and is given laxatives, rectal suppositories, and enemas. Enemas often are given until the solution returns free of fecal material. A poorly prepared

patient may delay the examination, which is an inconvenience to the x-ray department and results in additional expense to the patient.

After following the prescribed cleansing measures, the patient reports to the x-ray department at the scheduled hour and is given an enema of barium, a radiopaque substance, which the patient is asked to retain. Using the fluoroscope, the radiologist observes the filling of the colon, after which x-ray films are taken. The patient then is allowed to evacuate the barium. Sometimes the radiologist has the patient return for air-contrast studies after evacuating the barium. The colon is distended with air, and additional x-ray films are taken. The patient may feel exhausted after the examination, and therefore a period of rest is desirable. Because barium that has been retained in the bowel becomes difficult to expel, a warm oil retention enema or a laxative, such as magnesium citrate, may be ordered after the examination.

## Gastrointestinal Series

The gastrointestinal (GI) series is an x-ray examination of the upper GI tract using a radiopaque contrast medium. It is used to identify pathologic conditions in tissues of the stomach and duodenum. Because food in the stomach results in misleading x-ray films, the patient is told not to eat or drink for at least 6 to 8 hours before the examination. The patient reports to the x-ray department at the scheduled hour and is given a mixture of barium to drink. The fluoroscope is used to observe the barium as it passes through the esophagus and into the stomach. X-ray films are taken at specific intervals over several hours to study the movement of the barium from the stomach to the small intestine. The patient is not given any food until the x-ray department indicates that it is finished with the tests. Many patients, especially older adults, find the examination fatiguing, and the patient usually is hungry. He or she should be served a warm, appetizing meal, made comfortable, and allowed to rest undisturbed. In ambulatory settings the patient may remain in the area for observation and stabilization. A cathartic may be included in the barium mixture or ordered after the examination to hasten elimination of the barium from the intestines.

## Computed Tomography

Computed tomography (CT), also known as a CAT scan, is a computer-aided x-ray examination that has proven to be a major breakthrough in diagnostic technique. Conventional x-ray films can differentiate only bone, soft tissue, fat, and air with any precision. CT is

100 times more sensitive to differences in tissue densities, and individual organs and structures within organs can be seen. A narrow x-ray beam is rotated around the patient, and multiple exposures are made. Sensitive detectors record the results, which are processed by a computer. An image of the body section exposed to the x-ray beam, or tomogram, is constructed. Each image represents a horizontal cross-section, or "slice," of the body. This diagnostic device can be used to detect tumors and other pathologic conditions without performing special procedures that often are painful, complicated, invasive, or risky.

Because the x-rays are focused on a few thin layers of the body, the patient receives no more radiation than with a conventional x-ray examination. The patient lies on an adjustable hydraulic couch, and the scanner rotates around the chosen site. As the scanner rotates, it makes a clicking noise, which may frighten the unsuspecting patient. Patients must remain completely still because motion disturbs the image. Snug-fitting restraints often are used as appropriate. The procedure is safe and painless and usually requires no specific preparation or follow-up. Sometimes a contrast medium is given to highlight certain parts of the body. If the contrast medium is given intravenously, the patient is warned that it may cause a warm sensation. The x-ray staff should be alerted if the patient is allergic to iodine or contrast mediums. If an oral or intravenous (IV) contrast medium is to be used, the patient usually is told not to eat or drink for several hours before the test. The radiology department should be consulted for specific instructions for each test.

## Radioisotope Studies

Radioisotopes are elements that emit rays of energy. They occur naturally as radium or uranium or can be artificially produced from other elements. The most widely used radioisotopes in medicine are altered forms of iodine, phosphorus, cobalt, iron, and gold. The patient needs no specific preparation other than an explanation of the procedure. At a specified time the patient is given an intravenous injection of an isotope that has a tendency to accumulate in the organ to be studied. In the radioisotope laboratory, a sensing device charts or maps the areas of the organ that have picked up the radioactive material. Variations from normal are seen as lighter or darker areas and indicate abnormality of the organ, which often is a malignancy. For example, radioactive iodine is readily assimilated by the thyroid gland, and pathogenesis can be detected during a thyroid scan. It is now possible to scan most major organs, such as the brain, kidneys, liver,

pericardium, and bone. Because such minute amounts of radioactive material are used and because the material is eliminated so quickly, the patient is not considered radioactive.

## Magnetic Resonance Imaging

MRIs are relatively new. An MRI uses a magnetic field and radiofrequency sound waves to produce excellent images of the soft tissues, veins, arteries, brain, and spinal cord. The procedure is not invasive and poses no risk for radiation exposure. However, an MRI is costly ($700 or more) and may last up to 1½ hours. The patient must remove all metal objects and lie still for periods of up to 20 minutes on a narrow stretcher that is rolled into a shallow tunnel. Despite efforts to prevent claustrophobia by providing mirrors, a call button, and a voice-activated intercom, the procedure is frightening to many people. Teaching by the nurse is essential to reduce anxiety. Guided imagery and rhythmic breathing may be useful for distraction and for giving the patient control. As an alternative, the physician may order a light sedative. Some machines have been designed to allow the patient to be in a more open space during the examination—the so-called open MRI.

## Ultrasonography

Ultrasound techniques use high-frequency sound waves instead of x-rays to show the structure and function of internal organs. A sound wave transducer (transmitter and receiver) is moved over the skin. The sound waves pass through the skin and send echoes back to the transducer as they strike various organs. Each tissue produces a distinctive echo that can be identified by the transducer. The sound waves are changed into electrical energy that forms an image on a screen. With the advent of CT scans and MRIs, ultrasound has been used less but is still a good diagnostic test for some cancers and often is used to complement x-ray examinations. The advantages of ultrasound are that no radiation exposure or injections are involved and the patient feels no discomfort. Usually no special preparation is needed. The patient is asked to fast for several hours before a GI ultrasound and to drink fluids and keep the bladder full for pelvic ultrasounds.

## Laboratory Studies

Analyzing chemicals in the blood may help in diagnosing the type and extent of cancer. Some cancers produce substances called tumor markers. For example, carcinoembryonic antigen (CEA) is commonly found in metastatic colon cancer, and CA-125 usually is elevated in ovarian cancer. Elevated acid phosphatase and PSA levels may be found in people with prostate cancer. Most of these tests are not very useful in screening for cancer because these chemicals are also elevated in many benign conditions. PSA is now recommended as a screen for prostate cancer, but many experts do not consider it a cost-effective screening test. Tumor markers are most useful in evaluating responses to treatment.

# TREATMENT OF CANCER

Cancer may be treated in four ways: through surgery, radiotherapy, chemotherapy (including hormones), and biotherapy. Early diagnosis and treatment may result in a cure, whereas delayed diagnosis and treatment may result in treatment that is palliative only, with death the inevitable outcome. For many, cancer becomes a chronic illness, and nursing care focuses on rehabilitation and efforts to optimize the patient's quality of life.

## Surgery

Surgery often is the primary treatment for cancer, and it may be performed for various purposes. It may be preventive, diagnostic, curative, or palliative and may range from the removal of a small tumor to extensive surgical excision. Surgery is considered preventive if a premalignant lesion is removed, such as a suspicious mole or a colon polyp. Diagnosis of cancer in internal organs often requires a surgical procedure. In recent years laparoscopy has reduced the need for open surgical biopsies. Surgery is curative if a malignant tumor is completely removed before it spreads beyond the local area. If the cancer has metastasized, surgery usually is only palliative, such as for relieving intestinal obstruction or controlling pain. Palliative surgery contributes to the patient's comfort and may prolong life. Surgery that is performed early, before metastasis occurs, offers the best chance for cure.

Research is under way to find ways to increase the chances of cure by surgery. The effects of chemotherapy and/or radiation therapy administered before, during, or after surgery are being investigated; this type of therapy is called "adjuvant therapy." Some inoperable tumors have been reduced in size by drugs or radiation so that surgery can be performed. A course of chemotherapy or radiation therapy that is given after all visible tumor has been removed may reduce the risk of recurrence in some cancers, such as some stages of breast and colorectal cancer. Adjuvant chemother-

apy or hormonal therapy is commonly used for the treatment of early stage breast cancer after surgery and/or radiation therapy.

Newer surgical techniques and tools have been developed. Cryosurgery is used to treat some cancers of the skin and mouth, as well as other superficial lesions. Cryosurgery destroys tumors by freezing them with liquid nitrogen. Laser surgery uses intense light beams to vaporize some cancerous lesions such as those on the larynx or tumors that block the bronchi of the lung. Reconstructive or plastic surgery may be used to correct defects caused by the original surgical intervention. Many women are now choosing to have breast reconstruction after a modified radical mastectomy for breast cancer.

The preoperative and postoperative nursing care of patients undergoing surgical procedures for cancer is essentially the same as for any other type of surgery and is reviewed in the appropriate sections. However, psychosocial needs often are more intense because of the potential or actual diagnosis of cancer.

## Radiotherapy

Radiotherapy, or **radiation therapy,** refers to the use of ionizing radiation to treat tumors. Radiation is ionizing when it can break atoms of a substance into smaller parts that carry a positive or negative charge (ions). The most common types of radiation, such as heat and light, are not ionizing. X-rays, gamma-rays, and radioactive particles (electrons, neutrons, and protons) are types of ionizing radiation. When ionizing radiation passes through living tissue, it damages DNA molecules and disrupts cell function and division. The goal in using various forms of radiation to treat cancer is to give doses that are large enough to destroy cancer cells without causing irreparable damage to normal tissue that surrounds the tumor. Although both normal and malignant cells can be destroyed, most malignant cells are more susceptible to ionizing rays than are normal cells. Radiation therapy may be used to obtain a cure either alone or in combination with surgery or chemotherapy, or both, or it may be used for palliation of symptoms when a cure is impossible.

Ionizing radiation is considered hazardous material because both short-term and chronic exposure causes cellular changes that can lead to gene mutation, birth defects, and carcinogenesis. Whether the radiation is for diagnostic or treatment purposes, precautions must be taken to minimize patient and personnel exposure. People who work in radiation areas are carefully monitored to ensure that they do not receive more than the maximum permissible dose each year (5 rem). Nurses are most at risk for radiation exposure

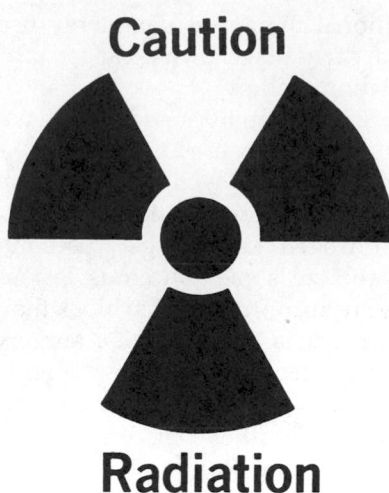

## Caution

## Radiation

**Figure 12-3** Radiation symbol.

when caring for patients receiving internal radiation therapy. Safety precautions are discussed later in this chapter. The symbol for a radiation area is shown in Figure 12-3.

Two general types of radiation therapy currently are used: external beam radiation (teletherapy) and internal radiation therapy (brachytherapy). External beam therapy is given from outside the body with various radiation-generating machines. Internal radiation therapy places a radiation source close to the tumor. Sealed radiation sources can be placed into the tumor-containing tissue or into a cavity close to the tumor. Unsealed internal radiation uses solutions of radioisotopes that emit ionizing radiation.

### External Beam Radiation Therapy

External beam radiation therapy uses machines that deliver ionizing radiation from outside the body. The most widely used radiation machine today is the linear accelerator, which generates supervoltage radiation that can be accurately directed to deep tumors, sparing the skin from damage. Before the first treatment is administered, the exact area to be irradiated is carefully mapped during a process called *simulation.* Indelible ink or tattoo marks are placed on the skin and are used to position the machine before each treatment. Shielding, in the form of lead blocks, is provided to protect the sites not being treated. Radiation generally is given in small doses over time, usually Monday through Friday each week for 4 to 8 weeks. Palliative radiation takes less time. This method of delivering radiation, which is called *fractionation,* may increase the destruction of cancer cells while minimizing damage

to normal tissues. Most of radiation treatment planning is now computerized.

**Assessment.** Before starting a course of external beam radiation therapy, the patient is assessed for knowledge level, including misconceptions or anxiety about the therapy. Any self-care deficits are noted, especially restrictions in mobility that would affect the patient's ability to get to the daily treatments or to get on and off the treatment table. Significant symptoms, such as pain, are noted and addressed. A baseline assessment is made of nutritional status and of skin integrity in the radiation field. The nurse should be aware of the location of the radiation field and the side effects that might result from damage to the underlying tissues (Dow, Hilderley, 1992; Strohl, 1996, Iwamoto, 1997).

> **NURSE ALERT**
>
> A patient who is receiving external beam radiation therapy is never a source of radiation." The nurse can help reduce patient anxiety by dispelling any misconceptions about radiation therapy.

**Nursing interventions.** External beam radiation therapy most often is given on an outpatient basis. The radiation oncologist usually explains the course of therapy prescribed for the patient. Nurses often can clarify uncertainties, answer questions, and explain the radiation procedure more fully. Teaching self-care measures to patients receiving external beam radiation therapy is essential, especially if the patient is receiving therapy as an outpatient. New patients usually are extremely apprehensive and need much reassurance and support. The term *radiation therapy* often incites fear in both the patient and the family, and this type of therapy often is viewed as the last resort when all else has failed.

It is helpful if the patient can be oriented to the radiation therapy department before the first treatment. It is important to explain to the patient that he or she will not become radioactive and that the treatments do not hurt. The nurse should explain that the patient lies very still on a table during the treatment and that the machine often rotates around the table making a clicking sound. Although the patient must be left alone during the 1- to 3-minute treatment, registered radiation therapists observe and are in constant communication with the patient from outside the shielded room.

The patient is informed that during the course of treatment, there may be some reddening of the treated skin, which may turn dark in color, become dry, itch, and slough (*dry* **desquamation**). The nurse should avoid referring to the reddening as a burn. When the radiation is directed close to the skin's surface or includes skin folds or prominences, the area may blister, crack, or weep (*moist desquamation*) (Strohl, 1988; Sitton, 1992).

Whether the patient may shower or bathe depends on the policies of the radiation therapy department. If permitted, the patient is instructed to use a mild, moisturizing soap such as unscented Dove, Ivory, Basis, or Neutrogena. The patient is also instructed to pat, not rub, the area dry. If ink markings are used, the patient must be careful not to remove them during bathing. Tattoo marks are permanent.

Ointments, medications, perfumes, cosmetics, powders, shaving lotions, and deodorants are not used in the treatment field unless approved by the radiation therapy department. These products may contain alcohol, oils, or metals that can react with the radiation and cause skin problems. These restrictions do not apply to the rest of the patient's skin. Cornstarch or unscented lotions usually are allowed to alleviate itching on unbroken skin. If moist desquamation occurs, great care must be taken to prevent infection. All routine skin products are withheld, and the radiation oncologist or nurse is consulted for further treatment. If ointments or dressings are ordered, they often must be removed and the skin cleansed before treatment is administered.

Extremes of heat or cold, such as ice packs, heat lamps, steam baths, whirlpools, or saunas, should be avoided in the irradiated area. The treated skin should not be exposed to the sun for the rest of the patient's lifetime. The patient is strongly urged to use protective clothing and sunscreen. Tight-fitting or rough clothes over the treatment area may cause irritation. Soft, loose-fitting cotton undergarments or shirts may be more comfortable next to the skin.

Because radiation therapy is more effective when the patient's nutritional status is good, a high-calorie, high-protein diet generally is recommended. Patients receiving external beam radiation may experience nausea, vomiting, and diarrhea. These reactions are most common when radiation is given to or near the GI tract. Several small feedings per day may be tolerated better than regular meals. If vomiting is severe, food intake may be reduced to liquids only and increased to 3000 ml/day to compensate for fluid loss. Several drugs, including prochlorperazine (Compazine) and trimethobenzamide (Tigan) may help control nausea and vomiting. Diarrhea usually can be controlled with loperamide (Imodium) or diphenoxy-late (Lomotil). Many radiation therapy departments have registered dietitians available to counsel patients and families about optimizing nutrition during therapy. Fatigue is common and peaks during the fourth and fifth weeks of therapy. Extra rest periods are encouraged throughout therapy, but some planned exercise may help restore energy levels.

The cumulative effects of radiation may involve damage to the bone marrow, where blood cells are formed. White blood cells are highly sensitive to radiation and may be destroyed. The resulting **leukopenia** produces an increased susceptibility to infection. Low platelet levels produce **thrombocytopenia,** and an increased tendency to hemorrhage may result, which necessitates that the patient be protected from injury. Anemia may also occur from the depression of red blood cell formation. Complete blood cell counts generally are done every week.

Additional symptoms may occur, depending on the site being treated. Radiation to the scalp may cause alopecia, or loss of hair. Cystitis may occur with radiation to the pelvis, and pneumonitis may occur with radiation to the lungs. Radiation to the mouth, throat, and neck often results in mouth soreness (stomatitis) and ulceration and a decrease in salivation, which may impair fluid and nutritional intake (Box 12-5).

Patients are encouraged to report any symptoms that may occur so that appropriate comfort measures can be started (Box 12-6). Symptoms gradually get worse during the treatment course and usually resolve within a few weeks after treatment ends. Although great care is taken during treatment planning to minimize radiation effects on normal tissues, damage can occur. Radiation effects can be divided into acute (those that arise during treatment to 6 months after) and chronic (those of variable onset after 6 months) (Table 12-3). Many of the acute changes have been discussed previously; these mostly involve tissues that contain many dividing cells, such as the skin, mucous membranes, bowel lining, hair follicles, and bone marrow. Acute reactions usually are reversible. Chronic changes involve tissues with cells that divide more slowly, such as muscles and the vascular system. Chronic effects include tissue fibrosis, tissue necrosis, fistula formation, and cataracts. These changes are rarely reversible.

## Sealed Internal Radiation Therapy

Sealed internal radiation therapy involves implantation or insertion of a radioactive substance directly into a tumor or in close proximity to a tumor (Strohl, 1996). Temporary radioactive sources (e.g., iridium-192 or cesium-137) are sealed inside applicators and placed into the tumor area for several days. They are

BOX 12-5

**Guidelines for Care of Patient with Mouth and Throat Problems**

The linings of the mouth and throat are among the most sensitive areas of the body. Cancer patients, especially those receiving chemotherapy or radiation treatments, often complain of soreness in these areas. These problems seem directly related to the treatment. Recent surgery in the head and neck area also may result in chewing and swallowing difficulties. Physicians may prescribe medicine to control mouth and throat pain or infection. Dentists also can give tips for mouth care. Remember that part of the healing process in this area of the body depends on eating well and drinking fluids. Eating food and drinking fluids are imperative for patients undergoing treatment for mouth and throat lesions.

*If the patient has a sore mouth or throat, suggest the following:*

1. Try soft foods that are easy to chew and swallow, such as milkshakes, soft fruits, cottage cheese, mashed potatoes, custards, puddings, gelatin, scrambled eggs, oatmeal, pureed foods, and liquids.
2. Cut food into small pieces.
3. Mix food with butter, thin gravies, and sauces to make it easier to swallow.
4. Use a blender or food processor to puree foods.
5. Use a straw to drink fluids.

6. Try foods cold or at room temperature. Hot and warm foods can irritate a tender mouth.
7. Avoid irritating foods such as citrus fruits or juices, spicy or salty foods, and rough, coarse, or dry foods.
8. Rinse the mouth often with water to remove food and bacteria.
9. Do not wear dentures if sores are present.
10. Consult the physician about numbing medications that permit anesthesia while eating.

*If the patient has a changed sense of taste, suggest the following:*

1. Choose and prepare foods that look and smell good.
2. Avoid foods that have an unpleasant taste.
3. Try tart foods, which may have more taste.

*If the patient has a dry mouth, suggest the following:*

1. Try very sweet or tart foods and beverages, such as lemonade. These foods help the mouth produce more saliva. Do not use these if the mouth is sore.
2. Suck on sugar-free hard candy or popsicles or chew sugar-free gum.
3. Eat foods with sauces and gravies.
4. Sip water often.
5. Keep the lips moist with lip salves.
6. Ask the physician or dentist about artificial saliva.

Modified from National Cancer Institute: *Eating hints,* NIH Pub No 92-2079, Washington, DC, 1992, The Institute.

TABLE 12-3

## Side Effects of External Radiation Therapy

| TIME OF OCCURRENCE | SIDE EFFECTS |
|---|---|
| Acute (during treatment and up to 6 months after treatment; usually reversible) | Skin reactions |
| | Erythema |
| | Dry desquamation |
| | Moist desquamation |
| | Nausea and vomiting |
| | Diarrhea |
| | Fatigue |
| | Bone marrow suppression |
| | Stomatitis |
| | Cystitis |
| | Pneumonitis |
| Chronic (6 months after radiation therapy; often permanent) | Fibrosis (lung, bladder, heart) |
| | Fistulas |
| | Necrosis (bone, nerve) |
| | Paresthesia |
| | Cataracts |
| | Cancer |

removed after a calculated dose of radiation has been delivered. Applicators come in a variety of forms. Needles, seeds, or wires may be implanted directly into tumors such as head and neck or prostate neoplasms. Tubes and capsules are used for internal radiation of the cervix and uterus. Permanent insertion of gold-198 or iodine-125 seeds may be used to treat some prostate, lung, and brain tumors. Because the radioactivity of these seeds decays rapidly, radiation exposure is minimal after the first few days and the seeds do not need to be removed.

**Nursing interventions.** A patient who is to have a radiation source implanted is assessed and prepared in the same way as most surgical patients. For a cervical or uterine implantation, a cleansing enema is given the night before treatment. A douche may also be given. During surgery the physician positions the applicator and either inserts the radioactive substance at that time (preloading) or waits until the patient has returned to the hospital bed (afterloading). Afterloading is often preferred because fewer hospital personnel are exposed to the radiation.

---

◄ **BOX 12-6** ► **NURSING PROCESS**

## EXTERNAL BEAM RADIATION THERAPY

**ASSESSMENT**

- Level of knowledge and understanding
- Anxiety level
- Restrictions in mobility and activities of daily living
- Skin condition in radiation field
- Presence and level of pain
- Nutritional status
- Area of body to be irradiated

**NURSING DIAGNOSES**

- Knowledge deficit related to treatment with external beam radiation
- Anxiety related to the procedures and effects of radiation
- Risk for impaired skin integrity related to radiation therapy
- Risk for altered nutrition related to effects of radiation therapy

**NURSING INTERVENTIONS**

- Observe for and manage radiation reactions (nausea, vomiting, diarrhea, skin reddening, skin breakdown, fatigue, weakness, anorexia, leukopenia, thrombocytopenia, anemia, and specific symptoms according to radiation site).

- Give reassurance and support.
- Include the following in patient teaching:
  Purposes and procedures
  Skin markings not to be removed
  Skin care instructions
  Diet high in calories, protein, and fluids
  Rest and exercise planning
  Reporting of infection and bleeding
  Site-specific symptom management (e.g., nausea, diarrhea, mucositis)

**EVALUATION OF EXPECTED OUTCOMES**

- Verbalizes understanding of the purposes of the therapy and procedures used
- Verbalizes less anxiety related to fear of the unknown or to misconceptions
- Verbalizes understanding of the importance and rationale of maintaining a high-calorie, high-protein diet and high fluid intake during therapy
- Skin markings present
- Cares for skin; follows measures for preventing skin breakdown and infection
- Reports signs and symptoms of radiation reactions
- Adjusts activities to compensate for fatigue

---

After returning to the unit, the patient is placed in a private room, and a sign is placed on the bed and door indicating that the patient is receiving radiotherapy. The patient is instructed to lie quietly to avoid displacing the radioactive source. After the patient's vital signs have stabilized, the temperature, pulse, and respiration are checked every 4 hours unless the nurse is directed otherwise.

When applicators are placed in the vagina and uterus, the patient is positioned with the head and chest fairly low. The patient is turned often and encouraged to breathe deeply. The legs are held close together and straight, and the patient is carefully rolled to the side when turning. No perineal care is given while the applicator is in place in the cervix. The treatment usually lasts for only 1 or 2 days. A Foley catheter may be inserted into the bladder to prevent distention, and it should be checked at intervals to ensure that it is draining properly. Patients are checked for any bleeding and leakage of urine around the Foley catheter, and the radiation oncologist should be notified if such complications occur. Patients usually are

given a low-residue diet and diphenoxylate to prevent bowel movements that might dislodge the implant. However, the patient should use the bedpan for bowel evacuation if necessary and should be instructed not to strain. The contents of the bedpan are inspected carefully before disposal. All clothing and bed linens are inspected before they are removed from the room.

Dark threads are attached to the vaginal applicator and brought to the outside, where they are fastened to the skin. The patient is cautioned to avoid pulling on the threads, which are counted every 4 hours and recorded on the patient's chart. Long forceps and a lead carrier are kept in the patient's room in case the applicator is accidentally displaced. Dislodged applicators should never be picked up with the hands. The forceps and carrier can also be used to remove the implant. If any radioactive source becomes dislodged, the radiation therapist should be notified immediately.

Head and neck cancer patients with implants have the head of the bed elevated to 30 to 45 degrees and are monitored for airway obstruction. Saline irrigation every 3 to 4 hours may be ordered (Iwamoto, 1997). Any vomitus is inspected for displaced implants. Talking is difficult and should be avoided. The nurse can provide a writing pad or flash cards to facilitate communication.

Any patient with sealed implants should be observed for symptoms of a radiation reaction. Nausea, vomiting, malaise, and anorexia may indicate that the treatment needs to be altered. An elevated temperature may indicate an infection. The physician must be notified of any unusual symptoms.

Psychologic preparation of a patient who is receiving an implant also is important. Personal care during the treatment is minimal, and the patient usually is in isolation. The nurse can provide quiet diversional activities and can help relieve the patient's anxiety by stopping often at his or her door or calling on the intercom or telephone.

When a sealed, temporary isotope is used, the radiation oncologist determines the exact length of time it should remain in place, and it must be removed at exactly the specified time. The physician uses long-handled forceps to remove the isotope, which is washed and placed in a lead-lined container. After the radioactive source has been removed, the patient should be given a warm cleansing bath and made comfortable on a freshly made bed. The equipment and utensils in the room are not radioactive and require only routine cleaning.

Postprocedural self-care instructions are given to the patient before discharge. Normal tissues in the area of the applicator often become irritated from the effects of the radiation. The patient is warned of the potential side effects and how to alleviate symptoms. Because mucositis may occur after implantation in the mouth area, mouth care instructions are given to such patients. Women who have had vaginal or uterine implantations may experience dysuria and vaginal dryness. Sexual intercourse can be resumed in a few weeks with the physician's approval. Because vaginal stenosis can occur, routine vaginal dilation usually is recommended. The patient may need the nurse's help in dealing with the physical and emotional impact of this procedure (Box 12-7).

It is important to realize that the patient does not become radioactive. When the sealed applicator is re-

---

> **BOX 12-7**

## NURSING PROCESS

### SEALED INTERNAL RADIATION THERAPY

**ASSESSMENT**

- Level of knowledge and understanding
- Anxiety level
- Area of body to receive sealed radiation

**NURSING DIAGNOSES**

- Knowledge deficit related to treatment with sealed internal radiation
- Anxiety related to the procedures and effects of radiation
- Risk for altered nutrition related to effects of radiation therapy

**NURSING INTERVENTIONS**

- Follow precautions as ordered.
- Attach radiation symbol to door of room.
- Check vital signs.
- Check position of applicator q 4 hr.
- Observe for symptoms of radiation reaction.
- Observe for specific symptoms according to radiation site.
- Maintain measures for self-protection.
- Limit amount of time spent in room; organize well.

- Approach patient only when necessary. Communicate from doorway.
- Use shielding if available.
- Never touch a radiation source with bare hands. If the applicator becomes dislodged, pick it up with long forceps, place it in a carrier, and notify the radiologist immediately.
- Provide support and opportunities to communicate using the principles of time, shielding, and distance.
- Patient education should include the following:
  Purpose and procedures
  Instructing patient to lie quietly
  Quiet diversional activities
  Encouraging high fluid intake
  Providing postprocedural self-care instructions

**EVALUATION OF EXPECTED OUTCOMES**

- Verbalizes understanding of the purposes of the therapy and procedures
- Verbalizes less anxiety related to fear of unknown or to misconceptions
- Radioactive applicator remains in place
- Describes appropriate postprocedural self-care

moved from the body, no radiation remains. Body fluids are not radioactive unless part of the source has become dislodged and is present in excretions. The sealed applicator *is* a source of radiation, and nurses and other hospital personnel are *exposed* to some radiation when caring for these patients but do not *become* radioactive. Radiation safety precautions must be taken by all who come in contact with the patient. Visitors should be instructed to limit their visits and to stay at least 1.8 m (6 feet) from the patient. Pregnant women and children should not be allowed to visit the patient.

**Self-protection.** Three main factors determine the amount of radiation the nurse receives while caring for the patient. The amount of *time* spent with the patient should be the absolute minimum required for whatever care is necessary. However, nursing care should be planned so that good care is provided without the nurse presenting a hurried appearance. As the *distance* from the source of radiation (the patient) is increased, the amount of radiation exposure significantly decreases (Hilderley, Dow, 1996). When caring for a patient with a cesium source in the pelvis, the nurse should plan care so that no more than 30 minutes a day is spent at a distance of no less than about 1 m (3 feet) from the source. At a distance of 1.8 m (6 feet), 2 hours a day is safe. This general guideline also applies to visitors. When a radioisotope has been placed in the pelvic area, it is safer to stand and work near the head of the bed. When the radioisotope has been placed in the head area, it is safer to stand near the foot of the bed.

Speaking often to the patient from the doorway provides him or her with reassurance and gives the patient the opportunity to communicate without exposing personnel to undue radiation. A bedside telephone helps the patient keep in touch with family. *Shielding* must also be considered for self-protection. Various materials, such as a lead sheet or shield, can be placed between the nurse and the patient to absorb the radiation. All personnel who spend considerable time in radiation areas must wear a personnel monitoring device such as a film badge or a pocket dosimeter. The film badge is developed at intervals and observed for fogging that might indicate overexposure. It is important to understand that these badges are to measure an *individual's* exposure to radiation. Therefore nurses should not use others' badges or lend their badge to others. Pocket dosimeters provide immediate exposure readings. The nurse reads and records the reading on the dosimeter before and after entering the room. Most hospitals that provide radiation therapy have radiation safety officers, who monitor patient safety and calculate safe working times and distances for each isotope and dose.

## Unsealed Internal Radiation Therapy

Unsealed internal radiation therapy involves administration of radioisotopes orally or by injection. Isotopes of iodine, phosphorus, cobalt, and gold can be used for this therapeutic purpose. Each has specific characteristics and necessitates various protective measures. Depending on the radioisotope used and its pattern of distribution in the body, the radioactivity may be localized or spread throughout the body.

**Nursing interventions.** Radioactive iodine (iodine-131) is commonly used to treat thyroid diseases. Like many other isotopes, radioactive iodine circulates in the bloodstream and is eliminated from the body by the kidneys. When large doses are given for treatment, patients are admitted to the hospital for a 2- to 3-day stay. Patients are placed in isolation, and special care must be taken in the handling and disposal of all body fluids (blood, urine, feces, saliva, sweat, and vomitus). Nurses should wear latex gloves and gowns while providing direct care or handling body waste and linens. Floors and other surfaces in the room will be covered with plastic-backed pads. Disposable diet trays are ordered. All linens and waste are stored in special containers inside the room and checked for radioactivity before removal. Patients are instructed to flush the toilet several times after each use, and male patients are asked to sit while urinating to reduce the risk of splashing. The radiation principles of time, distance, and shielding must be used while the patient is in isolation (Box 12-8). In the first day 50% of the radioactive iodine is excreted from the patient's body, and the radioactivity of the retained iodine decreases by one half every 8 days. Therefore precautions are rarely necessary after 1 week. The radiation safety officer will determine when the patient may safely be discharged and will check the room for residual radioactive contamination before releasing it for use. Discharge teaching includes instructions on drinking plenty of fluids to help excrete the remaining radioiodine more quickly, good hand washing after going to the toilet, and avoiding close contact with pregnant women and children for the next week.

It is important to note that the patient receiving therapeutic doses of any radioisotope does become a source of radioactivity as long as the radioisotope remains within the body and continues to emit radiation, and the radiation safety principles of time, distance, and shielding must be used. Nursing personnel must know which radioisotope was used, how and when it was administered, how long it will continue to emit radiation, and how it is distributed and excreted by the body.

A number of newer radiation techniques are being used in specialized radiation centers. These techniques

# NURSING PROCESS

## UNSEALED INTERNAL RADIATION THERAPY

### ASSESSMENT

- Level of knowledge and understanding
- Anxiety level
- Type of radioisotope, half-life, route of administration, distribution and excretion pattern

### NURSING DIAGNOSES

- Knowledge deficit related to treatment with unsealed internal radiation
- Anxiety related to the procedure and effects of radiation
- Risk for altered nutrition related to effects of radiation therapy

### NURSING INTERVENTIONS

- Follow precautions as ordered.
- Post radiation symbol on door of room when patient is receiving therapeutic doses of radioisotopes.
- Check patient's room for the following items:
    Solid waste container
    Soiled linen container
    Other containers as directed by hospital radiation safety officer

- Check that all meals are served on disposable items.
- Maintain visitor restrictions (no one under age 18, no pregnant women).
- Maintain measures for self-protection; use the principles of time, distance, and shielding.
- Wear gloves when handling any body fluids.
- Patient education includes the following:
    Purpose and procedure
    Reason to remain in the room
    Quiet diversional activities
    Use of the bathroom and waste containers
    Postprocedural instructions

### EVALUATION OF EXPECTED OUTCOMES

- Verbalizes understanding of the purposes of the therapy and procedures used
- Verbalizes less anxiety arising from fear of the unknown or from misconceptions
- Remains in isolation and uses containers for urine, feces, and vomitus
- Participates in maintaining nutrition and fluid intake

---

include intraoperative radiation therapy, hyperthermia, radiation sensitizers and proton beam treatment (Hilderley, Dow, 1996). High-dose rate remote afterloading brachytherapy is an innovative new method of delivering a high dose of radiation to a tumor in a short period. It reduces treatment time, eliminates the need for hospitalization, and reduces health care providers' exposure to ionizing radiation.

Strontium-89 (Megastron), another radioactive isotope, is now an option for palliative treatment of bone pain caused by metastases. After injection, strontium-89 is handled by the body like calcium and is carried into the bones, where it delivers radiation to the bony metastases precisely where it is needed. Pain relief may take 1 or 2 weeks to achieve, but it lasts several months. Side effects are minimal and mostly involve a drop in blood cell count. The effects of strontium-89 are confined within the patient's body, and other people are not harmed by bodily contact. However, in the first week after injection, the radioisotope is present in blood and urine. The patient must be instructed on precautions to take, such as flushing the toilet twice, washing hands after urination, and laundering urine-

or blood-stained clothing separately. Hospitalized patients do not need to be isolated, but body fluid precautions are strictly enforced.

## NURSE ALERT

A patient receiving any form of internal radiation therapy may be a source of radiation. Nurses caring for these patients must adhere to the safety principles of time, distance, and shielding.

## Chemotherapy

**Chemotherapy** is the use of cytotoxic drugs to control the growth and multiplication of malignant cells. This important method of treatment is used to cure, control, or palliate many types of cancer. Unlike surgery and radiation therapy, which are localized treatments, chemotherapy travels to all parts of the body and acts

**TABLE 12-4**

## Pharmacology of Selected Drugs Used to Treat Cancer

| DRUG (GENERIC AND TRADE NAME); ROUTE, AND DOSAGE | ACTIONS AND INDICATIONS | COMMON SIDE EFFECTS AND NURSING CONSIDERATIONS |
|---|---|---|
| **Bleomycin Sulfate** (Blenoxane) **Route:** SC, IM, IV **Dosage:** 10-20 U/m² weekly or twice weekly; intrapleural dose is usually 60 U; do not exceed total dose 400 U in lifetime | Antitumor antibiotic used for testicular cancer, squamous cell carcinoma, and Hodgkin's disease; also used as a sclerosing agent for pleural effusions | Stomatitis, anorexia, fever, chills, pulmonary fibrosis, and alopecia; fever can be controlled by premedication and around-the-clock administration of acetaminophen; skin changes include hyperpigmentation, erythema, nail changes and loss, and inflammation of the palms and hands; pulmonary fibrosis occurs more often with a cumulative dose >300 U; watch for dyspnea, dry cough, and rales; anaphylaxis can occur |
| **Carboplatin** (Paraplatin) **Route:** IV **Dosage:** 360-400 mg/m² q 4 wk | Alkylating-like agent used for ovarian malignancies | Bone marrow suppression, nausea, vomiting, mild renal toxicity, thrombocytopenia, and anemia |
| **Cisplatin** (Platinol) **Route:** IV **Dosage:** Dosage varies, from 20-40 mg/m²/day for 3-5 days q 3-4 wk or from 20-120 mg/m² as a single dose q 3-4 wk | Heavy metal, alkylating-like agent used for testicular, bladder, ovarian, and lung malignancies | Nausea, vomiting, renal toxicity, neurotoxicity, and anemia; at high doses, rigorous prehydration and mannitol (for osmotic diuresis) may be given to reduce risk of renal damage; monitor renal function, electrolytes, BUN, and creatinine; 24-hr urine collection for creatinine clearance may be evaluated before therapy; mild myelosuppression except at higher doses; ototoxicity is cumulative and may be permanent; anaphylaxis can occur |
| **Cyclophosphamide** (Cytoxan) **Route:** IV, PO **Dosage:** May be given as single dose or in several divided doses over a period of time, (e.g., 500-1500 mg/m² IV q 3 wk; 50-200 mg/m² (1-5 mg/kg/day) PO daily for 14 days q 28 days) | Alkylating agent used for lymphoma and for breast and ovarian malignancies | Bone marrow suppression, hemorrhagic cystitis, nausea, gonadal changes, and alopecia; push fluids (1.9-2.6 L [2-3qt]/day) to maintain urine output; check urine for blood at each void; administer drug early in day to prevent accumulation in bladder; encourage frequent voiding; cardiac damage and necrosis are possible with very large single doses |
| **Cytarabine** (Ara-C, Cytosar) **Route:** IV, SC, Intrathecal **Dosage:** Varies | Antimetabolite used for leukemia | Bone marrow suppression, nausea, stomatitis, and headaches; nausea, vomiting, and diarrhea increase in severity with increasing doses; stomatitis and anorexia very common; rash, palmar erythema and desquamation, conjunctivitis, and cerebellar toxicities occur with larger doses |

*BUN,* Blood urea nitrogen; *bid,* twice a day; *IM,* intramuscular; *IV,* intravenous; *PO,* oral; *SC,* subcutaneous; *tid,* three times a day.

*Continued*

systemically. Drugs may also be used in combination with surgery or radiotherapy. Since chemotherapeutic drugs were first used against cancer in the 1950s, more than 60 agents have been developed through research and approved for human use by the U.S. Food and Drug Administration (FDA).

Chemotherapeutic drugs disrupt the internal metabolism of cells so that they are either prevented from multiplying or are killed directly (Table 12-4). The drugs usually are classified according to their mechanism of action. *Alkylating agents* react with the nuclear material of cells to impair cell division and growth. *Plant alkaloids* disrupt the mechanics of cell division. *Antimetabolites* block the formation of normal nuclear material. *Antibiotics* used in cancer therapy are highly toxic drugs and are not used to treat infections. Antitumor antibiotics appear to destroy nuclear material, although their mechanisms of action vary. The action

**TABLE 12-4**

## Pharmacology of Selected Drugs Used to Treat Cancer—cont'd

| DRUG (GENERIC AND TRADE NAME); ROUTE, AND DOSAGE | ACTIONS AND INDICATIONS | COMMON SIDE EFFECTS AND NURSING CONSIDERATIONS |
|---|---|---|
| **Doxorubicin** (Adriamycin)<br>**Route:** IV<br>**Dosage:** 60-75 mg/m² daily, repeat q 21 days or 25-30 mg/m² daily for 2-3 days, repeat q 3-4 wk or 20 mg/m² wk; total cumulative dose should not exceed 550 mg/m² without monitoring of cardiac function | Antitumor antibiotic used for acute leukemia, breast cancer, and ovarian cancer | Bone marrow suppression, nausea, vomiting, stomatitis, cardiac toxicity, and alopecia; drug is a vesicant—avoid extravasation to prevent necrosis; myelosuppression and nausea and vomiting may be severe; cardiotoxicity is dose limiting; flare reaction (facial flushing and local flushing at IV site) may occur, especially during rapid infusion; alert patient that urine will turn red; radiation recall can occur |
| **Etoposide** (VePesid, VP-16)<br>**Route:** PO, IV<br>**Dosage:** Common doses are 50-120 mg/m² IV daily for 3-5 days, infuse over at least 30 min | Plant alkaloid used for lung and testicular cancer | Bone marrow suppression, neurotoxicity, and alopecia; orthostatic hypotension and bradycardia occur if drug is infused too rapidly |
| **5-Fluorouracil** (5-FU)<br>**Route:** IV, Topical<br>**Dosage:** Several regimens have been used, including 300-450 mg/m² IV daily for 5 days q 28 days; 600-750 mg/m² IV weekly; 1000 mg/m² IV over 24 hr for 4-5 days; 1%-5% topical cream or solution to lesions 1-2 times daily for 2-12 wk | Antimetabolite used for colon, stomach, breast, and pancreatic cancer | Diarrhea, bone marrow suppression, stomatitis; stomatitis and diarrhea are dose limiting and can be severe; skin changes include nail changes and loss, rash, darkening of the veins used for drug administration, and photosensitivity |
| **Flutamide** (Eulexin)<br>**Route:** PO<br>**Dosage:** 250 mg q 8 hr tid for a daily dosage of 750 mg | Antiandrogen used for prostate cancer | Hot flashes, decreased libido, impotence, gynecomastia, diarrhea, nausea, vomiting, and hepatitis; monitor liver function studies |
| **Ifosfamide** (Ifex)<br>**Route:** IV<br>**Dosage:** 1-1.2 g/m² daily for 5 days, q 3-4 wk | Alkylating agent used for lymphoma and testicular cancer | Hemorrhagic cystitis, nausea, vomiting, alopecia, somnolence, confusion, and neurotoxicity; cystitis can be prevented by concomitant administration of mesna, a uroprotective agent; maintain rigorous hydration (at least 2 L/day); myelosuppression may be dose limiting |
| **Megestrol Acetate** (Megace)<br>**Route:** PO<br>**Dosage:** 40-320 mg/daily in divided doses | Progestin hormone with antiestrogenic properties; used for breast cancer | Nausea, vomiting, hypercalcemia, and thrombophlebitis at drug administration site; do not use if pregnant |
| **Methotrexate** (MTX)<br>**Route:** PO, IV, IM, Intrathecal<br>**Dosage:** IV doses vary from 20-40 mg/m² q 1-2 wk (solid tumors) to 200-500 mg/m² q 2-4 wk (leukemias and lymphoma); large doses should be accompanied by leucovorin | Antimetabolite used for leukemia, breast cancer, and lymphoma | Stomatitis, bone marrow suppression, nausea, and renal toxicity; stomatitis and diarrhea may be severe and warrant interruption of treatment; photosensitivity may occur even without exposure to sunlight; patient may develop erythematous rash and must be cautioned to use sunscreen when outdoors |

**TABLE 12-4**

## Pharmacology of Selected Drugs Used to Treat Cancer—cont'd

| DRUG (GENERIC AND TRADE NAME); ROUTE, AND DOSAGE | ACTIONS AND INDICATIONS | COMMON SIDE EFFECTS AND NURSING CONSIDERATIONS |
|---|---|---|
| **Tamoxifen Citrate** (Nolvadex) **Route:** PO **Dosage:** 10-20 mg bid | Antiestrogenic hormone used for breast cancer | Thrombocytopenia, leukopenia, nausea, vomiting, hot flashes, headache, and lightheadedness |
| **Taxol** (Paclitaxel) **Route:** IV **Dosage:** 135-250 mg/m² q 3 wk; 1-, 3-, 24-, and 72-hr infusions have been used | Plant alkaloid used for ovarian, breast, and lung cancer | Bone marrow suppression, stomatitis, alopecia (universal and complete), peripheral neuropathies, joint and muscle pains; bradycardia and hypersensitivity reaction (flushing, hypotension, dyspnea, bronchospasm, urticaria) may occur during administration; premedication with dexamethasone, diphenhydramine, and ranitidine is recommended to prevent hypersensitivity reaction |
| **Vinblastine** (Velban) **Route:** IV **Dosage:** 0.1 mg/kg or 3.7 mg/m² weekly or q 2 wk, not to exceed 0.5 mg/kg or 18.5 mg/m² weekly | Plant alkaloid used for lymphoma | Bone marrow suppression, neurotoxicity, stomatitis, alopecia, mental depression; drug is a potent vesicant—avoid extravasation |
| **Vincristine** (Oncovin) **Route:** IV **Dosage:** 1-2 mg/m² wk, not to exceed 2 mg | Plant alkaloid used for acute leukemia and Kaposi's sarcoma | Renal and hepatic toxicity, skin rash, stomatitis, and alopecia; drug is a potent vesicant—avoid extravasation; no bone marrow toxicity; constipation, paralytic ileus, and abdominal pain can occur, as well as peripheral neuropathy (tingling and numbness in hands and feet) |

of *hormones* is largely unknown, but some block the action of the natural hormone, such as estrogen and testosterone, that stimulates tumor growth. Steroid therapy sometimes is used as cancer therapy, generally to alter certain hormones.

Although chemotherapeutic drugs are effective in destroying or preventing the multiplication of cancer cells, normal tissue also is affected. Tissues that multiply rapidly, such as cells in the GI tract, hair follicles, and bone marrow, are affected most. As a result, side effects can be expected from administration of these drugs. The type and severity of the side effects are determined by the class and dosage of the drug (Walters, 1990; Bender, Yasko, 1996; Guy, Ingram, 1996; Langhorne, 1997).

### Assessment

Chemotherapy may be given with the intent to cure, control, or palliate. It is important to determine the patient's expectations regarding the outcome of the therapy. Although the physician is responsible for

informing the patient of the risks and benefits of chemotherapy, the nurse needs to assess the patient's level of understanding and reinforce teaching. Patients generally dread receiving chemotherapy, and it is not uncommon for them to refuse treatment because they fear side effects such as vomiting and hair loss. Nurses play an important role in helping patients find ways to cope with the physical and emotional reactions to chemotherapy (Box 12-9).

### Nursing Interventions

Before treatment begins, the drug regimen is reviewed thoroughly, and the patient and family are given written information about the drugs and their side effects. The nurse can explain that the patient may or may not experience significant side effects but that those that do occur usually can be well controlled if treated promptly. Therefore the patient should report any symptoms as soon as possible. The patient should be given the physician's 24-hour phone number before discharge.

◁ BOX 12-9 ▷

# NURSING PROCESS

## CHEMOTHERAPY

### ASSESSMENT

- Level of knowledge and understanding
- Anxiety level
- Nutritional status
- Oral status
- Vital signs
- Baseline blood cell counts
- Prescribed drugs, route, dosage, and potential side effects

### NURSING DIAGNOSES

- Knowledge deficit related to treatment with chemotherapy
- Anxiety related to treatment with chemotherapy
- Altered nutrition: less than body requirements related to disease and treatment with chemotherapy
- Risk for infection related to leukopenia
- Risk for injury: bleeding, related to thrombocytopenia
- Risk for impaired skin/mucous membrane integrity related to treatment with chemotherapy

### NURSING INTERVENTIONS
### Immediate

- Explain all procedures.
- Observe for and manage adverse reactions during administration of chemotherapy:
    Nausea and vomiting
    Vital sign changes
    Fluid status changes
    Mental status changes
    Hypersensitivity reactions
    Infiltration at IV site

- Follow safe chemotherapy handling and disposal procedures.

### Ongoing

- Monitor patient for potential side effects of chemotherapy.
- Monitor blood cell counts weekly as ordered.
- Patient and family teaching should include:
    Verbal and written information about general and specific side effects
    Management of nausea and vomiting
    Nutritional information, dietitian consult
    Mouth care instructions
    Prevention of infection
    Prevention of injury that could lead to bleeding
    Signs and symptoms of infection and bleeding to report to physician
    Management of hair loss and skin changes
    Management of fatigue
- Give patient and family reassurance and support.

### EVALUATION OF EXPECTED OUTCOMES

- Verbalizes understanding of the purposes of the therapy and procedures
- Verbalizes less anxiety about chemotherapy
- Describes potential side effects of chemotherapy and how to manage side effects if they occur
- Promptly reports signs and symptoms of infection and bleeding
- Maintains adequate nutrition, stable weight
- Oral mucosa remains intact
- Maintains normal activities

Common GI reactions include nausea, vomiting, anorexia, diarrhea or constipation, and possibly distortion of taste. Nausea and vomiting occur most often within a few hours of administration of the drug, although they may not occur at all in some patients. When the physician orders an antiemetic medication, the nurse can encourage the patient to take it regularly before and after treatment to prevent nausea and vomiting. In the past few years antiemetics have been developed that block serotonin uptake (ondansetron [Zofran] and granisetron [Kytril]) (Distasio, 1993). These drugs have fewer side effects than previously used antiemtics and have significantly reduced the incidence and severity of chemotherapy-induced nausea and vomiting. Small, frequent feedings are suggested if nausea does occur, and patients are encouraged to increase their fluid intake. Most hospitals have registered dietitians, who are knowledgeable about the effect of chemotherapy on the nutritional status of the cancer patient. Whenever possible, a nutritional consult should be obtained for patients receiving chemotherapy.

Soreness and ulceration of the mouth also may occur a week or two after chemotherapy. Good oral hygiene, including frequent rinsing of the mouth, is encouraged. Dry, cracked lips may be soothed with petroleum jelly. Dietary changes may be indicated (see Box 12-5). Fungal, viral, and bacterial infections are common complications that can cause further discomfort when the mucous membranes are damaged by chemotherapy. Early detection of such infections leads to prompt medical treatment and better control of symptoms.

Alopecia, or loss of hair, may be a significant psychologic event. Wigs, scarves, and cosmetics can be effective at concealing the hair loss. The patient should be encouraged to buy a wig before the hair is lost, which usually is a few weeks after chemotherapy is first given. Some ACS units provide free wigs. The nurse should reassure the patient that the hair will grow back once treatment is discontinued but that it may have a different color and texture. Because not all chemotherapy drugs cause hair loss, the nurse should first check which drugs the patient will be receiving. Nursing research has shown that "icing" the scalp before chemotherapy reduces hair loss. Several commercial caps are available to "ice" the scalp. However, this procedure may be uncomfortable to the patient. The treatment also cannot be used for patients with tumors that can metastasize to the skin, because the ice cap will prevent the chemotherapy from reaching this area and will create a sanctuary for the cancer cells.

Suppression of bone marrow (**myelosuppression**) produces the most serious side effects. The bone marrow continually produces the three major types of blood cells: white blood cells, platelets, and red blood cells. Chemotherapy temporarily stops the division of blood cells in the marrow, which leads to a drop in the number of circulating blood cells (nadir counts) 1 to 2 weeks after chemotherapy is given. Complete blood cell counts should be checked weekly or more often if indicated. Leukopenia, the reduction in the number of white blood cells, can increase the risk of infection (Greifzu, 1991). To reduce this risk, patients undergoing chemotherapy should be instructed to do the following:

1. Inform the physician or nurse about any signs of infection (e.g., fever, chills, cough, sore throat, urinary frequency, or skin rashes).
2. Maintain good hygiene techniques (e.g., keep nails and hair clean, wash hands before meals).
3. Maintain good perineal care, including washing the genitalia after urination or bowel movements.
4. Avoid individuals with colds and flu and avoid crowds during the flu season.

> **NURSE ALERT**
>
> Fever is the most reliable indicator of infection in a patient with leukopenia. The nurse must ensure that the patient has a thermometer at home and knows how to use it.

Antibiotics are given at the first sign of infection. Patients with very low white blood cell counts may be hospitalized and placed on "reverse isolation," with good hand washing precautions and masks for visitors with colds. Uncooked fruits and vegetables are eliminated from the diet while the white cell count is low. Strict reverse isolation, using laminar airflow rooms or plastic bubbles, is used in bone marrow transplantation units for patients with extreme and prolonged bone marrow suppression.

Thrombocytopenia, a low platelet count, increases the chance of hemorrhage. If the platelet count is very low or the patient shows signs or symptoms of bleeding, platelet transfusions are needed. Bleeding precautions should be observed in patients with a platelet count below 50,000 cells/mm$^3$. Patients who receive chemotherapy are instructed on how to avoid bleeding and what signs and symptoms of bleeding to report. Anemia is more common in patients who have been receiving chemotherapy for several months. When anemia results in symptoms such as extreme fatigue, headache, or shortness of breath, packed red blood cell transfusions may be ordered.

> **NURSE ALERT**
>
> A patient with a platelet count of less than 50,000 cells/mm$^3$ should be on bleeding precautions, which include the patient avoiding trauma and reporting unusual bleeding promptly. Nurses should monitor patients' skin, mucous membranes, urine, and stool for unusual bleeding and should avoid invasive procedures such as intramuscular injections and rectal temperatures.

Hematopoietic growth factors now are often used to stimulate normal bone marrow recovery after chemotherapy. They have allowed the use of higher doses of bone marrow suppressive antineoplastic drugs. Growth factors are a form of biologic response modifier. Granulocyte colony-stimulating factor (G-CSF, filgrastim [Neupogen]) stimulates the bone marrow to produce more of the bacteria-fighting white blood cells, called neutrophils. The patient experiences less leukopenia, and the risk of infection is reduced. Erythropoietin (Procrit, EPO) is another growth factor available for use in chemotherapy patients who become anemic. It specifically stimulates red blood cell production in the bone marrow. Both G-CSF and erythropoietin are given by subcutaneous injection, and nurses are responsible for teaching patients how to give themselves the injection.

Other side effects of chemotherapy can occur that are specific to the type of drug given. For instance, cardiac toxicity can occur with some antitumor antibiotics, and altered functioning of the reproductive system can result from hormone therapy. Other organs that can be damaged by chemotherapeutic drugs include the kidneys, lungs, liver, and peripheral nerves. It is important for the nurse to determine the expected side effects of the drugs the patient is receiving and provide appropriate patient and family teaching (see Box 12-9) (Wujcik, 1993).

Chemotherapy usually is given intermittently to minimize side effects. Often a combination of several drugs is used to maximize the killing of tumor cells without causing unacceptable side effects. A variety of routes of administration are used: oral, intramuscular, intravenous, intraarterial, intrathecal, and intraperitoneal. IV administration is a relatively short and painless procedure and is the most common route of administration. Some drugs are vesicants and can cause tissue damage if they leak outside the vein. Intravenous sites must be observed carefully, and the integrity of the patient's veins must be preserved. Venous punctures should be done only when absolutely necessary. Blood for some tests can be obtained by fingerstick.

Most chemotherapy is administered in outpatient clinics or an oncologist's office. Regimens that involve high drug doses or multiple-day infusions may be given in the hospital, most often on **oncology** units, where the nurses are well educated in chemotherapy administration. A new technique for delivering chemotherapy is the use of ambulatory infusion pumps. These portable, battery-operated pumps are designed to deliver continuous drug therapy. The pump is small and light enough to attach to the patient's belt and enables the patient to receive continuous chemotherapy while engaged in daily activities in the community.

Because chemotherapeutic drugs have the potential to alter cell DNA, it is important for the nurse to prevent self-exposure when caring for a patient who is receiving chemotherapy. The nurse should wear disposable gowns and latex gloves when handling the patient's blood, vomitus, or excreta for 48 hours after drug administration because the drugs are circulated in body fluids and excreted in the urine and stool. Chemotherapy-contaminated bags, tubing, and other waste must be placed in special chemotherapy waste containers. Each facility where chemotherapy is given must have policies and procedures for proper handling of hemotherapeutic drugs during preparation, administration, and disposal (OSHA, 1995; Langhorne, 1997).

## Bone Marrow Transplantation

Chemotherapy and radiation therapy are used in **bone marrow transplantation.** Introduced in the 1980s as an important means of treating leukemia and its related cancers, transplantation is now being used in more than 15 different diseases, including leukemias, lymphomas, multiple myeloma, and advanced or resistant solid tumors, such as breast cancer (Leukemia Society of America, 1995). Bone marrow transplantation begins by using very large doses of drugs to kill all the cancer cells. The patient's bone marrow is then restored to prevent life-threatening bleeding or infection. High doses of chemotherapy and radiation are given to eradicate all tumor cells from the patient's body, as well as to suppress the patient's immunity to donor marrow. The patient's bone marrow is replaced by bone marrow from a compatible donor or from the patient. There are three basic types of bone marrow transplantation: *autologous* (the patient is his or her own donor), *allogeneic* (a person with compatible tissue, usually a sibling, is the donor), and *syngeneic* (an identical twin is the donor).

The donor marrow is obtained from the hip bone with a special syringe and needle. Because the procedure can be painful, it usually is performed using general anesthesia. The donor may be stiff for a few weeks. The donated bone marrow, which is infused into the patient's bloodstream, travels to the bone, where it begins to produce a new population of blood cells. If the marrow successfully grows (engraftment) and no malignant cells recur, the patient may be cured of the cancer.

For several weeks after transplantation, while the new marrow is developing, the patient is kept in the hospital in a bone marrow transplant unit. During this time he or she is very susceptible to infection and may bleed easily. Blood products, antibiotics, and antifungal medications can be used to support the patient. Germ-free precautions are strictly enforced. The patient stays in the hospital for 1 to 2 months and is followed very closely as an outpatient. The immune system can take as long as 9 months to recover. A complication of allogeneic transplants (but not of the autologous or syngeneic type) is graft-versus-host disease. This disease results when the donor T lymphocytes recognize the patient's cells as foreign and attack them. Symptoms, which can range from minor to severe, include skin rash and peeling, nausea, vomiting, diarrhea, liver dysfunction, photophobia, and dryness and burning of the eyes.

*Peripheral stem cell* transplants have become more common in the past few years. They are used instead of or in addition to autologous bone marrow transplants. Circulating blood contains some of the same stem cells that are harvested from the marrow. Peripheral stem cells are collected by apheresis, a process of separating blood into its different components. This collection procedure is better tolerated than bone marrow aspiration. Recovery from peripheral stem cell

## PATIENT/FAMILY TEACHING

### CHEMOTHERAPY SIDE EFFECTS

**GASTROINTESTINAL**

| | |
|---|---|
| Nausea | Eat small frequent meals when least nauseated. |
| | Avoid fatty, fried, sweet, and odorous foods. |
| | Try to maintain fluids. |
| Vomiting | Do not eat or drink until vomiting is under control and then drink clear liquids before progressing to full liquids. |
| | Use antiemetics regularly, as prescribed. |
| Anorexia | Increase protein, carbohydrate, and vitamin intake. |
| | Eat nutritional snacks, high-protein drinks, and pudding. |
| Diarrhea | Report persistent watery stools to physician. |
| | Drink plenty of fluids to replace losses. |
| | Take antidiarrheal medicine as prescribed by physician. |
| Constipation | Eat plenty of fruits and vegetables if possible. |
| | Drink plenty of fluids. |
| | Exercise regularly. |
| | Take stool softeners and stimulants as advised by physician. |

**SKIN/MUCOUS MEMBRANES**

| | |
|---|---|
| Alopecia (loss of hair) | Hair will grow back when chemotherapy finishes but may be different texture and color. |
| | Wigs, scarves, and turbans, which can be purchased in many stores, will improve body image. |
| | American Cancer Society can provide skin and hair advice through "Look Good Feel Better" program. |

| | |
|---|---|
| Stomatitis (mouth soreness) | Avoid smoking, drinking alcohol, and eating coarse or irritating foods. |
| | Brush teeth with soft toothbrush; use baking soda and salt mouth rinses at least twice a day. |
| | Use high-protein drinks or blenderized food until mouth heals. |
| | Report painful mouth sores, ulcers, and white patches to physician; medications may be necessary. |

**BONE MARROW DEPRESSION**

| | |
|---|---|
| Leukopenia (reduced white blood cells) | Avoid sources of infection such as unpeeled fruits and vegetables, persons with colds, and crowds. |
| | Practice good personal hygiene such as good hand washing and skin, mouth, and perineal care. |
| | Report fever, chills, and other symptoms of infection such as cough, sore throat, and urinary frequency promptly to physician. |
| Thrombocytopenia (reduced platelets) | Avoid physical trauma and contact sports. |
| | Use soft-bristled toothbrush. |
| | Use electric razor, no blades. |
| | Avoid medications such as aspirin or ibuprofen that may increase risk of bleeding. |
| | Report signs of bleeding such as nosebleeds, blood in urine, or stool promptly to physician. |
| Anemia (reduced blood cells) | Set priorities for activities and pace daily routine. |
| | Report symptoms of anemia such as fatigue, shortness of breath, headache, and dizziness to physician. |

transplants often is quicker, hospital stays are shorter, and complications are fewer.

As bone marrow transplantation becomes increasingly available in different parts of the country, nurses will be caring for more pretransplant and posttransplant patients. The nurse needs to be prepared to help the patient and family cope with both the physical and emotional reactions that result from such an intensive treatment.

## Biotherapy

Biotherapy is the fourth modality of cancer treatment. It is believed that the biggest achievements in this form of treatment are yet to come, and biotherapy is the focus of a great deal of research. Biotherapy, or biologic therapy, uses agents that are biologic in origin and includes but is not limited to immunotherapy, human growth factors, and **biologic response modifiers (BRMs).**

## History of Biotherapy

Treatment of cancer with biologic agents began in 1893 when William Coley, a New York surgeon, observed a complete remission of cancer in a patient with a metastatic sarcoma after two episodes of erysipelas, a streptococcal infection. He began to inject live and killed bacterial extracts, known as *Coley's toxins,* into the patient's tumors. The patient reacted with fever, chills, and other systemic effects that were believed to be essential to treatment. In spite of the fact that about one-fourth of Coley's patients had complete tumor regression, interest in toxin treatment was overshadowed by progress made in radiotherapy and chemotherapy. It is now believed that the active ingredient in Coley's toxins was endotoxin, a component in bacterial cell walls that generates tumor necrosis factor (TNF) and other cytokines (products of immune cells that coordinate and initiate effector defense functions) (Wheeler, 1997).

In the 1960s and 1970s, clinical trials were conducted using nonspecific immunopotentiators such as bacille Calmette-Guérin (BCG). BCG was originally developed as a vaccine for tuberculosis and showed evidence of increasing survival in children with acute lymphoblastic leukemia when used as adjuvant therapy after chemotherapy. This sparked interest in immunotherapy, but subsequent clinical studies showed little difference in cancer recurrence rates. Interest again faded (Wheeler, 1997).

In the early 1980s, advances in molecular biology, computerization, and genetic engineering provided a large number of new substances that were capable of modulating immune functions. These were called *BRMs,* which are the agents that will modify the relationship between tumor and host by modifying the host's biologic response to tumor cells. BRMs include agents that act on the host's antitumor immune mechanisms, cells or cell products that have direct antitumor effect, such as TNF, and biologic agents that have other biologic, antitumor effects such as interfering with the metastatic ability of the tumor. Recombinant DNA, the combining of genes from different sources to produce an organism with new qualities, is an important basic principle to biotherapy (Box 12-10) (Wheeler, 1997).

## Nursing Interventions, Biologic Response Modifiers

BRM therapy results in many of the same side effects as chemotherapy, but some nursing care problems are unique to the use of biologic agents. Because many BRMs stimulate the immune system to function more efficiently, patients receiving this therapy have symptoms similar to those suffered during a bacterial or viral infection. These flulike symptoms include chills, fever, headache, malaise, and fatigue. Comfort mea-

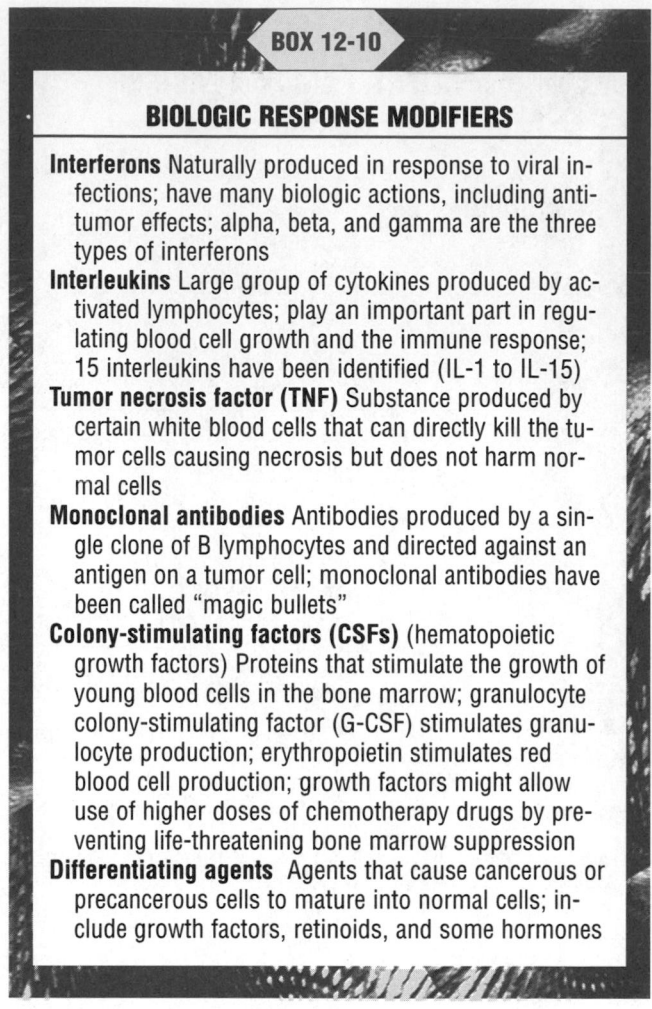

**BOX 12-10**

### BIOLOGIC RESPONSE MODIFIERS

**Interferons** Naturally produced in response to viral infections; have many biologic actions, including antitumor effects; alpha, beta, and gamma are the three types of interferons

**Interleukins** Large group of cytokines produced by activated lymphocytes; play an important part in regulating blood cell growth and the immune response; 15 interleukins have been identified (IL-1 to IL-15)

**Tumor necrosis factor (TNF)** Substance produced by certain white blood cells that can directly kill the tumor cells causing necrosis but does not harm normal cells

**Monoclonal antibodies** Antibodies produced by a single clone of B lymphocytes and directed against an antigen on a tumor cell; monoclonal antibodies have been called "magic bullets"

**Colony-stimulating factors (CSFs)** (hematopoietic growth factors) Proteins that stimulate the growth of young blood cells in the bone marrow; granulocyte colony-stimulating factor (G-CSF) stimulates granulocyte production; erythropoietin stimulates red blood cell production; growth factors might allow use of higher doses of chemotherapy drugs by preventing life-threatening bone marrow suppression

**Differentiating agents** Agents that cause cancerous or precancerous cells to mature into normal cells; include growth factors, retinoids, and some hormones

sures include body temperature stabilization with the use of acetaminophen (Tylenol), appropriate clothing, cooling blankets, and tepid baths. Attention should be paid to proper fluid and nutritional intake, and the patient should be allowed plenty of rest. GI effects of nausea, vomiting, anorexia, and altered taste should be treated in ways similar to those recommended for chemotherapy patients. BRMs may also cause skin rashes and itchiness, subtle mental status changes, and cardiac and blood circulation dysfunction. Nurses must be alert for any of these physiologic changes in patients receiving BRMs (Wujcik, 1993).

## Alternate Therapies

Beyond the standard treatment options described above, cancer patients may seek out alternate therapies. Most of these methods do not withstand scientific trials and have been referred to as quackery. Almost 20 years ago, *l*-mandelonitrile-b-glucuronic acid (Laetrile) received extensive publicity as a treatment that might cure cancer. Laetrile was studied by the National Cancer Institute for several years and was found to be a toxic drug that was *not* effective as a cancer treatment. Many other fad treatments have come and gone. However, alternative or complementary therapies, which include a wide array of methods, have continued to gain popularity with the general public and many health practitioners (Cassileth, Chapman, 1996).

In 1992 Congress mandated the creation of a National Institutes of Health Office of Alternative Medicine (OAM) to facilitate the evaluation of alternative medical treatments. OAM monitors and funds research studies, including several concerning cancer. Popular alternative therapies include such diverse approaches as special diets, herbs, bioelectromagnetics, traditional and folk remedies, shark cartilage, antineoplastons, prayer, therapeutic touch, support groups, massage, and relaxation techniques. Oncologists tend not to embrace alternative therapies, fearing that patients will refuse more traditional treatments that, while not a perfect solution, have been scientifically tested. But cancer patients are increasingly using alternative therapies, in part because of the frustratingly slow progress toward finding a cure for cancer. Because the immune system plays an important role in cancer, those therapies that have a positive effect on the immune system have the potential to enhance medical treatments. It is important that the patient fully describe all therapies so the physician will have a complete picture. The nurse must provide support and convey acceptance to patients if they are to feel comfortable in revealing alternative therapies. The exciting new approach of gene therapy, which is the introduction of normal genes into cells to prevent or cure diseases such as cancer, may revolutionize treatment but is still a long way from being perfected. In the future, it is likely that the best of both scientific and alternative therapies will be used to achieve optimal outcomes for cancer patients (Morra, Potts, 1994).

## EMOTIONAL CARE

One of the most important aspects of care of the patient with cancer is psychologic support. Often this aspect is more important than the patient's physical care. Anxiety and depression are common emotional reactions to cancer. Many patients suffer from feelings of guilt and see their illness as a punishment for their past. Overt anger also is a common behavior pattern in cancer patients and usually is accompanied by acute anxiety. Although they may not be verbalized, these feelings are close to the surface, and hope is the one indispensable aspect of treatment that must emanate from all those involved in the patient's care (National Cancer Institute, 1993).

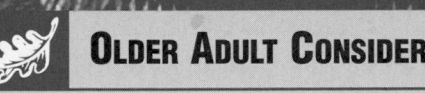

### OLDER ADULT CONSIDERATIONS

Cancer therapy may require modification for older adults. In elderly individuals the skin and mucous membranes, as well as bone marrow function, may be more vulnerable because of the normal functional declines associated with aging. Fatigue may be compounded by a disruption of life-style patterns. Anxiety and depression are expected psychologic reactions to cancer therapy. Referrals to community agencies can provide invaluable support for assistance in home care.

Public education has gone far in making people more conscious of the seriousness of cancer, and although many patients may know consciously or unconsciously that the diagnosis is cancer, they still hope that a cure may be found in time for them. Formerly, many physicians believed that patients should not be told that they had cancer. Education has resulted in a greatly enlightened public. The modern communication media have been used to present fictional dramas concerning cancer. These factors have helped bring changes in the knowledge and understanding of cancer.

It is believed that most patients suspect or know that they have cancer without being told. The nurse should be aware of statements made by the patient that indicate a need for some confirmation of the belief. The patient may say, "I'm sure that I have cancer" or may ask, "Did the doctor tell you that I have cancer?" Answers to such statements and questions may not be easy to give. The patient must be allowed to fully express his or her concerns and be given the opportunity to ask questions. It is essential that nursing personnel be aware of the patient's understanding. However, the individual's knowledge or understanding does not eradicate the emotional impact when the cancer diagnosis is given. Cancer is a threat to survival, and most people want to look forward to life, not death. The patient and family will need information during every phase of the illness (Table 12-5).

When caring for a cancer patient, the nurse must objectively examine personal attitudes and beliefs. The nurse's own feelings about cancer can be revealed both verbally and nonverbally to the patient and family. It is important that the nurse support the therapy offered to the patient and reassure the patient and family. It is best to stress the progress and events of the day rather than refer to the future optimistically. The nurse must realize that cancer can be cured and that patients can live with cancer under control for many years.

**TABLE 12-5**

## Information Needed by Cancer Patients and Spouses Over the Course of Illness

| DIAGNOSTIC PHASE | HOSPITAL PHASE | TREATMENT PHASE | ADAPTATION PHASE | RECURRENT PHASE |
|---|---|---|---|---|
| Type and purpose of diagnostic procedures to be performed | Type of surgery planned | Type and length of treatment planned | When follow-up examinations or tests are necessary | Type of treatment planned |
| When test results can be expected | When pathology report will be available | Anticipated side effects and when they may occur | The typical concerns during this phase (e.g., fear of recurrence) | Anticipated side effects and when they may occur |
| The person coordinating the patient's care | Expected length of hospitalization | Ways to minimize side effects | Importance of balancing needs of patient and family members | The typical feelings during this phase (e.g., uncertainty, sadness, fear) |
| The typical emotions that develop while awaiting diagnosis (e.g., anxiety, uncertainty) | Role limitations to anticipate when patient is discharged | Likelihood of temporary role changes | Availability of cancer education and support groups | Ways to maintain hope regardless of recurrence |
| | The effects of illness on other family members | Availability of cancer education and support groups | | Availability of support groups and community resources |

From Northouse LL, Peters-Golden H: *Semin Oncol Nurse* 9(2):77, 1993.

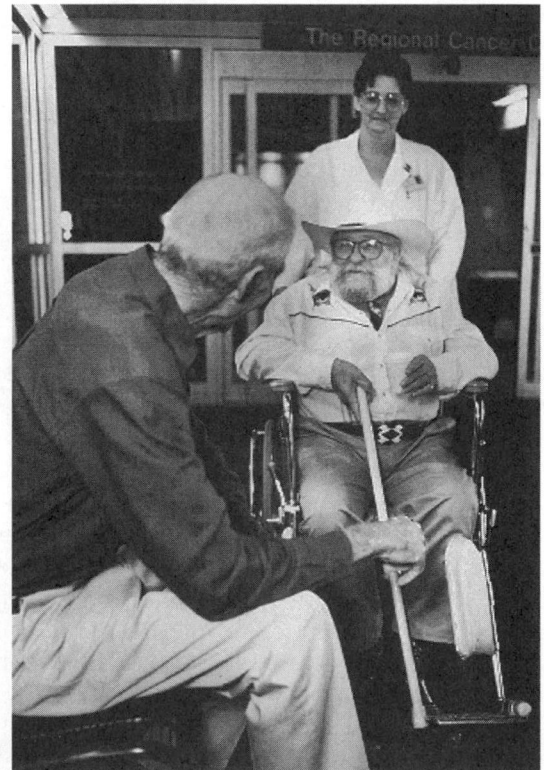

**Figure 12-4** Visits from a spiritual counselor can be important to the patient.

The ability to communicate with a cancer patient does not always involve the spoken word. A soothing back rub, a change of position, or a refreshing drink may be more meaningful to the patient than any conversation. Members of the patient's family also often need emotional support. Giving emotional support to the family may mean providing a blanket or a pillow at night or giving them a report of the patient's condition during surgery. Collaborative practice between the nurse and physician can be effective in gaining a joint understanding of the patient's fears and special problems. The patient with cancer, perhaps more than a patient with another condition, appreciates visits from the hospital chaplain, minister, or rabbi (Figure 12-4). The nurse can help arrange for such visits. When everything has been done for the patient that is humanly possible and the physician has terminated therapeutic measures, the nurse should continue to provide physical comfort and emotional support to the patient and family.

## REHABILITATION

Rehabilitation of a patient who has cancer is an obligation of those responsible for care. These patients are confronted with problems seldom experienced by patients with other diseases. Adjustments in body image and self-concept often must be made. The patient may have a permanent colostomy, a permanent tracheostomy, a loss of voice, or a ureterostomy. The thought of facing life with the loss of these normal functions may be overwhelming to the patient. If mutilating surgery is to be performed, the patient should know before the surgery what to expect and should be assured that care and information about self-care will be provided. Patients who are to undergo laryngectomies should be visited by the speech therapist, who can explain how they will be taught to speak

---

**BOX 12-11**

### SELF-HELP CANCER GROUPS*

**Reach to Recovery.** The American Cancer Society (ACS) sponsors this organization. On receiving a physician's referral, a trained ACS volunteer who has had breast cancer surgery visits a woman who has just had this surgery. The volunteer teaches the woman exercises to help her recover and offers practical advice about adjusting to a mastectomy.

**International Association of Laryngectomies.** Also sponsored by the ACS, this organization helps people who have had recent laryngectomies to make early adjustments to the loss of voice and to overcome psychosocial problems. Local clubs may be called "Lost Chord" or "New Voice."

**I Can Cope.** This ACS-sponsored educational program is designed to inform cancer patients and their families about the disease. Programs include classes on cancer and its treatments, how to live with the diagnosis of cancer, and the resources available to patients and families.

**US TOO.** A nonprofit organization that provides information, counseling, and educational meetings that help survivors of prostate cancer and their families lead healthy, productive lives. US TOO is administered for and by survivors of prostate cancer. Call or write: US TOO, International, Inc., 930 North York Road, Suite 50, Hinsdale, IL 60521-2993; phone: (630) 323-1002 or 1-800-80-USTOO (1-800-808-7866).

**United Ostomy Association.** Local chapters are composed primarily of people with ostomies and are formed for the purpose of providing mutual aid, moral support, and education to those who have had a colostomy, ileostomy, or urostomy. Write or call: United Ostomy Association, 36 Executive Park, Suite 120, Irvine, CA 92714; phone: 1-800-826-0826.

**Candelighters Childhood Cancer Foundation.** This national organization has local patient and family support networks. To find a nearby chapter, check local phone books or contact the national office: Candelighters Childhood Cancer Foundation, Suite 1011, 1901 Pennsylvania Avenue, NW Washington, DC 20006; phone: (202) 659-5136.

**National Coalition for Cancer Survivorship (NCCS).** This network of independent groups and individuals is concerned with survivorship and the support of cancer survivors and their loved ones. Address: NCCS, 323 Eighth Street SW, Albuquerque, NM 87102; phone: (505) 764-9956.

**Man to Man.** An ACS-sponsored education and support program to help men and their families cope with prostate cancer. Participation in the program provides education and promotes emotional support to assist in the recovery process.

*More information on ACS-sponsored groups can be obtained from local ACS units or by calling 1-800-ACS-2345.

---

again. In preparation for eventual hospital discharge, patients should be permitted to assist with procedures. These procedures may include management of the tracheostomy, suctioning, colostomy irrigations, oral irrigations, or gastrostomy feedings. Patients who have had mastectomies should be taught arm exercises (see Chapter 43). All patients should be encouraged to return to their normal activities as soon as possible.

If patients are in a terminal phase of illness, they should remain ambulatory and perform the daily activities of self-care as long as possible. Many patients are able to do this until the last stages of the illness. Although the prognosis may be poor and only a few months may remain, many patients return to their normal work for weeks or months. Most cancer patients remain at home and often are employed. Hospitalization is ordered intermittently and only when necessary. Nursing care can be given in the home by a community health nurse, and hospice programs are available in many communities, often as part of the nursing agency. While the patient is still hospitalized,

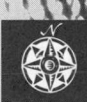

### ETHICAL DILEMMA

You have been caring for Mr. Edwards, a 90-year-old gentleman with a history of gastrointestinal cancer. He has been a resident for 2 years in the nursing home where you work. He has become increasingly confused and is refusing to eat. He is sleeping a great deal during the day and rouses only with stimulation. His wife, Emma, asks you to talk to the physician about writing an order for tube feedings. Discuss how you would respond to this request.

the home care nurse may visit the patient to plan with him or her the care needed after discharge.

Patients often are helped and encouraged by meeting and talking with a person who has had a similar cancer or cancer treatment, and the patient should be offered this opportunity. Such self-help groups can be very effective for the patient and family (Box 12-11).

# NURSING CARE PLAN

## PATIENT WITH LUNG CANCER

Mr. Halton is a 76-year-old male who has been admitted from home with the diagnosis of squamous cell cancer of the right lung. He is currently undergoing outpatient radiation therapy and had a treatment today. He has a known right pleural effusion secondary to the cancer. He has been dyspneic for several days, but tonight the dyspnea increased in severity, and Mr. Halton has come to the emergency room with markedly reduced breath sounds in the middle-to-lower lobes of the right lung, a low-grade fever, and dyspnea. His admitting diagnosis is pleural effusion and pneumonia/hypoxia secondary to cancer.

| Medical History | Psychosocial Data | Assessment Data |
|---|---|---|
| No known allergies | Has 4 brothers, deceased, and 2 sisters | Height: 5'6"; weight: 128 lb |
| Two- to three-pack-a-day smoker × 55 years | Widowed × 10 years; no children | Recent weight loss of 20 lb |
| Hypertension | Lives alone in mobile home | T 99.8; P 112; R 36, BP 156/86 |
| Peripheral vascular disease | Retired factory worker | *Mental status:* Alert and oriented; appears chronically ill |
| Non–insulin-dependent diabetes mellitus | Has several male friends who live in neighboring mobile homes; they gather together for "smoking and playing cards" | *Skin:* Warm, dry, intact; radiation markings on right anterior side of the chest |
| Chronic obstructive pulmonary disease | Verbalizes doubts about seeing them anymore since he is not able to smoke | *Eye, ear, nose, throat:* Mucous membranes dry; full upper and lower dentures; lips slightly cyanotic |
| Osteoarthritis of the spine | | *Respiratory:* Thoracentesis performed in emergency room with drainage of 500 ml of clear, serosanguinous fluid; rate 36-40, shallow, almost absent breath sounds in right middle-to-lower lobe before thoracentesis; rate remains diminished after thoracentesis; left lung field has scattered crackles |
| Younger sister with hypercholesteremia and arteriosclerotic heart disease | | *Cardiovascular:* Loud 3/6 holosystolic murmur; no gallop; peripheral pulses 1+ to lower extremities, 2+ to upper extremities; arterial pressure 112, irregular |
| Family history of heart disease | | *Abdomen:* Soft, nontender, nondistended; + bowel sounds |

*Laboratory data*

WBC 11.8, Hgb 7.3, Hct 23.2

Na 139, K 5.1, Cl 106, $CO_2$ 22

BUN 48, CR 1.3

ABGs: pH 7.45, $PCO_2$ 21, $PO_2$ 106, $HCO_3$ 24, $O_2$sat 95% on nonbreather $O_2$

CXR: preexisting right upper lobe effusion, wispy infiltrate right upper lobe

ECG: occasional PVC; left ventricle hypertrophy

*Medications*

Accucheck AC and HS

Regular insulin coverage

   150-200 2 U

   201-250 4 U

   251-300 8 U

   >300 12 U

ceftazidine (Fortax) 1 g IV q 8 hr

methylprednisolone (Solu-Medrol) 60 mg IV q 6 hr × 2 days

glyburide (DaBeta) 5 mg before breakfast

## NURSING CARE PLAN
## PATIENT WITH LUNG CANCER—cont'd

*Medications—cont'd*
enalapril maleate (Vasotec) 10 mg qd
alprazolam (Xanax) 0.5 mg tid
Transfuse 1 unit packed red blood cells

### NURSING DIAGNOSIS

Impaired gas exchange related to restricted lung expansion from pleural effusion; inflammation and tumor as evidenced by hypoxemia and dyspnea

| NURSING INTERVENTIONS | EVALUATION OF EXPECTED OUTCOMES |
| --- | --- |
| Assess respiratory status q 4 hr and prn. | No evidence of respiratory distress |
| Monitor pulse oximetry q 4 hr and prn. | Maintains an $O_2$ saturation of > 90% |
| Maintain high Fowler's position. | Experiences no dyspnea at rest; mild dyspnea on exertion |
| Maintain $O_2$ delivery to maintain $O_2$ saturation > 90%. (Recently changed from non-rebreather to ventimask at 35%) | Able to assist with self-care activities without dyspnea |
| Encourage coughing and deep breath q 2 hr. | Hgb is 10 or greater |
| Plan care in blocks of time and provide rest periods often. | |
| Increase activity as tolerated. | |
| Administer medications as ordered: | |
|   Corticosteroids to decrease inflammation | |
|   Antibiotics to decrease infection | |
| Administer blood transfusion according to hospital policy to increase oxygen-carrying components. | |
| Inform healthcare provider if respiratory status deteriorates. | |

### NURSING DIAGNOSIS

Risk for impaired skin integrity related to effects of radiation

| NURSING INTERVENTIONS | EVALUATION OF EXPECTED OUTCOMES |
| --- | --- |
| Assess skin condition in area of radiation. | Radiation marks on chest wall remain intact. |
| Bathe with mild soap. Avoid rubbing or using soap or lotion on chest area. Be careful not to wash the radiation marks placed on the skin to identify the area of radiation. | Skin of chest wall is maintained intact without redness, drying, or excoriation |
| Provide soft, loose clothing next to the chest area. | |
| Use mild water-based lubricant lotions. | |

### NURSING DIAGNOSIS

Altered nutrition: less than body requirements related to anorexia, dyspnea as evidenced by weight loss and inadequate consumption of meals

| NURSING INTERVENTIONS | EVALUATION OF EXPECTED OUTCOMES |
| --- | --- |
| Place in high Fowler's position for meals and provide $O_2$ at 5 L during meals. | No further weight loss |
| Provide soft foods that are high in calories and high in protein. | Able to consume 75% of the meals |
| Monitor percentage of meals and snacks consumed. | Verbalizes importance of adequate nutrition. |

*Continued*

# NURSING CARE PLAN
## PATIENT WITH LUNG CANCER—cont'd

| NURSING INTERVENTIONS | EVALUATION OF EXPECTED OUTCOMES |
|---|---|
| Provide rest periods before meals to minimize fatigue. | |
| Provide largest percentage of calories/protein for breakfast meal. | |
| Encourage sister to bring in favorite foods. Report this to dietician to plan subsequent American Dietetic Association meals. | |
| Weigh every third day. | |

**NURSING DIAGNOSIS**

Anticipatory grieving related to diagnosis of cancer and changes in life-style with friends as evidenced by patient statements

| NURSING INTERVENTIONS | EVALUATION OF EXPECTED OUTCOMES |
|---|---|
| Provide an atmosphere of care and concern. | Verbalizes feelings about diagnosis and changes in life-style |
| Establish rapport and develop relationship. | Expresses grief with staff and/or family |
| Encourage verbalization of anger, fear, sadness, and difficulties related to diagnosis and loss. | Uses available support systems |
| Provide realistic hope regarding prognosis and diagnosis. | |
| Explain the process of grieving to the patient and sister; encourage her support. | |
| Encourage and facilitate communication between patient and significant friends. | |
| Encourage honesty in discussing issues of smoking. | |
| Arrange a visit from clergy if desired by patient. | |

# KEY CONCEPTS

➤ Cancer is characterized by abnormal, unrestricted cell division and the spread of these cells into healthy tissues of the body.

➤ One out of 4 people and 3 out of 4 families in the United States will be affected by cancer at some time.

➤ The most common sites of cancer are the lungs, colon-rectum, breast, and prostate.

➤ Metastasis occurs when malignant cells break away from their original sites and are transported by the blood or lymph to new sites, where they begin to grow.

➤ The specific cause of cancer is unknown.

➤ Carcinogens are agents that can cause malignant genetic changes in healthy cells after prolonged exposure. Carcinogens include viruses, chemical agents, physical agents, hormones, and dietary factors. Hereditary factors are also important.

➤ Risk factors for the major cancers have been identified. Many of these factors are potentially avoidable, and risk declines as primary prevention is instituted and positive behaviors develop.

➤ Early detection and prompt treatment are secondary prevention goals.

➤ Several diagnostic tests can be used, depending on the site of the tumor.

➤ Cancer is treated by surgery, radiotherapy, chemotherapy, and biotherapy.

➤ In addition to meeting the physical needs of patients, nurses are responsible for clarifying uncertainties, answering questions, and explaining procedures fully.

➤ Patients receiving external beam radiation therapy are never sources of radiation.

➤ Time, distance, and shielding are important determinants of the amount of radiation health care workers receive when caring for patients undergoing internal radiation therapy. Self-protective measures should be used.

➤ A reduction in the number of white blood cells as a result of chemotherapy can increase the risk of infection. Fever is the most reliable indicator of this complication.

➤ Bleeding precautions should be observed in patients with a platelet count below 50,000 cells/mm$^3$.

➤ Patients undergoing immunotherapy and biotherapy may experience flulike symptoms.

➤ One of the most important aspects of care for the patient with cancer is psychologic support.

➤ Rehabilitation includes adjustments in body image and self-concept. Self-help groups may be very effective in the adjustment process.

# CRITICAL THINKING EXERCISES

1. How do American Cancer Society recommendations for early detection of cancer in a 20-year-old woman compare with those for a 60-year-old woman?
2. How does exfoliative cytology differ from biopsy?
3. Why does chemotherapy result in gastrointestinal and mucosal side effects?
4. Why do some scientists think immunotherapy will help the body fight cancer?
5. Which community resources could be used to help a cancer patient and his or her family cope with the disease?

## REFERENCES AND ADDITIONAL READINGS

American Cancer Society: *Taking control: 10 steps to a healthier life and reduced cancer risk,* Pub No 201915, Atlanta, 1994, The Society.

American Cancer Society: *Cancer facts and figures—1997,* Atlanta, 1997, The Society.

Bender CM, Yasko JM: Nursing role in management of cancer. In Lewis SM, Collier IC, Heitkemper MM, editors: *Medical-surgical nursing: assessment and management of clinical problems,* ed 4, St Louis, 1996, Mosby.

Cole P, Rodu B: Declining cancer mortality in the United States, *Cancer* 78:2045-2048, 1996.

Cassileth BR, Chapman CC: Alternative and complementary cancer therapies, *Cancer* 77(6):1026-1034, 1996.

Distasio SA: Zofran makes chemo bearable, *RN* 56(5):56-59, 1993.

Dow KH, Hilderley LJ: *Nursing care in radiation oncology,* Philadelphia, 1992, Saunders.

Greifzu S: Helping cancer patients fight infection, *RN* 54(7):24-29, 1991.

Guy JL, Ingram BA: Medical oncology: the agents. In McCorkle R et al, editors: *Cancer nursing: a comprehensive textbook,* ed 2, Philadelphia, 1996, Saunders.

Hilderley LJ, Dow KH: Radiation oncology. In McCorkle R et al, editors: *Cancer nursing: a comprehensive textbook,* ed 2, Philadelphia, 1996, Saunders.

Iwamoto R: Radiation therapy. In Otto SE, editor: *Oncology nursing,* ed 3, St Louis, 1997, Mosby.

Korinko A, Yurick A: Maintaining skin integrity during radiation therapy, *Am J Nurs* 97(2):40-44, 1997.

Langhorne M: Chemotherapy. In Otto SE, editor: *Oncology nursing,* ed 3, St Louis, 1997, Mosby.

Leukemia Society of America: *Bone marrow transplantation and peripheral blood stem cell transplantation,* New York, 1995, The Society.

Morra M, Potts E: *Choices: realistic alternatives in cancer treatment,* New York, 1994, Avon Books.

Nash JM: The enemy within, *Time* Fall 1996.

National Cancer Institute: *Eating hints,* NIH Pub No 92-2079, Washington, DC, 1992, The Institute.

National Cancer Institute: *Taking time: support for people with cancer and the people who care about them,* NIH Pub No 93-2059, Washington, DC, 1993, The Institute.

Occupational Safety and Health Administration (OSHA): Controlling occupational exposure to hazardous drugs, OSHA Instruction CPL 2-2.20B CH-4, Washington, DC, 1995, US Department of Labor.

Sitton E: Early and late radiation-induced skin alterations. II. Nursing care of irradiated skin, *Oncol Nurs Forum* 19(6):907, 1992.

Strohl RA: The nursing role in radiation oncology: symptom management of acute and chronic reactions, *Oncol Nurs Forum* 15(4):429-434, 1988.

Strohl RA: Nursing role in management: cancer. In Lewis SM, Collier IC, Heitkemper MM, editors: *Medical-surgical nursing: assessment and management of clinical problems,* ed 4, St Louis, 1996, Mosby.

Walters P: Chemo: a nurse's guide to action, administration, and side effects, *RN* 53(2):52-66, 1990.

Wheeler vs: Biotherapy. In Groenwald SL et al, editors: *Cancer nursing: principles and practice,* Sudbury, Mass, 1997, Jones and Bartlett.

Wujcik D: An odyssey into biologic therapy, *Oncol Nurs Forum* 20(6):879-887, 1993.

# CHAPTER 13

# Death and Dying

## KEY TERMS

| | |
|---|---|
| acceptance | euthanasia |
| anger | grief |
| anticipatory grief | hospice |
| assisted suicide | living will |
| bargaining | palliative care |
| bereavement | respite |
| denial | thanatology |
| depression | |

## DEATH

Until recently, Americans have had the reputation of being a death-denying society. Ministers, nurses, and physicians have experienced long-standing frustrations in attempting to support dying patients and their families who often deny the reality of the approaching death of their loved one.

In the 1960s and 1970s death, dying, grief, and bereavement became the focus of research in various disciplines. Through her writings concerning her work with dying patients, Elisabeth Kübler-Ross peaked the interest of the general public. **Thanatology,** the scientific study of death, found its way into the course offerings of many universities across the United States. Death has become a popular topic of books, articles, films, and videos. The hospice movement began in England and has rapidly developed in the United States as a support system for dying patients and their families.

Death and dying can be everyday realities of nursing practice and must be addressed. Kübler-Ross states that death is the final stage of growth and development. If death is accepted as the final stage, it should be faced and experienced fully. The nurse has a unique opportunity and a major responsibility to help the patient and his or her family through the experience of dying and death (Kübler-Ross, 1975). It is necessary to understand how the physiologic and psychologic factors that surround death affect the individual. Many of the physiologic processes are well known, and the nurse or physician may predict death with reasonable accuracy, however this is not always the case. The dying process is characterized by the slowing down of all organ functions until the maintenance of life processes can no longer occur. The pace and progression of the dying process depends on the patient's will to live, underlying organ function,

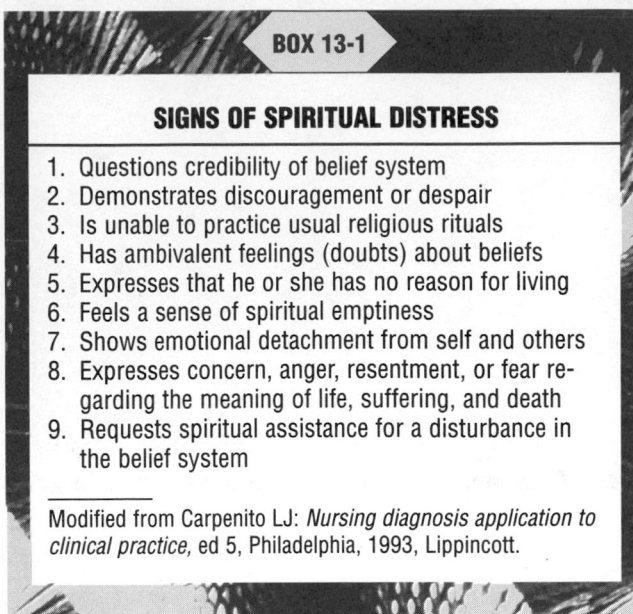

**BOX 13-1**

### SIGNS OF SPIRITUAL DISTRESS

1. Questions credibility of belief system
2. Demonstrates discouragement or despair
3. Is unable to practice usual religious rituals
4. Has ambivalent feelings (doubts) about beliefs
5. Expresses that he or she has no reason for living
6. Feels a sense of spiritual emptiness
7. Shows emotional detachment from self and others
8. Expresses concern, anger, resentment, or fear regarding the meaning of life, suffering, and death
9. Requests spiritual assistance for a disturbance in the belief system

Modified from Carpenito LJ: *Nursing diagnosis application to clinical practice,* ed 5, Philadelphia, 1993, Lippincott.

**BOX 13-2**

### SELECTED RELIGIOUS PRACTICES AT TIME OF DEATH

Christian Science: An autopsy is usually declined unless required by law. Donating organs is unlikely but is an individual decision.
Church of the Nazarene: Cremation is permitted, and stillborn infants are buried.
Islam: It is preferred that the family wash, prepare, and place the body in a position that faces Mecca. If necessary, health care providers may perform these procedures as long as they wear gloves. Burial is performed as soon as possible. Cremation is forbidden. An autopsy is also prohibited except for legal reasons, and no body part is to be removed. Donating body parts or organs is not allowed because beliefs indicate that the person does not own his or her body.
Mennonite: Prayer is important at times of crisis. Therefore contacting a minister is important.
Muslim: The family is contacted before any care of the deceased is performed. There are special procedures for washing and shrouding the body.
Reform Jews: The use of life support without heroic measures is advocated. Cremation is allowed, but it is suggested that ashes be buried in a Jewish cemetery.
Roman Catholics: Each Roman Catholic should participate in the sacraments of anointing of the sick, the Eucharist, and reconciliation before death. The body should not be shrouded until these sacraments have been performed. All body parts that retain human quality must be appropriately buried or cremated.

Modified from Carson VB: *Spiritual dimensions of nursing practice,* Philadelphia, 1989, Saunders.

degree of hydration, and severity of acute and chronic illnesses. The psychologic and spiritual impact of the impending death may also be difficult to predict and may vary widely according to the needs of each patient and family.

The needs of the dying patient are complex, but it is important to acknowledge and deal with them. The biologic needs include the need for adequate physical care, caring providers, prudent medical management, and comfort. The emotional and social aspects of death are closely tied with the spiritual needs of the dying patient and his or her family. Meeting the spiritual needs of the patient and family is as important as meeting the biologic needs (Gravely, 1993). Spiritual distress is a nursing diagnosis characterized by expression of concern with the meaning of life and death and by the questioning of belief systems that provide strength, hope, and meaning to life (NANDA, 1995) (Box 13-1). The nurse must remember that all people have a spiritual dimension despite whether they participate in formal religious practices (Carpenito, 1993). As each patient moves toward his or her own death, each views the experience and accepts death in a unique way. There is no specific pattern that is applicable to all persons. By studying death and dying, nurses and other members of the health care team can improve their ability to understand the terminally ill person and to support the family and their significant others. The nurse must be aware of his or her own personal beliefs and values and acknowledge that these values may not be effective for others. To meet the needs of the patients the nurse must be aware of the common religious and cultural practices regarding medical treatment and death in his or her area (Carson, 1989) (Box 13-2).

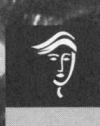 **PATIENT/FAMILY TEACHING**

**PAIN**
- Teach patient how to rate pain on a scale of 1 to 10.
- Teach family methods of comfort and relief such as massage.

## When Does Death Occur?

The question of when death occurs is highly controversial. A diagnosis of death is usually made when there is an absence of heartbeat and a cessation of respiration. The use of these signs as the only criteria for determining death was questioned when the first human heart transplant was accomplished in 1967. Physicians who were interested in organ transplants believed that a new definition was necessary, mainly because the donor organ must be removed as quickly as possible after death. Whether a person is actually dead, even though the heart may still be beating, is a question that has not yet been resolved.

In an effort to answer the question, "When does death occur?" physicians now use the electroencephalograph (EEG) to measure brain activity. They believe that the absence of brain activity on the EEG at three separate times indicates that death has occurred, even though the heart may still be beating. Most physicians accept a definition of death that is based on the absence of brain waves. The Uniform Determination of Death Act (1982) indicates that death has occurred when there is no spontaneous brain activity and no spontaneous respirations.

The use of the EEG in determining death is commonly used when a patient is being kept alive by extraordinary means and a decision to continue or discontinue life support must be made. In most situations in which life support has not been started, physicians determine death by the more traditional method: the absence of heartbeat and the cessation of respiration. Until recently this determination has been a medical responsibility and remains a medical responsibility within institutional settings.

## Prolonging Life

New technologies and drugs have made it possible to prolong the lives of some terminally ill patients. However, after transferring from home to the hospital, dying patients find themselves surrounded by technologically advanced equipment. Such an environment is often lonely and sterile for the patient without the support of friends or family.

The use of life support is a common subject of television programs, magazine articles, and health care ethics committees. The following question is posed: if death is inevitable, should care not be directed toward making the patient as comfortable as possible rather than toward prolonging life? This problem is dealt with on a daily basis in hospitals and nursing homes. Using extraordinary means to prolong the life of a terminally ill patient becomes a tangled web of ethical, religious, legal, and moral questions to which there are no decisive answers. The use of the physician's "No Code" or "Do Not Resuscitate" orders is becoming more common now. For the nurse this means that cardiopulmonary resuscitation or other "heroic" measures will not be started if the patient's heartbeat or respirations stop. Terminally ill patients and their families discuss these treatment options

with their nurse and physician before the order is written.

Studies (Gordon, Cheung, 1993; Schwenzer, Smith, Durbin, 1993; Tresch et al, 1993) have revealed that the type of patient who will probably not benefit from cardiopulmonary resuscitation (CPR) includes the following:
1. Those who have more than one or two medical problems
2. Those who do not live independently or who are living in long-term care facilities
3. Those who have a terminal disease
4. Those who have dementia

If CPR is begun outside the hospital, 911 should be called and the rescue squad will arrive. Once on the scene, the paramedics take over the care of the patient. They will then continue CPR until the patient has been transported to the nearest emergency room, where the staff will do everything in their power to restart the patient's heart. Measures could include continuing CPR or performing electric shock or mechanical ventilation. These efforts must continue until a physician stops the whole process by declaring the patient dead and further life prolonging efforts futile. Calling 911 automatically triggers these "heroic" responses because the rescue squad is trained to respond quickly and aggressively to save lives. Thus the nurse emphasizes education to families and to those working in long-term care facilities about the signs of approaching death and appropriate comfort measures so that panic does not occur and the patient is not subjected to CPR against his or her wishes.

It is important to note that assisted suicide and euthanasia are complicated issues and the subject of recent debate. **Assisted suicide** is defined as "the provision of equipment or medication by a care provider to a patient for the sole purpose of assisting that patient in ending his or her life." **Euthanasia** is the merciful killing of another who may be ill or in pain (Lynn et al, 1997). Nurses should be aware of the legal issues and public debate around these controversial issues.

## Living Wills and Advanced Medical Directives

The Patient Self-Determination Act became effective in December, 1991. It requires hospitals, nursing homes, hospices, and home health care and provider agencies to advise patients upon admission of their right to accept or refuse medical treatment and of their right to execute an advance directive. This step has become a routine part of many health care admission procedures. The advance directive can be in the form of a **living will** or a durable power of attorney.

Choice in Dying, a nonprofit educational council in New York, provides national leadership in addressing issues that involve the rights of the dying patient. The council has prepared a living will or advanced directive document that enables individuals to state in advance their wishes regarding the use of life-sustaining procedures in the event of terminal illness (Figures 13-1 and 13-2). Questions regarding the legality of a living will focus on when the will is drawn up and the patient's mental status. Therefore nationwide support for living will legislation is one of the main goals of the council. Living will legislation, although still controversial, is one of the first steps in an attempt to regulate and standardize the criteria on which life-and-death decisions are made for the terminally ill (Davies, Martens, Reimer, 1991). All 50 states and the District of Columbia have enacted a living will legislation that offers guidelines for health care professionals who are involved in making decisions about life and death.

A durable power of attorney allows the patient to designate an individual who will make treatment decisions should the patient be unable to make them. It is a stronger legal document and is more specific than the living will. Unlike the living will, the durable power of attorney covers all health care choices and is not limited to questions related to a terminal illness. It is not easy for most people to deal with this question, and hopefully public education will prepare individuals for this event. It is necessary for the patient to discuss with the individual who has been given durable power of attorney his or her wishes regarding treatment.

In situations in which the patient has not made and cannot make his or her wishes known, the physician is responsible for determining what measures to take. The patient's predetermined wishes (living will) and family input is sought whenever possible. The nurse's assessment of the patient and communication with the family contribute to the decision-making process. The nurse is not responsible for these decisions but should encourage communication between all parties so that they all agree to the plan of treatment. The decision to use any measure should be guided by what will contribute to the patient's comfort, safety, and well being. If the use of oxygen relieves labored respiration, it should not be considered a heroic measure; however, administering a new antibiotic drug that can in no way alter the outcome would be considered questionable.

## Fear of Dying and Death

A fear of dying may be present when an individual's health is so compromised that there is a distinct possibility that he or she may die. This fear may lead the person to seek or accept extraordinary measures to prolong his or her life and prevent death. When all life-preserving measures have failed and death is imminent, an individual may fear death. This fear focuses on the physical cessation of vital functions and what will happen when mortal life ceases. The fear of death may also be related to frequently overlooked psychologic and spiritual factors, which are often of primary importance to the dying patient (Box 13-3).

Once these fears are identified, the nurse should begin planning to alleviate these fears and record possible interventions in the nursing care plan. For instance, the patient who has unresolved or unfinished business may be assisted to contact family members or friends to discuss past events and clear up old resentments. The patient who is afraid to die alone can be moved to a room close to the nurse's station and scheduled for frequent visits and checking by the staff. Family members or hospice volunteers may be contacted to sit at home with dying patients. Some community and church groups have organized support programs for those wishing to die at home. Most dying patients feel a sense or relief when the nurse identifies and begins a plan to address the fears surrounding death and dying.

Although research into the fear of dying is limited, there is some evidence that not all people fear dying. Kastenbaum and Aisenberg (1992) report that the dying patient may experience fear and anxiety but that depression is far more commonly experienced. The patient with severe, painful physical symptoms may experience anxiety, whereas the patient who is aware of the terminal condition may experience a greater degree of depression.

Many variables are related to the fear of dying, including age, culture, social status, educational and occupational background, serious chronic diseases, and mental health status. The aged person who has undergone biologic changes that are characteristic of his or her age group appears to show less fear of dying than a younger person. Death means the end of everything that an individual has held dear and enjoyed. Although people mourn their losses, the fears are primarily related to the unknown. What happens after death? Is there an afterlife? Is death a painful experience? What will happen to the body after death? An individual who has well-developed spiritual or religious beliefs may have fewer fears about death. A dying person may also have concerns regarding the losses and grief that family members will experience at the time of his or her death. Family discussions regarding the future help alleviate these concerns. Kübler-Ross (1969) found that death could more easily be accepted when there is the opportunity for communication, counseling, and resolution of problems. As death approaches and the sensorium changes, the fears tend to subside and the individual often appears composed.

# FLORIDA LIVING WILL

**INSTRUCTIONS**

**PRINT THE DATE**
**PRINT YOUR NAME**

Declaration made this _____ day of _____, 19_____. I, _____,
willfully and voluntarily make known my desire that my dying not be artificially prolonged under the circumstances set forth below, and I do hereby declare:

If at any time I have a terminal condition and if my attending or treating physician and another consulting physician have determined that there is no medical probability of my recovery from such condition, I direct that life-prolonging procedures be withheld or withdrawn when the application of such procedures would serve only to prolong artificially the process of dying, and that I be permitted to die naturally with only the administration of medication or the performance of any medical procedure deemed necessary to provide me with comfort care or to alleviate pain.

It is my intention that this declaration be honored by my family and physician as the final expression of my legal right to refuse medical or surgical treatment and to accept the consequences for such refusal.

In the event that I have been determined to be unable to provide express and informed consent regarding the withholding, withdrawal, or continuation of life-prolonging procedures, I wish to designate, as my surrogate to carry out the provisions of this declaration:

**PRINT THE NAME, HOME ADDRESS AND TELEPHONE NUMBER OF YOUR SURROGATE**
© 1996
CHOICE IN DYING, INC.

Name: _____

Address: _____

_____ Zip Code: _____

Phone: _____

## FLORIDA LIVING WILL—PAGE 2 OF 2

I wish to designate the following person as my alternate surrogate, to carry out the provisions of this declaration should my surrogate be unwilling or unable to act on my behalf:

**PRINT NAME, HOME ADDRESS AND TELEPHONE NUMBER OF YOUR ALTERNATE SURROGATE**

Name: _____

Address: _____

_____ Zip Code: _____

Phone: _____

**ADD PERSONAL INSTRUCTIONS (IF ANY)**

Additional instructions (optional):

I understand the full import of this declaration, and I am emotionally and mentally competent to make this declaration.

**SIGN THE DOCUMENT**
**WITNESSING PROCEDURE**

Signed: _____

Witness 1:

Signed: _____

Address: _____

**TWO WITNESSES MUST SIGN AND PRINT THEIR ADDRESSES**
© 1996
CHOICE IN DYING, INC.

Witness 2:

Signed: _____

Address: _____

**Figure 13-1**    Sample Florida Living Will document. (Reprinted by permission of Choice in Dying, 1035 30th Street, NW, Washington, DC 20007, 800-989-9455. Choice in Dying strongly advises using documents specific to the state in which one resides.)

## FLORIDA DESIGNATION OF HEALTH CARE SURROGATE

**INSTRUCTIONS**

**PRINT YOUR NAME**

Name: _____

(Last)                              (First)                              (Middle Initial)

In the event that I have been determined to be incapacitated to provide informed consent for medical treatment and surgical and diagnostic procedures, I wish to designate as my surrogate for health care decisions:

**PRINT THE NAME, HOME ADDRESS AND TELEPHONE NUMBER OF YOUR SURROGATE**

Name: _____

Address: _____

_____ Zip Code: _____

Phone: _____

If my surrogate is unwilling or unable to perform his duties, I wish to designate as my alternate surrogate:

**PRINT THE NAME, HOME ADDRESS AND TELEPHONE NUMBER OF YOUR ALTERNATE SURROGATE**

Name: _____

Address: _____

_____ Zip Code: _____

Phone: _____

**ADD PERSONAL INSTRUCTIONS (IF ANY)**

© 1996
CHOICE IN DYING, INC.

I fully understand that this designation will permit my designee to make health care decisions and to provide, withhold, or withdraw consent on my behalf; to apply for public benefits to defray the cost of health care; and to authorize my admission to or transfer from a health care facility.

Additional instructions (optional):

### FLORIDA DESIGNATION OF HEALTH CARE SURROGATE—PAGE 2 OF 2

I further affirm that this designation is not being made as a condition of treatment or admission to a health care facility. I will notify and send a copy of this document to the following persons other than my surrogate, so they may know who my surrogate is:

**PRINT THE NAMES AND ADDRESSES OF THOSE WHO YOU WANT TO KEEP COPIES OF THIS DOCUMENT**

Name: _____

Address: _____

Name: _____

Address: _____

**SIGN AND DATE THE DOCUMENT**

Signed: _____

Date: _____

**WITNESSING PROCEDURE**

Witness 1:

Signed: _____

Address: _____

**TWO WITNESSES MUST SIGN AND PRINT THEIR ADDRESSES**

Witness 2:

Signed: _____

Address: _____

© 1996
CHOICE IN DYING, INC.

**Figure 13-2** Sample Florida Designation of Health Care Surrogate document. (Reprinted by permission of Choice in Dying, 1035 30th Street, NW, Washington, DC 20007, 800-989-9455. Choice in Dying strongly advises using documents specific to the state in which one resides.)

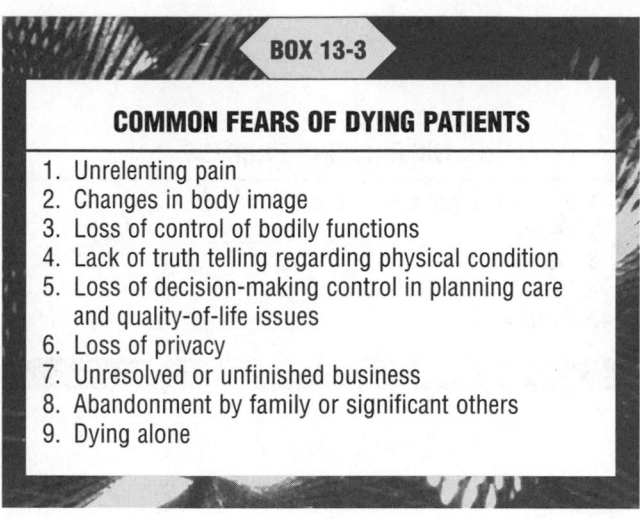

**BOX 13-3**

### COMMON FEARS OF DYING PATIENTS

1. Unrelenting pain
2. Changes in body image
3. Loss of control of bodily functions
4. Lack of truth telling regarding physical condition
5. Loss of decision-making control in planning care and quality-of-life issues
6. Loss of privacy
7. Unresolved or unfinished business
8. Abandonment by family or significant others
9. Dying alone

## Emotional Stages Experienced in the Dying Process

Observations of terminally ill patients indicate that patients experience stages of well-defined emotional feelings as they move through the dying process. These stages are identified as denial, anger, bargaining, depression, and acceptance (Kübler-Ross, 1969).

### Denial

When patients are unable to face the diagnosis of terminal illness, they often deny its existence. They are essentially saying, "No, not me." **Denial** is a defense mechanism that protects individuals from thoughts that they are unable to accept at that time.

### Anger

Patients who are not ready to accept that their illness is terminal become angry and displace that **anger** on those around them. Patients in this stage may be rude to their family, demanding of the nurse, and hostile to the physician. The patient who is experiencing anger asks, "Why me?"

### Bargaining

Anger may subside and patients may begin **bargaining,** or deciding how they can buy additional time. Such patients are saying, "Yes me, but. . . ." Their first approach may be to God, negotiating for an extension of time in exchange for leading a better life so that they can achieve a long-sought goal or attend a special event such as a wedding or graduation.

### Depression

**Depression** is marked by feelings of loss and despair. Depressed patients ask, "What is the use?" The ravages of disease and illness begin to take their toll. As the patient becomes weaker, the illness cannot be denied any longer. The patient becomes sad, may show less interest in visits from family and friends, may withdraw, and becomes uncommunicative.

### Acceptance

The final emotional stage is **acceptance.** The patient says, "I am ready." This stage may either be one of active acceptance or one of passive acceptance when the patient is too weak and tired to fight for life any longer. The struggle is over, and the patient longs for quiet and rest before the final journey (Kübler-Ross, 1969). However the patient still needs contact from family and friends. Touch is an important way to maintain contact and to support the patient during this time.

The sequence in which these emotions are experienced is varied. Some patients do not experience all of these emotional stages, and some do not exhibit the behavior characteristics of each stage. Not every patient will pass sequentially from denial to acceptance in the exact order. A patient often moves back and forth, entering the next stage and regressing to a previous stage. The patient's family and friends may experience the same stages but not necessarily in the same order or at the same time as the patient. Different family members may experience these stages at different times and in different orders. The patient may still be in the stage of anger when the family has progressed to the bargaining stage. This difference may cause problems in communication and make it more difficult for everyone to be supportive of one another. Both the patient and the family need the nurse's assistance to help them work through their individual stages.

The longer the period of dying, the more likely it is that the patient and family will move back and forth from one stage to another. Even if and when the patient reaches the stage of acceptance, hope still continues. Throughout the terminal illness the patient never loses hope that some new drug, treatment, or medical discovery will alter the outcome. Hope enables the patient to live as fully as possible despite weakness and vulnerability.

## GRIEF AND BEREAVEMENT

**Grief** is a normal emotional reaction to the loss of material possessions, self-identity, or a body function or part. A separation from loved ones such as in war or incarceration may also cause one to grieve. The death of a close relative or friend may cause an intense emotional response. The dying patient may grieve over the loss of life, independence, and meaningful experiences of the past; life work left unfinished; and the separation from loved ones.

After the patient dies, attention is focused on the significance of the death to the patient's family and friends. A period of **bereavement** is experienced by the family and friends of the deceased. More distant members of the family group and nurses who have had a long association with the patient may also grieve the death. Studies of bereavement indicate that a wide range of behavioral patterns may accompany grief. Some individuals are able to accept the situation and appear to have the emotional stability to adjust to the loss, whereas others may develop psychosomatic complaints. In some instances a physical illness may develop after the loss of a close friend or relative. If grieving is not experienced at the time of an individual's death, it may be experienced later, at the time of another loss.

The loss of a loved one rates high on the stress scale. Support from friends and the community is important when working through the grieving process. Recently, sources of help have become available in many communities and include bereavement support groups that are often affiliated with a hospital, funeral home, church, or hospice program.

According to the United States census, the number of widows far exceeds the number of widowers. Spouses who lose their partners are especially vulnerable to bereavement because of its consequences. An elderly person who loses a spouse may not experience the same problems as a younger person. Age, stage of development, and life experience affect how one adjusts to loss. When the loss of a loved one occurs, there is deprivation (Groenwald, 1991). Spiritually the individual is most acutely aware of the loss itself and may not think about deprivation until some time later. However, deprivation invariably follows loss. For example, the death of a mate can mean deprivation through loss of income, which lowers the standard of living to which the surviving spouse is accustomed. The surviving mate may also be left with the responsibility of raising a family alone. If the survivor is not already working, it may become necessary to seek employment to support the family.

Grieving is a psychologic process with three distinct phases. After the death of an individual, the survivor may be numb with grief and may protest the reality of the event. The survivor may experience physical changes such as loss of appetite, nausea, inability to sleep, weakness, and restlessness. A feeling of not be-

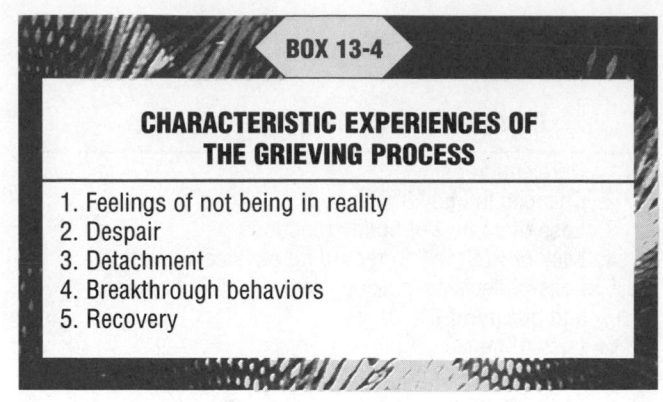

**BOX 13-4**

### CHARACTERISTIC EXPERIENCES OF THE GRIEVING PROCESS

1. Feelings of not being in reality
2. Despair
3. Detachment
4. Breakthrough behaviors
5. Recovery

ing in reality may exist, and the individual may be preoccupied with thoughts of the deceased. During this time the survivor is usually surrounded by friends and sympathizers. However, after the funeral the support systems often diminish. The individual is alone, and the second phase of grieving begins. This phase is characterized by despair. It is common to experience depression, decreased energy, a difficulty in making even simple decisions, and a sense of being slowed down in thought processes and actions. The final stage before recovery is characterized by detachment. Feelings of apathy, a loss of interest, and an absence of spontaneity may be present. The length of each of these stages varies and eventually culminates in some subtle "breakthrough" behaviors, such as reaching out to a new activity, interest, or person. These behaviors are accompanied by a fleeting sense of being able to enjoy some aspects of life once again (Box 13-4).

Many variables affect the grieving process, and no clear-cut pattern can be applied to every individual. The stages of grief are similar to the stages of dying. Grief is a response to a loss. Therefore it is logical that the bereaved person, like the dying person, moves along a similar path. For a few people the period of grief lasts only a few weeks, but for most others it may last more than a year. The progression through the grief process is not steady and is characterized by up and down periods rather than a gradual progression of feeling better. The process may vary if the death is sudden and unexpected or if it occurs after a prolonged terminal illness. If the family or loved ones have cared for and supported the patient, part of the grief work will have occurred before the death. This phenomenon is referred to as **anticipatory grief** and helps the individual move more quickly through the grieving process.

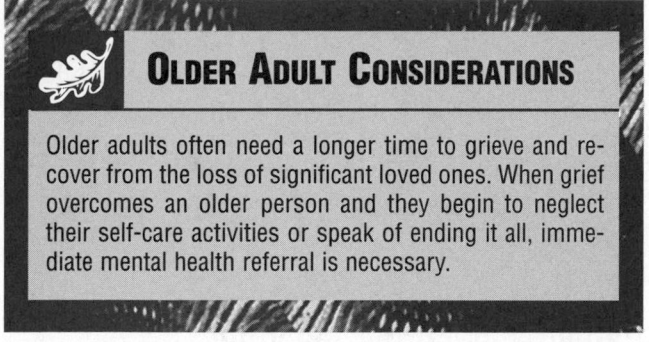

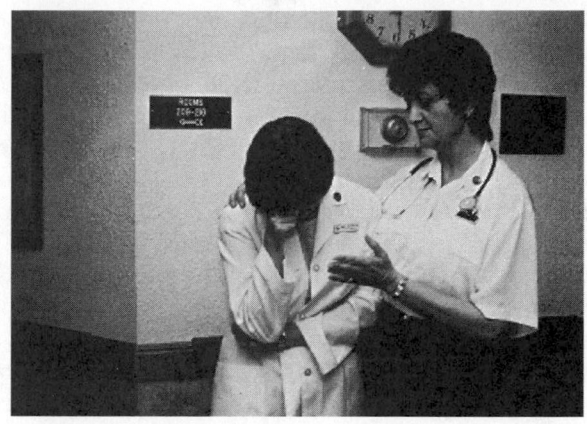

**Figure 13-3**   Colleagues can provide comfort for nurses. (Courtesy Michael S. Clement, MD, Mesa, Ariz. From Potter PA, Perry AG: *Basic nursing: theory and practice,* ed 3, St Louis, 1995, Mosby.)

---

| BOX 13-5 | **NURSING PROCESS** |
|---|---|

## CARE OF THE DYING

**ASSESSMENT**

- Presence and quality of pain and related unpleasant symptoms
- Need for food and fluids
- Elimination
- Skin integrity
- Social and spiritual needs
- Ability to communicate
- Need for family involvement

**NURSING DIAGNOSIS**

- Pain and symptom control related to the diagnosis of terminal disease

**NURSING INTERVENTIONS**

- Periodically assess pain and troublesome symptoms.
- Communicate with others on the health care team for medication adjustment.
- Provide pain medication as ordered and record outcome.

**EVALUATION OF EXPECTED OUTCOMES**

- Patient is pain and symptom free at time of death
- Family and friends are present at the time of death if desired by patient
- Dignity of the patient is maintained throughout the dying process

---

# NURSING CARE OF THE DYING PATIENT

The nurse is responsible for caring not only for a dying patient, but also for the patient's family and friends (Box 13-5). Several studies indicate that nurses sometimes avoid dying patients. It has been proposed that caring for a dying patient stimulates nurses to think about their own deaths or unresolved grief. For some nurses the avoidance may be from the frustration of being unable to "make everything right."

When working with the terminally ill, the nurse moves through the same stages of grieving as the family and patient. To fulfill this emotionally demanding role, the nurse must receive support from some other source (Figure 13-3). Individual sessions with more experienced nursing personnel and group sessions with pastoral care staff, social workers, and psychologists can provide support to the nurse. Expanding this type of support system is desirable to prevent burnout and to help nurses grow from their experiences. The nurse is urged to acknowledge and discuss her feelings, not repress them. Most nurses are caring people and often feel sadness and loss at the death of the patients they have cared for. Providing the best **palliative care,** which focuses on quality of life and symptom control, for the patient and emotional support for the family gives the nurse a feeling of accomplishment. The families of those who have died a comfortable and dignified death are usually grateful.

Caring for the terminally ill patient involves dealing with the physical, psychosocial, and spiritual health of the patient (Box 13-6). A terminal illness does not mean that the patient is facing immediate death. Many illnesses from which the patient is not expected to recover, such as acquired immunodeficiency syndrome and some types of cancer, are marked by long remissions that are punctuated by exacerbations.

During a patient's admission to the hospital, the nurse should get to know the patient and learn about his or her social and cultural background, religious or spiritual orientation, and personal problems that may be particularly concerning him or her. The nurse should assess how the patient is dealing with the illness and identify which emotional stages the patient and family are experiencing. In addition, the nurse can help the patient identify any unfinished business that the patient wishes to address before death.

Although many patients are aware of their prognosis, others may not be. Some patients who suspect that they have a terminal illness seek confirmation from the nurse. The nurse should be aware of this possibility and be prepared to handle it in a sensitive manner. It is especially important that the nurse know what the physician has told the patient and the family. Many experts in the field of death and dying believe that the patient always knows the truth, whether or not the family or physician has shared the prognosis. The nurse can be of greatest help to the patient by facilitating and encouraging open expressions of feelings and concerns. By conveying this information to the physi-cian and the family, the nurse can help all parties involved to openly face the subject of death.

If staffing patterns permit, the same nurse should be assigned to care for the patient on each admission. When this is possible, the patient and family develop a feeling of trust, security, and confidence. When the patient is admitted for the last time, the personal relationship that has been established may help to bridge the gap between living and dying.

## Patient and Family Teaching

The patient and family should be allowed to ask any questions they may have regarding treatments and the prognosis. The patient and family may repeat the same questions to different caregivers. They should be given as complete an explanation as they can deal with and understand.

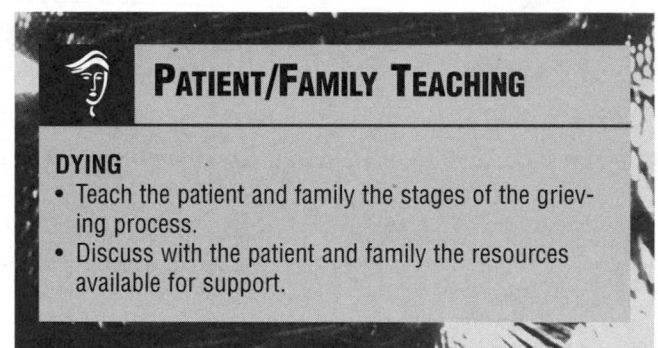

**PATIENT/FAMILY TEACHING**

**DYING**
- Teach the patient and family the stages of the grieving process.
- Discuss with the patient and family the resources available for support.

---

| BOX 13-6 | NURSING PROCESS |
| --- | --- |

## SPIRITUAL DISTRESS

**ASSESSMENT**
- Presence of anxiety, doubt, anger, and depression
- Rejection or neglect of previous religious practices
- Increased interest in spiritual matters

**NURSING DIAGNOSIS**
- Spiritual distress related to diagnosis of terminal disease

**NURSING INTERVENTIONS**
- Make time to listen actively to patient and family.
- Help the patient focus on successes and the value of the positive experiences in life.
- Offer to contact a religious leader if the patient wants counseling, or refer the patient to hospital chaplain services.

- Allow the patient to express feelings such as anger, guilt, and despair.
- Offer unconditional support to the patient and family.

**EVALUATION OF EXPECTED OUTCOMES**
- Verbalizes feelings concerning the diagnosis
- Talks with family and significant others about feelings
- Able to put this life event in perspective with the rest of life
- Works through the grief stages toward resolution
- Expresses feelings of acceptance of impending death

## Death Following Traumatic Injury

The nurse faces a special challenge when providing support to patients and families in the intensive care unit following a sudden and unanticipated traumatic injury in which death is imminent. In today's technologically advanced environment it is possible to lose sight of the patient as a person and to disregard what the patient considers to be in his or her best interests. Comfort and communication should be a high priority. The nurse is instrumental in ensuring that the family has the opportunity to stay with the patient as much as possible. These elements are crucial to ensuring a dignified death for the patient. Often the nurse's role is to ask questions to help the patient, family, and physician steer the situation toward responsible and appropriate treatment (Pelliter, 1992).

## Organ Donation

When death is inevitable, the patient and family have few choices. If the patient has the potential to be an organ or tissue donor, the option should be offered. Offering this option to a grieving family can be a final way to help them through their grief (Chabalewski, Gaedeke-Norris, 1994). It may be difficult for the family to understand and accept death when their loved one is being maintained on a ventilator and still has a heartbeat. The nurse should be supportive and answer any questions. The most common information that the nurse provides regarding organ donation includes the surgical recovery of donated tissue and organs, the fact that open caskets are still possible after donation, and the fact that the family does not assume the cost of the surgical recovery (Chabalewski, Gaedeke-Norris, 1994). To provide this information to the family the nurse must be well informed about the policies and procedures of the hospital. The nurse may also help determine which family member to approach when a potential donor is identified. This individual should be the one who has demonstrated emotional strength and clear thinking throughout the ordeal. The consent of the next of kin is also required. Organs presently used for transplant include the kidney, heart, liver, pancreas, and lung. Tissues that can be donated include the cornea, skin, bone, and heart valves (Chabalewski, Gaedeke-Norris, 1994).

## Hospice Movement

The special needs of the dying patient and his or her family are addressed by the concept of **hospice.** The term *hospice* originally referred to a resting place for travelers on a difficult journey. The concept of care for the dying patient began in England and has rapidly spread throughout the United States in the last decade. There are three basic types of hospices: (1) home-based, which provides a support system that enables a patient to die at home; (2) freestanding, which is available as a haven for the terminally ill to come to die; and (3) defined areas or teams, which exist in the general hospital setting. The hospice concept requires the cooperation of various disciplines, including nurses, physicians, pharmacists, social workers, dietitians, clergy, and volunteers. All of these people work together around the clock to address the patient's physical, emotional, and spiritual needs (Figure 13-4). The basic goals of hospice care are as follows:

1. To maintain the patient in as symptom-free a state as possible. In many cases this means addressing the problem of pain control. The nurse, physician, and pharmacist work together to keep the patient as nearly free of pain as possible and at a level of alertness that enables him or her to interact with family and friends.
2. To encourage the patient to continue to define quality of life, maintain control, and make decisions about care.
3. To encourage the patient to live fully and support his or her own efforts to communicate with family and friends to complete the unfinished business of life. The nurse, social worker, and clergy often work together to attain this goal.
4. To be available to the family and provide them with individualized and appropriate support. Volunteers are important members of the hospice team and provide **respite** care for family members, help with household chores, and run errands.

If nurses are in tune with the patient's needs, many of these goals can be accomplished at home or in the hospital.

### ETHICAL DILEMMA

1. Should a dying patient be told of his or her condition? Justify your answer and give reasons.
2. Should limited health care resources such as intensive care unit beds and dialysis machines be restricted to patients who have a chance of recovery?
3. Is a patient's refusal of life-sustaining treatment the same as suicide?
4. Who makes the decisions regarding life-sustaining treatment if the patient cannot?
5. How might a nurse's personal view of death affect the care of dying patients? Should personal views affect the care provided?

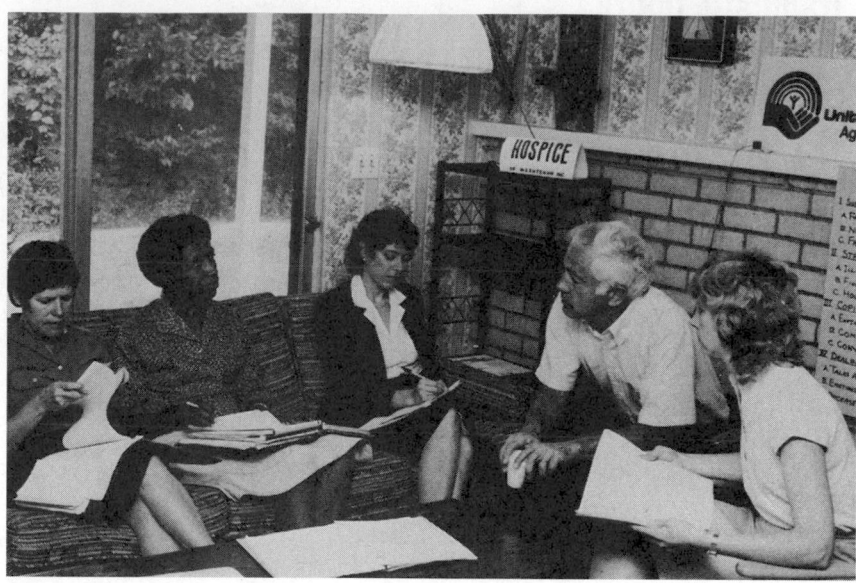

**Figure 13-4**    Hospice teams meet to plan care for their terminally ill patients and families. (Courtesy of Hospice of Washtenaw, Ann Arbor, Mich.)

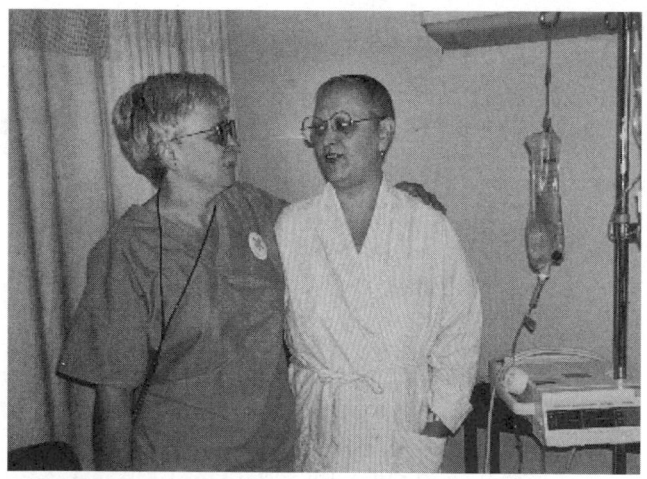

**Figure 13-5**    The nurse serves as a role model for the family by demonstrating appropriate methods of comfort and support.

Each patient faces death in a unique way. In most cases the patient does not want to feel abandoned and desires the company of a close friend or relative. The family should be encouraged to spend as much time with the patient as possible. A nurse's frequent visits to the patient's room, a gently placed hand on the patient's shoulder, and a kind word convey to the patient that he or she is not alone (Figure 13-5). The nurse should serve as a role model for the family by demonstrating appropriate methods of comfort and support. Small objects belonging to the patient, such as family pictures, should be placed within easy viewing distance. The creative use of light, flowers, and music can provide a comforting atmosphere. The patient should be placed in an area where he or she can hear people and not feel alone.

## Nursing Interventions
### Physical Care

The physical care of the patient must continue to the end. Such care is supportive and maintains the patient's comfort. As with all patients, it is appropriate to use universal and body substance isolation precautions when providing care. The patient may be unable to care for his or her personal hygiene needs. Bathing, including perineal and skin care, is essential. It is also important to establish a regular schedule for turning the patient. The dying patient may experience edema, muscle atrophy, or decreased mobility, which makes good skin care essential for the patient's comfort. Oral care must not be neglected. Many terminally ill patients breathe through their mouths, which causes mucous membranes to become dry and sore. A poor oral condition interferes with speech and swallowing. When dentures cannot be worn, drooling occurs. Pathogenic organisms and oral secretions may cause stomatitis and maceration of tissues around the mouth, which may cause the patient pain. Oral care should be given regularly and should be sufficient to keep the tissues clean and free of odor.

Studies have shown that terminally ill patients experience hunger and thirst only briefly or not at all (McCann, Hall, Groth-Juncker, 1994). The symptoms of hunger and thirst can be relieved with small amounts of food, fluids, ice chips, and lubrication to

---

| BOX 13-7 | **NURSING PROCESS** |
| --- | --- |

## PAIN

**ASSESSMENT**

- Physical pain
- Levels of pain
- Previous successful and unsuccessful pain relief measures

**NURSING DIAGNOSIS**

- Pain related to physiologic processes

**NURSING INTERVENTIONS**

- Administer pain relief medications as per orders; assess effectiveness frequently.

- Reposition patient to a more comfortable position.
- Attend to patient's personal hygiene needs.
- Provide back rubs and massages as needed for relief of muscular discomfort resulting from immobility.

**EVALUATION OF EXPECTED OUTCOMES**

- Verbalizes that pain is decreased or absent
- Family participation in providing effective pain relief measures to patient

---

the lips. Sometimes administration of larger amounts of fluids to dying patients (including intravenous fluids) increases their level of discomfort because secretions build in the lungs, thus frequent suctioning may be necessary. Of course the symptoms of pain and shortness of breath must be controlled and are usually done so with narcotics.

Because a terminal illness is often accompanied by pain, ongoing assessment of pain is important (Box 13-7). Pain medication can be administered by intravenous route, orally, by subcutaneous injection, or by a transdermal patch. Often the dose of pain medication given to a terminally ill patient far exceeds the normal ranges for the drug because the patient needs greater amounts to control the increasing pain. It is important for the nurse to recognize this need and to be willing to adjust the dosage according to the patient's need for pain control. Pain medication should not be administered on an "as needed" (prn) basis because it necessitates the patient experiencing pain, calling for medication, and awaiting relief from the medication. Pain medication should be administered routinely around the clock to prevent the pain from recurring and causing physical and emotional distress to the patient and his or her family. The dosing schedule is dependent on the therapeutic effectiveness of the drug. Drugs with a short half-life (subcutaneous morphine sulfate) may be administered every 3 to 4 hours in the dying patient to control symptoms and provide effective pain control.

Pain and the effects of pain medications affect the patient's appetite, which leads to poor nutritional status and further debilitation. A stool softener is an important adjunct to pain control medication and prevents the additional discomfort of constipation. The sensory effects of the pain medication can make it im-

possible for the patient to think clearly and to deal effectively with loved ones.

Recent developments in pain control include new methods of morphine use. The use of oral morphine has increased. Concentrated oral morphine may be administered under the tongue via an eyedropper so that even the patient with swallowing difficulties may benefit from concentrated oral solutions absorbed sublingually. Higher concentrated solutions of morphine and sustained-release morphine tablets are also available for oral use. Transdermal patches with analgesics are also being used for pain control. However, transdermal patches have a slow onset of effectiveness (up to 72 hours), and the patient may need some supplemental short-acting analgesics while waiting for the patch medication to reach effective levels.

Effective pain control is possible if medications are given around the clock. The dosage should be adjusted according to the patient's unique and changing needs. This method of medication administration replaces the demand, or prn, method and is more successful in controlling pain breakthrough and erasing pain memory. The nurse should check frequently with the patient or the patient's family to make sure the pain is being controlled effectively. Nonverbal patients should be carefully observed for signs of pain including moaning, rigidity, rapid gasping breathing, and facial grimacing.

### Emotional Support

The patient or family may be demanding and angry, tearful, or withdrawn. It is important that the patient express his or her feelings. The nurse can best facilitate the expression of feelings by being an attentive, nonjudgmental listener. The nurse's continued presence and support conveys feelings of care and concern and lessens the fear of abandonment. Attentive listening enables the nurse to identify the family's and the patient's specific concerns or unfinished business. If the nurse cannot assist in problem solving, the patient and family may be referred to a social worker, minister, or psychiatrist as appropriate.

Reminiscence therapy and relaxation techniques may also help provide emotional support to the patient and family. Humor also plays an important role in interacting with the terminally ill and is thought to provide a sense of power and self-worth when emotional pain is overwhelming. Herth (1990) states that humor is closely related to self-concept and provides a sense of perspective, hope, and joy, which empowers the individual and results in a sense of control. Shared humor also serves as a connecting mechanism and diminishes the feelings of isolation that are associated with dying.

## Spiritual Support

Before providing spiritual support to patients and their families, nurses must assess their feelings regarding their own death and dying experiences. The process of identifying personal spiritual beliefs continues throughout a nurse's lifetime and enables continued improvement in the nurse's supporting skills.

If the nurse can suspend judgment, interpretation, and analysis, an atmosphere of openness can be created and the patient and family may feel more comfortable sharing their spiritual philosophy or religious beliefs. It is essential to listen, affirm beliefs, and help the patient and family participate in familiar religious rituals. When requested to do so, the nurse may pray with or read to the patient and family from the patient's personal religious text. If the nurse feels uncomfortable in this role, a member of the clergy may be contacted to visit the patient and provide this valuable service.

### NURSE ALERT

**Regardless of the nurse's beliefs, support should be provided within the patient's own spiritual or religious framework. With the patient's and the family's permission, referrals can be made to the patient's minister or to the hospital pastoral care staff.**

## Family Support

Attending to the family's needs is an extension of caring for the dying patient. Emotional support includes providing the family with as much uninterrupted time

with the patient as possible. Providing a quiet and private place for the family to be together is also important. Family members should be given the opportunity to express their feelings as death approaches (Box 13-8)

## Following Death

In addition to the legal requirements for autopsy, death certificates, and interstate transport of bodies, each hospital, county, and state has its own policies and procedures regarding death. The nurse should become familiar with these policies and procedures. When the patient dies, the family should have the opportunity to view and spend time with the deceased family member. If possible, the nurse should straighten the bedclothes and surroundings and place the deceased in a composed position before the viewing.

---

**BOX 13-8**

### Guidelines for the Care of the Dying Patient and His or Her Family

1 Decisions concerning the use of extraordinary means to prolong life are the responsibility of the patient, the family, and the physician. Input from other members of the health care team may often be helpful.

2 Encouraging the patient to be a decision maker regarding his or her care and treatment for as long as the condition permits is basic to maintaining dignity and feelings of self-worth.

3 It is the nurse's responsibility to see that physical care and emotional and spiritual support are available to the dying patient. The nurse plays an important part in this care and should involve others in the health care team as appropriate.

4 The patient may identify one or two members of the family or the hospital staff with whom he or she feels most comfortable discussing feelings. The choices of individuals should be respected.

5 The nurse should assess how the patient's family members and friends are dealing with the impending loss of their loved one, encourage them to express their feelings, and direct them toward additional support from the health care team as necessary.

6 Various cultures and religions have ritualistic practices that help a bereaved individual move through the grieving process. These practices should be encouraged and respected.

7 It is common for the bereaved to express feelings of guilt in regard to past life experiences with the deceased.

8 Family and friends should be made aware of local bereavement support groups.

After the family has finished viewing the deceased family member, the body is prepared for removal. Unless there is to be an autopsy, all invasive tubes are removed. The eyes and mouth should be closed. To secure the jaw closed it may be necessary to place a roll of gauze under the chin and tie another piece of gauze under the chin and over the top of the head. Tags with identifying information are usually placed on the wrist, ankle, and shroud. After the body has been removed, the nurse should help the family gather the patient's belongings. Handling the patient's body and belongings with dignity conveys to the family respect for the deceased and concern for their feelings. Emotional support for the family should continue.

---

## NURSING CARE PLAN

## DEATH AND DYING

Mr. Duffy is a 66-year-old man who was diagnosed with oat cell carcinoma of the lungs 2 months ago. He has been hospitalized for 7 days because of recurring high fever, cachexia, and a persistent, debilitating cough. For several days Mr. Duffy has refused inhalation therapy and other treatments. He has requested that the blinds be drawn in his room during the day shift and has spent the last 2 days lying with his eyes closed and facing the wall when awake. Today he refused to eat his breakfast and lunch. When the nurse expressed concern he stated, "I feel sad and empty. How can God let this happen to me?" He asks the nurses to tell his family that he prefers not to see them during visiting hours.

| Medical History | Psychosocial Data | Assessment Data |
|---|---|---|
| No previous surgeries | Married for 29 years | Alert and oriented ×3 |
| History of smoking x 40 years | Has four living children; closest is living 5 hours away; other children live out of state | Vital signs stable and within normal limits |
| Has had recurrent respiratory infections, but none serious enough to warrant hospitalization | Owns three-story house with large yard | Coughing productively at times; producing thick, white sputum tinged with blood |
| No current medications except pain medications and cough suppressants | Retired attorney | Respirations somewhat labored; nasal $O_2$ at 2 L/min administered via nasal cannula |
| Has poor vision corrected somewhat by glasses | Recreational activities include fishing, reading, working crossword puzzles, and gardening | |

### NURSING DIAGNOSIS
Spiritual distress related to terminal disease diagnosis

### NURSING INTERVENTIONS

Take time to sit with the patient and listen in a nonjudgmental manner.

Encourage the patient to reminisce about past experiences and their significance to his life. Help him focus on successes and the value of positive experiences.

Help the patient place the illness experience into the context of the total life experience. Pray with the patient as he desires.

Discuss the patient's significant family relationships and ways to maintain and strengthen them. Provide for privacy needs during visiting hours. Be available to the family with ideas regarding how to best support the patient, such as hospice or pastoral referral.

Help the patient with relaxation techniques. Suggest music therapy, meditation, and prayer.

### EVALUATION OF EXPECTED OUTCOMES

Expresses anger and other feelings

Increases his level of acceptance of self, God, and others

Experiences an increased sense of meaning in living with an illness

Maintains communication with and accepts support from his family

Develops an increased sense of hope and inner peace

Describes what loss and death mean to him

Shares his feelings and grief with his family and significant others

## KEY CONCEPTS

➤ The nursing care of terminally ill patients deals with the physical, psychosocial, and spiritual health of the patients.

➤ The nurse can facilitate communication between the patient and family members during these emotional times and provide for the physical needs of the patient.

➤ In working with terminally ill patients and their families, the nurse often moves along the same stages of grief as the families and the patients do.

➤ Supporting patients and families following a sudden and unanticipated traumatic injury in which death is imminent provides a special challenge.

➤ The nurse should serve as a role model for the family by demonstrating appropriate ways to comfort and support the patient.

➤ The physical care of the dying patient focuses on maintaining the comfort of the patient. This includes not only personal hygiene needs but also adequate pain control.

➤ The nurse can best provide emotional support by being an attentive listener.

➤ The nurse needs to provide the patient and family with an atmosphere of acceptance and openness in which to discuss spiritual concerns.

➤ Grief is the emotional response to loss.

➤ When moving through the dying process, terminally ill patients experience stages of denial, anger, bargaining, depression, and acceptance. Friends and families also experience these emotional stages.

➤ Terminally ill patients now discuss options with their physicians regarding prolonging life with extraordinary means. Advanced directives or living wills are documents that allow other individuals to state a patient's health care wishes if the patient is unable to do so.

➤ The nurse should discuss organ donation with the families of potential donors.

➤ The hospice movement developed as a support system for dying patients and their families.

➤ The use of technology to prolong life has made the definition of death more difficult. Death is defined as the absence of spontaneous brain activity and spontaneous respirations.

➤ Using extraordinary means to prolong the life of terminally ill patients becomes a tangled web of ethical, religious, legal, and moral questions that have no clear answers.

## CRITICAL THINKING EXERCISES

1. What factors have influenced the change in American society's attitudes regarding death?

2. How does anticipatory grief affect the period of bereavement?

3. What factors must be considered in selecting treatment measures for the patient who has completed an advance directive and designated a durable power of attorney for health care?

## REFERENCES AND ADDITIONAL READINGS

Bersford J: *Hospice handbook,* Boston, 1993, Little, Brown.

Boutell K, Bozett F: Nurses' assessment of patients' spirituality: continuing education implications, *J Contain Educ Nubs* 21(4):172-176, 1990.

Carpenito LJ: *Nursing diagnosis application to clinical practice,* ed 5, Philadelphia, 1993, Lippincott.

Carson VB: *Spiritual dimensions of nursing practice,* Philadelphia, 1989, Saunders.

Chabalewski F, Gaedeke-Norris MK: The gift of life: talking to families about organ and tissue donation, *Am J Nurs* 94(6):28-33, 1994.

Clark C et al: Spirituality: integral to quality care, *Holist Nurs Pract* 5(3):67-76, 1991.

Clarke J: The day after a death, *Nurs Time* 89(12):46-47, 1993.

Claxton JW: Paving the way to acceptance: psychological adaptation to death and dying in cancer, *Prof Nurse* 8(4):206-211, 1993.

Dart S, Taylor E: Talking it through, *Nurs Time* 89(16):50-52, 1993.

Enck RE: The last few days, *Am J Hospice Palliat Care* 9(4):11-13, 1992.

Gordon M, Cheung M: Poor outcome of on-site CPR in a multi-level geriatric facility: three and a half years experience at the Baycrest Centre for Geriatric Care, *J Am Geriatr Soc* 41:163-166, 1993.

Gravely JN, Jr: *Spirituality as a nursing diagnosis in the plan of care for terminally ill clients,* unpublished master's thesis, Radford, Va, 1993, Radford University School of Nursing.

Groenwald SL: *Psychosocial dimensions of cancer,* Boston, 1991, Jones & Bartlett.

Hallal JC, Walsh MB: Loss, bereavement, and care of the dying person. In Burke MM, Walsh M, editors: *Gerontologic nursing: wholistic care of the older adult,* St Louis, 1993, Mosby.

Herth K: Contributions of humor as perceived by the terminally ill, *Am J Hospice Care* 7(1):36-40, 1990.

Irvine B: Teaching palliative care to nursing students, *Nurs Stand* 7(50):37-39, 1993.

Johnson SH: Saying "goodbye" . . . when a family member is near death, *Dimens Crit Care Nurs* 12(6):319, 1993.

Kastenbaum R, Aisenberg RB: *The psychology of death,* ed 2, New York, 1992, Springer.

Kübler-Ross E: *On death and dying,* New York, 1969, Macmillan.

Kübler-Ross E: *Death: the final stage of growth,* Englewood Cliffs, NJ, 1975, Prentice Hall.

Lynn J et al: American Geriatrics Society on physician-assisted suicide, *J Am Geriatr Soc,* 45(4):491-499, 1997.

MacInnis K: Making good-byes, *Am J Nurs* 92(3):120, 1992.

Madden E: *Carpe diem . . . enjoying every day with a terminal illness,* Boston, 1993, Jones & Bartlett.

Maher MF, Smith DC: Achieving a healthy death: the dying person's attitudinal contributions, *Hospice J* 9(1):21-32, 1993.

Mallison MB: Decoding the messages of the dying, *Am J Nurs* 93(1):7, 1993.

Marks M: Palliative care, *Nurs Stand* 6(33):9-16, 1992.

McCaffery M, Wolff M: Pain relief using cutaneous modalities, positioning, and movement, *Hospice J* 8(1,2):121-153, 1992.

McCann RM, Hall WJ, Groth-Juncker A: Comfort care for terminally ill patients: the appropriate use of nutrition and hydration, *JAMA,* 272(16): 1263-1266, 1994.

McFarland G, McFarland E: *Nursing diagnosis and intervention,* ed 2, St Louis, 1993, Mosby.

McMillam CL, Burdock J, Wamsley J: The challenging experience of palliative care support-team nursing, *Oncol Nurs Forum* 20(5):779-785, 1993.

Mendyka BE: The dying patient in the intensive care unit: assisting the family in crisis, *AACN Clin Issues Crit Care Nurs* 4(3):550-557, 1993.

Moore FD: Ethics at both ends of life. In Moore FD: *A miracle and a privilege: recounting a half century of surgical advances,* Washington, DC, 1995, Joseph Henry Press.

Murphy PA, Price DM: "ACT": taking a positive approach to end-of-life care, *Am J Nurs* 95(3):42-43, 1995.

North American Nursing Diagnosis Association: *NANDA nursing diagnoses: definitions and classification 1995-1996,* Philadelphia, 1995, The Association.

Nystanga B: Emotional pain in terminal illness: a dilemma for nurses, *Senior Nurse* 13(3):46-48, 1993.

Pelliter M: The organ donor family members' perception of stressful situations during the organ donation experience, *J Adv Nurs* 17(1):90-97, 1992.

Schwenzer KJ, Smith WT, Durbin CG, Jr: Selective application of cardiopulmonary resuscitation improves survival rates, *Anesth Analg,* 76:478-484, 1993.

Teno J, Lynn J, Connors AF: The illusion of end-of-life resource savings with advanced directives, *J Am Geriatr Soc* 45(4):513-518, 1997.

Tresch DD et al: Outcomes of cardiopulmonary resuscitation in nursing homes: can we predict who will benefit? *Am J Med* 95:123-130, 1993.

United States Department of Health and Human Services: *Clinical practice guidelines: management of cancer pain,* Washington, DC, March 1994, Agency for Health Care Policy and Research.

Zerwekh J: Do dying patients really need IV fluids? *Am J Nurs* 97(3):26-31, 1997.

# CHAPTER 14

# Community-Acquired Infections

## CHAPTER OBJECTIVES

1 Discuss the interrelationships between the agent, host, and environment in the development of infectious disease.
2 Describe the major means of transmission of communicable diseases.
3 Explain the role of immunization in the prevention of communicable diseases.
4 Differentiate among the common infectious diseases in the community setting according to agent, host, and environmental characteristics.
5 Define the nurse's role in treatment, prevention, and control of communicable disease.

## KEY TERMS

acquired active immunity
agent
antitoxin
biologic
carrier
communicable disease
environment
epidemiologic surveillance
fomite
host
immunogenicity
immunoglobulins
incubation period
infectious disease
infectivity
infestation
natural passive
  immunity
passive immunity
pathogen
pathogenicity
physical
primary prevention
secondary prevention
socioeconomic
tertiary prevention
toxoid
vaccine
vectorborne
virulence

One of the greatest accomplishments of the twentieth century has been the control of communicable diseases in humans. There are remarkable contrasts when one examines health trends during the past 100 years. Those born at the beginning of the century had an average life expectancy of 47.5 years. In 1900 tuberculosis accounted for 25% of all deaths. Of all major illnesses, 75% resulted from acute infectious diseases. These diseases took a particularly devastating toll on infants.

Public health measures, such as clean drinking water, effective waste control, availability of a variety of foods, better methods of food handling, and public enlightenment have been largely responsible for the remarkable decrease in these illness burdens. Medical advances have produced immunizing agents, such as serums and vaccines, that aid human immune processes in preventing disease or in modifying its severity. Antibiotics have reduced the impact of many diseases and have enhanced recovery with minimal complications. The result, over what is a relatively short period, has been a decline in disease-related deaths, particularly infant deaths, and an increase in life span.

Life expectancy is currently more than 75 years, and the population is not only increasing but is also growing older. Illnesses have changed. With the exception of acquired immunodeficiency syndrome (AIDS), chronic noninfectious diseases have replaced most infectious diseases as the leading causes of morbidity and mortality in the United States. Atherosclerosis, the underlying disease process in heart attacks and strokes, and conditions such as cancer, diabetes, emphysema, and arthritis now comprise the majority of the health burdens in the United States. These illnesses are long lasting, demand continuous monitoring and care, and have contributed, in part, to the increase in medical costs during the latter part of the century.

Despite the remarkable success in reducing the impact of infectious diseases on society, an ongoing program of infectious disease prevention and control must be maintained. Infectious processes continue to account for a major proportion of acute illnesses. Pneumonia has consistently remained among the ten highest causes of death. Lost schooldays and workdays per year from infectious diseases are significant. AIDS continues to be a major cause of morbidity and mortality. From 1981 through 1996 a total of 573,800 AIDS cases in persons 13 years old and older were reported to the Centers for Disease Control and Prevention (CDC). In the first 6 months of 1996 there were 22,000 AIDS deaths reported (CDC, 1997).

In addition, the emergence of drug-resistant bacteria such as penicillin-resistant *Streptococcus pneumoniae* and multiple-resistant *Mycobacterium tuberculosis* has created new challenges for health care.

## CHARACTERISTICS OF THE INFECTIOUS PROCESS

A communicable disease is an **infectious disease** in which the causative organism is transmitted from where it lives and multiplies to another person or place. It can be transmitted directly from one person to another or indirectly through contaminated objects or infected insects or animals. The development of the infection depends on the interaction of the causative **agent, host,** and the **environment** (Figure 14-1). The interaction among the agent, the host, and the environment must be optimal for an infectious disease to develop. For instance, organisms such as tetanus spores cannot grow and multiply in oxygen-rich environments. Other organisms, such as the tubercle bacillus, thrive in persons who are malnourished, fatigued, and exposed to poor sanitary conditions (e.g., homeless persons).

## Agent

The infectious agent is usually a microorganism called a **pathogen.** Parasites such as helminths (small worm-like animals) and insects such as lice are communicable **infestations.** Infectious agents are classified as bacteria, viruses, fungi, protozoa, and helminths (see Chapter 7). All infectious agents have intrinsic properties that are unique to the microorganism or parasite. These characteristics include size, chemical character, growth requirements, antigenic properties, ability to produce toxin, ability to become resistant to chemicals, ability to live outside of the host, and other factors. Some organisms require moist, warm, dark breeding grounds. Others can survive in dry, warm, or cold settings until the proper conditions exist for them to grow and multiply. The virulence of the organism can vary, particularly in those organisms that are subject to change, such as the influenza viruses. Some organisms can exist in a dormant state. Knowledge of these intrinsic properties is essential to the prevention and control of infectious agents.

Some properties of infectious agents are not necessarily intrinsic to the agent but result from an interaction among the agent, the host, and the environment. These properties include the **infectivity, pathogenicity, virulence,** and **immunogenicity** of a specific infectious agent (Box 14-1). There are normal ranges of these properties for all infectious agents. However, host factors such as age, nutritional status, and underlying illness can result in an increased or decreased resistance to the agent. Similarly, environmental conditions can affect such factors as the amount of the dose and the ability of the agent to be transmitted to the host.

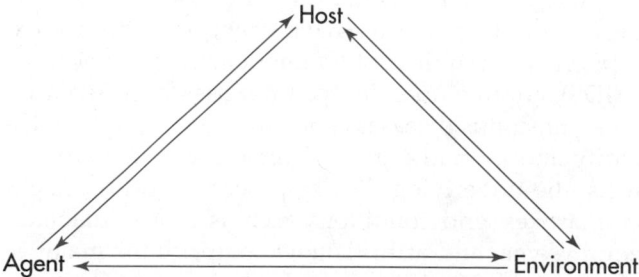

**Figure 14-1** Interactions among the agent, host, and environment must be optimal for an infectious disease to develop.

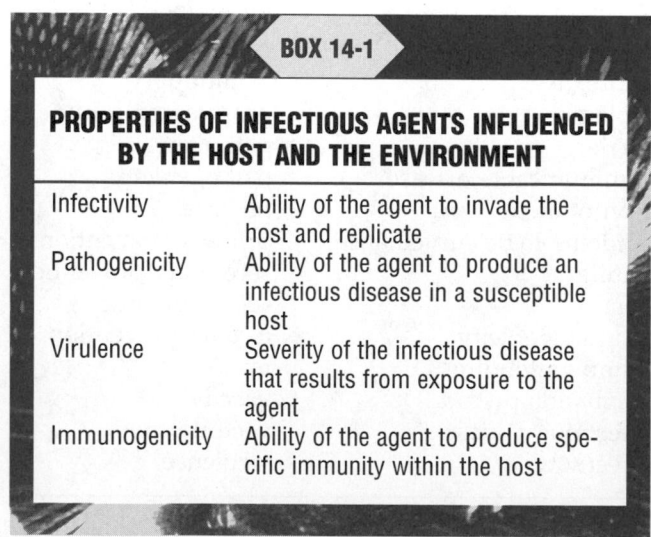

**BOX 14-1**

**PROPERTIES OF INFECTIOUS AGENTS INFLUENCED BY THE HOST AND THE ENVIRONMENT**

| | |
|---|---|
| Infectivity | Ability of the agent to invade the host and replicate |
| Pathogenicity | Ability of the agent to produce an infectious disease in a susceptible host |
| Virulence | Severity of the infectious disease that results from exposure to the agent |
| Immunogenicity | Ability of the agent to produce specific immunity within the host |

## Host

The presence of an infectious agent does not always produce disease. A susceptible host must also be present. Many underlying host factors determine whether the person develops the infection. Factors that contribute to susceptibility include the person's general health, immune status, and age; the amount or dose of the infectious agent; and the duration of exposure.

Infectious processes can produce a variety of clinical effects in the host, ranging from inapparent (subclinical) infection to mild, moderate, or severe clinical illness or death. Inapparent infection can occur when the infectious agent invades the host and begins to grow and multiply but does not produce symptoms of illness. The host's immune system is able to combat the infection without visible effects. Such a person may become a **carrier** who is capable of infecting others without having evidence of the disease. This characteristic of early human immunodeficiency virus (HIV) infection, the causative agent in AIDS, has produced great problems for the prevention and control of its spread. Depending on the agent characteristics, people with active infections are communicable for varying periods, but an average for common infectious diseases is from 3 to 7 days.

## Environment

The interaction between the agent and the host occurs in the environment. The environment includes all external influences that affect living organisms. The **physical** environment includes the characteristics of the place (geography), the climate, and the seasons. The **biologic** environment is comprised of the living plants and animals that surround the host. The **socioeconomic** environment refers to the social and economic conditions that have an impact on the quality of life. These conditions determine the availability of safe drinking water, sanitary facilities, a variety of food, and medical care. Poor socioeconomic conditions commonly contribute to the spread of infectious diseases.

Modification of the environment is one way that the agent-host-environment interaction may be changed to prevent or control an infectious disease. Changing environmental conditions can alter the infectivity, pathogenicity, virulence, and immunogenic properties of the agent and decrease its ability to cause illness in human beings. For example, placing contaminated objects in boiling water has long been used to destroy organisms and prevent their spread.

## Transmission

The transmission of infectious agents to a susceptible host occurs in the environment. The transmission of microorganisms involves many factors (Figure 14-2). There are four main modes of transmission: contact, airborne, vehicle, and vectorborne. A single microorganism may be transmitted by more than one route. For example, the varicella-zoster virus (VZV) (chickenpox) can be spread either by the airborne route or by direct contact.

Contact transmission is the most common method by which microorganisms are transmitted from one person to another. Contact transmission can be divided into three subgroups: direct contact, indirect contact, and droplet contact. Direct contact involves person-to-person spread and occurs when there is physical contact between the source and the susceptible person. Contact occurs constantly during daily patient care, with hands having the most contact with the patient. Therefore thorough handwashing is the best way to prevent transmission by direct contact. Indirect contact involves personal contact of the susceptible host with a contaminated intermediate object, or a **fomite**. For example, an inadequately disinfected endoscope can indirectly transfer organisms. Droplet contact occurs when an infectious agent briefly passes through the air. The infected sources and the susceptible host are usually within a few feet of each other. This is considered "contact" transmission rather than airborne because droplets usually travel no more than 3 feet. Organisms are usually dispersed when an infected person coughs, sneezes, or talks.

*Airborne transmission* occurs when infectious agents remain suspended in the air for long periods. The organisms can be widely dispersed by air currents before being inhaled by or deposited on the susceptible host. Tuberculosis is a disease transmitted by this route.

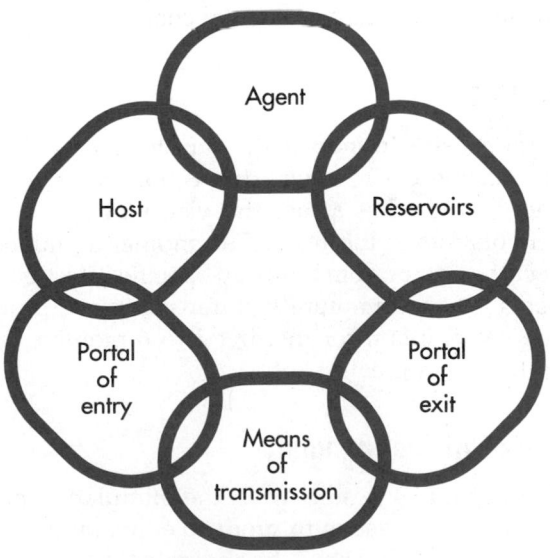

**Figure 14-2**   Chain of infection.

Good ventilation systems help prevent the transmission of infectious agents by the airborne route.

*Vehicle transmission* occurs when contaminated items such as blood, blood products, food, water, or drugs serve as the vector of transmission to multiple persons. An example of this type of transmission is the spread of salmonellosis from contaminated dairy products and poultry.

> **NURSE ALERT**
>
> **Handwashing is the best way to prevent person-to-person direct transmission of infectious organisms.**

**Vectorborne** *transmission* occurs when insects or other animals serve as intermediate hosts for an infectious agent. Malaria, transmitted by mosquitos, and Rocky Mountain spotted fever and Lyme Disease, transmitted by ticks, are examples of diseases transmitted by vectors.

# CONTROL OF COMMUNICABLE DISEASE

Prevention and control of **communicable disease** involves interfering with the normal pattern of transmission of the organism. This may be done by altering characteristics of the agent, the host, or the environment. One of the most common methods of breaking the chain of infectious events is to enhance the immunity of the host. Other methods involve altering or destroying the agent or interrupting the life cycle of the organism through environmental changes.

## Immunity

**Natural passive immunity** is not produced by the immune response. It results from the passage of a mother's antibodies across the placental barrier into the circulation of the fetus. The mother's antibodies protect the newborn infant from specific infectious organisms. Natural immunity is transitory and protects the newborn infant for the first 3 to 6 months, when mortality is the greatest.

## Acquired Active Immunity

**Active immunity** results from the stimulation of the body's immune system to produce either *antibodies* or specialized cells that have the ability to destroy or neutralize foreign microorganisms (see Chapter 7). Active natural immunity occurs after an infectious agent is introduced into the body, producing either an illness or an inapparent illness, or through active artificial *immunization*. Immunity is most durable if the person actually acquires the infectious disease. However, severe or fatal complications can result from some infections. It is also possible for a recovered person to become a carrier and harbor microorganisms and transmit them to others unknowingly.

Following exposure, part of the microorganism acts as an *antigen*, a substance that is usually comprised of large protein or polysaccharide molecules and is capable of inducing a specific immune response (see Chapter 7). The body responds with the production of antibodies **(immunoglobulins),** which are protein molecules that are specific to the antigen and can interact with the antigen to interfere with the infectious process.

> **NURSE ALERT**
>
> **All healthy children should received immunizations early in life and as recommended throughout their life span.**

Immunizations produce artificially acquired active immunity. The immunizing agents are **vaccines** or **toxoids.** Vaccines are suspensions of killed microorganisms or live, attenuated (altered) microorganisms. Toxoids are toxins produced by microorganisms that have been treated with chemicals or heat to decrease their toxic effect while retaining their ability to stimulate the immune system. Immunizations are usually given before the person has been exposed to the illness. Because the immune response that results from a vaccine or toxoid is not as strong as that which results from acquiring the acute illness, boosters may be given periodically to maintain immunity.

Most immunizations are given early in life because young children can suffer severe complications from many infectious diseases (Table 14-1). These immunizations prevent diphtheria, pertussis, tetanus, polio, measles, mumps, rubella, *Haemophilus influenzae* type B (HIB), and hepatitis B (HB). Vaccines are available either singly or in combinations such as measles and rubella (MR).

Measles is a serious contagious disease. Every child and young adult should receive protection from this disease because complications can lead to encephalitis, mental retardation, pneumonia, blindness, and death. Side effects of the vaccine do not occur often, but a mild temperature elevation may occur or a skin rash may appear.

**TABLE 14-1**

# Recommended Childhood Immunization Schedule[a]—United States, 1997

| VACCINE | BIRTH | 1 MO | 2 MO | 4 MO | 6 MO | 12 MO | 15 MO | 18 MO | 4–6 YR | 11–12 YR | 14–16 YR |
|---|---|---|---|---|---|---|---|---|---|---|---|
| Hepatitis B[b,c] | Hep B-1 | Hep B-1 | Hep B-2 | | Hep B-3 | | | | | Hep B[c] | |
| Diphtheria and tetanus toxoids and pertussis[d] | | | DTaP or DTP | DTaP or DTP | DTaP or DTP | | DTaP or DTP[d] | | DTaP or DTP | Td | |
| *Haemophilus influenza* type b[e] | | | Hib | Hib | Hib | Hib | | | | | |
| Poliovirus[f] | | | Polio | Polio | Polio[f] | | | | Polio | | |
| Measles-mumps-rubella[g] | | | | | | MMR | | | MMR | MMR | |
| Varicella virus[h] | | | | | | Var | | | | Var | |

From Advisory Committee on Immunization Practices (ACIP), American Academy of Pediatrics (AAP), and American Academy of Family Physicians (AAFP).

▬▬▬ Range of acceptable ages for vaccination.

⬭ Vaccines to be assessed and administered if necessary

[a] This schedule indicates the recommended age for the routine administration of currently licensed childhood vaccines; vaccines are listed under the ages for which they are routinely recommended. Catch-up immunization should be done during any visit when feasible. Some combination vaccines are available and may be used whenever administration of all components of the vaccine is indicated. Providers should consult the manufacturers' package inserts for detailed recommendations.

[b] **Infants born to hepatitis B surface antigen (HBsAg)-negative mothers** should receive 2.5 μg of Merck vaccine (Recombivax HB) or10 μg of SmithKline Beecham (SB) vaccine (Engerix-B). The second dose should be administered at least 1 month after the first dose. The third dose should be administered at least 2 months after the second but not before 6 months of age. **Infants born to HBsAg-positive mothers** should receive 0.5 ml hepatitis B immune globulin (HBIG) within 12 hours of birth, and either 5 μg of Merck vaccine (Recombivax HB) or 10 μg of SB vaccine (Engerix-B) at a separate site. The second dose is recommended at age 1–2 months and the third dose at age 6 months. **Infants born to mothers whose HBsAg status is unknown** should receive either 5 μg of Merck vaccine (Recombivax HB) or 10 μg of SB vaccine (Engerix-B) within 12 hours of birth. The second dose of vaccine is recommenced at age 1 month and the third dose at age 6 months. Blood should be drawn at the time of delivery to determine the mother's HBsAg status; if it is positive, the infant should receive HBIG as soon as possible (no later than age 1 week). The dosage and timing of subsequent vaccine doses should be based on the mother's HBsAg status.

[c] Children and adolescents who have not been vaccinated against hepatitis B in infancy may begin the series during any visit. Those who have not previously received three doses of hepatitis B vaccine should initiate or complete the series during the routine visit to a health-care provider at age 11–12 years, and unvaccinated older adolescents should be vaccinated whenever possible. The second dose should be administered at least 1 month after the first dose, and the third dose should be administered at least 4 months after the first dose and at least 2 months after the second dose.

[d] Diphtheria and tetanus toxoids and acellular pertussis vaccine (DTaP) is the preferred vaccine for all doses in the vaccination series, including completion of the series in children who have received one or more doses of whole-cell diphtheria and tetanus toxoids and pertussis vaccine (DTP). Whole-cell DTP is an acceptable alternative to DTaP. The fourth dose (DTP or DTaP) may be admistered as early as age 12 months, provided 6 months have elapsed since the third dose and if the child is unlikely to return at age 15–18 months. Tetanus and diphtheria toxoids, adsorbed, for adult use (Td), is recommended at age 11–12 years if at least 5 years have elapsed since the last dose of DTP, DTaP, or diphtheria and tetanus toxoids, adsorbed, for pediatric use (DT). Subsequent routine Td boosters are recommended every 10 years.

[e] Three *Haemophilus influenzae* type b (Hib) conjugate vaccines are licensed for infant use. If *Haemophilus* b conjugate vaccine (meningococcal protein conjugate) (PRP-OMP) (PedvaxHIB [Merck]) is administered at ages 2 and 4 months, a dose at age 6 months is not required.

[f] Two poliovirus vaccines are currently licensed and distributed in the United States: inactivated poliovirus vaccine (IPV) and oral poliovirus vaccine (OPV). The following schedules are all acceptable to the ACIP, AAP, and AAFP. Parents and providers may choose among these options: 1) two doses of IPV followed by two doses of OPV; 2) four doses of IPV; or 3) four doses of OPV. ACIP recommends two doses of IPV at ages 2 and 4 months followed by a dose of OPV at age 12–18 months and at age 4–6 years. IPV is the only poliovirus vaccine recommended for immunocompromised persons and their household contacts.

[g] The second dose of measles-mumps-rubella vaccine (MMR) is recommended routinely at age 4–6 years but may be administered during any visit, provided at least 1 month has elapsed since receipt of the first dose and that both doses are administered beginning at or after age 12 months. Those who have not previously received the second dose should complete the schedule no later than the routine visit to a health care provider at age 11–12 years.

[h] Susceptible children may receive varicella vaccine (Var) at any visit after the first birthday, and those who lack a reliable history of chickenpox should be vaccinated during the routine visit to a health care provider at age 11–12 years. Susceptible children aged ≥13 years should receive two doses at least 1 month apart.

Use of trade names and commercial sources is for identification only and does not imply endorsement by CDC or the U.S. Department of Health and Human Services.

The measles vaccine is a live virus vaccine that has been attenuated, or reduced, in virulence. It is believed that one dose is sufficient to produce long-lasting immunity, although some states require a second dose before entering school. Because egg protein is used in the manufacturing of measles vaccine, the few children who have sensitivity to eggs should not receive this vaccine. Contraindications for the administration of the measles virus vaccine include leukemia or other malignant disorders. Children whose resistance is low as a result of receiving steroid therapy, radiation, alkylating drugs, and antimetabolites should not be given the measles vaccine. Administration of the vaccine during pregnancy should be avoided.

Mumps can be a serious disease and lead to deafness and encephalitis in children and orchitis and oophoritis in adults. Sterility can occur. Administration of live mumps virus vaccine provides an active immunity against mumps. The vaccine is prepared in a chick embryo cell culture and therefore should not be given to the few persons sensitive to the proteins of eggs. Contraindications for its use are the same as for the measles vaccine.

A live rubella virus vaccine provides active immunity against rubella (German measles). The vaccine should not be given to pregnant women because of the possibility of producing the disease in the unborn child. Rubella has caused defects of the heart, brain, eye, and ears in children whose mothers have had rubella during the first trimester of pregnancy. The rubella vaccine is given to all children to prevent the spread of the disease to pregnant women and their unborn children. The CDC in Atlanta recommends that educational and training institutions seek proof of rubella immunity from all female students and employees. The vaccine may be given to women of childbearing age only if pregnancy will be avoided for at least 2 months. It should not be given during a major febrile illness. However, minor febrile episodes are not a contraindication for vaccine administration. Other contraindications are the same as for the measles and mumps vaccines. To prevent hypersensitivity reactions, the label on the bottle should be read before administering the vaccine to determine the type of cells from which the vaccine has been prepared. Box 14-2 presents a summary of the contraindications for immunization.

Poliomyelitis is an acute viral infection with a severity that ranges from a nonapparent, subclinical infection to paralytic disease and death. It occurs worldwide and is transmitted by close direct contact through a fecal-oral route. It is currently targeted for elimination, similar to the eradication of smallpox from the world as announced by the World Health Organization in 1980. Both a live attenuated oral po-

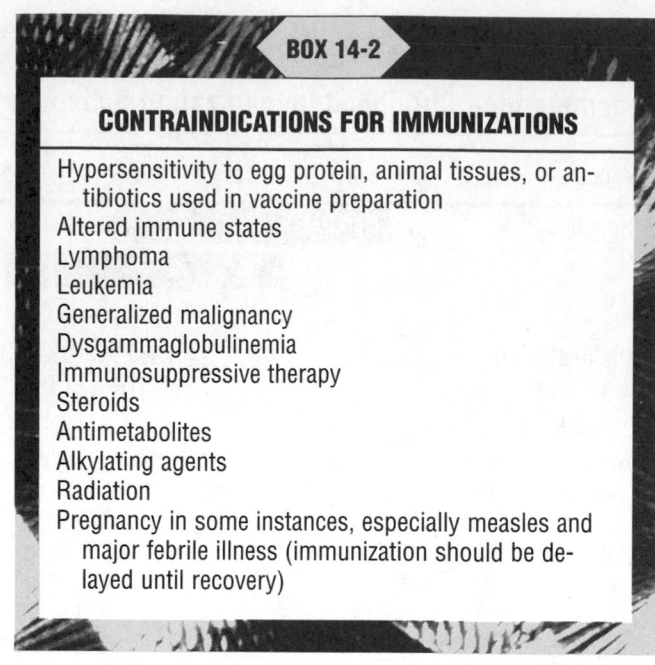

**BOX 14-2**

**CONTRAINDICATIONS FOR IMMUNIZATIONS**

Hypersensitivity to egg protein, animal tissues, or antibiotics used in vaccine preparation
Altered immune states
Lymphoma
Leukemia
Generalized malignancy
Dysgammaglobulinemia
Immunosuppressive therapy
Steroids
Antimetabolites
Alkylating agents
Radiation
Pregnancy in some instances, especially measles and major febrile illness (immunization should be delayed until recovery)

liovirus vaccine (OPV) and an inactivated poliovirus vaccine (IPV) are available and are administered by subcutaneous injection. Contraindications of the OPV are pregnancy and immunocompromised states. However, IPV can be administered in these instances.

In recent years, HIB and HB have been added to the recommended schedule for routine vaccinations. HIB occurs worldwide and in the United States has been the most common type of bacterial meningitis in children under 5 years of age. Since 1988, when the vaccine was licensed, the incidence of HIB has decreased markedly. HB is also found worldwide, and the severity of this disease ranges from mild to severe liver disease. The vaccine is contraindicated for persons who have an allergy to yeast.

## Acquired Passive Immunity

**Passive immunity** is acquired by introducing a serum that contains antibodies to the infectious organism into the susceptible host. Because the person receives antibodies that have been formed elsewhere, there is no direct stimulation of the person's own immune system. The immunity that is acquired is temporary and rarely lasts longer than a few weeks. It is useful in emergency situations and in the treatment of specific diseases. Administration of Ig (gamma globulin) to prevent hepatitis A in exposed people is an example.

**Antitoxins** contain antibodies that react against the toxin that is produced by the particular microorganism infecting the body. An antitoxin is administered to neutralize the poisons produced by pathogens and does not have any effect on the organism itself. Chemotherapeutic drugs may be given to the individual to destroy the organism. Examples of antitoxins include diphtheria antitoxin, tetanus antitoxin, and antisnake (antivenom) serum.

Immunoglobulin (immune gamma globulin) is the fraction of the plasma of human blood that contains antibodies against certain diseases. It is occasionally used to treat or modify measles in a nonimmune person. It may also be used to prevent infectious hepatitis in exposed persons. Immunoglobulin is prepared in a sterile solution for administration. Emphasis should be placed on active immunization to prevent those diseases for which vaccines are available.

## Public Education

Today people are less concerned about communicable childhood diseases than they were in previous decades. The incidence of these diseases has decreased to such an extent that fear of them or their consequences has been lessened. Although this decrease in incidence has contributed to an increased quality of life, problems still exist. Immunization rates throughout the United States have gradually declined, especially among some religious groups. As a result there has been a rise in the incidence of some diseases such as measles.

Many states have attempted to remedy this situation by passing laws that require immunizations for children before attending school. However, these laws do not reach all segments of the population. Preschool children and elderly people are not included. Some local health departments operate well-child clinics for the purpose of monitoring immunization status and general wellness. The United States has launched a nationwide campaign to increase the levels of immunity throughout the country. In some communities immunization levels have fallen to 50% or less. There is a continual need for study and development of programs that will reach all members of the population.

There also is a need for public education programs regarding positive health practices that are important in the prevention of disease. Sociologic factors may have a profound effect on the incidence of certain infectious diseases. Reservoirs of infection may exist in areas that have a low socioeconomic status, inadequate access to good medical care, inadequate housing, poor sanitary facilities, inadequate refuse collection, and possibly even contaminated water supplies.

Poor nutritional standards also decrease resistance to disease and provide the opportunity for pathogens to invade the human body. The social picture is often one of apathy and lack of motivation coupled with lack of transportation and inaccessible medical and

---

**BOX 14-3**

### *HEALTHY PEOPLE 2000* OBJECTIVES FOR IMMUNIZATION AGAINST INFECTIOUS DISEASES

- Eliminate diphtheria, tetanus, polio, measles, and rubella among people age 25 and younger
- Reduce cases of mumps to 500 per year
- Reduce cases of pertussis to 1000 per year
- Increase the levels of basic immunization series among children under age 2 to at least 90%
- Increase the levels of basic immunization series among children in licensed child care facilities and kindergarten through postsecondary education institutions to at least 95%
- Increase immunization levels for pneumococcal pneumonia and influenza among institutionalized, chronically ill, or older people to at least 80%
- Increase immunization levels for pneumococcal pneumonia and influenza among noninstitutionalized high-risk populations to at least 60%
- Increase hepatitis B immunization among high-risk populations to at least 90%
- Reduce postexposure rabies treatments to no more than 9000 per year

---

clinical services. Such conditions contribute to a failure to secure immunization of young children and produce conditions for a potential epidemic of infectious disease.

The high mobility of some segments of the population means that a person who has been exposed to an infectious disease or who is a possible source of disease may be hundreds of miles away from the point of contact within a few hours. Therefore the worldwide spread of infectious diseases is more of a problem now than ever before.

*Healthy People 2000* is a visionary agenda for the health of the nation that grew out of a health strategy that the federal government initiated in 1979 (Healthy People 2000, 1991). It reflects a consensus of a consortium of almost 300 national organizations, the U.S. Public Health Service, state health departments, and the Institute of Medicine of the National Academy of Sciences. On the basis of measurable objectives, the report presents goals that will increase the span of healthy life and reduce health disparities for the American people. One of the goals to be achieved includes reducing the risk for infectious diseases (Box 14-3). To achieve this goal, several types of activities are recommended, including expanding immunization laws; increasing the proportion of primary care providers who provide information, counseling, and immunizations; and removing financial barriers to receiving immunizations. The CDC and state health departments monitor the accomplishment of these objectives through a series of surveillance activities.

## Nursing's Role in Prevention

The development of an infection is multifactorial and results from complex interactions among many factors that are related to the agent, the host, and the environment. The development of appropriate interventions requires a complete analysis of these factors. The goal is to prevent the spread of the infectious agent from its reservoir, or source, to susceptible hosts and thereby break the chain of infection (see Figure 14-2). Interventions should be based on the natural history of the disease and directed toward the link in the chain of infection that is the most susceptible to interruption.

Nurses are constantly involved with assessing patients for factors that indicate whether a patient requires preventive intervention, is at high risk for infection, or is experiencing an infection. **Primary prevention** strategies that prevent diseases from occurring include immunizations, healthy life-style behaviors (e.g., proper nutrition and exercise), and patient education. Nurses have a primary role in encouraging all people to keep immunizations current and to maintain proper records of their immunization history. Every nurse should engage in public information or education programs and provide information to individuals in their health practices whenever possible. For example, prevention of HIV infection should be a consideration of all nurses. Nurses often observe human behavior as it relates to health and illness and can offer solutions to problems that are related to disease prevention.

**Secondary prevention** measures are designed to detect disease and initiate early treatment to limit the spread and severity of infectious disease and to prevent complications. These activities include the assessment of individuals for signs and symptoms that indicate infectious disease, periodic examinations, and screening procedures. Nurses should encourage patients to seek medical attention whenever they observe unusual physical symptoms. Diagnosing a disease when early physiologic changes are occurring limits the complications. Too often the infections are well advanced before treatment is sought.

**Tertiary prevention** involves treatment to arrest the infectious process and minimize disability. Nurses are often responsible for the administration of medications and are expected to maintain proper handwashing techniques, as well as precautions with excretions, secretions, trash, and waste. These measures are specific to the characteristics of the infectious process and the limitations that face the patient (see Chapter 15).

Residual disabilities do occur with some infections. For example, repeated ear infections can result in hearing loss, and chronic Lyme disease can produce cardiovascular problems.

# PATIENT WITH A BACTERIAL INFECTION

Because of improved public health standards and the widespread use of immunizations, many infectious diseases have a less significant impact on the population now than at the beginning of the century. Four bacterial infectious diseases caused significant morbidity in the past: diphtheria, pertussis, tetanus, and typhoid fever. Other infectious diseases are prevalent among certain groups in specific geographic locations or on a seasonal or cyclic basis.

## Staphylococcal Infections

In many people, staphylococcal organisms are normal inhabitants of the upper respiratory tract, skin, and gastrointestinal (GI) tract. It is estimated that about 30% of all persons are asymptomatic carriers of *Staphylococcus aureus*, which provides a source of infection for themselves and for others when host resistance is lowered. Transmission usually occurs through direct contact with an infected or colonized person. Transmission through fomites or airborne particles is rare. The **incubation period** is 4 to 10 days. The organism is communicable as long as purulent lesions continue to drain or the carrier state persists. Staphylococcal infections occur worldwide but are more prevalent in overcrowded areas where personal hygiene is poor. There are no specific preventive measures other than cleanliness and adherence to strict aseptic technique where appropriate.

In the community, *S. aureus* infections usually manifest as skin lesions such as impetigo, boils, carbuncles, abscesses, wound infections, and conjunctivitis. Some toxin-producing strains can cause a distinctive scalded skin syndrome. Infection around the nose and mouth can spread backward into the cranial vault, where there are no mechanical barriers to halt the spread. Systemic disease is rare and usually occurs in those who are immunosuppressed or suffering from a debilitating illness. However, septicemia, lung and brain abscesses, pneumonia, endocarditis, osteomyelitis, and other complications can occur. Staphylococcal pneumonia can occur as a complication of influenza. However, this condition rarely occurs except during influenza outbreaks.

Prevention is best accomplished through education in personal hygiene, especially in handwashing. Prompt treatment with topical antibiotics (or systemic antibiotics if the infection has disseminated) reduces transmission. Contaminated articles should be disinfected appropriately. Outbreaks in schools, camps, and other population groups should be reported to public health authorities.

## Toxic Shock Syndrome

During 1980 and 1981 an epidemic of toxic shock syndrome (TSS) occurred that was associated with toxin-producing strains of *S. aureus*. TSS is a severe illness that is characterized by sudden onset of high fever, vomiting, profuse diarrhea, and myalgia. It can lead to hypotension, shock, and death. A deep red "sunburn" rash develops within a few hours and is followed by desquamation of the skin approximately 10 days after onset, especially on the palms of the hands and soles of the feet. Approximately 95% of the reported cases in women occurred during the menstrual period, and most cases were associated with use of certain vaginal tampons. In cases of TSS that are not associated with menstruation, including cases in men, *S. aureus* has been isolated from focal lesions of skin, bone, lung, and stool. Aggressive fluid, electrolyte, and anti-staphylococcal antibiotic therapy are required.

Nurses in community and school settings should communicate information regarding the risk of TSS. Menstrual TSS can be prevented by using tampons intermittently, changing them often, and avoiding products that have the potential to irritate mucous membranes.

## Streptococcal Infections

Streptococci, like staphylococci, are found almost everywhere in the environment. These infections probably cause more illnesses than any other group of organisms. They can attack any part of the body and cause both primary and secondary disease. Many distinct strains exist, but not all are pathogenic. Streptococci are normal inhabitants of the human respiratory tract. Group A beta-hemolytic *Streptococcus pyogenes* produces the most significant variety of diseases in humans. Streptococcal sore throat and skin infections are the most common. Cellulitis, mastoiditis, otitis media, pneumonia, wound infections, septicemia, scarlet fever, and other diseases can also occur. These conditions can be particularly severe in the elderly.

Streptococcal sore throat is prevalent in temperate and semitropical regions. In the United States epidemics in New England and in the Great Lakes region are common. Transmission results from direct contact with another infected person or object. Organisms usually enter the body through the respiratory tract or through a wound. Nasal carriers are often transmitters of the organism. Outbreaks of streptococcal sore throat rarely follow ingestion of contaminated foods, partic-

ularly milk and milk products. Following a short incubation period of 1 to 3 days, the organism becomes established in the lymphoid tissues, causing local cellulitis. The infectious process can easily spread because toxins released by the organism prevent the normal inflammatory process from walling off the lesion.

Infected persons exhibit fever, sore throat, exudative tonsillitis or pharyngitis, and tender anterior cervical lymph nodes. However, symptoms can be minimal. Repeated attacks of streptococcal sore throat or other illnesses as a result of different types of streptococci are also relatively common. With antibiotic therapy, transmission is generally limited to 24 to 48 hours, but untreated cases can transmit the organisms for an indefinite period. Complications such as scarlet fever, rheumatic fever, or acute glomerulonephritis may appear in 1 to 5 weeks following infection, but this is rare and is usually related to the host immune response.

Scarlet fever includes all of the symptoms that occur with a streptococcal sore throat, although it may be associated with infections at other sites. It has an abrupt onset with chills, vomiting, headache, and high temperature. In approximately 24 hours a fine, erythematous rash occurs that blanches on pressure and feels like sandpaper. The rash occurs most often on the neck, chest, axillary folds, elbows, groin, and the surface of the inner thighs. Usually it does not affect the face. The tongue has a furred appearance that gradually disappears and becomes characteristically red (strawberry tongue). The incidence and severity of scarlet fever has decreased in recent years, although the mortality rate in some parts of the world has been as high as 3% (Beneson, 1990).

One of the most important factors in control of these infections is the identification and treatment of streptococcal infections before serious complications result. The treatment of choice is penicillin therapy for at least 10 days. Treatment that is initiated within the first 24 to 48 hours decreases severity, reduces complications, and prevents the development of most cases of acute rheumatic fever. Infected people should be observed carefully for complications that may appear throughout the course of the illness. Preventive measures that nurses should convey include education of the public regarding the transmission of the organism and the relationship of streptococcal infections to scarlet fever, acute rheumatic fever, and other complications.

## Pulmonary Tuberculosis

Tuberculosis is one of the oldest known diseases and is one of the most devastating worldwide diseases of all time. It can attack any organ or tissue and can result in years of chronic invalidism or death if not diagnosed and treated. In 1882 Robert Koch discovered *M. tuberculosis* as the causative organism, and modern treatment became possible. Significant advances have been made in the treatment, prevention, and control of the disease, which has resulted in downward trends in morbidity and mortality in many countries. In 1996 the incidence rate in the United States was 8.04 new cases per 100,000 (CDC, 1997). The incidence has risen in recent years, primarily as a complication of the immunosuppression that accompanies persons infected with the HIV virus. An increase in immigration from countries where the disease is widespread has also contributed to the increased incidence of tuberculosis. Resistant strains of the organism have also emerged. Morbidity and mortality increase with age, are higher in men than women, and are higher in nonwhite people than in white people (CDC, 1994). Tuberculosis is also more common among people of a lower socioeconomic status, in which factors such as overcrowding increase the risk of infection.

## Transmission

Transmission of *M. tuberculosis* occurs when a susceptible person inhales airborne droplet nuclei. When a person with active tuberculosis coughs or sneezes, the infectious organisms are carried into the air as droplets, or droplet nuclei. Droplet nuclei are particles that contain the microorganisms that become suspended in the air. However, prolonged contact is usually necessary for infection to occur, and transmission through indirect contact is rare.

The incubation period for a primary tuberculosis lesion is approximately 4 to 12 weeks. Persons who have the microorganisms in their system react positively to a tuberculin skin test (10 mm or greater), although the disease may not be present. People can transmit the organism to others as long as the organism is being discharged from their bodies. Progressive development of the disease is greatest within 1 to 2 years after infection, although it may remain as a latent infection throughout a lifetime. Pulmonary tuberculosis is most common, although dissemination of the organism through lymphatic drainage and circulation can lead to involvement of many parts of the body.

## Assessment

Primary pulmonary infections usually go unnoticed by the individual. As a result of the stimulation of the immune system of the body, lesions containing the tubercle bacillus often become walled off and calcified, which isolates the organism and prevents spread of the disease. However, reactivation of the disease may occur later in life or if medical conditions or their treatment results in immunosuppression of the host.

Clinical manifestations of active tuberculosis include infection, cavitation of lung tissue, and tissue de-

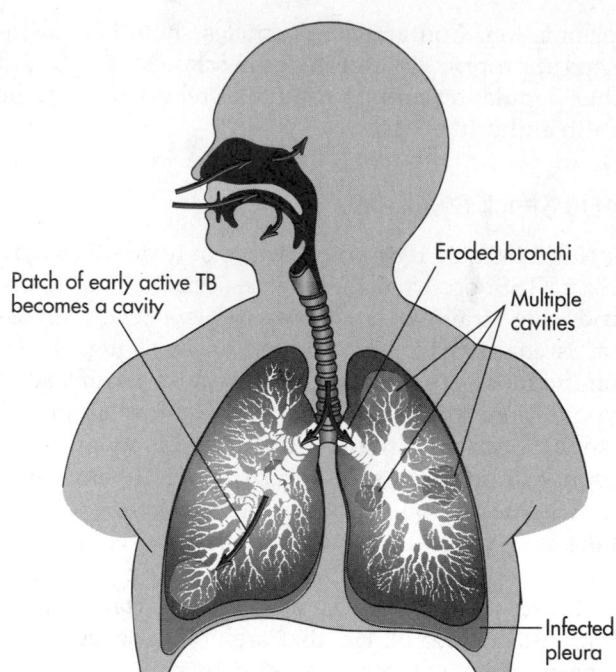

**Figure 14-3**   Infection, cavitation, and tissue destruction are characteristic of active tuberculosis infection. (From Beare P, Myers J: *Principles and practice of adult health nursing*, ed 3, St Louis, 1998, Mosby.)

struction (Figure 14-3). Symptoms are often the result of toxic manifestations produced by the infection. Mild fever, fatigue, and gradual weight loss can occur early, whereas cough, chest pain, dyspnea, and hemoptysis become prominent only when the disease has progressed. Profuse sweating may occur late in the day and at night. The spitting of blood (hemoptysis) may occur when cavitation extends into a blood vessel. A wide variety of symptoms can accompany tuberculosis, and there is no specific pattern in which they occur.

## Case Finding

When tuberculosis is suspected, the patient must have a complete history and physical examination, including routine laboratory examinations. A history of exposure or a family history of infection or disease is of special significance. A definitive diagnosis of active tuberculosis is made by culturing *M. tuberculosis* from sputum or other body fluids or tissues. Finding acid-fast bacilli in smears of sputum or other specimens support the diagnosis, but the diagnosis is confirmed only by culture or molecular techniques such as gene probes. Regular sputum examinations are required to isolate the tubercle bacillus, and failure to find it does not always rule out the diagnosis of tuberculosis. Under some conditions it may be impossible to secure sputum for examination. In this case a gastric lavage is performed, and the gastric contents are examined. A bronchoscopic examination is often done to secure secretions from the bronchial tree or directly from portions of the lung. X-ray films visualize calcified nodules in the lung and can be used to follow the progression of the disease following diagnosis.

The tuberculin test is a diagnostic aid that indicates the presence of infection but does not necessarily indicate the presence of the disease. The tuberculin test is presently used as a screening method to detect persons with infection.

The Mantoux test is the skin test of choice for identifying infected persons. It involves inoculation of tubercle bacillus extract (tuberculin) intradermally on the inner surface of the forearm. Purified protein derivative is usually used. The reaction is an example of a delayed (cellular) hypersensitivity reaction. The test is read between 48 and 72 hours after administration. Different cut-points are used to separate positive reactions from negative reactions for different populations, depending on the risk for TB infection in that population. For example, a reaction of 5 mm is considered positive for a person with HIV infection, whereas a person with no risk factors would be read as a nonreactor. An induration of ≥15 mm is classified as a positive reaction in normal, healthy persons with no increased risk for tuberculosis. The amount of induration, or hardness, is important, not the amount of redness present. A positive reaction indicates that a patient has had contact and has become infected with the tubercle bacillus, but active tuberculosis may not be present. Generally, the more intense the reaction to the test, the greater the likelihood that an infection with *M. tuberculosis* has occurred. Positive reactions may be suppressed in patients who are acutely ill with tuberculosis, receiving corticosteroid drugs, or infected with certain other infectious diseases such as measles.

Ideally, everyone should have an annual tuberculin skin test. All health care personnel should participate in an annual screening program. X-ray examinations should be restricted to those persons with symptoms suggestive of tuberculosis. The greatest emphasis in screening should be on high-risk groups, such as contacts of active tuberculosis cases, patients in general hospitals and mental institutions, immigrants from areas in which tuberculosis is common, and populations of lower socioeconomic status. All active cases must be reported to local health departments so that contacts may be examined and monitored.

## Drug Therapy

Following diagnosis, the stage of the patient's disease is evaluated and an individual schedule of treatment is planned. Effective chemotherapy reverses the infectiousness of tuberculosis within 2 weeks of initiation

and prevents progression of the illness. A combination of agents is used to affect the organism in different stages of growth. Primary drugs include isoniazid (INH), rifampin (RIF), streptomycin (SM), pyrazinamide (PZA), and ethambutol (EMB) in varying combinations. The standard treatment is INH, RIF, and PZA for 2 months followed by INH and RIF for an additional 4 months. Because of the recently increasing problem of multiple drug resistance, EMB may be added to the regimen until sensitivity reports are available (CDC, 1994). Secondary drugs are available for cases that are resistant to the primary drugs. Any treatment considers the stage of the disease, its activity, and the patient's resistance to the drug.

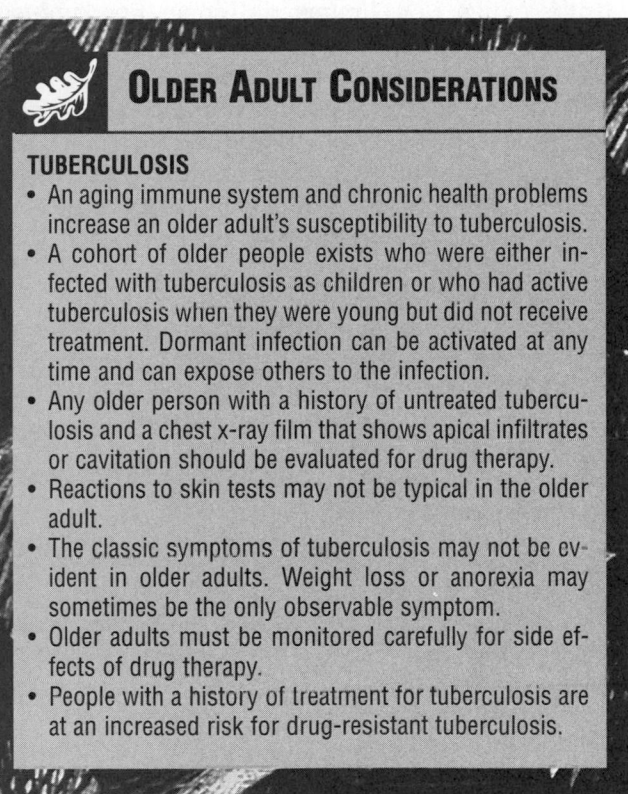

## OLDER ADULT CONSIDERATIONS

**TUBERCULOSIS**
- An aging immune system and chronic health problems increase an older adult's susceptibility to tuberculosis.
- A cohort of older people exists who were either infected with tuberculosis as children or who had active tuberculosis when they were young but did not receive treatment. Dormant infection can be activated at any time and can expose others to the infection.
- Any older person with a history of untreated tuberculosis and a chest x-ray film that shows apical infiltrates or cavitation should be evaluated for drug therapy.
- Reactions to skin tests may not be typical in the older adult.
- The classic symptoms of tuberculosis may not be evident in older adults. Weight loss or anorexia may sometimes be the only observable symptom.
- Older adults must be monitored carefully for side effects of drug therapy.
- People with a history of treatment for tuberculosis are at an increased risk for drug-resistant tuberculosis.

Patients must be monitored for the onset of toxic symptoms that would necessitate a change or discontinuance of the drug. Numbness, tingling, and weakness of the extremities are toxic signs that may be observed when INH is being given. SM may cause deafness, dizziness, unsteadiness of gait, ringing in the ears, or severe headache. Toxic symptoms are more likely to occur in older persons. Because patients with tuberculosis often receive chemotherapeutic drugs over a prolonged time, regular laboratory examinations are important. In addition, visual acuity and hearing tests should be done at intervals if indicated. Patients receiving INH should avoid drinking alcohol while taking the drug.

## Nursing Interventions

Tuberculosis is not a highly infectious disease, and prompt specific chemotherapy limits the release of tubercle bacilli into the air within a few days after effective therapy is initiated. The patient needs instruction regarding the proper handling of sputum to prevent organisms from becoming airborne. When the patient coughs or sneezes, moist droplets are carried into the air. Some droplets fall into the immediate environment, whereas others remain suspended in the air as droplet nuclei. Good ventilation carries droplet nuclei on air currents, where they may be killed by sunlight or ultraviolet light. When the patient is taught to cover his or her nose and mouth when coughing or sneezing, the dissemination of moist droplets into the environment is reduced or eliminated. Cooperation can usually be expected when the patient understands the importance of this procedure.

Nurses should emphasize the importance of continuing to take the prescribed medications (Box 14-4). One of the main factors in the continued transmis-sion of tuberculosis is lack of adequate patient education and follow-up to ensure that therapy is completed. Pa-

tients should understand the nature and extent of the illness and recognize that medications must be continued as prescribed. Failure to take medications regularly impedes the healing process and contributes to the development of resistant strains of the organism. For this reason, directly observed therapy (DOT) should be considered for any patient with a potential for noncompliance. DOT is especially indicated for alcohol- or other substance-using patients.

## Prevention and Control

In addition to drug therapy, a variety of other prevention and control measures are recommended that interfere with transmission patterns in other ways. A vaccine known as bacille Calmette-Guérin (BCG) is available. However, the amount of protection that it produces against tuberculosis is variable. In the United States, where the risk of infection is low, immunization is not generally indicated. It may be used for medical personnel who risk exposure to undiagnosed cases, for contacts of active tuberculosis cases, and for newborns whose mothers have active tuber-

---

> **BOX 14-4**

# NURSING PROCESS

## TUBERCULOSIS (COMMUNITY)

### ASSESSMENT

- Understanding of disease process and transmission
- Compliance with medical therapy
- Respiratory status (breath sounds, dyspnea, cough)
- Hemoptysis
- Temperature
- Laboratory studies (sputum acid-fast bacillus (AFB), urinalysis, blood urea nitrogen, creatinine, alanine aminotransferase/aspartate aminotransferase)

### NURSING DIAGNOSES

- Risk for infection related to *Mycobacterium tuberculosis* in respiratory secretions
- Impaired home maintenance management, noncompliance, and inadequate handling of secretions related to long-term therapy
- Noncompliance related to lack of understanding, financial resources, emotional support, and substance abuse, including alcohol and drugs
- Knowledge deficit related to new medical condition and treatment
- Ineffective breathing pattern related to respiratory secretions

### NURSING INTERVENTIONS

- Maintain/teach AFB isolation until antimicrobial therapy is initiated.
- Maintain adequate nutrition and fluid intake.
- Encourage rest and progressively increase activity as tolerated.
- Administer or supervise medication use.
- Monitor for symptoms of toxic side effects of medications.
- Reinforce the importance of compliance with therapy.
- Refer to Visiting Nurse Association for follow-up.
- Examine close contacts at time of treatment and in 3 months.

### EVALUATION OF EXPECTED OUTCOMES

- No evidence of active infection or complications of tuberculosis
- Self-administers medications as prescribed
- No transmission of infection to close contacts
- No evidence of dyspnea or hypoxia

culosis. If BCG is used, it is given only to persons who have a negative tuberculin test. Improving social conditions and educating the public about prevention of the spread of tuberculosis organisms can help control the transmission of the organisms. Tuberculin testing in high-risk groups, increased availability and accessibility of medical diagnosis and treatment, and nursing case management are important methods for case finding and controlling the spread of tuberculosis. The use of chemotherapeutic drugs is now recommended for known contacts who have been exposed to tuberculosis and tested positive but do not have the disease.

Tuberculosis has occurred among persons infected with the HIV virus. HIV infection causes immunosuppression, which allows latent tuberculosis infection to progress to a clinically apparent disease. *M. tuberculosis* infection in the presence of laboratory evidence for HIV infection and involving at least one site outside the lung is now diagnostic of AIDS. Prevention and control efforts need to focus on those with or at risk for HIV infection.

The U.S. Department of Health and Human Services released a strategic plan for the elimination of tuberculosis in the United States by the year 2010. The report also established an interim target case rate of 3.5 per 100,000 by the year 2000. The three-step plan includes (1) more effective use of existing prevention and control measures, especially for high-risk populations; (2) development and evaluation of new technologies for diagnosis, treatment, and prevention; and (3) rapid assessment and transfer of newly developed technologies into health care practices (CDC, 1989). An effective tuberculosis elimination effort such as this requires good **epidemiologic surveillance** data that target the affected populations and geographic areas. The emergence of resistant organisms and the increased incidence linked to HIV infection are barriers to achieving this goal.

## Lyme Disease

Lyme disease was first identified by a Yale rheumatologist in 1975 when he analyzed an unusual cluster of arthritis cases that occurred in Lyme, Connecticut. Cases have spread rapidly in the Northeast, the Midwest, and the California coast and have reached epidemic proportions. Cases have been diagnosed in almost every state and in many other countries throughout the world. Cases have been recorded in Europe for several decades. The true incidence is unknown because health care workers are not required to report the disease to public health authorities.

The organism *Borrelia burgdorferi* is the causative agent. The bacterial spirochete is transmitted to humans through the bite of a small tick vector the size of

a poppy seed. Studies of the life cycle of the tick indicate that it commonly feeds on an infected white-footed mouse in its larval stage, medium-size mammals including people in its nymph stage, and white-tailed deer as adults (Hudacek, 1990) (Figure 14-4). The tick deposits the organism in the capillary system as it feeds on the host's blood, often from 12 to 24 hours. The incubation period is from 3 to 21 days after tick exposure. The human immune system responds weakly to the infection, and antibodies do not appear in any quantity for 4 to 6 weeks. Because of this, laboratory tests are not helpful in early stages and may produce false-negative results.

Like other spirochete infections such as syphilis, symptoms of Lyme disease resemble many other diseases. The majority of people may first realize they were bitten when a characteristic "bulls-eye" rash at the site of the bite appears. It is an expanding red circle that often has a white center. Flulike symptoms such as fever, headache, fatigue, a stiff neck, and swelling of the knee joints are common. If Lyme disease is not treated promptly, generalized arthritis, severe fatigue, arrhythmias, and symptoms of central nervous system involvement such as numbness, facial paralysis, visual disturbance, and seizures may occur. Permanent structural damage to joints may develop. Early treatment with antibiotics usually prevents complications. Advanced cases may require prolonged intravenous or intramuscular antibiotics. Ceftriaxone (Rocephin) penetrates the blood-brain barrier and is used in people with central nervous system involvement.

Various measures have been used to interfere with the transmission of Lyme disease. However, the most effective measures so far involve preventing the bite of the tick. People are advised to (1) check their bodies for "moving freckles" when in an area known to be tick infested, (2) wear a hat and tuck pants into long socks and wear a long-sleeved shirt when in tick-infested areas, (3) wear light colors and tightly woven fabrics, (4) spray insect repellent containing the ingredient DEET on the clothes, (5) avoid tall grass and low brush, (6) keep pets free of ticks, and (7) remove ticks with tweezers. Large-scale spraying has been ineffective in reducing the tick population, and efforts to treat infestations in mice with cotton-soaked insecticides are expensive and practical only in small areas (Hudacek, 1990).

## Meningococcal Meningitis

Meningococcal meningitis is an acute bacterial infection of the membranes that cover the brain and spinal cord. The causative organism is *Neisseria meningitidis*. It occurs worldwide, most commonly in the winter and in the spring. Children and young adults are usually the victims, although outbreaks have occurred in

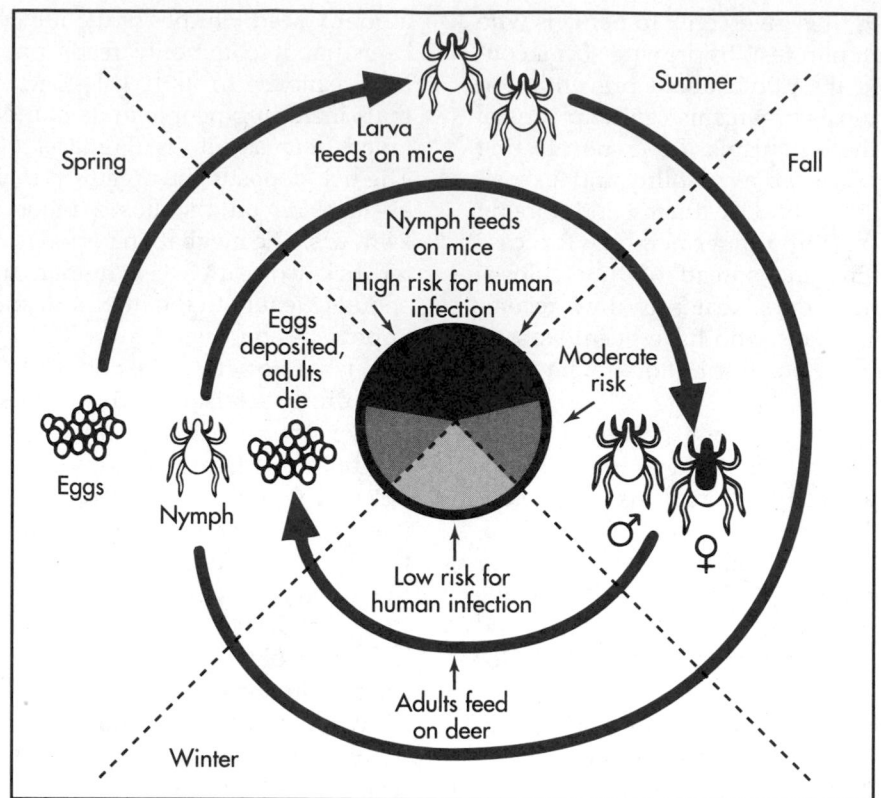

**Figure 14-4** Life cycle of the *Ixodes dammini* tick. Tick is a vector and reservoir for *Borrelia burgdorferi*, agent that produces Lyme disease in humans. (From Harkness GA: *Epidemiology in nursing practice*, St Louis, 1995, Mosby.)

adults who live in crowded conditions. Meningococcal infections may be asymptomatic or may exhibit respiratory tract symptoms. The disease can cause community outbreaks. A vaccine against certain serotypes of the organism is available and can be used under special circumstances such as community outbreaks. It is generally recommended for military personnel in the United States and for civilians who travel to areas of the world where the organism is prevalent. The treatment of choice is penicillin (see Chapter 30). However, rifampin is used prophylactically to eradicate the carrier state in close family and intimate contacts of an index case.

## Legionellosis

Legionellosis (legionnaires' disease) is primarily a respiratory infection that is caused by bacterium named *Legionella pneumophila*. Although occasional outbreaks occur, it is not considered a significant health problem in the United States. Recently nosocomial outbreaks of legionellosis have been documented (see Chapter 15). It is believed to be transmitted by airborne droplets from contaminated water sources including contami-

nated shower heads. The sources of several outbreaks have involved various types of air-conditioning systems, although the organism has been isolated from a creek near a contaminated water-cooling system. It is believed that the organism is free-living in soil. Symptoms of infection include fever, malaise, a nonproductive cough, and respiratory difficulty. Some patients have complained of chest pain, abdominal pain, and other GI symptoms. Complications have included renal damage and encephalitis. The organism is sensitive to erythromycin.

## Clostridium Infections

The *Clostridium* organisms include all anaerobic, grampositive, spore-forming bacterial bacilli. They are widely distributed in nature and are found in soil, decaying vegetation, marine sediment, and the intestinal tract of humans and animals. Several species produce toxins that are responsible for illness in humans.

Strains of *Clostridium perfringens* are common sources of food poisoning (Table 14-2), which is an intestinal disorder that is characterized by abdominal cramps, diarrhea, and nausea. Fever and vomiting are

**TABLE 14-2**

## Overview of Food Poisoning: Intoxications and Enteric Infections

| | INTOXICATIONS | | ENTERIC INFECTIONS | | |
| --- | --- | --- | --- | --- | --- |
| | **STAPHYLOCOCCAL FOOD POISONING** | **BOTULISM** | **CLOSTRIDIUM PERFRINGENS** | **VIBRO PARAHAEMOLYTICUS** | **BACILLUS CEREUS** |
| **Occurrence** | Widespread and frequent; one of the principal acute food poisonings in the United States | Sporadic; family-grouped cases occur | Widespread and frequent in countries with cooking practices that favor growth of organism | Sporadic cases and outbreaks occur in warm months of the year | Outbreaks in Europe and United States |
| **Etiologic agent** | Several enterotoxins of staphylococci; stable at boiling temperature | Toxins produced by *Clostridium botulinum* in anaerobic conditions; destroyed by boiling | Type A strains of *C. perfringens (C. welchii)* | *V. parahaemolyticus* (many types) | *B. cereus*, an aerobic spore former that produces two enterotoxins—one heat stable, causing vomiting, and one heat labile, causing diarrhea |
| **Reservoir** | Humans; cows with infected udders; dogs and fowl | Soil, water, and intestinal tract of animals and fish | Soil and gastrointestinal tract of humans and animals | Marine silt, coastal waters, fish, and shellfish | Soil; commonly found in raw, dried, and processed foods |
| **Transmission** | Ingestion of food containing staphylococcal toxin, which formed while food was held at room temperature | Ingestion of food in which toxin has formed; generally home-canned vegetables, fruits, and meats; also onions and potatoes cooked and held at room temperature | Ingestion of food, especially meat, contaminated by soil or feces; spores survive normal cooking temperatures, germinate, and multiply during cooking and reheating | Ingestion of raw or undercooked seafood; food contaminated with seawater | Ingestion of food that has been kept at ambient temperatures after cooking, permitting multiplication of the organism |
| **Incubation period** | 30 min–7 hr; usually 2–4 hr | 12–36 hr | 6–24 hr; usually 10–12 hr | 4–96 hr; usually 12–24 hr | 1–6 hr for disease causing vomiting; 6–20 hr for disease causing diarrhea |
| **Period of communicability** | Noncommunicable | Noncommunicable | Noncommunicable | Noncommunicable | Noncommunicable |
| **Susceptibility and resistance** | General; no immune response | General; no immune response | General; no resistance develops from exposure | General | Unknown |
| **Report to local health authority** | Prompt report of outbreaks | Report of cases and outbreaks | Prompt report of outbreaks | Report of outbreaks | Report of cases and outbreaks |

Data from Benenson A, editor: Control of communicable diseases in man. In Grimes D: *Infectious diseases: Mosby's clinical nursing series*, St Louis, 1991, Mosby.

usually absent. Almost all outbreaks are associated with inadequately heated or reheated beef, chicken, or turkey. The spores can survive normal cooking temperatures and germinate and multiply with inadequate storage or rewarming. The illness is produced by the toxins released from the bacteria. *Clostridium botulinum* intoxication occurs sporadically and produces severe neurologic symptoms, including flaccid paralysis. It occurs predominantly from inadequate heating in home canning of fruits and vegetables. *C. perfringens* and other clostridial species can also cause myonecrosis or gas gangrene. Organisms may find their way into a wound that is contaminated with dirt or through soiled clothing. Penetrating wounds such as gunshot wounds, compound fractures, or lacerated wounds present the greatest risk because these bacilli live and multiply in the absence of air.

The onset of symptoms is usually sudden and may occur 1 to 4 days after injury. Severe pain and edema develop and, although there may be little fever, the pulse rate may be rapid, weak, and thready. The respiratory rate is increased, and the blood pressure may fall. The wound may have a peculiar odor, which often is the first indication of the infection. The slightest unusual odor should be reported immediately to the physician. As the infection extends into the surrounding muscles, skin color change and gas bubbles may be seen at the site of the wound or may be expressed from the muscles. Unless it is treated promptly, the disease is fatal.

The most important aspect of treatment is the excision of all infected tissue. Antibiotic therapy is also started. Supportive treatment may include blood transfusion and intravenous fluids. When an extremity is involved, amputation may be necessary to save the patient's life. If the wound is large and drainage cannot be contained in a dressing, the patient must be placed on Contact Isolation. Equipment used during surgical procedures or for wound care is sterilized or discarded.

*Clostridium difficile* is a common organism in the GI tracts of children and is carried in the GI tract of approximately 5% of all adults. It does not normally result in illness. However, disease can occur when the organism is present and the normal flora of the bowel is disturbed. Disease can occur during antibiotic therapy, and colitis can result because of the effects of a toxin secreted by the organism. *C. difficile* has become an increasing problem in institutions in which organisms can be transmitted from person to person by the hands of health care workers. Infections can be treated with metronidazole for 10 days.

Tetanus (lockjaw) is an acute neurointoxication induced by *Clostridium tetani*. Tetanus spores can enter the body through a trivial cut or an extensive wound.

The anaerobic organism multiplies in the wound and produces a lethal toxin. Early symptoms of headache, restlessness, and irritability progress to opisthotonos (arching of the spine), generalized muscle spasms, and convulsions. Because most people have been immunized for this infectious disease, the incidence is low in the United States. However, adults who have never received a primary series of immunization are at risk for the infection.

## Food Poisoning

Food poisoning refers to illnesses that are acquired through consumption of food or liquids contaminated with chemicals, bacteria, viruses, bacterial toxins, or organic poisons that are naturally present in some edible substances. The bacteria often multiply in food that has been stored at improper temperatures. Food poisonings resulting from bacterial contamination occur shortly after ingestion of food. These illnesses are infectious but not communicable diseases and are not usually transmitted from one person to another (Box 14-5 and see Table 14-2).

### Staphylococcal Enteric Intoxication

The *S. aureus* enterotoxin is one of the more common causes of food poisoning in the United States. The foods commonly involved are those touched by the food handler without subsequent cooking or those that are improperly heated. Foods such as pastries, custards, salad dressings, and sliced meats can be contaminated by purulent discharges. If the food stands at room temperature for several hours before eating, an environment favorable to reproduction of the organism and subsequent enterotoxin production is created. Acute gastroenteritis occurs approximately 1 to 6 hours after ingestion of the food. Severe nausea, cramps, vomiting, and diarrhea can occur and last for several hours. The duration of the illness is 1 or 2 days, and hospitalization may be required. Deaths are rare.

The food is often consumed by large groups of people, which causes an outbreak that is reportable to public health authorities. Individual cases are rarely identified. An epidemiologic investigation can determine the population at risk, the place and time of exposure, and ultimately the food item responsible for the attack. The implicated food will have the highest attack rates. Most of the ill patients will have eaten the food, and most of the well will have not eaten the food.

Prevention includes the reduction of food-handling time, with no more than 4 to 5 hours at room temperature, refrigeration of perishable foods at 4.4° C (40° F) or lower, and maintenance of hot foods above 60° C (104° F). Nurses should promote these practices as

---

<< BOX 14-5 >>                     **NURSING PROCESS**

**ACUTE FOOD POISONING**

**ASSESSMENT**

- History of eating high-risk foods or under high-risk conditions
- Nausea, vomiting, diarrhea, vertigo, abdominal pain, paralysis
- Vital signs
- Fluid volume status

**NURSING DIAGNOSES**

- Fluid volume deficit related to prolonged vomiting and diarrhea
- Diarrhea related to pathogens in intestinal tract
- Ineffective breathing pattern related to neurologic effect
- Impaired physical mobility related to neurologic effect

**NURSING INTERVENTIONS**

- Encourage sips of clear fluids as tolerated.
- Progress diet as tolerated.
- Instruct patient to wash hands and lubricate anal opening after diarrhea.
- Instruct patient to report and seek medical treatment immediately if having difficulty breathing or swallowing or if experiencing paralysis.
- Report to local health authority, if indicated.

**EVALUATION OF EXPECTED OUTCOMES**

- No evidence of dehydration
- Returns to previous pattern of elimination
- Verbalizes understanding of preventive measures
- No respiratory compromise or neurologic deficits

---

everyday concerns in all households. Persons with boils, abscesses, and other purulent lesions of the hands and face should be prohibited from handling food. All food handlers should be educated in proper hygiene techniques. These techniques include washing hands, cleaning fingernails, keeping the food preparation area clean, and using proper temperature control, therefore reducing the danger of infections.

## Salmonella Infections

Salmonellosis is an acute gastroenteritis caused by certain species of the genus *Salmonella*. It is usually classified with food poisoning because food is the most common vehicle of infection. The proportion of cases that are recognized and reported are probably very small. Outbreaks that are reported usually involve hospitals, schools, restaurants, and nursing homes. Infections usually occur as a result of food that has been contaminated at its source, cross-contaminated during processing, or contaminated at some point by an undetected carrier. Most poultry should be considered contaminated and should be handled and cooked accordingly. The organism is also found in eggs, meat, and meat products. Infection is prevented by thoroughly cooking all foodstuffs derived from animal sources and by educating all food handlers.

The incubation period is from 6 to 72 hours, usually from 12 to 36 hours. It is followed by a sudden onset of frequent, bulky stools and then watery diarrhea. Abdominal pain, nausea and vomiting, headache, and

fever may occur. Anorexia and loose stools may persist for several days. The organism may localize in any part of the body and cause a variety of complications. Generally deaths are uncommon and occur only in the very young and the elderly.

Treatment is supportive. The infection is usually self-limiting, and antibiotic treatment may prolong the carrier state. However, antibiotics are indicated when complications occur. The primary objective in care is to maintain hydration. Lost fluids and electrolytes may need to be replaced intravenously.

## Shigellosis

Shigellosis, caused by the *Shigella bacillus* bacterium, may be mild or severe. In mild infections the clinical symptoms consist of watery or loose stools for several days. More severe cases of shigellosis (bacillary dysentery) are characterized by fever, headache, and profuse watery diarrhea. The inflammatory condition, which may also involve portions of the ileum, may result in severe ulceration and, if sufficiently intense, may destroy the mucous membrane of the colon, although perforation may not occur. The disease is spread by the fecal-oral route, often through contaminated water, food, or feces. The organism has been isolated from milk products and shrimp. It usually occurs in crowded areas where sanitary conditions are poor.

The incubation period is usually between 1 and 7 days, with an abrupt onset. The diarrhea results in loss of fluids and electrolytes, and the patient becomes severely dehydrated. The stools may contain blood, pus, and mucus. The temperature may range from low-grade elevation to between 39° C and 40° C (102° F and 104° F) in the afternoon.

A problem in the treatment of bacillary dysentery has been the resistance of the organisms to various antimicrobial drugs. Tetracycline, ampicillin, and trimethoprim-sulfamethoxazole are considered to be effective. Intravenous fluids and electrolytes are given to combat dehydration. The disease is considered to be self-limiting, and mortality is low when treatment is secured.

## Rickettsial Infections

The rickettsia are small, round, or rod-shaped specialized bacteria that live as intracellular parasites in fleas, lice, ticks, and mites. They are transmitted to humans by bites from these insects. Illnesses resulting from rickettsial infections are infectious but not communicable diseases. Rickettsial diseases have been responsible for many severe epidemics, such as epidemic typhus. However, in parts of the world where insect and rodent populations are well controlled, rickettsial diseases are uncommon.

### Rocky Mountain Spotted Fever

Rocky Mountain spotted fever is caused by *Rickettsia rickettsii* and is the most common rickettsial disease in the United States. The incidence of Rocky Mountain spotted fever is low and is greater along the eastern seaboard and in the southeastern states than in the Rocky Mountain area. Three types of ticks may be responsible for the disease: the American dog tick, the Rocky Mountain wood tick, and the Lone Star tick. The disease is seasonal and is more common from April to August. In some areas the disease presents an occupational hazard. When occupations take persons into areas that are heavily infested with ticks, the risk is greater. The disease is commonly contracted by persons vacationing or picnicking in areas where ticks exist. The fatality rate is high if the disease is untreated. The incubation period is 3 to 14 days.

**Assessment.** The disease may be mild, with the person remaining ambulatory, or may be severe, with death occurring within a few days after its onset. Early symptoms may be loss of appetite, malaise, irritability, and vague aches and pains. The disease may have an abrupt onset, beginning with chills, a severe headache, an elevation of temperature to 40° C (104° F) or higher, and severe muscle aching. There may be an unproductive cough, nosebleeds, and abdominal pain with nausea and vomiting. The face is flushed, there is profuse sweating, the mouth is dry,

and the tongue is coated. In severe cases there may be rigidity of the neck, mental confusion, delirium, incontinence, constipation, and severe prostration, and convulsions and coma may occur. On the third or fourth day a rash appears that begins on the wrists and ankles but gradually spreads over the body and may include the scalp and mucous membranes of the mouth and throat. The rash is petechial in type and tends to fade on pressure. It is rose colored in the beginning but darkens as the disease continues. The acute illness may last for 2 or 3 weeks with the temperature remaining high for as long as 10 days. The pulse rate is usually slow in relation to the amount of fever present, but in persons with severe cases it may become weak and rapid.

**Intervention.** The treatment of Rocky Mountain spotted fever is with chloramphenicol (Chloromycetin) or tetracycline and should be administered early in the disease, preferably with the beginning of the skin rash. The use of antibiotic therapy may remarkably improve the symptoms and reduce the febrile period. Other treatment consists of administering intravenous fluids if sufficient fluid is not taken orally. Blood transfusions may sometimes be indicated.

Care is the same as that for any patient with a febrile disease. The patient is on a regimen of bed rest, and measures to control the temperature, such as sponge baths and antipyretic drugs, are instituted. Special mouth care and eye irrigations may be necessary. The diet should be high in protein with extra between-meal feedings that are also high in protein.

**Prophylaxis.** No vaccine is currently licensed in the United States. Preventive measures are similar to Lyme disease. Persons who work in tick-infested areas and persons who go camping or picnicking in areas in which they may be exposed to ticks should use tick repellents, avoid sleeping on the ground, wear long pants tucked into socks, and inspect clothing and skin carefully. Areas such as the hairline and under the arms should be given special attention. When removing ticks it is important to avoid crushing them or leaving their heads embedded in the skin. The greatest danger of infection occurs after the tick has fed for 6 to 8 hours.

## PATIENT WITH A VIRAL INFECTION

### Measles

Measles (rubeola) is a highly infectious and often severe viral disease that occurs in young children. Although measles is preventable through active immunization, the disease has occurred in a significant number of people in recent years. Before the measles vaccine was available, more than 400,000 cases were reported annually in the United States. Since the introduction of the vaccine in 1963, the incidence of cases per year has decreased by more than 90%. However, the incidence of measles has increased somewhat in all age groups, with the highest incidence in preschoolers who were never immunized. In 1990 11.2 cases of measles occurred per 100,000 people (CDC, 1994). This rate contrasts with 1.4 cases per 100,000 people in 1988. This remarkable increase stimulated federal- and state-funded primary prevention programs to immunize children throughout the United States. In 1996 the rate dropped to 0.2 cases per 100,000 people (CDC, 1997). Measles control in the future depends on the success of continuing programs to immunize all susceptible persons who can tolerate the vaccine.

The onset of measles is usually sudden after an incubation period of 7 to 14 days. It occurs most often in the late winter or early spring. In the beginning the disease is often mistaken for a severe cold. Coryza; lacrimation of the eyes, which are red and sensitive to light; sneezing; and a bronchial cough appear. The patient may have a fever, with temperatures ranging from 39.5° C to 40.5° C (103° F to 105° F) and often appears severely ill. During this period, examination of the throat will reveal small white spots with a reddened base (Koplik's spots). In approximately 4 days a macular type of rash begins to appear around the face and gradually extends over the entire body. The rash gradually coalesces to form a slightly elevated eruption that reaches its height in approximately 48 hours, after which it begins to fade. After the rash disappears, a fine desquamation of the skin occurs.

With the development of the rash, the acute symptoms begin to subside. If complications do not develop, recovery may be expected in 10 to 14 days. Measles is often complicated by bronchopneumonia, otitis media, and encephalitis. Encephalitis accompanies rubeola in approximately 1 of every 1000 children affected and may cause brain damage and mental retardation.

## Intervention

There is no specific treatment for measles. The child with measles should be isolated from other children, and care should be taken in the disposal of nose and throat secretions. The patient is usually more comfortable in a darkened room because of the sensitivity to light. Sponge baths may be given to reduce fever, and fluids should be encouraged. Bed rest is indicated, and exposure to drafts or respiratory infections should be avoided. The nurse should be alert to complaints of earache or enlargement of the cervical lymph nodes, and the physician should be notified if these symptoms occur. During the febrile period, the diet should be liquid or soft. Cough medications have little effect on the cough. Antibiotic therapy is not indicated.

## Prophylaxis

For children who have not had measles, active immunization should be given at 15 months of age. A second dose is recommended at school entry or middle school entry. Maternal measles antibodies in the serum of a child under age 1 limit the effectiveness of the measles vaccine in producing an active immunity. If an unvaccinated child has been exposed to measles, an immunization given within 72 hours may provide protection.

The measles vaccine produces a mild or subclinical, noncommunicable infection in 95% of susceptible children. It is recommended that persons who were immunized with a live measles vaccine before 12 months of age and those who received an inactivated vaccine that was available between 1963 and 1967 be reimmunized.

## Rubella

Rubella (German measles) is sometimes called *3-day measles* because of the short duration of the disease. The symptoms may be similar to those of rubeola but are usually much milder, and Koplik's spots are absent. Some cases may be so mild that the rash is the first and only significant indication of the disease. The lymph nodes behind the ears are almost always enlarged.

The incubation period of rubella is from 12 to 23 days. Isolation and careful handling and disposal of respiratory secretions are important during the course of the disease.

## Pregnancy

The occurrence of rubella during pregnancy has been found to present a major hazard to early fetal development. The rubella virus infects the placenta and spreads to the fetal circulation. The time of gestation and the length of time that the virus survives and continues to grow in fetal tissue determine the effects on the fetus. The greatest incidence of defects takes place between the second and the sixth week of gestation. After 8 weeks, the chance of developing heart defects, cataracts, and glaucoma decreases, but brain and ear defects may continue to occur into the second trimester of pregnancy. Fetal defects do not develop during late pregnancy. Because 75% of rubella cases occur in school-age children, they represent the reservoir of infection for pregnant women and women of childbearing age.

## Prophylaxis

In 1969 the U.S. government licensed a live rubella virus vaccine for general distribution. Children in kindergarten and early grades may be the source of community epidemics and should be high on the priority list for immunization. A single dose of rubella vaccine produces protective antibodies in approximately 95% of susceptible persons. It is often combined with measles or measles-mumps vaccines and given at 15 months of age.

The vaccine should not be given to pregnant women or to women who may become pregnant within 3 months of receiving the vaccine. Persons with major febrile illness should not be immunized until they have recovered from their illness. The vaccine has not been reported to be associated with allergic reactions. However, some vaccines do contain trace amounts of antibiotics. Therefore label information on the vaccine bottle should be reviewed carefully before administering the vaccine to patients who are allergic to antibiotics.

The immunization of male adolescents and adults is useful in preventing and controlling epidemics. Because the rubella vaccine is in general use, several factors are important: (1) surveillance of epidemics, (2) accurate diagnosis and reporting of cases, and (3) reporting of all birth defects related to rubella.

## Chickenpox

Chickenpox (varicella) is the second most commonly reported communicable disease (following gonorrhea) in the United States. The herpes VZV is the causative agent and is transmitted by direct contact with skin lesions or by airborne transmission of respiratory tract secretions. The incubation period is 2 to 3 weeks, and the period of communicability is usually 1 to 2 days before onset of the characteristic rash.

There is a sudden onset of slight fever with a maculopapular rash. The rash is superficial and first appears on the chest, abdomen, and back. It gradually extends to other parts of the body. The lesions appear in crops, and small reddened spots are often observed in the throat before the rash appears on the skin. The rash goes through a series of stages, beginning with a macule and progressing to a papule, vesicle, and crust. Headache, loss of appetite, and malaise are also common symptoms. Scratching the lesions may lead to secondary infections, and scar formations may result. The disease is self-limiting, and there is no specific treatment. Contact and airborne isolation are indicated for hospitalized cases. In the community isolation is generally considered unnecessary, but items contaminated with nose and throat discharges should be carefully discarded.

Although chickenpox is usually a relatively benign disease, infection in a child who has leukemia may result in a widely disseminated infection. More children are surviving with leukemia because of the use of chemotherapeutic drugs. However, infection with chickenpox may be fatal.

A live, attenuated varicella virus vaccine was licensed in March 1995 for use in healthy persons at or more than 12 months of age. It is not licensed for use in persons who have altered immunity. However, patients with leukemia who meet certain criteria may be vaccinated if entered into a research protocol (CDC, 1996). Varicella zoster immune globulin is available and is used primarily for passive immunization of susceptible, immunocompromised children after exposure to chickenpox or herpes zoster.

## Herpes Zoster

Herpes zoster (shingles) is a local manifestation of a recurrent infection that occurs with the chickenpox virus, usually in an older adult. Vesicles erupt on the skin in crops or in irregular patterns along a sensory nerve. Eruptions commonly appear along the chest wall and, occasionally, the ophthalmic branch of the trigeminal nerve may be involved. Severe pain and paresthesias can occur over the infected nerve. The pain is controlled with analgesics. Antiviral drugs such as acyclovir, famciclovir, and valacyclovir have been shown to shorten the coarse of the disease and to reduce the duration of postherpetic pain, especially in the older patient.

## Mumps

Mumps (parotitis) is an infectious disease caused by a specific virus that primarily affects children. However, susceptible adults may contract the disease. It has continued to decrease in incidence since the vaccine was licensed in December 1967. In 1996 0.29 cases per 100,000 people occurred (CDC, 1997). Mumps is characterized by inflammation and swelling of the parotid glands on one or both sides, and the salivary glands may be affected. However, 40% of the cases are believed to be subclinical. The incubation period is 14 to 21 days but may extend beyond 21 days. The disease is transmitted through droplet infection from the upper respiratory tract.

Symptoms depend on the severity of the attack, and may include a slight to moderate temperature elevation, general malaise, and pain on moving the jaw or opening the mouth. A characteristic condition associated with mumps is an acute sensitivity to acidic substances.

Other glands in the body occasionally become involved, the most common being the testes in men who have been through puberty. Encephalitis, aseptic meningitis, and unilateral nerve deafness are the most serious complications. The question of mumps occurring during early pregnancy as a possible cause of fetal malformations has come under investigation.

## Intervention

The patient should be isolated until all symptoms of the mumps infection have subsided. Warm or cold packs may be applied to swollen, tender salivary glands. The diet should be liquid or soft, and any food or drink with a tart or acidic taste should be avoided. If orchitis develops, bed rest, narcotic analgesics, support of the inflamed testis with a bridge, and ice packs may make the patient feel more comfortable. If the illness remains uncomplicated, it may run a course of approximately 7 to 10 days.

## Prophylaxis

Although it is available independently, the mumps vaccine is usually combined with a MR vaccine and administered at age 15 months. Administration of the vaccine within 1 to 2 days after exposure offers some protection to the susceptible person.

## Infectious Mononucleosis

Infectious mononucleosis is an acute infection caused by the Epstein-Barr virus (EBV), which is closely related to the herpes viruses. The name *mononucleosis* was derived from the atypical lymphocytes among the white blood cells. Infection with the virus is worldwide, but infectious mononucleosis occurs primarily in developed countries where contact with the virus is delayed from early childhood until the age of 15 to 25. Infection with the virus at an early age results in a subclinical infection that usually goes unnoticed. A syndrome resembling infectious mononucleosis may be caused by herpesvirus type 6 or cytomegalovirus (CMV), another member of the herpesvirus group of organisms.

The disease often occurs among groups of young people living together, as in college dormitories. The disease has been referred to as the "kissing disease," because transmission appears to be by the oral route and the exchange of saliva. Infection with EBV is very common and by the time adulthood is reached, 90% of individuals have antibodies. However, disease from the infection is unusual and only about 10% of those infected develop clinically apparent infectious mononucleosis.

The disease is characterized by sore throat, fever, enlarged lymph nodes, headache, and vomiting. In persons with severe cases the spleen may be enlarged or jaundice may occur. The incubation period is believed to be 4 to 14 days but may be as long as 6 weeks.

There is no specific treatment for the disease, which is self-limiting. During the acute phase the patient should be confined to bed. Mild analgesics may be given to relieve the discomfort from the sore throat and enlarged glands. Antibiotics have no effect on the course or the outcome of the disease. In severe cases, steroid therapy may be recommended. Although serious complications, including neurologic problems, are possible, they are rare.

## Influenza

Influenza is an acute viral disease of the respiratory tract. Epidemics and pandemics of influenza have been known since the sixteenth century. The worst pandemic of modern times occurred in 1918 and 1919, when it was estimated that 20 million people died. More than half of these deaths occurred in the United States. Several serious epidemics have occurred since then. The disease occurs in cycles, but sporadic illness occurs during nonepidemic years. Each year, most states report cases of influenza to the CDC, although only epidemics are required to be reported. Attack rates during epidemics have been estimated from less than 15% of the population to 25% in large communities. True incidence data is difficult to obtain.

Three types of influenza viruses have been identified: A, B, and C. Types A and B have long been associated with epidemics. Type C has appeared only sporadically and in localized outbreaks. Strains of influenza A are described by geographic origin, strain number, year of isolation, and an index that identifies the antigenic characteristics of the strain. Hemagglutinin (H) and neuraminidase (N) are surface antigens of the virus that stimulate antibody production. Each strain has specific configurations. For instance, the viral strain that caused the Hong Kong influenza epidemic in 1968 is described as A/Hong Kong/1/68 (H3N2).

The mode of transmission is by direct contact through droplet infection, which is often airborne in crowded, enclosed areas. The incubation period is short, usually from 24 to 72 hours, and the period of communicability is limited to 3 days from the onset of clinical symptoms. The typical onset is sudden with shaking chills (rigors); a temperature of (38.8° C [102° F]) or above; aching of the head, back, and extremities; sore throat; coughing; sneezing; and weakness. In uncomplicated cases the acute period usually lasts from 3 to 5 days. Influenza is especially hazardous for the elderly, and mortality from influenza-related pneumonia is high. Generally the treatment is symptomatic. Antibiotics may be given if a secondary infection such as a bacterial pneumonia occurs.

Susceptibility to the influenza viruses is universal. Infection produces immunity to the specific infecting virus, and infections with related viruses broadens immunity. However, type A influenza viruses undergo "antigenic shifts" in which distinctive new hemagglutinin or neuraminidase surface antigens are formed. These shifts result from changes in the genetic material of the virus. These new variants of influenza create new epidemics when enough of the population is susceptible.

Vaccines have been created to immunize people at high risk, including health care workers. Because the antigenic characteristics of the current strains provide the basis for selecting the virus strains included in each year's vaccine, the vaccines may not be effective if new strains appear. Because the proportion of elderly people in the United States is increasing and chronic diseases are more prevalent, an increased emphasis on control measures is necessary for the future. It is recommended that the following groups be targeted for vaccination programs (in order of priority):

1. Children and adults with chronic disorders of the cardiovascular or pulmonary system
2. Residents of chronic care facilities
3. Healthy individuals who are 65 years old or older
4. Children and adults with chronic metabolic diseases, renal dysfunction, anemia, or immunosuppression
5. Children and teenagers who are receiving long-term aspirin therapy because they are at risk of Reye's syndrome following influenza infection
6. Physicians, nurses, and other personnel that have extensive contact with high-risk patients because they may transmit the virus and cause nosocomial infections in patients
7. Providers of care to high-risk people in the home

Local health planning and education in schools and institutions and surveillance of the extent and progress of outbreaks are other means of prevention and control.

## Hepatitis

Viral hepatitis is an infectious disease that attacks the liver and causes a diffuse inflammatory reaction. Several distinct infections actually occur and differ in etiologic and pathologic characteristics. Their prevention and control measures also vary (see Chapter 35).

The virus is transmitted from person to person by the fecal-oral route, and contaminated food is a common vehicle. The incubation period is from 15 to 50 days and averages from 28 to 30 days. The virus is excreted in the feces long before clinical symptoms appear, although the carrier is thought to be most infectious just before the onset of symptoms. Because the disease has a low incidence in infants and preschool-aged children, mild, inapparent, and asymptomatic infections are probably common.

The onset of viral hepatitis is abrupt, with fever, malaise, nausea, and abdominal discomfort followed by jaundice within a few days. The illness varies from clinically asymptomatic infection to mild symptoms to a severely disabling disease that lasts several months. Severity increases with age, although complete recovery is normal. A vaccine for hepatitis A has recently become available. Immunoglobulin may be given as a prophylactic measure to exposed persons or to those who anticipate travel to highly endemic areas. All feces, blood, and body fluids from the infected individual should be treated as potentially infectious. Prevention and control measures focus on education of the public regarding good sanitation, personal hygiene, and handwashing.

HB has a similar incidence to hepatitis A: 5.18 cases per 100,000 people in 1993 (CDC, 1994). The infection occurs worldwide with little seasonal variation. The virus is comprised of a core surrounded by an outer coat that contains the surface antigen. Transmission occurs when blood, serum, or plasma from an infected person is introduced parenterally, often through venipuncture equipment or needle sticks. The infection can also be transmitted through contamination of open wounds or through exposure of mucous membranes to infected body fluids. Fecal-oral transmission has not been demonstrated. The average incubation period is 60 to 90 days. Blood is infectious weeks before the onset of symptoms, through the clinical course of the illness, and during the chronic carrier state, which may last for years. Surface antigens can be detected in the serum several weeks before onset of symptoms and into the carrier state.

The onset is usually insidious, with vague abdominal discomfort, anorexia, malaise, nausea and vomiting and joint pain. Fever may be mild or absent. Jaundice is common and is accompanied by dark urine, clay-colored stools, and pruritus. The illness ranges from inapparent infection to acute hepatic necrosis, which may be fatal. Treatment is symptomatic only and is planned to strengthen the patient's resistance to infection. The patient's contacts and those who are accidentally exposed can be immunized with an inactive viral antigen (HB). Preventive measures include strict discipline in blood banks, use of blood and blood products only when essential, and sterilization of all reusable equipment. A vaccine for HB has been available in the United States since 1982.

Hepatitis C resembles HB clinically and epidemiologically. It is usually less severe in the acute stage, but asymptomatic or symptomatic chronicity is common. The incubation period is from 2 weeks to 6 months. Treatment, control, and prevention measures are similar to those for HB.

# PATIENT WITH A PROTOZOAL DISEASE

There are approximately 30 known protozoal diseases. Most of them have a low incidence in the United States but are prevalent in other parts of the world. Most cases occur in travelers who have been to countries where the infections are endemic. Examples include amebiasis and giardiasis, which affect the intestine; toxoplasmosis and malaria, which are systemic diseases; and trichomoniasis, which affects the genitourinary tract and is considered to be a sexually transmitted disease (STD). Trichomoniasis is widespread throughout the world. Malaria is a serious, worldwide disease and is reportable to the CDC.

Malaria is transmitted from person to person by a mosquito known as the *Anopheles quadrimaculatus.* Control of the disease in the United States has been brought about primarily through destruction of mosquito-breeding places and adequate treatment of persons with malaria. Most cases in the United States have been in persons returning from areas of the world where the disease still exists.

Four species of the parasite cause malaria in humans. The most serious is known as *Plasmodium falciparum.* The parasite is injected into the body by a female mosquito that is seeking a blood meal before ovulation. The parasites invade the liver, where they grow and multiply. After 12 to 14 days (the incubation period), they enter the bloodstream and invade red blood cells. The symptoms that result are caused by the continual lysis of red blood cells.

Symptoms of malaria begin with a headache and a gradually increasing fever. The typical malaria pattern soon develops: severe chills followed by a high fever, with temperatures ranging from 39.5° C to 40.5° C (103° F to 105° F), followed by a rapid fall in temperature and profuse sweating. This sequence may repeat itself every 48 hours, and between the episodes the patient may be reasonably well. However, without adequate treatment, anemia and enlargement of the spleen gradually develop.

Oral administration of chloroquine (Aralen) is the treatment of choice for most cases of malaria. However, in areas where *P. falciparum* has become resistant to chloroquine, quinine sulfate is given along with tetracycline (Beneson, 1990). Travelers to Asia, Africa, or South America, where the chloroquine-resistant organisms are present, are advised to take mefloquine for prophylaxis. This drug is contraindicated for preg-

nant women, and other drug therapy is recommended. Administration of the drug should begin 2 weeks before departure and continue for 6 weeks after leaving the malarious area.

# PATIENT WITH HELMINTHIC INFESTATIONS

Metazoa are parasites that belong to the animal kingdom. When they invade the human body, this is referred to as a *helminth infestation.* The Metazoa are divided into two groups: (1) Platyhelminthes, which includes tapeworms; and (2) Nematoda, or roundworms. Nematoda include Ascaris parasites, hookworms, pinworms, and *Trichinella* parasites.

Parasites often ingest nutrients in the GI tract of the infected person, which causes a state of malnutrition even though the person is eating a balanced diet. Irritation and tissue damage can occur. If the parasites grow or increase in number, blood vessels, ducts, and even the GI tract can be blocked. Pinworms are sometimes found in the appendix when acute appendicitis has necessitated its removal. Some parasites produce toxins that injure tissue or cause severe allergic tissue reactions.

## Platyhelminthes (Flatworms)

Tapeworms (Cestoda) are flatworms, and nearly all flatworms are segmented. At one end there is a head and a neck called the *scolex.* The head is tiny in relation to the size of the worm. The scolex contains a mechanism that enables the worm to attach itself to the mucous membrane of the intestinal tract. Three forms of the worm are known to infect humans in the United States: (1) the dwarf tapeworm, (2) the beef tapeworm, and (3) the fish tapeworm.

The dwarf tapeworm is the smallest of the tapeworms. It is most prevalent in areas where sanitation is extremely poor. Infection occurs after ingesting the eggs of the worm, which hatch in the human intestinal tract. The cycle begins when the worms produce eggs that are discharged in the feces. Improper handwashing after using the toilet is the medium by which the eggs are conveyed to the mouth and thus to the intestinal tract.

The beef tapeworm, the most commonly found tapeworm in the United States, reaches the human intestinal tract through the ingestion of raw or insufficiently cooked beef that contains the larvae of the worm. The cycle begins when the larvae produce worms. The eggs produced by the worms are present in human feces and are deposited onto soil where cattle graze. A cow ingests the eggs, which hatch in the small intestine. The larvae (an intermediate stage in the development of the worm) lodge in the animal's tissues. A person who eats raw or undercooked beef that contains the larvae may become infected. The beef tapeworm is known to grow to a length of 25 feet, and as long as the head remains attached to the mucous membrane of the intestinal wall, it continues to grow and produce eggs.

The fish tapeworm, like the beef tapeworm, requires an intermediary host, and human infection occurs in a similar way. Human feces containing the eggs are deposited into fresh water, where the eggs mature into tiny embryos. The embryos are usually eaten by small shellfish, which are ultimately eaten by larger fish. The embryo then matures in the tissues of the fish. Infection may occur in areas where fish is eaten raw or is insufficiently cooked. The fish tapeworm may grow to 30 feet in length and may live for many years in the human intestine. Fish tapeworm infection is believed to be more prevalent than previously thought. Infection is known to result in severe anemia, and it is reported that the worm absorbs large amounts of vitamin B12 from the intestinal tract. Praziquantel (Biltricide) or niclosamide (Niclocide) is the drug of choice for both beef and fish tapeworm infestations.

## Nematoda (Roundworms)

*Ascaris* is a genus of large roundworms that resemble the common earthworm (fishworm). Roundworms vary in length from 4 to 12 inches, and the female worm may produce as many as 27 million eggs. When human feces are deposited on the ground, they become mixed with the soil, where the eggs may live for indefinite periods. Infection results from ingestion of the eggs containing the larvae. The larvae reach the small intestine, where they mature. Infection with *Ascaris* may be serious and cause complications such as intestinal obstruction, perforation of ulcers, appendicitis, and similar conditions. Administration of mebendazole (Vermox), pyrantel pamoate (Antiminth), or piperazine salts provides effective treatment.

## Hookworms

There are two species of hookworm, and both may cause human infection. One species is most common in the southern United States, and the other species is most prevalent in Europe and Asia. As with many other types of worms, the source of infection is soil that has been contaminated with human feces that contain the eggs. The larva of the hookworm penetrates the unbroken skin of the feet and legs and enters the body by way of the hair follicles and sweat glands. It penetrates lymph and blood vessels and may reach the lungs, where it is often coughed up and expectorated.

If larvae are swallowed, they reach the small intestine, where the worms mature. The worm attaches itself to the intestinal mucosa by a pinching kind of hook. A mature worm produces from 5000 to 10,000 eggs daily. The hookworm is reported to ingest as much as 50 ml of the host's blood daily, which results in a severe iron-deficiency anemia. It also damages and ingests bits of tissue from the intestinal mucosa and commonly causes allergic reactions. Mebendazole (Vermox) and thiabendazole (Mintezol) are effective in testing the infestation. Examination of stool specimens should be repeated after 2 weeks.

## Pinworms (Threadworms, Seatworms)

Pinworms are found worldwide and represent the most common helminth infection in the United States. Prevalence is highest in school-age children and lowest in adults. Often entire families are infected at the same time. The pinworm is a tiny worm, and infection is self-induced by the anal-oral route. The ingested eggs pass into the stomach, and the worm matures in the large intestine. When the mature worm is ready to lay its eggs, it crawls to the outside and deposits its eggs in folds around the rectum and anus, after which it dies. The life cycle is approximately 4 to 6 weeks. Severe itching occurs around the area. Through scratching, the hands become infected with the eggs, which are then carried to the mouth, and the entire cycle begins again. Reinfection may cause the number of worms present in the GI tract to increase over several months.

Several drugs are effective in eliminating the infestation, among them pyrantel pamoate, mebendazole, albendazole, and pyrvinium pamoate (Povan). Treatment is repeated after 2 weeks. Taking daily showers, changing underclothes and bed sheets often, washing hands often, discouraging nail biting, and providing education in personal hygiene help prevent outbreaks.

## Trichinellosis (Trichinosis)

Trichina is a parasitic organism of the genus *Trichinella* and is responsible for trichinosis. The primary source of trichinosis is insufficiently cooked pork and pork products that are infected with the worm. The larva that is present in the meat passes into the intestinal tract, and the worm matures in the intestine, where it becomes embedded in the mucosa. The larva is then released and eventually reaches the bloodstream. After entering the general circulation, the larva is carried to skeletal muscle tissue and becomes encased in a cyst. There are several stages of infection during the development of the worm and its passage through the body. During the various stages of the infection, symptoms may be acute, with fever, increased leukocyte count, allergic manifestations, and psychologic symptoms. After encasement, the primary symptom is rheumatic-like pain. The disease is serious, and 5% to 10% of the persons infected die.

Thiabendazole has been effective in treatment of the infestation when given during the very early intestinal stage of the disease. Mebendazole is used in the muscular stage of the disease. Corticosteroids are indicated only in severe cases.

## SEXUALLY TRANSMITTED DISEASES

Six diseases are classified as STDs and are reportable to public health authorities: AIDS, syphilis, gonorrhea, chancroid, lymphogranuloma venereum, and granuloma inguinale. AIDS is the epidemic of the twentieth century (see Chapter 16). Syphilis and gonorrhea remain significant health problems in the United States. The incidence rates of chancroid, lymphogranuloma venereum, and granuloma inguinale are less than 0.2 cases per 100,000 people (CDC, 1997).

Trichomoniasis, venereal warts, herpes simplex type 2, and some chlamydial infections can also be sexually transmitted, but reporting these conditions is not required. The most common conditions are discussed in the following sections. Table 14-3 outlines the characteristics of the less prevalent or less serious venereal diseases, and Box 14-6 outlines the care for patients with STDs.

**TABLE 14-3**

## Characteristics of Sexually Transmitted Diseases

| DISEASE (PATHOGEN) | TRANSMISSION/INCUBATION | SYMPTOMS | PREVENTION AND CONTROL |
|---|---|---|---|
| Chancroid (Haemophilus ducreyi) | Direct contact; 3-5 days, up to 14 days | Painful ulcers at site; painful regional lymph nodes | Ceftriaxone or erythromycin; report to health authorities; prophylactic treatment of contacts |
| Condyloma acuminatum, genital warts (human papillomavirus) | Direct contact; 2-3 months average | Fleshy, cauliflower-like growths around genitalia | 10%-25% podophyllin in tincture of benzoin; intralesional recombinant interferon alfa-2b (Intron A); sexual contacts should be examined and treated, if indicated |
| Granuloma inguinale (Calymmatobacterium granulomatis) | Direct contact through sexual activity; 8-80 days | Small, beefy-red nodule, slowly spreads; often painless; can spread to other parts of the skin, mucous membranes | Tetracycline, co-trimoxazole, or chloramphenicol for 3 weeks; report to health authorities; examine sexual contacts |
| Lymphogranuloma venereum (Chlamydia trachomatis) | Direct contact, usually sexual intercourse; 4-21 days, usually 7-12 days | Small, painless papule or nodule often unnoticed; suppuration of regional lymph nodes and invasion of adjacent tissues; fever, chills, headache, joint pain | Tetracycline; doxycycline; treatment of recent contacts; report to health authorities |
| Molluscum contagiosum (Molluscipoxvirus) | Direct sexual contact and indirect contact; 2-7 weeks | Smooth-surfaced, firm, spherical papules, white translucent or yellow; 2-5 mm in diameter | No drug therapy available; curettage with local anesthesia |
| Other chlamydial infections | Direct contact through sexual intercourse; 7-14 days or longer | Males: urethritis; females: mucopurulent cervicitis; itching, burning on urination | Tetracycline or doxycycline; prophylactic treatment of sexual partners; reportable in some states |
| Trichomoniasis (Trichomonas vaginalis) | Direct contact with vaginal and urethral discharges or contaminated articles; trnasmitted to infants during birth; 4-20 days, average 7 days | Petechial lesions; profuse, thin, foamy, yellow discharge with foul odor; sometimes asymptomatic vaginitis, or urethritis | Metronidazole (Flagyl); sexual partners should be treated concurrently |

---

| BOX 14-6 | NURSING PROCESS |
| --- | --- |

## SEXUALLY TRANSMITTED DISEASE

**ASSESSMENT**

- Sexual history
- Dysuria, discharge, rectal irritation, malaise
- Posterior pharynx for inflammation, exudate
- Temperature
- External genitalia
- Inguinal lymphadenopathy

**NURSING DIAGNOSES**

- Risk for infection (patient contacts) related to pathogens in lesions and mode of transmission
- Risk for infection (patient) related to untreated or inadequately treated disease
- Anxiety or fear related to social stigma of venereal disease
- Knowledge deficit related to new condition, transmission, prevention, and treatment

**NURSING INTERVENTIONS**

- Administer medications (antivirals, antibiotics) as prescribed.
- Monitor for symptoms of pelvic inflammatory disease with gonorrhea and chlamydia.
- Keep lesions clean and dry.
- Report to local health authority, if indicated.
- Reexamine and treat pregnant women before delivery.
- Examine and treat patient contacts.
- Provide emotional support.

**EVALUATION OF EXPECTED OUTCOMES**

- Describes medication regimen
- Describes correct use of condom
- Verbalizes avoidance of sexual contacts until lesions are healed
- Infection resolved

---

### NURSE ALERT

**Acquired immunodeficiency syndrome, syphilis, gonorrhea, chancroid, lymphogranuloma venereum, and granuloma inguinale are reportable sexually transmitted diseases.**

## Syphilis

Syphilis (lues) is a widespread communicable disease. Syphilis primarily involves people between 15 and 30 years of age. Social factors are significantly related to the disease. It is more common in urban settings and among male homosexuals in some areas. It also is more common in males than females.

Syphilis is contracted almost exclusively through direct sexual contact with exudates from a person infected with the bacterial spirochete *Treponema pallidum*. Susceptibility is universal. Saliva, semen, blood, and vaginal discharges may carry the organism. Fetal infection may occur through transfer of the organism through the placenta. The incubation period is from 10 days to 10 weeks but is usually 3 weeks. Four stages of development have been identified: the pri-

mary, secondary, latent, and late stages. The period of communicability of untreated patients is variable and indefinite.

### Primary Syphilis

The primary lesion appears as a painless papule that occurs on the male prepuce or female vulva, vagina, or cervix. It may become an indurated chancre. The serologic blood test is usually negative at this time. During the primary stage the disease is highly infectious. The primary lesion disappears in 3 to 4 weeks with or without treatment, and no topical application will hasten its healing. Positive identification of the specific spirochete may be made at this time by a dark-field examination (a special attachment on the microscope). When adequate treatment is given early during the primary stage, the serologic test may remain negative. Without treatment the disease progresses to the secondary stage. The secondary stage usually begins 2 to 8 weeks after the appearance of the chancre.

### Secondary Syphilis

As a result of the invading organisms, several symptoms develop, including a rash. The rash may be a slight erythema or may be extensive, with macular, papular, or pustular lesions. The rash may involve the entire body and especially the palms and soles, which are locations that strongly suggest the diagnosis. Lesions called *mucus patches* appear around the mouth and lips, and the throat may be sore. A papular type of lesion (condyloma latum) appears around the genitals. All moist lesions are infectious, and positive dark-field examination may often be secured from these secondary lesions. Other symptoms include alopecia, pain in the bones, gastric disturbances, inflammation of the eyes, loss of appetite, and malaise. Without treatment, the symptoms of secondary syphilis may disappear slowly and recur at intervals for as long as 2 years. The disease is considered highly infectious during this stage.

## Latent Syphilis

The latent stage is generally considered to cover 4 years or more from time of onset of the disease. During this period, there is no clinical evidence of the disease after the disappearance of secondary lesions, except for the reactive serologic test. However, it is during this time that the organism attacks the vital structures and causes an inflammatory condition. The body's defenses may be sufficient to overcome the destructiveness of the organism. However, there is no way to determine which individuals may ultimately suffer severe disability. The serologic test remains reactive, and the disease is potentially infectious through sexual contact. Latency sometimes continues throughout life, and spontaneous recovery may occur.

## Late Syphilis

The late stage occurs 5 to 20 years after initial infection. Disabling lesions occur in the cardiovascular system and central nervous system. This stage is often referred to as neurosyphilis, cardiovascular syphilis, or gummatous syphilis. These late manifestations impair health, limit occupational efficiency, and shorten life.

## Congenital Syphilis

Mothers with untreated syphilis often have a history of repeated abortions. If the pregnancy is completed, the fetus may be stillborn. If the infant survives, he or she may have syphilis. An infant with congenital syphilis may have a rash on the face, palms, soles, and buttocks, with the latter often mistaken for diaper rash. There may be nasal stuffiness and rhinitis (snuf-

fles). The bones and abdominal organs are often involved. The syphilitic lesions of the infant are infectious, just as are those of the adult. The child who survives may develop complications at any time before 16 years of age. These complications include changes in the bones, deformed permanent teeth, interstitial keratitis, and eighth nerve deafness. The central nervous system may be involved, and mental retardation may occur in a small number of children.

### Intervention

The present treatment of syphilis is administration of long-acting penicillin G. There is no evidence that the syphilitic organism is becoming resistant to penicillin. However, caution must be exercised because more individuals are becoming sensitive to penicillin. The same care should be exercised as when administering penicillin to a patient for any condition. Treatment may extend over a period of several days or may be given in one initial dose. Patients who are sensitive to penicillin may be treated with tetracycline or erythromycin.

The fundamental approach to controlling syphilis is to interview patients to identify contacts. All identified contacts of confirmed syphilis cases should receive preventive penicillin therapy and should be educated about the disease. The privacy of the individual must be protected. Preventive measures assumed by nurses include health and sex education, discouragement of sexual promiscuity, and encouragement of syphilis serology during prenatal examination. Control of prostitution and ensuring availability and accessibility of care are broader goals for health care personnel.

## Gonorrhea

Gonorrhea remains an epidemic in the United States. It is an infection of the genitourinary tract with the organism *Neisseria gonorrhoeae* (gonococcus bacterium). Gonorrhea is the most commonly reported infectious disease. It is common in the United States among sexually promiscuous male homosexuals. With the introduction of resistant strains of the organism, the incidence has increased worldwide (CDC, 1994).

Transmission of the organism occurs through direct contact with exudates from the mucous membranes of infected people. The incubation period is 2 to 7 days. Without treatment, the infection may be self-limiting or result in a chronic carrier state. In females, urethritis or cervicitis initially occurs. It is often mild and may go unnoticed. Chronic endocervical infection is common, and the uterus may be invaded as the infection progresses. Because of the sometimes mild nature of the disease in women, many cases go untreated and the infection is spread to others. The period of communicability may extend for months if untreated. A disseminated gonococcal infection develops in approximately 5% of those infected and causes arthritis, fever, and skin lesions (Beneson, 1990).

The characteristic symptoms begin with burning, urgent, and painful urination. There may be redness and edema of the urinary meatus. After the initial symptoms, a purulent urethral discharge occurs in men, and a discharge may be expressed from the vaginal glands, ducts, and the urethra in women. In the absence of treatment or with inadequate treatment, the disease may become chronic and lead to complications. Epididymitis and prostatitis may occur in men, and salpingitis and pelvic inflammatory disease may occur in women. An acute inflammatory condition in the fallopian tubes leads to occlusion and sterility.

The usual treatment for gonorrhea consists of Ceftriaxone 125 to 250 mg IM in a single dose. Because coinfection with *Chlamydia trachomatis* is common, 100 mg of doxycycline taken orally twice a day for 7 days is given in addition to the Ceftriaxone. Interviewing patients and tracing contacts are fundamental elements of a control program. Preventive measures are the same as for syphilis.

## Herpes Simplex

There are several types of herpes viruses. The herpes simplex virus types 1 (HSV-1) and 2 (HSV-2) cause both genital and oral infections. Other viruses included in this family are the EBV, which causes mononucleosis; the VZV, which causes chickenpox and shingles; and CMV, which can result in severe congenital abnormalities. The majority of oral HSV infections are caused by type 1, and most genital lesions are caused by type 2. However, either strain can be found in the oral and genital areas, as well as on other parts of the body as skin lesions. Recurring cold sores around the external surface of the mouth are considered oral herpes. HSV-1 and HSV-2 infections can be distinguished only by tissue culture.

Most people have been infected with HSV-1 or HSV-2 infections. Random sampling of various populations for the presence of antibodies to the virus has estimated that 40% to 100% of the general population has been exposed at some time to the viruses.

### Pathophysiology

HSV infections are believed to be transmitted by skin-to-skin contact with an infected lesion. The virus enters the body through a break in the skin or mucous membrane, and transmission is not necessarily sexual in nature. Incubation is from 2 to 12 days. The virus enters the nervous system at the site of infection, resides in that area permanently, and can remain dormant indefinitely. An outbreak of active infection can be triggered by such things as local trauma, sunlight, emotional stress, and the presence of other debilitating diseases. Asymptomatic transmission can also occur, which causes extensive problems for prevention and control of the infection.

The initial or primary infection is usually the most severe and lasts from 7 to 21 days. An initial infection in the mouth causes severe stomatitis, but the lesions do not recur. A fluid-filled vesicle forms first, followed by shallow ulcerations. When this occurs in the genital area, itching, burning, tingling, and sometimes severe pain may be present. Edema, swollen lymph glands, and a thin, white discharge may occur. The number of lesions may vary considerably. Moist lesions heal more slowly than dry lesions. Outbreaks may recur, although they become progressively more mild and less common, and lesions last from 4 to 10 days.

### Prevention and Control

There is no cure for oral or genital herpes. Acyclovir (Zovirax), famciclovir, or valacyclovir may diminish pain and accelerate healing time. Keeping lesions dry and clean is essential. A vaccine for HSV is under study but will have little effect for those who have already been infected. Prevention of herpes focuses on the avoidance of contact with open lesions. Health care personnel should wear gloves when in contact with mucous membranes that may be infected with HSV. Using a condom during sexual activity may decrease the risk of infection.

HSV infections during pregnancy may have devastating effects on the fetus, particularly if it is an initial infection. The infection in the infant can be systemic and result in death. A cesarean section may be performed to prevent infection in the newborn when the mother has an active infection.

The emotional problems associated with a herpes infection can be severe. Guilt and despair can result when a mother unknowingly infects her infant or when a person passes the infection to a sexual partner. The social stigma of venereal disease may be very destructive. Empathy and acceptance are imperative.

◆ ◆ ◆

STDs have commonly been termed *social diseases* because of the factors in society that contribute to

---

**BOX 14-7**

### SUMMARY OF *HEALTHY PEOPLE 2000* OBJECTIVES FOR SEXUALLY TRANSMITTED DISEASES

- Confine annual incidence of diagnosed acquired immunodeficiency syndrome cases to no more than 98,000 cases.
- Confine the prevalence of human immunodeficiency virus infections to no more than 800 per 100,000 people.
- Reduce gonorrhea to an incidence of no more than 225 cases per 100,000 people; reduce repeat gonorrhea infections to no more than 15% within the previous year.
- Reduce *Chlamydia trachomatis* infections to no more than 170 cases per 100,000 people.
- Reduce primary and secondary syphilis to an incidence of no more than 10 cases per 100,000 people.
- Reduce the annual number of first-time consultations with a physician for genital herpes and genital warts to 142,000 and 385,000, respectively.
- Reduce sexually transmitted hepatitis B infections to no more than 30,500 cases

---

**BOX 14-8**

### PATIENT/FAMILY EDUCATION GUIDE FOR PREVENTION OF SEXUALLY TRANSMITTED DISEASES

- Reduce the number of sexual partners, preferably to one person.
- Avoid sexual contact with people who have multiple partners or other high-risk behaviors, such as drug abuse.
- Know partner's present and past sexual activities.
- Avoid sexual contact with individuals known to be infected.
- Examine genital areas for sores, rashes, or pus before having sex, and avoid sexual contact if these signs are present.
- Use a water-based lubricant.
- Use latex condoms whenever having sex.
- Wash hands and genital area before and after sex.
- Use mouthwash or gargle with hydrogen peroxide or an antiseptic to reduce the risk of oropharyngeal infection.
- Urinate after intercourse.
- Avoid excessive douching.
- Seek medical help whenever there is any suspicion of a sexually transmitted disease, and have periodic examinations.

---

their existence, including poverty, poor housing, low income, ignorance, and in more recent times the high mobility of people, increased alcohol consumption, ease of treatment, and a change in value systems. All these factors contribute to the incidence of STDs.

Prevention and control continues to be a major health focus. *Healthy People 2000* has created a list of objectives (Box 14-7). Preventive measures include educational programs, especially in schools, on general health, sex education, and preparation for marriage (Box 14-8).

Some states require premarital and prenatal examinations, including blood serology. Discouraging sexual promiscuity and teaching methods of personal prophylaxis will help protect members of the community. Facilities for early diagnosis and treatment should be available in all communities.

## EMERGING INFECTIONS

The CDC maintains an ongoing surveillance system for the detection of emerging infectious diseases. *Emerging infectious diseases* refers to those infectious diseases that have an incidence in humans that has increased within the past two decades or threatens to in-

crease in the near future. These diseases may be new, previously unrecognized, reemerging, or those that have developed a resistance to previously effective antimicrobial drugs. Several of these diseases are posing an increasing threat to public health. Strains of *Escherichia coli, Streptococcus,* and Hantavirus are examples (CDC, 1994).

### *Escherichia coli*

An outbreak of a specific strain of *E. coli* found in contaminated meat affected more than 500 people in four western states and resulted in 56 cases of hemolytic uremic syndrome and four deaths. It is believed that the prevalence of this infection is much higher. It is recommended that this infection be made reportable by all states and territories.

### Streptococcal Diseases

The prevalence of *S. pneumoniae* (pneumococcus) strains that are highly resistant to penicillin has increased significantly in recent years. This organism is the agent for much of the community-acquired pneumonia, particularly in the elderly. The CDC and other organizations are developing recommendations for the surveillance of these infections along with optimal treatment regimens. Surveillance for group A streptococcal disease is also being expanded. This organism is responsible for invasive diseases such as TSS and necrotizing fasciitis. The incidence of these diseases appears to be increasing, particularly in the very young and the elderly.

## Hantavirus Pulmonary Syndrome

Hantavirus pulmonary syndrome (HPS) is a newly recognized illness that is characterized by influenza-like symptoms followed by an acute onset of respiratory failure. It was first identified in the southwestern United States in 1993 following a cluster of unexplained deaths. A new Hantavirus was found to reside primarily in the deer mouse, and contact with mouse excreta has produced illness in humans. It has now been found in 20 states and has a case fatality rate of 53%.

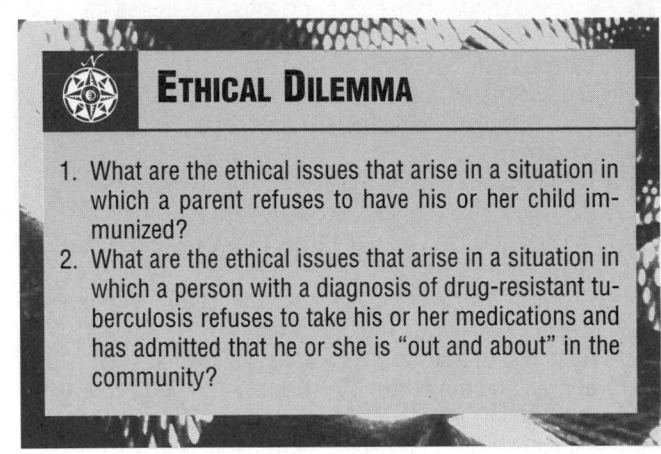

**ETHICAL DILEMMA**

1. What are the ethical issues that arise in a situation in which a parent refuses to have his or her child immunized?
2. What are the ethical issues that arise in a situation in which a person with a diagnosis of drug-resistant tuberculosis refuses to take his or her medications and has admitted that he or she is "out and about" in the community?

## NURSING CARE PLAN
## PATIENT WITH A COMMUNITY-ACQUIRED INFECTION

Mrs. Johnson is an 84-year-old woman who lives independently in a senior citizen housing project. She tends to avoid physician visits and does not believe in immunizations. She refuses the influenza vaccine each year on the basis that she is allergic to eggs because she suffers from diarrhea when she drinks eggnog. Until one week ago, Mrs. Johnson was alert, oriented, continent, and able to enjoy social activities with her friends and family.

One week ago her son noticed that she was increasingly lethargic, spent more time in bed, and had occasional urinary incontinence. Her appetite was markedly decreased. Mrs. Johnson stated that she felt very weak but had no complaints of pain or shortness of breath. Her son took her to see her physician who, after physical examination, diagnosed her as having pneumonia, probably caused by *Streptococcus pneumoniae.*

| Medical History | Psychosocial Data | Assessment Data |
|---|---|---|
| Cerebrovascular accident 9 years ago with resultant left hemiparesis | Parents deceased of unknown causes | Height 5′ 1″, weight 110 lb |
| Osteoporosis with loss of height | Two sons both healthy | Quiet, withdrawn, drowsy |
| Decreased vital capacity related to vertebral shortening | Lives in small apartment and manages well with the assistance of her son, who lives nearby and visits her 3 to 4 times a week | *Skin:* Intact, overall coloring is very pale |
| | | *Respiratory:* Diminished breath sounds bilaterally; crackles in the right lower lobe; rate 22-26, slightly shallow, symmetrical; infrequent, dry, nonproductive cough |
| | | *Cardiovascular:* Apical pulse 90 and regular; strong peripheral pulses |

## NURSING CARE PLAN

### PATIENT WITH A COMMUNITY-ACQUIRED INFECTION—cont'd

| Medical History | Psychosocial Data | Assessment Data |
|---|---|---|
| Hypertension | Eats one meal a day in a communal dining room and attends many social activities sponsored by the housing project; approximately 300 other residents live in the building and 50 to 75 residents typically congregate for social events | *Abdominal:* Soft, nontender, nondistended abdomen; normoactive bowel sounds<br>*Musculoskeletal:* Full range of motion right side; weakened active ROM left side; full passive ROM left side; ambulates with quad cane; gait slightly unsteady<br>**Laboratory data**<br>WBC 18,000<br>*Sputum:* Unable to obtain<br>*Urinalysis:* Within normal limits<br>*Chest x-ray:* Consistent with right lower lobe pneumonia<br>**Medications**<br>furosemide (Lasix) 40 mg qd<br>amoxicillin 500 mg tid |

### NURSING DIAGNOSIS

Ineffective airway clearance related to secretions, advanced age, decreased vital capacity as evidenced by increased respiratory rate, crackles in the right lower lobe, nonproductive cough

| NURSING INTERVENTIONS | EVALUATION OF EXPECTED OUTCOMES |
|---|---|
| Teach proper self-administration of antibiotic.<br>Encourage liberal fluid intake, adequate nutrition, and frequent rest periods and explain rationale.<br>Encourage use of humidifier in home.<br>Encourage visits from family to ensure ability to take medication, to take adequate fluid and diet, and to monitor for improvement in status.<br>Instruct patient and family to contact physician in 2 days if condition does not improve. | No evidence of respiratory distress<br>Respirations <24/min<br>No dyspnea<br>Able to consume previous dietary intake and adequate fluid intake<br>Energy and activity restored to level before illness |

### NURSING DIAGNOSIS

Risk for injury related to weakness, acute illness, advanced age, and hemiparesis

| NURSING INTERVENTIONS | EVALUATION OF EXPECTED OUTCOMES |
|---|---|
| Identify effects of illness on ability to perform self-care activities.<br>Assess ability to care for self independently.<br>Explore possibility of family staying with patient until acute aspect of illness is resolved.<br>Encourage provision of safe environment (e.g., use of quad cane, removal of throw rugs). | Patient/family able to identify potential for injury<br>Safe environment<br>Patient/family comfortable with assistance required during acute illness<br>Recuperates from illness without further injury |

*Continued*

---

## NURSING CARE PLAN

### PATIENT WITH A COMMUNITY-ACQUIRED INFECTION—cont'd

**NURSING DIAGNOSIS**
Knowledge deficit related to acute illness and possible preventive measures

| NURSING INTERVENTIONS | EVALUATION OF EXPECTED OUTCOMES |
|---|---|
| Explain the rationale for rest, increased fluids, and adequate nutrition during recuperation. | Verbalizes understanding of disease prevention and treatment |
| Teach the action, dosage, and side effects of antibiotic. | Verbalizes reportable symptoms |
| Discuss preventive strategies to avoid recurrence; discuss the importance of seeking early medical attention for subtle changes that may signify onset of pneumonia or worsening of condition. | Verbalizes understanding of influenza vaccine |
| Reeducate patient regarding the influenza vaccine and pneumococcal vaccine. | |
| Teach patient to avoid persons with coughs and colds during flu season. | |

---

## KEY CONCEPTS

➤ Infectious diseases result from a complex interaction among the agent, the host, and the environment.

➤ Properties of infectious agents that are influenced by characteristics of the host and the environment include infectivity, pathogenicity, virulence, and immunogenicity.

➤ Transmission of infectious agents occurs through contact, airborne, vehicle, and vectorborne routes.

➤ Immunizations with vaccines or toxoids produce artificially acquired active immunity.

➤ Routine vaccination of infants and children include immunizations for diphtheria, tetanus, pertussis, polio, measles, mumps, rubella, *Haemophilus influenzae* type B, and hepatitis B.

➤ *Healthy People 2000* is a visionary agenda to increase the span of healthy life and to reduce health disparities for the American people.

➤ The nurse's role in prevention is multifaceted and includes primary, secondary, and tertiary prevention strategies.

➤ Common bacterial infections include staphylococcal and streptococcal infections, tuberculosis, and Lyme disease.

➤ Meningococcal infections, legionellosis, and clostridium infections are less prevalent but serious conditions.

➤ Food intoxications and infections are prevalent but are often not diagnosed.

➤ Measles, mumps, rubella, and chickenpox are viral infections that have a relatively low incidence in the United States.

➤ Infectious mononucleosis, influenza, and hepatitis B are viral infections and are found worldwide.

➤ With the exception of pinworms, helminthic infestations are not common in the United States.

➤ Six sexually transmitted diseases are reportable to public health authorities: acquired immunodeficiency syndrome, syphilis, gonorrhea, chancroid, lymphogranuloma venereum, and granuloma inguinale.

➤ Emerging community-acquired infections include strains of *Escherichia coli*, resistant strains of *Streptococcus pneumoniae*, invasive group A streptococcal infections, and the Hantavirus.

## CRITICAL THINKING EXERCISES

1. What sociologic factors contribute to the spread of infectious disease?
2. Why is it a mistake to wait until a child begins school before having him or her immunized?
3. What is the danger of making pets of wild animals?
4. Why are sexually transmitted diseases the most difficult to prevent and control?
5. What social factors are contributing to the emergence of new and resistant strains of microorganisms?

## REFERENCES AND ADDITIONAL READINGS

Alder MB et al: Health promotion and disease prevention for the international traveler, *Nurse Pract* 16(5):10, 12-14, 16-18, 1991.

American Thoracic Society: Control of tuberculosis in the United States, *Am Rev Resp Dis* 146(6):1623-1633, 1992.

Beneson AS: *Control of communicable diseases in man,* ed 15, Washington, DC, 1990, American Public Health Association.

Bentley DW: Tuberculosis in long-term facilities, *Infect Control Hosp Epidemiol* 11(1):42-46, 1990.

Biester DJ: Childhood immunization: nursing's role and responsibility, *J Pediatr Nurs* 7(1):65-66, 1992.

Blaylock B: The aging immune system and common infections in elderly patients, *J Enter Nurs* 20(2):63-67, 1993.

Boley T et al: Herpes zoster: etiology, clinical course, and suggested management, *J Am Acad Nurse Pract* 2(2):64-68, 1990.

Boskovich SJ: New concepts in nursing management of the TB patient: a community training program, *J Community Health Nurs* 11(1):45-49, 1994.

Burgess W: The great white plague and other epidemics: lessons from early visiting nursing, *J Home Health Care Pract* 6(1):12-17, 1993.

Centers for Disease Control and Prevention: A strategic plan for the elimination of tuberculosis in the United States, *MMWR* 38(suppl S-3):1-25, 1989.

Centers for Disease Control and Prevention: Summary of notifiable diseases: United States, 1996, *MMWR* 44(53):1-88, 1996.

Centers for Disease Control and Prevention: *Guidelines for preventing the transmission of mycobacterium tuberculosis in health care facilities,* 1994, Federal Register, 59, October 28, 1994.

Centers for Disease Control and Prevention: Prevention of varicella: recommendations of the Advisory Committee on Immunization Practices (ACIP), *MMWR* 45(RR-11):1, 1996.

Centers for Disease Control and Prevention: Recommended childhood immunization schedule—United States, 1997, *MMWR* 47(1):8-12, 1998.

Centers for Disease Control and Prevention: Update: trends in AIDS incidence, deaths and prevalence—United States, 1996, *MMWR* 46(8):165-173, 1997.

Committee on Infectious Diseases. *1994 Red Book Report of the Committee of Infectious Diseases,* Elk Grove Village, Ill, 1994, American Academy of Pediatrics.

Cuzzell JZ: Clues: pain, burning, and itching, *Am J Nurs* 90(7):15-16, 1990.

Czurylo KT et al: Dealing with a hidden hazard: methicillin-resistant *Staphylococcus aureus, Nursing* 21(12):68-69, 1991.

Dawkins BJ: Genital herpes simplex infections, *Prim Care* 1(17):95-113, 1990.

Embry FC: A guide through the maze of viral hepatitis, *J Home Health Care Pract* 6(1):18-26, 1993.

Falco V et al: *Legionella pneumophila:* a cause of severe community-acquired pneumonia, *Chest* 100(4):1007-1011, 1991.

Ferreing N: Sexually transmitted *Chlamydia trachomatis, Nurse Pract Forum* 7(1):40-46, 1996.

Gaffney KF et al: "Think TB": new focus for family assessment, *Pediatr Nurs* 20(1):36-38, 1994.

Glittenberg JE: Problems of global control of tuberculosis, *J Prof Nurs* 6(2):73, 1990.

Goldman DA et al: Strategies to prevent and control the emergence and spread of antimicrobial-resistant microorganisms in hospitals, *J Am Med Assoc* 275(3):234-240, 1996.

Graham JM et al: Chlamydial infections, *Prim Care* 17(1):85-93, 1990.

Gurevich I: Counseling the patient with herpes, *RN* 53(2):22-28, 1990.

Gurevich I: Varicella zoster and herpes simplex virus infections, *Heart Lung* 21(1):85-93, 1992.

Harkness GA et al: Streptococcus pyogenes outbreak in a long-term care facility, *Am J Infect Control* 209(3):142-148, 1992.

Harning AT: Stirring up trouble: food-related emergencies, *JEMS* 17(8):24-30, 79-83, 1992.

Healthy People 2000: *National health promotion and disease prevention objectives,* Washington, DC, US Government Printing Office, 1991, Pub No (PHS) 91-50213, Department of Health and Human Services.

Hudacek SS: Lyme disease: facts & essential assessments, *Adv Clin Care* 5(4):6-9, 1990.

Igoe JB et al: Meeting the challenge of immunizing the nation's children, *Pediatr Nurs* 17(6):583-585, 1991.

Ismeurt RL et al: Tuberculosis: a new threat from an old nemesis, *Home Health Nurse* 11(4):16-23, 1993.

Kamper C: Treatment of Rocky Mountain spotted fever, *J Pediatr Health Care* 5(4):216-222, 1991.

Lippman H: Taking the fight to the streets, *RN* 56(9):34-39, 1993.

Lisanti P et al: An overview of viral hepatitis: A through E, *AORN J* 59(5):997-998, 1000-1005, 1994.

Long CO et al: The tuberculin skin test, *Home Health Nurse* 11(3):13-18, 1993.

Mason JO: Food irradiation—promising technology for public health, *Public Health Rep* 107(5):489-490, 1992.

Melvin SY: Syphilis: resurgence of an old disease, *Prim Care* 17(1):47-57, 1990.

Nettina SL: Syphilis: a new look at an old killer, *Am J Nurs* 90(4):68-70, 1990.

Nettina SL et al: Diagnosis and management of sexually transmitted genital lesions, *Nurse Pract* 15(1):20, 1990.

Noble RC: Sequelae of sexually transmitted diseases, *Prim Care* 17(1):173-181, 1990.

Powell MA: Question and answer: infectious mononucleosis, *J Am Acad Nurse Pract* 5(2):89-91, 1993.

Rapini RP: Venereal warts, *Prim Care* 17(1):127-144, 1990.

Richards MS et al: Investigation of a staphylococcal food poisoning outbreak in a centralized school lunch program, *Public Health Rep* 108(6):24-30, 79-83, 1993.

Richardson JP: Tetanus and tetanus immunization in long-term care facilities, *Infect Control Hosp Epidemiol* 14(10): 591-594, 1993.

Robinson KR: The role of nursing in the influenza epidemic of 1918-1919, *Nurs Forum* 25(2):19-26, 1990.

Semonin-Holleran R: Taking the sting out of summer, *RN* 56(7):40-46, 1993.

Sharts-Engel NC: An overview of maternal-child infectious diseases (1976-1990), *Am J Matern Child Nurs* 16(1):58, 1991.

Swanson JM et al: Psychosocial aspects of genital herpes: a review of the literature, *Public Health Nurs* 7(2):96-104, 1990.

Walsh ML et al: Update on antimicrobial agents, *Nurs Clin North Am* 26(2):341-360, 1991.

Weingarten CT et al: Measles: again an epidemic, *Pediatr Nurs* 18(4):369-371, 1992.

White MC: Infections and infection risks in home care settings, *Infect Control Hosp Epidemiol* 13(9):535-539, 1992.

Willis D: Lyme disease, *J Neurosci Nurs* 23(4):211-219, 1991.

Yu VL: Legionnaire's disease: new understanding of community-acquired pneumonia, *Hosp Pract* 28(10A):63-67, 1993.

# CHAPTER 15

# Hospital-Acquired Infections

## CHAPTER OBJECTIVES

1 Differentiate between nosocomial and community-acquired infections.
2 Name the most common sites, hospital services, and types of organisms associated with hospital-acquired infections.
3 List the risk factors that increase a patient's susceptibility to infection.
4 Identify measures to prevent and control urinary tract infections, surgical site infections, pneumonia, and bloodstream infections.
5 Define the terms *antiseptic* and *disinfectant.*
6 Describe effective surveillance methods for hospital-associated infections.
7 Explain the two-tier system of isolation.
8 Discuss the possible emotional responses of patients with nosocomial infections.

## KEY TERMS

| | |
|---|---|
| Airborne Precautions | Droplet Precautions |
| airborne transmission | endemic |
| antiseptic | endogenous |
| bacteremia | etiologic |
| bloodstream infection | exogenous |
| colonization | fomite |
| community acquired | high risk |
| compromised host | indirect contact |
| Contact Precautions | infection |
| contact transmission | isolation |
| control | nosocomial |
| direct contact | pathogens |
| disinfection | reservoir |
| source | surveillance |
| spores | Universal Precautions |
| Standard Precautions | vector-borne transmission |
| sterilization | vehicle transmission |

## HOSPITAL INFECTIONS

Infections have always been associated with hospitalization. A **nosocomial** infection is defined as an **infection** that occurs in a hospitalized patient that was not present or incubating at the time of admission. Infections that are acquired in the hospital but that appear after discharge are also classified as nosocomial. The term *nosocomial* is derived from the Greek word *nosos* (illness or disease) and *komeo* (to take care of). One of the first private hospitals in ancient Greece was called a nosocomium.

In contrast to nosocomial infections, **community-acquired** infections are known or incubating infections already present in patients who enter the hospital. In these cases the symptoms of infection may be apparent or may appear during hospitalization. Any infection, whether hospital acquired or community acquired, may be spread to other susceptible individuals.

The hospital is an environment contaminated by patients, visitors, and hospital personnel. People admitted to hospitals are exposed to a wide variety and a higher concentration of microbial organisms. A **reservoir** is the location where an infection-causing microorganism is usually found. Patients, health care personnel, health care equipment, and the environment are reservoirs that have been associated with nosocomial infections. A **source** is the location from which the organism is transmitted to a host. The reservoir and the source may be the same location, such as an infected wound, or the source may be a piece of equipment that becomes contaminated and subsequently comes into contact with a susceptible host. In human beings, portals of exit for infectious agents include the respiratory, gastrointestinal (GI), and genitourinary (GU) tracts. Skin, wounds, and blood also can serve as portals of exit.

All people, as well as the environment, are colonized with a multitude of microorganisms. Human beings live in harmony with a family of microorganisms referred to as normal flora. However, when these normal flora invade a body part in which they are not "normal," an infection may occur. For example, a serious **bloodstream infection** may occur if *Staphylococcus epidermidis*, a component of the normal skin flora, invades the vascular system by way of a intravenous (IV) catheter. Patients often are exposed to new organisms that are peculiar to the hospital environment and that have developed increased virulence and drug resistance. Methicillin-resistant *Staphylococcus aureus* (MRSA), aminoglycoside-resistant gram-negative organisms, penicillin-resistant pneumococci and, most recently, vancomycin-resistant enterococci (VRE) and multiple drug–resistant tuberculosis (MDRTB) are examples of such organisms. Illness decreases the body's resistance and therefore increases the patient's susceptibility to infection.

Diagnostic and treatment techniques also may weaken or bypass normal defense barriers and place patients at **high risk** for nosocomial infections. Medical-surgical supplies and equipment may become contaminated during use. Ventilators, respiratory therapy equipment, pressure monitoring devices, IV catheters, and urinary catheters are examples of equipment that bypass normal body defenses and that can become a source of infection. Even prepackaged sterile supplies designed to protect the patient can become contaminated and serve as a source of nosocomial infection.

## Incidence of Nosocomial Infections

In 1969 the Centers for Disease Control and Prevention, commonly known as the CDC, initiated the National Nosocomial Infections Study (NNIS) to gather ongoing data from a variety of hospitals in the United States. Their statistics indicated that when all infections from all types of hospitals were considered, there were approximately 3.4 nosocomial infections per 100 discharged patients, or an infection rate of 3.4%. Infection rates appear to be associated with the type of facility and the type of service offered. Large teaching hospitals have the highest reported incidence of nosocomial infections, and small, nonteaching hospitals have the lowest. It has been suggested that the latter finding is partly a result of the severity of the illnesses

and the longer hospitalizations that often are factors in larger hospitals (CDC, 1986).

The Study of the Efficacy of Nosocomial Infection Control (SENIC) was a large-scale study conducted by the CDC in 1975 and 1976. A statistical sample of all U.S. hospitals was used. The national nosocomial infection rate was determined to be 5.7 nosocomial infections per 100 admissions (Haley et al, 1981).

Before 1986 NNIS calculated and reported infection rates by service, using hospital admissions, discharges, or patient-days as a denominator. However, these rates did not adjust for specific infection risks and, therefore, were not appropriate for interhospital comparison. Therefore in October, 1986, the CDC added three components to the NNIS database:

1. Adult and pediatric intensive care unit (ICU) surveillance, in which site-specific infection rates are calculated using as a denominator the total number of patient-days and the number of device-days for indwelling urinary catheters, central vascular devices, and ventilators. Table 15-1 summarizes data from January 1992 to April 1996.
2. High-risk nursery (HRN) surveillance, in which the site-specific infection rates are divided into four birth weight categories.
3. Surgical site surveillance, in which infection rates are reported by specific surgical procedure categories, which in turn are risk stratified by wound class, anesthesia score, and duration of the surgical procedure.

These risk-stratified rates of nosocomial infection are more appropriate for interhospital comparisons than are the rates based only on admissions, discharges, or patient-days (CDC, 1996).

## High-Risk Patients

Nosocomial infections can be classified as either exogenous or endogenous. **Exogenous** infections are ac-

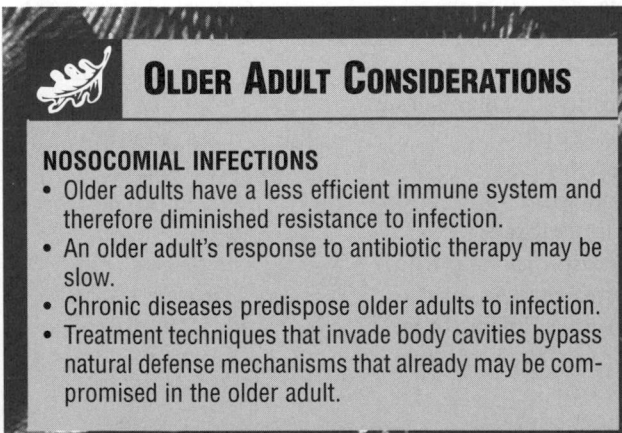

**OLDER ADULT CONSIDERATIONS**

**NOSOCOMIAL INFECTIONS**
- Older adults have a less efficient immune system and therefore diminished resistance to infection.
- An older adult's response to antibiotic therapy may be slow.
- Chronic diseases predispose older adults to infection.
- Treatment techniques that invade body cavities bypass natural defense mechanisms that already may be compromised in the older adult.

**TABLE 15-1**

## Intensive Care Unit Surveillance Component. Pooled Means and Percentiles of the Distribution of Device-Associated Infection Rates, by Type of ICU, NNIS System, January 1992–April 1996

### Urinary Catheter–Associated UTI Rate*

| TYPE OF ICU | NO. OF UNITS | URINARY CATHETER DAYS | POOLED MEAN | PERCENTILE 10% | 25% | 50% (MEDIAN) | 75% | 90% |
|---|---|---|---|---|---|---|---|---|
| Coronary | 100 | 246,232 | 7.1 | 1.1 | 3.6 | 6.3 | 10.6 | 14.0 |
| Medical | 107 | 468,394 | 8.0 | 2.2 | 4.8 | 7.4 | 9.7 | 12.7 |
| Medical/surgical | 188 | 944,202 | 5.4 | 1.3 | 3.0 | 5.1 | 7.5 | 10.1 |
| Neurosurgical | 40 | 126,060 | 8.5 | 1.7 | 5.0 | 8.0 | 10.4 | 14.9 |
| Pediatric | 55 | 119,917 | 5.3 | 1.0 | 3.1 | 5.1 | 8.0 | 12.1 |
| Surgical | 163 | 908,414 | 5.3 | 0.7 | 2.4 | 4.4 | 6.7 | 9.2 |
| Burn | 14 | 17,191 | 10.5 | — | — | — | — | — |
| Respiratory | 6 | 16,844 | 7.1 | — | — | — | — | — |
| Trauma | 16 | 91,879 | 8.3 | — | — | — | — | — |

### Central Line–Associated BSI Rate**

| TYPE OF ICU | NO. OF UNITS | CENTRAL LINE DAYS | POOLED MEAN | PERCENTILE 10% | 25% | 50% (MEDIAN) | 75% | 90% |
|---|---|---|---|---|---|---|---|---|
| Coronary | 98 | 154,300 | 5.0 | 0.0 | 1.4 | 4.3 | 6.7 | 10.3 |
| Medical | 107 | 340,172 | 6.1 | 1.7 | 3.4 | 5.3 | 7.3 | 12.1 |
| Medical/surgical | 186 | 600,367 | 4.5 | 0.0 | 2.2 | 4.5 | 6.3 | 8.2 |
| Neurosurgical | 39 | 67,590 | 5.7 | 0.0 | 2.3 | 4.4 | 8.2 | 9.9 |
| Pediatric | 56 | 168,960 | 8.1 | 1.3 | 5.0 | 7.5 | 10.0 | 13.7 |
| Surgical | 163 | 766,964 | 4.9 | 0.8 | 2.0 | 3.7 | 6.5 | 9.2 |
| Burn | 14 | 12,934 | 14.6 | — | — | — | — | — |
| Respiratory | 6 | 7,661 | 4.6 | — | — | — | — | — |
| Trauma | 16 | 68,729 | 7.2 | — | — | — | — | — |

### Ventilator-Associated Pneumonia Rate***

| TYPE OF ICU | NO. OF UNITS | VENTILATOR DAYS | POOLED MEAN | PERCENTILE 10% | 25% | 50% (MEDIAN) | 75% | 90% |
|---|---|---|---|---|---|---|---|---|
| Coronary | 94 | 102,220 | 10.2 | 0.0 | 3.5 | 8.1 | 12.9 | 19.1 |
| Medical | 105 | 320,163 | 8.9 | 1.6 | 4.5 | 7.7 | 11.7 | 17.6 |
| Medical/surgical | 185 | 475,628 | 11.8 | 3.6 | 6.8 | 10.9 | 14.5 | 18.3 |
| Neurosurgical | 39 | 59,316 | 18.3 | 2.6 | 9.5 | 14.3 | 21.1 | 30.2 |
| Pediatric | 56 | 177,718 | 5.8 | 0.0 | 1.3 | 5.0 | 7.4 | 10.7 |
| Surgical | 163 | 500,412 | 14.5 | 4.2 | 7.6 | 12.7 | 17.9 | 23.8 |
| Burn | 14 | 10,041 | 24.1 | — | — | — | — | — |
| Respiratory | 6 | 14,877 | 6.7 | — | — | — | — | — |
| Trauma | 16 | 60,481 | 17.2 | — | — | — | — | — |

From National Nosocomial Infections Surveillance (NNIS) report, data summary from October 1986-April 1997, issued May 1997: a report from the NNIS System, *Am J Infect Control* 25(6):477-487, 1997.

* $\dfrac{\text{Number of urinary catheter-associated UTIs}}{\text{Number of urinary catheter days}} \times 1000$

** $\dfrac{\text{Number of central line-associated BSIs}}{\text{Number of central line days}} \times 1000$

*** $\dfrac{\text{Number of ventilator-associated pneumonias}}{\text{Number of ventilator days}} \times 1000$

quired from sources outside the patient; **endogenous** infections result when circumstances enable the host's normal but potentially virulent flora to multiply, causing a pathologic condition. Endogenous infections occur when the host's normal defense mechanisms are deficient or compromised. A person with deficient defense mechanisms is known as a **compromised host.**

Many underlying host factors determine whether a person develops an infection. Age and underlying disease are two of the most important determinants. Newborn infants, especially those of low birth weight, have immature immune systems and therefore have fewer physical resources for combating infectious microorganisms. The elderly have less efficient immune systems and thus their resistance to infection is diminished. Chronic diseases, such as renal failure, diabetes, or cancer, and conditions such as burns, malnutrition, or shock all can predispose a patient to infection. Treatment measures that invade body cavities bypass natural defense mechanisms and create a direct route for microorganisms to gain entrance to body organs and

cause infection (Box 15-1). Urinary catheterization, IV infusions, peritoneal dialysis, and surgical incisions of the skin are examples of treatment interventions that can allow microbial access. Ionizing radiation and immunosuppressive drug therapy can depress the immune response and place the patient at high risk for infection. The extensive use of antibiotics also may be responsible for the decline in host resistance and the development of more virulent and resistant strains of organisms.

## Methods of Transmission

Microorganisms are transmitted by various routes, and a single microorganism may be transmitted by more than one route. For example, the varicella-zoster virus (chickenpox) can spread by the airborne route and by direct contact. Organisms are transmitted to a susceptible host by four main routes: contact transmission, airborne transmission, vehicle transmission, and vector-borne transmission.

**Contact transmission** is the most common method by which microorganisms are transmitted from one person to another. Contact transmission can be divided into three subgroups: direct contact, indirect contact, and droplet contact. **Direct contact** involves person-to-person contact between the source and the susceptible individual. Contact occurs constantly during daily patient care, with hands having the most contact with the patient; therefore thorough hand washing, even when gloves have been worn, is the best means of preventing transmission by direct contact. **Indirect contact** involves personal contact of the susceptible host with a contaminated intermediate object, or **fomite**. For example, an inadequately disinfected endoscope can indirectly transfer organisms. Droplet contact occurs when an infectious agent passes briefly through the air. The infected sources and susceptible host usually are within a few feet of each other. This is considered contact, rather than airborne, transmission because droplets usually travel no more than approximately 1 m (about 3 feet). Organisms usually are dispersed when an infected person coughs, sneezes, or talks and during the performance of certain procedures, such as suctioning.

**Airborne transmission** occurs when infectious agents remain suspended in the air for long periods. Organisms carried in this manner can be widely dispersed by air currents before they are inhaled by or deposited on the susceptible host. Tuberculosis (TB) is transmitted by this route. Good ventilation systems help prevent airborne transmission of infectious agents.

**Vehicle transmission** occurs when contaminated items such as blood, blood products, food, water, or drugs serve as the vector of transmission to several individuals. Examples of this type of transmission are

---

**BOX 15-1**

## FACTORS THAT COMPROMISE A HOST

### DISEASE OR DISORDER
Burns
Chronic disease
Circulatory impairment
Cirrhosis
Diabetes mellitus
Extensive dermatitis
Hepatitis
Immune deficiencies
Malignancies
Malnutrition
Open wounds
Persons receiving immunosuppressant drugs
Renal failure
Shock
Transplant recipient
Trauma

### THERAPEUTIC TECHNIQUES
Bladder catheterization
Central nervous system shunts
Decubitus care
Hyperalimentation
Immunosuppressive therapy
Intravenous cannulation
Radiation therapy
Respiratory therapy
Surgery
Tracheostomy

the spread of salmonellosis from contaminated dairy products or hepatitis A from contaminated food.

**Vector-borne transmission** occurs when insects or other animals serve as intermediate hosts for an infectious agent. For example, malaria is transmitted by mosquitoes, and Rocky Mountain spotted fever is transmitted by ticks. Vectors have not played a significant role in the transmission of nosocomial infections in the United States.

# TYPES OF NOSOCOMIAL INFECTIONS

## Urinary Tract Infections

Urinary tract infections (UTIs) are the most common nosocomial infections found in hospitalized patients, and most nosocomial UTIs are associated with urinary tract manipulation (Mayhall, 1996). Nosocomial UTIs account for 40% of hospital-acquired infections. Annual costs exceeding $1.8 billion have been attributed to UTIs (Burke, 1993). Catheter-associated UTIs are caused by a variety of pathogens, including *Escherichia coli*, enterococci, *Pseudomonas aeruginosa*, *Klebsiella pneumoniae*, *Candida albicans*, and *Enterobacter* species (CDC, 1996). Many of these microorganisms are part of the patient's endogenous bowel flora, but they also can be acquired by cross-contamination from other patients, the hands of hospital personnel, contaminated solutions, or contaminated equipment (see Table 15-1).

Host factors that appear to increase a person's susceptibility to catheter-associated UTIs include debilitation, chronic disease, and the presence of pathogenic bacteria in the periurethral area. Women and the elderly have higher rates of such infections. Although most UTIs are of low morbidity and mortality, infections occasionally can lead to such complications as prostatitis, epididymitis, cystitis, pyelonephritis, and **bacteremia**.

Infecting microorganisms gain access by several routes. Microorganisms that colonize in the meatus or distal urethra can be introduced directly into the bladder when the catheter is inserted. Infecting microorganisms also can migrate to the bladder along the outside of the catheter and the periurethral mucous sheath or along the internal lumen of the catheter after the collection bag or catheter drainage tube junction has been contaminated.

Nursing measures that can prevent or control urinary catheter–associated infections involve optimal catheter care for patients who require indwelling catheterization. The most direct way to prevent catheter-associated bacteriuria is to avoid catheterization. Urinary catheters should be inserted only when necessary and should be left in place only as long as necessary. Indications for an indwelling catheter include relief of urinary obstruction, a neurogenic bladder, and a need for accurate measurement of output. Aseptic technique and sterile equipment must be used when inserting a catheter. Routine use of indwelling catheters for incontinence is not appropriate unless massive skin breakdown is a concern (Box 15-2).

---

| BOX 15-2 | NURSING PROCESS |
| --- | --- |

### URINARY TRACT INFECTION (UTI)

**ASSESSMENT**

- Frequency, urgency, burning on urination
- Fever and chills
- History of previous infections
- Urine culture results
- Presence of occult blood

**NURSING DIAGNOSES**

- Altered urinary elimination related to urinary tract infection
- Pain related to inflammation
- Knowledge deficit related to causes of urinary tract infection and prevention measures

**NURSING INTERVENTIONS**

- Remove the indwelling urinary catheter as soon as possible.

- Use aseptic technique for inserting or manipulating the urinary catheter.
- Maintain an unobstructed urinary flow.
- If ordered, give antibiotic therapy on schedule until course of treatment has been completed.
- Ensure that patient gets 3-4 L of fluids per day if possible.
- Teach the patient to recognize the signs and symptoms of UTI.

**EVALUATION OF EXPECTED OUTCOMES**

- No indication of infection seen in urine bacteria count
- States that urinary symptoms have been relieved
- Correctly describes the signs and symptoms of UTI, the risk factors, the rationale for increasing fluids, the routine for taking medications, and the need for follow-up care

Once a urethral catheter is in place, UTIs are best avoided by maintaining a closed system and by minimizing the duration of catheterization. Urine specimens should be obtained without opening the catheter collection tube junction. Special ports in the system allow for aseptic collection of urinary specimens. These ports should be cleansed with a disinfectant before a sterile needle and syringe are used to aspirate the urine.

Urinary flow should be unobstructed. The catheter and collecting tubing should be free of kinking, and the collecting bag should be emptied regularly, with a separate collecting container used for each patient. Nosocomial transmission has occurred between patients when contaminated urine-collecting devices have been used for more than one patient. Routine changing of indwelling catheters, continuous irrigation of the bladder, and application of antimicrobial ointment to the urethral meatus have not been shown to prevent nosocomial UTIs (Batt, Galaviz, 1996).

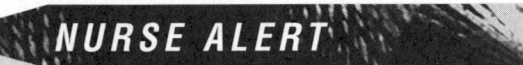

**NURSE ALERT**

UTIs can best be avoided by maintaining an undisturbed closed drainage system and by minimizing the duration of catheterization.

Hand washing is extremely important and should be done immediately before and after any manipulation of the catheter, even if gloves have been worn. It is imperative that hands be washed between handling the catheters of different patients (Box 15-3).

## Nosocomial Pneumonia

Nosocomial pneumonia is the second most common nosocomial infection, accounting for 15% of all nosocomial infections in U.S. hospitals. Nosocomial pneumonia is associated with mortality rates that range from 20% to 50% and is the most common fatal nosocomial infection (Mandell, Douglas, Bennett, 1990).

The estimated overall incidence of nosocomial pneumonia in U.S. hospitals is 0.6% of admitted patients. The disease can prolong hospitalization 4 to 9 days and result in an estimated total of $1.3 billion in extra hospital charges (Tablan, 1996). Most of these cases of pneumonia occur in ICUs or postanesthesia care units (see Table 15-1). The predominant organisms in cultures of respiratory secretions of patients with nosocomial pneumonia are *S. aureus, P. aeruginosa, Enterobacter* species, *K. pneumoniae, C. albicans,* and *Haemophilus influenzae* (CDC, 1996). In immuno-

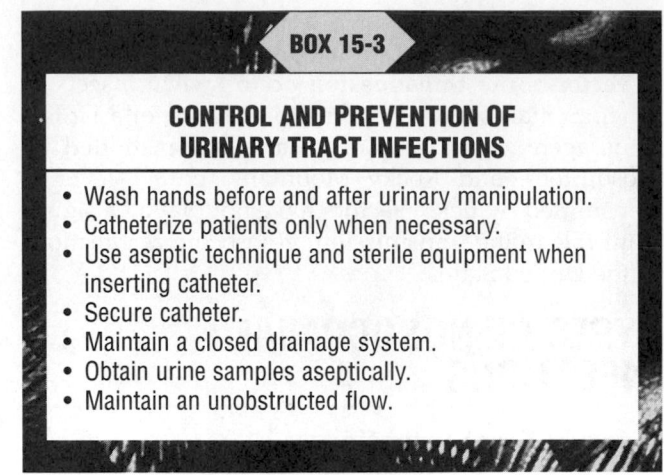

**BOX 15-3**

### CONTROL AND PREVENTION OF URINARY TRACT INFECTIONS

- Wash hands before and after urinary manipulation.
- Catheterize patients only when necessary.
- Use aseptic technique and sterile equipment when inserting catheter.
- Secure catheter.
- Maintain a closed drainage system.
- Obtain urine samples aseptically.
- Maintain an unobstructed flow.

compromised patients, *Aspergillus* and *Legionella* organisms may be **etiologic** agents (Tablan, 1996).

Some hospitals have experienced clusters of nosocomial *Legionella* pneumonia, which usually are related to environmental factors such as contamination of water or air conditioning systems.

Nosocomial lower respiratory viral infections can occur and often reflect the occurrence of a virus in the community. During community outbreaks, viruses are introduced into the hospital by patients, employees, and visitors. These viral infections may be particularly severe in high-risk, debilitated patients. Respiratory syncytial virus (RSV), parainfluenza virus, and influenza are responsible for a large proportion of cases of viral nosocomial pneumonia.

A number of factors predispose patients to hospital-acquired pneumonia. Intubation of the respiratory tract is associated with a high incidence of nosocomial pneumonia because endotracheal tubes bypass the protective defense mechanisms of the upper respiratory tract. Hospitalized patients also often have impaired host defenses as a result of clinical conditions such as chronic obstructive pulmonary disease (COPD), cystic fibrosis, leukemia, central nervous system (CNS) depression (coma), and electrolyte imbalances. These patients can become colonized with potential pathogens from their own endogenous flora or from exogenous sources, such as contaminated respiratory therapy equipment and the hands of hospital personnel. A colonized patient may become infected through aspiration of upper respiratory tract secretions.

Diagnosing nosocomial pneumonia may be difficult. A positive result on culture of respiratory tract secretions does not distinguish between oropharyngeal **colonization** and the true **pathogens** that cause pneumonia. Therefore, to make a diagnosis, the clinician must rely on a change in clinical symptoms, such as altered mental status, fever, results of chest x-ray films, cough, sputum production, and an elevated leukocyte count.

However, these clinical conditions may be found without pneumonia.

The prevention of nosocomial respiratory tract infections is based on reducing the acquisition of potential bacterial pathogens in the upper airways and thereby reducing the risk of aspiration of these organisms. Gloves should be worn during all contact with respiratory secretions. Hands should be washed after contact with respiratory secretions even if gloves have been worn. Hands must be washed before and after contact with a patient who is intubated or who has had a recent tracheostomy.

General nursing techniques such as maintaining an open airway; having the patient turn, cough, and deep breathe; and early ambulation after surgery are important interventions for preventing postoperative pneumonia. Before surgery, patients should be taught measures to reduce the risk of nosocomial pneumonia. They should be able to demonstrate and practice adequate coughing and deep breathing. It is important to control pain in a postoperative patient so that it does not interfere with coughing and deep breathing (Box 15-4).

Closely adhering to the guidelines for use of respiratory therapy equipment also reduces the incidence of nosocomial pneumonia. Only sterile fluids should be nebulized or used in a humidifier. Nebulizers (including medication nebulizers) and their reservoirs and cascade humidifiers should be changed or replaced with sterilized or disinfected equipment every 24 hours. Warm humidifiers that create droplets to humidify should not be used. Ventilator tubing once was changed routinely every 24 hours, but data now suggest that circuit changes every 48 hours or at even longer intervals do not increase the risk of nosocomial pneumonia.

Sterile technique should be used for suctioning of patients who have a tracheostomy. Because the risk of cross-contamination and excessive trauma increases with frequent suctioning, the procedure should be done with a "no touch" technique and with sterile gloves on both hands. A new, sterile catheter should be used for each series of suctioning. If the catheter must be flushed because of tenacious mucus, sterile fluid should be used to remove the secretions. Fluid used for one series of suctioning should be discarded. Many hospitals now use closed system, multiuse catheters. After the catheter is used, a sheath slides over it to protect it from environmental contamination. These catheters usually are changed every 24 hours.

Enteral feeding may increase the risk of aspiration and pneumonia. Using continuous rather than bolus feeding, maintaining and removing residua, and keeping the patient in an upright position may reduce the risk of aspiration and subsequent pneumonia.

---

**BOX 15-4**

## CONTROL AND PREVENTION OF NOSOCOMIAL PNEUMONIA

- Wear gloves for all contact with respiratory secretions.
- Wash hands after contact with respiratory secretions, even if gloves have been worn.
- Maintain open airways.
- Teach patient how to cough and deep breathe before surgery.
- Control pain.
- Follow guidelines for use of respiratory therapy equipment.
- Use sterile technique when suctioning a tracheostomy.
- Wear sterile gloves on both hands and use "no touch" technique when suctioning.
- Elevate the patient's head if he or she is receiving enteral feedings.
- Isolate patients with potentially transmissible respiratory infections.

---

Patients in intensive care units are given one of several prophylactic regimens to prevent stress bleeding. Data suggest that patients receiving sucralfate have a lower risk of pneumonia than those receiving $H_2$-blockers or antacids but have the same protection against stress bleeding.

Patients with potentially transmissible respiratory infections should be isolated from other patients according to the hospital's isolation guidelines. To prevent acquisition of nosocomial viral infections from employees, health care workers with acute respiratory infections should not be assigned to direct care of high-risk patients. In addition, all health care workers assigned to care for high-risk patients should receive an influenza vaccine annually to reduce the risk of transmission to patients.

## Surgical Site Infections

In most hospitals, surgical site infection (SSI) is the third most common type of nosocomial infection. The term *surgical site infection* has replaced surgical wound infection. For the purposes of nosocomial studies, SSIs are divided into three categories (Horan, Gaynes, Martone et al, 1992):

- *Superficial SSIs*, which involve only the skin or subcutaneous tissue.
- *Deep incisional SSIs*, which involve deep soft tissues of the incision (e.g., fascial and muscle layers).

- *Organ/space SSIs*, which involve any part of the anatomy other than the incision. This category includes deep abscesses, osteomyelitis, mediastinitis, endocarditis, and other deep infections associated with a surgical procedure.

A wound is considered infected if purulent material drains from it, even without a positive result on wound culture. Wounds are classified according to the likelihood and degree of wound contamination at the time of the operation. A widely accepted classification scheme outlined by the American College of Surgeons (1984) predicts the relative probability that a wound will become infected. The classifications are clean wounds, clean-contaminated wounds, contaminated wounds, and dirty wounds.

*Clean wounds* are those in which neither the gastrointestinal, respiratory, and genitourinary tracts nor the pharyngeal cavity has been entered and in which no inflammation is found during surgery. Clean wounds are also cases in which no breaks in aseptic technique have occurred. These wounds have a 1% to 5% risk of infection.

*Clean-contaminated wounds* are those in which the gastrointestinal, respiratory, or genitourinary tract is entered but in which significant spillage did not occur during the procedure. These wounds have a 3% to 11% risk of infection.

*Contaminated wounds* result from surgical procedures involving a major break in aseptic technique or gross spillage from a contaminated system, or in which acute inflammation without pus is encountered. Fresh traumatic wounds also fit into this category. Contaminated wounds have a 10% to 17% risk of infection.

---

**BOX 15-5**

### CONTROL AND PREVENTION OF SURGICAL SITE INFECTIONS

- Assess for infections that may need treatment before surgery.
- Instead of a razor, use a depilatory or clip hair before surgery.
- Wash hands before and after changing a surgical wound dressing.
- Maintain aseptic technique and a "no touch" technique when changing surgical wound dressings.
- Wear gloves for changing surgical dressings. Wear a gown if soiling of clothing is likely.
- Contact precautions are indicated for infected wounds with a large amount of drainage that is not contained.

---

*Dirty wounds* are old traumatic wounds or wounds with pus or a perforated viscus. The risk of infection in these wounds is over 27% (CDC, 1985) (Box 15-5).

A multivariate index for predicting the likelihood of surgical site infection was developed and tested during the SENIC study.

NNIS has developed an index for the risk of surgical site infection that includes the following elements: (1) if the patient's wound was classified as contaminated or dirty, (2) if the patient was assigned an American Society of Anesthesiology (ASA) score, and (3) the duration of the surgical incision time. Investigators believe that this index is a better indicator of patients at risk for SSI than wound class alone.

Age is one host factor that may influence the risk of infection. People over 65 years of age have twice the risk of contracting nosocomial SSIs as younger people. Obesity, severe malnutrition, infection at other sites, and extended preoperative stays in the hospital are other host factors associated with a greater risk of infection.

Gram-negative aerobic bacteria account for approximately 40% of the pathogens isolated from surgical wounds. However *S. aureus* is the species most commonly isolated from these wounds. Microorganisms that infect surgical wounds can be acquired from the patient, the hospital environment, or hospital personnel, but the patient's own flora are responsible for most infections. Sources of infection include the gastrointestinal, respiratory, genital, and urinary tracts, as well as the skin and anterior nares. Whether acquired from the environment or the patient's own flora, most infections appear to be acquired in the operating room. Few infections are acquired after surgery with primary closure of the wound. Open wounds and the presence of drains increase the risk of infection in the postoperative period.

Measures to prevent SSI actually begin before the operation. An important preoperative measure is treatment of any active infection. Shortening the patient's preoperative hospital stay also reduces the risk of infection. Historically, hair adjacent to or in the area of the proposed surgery has been removed to prevent it from contaminating the wound during the operation. However, several recent studies suggest that shaving with a razor can injure the skin and increase the risk of infection. Therefore clipping hair, using a depilatory, or not shaving at all have been suggested in place of shaving.

Before surgery, the skin at the operative site should be cleaned thoroughly with an **antiseptic** solution to remove all superficial skin flora, soil, and debris. The surgical team must scrub their hands to minimize the normal flora on their skin. The surgical scrub is designed to kill and remove as many bacteria as possible, including resident bacteria. After scrubbing their hands, the surgical team dons sterile gloves, which act as an additional barrier against the transfer of microorganisms to the surgical wound.

To reduce airborne contamination, modern operating rooms have ventilation systems that produce 20 changes of highly filtered air per hour. Some operating rooms, especially those used for orthopedic operations involving joint replacement, have installed laminar flow ventilation units.

Surgical technique is the most important measure for preventing wound infection. For example, perforation of the bowel during surgery prolongs the operation and increases the risk of postoperative infection.

Another approach to preventing SSI is use of prophylactic antimicrobial therapy. Prophylactic antibiotics are recommended for operations associated with a high risk of infection or considered severe or life-threatening. Antibiotics used for prophylaxis should be started shortly before the operation and promptly discontinued after the surgery. The area also may be irrigated with antibiotic solutions during surgery. One highly recommended preventive measure, which arose from the findings of the SENIC study, is to report the SSI rate to individual surgeons.

The postoperative period usually does not contribute greatly to the risk of surgical site infection. However, wounds can become contaminated and infected if they are not handled with aseptic technique, which is especially important if the wound is not closed completely. Wounds should be kept covered with a sterile dressing until they are sealed, which usually occurs within 24 hours after the operation. Nursing personnel can reduce the risk of SSI by washing their hands and by using a "no touch" technique when changing surgical wound dressings. If the wound becomes infected, either drainage-secretion precautions or contact isolation should be instituted.

## Nosocomial Bloodstream Infections

Nosocomial bloodstream infection (BSI) is defined as the isolation of an organism from a properly obtained blood culture specimen in a patient who has clinical signs of sepsis and who was admitted with without signs or symptoms of infection and without a positive result on blood culture. Nosocomial BSI (bacteremia) can be divided into two categories. *Primary bacteremia* occurs without any recognizable focus of infection with the same organism at another site. These infections are believed to be related to IV fluid therapy when an IV line is present. Concordant growth between cultures obtained from the catheter or insertion site exudate further confirm the presence of a intravascular device–related BSI (Mermel, 1996). *Secondary bacteremia* results from an infection at another site. This section focuses on primary nosocomial bacteremia associated with in-

travascular devices. Secondary bacteremia is reduced by giving attention to the prevention and control of infections at other body sites.

Intravascular-related BSIs arise from microbial contamination of the cannula, the cannula wound, or the intravenous solution (infusate). Most of these infections are cannula related. Factors that influence a patient's risk of acquiring cannula-related infection include the patient's susceptibility, the type of cannula used, the method of insertion, the duration of cannulation, and the purpose of the cannula. Plastic cannulas have been associated with a higher risk of infection than steel cannulas. Peripheral catheters that remain in place longer than 72 hours are associated with a marked increase in infection rates. Central cannulas, which are used for monitoring central venous pressure, are also associated with high rates of infection.

Coagulase-negative staphylococci, particularly *S. epidermidis*, have become the pathogens most frequently isolated in catheter-related bloodstream infections; they accounted for 31% of nosocomial BSIs reported to NNIS from 1990 to 1996 (CDC, 1996). Before 1986, *S. aureus* was the pathogen most often reported as the cause of nosocomial BSI. *S. aureus* currently accounts for 16% of the cases reported to NNIS. Other significant pathogens are enterococci (9%), *E. coli* (5%), *C. albicans* (5%), and *K. pneumoniae* (5%) (CDC, 1996). Infections related to microbial contamination of infusate are far less common than cannula-related infections. Contamination can occur during the manufacturing process or during hospital preparation. Infections caused by contaminated infusate usually are caused by gram-negative bacilli.

Nursing interventions are important in preventing vascular-related infections. As with other nosocomial infections, hand washing is of major importance. Hands should always be washed before inserting an IV cannula and before performing any manipulation of the cannula or line. Gloves should be worn for cannula insertion.

In adults, it is preferable to insert a cannula into the upper extremity rather than the lower one. The IV site should be scrubbed with antiseptic before venipuncture. Tincture of iodine is the antiseptic of choice in the United States; however, because iodine may irritate the skin, povidone-iodine is the antiseptic most often used for preparation of the site (Mermel, 1996). After insertion, the cannula should be secured to stabilize it at the insertion site, and a sterile dressing should be applied over the insertion site. Use of an antibiotic ointment at the insertion site is not recommended (CDC, 1996). The date of the insertion should be recorded in a place where it can be found easily. Many institutions record the date of insertion in both the medical record and on the dressing or tape at the IV site.

Patients with IV devices should be evaluated at least every 8 hours for evidence of cannula-related complications. An evaluation can be performed by palpating the insertion site through the dressing or by visually examining the site through a transparent polyurethane dressing. Pain or tenderness warrants removal of the dressing and inspection of the site. Catheter dressings should be replaced when the dressing becomes damp, loosened, or soiled. In patients who have large, bulky dressings that prevent palpation or direct visualization of the catheter insertion site, the dressing should be removed, the site inspected, and the dressing replaced every day (CDC, 1996).

Hospital policies usually require peripheral cannulas to be replaced every 48 to 72 hours. Current CDC guidelines recommend changing peripheral venous catheters every 48 to 72 hours. Catheters inserted under emergency conditions should be changed within 24 hours (CDC, 1996). A silver-impregnated, cuffed catheter and an antiseptic-impregnated catheter are now available and may be beneficial in preventing catheter-associated BSI. Any cannula that has been inserted without proper asepsis, such as in an emergency setting, should be replaced at the earliest opportunity. If purulent thrombophlebitis, cellulitis, or IV-related bacteremia is diagnosed or strongly suspected, the entire IV system should be changed. No general guidelines are available that recommend a specific interval for changing central lines, but many hospitals require routine changes as a means of reminding the physician to reassess the need for the line (Widmer, 1997). All intravascular lines should be removed as soon as they are no longer medically indicated. Insertion and removal of all intravascular lines should be documented in the patient's medical record.

IV administration tubing usually is changed every 72 hours. Tubing used for hyperalimentation sets should be changed every 24 to 48 hours. The tubing should be changed immediately after administration of blood, blood products, or lipid emulsions. Once started, all parenteral fluids should be completely used or discarded within 24 hours. When lipid emulsions are given alone, the infusion should be completed within 12 hours of the time it was started (CDC, 1996).

Nurses caring for patients with intravascular devices must always remember to follow strict aseptic technique. Although nosocomial bacteremia does not occur often, it can be life-threatening (Box 15-6).

## Other Sites of Nosocomial Infections

Although the previously discussed sites of infection account for most nosocomial infections, approximately 10% to 15% fall into the category of "other nosocomial infections." These infections include skin and subcutaneous infections, CNS infections, gastroenteritis, and endometritis. In preventing these infections, the nurse must always remember the routes of transmission, the practice of good hand washing, the use of adequate aseptic technique in all procedures, and the importance of general skin care for all hospitalized patients.

# PREVENTION AND CONTROL

The first recommendations regarding hospital-acquired infections were developed by the American Hospital Association (AHA) and published in 1958. Since that time, the Joint Commission on Accreditation of Healthcare Organizations (JCAHO), the CDC, the U.S. Department of Health and Human Services, and various state licensing laws have established standards for infection control in hospitals. The general recommendations of these organizations include (1) establishment of an active, hospital-wide infection control program; (2) establishment of a multidisciplinary committee responsible for monitoring the infection control program; (3) development of specific, written infection control policies and procedures for all services in the hospital; and (4) development of a practical system for reporting and evaluating infections among patients and personnel.

## Infection Control Committee

The primary function of the infection control committee is to establish and implement hospital policy regarding the investigation, control, and prevention of

---

**BOX 15-6**

### CONTROL AND PREVENTION OF BACTEREMIA FROM AN INTRAVENOUS DEVICE

- Wash hands before inserting an intravenous (IV) cannula and before manipulating the cannula or line.
- Wear gloves and use strict aseptic technique for cannula insertion.
- Place sterile occlusive dressings over cannula insertion sites.
- Record the date of insertion in the medical record and where it can be easily found, such as on the dressing or tape at the IV site.
- Evaluate patients with IV devices at least q 8 hr.
- Inspect and care for peripheral IV sites often.
- Pain or tenderness at the IV site requires removal of the dressing and inspection of the site.
- Change dressing when it is loose, soiled, or damp.

infections within hospitals. Standards of care must be developed that reduce the risk of hospital-associated infections among both patients and personnel. The committee is responsible for establishing mechanisms for effective surveillance of nosocomial infections, instituting control measures (e.g., isolation techniques and aseptic procedures), reviewing bacteriologic services, monitoring antibiotic therapy, providing educational programs, and establishing techniques for discovering infections that are not manifest until after the patient has been discharged.

The composition of infection control committees varies with individual hospitals. However, membership should include the hospital epidemiologist, physician representatives of the major clinical departments, the infection control practitioner, a hospital administrator, a pathologist, a nursing service representative, and representatives from other departments of the hospital as appropriate for the individual facility. A representative from the local health department often is invited to become a member. The 1995 JCAHO standards do not require an infection control committee, but most hospitals are opting to maintain the committee to ensure active, continual infection control programs (JCAHO, 1995).

## Infection Control Practitioner

The infection control practitioner is the member of the infection control team who is primarily responsible for the development, coordination, and supervision of the entire infection control program within the hospital. Most infection control practitioners are nurses, although some are medical technologists, public health professionals, or members of other allied health care disciplines. Regardless of their background, most infection control practitioners belong to the Association for Professionals in Infection Control and Epidemiology (APIC). The organization provides its members with guidance and leadership through materials and programs that include an annual educational conference, a professional journal, and published guidelines for various aspects of practice.

One function of the infection control practitioner is to collect, analyze, and report data regarding nosocomial infections; this activity is called **surveillance**. Other functions of the infection control practitioner include monitoring patient care activities, developing and updating specific prevention and control policies, participating in educational programs, conducting special studies, and collaborating with all disciplines and departments in the facility. Probably the most important attributes of an effective infection control practitioner are an understanding of human nature and the ability to develop effective interpersonal relationships.

The APIC and CDC have recommended a ratio of one infection control practitioner for every 250 beds in an acute care facility and one for every 500 beds in a long-term health care facility.

## Surveillance

The purpose of a surveillance program is to detect, record, and report hospital-associated infections in a systematic fashion so that effective, practical control measures can be instituted. In the past, surveillance centered on reports from the bacteriology laboratory and observations made by nursing personnel or house staff, whose time was devoted primarily to the care of patients. As a result, underreporting of nosocomial infection was a serious problem. Because no single surveillance system provides complete information on the occurrence of hospital-associated infections, a combination of techniques appropriate for the individual institution are used.

Laboratory reports remain an important source of information. Urine, chemistry, culture, and postmortem reports are checked. The criteria for identifying nosocomial infections at various body sites must be established by the infection control committee. The patient's medical record is reviewed to determine if a nosocomial infection is present. Radiology report summaries, especially those involving the respiratory and GI tracts, may provide evidence of infection. If the surveillance system includes identification of all community-acquired infections for control purposes, patients admitted with known infections or suggestive symptoms should be investigated.

Most of the data can be gathered through daily rounds on patient units. The nursing staff, physicians, and others often offer information that can provide clues to possible nosocomial infections or identify possible sources of infection. Observing individual patient nursing care plans may provide clues as to whether a patient may be at high risk of developing a nosocomial infection. Patients who have one of the risk factors are noted, and their charts are reviewed.

Two areas often neglected when surveying for nosocomial infections are infections that appear in hospital personnel and those that appear in discharged patients. Physicians should be encouraged to notify the infection control practitioner when infections develop after a patient has been discharged from the hospital. Employees with infections such as open or draining skin infections or enteric disease should not be allowed to handle food, equipment, or other objects that come in direct contact with patients, and they should not be allowed to participate in patient care. Nosocomial infections in health care personnel should be monitored.

Knowing the usual prevalence, or **endemic** rate, of infection in a hospital allows the infection control practitioner to identify areas that require investigation, to institute more specific control measures, or to detect epidemics, should they occur. Surveillance information also can be used for educating staff members, evaluating new control measures, or establishing goals to reduce nosocomial infections.

Not all hospital-associated infections can be prevented. The patient's underlying disease, condition, or therapy may increase his or her vulnerability to both exogenous and endogenous microorganisms. Hospitals with well-developed surveillance systems have demonstrated that after an initial reduction of nosocomial infection rates (presumably as a result of the impact of surveillance activities), a relatively stable endemic level of infection remains.

## Preventive Policies and Procedures

The best basic way to prevent and control infectious diseases is to use general sanitary practices and aseptic techniques. *Prevention* refers to the elimination of the occurrence of an infectious process, whereas **control** pertains to restricting the spread of an infectious process. The single most important technique in both prevention and control is proper hand washing.

## Hand Washing

Every person has a relatively stable, resident bacteria population on the skin. New bacteria may be added and, unless removed, may become part of the resident populations and be spread to other people. Nurses constantly come in contact with contaminated equipment and material. In providing nursing care, they often move from patient to patient and may unconsciously transfer pathogenic organisms from one patient to another and even endanger their own health. The safest way for nurses to protect themselves and their patients is thorough, careful hand washing.

Ideal facilities for proper hand washing include a sink with knee, foot, or sensor controls; hot and cold running water; soap; and paper towels. Antiseptic agents should be used for hand washing when the nurse is participating in an invasive procedure. The hands should be washed between all patient contacts, even if gloves have been worn (Figure 15-1). Soap, running water, friction, and time are the essential factors in good hand washing procedure. The fingernails and the areas between the fingers should be given special attention. Hands should be thoroughly rinsed and kept in a downward position to prevent water from running up the arms, draining back again, and con-

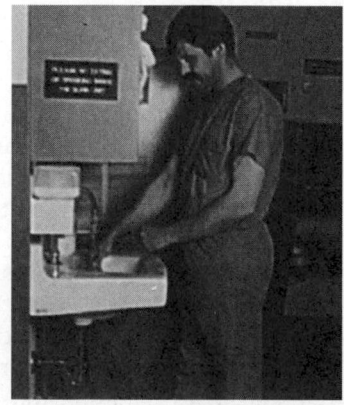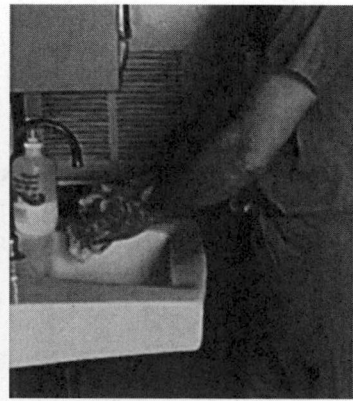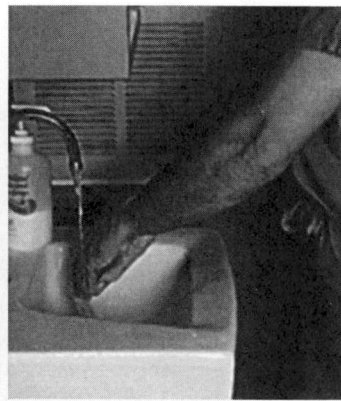

**Figure 15-1**   Good hand washing procedure involves a combination of soap, running water, friction, and time. Note that the hands are kept in a downward position until dried. (From Perry AG, Potter PA: *Clinical nursing skills and techniques*, ed 3, St Louis, 1994, Mosby.)

taminating the hands. The hands should be thoroughly dried, and a dry paper towel should be used to turn off the faucets to prevent recontamination of the hands. The times when hand washing should be performed are listed in Box 15-7. Failure of hospital personnel to wash their hands is a common cause of hospital-acquired infections.

## Sterilization and Disinfection

Sterilization and disinfection procedures are crucial to prevention of nosocomial infections. Inanimate objects used in patient care must be sterilized or disinfected between patients. **Sterilization** is the complete elimination or destruction of all microbial life, including large numbers of bacterial **spores**. Sterilization is accomplished by means of steam under pressure (autoclave), ethylene oxide (gas), dry heat, or liquid chemicals. **Disinfection** eliminates many or all pathogenic organisms except for bacterial spores. Liquid chemicals are used for disinfection. Whether a device should be sterilized or disinfected between patients is determined by the degree of risk of infection. Four categories of medical devices have been defined: (1) critical instruments or devices, (2) semicritical instruments or devices, (3) noncritical instruments or devices, and (4) environmental surfaces (Favero, Bond, 1991; Rutala, 1996).

A substantial risk of infection exists if critical instruments or devices are contaminated with any microorganism. Because critical instruments enter the bloodstream or normally sterile body areas, they must be sterile. Such devices include surgical instruments, cardiac catheters, implants, needles, and transfer forceps.

Biopsy forceps that penetrate mucosal barriers also fall into this category.

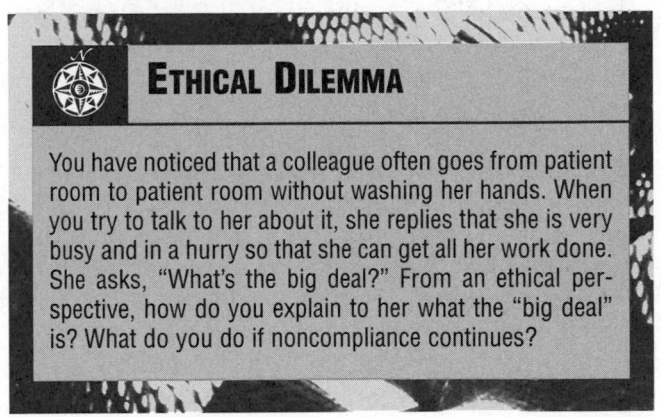

**ETHICAL DILEMMA**

You have noticed that a colleague often goes from patient room to patient room without washing her hands. When you try to talk to her about it, she replies that she is very busy and in a hurry so that she can get all her work done. She asks, "What's the big deal?" From an ethical perspective, how do you explain to her what the "big deal" is? What do you do if noncompliance continues?

Semicritical instruments or devices are those that come in contact with mucous membranes or nonintact skin. Such instruments include flexible fiberoptic endoscopes, endotracheal tubes, bronchoscopes, respiratory therapy equipment, anesthesia breathing circuits, ophthalmic devices, and vaginal speculums. Items in this category must be manually and meticulously cleaned and submitted to a disinfection process that eradicates all microorganisms except for high numbers of bacterial spores.

Noncritical instruments or devices have contact only with unbroken skin. Examples of these devices may include blood pressure cuffs, face masks, most neurologic and cardiac diagnostic electrodes, and bedpans. Sterility is not critical for these items. In today's hospital most such items are disposable and are discarded after use.

As described by Favero and Bond (1991), environmental surfaces include medical equipment surfaces such as adjustment knobs on dialysis machines, ventilators, x-ray machines, and IV pumps. A second group of environmental surfaces includes housekeeping surfaces such as floors, walls, tabletops, and curtains. Although items in this category are not usually in direct contact with patients, hand contact with these surfaces may lead to cross-contamination among patients. Cleaning these surfaces with a detergent or hospital-grade disinfectant detergent is adequate for environmental surfaces.

The disinfectant process has been divided into three levels of germicidal actions: high level, intermediate level, and low level. High-level disinfection (HLD) destroys all microorganisms except for bacterial spores. All semicritical medical devices should be subjected to HLD. HLD may be accomplished with glutaraldehyde, chlorine dioxide, 6% hydrogen peroxide, or formulations with a peracetic acid base. These same

---

**BOX 15-7**

### WHEN TO WASH HANDS

- Before and after the workday
- After direct care of any patient
- After handling any equipment
- Before performing invasive procedures, even if sterile gloves will be worn
- Before and after contact with any wound
- Before contact with a patient at high risk for infection
- After contact with a source likely to be contaminated with virulent microorganisms (e.g., secretions or excretions)
- Between contact with different patients in special care units
- After removing gloves

agents can be used to achieve sterilization. The single most important variable in achieving HLD and sterilization is contact time (Rutala, 1996).

Intermediate-level disinfection (ILD) destroys *Mycobacterium tuberculosis*, vegetative bacteria, most viruses, and most fungi but not necessarily bacterial spores. Examples of agents used for ILD include alcohol (70% to 90% ethyl or isopropyl), chlorine compounds (sodium or calcium hypochlorite, chlorine dioxide), certain phenolics, and certain iodophor preparations. Sodium hypochlorite (bleach) in a concentration of 0.5% has broad germicidal activity and is the most common disinfectant used worldwide.

Small, nonlipid viruses such as enterovirus and rhinovirus may be more resistant to germicides. However, medium and large lipid-containing viruses, including adenovirus, human immunodeficiency virus (HIV), and hepatitis B virus (HBV), are more sensitive to germicides. HBV and non-A, non-B hepatitis are difficult to test in the laboratory. However, no evidence exists that these viruses are unusually resistant to disinfectants. HIV is relatively unstable in the environment. Any disinfectant used in a health care environment should be approved by the Environmental Protection Agency (EPA). An EPA registration number can be found on the label of all approved disinfectants.

Low-level disinfection (LLD) destroys vegetative forms of most bacteria and fungi, as well as medium to large lipid-containing viruses. LLD does not destroy bacterial endospores, mycobacteria, small nonlipid viruses, or some fungi. Low-level disinfectants include the quaternary ammonium compounds, certain iodophors, and certain phenolics.

A number of factors must be considered when using disinfectants. One factor is the length of time for the process. Medical items with smooth, nonporous, and cleanable surfaces are the easiest to disinfect. Instruments with crevices, joints, and pores in the surfaces represent potential barriers to cleaning and to subsequent penetration of the germicide. Even sterilization methods can fail if organisms are trapped in organic materials. When medical devices are evaluated for purchase, the manufacturer's recommendations for cleaning and disinfection should be reviewed. The manufacturer's guidelines should be consistent with the disinfection level required for that category of equipment. The type and level of microbial decontamination influences the effectiveness of the disinfectant, and the number of microorganisms present also influences the time necessary to achieve disinfection. For example, it takes longer to kill 1000 bacterial spores than to kill 1 million cells of *S. aureus* (Favero, Bond, 1991). The amount of serum, blood, mucus, pus, or feces present on the device is a significant factor. Some disinfectants, such as chlorine and iodine, are inacti-

vated in the presence of organic material; therefore, cleaning is required before disinfection.

Most disinfectants do not act quickly. Generally, the higher the concentration of the germicide, the shorter the time required to kill the microorganism. The longer the time of exposure, the greater the effectiveness of the disinfectant process. For example, glutaraldehydes achieve HLD in 20 minutes of exposure but can achieve sterilization if the exposure time is extended to 10 to 12 hours. All surfaces of the equipment must have contact with the disinfectant for the entire exposure time. Temperature, pH, water hardness, and the presence of other chemicals, such as soaps, also may affect the activity of the disinfectant. Because of these variables, it is essential that hospital personnel read and follow the manufacturer's directions for use of the disinfectant.

## Antisepsis

Antiseptics are preparations used on the skin to inhibit or destroy microorganisms. The antimicrobial ingredient may be alcohol, chlorhexidine, hexachlorophene, iodine, iodophors, chloroxylenol (PLCMX), or triclosan. Some of these ingredients are also found in disinfectants. However, because the formulations usually are different, it is crucial that the product's directions for use be strictly followed. Antiseptics are used for personal hand washing, surgical scrubs, and skin preparation for surgery or for insertion of invasive devices. A guideline for hand washing and hand antisepsis in health care settings has been published by APIC (Larson, 1995).

## Personnel

Personnel in charge of direct patient care should be free of infection and are responsible for maintaining personal hygiene and grooming. All hospital personnel should maintain their immunization levels, report and treat all illnesses promptly, and refrain from patient care when they are ill. Employee health services are available and must be consulted for work-related injuries, illnesses, or exposures.

## High-Risk Areas

Delivery, operating, and recovery rooms, intensive care units, and other specialized units, such as the hemodialysis unit, are considered high-risk areas. Patients in these areas are usually considered compromised hosts and therefore are highly susceptible to infection or disease.

If a patient is identified as being at high risk for infection, protective measures should be implemented as part of his or her care. Attempts should be made to minimize the patient's contact with infectious agents. Catheters and tubes that bypass normal defense mechanisms should be used judiciously. Special instructions should be given to the patient and family about health maintenance and avoiding contact with other infected people. Thorough hand washing must be practiced between each patient contact.

## Control Policies and Procedures
### Isolation

Nursing care of a patient with an infectious disease involves two basic principles of medical asepsis: (1) confining all pathogens to a given area, which prevents their spread from an infected patient to others; and (2) protecting susceptible people from pathogens present in the environment or carried by others. **Isolation** is a means of interrupting the transmission of infectious organisms, because sources of infection and susceptible hosts are more difficult to control. The procedure establishes a barrier around the patient in an attempt to prevent the spread of infection either to or from the patient. Nurses assigned to the care of a patient in isolation should have a basic knowledge of the infectivity of the disease and its mode of transmission, as well as an understanding of the high-risk factors involved with susceptible patients.

The *CDC Guidelines for Isolation Precautions in Hospitals* recommends two tiers of precautions (Hospital Infection Control Practices Advisory Committee, 1996). The first tier comprises precautions designed for the care of all hospital patients regardless of their diagnosis or presumed infection status. These precautions, called Standard Precautions, are the primary strategy for successful control of nosocomial infections. The second tier is designed for the care of patients with a specific diagnosis; these precautions are called Transmission-Based Precautions. The categories included in this second tier are Airborne Precautions, Droplet Precautions, and Contact Precautions.

The 1996 guideline replaced the 1983 guideline, which contained the following categories of isolation: Strict Isolation, Contact Isolation, Respiratory Isolation, Tuberculosis (AFB) Isolation, Enteric Precautions, Drainage-Secretion Precautions, and Blood and Body Fluid Precautions.

### Standard Precautions

**Standard Precautions** synthesize the major features of Universal Precautions and Body Substance Isolation. Standard Precautions apply to blood and all other body fluids, secretions and excretions, nonintact skin, and mucous membranes. Standard Precautions are designed to reduce the risk of transmission of microorganisms from both known and unknown sources of infection (Boxes 15-8 and 15-9 and Figure 15-2).

---

**BOX 15-8**

### STANDARD PRECAUTIONS

1. Wash hands after touching blood, body fluids, secretions, excretions, mucous membranes, nonintact skin, and contaminated items.
2. Wear gloves when touching blood, body fluids, secretions, excretions, mucous membranes, nonintact skin, and contaminated items. Remove gloves promptly after use and *wash hands*.
3. Wear a mask and eye protection when performing procedures or patient care activities likely to generate spray or splashes.
4. Wear a gown during procedures or patient care activities that may generate spray or splashes of blood or other body fluids.
5. Disinfect or sterilize all reusable equipment between patients. Handle contaminated equipment in a manner that prevents contamination of skin, clothing, or the environment.
6. Disinfect environmental surfaces, beds, and bedside equipment.
7. Prevent injuries by safe handling of sharps (Box 15-9).
8. Use mouthpieces, resuscitation bags, or other ventilation devices as an alternative to mouth-to-mouth resuscitation.

From Centers for Disease Control and Prevention (CDC): *Am J Infect Control* 24(5):380-388, 1996.

---

**BOX 15-9**

### PREVENTING INJURIES FROM CONTAMINATED NEEDLES AND OTHER SHARPS

1. Never recap needles using two hands.
2. Use a one-handed "scoop" technique or a resheathing device.
3. Do not remove needles from disposable syringes.
4. Place used needles and sharps in puncture-resistant containers kept as close as possible to the point of use.
5. Use needleless intravascular system components whenever possible.

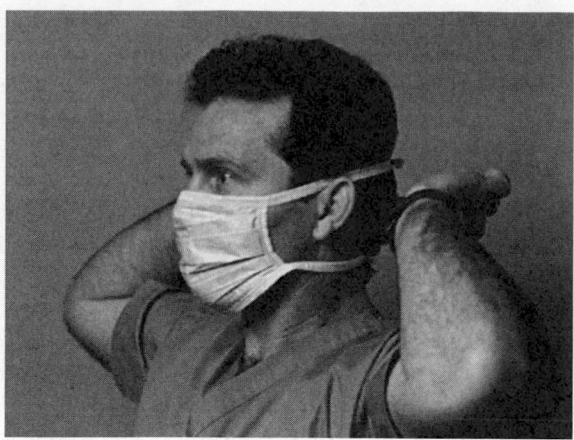

**Figure 15-2** Masks should cover the nose and mouth and should be used only once. (From Potter PA, Perry AG: *Fundamentals of nursing: concepts, process, and practice*, ed 4, St Louis, 1997, Mosby.)

## Airborne Precautions

**Airborne Precautions** are implemented in addition to Standard Precautions to reduce the risk of airborne transmission of infectious agents. Airborne transmission occurs by dissemination of airborne droplet nuclei (5 mm or smaller) that remain suspended in the air for long periods, or by dust particles that contain the infectious agent. Special air handling and ventilation are required to prevent airborne transmission (Box 15-10).

## Tuberculosis

Airborne Precautions should be instituted for patients with a positive sputum smear for acid-fast bacilli (AFB) or a chest x-ray film that suggests active TB. In general, infants and young children with pulmonary TB do not require isolation because they rarely cough, and their bronchial secretions excrete few AFB.

Because of the increase in the number of TB cases, especially cases of drug-resistant TB, the CDC has published recommendations for isolation of patients with TB or suspected of having TB. Room requirements include that the room be under negative air pressure in relation to the corridor, that it have six air exchanges per hour, and that it exhaust to the outside (CDC, 1990, 1994). High-efficiency particulate air (HEPA) filters and ultraviolet light may be used in some areas. The federal Occupational Safety and Health Administration (OSHA) initially required the use of particulate respirators with HEPA filters as the minimum respiratory protection for those providing direct care to infectious TB patients. More recently the use of N95 particulate respirators has been approved. The need for a level of protection is controversial, because epidemiologic data do not exist to demonstrate

---

**BOX 15-10**

### AIRBORNE PRECAUTIONS

Use in addition to Standard Precautions.
1. Use private room with:
   - Monitored negative air pressure
   - 6-12 air changes per hour
   - Discharge of air outdoors or HEPA filtration before air is recirculated. *Keep room door closed and patient in room.*
2. Ensure respiratory protection:
   - Wear an N95 respirator mask for known or suspected cases of tuberculosis.
   - Susceptible individuals should not enter the room of patients with known or suspected cases of measles (rubeola) or varicella (chickenpox) if immune caregivers are available.
   - If susceptible individuals must enter the room, a mask is required.
3. Limit the movement and transportation of patients outside the room to essential purposes only. During transport, minimize the spread of droplet nuclei by placing a surgical mask on the patient if possible.

**ILLNESSES REQUIRING AIRBORNE PRECAUTIONS**
- Measles
- Varicella (chickenpox and disseminated zoster)
- Tuberculosis

From Centers for Disease Control and Prevention (CDC): *Am J Infect Control* 24(5):380-388, 1996.

---

its effectiveness. Data show that hospitals with programs for early detection and isolation of patients in properly ventilated rooms have not had nosocomial transmission of TB (Adal et al, 1994).

## Droplet Precautions

**Droplet Precautions** are used in addition to Standard Precautions for patients known to be or suspected of being infected with microorganisms transmitted by droplets (larger than 5 mm) that can be generated by the patient during coughing, sneezing, talking, or the performance of procedures (Box 15-11).

## Contact Precautions

**Contact Precautions** are used in addition to Standard Precautions for patients known to be or suspected of being infected or colonized with epidemiologically significant microorganisms that can be transmitted by

## DROPLET PRECAUTIONS

Use in addition to Standard Precautions
1. Place the patient in a private room. If a private room is not available, cohort with patients who have an active infection with the same microorganism but who have no other infection. Maintain spatial separation of at least 1 m (about 3 ft) from other patients and visitors if cohorting or if private room is not available. Room door may remain open. Special ventilation is not required.
2. Mask is required when working within 1 m (about 3 ft) of patient or when entering the room; check hospital's policy.
3. Limit the movement and transportation of patients outside the room to essential purposes only. During transport, minimize the spread of droplets by placing a surgical mask on the patient if possible.

### ILLNESSES REQUIRING DROPLET PRECAUTIONS
- Invasive *Haemophilus influenzae* type b disease (meningitis, pneumonia, epiglottitis, and sepsis)
- Invasive *Neisseria meningitidis* disease (meningitis, pneumonia, and sepsis)
- Invasive multidrug-resistant *Streptococcus pneumoniae* disease (meningitis, pneumonia, sinusitis, and otitis media)
- Other serious bacterial respiratory infections spread by droplet transmission, including:
  Diphtheria (pharyngeal)
  *Mycoplasma* pneumonia
  Pertussis
  Pneumonic plague
  Streptococcal pharyngitis, pneumonia, or scarlet fever in infants and young children
- Serious viral infections spread by droplet transmission, including:
  Adenovirus
  Influenza
  Mumps
  Parvovirus B19
  Rubella

From Centers for Disease Control and Prevention (CDC): *Am J Infect Control* 24(5):380-388, 1996.

direct contact with the patient or indirect contact with environmental surfaces or patient care items in the patient's environment (Box 15-12).

Instruction cards have been designed to give concise information about appropriate precautions. These cards should be posted where they are visible to all personnel providing care to the patient. Cards must be designed in such a manner that the patient's right to confidentiality is maintained. The patient and family should be informed that an isolation card has been posted.

## Universal Precautions

In August 1987, the CDC published a set of recommendations for preventing HIV transmission in health care settings. The recommendations are referred to as Universal Blood and Body Fluid Precautions, or simply **Universal Precautions**. Because it is impossible to recognize all patients who are infected with bloodborne pathogens when giving care, Universal Precautions need to be implemented for all patients undergoing medical care.

The body fluids to which Universal Precautions should apply include blood, semen, vaginal secretions, cerebrospinal fluid (CSF), synovial fluid, and amniotic fluid. Universal Precautions do not apply to feces, nasal secretions, sputum, sweat, tears, urine, or vomitus unless they contain visible blood. As written, Universal Precautions are designed to protect health care workers from exposure to bloodborne pathogens, but they do not address the prevention of cross-contamination between patients (CDC, 1986, 1987). In the current isolation system, Universal Precautions have been integrated into Standard Precautions, which address cross-contamination between patients as well as protection of the health care worker.

Health care employers are now being regulated by OSHA and are being charged with providing a safe working environment for all health care workers. OSHA issued regulations in 1991 that obligate hospitals to implement Universal Precautions in the care of all patients. In addition to these precautions, the regulations require health care employers to provide hepatitis B vaccine to employees who are often exposed to blood and potentially infectious materials, to provide postexposure evaluation and medical follow-up, to train all employees in the use of Universal Precautions, and to maintain records of training and occupational exposure (U.S. Department of Labor, 1991).

## Body Substance Isolation

A system of isolation proposed by Lynch and others (1987) departs from the standard CDC isolation systems. This system is referred to as Body Substance Isolation (BSI) and is used for all patients. Gloves are worn for any anticipated contact with blood or body fluids. Gloves are changed between all patients, and hand washing after patient contact is indicated. Gowns, aprons, masks, or goggles are worn when blood or body fluids are likely to touch the clothing, skin, or face. Private rooms may be necessary for patients with airborne infections or those who soil the environment with body substances.

Under this system of isolation, a BSI card is placed in all patient rooms. A separate "stop sign alert" card with instructions is placed outside the rooms of patients who have airborne infections, and masks are worn for these particular patients. Other forms of isolation are not used under this system. BSI is intended to prevent both the exposure of health care workers to pathogens and cross-contamination between patients. This system also has been integrated into Standard Precautions as described by the CDC.

## EMOTIONAL SUPPORT

Hospital-acquired infections cannot help but evoke feelings of anxiety, frustration, and hostility in the patient and family. Through no fault of his or her own, the patient has acquired an infection that may mean additional hospital days, increased hospital costs, time away from work, or disruption of home life. Isolation

---

**BOX 15-12**

### CONTACT PRECAUTIONS

Use in addition to Standard Precautions.
1. Place the patient in a private room. If a private room is not available, cohort with patients who have active infection with the same microorganism but who have no other infection.
2. Wear gloves when entering the room. Change gloves after contact with infective material. Remove gloves before leaving the patient's room.
3. *Wash hands immediately* with antimicrobial agent before leaving the patient's room. After removing gloves and washing hands, ensure that hands do not touch possibly contaminated environmental surfaces or items in the patient's room to avoid transferring microorganisms to other patients or environments.
4. Wear a gown if you anticipate that your clothes will have substantial contact with the patient, environmental surfaces, or items in the patient's room or if the patient has any of the following:
    Colostomy
    Diarrhea
    Ileostomy
    Incontinence
    Wound drainage not contained by a dressing
5. Remove gown before leaving the patient's environment.
6. Limit the movement and transportation of patients outside the room to essential purposes only. During transport, ensure that all precautions are maintained at all times.
7. When possible, dedicate the use of noncritical patient care equipment for each patient.

### ILLNESSES REQUIRING CONTACT PRECAUTIONS
- Gastrointestinal, respiratory, skin, or wound infections or colonization with multidrug-resistant bacteria as judged by the infection control program, based on current state, regional, or national recommendations, to be of special clinical and epidemiologic significance
- Enteric infections with a low infectious dose or prolonged environmental survival, including:
    *Clostridium difficile*
    For diapered or incontinent patients: enterohemorrhagic *Escherichia coli* O157:H7, *Shigella* infections, hepatitis A, or rotavirus
- Respiratory syncytial virus, parainfluenza virus, or enteroviral infections in infants and young children
- Skin infections that are highly contagious or that may occur on dry skin, including:
    Diphtheria (cutaneous)
    Herpes simplex virus (neonatal or mucocutaneous)
    Impetigo
    Major (noncontained) abscesses, cellulitis, or decubiti
    Pediculosis
    Scabies
    Staphylococcal furunculosis in infants and young children
    Staphylococcal scalded skin syndrome
    Zoster (disseminated or in immunocompromised individual)
- Viral or hemorrhagic conjunctivitis
- Viral hemorrhagic fevers (Lassa fever or Marburg virus)

From Centers for Disease Control and Prevention (CDC): *Am J Infect Control* 24(5):380-388, 1996.

procedures are time-consuming and costly and may discourage personnel from spending extra time with these patients. The solitude that usually accompanies isolation deprives the patient of normal social relationships, and emotional reactions are likely to occur.

A wide range of emotional reactions can be seen in patients subject to isolation precautions. They may exhibit overt abusive or aggressive behavior or show signs of withdrawal and depression. The excessive demands made by some patients can be extremely frustrating to nursing personnel. Family members may fear the possibility of developing the infection themselves and may avoid contact with the patient. The

procedures of donning a gown and mask and proper hand washing may convey feelings of rejection.

Every patient in isolation should have a basic understanding of what to expect. Both the patient and family should be given a thorough explanation of the way in which the infection is transmitted and the procedures of isolation that tend to interrupt transmission. When they realize the significance of isolation and their roles in preventing further transmission, their cooperation and acceptance can be achieved. Much can be done to relieve the patient's anxiety by maintaining a friendly, understanding, sympathetic, and reassuring manner.

# NURSING CARE PLAN
## PATIENT WITH A NOSOCOMIAL INFECTION

Mr. Jackson is a 48-year-old male who was admitted from the emergency department with severe abdominal pain, abdominal rigidity, nausea, and vomiting. He had been experiencing vague abdominal discomfort for 3 days, but the pain became increasingly severe over the 6 hours before admission. An abdominal x-ray film indicated free air in the peritoneum, and an emergency exploratory laparotomy was done. He was found to have a ruptured diverticulum, and a temporary colostomy was performed.

Mr. Jackson developed a wound infection 3 days after surgery, as evidenced by purulent drainage from the inferior aspect of the incision and erythema and warmth around the incision. Infection was confirmed by a wound culture. The staples were removed from the inferior portion of the incision, the wound was irrigated, and dressing changes have been prescribed every 8 hours.

| Medical History | Psychosocial Data | Assessment Data |
|---|---|---|
| No known allergies to food or drugs<br>Has smoked two packs of cigarettes a day for 20 yr<br>Hypertension for approximately 5 yr; reports it is well controlled with medications<br>Diverticulitis (hospitalized 2 yr ago for an acute episode); has had difficulty following prescribed dietary changes as a result of his life-style; work requires meals on the road; dislikes fruits and vegetables | Married for 22 years; has three children, ages 10, 13, and 16; wife is very supportive and has been trying to make dietary changes, without much success<br>Wife is a homemaker and is in excellent health<br>Employed as an advertising executive in a large firm; enjoys his work, but recently work environment has become tense and stressful as a result of layoffs and restructuring of departments<br>Works 12- to 14-hr days<br>Gets minimal exercise<br>Involved in children's activities on weekends<br>Watches television every evening | Height 5′ 9″; weight 110.25 kg (245 lb)<br>*Vital signs:* Temp, 38.2° C (100.9° F); Pulse, 96; Respir, 22; BP, 152/88<br>Alert and oriented × 3; appears stated age<br>*Skin:* Warm, dry, intact (other than incision)<br>*Eye ear, nose, throat:* Mucous membranes moist; teeth in good repair; lips pink<br>*Respiratory:* 22-26/min, shallow, symmetric; diminished breath sounds; bilateral bases; scattered rhonchi and crackles; occasional loose cough that produces white sputum; using incentive spirometer, approximately 1000 ml inspiratory volume<br>*Abdominal:* Protuberant, soft abdomen; hypoactive bowel sounds; colostomy producing scant, serosanguineous drainage; no stool output yet; started on sips of clear liquids today; vertical abdominal incision; superior portion of incision with staples intact and well approximated; slight erythema around staple insertion site; inferior portion approximately 6 cm (2.4 in) open with moderate amount of serosanguineous and purulent drainage; erythema around wound margin<br>*Cardiovascular:* AP 96 and regular; peripheral pulses strong bilaterally; no peripheral edema |

*Continued*

# NURSING CARE PLAN

## PATIENT WITH A NOSOCOMIAL INFECTION—cont'd

| Medical History | Psychosocial Data | Assessment Data |
|---|---|---|
| | | *Laboratory data* |
| | | RBC, 3.8; Hgb, 11.4; Hct, 36; WBC, 14,000; Na, 132; K, 4.1; Cl, 96; $CO_2$, 26 |
| | | *Blood gases:* pH, 7.37; $P_{CO_2}$, 45; $P_{O_2}$, 88; $HCO_3$, 26; $O_2$ sat, 91% |
| | | *ECG:* Normal sinus rhythm |
| | | *Chest x-ray:* Atelectasis bilateral lower lobes |
| | | *Urinalysis:* Within normal limits |
| | | *Wound culture:* S. aureus |
| | | ***Medications*** |
| | | Meperidine (Demerol), 75-100 mg |
| | | Hydroxyzine (Vistaril), 25-50 mg IM q 3-4 hr prn pain |
| | | Enalapril (Vasotec), 10 mg bid |
| | | Cefazolin (Ancef), 1 g IV q 6 hr |
| | | $D_5$ 1/2 NS with 20 mEq KCl at 100 ml/hr |
| | | $O_2$ 2 L/min via nasal cannula |

### NURSING DIAGNOSIS

Risk for infection related to ruptured diverticulum, invasive procedure, obesity, inadequate nutrition as evidenced by wound culture, purulent wound drainage, and elevated temperature

| NURSING INTERVENTIONS | EVALUATION OF EXPECTED OUTCOMES |
|---|---|
| Assess wound q 8 hr for evidence of healing, drainage, erythema, and warmth. | Afebrile; vital signs within normal limits for patient |
| Monitor vital signs q 4 hr. | Absence of purulent drainage from wound |
| Monitor laboratory values, especially WBC. | Evidence of wound healing |
| Maintain aseptic technique in dressing changes. | |
| Change dressing q 8 hr; dampen dressing with sterile normal saline. | |
| Administer antibiotics as prescribed. | |
| If patient does not advance diet in 1-2 days, discuss nutritional concerns with physician. | |
| Teach patient and family the signs and symptoms of infection and the techniques for current treatment. | |
| Consult with infection control nurse if indicated. | |

### NURSING DIAGNOSIS

Ineffective breathing pattern related to smoking history, pain, immobility, and sedation for analgesics

| NURSING INTERVENTIONS | EVALUATION OF EXPECTED OUTCOMES |
|---|---|
| Assess respiratory rate, depth, and breathing pattern q 8 hr. | Respiratory rate 20-24/min without $O_2$ |
| Assess for dyspnea at rest and with exertion. | Breath sounds clear |
| Auscultate breath sounds q 8 hr. | Skin and nail beds pink |
| Monitor for changes in orientation, increased restlessness, and anxiety. | Able to perform incentive spirometry to 1500 ml inspiratory volume |
| Monitor sputum for quantity, color, and consistency. | No evidence of dyspnea or respiratory distress |

## NURSING CARE PLAN

### PATIENT WITH A NOSOCOMIAL INFECTION—cont'd

| NURSING INTERVENTIONS | EVALUATION OF EXPECTED OUTCOMES |
|---|---|
| Maintain patient in a position that supports optimal breathing, with head of bed elevated.<br>Maintain $O_2$ at 2 L/min via nasal cannula; monitor $O_2$ sat as indicated.<br>Encourage coughing and deep breathing and/or incentive spirometry q 2 hr.<br>Provide a dose of analgesic that controls pain but does not oversedate.<br>Encourage out-of-bed activity, sitting in chair tid for 1 hr and ambulating in hall qid.<br>Instruct in splinting of abdominal incision when coughing and deep breathing and during other activities. | |

**NURSING DIAGNOSIS**

Pain related to surgical incision as evidenced by verbal complaints and pain behavior with movement

| NURSING INTERVENTIONS | EVALUATION OF EXPECTED OUTCOMES |
|---|---|
| Assess pain characteristics q 4 hr and prn.<br>Monitor vital signs.<br>Administer analgesics as prescribed; evaluate effectiveness.<br>Promote activity 30 min after administration of analgesic.<br>Teach diversion, relaxation, splinting, and guided imagery.<br>Help patient assume a comfortable position and provide comfort measures. | Verbalizes pain relief<br>Able to perform respiratory exercises and activity without severe pain<br>Uses alternative pain control measures |

**NURSING DIAGNOSIS**

Knowledge deficit related to necessary life-style changes, new ostomy as evidenced by numerous questions and verbalized difficulty with following previous dietary recommendations

| NURSING INTERVENTIONS | EVALUATION OF EXPECTED OUTCOMES |
|---|---|
| Assess patient's understanding of disease.<br>Review cause of disease and factors that may aggravate condition.<br>Teach patient the purpose and care of the ostomy; obtain an enterostomal therapy consult.<br>Include wife in all teaching.<br>Allow for return demonstrations and provide appropriate positive feedback.<br>Provide dietary instruction (e.g., importance of adequate fluids, moderate use of high-fiber foods and foods that cause flatus).<br>Discuss effect of ostomy on body image and sexuality.<br>Identify appropriate community resources (e.g., local ostomy support group, Visiting Nurse Association, medical supply company). | Patient and wife verbalize understanding of disease, surgery, and treatment<br>Able to care for ostomy<br>Knowledgeable about available community resources |

# KEY CONCEPTS

➤ A nosocomial infection is a clinically active infection that occurs in a hospitalized patient that was not present or incubating at the time of admission to the health care facility.

➤ A reservoir is the location where microorganisms that cause infections usually are found, such as patient, health care personnel, health care devices, and the environment.

➤ The rates for nosocomial infection range from 3% to 15% of all patients admitted to hospitals.

➤ The urinary tract is the most common site for nosocomial infections, followed by the lower respiratory tract and surgical site infections.

➤ Exogenous infections are acquired from sources outside the patient or from the environment.

➤ Endogenous infections occur when potentially virulent microorganisms that normally reside in the patient begin to multiply and cause a pathologic condition.

➤ Microorganisms are transmitted to a susceptible host by contact, airborne, vehicle, or vector-borne routes.

➤ Primary nosocomial bacteremia associated with intravascular devices is a growing problem in health care facilities.

➤ The infection control committee establishes and implements hospital policy concerning the investigation, control, and prevention of infection within health care facilities.

➤ The infection control practitioner is primarily responsible for developing, coordinating, and supervising the infection control program throughout the health care facility.

➤ Surveillance programs detect, record, and report hospital-associated infections in a systematic fashion so that effective, practical control measures can be instituted.

➤ The single most important technique in both preventing and controlling infection is proper hand washing.

➤ Sterilization and disinfection procedures are crucial to the control and prevention of nosocomial infections.

➤ Principles of medical asepsis include (1) confining all pathogens to a given area, which prevents their spread from an infected person to others; and (2) protecting susceptible people from pathogens that are present in the environment or are carried by other people.

➤ Isolation may produce a wide range of emotional reactions in patients.

# CRITICAL THINKING EXERCISES

1. Why are elderly hospitalized patients considered to be at high risk for nosocomial infections?
2. Outline a plan for preventing urinary tract infections, surgical site infections, pneumonia, and bacteremia in acute and long-term care settings.
3. How can the staff nurse assist the infection control practitioner in surveillance for infections?
4. What is the rationale for the two-tier isolation system and each of the three transmission-based categories?

# REFERENCES AND ADDITIONAL READINGS

Adal K et al: The use of high-efficiency particulate air filter respirators to protect hospital workers from tuberculosis, *N Engl J Med* 331(3):169-173, 1994.

American College of Surgeons: *Manual on control of infection in surgical patients,* ed 2, Philadelphia, 1984, Lippincott.

Batt MD, Galaviz CJ: Urinary tract infections. In APIC: *APIC infection control and applied epidemiology,* St Louis, 1996, Mosby.

Burke JP: Nosocomial urinary tract infections. In Wenzel RP, editor: *Prevention and control of nosocomial infections,* ed 2, Baltimore, 1993, Williams & Wilkins.

Centers for Disease Control and Prevention (CDC): *Guidelines for the prevention of surgical wound infections,* Atlanta, 1985, US Department of Health and Human Services.

Centers for Disease Control and Prevention (CDC): *National nosocomial infections study report: annual summary—1984,* Atlanta, 1986, US Department of Health and Human Services.

Centers for Disease Control and Prevention (CDC): Recommendations for prevention of HIV transmission in health care settings, *MMWR* 36(suppl 25):1S-18S, 1987.

Centers for Disease Control and Prevention (CDC): Update: universal precautions for prevention of transmission of human immunodeficiency virus, hepatitis B virus, and other bloodborne pathogens in health care settings, *MMWR* 37(24):377-388, 1988.

Centers for Disease Control and Prevention (CDC): Guidelines for preventing the transmission of tuberculosis in health care settings, with special focus on HIV-related issues, *MMWR CDC Surveill Summ* 39(No RR-17):1-29, 1990.

Centers for Disease Control and Prevention (CDC): Nosocomial infection rates for interhospital comparison: limitations and possible solutions, *Infect Control Hosp Epidemiol* 12(10):609-621, 1991.

Centers for Disease Control and Prevention (CDC): Guidelines for preventing the transmission of *Mycobacterium tuberculosis* in health care facilities, 1994, *Fed Reg* 59, October 28, 1994.

Centers for Disease Control and Prevention (CDC): National nosocomial infections surveillance (NNIS) report: data summary from October 1996–April 1996, *Am J Infect Control* 24(5):380-388, 1996.

Favero MS, Bond WW: Chemical disinfection of medical and surgical materials. In Block SS, editor: *Disinfection, sterilization, and preservation,* ed 4, Philadelphia, 1991, Lea & Febiger.

Garner JS: Hospital Infection Control Practices Advisory Committee: Guidelines for isolation precautions in hospitals, *Am J Infect Control* 24(1):24-45, 1996.

Haley RW: *Managing hospital infection control for cost-effectiveness,* Chicago, 1986, American Hospital Publishing.

Haley RW et al: Nosocomial infections in U.S. hospitals, 1975-1976: estimated frequency by selected characteristics of patients, *Am J Med* 70(4):947-959, 1981.

Horan TC, Gaynes RP, Martone WJ et al: CDC definitions of surgical site infections, 1992: a modification of CDC definitions of surgical wound infections, *Am J Infect Control* 20:271-274, 1992.

Hospital Infection Control Practices Advisory Committee: Guidelines for isolation precautions in hospitals. Part II. Recommendations for isolation precautions in hospitals, *Am J Infect Control* 24:32-52, 1996.

Joint Commission on Accreditation of Healthcare Organizations (JCAHO): *Accreditation manual for hospitals,* Chicago, 1995, The Commission.

Larson E: APIC guideline for hand washing and hand antisepsis in health care settings, *Am J Infect Control* 23(4):251-269, 1995.

Mayhall CG: *Hospital epidemiology and infection control,* Baltimore, 1996, Williams & Wilkins.

Mermel L: Infections related to intravascular devices. In APIC: *APIC infection control and applied epidemiology,* St Louis, 1996, Mosby.

Pearson ML: CDC guideline for prevention of intravascular device–related infections, *Infect Control Hosp Epidemiol* 17(7):438-473, 1996.

Rutala WA: APIC guideline for selection and use of disinfectants, *Am J Infect Control* 4(4):313-342, 1996.

Tablan O: Nosocomial pneumonia. In APIC: *APIC infection control and applied epidemiology,* St Louis, 1996, Mosby.

Widmer A: Intravenous-related infections. In Wenzel RP, editor: *Prevention and control of nosocomial infections,* Baltimore, 1997, Williams & Wilkins.

# CHAPTER 16

# HIV Infection and AIDS

## CHAPTER OBJECTIVES

1 Discuss the role of viral replication in HIV infection.
2 Explain the role of the CD4 cell in the immune system.
3 Identify the symptoms associated with primary HIV infection.
4 Discuss the stages of HIV infection.
5 Define HIV/AIDS.
6 Explain the role of viral load testing in the management of HIV.
7 Identify the major opportunistic infections and other complications that occur in people with AIDS.
8 List the modes of transmission of HIV infection.
9 Discuss the components of occupational exposure management.
10 Discuss the major therapies used to manage HIV infection.

## KEY TERMS

acquired immunodeficiency syndrome (AIDS)
antiretroviral therapy
candidiasis
CD4 lymphocyte
clinical latency
HIV antibody
human immunodeficiency virus (HIV)
human papillomavirus (HPV)

Kaposi's sarcoma (KS)
occupational exposure
opportunistic infection
*Pneumocystis carinii* pneumonia (PCP)
primary infection
prophylaxis
Universal Precautions
viral load
viral resistance

The **human immunodeficiency virus (HIV)** is a complex virus that leads to progressive destruction of the immune system, leaving its host vulnerable to opportunistic infections, malignancies, and other conditions. The spectrum of illness with HIV begins at the moment of infection and continues through the diagnosis of **acquired immunodeficiency syndrome (AIDS)** as a chronic disease. Researchers have learned a great deal about HIV infection since the first cases were identified in 1981. Information about the structure of the virus, how it affects the immune system, and ways to suppress the viral mechanisms have led to the development of effective therapies that have enabled people to live for many years. Nurses have played vital roles in the AIDS epidemic since its inception, serving as caregivers, advocates, and educators.

## EPIDEMIOLOGY

By the end of 1996, it was estimated that 8.4 million people worldwide had been diagnosed with AIDS. It also has been estimated that since the beginning of this epidemic, more than 29 million people have been infected with HIV and more than 6.4 million have died. According to 1996 estimates alone, 3.1 million new HIV infections occurred that year; this works out to 8500 new infections a day—7500 in adults and 1000 in children (Global AIDS Policy Coalition, 1996).

Experts have predicted that, given current infection rates, 60 million to 70 million adults will have been infected worldwide by the end of the year 2000 (Global AIDS Policy Coalition, 1996). The epidemic continues to spread in all countries, and more than 75% of cases are transmitted through unprotected sexual intercourse (Global AIDS Policy Coalition, 1996). Almost 70% of AIDS cases have occurred in Africa; in some sub-Saharan areas, as many as 25% to 30% of women of childbearing age are infected. Current trends show increasing HIV infection among women, accounting for approximately 42% of all those living with AIDS (Broder, Merigan, Bolognasi, 1994).

In the United States, the HIV epidemic is tracked by the Centers for Disease Control and Prevention (CDC). All states report confirmed cases of AIDS, and many states now report cases of HIV infection. The cumulative total of cases reported in adults in the United States has risen to almost 600,000 since 1981. AIDS is now the leading cause of death among adults in the United States age 25 to 44 (CDC, 1995a). As of December, 1996, 362,004 people had died of AIDS in the United States; of those, 357,598 were adults and 4406 were children (CDC, 1995a). However, the CDC has identified a hopeful trend: thanks to highly active antiretroviral therapy (HAART), 1996 marked the first year of decline in AIDS deaths in the United States since the epidemic began.

Early in the epidemic, AIDS was thought to be a disease that affected only gay men. However, the HIV epidemic in the United States has transcended all racial, ethnic, and class differences. The disease affects people from all walks of life, although the poor and disenfranchised individuals living in inner cities have been particularly vulnerable to the devastation of HIV. Also, the number of HIV cases among older adults is rising. The Older Adult Considerations box presents some important points to remember in addressing this growing HIV-positive population.

## OLDER ADULT CONSIDERATIONS

- Approximately 10% of all people with acquired immunodeficiency syndrome are 50 years of age or older.
- Older adults engage in sexual activity.
- When taking a history from older adults, the nurse should ask open-ended questions rather than make assumptions. For example, the nurse should ask, "When was the last time you had sex?" rather than "Do you ever have sex?"
- Human immunodeficiency virus (HIV) encephalopathy (dementia) can be mistaken for Alzheimer's disease.
- Older adults may have different, enhanced, or delayed reactions to drug therapy.
- Renal and hepatic function tests should be evaluated before any new medications are started.
- Older adults may progress faster when infected with HIV.

### TABLE 16-1

### Distribution of AIDS Cases in the United States by Transmission Category

| TRANSMISSION CATEGORY | NUMBER IN THE U.S. | PERCENTAGE |
|---|---|---|
| Gay/bisexual male | 287,576 | 50 |
| Injection drug user | 146,359 | 25 |
| Gay/bisexual male and IDU* | 37,152 | 6 |
| Adult hemophiliac | 4443 | 1 |
| Heterosexual contact | 49,764 | 9 |
| Transfusion | 7888 | 1 |
| Undetermined† | 40,618 | 7 |
| Pediatric | 7629 | 1 |
| **Total** | **581,427** | **100** |

From Centers for Disease Control and Prevention (CDC), Department of HIV/AIDS Prevention: *Joint United Nations programme on HIV/AIDS*, December, 1996.

*Individuals who have identified exposure to human immunodeficiency virus through both sexual practices and injection drug use.

†Individuals who are in the process of being reported, who died before their risk was identified, or who could not identify their risk.

The behaviors that have resulted in transmission of HIV infection are known as transmission categories. Table 16-1 shows the distribution of diagnosed AIDS cases across transmission categories from 1981 through December, 1996 (CDC, 1996b). The transmission categories generally have remained stable, although three trends can be seen: (1) an increase in the number of women who have acquired HIV through sexual contact, (2) an increase in the proportion of people who have acquired HIV through injection drug use, and (3) a decline in the percentage of gay men who contribute to the total of AIDS cases.

## Viral Structure

Each HIV virion (a single virus particle) contains at least nine genes that govern the action of HIV in the body (Figure 16-1). These genes have been identified as gag, pol, env, vif, vpu, vpr, tat, rev, and nef. The nine genes are linked, forming a single strand of RNA that lies within the core of the virus. Also in the core are three important enzymes—reverse transcriptase, protease, and integrase—that assist in different phases of the replication cycle.

The viral core is enclosed by a capsid covering made up of proteins and glycoproteins, which are identified by their molecular weight measured in nanograms (e.g., the protein p9 has a molecular weight of 9 ng). The major capsid protein is called p24. Encasing the capsid is a glycoprotein envelope with 72 external spikes (formed by two envelope proteins, gp120 and gp41).

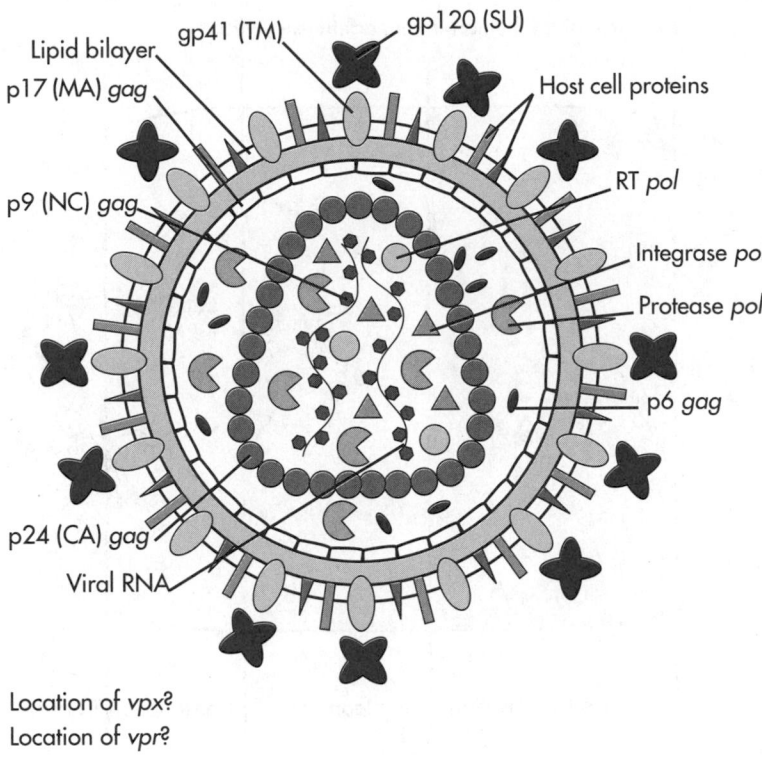

**Figure 16-1**   Structure of the human immunodeficiency virus.

## HIV Life Cycle

Like all viruses, HIV is totally parasitic. It cannot reproduce independently; rather, it must invade a host cell and use that cell's machinery to replicate. The process of viral replication in various host cells in the body is called the *viral life cycle* (Figure 16-2). The single strand of RNA in the core of the virus must be transcribed into DNA in order to infiltrate the host cell's DNA and in order for viral replication to occur. This transformation from RNA to DNA occurs with the help of reverse transcriptase, one of the enzymes found in the viral core. The viral DNA then is able to infiltrate the host cell's DNA in order to replace the host cell's genetic instructions with its own. The host cell thus is transformed into an HIV factory, which produces viral proteins instead of the cell's normal regulatory proteins.

## Immune System

Four types of cells in the immune system, T cells (lymphocytes), monocytes and macrophages, and follicular dendritic cells (FDCs), are primary targets for HIV because of the virus' affinity for the CD4 molecule on the surface of each of these cells.

T cells, or lymphocytes, begin as white blood cells. These cells develop in the bone marrow but mature and differentiate in the thymus gland into subsets of T cells (the "T" of T cell stands for thymus). Each of these subset T cells plays a unique and important role in the immune system. They detect specific antigens and orchestrate a complex immune response, which includes stimulating B lymphocytes (which mature in the bone marrow) to secrete antibody, signaling killer T cells to destroy infected cells, and alerting inflammatory T cells to call in phagocytes to devour the invader. Once the infection is under control, the remaining helper T cells persist as memory cells, which stand ready to counter future attacks by the same antigen.

Two kinds of T cells are particularly important in HIV infection. The helper T cells (also known as T4 cells or **CD4 lymphocyte**) have been identified as the master coordinator of the body's immune response. One of its roles is signaling the production of antibodies. HIV has a high affinity for CD4 cells, particularly when the cell has been activated (i.e., has been turned on and is reproducing in order to fight infection). Ironically, the very cell that directs the body's fight against HIV is the cell that is most vulnerable to the virus. Suppressor T cells (also known as T8 cells, CD8 cells,

Life cycle of the human immunodeficiency virus

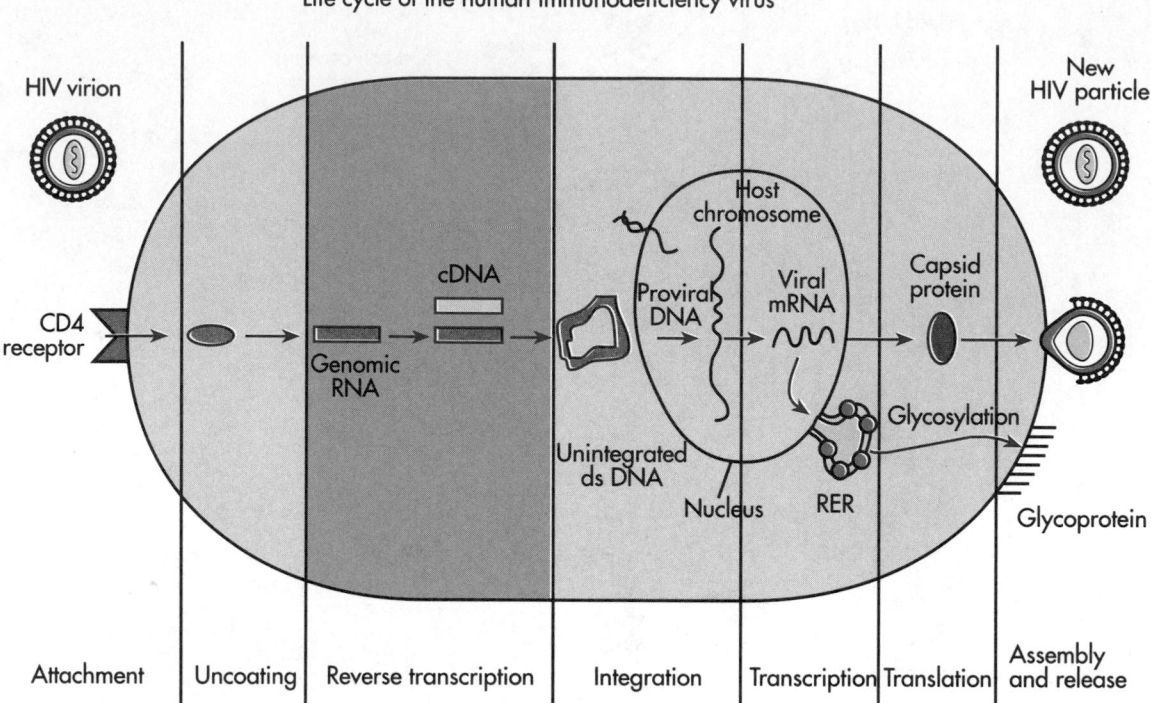

**Figure 16-2** The life cycle of the human immunodeficiency virus (HIV) begins with attachment of the virus to at least two receptors on the outside of the cell, the CD4 molecule and the CCR-5 molecule. The outer membranes of the virus and the host fuse; this step immediately precedes entry of the viral RNA into the cell. After entering the cell, the virus partially sheds its coat so that the RNA can be transcribed into a double-stranded DNA. Another enzyme, integrase, facilitates insertion of the viral DNA into the host cell's nucleus, where it infiltrates the host cell's DNA. Because DNA is unable to leave the nucleus (the center of a cell), it must be transcribed back into RNA; however, the RNA is now *viral* RNA, not *host cell* RNA. The RNA carries the genetic code to the ribosome, located in the cytoplasm (the intracellular fluid of the cell). The ribosome "reads" the code on the RNA and follows those genetic instructions to manufacture long strips of new *viral* proteins, including enzymes, which enable the virus to reproduce. The long strips are then chopped into usable pieces by the enzyme protease and reassembled as new viral particles, which bud from the host cell and are released.

or cytotoxic T lymphocytes) signal the helper cells and antibodies to deactivate after infection has been brought under control. These cells are important because research has proved their ability to control HIV replication in the cells. Individuals with a high number of CD8 cells may have a better chance of internal control of the virus and therefore may progress more slowly. Ironically, immune activation is a mixed blessing; it can control HIV through the activation of CD4 and CD8 cells, but it also facilitates infection of new CD4 cells through that very activation.

Monocytes and macrophages are large white blood cells that devour foreign material in blood and tissue, respectively, by phagocytosis. They also present antigens to T cells. Macrophages are important targets for HIV because they may serve as reservoirs for the virus,

supporting replication for months or years without being destroyed.

FDCs are present in lymph tissue (e.g., lymph nodes), where they trap antigens. HIV particles become trapped by dendritic cells particularly in the early and intermediate stages of HIV infection. This trapping in an area to which T cells regularly migrate greatly enhances the T cells' exposure to HIV and facilitates their infection.

Although they do not become infected with the virus, cytokines must be mentioned because they are chemical messengers, secreted by macrophages and T cells to communicate with other cells in the immune system. Cytokines give directions that regulate the growth, function, and differentiation of other immune system cells. Because HIV causes T cells and macrophages to

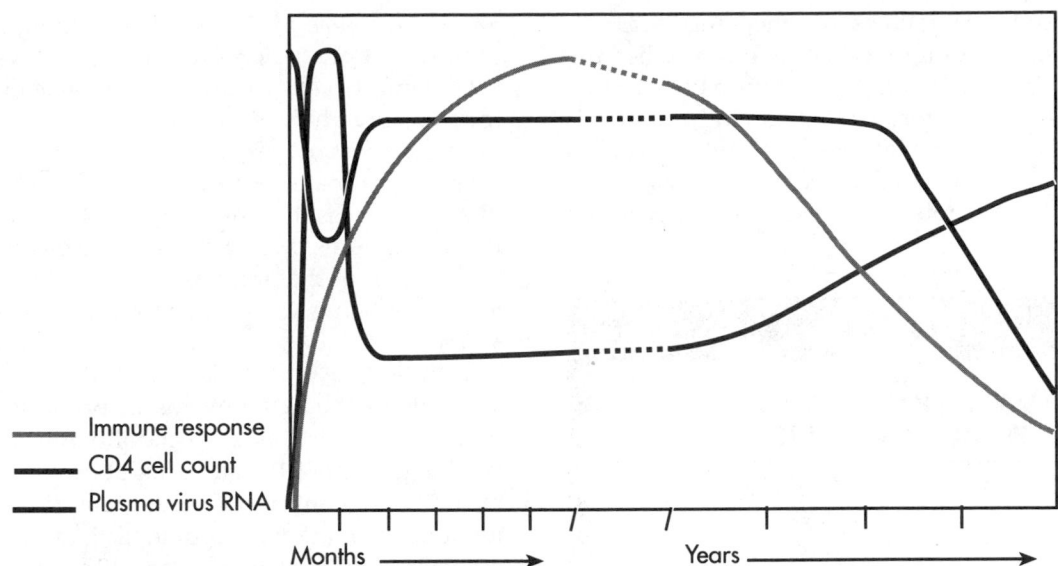

**Figure 16-3**  Generalized virologic and immunologic course of HIV disease: natural history of untreated HIV disease. (From Saag M et al: *Nat Med* 2(6):625-629, 1996.)

malfunction, cytokine production by these cells may be diminished or increased. This contributes to the progression of HIV by many different mechanisms, including activation of otherwise latent (inactive) CD4 cells, which can then serve as hosts for replication. Interferons (IF), interleukins (IL), tumor necrosis factor (TNF), and erythropoietin (EPO) are cytokines.

## Pathogenesis
### Viral Replication

Relentless viral replication in susceptible cells is the primary mechanism of immune system destruction. The amount of virus in the body is referred to as the **viral load**. Current research shows that each day more than a billion new virus particles may be manufactured in the body; the immune system tries to counter this attack, daily replacing more than a billion T cells (Ho et al, 1995). Over time the T-cell replenishing system tires, whole populations of T cells, such as the memory cells that recognize antigens, are wiped out, and HIV gains control.

Because of the high viral turnover and the error-prone enzyme reverse transcriptase, slight changes in the structure of the virus occur frequently. These changes, known as mutations, present a substantial challenge because they produce a virus that is no longer sensitive to treatment.

### Natural History

The course of HIV infection is referred to as its natural history. The four stages of HIV infection can be described as (1) primary infection, (2) clinical latency, (3) symptomatic HIV disease, and (4) AIDS. Each of these phases corresponds with a typical level of CD4 cells and of virus in the body (Figure 16-3). Especially noteworthy is the inverse relationship between the amount of virus and the number of CD4 cells. The needs of a person with HIV vary, depending on the stage of disease. In each of these phases, the nurse's role includes teaching the patient about the disease or the particular phase and the medications required, managing symptoms, and supporting the therapeutic program by overseeing medication adherence, providing resource referrals, and offering psychosocial support. Each patient must be assessed carefully so that interventions appropriate to his or her needs can be chosen.

**Primary infection.** Within the first few weeks of infection, a period of intense, uncontrolled viral replication occurs with a burst of virus in the blood. This period is known as **primary infection**. The viral load may measure in the millions, higher than at any other time during infection. During this time the CD4 cell count may drop acutely. The viral protein p24 is detectable in the blood within 1 to 2 weeks of infection.

Monocyte and macrophage cells become infected early, presenting HIV to CD4 cells, which alert B cells to produce antibody. The production of HIV antibodies is referred to as seroconversion. Seroconversion occurs an average of 6 to 12 weeks after infection, but in rare cases it can take as long as a year or longer.

Shortly after exposure and infection, the level of virus in the blood drops, largely through CD8 control and FDC trapping of the virus in the lymph nodes. The amount of virus present after the initial burst and the immune control that follows is called the viral setpoint. The viral setpoint reflects a balance reached between the virus and the immune system, a balance that usually is maintained for years. The viral setpoint is known to predict survival. Mellors and colleagues (1995) found that 62% of those with a viral setpoint above 36,270 copies/ml developed AIDS within 5 years, whereas of those with a setpoint below 4530 copies/ml, only 8% progressed within 5 years.

HIV infects cells of the nervous system, bone marrow, and lymphoid tissue. The clinical picture during primary infection can vary greatly (Box 16-1). However, approximately 80% of those infected experience a viral-like illness that may last 1 to 4 weeks. The severity of symptoms during this time also is thought to be an indicator of the prognosis, with more severe symptoms correlating with faster progression (Pederson et al, 1989).

**Clinical latency.** A period of **clinical latency** generally follows the acute events of primary infection. It may begin as early as 12 weeks after infection and may last longer than 10 years. This phase is characterized by a cycle of continuous viral replication and chronic immune activation. Immune activation provides a constant supply of new, susceptible targets for viral replication in the form of uninfected but activated T cells. Even though no obvious signs of infection may be seen during this time, viral replication continues at a constant rate in the lymph nodes. Early seeding of monocyte and macrophage cells also creates a long-term reservoir for replicating virus. As mentioned ear-

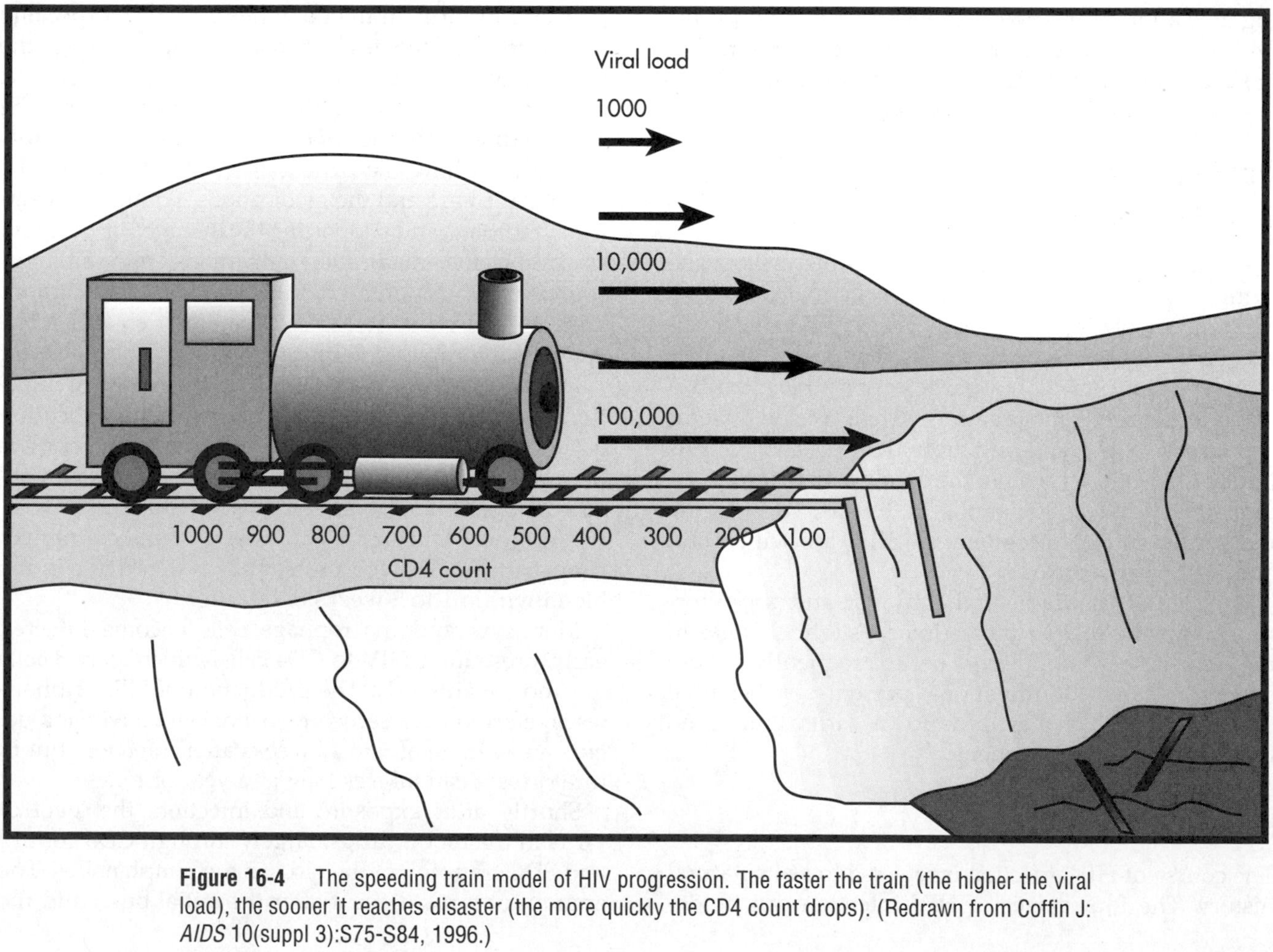

---

**BOX 16-1**

## SIGNS AND SYMPTOMS OF PRIMARY HIV INFECTION

| MOST COMMON | LESS COMMON |
|---|---|
| • Fever | • Anorexia |
| • Rash | • Nausea |
| • Fatigue | • Vomiting |
| • Sore throat | • Diarrhea |
| • Body aches | • Oral ulcers |
| • Lymphadenopathy (swollen lymph glands) | • Oral candidiasis (thrush) |

---

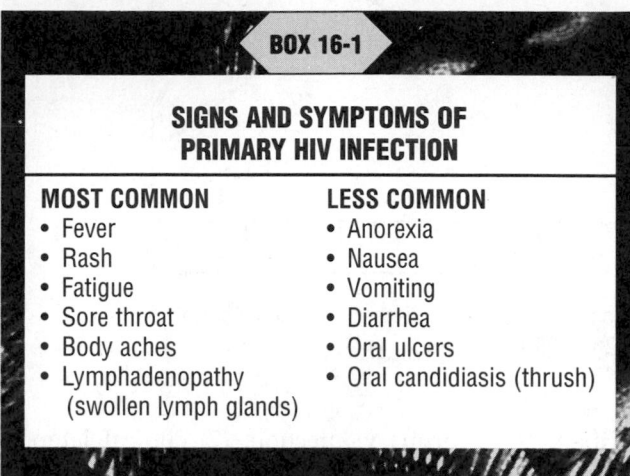

**Figure 16-4** The speeding train model of HIV progression. The faster the train (the higher the viral load), the sooner it reaches disaster (the more quickly the CD4 count drops). (Redrawn from Coffin J: *AIDS* 10(suppl 3):S75-S84, 1996.)

lier, infected macrophages contribute to the infection of new CD4 cells through their normal presentation of antigens to CD4 cells.

As T cells pass through the lymph system during the normal course of the day, they are continuously exposed to and infected with the virus. Within a few months of infection, 5 to 10 times more virus is found in the lymphoid tissue than in the peripheral blood. Infected individuals may develop persistent general lymphadenopathy (PGL), which can last for years, as a result of the vigorous activity occurring in the lymph nodes.

Increased secretion of some cytokines and depletion of others contribute to progression during this phase.

Even when a patient is asymptomatic, the level of virus in the blood may range from undetectable to hundreds of thousands. The CD4 cell count generally is over 500 in this phase of infection, but each time the viral life cycle occurs in a CD4 lymphocyte, the CD4 cell dies, resulting in a gradual decline in the number of these cells. Ho (1996) has identified the time interval between infection of a new cell and its death as about 53 hours (2.2 days). Monitoring the amount of virus in the plasma (the viral load) during this stage of infection is important because maintaining undetectable or low levels of virus can forestall progression to the next stage of infection (Mellors et al, 1996). Viral load measurements also provide a guide for predicting progression because the amount of virus in the blood correlates with the destruction and decline of T cells. The analogy of a train speeding down a track has been used to underscore the relationship of the virus and the rate of T cell loss (Coffin, 1996). In this model, the amount of virus determines the speed of the train, and the number of T cells left represents the nearness of the train to destruction (Figure 16-4).

**Symptomatic HIV disease.** Eventually viral replication in the lymph nodes destroys the lymph node structure, and large amounts of virus are released back into the plasma. Lymphadenopathy disappears as the lymph nodes are destroyed. The destruction of the lymph node architecture severely cripples the body's ability to mount an immune response. As viral replication continues and the viral load climbs, the immune system's ability to maintain effective control of the virus diminishes. The numbers of CD4 and CD8 cells also steadily decline. All these factors contribute to an increasing inability by the body to protect itself from infection.

During this phase the viral strain actually may become more virulent or powerful. Infected cells may begin to infect uninfected cells by fusing to the CD4 receptor on the outside of a cell, forming one large, infected cell. This process, by which a few infected cells infect a large number of cells, is called syncytia formation, and it results in the death of all cells involved. The virus generally is not able to cause syncy-

tia formation early in the disease but may switch to a syncytia-forming virus later.

After years of assault on the immune system, the virus begins to take a clinical toll. Symptoms begin to appear when the CD4 count falls between 200/mm$^3$ and 500/mm$^3$ (Figure 16-5). These symptoms may include oral candidiasis, oral hairy leukoplakia, shingles, and chronic lymphadenopathy. Lean body muscle mass may be depleted despite a normal appearance and normal body weight.

**Acquired immunodeficiency syndrome.** The actual loss of the body's ability to continue making a stable population of T cells is not completely understood. A variety of mechanisms probably contribute to the demise of the T-cell replenishing system. As the viral load increases and the number of T cells falls to a dangerously

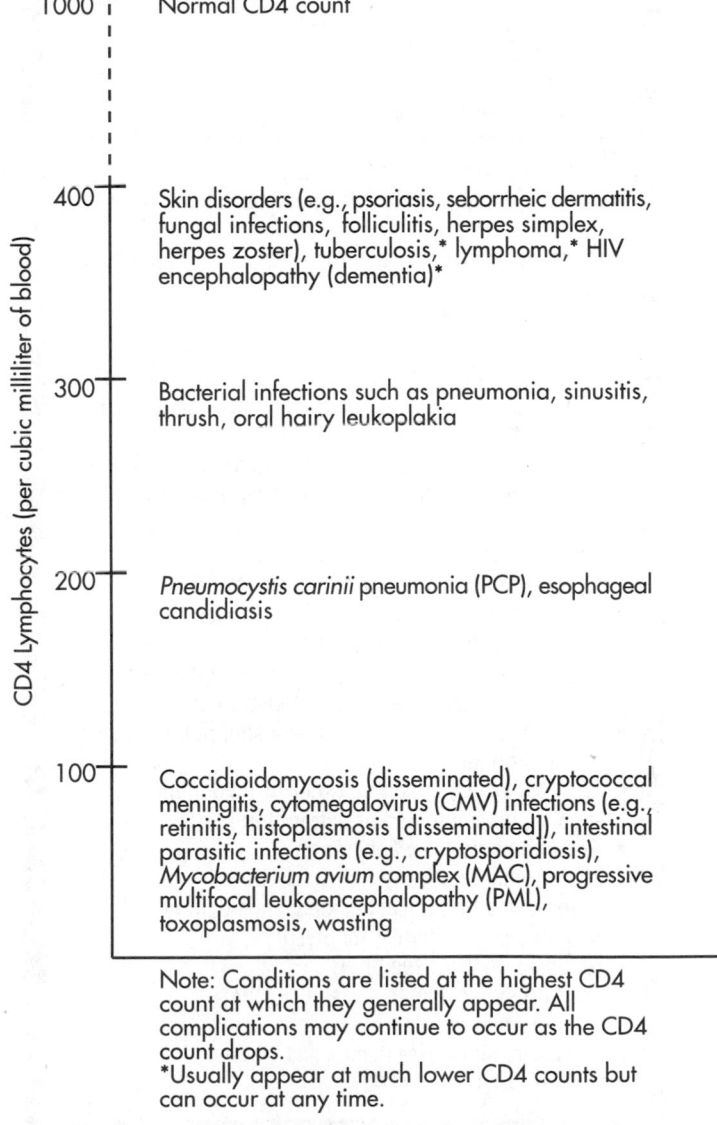

Figure 16-5  Risk of HIV-related complications based on CD4 cell count.

low level, patients become susceptible to opportunistic infections. An **opportunistic infection** is an infection that takes the opportunity to strike individuals without an intact immune system. The CDC has set the criteria for the diagnosis of AIDS. Box 16-2 presents a list of AIDS-defining conditions that meet these criteria. The diagnosis of AIDS can be made only when at least one AIDS-defining illness occurs. Most AIDS-defining illnesses do not occur until the CD4 count is less than $200/mm^3$; however, several of these conditions may be seen earlier. (Also see AIDS-Defining Conditions and

---

**BOX 16-2**

### AIDS-DEFINING CONDITIONS

By CDC criteria, the diagnosis of AIDS can be made only if at least one AIDS-defining condition occurs.

- Candidiasis of bronchi, trachea, or lungs
- Candidiasis, esophageal
- CD4 cell count <$200/mm^3$ in an individual with HIV
- Cervical cancer, invasive
- Coccidioidomycosis, disseminated or extrapulmonary
- Cryptococcosis, extrapulmonary
- Cryptosporidiosis, chronic intestinal (over 1 month's duration)
- Cytomegalovirus disease (other than liver, spleen, or nodes)
- Cytomegalovirus retinitis (with loss of vision)
- Encephalopathy, HIV related
- Herpes simplex: one or more chronic ulcers (over 1 month's duration) or bronchitis, pneumonitis, or esophagitis
- Histoplasmosis, disseminated or extrapulmonary
- Isosporiasis, chronic intestinal (over 1 month's duration)
- Kaposi's sarcoma
- Lymphoma, Burkitt's (or equivalent term)
- Lymphoma, immunoblastic (or equivalent term)
- Lymphoma, primary, of the brain
- *Mycobacterium avium* complex or *Mycobacterium kansasii*, disseminated or extrapulmonary
- *Mycobacterium tuberculosis*, any site, pulmonary or extrapulmonary
- *Mycobacterium* infection, other or unidentified species, disseminated or extrapulmonary
- *Pneumocystis carinii* pneumonia
- Pneumonia, recurrent
- Progressive multifocal leukoencephalopathy
- *Salmonella* septicemia, recurrent
- Toxoplasmosis of the brain
- Wasting syndrome as a result of HIV

From Centers for Disease Control and Prevention (CDC): *MMWR* 44(RR-17):1-19, 1993.

---

Opportunistic Infections, p. 370.) Nursing considerations for patients with AIDS are presented in Box 16-3.

*Long-term nonprogressors and exposed uninfected individuals.* Approximately 5% to 10% of people infected with HIV appear to progress slowly or not at all. Slow progression is defined as 10 to 15 years of infection, no symptoms, and a stable CD4 count. Certain factors have been identified that appear to correlate with slowly progressing HIV infection (Panateleo et al, 1995). Individuals who progress slowly generally have an effective CD8 response, a low viral burden, intact lymph node architecture, little activation of immune system cells, and a non-syncytia-forming viral strain.

Recently several additional sites of viral attachment on the CD4 molecule were identified. Two of these receptor sites, CCR-5 and CXCR-4, have been implicated as having a role in HIV transmission and disease progression. The CCR-5 molecule is thought to be necessary for the virus to gain entry into the cell. Therefore, it is postulated that a defective CCR-5 molecule on an individual's CD4, CD8, and monocyte cells makes that individual immune to infection. Several such individuals have been identified in research studies; they are known as exposed uninfected persons because they remain HIV negative despite repeated exposure to the virus. The CXCR-4 molecule is thought to be necessary to syncytia formation and more rapid progression. Therefore individuals who have the CXCR-4 molecule on their CD4 cells tend to be more rapid progressors (Eron, 1997).

## CLINICAL MANIFESTATIONS OF HIV INFECTION AND AIDS

This section has been divided into Clinical Manifestations of Symptomatic HIV Disease (conditions that may occur when the CD4 count is between $200/mm^3$ and $500/mm^3$) and AIDS-Defining Conditions and Opportunistic Infections. It is difficult to summarize all the conditions that may occur in HIV disease because people with HIV are subject to every infirmity to which the general population is vulnerable. The first and foremost thing the nurse must remember is that the patient is a human being, and having HIV does not mean that every ailment will be strange and unusual. Few illnesses are unique to HIV disease. Even most AIDS-defining illnesses at times infect HIV-negative people.

Also, the HIV-related conditions cannot all be assigned a particular CD4 count. It generally can be said that most AIDS-defining illnesses occur at lower CD4 counts (usually under $100/mm^3$). But for many conditions, there is no magic number above which the condition never occurs and below which it always occurs. The nurse must keep these considerations in mind when reading about HIV and while caring for HIV-positive patients.

Nurses care for patients in many stages of HIV infection. Some patients may have just learned that they have HIV. The illnesses that brought them into medical care may be the first clinical manifestation of HIV they have had. Thus these patients may be dealing with the enormity of an HIV diagnosis at the same time their bodies are fighting a serious infection such as pneumonia or meningitis. Once the medical crisis is over, a social services or psychiatric consult may be appropriate for such a patient. The nurse also may be caring for a patient who has known for years that he or she is HIV positive but who is just now facing the first

---

◁ **BOX 16-3** ▷              **NURSING PROCESS**

## PATIENT WITH AIDS

### ASSESSMENT

- General appearance
- Signs and symptoms of infection
- Knowledge of disease, transmission, and complications
- Nutritional status (weight, serum albumin, stomatitis)
- Coping mechanisms
- Social support
- Tolerance to activity
- Respiratory status
- Oral mucosa (for lesions or ulcers)
- Musculoskeletal system (for muscle wasting, weakness)

### NURSING DIAGNOSES

- Powerlessness related to poor prognosis and perceived lack of control
- Risk for infection related to inadequate immune system
- Social isolation related to stigma attached to AIDS diagnosis
- Altered nutrition: less than body requirements related to loss of appetite, oral discomfort, or high metabolic needs
- Activity intolerance related to weakness, fatigue, and malnutrition
- Knowledge deficit related to new condition

### NURSING INTERVENTIONS

- Reduce the stigma of isolation by respecting the patient's dignity; encourage the patient to express his or her feelings of isolation; provide feedback and support.
- Assure the patient and significant others that AIDS does not spread by ordinary physical contact; encourage casual interaction.
- Assess and chart behaviors indicative of social isolation; confer with other experts to establish a plan to reduce social isolation; specify plan; make local and national support groups or hot lines available

to the patient (AIDS information number: 1-800-342-AIDS).
- Explain the rationale for protective isolation to the patient and family; encourage telephone contact with significant others.
- Monitor and document food intake; confer with the health care provider about the need for supplements, tube feeding, and total parenteral nutrition; develop the meal plan with the patient (meal schedules, eating environment, likes, dislikes, food temperature); encourage high-protein, high-carbohydrate foods.
- Assess oral mucous membranes q 8 hr and provide appropriate interventions to ease pain.
- Weigh the patient every other day.
- Provide for periods of rest by scheduling treatments, minimizing room noise, and limiting visitors.
- Instruct the patient in energy-saving techniques and improving nutritional status to increase activity tolerance; encourage progressive activity as tolerated; assess pulse, respiration, blood pressure, presence of dyspnea, cyanosis, and pain as indicators of overexertion.
- Assist the patient with hygiene as needed.

### EVALUATION OF EXPECTED OUTCOMES

- Free of opportunistic infections
- Verbalizes factors that may increase risk of infection
- Verbalizes a decrease in loneliness and sense of isolation
- Maintains relationships with significant others
- Maintains a desirable weight
- Tolerates prescribed diet
- Has healthy gums and oral mucous membranes
- Demonstrates ability to alternate activity with appropriate rest periods
- Verbalizes increased comfort while performing activities

serious illness arising from the disease; or for a patient who has been in and out of the hospital with various infirmities; or for one who is HIV positive but essentially well—all these patients are people, and they must be treated with compassion and respect by their health care providers.

## Clinical Manifestations of Symptomatic HIV Disease

Clinical manifestations of symptomatic HIV disease may occur with a CD4 count of 200/mm³ to 500/mm³.

### Bacterial Infections

Bacterial pneumonias are so common in HIV disease that in 1993 the CDC added recurrent pneumonia as a criterion for defining AIDS (two or more episodes in 1 year) (CDC, 1993a). *Streptococcus pneumoniae, Haemophilus influenzae*, and *Staphylococcus aureus* are the usual etiologic agents (Sande, Volberding, 1997). The nurse should obtain vital signs, especially temperature, respiratory and heart rates, and at least a baseline pulse oximetry in any patient who has a cough. Bacterial pneumonias are treated with antibiotics, but the patient may have a prolonged, severe, and recurrent illness.

**Nursing implications.** It is particularly important in preventing pneumococcal pneumonia that *all* HIV-positive patients receive the pneumococcal vaccine (Pneumovax) as early as possible in the course of HIV infection.

Sinusitis is common in HIV disease, causing frontal or maxillary headache, nasal congestion, nasal drainage and postnasal drip. It is treated with antibiotics but may require a longer than usual course of medication (Zurlo et al, 1992).

### Dermatologic Manifestations

(Also see Dermatologic Conditions, p. 371.)

As was indicated earlier, HIV-positive individuals are subject to every illness that affects the rest of the population, and this is probably most true for dermatologic conditions. An HIV-positive individual often has chronic and severe forms of common skin conditions, which worsen as the CD4 count drops.

Drug reactions, particularly to the sulfonamides and penicillins, occur often in HIV disease. Any new rash should be evaluated with this diagnosis in mind. The patient's medication regimen should be reviewed for any new drugs and to determine if the patient is taking any sulfa drugs or penicillins. Such rashes usually are generalized, erythematous, and maculopapular, as well as quite pruritic. The rash is treated by withdrawing the causative medication. Antihistamines often are adequate pharmacologic treatment.

**Folliculitis.** Folliculitis can occur in both HIV-positive and HIV-negative individuals. The disorder, a follicular inflammation or infection usually caused by *S. aureus*, responds to antibiotics such as the cephalosporins. *S. aureus* can cause other skin infections as well, such as impetigo and cellulitis. An intensely pruritic form of folliculitis called *eosinophilic folliculitis* is unique to HIV. It is not caused by *S. aureus*. With eosinophilic folliculitis, a skin biopsy shows inflammation and the presence of eosinophils. The etiology of eosinophilic folliculitis is unknown, and treatment varies. Antihistamines, emollients, oatmeal baths, topical corticosteroids, itraconazole, ultraviolet light therapy with oral psoralen (PUVA), permethrin cream, and isotretinoin all have been used, with varying degrees of success.

**Topical fungal and yeast infections.** Tinea versicolor manifests as slightly scaly, hyperpigmented or hypopigmented macules that usually are more visible during the summer months, when the surrounding skin tans. It usually is asymptomatic but can be a cosmetic concern to the patient. Tinea pedis (athlete's foot) and tinea cruris (jock itch) are quite pruritic, usually erythematous and, particularly on the feet, scaly. All these conditions are treated with topical antifungal creams or lotions. Systemic antifungal agents may be required in cases of severe topical infection. The nurse should instruct the patient to keep the affected area dry and to continue treatment for 1 to 3 weeks (depending on the thickness of the skin in the treated area) after the rash has cleared up. As the epithelium normally sloughs off, the medication continues to treat the newly exposed layers of skin. (Also see HIV in Women, p. 379.)

**Herpes simplex virus.** Herpes simplex virus (HSV) can cause ulcerative lesions, primarily in the oral cavity and on the genitals (see Genital Tract Manifestations, p. 368; Oral Manifestations, p. 369; Esophagitis, p. 371; and HIV in Women, p. 379).

**Molluscum contagiosum.** Molluscum contagiosum is a viral infection that can cause small, scattered, umbilicated papules (having a small central depression). usually on the face but sometimes in the perianal and genital areas. These papules may be asymptomatic or pruritic. They can be treated with cryosurgery but may recur. Corticosteroid creams may be prescribed to relieve itching.

**Nails.** Dermatophytes (fungal parasites) can cause onychomycosis, a fungal infection that causes thickening and sometimes yellowing of the nails, which may crumble at the tips. Hyperpigmented blue or black horizontal bands may appear on the nails as a harmless side effect of zidovudine (AZT). This condition is more common in dark-skinned people and generally is reversible if AZT is withdrawn (Casey, Cohen, Hughes, 1996). Similar hyperpigmented macules may appear in the mouth (buccal mucosa, gingiva, and tongue).

***Nursing implications.*** Onychomycosis can be cosmetically bothersome to patients. It can be treated with a long course of systemic antifungal medications, but often the decision is made not to treat the condition because resistance to these medications can develop as a result of prolonged exposure. This can have serious implications for the future because not only the dermatophytes, but also the small population of *Candida* organisms normally present in the gastrointestinal (GI) tract (in everyone), can develop resistance. If the patient later develops esophageal candidiasis, his or her "native" *Candida* species may already be resistant to the best available medication. For this reason, treatment for onychomycosis often is deferred. Some patients prefer to cover their nails with nail polish or to keep their nails trimmed very short.

**Prurigo nodularis.** Prurigo nodularis is a dermatologic condition of unknown origin. It causes intense, widespread pruritus (itching) with the formation of excoriations and papules or nodules on the skin. The condition is difficult to treat. First-line treatment consists of emollients or antihistamines (or both) for itching. If this approach is unsuccessful, small doses of oral steroids (e.g., 15 mg of prednisone) sometimes give some relief.

**Pruritus.** Pruritus is extremely common in HIV disease and often is exacerbated by xerosis (abnormally dry skin). The nurse should inquire about this and suggest that the patient use emollients, oatmeal baths, and other strategies for hydrating the skin. The nurse should make sure that the patient is not bathing more than once a day because frequent hot baths or showers can remove natural oils from the skin, exacerbating pruritus.

**Psoriasis.** Psoriasis is a chronic skin condition that causes scaly patches to form, typically in the scalp and on the extensor surfaces of the elbows and knees. The lesions can be quite erythematous, and the scales may have a silvery appearance. Patients who are HIV positive may have widespread, more severe psoriasis. Cure is not always possible, but treatment can afford some improvement. Topical corticosteroids are the cornerstone of therapy; other treatments may include topical coal tar solution, anthralin cream, ultraviolet light therapy (UVB), PUVA, etretinate, and methotrexate (Sauer, Hall, 1997).

**Scabies.** Scabies also is not unique to HIV infection. Scabies is caused by a mite, *Sarcoptes scabiei*, which burrows into the skin. The fecal pellets of these mites cause intense itching, which usually is worse at night and when the patient is hot (e.g., during a hot shower).

The condition appears as tiny red papules, usually excoriated, on the trunk and extremities; the papules may cluster in the axillae and groin (Sauer, Hall, 1997). The mites' burrows (thin, linear ridges less than 1 cm long) may be seen in the web spaces between the fingers and toes; these burrows are considered diagnostic of scabies. Several scabicides are available for treatment. Lindane (Kwell) and permethrin (Elimite) are the ones most commonly used.

***Nursing implications.*** Scabicides must be applied and left on overnight. A toothbrush should be used to apply the lotion under the nails. When the cream is washed off the next morning, freshly laundered clothes must be put on and all clothes, linens, and towels must be washed in hot water and dried in a hot dryer. Patients should be informed that the pruritus may not resolve for 1 to 2 weeks. A second application usually is not needed. Scabies generally is spread by direct skin-to-skin contact, although it can survive for short periods on fomites (hence the rationale for washing sheets and towels). Close household contacts should be examined. Because it may take a month before an infected person develops symptoms, some health care providers routinely treat all members of a household.

**Seborrheic dermatitis.** Seborrheic dermatitis causes dry, greasy scales on the scalp and in the eyebrows and nasolabial folds on the face. It generally responds well to topical corticosteroids. Because the yeast *Pityrosporum ovale* has been implicated in seborrheic dermatitis, an antifungal shampoo (e.g., ketoconazole shampoo) with or without a topical corticosteroid often is beneficial.

**Herpes zoster.** Varicella-zoster virus (VZV, or herpes zoster), which is common to all populations, causes an eruption of painful red vesicles in an dermatomal distribution (dermatomes are areas of skin innervated by a particular segment of the spinal cord). The appearance of vesicles often is preceded by a prodrome of pain in the affected dermatome for 1 or 2 days. This infection, commonly called shingles, is a reactivation of a previous VZV infection, chickenpox.

Herpes zoster should be treated with acyclovir or a similar drug (e.g., famciclovir). Analgesics are almost always required because shingles usually is exquisitely painful. The patient should keep the lesions clean to prevent secondary bacterial infection and as dry as possible. Patients should avoid contact with others who have not had chickenpox because a minute risk exists that VZV can become aerosolized and transmitted from zoster lesions to a person who has no varicella antibodies, causing chickenpox. Herpes zoster can cause postherpetic neuralgia, meaning the patient suffers unremitting pain in the affected dermatome for days, months, or sometimes even years after the acute infection has resolved. Postherpetic neuralgia may respond to treatment with acetaminophen, nonsteroidal antiinflammatory drugs (NSAIDs), tricyclic antidepressants such as amitriptyline, antiseizure drugs, and other medications. Narcotic analgesics are avoided if possible in the management of chronic pain.

*Nursing implications.* In the course of providing care to a patient with shingles, the nurse should always wear gloves. If the nurse has small breaks in his or her skin, direct contact with oozing lesions can result in transmission of VZV to the nurse.

**Nursing implications for dermatologic care of the HIV-positive patient.** Remember that HIV-positive patients must tolerate a great deal of ignorance on the part of people with whom they come in contact. This ignorance often takes the form of fear of touching the HIV-positive person. *HIV is not transmitted through touching.* The nurse should wear gloves only if there is a possibility of contact with bodily fluids. When caring for a patient whose skin is not intact because of dermatitis, it is appropriate for the nurse to wear gloves. If the skin is not broken, the nurse need not wear gloves when caring for a dermatology patient.

## Gastrointestinal Manifestations

Men and women who practice receptive anal intercourse are at risk for a variety of anorectal infections caused by bacteria, parasites, viruses, or yeast (*Candida albicans*). Bacterial infections can be caused by *Chlamydia trachomatis* (lymphogranuloma venereum) or *Neisseria gonorrhoeae* (gonorrhea). Infecting viruses include HSV and human papillomavirus (HPV). All these can occur at any level of the CD4 count. Treatment depends on the causative organism.

**Diarrhea.** Diarrhea that occurs when the CD4 count is over $100/mm^3$ probably is caused by a pathogen that could affect anyone regardless of HIV status. Such pathogens comprise bacterial, parasitic, and viral organisms. Bacterial organisms include *Shigella, Salmonella, Campylobacter,* and *Clostridium difficile* species. *Giardia* organisms cause the most common parasitic infection. The agents that usually cause self-limited viral gastroenteritis are rotavirus and Norwalk virus. Lactose intolerance also can cause chronic intermittent diarrhea, and patients should be asked about their intake of dairy foods. The diagnosis of diarrhea hinges on proper collection of several stool specimens, and treatment, of course, depends on the diagnosis.

*Nursing implications.* Nonspecific treatment for diarrhea includes maintaining a good fluid intake, eliminating aggravating foods or supplements, and possibly pharmacologic treatment as well (e.g., kaopectate, loperamide [Imodium], or atropine sulfate/diphe-

**BOX 16-4**

### Guidelines for Easy Interpretation of Hepatitis Serologies

| Serologic factor | Meaning |
|---|---|
| Hepatitis B surface antigen (HBsAg) | Positive result means that the patient is newly infected with acute hepatitis B *or* if HBsAg is positive for 3 months, the patient is a chronic carrier and at risk for chronic active hepatitis B. In acute infection, HBsAg usually is positive in the blood for 1 to 2 weeks before and for 2 months after clinical symptoms appear. Persistently elevated liver enzymes indicate that the patient has chronic active hepatitis B. |
| Hepatitis B core antibody (HBcAb, anti-HBc) | *Not to be confused with hepatitis C antibody (HCVAB).* HBcAb tests positive after HBsAg and coincides with onset of clinical symptoms of hepatitis. Levels usually decline to undetectable over the course of a year. HBcAb sometimes is useful in diagnosing acute infection in the "window period" during which HBsAg already is negative but HBsAb has not yet become positive. |
| Hepatitis B surface antibody (HBsAb, anti-HBs) | Positive result means that the patient has had hepatitis B or hepatitis B vaccine in the past and is immune. |
| Hepatitis C antibody (HCVAB, anti-HC) | *Not to be confused with HBcAb.* Positive result means the patient has acute hepatitis C or has had hepatitis C in the past. Hepatitis C testing is not as sophisticated as that for hepatitis B and there is no way to know if an individual is a chronic carrier; therefore it must be assumed that all who are HCVAB positive are carriers. If liver enzymes remain elevated, the patient probably has chronic active hepatitis C, although chronic active hepatitis C disease may be present even if liver enzymes are not elevated. |

noxylate hydrochloride [Lomotil]) (Andrews, Novick, 1995).

**Hepatitis.** Hepatitis B virus (HBV) and hepatitis C virus (HCV) are transmitted in the same way as HIV and consequently often coexist with HIV (Spencer, Ross, 1996). Care for patients with active viral hepatitis is directed toward management of symptoms (see Chapter 14). Exactly how viral hepatitis and HIV affect each other is unclear. Some patients with a history of hepatitis B become chronic carriers, and all patients with hepatitis C should be considered chronic carriers. (See Box 16-4 for guidance in determining if patients are chronic carriers based on their hepatitis serologies.) Patients with hepatitis B or C or who have a history of hepatitis are at risk of developing chronic active hepatitis (CAH); this risk is much greater with hepatitis C than with hepatitis B.

Chronic active hepatitis B or C can lead to cirrhosis and liver cancer. CAH can be treated with interferon-alpha (IF-alpha). IF-alpha normalizes liver enzymes in about one third of patients who are hepatitis B positive but HIV negative (Barker, Randol, Zieve, 1995). Treatment of chronic active hepatitis C with IF-alpha results in normal liver enzymes in 15% to 20% of patients who are hepatitis C positive but HIV negative (Dusheiko et al, 1996). Whether treatment with IF-alpha is beneficial in the presence of HIV infection is still a matter of debate. Some clinicians recommend a trial of IF-alpha for patients coinfected with HIV and HCV. IF-alpha must be given three times a week for 4 months for hepatitis B and for 6 months for hepatitis C, and it is not well tolerated (Table 16-2).

**Malabsorption.** Malabsorption occurs when HIV infects the cells of the intestinal villi, impairing their

*Text continued on page 368.*

## TABLE 16-2

## Pharmacology of Drugs Used in HIV Infection and AIDS

| DRUG (GENERIC AND TRADE NAME); ROUTE AND DOSAGE | ACTION/INDICATION | COMMON SIDE EFFECTS AND NURSING CONSIDERATIONS |
|---|---|---|
| **Acyclovir** (Zovirax) **Route:** PO, Topical, IV (rare) **Dosage:** For genital herpes 200 mg q 4 hr (5 times daily) for 10 days; for recurrent herpes 400 mg bid-tid maintenance; for herpes zoster 800 mg q 4 hr (5 times daily) for 7-10 days; for chickenpox (pediatric and adult) 20 mg/kg (not to exceed 800 mg/dose) qid for 5 days | Antiviral used in the prophylaxis and management of genital herpes and herpes zoster; also used for chickenpox; has been associated with longer survival in those with HIV disease | Generally well tolerated, but some patients may have nausea, vomiting, headache, diarrhea, itching, rash, and hives; dose must be adjusted with renal impairment |
| **Amphotericin B** (Fungizone) **Route:** Topical, PO **Dosage:** Give initial test dose of 1 mg PO and observe for reaction; continue with dosage of 0.25 mg/kg slowly; increase daily dosage slowly to 0.5 mg/kg (can give up to 1 mg/kg or 1.5 mg/kg every other day); topical 2-4 times daily | Antifungal used to treat multiple yeast and fungal infections in HIV/AIDS | Anemia, anorexia, fever, chills, headache, hypotension, hypokalemia, dyspepsia, nausea, vomiting, diarrhea, cramping, epigastric pain, muscle and joint pain, paresthesia, seizures, nephrotoxicity, tachypnea, leukopenia, thrombocytopenia; use with caution in patients with renal impairment and electrolyte abnormalities; drug is very irritating to tissues, and site must be monitored |
| **Atovaquone** (Mepron) **Route:** PO **Dosage:** 750 mg tid | Antiprotozoal used for mild to moderate cases of PCP; also used to treat toxoplasmosis | Rash, nausea, diarrhea, headache, vomiting, fever, insomnia, asthenia, pruritus, anemia, increased liver enzymes (LFTs), hyponatremia; must be taken with food; fatty food best increases absorption |

*bid,* Twice daily; *CMV,* cytomegalovirus; *DS,* double-strength tablet; *GI,* gastrointestinal; *IV,* intravenous; *MAC, Mycobacterium avium* complex; *NRTI,* nucleoside reverse transcriptase inhibitor; *NNRTI,* nonnucleoside reverse transcriptase inhibitor; *PCP, Pneumocystis carinii* pneumonia; *PI,* protease inhibitor; *PO,* oral; *qhs,* hourly; *qid,* four times a day; *RBCs,* red blood cells; *SC,* subcutaneous; *SOB,* shortness of breath; *SS,* single-strength tablet; *tid,* three times a day; *TMP-SMX,* trimethoprim-sulfamethoxazole; *WBCs,* white blood cells. *Continued*

**TABLE 16-2**

## Pharmacology of Drugs Used in HIV Infection and AIDS—cont'd

| DRUG (GENERIC AND TRADE NAME); ROUTE AND DOSAGE | ACTION/INDICATION | COMMON SIDE EFFECTS AND NURSING CONSIDERATIONS |
|---|---|---|
| **Clarithromycin** (Biaxin)<br>**Route:** PO<br>**Dosage:** 250-500 mg q 12 hr | Antibiotic used for some upper and lower respiratory tract infections, including bronchitis and pneumonia; also used in MAC treatment and prophylaxis | Diarrhea, vomiting, nausea, dyspepsia, taste changes, abdominal pain and discomfort, headache; use with caution in patients with severe liver and renal impairment |
| **Dapsone** (Avlosulfon)<br>**Route:** PO<br>**Dosage:** 50-100 mg/day or 100 mg 2-3 times a week | Antibiotic/antiprotozoal originally used for leprosy; now also used for prophylaxis against PCP | Nausea, vomiting, abdominal pain, pancreatitis; severe anemia resulting from hemolysis at doses over 100 mg/day in patients with G6PD deficiency; drug should be taken 1 hr before or 2 hr after didanosine (the buffer in didanosine reduces absorption); antacids should not be taken for 1-2 hr after taking dapsone; use with caution in patients with anemia or renal or liver disease |
| **Delavirdine** (Rescriptor)<br>**Route:** PO<br>**Dosage:** 400 mg tid | Antiretroviral; NNRTI used in combination therapy against HIV | Rash; must be taken on an empty stomach with no other medications; avoid alcohol |
| **Didanosine** (ddI, Videx)<br>**Route:** PO<br>**Dosage:** >60 kg: 200 mg bid<br>        <60 kg: 125 mg bid | Antiretroviral; NRTI used against HIV | Pancreatitis, peripheral neuropathy, nausea, diarrhea; patients often do not like the taste, but powdered form can be mixed into cold juice; must be taken on an empty stomach; reduces ganciclovir level by 20% |
| **Erythropoietin** (EPO, Epogen, Procrit)<br>**Route:** SC, IV<br>**Dosage:** 50-100 U/kg 3 times a week | Naturally occurring hormone that stimulates bone marrow to produce RBCs; used to treat anemia secondary to bone marrow suppression | Hypertension, headache, arthralgia, nausea, edema, fever, fatigue, diarrhea, vomiting, chest pain, asthenia, rash, SOB, dizziness, iron deficiency anemia; should not be used in patients with uncontrolled hypertension; EPO is not effective if anemia is caused by iron deficiency, infection, or blood loss |
| **Filgrastim** (granulocyte colony-stimulating factor, neupogen, G-CSF)<br>**Route:** SC, IV<br>**Dosage:** 100-300 $\mu$g 3 times a week (based on WBC count) | Growth factor used to stimulate bone marrow to make WBCs | Bone pain, elevated alkaline phosphatase |
| **Fluconazole** (Diflucan)<br>**Route:** PO, IV<br>**Dosage:** 100-400 mg/day | Antifungal used for prophylaxis and treatment of multiple yeast and fungal infections ins HIV/AIDS | Nausea, headache, rash, vomiting, abdominal pain, diarrhea; hepatotoxicity and exfoliative skin disorders are less common; rare cases of anaphylaxis have been reported; when used in combination with oral hypoglycemic agents may increase the risk of low glucose levels; use with caution in patients with renal and liver impairment |
| **Folinic Acid** (leucovorin calcium)<br>**Route:** PO, IM, IV<br>**Dosage:** 10-20 mg qd | Vitamin given to prevent aplastic anemia in patients taking pyrimethamine | Thrombocytosis, allergic reactions; use with caution in patients with renal failure |

| TABLE 16-2 | | |
| --- | --- | --- |

## Pharmacology of Drugs Used in HIV Infection and AIDS—cont'd

| DRUG (GENERIC AND TRADE NAME); ROUTE AND DOSAGE | ACTION/INDICATION | COMMON SIDE EFFECTS AND NURSING CONSIDERATIONS |
| --- | --- | --- |
| **Foscarnet** (Foscavir)<br>**Route:** IV<br>**Dosage:** 60 mg/kg q 8 hr for 14-21 days, then 90-100 mg/kg/day maintenance | Antiviral used to treat CMV infections and for ganciclovir-resistant herpes infections | Nephrotoxicity, electrolyte imbalance, fever, seizures, nausea, anemia, diarrhea, vomiting, headache, bone marrow suppression, fatigue, rigors, asthenia, malaise, pain, paresthesia, dizziness, muscle contractions, anorexia, depression, confusion, anxiety, rash, sweating; must be injected by infusion pump to ensure slow infusion; patient must be well hydrated before infusion; **do not administer as a bolus infusion** |
| **Ganciclovir** (Cytovene, DHPG)<br>**Route:** IV, PO, Ocular Implant<br>**Dosage:** 5 mg/kg q 12 hr IV; PO 1 g tid; intraocular implant 1 $\mu$g/ml q mo | Antiviral used to treat CMV infections | Neutropenia, leukopenia, thrombocytopenia, anemia, fever, abdominal pain, chills, sepsis, diarrhea, nausea, anorexia, vomiting, neuropathy, paresthesia, rash, sweating, pruritus, vitreous disorders; ganciclovir elevates didanosine levels up to 70%, increasing the risk of pancreatic disease; oral ganciclovir is not as effective as IV administration but offers better quality of life; ganciclovir implants are very effective in the treatment of CMV retinitis but do not prevent CMV from spreading to other parts of the body; oral ganciclovir has been used in CMV prophylaxis |
| **Indinavir** (Crixivan)<br>**Route:** PO<br>**Dosage:** 800 mg q 8 hr | Antiretroviral; PI used against HIV | Nausea, vomiting, headache, nephrolithiasis, hyperbilirubinemia; must be taken on an empty stomach 1 hr apart from didanosine or with a light, low-fat snack; patient must drink at least 48 oz (6 cups) of water daily |
| **Interferon Alfa-2a** (Roferon-a)<br>**Route:** IM, SC<br>**Dosage:** 36 million IU for 10-12 wk (reduce dosage if severe adverse reactions occur) | Immune-based therapy used in the treatment of hepatitis B and C and AIDS-associated Kaposi's sarcoma | Dizziness, fatigue, fever, myalgia, headache, chills, arthralgia, anorexia, nausea, vomiting, diarrhea, abdominal pain, diminished mental status, depression, confusion, paresthesia, diaphoresis, visual disturbances, sleep disturbances, coughing, alopecia, rash, weight loss, altered taste, dry mouth, night sweats, neutropenia, leukopenia, anemia, thrombocytopenia, increased LFTs |
| **Isoniazid** (INH)<br>**Route:** PO, IM<br>**Dosage:** 5-10 mg/kg/day (usually 300 mg) or 15 mg/kg 2-3 times a week after 2 mo at 300 mg/day | Antitubercular used as a first-line drug in combination with other agents in the treatment of active TB; used for prevention of TB in patients exposed to the disease | Peripheral neuropathy, nausea, vomiting, aplastic anemia, fever, increased LFTs; must be taken on an empty stomach; do not take with antacids; use with caution in patients with hepatic impairment (e.g., chronic alcohol abuse, renal disease, malnutrition, diabetes); commonly prescribed with pyridoxine (vitamin $B_6$) to prevent isoniazid-induced peripheral neuropathy |
| **Itraconazole** (Sporanox)<br>**Route:** PO<br>**Dosage:** 200-400 mg/day | Antifungal used for prophylaxis and treatment of many yeast and fungal infections in HIV/AIDS | Nausea, vomiting, rash, headache, pruritus, diarrhea, elevated liver enzymes, hypertension; should be taken with food; do not take with antacids or $H_2$ antagonists; use with caution in patients with hepatic impairment |
| **Ketoconazole** (Nizoral)<br>**Route:** PO, Topical, Shampoo<br>**Dosage:** PO 200-400 mg/day; topical 2% 1-2 times daily; shampoo 3 times a week for 1 mo | Antifungal used for treatment of many yeast and fungal infections in HIV/AIDS | Nausea, vomiting, abdominal pain, pruritus, elevated LFTs; Use with caution in patients with hepatic impairment |

*Continued*

**TABLE 16-2**

## Pharmacology of Drugs Used in HIV Infection and AIDS—cont'd

| DRUG (GENERIC AND TRADE NAME); ROUTE AND DOSAGE | ACTION/INDICATION | COMMON SIDE EFFECTS AND NURSING CONSIDERATIONS |
|---|---|---|
| **Lamivudine** (Epivir, 3TC)<br>**Route:** PO<br>**Dosage:** 150 mg bid | Antiretroviral; NRTI used against HIV | Nausea, headache, neutropenia, musculoskeletal pain, peripheral neuropathy |
| **Nelfinavir** (Viracept)<br>**Route:** PO<br>**Dosage:** 750 mg tid | Antiretroviral; PI used against HIV | Diarrhea, nausea, flatulence, headache, asthenia, rash |
| **Nevirapine** (Viramune)<br>**Route:** PO<br>**Dosage:** 200 mg qd for 14 days, then 200 mg bid | Antiretroviral; NNRTI used against HIV | Rash, Stevens-Johnson syndrome, fever, headache, nausea, hepatitis; must be taken 1 hr apart from indinavir |
| **Nystatin** (Mycostatin)<br>**Route:** Oral suspension, intravaginal tablet<br>**Dosage:** Oral suspension 400,000-600,000 U 4 times daily (usually swish and swallow); vaginal tablets 1/day for 2 wk | Antifungal used in local treatment of candidal infections (e.g., thrush) | Generally well tolerated; suspension contains sugar and may promote development of caries; must be used with caution in patients with diabetes |
| **Pentamidine** (Nebupent)<br>**Route:** IV, Aerosolized<br>**Dosage:** IV 4 mg/kg once a day for 14-21 days (longer treatment may be required); inhaler via nebulizer 300 mg q 4 wk | Antiprotozoal used in the treatment and prophylaxis of PCP | Nausea, vomiting, renal impairment, hypoglycemia, hyperglycemia, pancreatitis, cough (aerosol), bad taste in the mouth, elevated LFTs, leukopenia, nausea, anorexia, hypotension, fever, rash, confusion, hallucinations, anemia; *aerosolized* pentamidine cannot treat or prevent extrapulmonary PCP |
| **Pyridoxine** (Vitamin $B_6$)<br>**Route:** PO, IM, IV<br>**Dosage:** 10-50 mg/day; if peripheral neuropathy already exists, higher doses will be needed | Water-soluble vitamin used for the treatment and prevention of isoniazid-induced peripheral neuropathy | Generally well tolerated |
| **Pyrimethamine** (Daraprim)<br>**Route:** PO<br>**Dosage:** 50-75 mg starting dose; cut in half after 1-3 wk | Antiprotozoal used in combination with a sulfonamide for the treatment and prophylaxis of toxoplasmosis | Hypersensitivity reaction, anorexia, vomiting, megaloblastic anemia, leukopenia, thrombocytopenia, atrophic glossitis, hematuria, arrhythmias; use with caution in patients taking phenytoin or who have underlying anemia, bone marrow suppression, or impaired liver or kidney function; should be given with folinic acid to prevent hemolytic anemia |
| **Rifabutin** (Mycobutin)<br>**Route:** PO<br>**Dosage:** 300 mg once a day; if GI upset occurs, may give 150 mg twice daily with food | Antimycobacterial used to prevent or treat MAC disease in patients with advanced HIV infection | Brown-orange discoloration of tears, saliva, urine, and other bodily fluids; rash, leukopenia, anorexia, diarrhea, dyspepsia, nausea, vomiting, abdominal pain, eructation, fever, headache, myalgia, altered taste, neutropenia, thrombocytopenia, eosinophilia, increased liver enzymes; contraindicated in patients with active TB; patient should be warned in advance about discoloration of bodily fluids |

**TABLE 16-2**

## Pharmacology of Drugs Used in HIV Infection and AIDS—cont'd

| DRUG (GENERIC AND TRADE NAME); ROUTE AND DOSAGE | ACTION/INDICATION | COMMON SIDE EFFECTS AND NURSING CONSIDERATIONS |
|---|---|---|
| **Rifampin** (Rifadin) **Route:** PO, IV **Dosage:** 600 mg/day; may also be given 2-3 times a week | Antimycobacterial used in combination with other agents in the management of active TB or MAC; may be used to prevent TB in those exposed to the disease who cannot tolerate isoniazid | Nausea, vomiting, heartburn, abdominal pain, flatulence, diarrhea, brown-orange discoloration of tears, saliva, urine, and other bodily fluids; hypersensitivity reaction, pruritus, rash; use with caution in patients with liver disease; contraindicated in patients with hypertension |
| **Ritonavir** (Norvir) **Route:** PO **Dosage:** 600 mg bid | Antiretroviral; PI used against HIV | Circumoral paresthesia, asthenia, nausea, vomiting, diarrhea, anorexia, abdominal pain, altered taste, headache, hypersensitivity reaction, hepatic toxicity; must be taken with high-fat, high-protein food; dosage may be titrated slowly to therapeutic levels over 14 days or can be reduced to 400 mg bid given with saquinavir 400 mg bid to minimize side effects and increase potency of saquinavir |
| **Saquinavir** (Invirase) **Route:** PO **Dosage:** 600 mg tid | Antiretroviral; PI used against HIV | Nausea, diarrhea, abdominal pain, photosensitivity; should be taken with food or within 2 hr of a meal; grapefruit juice increases absorption; must be taken 1 hr apart from didanosine |
| **Stavudine** (d4T, Zerit) **Route:** PO **Dosage:** >60 kg: 40 mg bid <60 kg: 30 mg bid | Antiretroviral; NRTI used against HIV | Peripheral neuropathy, hepatitis, pancreatitis; do not use with AZT; dose must be adjusted in patients with renal failure |
| **Trimethoprim and Sulfamethoxazole** (TMP/SMX, Bactrim, Septra) **Route:** PO, IV **Dosage:** PCP prophylaxisis 1 DS qd or 1 DS 3 times a week Toxoplasmosis 1 DS qd; PCP treatment 6 DS qd or 5 mg/kg (TMP) IV q 6-8 hr for 21 days | Antibacterial used in the prevention of *P. carinii* pneumonia and toxoplasmosis; also used in the treatment of PCP and many other infections commonly seen in HIV | Nausea, vomiting, rash, pruritus, elevated liver enzymes, neutropenia, leukopenia, anemia, thrombocytopenia; photosensitive rash can occur in direct sunlight; use with caution in patients with renal and hepatic impairment; increased incidence of allergy and hematologic side effects in patients with HIV |
| **Zalcitabine** (ddC, Hivid) **Route:** PO **Dosage:** 0.75 mg bid | Antiretroviral; NRTI used in combination therapy against HIV | Peripheral neuropathy, oral aphthous ulcers, fever, rash; pancreatitis is rare, but the incidence is higher in patients with a history of pancreatitis |
| **Zidovudine** (Retrovir, AZT) **Route:** PO, IV **Dosage:** PO 200 mg tid; IV 1-2 mg/kg infused over 1 hr q 4 hr; change to PO therapy as soon as possible | Antiretroviral; NRTI used against HIV | Headache, weakness, nausea, insomnia, myalgia, asthenia, discolored nails, abdominal pain, diarrhea, anemia, granulocytopenia; use with caution in patient with decreased bone marrow or severe hepatic or renal disease |

normal functioning and the absorption of nutrients. The presence of HIV in the intestinal walls may result in a loss of lactase, the enzyme needed to digest lactose (the sugar found in dairy foods). This causes a lactose intolerance, which in turn may cause flatulence, a feeling of being bloated, and sometimes diarrhea (Romeyn, 1995).

## Genital Tract Manifestations

Sexually transmitted diseases (STDs) may or may not appear with increasing frequency in individuals who are HIV positive, depending on their sexual practices. HSV and HPV cause sexually transmitted diseases that may recur at any time after initial infection regardless of current sexual practices, and the frequency of recurrence is likely to increase as the CD4 count drops.

HSV causes both oral and genital ulcers (see Oral Manifestations, p. 369) and is present in many people regardless of HIV status. Historically, herpes simplex virus type 1 (HSV-1) has been implicated as the cause of oral herpes and herpes simplex virus type 2 (HIV-2) has been thought to be the cause of genital herpes. However, significant "cross-fertilization" has occurred, and both HSV-1 and HSV-2 now affect both areas of the body. HSV-1 and HSV-2 cause similar patterns of recurrent genital lesions (although HSV-1 infections tend to be less severe). Primary genital HSV infection may be asymptomatic or may cause extensive painful genital lesions and produce systemic symptoms such as fever and malaise. Recurrent herpes lesions tend to be fewer in number and milder in course. In an HIV-positive patient, recurrent episodes can become severe and frequent, especially as the CD4 count declines. Genital herpes can be treated with acyclovir, and patients with recurrent HSV may need to be maintained on a prophylactic regimen.

HPV lesions (venereal warts, or condylomata acuminata) often recur after removal. They are considered precancerous lesions.

Syphilis may be difficult to eradicate in an HIV-positive patient, and it is unclear whether HIV-positive status makes the patient with syphilis more likely to develop neurosyphilis. A note about HIV transmission: An open lesion (e.g., a genital herpes ulcer or a primary syphilitic chancre) on an HIV-negative person increases that person's risk of contracting HIV from sexual contact with an HIV-positive person because of the break in the genital mucosa.

**Nursing implications.** Many patients have heard of "herpes" as an incurable sexually transmitted disease. It is important to inform them that herpes is simply a virus that can cause "cold sores" and that although it cannot be cured (just as the common cold cannot be cured), it can be treated. The patient is contagious from the time of the first symptom of genital HSV until all ulcers are completely healed. Also, physical abrasion of the lesions during intercourse can inoculate new areas of the patient's genitalia with HSV. For these reasons, the patient should avoid sexual activity during an outbreak of HSV. Additionally, asymptomatic shedding of the virus is common; therefore condoms should be used during all sexual contact even if no lesions present. Women with HPV should have Papanicolaou (Pap) smears every 6 months.

## Hematologic Manifestations

The blood has three kinds of cells: red cells (RBCs); white cells (WBCs); and platelets, which actually are cell fragments. All three types are made in the bone marrow, and disturbances in the marrow can result in low numbers of any of these cells. HIV itself can infect the marrow, as can some AIDS opportunistic infections such as *Mycobacterium avium* complex (MAC) and histoplasmosis. Malignancies can infiltrate the marrow, and many different medications can cause bone marrow depression. Anemia refers to a low number of red blood cells, leukopenia refers to a low number of white blood cells, neutropenia refers to a low number of neutrophils (a kind of WBC also called "polys" or "segs"), and thrombocytopenia refers to a low number of platelets. Pancytopenia refers to low numbers of all three types of cells. If any of these conditions is present, further tests must be done to determine the cause so that appropriate treatment can be instituted. Sometimes, when the cause cannot be treated adequately or if the condition is a side effect of a necessary medication, the patient may be given injections of erythropoietin (Epogen) to stimulate the marrow to produce more RBCs, or injections of filgrastim (Neupogen) to stimulate production of more WBCs.

**Nursing implications.** The complete blood count (CBC) must be monitored when a patient is undergoing treatment with erythropoietin or filgrastim. The blood pressure also is monitored because erythropoietin can cause hypertension. Bone pain may be a side effect of filgrastim. Patients with severe neutropenia may require reverse isolation because they are extremely vulnerable to infection.

## Musculoskeletal Manifestations

Patients who are HIV positive often have joint or muscle pain, or both. They may have arthritis of various origins (e.g., Reiter's syndrome) or simply arthralgia (joint pain) of unknown cause. Myositis, or inflammation of the muscles, can occur as a result of HIV itself or as a side effect of AZT. In true myositis, the enzymes aldolase and creatine kinase (CK or CPK) are elevated.

The first step of treatment is to discontinue the possible causative medication. The patient may simply have myalgia (muscle pain) as a result of decreased mobility or unknown causes. The nurse should ask the patient about "aches and pains." Although it may not be possible to diagnose the cause of these syndromes, it usually is possible to treat them with some degree of success with NSAIDs and nonnarcotic analgesics.

## Neurologic Manifestations

Peripheral neuropathy may be caused by HIV itself or, more commonly, may occur as a side effect of antiretroviral medications, particularly didanosine, zalcitabine, or stavudine. Symptoms include numbness or burning pain, which usually starts in the feet and can progress to a "glove and stocking" distribution. If the feet are affected, the patient may have difficulty walking because of pain. Treatment consists of withdrawing any medications that may be responsible and observing for abatement of symptoms. If symptoms persist, the patient's vitamin $B_{12}$ level should be checked, since a deficiency can cause peripheral neuropathy. Tricyclic antidepressants usually give good pain relief; if not, the same medications given for postherpetic neuralgia can be used.

## Oral Manifestations

Aphthous stomatitis causes lesions commonly known as canker sores in the oropharynx of many people regardless of HIV status. These ulcers are thought to be autoimmune in origin, and they usually respond to treatment with corticosteroids (topical in mild cases or oral prednisone in more severe cases). Aphthous ulcers can be recurrent and also can cause esophagitis. In extremely recalcitrant cases, thalidomide may be useful, although special arrangements must be made to obtain it through the Compassionate Use Program of the U.S. Food and Drug Administration (FDA).

**Nursing implications.** Alert the patient to the fact that systemic corticosteroids increase the patient's risk for candidiasis. Patients should examine their mouths daily for white patches, and women should report any unusual vaginal itch or discharge. Aphthous ulcers can be quite painful, and topical viscous lidocaine may give temporary relief. Thalidomide is absolutely contraindicated in pregnancy.

**Candidiasis.** Mucocutaneous **candidiasis**, the most common fungal infection in HIV patients, can appear as oral thrush, esophagitis, or vaginitis. Nurses may see a whitish coating on the patient's tongue, gums, or other mucous membranes. This coating appears as patches that can be wiped off. Candidiasis also may appear as flat, bright red areas on the hard palate, buccal mucosa, or tongue. Nystatin suspension (Mycostatin) and clotrimazole troches (Mycelex) are commonly used topical therapies with few side effects. Itraconazole (Sporanox) and amphotericin B oral suspensions (Fungizone) also are very effective, and fluconazole oral suspension (Diflucan) probably will be approved soon. Less conventional but quite efficacious are nystatin or clotrimazole vaginal troches used orally (Greenspan, Greenspan, 1997). If topical treatment fails, systemic oral antifungals are indicated, such as fluconazole, itraconazole, or terbinafine (Lamisil). The patient must take these oral medications exactly as prescribed; otherwise, resistance is more likely to develop. Treatment of resistant candidal infection is difficult and involves toxic medications such as intravenous (IV) amphotericin B. Angular cheilitis, another form of candidiasis, forms cracks or fissures at the corners of the mouth. It usually responds to topical antifungal cream, such as clotrimazole or ketoconazole.

**Nursing implications.** In a patient who is not known to have HIV, the presence of oral candidiasis should alert the nurse to consider HIV as a possible underlying cause. Patients with oral candidiasis should be urged to practice good oral hygiene.

**Gingivitis and periodontitis.** Gingivitis and periodontitis are extremely common in people with HIV. In asymptomatic, HIV-positive patients, gingivitis (inflammation of the gingiva, or gums) may simply be a result of poor dental hygiene and inadequate dental care (many dentists do not want to work on patients with HIV, and many health insurance plans do not include dental care). Meticulous dental hygiene (e.g., frequent brushing, regular flossing) is essential, and chlorhexidine gluconate (Peridex) mouthwash may effect some improvement. Periodontitis (inflammation or degeneration, or both, of the membrane that covers dental bone) is more likely to occur in patients with AIDS than in those who are simply HIV positive. It requires dental care. Signs of gingivitis and periodontitis are halitosis, redness at the margin where the teeth meet the gingiva, gingival puffiness, and receding of gingival tissue.

**Nursing implications.** The nurse should ask about routine dental care and any dental pain, and if the patient's gums bleed when brushing the teeth. The nurse should be an advocate for the patient in need of proper dental care.

**Hairy leukoplakia.** Hairy leukoplakia is another common oral manifestation of HIV. It appears as white thickening on the buccal mucosa, soft palate, or tongue. Unlike candidiasis, it cannot be scraped off. On the lateral margins of the tongue it typically has a corrugated or fissured appearance (Bolan, 1997). Oral hairy leukoplakia has been associated with Epstein-Barr virus (EBV). It does not usually require treatment, but, if the patient is uncomfortable, the condition may respond to treatment with acyclovir or one of acyclovir's sister drugs (samciclovir or valacyclovir).

**Herpes simplex virus.** HSV causes vesicles and ulcers, commonly called cold sores or fever blisters, on the lips and oral mucosa of many people regardless of HIV status. The usual course of HSV, in anyone, is one of recurrent lesions, which may occur frequently or only very occasionally. Individuals with HIV may have more frequent and more severe recurrences than people without HIV. Treatment with acyclovir or one of its sister drugs usually is quite effective and rarely causes side effects. (See Genital Tract Manifestations, p. 368, for a discussion of genital HSV.)

***Nursing implications.*** The patient with HSV lesions should be careful not to kiss anyone while an active lesion is present. Nurses should wear gloves when suctioning or providing mouth care to these patients.

**Human papillomavirus. Human papillomavirus (HPV)** can cause oral as well as anogenital warts. These warts may have a cauliflower-like surface or may be slightly raised and smooth. They can be removed by laser or surgical excision, but because they are likely to recur, treatment usually is not recommended unless the warts are numerous or unsightly or interfere with function.

# AIDS-Defining Conditions and Opportunistic Infections
## Coccidioidomycosis*

Coccidioidomycosis is caused by the fungus *Coccidioides immitus,* which lives in the soil of some deserts. It is endemic in parts of Arizona, California, New Mexico, and western Texas and in parts of Central and South America. The fungus, which can infect human beings regardless of HIV status, becomes aerosolized and enters the body via the respiratory tract. In 33% of those infected, it causes a self-limited pulmonary infection; 66% of cases are asymptomatic. Besides respiratory symptoms, joint effusions and skin rashes are common. In an immunocompetent host, the immune system usually contains the organism, which remains quiescent (Bennet, Plum, 1996). In an immunocompromised host, especially an HIV-positive person with a CD4 count under 250/mm³, disseminated coccidioidomycosis occurs, either as a primary infection or, less commonly, as a reactivation of latent infection. The disease can cause pneumonitis, meningitis, bone marrow infection, and skin lesions. The diagnosis is

made by culturing blood and infected body tissues. The initial treatment is IV amphotericin B, followed by maintenance doses of itraconazole or fluconazole (Sande, Volberding, 1997).

**Nursing implications.** Nurses must teach the patient the importance of lifelong maintenance therapy. If the patient discontinues the antifungal medication, the disease will recur.

## Cryptococcosis

Cryptococcosis is caused by the yeast *Cryptococcus neoformans,* which typically infects the central nervous system (CNS), causing cryptococcal meningitis. Infection occurs through the respiratory tract, yet it can affect many other areas of the body as well, such as the joints and skin. Patients with a CD4 count less than 200/mm³ are at risk for this infection. Cryptococcal meningitis has a very slow onset, with weeks of intermittent fever, headache, and malaise; other symptoms may include photophobia, cough, stiff neck, nausea, or vomiting. Because of its waxing and waning course, the disease typically is diagnosed as long as a month after onset. The patient's mental status at the time of presentation is prognostic (Sande, Volberding, 1997).

Patients suspected of having cryptococcal meningitis should be prepared for a lumbar puncture, since this procedure must be performed to obtain cerebrospinal fluid (CSF) for culture. An india ink preparation of the CSF often is examined on a slide under a microscope for a quick, tentative diagnosis while the culture is incubating. Of patients with cryptococcal meningitis, 74% to 88% have a positive result on the CSF india ink test. CSF and serum should be examined for cryptococcal antigen. This test is very sensitive; it is positive in 93% to 99% of patients with cryptococcal meningitis. Almost always, a computed tomography (CT) or magnetic resonance imaging (MRI) scan is done before the lumbar puncture to rule out a mass lesion in the brain. Nurses should ask the patient about any allergies to contrast media dyes before the CT scan is done.

After the lumbar puncture, the patient should be kept supine (lying on the back) and quiet for 6 hours to minimize postprocedural headache. Cryptococcal disease usually is treated in two stages: a 2-week "induction period," during which the patient receives IV amphotericin B (with or without flucytosine), followed by a "consolidation period," during which the patient usually receives fluconazole, 400 mg twice a day for 2 days, then daily for 8 weeks. Cultures are then repeated to make sure the result is negative. As with cytomegalovirus, the patient must take medication for life after acute cryptococcal infection. The medication

*Conditions marked with an asterisk (*) may occur at CD4 counts below 200/ml³.

usually given is fluconazole, 200 to 400 mg daily. As previously mentioned, amphotericin B often causes renal impairment.

**Nursing implications.** Patients with cryptococcal meningitis may have altered mental status, which may manifest subtly. Patient education about lifetime treatment and the importance of medication adherence to prevent relapse is important. Left untreated, cryptococcal meningitis is a fatal disorder.

## Cytomegalovirus

Cytomegalovirus (CMV) may affect the eyes, GI tract, lungs, and adrenals, as well as many other tissues. It can cause esophagitis, colitis, pneumonia, encephalitis, and other infections. However, it most notably causes retinitis through a reactivation of latent infection. Patients at risk are those with a CD4 count under 50/mm$^3$; these patients should see a ophthalmologist every 6 months for an eye examination. Symptoms include "floaters" and visual field deficits. The nurse should ask any patient with a CD4 count under 50/mm$^3$ about vision changes because CMV can cause blindness if not treated and can progress very quickly.

> **NURSE ALERT**
>
> A vision examination (with an eye chart) should be administered to any patient with any visual complaint and on a regular basis to patients with lower CD4 cell counts.

Diagnosis of CMV retinitis is made by fundoscopic examination, which will reveal whitish exudates and hemorrhages on the retina. Intravenous ganciclovir is the most commonly prescribed medication for CMV infections; foscarnet may be given either with ganciclovir or alone if ganciclovir resistance develops. Both medications require central venous access such as a Hickman catheter or a Port-A-Cath, and patients need to be taught how to maintain the "line" and administer the medications. Bone marrow suppression is common with ganciclovir; the CBC must be monitored, particularly for leukopenia. Foscarnet can cause nephrotoxicity, hypocalcemia or hypercalcemia, and seizures (Casey, Cohen, Hughes, 1996). Both drugs are virustatic, not virucidal, therefore relapses occur if therapy is not continued. Patients need to understand the importance of lifetime treatment.

Many new treatments are available for CMV retinitis, but they all are problematic in one way or another.

The ganciclovir intraocular implant carries with it postoperative complications (e.g., retinal detachment). Furthermore, it does not protect the patient from other systemic manifestations of CMV disease. Oral ganciclovir has the same drawback. New drugs for the treatment of CMV disease are in development.

**Nursing implications.** Patients with CMV retinitis may be a safety risk because of impaired vision. The nurse should evaluate this with the family and make a home care nurse referral to evaluate the home for safety. Individuals with CMV of the GI tract should have a consultation with a registered dietitian and receive close nutritional supervision (see Nutrition, p. 380.)

## Dermatologic Conditions

Dermatologic conditions may worsen in AIDS. Rashes of many different etiologies (e.g., dermatophytes, psoriasis, seborrheic dermatitis) often spread. Disseminated herpes may occur, usually caused by VZV but sometimes by HSV. The rash manifests as small ulcers or hyperkeratotic lesions scattered over the trunk and limbs (Buchness, 1995). It is treated with acyclovir or a similar drug.

## Diarrhea

(Also see Gastrointestinal Manifestations, p. 362.) At CD4 counts under 100/mm$^3$ (usually at 50/mm$^3$ or lower), opportunistic pathogens enter the list of possible causes of diarrhea. These pathogens include *Cryptosporidium* and *Microsporidium* species, *Isospora belli*, MAC, and CMV. Kaposi's sarcoma and lymphoma of the GI tract can cause diarrhea as well, and HIV itself can cause an enteropathic condition. If a causative organism cannot be identified by the means described above, a GI consult should be obtained because the patient will require colonoscopy with biopsy to detect organisms such as *Cryptosporidium* species and MAC that may have eluded detection in stool specimens (Sande, Volberding, 1997). In patients with very low CD4 counts, diarrhea may be treatable but not curable, particularly when it is caused by cryptosporidiosis or microsporidiosis. Lifelong use of medications may be required, and exacerbations can be expected.

## Esophagitis

Esophagitis can be caused by *Candida* organisms, CMV, HSV, or aphthous ulcers. The symptoms are dysphagia or odynophagia, or both. The diagnosis sometimes is made presumptively, depending on findings in the oral cavity. For example, dysphagia in the presence of thrush is most likely to be caused by candidal esophagitis. A definitive diagnosis can be made by endoscopy. Sometimes radiologic tests are used, such as the barium swallow or upper GI studies. Treatment depends on the causative organism. *Candida* infection is treated with systemic antifungals, CMV with ganciclovir, HSV with acyclovir or a similar drug, and aphthous esophagitis with prednisone.

**Nursing implications.** Patients with esophagitis need high-protein, high-calorie soft foods that are not acidic. If the esophagitis is severe, a liquid diet may be necessary at the beginning of treatment.

## Hematologic Manifestations

Hematologic manifestations such as anemia, leukopenia, thrombocytopenia, and pancytopenia are more likely to occur in AIDS than in HIV alone (see Hematologic Manifestations, p. 368).

## Histoplasmosis

Histoplasmosis is caused by the fungus *Histoplasma capsulatum*, which grows in soil and is endemic in the northern and south central United States, particularly in the Mississippi, Tennessee, Missouri, Ohio, and St. Lawrence river valleys, as well as in some areas of the eastern United States (Bennet, Plum, 1996). It is also endemic in Puerto Rico, Mexico, and Central and South America. *H. capsulatum* enters the body through the respiratory tract. The immune system of an immunocompetent host usually contains the infection successfully. It may lie quiescent for years but is reactivated when an immunocompromised state develops. In a patient with AIDS, especially one with a CD4 count under 50/mm³, initial infection cannot be contained and widespread disease ensures. Whether arising as a reactivation of latent infection or as a new infection, histoplasmosis disseminates in the AIDS patient, causing constitutional symptoms such as fever, chills, malaise, and weight loss. It can affect many parts of the body, causing respiratory infection, oral lesions, skin rash, hepatosplenomegaly, lymphadenopathy, bone marrow suppression, and adrenal insufficiency. Most seriously, it can infect the central nervous system, causing meningitis. It is diagnosed by culturing the fungus from blood or infected tissues. A *Histoplasma* antigen test also may be used. Histoplasmosis is treated with IV amphotericin B or with oral itraconazole (Sande, Volberding, 1997).

**Nursing implications.** Antifungal therapy for histoplasmosis must be continued for life, or relapse occurs. The nurse plays a critical role in patient education in this matter.

## HIV Encephalopathy*

HIV encephalopathy (dementia) can affect cognitive, motor, and behavioral functioning. It was more common in the days before antiretroviral therapy. Now, mild or early HIV dementia in the form of poor memory, difficulty concentrating, and cognitive slowing frequently occurs in those with symptomatic HIV disease. Subtle personality changes may occur, but severe behavioral and motor manifestations are not as common as in the past. Dementia may occur at CD4 counts under 500/mm³. In severe or late dementia, the patient may develop clumsiness, ataxia, and even paraplegia and mutism (Andrews, Novick, 1995).

**Nursing implications.** The nurse may be the first to recognize the effects of dementia in the patient. The patient may be having difficulty performing simple tasks such as bathing or eating or even tying a shoelace. It is important to ask patients in the middle or late stages of HIV disease if they are having difficulty remembering. Sometimes the patient is in fact having trouble but is not conscious of it and needs support. The nurse can coach the patient who has memory and cognitive deficits on strategies for aiding memory. Writing appointments down in a date book and telephone numbers in address books may be helpful. Medication boxes and alarm wristwatches can help the patient keep track of which medications must be taken that day. Family members, friends, volunteers, case managers, and home care nurses all may be enlisted to offer the patient appropriate assistance.

## Malignancies

HPV infection, a sexually transmitted disease that causes anogenital warts (condylomata acuminata), is considered a precancerous condition. Lesions may be few and may resolve spontaneously, especially in those with a high CD4 count and in HIV-negative individuals. However, as the CD4 count drops and immunodeficiency becomes more profound, HPV can cause multiple lesions, which often recur after excision by chemical, surgical, electrocautery, or cryosurgical techniques. These patients must be screened carefully for cervical or anal neoplasia. Some clinicians recommend that women with a history of HPV have a Pap smear every 6 months and that men and women with HPV have a careful genital and anal examination every 6 months. Studies are underway to assess the efficacy of anal Pap smears as a screening tool.

**Nursing implications.** Patients who have a history of HPV in the form of genital or anal warts probably

---

*Conditions marked with an asterisk (*) may occur at CD4 counts below 200/ml³.

should be examined for anogenital neoplasia every 6 months, especially patients with lower CD4 counts.

## Kaposi's Sarcoma*

**Kaposi's sarcoma (KS)** was a relatively rare malignancy in the United States before the advent of AIDS. Before that time, it was seen almost exclusively in older men of Mediterranean origin. It was a fairly benign malignancy, and the patient usually died of other causes. Kaposi's sarcoma in HIV occurs almost exclusively in men who have had sex with men and, less commonly, in their female sexual partners. It is thought to be caused by human herpes virus-8 (HHV-8). It usually appears as pink-to-purple lesions on the skin (it may look like an ecchymosis, or bruise); it is rarely painful but can be disfiguring. KS also can involve the lungs, lymph nodes, brain, and GI tract, including the mouth and esophagus. Its course varies considerably; it may be quiescent for years or may progress very rapidly. For this reason and because treatment is not very effective, it is reasonable at first simply to monitor the lesions until it becomes clear that therapy is indicated for cosmetic or palliative reasons (Levine, 1997). Treatment may be given in the form of local injections of IF-alpha, vinblastine or vincristine, local therapy with liquid nitrogen or argon laser, radiation therapy, or systemic chemotherapy with medications such as vincristine, vinblastine, doxorubicin, or paclitaxel. Patients should be assessed for nausea, vomiting, and other potential reactions to these very potent medications.

**Nursing implications.** Nurses should be aware that KS could be disfiguring. It can cause altered body image and low self-esteem because it is an obvious sign of HIV and a constant reminder to others of the illness. The patient may need referral to support services. If KS affects the GI tract, the patient will have impaired nutrition and weight loss.

## Lymphoma*

Lymphoma is cancer of the lymphoid tissues, which includes, naturally, T and B cells. Both Hodgkin's lymphoma and non-Hodgkin's lymphoma (NHL) occur more frequently in HIV-positive individuals than in those who are HIV negative. The most common type in the HIV-positive patient is non-Hodgkin's lymphoma of the B cells. NHL typically is widespread throughout the body (extranodal) at the time of diagnosis. Common sites are the central nervous system,

*Conditions marked with an asterisk (*) may occur at CD4 counts below 200/ml³.

bone marrow, GI tract, and liver. Peripheral NHL can occur even when the CD4 count is over 200/mm³. Lymphoma affects the CNS at lower CD4 counts (under 100/mm³ and usually under 50/mm³).

The onset of lymphoma symptoms may be insidious, with nonspecific symptoms of night sweats, fever, and weight loss, or it may be acute, as with seizures in a patient with CNS lymphoma. Other symptoms are related to the organs affected (e.g., nausea and abdominal pain from GI tract disease or pancytopenia from bone marrow infiltration). CNS lymphoma may cause confusion, lethargy, and memory loss, as well as hemiparesis, aphasia, seizures, and headache (Sande, Volberding, 1997).

The diagnosis usually is made by CT scan or MRI, or both. Other possible tests include a lumbar puncture and cryptococcal antigen and toxoplasmosis titers (the two titers are done to rule out these diseases). Tests required to properly stage NHL may include a CT scan of the chest, abdomen, and pelvis; a gallium scan; and bone marrow aspiration with biopsy (Levine, 1997).

Treatment of NHL is difficult because of the poor baseline bone marrow reserves in the AIDS patient. Also, chemotherapy almost always has the side effect of bone marrow suppression, resulting in diminished immunity; it therefore exacerbates the AIDS patient's already-existing vulnerability to opportunistic infection. No standard chemotherapeutic regimen has been recommended for NHL in the HIV-positive patient. The response usually is poor, and even in those who do respond, life expectancy may be as short as 2 to 5 months (Sande, Volberding, 1997). Factors associated with a poor prognosis are elevated lactase dehydrogenase (LDH), advanced-stage disease (stage III or IV), age over 35 years, a history of an AIDS-defining illness, and poor performance status on the Karnofsky Scale (a tool used to estimate a patient's physical state). The prognosis is better if the CD4 count is over 100/mm³, if the patient has had no previous AIDS diagnosis or extranodal disease, and if the Karnofsky performance score is 70% or higher (Straus et al, 1995.)

## *Mycobacterium avium* Complex

*Mycobacterium avium* complex (MAC, used interchangeably with MAI) refers to *Mycobacterium avium* and *Mycobacterium intracellulare*. These mycobacteria are ubiquitous in the soil and water. They probably gain entry into the human host through the respiratory or GI tract. MAC has been implicated as the cause of lower respiratory tract or GI infections, but it is best known for causing disseminated disease (DMAC). It has been estimated that one third or more of those with a CD4 count under 100/mm³ will develop MAC unless they receive prophylaxis to prevent it. DMAC infects several organs; in autopsy studies it has been isolated from the spleen, lymph nodes, liver, lung, adrenals, colon, kidney, and bone marrow (Sande, Volberding, 1997).

Signs and symptoms of dissemination usually are nonspecific and include fever, malaise, weight loss, and often anemia and neutropenia. MAC must be treated with several medications because bactericidal levels of medication cannot be achieved in vivo. For the same reason, treatment must continue for life. The medication regimen usually includes a macrolide antibiotic (e.g., clarithromycin or azithromycin) and at least one other medication, usually ethambutol, rifabutin, clofazimine, or ciprofloxacin. Nurses should be aware that most of these medications can have GI side effects (nausea, vomiting, diarrhea, abdominal pain). In addition, ethambutol has the rare but serious side effect of optic neuritis. Patients should have baseline and periodic eye examinations, and the nurse should advise the patient to report immediately any decline in vision. Ciprofloxacin is generally well tolerated; however, antacids containing magnesium hydroxide or aluminum hydroxide reduce absorption by up to 90%; therefore the drug should be taken 1 hour before or 2 hours after an antacid. (*Note*: ddI [didanosine, or Videx] contains an antacid.) Clofazimine almost always causes skin discoloration (pink to brownish black) and often causes GI symptoms as well (Petrow, 1995).

**Nursing implications.** The causative organism in MAC is a mycobacterium, as is the causative organism in tuberculosis (TB). Mycobacteria show up as positive on acid-fast stains. If a patient is symptomatic with cough and sputum specimens are sent for acid-fast bacilli (AFB) smears, the test will be positive if either MAC or TB is the causative organism. Therefore AFB-positive patients must be treated as if they have TB (with three or four medications) until a DNA probe or similar quick test or culture distinguishes between the two mycobacteria. Patients with MAC bronchitis or pneumonia do not require respiratory isolation.

## Mycobacterium tuberculosis*

The disease caused by *Mycobacterium tuberculosis*, commonly known as TB, has been on the rise in the United States over the past several years. This is partly attributable to the fact that AIDS patients are especially vulnerable to TB, but it also is a result of the increase in immigration from countries that have a high preva-

lence of TB and to the growth of the socioeconomic underclass in our country. The crowded, poorly ventilated environment of homeless shelters and substandard housing in our cities replicate the conditions of the poorhouses and tenements of the eighteenth and nineteenth centuries, which were breeding grounds for TB.

TB is spread by airborne droplet transmission. The organism is carried on tiny droplet nuclei that are expelled into the air when a person with pulmonary TB coughs, sneezes, or even sings. It is breathed into the lungs of other people, and over the next several weeks, it "seeds" to other organs such as the bone and kidneys. This process of exposure is called TB infection. In an immunocompetent host, an immune response develops in which the tubercular bacilli in the lung (and in the other tissues to which the bacilli have seeded) are walled off within granulomatous tissue. People who have TB infection but not TB disease are asymptomatic and are not infectious. For those who have TB infection and are HIV negative, the lifetime risk of developing TB disease is about 10%. Of these, 5% develop the disease in the first year after infection, and 5% at a later time when the immune system fails to contain the TB infection (CDC, 1994a). People who have TB infection and are HIV positive are known to have a higher lifetime risk of developing TB disease. But the data from different groups vary so greatly that an exact percentage cannot be assigned to that risk (Sande, Volberding, 1997).

Infection with TB is detected by using the purified protein derivative (PPD) skin test. Box 16-5 presents guidelines for reading the test and explains how it works and what information can be obtained. If the PPD test is positive or if the patient has a history of a positive PPD result and was never treated for TB infection, a chest x-ray should be performed to rule out active pulmonary TB. If the chest x-ray is negative, most patients should receive prophylactic treatment, usually with isoniazid (INH), for 6 to 12 months (recommendations vary). This should kill the latent TB; however, it does not protect the patient from future reinfection. The nurse should be aware that INH can cause hepatitis and should teach the patient to report nausea, vomiting, anorexia, malaise, dark urine, or icterus that lasts 3 days or longer. Liver function tests should be done before INH therapy is begun and at any time during therapy that hepatitis becomes a question. INH also can cause paresthesia, particularly in the hands and feet. Some health care providers routinely prescribe pyridoxine (vitamin $B_6$) to prevent this side effect.

TB disease refers to active infection, usually in the lungs, but sometimes in extrapulmonary sites such as those mentioned above. TB disease almost always is a

---

*Conditions marked with an asterisk (*) may occur at CD4 counts below 200/ml³.

BOX 16-5

### Guidelines for Reading the Purified Protein Derivative (PPD) Test

Inoculation with foreign protein (e.g., tetanus) results in the formation of antibodies; this is the way in which vaccines work. The antibodies circulate in the bloodstream and attack when that antigen (foreign protein) next enters the body. Therefore exposure to an antigen results in circulating, or humoral, immunity.

A similar process occurs at a cellular level. As explained in the text discussion on *Mycobacterium tuberculosis*, when an immunocompetent person is infected with tuberculosis by inhaling droplet nuclei, a local response occurs in the lung in which the tubercular bacilli are walled off within granulomatous tissue. The body retains a "cellular memory" of this exposure, and if in the future a small amount of TB protein is injected intradermally, a localized cellular response occurs in the form of erythema and induration. Thus injection of PPD in the Mantoux tuberculin skin test produces a reaction if the individual has TB infection *and* if the individual's cellular immunity is intact. (Failure to respond to an antigen of which the body should have a "cellular memory" is called *anergy*.)

The PPD most commonly is placed on one forearm, and it should be read 48 to 72 hours after placement. Induration (palpable swelling) constitutes a positive result. Erythema (redness) should *not* be measured. The indurated area is outlined carefully in ink and measured *across* the forearm (perpendicular to the long axis). **A PPD reading ≥5 mm is considered positive in HIV-positive patients.** A positive PPD result indicates that the patient has a TB infection, which may or may not be manifested clinically in the form of TB disease.

reactivation of latent infection. The infection may have occurred years in the past and is most likely to reactivate when the host's immune system is compromised. In HIV disease TB may occur with CD4 cell counts of $400/mm^3$ or lower, or at any CD4 count, as it can with HIV-negative individuals.

Patients with AIDS may develop TB disease at the time of primary TB infection because they are unable to mount the initial immune response required to contain the tubercular bacilli. Patients with TB disease may have fever, weight loss, night sweats, and cough, sometimes with hemoptysis. In the outpatient setting, any HIV-positive patient with a cough should be immediately taken from the waiting room, masked, and moved to an examining room to wait until he can be seen. According to the guidelines of the U.S. Occupational Safety and Health Administration (OSHA),

health care professionals who are in contact with the patient should wear a mask equipped with a high-efficiency particulate air (HEPA) filter, which filters out particles 1 $\mu$m or larger (droplet nuclei measure 1 to 5 $\mu$m). In the outpatient setting, rooms where the patient has been, such as the examining room and the waiting room, should be treated with a HEPA filter—equipped "air scrubber" or with an ultraviolet light, or both. The nurse should contact the designated infection control resource in her agency for more detailed guidance. A hospitalized patient suspected of having or known to have TB disease must be placed in isolation in a negative pressure room, which vents all room air to the outside. In addition, health care personnel must wear HEPA-filter masks while in the room.

The nurse has several responsibilities toward a patient who is symptomatic for TB. The nurse should:

1. Institute respiratory isolation.
2. Plan a PPD and anergy panel, unless the patient is already known to be anergic.
3. Obtain three sputum samples for AFB smear and culture.
4. Initiate pharmacologic treatment if suspicion is high for TB disease. If the AFB smears are positive, tests must be done to determine if TB or MAC is the causative organism. Tests such as a DNA probe can distinguish between these two in a matter of about 2 weeks, but cultures are still needed so that sensitivity tests can be conducted to determine the medications to which the organism is sensitive or resistant (also see Nursing Implications under *Mycobacterium avium* complex, p. 374). This can take up to 6 weeks (Leiner, Mays, 1996).

Treatment for TB disease involves three or four medications (usually isoniazid, rifampin, pyrazinamide, and ethambutol or streptomycin), and protocols vary for dosing, frequency, and duration of different drug combinations. HIV-positive patients probably should be treated for at least 9 months (Pulido et al, 1997). Multiple drug–resistant TB (MDRTB) develops when patients take their TB medication (prophylaxis or treatment) erratically. There are many reasons for nonadherence in all patient populations. AIDS patients may already be taking dozens of medications and may find it difficult to add still more pills to their regimen. Added to that are drug-drug and drug-food interactions, NPO requirements versus medications that must be taken with food, and social factors such as poverty and homelessness, all of which make adherence an arduous task. The result of nonadherence can be relapse with MDRTB, which is seen with increasing frequency, especially in cities. MDRTB is extremely difficult to treat, and the mortality rate in AIDS patients with MDRTB is high.

One strategy for ensuring adherence is directly observed therapy (DOT), which involves having the patient take the medication on a twice weekly schedule in the presence of a health care worker. DOT has proved effective, and research has demonstrated that it is the *least* expensive approach to treatment of TB disease once factors such as hospitalization, relapses, medications, contact investigations, prophylaxis, and treatment of contacts are factored in (Moore et al, 1996). DOT also is cost-effective compared with self-administered therapy for TB (Bass et al, 1994). However, because of inadequate funding, most public health departments do not have the resources to commit to an effective DOT program.

Patients with TB disease are considered noninfectious when they have been undergoing anti-TB therapy for 2 weeks, when the symptoms (especially cough) have improved, and when three sputum samples test negative for AFB (CDC, 1994a). Patients must be taught about transmission, the rationale for isolation, and treatment of the disorder. Close contacts, such as family members, should be given the PPD test.

**Nursing implications.** With both TB prophylaxis and treatment, patients should be seen monthly. They should be asked about medication side effects and adherence to the medications. No more than 1 month's supply of medication should be dispensed at any given time. Patient teaching about the rationale for taking all the medications for as long as prescribed should be reinforced at each visit. Patients who are not on DOT may benefit from the help of a home health nurse to ensure adherence. Nurses should review signs and symptoms of medication side effects. INH can cause hepatitis (malaise, anorexia, nausea, possibly vomiting, and dark urine). Nurses should be aware that rifampin may reduce blood levels of methadone, Coumadin derivatives, glucocorticoids, estrogens (including oral contraceptive pills), some oral hypoglycemic agents (sulfonylureas), digitalis, anticonvulsants, ketoconazole, fluconazole, and cyclosporine. Patients taking these medications are likely to require a higher dose. Women taking rifampin should not rely on oral contraceptives or implanted contraceptives, such as Norplant; another method of contraception is required (CDC, 1994a).

### Pneumocystis carinii Pneumonia

*Pneumocystis carinii* **pneumonia (PCP),** formerly the most common opportunistic infection seen in AIDS, occurs less often now that PCP prophylaxis (usually in the form of trimethoprim-sulfamethoxazole [TMP/SMX, Bactrim]) is routinely prescribed (Hoover et al, 1993) and now that effective new antiretroviral therapies are available. As indicated before, combination antiretroviral therapy can strongly suppress the virus, allowing the body to maintain a higher count of CD4 cells. This enhanced immune response also enables the patient to better fight off infections such as PCP.

Patients with PCP may have nonspecific signs or symptoms (e.g., nonproductive cough or malaise) for several weeks, or they may have severe symptoms, such as dyspnea and fevers. The nurse should ask how long the patient has been sick and whether the cough is productive. Nurses should assess respirations, examine for use of accessory muscles of respiration, and, at least on initial examination, perform pulse oximetry. Auscultation of the lungs may reveal the presence of crackles (rales). The chest x-ray over time shows a progression from normal to diffuse interstitial infiltration. Blood tests usually reveal an elevated lactase dehydrogenase (LDH). The diagnosis is made on the basis of the clinical presentation and testing of an induced sputum specimen. If the sputum is negative, a definitive diagnosis can be made by recovering the organism through bronchoscopy.

Several drug therapies are used to treat PCP, the most common of which is TMP/SMX. Before administering TMP/SMX, nurses should determine if a patient is allergic to sulfa, and after administration they should observe for rash or fever. Patients should be cautioned to avoid direct sunlight, which can trigger a photosensitive rash. Several other treatment options also are available. Atovaquone should be given with a high-fat meal to enhance absorption and reduce GI side effects. Pentamidine usually is given parenterally for PCP treatment, but it is less effective than TMP/SMX and carries the risk of renal toxicity, hypoglycemia, and pancreatitis, sometimes followed by diabetes mellitus. In rare cases patients may be treated with aerosolized pentamidine in a special contained booth or room; however, aerosolized pentamidine is not the first-line treatment for several reasons; it does not treat the apices of the lungs well, and it will not treat extrapulmonary sites of PCP infection. Trimetrexate with folinic acid, trimethoprim with dapsone, and clindamycin with primaquine are other alternative regimens that may be used to treat PCP (Casey, Cohen, Hughes, 1996).

**Nursing implications.** Nurses should make sure that the CBC is monitored for neutropenia and thrombocytopenia from the trimethoprim in TMP/SMX. A blood test for glucose-6-phosphate dehydrogenase (G6PD) should be obtained before dapsone is administered because this medication can cause hemolytic anemia in G6PD-deficient patients. The nurse also should be alert for diarrhea secondary to clindamycin, which is a major cause of pseudomembranous colitis resulting from *C. difficile.*

In the care of patients with PCP pneumonia, nurses must be aware that patients must maintain adequate oxygenation. Restriction of the patient's activities to reduce oxygen requirements is appropriate.

## Progressive Multifocal Leukoencephalopathy

Progressive multifocal leukoencephalopathy (PML) is a neurologic infection caused by the JC virus (named after a patient with the disease). It is a reactivation of an old asymptomatic infection with this virus, which never causes a pathologic condition unless immunosuppression is present. The JC virus causes extensive demyelination of the white matter of the brain, the brainstem, and the cerebellum. Its onset occurs over the course of weeks, with the development of neurologic symptoms such as visual field disturbances, ataxia, aphasia, confusion, or seizures. The time from onset to death usually is about 3 to 12 months; occasionally the disease follows a fluctuating course in which initial improvement is followed by a slower period of decline over 12 to 18 months. Treatment is symptomatic only.

**Nursing implications.** The onset of PML is so sudden and the prognosis is so poor that patients and their significant others need much support. Because patients may be confused and aphasic, their behavior often is different and alarming to the family. Trying to make patients talk may only exacerbate their frustration. The family may benefit from a referral to social services, a clergy member, or a support group for families of the terminally ill. The nurse must evaluate the patient for safety because patients with PML can be at risk for wandering or falling. If the patient is to be discharged home, a home care nurse must do a home safety evaluation. The nurse also should assess the patient for bowel and bladder incontinence and, if needed, develop a plan for managing these problems.

## Toxoplasmosis Encephalitis

Toxoplasmosis encephalitis is caused by the protozoa *Toxoplasma gondii*. This organism is found in many birds and mammals (Box 16-6). People can become infected through the fecal-oral route after direct contact with the oocysts (e.g., in cat feces) or through ingestion of oocysts in undercooked meat or on foods grown in contaminated soil. Toxoplasmosis is caused by a reactivation of a previously acquired latent infection. The information in the Patient/Family Teaching box below can be given to patients to help prevent transmission of toxoplasmosis. Toxoplasmosis encephalitis usually has a subacute onset of focal neurologic symptoms. The patient may have altered mental status, including confusion, lethargy, and anomia, as well as neuropsychiatric

---

**BOX 16-6**

### PETS AND HUMAN IMMUNODEFICIENCY VIRUS

These recommendations may be useful for human immunodeficiency virus (HIV)-positive individuals who are considering keeping a pet. Pets can carry many different infections that can be transmitted to human beings. These strategies can help reduce the risk of transmission:

- Always seek veterinary care for any pet with diarrhea. Animals can carry enteric pathogens such as *Cryptosporidium*, *Salmonella*, and *Campylobacter* organisms.
- New pets should be over 6 months of age and free of diarrhea.
- Always wash hands after handling pets—especially before eating.
- Avoid contact with reptiles (e.g., iguanas, lizards, snakes, and turtles); they often carry *Salmonella* organisms.
- Wear gloves while washing aquariums to reduce exposure to *Mycobacterium marinum*.
- Avoid contact with exotic pets, such as nonhuman primates.

**CAT OWNERS**

- Cats should be over 1 year of age.
- Cat feces can transmit toxoplasmosis, which can cause encephalitis in AIDS patients and congenital defects in neonates infected in utero. An HIV-negative person who is not pregnant should change the litter box. If an HIV-positive person must change the litter box, he or she should wash hands before and after doing so.
- To reduce the risk of toxoplasmosis, keep cats indoors and do not feed them raw or undercooked meat.
- Try to avoid cat scratches, and wash any scratches promptly (cats can transmit *Bartonella* organisms, which cause "cat-scratch disease"). Seek medical care promptly for any cat scratches that do not heal.

Modified from Centers for Disease Control and Prevention (CDC): *MMWR* 44(RR-8):1-33, 1995.

symptoms such as delusions or psychosis, ataxia, seizures, and hemiparesis (Sande, Volberding, 1997).

If an AIDS patient has focal neurologic findings such as acute mental status changes or seizures, it is useful to check the patient's record to see if the baseline toxoplasmosis titer was positive. If so, the patient may well be experiencing a reactivation of latent *Toxoplasma* infection. If not, the symptoms are extremely unlikely to be caused by toxoplasmosis. The diagnosis is made presumptively by a CT or MRI scan, which will show multiple ring-enhancing lesions. Several different treatment regimens are available, which typically include two or three medications. The regimen may include pyrimethamine (which must always be given with folinic acid, or bone marrow suppression will result), sulfadiazine, clindamycin, TMP/SMX, clarithromycin, atovaquoné, azithromycin, and dapsone. In rare cases the patient may require further short-term systemic corticosteroids to reduce intracranial pressure. Once the patient has improved clinically and radiographically, the medication is reduced to a maintenance dosage. This must be continued for life, or the infection will reoccur.

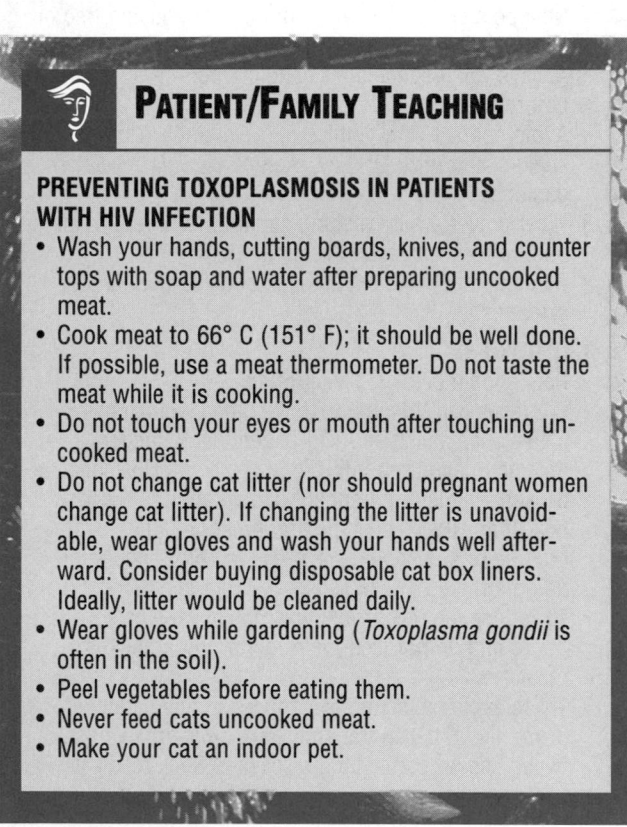

### PATIENT/FAMILY TEACHING

**PREVENTING TOXOPLASMOSIS IN PATIENTS WITH HIV INFECTION**
- Wash your hands, cutting boards, knives, and counter tops with soap and water after preparing uncooked meat.
- Cook meat to 66° C (151° F); it should be well done. If possible, use a meat thermometer. Do not taste the meat while it is cooking.
- Do not touch your eyes or mouth after touching uncooked meat.
- Do not change cat litter (nor should pregnant women change cat litter). If changing the litter is unavoidable, wear gloves and wash your hands well afterward. Consider buying disposable cat box liners. Ideally, litter would be cleaned daily.
- Wear gloves while gardening (*Toxoplasma gondii* is often in the soil).
- Peel vegetables before eating them.
- Never feed cats uncooked meat.
- Make your cat an indoor pet.

## Wasting

The CDC (1992) defines wasting as profound, involuntary weight loss of more than 10% of the baseline body weight, plus either chronic diarrhea (at least two loose stools a day for more than 30 days) or chronic weakness and documented fever for 30 days or longer (intermittent or constant) in the absence of a concurrent illness or condition other than HIV infection that could explain the findings (e.g., cancer, TB, cryptosporidiosis, or other specific enteritis). According to the CDC, wasting was the third most common AIDS-indicating condition in 1995, after a CD4 count under 200/mm$^3$ and PCP (Reiter, 1996). Death from starvation occurs

### BOX 16-7

### CAUSES OF WASTING

**POSSIBLE FACTORS**
- *Metabolic alteration.* HIV infection *at all stages* increases the body's resting energy expenditure (REE). The REE of asymptomatic HIV-positive individuals is 9% to 12% higher than that of seronegative controls. The REE of people with AIDS is 25% to 35% higher than that of seronegative controls. This indicates a faster metabolic rate, which means that calories are burned more quickly. Normally, if we caloric intake declines, the REE drops to accommodate it. But in AIDS wasting, the REE does not slow down even when the person's nutrition is poor (Reiter, 1996). This means that people with AIDS waste more quickly than people suffering from starvation. Also, in starvation, fat is burned preferentially before muscle, whereas in HIV disease muscle is used first to satisfy caloric requirements.
- *Inadequate oral intake.* This problem can have a number of causes such as hippus stomatitis or decreased appetite.
- *Malabsorption.* HIV damages the intestinal villi, impairing absorption of nutrients. Diarrhea also may contribute to malabsorption.
- *Endocrine dysfunction.* Approximately half of men with AIDS have low levels of androgenic hormones, especially testosterone. The effects of HIV on female androgen levels have not been well studied. Androgens contribute to muscle anabolism and hence to the restoration and maintenance of lean body mass (Reiter, 1996).
- *Cytokine effects.* Cytokines, especially tumor necrosis factor (TNF) and interferon-alpha, appear to act synergistically in causing lipogenesis, muscle catabolism, and a negative nitrogen balance. They also contribute to the increase in the metabolic rate.
- *Concomitant infection.* Infection of any kind alters the absorption and use of nutrients and the metabolism of lipids, carbohydrates, protein, vitamins, and trace elements. Infection also raises the REE and accelerates metabolism.

when a person reaches 66% of his or her ideal body weight.

Some of the factors that cause wasting are presented in Box 16-7. However, other factors involved in this condition remain unclear.

Contributing factors may trigger or exacerbate wasting. For example, infections of the mouth or esophagus caused by *Candida* organisms, aphthous ulcers, CMV, or HSV can make eating painful or difficult.

Many GI infections (CMV, cryptosporidiosis, salmonellosis, giardiasis) cause diarrhea and subsequent malabsorption. Systemic infections (TB, MAC, histoplasmosis) commonly cause anorexia. Regimens involving several medications can cause nausea. Fatigue can rob a patient of the energy it takes to prepare and eat a meal, or the patient simply may not have enough money to buy adequate food.

**Treatment for wasting.** Also see Nutrition, p. 380.

***Treatment of pathogens.*** Aggressive antiretroviral therapy is used to reduce the total body viral burden. In addition, any other infection, such as those referred to above, must be treated, as well as other effects of those infections. For example, for diarrhea caused by *Giardia* organisms, treatment may include an antidiarrheal medication in addition to metronidazole to treat the giardiasis.

***Symptom management.*** Appetite stimulants may be used in the treatment of wasting. If the patient is anorexic, cyproheptadine (Periactin), an antihistamine with the side effect of appetite stimulation, sometimes is used, and anecdotal evidence indicates that it can be effective. Megestrol acetate (Megace) stimulates appetite, but the weight gained is mostly adipose tissue. Megestrol acetate also diminishes testosterone levels. Dronabinol (Marinol) is tetrahydrocannabinol, the active ingredient in marijuana. It stimulates the appetite but also can cause drowsiness and confusion. Marijuana itself, either smoked or used in baked goods, stimulates the appetite but has the disadvantage of being illegal in most states.

Antiemetics may be required for nausea. If the nausea may be related to the patient's medications, consultation with a clinical pharmacologist often produces strategies for reducing this discomfort (e.g., changing the medication schedule, changing a medication).

***Nutritional support.*** The nurse should remind the patient that food, if tolerated, is better than supplements. Many patients believe that certain supplements will have a dramatically beneficial effect, a belief that has led to a black market in Ensure in some cities.
- *Oral nutritional support*
  1. If the patient is not lactose intolerant, recommend milkshakes or Carnation Instant Breakfast, which is similar to some supplements in nutritional quality but much more palatable. Recommend that these calorie boosters be taken between meals, not in place of them.
  2. Calorie-dense and lactose-free nutritional supplements such as Ensure, Sustacal, and Advera can be used as recommended above.
  3. If the patient is intolerant of fats and lactose, supplements containing medium-chain triglycerides

(MCTs), such as Lipisorb and Peptamen, may be better tolerated (Anastasi, Lee, 1994).
  4. Complete elemental formulas, such as Vivonex TEN, which are made up of free amino acids, are low in fat and highly absorbed but are expensive and unpalatable (Anastasi, Lee, 1993).
- *Enteral feedings*
  If the patient is unable to take food by mouth, an alternate route can be established by using such devices as a nasogastric tube, a nasoenteric tube, or a percutaneous endoscopic gastrostomy (PEG) tube.
- *Parenteral nutrition*
  Total parenteral nutrition (TPN) should be used as a last resort in patients who cannot absorb even elemental formulas and who have intractable diarrhea. TPN is expensive, requires sterile technique, and carries with it the risk of sepsis arising from the disruption in skin integrity. TPN should not be used for intravenous drug users.

***Treatment of underlying defects.*** Androgenic hormones (e.g., testosterone, nandrolone, oxandrolone) are being used in some cases to promote the production of lean body mass. Thalidomide and pentoxifylline sometimes are used for their antichemokine effect, particularly their ability to inhibit the production of TNF-alpha, which has been implicated as a factor in wasting.

# HIV IN WOMEN

It is clear that women constitute the fastest growing population in the HIV epidemic (CDC, 1995a). In the United States, AIDS is the third leading cause of death among women between the ages of 25 and 44 and the leading cause of death in African-American women in that age group (Squires, 1997). The strain of HIV that predominates in the United States is much more easily transmitted from men to women than vice versa. In other parts of the world where different viral strains predominate, the risk of heterosexual transmission between men and women is equal. For many reasons, most research studies of all types done in the field of HIV have underrepresented women. Therefore it is possible that HIV may affect women differently from men in ways that are not yet known. We do know that HIV-positive women are at risk for cervical cancer, abnormal Pap smears, pelvic inflammatory disease, and vaginal candidiasis. Pregnancy also may have a negative effect in women who are HIV positive.

## Cervical Cancer and Abnormal Pap Smears

Although statistics vary from study to study, HIV-positive women are indisputably more at risk for abnormal Pap smears and cervical cancer than are HIV-negative women. The risk increases as the CD4 count declines. Cervical cancer is closely linked to HPV, a sexually transmitted disease (see Malignancies, p. 372). If a patient is known to have HPV, she should have a Pap smear every 6 months. If she does not have HPV, the CDC recommends two baseline Pap smears 6 months apart and, if the second one is normal, an annual Pap smear thereafter (CDC, 1993b). If at any time reactive atypia (probably occurring secondary to inflammation) appear on the Pap smear, the test should be repeated in 3 months. Any cervical dysplasia (abnormal cell division), squamous intraepithelial lesions (SIL), abnormal squamous cells of uncertain significance (ASCUS), or carcinoma should be referred for colposcopy and treatment. (Colposcopy is a procedure in which the cervix is closely examined under high magnification and can be biopsied.) Because some studies have found that HIV-positive women with normal Pap smears have had abnormal colposcopic findings, many HIV care providers have a low threshold for referring patients for gynecologic evaluation. Cervical cancer is an AIDS-defining illness (see Malignancies, p. 372).

## Pelvic Inflammatory Disease

Pelvic inflammatory disease (PID) may be more prevalent and more severe in HIV-positive women; studies are continuing. Physicians and nurse practitioners may be quick to hospitalize an HIV-positive woman with PID, especially if she has a low CD4 count. Patients usually respond well to antibiotic treatment.

### Nursing Implications

PID usually is a sexually transmitted disease. A woman who has HIV should be sure that her partner wears a condom. If he will not, the female condom is now available in many pharmacies. Some HIV-positive women want to know if their partner must use a condom if he also is HIV-positive and the couple is monogamous. The answer is yes. Each ejaculation exposes the woman to an extra bolus of HIV. Furthermore, HIV can mutate into more virulent strains in any HIV-positive person, especially as the CD4 count declines. If a woman's partner has developed a more virulent strain and she has not, unprotected intercourse will inoculate her with a more destructive virus.

## Pregnancy

It is now well known that HIV can be transmitted from mother to baby during pregnancy, birth, and breastfeeding (see Perinatal [Vertical] Transmission, p. 382).

What is not known, however, is whether pregnancy adversely affects the course of the mother's HIV infection. Several flawed studies have suggested that CD4 counts decline during pregnancy and do not rebound postpartum. More data are needed to determine if pregnancy does indeed have a negative effect on the mother's HIV disease. Research in this area continues (Sande, Volberding, 1997).

### Nursing Implications

The CDC recommends that all pregnant women be offered HIV testing. Some state health departments recommend that all women of childbearing age be offered HIV testing. All HIV-positive women should be counseled about the risk of perinatal transmission and should be offered contraception. The nurse should emphasize that the woman may need two methods: one to prevent pregnancy (e.g., oral contraceptives) and one to prevent sexually transmitted disease.

## Vaginal Candidiasis

Vaginal candidiasis, the simple "yeast infection" that can affect all women, is extremely common in HIV. It usually is caused by the yeast *C. albicans* or another *Candida* species. Because of the risk of development of resistant strains of *Candida*, vaginal candidiasis is treated topically as long as topical treatment works (see Nails, p. 360, for a discussion of resistance). Vaginal creams or suppositories such as clotrimazole and terconazole generally are effective. If these methods fail, oral antifungal agents such as fluconazole may be needed. Severe recurrent vaginal candidiasis may require lifelong prophylactic medication to prevent recurrences.

### Nursing Implications

Any woman with recurrent severe vaginitis whose HIV status is unknown should be offered the option of HIV testing.

# NUTRITION

It has been clearly established that nutrition plays an important role in HIV disease. Poor nutritional status influences the length of survival by adversely affecting the immune response, damaging visceral tissue (particularly in the GI tract), interfering with absorption of medications and food, and contributing to debilitation (Severson et al, 1996). However, it is not always appreciated that loss of nutritional status occurs early in HIV disease. HIV-positive individuals begin to lose lean body mass (primarily muscle), without necessarily losing weight, even when they are asymptomatic and have a high CD4 count. The loss of lean body mass (LBM) is associated with quicker progression to AIDS and death, and, once lost, LBM is difficult to regain. Furthermore, patients with asymptomatic HIV disease have been found to be deficient in vitamins A, $B_6$, $B_{12}$, E, and riboflavin and in trace elements such as copper, selenium, and zinc (Anastasi, Lee, 1993). These vitamins and micronutrients are essential to normal immune function. Often, however, nutritional interventions are not initiated until the patient is losing weight, by which time much ground already has been lost. Nutritional assessment should be done early and often to prevent loss of LBM and to maintain adequate levels of nutrients.

## Nursing Nutritional Assessment

A nutritional assessment should be part of routine care of the HIV-positive patient. With the improvement in treatment of HIV, many patients are followed in the ambulatory care setting for years before they are hospitalized. By the time the patient is sick enough to be hospitalized, he or she is nutritionally compromised. It makes sense, then, to address nutritional status routinely in the outpatient setting. The nurse can contribute greatly to maintenance of the patient's weight and preservation of lean body mass with a few simple nutritional interventions: (1) Patients should be weighed at each visit, and height should be measured at the initial visit; (2) the patient should be asked about his or her usual body weight; (3) the nurse should take an abbreviated diet history (e.g., food intake for the past 2 days) to form an impression about the patient's intake; if it is questionable, a food diary may be helpful; (4) the nurse should ask about appetite and GI symptoms such as altered taste perception, nausea, vomiting, and diarrhea. The nurse also should ask if dairy products cause flatulence or loose stools (lactose intolerance may be a possibility).

Socioeconomic circumstances also can affect nutrition. Can the patient afford to buy food? Does the patient have transportation to the store? Is the patient strong enough to carry groceries? Who does the shopping? Are refrigeration and cooking facilities available? Does the patient understand the principles of good nutrition? The nurse also should assess other factors that may affect nutrition. Is the patient too tired to prepare food? Is cognitive impairment an issue, causing the patient to forget to eat? The use of alcohol can result in diminished food intake, as well as folate and thiamine deficiencies. Illicit drug use may affect appetite, priorities, and budget. The patient's nutritional laboratory values should be checked for clues to nutritional status (Box 16-8).

---

**BOX 16-8**

### LABORATORY TESTS FOR ASSESSING NUTRITIONAL STATUS

- **Albumin** is a measure of lean body mass but a rather late indicator of nutritional compromise; 3.2 to 4.5 g/dl is considered normal, 2.8 to 3.1 g/dl indicates mild protein depletion, 2.1 to 2.7 g/dl indicates moderate protein depletion, and <2.1 g/dl indicates severe protein depletion (Anastasi, Lee, 1993).
- **TIBC (total iron-binding capacity)** is an indirect measure of the protein transferrin. Because transferrin has a shorter half-life, it shows protein depletion earlier than albumin.
- **Prealbumin** has an even shorter half-life than transferrin and is a very sensitive indicator of acute protein loss. It can be useful in assessing acutely ill patients (Romeyn, 1995).
- **Triglycerides** are lipids that the body uses primarily to assist in the storage of fats. Because of the derangement of fat metabolism, triglycerides often are elevated in HIV disease.
- **Cholesterol,** which is also a lipid, is essential for the production of steroid hormones such as cortisol. A below-normal cholesterol level indicates nutritional compromise.
- **24-hour urine creatinine** can be used with the patient's height to calculate the creatinine-height index. Creatinine is a byproduct of muscle anabolism (production); therefore if low levels are excreted, little muscle is being produced.
- **Hemoglobin** and **hematocrit** are used to assess for anemia, which may arise from a deficiency state.
- **Vitamin $B_{12}$** and **folate** deficiencies cause a macrocytic anemia, that is, anemia in which the mean corpuscular volume (MCV) in the complete blood count is below 100. A vitamin $B_{12}$ deficiency can result in neuropathy.

---

In the acute care setting, the nutritional status of an acutely ill patient should be assessed more often. Patients should be weighed on admission and at least every 3 days. The nurse should ask (or observe) whether the patient is eating all meals. If not, the nurse should note how much and ask the patient why he or she is not eating (Anastasi, Lee, 1993). Another consideration is how the patient's current medical problems affect his or her nutritional status. For example, fever increases the metabolic rate, meaning that calories are burned faster. Infection can cause weakness and anorexia. Oral lesions can make eating painful. Diarrhea causes inadequate absorption of nutrients and fluid loss.

The registered dietitian can perform anthropometric testing and calculate LBM from triceps skin fold and midarm circumference measurements. The dietitian should calculate the appropriate number of calories for the patient (a number that can vary widely, from 25 to 60 kcal/kg/day, with at least 20% of calories from protein) (Anastasi, Lee, 1993). A workable meal plan that takes into consideration the patient's food preferences can then be developed.

## Nursing Nutritional Interventions

After consultation with the dietitian, the patient should have a clear diet plan. In addition, he or she daily should take two multivitamins that contain antioxidants and trace minerals (the Recommended Daily Allowance [RDA] describes the amount of nutrients required to keep healthy people from developing deficiencies). Exercise, particularly weight-bearing exercise, is important for HIV-positive patients because, in addition to promoting a feeling of well-being, it helps build lean body mass. HIV-positive people in the early years of their illness should incorporate regular exercise into their daily lives. Those who are symptomatic should do what they can without causing excess fatigue. Maximizing antiretroviral therapy to minimize the body's total viral burden also is critical, since HIV has damaging effects on nutritional status at all stages of infection (see Box 16-7 for strategies for patients who have already lost weight). The nurse should be actively involved in teaching patients strategies to maximize nutritional status.

High-calorie, high-protein diets can help prevent and reverse loss of lean body mass. HIV-positive patients should be encouraged to include high-protein foods in all meals and snacks.

## TRANSMISSION

The Centers for Disease Control and Prevention has overseen the surveillance of AIDS cases since HIV was first identified. The modes of transmission identified have remained constant over the course of the epidemic. HIV can be transmitted through exposure to blood, semen, vaginal, or cervical secretions during sexual intercourse. It can be transmitted through exposure to blood through needle sharing among injection drug users, through an occupational exposure, or through an infected transfusion of blood or blood products. It also can be transmitted from mother to baby in utero, at the time of birth, or during breast-feeding.

Successful infection may depend on the amount of virus to which the recipient is exposed, the route of exposure, the recipient's health status, and the donor's stage of disease. Variables that affect transmission have been identified for all routes of exposure. For example, transmission from male to female is estimated to be approximately a 20 times greater risk than female to male transmission. The explanation for this seems to be the greater surface area of mucosal tissue in a woman's vagina that is exposed to infectious HIV compared with the amount of mucosal tissue in the male urethra that is exposed to vaginal secretions (Sande, Volberding, 1997). Inflammation present during genital infections also is known to facilitate transmission, as is exposure to larger amounts or more virulent viral strains from a donor who is in the primary infection stage or in advanced-stage disease.

## Perinatal (Vertical) Transmission

Perinatal transmission can occur in utero, intrapartum, or postpartum through breast-feeding. Perinatal transmission is the identified route of transmission for approximately 90% of children infected with HIV in the United States. Perinatal transmission has its own variables, which include the mother's stage of disease, including her CD4 count and viral burden; the type of delivery; whether a cesarean section was performed; prematurity; and prolonged rupture of membranes. HIV is also carried in breast milk. Breast-feeding carries a 14% increased risk of transmission compared with bottle feeding (Sande, Volberding, 1997). HIV-positive women in the United States are discouraged from breast-feeding their infants. Studies have shown that antiretroviral therapy can significantly reduce the risk of perinatal transmission. The AIDS Clinical Trials Group (ACTG) Study 076 compared pregnant women taking AZT to those taking a placebo. For the women taking AZT, the risk of transmission was reduced from 25% to 8%. Subsequent recommendations from the federal Public Health Service have encouraged the use of AZT during pregnancy and at the time of birth to reduce transmission and in the infant until 6 weeks of age (CDC, 1995b).

All women of childbearing age should be evaluated for HIV risk, counseled about HIV, and offered antibody testing so that they can make informed decisions about pregnancy.

## Occupational Transmission

**Occupational exposure** to HIV leads to transmission of infection overall in 0.3% of exposures in the health care setting (1 in 200 to 1 in 400 exposures). A case control study performed by the CDC (1996a) identified risk factors for infection after exposure. The risk increased with (1) exposures involving deep perforation of the skin, (2) visible blood on the device causing injury, (3) exposure to a device previously placed in the source patient's vein or artery (e.g., a needle used for phlebotomy), and (4) a source patient who died of AIDS within 60 days of exposure (who was presumed to have a high viral burden). The risk of infection may exceed 0.3% in exposures involving high viral loads or larger volumes of blood. Risk involving mucous membranes is approximately 0.1% and less than 0.1% for skin exposures to HIV-infected blood. These also may vary by HIV titer, volume of blood, and duration of exposure. In June, 1996, the CDC published its guidelines in the article, "Recommendations for Post-Exposure Prophylaxis for Health Care Workers" (CDC, 1996c). Postexposure prophylaxis with AZT was associated with a 79% decrease in the risk of infection from percutaneous exposure.

Current recommendations suggest that postexposure prophylaxis should be used in cases in which the risk of HIV transmission is highest. AZT should be used in postexposure regimens with lamivudine to increase antiretroviral potency. A protease inhibitor may be added when the highest risk of transmission exists, as described above (indinavir generally is used because of its potency and favorable side effect profile). All institutions should have a protocol for handling exposure to HIV. The nurse should familiarize herself with the steps involved in this protocol. See Box 16-9 for general recommendations for postexposure management.

## Universal Precautions

Prevention of accidental exposures is the most effective tool against transmission in the health care setting. Occupational exposure to HIV refers to contact with blood, needle sticks, punctures with other sharp objects, and contact with mucous membranes or open skin.

To prevent occupational exposures, all health care workers must practice **Universal Precautions**. This assumes that all patients are potentially infectious. Extreme care must be taken in handling sharp instruments, needles should never be recapped, and all sharps must be disposed of in an approved container. Universal Precautions apply to blood or other potentially infectious material such as semen, vaginal secretions, CSF, synovial fluid, saliva in dental procedures,

---

**BOX 16-9**

### COMPONENTS OF POSTEXPOSURE MANAGEMENT

- Rapid reporting of exposure incident
- Rapid evaluation
  Details of exposure (depth of stick, amount of inoculum)
  History of source patient (CD4 count, viral load, antiretroviral history)
- If appropriate, prophylaxis should be started within 24 hours or sooner
- Anxiety control
  Instruction on transmission and incidence of seroconversion
  Mental health consultation or referral if appropriate

---

any body fluid that is visibly contaminated with blood, and all body fluid situations in which it is difficult or impossible to differentiate body fluids. Other guidelines are:

- Hands must be washed after gloves are removed or if contamination with blood or other infectious material may have occurred.
- Gloves should be worn when the nurse can reasonably anticipate contact with blood or other potentially infectious materials, or with mucous membranes or nonintact skin, or in other such conditions when performing vascular access procedures.
- Gloves should be replaced if contaminated, torn, or punctured or when their ability to function as a barrier is compromised.
- Gloves should be changed between contact with different patients.
- Masks, eye protection, and face shields should be worn whenever splashes, spray, splatter, or droplets of blood or other infectious material may be generated and when eye, nose, or mouth contamination can be reasonably anticipated.
- Gowns, aprons, and other protective body clothing should be worn in situations or for procedures that may involve occupational exposure. The type of protective garments depends on the task and the degree of potential exposure to infected bodily fluids.
- Surgical caps or hoods and shoe covers or boots should be worn when gross contamination can be reasonably anticipated.
- Contaminated needles and other contaminated sharps should not be bent or sheared. Recapping is prohibited unless no alternative is available;

then a recapping device or one-handed technique may be used.

• Immediately after use, contaminated needles or sharps should be placed in puncture-resistant, leak-proof containers as close to the site of use as possible.

• Specimens should be placed in a leak-proof container. Care must be taken to avoid contaminating the outside of the container.

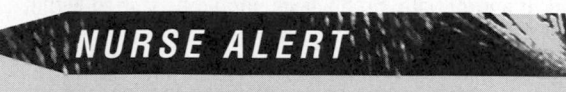

**NURSE ALERT**

Proper disposal of sharps protects the nurse and other health care workers at risk.

## LABORATORY TESTS

### Obtaining Informed Consent

Finding out that one is HIV infected can have enormous emotional and personal consequences. Therefore in most cases individuals cannot be tested without their consent. Most states have a law requiring that informed consent be obtained before a person is tested for HIV infection. These laws often specify what information must be disclosed before testing and who may be privy to the information after it is received. Health care workers must obtain a release of information from the patient before disclosing the patient's HIV status.

### HIV Antibody Testing

**HIV antibody** testing was developed in 1985 with the primary goal of screening the nation's blood supply. It soon became widely used as an indicator of infection. Antibody testing reflects the fact that antibodies are produced against viral proteins in the envelope and the core of the virus and against regulatory gene proteins. The body generally takes 6 to 12 weeks to produce these antibodies but may take longer. The period of time required for antibodies to become detectable is called the window period. If a person is tested for HIV antibodies during the window period, the result could be negative when in fact the individual is truly infected but has not yet produced antibodies. This could falsely lead an individual to believe that he or she is not infected. The antibody testing most frequently used is the enzyme-linked immunofluorescence assay (ELISA) screening and the Western blot confirmatory test. If the ELISA result is positive, the Western blot test is performed to confirm the presence of antibodies. In general, a positive result means that the patient has made antibody to at least two of the viral proteins p24, gp41, or gp160/120. If both the ELISA and the Western blot test are positive, the patient is HIV infected.

If the antibody testing is negative, the patient may still be in the window period and may not have produced antibodies yet but nevertheless is truly infected. For this reason it is prudent to repeat the test if the index of suspicion for HIV is high.

Recently, home HIV antibody tests have been developed so that those who are not comfortable being tested will have access to private testing. Although these tests appear to have the same accuracy as testing done in physicians' offices or counseling and testing sites, they do not offer the benefits of in-person counseling and support. Those who find out that they are HIV positive may receive information on the phone from staff employed by home testing companies. Nurses may encounter individuals who need support and resource referral after finding out at home that they are HIV positive.

### Absolute CD4 Cell Count and CD4 Percentage

CD4 cell measurements are used as part of the evaluation to determine a patient's stage of disease. They also are used as a guide to determine a patient's risk for HIV complications and the need for prophylaxis against opportunistic infections. Figure 16-5 shows the relationship between the CD4 count and HIV/AIDS-related complications. When combined with viral load testing, CD4 counts also provide useful information for the decision on when to initiate antiretroviral therapy. Normal CD4 values range from $700/mm^3$ to $1100/mm^3$ but may be slightly higher or lower even in uninfected individuals.

CD4 cells vary diurnally, with lowest levels occurring at 12:30 PM and the highest levels at 8:30 PM (Malone et al, 1990). CD4 values also decline with concurrent illness, particularly with acute CMV infection, hepatitis B infection, and TB, and sometimes after surgery. Administration of corticosteroids can reduce CD4 levels significantly. Values also can differ significantly between laboratories.

It is important to obtain serial CD4 measurements so that trends can be identified. The value of a single CD4 count is limited. These values generally are measured several months apart.

### CD4 Percentage

Some clinicians prefer to monitor the CD4 cell percentage because it is less subject to variation than the absolute CD4 count and over time remains more consistent. The proportion of all lymphocytes that have the CD4 cell surface markers normally is 40% to 70%. When an absolute CD4 count is different from that expected, it may be useful to compare serial CD4 percentages to determine if the change in the absolute count is meaningful.

As discussed under Natural History, CD4 values also correlate closely with the risk for various opportunistic infections; therefore decisions on prophylaxis and diagnosis of opportunistic infections can be aided by CD4 testing. For example, if a patient with pneumonia has a CD4 count that has consistently been 500/mm³, PCP can be ruled out because it occurs mostly with CD4 counts around 200/mm³ or lower.

---

**NURSE ALERT**

Patient teaching should include information about the CD4 count so that the patient knows his or her risk for opportunistic infections. Encouraging patients to get the CD4 test at the same time of day and in the same laboratory helps make comparison of results useful.

---

## Viral Load

The amount of virus found in the plasma of the blood is known as the viral load. Viral load measurements provide valuable insight into the effectiveness of treatment (Kappes et al, 1995), as well as the rate of progression (Mellors et al, 1996). Since the amount of virus found in the plasma at a given moment is a result of the struggle between viral replication and the immune response, the viral load measurement reveals how actively the virus is reproducing and correlates closely with the rate of CD4 cell destruction.

Additionally, the viral load is predictive of the number of years until the patient develops AIDS. Mellors and colleagues separated viral loads into five categories to see if they could predict progression to AIDS or death by viral load. Their findings were startling. They found that the following percentages of patients in each category developed AIDS within 6 years: 5.4% of those with 500 copies/ml or less; 16.6% of those with 501 to 3000 copies/ml; 31.7% of those with 3001 to 10,000 copies/ml; 55.2% of those with 10,001 to 30,000 copies/ml; and 80% of those with more than 30,000 copies/ml. They also found that the following percentages of patients in each category died of AIDS within 6 years: 0.9% of those with 500 copies/ml or less; 6.3% of those with 501 to 3000 copies/ml; 18.1% of those with 3,001 to 10,000 copies/ml; 34.9% of those

with 10,001 to 30,000 copies/ml; and 69.5% of those with more than 30,000 copies/ml.

Currently two different measures of viral load are used, the HIV ribonucleic acid polymerase chain reaction (RNA PCR) and the branched DNA assay (bDNA). Both of these tests actually measure the molecules of RNA found in one milliliter of plasma. It is important to note that standard viral load testing measures only the amount of virus detectable in the plasma and not in other important viral compartments such as the lymph nodes. Although both tests measure the viral RNA, they use different methods. Unfortunately, the results are difficult to compare; therefore it is important to be consistent about which test is used for an individual patient. The HIV RNA PCR involves taking the patient's viral sample and adding a set amount of virus to it so that the amount of virus can be detected. After the virion have been counted, the multiplier is subtracted to quantify the remaining virus. Branched DNA also measures the amount of RNA by attaching a signal amplifier to the virus that actually lights the virus so that it can be easily identified and measured. According to data obtained in the Multicenter AIDS Cohort Study (MACS), HIV RNA PCR values are approximately two times higher than those obtained by bDNA (Mellors et al, 1997), so that if a patient has used both assays, the RT-PCR result can be divided by two to make an approximate comparison of the two measurements. The results of either bDNA or RNA PCR can be greatly affected if the tests are not performed properly. Box 16-10 presents a summary of important points.

Viral load is reported in "copies per milliliter" (one "copy" equals one virion, or particle of virus)

---

**BOX 16-10**

### POINTS TO REMEMBER ABOUT VIRAL LOAD TESTING

- Viral load measurements obtained approximately 6 months after seroconversion predict progression.
- Measurements from the same patient may vary, sometimes greatly.
- Significant transient increases can occur after immunization and during concurrent illness.
- Collecting blood in test tubes containing heparin will distort the viral load results.
- Specimens for viral load testing must be processed within 6 hours of being drawn.
- Reducing the viral load is a key factor in improving survival.

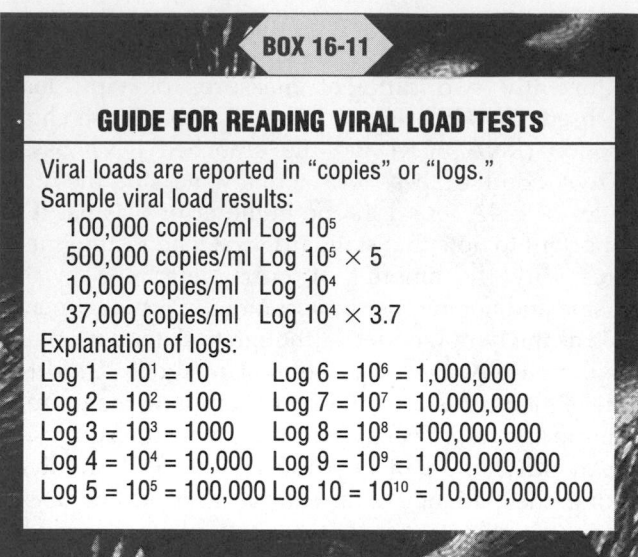

BOX 16-11

**GUIDE FOR READING VIRAL LOAD TESTS**

Viral loads are reported in "copies" or "logs."
Sample viral load results:
  100,000 copies/ml Log $10^5$
  500,000 copies/ml Log $10^5 \times 5$
  10,000 copies/ml  Log $10^4$
  37,000 copies/ml  Log $10^4 \times 3.7$
Explanation of logs:
Log 1 = $10^1$ = 10       Log 6 = $10^6$ = 1,000,000
Log 2 = $10^2$ = 100      Log 7 = $10^7$ = 10,000,000
Log 3 = $10^3$ = 1000     Log 8 = $10^8$ = 100,000,000
Log 4 = $10^4$ = 10,000   Log 9 = $10^9$ = 1,000,000,000
Log 5 = $10^5$ = 100,000  Log 10 = $10^{10}$ = 10,000,000,000

(Box 16-11). Measuring a baseline viral load at the start of treatment and then remeasuring 3 to 4 weeks later provides essential information on the effectiveness of the treatment regimen. The viral load on a new treatment should begin to drop after several weeks of therapy. The maximum drop on a particular regimen may not occur for months. The results usually come back from the laboratory in absolute copy numbers and in "log" numbers.

According to guidelines published by the federal Department of Health and Human Services (1997), effective treatment should reduce the viral load minimally by 1 log. The optimal goal in any treatment regimen is to reduce the amount of virus in the plasma to below the limit of detection, which at this time varies depending on which method is used. New ultrasensitive testing measures viral load down to 20 to 50 copies. Reducing the amount of virus to below the limit of the tests' detection is *not* synonymous with eliminating the virus; it means that the level of remaining virus in the blood is too low to measure. Furthermore, it must be remembered that viral load testing measures only the virus in the blood and not in other places where the virus lives, such as the lymph nodes. This is important information to convey to patients who may confuse undetectable with eliminated.

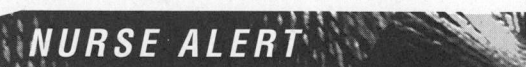

**NURSE ALERT**

Stress to the patient that although the viral load may be undetectable, this does not mean the virus has been eliminated from the body.

## TREATMENT

Medications used to interfere with the viral life cycle and replication process are known as antiretrovirals. Several classes of **antiretroviral therapy** currently are available for treating HIV. The basis for each class of medication is that viral replication is the primary mode of immune system destruction. Thus it is imperative that viral replication be stopped or at least limited if survival is to be improved. Each medication is designed to interrupt the virus' ability to produce mature virus particles that are able to infect other cells. Information learned about the viral life cycle has provided insight into possible points of interruption and hence viral suppression.

The field of HIV treatment has evolved rapidly since the FDA approved the first HIV medication, AZT, in 1986. The development of numerous other medications for HIV have raised questions of treatment strategy; when to start treatment, what to start with, when to switch treatment, and what to switch to. Concerns about the impact of drug resistance on treatment options have fueled these discussions. Table 16-3 shows a detailed list of the risks and benefits of initiating antiretroviral therapy early (U.S. Department of Health and Human Services, 1997). The development of more potent therapies and the means to evaluate these therapies have shaped the current strategy, "Hit early, hit hard." *Hit early* implies that treatment should be initiated early in the disease so that the damage from uncontrolled replication can be minimized and the immune system spared. *Hit hard* implies that the treatment regimen should include the most potent medications possible within side effect, resistance, and drug interaction limitations (see drug resistance and drug interaction in the following sections). Numerous studies have shown that treatment delays the onset of progression to symptomatic disease or AIDS (Walthen et al, 1996).

Currently three different classes of antiretroviral therapy are used against HIV infection. They are the nucleoside reverse transcriptase inhibitors (NRTIs), which are also called nucleoside analogs; the nonnucleoside reverse transcriptase inhibitors (NNRTIs), and the protease inhibitors (PIs). Although each of the medications in these classes works against the virus, each has a different mechanism of action; these mechanisms of action are outlined in Table 16-4.

An analog is a substance that closely resembles another substance; hence nucleoside analogs resemble nucleosides, which are the chemicals that form DNA. The nucleoside analogs, or NRTIs, work very early in the viral life cycle by "fooling" the virus into using the artificial nucleosides to form DNA as if they were viral nucleosides. Thus the viral genetic code is altered, and successful replication cannot occur. NNRTIs work

---

**TABLE 16-3**

## Risks and Benefits of Early Initiation of Antiretroviral Therapy in the Asymptomatic HIV-Infected Patient

| POTENTIAL BENEFITS | POTENTIAL RISKS |
|---|---|
| Control of viral replication and mutation, reduction of viral burden | Reduction in quality of life from adverse effects of drug |
| Prevention of progressive immunodeficiency; potential maintenance of a normal immune system | Earlier development of drug resistance |
| | Limitation in future choices of antiretroviral agents |
| | Dissemination of drug-resistant virus |
| Delayed progression to AIDS and prolongation of life | Unknown long-term toxicity of certain drugs |
| Reduced risk of developing resistant virus | Unknown duration of effectiveness of current antiretroviral therapies |
| Reduced risk of drug toxicity | |

From US Department of Health and Human Services: *Fed Reg* 62(118):33417, 1997.

---

**TABLE 16-4**

## Classes of Antiretroviral Agents

| CLASS | ACTIVITY | AGENTS |
|---|---|---|
| Nucleoside reverse transcriptase inhibitors (NRTIs)—*thymidines* | Work in *activated* CD4 cells to prevent HIV RNA from becoming DNA | AZT (zidovudine, Retrovir) |
| | | d4T (stavudine, Zerit) |
| Nucleoside reverse transcriptase inhibitors (NRTIs)—*nonthymidines* | Work in *resting* CD4 cells to prevent HIV RNA from becoming DNA | ddI (didanosine, Videx) |
| | | ddC (zalcitabine, Hivid) |
| | | 3TC (lamivudine, Epivir) |
| Nonnucleoside reverse transcriptase inhibitors (NNRTIs) | Bind to enzyme reverse transcriptase to prevent HIV RNA from becoming DNA | Nevirapine (Viramune) |
| | | Delavirdine (Rescriptor) |
| Protease inhibitors (PIs) | Prevent newly made HIV particles from being assembled and released from infected CD4 cell | Saquinavir (Invirase) |
| | | Indinavir (Crixivan) |
| | | Ritonavir (Norvir) |
| | | Nelfinavir (Viracept) |

---

later in the viral life cycle by binding to the enzyme reverse transcriptase, which is necessary for the transcription of HIV RNA to HIV DNA. Without reverse transcriptase, the viral RNA cannot be changed into DNA and thus cannot replicate. The protease enzyme is required for successful assembly of viral proteins at the end of the viral life cycle so that mature viral particles are produced. PIs act by binding to protease and preventing it from assembling viruses. The PIs are thus far the most potent medications against HIV. However, none of these medications should ever be used alone.

Two studies performed by the ACTG and analyzed in 1996 and 1997 have guided the principles of HIV treatment. ACTG 175 showed that combining different antiretroviral agents is far more effective in suppressing viral replication than using any single agent. ACTG 320 then showed that three drugs are more potent than two and therefore should be the standard of care in most cases.

Depending on the level of illness, all patients who choose to be treated for HIV generally are treated with three to four medications that have been shown to work well together. Combining medications has the benefit of synergy (two or more drugs used together have a greater benefit than any drug used alone); a decrease in side effects because sometimes lower doses of each drug can be used, which minimizes toxicity; and diminished resistance to each of the medications. Treatment is guided by viral load measurements and CD4 cell counts, which should be obtained at the start of treatment. A second viral load measurement should be obtained 2 to 4 weeks after the start of treatment. Viral load measurements should then be measured every 3 to 4 months during therapy as a surrogate marker for loss of drug effectiveness resulting from viral resistance. In the past a viral load decrease of 1 log was considered an acceptable response to therapy. However, it is now known that the development of resistance to medication is inevitable unless viral replication is completely suppressed. The treatment goal, then, is to bring the viral load down to a nondetectable level (i.e., less than 20 to 50 copies/ml). At this time actual resistance testing, although available, is not standardized and is very costly, and its results are difficult to interpret.

Although substantial progress has been made in HIV since the beginning of the epidemic, many questions remain unanswered. Is complete eradication of the virus within the body possible? Will discontinuation of treatment ever be possible? What is the role of immune system–boosting therapies in HIV care? What is the real value of increasing T-cell counts? Is a vaccine possible?

## Viral Resistance

**Viral resistance** means that the structure of the virus has changed sufficiently to render the antiretroviral medication less effective or ineffective against the virus. During the HIV replication process, mistakes in translation of the viral strands occur regularly. This happens because of the intense rate of viral replication and because the enzyme reverse transcriptase is very error prone. As a result of these mistakes, the amino acids that form the HIV RNA strands are substituted for other amino acids at various locations on the RNA strand, changing its structure. These substitutions in amino acids are called *mutations*. The locations of individual amino acids on the RNA strand are called codons. The codons are identified by number, and mutations occur at specific codons. For example, AZT resistance occurs because of mutations at several codons, including codon 215.

The most important factor in the development of resistance to HIV medications is incomplete suppression of viral replication. This can occur because of an inadequate treatment regimen or because of suboptimal adherence to treatment (i.e., patients do not take their medications exactly as prescribed). Even when the patient takes all doses of medication, resistance eventually emerges if viral replication is not completely suppressed. Also, cross-resistance can occur with different HIV medications, so that the development of resistance to one medication means the virus automatically is resistant to other medications in the same class that act in similar ways.

## Adherence to Antiretroviral Regimens

The ability to comply with current medication regimens has become quite complex for people with HIV. Drug-drug interactions and food-drug interactions lay the foundation of difficult medication schedules. Instructions such as "Take one pill with food, take an-

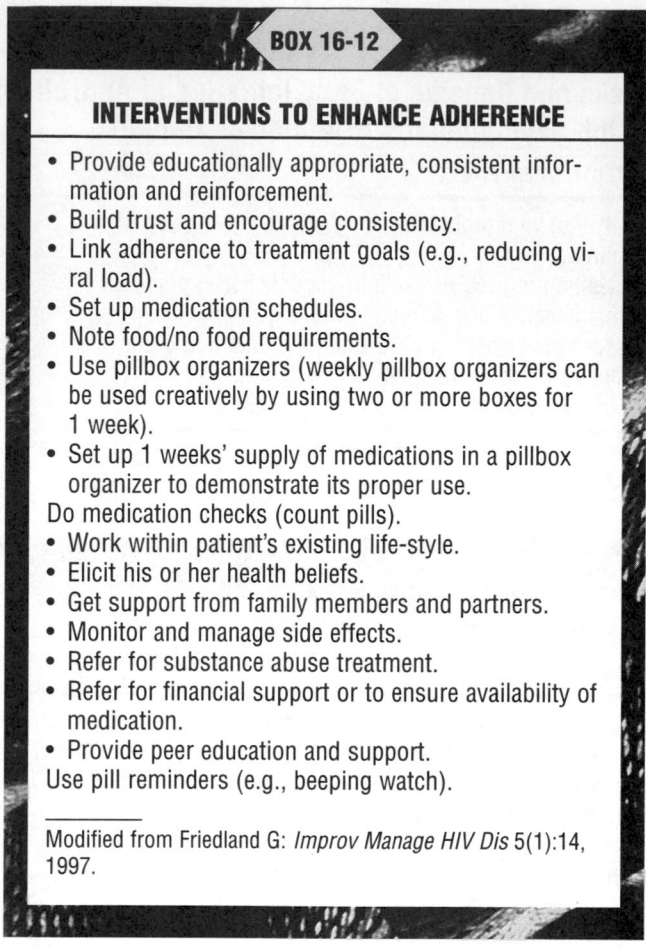

**BOX 16-12**

### INTERVENTIONS TO ENHANCE ADHERENCE

- Provide educationally appropriate, consistent information and reinforcement.
- Build trust and encourage consistency.
- Link adherence to treatment goals (e.g., reducing viral load).
- Set up medication schedules.
- Note food/no food requirements.
- Use pillbox organizers (weekly pillbox organizers can be used creatively by using two or more boxes for 1 week).
- Set up 1 weeks' supply of medications in a pillbox organizer to demonstrate its proper use.

Do medication checks (count pills).

- Work within patient's existing life-style.
- Elicit his or her health beliefs.
- Get support from family members and partners.
- Monitor and manage side effects.
- Refer for substance abuse treatment.
- Refer for financial support or to ensure availability of medication.
- Provide peer education and support.

Use pill reminders (e.g., beeping watch).

Modified from Friedland G: *Improv Manage HIV Dis* 5(1):14, 1997.

other on an empty stomach, but take neither within 2 hours of each other or of certain other pills" easily overwhelm even sophisticated consumers. Large numbers of pills (sometimes more than 25 a day) and side effects of these drugs also demotivate patients from adhering to difficult regimens. Patient factors also contribute to the success or failure of adherence. Knowledge and understanding of medications, personal beliefs about treatment and illness, and trust in the provider, as well as a nonstructured environment (from homelessness or drug or alcohol addiction), heavily influence individuals.

The nurse's role in patient compliance is a vital one that begins with evaluating the likelihood of compliance. Time spent with the patient in the home, the hospital, or the clinic can give the nurse the opportunity to ask focused questions, the answers to which can provide insight into compliance. Vague or unsure answers in response to questioning about regimens may offer insight. Pill counts have proved to be only a moderately reliable indicator of compliance. Social support and a consistent provider can improve the likelihood of adherence. The Patient/Family Teaching box below lists some points that patients should be taught about HIV medication, and Box 16-12 presents interventions for enhancing adherence to these recommendations.

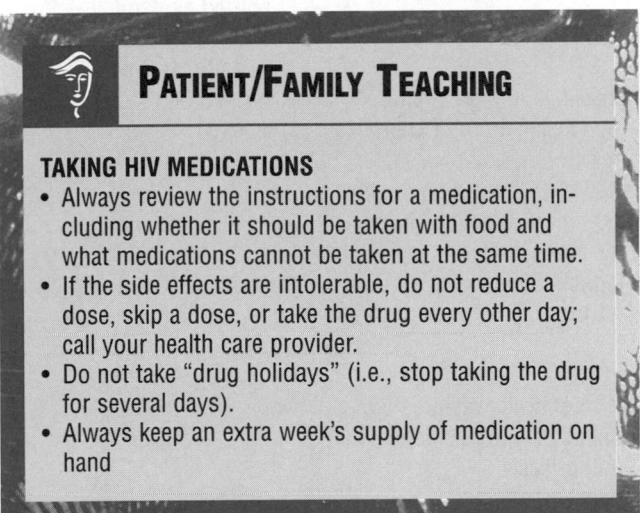

## NURSE ALERT

**The nurse must stress the importance of adherence to medication regimens in order to delay resistance to treatment.**

## PATIENT/FAMILY TEACHING

**TAKING HIV MEDICATIONS**
- Always review the instructions for a medication, including whether it should be taken with food and what medications cannot be taken at the same time.
- If the side effects are intolerable, do not reduce a dose, skip a dose, or take the drug every other day; call your health care provider.
- Do not take "drug holidays" (i.e., stop taking the drug for several days).
- Always keep an extra week's supply of medication on hand

## Summary of Principles of HIV Infection Therapy

Box 16-13 presents a summary of the principles of HIV infection therapy drawn from the 1997 guidelines published by the U.S. Department of Health and Human Services.

## Prophylaxis

It is possible to prevent many opportunistic infections through medication **prophylaxis**. The word *prophylaxis* comes from the Greek word meaning "to guard against." The CDC issues recommendations for specific medications to be prescribed at different CD4 counts to prevent designated opportunistic infections. Primary prophylaxis refers to medication given to prevent the first episode of a particular infection. Secondary prophylaxis refers to medication given to prevent recurrence once a particular infection has occurred. See Tables 16-5 and 16-6 for the CDC's recommendations on prophylaxis.

---

**BOX 16-13**

### SUMMARY OF THE PRINCIPLES OF THERAPY FOR HIV INFECTION

1. HIV replication leads to immune system damage and progression to AIDS. HIV infection is always harmful, and true long-term survival free of clinically significant immune dysfunction is unusual.
2. Plasma HIV RNA levels indicate the magnitude of HIV replication and its associated rate of CD4 cell destruction. CD4 cell counts indicate the extent of HIV-induced immune damage already incurred. Regular periodic measurement of plasma HIV RNA levels and CD4 T cells is necessary to determine the risk of disease progression in an HIV-infected individual and to determine when to initiate or modify antiretroviral treatment regimens.
3. Just as the rate of disease progression differs among individuals, treatment decisions should be individualized and should be based on the level of risk indicated by plasma HIV RNA levels and the CD4 cell counts.
4. Resistance is the major factor limiting the ability of antiretroviral drugs to inhibit viral replication and delay the progression of disease. Using potent combination antiretroviral therapy to suppress HIV replication to levels below detection limits the potential for emergence of HIV strains resistant to medications. Therefore the goal of therapy should be the maximum achievable suppression of HIV replication.
5. The most effective way to accomplish durable suppression of HIV replication is simultaneous initiation of combinations of effective anti-HIV drugs that the patient has not been treated with previously *and* that are not cross-resistant with antiretroviral agents that the patient has been treated with previously.
6. Each of the antiretroviral drugs used in combination therapy regimens should always be used according to optimum schedules and dosages.
7. The available effective antiretroviral drugs are limited in number and mechanism of action, and cross-resistance between specific drugs has been documented. For this reason, any change in antiretroviral therapy tightens future therapeutic constraints.
8. Women should receive optimum antiretroviral therapy regardless of pregnancy status.

---

Modified from US Department of Health and Human Services: *Fed Reg* 62(118):33417, 1997.

**TABLE 16-5**

## Recommended Prophylaxis against Opportunistic Infections in HIV-Positive Adults*

| PATHOGEN | INDICATION | FIRST-CHOICE PROPHYLAXIS | SECOND-CHOICE PROPHYLAXIS |
|---|---|---|---|
| **Strongly Recommended as Standard of Care** | | | |
| *Pneumocystis carinii* | CD4 count <200/$\mu$l, or unexplained fever for 2 wk or longer, or oropharyngeal candidiasis | TMP-SMX, 1 DS PO qd | TMP-SMX, 1 SS PO qd or 1 DS PO 3 times/wk; dapsone, 50 mg PO bid or 100 mg PO qd; dapsone 50 mg PO qd *plus* pyrimethamine, 75 mg PO weekly *plus* leucovorin, 25 mg PO weekly; aerosolized pentamidine, 300 mg monthly via Respirgard II nebulizer |
| *Mycobacterium tuberculosis* (isoniazid sensitive) | TST reaction ≥5 mm or previous positive TST result without treatment or contact with case of active tuberculosis | Isoniazid, 300 mg PO plus pyridoxine 50 mg PO qd for 12 mo; or isoniazid, 900 mg PO *plus* pyridoxine 50 mg PO 2 times/wk for 12 mo | Rifampin, 600 mg PO qd for 12 mo |
| *Mycobacterium tuberculosis* (isoniazid resistant) | Same as above; high probability of exposure to isoniazid-resistant tuberculosis | Rifampin, 600 mg PO qd for 12 mo | Rifabutin, 300 mg PO qd for 12 mo |
| *Mycobacterium tuberculosis* (multidrug resistant) | Same as above; high probability of exposure to multidrug-resistant tuberculosis | Choice of drugs requires consultation with public health authorities | None |
| *Toxoplasma gondii* | IgG antibody to *Toxoplasma* and CD4 count <100/$\mu$l | TMP-SMX, 1 DS PO qd | TMP-SMX, 1 SS PO qd or 1 DS PO 3 times/wk; dapsone, 50 mg PO qd *plus* pyrimethamine, 50 mg PO weekly *plus* folinic acid, 25 mg PO weekly |
| **Recommended for Consideration in All Patients** | | | |
| *Streptococcus pneumoniae* | All patients | Pneumococcal vaccine 0.5 ml IM once, then q 6 yr | None |
| *Mycobacterium avium* complex | CD4 count of <75/$\mu$l | Rifabutin 300 mg PO qd | Azithromycin 1200 mg PO weekly; clarithromycin, 500 mg PO bid |
| **Not Recommended for Most Patients; Indicated for Consideration only in Selected Populations or Patients** | | | |
| Bone marrow infections or malignancy | Neutropenia | Granulocte colony-stimulating factor (G-CSF or filgrastim) 5-10 $\mu$g/kg SC qd for 2-4 wk; or granulocyte-stimulating factor, 250 $\mu$g/m$^2$, IV over 2 hr qd for 2-4 wk | None |

Modified from Centers for Disease Control and Prevention (CDC): *MMWR* 44(RR-8):1-33, 1995.
*Not all the recommended regimens reflect current U.S. Food and Drug Administration–approved labeling.
*Anti-HBc,* Antibody to hepatitis B core antigen; *bid,* twice daily; *CMV,* cytomegalovirus; *DS,* double-strength tablet; *IM,* intramuscular; *IV,* intravenous; *PO,* oral; *qd,* daily; *qid,* four times a day; *SC,* subcutaneous; *SS,* single-strength tablet; *tid,* three times a day; *TMP-SMX,* trimethoprim-sulfamethoxazole; *TST,* tuberculin skin test.

| TABLE 16-5 |
| --- |

## Recommended Prophylaxis against Opportunistic Infections in HIV-Positive Adults*—cont'd

| PATHOGEN | INDICATION | FIRST-CHOICE PROPHYLAXIS | SECOND-CHOICE PROPHYLAXIS |
| --- | --- | --- | --- |
| *Candida* species | CD4 count <50/$\mu$l | Fluconazole 100-200 mg PO qd | Ketoconazole 200 mg PO qd |
| *Cryptococcus neoformans* | CD4 count <50/$\mu$l | Fluconazole 100-200 mg PO qd | Itraconazole 200 mg PO qd |
| *Histoplasma capsulatum* | CD4 count <50/$\mu$l; endemic geographic region | Itraconazole 200 mg PO qd | Fluconazole 200 mg PO qd |
| *Coccidioides immitis* | CD4 count <50/$\mu$l; endemic geographic region | Fluconazole 200 mg PO qd | Itraconazole 200 mg PO qd |
| Cytomegalovirus (CMV) | CD4 count <50/$\mu$l and CMV antibody positivity | Ganiciclovir, 1 PO tid; only preliminary data available | None |
| Unknown (herpes viruses?) | CD4 count <200/$\mu$l | Acyclovir 800 mg PO qid | Acyclovir 200 mg PO tid-qid |
| **Recommended for Consideration** | | | |
| Hepatitis B virus | All susceptible (anti-HBc–negative patients) | Engerix-B 20 $\mu$g IM, 3 doses; or Recombivax HB 10 $\mu$g IM, 3 doses | None |
| Influenza virus | All patients (annually, before influenza season) | Whole or split virus 0.5 ml IM annually | Rimantadine 200 mg PO bid or amantadine 100 mg PO bid |

| TABLE 16-6 |
| --- |

## Recommended Prophylaxis against Recurrent Opportunistic Infection* in HIV-Infected Adults†

| PATHOGEN | INDICATION | FIRST-CHOICE PREVENTIVE REGIMEN | SECOND-CHOICE PREVENTIVE REGIMEN |
| --- | --- | --- | --- |
| **Recommended for Life as Standard of Care** | | | |
| *Pneumocystis carinii* | Previous *P. carinii* pneumonia | TMP-SMX, 1 DS PO qd | TMP-SMX, 1 SS PO qd *or* 1 DS 3 times/wk; dapsone 50 mg PO bid *or* 100 mg PO qd; dapsone 50 mg PO qd *plus* pyrimethamine 75 mg PO weekly *plus* folinic acid 25 mg PO weekly; dapsone 200 mg PO weekly *plus* pyrimethamine 75 mg PO weekly *plus* leucovorin 25 mg PO weekly; aerosolized pentamidine 300 mg monthly via Respirgard II nebulizer |
| *Toxoplasma gondii* | Previous toxoplasmic encephalitis | Sulfadiazine 1-1.5 g PO q 6 hr *plus* pyrimethamine, 25-75 mg PO qd, *plus* folinic acid 10-25 mg PO qd-qid | Clindamycin 300-450 mg PO q 6-8 hr *plus* pyrimethamine 25-75 PO qd *plus* leucovorin 10-25 mg PO qd-qid |

Modified from Centers for Disease Control and Prevention (CDC): *MMWR* 44(RR-8):1-33, 1995.
*Patient has had at least one previous episode of opportunistic infection.
†Not all the recommended regimens reflect current U.S. Food and Drug Administration–approved labeling.
*bid*, Twice daily; *CMV*, cytomegalovirus; *DS*, double-strength tablet; *IV*, intravenous; *PO*, oral; *qd*, daily; *qid*, four times a day; *SS*, single-strength tablet; *tid*, three times a day; *TMP-SMX*, trimethoprim-sulfamethoxazole.

*Continued*

**TABLE 16-6**

## Recommended Prophylaxis against Recurrent Opportunistic Infection in HIV-Infected Adults—cont'd

| PATHOGEN | INDICATION | FIRST-CHOICE PREVENTIVE REGIMEN | SECOND-CHOICE PREVENTIVE REGIMEN |
|---|---|---|---|
| **Recommended for Life as Standard of Care—cont'd** | | | |
| *Mycobacterium avium* complex | Documented disseminated disease | Clarithromycin 500 mg PO bid *plus* one or more of the following: ethambutol 15 mg/kg PO qd; clofazimine 100 mg PO qd; rifabutin 300 mg PO qd; ciprofloxacin 500-750 mg PO bid | Azithromycin 500 mg PO qd *plus* one or more of the following: ethambutol 15 mg/kg PO qd; clofazimine 100 mg PO qd; rifabutin 300 mg PO qd; ciprofloxacin 500-750 mg PO bid |
| Cytomegalovirus (CMV) | Previous end-organ disease | Ganciclovir 5-6 mg/kg IV 5-7 days/wk or 1000 mg PO tid; *or* foscarnet 90-120 mg/kg IV qd | Sustained-released ocular implants with PO ganciclovir |
| *Crypotcoccus neoformans* | Documented disease | Fluconazole 200 mg PO qd | Itraconazole 200 mg PO qd; amphotericin B, 0.6-1 mg/kg IV 1-3 times/wk |
| *Histoplasma capsulatum* | Documented disease | Itraconazole 200 mg PO bid | Amphotericin B, 1 mg/kg IV weekly; fluconazole 200-400 mg PO qd |
| *Coccidioides immitis* | Documented disease | Fluconazole 200 mg PO qd | Amphotericin B, 1 mg/kg IV weekly; itraconazole 200 mg PO bid; ketoconazole 400-800 mg PO qd |
| *Salmonella* species (nontyphi) | Bacteremia | Ciprofloxacin 500 mg PO bid for several months | None |
| **Recommended only if Subsequent Episodes Are Frequent and Severe** | | | |
| Herpes simplex virus | Frequent/severe recurrences | Acyclovir 200 mg PO tid *or* 400 mg PO bid | None |
| *Candida* species (oral, vaginal, or esophageal) | Frequent/severe recurrences | Fluconazole 100-200 mg PO qd | Ketoconazole 200 mg PO qd; itraconazole 100 mg PO qd; clotrimazole troche 20 mg PO 5 times daily nystatin 500,000 U PO 5 times daily |

# HIV INFECTION/AIDS AND THE NURSING PROCESS

The nursing assessment is a systematic method of obtaining information about an individual's needs, status, and perception of health. The nurse must assess through observation, review of the record, careful history taking, and physical examination.

The history is the starting point of the assessment. It includes the patient's physical and mental health, sexual history, and patterns of taking medication and receiving care. Questions pertaining to patient and family coping skills in times of stress also provide valuable insight. If a release of information is obtained, collaboration with other caregivers can be helpful in developing an accurate assessment.

The health history should begin with specific questions about the patient's HIV infection. If a health history has already been obtained by another health care professional, the nurse should review it before the interview with the patient. A health history should cover unexplained weight loss, fever, loss of appetite, shortness of breath, skin lesions, cough, night sweats, swollen lymph nodes, diarrhea, history of sexually transmitted diseases, and CNS changes such as headaches, seizures, or changes in mental status.

It is important to assess the patient's risk for HIV. Important clues can come from sexual or drug histories and from reports of previous blood transfusions. Many times, however, patients are reluctant to discuss this information during the initial interview.

It is essential that the nurse determine the patient's psychologic state and ability to cope with the disease. The nurse should explore the patient's knowledge of AIDS and his or her perceptions of the outcome of the disease. What changes in body image does the patient perceive? Are there outward expressions of fear, denial, grief, or loss? Does the patient have an adequate support system? What about family and friends? Who can the patient tell about the diagnosis? What coping strategies seem to work for the individual? Is there a real or perceived financial problem?

The nurse should ask open-ended questions and include, to the degree possible, family or significant others. From this assessment, a nursing diagnosis can be formed.

## Patient Education

Nurses play a valuable role in the education of patients about HIV infection. This teaching function can be integrated into the nurse's encounters with patients in outpatient or inpatient settings or in the home.

It is important to understand just how overwhelming a new HIV diagnosis can be. Individuals with HIV may have concerns about the finality of their life, their finances, their medical care, housing, and discrimination on the job or by their friends or family. Many in America still do not accept people with HIV with compassion and understanding. Judgments about how individuals were infected and their life-styles and misinformation about transmission contribute to the continuing stigma of HIV.

When educating patients about their disease, the nurse must be sensitive to cultural, ethnic, and linguistic differences. Information about HIV must be given in the patient's primary language; therefore every attempt must be made to use a translator. Also, information should be given at a level the patient can understand. Some of the information that needs to be given to individuals with HIV can make both the nurse and the patient quite uncomfortable. Patients sense the nurse's level of comfort with subjects such as sex and drugs. They generally feel as at ease as the nurse does. Therefore if either of these subjects make the nurse so uncomfortable that he or she is apt to skip the information, it would be better to find someone else who can provide the information.

The following five Patient/Family Teaching boxes provide the nurse with educational information that needs to be covered in the suggested simplified language. If the patient is being seen by the nurse over time, these points do not need to be reviewed all at once; in fact, a slower approach that allows the patient to digest the information may be more effective.

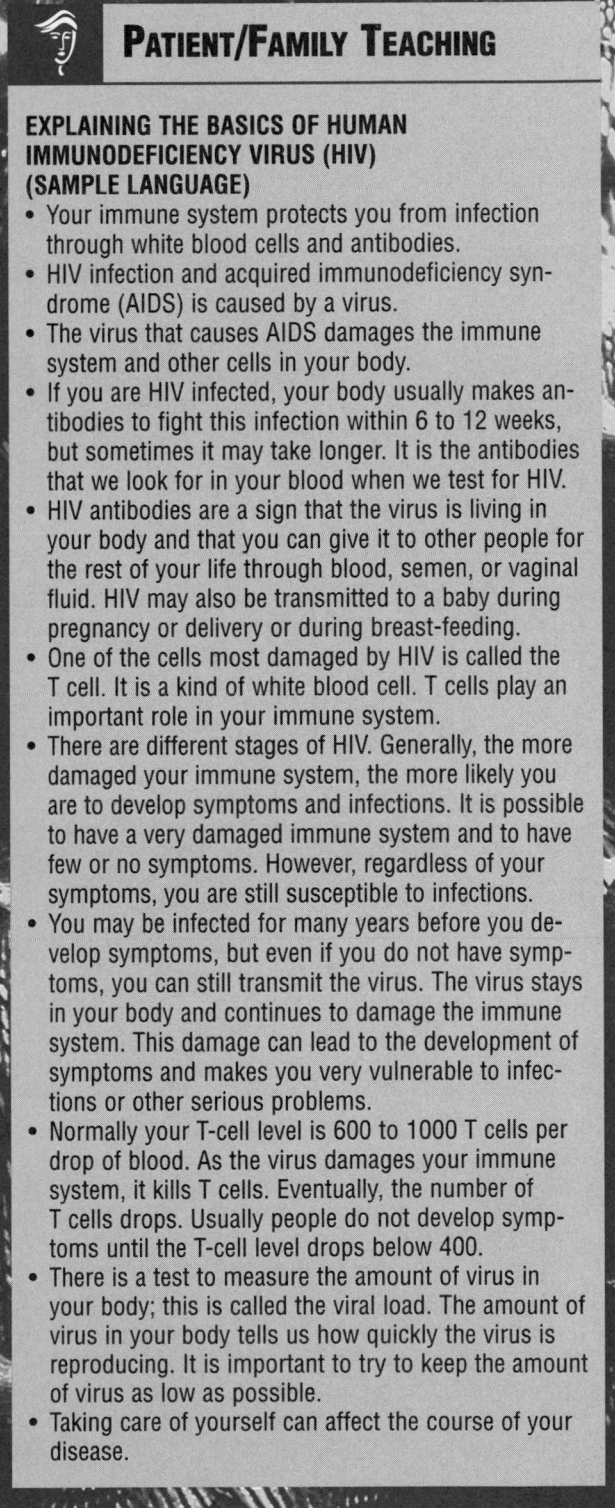

**PATIENT/FAMILY TEACHING**

**EXPLAINING THE BASICS OF HUMAN IMMUNODEFICIENCY VIRUS (HIV) (SAMPLE LANGUAGE)**

- Your immune system protects you from infection through white blood cells and antibodies.
- HIV infection and acquired immunodeficiency syndrome (AIDS) is caused by a virus.
- The virus that causes AIDS damages the immune system and other cells in your body.
- If you are HIV infected, your body usually makes antibodies to fight this infection within 6 to 12 weeks, but sometimes it may take longer. It is the antibodies that we look for in your blood when we test for HIV.
- HIV antibodies are a sign that the virus is living in your body and that you can give it to other people for the rest of your life through blood, semen, or vaginal fluid. HIV may also be transmitted to a baby during pregnancy or delivery or during breast-feeding.
- One of the cells most damaged by HIV is called the T cell. It is a kind of white blood cell. T cells play an important role in your immune system.
- There are different stages of HIV. Generally, the more damaged your immune system, the more likely you are to develop symptoms and infections. It is possible to have a very damaged immune system and to have few or no symptoms. However, regardless of your symptoms, you are still susceptible to infections.
- You may be infected for many years before you develop symptoms, but even if you do not have symptoms, you can still transmit the virus. The virus stays in your body and continues to damage the immune system. This damage can lead to the development of symptoms and makes you very vulnerable to infections or other serious problems.
- Normally your T-cell level is 600 to 1000 T cells per drop of blood. As the virus damages your immune system, it kills T cells. Eventually, the number of T cells drops. Usually people do not develop symptoms until the T-cell level drops below 400.
- There is a test to measure the amount of virus in your body; this is called the viral load. The amount of virus in your body tells us how quickly the virus is reproducing. It is important to try to keep the amount of virus as low as possible.
- Taking care of yourself can affect the course of your disease.

## PATIENT/FAMILY TEACHING

**TIPS FOR TAKING CARE OF YOURSELF**
- Be sure you have a healthy diet.
- Exercise regularly.
- Cook meat and eggs well.
- Avoid alcohol and drugs; they can contribute to disease progression.
- Get adequate sleep.
- Reduce stress if possible.
- Wear gloves when changing cat litter or bird cages (see Box 16-6).
- Do not miss any doses of medications you are taking.

## PATIENT/FAMILY TEACHING

**RISK-REDUCING PRACTICES**
- Do not share your toothbrush or razor. They may have blood on them.
- It is OK to wash your clothes and dishes with others'.
- Use bleach to clean blood spills.
- Do not donate blood, sperm, organs, or other body tissues.

## PATIENT/FAMILY TEACHING

**MINIMIZING HARM FOR INJECTION DRUG USERS**
The harm reduction theory is based on meeting individuals at their own level. Thus, recognizing that not all injection drug users will be able to become abstinent, it is important that they minimize the harm to themselves and others. They should be educated concerning the following:
- Do not share needles, cookers, or other works.
- Works and syringes should be flushed with chlorine bleach twice and water twice.
- Use needle exchange programs if available. These programs provide clean needles at no cost to injection drug users, they remove dirty needles from the street, and they have proved effective in reducing the pool of HIV among injection drug users.
- Inform sexual and needle-sharing partners of your HIV status

## PATIENT/FAMILY TEACHING

**SAFE SEXUAL PRACTICES**
- Keep blood, semen, preejaculate, and vaginal secretions from entering another's body.
- Different sexual behaviors carry different levels of risk, depending on how likely they are to allow blood, semen, preejaculate, and vaginal secretions to enter a partner's body.
- Understanding the levels of risk is important for making informed choices about how much risk is acceptable.
- Wear latex condoms for both anal and vaginal sex even if your partner also has HIV. Space should be left at the condom tip so that it does not break after ejaculation. Air should be squeezed out of the tip when you put on the condom.
- The condom should be removed immediately after ejaculation.
- Using condoms with a spermicide containing nonoxynol-9 may offer additional protection. However, nonoxynol-9 can cause irritation in some people, increasing the risk of transmission. For this reason, a small amount should be applied to the wrist before use to check for irritation, and it should not be used if irritation occurs.
- Although oral sex carries less of a risk than anal or vaginal sex, it is wise to wear condoms for this practice as well.
- Use water-based lubricants, such as KY Jelly; never use a lubricant that is oil-based, such as hand lotion, Vaseline, or Crisco.

**Levels of Safer Sex Practices**
- **Absolutely safe:** Kissing; masturbating; "humping"; performing oral sex on a man with a condom, oral sex on a woman with a dental dam or plastic wrap, finger sex with latex gloves or finger cots, or external water sports (urinating on someone); rimming (oral-anal) with a dental dam or plastic wrap, touching, massaging, fantasizing.
- **Reasonably safe:** Vaginal intercourse with a condom, anal intercourse with a condom.
- **Risky:** Oral sex on a man without a condom, masturbation on open sores or broken skin, oral sex on a woman without a barrier, rimming without a barrier.
- **High risk:** Vaginal or anal intercourse without a condom, oral sex without a barrier on a woman while she is menstruating, internal water sports, "fisting" (inserting a fist into the vagina or anus) without gloves and a lubricant.

## Psychosocial Issues

Understanding the psychosocial concerns of a person with HIV enhances your ability to provide effective care. Patients' responses to a diagnosis of HIV affect their ability to take care of themselves, to engage in treatment, and to follow through on medication regimens. Your psychosocial assessment can be used to help you intervene in meaningful ways. The life-threatening nature of the disease, its unpredictable course, the stigma that still exists about HIV in our society, and the life-altering medication regimens elicit intense and varied reactions. The responses likely to occur in any individual include denial, self-blame, fear, anxiety, anger, guilt, depression, dependent behavior, and ambivalence. Some may respond by withdrawing from friends, family, and their significant other.

Observing the interaction between the patient and his or her family, friends, and significant other can offer insights into the need for support.

After diagnosis, a feeling of being overwhelmed often sets in; the patient must consider whom to tell, what to do, where to get care, how to pay for it, and how to live with HIV. The nurse can be most helpful during this period by encouraging a "one step at a time" approach. Addressing issues one by one, giving permission not to figure everything out at once, and helping to prioritize may feel lifesaving for a newly diagnosed individual. The nurse must work with patients to identify support. The patient must plan whom to tell about the HIV infection and how to tell them (Box 16-14).

For those who have known about their diagnosis for years, the issues are different. An emerging issue for

---

◀ **BOX 16-14** ▶ | **NURSING PROCESS**

### PATIENT WITH NEWLY DIAGNOSED HIV INFECTION

**ASSESSMENT**

- General appearance
- HIV-focused history
- Nutritional status (height, weight, dietary history)
- Knowledge of disease, transmission, and complications, as well as resources
- Coping mechanisms
- Perception of illness and treatment
- Social support
- Activity level
- Sleeping patterns
- Drug and alcohol history
- Psychiatric history
- Current medications, including over-the-counter vitamins, herbs, and supplements

**NURSING DIAGNOSES**

- Ineffective coping caused by feeling overwhelmed by diagnosis and its implications
- Social isolation related to stigma of HIV
- Feelings of shame and guilt
- Knowledge deficit as a result of new diagnosis
- Denial
- Decreased self-esteem
- Anxiety resulting from uncertain prognosis
- Risk for malnutrition because of loss of appetite, altered metabolism, or other reasons
- Altered activity level

**NURSING INTERVENTIONS**

- Encourage a step-by-step approach to dealing with issues.

- Provide support and resources as necessary.
- Provide information in the patient's primary language at a level he or she can understand.
- Assess interactions with family, friends, and significant other.
- Make referrals to support group for individuals newly diagnosed with HIV.
- Monitor and document food intake and weight; educate patient about nutritional needs and concerns.
- Refer patient to a registered dietitian for nutritional consult if available.
- Encourage and validate expression of feelings.
- Assist in procurement of financial, medical, and legal resources.
- Educate patient about sleep hygiene.
- Collaborate with others on the health care team as appropriate (e.g., substance abuse counselor, psychiatrist, social services).

**EVALUATION OF EXPECTED OUTCOMES**

- Becomes knowledgeable about HIV pathogenesis, transmission, and treatment
- Begins to come to terms with HIV diagnosis
- Understands the importance of taking good care of himself or herself
- Maintains good nutritional status
- Develops a positive attitude about staying healthy
- Participates actively in care and treatment
- Receives essential support and services

many who were critically ill is how to go on living. In an era of effective treatment, they may be contemplating going back to work after years on disability and wondering how they will explain prolonged absences from the workforce without disclosing their HIV status. They may have spent their entire savings and already have cashed in their insurance policies. They may be perplexed by their own hesitation to feel joy, which is overshadowed by the enormity of planning their life instead of planning their death. The nurse should be aware of predictable crisis points so that appropriate interventions can be made (Table 16-7).

**TABLE 16-7**

## Crisis Points and Emotional Responses

| CRISIS POINT | EMOTIONAL RESPONSE | INTERVENTIONS |
|---|---|---|
| Initial diagnosis | Anxiety, fear, anger, guilt, suicidal ideation, impulsive behavior, feeling out of control | Crisis intervention, suicide assessment, education, referrals for peer counseling, psychotherapy, support group |
| Initiation of treatment | Can range from depression, loss of control, and feeling overwhelmed to feeling optimistic at controlling the virus | Adherence assessment and support, patient education, resource referral |
| New symptoms | Anxiety, fear, sense of defeat | Education, emotional support |
| First hospitalization | Fear, anger, depression | Intrahospital resource referrals, support |
| Recurrence of complications | Depression; apathy; fear of abandonment, suffering, and death | Emotional support, referrals for psychotherapy, pastoral counseling |
| Improvement of health | Conflicting emotions ranging from renewed optimism and hope to confusion and guilt | Emotional support, referrals for job retraining programs |

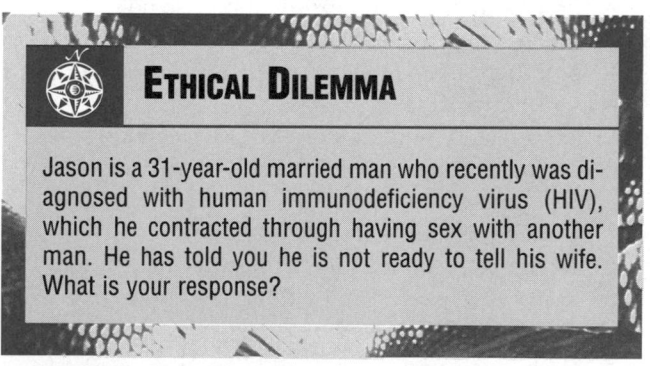

## ETHICAL DILEMMA

Jason is a 31-year-old married man who recently was diagnosed with human immunodeficiency virus (HIV), which he contracted through having sex with another man. He has told you he is not ready to tell his wife. What is your response?

## CASE STUDY

Victoria T. is a 26-year-old woman who is admitted to the hospital with PCP. She was diagnosed as HIV positive in 1994, when she was pregnant with her second child, a son. She did not receive zidovudine (AZT) during the pregnancy, and her son is also HIV positive. Her older daughter, now age 11, is HIV negative. Ms. T. has been diligent about keeping her son's medical appointments and ensuring that he gets proper care, but she has not sought treatment for herself. When asked about this, she tells the nurse that her son's care is more important than her own. She is a single mother without a car and is too ashamed to request regular help from her mother, who is the only one who knows Ms. T's diagnosis. The nurse organizes a multidisciplinary team meeting, which includes a home care nurse, a social worker, an HIV case manager, and a nurse from the outpatient clinic. The team schedules a posthospitalization follow-up appointment for Ms. T. and arranges for transportation to the appointment, as well as baby-sitting during that time. Each team member introduces herself to Ms. T. over the next few days. A home care referral is made. Ms. T. is then receptive to following through with treatment for herself.

# NURSING CARE PLAN

## PATIENT WITH ACQUIRED IMMUNODEFICIENCY SYNDROME

The patient is a 37-year-old man who reenters the medical unit after having been discharged 3 months ago. He is diagnosed as having acquired immunodeficiency syndrome (AIDS) and has been receiving outpatient therapy for chronic symptoms, including fever, night sweats, diarrhea, fatigue, and weight loss. He is experiencing dyspnea, shortness of breath (SOB), and cough, which began 2 days ago. The SOB has intensified, causing him to become anxious and at times confused. *Pneumocystis carinii* infection is confirmed by assessments, x-ray studies, and cultures. He is admitted for further evaluation, nursing care, and treatment. He has no known food or drug allergies, does not smoke or tolerate secondhand smoke, and denies use of alcohol or drugs.

| Medical History | Psychosocial Data | Assessment Data |
|---|---|---|
| Generally healthy until 1 yr ago, when he developed generalized lymphadenopathy; sought medical advice immediately<br>Blood test confirmed the presence of human immunodeficiency virus antibodies; started on zidovudine (AZT) and Bactrim DS on an outpatient basis<br>Progress monitored by a private medical doctor<br>22.5 kg (50 lb) weight loss in 6 mo<br>Depression for 3 mo; receiving psychotherapy weekly<br>Homosexual activity began at age 18 | Has significant other (SO) with whom he has had a 6-yr relationship; partner unwilling to be tested for AIDS at this time; supportive relationship with lover<br>Both parents well, in their early 60s, live out of state and plan to retire soon from professional careers; said to be adjusting to son's homosexual disclosure and illness; have been to visit twice; patient considers SO as present family<br>One brother age 35 and a sister age 30; both well; no family history of hypertension, diabetes, or renal disease; cancer history in both sets of grandparents (now deceased)<br>Self-employed as a dentist; has been unable to maintain practice and is in the process of selling practice and applying for disability benefits under Social Security<br>Confidentiality requested by patient; believes that "giving up" license to practice denotes surrendering to illness<br>Owns own home; easy access to entrance | Frail, thin male who appears much older than his stated age<br>Flat affect with very little verbal exchange; responds to questions but offers no extra information; some eye contact<br>Height 5' 10"; weight 58.5 kg (130 lb)<br>Oriented to time, place, and person; color pale<br>*Vital signs:* T 100.6, P 92, R 38, BP 140/70<br>*Skin:* Warm, dry, and intact; no signs of rashes, bruises, or decubiti<br>*Eye, ear, nose, throat:* Mucous membranes moist; no mouth lesions; extraocular motions intact; both nares patent; prominent cheek bones from apparent weight loss; generalized lymphadenopathy: cervical, postauricular, and axillary nodes enlarged bilaterally<br>*Respiratory:* Rate 36-40; labored with increased use of accessory muscles; dyspnea on exertion; bilateral wheezes heard in both lower lobes, greater on expiration than inspiration; adventitious sounds heard in all lung fields; "guarding" of chest while coughing; productive cough<br>*Abdominal:* Wasted appearance, decreased tone; hypotonic bowel sounds heard in all four quadrants<br>*Musculoskeletal:* Range of motion in all joints, with some obvious degree of discomfort; unsteady gait; positive peripheral pulses; no edema in ankles or feet<br>***Laboratory data***<br>RBC 3.09, Hgb 8.1, Hct 29, WBC 18,000, Cholesterol 105<br>Platelets 300,000; Electrolytes: Na 145, K 4.2<br>Chloride 108, $CO_2$ 24<br>*Blood gases:* pH 7.36, $pCO_2$ 47, $HCO_3$ 28, $Po_2$ 78, $O_2$ sat 82%<br>*ECG:* Within normal limits<br>*Chest x-ray:* Shows infiltration, both lungs<br>*Urinalysis:* Within normal limits<br>*Stool culture:* Positive for *Giardia lamblia* |

*Continued*

# NURSING CARE PLAN

## PATIENT WITH ACQUIRED IMMUNODEFICIENCY SYNDROME—cont'd

Has private medical insurance through group practice; anxious over continuing coverage once illness progresses

*Religion:* Protestant; attends services only on holidays; has discussed illness with minister

*Hobbies:* Likes listening to classical music; watches sports on television; interested in antique cars

*Medications*

AZT (Retrovir) 100 mg PO 4 times a day

Metronidazole (Flagyl) 400 mg IVPB q 6 hr (infuse over 1 hr)

Trimethoprim/sulfamethoxazole (Bactrim DS) 2 tabs PO q 8 hr

Diazepam (Valium) 5 mg PO q 4-6 hr prn anxiety

1000 ml D5W with 10 mEq KCl q 8 hr

Oxygen at 6 L via nasal cannula

*Universal Precautions maintained*

### NURSING DIAGNOSIS

Ineffective airway clearance related to *Pneumocystis carinii* pneumonia as indicated by dyspnea, cough, and increased respiration

### NURSING INTERVENTIONS

Monitor vital signs q 4 hr and prn.

Assess breath sounds.

Have patient turn, cough, and deep breathe q 4 hr.

Demonstrate and assist with splinting technique during coughing and deep breathing.

Offer cough medication q 4 hr (not prn); not to be given with meals.

Encourage use of cough drops and tea with lemon and honey.

Offer warm saline mouthwash and gargle for sore throat.

Provide 2.5 L of fluids per day for adequate hydration; offer 8-12 oz of fluids q 4 hr during waking hours (likes ginger ale and apple juice); monitor intake and output.

Encourage use of assistance devices such as trapeze, wheelchair, and walker.

Assist patient and family in planning care to conserve energy, such as shower chair while bathing, sitting down while dressing.

### EVALUATION OF EXPECTED OUTCOMES

Vital signs and breath sounds within normal limits

Verbalizes improved respiratory functioning

Patient and family able to demonstrate use of pillow as splint during coughing

Regulates own medication

Has decreased cough symptoms

Does not have a sore throat

Identifies preferred fluids, maintains intake at 2.5 L, keeps self-record of intake at bedside

Able to use assistance devices to conserve energy

Patient and family able to plan 24 hr of care

## NURSING CARE PLAN
## PATIENT WITH ACQUIRED IMMUNODEFICIENCY SYNDROME—cont'd

**NURSING DIAGNOSIS**

Anticipatory grieving related to advancement of illness as evidenced by behavior manifestations

| NURSING INTERVENTIONS | EVALUATION OF EXPECTED OUTCOMES |
|---|---|
| Help patient to understand the grieving process and to accept feelings as normal. | Uses healthy coping mechanisms |
| Emphasize patient's identified strengths; provide positive reinforcement for effective coping behaviors. | Contacts support group within 2 wk of hospitalization |
| Inform him of existing support groups in the facility or community; offer to contact clergy of choice; accept the way of responding to the illness; provide privacy, dignified care, and acceptance on a daily basis. | Shares feelings with significant other, family, friends, and clergy |
| | Expresses feelings about illness |
| Help patient discuss fears by establishing a trusting relationship. | Communicates an understanding about the stages of grief |
| Plan time during each shift to sit with and actively listen to the patient. | Accepts feelings and behavior brought on by potential loss |
| Give private time with significant other and family. | |

**NURSING DIAGNOSIS**

Decisional conflict related to surrender of dental practice and license as evidenced by delayed decision making and vacillation between choices

| NURSING INTERVENTIONS | EVALUATION OF EXPECTED OUTCOMES |
|---|---|
| Acknowledge patient's feelings; be supportive and use a nonjudgmental approach. | Openly expresses feelings |
| Help patient identify available options and their possible consequences. | Describes conflicts related to illness, disclosure, and treatment |
| Help patient make decisions about daily activities; keep patient oriented to reality. | Identifies consequences of potential choices |
| Encourage visits with family, friends, clergy, and peers. | Makes at least two care-related decisions daily |
| Demonstrate respect for the patient's right to make choices based on his or her own values and beliefs. | Expresses increased comfort in dealing with conflicts |

*Continued*

# NURSING CARE PLAN

## PATIENT WITH ACQUIRED IMMUNODEFICIENCY SYNDROME—cont'd

**NURSING DIAGNOSIS**

Powerlessness related to chronic illness as evidenced by sadness, crying, and passivity

| NURSING INTERVENTIONS | EVALUATION OF EXPECTED OUTCOMES |
|---|---|
| Encourage patient to express feelings; set aside time for discussion; allow silence; listen for clues of expression. | Verbalizes both positive and negative feelings about current situation |
| Accept patient's feelings of powerlessness as normal; try to be present during situations when feelings of powerlessness are likely to be greatest, to help patient cope in a positive way. | Describes strategies for reducing anxiety |
| Identify and develop patient's coping mechanisms, strengths, and resources. | Demonstrates control by participating in decision making related to care |
| Discuss situations that provoke feelings of anger, anxiety, or powerlessness. | Actively plans and executes aspects of decision making regarding future of dental practice |
| Encourage participation in self-care as much as possible. | Includes significant other in a discussion of his feelings and needs |
| Provide as many opportunities as possible for patient to make decisions about care (positioning, rest, choosing an IV site, visiting, fluid and food choices). | Identifies the potential for appointing a "power of attorney" as the illness progresses |
| Modify the environment when possible to meet self-care needs (commode, lounge chair). | |
| Encourage family and significant other to support patient without taking control. | |
| Reinforce patient's rights as stated in the "Patient's Bill of Rights." | |
| Identify and arrange to accommodate the patient's spiritual needs. | |

# KEY CONCEPTS

➤ The pathogenesis of HIV infection is directly related to the relentless replication of the human immunodeficiency virus. This replication is responsible for damage to the immune system and progression of the disease.

➤ The CD4 cell is the orchestrator of the immune response. It directs other cells of the immune system in fighting infection. The CD4 cell is the cell most profoundly damaged by HIV.

➤ HIV disease begins at the moment of primary infection, which often manifests as a viral-like syndrome. The disease course continues through a period of clinical latency, during which time active viral replication continues and the patient usually is asymptomatic. As the number of CD4 cells drops, the patient may become symptomatic with many HIV-related illnesses. The diagnosis of AIDS is made only when the CD4 count drops under $200/mm^3$ or when the patient develops one of the following disorders: opportunistic infection, HIV encephalopathy, malignancy (e.g., Kaposi's sarcoma, lymphoma, or invasive cervical cancer), tuberculosis, wasting, or two or more episodes of pneumonia within 10 months.

➤ The amount of virus in the blood can be measured using the viral load test. Higher viral loads indicate a rapidly replicating virus, and higher loads have been linked to more rapid progression of disease. Viral load testing is used to guide decisions about starting or changing antiretroviral treatment.

➤ Opportunistic infections and other HIV-related complications occur as a direct result of immune system destruction. Major opportunistic infections seen in people with AIDS are candidiasis, *Pneumocystis carinii* pneumonia, cytomegalovirus, HIV encephalopathy, *Mycobacterium avium* complex, toxoplasmosis encephalitis, and wasting.

➤ HIV is transmitted via blood, semen, vaginal secretions, and breast milk. Behaviors such as unprotected sex and intravenous drug use, which allow these fluids to enter another person's body, can result in transmission of HIV. HIV can be transmitted from mother to baby (perinatal transmission) in utero, during birth, or through breastfeeding. Transmission in the health care setting (occupational exposure) usually is the result of a needle stick or other exposure to blood by means of sharp instruments.

➤ Combination antiretroviral therapy is the standard of care for HIV infection. Effective combinations have been shown to suppress viral loads to undetectable levels in the plasma. This correlates with improved survival rates. Currently, antiretroviral drugs are divided into three categories: The nucleoside reverse transcriptase inhibitors (NRTIs) are zidovudine (AZT), zalcitabine (ddC), didanosine (ddI), lamivudine (3TC), and stavudine (d4T); the nonnucleoside reverse transcriptase inhibitors (NNRTIs) are delavirdine and nevirapine; the protease inhibitors (PIs) are indinavir, ritonavir, saquinavir, and nelfinavir.

# CRITICAL THINKING EXERCISES

1. What information would you give a patient who tells you that he takes his pills only about half the time because the pills make him feel bad?

2. What would you discuss with a woman who has HIV and is contemplating pregnancy?

3. What information should an individual who is newly diagnosed with HIV be given about the virus and how it works?

4. Your closest colleague at work has just been stuck by a needle. Since you want to be supportive, what instruction do you give?

## REFERENCES AND ADDITIONAL READINGS

Anastasi J, Lee V: HIV wasting: how to stop the cycle, *Am J Nurs* 94(6):18-24, 1994.

Andrews L, Novick L, editors. *HIV care: a comprehensive handbook for providers*, Thousand Oaks, Calif, 1995, Sage.

Barker L, Randol BJ, Zieve PD, editors. *Principles of ambulatory medicine*, Baltimore, 1995, Williams & Wilkins.

Bass J et al: Treatment of tuberculosis and tuberculosis infection in adults and children, *Am J Respir Crit Care Med* 149:1359-1374, 1994.

Bennet J, Plum F, editors: *Cecil's textbook of medicine*, Philadelphia, 1996, Saunders.

Bolan G: Management of syphilis in HIV-infected persons. In Sande M, Volberding P, editors: *The medical management of AIDS*, Philadelphia, 1997, Saunders.

Bristol-Myers Squibb: *The war on HIV*, Wallingford, Conn, 1997, Bristol-Myers Squibb.

Broder S, Merigan TC Jr, Bolognasi D, editors: *Textbook of AIDS medicine*, Baltimore, 1994, Williams & Wilkins.

Buchness MR: Treatment of skin diseases in HIV-infected patients, *Dermatol Clin* 13(1):231-238, 1995.

Casey KM, Cohen F, Hughes A: *ANAC's core curriculum for HIV/AIDS nursing*, Philadelphia, 1996, Nursecom.

Centers for Disease Control and Prevention (CDC): 1993 revised classification system for HIV infection and expanded surveillance case definition for AIDS among adolescents and adults, *MMWR* 44(RR-17):1-19, 1993a.

Centers for Disease Control and Prevention (CDC): Sexually transmitted disease treatment guidelines, *MMWR* 42(RR-14):91, 1993b.

Centers for Disease Control and Prevention (CDC): *Core curriculum on tuberculosis: what the clinician should know*, Atlanta, 1994a, Public Health Service, US Department of Health and Human Services.

Centers for Disease Control and Prevention (CDC): Guidelines for preventing the transmission of *Mycobacterium tuberculosis* in health care facilities, *MMWR* 43(RR-13):1-132, 1994b.

Centers for Disease Control and Prevention (CDC): HIV/AIDS surveillance report: year end edition, *HIV/AIDS Surveill Rep* 7(2):1, 1995a.

Centers for Disease Control and Prevention (CDC): Recommendations of the Public Health Service Task Force on the Use of Zidovudine to Reduce Perinatal Transmission of Human Immunodeficiency Virus, *MMWR* 43:1, 1995b.

Centers for Disease Control and Prevention (CDC): USPHS/ISDA guidelines for the prevention of opportunistic infections in persons infected with human immunodeficiency virus: a summary, *MMWR* 44(RR-8):1-33, 1995c.

Centers for Disease Control and Prevention (CDC): HIV/AIDS surveillance report: mid-year edition, *HIV/AIDS Surveill Rep* 8(1):1, 1996a.

Centers for Disease Control and Prevention (CDC): HIV/AIDS surveillance report: year end edition, *HIV/AIDS Surveill Rep* 12:1, 1996b.

Centers for Disease Control and Prevention (CDC): Recommendations for postexposure prophylaxis for health care workers, *MMWR* 45(22):468, 1996c.

Centers for Disease Control and Prevention (CDC), Department of HIV/AIDS Prevention: Joint United Nations programme on HIV/AIDS, *HIV/AIDS Surveill Rep* December, 1996d.

Coffin J: HIV population dynamics in vivo: implications for genetic variation, pathogenesis, and therapy, *Science* 267:483-489, 1995.

Coffin J: HIV viral dynamics, *AIDS* 10(suppl 3):S75-S84, 1996.

Dannemann BR et al: Treatment of toxoplasmic encephalitis patients with AIDS: a randomized trial comparing pyrimethamine plus clindamycin to pyrimethamine plus sulfonamides, *Ann Intern Med* 116:33-43, 1992.

Dusheiko GM et al: A rational approach to the management of hepatitis C infection, *BMJ* 312(7027):357-364, 1996.

Eron JJ: Viral dynamics: what the virus does and how it does it! Fourth Conference on Retroviruses and Opportunistic Infections, Washington, DC, 1997, Healthcare Communications Group, LLC (from the conference's Internet homepage).

Friedland G: Adherence: the Achilles heel of highly active antiretroviral therapy, *Improving the Management of HIV Disease* 5(1):14, 1997.

Greenspan D, Greenspan JS: Oral manifestations of HIV infection, *AIDS Clin Care* 9(4):29-33, 1997.

Ho DD: Viral counts in HIV infection, *Science* 272:1124-1125, 1996.

Ho D et al: Rapid turnover of plasma virions and CD4 lymphocytes in HIV-1 infection, *Nature* 373(6510):123-126, 1995.

Hoover D et al: Clinical manifestations of AIDS in the era of *Pneumocystis* prophylaxis, *N Engl J Med* 329:1922-1926, 1993.

Kahn J, Hecht F: Treating primary infection, *HIV Newsline* 2(6):135-141, 1996.

Kaplan LD, Norfelt DW: Malignancies associated with AIDS. In Sande M, Volberding P, editors: *The medical management of AIDS*, Philadelphia, 1997, Saunders.

Kappes JC et al: Assessment of antiretroviral therapy by plasma viral load testing: standard and ICD HIV-1 p24 antigen and viral RNA (QC-PCR) assays compared, *J Acquir Immune Defic Syndr Hum Retrovirol* 10:139-149, 1995.

Landers DV, Shannon M: Management of pregnant women with HIV infection. In Sande M, Volberding P, editors: *The medical management of AIDS*, Philadelphia, 1997, Saunders.

Leiner S, Mays M: Diagnosing latent and active pulmonary tuberculosis, *Nurse Pract* 21(2):86-106, 1996.

Levine A: AIDS-related malignancies, Fourth Conference on Retroviruses and Opportunistic Infections, Washington, DC, 1997, Healthcare Communications Group, LLC, 1997 (from the conference's Internet homepage).

Malone JL et al: Sources of variability in repeated T-helper lymphocyte counts from human immunodeficiency virus type 1 infected patients: total lymphocyte count fluctuations and diurnal cycle are important, *J Acquir Immune Defic Syndr* 3:144-151, 1990.

Mellors JW et al: Quantitation of HIV-1 RNA in plasma predicts outcome after seroconversion, *Ann Intern Med* 122(8):573-579, 1995.

Mellors JW et al: Prognosis in HIV-1 infection predicted by the quantity of virus found in plasma, *Science* 272:1167, 1996.

Mellors JW et al: Plasma viral load and CD4 lymphocytes as prognostic markers of HIV infection, *Ann Intern Med* 126:846-954, 1997.

Moore RD et al: Cost-effectiveness of directly observed therapy versus self-administered therapy for tuberculosis, *Am J Crit Care Med* 154:1013-1019, 1996.

Panteleo G et al: Studies in subjects with long-term nonprogressive human immunodeficiency virus infection, *N Engl J Med* 332(4):209-216, 1995.

Pederson C et al: Clinical course of primary HIV infection: consequences for subsequent course of infection, *BMJ* 299:154-157, 1989.

Perelson A et al: HIV-1 dynamics in vivo: virion clearance rate, infected cell life span, and viral generation time, *Science* 271:1582-1586, 1995.

Petrow S, editor: *Project inform: the HIV drug handbook*, New York, 1995, Pocket Books.

Piot P, Laga M: Epidemiology of AIDS in the developing world. In Broder S, Merigan TC Jr, Bolognasi D, editors: *Textbook of AIDS medicine*, Baltimore, 1994, Williams & Wilkins.

Pulido F et al: Relapse of tuberculosis after treatment in human immunodeficiency virus–infected patients, *Arch Intern Med* 157:227-232, 1997.

Reiter G: The HIV wasting syndrome, *AIDS Clinical Care* 8(11):89-96, 1996.

Romeyn M: *Nutrition and HIV: a new model for treatment*, San Francisco, 1995, Jossey-Bass.

Sande M, Volberding, H: *The medical management of AIDS*, Philadelphia, 1997, Saunders.

Sauer G, Hall J: *Manual of skin diseases*, Philadelphia, 1997, Lippincott.

Severson JS et al: Nutritional status assessment and intervention in early stage HIV infection in an urban,

hospital-based outpatient clinic population, Proceedings of the Eleventh International Conference on AIDS, Vancouver, 1996, WeB.3273.

Spencer M, Ross J: Hepatitis C prevalence, demographics, and selection criteria for interferon therapy in an urban HIV-positive cohort, Proceedings of the {Eleventh} International Conference on AIDS, 1996, MoB.1242.

Squires K: Ninth National Conference on Women and HIV, New York, May 12, 1997, Health Information Network, World Health Communications (from the Internet).

Stein D, Korvick J, Vermund S: CD4 lymphocyte cell enumeration for prediction of clinical course of human immunodeficiency virus disease: a review, *J Infect Dis* 165:352-363, 1992.

Straus D et al: Prognostic factors in the treatment of HIV-associated non-Hodgkin's lymphoma: analysis of ACTG-142 (low dose vs standard dose in BACOD and BC-CSF), *Blood* 86:604a, 1995.

UNSAIDS/WHO: *Report on the global HIV/AIDS epidemic*, Geneva, Switzerland, 1996, World Health Organization.

US Department of Health and Human Services: Availability of report of NIH panel to define principles of therapy of HIV infection and guidelines for the use of antiretroviral agents in HIV-infected adults and adolescents, *Fed Reg* 62(118):33417, 1997.

US Department of Health and Human Services: Guidelines for the use of antiretroviral agents in HIV-infected adults and adolescents, *Fed Reg* 62(118): 33417, 1997.

Walthen LK et al: HIV RNA viral burden at baseline or its reduction following antiretroviral therapy is highly correlated with reduced HIV-1 progression. Paper presented at the Third Conference on Retroviruses and Opportunistic Infections, Washington, DC, 1996.

Whipple B, Scura K: The overlooked epidemic: HIV in older adults, *Am J Nurs* 96(2):22-28, 1996.

Zurlo JJ et al: Sinusitis in HIV-1 infection, *Am J Med* 93:157-162, 1992.

## CHAPTER 17

# Rehabilitative Care

## CHAPTER OBJECTIVES

1 Identify the goals of rehabilitation.
2 Describe the application of rehabilitation principles to the practice of nursing.
3 Define disability and theoretic models of disability.
4 Discuss the concept of an interdisciplinary rehabilitation team, its members, and their roles.
5 Identify types of facilities and agencies that provide rehabilitation services.
6 Discuss the rehabilitative aspects of each phase of patient care: primary, secondary, and tertiary.
7 Identify the emotional responses to disability and discuss related nursing interventions.
8 Identify nursing activities that promote mobility and movement: range of joint motion, positioning, transfers, and participation in self-care.
9 Discuss nursing interventions for incontinence, skin breakdown, and impaired swallowing.
10 Discuss the role of the rehabilitation nurse as a motivator and teacher.
11 Discuss the use of prostheses, braces, and crutches.
12 Give examples of assistive and adaptive devices.

## KEY TERMS

| | |
|---|---|
| activities of daily living | impairment |
| adaptation | interdisciplinary team |
| body image | motivation |
| continuity | range of joint motion |
| disability | (ROJM) |
| dysphagia | rehabilitation |
| functional assessment | rehabilitation nursing |
| functional limitations | |

## REHABILITATION

**Rehabilitation** is a fundamental process of total patient care. The concept of rehabilitation has many definitions and interpretations, but all share a common meaning: rehabilitation is the process of assisting individuals with disability or chronic illness in recovering to the highest possible level of independence and well-being. The need for rehabilitation arises when a person's previous way of life is changed by illness or injury. Depending on the type of disability, the physical, mental, vocational, social, and economic aspects of a person's life may be altered (Box 17-1). Some disabling events may be minor, presenting only a limited need for rehabilitation; others may require extensive rehabilitation that involves many facets of a person's life.

An important principle of rehabilitation is the restoration of an individual to his or her fullest capability in all areas. Rehabilitation helps the individual to live the most productive life possible. Instead of the classic emphasis on disease, diagnosis, and therapeutic procedure, rehabilitation stresses restoration of normal function, prevention of complications, education of patient and family, and adaptation.

**Adaptation** is the process of adjusting to life changes that occur with disability. Adapting to the changes imposed by illness or injury may be difficult for some patients, yet may seem relatively stress free for others. Patients need to make some degree of adaptation, otherwise rehabilitation may be incomplete or unsuccessful. Patients adapting to a disability show a wide range of personal styles; some respond with anger and rage, whereas others use humor to cope with the changes in their lives. Some disabled individuals may deny their experience totally even while participating in an active rehabilitation program.

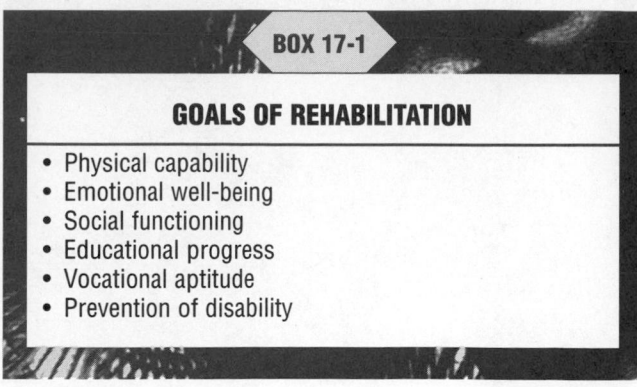

**BOX 17-1**

**GOALS OF REHABILITATION**

- Physical capability
- Emotional well-being
- Social functioning
- Educational progress
- Vocational aptitude
- Prevention of disability

**CASE STUDY**

Mr. Jones is 35 years old, married, and the father of five. He was driving his truck on a rain-slicked expressway when a large truck suddenly crossed the highway and crashed into his vehicle. Mr. Jones was rushed by ambulance to the hospital. Both legs were so badly injured that above the knee amputations were necessary. Soon thereafter Mr. Jones was admitted to a rehabilitation hospital. After evaluation by the nursing, therapy, social service, and medical team members, Mr. Jones' rehabilitation began. He participated in therapy, and he was fitted with artificial limbs and learned how to walk with them. He and his family were taught the care of his amputation sites and of the prostheses, and they were given the opportunity to discuss how the accident affected their lives and their expectations for the future. Plans were made for Mr. Jones to be trained for a new kind of work. He now lives at home and is in an outpatient rehabilitation program. He is anxious to progress with his rehabilitation. At times he is fearful and sad, yet he is ready to proceed with his training and is looking forward to complete independence and to being able to care for his family.

## DEFINITION OF DISABILITY

A variety of terms are used to describe loss of independent functioning. It is important to have clarity about these terms because of the stigma often associated with such words as "handicapped" or "crippled." Over the past 25 years conceptual models of disability have been developed that help define these terms. The two main theorists of disability models are Saad Nagi and Philip Wood (Kelly-Hayes, 1991).

Nagi describes three potential consequences of pathologic conditions or disease: **impairment**, or physiologic alteration; **functional limitations**, which are limitations on activities such as walking and dressing; and **disability**, which is a limitation in performing so-cial roles and activities (e.g., work, family life, and independent living) (Nagi, 1969).

Philip Wood continued the work of Nagi. He developed for the World Health Organization (WHO) International Classification of Impairments, Disabilities, and Handicaps a model that included the concept of handicap. A handicap was described as a disadvantage for a given individual, resulting from an impairment or disability, that limits or prevents fulfillment of a role that is normal for that individual (WHO, 1980). In this model the term *handicap* is similar to Nagi's use of the term *disability*. However, because of the stigma associated with the word *handicap*, the Nagi model is the one most often used by rehabilitation professionals, and the term *handicap* is discouraged.

The definition of disability set forth by the Americans with Disabilities Act, which was passed in 1990, requires an individual to meet at least one of three criteria: the individual must have a physical or mental impairment that substantially limits one or more of the major life activities; the person must have a record of such an impairment; and he or she must be regarded as having such an impairment (Americans with Disabilities Act, 1992). The act defines physical or mental impairment as follows:

- Any physiologic disorder or condition, cosmetic disfigurement, or anatomic loss that affects one or more of the body systems
- Any mental or psychologic disorder (e.g., mental retardation, organic brain syndrome, or emotional or mental illness)
- Specific learning disabilities

## REHABILITATION NURSING

Rehabilitation can be viewed as an underlying theme of all nursing care. Regardless of the care setting, be it an acute care hospital, a long-term care facility, a rehabilitation facility, or the community, nurses use rehabilitative patient care practices and techniques that focus on restoring function and preventing complications. These approaches form some of the basic tenets of nursing practice. For example, a nurse caring for a bedridden patient uses methods to position the patient in bed and provide movement and exercise to prevent skin breakdown, respiratory complications, and joint deformity. As the patient improves, the nurse uses a range of techniques. Methods to improve mobility through transfer training, strengthening exercises, and ambulation are planned in coordination with the physical therapist. The emphasis is on improving the patient's ability to participate in **activities of daily living (ADL)** such as bathing, grooming, dressing, feeding, walking, and toileting. And, if needed, the nurse uses methods to assess and correct such problems as poor nutritional intake and incontinence.

Although principles of rehabilitation are integral to all nursing practice, **rehabilitation nursing** is viewed as a specialty practice in nursing. In 1988 the Association of Rehabilitation Nurses, in cooperation with the American Nurses Association, defined rehabilitation nursing and stated its goals as follows:

Rehabilitation nursing is a specialty practice area within the scope of professional nursing practice. Rehabilitation nursing is the diagnosis and treatment of human responses of individuals and groups to actual or potential health problems stemming from altered functional ability and altered lifestyle. The goal of rehabilitation nursing is to assist the individual with disability and chronic illness in the restoration and maintenance of maximal health. The rehabilitation nurse should be skilled at treating alterations in functional ability and life-style resulting from physical disability and chronic illness (American Nurses Association, Association of Rehabilitation Nurses, 1988).

Rehabilitation nurses care for patients with a wide range of disabling conditions, including stroke, spinal cord injury, brain injury, amputation, cancer, congenital deficits, and addiction problems. In addition to providing nursing care based on the rehabilitation philosophy of maximizing function and preventing complications, rehabilitation nurses understand the impact of these conditions on a person's life and are knowledgeable about the specific nursing interventions these patients need. For example, in caring for a person with a brain injury, the rehabilitation nurse must have the ability to assess behavioral and communication problems that occur as a consequence of the injury. In caring for a person with a spinal cord injury, the rehabilitation nurse develops specialized approaches to bowel and bladder care.

This chapter describes some of the basic techniques of rehabilitation nursing. More detailed descriptions of rehabilitation nursing care of patients with specific disabilities can be found in a rehabilitation nursing textbook (Kelly-Hayes, 1995; Dittmar, 1989; McCourt, 1993).

# REHABILITATION IN EACH PHASE OF HEALTH CARE

Health care can be divided into three phases or stages: *primary* health care refers to preventive efforts, *secondary* health care deals with the period of acute illness, and *tertiary* health care involves recovery and rehabilitation from an illness or accident. The philosophy and practices of rehabilitation nursing are part of all aspects of health care and are integral to each phase of nursing care.

## Primary Health Care

In this phase emphasis is placed on *preventing* disease and accidents. One aspect of prevention is protection of all susceptible individuals against diseases for which positive immunizing agents are available. The crippling conditions of poliomyelitis have nearly been eliminated by administration of the polio vaccine. Another preventive approach uses early assessment and education about chronic conditions to reduce long-term disability. Hypertension, when detected early, can be managed through a variety of approaches, including dietary management, eliminating smoking, exercise, meditation, and, when needed, medications. If hypertension is carefully managed, the long-term risks associated with it (e.g., heart and renal disease and stroke) can be reduced.

The prevention of injury is another focus of primary health care. Methods to promote safety in the work place, enhanced driving safety through reducing speed and using seat belts, and reduction of pollutants in the environment are examples of these preventive health practices.

Nurses working in primary health care and in all other health care settings have the opportunity to educate individuals and groups in many preventive practices. These include the importance of regular health and dental evaluation, well-balanced nutrition, exercise, eliminating smoking, approaches to management of chronic disease, and appropriate use of medications. The goal of these practices is to keep the individual at a maximum level of health and well-being. From this perspective, these practices can be said to be rehabilitative in focus.

## Secondary Health Care

Rehabilitation nursing concepts are essential aspects of the care of acutely ill patients. During the patient's hospital stay, the nurse must recognize the potential impact of illness and disability on the individual's physical function and emotional state. Through continual nursing assessment, the extent of a patient's functional limitations such as limitation in the ability to care for himself or herself, level of mobility, and continence status can be determined and interventions can be planned to support and maintain recovery of these functions. Even at the earliest stages of illness and disability, realistic short-term and long-term goals should be established with the patient that reflect the person's potential for participating in a rehabilitation approach. The nurse uses these goals in planning daily care.

By planning with the physician and other members of the health care team, the nurse helps the patient participate in a program of increased activity, and the nurse needs to continually assess the effects of this increased activity on the patient. For example, in the elderly, fatigue likely will have a greater effect on recovery and the effort to increase activity than it does in younger patients. As a result, activity tolerance must be carefully assessed in an acutely ill older person. Checking vital signs, observing respiratory and skin color changes during activity, and determining endurance for participation in sitting, transferring, and walking are a few of these assessment parameters (Mol, Baker, 1991).

During this time it is especially important to prevent *secondary complications,* such as pressure ulcers or contractures, that may develop because of the patient's immobility and altered physical and medical status. Keeping the patient as mobile and well nourished as possible is the goal. Maintaining body alignment, providing **range of joint motion (ROJM)** exercises, preventing excessive pressure on the patient's skin, and getting the patient out of bed and mobile as soon as possible helps reduce the incidence of secondary complications.

## Tertiary Health Care

Tertiary health care is provided outside the acute hospital setting. As soon as the acute phase of illness has passed, the patient's need for continued care should be evaluated carefully, and, if necessary, an appropriate rehabilitation setting should be identified. Rehabilitation programs are based in a variety of settings, including acute care hospitals, free-standing facilities, long-term care facilities, and the community. Centers are operated by for-profit and nonprofit organizations, state vocational agencies, insurance companies, private agencies, and a variety of community agencies. The setting selected depends on the severity of the disability, the limitations on self-care, and the potential for some level of recovery.

A patient in need of an intense, comprehensive rehabilitation program may be admitted to an inpatient rehabilitation unit in an acute hospital or to an inpatient free-standing rehabilitation hospital. These programs provide a multitude of comprehensive interdisciplinary services. Patients in these programs must be able to participate in an active rehabilitation schedule that involves 3 hours of therapy a day, must be able to comprehend the instructions and teaching that are part of therapy, must have sufficient endurance to be out of bed and sitting for at least 1 hour at a time, and must have no other medical problems that would be contraindicated by this level of physical activity (Box 17-2). After members of the interdisciplinary team have assessed the patient, they, the patient, and the family become involved in setting goals and planning for discharge.

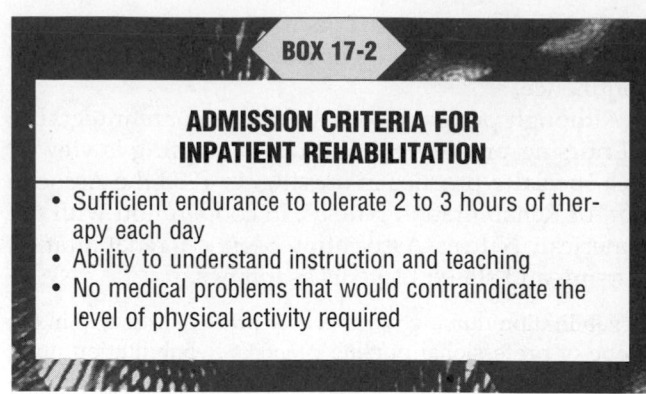

**BOX 17-2**

**ADMISSION CRITERIA FOR INPATIENT REHABILITATION**

- Sufficient endurance to tolerate 2 to 3 hours of therapy each day
- Ability to understand instruction and teaching
- No medical problems that would contraindicate the level of physical activity required

Rehabilitation programs also are offered in skilled nursing facilities. Some of these programs are as comprehensive as the inpatient regimens, whereas others are less intense. Often these programs are designed for the more elderly, frail patient. Rehabilitation of the aged and chronically ill may be a long process. The short-term and long-term goals have to be adjusted to fit the individual's potential. An older person may take longer to attain certain skills; fatigue and diminished endurance and stamina may be more of a factor for an older person than for a younger one. Dependency and low self-esteem may cause an older person to reject participation in rehabilitation (Hesse, Campion, 1983). However, recent studies have documented the positive impact of exercise and increased activity on strength and endurance in the elderly (Fiatarone et al, 1993, 1994).

More recently, home rehabilitation programs have been developed. A full range of interdisciplinary services is available through these programs and is provided on a regular basis in the patient's home. Staff members have the benefit of observing the patient in his or her own home and may be able to determine more exactly what is needed for independence in that setting. For some patients the desire to be in their own home and out of the hospital makes rehabilitation efforts in the home setting more successful. Determining the patient's level of safety before discharge home, particularly in the area of preventing falls, is an important consideration in this type of program (Box 17-3). To be successful, most home rehabilitation programs need sufficient support from family or friends. Home rehabilitation programs lack the shared experience with other patients and families with similar disabilities that is a benefit of some inpatient programs.

In other cases, some patients are able to obtain rehabilitation services on an outpatient basis. Patients who participate in this type of program usually are more independent and need the services of fewer rehabilitation professionals. Having the necessary transportation and the support of family and friends are important aspects of participation in outpatient rehabilitation services.

In some disabled or chronically ill individuals, full participation in the level of activity required by a rehabilitation program may be diminished by physical, cognitive, and emotional limitations. It may not be possible to restore all patients to the level of independence they desire; severe disability may limit the potential for total independence. Options for safe, supportive living situations may be limited by the patient's need for care, by financial constraints, and by lack of family support. Continued guidance and support from the interdisciplinary team are needed when the patient's disabilities require a long-term care setting.

### NURSE ALERT

**Rehabilitation programs require a team of experts from many areas, depending on the restorative needs of the patient.**

If a patient becomes acutely ill while participating in a rehabilitation program, returning the patient to the acute care hospital may be necessary. Most inpatient rehabilitation programs, skilled nursing facilities, and home services do not have the diagnostic and treatment capabilities of such hospitals. Acute cardiac, respiratory, and infectious processes must be treated in the acute care hospital. If the acute illness is protracted, the disabled person may lose the gains made in a rehabilitation program. Communication between referring agencies is particularly important in attempting to maintain the gains the patient has made while in an active rehabilitation program.

Of particular importance in the transition between the acute care hospital and the tertiary setting is communication between the hospital and the rehabilitation staff. A copy of pertinent parts of the hospital record and clearly written, detailed referral information is necessary for the patient's smooth transition into the new setting. Nursing data are essential components of this information and should include the patient's level of independence, nutritional status, sleep pattern, continence status, medication regimen, and social and family status, as well as specific nursing interventions needed. Nurses in the new setting need this information to begin care of the patient safely.

## REHABILITATION TEAM

Any comprehensive rehabilitation program requires a group of experts in various areas of restorative care because no single profession can provide all the necessary services for a complete rehabilitation program. This group, an **interdisciplinary team**, meets regularly to establish goals for the patient, to evaluate progress, and to revise the treatment plan (Figure 17-1). In more comprehensive rehabilitation programs a full spectrum of rehabilitation professionals may be available, whereas the less intense programs may have only a limited staff.

### The Patient

The most important member of the rehabilitation team is the patient. Success in a rehabilitation program can occur only if the patient has an understanding of his or her disability, is involved in setting goals, and participates in the plan of care. Because of the stress of adapting to all the life changes imposed by the disability, the patient may have lost motivation for this level of participation. Involving the family and significant others often is pivotal in helping the patient find such motivation. Family and friends often can provide the impetus for participation that the patient is unable to find

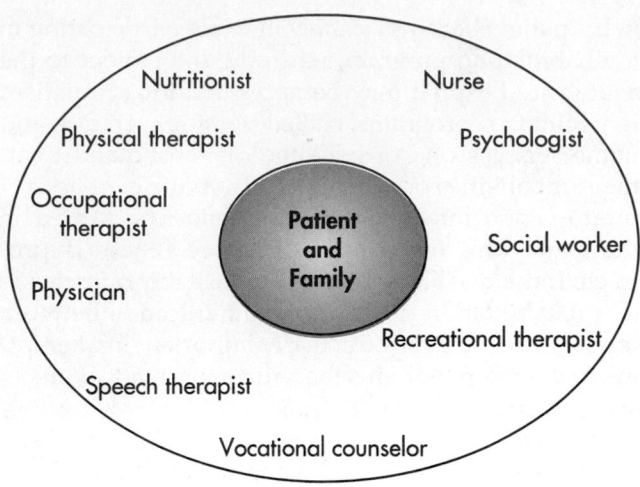

**Figure 17-1** The interdisciplinary team.

on his or her own. Meetings with the patient, family, and members of the team provide the information necessary for a more successful outcome. Such meetings should occur during the early part of the program to aid the patient in adjusting, then should be scheduled on a regular basis, and finally should be held in preparation for discharge.

## The Nurse

The role of the nurse in a rehabilitation setting is a diverse one. The nurse functions as caregiver, teacher, coordinator, evaluator, and facilitator for the patient and family members. The nursing staff spends the most time with the patient, being present 24 hours a day. This affords nurses the opportunity to observe, assess, teach, reinforce, and evaluate the effects of the total rehabilitation program. Nurses use assessment criteria to determine the patient's level of disability, stage of adaptation and adjustment, and learning needs; nursing care is based on these findings. In some settings the nurse coordinates the meetings of the interdisciplinary team. The nurse, as well as other team members, contributes pertinent information that provides a clear picture of the patient's progress over time. Assessment and documentation of the patient's progress are important aspects of rehabilitation.

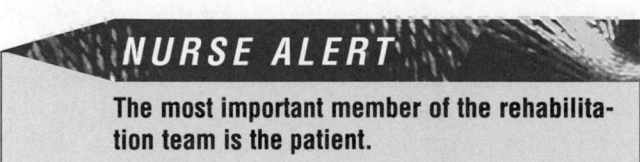

**NURSE ALERT**

**The most important member of the rehabilitation team is the patient.**

Outside of established rehabilitation programs, the team may consist of the physician, the nurse, the patient, and the family. The nurse with a basic understanding of rehabilitation is a key person in this type of team approach. In the acute care setting, it often is the nurse's responsibility to plan and coordinate the patient's rehabilitation program and to initiate early interventions. In extended care facilities, it usually is the nurse who works with the patient in performing the activities or exercises prescribed by the physical therapy department. The patient being cared for at home may benefit from the services of a physical therapist, speech therapist, or occupational therapist, provided through private agencies or public health departments. In a rehabilitation center the patient may participate in therapy sessions daily, whereas visits in the home may occur less frequently. The community-based nurse often is responsible for supervising and conducting ongoing therapy as prescribed by each therapist and for reporting the patient's progress.

## The Physician

The physician on the rehabilitation team may be a *physiatrist*, a physician trained in the specialty practice of physical medicine and rehabilitation. In other settings the physician may be a member of another medical specialty, such as neurology, orthopedics, oncology, cardiology, surgery, medicine, or pediatrics. Physicians trained in these areas who choose to practice in a rehabilitation setting often have a special interest in this phase of care. The physician assesses the patient's medical status, prescribes various evaluative procedures, medications, consultations, and therapies, and provides important information about the patient's status to other staff members, the patient, and the family.

## The Occupational Therapist

The occupational therapist (OT) evaluates the impact of the disability on the patient's physical and cognitive abilities in a variety of domains. An occupational therapist assesses (1) the patient's ability to perform a variety of ADL (e.g., bathing, dressing, eating), (2) the patient's cognitive ability to perceive and understand the environment so that he or she may function in a safe, meaningful way, and (3) movement problems. With the nurse, physician, and speech therapist, the OT may assist with evaluation and treatment of chewing and swallowing problems. An OT's treatment approach may include exercise regimens; therapies such as heat, cold, or vibration; and craft activities to strengthen the patient's muscles and improve coordination and balance. Methods to improve the patient's ability to concentrate and the prescription of assistance devices (e.g., splints, adapted eating utensils, dressing aids) may be included. The OT also may be involved in driving evaluations and in planning for the patient's return to work.

## The Physical Therapist

The physical therapist (PT) deals with problems of mobility, muscle strength, and exercise. After an initial assessment of functions such as muscle strength and tone, ROJM, sitting and standing balance, gait, stability of gait, and endurance, the PT selects exercises and therapeutic techniques for the patient. Assessment and evaluation results are reported regularly to the team, as are specific approaches that work well for the particular patient. The physical therapist also implements prescriptions for splints, braces, prostheses, and wheelchairs and is an excellent resource for the nurse when problems arise with this equipment.

## The Social Worker

The social worker addresses the stress of adapting to disability experienced by the patient, family, and friends. The problems of family relationships, housing, finances, and transportation also are addressed by the social worker. This team member often is the link between the institution and the community, helping the patient and family to solve the problems of transition and to meet the needs for placement in another setting or for home support.

## The Speech Therapist

Patients who suffer brain damage from conditions such as stroke, brain injury, tumors, or progressive neurologic disease may develop problems with the use of language and the ability to communicate. The speech therapist assesses patients with communication deficits and develops therapeutic interventions to return as much communication ability to the patient as possible. The speech therapist works with other members of the team and with the family to identify the best approach to communicating with the patient. The speech therapist also assists with evaluation and treatment of patients with swallowing problems.

## The Psychologist

Emotional problems are bound to arise in a crisis situation such as the sudden occurrence of disability. Disruptions of life-style, family structure, and body image may result in profound psychologic stress. The psychologist may use specific testing and interviews with the patient and family to identify problems; he or she then works with the patient and family to develop coping mechanisms and approaches for adjusting to

the disability. Advising other team members on ways to deal with patients undergoing emotional distress is an important role of the psychologist.

## The Recreational Therapist

Recreation and play are as important to total patient care as physical and emotional support. The recreational therapist assesses the patient's interests and provides for involvement in games, sports, hobbies, music, and other forms of diversion. Structured programs in the institution are implemented to meet the patient's needs, and trips outside the facility to movies, shopping, restaurants, and plays, as well as other activities, help the person apply some of the adaptation skills he or she has learned in the rehabilitation process.

## The Vocational Counselor

The vocational counselor or therapist assesses the patient's job skills, educational needs, interests, and motivation. If the disability results in the need to change occupation, the vocational therapist counsels the patient about vocational opportunities and arrangements for return to work.

## Other Team Members

Often the rehabilitation team will include a dietitian, orthopedist, dentist, teacher, the clergy, and members of other professions, depending on the type of disability.

## The Work of the Interdisciplinary Team

The interdisciplinary team approach to patient care is an important concept of rehabilitation (Figure 17-2). Often the expertise of many professionals is needed in the care of a disabled person, and the team approach is a means of coordinating this care. On admission to a rehabilitation program, a patient is assessed by each member of the team and plans of care are developed. The interdisciplinary team meets regularly to discuss both current and new patients. For newly admitted patients, assessment data are shared, short- and long-term goals are defined, interventions are outlined, and emotional, social, and educational needs are identified. For patients already enrolled in the program, progress toward goals, adaptation to disability, and discharge planning are discussed.

Soon after the patient is admitted, members of the interdisciplinary team may meet with the patient and family to discuss the rehabilitation plan and the expected length of stay, to begin discussion of the patient's discharge and the need for follow-up, and to address the concerns of the patient and family. Subsequent meetings may be held during the patient's stay

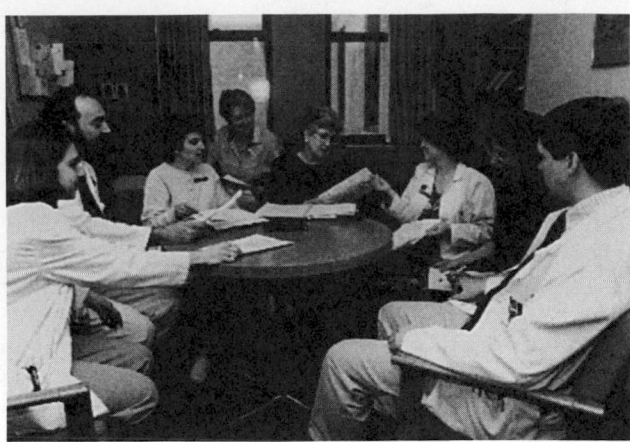

**Figure 17-2** Rehabilitation team participating in interdisciplinary team conference. (Courtesy Beth Israel Deaconess Medical Center, Boston.)

and in preparation for discharge (Glennon, Smith, 1990).

## REHABILITATION LEGISLATION

The number of personal disability cases that resulted from World War II placed emphasis on the need to establish programs and centers for rehabilitation treatment. Over the past 40 years such programs have grown rapidly. During this same period, Congress passed legislation affecting services to the disabled.

In 1954 the Vocational Rehabilitation Act was approved. It provided funds to state agencies for improving and expanding rehabilitation services. The act was updated in 1973 and amended in 1978 to include a comprehensive definition of independent living and an improved definition of funding for disabled individuals. The amendment required any institution receiving federal funds to make its facilities open and accessible to the disabled; this includes not only government buildings but also institutions of higher learning, medical facilities, public schools, national parks and recreation areas, and local programs funded by the federal government.

In July 1990 Congress passed the Americans with Disabilities Act. This law gives disabled people uniform protection against discrimination throughout the United States. It prohibits discrimination on the basis of disability in employment, activities of state and local governments, public and private transportation, and telecommunications. It is much broader than the 1973 update of the Vocational Rehabilitation Act; the law requires that all individuals with disabilities be allowed to participate in all services and programs in an integrated way. For example, in the past, public school systems provided special classes for children with disabilities, and schools were established for children with specific disabilities. The 1990 law requires public schools to integrate children with disabilities into the regular classroom (Americans with Disabilities Act, 1992).

The primary objectives of the Social and Rehabilitation Service (formerly called the Vocational Rehabilitation Department) are to educate and train disabled people for employment. By participating in rehabilitation programs, many disabled people can find jobs and become economically independent and self-sufficient. The programs created under the Social and Rehabilitation Service have been expanded to cover many more types of disability. The developmental disabilities program now offers services to people afflicted by mental retardation, cerebral palsy, convulsive disorders, and other neurologic conditions. A primary problem has been the shortage of trained personnel. In an effort to overcome this problem, the agency has provided grants to universities and certain institutions to train individuals in vocational rehabilitation. Medicare, which is administered by the Social Security Administration, now includes rehabilitative services for hospitalized patients and for those recuperating elsewhere. The Veterans Administration provides rehabilitation services for veterans.

Other areas of concern are being discussed at both the local and federal levels. Concern is growing about the problems of chronic alcoholism and drug addiction. Centers, public and private, are available to treat and rehabilitate addicted people. Also, federal and state governments are developing programs for research in mental retardation and mental illness. It is important not only to learn more about the causes of these conditions, but also to learn how many of these individuals can be rehabilitated to lead productive lives. Physical, psychologic, and developmental disabilities are not the only areas in which rehabilitative services are needed. There is a growing awareness that other factors can lead to disability in our society, including poverty, the health problems of the poor (e.g., migrant workers, the poor elderly), the impact of violent crime, and the lack of support systems for women and children. Some rehabilitative efforts are being made in these areas, but much remains to be done.

## EMOTIONAL RESPONSE TO DISABILITY

A disabling event often creates a period of crisis for the patient. With loss of body function, loss of ability to work, or loss of ability to function independently, a person's sense of self-worth may be changed for a limited period or for a long time. The individual's **body image,** one's personal view of his or her own body, may undergo significant change. The person gradually may realize that he or she is different and that life probably will be changed forever. The individual may wonder how he or she will be accepted by family, friends, and colleagues. Fear, worry, anxiety, and apprehension increase, and the person may enter a period of shock and dismay. Discouragement and depression are common during this early time.

Many factors can influence a person's ability to cope with a disabling event. Some of these factors are age, type and severity of disability, and what the loss means to the person. The age at onset of disability and the needs at certain periods of life may have an impact on how well the person copes. For example, a person born with a physical disability may adjust to the limitations in life but experience difficulty at certain times. Adolescence may be such a time because the adolescent goal of independence from family may be limited by the need for physical care. A disabled adolescent may refuse to participate in long-established care routines as a way of seeking independence. The impact of age on the reaction to disability also may be seen in the elderly. An older individual may be reluctant to accept the rationale for participating in the difficult work of recovery, feeling that he or she is just "too old" for such an effort.

A person who becomes disabled through a traumatic event may experience an acute emotional reaction to the loss and changes that occur, and this reaction may be severe enough to limit the person's ability to participate in rehabilitation. Individuals with chronic progressive disease may adapt to the gradual changes in function but experience emotional distress if acute medical problems require hospitalization or if care supports cannot meet their needs. When a person with a chronic progressive disease reaches a point where independent living is no longer possible, the need for placement in an extended care facility may create great distress.

The meaning of the loss of function that has resulted varies among individuals. Loss of an arm may affect a professional pianist or carpenter more severely than a schoolteacher or chemist. Much depends on how the loss affects the patient's everyday life. Personality problems that develop after a disability occurs may arise as a result of the patient's personality characteristics before the injury. A person who could easily be made to feel inadequate before the injury may have these feelings compounded by the emotional stress of the injury.

The initial reaction to a physical injury may be shock. The patient experiences disbelief, anxiety, and fear, which are considered part of the mourning

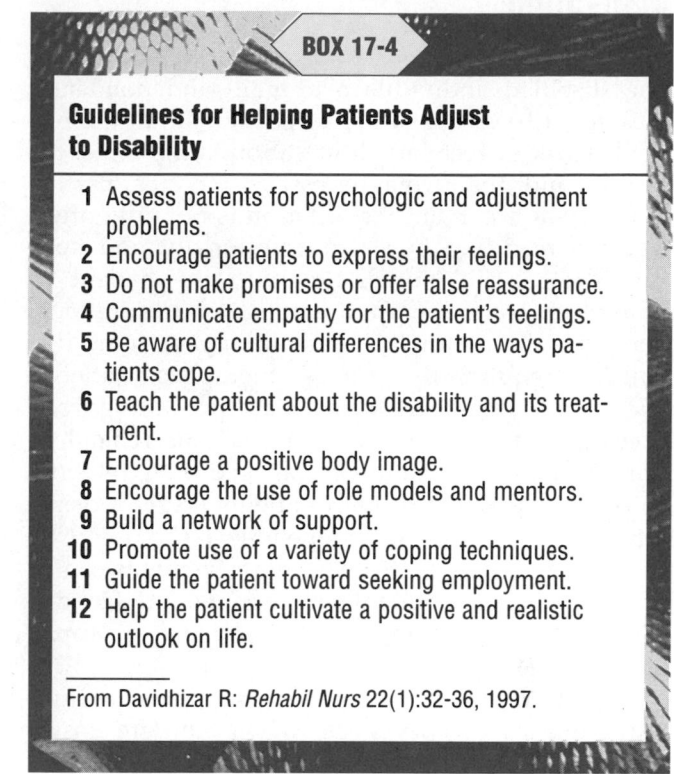

**BOX 17-4**

### Guidelines for Helping Patients Adjust to Disability

 1  Assess patients for psychologic and adjustment problems.
 2  Encourage patients to express their feelings.
 3  Do not make promises or offer false reassurance.
 4  Communicate empathy for the patient's feelings.
 5  Be aware of cultural differences in the ways patients cope.
 6  Teach the patient about the disability and its treatment.
 7  Encourage a positive body image.
 8  Encourage the use of role models and mentors.
 9  Build a network of support.
10  Promote use of a variety of coping techniques.
11  Guide the patient toward seeking employment.
12  Help the patient cultivate a positive and realistic outlook on life.

From Davidhizar R: *Rehabil Nurs* 22(1):32-36, 1997.

process. Loss of anything that is meaningful to the patient may produce a period of grief (Werner-Beland, 1980). The patient may be unable to look at the changed body part, attempting to deny its existence. Gradually the patient will begin to talk about the change, and often nurses are the first to be questioned about the disability. The patient may ask to see the disabled part and may seem both fascinated and revolted.

During this stage of adjustment, depression and anger may be present. Eventually the patient may realize that life cannot be as it was before and will begin to examine the values placed on conventional "normality." He or she may realize that the disability need not alter one's entire life and may begin to react more openly with others. Time is essential for the process of adaptation and adjustment to disability. The amount of time needed for this is a most personal and individual phenomenon.

The initial nursing assessment of the patient's and family's ability to cope is important. A psychosocial history, obtained on admission and updated over time, helps the nurse plan therapeutic interventions geared to the specific patient and family. Davidhizar (1997) has suggested a number of approaches for helping patients adjust to disability (Box 17-4).

## Motivation

**Motivation** is an important aspect of rehabilitation. For disabled individuals to gain independence, they must have the desire to participate in the difficult work of recovery. Motivation is the force, the desire, and the drive necessary for this participation. The work of rehabilitation is not only physically demanding but also emotionally and spiritually stressful. Nurses are with the patient 24 hours a day, and therapy treatments often are long. During the term of hospitalization that some disabilities require, the nurses, therapists, patients, and family members often develop strong relationships that become a vital part of rehabilitation. Nurses and therapists can use their relationships with patients to help patients create a desire for self-sufficiency and independence (Banja, 1990). Emphasizing capabilities and improvements can be of great value at a time when patients may feel discouraged and lacking in self-confidence (Learman et al, 1990).

Patients may have periods of regression as they move toward independence. When they are unsuccessful in their efforts to learn new skills or tasks, they may begin to feel "what's the use?" and frustration and depression may result. At these times, the nurse's gentle reminder of what has been accomplished, no matter how small, and encouragement to talk about frustrations and fears can be of great value to the patient. Acknowledging the fact that rehabilitation is hard work expresses an understanding of this to the patient.

Some patients may have received maximum benefit from rehabilitation but achieved only partial recovery. The goal of independence may be limited by the degree of disability. As a result, the patient may be resentful, angry, and depressed. The need for long-term follow-up care and continued support is essential. Being constantly alert to the patient's emotional stress and pain and encouraging the expression of feelings may help relieve some of the pressure the patient feels. Stress may become so great that the patient is unable to find the energy to participate in the work of rehabilitation. In this case, the entire interdisciplinary team must be involved in the discussion of assisting the patient through this period. Psychiatric counseling often can help the patient identify ways to cope and adapt. Group counseling with patients with similar disabilities and group leaders (psychiatric therapists, social workers, nurses, OTs, or PTs) can be most helpful. Some patients may need the assistance of psychotropic medications to deal with the depression and hopelessness they feel as a result of their illnesses and disabilities.

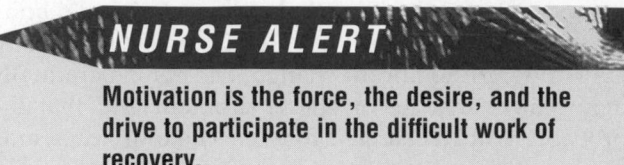

**NURSE ALERT**

Motivation is the force, the desire, and the drive to participate in the difficult work of recovery.

## The Patient's Family

A family's response to a patient's illness and loss of function is based on many factors. The relationships of the individuals involved, the methods of family coping, the role of the patient in the family, and economic issues all may have an impact on this response. During the acute phase of care, the family suffers from anxiety, apprehension, and fear. They should be given emotional support, comfort, and all the information possible during this critical period. If the patient is the breadwinner, the spouse may be distressed about how medical and hospital bills will be paid or how to provide for the family. A serious disability may mean social isolation for the family as well as the patient, and this isolation may lead to loneliness and depression. As soon as the prognosis can be made, long-term goals should be established for the patient. The family should be given information about sources of help in rehabilitation and economic assistance. A social worker may help the family, but if a social worker is not available, nurses should be familiar with community agencies and organizations for people with disabilities. Specific support groups are available for families of disabled people. For example, the National Head Injury Foundation provides information, education, resources, and peer support for patients and their families; the foundation's address is 33 Turnpike Road, Southboro, Massachusetts 01772.

## Sexuality

In considering all the needs of the patient and his or her family, the area of sexuality must be addressed. To discuss this sensitive subject with their patients, nurses must understand their own feelings about sexuality, and they must be knowledgeable about the effects of disability on sexual function. The patient may be hesitant to ask questions or to bring up the subject of sex, but if the nurse lets it be known that it is an appropriate topic, the patient may initiate discussion. Experts in this field, often disabled individuals themselves, are available for referral, and literature is available in nursing journals and from rehabilitation hospitals and state rehabilitation departments.

If the nurse feels unqualified or uncomfortable with the topic of sexuality, he or she should let the patient know that it is an appropriate topic to raise but that another team member could better address these concerns. In a rehabilitation setting, there is often a team member who is an expert in the area of sexuality and sexual counseling who can assist the patient or help others on the team counsel the patient. In other types of settings the sexual concerns of patients are not always discussed. Across the country, many training programs have been instituted to help health care professionals become more knowledgeable in this important area.

# NURSING APPROACHES TO REHABILITATION CARE

As a member of the rehabilitation team, the nurse must assume a share of responsibility for guiding the disabled patient toward health and independence. In some situations the nurse will be working with the physician without the services of other persons who contribute to a comprehensive rehabilitation program. Therefore it is increasingly important for the nurse to become familiar with the local and state agencies that provide rehabilitation services and also with agencies, societies, and foundations that provide educational materials and information about specific disabilities.

## Assessment

Nursing care begins with assessment of the patient. The initial assessment is the time for the nurse to gather information about the patient to establish goals of care and to plan interventions. Many institutions and agencies have established admission nursing assessment guidelines. Assessment occurs with every interaction between the nurse and patient.

In the rehabilitation setting an interdisciplinary approach to assessment usually is taken, and a variety of assessment tools are available to document the patient's status. Some of the tools specific to rehabilitation measure functional status or the patient's ability to perform basic ADL. Others measure more complex activities, known as instrumental activities of daily living (IADL), such as shopping and money management. Still other tools measure emotional state or quality of life. **Functional assessment** is completed to determine the patient's physical functional status, to document the need for intervention, to plan treatment, and to measure progress (Kelly-Hayes, 1991).

Nurses may use these tools as part of their own practice or as part of the work of the interdisciplinary team. The information obtained from this form of assessment may assist the nurse in many ways, includ-

ing providing a baseline measure of the patient's status, serving as a means to communicate the patient's status to other caregivers, assessing a patient's need for rehabilitation, identifying the need for support services in the home, and measuring outcomes of care. In some settings functional assessment may be included as a measure of the intensity of nursing care needs on a nursing unit.

> ## NURSE ALERT
> All patients need a thorough physical, emotional, and social assessment before an individualized rehabilitation program can be established.

Functional data are obtained by observing the patient participate in self-care activities. The two functional assessment tools commonly used in the rehabilitation setting are the Barthel Index and the Functional Independence Measure (FIM). The Barthel Index measures performance in mobility, self-care, and continence (Mahoney, 1965). The FIM measures function in feeding, grooming, bathing, dressing the upper body, dressing the lower body, toileting, bladder and bowel management, transfer ability, locomotion, communication, and social cognition (Figure 17-3) (Kelly-Hayes, 1991; Gyde for the Uniform Sets for Medical Rehabilitation (Adult FIM), 1993).

## Nursing Interventions

In caring for patients, particularly immobilized individuals, the nurse must use rehabilitation techniques to promote maximum functioning and to prevent secondary complications. These techniques include (1) methods to improve movement and mobility (ROJM, positioning and transferring of the patient in bed and in a chair, and encouraging the patient to participate in self-care); (2) approaches to preventing complications (bladder and bowel care, skin care, care of the patient with swallowing difficulty); and (3) use of adaptive equipment, mobility aids, and prosthetic equipment (Box 17-5). Teaching the patient the implications of his or her diagnosis, reinforcing aspects of self-care, and providing for **continuity** of care are additional important themes of nursing care of the disabled.

### Methods to Improve Mobility

**Range of joint motion.** Each joint of the human body has a potential range of motion that is normal for that

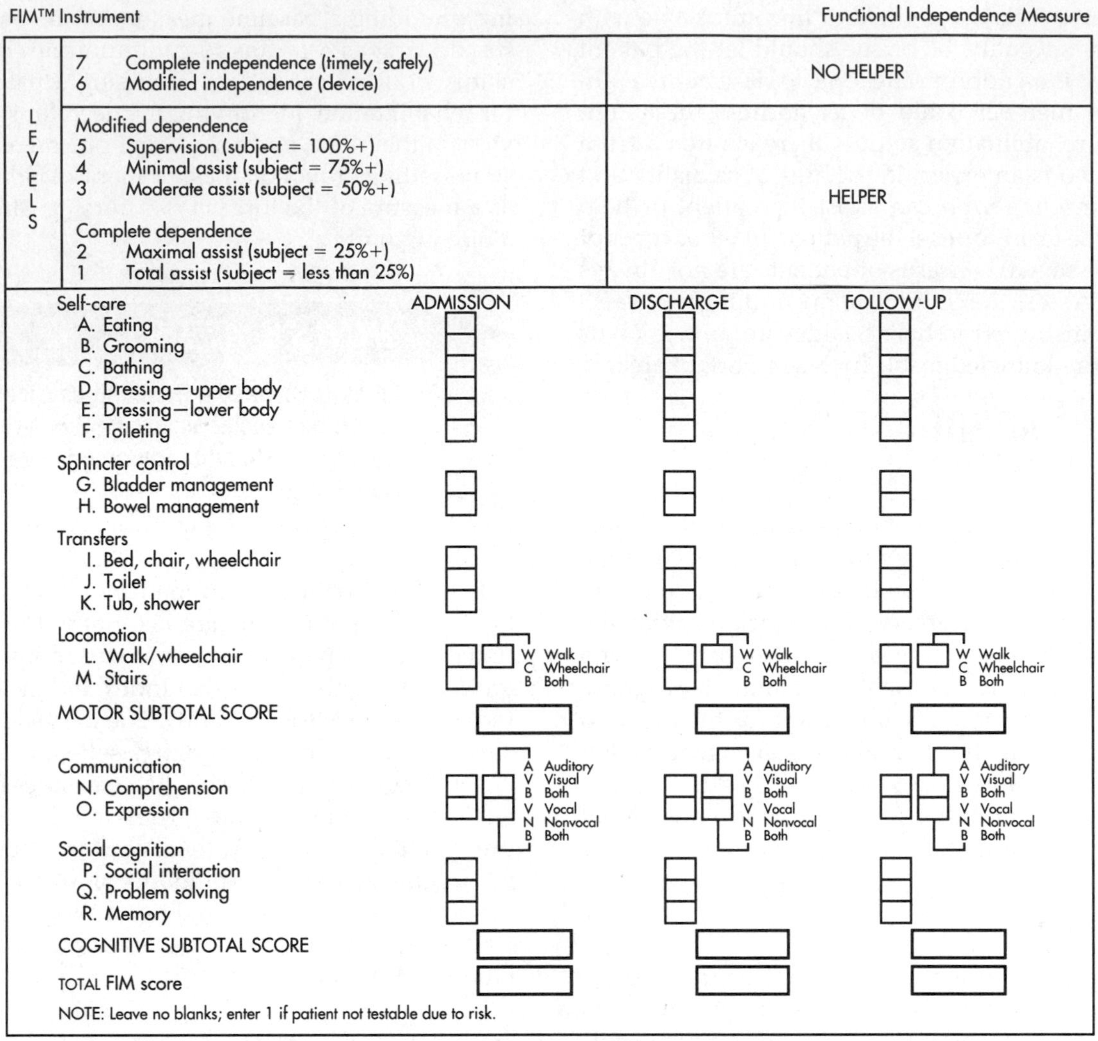

FIM™ Instrument                                                                                    Functional Independence Measure

| | | ADMISSION | DISCHARGE | FOLLOW-UP |
|---|---|---|---|---|

L E V E L S

| 7 Complete independence (timely, safely)<br>6 Modified independence (device) | NO HELPER |
|---|---|
| **Modified dependence**<br>5 Supervision (subject = 100%+)<br>4 Minimal assist (subject = 75%+)<br>3 Moderate assist (subject = 50%+)<br><br>**Complete dependence**<br>2 Maximal assist (subject = 25%+)<br>1 Total assist (subject = less than 25%) | HELPER |

**Self-care**
A. Eating
B. Grooming
C. Bathing
D. Dressing—upper body
E. Dressing—lower body
F. Toileting

**Sphincter control**
G. Bladder management
H. Bowel management

**Transfers**
I. Bed, chair, wheelchair
J. Toilet
K. Tub, shower

**Locomotion**
L. Walk/wheelchair   W Walk  C Wheelchair  B Both
M. Stairs

**MOTOR SUBTOTAL SCORE**

**Communication**
N. Comprehension   A Auditory  V Visual  B Both
O. Expression   V Vocal  N Nonvocal  B Both

**Social cognition**
P. Social interaction
Q. Problem solving
R. Memory

**COGNITIVE SUBTOTAL SCORE**

**TOTAL FIM score**

NOTE: Leave no blanks; enter 1 if patient not testable due to risk.

**Figure 17-3**   The Functional Independence Measure. FIM™ is a trademark of the Uniform Data System for Medical Rehabilitation, a division of UB Foundation Activities, Inc. (From *Guide for the Uniform Data Set for Medical Rehabilitation (including the FIM™ instrument)*, Version 5.1: Buffalo, NY, 1997, State University of New York at Buffalo.)

joint. For movement to be maintained, the limbs of the body must be moved to stretch the muscles, ligaments, and tendons that surround and support each joint. This stretching occurs with normal daily activity. However, when illness or injury limits normal movement, movement in joints and muscle strength may be lost. Without the stretching associated with normal movement, the muscles, tendons, and ligaments surrounding joints can become shortened, limiting the amount of movement possible. When this occurs, a *contracture*, or fixed movement of the joint, may develop. With loss of muscle strength or paralysis, a contracture can develop within a relatively short period. Spasticity, an excessive amount of muscle tone, also can cause a contracture to develop quickly. A contracture can limit function in a joint and cause secondary complications. For example, a foot contracted in a position of footdrop may not be able to support the leg

for walking, or an elbow severely contracted in the flexed position may cause skin breakdown in the antecubital space because of pressure and maceration of the skin.

When a patient is unable to move, nurses need to provide the motion necessary to keep the patient's joints as mobile as possible. This type of motion regimen, ROJM, needs to be provided several times a day to each joint to prevent stiffness and contractures. Joints that should be exercised include the neck, shoulders, elbows, wrists, fingers, hips, knees, ankles, and toes. For patients unable to move, the exercises are passive; the nurse exercises the joints without assistance from the patient. Passive exercise helps keep joints mobile, promotes venous return and lymphatic flow, and helps prevent excess demineralization in the bone, a condition exacerbated by inactivity. If the patient is able to move, he or she can perform active

---

BOX 17-5

## NURSING PROCESS

### REHABILITATION OF THE IMMOBILE PATIENT

**ASSESSMENT**

- Mobility deficits
- Range of motion
- Ability to perform activities of daily living
- Skin integrity
- Nutritional status
- Respiratory status
- Complications (e.g., thrombophlebitis, constipation)
- Coping mechanisms
- Laboratory studies (albumin, transferrin, hemoglobin, hematocrit)

**NURSING DIAGNOSES**

- Impaired physical mobility related to musculoskeletal or neuromuscular impairment, weakness, or pain
- Constipation related to immobility
- Self-care deficit related to physical impairment or weakness
- Impaired skin integrity related to immobility, incontinence, or poor nutritional status
- Powerlessness related to dependence on others

**NURSING INTERVENTIONS**

- Perform or assist with active or passive range-of-motion exercises to all extremities 3 or 4 times a day.
- Reposition every 2 hours, maintaining proper body alignment.

- Support feet with foot board or firm pillows to prevent footdrop.
- Encourage and assist with early mobilization.
- Assist with transfer, using appropriate devices and help.
- Allow patient to perform tasks at his or her own rate.
- Encourage participation in self-care activities.
- Obtain pressure-relieving bed and cushions for chair as indicated.
- Avoid pressure on heels with pillows, splints, or boots.
- Keep skin clean and dry; lubricate as necessary.
- Encourage optimum nutrition.
- Encourage coughing and deep breathing.
- If not contraindicated, encourage fluid intake to 2000 ml every 24 hours.
- Encourage verbalization of feelings and frustrations.
- Emphasize ability rather than disability.

**EVALUATION OF EXPECTED OUTCOMES**

- Able to perform physical activities with assistive devices as needed
- No evidence of complications of immobility
- Skin integrity intact
- No signs or symptoms of thrombophlebitis
- Bowel pattern shows previous level of functioning

---

range of motion by taking the limbs through all the potential degrees of movement.

Areas of assessment the nurse should consider before initiating ROJM exercises include the muscle strength of the involved limbs, the muscle tone, the degree of possible joint motion, and the presence of pain, stiffness, bony deformities, or edema. This assessment is made as the nurse moves the patient or observes the patient moving and can be done as part of routine care, such as bathing.

The normal range of motion for joints is as follows (Figure 17-4):

- *Neck*—The neck is able to rotate from side to side, flex toward the chest and extend toward the back, and extend away from the flex toward the shoulders on each side.
- *Shoulders*—The shoulders are able to rotate (with arms moving in a circular motion), flex forward, extend backward, move away from the body (abduction), and move toward the body (adduction).

- *Elbows*—The elbows are able to flex toward the upper arm and extend away from the upper arm.
- *Hips*—The hips are able to rotate in a circular motion, flex toward the body, extend and hyperextend away from the body, and move toward the body (adduction) and away from the body (abduction).
- *Knees*—The knees are able to bend (flex) and straighten (extend).

When providing ROJM exercises, the nurse should never push or stretch the joint beyond the point of stiffness, pain, or discomfort (Box 17-6). A PT or OT can assist with care of tight, painful joints. When providing such exercises, the nurse should support the limb and the joints involved. For example, if a nurse is flexing a patient's hip, the leg should be cradled in the nurse's arm at the knee. The nurse gently holds the hip down with the other hand to prevent lifting of the hip. Use of the principles of body mechanics is important while lifting or moving the patient during

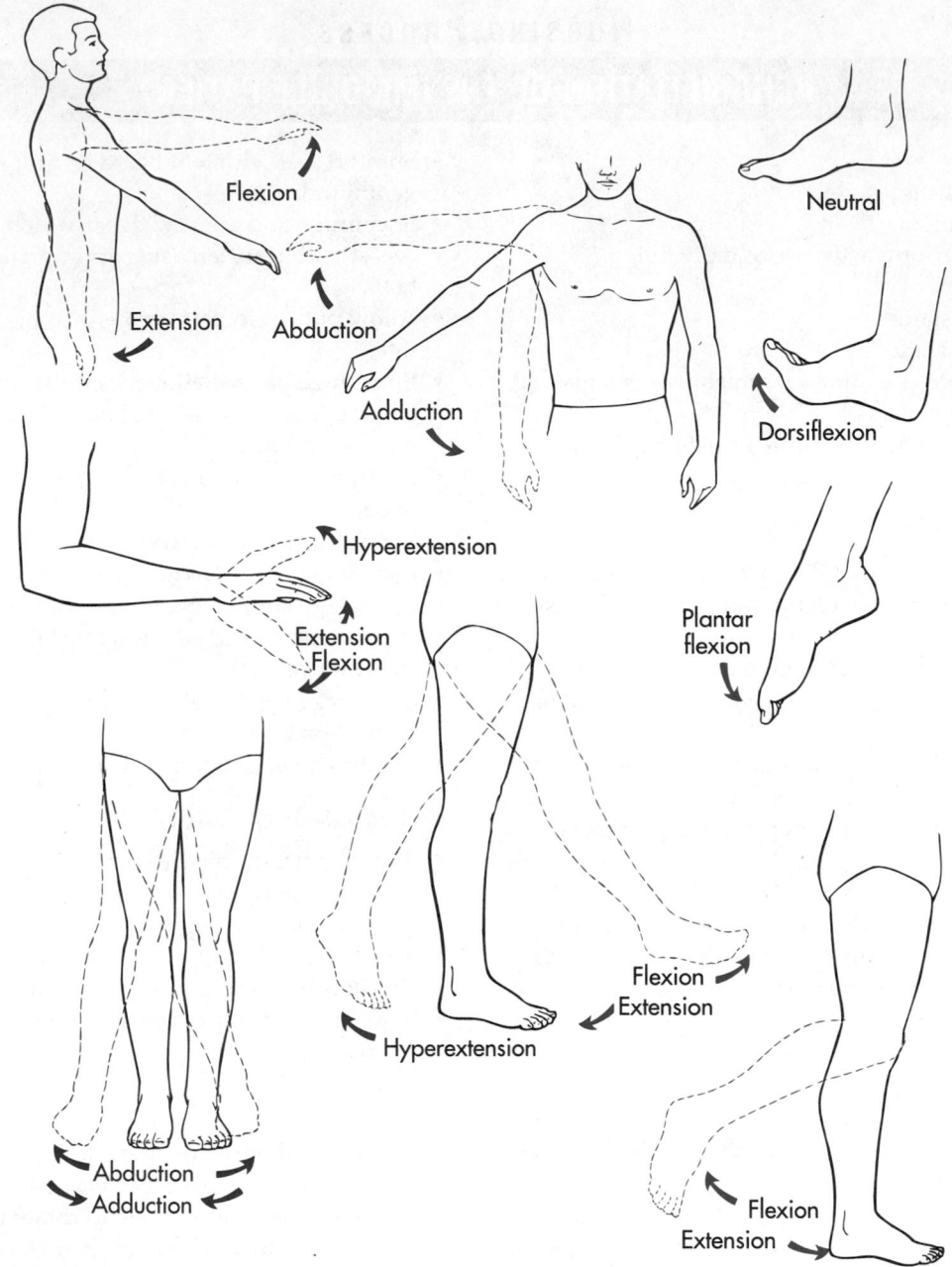

**Figure 17-4** Range of joint motion. Methods of exercising joints to prevent contractures and to stimulate circulation.

range-of-motion exercises (Box 17-7). The nurse should stand as close as possible to the patient, with the height of the bed adjusted to prevent the nurse from having back, shoulder, or arm strain. Also, the patient's family can be taught these exercises. Having the family perform range-of-motion exercises often is an initial approach to including the family in the patient's care.

If the patient has weakness or paralysis in one limb or on one side of the body and has normal strength on the other side, the patient can be taught to perform self–range-of-motion exercises. The nurse or therapist can instruct the patient to cradle and lift the weaker limb with the strong limb. A stroke patient can use the strong arm to lift and exercise the weak arm and can use the strong foot and leg by pushing it under the weak leg and lifting. In acute care hospitals, nursing homes, rehabilitation hospitals, and adult day care programs in the community, nurses and therapists or-

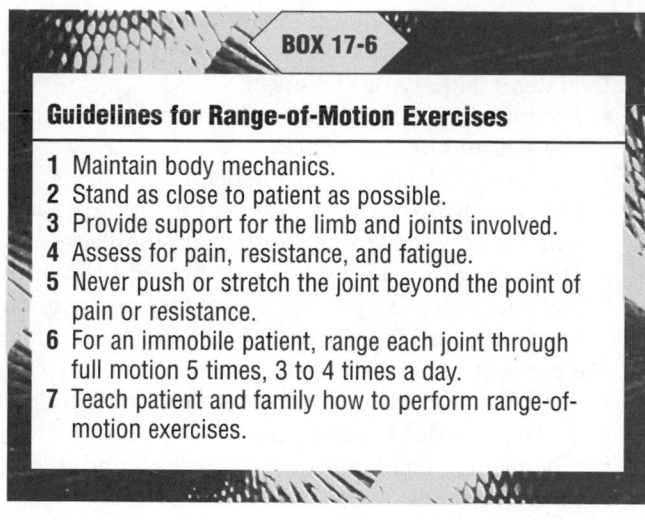

**BOX 17-6**

**Guidelines for Range-of-Motion Exercises**

1 Maintain body mechanics.
2 Stand as close to patient as possible.
3 Provide support for the limb and joints involved.
4 Assess for pain, resistance, and fatigue.
5 Never push or stretch the joint beyond the point of pain or resistance.
6 For an immobile patient, range each joint through full motion 5 times, 3 to 4 times a day.
7 Teach patient and family how to perform range-of-motion exercises.

**BOX 17-7**

**PRINCIPLES OF BODY MECHANICS IN MOVING PATIENTS**

• Communicate your plan to the patient.
• Decide if you are able to move the patient by yourself or if you need assistance.
• Give yourself a broad base of support and good balance by keeping your feet apart.
• Get as close to the patient as possible.
• Keep your back straight and bend at the knees.
• Turn your body in the direction you are moving the patient.
• Straighten your legs as you lift.
• Do not twist your back; shift your feet and the direction of your body as you turn.
• Lift smoothly and in coordination with others.
• Push and pull the patient on a draw sheet rather than lifting.

ganize patients to participate in group exercise programs. Some of these programs incorporate self range of motion and active range of motion as part of the program. These programs have been found to have additional benefits, such as increased tolerance of activity and socialization opportunities (Paillard, Nowak, 1985). Recent evidence suggests that resistance exercises are effective in increasing strength, even in the oldest old, those in their 90s (Fiatarone et al, 1993, 1994).

## Positioning

In addition to ROJM exercises, proper positioning of the immobile patient in a lying or sitting position is necessary to prevent joint deformities, skin breakdown, and impaired respiratory function. Continual nursing assessment is a necessary aspect of determining the patient's positioning needs. Pressure sores, paralysis or weakness, edema, pain, restricted respiratory status, joint deformity, an unstable fracture, or an acute medical problem such as cardiopulmonary distress may limit the positions possible and influence the timing of position changes.

The scheduling of position changes depends on the patient's needs. A patient in severe pain or one with fragile skin may have to be turned every hour or even more often. Patients who are completely unable to move because of paralysis, coma, edema, or loss of sensation may have to be turned every 2 hours. A patient who has some degree of movement may not have to be turned as often (Panel for Prediction and Prevention of Pressure Ulcers in Adults, 1992). Determining the priorities of care is another factor in planning a turning schedule. For example, the need to wake a sleep-deprived patient for turning should be weighed carefully. The nurse needs to determine if the greater

priority of care for this patient is the need to be repositioned or the need for sleep.

Assessment areas the nurse may consider in planning a position schedule include (1) examination of bony prominences for redness and discoloration, (2) examination of edematous extremities for indentations of the skin and weeping of fluid through the skin, (3) development of tightness around joints or a contracted position that is difficult to correct, and (4) patient complaints of pain, stiffness, and soreness. Contraindications for specific positions are considered, including the presence of an unstable fracture, increased intracranial pressure or poor cerebral perfusion, and cardiac or pulmonary restrictions.

The following are some positioning guidelines. In the supine (back-lying) position:

• A small pillow should be placed under the head, neck, and shoulders. A large pillow under the head places the head in an excessively flexed position.
• Arms and hands should be positioned to provide support and comfort. A neutral position with the arms at the side of the body may be comfortable for some patients, although edema or pain may require supporting the arms and hands on pillows. Hand rolls can be used to maintain a functional position of the hand and to prevent wrist-drop if paralysis is present. In some situations the OT may be of assistance in selecting the type of hand roll needed. Patients with spasticity of the hand muscles may require a firm hand roll

because use of a roll made of soft material is thought to increase spasticity (Jamison, 1980).

• Excessive hip flexion and outward rotation of the hips and legs should be avoided. A firm mattress reduces hip flexion. Immobile patients who use a soft bed surface or who have had an above-the-knee amputation and who remain for long periods in a supine position are at risk of developing a hip flexion contracture that can severely limit ambulation and mobility. A sagging bed makes it difficult to maintain body alignment; a bed board placed between the springs and mattress helps provide firmness. To prevent outward rotation of the hip and leg, a rolled towel or trochanter roll can be placed along the side of the body between the hip and the knee (Figure 17-5).

• Legs and feet should be kept in line with the torso of the body, and an adjustable foot board that extends above the toes can be used to help prevent footdrop and to keep covers off the feet. Pillows, splints, or protective boots should be used to keep the heels free of pressure (Panel for Prediction and Prevention of Pressure Ulcers in Adults, 1992). If the mattress has removable sections, the foot section can be removed to reduce pressure over the heels.

> ### NURSE ALERT
> **Proper scheduling of position changes depends on a thorough assessment of need.**

• The feet should be kept at a right angle to the legs. Foot splints or high-topped tennis shoes worn with socks can be used intermittently (3 hours on, 1 hour off) to prevent footdrop (Figure 17-6). Unlike a foot board, these shoes and splints maintain proper alignment when the patient is positioned on either side. The bony prominences of the foot must be inspected when these devices are re-

moved to ensure that they are not causing excessive pressure, which can lead to skin breakdown.

In the lateral (side-lying) position:
• The patient is supported in this position by a pillow placed along the back.
• A pillow is placed under the head.
• The downward arm lies along the side of body, and the upward arm is supported by pillows.
• The upward leg may be flexed, brought forward, and supported by pillows to prevent pressure on the downward leg (Figure 17-7).

In the prone (front-lying) position:
• The head is turned to one side and a small pillow is placed under it for support.
• Pillows may be placed under the chest and thighs for comfort and to support the legs.
• A pillow placed under the lower legs may keep the feet at right angles to the legs, or the patient may be positioned lower in the bed so that the feet can be placed over the bottom edge of the bed.

In the sitting position in a chair:
• Placement in a chair depends on the patient's height, weight, posture, sitting balance, strength, and muscle tone.
• The type of chair used is selected for safety, support, mobility, and independence.
• The patient should sit in the middle of the seat with the buttocks against the back of the chair. The arms and head are supported. The feet are supported without placing excessive pressure on the knees and hips, which should be flexed at a 90-degree angle.

**Patient transfers.** The patient's level of independence in transfer ability should be assessed by the PT and the nurse (Box 17-8). During an acute illness, especially one requiring bed rest, patients may become debilitated and weak. Even the most basic movements, such as turning in bed or getting out of bed, may be impossible for a severely debilitated person. With recovery, as a patient's strength and endurance increase, the ability to lift himself or herself out of bed into a chair

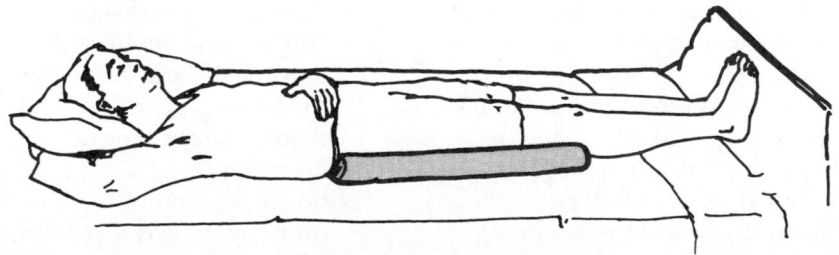

**Figure 17-5**   Trochanter roll is placed against patient's body between the hip and knee to prevent external rotation of the hip and excessive pressure against the hip and side of the ankle.

or onto a commode increases. Patients with a disability may be completely dependent in this area or may need moderate to minimum assistance.

Safety is of prime importance in transferring a patient. Ways to prevent injury to the patient and the nurse must be considered before the patient is moved. Patient assessment areas include (1) ability to compre-hend instructions; (2) weight and height; (3) ability to stand; (4) ability to bear weight; (5) presence of medical or orthopedic instability; (6) and presence of orthostatic hypotension. To reduce the risk of injury, the nurse needs to plan the transfer and describe each step to the patient and any other care providers involved before the patient is moved. If the patient is completely

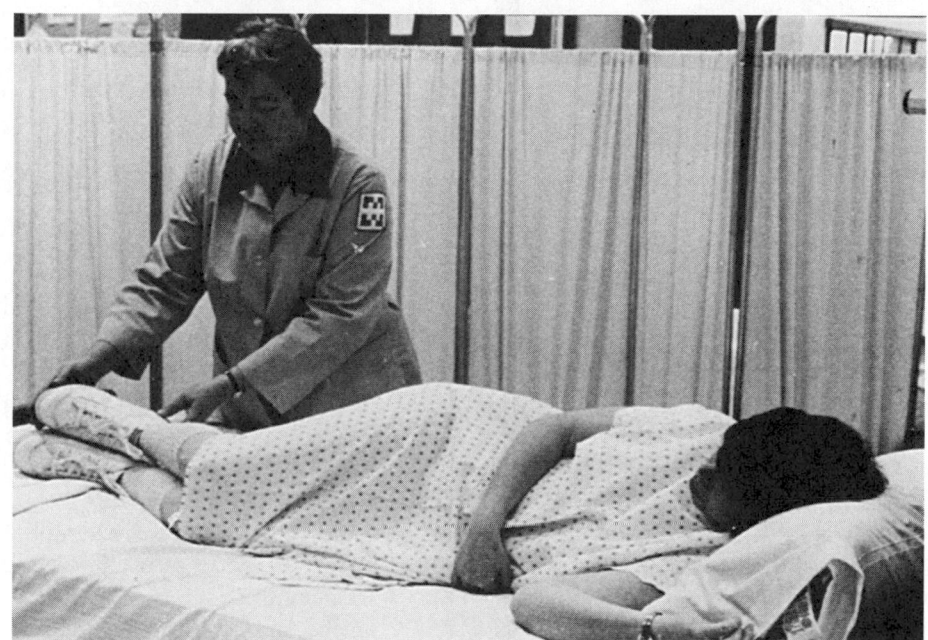

**Figure 17-6**    High-topped canvas shoes maintain foot alignment regardless of patient's position in bed. Shoes are worn with socks for 3 hours, removed for 1 hour, and then put back on. (Courtesy William Rainey Harper College, Palatine, Ill.)

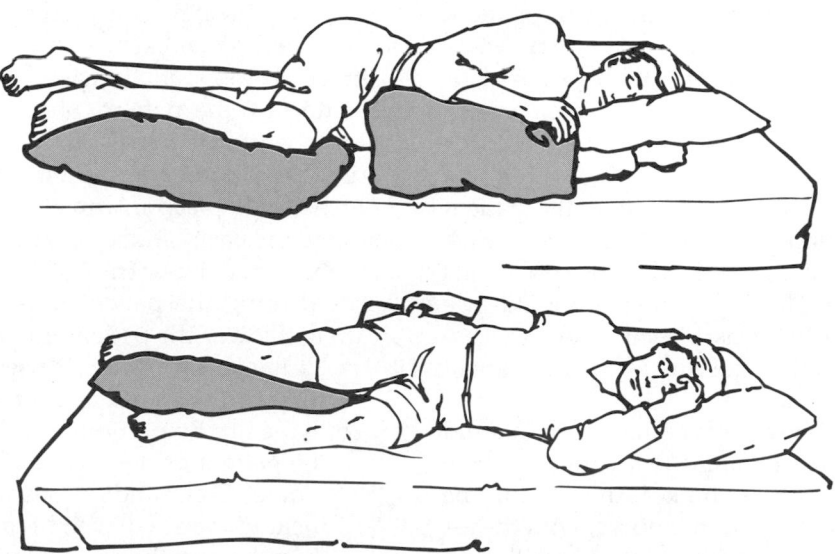

**Figure 17-7**    In the side-lying position, the arm and leg should be supported with pillows. The patient's trunk and limbs can be positioned toward the front of the body or toward the back.

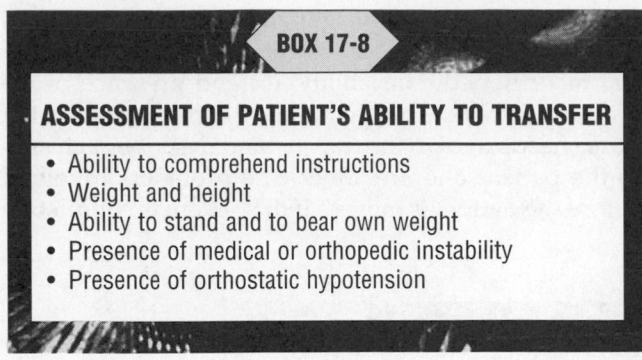

**BOX 17-8**

### ASSESSMENT OF PATIENT'S ABILITY TO TRANSFER

- Ability to comprehend instructions
- Weight and height
- Ability to stand and to bear own weight
- Presence of medical or orthopedic instability
- Presence of orthostatic hypotension

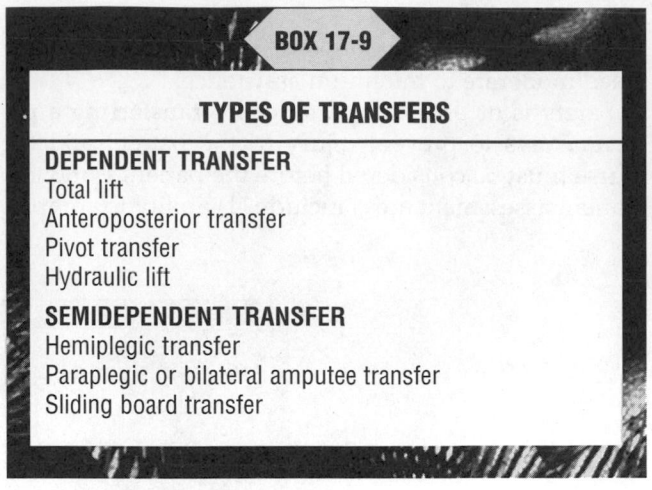

**BOX 17-9**

### TYPES OF TRANSFERS

**DEPENDENT TRANSFER**
Total lift
Anteroposterior transfer
Pivot transfer
Hydraulic lift

**SEMIDEPENDENT TRANSFER**
Hemiplegic transfer
Paraplegic or bilateral amputee transfer
Sliding board transfer

dependent and several staff members are involved in the transfer, one staff person should be designated the leader and assigned to direct all steps of the process. Transfer activity may be described as bed to chair; bed to wheelchair, toilet, bath, or shower; or wheelchair to car.

Use of a transfer belt may make transferring the patient safer and easier. Transfer belts are strongly constructed and made of leather or nylon with sturdy loops on the sides and back of the belt. In preparing for transfer, the belt is placed securely around the patient's waist. The nurse bends at the knees and places his or her hands through the side loops and holds onto the back loop; this gives the nurse a secure hold on the patient as the patient stands. As the patient comes into a standing position, the nurse brings him or her as close as possible; this makes the transfer more stable because the patient's center of gravity is close to the nurse's center of gravity. The nurse then guides the patient into a chair.

Several types of transfers can be used (Box 17-9).

**Dependent transfer.** The patient is unable to assist with any aspect of this activity. Moving the patient may require lifting him or her through a total lift or pivot transfer or use of a lift sheet, a transfer board, or a hydraulic lift. Lifts for the totally dependent patient include the following:

- *Total lift.* At least two nurses are involved in this lift. One nurse should stand behind the patient with the arms placed under the patient's arms and around the chest, with the nurse's hands gripped together. The second nurse should face the patient with the arms placed under the patient's knees. Together the nurses lift the patient up into bed or onto a chair.
- *Anteroposterior (AP) transfer.* The nurse should place the chair at a right angle to the middle of the bed and, if the chair has brakes, they should be locked. Using a pull sheet, the nurse, with the assistance of another if needed, should turn the patient across the bed so that his or her back is to the chair. Next, the nurse, again with assistance if

needed, slides the patient on the pull sheet into the chair. This procedure should be reversed to return the patient to bed.

- *Pivot transfer.* This transfer requires one or two people to assist the patient. In a one-person pivot transfer, the patient should be placed in a sitting position on the side of the bed. The nurse should stand in front of the patient, bending the knees to lower the body and center of gravity for greater stability and safety. The nurse's arms should be placed under the patient's arms and around the back. At the same time, the patient should wrap his or her arms around the nurse's shoulders. Through a gentle rocking motion, the nurse should lift the patient to a standing position and then slowly turn the patient toward the chair and lower him or her into the chair.

A two-person pivot transfer may be used for a more debilitated patient. The patient should be placed in a sitting position on the side of the bed. Each nurse should face the patient, one on each side of the patient's body. The nurses should bend their knees, lowering their bodies and their centers of gravity. One nurse should place an arm under the patient's arm and around the back. The second nurse should do the same on the other side. Through a rocking motion, they should bring the patient to a standing position and turn and lower the patient into the chair.

- *Hydraulic lift.* This lift uses a one- or two-piece sling that is placed under the patient and attached to the lift. By pumping the lift, the nurse can raise the patient off the bed and easily move the individual. Contraindications for use of such devices include excessive weight or height, agitation, and medical or orthopedic instability.

**Semidependent transfer.** The patient is able to assist the nurse to some degree with this lift (Dittmar,

1989). Lifts for the semidependent patient include the following:

- *Hemiplegic transfer.* The wheelchair should be placed at the side of bed on the patient's unaffected side of body. The nurse should then remove the armrest and lock the brakes. Next, the patient should be helped to sit on side of bed and then to stand, turn, and back up to the chair. The nurse may need to assist the patient to move the hemiplegic leg by placing her foot at right angles to the patient's involved foot and bracing a knee against the patient's involved knee. The patient should place the strong arm on the wheelchair arm, while pushing back into the chair.
- *Paraplegic or bilateral amputee transfer.* This is the same as the AP transfer described previously, except that the patient should have enough arm strength to hold himself or herself up in bed and scoot back into the chair.
- *Sliding board transfer.* A chair sliding board is a rectangular piece of wood or plastic, usually measuring about $2\frac{1}{2}$ feet by 1 foot. It is used to assist patients when moving between the bed and the chair, the chair and the toilet, and the chair and the car. The nurse should place the wheelchair at the side of the bed, lock the brakes, and remove the armrest of the chair. The height of the bed should be at the same height as the chair seat. The nurse should assist the patient to sit on the side of the bed. One end of the chair sliding board should be placed under the patient's buttocks and the other end is placed on the chair seat. The patient should reach for the wheelchair arm and pull across the board into the chair.

Not all patients are able to sit in a wheelchair. A debilitated patient may need a recliner chair for comfort, support, and safety, particularly the style of chair that can be fitted with a tray. Recliner chairs are used widely across the country, yet this chair design makes patient transfers most difficult and, with some patients, is unsafe. It is important to make sure that the chair is in good working order. If brakes are not operational, the chair should be placed against a wall. Most of these chairs do not have removable arms, and nurses need to help the patient over the arm and into the chair. With a frail patient, two nurses using a two-person pivot transfer may be needed. However, if the patient has difficulty bearing weight or is confused, it is safer to use the AP transfer, a total lift with a sheet, or a hydraulic lift.

## Patient Participation in Self-Care

The nurse can promote activity, mobility, and exercise by encouraging the patient to participate in his or her own care. If the patient has been acutely ill, this activity may be limited. Turning independently in bed and balancing oneself while sitting on the side of the bed may increase strength, endurance, and balance.

While the patient sits on the side of the bed or in a chair, the nurse should have him or her raise one leg for a few seconds, lower that leg, and raise the other. This simple exercise helps strengthen the quadriceps muscles, a major muscle group involved in standing and walking (Lewis, 1989). Brushing one's own hair or teeth may promote upper extremity strength and trunk balance. Gradually the patient should engage in more activities. The nurse and the PT must work together to reinforce the patient's independence in transfers in and out of bed, standing, and walking. As the patient's activity level increases, strength and endurance increase. Recent studies on the impact of exercise in the elderly indicate that resistance exercise, with use of weights, is the most effective means of increasing strength. Patients in their 90s made improvements through participation in regular resistance training (Payton, Poland, 1983; Fiatarone et al, 1994).

## Preventive Approaches to Care

**Skin breakdown.** Preventing skin breakdown is another aspect of care of the immobile or disabled person. Skin breakdown occurs when excessive pressure is exerted by bed or chair surfaces against the bony prominences of the body when the patient is lying or sitting (Figure 17-8). The common names for this problem, *bedsore* or *decubitus ulcer,* are inaccurate terms. The correct term is *pressure ulcer.* The word *decubitus* comes from the Latin meaning lying down. However, the source of the problem is not solely lying down or being in bed; the real culprit is pressure. Pressure that is excessive and of long duration occludes capillary blood flow to the tissue overlying the bony prominences, depriving that tissue of oxygen. This hypoxic tissue cannot survive, and a wound forms. The size and depth of the wound depend on the intensity of pressure and the length of time the pressure goes unrelieved. Healthy people feel discomfort from sitting in one position too long and simply change position, but people who are unable to move or who cannot feel painful sensations cannot relieve this pressure on their own, and they run a much greater risk of developing pressure ulcers.

Other factors play an important role in skin health, including nutritional status, mobility, sensory ability, medical status, continence, and circulatory status. Age-associated changes in the skin make older patients more susceptible to skin breakdown. The skin of an older person is drier and less elastic and has less subcutaneous tissue. When a patient is admitted, the nurse needs to determine if he or she is at risk for

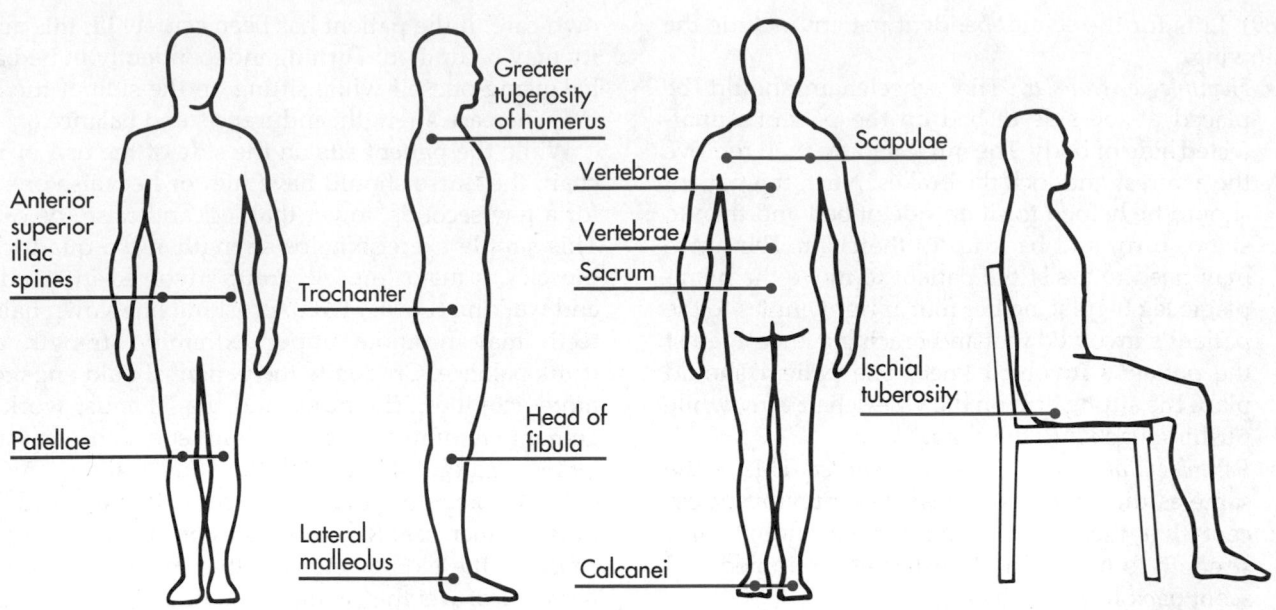

**Figure 17-8**   Bony prominences of the body.

### TABLE 17-1

## Norton Scale

| | | PHYSICAL CONDITION | | MENTAL CONDITION | | ACTIVITY | | MOBILITY | | INCONTINENT | | TOTAL SCORE |
|---|---|---|---|---|---|---|---|---|---|---|---|---|
| | | Good | 4 | Alert | 4 | Ambulant | 4 | Full | 4 | Not | 4 | |
| | | Fair | 3 | Apathetic | 3 | Walk/help | 3 | Slightly limited | 3 | Occasionally | 3 | |
| | | Poor | 2 | Confused | 2 | Chairbound | 2 | Very limited | 2 | Usually/urine | 2 | |
| | | Very bad | 1 | Stupor | 1 | Bed | 1 | Immobile | 1 | Doubly | 1 | |
| Name | Date | | | | | | | | | | | |
| | | | | | | | | | | | | |
| | | | | | | | | | | | | |

From Centre for Policy on Aging, London, England.

developing a pressure ulcer. The federal Department of Health and Human Services' Clinical Practice Guideline for preventing pressure ulcers recommends that a risk assessment tool be used to identify such patients (Panel for Prediction and Prevention of Pressure Ulcers in Adults, 1992). Two such tools recommended are the Braden Scale (Figure 17-9) and the Norton Scale (Table 17-1) (Norton, McLaren, Exton-Smith, 1962; Bergstrom et al, 1987; Braden, Bergstrom, 1989).

If a patient is identified as being at risk of pressure ulcers, several nursing interventions should be instituted to prevent them. Pressure can be relieved by several methods, including turning the patient as needed, using pressure-reducing bed and chair surfaces, and protecting the heels with pillows, splints, or boots or removing heel blocks from the mattress. Careful attention must be paid to the patient's nutritional and fluid

intake. Laboratory values that indicate the patient's nutritional and medical status must be obtained and monitored. Albumin and transferrin levels provide data on the visceral protein stores available for promoting tissue integrity and wound healing. The total lymphocyte count, hematocrit, hemoglobin, and body chemistries also must be monitored because they reflect the patient's state of health. Vitamin and mineral levels are important because these elements play a vital role in healing.

Nutritional consultation is needed for a malnourished patient at risk of developing a pressure ulcer. Measuring the patient's caloric and fluid intake is helpful in trying to assess adequacy of nutrition. The nutritionist can complete a more comprehensive nutritional assessment and can advise the nursing staff on ways to supplement an inadequate diet. Protein, fat,

**Note**: Bed- and chairbound individuals or those with impaired ability to reposition should be assessed upon admission for their risk of developing pressure ulcers. Patients with established pressure ulcers should be reassessed periodically.

PATIENT NAME _____

ROOM NUMBER _____ DATE _____

| **Sensory perception**<br>Ability to respond meaningfully to pressure-related discomfort | **1. Completely limited:** Unresponsive (does not moan, flinch, or gasp) to painful stimuli, due to diminished level of consciousness or sedation **Or** Limited ability to feel pain over most of body surface | **2. Very limited:** Responds only to painful stimuli; cannot communicate discomfort except by moaning or restlessness **Or** Has a sensory impairment that limits the ability to feel pain or discomfort over ½ of body | **3. Slightly limited:** Responds to verbal commands but cannot always communicate discomfort or need to be turned **Or** Has some sensory impairment that limits ability to feel pain or discomfort in one or two extremities | **4. No impairment:** Responds to verbal commands; has no sensory deficit that would limit ability to feel or voice pain or discomfort | (Indicate appropriate score) |
|---|---|---|---|---|---|
| **Moisture**<br>Degree to which skin is exposed to moisture | **1. Constantly moist:** Skin is kept moist almost constantly by perspiration, urine, etc.; dampness is detected every time patient is moved or turned | **2. Very moist:** Skin is often, but not always, moist; linen must be changed at least once a shift | **3. Occasionally moist:** Skin is occasionally moist, requiring an extra linen change approximately once a day | **4. Rarely moist:** Skin is usually dry; linen only requires changing at routine intervals | |
| **Activity**<br>Degree of physical activity | **1. Bedfast:** Confined to bed | **2. Chairfast:** Ability to walk severely limited or nonexistent; cannot bear own weight and/or must be assisted into chair or wheelchair | **3. Walks occasionally:** Walks occasionally during day, but for very short distances, with or without assistance; spends majority of each shift in bed or chair | **4. Walks frequently:** Walks outside the room at least twice a day and inside room at least once every 2 hours during waking hours | |
| **Mobility**<br>Ability to change and control body position | **1. Completely immobile:** Does not make even slight changes in body or extremity position without assistance | **2. Very limited:** Makes occasional slight changes in body or extremity position but unable to make frequent or significant changes independently | **3. Slightly limited:** Makes frequent though slight changes in body or extremity position independently | **4. No limitations:** Makes major and frequent changes in position without assistance | |
| **Nutrition**<br>Usual food intake pattern | **1. Very poor:** Never eats a complete meal; rarely eats more than ⅓ of any food offered; eats two servings or less of protein (meat or dairy products) per day; takes fluids poorly; does not take a liquid dietary supplement **Or** Is NPO and/or maintained on clear liquids or IVs for more than 5 days | **2. Probably inadequate:** Rarely eats a complete meal or generally eats only about ½ of any food offered; protein intake includes only three servings of meat or dairy products per day; occasionally will take a dietary supplement **Or** Receives less than optimum amount of liquid diet or tube feeding | **3. Adequate:** Eats over half of most meals; eats a total of four servings of protein (meat, dairy products) each day; occasionally will refuse a meal, but will usually take a supplement if offered **Or** Is on a tube feeding or TPN regimen which probably meets most of nutritional needs | **4. Excellent:** Eats most of every meal; never refuses a meal; usually eats a total of four or more servings of meat and dairy products; occasionally eats between meals; does not require supplementation | |
| **Friction and shear** | **1. Problem:** Requires moderate to maximum assistance in moving; complete lifting without sliding against sheets is impossible; frequently slides down in bed or chair, requiring frequent repositioning with maximum assistance; spasticity, contractures, or agitation lead to almost constant friction | **2. Potential problem:** Moves freely or requires minimum assistance; during a move, skin probably slides to some extent against sheets, chair, restraints, or other devices; maintains relatively good position in chair or bed most of the time but occasionally slides down | **3. No apparent problem:** Moves in bed and in chair independently and has sufficient muscle strength to lift up completely during move; maintains good position in bed or chair at all times | | |
| **Note:** patients with a total score of 16 or less are considered to be at risk of developing pressure ulcers. (15 or 16 = low risk, 13 or 14 = moderate risk, 12 or less = high risk). | | | | **Total score** | |

**Figure 17-9**   Braden Risk Assessment Scale. (Copyright 1988 Barbara Braden and Nancy Bergstrom.)

carbohydrates, minerals, and vitamins all are necessary to promote skin integrity and wound healing.

Cleansing of the skin and close attention to its condition are important. If the skin is too dry, lubricating creams and ointments should be applied. If the skin is too moist, a light application of a drying powder may be beneficial. A bladder and bowel program should be planned for incontinent individuals to prevent skin maceration. If incontinence cannot be corrected, measures to protect the skin include skin barrier creams and ointments, fecal incontinence devices, and, for men, condom drainage systems.

A patient who sits in a wheelchair or other type of chair should be protected from pressure on the sitting surfaces of the body by use of a wheelchair cushion. A bed pillow does not provide adequate pressure relief. A 10-cm (4-inch) foam cushion may be fine for most patients, although those who are unable to move or who have poor sensation may require a more therapeutic cushion.

If the patient already has a pressure ulcer, many of the previously mentioned interventions need to be initiated. The treatment of a pressure ulcer is based on the size and depth of the wound. Many hospitals have developed protocols for care of such wounds. Based on the size and depth of the wound and the appearance of the wound bed, cleaning agents, dressings for the wound, and bed surface selection are recommended (Phipps, Bauman, 1984). The Agency for Health Care Policy and Research (AHCPR) has developed national practice guidelines for the treatment of pressure ulcers (Bergstrom et al, 1994).

Some pressure ulcers extend to bone and can put the patient at risk of death from infection and sepsis. For the most part, pressure ulcers are a preventable problem. If there is no pressure, an ulcer does not form. Scrupulous attention must be paid to the patient at risk to prevent the formation of pressure ulcers. If pressure goes unrelieved in an at-risk patient, a pressure ulcer can develop within a few hours. All at-risk patients, especially older ones, should be gotten out of bed as much as possible. Besides relieving pressure, moving from bed to chair provides activity for muscles that otherwise receive little exercise. It also allows for better ventilation of the lungs by helping prevent accumulation of fluid at the base of the lung (Box 17-10).

---

**BOX 17-10**

## NURSING PROCESS

### PRESSURE ULCER

**ASSESSMENT**

- General condition of skin
- Skin over body prominences
- Awareness of pressure sensation
- Ability to move
- Nutritional status
- Urinary or fecal incontinence
- Amount of shear and friction on skin
- Pressure ulcer staging (color, odor, presence of necrotic tissue, exudate, condition of surrounding skin)
- Vital signs (temperature)
- Laboratory values (albumin, ferritin, wound culture, whole blood cell count)
- Family's ability to provide associated care

**NURSING DIAGNOSES**

- Impaired skin integrity related to friction, shear, or pressure
- Risk for infection related to open pressure sore or poor nutritional status
- Impaired home maintenance management related to long-term therapy
- Risk for caregiver role strain related to long-term therapy

- Altered nutrition: less than body requirements related to chronic illness

**NURSING INTERVENTIONS**

- Maintain preventive measures, including reduction or relief of pressure.
- Maintain nutritional regimen and management of incontinence.
- Provide aseptic local wound care as ordered.
- Keep pressure off sore while it is healing.
- Provide perineal hygiene after incontinence episode.
- If not contraindicated, encourage high-protein, high-calorie diet.
- Administer antibiotics as prescribed.
- Refer patient to social worker to assist with discharge planning.
- Discuss possible need for respite care.

**EVALUATION OF EXPECTED OUTCOMES**

- Pressure ulcer shows evidence of healing
- No evidence of local or systemic infection
- Verbalizes necessary home care measures
- Verbalizes available resources

### Incontinence

***Urinary incontinence.*** Urinary incontinence is a major health care problem. It has been estimated that 15% to 30% of noninstitutionalized adults over 60 years of age and as many as half of the 1.5 million Americans in long-term care facilities experience urinary incontinence. The impact of this problem is felt not only in financial terms, which are great, but also in the disruption of the incontinent person's social and personal life. In the elderly, urinary incontinence is one of the three major causes of placement in long-term care. Urinary incontinence also can lead to secondary problems such as skin breakdown or falls from slipping in urine.

Care of the incontinent patient involves assessing the underlying cause of the incontinence and developing approaches to improve the condition. The nurse must work closely with the patient and family, the physician, and other health care team members to find methods to improve the patient's incontinence or to determine alternative safe and convenient interventions (Box 17-11). In caring for an elderly incontinent patient, it is particularly important to recognize that urinary incontinence is not normal in old age, but rather is an abnormal development that often has more than one identifiable cause. Urinary incontinence is a symptom, not a disease or a condition.

Urinary incontinence can be described in a variety of ways. One of the more useful approaches is to categorize incontinence as either a transient condition that can be corrected or as an established or fixed condition that cannot be corrected. Nursing assessment and interventions are important aspects of the care of patients with either type of urinary incontinence. The AHCPR has developed a national practice guideline for urinary incontinence in adults (Urinary Incontinence Guideline Panel, 1992; Fantl et al, 1996). The goals of this guideline are to develop national recognition of the scope of the problem of urinary incontinence and to offer research-based approaches to intervention.

Transient or temporary incontinence has been described as an uncontrolled leakage of urine that may be reversible once the underlying causes have been corrected. Recognized causes of temporary incontinence include confusion, infection, medication side effects, immobility that may limit the patient's access to toilet facilities, constipation, depression, inadequate fluid intake, and medical conditions that lead to excessive production of urine. Elderly women may develop urinary incontinence because of cellular changes that occur in the lower urinary tract after menopause. This condition, known as *atrophic urethritis*, may be corrected with medicated creams.

Often a combination of factors leads to temporary urinary incontinence. For example, elderly patients admitted to an acute care hospital for pneumonia or a hip fracture may experience fever, a decrease in fluid intake, confusion, immobility, and constipation.

---

**BOX 17-11** **NURSING PROCESS**

## REHABILITATION OF THE INCONTINENT PATIENT

**ASSESSMENT**
- Episodes and frequency of incontinence
- Pain or burning with urination
- Ability to manage clothes
- Ability to get to the bathroom
- Mental status
- Fluid volume status
- Bladder distention

**NURSING DIAGNOSES**
- Altered urinary elimination: incontinence related to trauma, musculoskeletal, neurologic injury, infection, injury to urinary system, or impaired cognition
- Body image disturbance related to incontinence
- Impaired skin integrity related to incontinence
- Self-care deficit: toileting related to neuromuscular or musculoskeletal disorder or cognitive impairment

**NURSING INTERVENTIONS**
- Offer bedpan or urinal or assist to bathroom every 2 to 3 hours; gradually lengthen time interval.
- Assist with normal position for voiding.
- Instruct in and encourage patient to perform perineal exercises.
- Space fluid intake throughout the day.
- Limit oral intake in the evening.
- Instruct patient to avoid beverages with caffeine.
- Use behavior modification as indicated.
- Administer medications as prescribed.

**EVALUATION OF EXPECTED OUTCOMES**
- Remains continent of urine
- Verbalizes management strategies

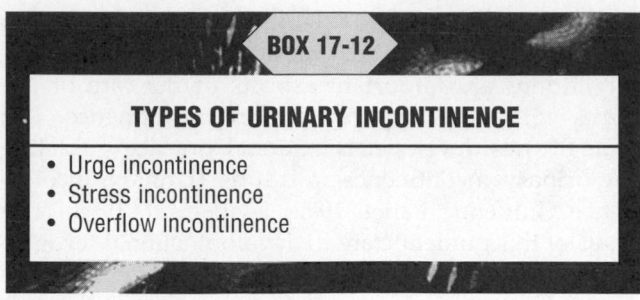

**BOX 17-12**

**TYPES OF URINARY INCONTINENCE**

- Urge incontinence
- Stress incontinence
- Overflow incontinence

Urinary incontinence may be an outcome of these factors. Once the medical problems have been corrected, the incontinence usually improves.

Fixed urinary incontinence is not reversible. However, like temporary incontinence, it may have several causes. Pathologic, physiologic, or anatomic changes in the urinary tract and its supporting structures or in the nervous system pathways that integrate bladder function lead to this problem. Some neurologic disorders, such as multiple sclerosis or spinal cord injury, leave a patient with fixed urinary incontinence. The care of patients with fixed incontinence requires medical assessment to identify the cause and to define the specific type. The physician and nurse work closely with the patient and family to plan the best method to manage the incontinence. The medical evaluation may include specific procedures, such as a cystometrogram and urine flow studies, to describe the type of fixed urinary incontinence.

The AHCPR practice guideline describes three types of incontinence: urge, stress, and overflow incontinence (Box 17-12). Urge incontinence is the involuntary loss of urine associated with an abrupt, strong desire to void (Urinary Incontinence Guideline Panel, 1992; Fantl et al, 1996). If no associated neurologic disorder is present, this condition may be defined as detrusor instability. The detrusor is the muscle mass that forms the urinary bladder. If the patient has a neurologic disorder, this type of bladder dysfunction may be classified as detrusor hyperreflexia. Stress incontinence is the involuntary loss of urine during coughing, sneezing, laughing, or other activities that increase abdominal pressure (Wells, 1988). Overflow incontinence occurs when the bladder becomes overdistended. Both stress and overflow incontinence have many causes. The importance of a complete, thorough medical evaluation for any type of urinary incontinence cannot be overemphasized because in many situations this is a treatable condition.

Nursing assessment of a patient with urinary incontinence involves obtaining a patient history and performing a physical assessment. Interviewing the patient and family about the incontinence may bring to light important information. The nurse might ask specific questions of the patient and family, such as the following:

- What problems are you having with urination?
- Can you feel when your bladder is full?
- How long can you wait to get to the bathroom after you feel the need to empty your bladder?
- Do you need to get out of bed at night to urinate?
- Do you have any dribbling of urine when you laugh, cough, or sneeze?
- Do you have pain or burning with urination?
- Have you noticed a change in the color or odor of your urine?

The nurse may need to assess the patient's mental status because confusion can lead to incontinence. A limited mental status evaluation includes the patient's orientation to person, place, and time, as well as long- and short-term memory. If possible, the nurse should assess the patient's ability to get in and out of bed, in and out of the bathroom, and on and off the toilet, as well as his or her ability to manage clothing and toilet tissue. With a bedbound patient, the nurse may assess the patient's ability to manipulate a urinal or bedpan.

A 48-hour record of the patient's fluid intake and urinary output is helpful in determining fluid balance. A 48-hour history of urinary incontinence is best recorded by using an incontinence chart that indicates the patient's condition (wet or dry) at 2-hour intervals (Figure 17-10). Keeping this chart may help reveal a possible pattern of urinary incontinence.

The physician and nurse should work together in assessing the patient's physical status to determine bladder fullness or distention and to determine if the bowel is impacted with stool. The physician may decide to perform a neurologic examination, including an evaluation of the reflex activity needed for normal bladder function. The patient's medical record should be reviewed to identify important factors that could be relevant to bladder problems, such as a medical diagnosis, medications, laboratory values, or previous operations.

Once this information has been collected and documented, the nurse and other members of the health care team should plan specific interventions. All reversible causes of incontinence need to be identified. Once such factors as confusion, fever, constipation, dehydration, immobility, and decreased fluid intake have been corrected, incontinence may diminish. If incontinence persists or is unrelated to these factors, the assessment should continue.

Interventions for urinary incontinence include medication, surgery, or behavioral approaches. The first two interventions are beyond the scope of this chapter, but extensive literature on these subjects is available (Wells, 1988; Urinary Incontinence Guideline Panel, 1992; Fantl et al, 1996). Behavioral approaches, which often are the domain of the nurse, include bladder training (retraining), habit training (timed voiding), prompted voiding,

## INCONTINENCE RECORD

Patient's name _____

Room number _____

| Date: | | Date: | | Date: | |
|---|---|---|---|---|---|
| Time | Wet or dry | Time | Wet or dry | Time | Wet or dry |
| 8 am | | 8 am | | 8 am | |
| 10 am | | 10 am | | 10 am | |
| 12 N | | 12 N | | 12 N | |
| 2 pm | | 2 pm | | 2 pm | |
| 4 pm | | 4 pm | | 4 pm | |
| 6 pm | | 6 pm | | 6 pm | |
| 8 pm | | 8 pm | | 8 pm | |
| 10 pm | | 10 pm | | 10 pm | |
| 12 MN | | 12 MN | | 12 MN | |
| 2 am | | 2 am | | 2 am | |
| 4 am | | 4 am | | 4 am | |
| 6 am | | 6 am | | 6 am | |

**Figure 17-10**    Example of 48-hour incontinence record.

and pelvic floor (Kegel) exercises (Box 17-13). Bladder training is based on clear patterns of communication between staff and patients to regulate fluid intake and to develop a pattern or schedule of urinary elimination. The patient's voiding history, fluid intake record, and incontinence chart are reviewed to establish this schedule. If no pattern of incontinence can be identified from the incontinence chart, the nurse establishes a bladder emptying schedule. The voiding schedule includes a plan for progressively increasing the time between scheduled voidings. The patient's schedule and expected outcome should be clearly documented and understood by all staff members and by the patient and family. The patient's response to the bladder program must be documented and communicated to all involved.

The following is an example of a bladder program developed for a patient who is consistently incontinent after meals.

- *Fluid intake*: 2000 to 3000 ml/day; 200 ml every 2 hours beginning at 6 AM and ending at 8 PM. Fluids are restricted at night. A variety of fluids preferred by the patient should be offered.
- *Voiding routine*: On arising, ½ hour after each meal, and ½ hour before going to bed. If the patient is incontinent between voiding times, the times and surrounding events should be noted. The time between voidings is increased gradually, and the patient is encouraged to delay voiding.

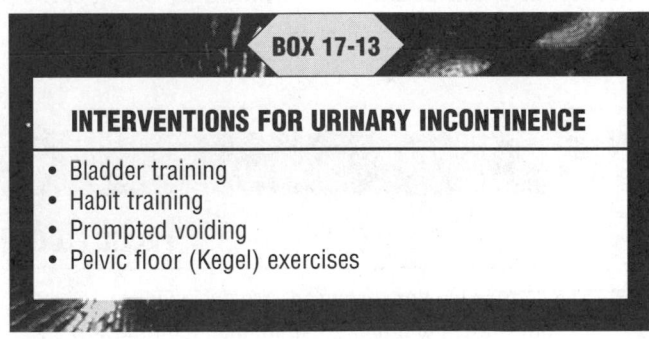

### BOX 17-13

### INTERVENTIONS FOR URINARY INCONTINENCE

- Bladder training
- Habit training
- Prompted voiding
- Pelvic floor (Kegel) exercises

Habit training generally is used for patients who have no clear pattern of incontinence. A bladder program might include a fluid regimen similar to that described previously with a planned voiding routine of every 2 hours, or whatever time interval allows the patient to remain dry. When the patient attempts to void, he or she should have privacy and should be placed in a comfortable position.

Prompted voiding often is used with cognitively impaired patients. This type of program involves monitoring the patient's state of dryness, prompting the person to use the toilet, and praising the patient when he or she is continent (Wells, 1988). Success in bladder training depends on patient cooperation. Prompted voiding is a form of behavior modification used to motivate patients to cooperate with the program. Behavior modification is a therapeutic program that involves rewards or positive reinforcement for desired behavior. Patients, of course, vary in their likes and dislikes; an action or reward that is positive for one patient may be negative for another. The desired behavior, in this case continence, is more likely to be repeated if the patient experiences some reward for that behavior. The reward may be material or it may be in the form of praise, but it must be seen as a reward by that individual patient if it is to be effective. The patient is checked every 2 hours; if he or she is dry, a reward is given. If the patient is incontinent, no reward is given. Appropriate use of the toilet or commode also is rewarded. The short-term goal of staying dry or using the commode appropriately leads to the long-term goal of independent use of bathroom facilities and continence. The entire staff must fully understand the program and its methods and implement it appropriately.

The goal of pelvic floor, or Kegel, exercises is to strengthen the muscles that aid in closing the urethra. This is accomplished through contraction and relaxation of the perivaginal muscles (Box 17-14) (Wells, 1988).

An indwelling catheter should not be used as a means of treating incontinence because a patient with an indwelling catheter has a high probability of developing a urinary tract infection (UTI). Some estimates indicate that 70% of patients develop a UTI within 72 hours of insertion of a catheter. However, an indwelling catheter is necessary for some individuals, such as those with an acute illness, patients who have had surgery, incontinent patients in such severe pain that changing linen is difficult, or patients who cannot urinate.

Bladder training of a patient with an indwelling catheter is controversial. If the patient has a UTI, the physician may decide to treat the infection with medication. Another approach is simply to remove the catheter as the source of infection rather than treating the patient with medication. There also is some disagreement about the benefit gained by clamping and unclamping the indwelling catheter before removal. Some authorities believe it is necessary to clamp the catheter periodically to increase bladder capacity and sensation; others believe that clamping has no effect on the outcome (Gross, 1990). Whether the catheter is clamped or removed abruptly, the patient's attention should be directed to the sensation caused by expansion of the bladder as it fills and contraction of the bladder as it empties.

---

### NURSE ALERT

Behavioral approaches to urinary incontinence often are the domain of the nurse. These techniques include bladder training, habit training, prompted voiding, and pelvic floor (Kegel) exercises.

---

**BOX 17-14**

## PELVIC FLOOR (KEGEL) EXERCISES

Kegel, or pelvic floor, exercises are designed for use by both women and men to strengthen the muscles, ligaments, and tendons of the pelvic floor that support the bladder and lower bowel. Strengthening and toning these muscles may diminish or relieve symptoms of stress urinary incontinence (i.e., involuntary loss of urine when sneezing, coughing, or laughing). The nurse should review the following points with the patient.

### IDENTIFYING THE CORRECT MUSCLES

1. To find the muscle, place your finger inside your vagina or rectum. Try to squeeze around your finger; that's the muscle you want to exercise. This is the same muscle you use to hold back a bowel movement or gas.
2. Never use your stomach, leg, or buttocks muscles. The most common mistake people make is using too many muscles. To find out if you are contracting your stomach muscles, place your hand on your abdomen while you squeeze your pelvic floor muscles. If you feel your abdomen move, you are also using these muscles.
3. These exercises can be practiced anytime, in any place. Because the muscle is internal, no one can see you exercising these muscles.

### PERFORMING THE EXERCISE

1. Squeeze the muscle that you identified earlier and hold for a count of 10, or for 10 seconds. Then relax for a count of 10. Remember, it is as important to relax as it is to contract the muscle.
2. Choose one of the following schedules:
   - Do 15 exercises in the morning, 15 in the afternoon, and 15 at night.
   - Exercise for 10 minutes 3 times a day

You may notice a change after about 2 weeks of consistent daily exercise; in 1 month you may notice even greater improvement.

Behavioral techniques may help patients with either temporary or fixed incontinence. However, other approaches may be necessary because of the extent and type of bladder dysfunction. If the patient has no sensation of bladder fullness and no ability to empty the bladder, a program of intermittent catheterization may be initiated. The scheduling of this program is based on fluid intake and the volume of catheterized urine. Initially the patient is catheterized every 4 hours, then every 6 to 8 hours while the patient is awake. Depending on the type of bladder dysfunction, this program eventually may allow for reflex bladder emptying without catheterization. For some patients intermittent catheterization becomes the only method of urinary elimination, and the patient may be taught self-catheterization. A patient performing self-catheterization at home may use a clean rather than sterile technique. The clean technique allows the patient to reuse catheters after washing them with soap and water. Sterile techniques should be used for self-catheterization in the hospital.

Some individuals may need to use an indwelling catheter on a long-term basis. UTI is a constant threat with long-term catheterization, and these individuals should be followed up on by a physician if they are discharged home with the catheter. Adequate fluid intake, care of the catheter and collecting bags, and attention to skin care must become part of the daily routine.

Urine collecting devices are another means of managing incontinence. A condom collecting system may be beneficial to some men. The condom should be changed daily, with close attention given to skin care and cleaning. Several urine-collecting devices are available for women. These products fit over the perineum and are connected to a drainage bag. Proper fit is a problem for many women; if the fit is not tight, the urine leaks. Close attention to skin care also is essential with these devices.

Some individuals may choose diapering to manage their urinary incontinence, particularly if soiling of clothing or slipping in urine are problems. However, a complete assessment and all other treatment interventions should be evaluated before this method is adopted. Preventing skin problems caused by wet diapers becomes an important aspect of care. Many diapering products are available, and the type chosen should be selected according to the individual's specific needs. In bedbound patients, diapers must be changed when wet because of the high potential for skin breakdown. Some disposable diapers are made to keep the layer next to the skin dry, the urine being absorbed in other layers.

**Approaches to altered bowel function.** A patient with altered bowel function requires an in-depth nursing assessment before intervention can begin. The patient's history is taken and should include information about any medical condition that would lead to changes in bowel function, as well as the pattern of elimination, dietary habits, difficulty with bowel elimination, a review of medications, abdominal surgical procedures, problems with dentition that would limit dietary intake, and problems with mobility.

Changes in bowel pattern may develop as constipation, diarrhea, or fecal incontinence. It is beyond the scope of this chapter to review all the factors that can lead to the development of these problems. However, disabled individuals may develop altered bowel function and may need specialized approaches to bowel care. The bowel pattern may need to be "retrained" because of the consequences of neurologic disease, immobility, altered nutritional intake, medication, and altered mobility. This training involves developing a pattern of scheduled elimination.

Bowel function is aided by adding high-residue foods to the diet. Whole-grain breads, bran cereal, prune juice, and fresh fruits have proven effective in stimulating bowel function. An adequate fluid intake also is essential to normal bowel function. Medication may be prescribed to soften the stool or increase peristalsis. Harsh laxatives and enemas should not be used to regulate bowel function. Dietary restrictions and other physician orders should be considered, and the physician should be consulted in planning a retraining program for an incontinent patient.

A bowel program is an individualized approach to scheduled elimination (Venn et al, 1992). Some important points are presented in Box 17-15. When a patient begins such a schedule, fecal impaction can be a problem, but it usually can be corrected by adjusting the fluid intake. In some cases stronger laxatives or enemas may be necessary. A 3- or 4-day trial of any pharmacologic agent is necessary to determine its effect on the patient. A routine can be established that prevents accidental elimination. Patients with certain neurologic disorders may require digital stimulation for evacuation to occur. This requires placing a gloved, lubricated finger into the rectum and moving the finger in a circular motion to stimulate the anal sphincter to relax. Some patients are able to do this independently or with an adaptive device.

## Impaired Swallowing Ability

The term **dysphagia** describes disorders of swallowing mechanisms caused by anatomic impairment or neurologic disorders (Kohler, 1991). Early assessment and identification of impaired ability to swallow is necessary to prevent aspiration and malnutrition (Box 17-16). Aspiration has been described as the entry of material into the airway below the true vocal cords (Logemann, 1986), which can lead to the development of pneumonia and sepsis. Malnutrition may result from the patient's inability to take in sufficient nutri-

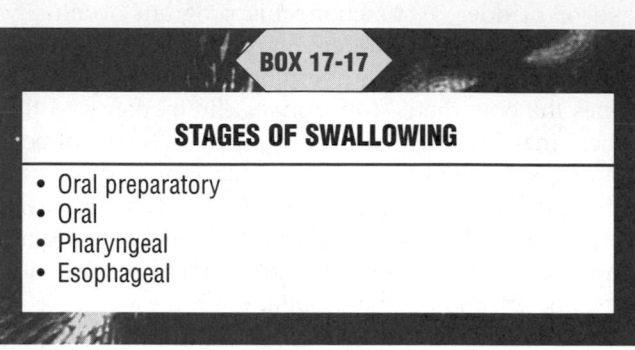

**BOX 17-15**

**Guidelines for Establishing a Bowel Program**

1 Before a bowel program can be started, any fecal impaction must be cleared. If impaction is present, a Fleet's enema or soapsuds enema may be necessary.
2 If possible, the patient should eat a high-fiber diet and, if medically possible, take in at least 2000 ml of fluid a day.
3 Consider bowel medications if indicated. A mild laxative increases peristaltic activity. It takes about 8 hours for this medication to take effect, so plan the dose accordingly. If elimination is scheduled for the morning, the laxative should be given the evening before. A mild suppository stimulates the rectum. It must be placed into the rectum, beyond the anal sphincter, and against the rectal wall. Suppositories require about 15 to 30 minutes to take effect.
4 If possible, get the patient out of bed and sitting on a toilet or commode because the squatting position is the most effective for evacuation. The abdominal muscles contract when the thighs are flexed against the abdomen, which increases intraabdominal pressure and aids in expelling feces. If the toilet seat is too high to allow this position, a footstool or sturdy box should be placed under the patient's feet. A patient who cannot assume this squatting position will have more difficulty establishing regular bowel patterns. Exercises that strengthen the abdominal muscles aid evacuation, and the contraction and relaxation of perineal muscles assist in the control of bowel evacuation.
5 A regular time for evacuation should be established. The gastrocolic reflex, the increase in intestinal peristaltic activity that occurs when food enters the stomach, reaches its maximum effect 30 minutes after eating. For some patients, the most effective evacuation time is 30 minutes after breakfast. However, this is not true for everyone, and the time for evacuation is best scheduled on the previous elimination pattern.
6 Privacy must be ensured, and the patient should feel relaxed.

**BOX 17-16**

**CONSEQUENCES OF DYSPHAGIA**

- Aspiration pneumonia
- Malnutrition
- Dehydration

**BOX 17-17**

**STAGES OF SWALLOWING**

- Oral preparatory
- Oral
- Pharyngeal
- Esophageal

tongue squeezes the bolus against the hard palate and toward the pharynx. In the pharyngeal phase the bolus passes through the pharynx and toward the esophagus while the protective mechanisms of laryngeal elevation and vocal cord closure prevent food from entering the airway. In the esophageal phase, peristaltic activity allows food to pass from the pharynx and enter the stomach via the cardiac sphincter. Problems with swallowing can occur in any of these four stages.

> **NURSE ALERT**
>
> **Prevention of aspiration is essential in the rehabilitation of a dysphagic patient.**

A patient may overtly demonstrate difficulty with swallowing by the following symptoms: dribbling food out of the mouth, holding food in the mouth for a long time without swallowing, pocketing food in one side of the mouth, showing little appetite, having food draining from the nose, and coughing or choking while eating (Box 17-18) (Phipps, 1991b). However, the patient may not demonstrate any symptoms that would suggest swallowing problems. This difficulty may first be identified when the patient develops aspiration pneumonia, which is diagnosed by the presence of a particular pattern on the chest x-ray. This lack of symptoms is referred to as *silent aspiration* (Horner, Massey, 1988). The patient's medical diagnosis may be

ents to support metabolic needs. Elderly debilitated patients are considered to be at risk. It has been found that as many as 74% of patients in skilled nursing homes have difficulty eating (Kohler, 1991).

The act of swallowing can be divided into four stages: oral preparatory, oral, pharyngeal, and esophageal (Box 17-17). During the first two stages, food is chewed and then formed into a bolus by the action of the tongue. The lips are closed tightly to keep the food and fluid in the mouth. In a sequential manner the

## BOX 17-18

### SIGNS AND SYMPTOMS OF DYSPHAGIA

Any of the following symptoms or combination of symptoms may indicate a problem with swallowing:
- Diminished appetite
- Loss of taste
- Nasal burning and dripping
- Burning or itching at the back of the throat
- Coughing after ingesting food or fluids
- Holding food in the mouth
- Gurgly, wet voice
- Nasal-sounding voice
- Pocketing food in the cheek
- Drooling, asymmetry of face
- Loss of oral secretions
- Untouched food
- Eating very quickly or slowly
- Terrible taste in the mouth

## BOX 17-19

### ASSESSING THE PATIENT AT RISK FOR DYSPHAGIA

**FACIAL-MUSCLE TESTING**
- Ask the patient to clench the teeth; palpate masseter muscle function on both sides of the face.
- Ask the patient to smile, frown, and whistle; observe for bilateral function.

**TONGUE FUNCTION**
- Ask the patient to stick out his or her tongue and move it to the left and to the right.
- Ask the patient to stick out his or her tongue and resist pressure from a tongue blade on lateral movements of the tongue.

**COUGH REFLEX**
- Ask the patient to cough two times in rapid succession.

**SWALLOWING REFLEX**
- Gently place your thumb and forefinger on the patient's laryngeal protuberance. Ask the patient to swallow; feel for laryngeal elevation.

**GAG REFLEX**
- Do not test unless the cough and swallow reflexes are intact
- With a throat swab, gently stroke the posterior pharyngeal wall on each side, observing for gag. Traditionally, the gag reflex has been used as the sole initial assessment of swallowing ability. However, it is only one aspect of the process. The swallowing reflex is the most protective mechanism in the swallowing process.

**QUALITY OF PATIENT'S VOICE**
- Dysphonia
- Wet or hoarse
- Changes in speech fluency while eating

**ORAL MOTOR OR SENSORY PROBLEMS, APRAXIA, AND PERCEPTUAL PROBLEMS THAT AFFECT EATING**
- Condition of the mouth and teeth

the only indication that he or she is at risk of silent aspiration. Patients at risk include those suffering from stroke, multiple sclerosis, Parkinson's disease, brain tumor, dementia, cranial nerve damage, or structural or anatomic changes in the swallowing mechanisms.

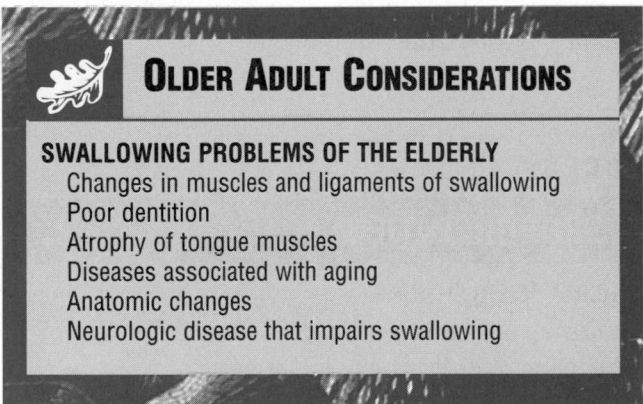

### OLDER ADULT CONSIDERATIONS

**SWALLOWING PROBLEMS OF THE ELDERLY**
Changes in muscles and ligaments of swallowing
Poor dentition
Atrophy of tongue muscles
Diseases associated with aging
Anatomic changes
Neurologic disease that impairs swallowing

Early assessment of dysphagia (Box 17-19), early initiation of interventions to prevent aspiration, and use of therapeutic techniques and feeding methods designed to fit the specific deficit in swallowing are essential aspects of care. Additional assessment points include checking the condition of the mouth and teeth and inspecting the patient's mouth after he or she has swallowed for food or medication (DiIorio, Price, 1990; Phipps, 1991).

If a patient demonstrates any difficulty through this initial assessment or is considered to be at risk of aspiration pneumonia because of his or her medical condi-

tion, a more detailed swallowing evaluation must be done. Videofluoroscopy, using the modified barium swallow method developed by Logemann (1986), is recommended for assessing swallowing ability and identifying aspiration (Horner, Massey, 1988; Horner et al, 1988; Chen et al, 1990). The patient must be able to sit in a chair and cooperate with instructions for this examination. The patient is given barium-enhanced liquid and foods of different consistencies, and swallowing is observed and recorded through videofluoroscopy.

A wide variety of interventions for dysphagia and methods of preventing aspiration are described in the literature (Boxes 17-20 and 17-21). If a patient is suspected of having a swallowing problem, suctioning equipment should be available during eating. Mouth care before and after eating may enhance the patient's ability to eat. Some nursing approaches include the following:

- *Positioning*
Ensure that the patient is out of bed and sitting up straight in a chair.
Position the patient's head so that it tilts forward (to enlarge the vallecular space).
- *Eating techniques*
Identify the appropriate food consistency, temperature, and texture (some patients are more successful with foods of a thicker consistency).
Feed the patient in smaller bolus amounts

---

**BOX 17-20**

### NURSING CONSIDERATIONS FOR DYSPHAGIA

- Patient in upright position
- Quiet environment
- Food consistency and temperature
- Size of bolus
- Swallowing techniques
- Individual therapeutic interventions
- Group therapeutic interventions
- Patient and family education

---

Identify the most effective method of feeding the patient (e.g., a teaspoon may be more successful than a fork)
Teach the patient to cough and clear before inhaling after swallowing.
Teach the patient to swallow again after swallowing food (the "double swallow" technique)
- *Group dysphagia program* (Emick-Herring, Wood, 1990)
Use a feeding program in a group with close supervision; the program should include proper positioning, patient teaching and assessment, monitoring of eating ability, and teaching about adaptive equipment.
- *Patient and family instruction*
Describe dysphagia.
Discuss the complications of the condition.
Explain the approaches to feeding.

### Adaptive Equipment

Adaptive equipment and assistive devices are selected for patients who need a piece of equipment or a device to perform self-care activities (Box 17-22 and Figures 17-11 and 17-12). When an interdisciplinary team is available, the PT, OT, prosthetist, and orthotist assist the nurse in assessing and teaching the patient. However, some parts of the country do not have such a wealth of rehabilitation professionals, and in these areas the nurse plays a more central role in teaching the patient the use of this equipment.

---

**BOX 17-21** — NURSING PROCESS

## REHABILITATION OF THE DYSPHAGIC PATIENT

**ASSESSMENT**
- Gag reflex
- Facial muscle strength, tongue function, ability to swallow
- Residual food in mouth after eating
- Choking or coughing with eating and drinking
- Respiratory status
- Condition of mouth and teeth

**NURSING DIAGNOSES**
- Impaired swallowing related to neuromuscular or mechanical factor, fatigue, or decreased cognition
- Risk for aspiration related to depressed cough and gag reflex and impaired swallowing

**NURSING INTERVENTIONS**
- Keep suction equipment at bedside.
- Maintain quiet environment for meals.
- Help patient into an upright position, preferably in a chair.
- Provide foods of thick consistency.
- Encourage only small amounts of food at one time.
- Instruct patient not to talk while eating.
- Encourage thorough chewing and double swallowing.
- Supervise all meals and fluid intake.

**EVALUATION OF EXPECTED OUTCOMES**
- Maintains stable weight
- Shows no evidence of aspiration
- Verbalizes techniques that prevent choking
- Demonstrates emergency measures

The patient's functional level and level of adaptation to disability, as well as the architecture of his or her living environment, need to be considered when selecting equipment. If these factors are not considered, the equipment ordered may be unnecessary or inadequate to meet the patient's needs. Equipment selected without consulting the patient and family may not be used or may be discarded. Much of this equipment is expensive; the patient's insurance coverage and financial situation need to be considered before a decision is made on what to buy (Lowman, Klinger, 1969). Some types of assistive equipment are described in Box 17-23.

**Prostheses.** A *prosthesis* is an artificial substitute for some part of the body. Prosthetic limbs and eyes are discussed in this section.

Prostheses for amputees must be fitted for the individual patient and adapted to the patient's weight and size. Prostheses are made of various materials. Those made of plastic are lightweight, easy to keep clean, and do not absorb body odors. Prostheses for legs are held in place by pelvic belts, waistbands, or suction cups. If the patient's condition allows, temporary prostheses for above-the-knee and below-the-knee amputations can be fitted immediately after surgery; however, this may not be possible with severely debilitated or medically unstable patients.

Leg prostheses are made of casting materials contoured to the amputation stump. They provide a rigid dressing that controls bleeding and swelling after surgery. A temporary peg, or pylon, and foot are attached to the cast, which allows the patient to dangle and stand within a few days after surgery. There are many advantages to this procedure. The patient is more active, muscle activity and circulation are

---

**BOX 17-22**

### EXAMPLES OF PRODUCTS MORE EASILY USED BY DISABLED

- Sponge rather than washcloth for bathing
- Sponge attached to a long handle with a pocket for soap
- Loose clothing with large armholes
- Front closing for clothing, with grippers rather than buttons
- Neckties already tied
- Elastic shoelaces and long-handled shoehorns
- Suction cups or sponge rubber mats for dishes
- Runways and ramps for wheelchair use
- Handrails, particularly in hallways and bathrooms
- Toilet seat to fit over toilet
- Lavatories, sinks, appliances, and electrical outlets placed at a height the patient can reach easily
- Special eating utensils (e.g., silverware with padded or curved handles, glass holders, and place guards)
- For a blind patient, food arranged clockwise on the plate and tray

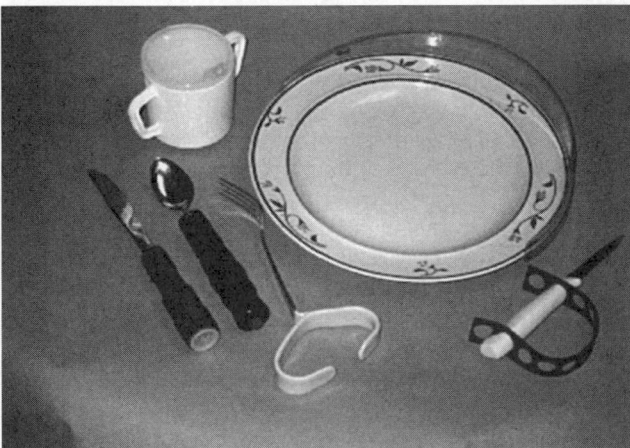

**Figure 17-11**   Special eating utensils. (From Elkin M et al: *Nursing interventions and clinical skills,* St Louis, 1996, Mosby.)

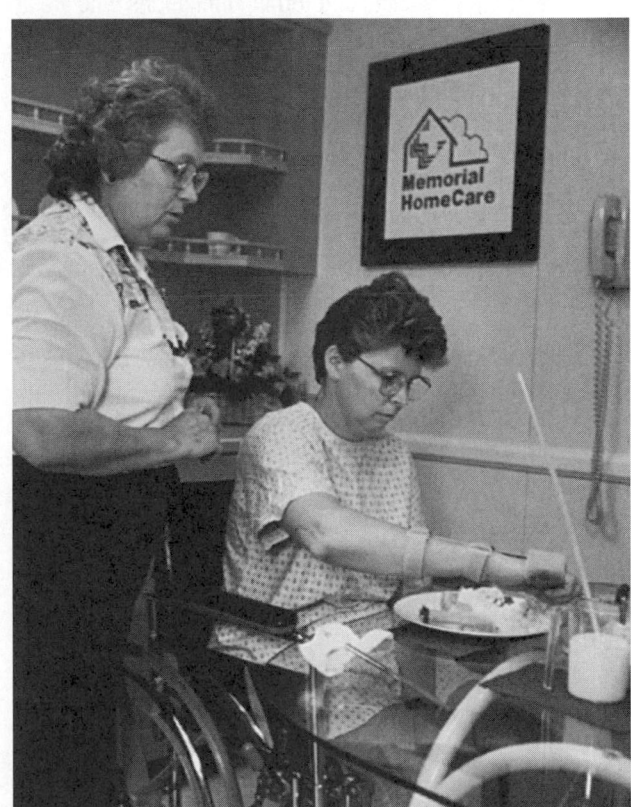

**Figure 17-12**   Assistive devices foster independence for people with functional disabilities.

BOX 17-23

## ASSISTIVE DEVICES

### EATING DEVICES
- Built-up handles on utensils (for weak or incomplete grasp)
- Universal cuff on utensils (for weak or incomplete grasp)
- Rocking knife (for one-handed cutting)
- Nonskid mats to stabilize plate (for eating with one hand)
- Plate guards or scoop dishes for scooping food off plate (for weakness or incoordination in the arm or hand)
- Cuff-type holder to assist with lifting a cup
- Specially designed cups to hold liquid in the upper part of the cup, to prevent excessive back tilting of the head when drinking (for patients at risk of aspiration because of difficulty swallowing)

### BATHING AND GROOMING DEVICES
- Long-handled sponge (for limited reach)
- Washcloth or sponge mitt (for diminished grasp)
- Toothbrush, hairbrush, and comb with built-up handle or universal cuff (for diminished or weakened grasp)
- Adapted shaving equipment
- Hand-held shower nozzle
- Long-handled mirror for inspecting the skin (for patients with reaching and turning limitations who are at risk for skin breakdown)

### TUB AND SHOWER TRANSFER EQUIPMENT
- Nonskid mats in tub or shower to prevent slipping and falling
- Grab bars in tub or shower, if possible
- Shower and tub seats designed for diminished ability to stand in shower or sit in tub
- Shower and tub transfer seats (for difficulty getting into shower or tub)
- Shower chairs that can be pushed into wheelchair-accessible shower (for inability to transfer or stand while showering)
- Depending on architecture of bathroom, hydraulic and motorized tub lifts (for inability to get into or out of tub)

### DRESSING EQUIPMENT
- Velcro closures (for one-handed dressing)
- Button hooks, zipper pulls, elasticized shoestrings (for one-handed dressing)
- Long-handled reachers to pull up clothing (for limited reaching ability)
- Long-handled shoehorn (for limited reach)

### WALKING DEVICES
- Canes that provide a single point of contact with the floor, to improve stability of gait when the lower extremity muscles are minimally or moderately involved. The cane should be fitted to the patient, who should be instructed in its use. The cane should be equipped with a rubber tip to provide traction and safety.
- Tripod or quadripod (quad) canes, which provide three or four points of contact with the ground. These canes provide greater stability than a regular cane but are bulkier to handle.
- Walkers, which differ according to structure and purpose (Dittmar, 1989):(1) adjustable, pick-up walkers are used for patients who can lift the walker and maintain balance; (2) reciprocal walkers are designed for patients who might lose their balance when lifting a regular walker; and (3) rolling walkers increase energy-efficient walking but may be too unstable for some patients.

### WHEELCHAIRS
- May be selected for a disabled patient who is unable to walk because of the severity of motor deficits or because of fatigue, medical complications, or other functional problems
- Selection may be a joint decision of the interdisciplinary team, with direction from physical and occupational therapy
- Selection is based on the patient's dimensions, need for modifications, wheelchair weight requirements, and the patient's need for safety, comfort, and maneuverability

#### Wheelchair Cushions
- Should be used by any patient who spends time sitting in a wheelchair, for comfort and to prevent skin breakdown
- Type is based on the patient's mobility status, body build, nutrition, and skin care status

### TRANSFER DEVICES
- Transfer boards, plastic or wooden boards for the patient who cannot stand, to perform sliding transfer from bed to wheelchair or from wheelchair to and from car
- Hydraulic lifts for bed-to-chair, chair-to-tub, or chair-to-car transfers (for patients unable to stand to transfer)
- Hydraulic or electric stair lifts (for patients unable to climb stairs)
- Chairs with seats that raise electrically or mechanically (for patients unable to lift out of seat)

stimulated, and the process of physical rehabilitation begins immediately. Being able to assume an upright position soon after surgery encourages the patient and helps in his or her adjustment to an altered body image. Applying this device at the time of surgery may diminish phantom pain, an unpleasant sensation that arises from the area of the amputated limb. This first prosthesis is temporary. The permanent prosthesis is not fitted until stump shrinkage has occurred.

The amputee is confronted not only with a physical problem, but also with social, vocational, and psychologic problems that require the services of the entire rehabilitation team, as well as a skilled prosthetist, the designer and maker of the prostheses. When healing is underway, the stump must be molded to a conical shape to fit into the prosthesis. Compression bandages generally are used for this purpose, and wrapping of the stump to achieve this shape becomes part of the patient's daily care. Elastic stump-shrinking socks also can be used. Careful washing of the stump is important, and the bandages should be removed and rewrapped several times a day. The skin should be completely dry before the bandages are reapplied; careful skin care prevents maceration of the suture line.

A greater variety of prostheses are available for patients who have had a lower extremity amputation than for patients who have undergone upper extremity amputation. The function of the arm and hand is complex, and designing an upper extremity prosthesis that is both cosmetically acceptable and functional is a difficult task. The hook-type hand is used most often; on some models, cosmetic hands are available to fit over the hook. This prosthesis is difficult to master. The myoelectric prosthesis is more acceptable cosmetically and has capabilities not previously available. It is capable of gross hand motion, index finger—thumb opposition, grasp, and wrist pronation and supination. However, it does not provide fine movements of the fingers and hand. It is most effective when the lost extremity is on the nondominant side. A right-handed person who loses the left arm does not require as much fine movement in the prosthesis. When the prosthesis arrives and the patient begins to wear it, the patient and the family should be instructed in the care of the stump and the appliance. Not all patients are suitable candidates for an artificial extremity, and numerous factors must be considered, along with careful examination of the individual patient.

In teaching a patient to care for a prosthesis, the nurse should stress these points:
- Cleanliness is important in preventing skin problems. The socket of the prosthesis should be washed, rinsed, and dried daily. Once a week, lint

and dirt should be removed and the joints lightly oiled. The joints should be inspected for loose or worn parts, and replacements should be made promptly by a prosthetist. Any problems or changes in the fit, which may occur normally as the stump shrinks, should be identified and the patient referred for evaluation.
- The skin beneath the prosthesis is prone to irritation and breakdown if not cared for and inspected carefully. Daily hygiene is essential; washing the skin with soap and water and rinsing thoroughly is adequate. The patient should not use creams or preparations containing alcohol. If the patient uses a stump sock, it must fit well and be free of wrinkles or mended areas. The sock should be washed daily in cool water and mild soap.
- A lower extremity stump shrinks over time, requiring adjustments in the socket of the prosthesis. The patient should be warned against padding the stump or socket with cotton or washcloths because this causes an uneven distribution of pressure, resulting in pressure areas on the skin and possibly subsequent infection. A change in stump size requires a visit to the prosthetist for adjustment of the prosthesis. The fit of the prosthesis also can be affected by a change in the patient's weight.

An artificial eye is made of glass or plastic and is painted by a skilled artist to match the patient's other eye. Eyes made of glass are heavier and break easily if dropped. Those made of plastic are less durable and may become scratched unless care is taken. The prosthesis may be used as soon as the socket has healed, which can be 3 to 6 weeks after surgery.

The artificial eye can be removed for cleaning by pulling down on the lower eyelid and letting the prosthesis slip out of the eye socket. The prosthesis can be washed with soap and water and stored in a clean piece of gauze or a labeled envelope. It must be moistened before it is reinserted, and sterile saline generally is used for this purpose. To replace the prosthesis, the patient pulls down on the lower eye lid, slips the artificial eye into the eye socket, lifts up the upper lid, and positions the prosthesis. Patients must be taught to remove and insert the prosthesis because they may be nervous at first, but most soon master the technique and develop skill and confidence. When a patient with an eye prosthesis is admitted to the hospital, the nurse should realize that the patient has a special method of caring for the eye and should supply whatever equipment is needed so that the patient's procedure need not be altered.

**Braces.** The overall purpose of braces is to improve the patient's mobility. Specifically, braces may be used to support the body weight, to limit involuntary movement of the body, and to prevent and correct deformities. Leg braces may be of the short leg or long leg type and may have attachments, depending on their purpose. Braces usually consist of a steel frame with joints, hinges, and straps; belts are used to secure them in place. Braces generally are attached to the heel of the shoe. An inside lining on the straps protects the body from friction.

The patient must be taught the proper care of the brace. All locks should be opened regularly and lint and dirt removed. A drop of machine oil should be placed in each joint and the excess wiped away because any oil left on the leather causes deterioration. The leather parts may be washed with warm water and saddle soap, then dried and polished. Shoes should be kept in good repair and should have rubber heels. If knee pads are part of the brace, they should be worn with it. The skin under the brace should be inspected daily for discoloration, bruises, abrasions, or evidence of friction.

Children who wear braces during the growth period should have them checked at regular intervals by the physician, and any change indicated should be made properly. A brace that is too small for a growing child may do harm. Braces may be used to support the torso, and these should be put on with the patient lying down, with the body in good alignment. A cotton shirt worn beneath the brace helps absorb perspiration and body odor and contributes to the patient's comfort.

The patient needs to be prepared for use of a brace. He or she should be taught range-of-motion and other prescribed exercises, and these should be done regularly before the brace is put on. The patient also needs to be instructed in the proper position to assume when putting on a brace. A back brace is more easily put on while the patient is in bed. To be prepared psychologically, the patient should understand why the braces are necessary, how they will help, and how to care for them. Unless the patient is prepared for this device, he or she may resent it and develop negative attitudes, in which case its value may be minimized. Young people may be concerned with the cosmetic effect and must be given the chance to express their feelings.

**Crutches.** Crutches are assistive walking devices (Figure 17-13). They may be used temporarily or permanently, but in either case both the nurse and the physical therapist play an important role in helping prepare the patient for crutch walking (Box 17-24). If the patient is on bed rest, exercises can be started in bed to strengthen the muscle groups involved in the use of crutches; these include the muscles of the neck, arms, shoulders, chest, and back. Resistance exercise with weights is the most effective way to increase strength; weights can be

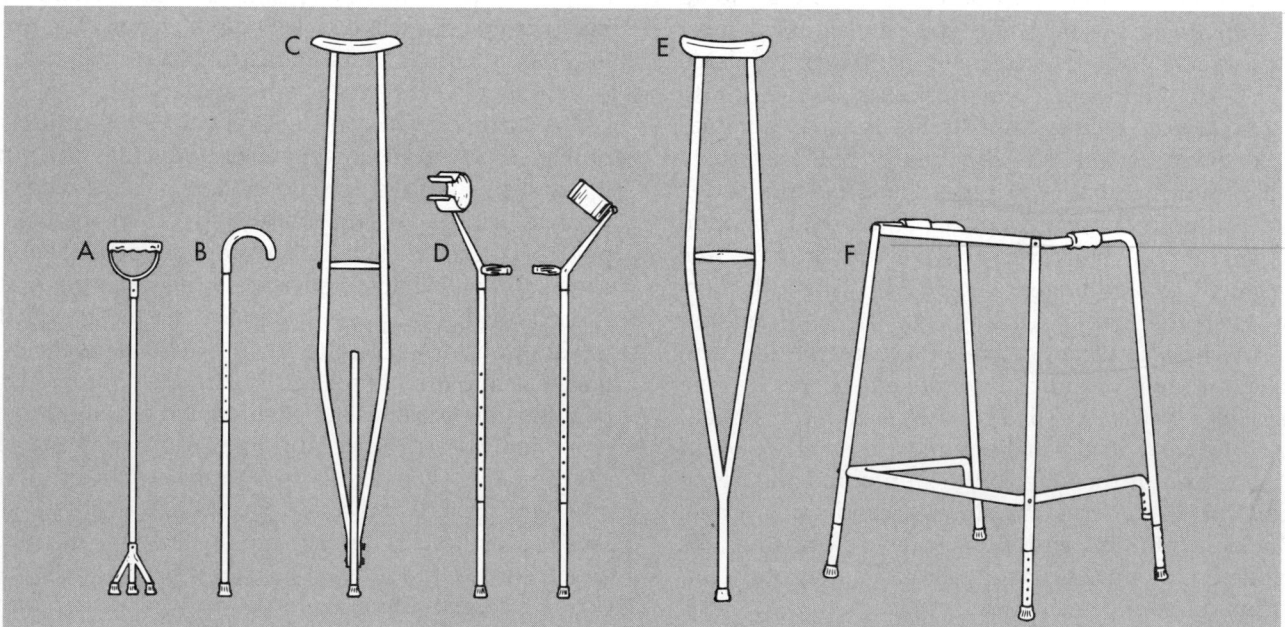

**Figure 17-13**  Types of crutches and canes. *A,* Quadripod cane. *B,* Adjustable aluminum cane. *C,* Adjustable aluminum crutch. *D,* Adjustable aluminum Canadian crutch. *E,* Nonadjustable wooden crutch, available in various lengths. *F,* Walker.

attached to the overhead trapeze or to a rope fastened to a pulley at the foot of the bed. The patient can be taught to do pushups by placing the palms flat on the bed.

The patient's ability to stand and the status of standing balance are important areas to assess before initiating crutch training. Older patients may have a poor sense of balance and coordination. They may be fearful and find it difficult to strengthen muscles before walking. Ideally, parallel bars should be used to help the patient stand and achieve balance before attempting crutch walking. The physical therapist usually fits the patient with crutches and assists the patient with standing and balancing during his or her initial attempts to walk with crutches. However, in many areas this may be the responsibility of the physician and the nurse (Figure 17-14).

There are several types of gait, and the type used depends on the disability. The most common types of gait are the four-point gait, the two-point gait, and the swing-to or swing-through gait (Figure 17-15). In the four-point gait the patient bears weight on both legs, one at each step, so that he or she always has three points of contact with the floor—the crutch tips and one foot. This gait requires constant shifting. In the two-point gait the patient has two points of contact with the floor; this method is similar to the four-point gait but faster. In the swing-to gait the patient places the crutches ahead, then lifts his or her weight on the crutches and swings the body to the crutches. The swing-through gait is similar except that the patient lifts his or her weight and swings beyond the crutches. In the three-point gait, the weight is placed on the crutches and unaffected leg; this gait may be used when partial weight bearing is permitted.

A patient who has been taught to use crutches should have mastered sufficient daily care activities to be independent when leaving the hospital and also should have been taught how to get up and down steps and into and out of cars.

---

**BOX 17-24**

### Guidelines for Patients Using Crutches

**1** The patient should be measured for crutches so that the right length will be used. Crutches should be adjustable and must have heavy rubber tips.

**2** Padding of the axillary bar generally is discouraged because it encourages the patient to place weight or lean on it. In doing so, the patient is at risk of developing a paralysis of the radial nerve (crutch paralysis). Crutches that are too long or too short may also cause crutch paralysis. Crutch length should be adjustable so that the patient bears *no* weight in the axillae.

**3** The patient should be taught from the beginning to maintain good posture. The head should be held high and straight, with the pelvis over the feet (Figure 17-14).

**4** Crutch walking must be taught, and several short lessons a day are of more value to the patient than a long one that causes fatigue.

**5** When beginning ambulation, it is desirable to have an attendant in front of the patient and one behind; however, they should not touch the patient.

**6** Whether the patient can bear weight or shift weight will depend on his or her disability and the physician's order. Some patients, especially elderly ones, may learn to use a walker before using crutches.

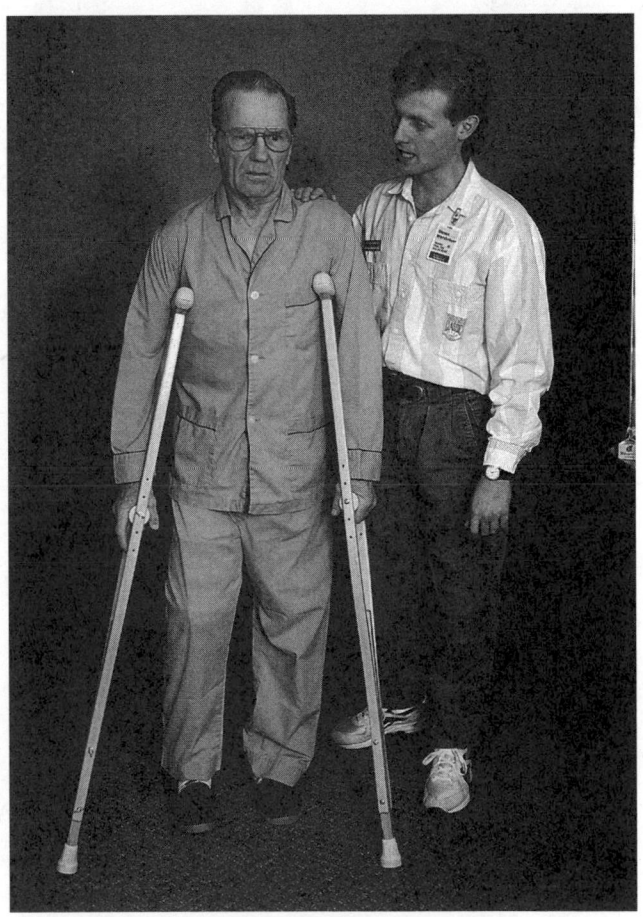

**Figure 17-14** In assessing a patient using crutches, the nurse observes fit, posture, and gait. (From Potter PA, Perry AG: *Basic nursing: theory and practice,* ed 3, St Louis, 1995, Mosby.)

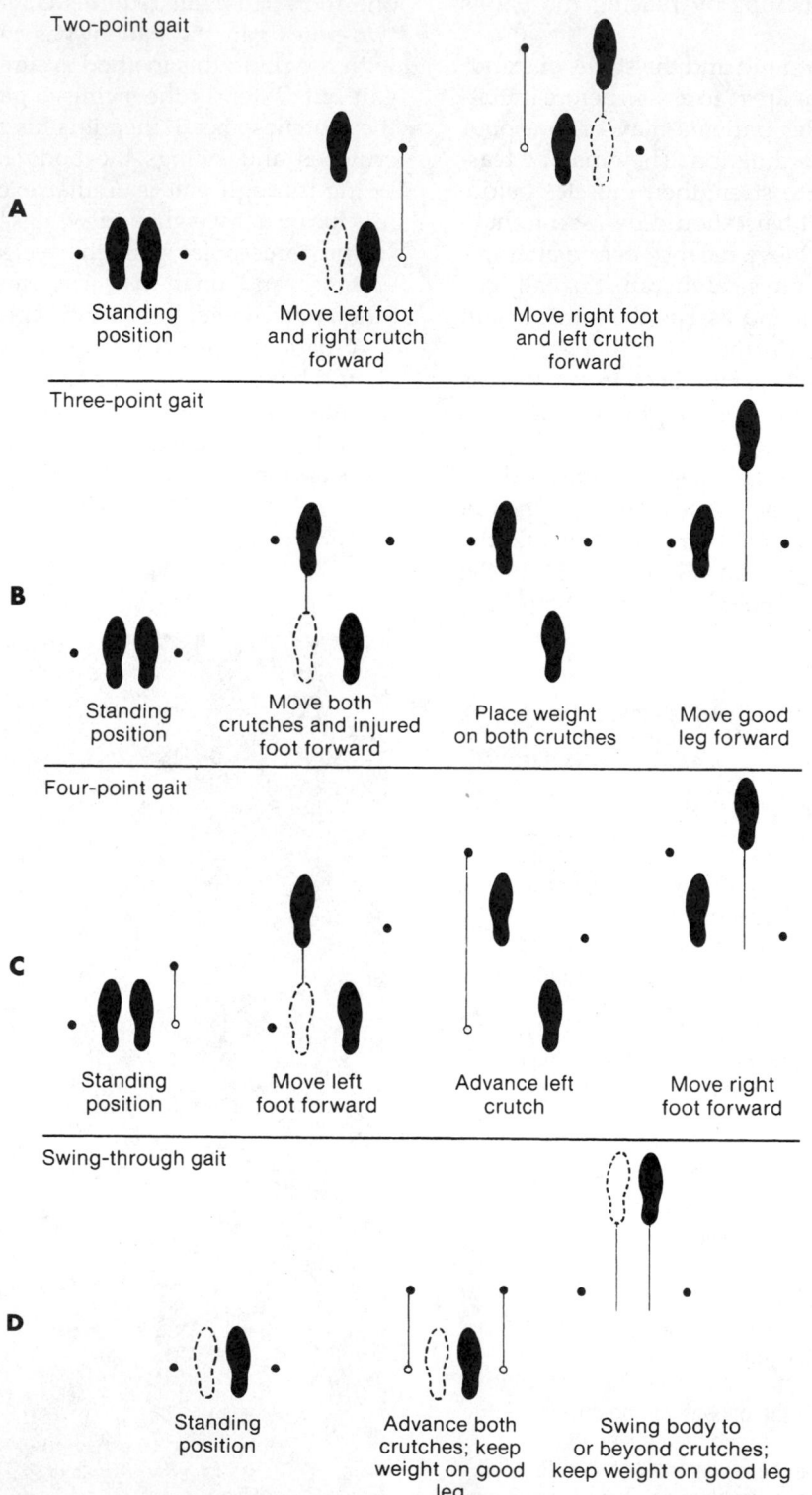

**Figure 17-15**   Crutch walking. **A,** Two-point gait. **B,** Three-point gait. **C,** Four-point gait. **D,** Swing-through gait.

# PATIENT TEACHING IN REHABILITATION

The nurse assumes a major role in teaching patients. For a patient participating in a rehabilitation program, this teaching might include the following:

- Reinforcement of skills taught in therapy sessions, such as self-care activities, transfers, and crutch walking
- A description of the illness or disability and a description of the expected course of the disease
- Health practices the patient needs to incorporate into daily living to stay healthy
- Symptoms that indicate a health problem has developed and medical care is needed
- Methods of finding health care when needed
- An explanation of the medications prescribed and the reason for them, as well as their possible side effects
- Approaches to finding home support when needed

The nurse assesses the patient's learning needs and learning ability before establishing a teaching plan. An important question to ask is, "What does the patient and family need to know to have an easier transition at the time of discharge?" In teaching a patient an activity or providing some important information, the environment should be as conducive to learning as possible. Teaching should be done during a nonstressful time of day, in a quiet place, and without any sense of haste. This is especially true for the elderly, who generally do not have difficulty learning new material but who do have difficulty learning new skills within a limited period (Katzman, Terry, 1983). Finding a quiet environment in a busy hospital may be difficult but, with planning, is not impossible. Some patients tire easily and need frequent rest periods.

Along with teaching, the nurse should provide the patient and family members with educational materials. The stress of learning new information may reduce retention. Having reference materials available to reinforce the new information may help the patient and family understand and apply the new ideas. Not all educational materials contain correct information or are appropriate for the needs of all patients. In some hospitals or agencies, nurses participate in patient education committees. One task of such a committee is to review patient educational materials for acceptability, readability, and accuracy.

A basic principle of teaching-learning is progressing from the simple to the complex. Simple activities should be taught first and each mastered before a new one is introduced. The patient may become discouraged and need much encouragement; even the slightest progress should be noted. Adult patients need to be treated as adults, and no patient should ever be belit-

## PATIENT/FAMILY TEACHING

### REHABILITATION
**Considerations**
- Assess the learning needs and learning ability of the patient and family members.
- Provide an environment conducive to learning.
- Review educational materials before giving them to the patient and family.
- Progress from the simple to the complex.
- Treat adult patients and family members as adults.
- Provide time for practice, discussion, and feedback.
- Evaluate the need for a group teaching program.
- Evaluate the impact of teaching; continually assess the patient's and family's understanding of the information provided.
- Involve the patient and family in setting the goals of rehabilitation and in the discharge planning.
- Make sure that patient and family education is continual and part of the patient's care as he or she progresses toward discharge.
- Encourage the family to participate in family education programs.
- Provide the family with as much information as possible about rehabilitation programs and services.
- Schedule follow-up appointments with therapists and physicians before the patient is discharged.
- Prepare referrals for the patient's discharge.

**Possible Content**
- Describe the illness or disability and the expected course of the disease and recovery.
- Reinforce of skills taught in therapy sessions (e.g., self-care activities, transfers).
- Review health practices the patient needs to incorporate into daily living to stay healthy.
- Identify of symptoms that indicate a health problem has developed and further health care is needed.
- Review methods to find health care when needed.
- Review rationale for medication and potential side effects.
- Explain approaches for locating home support when needed.
- Explain approaches for instructing others in the care of the patient and for the patient in ways he or she can ask others for assistance.
- Discuss sexuality.
- Discuss mental health and spiritual concerns.

tled or demeaned for being unable to master a new skill or retain new information. Patients who become frustrated and overwhelmed by the amount of detail needed to complete some skills may need to learn patience. Some patients may never develop this degree of patience, and for these individuals, participation in rehabilitation will remain a difficult task.

Giving a patient the opportunity to practice a task or discuss information is another important aspect of teaching. In teaching the patient to be independent, the nurse may need to sit back and watch the patient struggle with a new task. After demonstrating the task and giving the patient the opportunity to return the demonstration and to practice, the nurse must let the patient do the work or task alone. Nurses who work in rehabilitation must learn to "hold their hands behind their backs" and let the patients do for themselves, even if that involves discomfort for the patient and the nurse.

Another approach to teaching new skills or new information is the use of group teaching sessions for patients and families. Bringing together patients with like disabilities gives the nurse the opportunity to reach a larger audience and gives patients a chance to share their insights, questions, and frustrations with each other. In these group situations, patients often develop close relationships with each other and can learn new ways of coping. Laughter, one of the most important coping skills, often becomes an important part of these group activities (Schmitt, 1990). Group teaching programs for families also can provide information, support, and coping strategies.

The educational needs of family caregivers of disabled individuals are important, and research in this area has expanded in recent years. With the aging of our society, interest has increased in determining the health care needs of the disabled elderly and the impact this has on families and on both formal and informal support systems. In interviewing the families of

## KEY CONCEPTS

➤ Rehabilitation is the process of assisting individuals with a disability or chronic illness to the highest possible level of independence and well-being.

➤ Rehabilitation programs are designed to restore an individual's ability to function physically, emotionally, socially, educationally, and vocationally.

➤ Rehabilitation stresses restoration of normal function, prevention of complications, education of the patient and family, and adaptation.

➤ Short- and long-term care plans are developed with the patient according to his or her values, beliefs, life-style choices, and culture.

➤ Application of all the components of the nursing process is an integral part of the rehabilitation program.

➤ Communication with the rehabilitation team is essential at all levels of health service.

➤ An individual's body image may undergo significant changes as a result of disability or chronic illness.

➤ The success of a rehabilitation program depends on the individual's motivation.

➤ Plans that incorporate range of motion are integral activities for the nurse and patient during all phases of care.

➤ Pressure sores can be prevented through a disciplined plan of movement, frequent repositioning, and use of appropriate equipment.

➤ Urinary incontinence can be reduced or prevented through bladder and habit training, prompt voiding, and practice of the Kegel exercises.

➤ Aspiration can be reduced or prevented by positioning the patient properly for eating, adjusting the consistency of foods, and using appropriate eating techniques.

➤ Adaptive equipment is chosen on an individual basis with consideration given to need, cost, and usefulness in different settings.

➤ Aspects of patient education are incorporated into the rehabilitation program.

## CRITICAL THINKING EXERCISES

1. Why is it important to consider the whole patient (including the family and community) in attempting to restore an individual to a productive life?

2. What factors make rehabilitation of the elderly and chronically ill more difficult than rehabilitation of other patient groups?

3. How do race and culture affect an individual's plan of care?

newly disabled individuals, Weeks (1995) found that these families not only were concerned about learning about the disability and the patient's physical care requirements, but also needed education in the financial aspects of caregiving, such as insurance coverage and applying for disability insurance.

## REFERENCES AND ADDITIONAL READINGS

American Nurses Association and Association of Rehabilitation Nurses: *Rehabilitation nursing*, Kansas City, Mo, 1988, American Nurses Association.

*Americans with Disability Act: a guide to provisions affecting persons with seizure disorders*, Landover, Md, 1992, Epilepsy Foundation of America.

Banja JD: Rehabilitation and empowerment, *Arch Phys Med Rehabil* 71(8):614-615, 1990.

Bergstrom N et al: The Braden Scale for predicting pressure sore risk, *Nurs Res* 36(4):205-210, 1987.

Bergstrom N et al: Treatment of pressure ulcers, Clinical Practice Guideline No 15, AHCPR Pub No 95-0652, Rockville, Md, 1994, US Department of Health and Human Services.

Braden BJ, Bergstrom N: Braden scale for predicting pressure sores at risk, *Decubitus* 2:44-51, 1989.

Chen M et al: Oropharynx in patients with cerebrovascular disease: evaluation with videofluoroscopy, *Radiology* 176:641-643, 1990.

Davidhizar R: Disability does not have to be the grief that never ends: helping patients adjust, *Rehabil Nurs* 22(1):32-36, 1997.

DiIorio C, Price M: Swallowing: an assessment guide, *Am J Nurs* 90(7):38-41, 1990.

Dittmar S, editor: *Rehabilitation nursing: process and application*, St Louis, 1989, Mosby.

Emick-Herring B, Wood P: A team approach to neurologically based swallowing disorders, *Rehabil Nurs* 15(3):126-131, 1990.

Fantl JA et al: Urinary incontinence in adults: acute and chronic management, Clinical Practice Guideline No 2, AHCPR Pub No 96-0682, Rockville, Md, 1996, US Department of Health and Human Services.

Fiatarone M et al: The Boston FICSIT study: the effects of resistance training and nutritional supplementation on physical frailty in the oldest old, *J Am Geriatr Soc* 41:333-337, 1993.

Fiatarone M et al: Exercise training and nutritional supplementation for physical frailty in elderly people, *N Engl J Med* 330(25):1769-1775, 1994.

Glennon TP, Smith BS: Questions asked by patients and their support groups during family conferences on inpatient rehabilitation units, *Arch Phys Med Rehabil* 71(8):699-702, 1990.

Gross J: Bladder dysfunction after stroke, *J Gerontol Nurs* 16(4):20-25, 1990.

Gyde for the Uniform Sets for Medical Rehabilitation (Adult FIM), version 4.0, Buffalo, NY, 1993, State University of New York at Buffalo.

Hesse K, Campion E: Motivating the geriatric patient for rehabilitation, *J Am Geriatr Soc* 31(10):586-589, 1983.

Horner J, Massey E: Silent aspiration following stroke, *Neurology* 38:317-319, 1988.

Horner J et al: Aspiration following stroke: clinical correlates and outcome, *Neurology* 38:1359-1362, 1988.

Jamison S: A hand-held positioning device to reduce wrist and finger hypertonicity, *Nurs Res* 29(5):285-289, 1980.

Jette A, editor: Functional disability and rehabilitation of the aged, *Top Geriatr Rehabil* 1(3):1-9, 1986.

Katzman R, Terry R: *The neurology of aging*, Philadelphia, 1983, Davis.

Kelly-Hayes M: A preventative approach to stroke, *Nurs Clin North Am* 26(4):931-943, 1991.

Kelly-Hayes M: Functional evaluation. In Hoeman S, editor: *Rehabilitation nursing: process and application*, ed 2, St Louis, 1995, Mosby.

Kohler E: A dysphagia model for rural elderly, *Phys Occup Ther Geriatr* 10(1):81-95, 1991.

Kowalsky E: Grief: a lost life-style, *Am J Nurs* 78(3):418-420, 1978.

Learman LA et al: Pygmalion in the nursing home: the effect of caregiver expectations on patient outcome, *J Am Geriatr Soc* 38(7):797-803, 1990.

Lewis C: *Improving mobility in older patients*, Rockville, Md, 1989, Aspen.

Logemann J: Treatment for aspiration related to dysphagia: an overview, *Dysphagia* 1:34-38, 1986.

Lowman E, Klinger J: *Aids to independent living*, New York, 1969, McGraw-Hill.

Mahoney FI: Functional evaluation: the Barthel Index, *Md Med J* 14:56-61, 1965.

Martin N, Holt N, Hicks D: *Comprehensive rehabilitation nursing*, New York, 1981, McGraw-Hill.

McCourt A, editor: *The specialty practice of rehabilitation nursing: a core curriculum*, ed 3, Skokie, Ill, 1993, Rehabilitation Nursing Foundation.

Mol V, Baker C: Activity intolerance in the elderly stroke patient, *Rehab Nurs* 16(6):337-343, 1991.

Nagi S: Disability concepts revisited. In *Sociology and rehabilitation*, Washington, DC, 1969, American Sociological Association.

Nagi S: *Disability and rehabilitation*, Columbus, 1969, Ohio State University Press.

Nagi S: An epidemiology of disability among adults in the United States, *Milbank Q* 54:439-467, 1976.

Norton D, McLaren R, Exton-Smith A: *Investigation of geriatric nursing problems in the hospital*, London, 1962, National Corporation for Care of Old People.

Paillard M, Nowak K: Use of exercise to help older adults, *J Gerontol Nurs* 11(7):36-39, 1985.

Panel for Prediction and Prevention of Pressure Ulcers in Adults. Pressure ulcers in adults: prediction and prevention, Clinical Practice Guideline No 3, AHCPR Pub No 92-0047, Rockville, Md, 1992, US Department of Health and Human Services.

Payton O, Poland J: Aging process: implications for clinical practice, *Phys Ther* 63(1):41-47, 1983.

Phipps M: Assessment of neurologic deficits in stroke: acute care and rehabilitation implication, *Nurs Clin North Am* 26(4):957-971, 1991.

Phipps M, Bauman B: Staging care for pressure sores, *Am J Nurs* 84(8):999-1003, 1984.

Phipps M, Kelly-Hayes M: Rehabilitation of older adults. In Baines E, editor: *Perspectives in gerontological nursing*, Newbury Park, Calif, 1991, Sage.

Resnick N: Urinary incontinence in the elderly, *Med Grand Rounds* 3:281-290, 1984.

Schmitt N: Patients' perception of laughter in a rehabilitation hospital, *Rehabil Nurs* 15(3):143-147, 1990.

Smith E, editor: Exercise and aging, *Top Geriatr Rehabil* 1(1):1-88, 1985.

Sudarsky L: Geriatrics: gait disorders in the elderly, *N Engl J Med* 322(20):1441-1446, 1990.

Umhuauer MK: Movement. In Hoeman S, editor: *Rehabilitation nursing: process and application*, ed 2, St Louis, 1995, Mosby.

Urinary Incontinence Guideline Panel: Urinary incontinence in the adult: clinical practice guideline, AHCPR Pub No 92-0038, Rockville, Md, 1992, US Department of Health and Human Services.

Urinary Incontinence Guideline Panel: Urinary incontinence in the adult: update, Pub No 95-062, Rockville, Md, 1996, US Department of Health and Human Services.

Venn R et al: The influence of timing and suppository use on efficiency and effectiveness of bowel training after stroke, *Rehabil Nurs* 17(3):116-120, 1992.

Weeks SK: What are the educational needs of prospective family caregivers of newly disabled adults? *Rehabil Nurs* 20(5):256-272, 1995.

Wells T: Additional treatments for urinary incontinence, *Top Geriatr Rehabil* 3(2):48-58, 1988.

Werner-Beland J: *Grief responses to long-term illness and disability*, Reston, Va, 1980, Reston Publishing.

World Health Organization (WHO): International classification of impairments, disabilities, and handicaps: a manual of classification relating to the consequences of disease, Geneva, Switzerland, 1980, World Health Organization.

# CHAPTER 18

# Long-Term Care

## CHAPTER OBJECTIVES

1 Explain the relationship of a nursing home to long-term care.
2 Explain how the concepts of autonomy, independence, and maintenance or improvement of function guide the care of the nursing home resident.
3 Define medical ethics.
4 Explain differences between life-sustaining measures and *do not resuscitate* orders.
5 Discuss general areas important for a nursing assessment of the older person.
6 Discuss risk factors and preventive measures for falls among the elderly nursing home resident.
7 Discuss problems associated with the use of restraints and identify alternatives.
8 Discuss assessments and interventions for the nursing home resident with urinary incontinence.
9 Discuss assessment of the nursing home resident with constipation.
10 Explain risk factors for preventive measures and interventions for skin breakdown among nursing home residents.
11 Discuss behavioral interventions for the cognitively impaired nursing home resident.

## KEY TERMS

| | |
|---|---|
| autonomy | ethical dilemma |
| chemical restraints | functional assessment |
| delirium | long-term care |
| dementia | mental status assessment |
| depression | minimum data sets |
| do not resuscitate | physical restraints |

At one time the words **long-term care** or *nursing home* might have conjured up images of very old, confused people living out their last days in sadness and neglect. Today long-term care encompasses a variety of services within the health care system that enables people in all stages of chronic illness and all levels of ability to live as fully and independently as possible. In the near future, more people age 65 and older will need a variety of long-term care services, and new models of health care are being developed to accommodate this expected increase. For a complete discussion of the long-term care continuum, see Chapter 17.

The nursing home is only one of many types of long-term care available today. The older person who moves into a nursing home generally cannot live independently. This does not mean that the person is totally dependent, but the person has deficits in functional ability when compared with older people living independently. Approximately 50% of all nursing home residents have impairment of six activities of daily living (ADL) (Ebersole, Hess, 1994). These residents may need assistance with eating, transferring, toileting, dressing, bathing, or mobilization. The source of their deficit may be the result of a physical or cognitive impairment. About 50% of all nursing home residents are diagnosed with Alzheimer's disease or some other cognitive impairment.

The typical nursing home resident is about 84 years old, white, female, widowed, and has few financial resources. In addition, the resident has age-related physiologic changes and multiple chronic diseases that require a wide variety of medications and health services. The older person in a nursing home may require complex health care to meet all of his or her needs. When families are choosing a nursing home, the nurse may be consulted for advice. The family should be urged to look carefully for an institution that best meets the needs of the older loved one. Some area agencies on aging publish comprehensive guides to local nursing homes, including those offering special Alzheimer's units. Additional information may be found at a local branch of the Alzheimer's Association, a community visiting nurse association, and a geriatric program at a local hospital. In general, when choosing a nursing home, a convenient location is important, as most families prefer to make more frequent short visits rather than extended visits. Families should be encouraged to also consider the following:

1. *Physical environment.* Is the nursing home clean? What is the noise level? Are there unpleasant odors? Are there lounges and places for residents to gather? Are the meals served in a pleasant dining room? Is the food palatable?

2. *Daily activities.* Are the residents up and dressed? Are residents parked around the nurses' station with nothing to do? Are the residents treated respectfully by staff? Is there an activities program appropriate to the needs and likes of the loved one?

3. *Staff qualifications.* Are the units staffed by licensed nursing personnel? What are the qualifications of the medical director? Are consultants such as podiatrists, dietitians, dentists, social workers, and pharmacists available?

4. *Policies and procedures.* What is the policy of the nursing home toward resident privacy, use of physical restraints, wandering, and use of sedative or hypnotic drugs?

Many families feel strongly about the care their family member will receive. They should be urged to communicate their preferences clearly before placing their loved one in the nursing facility. Families may have preferences regarding where meals are served, the time residents are put to bed, the policy toward the use of physical and chemical restraints, and policies guiding the use of outside consultants such as dentists, podiatrists, and mental health professionals.

Most nursing homes welcome visits from families of potential residents. These visits should be planned at various times of the day to get an accurate picture of the life-style offered by each facility.

Caring for a nursing home resident is one of the most rewarding and challenging areas of nursing practice. The nurse working in long-term care has the opportunity to be creative and independent, acting as a case manager and promoting multidisciplinary care. Additionally, the nurse has the opportunity to really get to know the patients and their families. Unlike acute care hospitals where the length of stay is often very short, the residents in an extended care facility often develop close relationships with their caregivers. When successes are achieved and a resident's condition improves or stabilizes, most nurses share in the joy with the resident and family.

There are three related concepts that guide the care of the nursing home resident: autonomy, promotion of independence, and maintenance or improvement of function. **Autonomy** can be defined simply as either self-governance or not being controlled by outside forces or individuals. An autonomous person makes decisions about his or her care, chooses activities and organizes care according to his or her preferences, and generally takes charge of any situations that arise. Although complete autonomy is not always possible, each nursing plan of care must be established with the input of the resident and the family, as appropriate. It is important for the nurse to remember that the older person is a special type of survivor who is usually capable of decision making if given the chance. If the nurse promotes autonomy and independence, maintenance or improvement of function is likely to follow.

By recognizing the need for autonomy in the nursing home resident, including those with cognitive impairment, the nurse often serves as an advocate. Many nursing home residents feel as though they have lost control of their lives and can no longer make decisions for themselves. The nurse may be tempted to "do for" the resident rather than teach, encourage, and arrange things so that the resident can do things for himself or herself. It may take longer to assist a frail resident with dressing, but the resident will feel tremendous satisfaction from choosing the appropriate clothing, working at his or her own pace, and dressing himself or herself. Increasing self-care ability helps the older resident feel a sense of autonomy.

---

### CASE STUDY

Mrs. Allen had been a resident in the nursing home for several months and had been known as a "good eater." Her weight had been stable at about 126 pounds since her admission. However, a few weeks ago she stopped eating well and began to "pick at her food." The chart documented a 4-pound loss in a 2-week period, and Mrs. Allen's daughter was concerned. The nurse, after watching Mrs. Allen eat, carefully checked the fit of her dentures and noted an area of ulceration on the lower gum. A dentist was consulted, and the dentures were adjusted for a better fit. A few days later, Mrs. Allen began eating as well as she had before. Mrs. Allen's daughter called the nurse to thank her and nicknamed her "Nurse Sherlock Holmes" because she had solved the mystery.

# ETHICAL DILEMMAS IN LONG-TERM CARE

When promoting autonomy, ethical issues will arise. Ethics is a philosophic discipline, and medical ethics is a unique field within ethics. Medical ethics explores grounds for deciding moral actions. Medical ethics asks questions such as, "What is informed consent?" "When is a person considered informed?" "What is quality of life?" "When is it morally right to make decisions for someone else?"

There are, of course, no absolute answers to these and other ethical questions. The purpose of asking questions is to clarify thoughts and values, to specify the dilemma, and to identify information needed to make decisions. An **ethical dilemma** occurs when there are conflicting values and answers to questions.

Ethical dilemmas typically arise when the resident's competence is diminished and there is a conflict between protecting safety and preserving autonomy (Freeman, 1990). Nurses, like others in the health care system, often have erred on the side of excessive safety. For instance, it is not possible to prevent all falls in the nursing home unless each resident is restrained 24 hours a day and not permitted to walk at all. Policies and nursing interventions that attempt to find a balance between safety and autonomy should be developed, even if there is some risk.

The Patient Self-Determination Act requires the development of advance directives at the time of a hospital admission. Its purpose is to involve patients in the care they receive. Some older people discuss these issues with their caregivers and families, and others do not. Nurses need to assess if there has been any discussion about life-sustaining measures. Often little or no information is available. Many times the **do not resuscitate** order has been written, but there is no mention of other life-sustaining measures. Cardiopulmonary resuscitation (CPR) is only one of many life-sustaining measures and generally has an unfavorable outcome in the elderly nursing home resident. The

very frail; those with serious illness such as pneumonia, cancer, or renal failure; and those with severe functional disabilities have a survival rate of 5% or less (Eisenberg et al, 1990). Often frail older people who receive CPR suffer broken ribs, cognitive deficits from hypoxia to the brain, and subsequent cardiac arrhythmias that are life threatening.

Other life-sustaining measures in the nursing home include artificial feedings (gastric and nasogastric feedings), ventilators, antibiotics, and even transfer to an acute care hospital for an acute illness. Many nursing homes have checklists that state the residents and families' preferences for each intervention. These decisions are best made in nonemergency situations, when the resident and family have the opportunity to ask questions, receive accurate information regarding the various interventions, and weigh the risks and benefits of each decision. All long-term care facilities need specific policies and procedures relating to all aspects of life-sustaining measures.

Although end-of-life decision making is of major importance, it is not the only decision to be made in long-term care. Although independence and decision-making abilities in the older patient are valued by health care professionals, the patient is commonly excluded from decisions about treatment and care. It is often assumed that the older person is cognitively impaired or should be spared difficult decisions. Involvement in discussions about goals and interventions promotes feelings of self-determination. The older person values independence, as does the health care professional.

## GENERAL ASSESSMENT GUIDELINES

Nursing assessments are crucial for identifying barriers to autonomy, independence, and functional abilities. The combination of changes in physiology, multiple chronic illnesses, multiple medications, and years of life experience makes assessment difficult. Signs and symptoms of acute illness are often vague or seem unrelated to a particular illness. Because of this, the initial nursing assessment must be complete so that even subtle changes will be recognized.

Each nursing home completes a holistic assessment of new residents called the **minimum data set.** This assessment includes information on health practices, activities, exercise, elimination patterns, coping styles, nutrition, sleep patterns, sexuality, support systems (including family and friends), cognition and perception, spirituality, and self-concept. When gathering this data the nurse must remember that the person admitted to the nursing home has had an average of 84 years of experience. It is important to find out what the person was like as a youth, young adult, adult, and older person. Questions about childhood activities, family relationships, household responsibilities, education, leisure activities, activities with family and

friends, occupation, and roles and relationships add to the understanding of who the person is today. Previous behavior patterns, learning styles, interaction styles, and coping styles will continue in some form. Using this information, nursing interventions can be creative and individualized to maintain the resident's autonomy as much as possible.

In addition to a general assessment, specific assessment data regarding functional status, mental status, and depression must be gathered on each nursing home resident.

## Functional Assessment

A **functional assessment** identifies the person's level of independence, focusing on abilities rather than disabilities. Each person's ability to perform ADL is often assessed upon admission and periodically thereafter. An accurate representation of each resident's functional ability allows the nurse to devise a nursing care plan consistent with the resident's abilities. Abrupt changes in functional status may also be a key indicator when a cognitively impaired resident becomes ill. Residents who usually walk with minimal assistance and then suddenly become unable to walk may be injured or constipated, may have the beginnings of pneumonia or another infection, or may have suffered a cerebrovascular accident (CVA) or heart attack. Functional status is the chief indicator of a resident's health in the nursing home and requires careful assessment. Refer to Chapter 17 for a more complete discussion of instruments and measures of functional assessment.

Both physical ADL and instrumental ADL need to be assessed. Physical ADL are bathing, dressing, eating, ambulating, managing a wheelchair, and using the toilet. Instrumental ADL involve balancing a checkbook, housekeeping, going to the store, doing laundry, answering the telephone, and managing medications. Most often, physical ADL are assessed in the nursing home and the staff performs instrumental ADL.

The nurse may identify other members of the health care team who can assist the resident in reaching goals. The resident and health care team may then establish a contract that clearly outlines the strategies to be used in achieving those goals. For instance, a person may need to improve muscle strength. The nurse or physical therapist may design an individualized exercise program that the resident can perform independently on a routine basis. In this way, both the health care provider and the patient play a role in improving functional status.

Instrumental ADL provide insights into abilities. The resident can be encouraged to continue activities according to abilities and goals within the constraints of the facility. It may be possible for the resident to keep some medications at the bedside. Nursing interventions may also include encouraging the person to make decisions, keep plants in the room, make his or her own bed, or rearrange his or her room. There are a number of creative approaches to the care of the older person that can be developed using the functional assessment as a base.

## Mental Status Assessment

Every person entering a nursing home needs a **mental status assessment.** A mental status assessment examines cognitive functions such as the ability to think and make decisions. In addition to this admission assessment, it is important to ascertain previous mental status and mental status after 3 months of institutionalization. Many times the nursing home resident is first admitted to an acute-care hospital, treated for an acute illness, and then transferred to the long-term care facility.

Before the acute episode, the person may have had no problems with mental status. But the acute episode and the change in environment may cause changes in mental status that have not resolved on admission to the nursing home. Knowledge of past function helps identify recent changes and give direction for care. Often when the person adjusts to the new environment, intact mental status returns. A mental status assessment is also performed any time the nurse believes that there has been a change in cognitive function. It is best to avoid labeling someone as "confused" because this general term gives little information. When describing someone with deficits in mental status, it is important that the nurse be as specific as possible. For instance, the notation may read: "Mr. Jones has deficits in short-term memory but is oriented to time, place, and person" or, "Mrs. Lawry has intact long- and short-term memory but exhibits deficits in ability to perform calculations and abstract thinking."

The mental status assessment serves three purposes. The first is to give baseline information about the person's cognitive state so that changes can be identified. The second purpose is to screen for problems or potential problems. And the third is to identify areas of strength and weakness and areas in need of additional evaluation.

There are a number of mental status questionnaires useful in long-term care. Because altered mental status can involve many parts of the central nervous system, the mental status assessment uses a variety of questions aimed at identifying specific areas of dysfunction. Thus assessment of mental status is more than an examination of orientation. Refer to Chapter 9 for a complete discussion of instruments and scoring of mental status.

## Depression Assessment

Because **depression** affects many older people but is often not diagnosed or treated, all nursing assessments should include a measure of depression. See Chapter 9 for a discussion of instruments and ways to measure depression in the elderly. Rates of depression are highest in physically ill older adults and those in long-term care facilities in which 40% to 50% of residents are found to be depressed (Cornacchione, Slusser, 1994). Depression in the nursing home is found to be related to physical illness, medication, and psychosocial losses. Physical illnesses linked to depression include liver disease, diabetes, chronic obstructive pulmonary disease, CVA, Alzheimer's disease, congestive heart failure, and anemia. Signs and symptoms of these diseases include decreased energy, anorexia, sleep disturbances, and other somatic symptoms that mimic depression. The relationship between physical illness and depression is unknown, but it is difficult to enjoy life when symptoms of physical illness exist. Improvement of physical status may relieve some of the symptoms of depression.

Research indicates that depression and dementia coexist in approximately 23% of cognitively impaired older adults (Cornacchione, Slusser, 1994). Many older people with Alzheimer's disease realize they are losing their ability to function and feel great sadness and loss over their state of health and their prognosis. The nurse should take time to talk with the depressed resident and his or her family, listen carefully for clues of depression, and address any concerns promptly. The multidisciplinary team can assist in evaluating the presence of depression and in planning care. Medications, psychotherapy, support groups, and involvement in social activities may all be appropriate interventions.

Medications associated with depression in the elderly include antihypertensives (especially beta-blockers), narcotic analgesics, antiparkinson drugs, sedatives, and alcohol. A careful assessment of all prescription and nonprescription drugs should be obtained from all residents on admission to the nursing home. If the onset of depression is associated with a new medication, the physician should be notified so that new medications can be substituted.

Psychosocial losses can contribute to depression in the nursing home. Lack of contact with family and friends, isolation from pleasurable activities, and changes in health status often are associated with nursing home admission. Despite everyone's best efforts to provide a loving, homelike environment in the nursing home, it is never the same as living independently in one's own home. It may be especially difficult around the holidays, when residents think back to the days when they were younger, healthier, and surrounded by family and friends. Many elderly people have little time to grieve between losses. The following is part of an account written by Anna Mae Halgrim Seaver, an 84-year-old nursing home resident (Seaver, 1994).

This is my world now. It's all I have left. You see, I'm old. And, I'm not as healthy as I used to be. I'm not necessarily happy with it, but I accept it. Occasionally, a member of my family will stop in to see me. He or she will bring me some flowers or a little present. Maybe a set of slippers, I've got eight pair. We'll visit for awhile and then they will return to the outside world and I'll be alone again . . .

# RISK AND SPECIFIC CARE ISSUES

## Falls

Falls and associated morbidity and mortality represent a major problem for the elderly. Sequelae include fractures, decreased mobility, loss of confidence, psychologic distress, and self-imposed isolation because of a fear of falling. Resulting disability leads to loss of function and independence. Autonomy is threatened.

There are intrinsic and extrinsic risk factors for falls (Figure 18-1). Intrinsic factors involve age-related changes such as altered gait and balance, visual and hearing changes, osteoporosis, loss of muscle mass, and degenerative joint disease. These factors may be the result of aging or the presence of acute or chronic disease or the side effects of medications or treatments.

Extrinsic factors include hazards in the environment, including scatter rugs, poorly fitting slippers, waxed floors, dimly lit hallways, and dangling electric cords. Many nursing homes are bustling with activity and movement, and residents, staff, and families congregate around the nurses' station. It may be difficult for residents with walkers, wheelchairs, and poor vision or hearing to pass up and down the corridor safely. The nurse should always be alert for hazards such as congested areas, wet floors, light bulbs needing to be replaced, and other extrinsic factors that could be dangerous for residents. If a resident should fall, the nurse should carefully examine the area where the fall occurred to assess for environmental hazards. Such information will be helpful when deciding on what changes, if any, should be made in the nursing care plan.

## Gait and Balance

Elderly persons at risk for falls may have a gait that is slow with short, irregular shuffling steps, and they

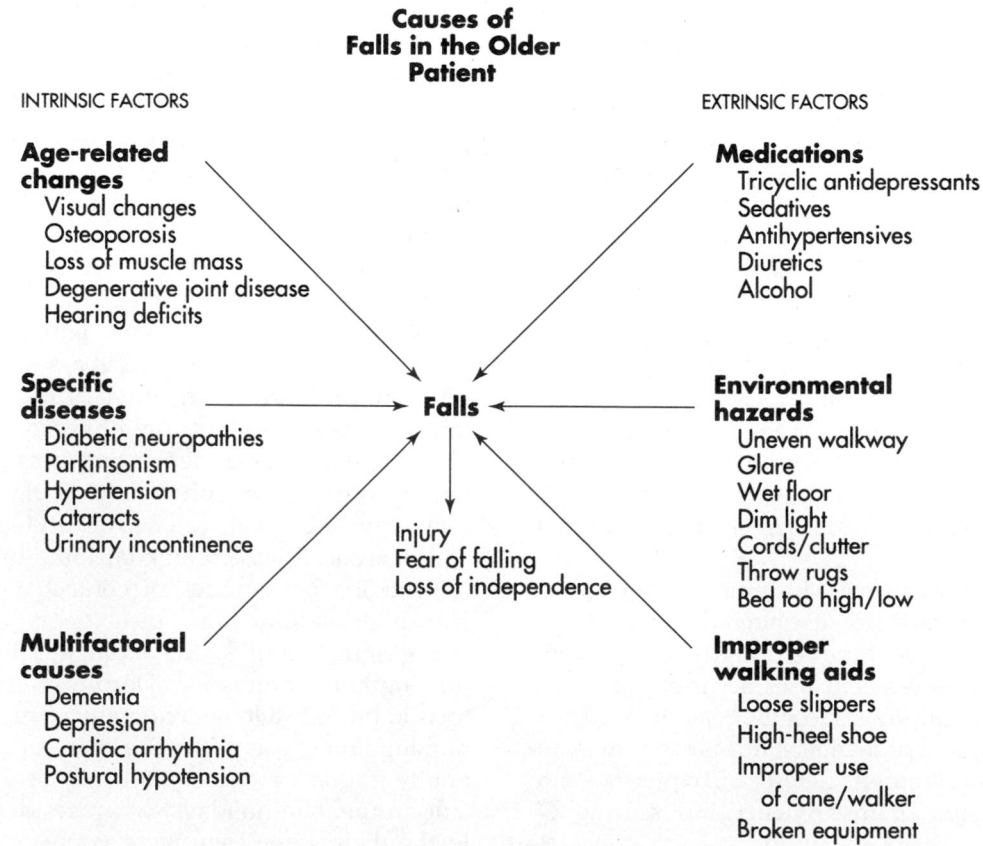

**Figure 18-1**  Causes of falls in older adults.

may place their feet widely apart. A change in gait produces a less secure base of support and an inability to recover from a change in balance. Balance is a function of vision, proprioception, stabilizing muscles, and vibratory senses. Problems may be caused by vestibular (inner ear) alterations resulting in vertigo and dizziness. Proprioception is knowing where extremities are in space. Changes in proprioception result in errors in placing the feet.

## Muscle Strength

Muscle strength may also put the elderly person at risk of falling. It was once thought that muscle weakness and atrophy were normal consequences of aging. Biology-of-aging researchers find, however, that the person who exercises regularly does not lose strength and endurance. In addition, older people who have not exercised but who begin a regular exercise program have increased strength and endurance.

Aging muscle that is not exercised loses lean mass, strength, and endurance, particularly in the essential weight-bearing muscles of the legs. Immobility produces progressive loss of muscle tone and weakness and may be associated with psychogenic vertigo and dizziness. Immobility also contributes to loss of calcium from the long bones, resulting in an increased risk of fractures.

Balance, gait, and muscle strength are probably the most important risk factors for falls. However, numerous contributory factors must be assessed.

## Sensory Changes

Sensory changes in vision and hearing in the older person contribute to altered depth perception. Visual acuity decreases, and the ability to distinguish blues and greens diminishes. Glare, especially from highly waxed floors, disturbs depth perception and may actually "blind" the person, so perception of surroundings becomes difficult, if not impossible. Glaucoma alters peripheral vision. Cataracts, dirty or out-of-date prescription glasses, and dim lighting alter direct vision. Impaired hearing places the older person at risk because he or she may not hear approaching food carts, the warnings of other residents, or the approach of other environmental hazards.

## Medications

Medications produce a variety of risk factors including orthostatic hypotension, dizziness, and confusion. Each medication must be evaluated by the pharmacist for possible interaction with other drugs being taken simultaneously and keeping in mind the physiologic state of the resident. Diuretics tend to dehydrate older persons and place them at risk for orthostatic hypotension. Beta-blockers suppress cardiac output and can induce heart failure. Sedative hypnotics tend to impair balance and make the older person less attentive to the environment. Careful assessment of vital signs, a complete medication history, and discontinuation of all nonessential medications are appropriate nursing measures for the older person at risk for falling in the nursing home.

## Incontinence

Incontinence is another major risk factor for falls. The older person may attempt to get to the bathroom in a hurry and fall or may dribble urine and slip and fall. Placing a commode by the bedside and assessing and treating urinary incontinence may reduce the risk of falling.

## Age and Gender and History of Falls and Confusion

Age and gender are associated with falls. The older the person, the higher the risk. Women are more likely to fall than men. This gender difference reflects the fact that there are more older women than older men, that older women have more chronic diseases than older men, and that older women take more medications than older men.

A history of falls represents yet another important risk factor. An assessment must include information on incidents of falling at home or in the nursing home. Residents who fall tend to fall again. Impaired cognitive status also places the person at risk for falls and tends to form a dangerous combination with all risk factors.

The risk of falling is complex and requires careful evaluation. Table 18-1 lists risk factors that should be part of the nursing assessment and used to explore additional assessments or plan interventions.

## Interventions

Examining the list of risk factors associated with falls helps identify possible interventions. A change in environment, stressful life events, or a change in medications places the person at risk. Additional orientation to the new facility and extra supervision and observation, particularly at night, will decrease the risk. Evaluation of mental status and depression helps identify the extent of the problem. Taking time to listen to concerns and offer support helps the person gain an understanding of events. Autonomy and independence should be encouraged.

| TABLE 18-1 | | | | | |
| --- | --- | --- | --- | --- | --- |
| **Assessment of Risk Factors for Falls** | | | | | |
| **RISK FACTOR** | **YES** | **NO** | **RISK FACTOR** | **YES** | **NO** |
| Admission (within 2 weeks) | | | Incontinent (urine) | | |
| Transfer to unit or room change | | | Hearing deficit | | |
| Medication change (within 30 days) | | | Visual deficit | | |
| Cardiac medications | | | Confusion | | |
| Antihypertensives | | | Head injury | | |
| Diuretics | | | Cerebrovascular accident | | |
| Tranquilizers | | | Amputee | | |
| Sleeping medications | | | Diabetic | | |
| Pain medication | | | Metastatic disease | | |
| More than five medications | | | Degenerative neuromuscular disease | | |
| | | | Previous falls | | |
| | | | Proper use of cane or walker | | |
| | | | Environmental hazards | | |
| | | | Safe shoes or footwear | | |

Medications are the culprit in many problems of elderly patients. A patient's blood pressure should be taken when he or she is reclining and again upon standing to identify orthostatic hypotension. Periods of dizziness, disorientation, or change in mental status should be observed and related to routine medications or medications taken as needed.

The resident should be referred to physical and occupational therapy for a thorough evaluation of function, with an emphasis on potential for falls. The treatment plan should address individual risk factors for falls. Group and individual exercises should be encouraged. Even the person in a wheelchair can benefit from regular exercise. The nurse should ensure that lighting is adequate and that glare is kept to a minimum. Bright colors for bedspreads and walls help perceptual problems.

Records of incontinence and bladder and bowel patterns help identify when the person should be taken to the bathroom. A common time for falls is at night when the person tries to climb over the side rails of the bed to get to the bathroom. If used at all, half side rails are best. These assist the person in moving in bed and provide a means of stabilization when the person sits up on the edge of the bed.

**Physical and chemical restraints.** One of the most common, but incorrect, methods of preventing falls is the use of physical restraints. Interestingly, a high percentage of falls occur when restraints are in place and side rails are up (Mion, Strumpf, 1994). **Physical restraints** are any manual method or physical device that the resident cannot remove; that restricts the resi-

dent's physical activity; and that is not a usual and customary part of a medical, diagnostic, or treatment procedure. Further, a physical restraint does not serve to promote the resident's independent functioning (Stumpf, Evans, 1988). Vest restraints, waist restraints, seat belts, and gerichairs are all types of physical restraints. Cognitively impaired residents often untie or attempt to slide out of the restraints and become entangled, choke, fall, or seriously injure themselves. Morbidity and mortality risks associated with physical restraints include nerve injury, pressure sores, pneumonia, incontinence, increased confusion, inappropriate drug use, strangulation, and asphyxiation (Evans, Strumpf, 1987). When a person with a cognitive impairment is put to bed with side rails up, they often attempt to climb over them, becoming entangled and causing injury. Of all possible interventions, restraints are the most harmful to the person's sense of autonomy, independence, function, and self-esteem. Federal regulations under the Omnibus Reconciliation Act (OBRA '87) mandate against using restraints that are (1) used for discipline or convenience of the staff, (2) used without a trial of less-restrictive measures, or (3) used without the consent of the resident or his or her legal representative. Residents who are restrained should be released, exercised, toileted, and checked for skin redness every 2 hours. The need for the restraint should be reevaluated periodically. It is the responsibility of the medical director and nursing home administrators with the input of nursing staff to develop policies and procedures for the appropriate use of restraints. This ensures the highest quality of life and promotes autonomy of the residents.

Many nurses and long-term care administrators are concerned because they fear they will be held liable for injuries from a fall. Although the move to restraint-free environments is relatively new in the United States, it is not new in England and other European countries. In England and the Scandinavian countries, restraints are not used at all. In the United States, pilot projects have shown that the number of falls and injuries from falls has not increased when restraints are removed (Evans, Strumpf, 1987). Careful environmental assessment, reduced psychotropic drug use, and supervision of patients who frequently fall are all effective in reducing the risk of falls and avoiding restraints.

OBRA '87 also sets standards for the use of **chemical restraints,** which are defined as sedative and antipsychotic drugs. Studies done in the 1980s in nursing homes revealed that there had been excessive, often inappropriate use of these drugs and that they were associated with significant risk for injury (Rader, Donius, 1991). Conditions that are considered inappropriate for antipsychotic drug treatment include wandering, anxiety, fidgeting nervousness, agitation, and anxiety. Use of antipsychotic drugs is limited to specific conditions such as psychotic mood disorder and schizophrenia. Behaviors that make the resident a danger to himself or herself or others, as well as behaviors that make the delivery of nursing care impossible, are considered justifiable reasons for the use of psychotropic drugs. If these drugs are used, the nurse should carefully document the need for the medication, using a 24-hour behavior log. Once the medication is administered, the behavior log should reflect an improvement in the troublesome behaviors. If not, the medication should be discontinued. Regulations further state that trial dose reductions and discontinuation of these drugs should be instituted on a regular basis.

Identifying alternatives to physical and chemical restraints should occur after exploring the need for restraints. If the reason is the potential for falls, an evaluation of the risk factors and the measures to correct them can provide the nurse with alternatives. Exercise programs, activity programs, lower bed height, and relocation closer to the nurses' station are possible interventions to permit the removal of restraints. Bed monitors signal the nurses' station when a patient who frequently falls arises from bed and may need supervision. Nonskid mats placed on the path to the bathroom keep the floor dry for incontinent patients. Behavioral interventions are suggested for dealing with the cognitively impaired resident who refuses care, exhibits symptoms of agitation, or presents a danger to himself or herself or others (Box 18-1) (Besdine et al, 1996).

---

**BOX 18-1**

**Guidelines for Dealing with the Cognitively Impaired Nursing Home Resident**

1 Prevention is the most effective approach for reducing behavior problems. Be aware of the person's history, strengths, and weaknesses. There may be a better time to approach the resident. Do not force a confrontation.

2 Be objective when assessing problems. If the problem is more of an inconvenience to caregivers than it is to the resident, no intervention may be necessary.

3 Determine the reason for the behavior. If the resident is not cooperating with care, is it the way he or she was approached? Is the resident overwhelmed with sensory stimulation? Is the resident ill, constipated, or fatigued? Is it the time of the day?

4 Assess problems as a team. Seek input from all team members involved, including other nurses, therapists, social workers, activities therapists, families, and nurses aides. Remember that others see the resident from a different perspective and that all information is helpful.

5 Do not blame the resident for the behavior. Cognitively impaired residents have a disease that inhibits their ability to think clearly. It is the responsibility of nurses to devise the best environment that supports maximum function. Sleep, appetite, bowel function, and personality are all affected by the degenerative brain changes that occur in Alzheimer's disease.

6 Be creative in your approach. Use calming music (Tabloski et al, 1995), pictures of family members, favorite foods, and a flexible approach to bathing, sleeping, and eating routines. Your efforts will be well worth it, and the older person's dignity will be respected. When you find something that works, share it with others. You will be a role model for others, and the resident will benefit from a consistent approach.

---

## Urinary Incontinence

Urinary incontinence, the involuntary loss of urine, is a problem for at least 10 million noninstitutionalized American adults and accounts for approximately $10 billion spent on products to manage the problem. Urinary incontinence causes significant disability and dependency and is a leading cause of institutionalization.

It is often assumed that urinary incontinence is a consequence of aging, that there is no treatment, and that therefore one must learn to live with it. There is a large market for incontinence pads and adult diapers. Urinary incontinence, however, is a symptom rather than a disease, and it is not a normal part of the aging process. Unfortunately, the evaluation and treatment of urinary incontinence is often neglected by health care professionals. When treated appropriately, however, mobility, function, and independence improve significantly.

In long-term care facilities, 50% or more of the residents probably will have urinary problems. Urinary incontinence is complex, with multiple causative factors. There are three main types: stress incontinence, urge incontinence, and overflow incontinence. Although there are three distinct types, older people may experience two or all types at the same time. The nurse plays a vital role in the treatment of the patient with urinary incontinence that begins with a complete assessment, which includes a mental status examination, functional assessment, documentation of the pattern of incontinence, and assessment aimed at identifying the type of

incontinence. Table 18-2 illustrates important diagnostic criteria for the three types of incontinence.

## CASE STUDY

Mr. Alcott is a 78-year-old nursing home resident with Alzheimer's disease. He often attempts to strike the nurses when he receives his weekly bath. The nurses and aides are frightened of him and approach him with fear. Ms. Bradley, the new staff nurse, suggests the following approach: (1) Mr. Alcott seems to like one nurse better than the others. Therefore she should arrange for his bath. (2) Mr. Alcott seems calmer in the early morning rather than the afternoon. His bath time should be rescheduled to the morning. (3) Mrs. Alcott should be asked to bring in a tape recording of some of Mr. Alcott's favorite music to play in the background during the bath. These measures greatly reduce Mr. Alcott's fear, and he becomes less combative during bath time.

## TABLE 18-2

## Urinary Incontinence Analysis

| DATA OBTAINED FROM HISTORY OR INCONTINENCE ASSESSMENT TOOL | TYPE OF INCONTINENCE | | |
|---|---|---|---|
| | STRESS | URGE | OVERFLOW |
| Amount of leakage | + Small squirts | + Large | + Dribbling |
| Time of day of leakage | + Day | + Day and night | + Day |
| Associated events | + Coughing; laughing; sneezing; bending; changing position | + Strong urge to void, unable to hold it until toilet reached | + None |
| Stream of urine | Normal | Normal | + Hesitancy, interruption, weak |
| Awareness of urge to void at time of incontinent episode | − | + | − |
| Feeling of incomplete emptying after void | − | − | + |
| **Physical Findings** | | | |
| Fecal impaction or incontinence | − | − | + |
| Enlarged prostate | − | − | + |
| Palpable bladder postvoid | − | − | + |
| Cystocele, rectocele, uterine prolapse, urethral prolapse | + | − | − |
| Atrophic vaginitis | + | + | − |
| Leakage of urine after cough (full bladder) | + Immediate | + 3-5 seconds after cough | − |
| Catheter for residual | <100 ml | <100 ml | >100 ml |
| Obesity | + | − | − |
| Presence of girdle | + | − | − |

## Stress Incontinence

Stress incontinence, the involuntary leakage of small amounts of urine usually in response to increased intraabdominal pressure, accounts for about 35% of incontinence in older people. The person complains of losing small amounts of urine, usually during the day, when coughing, laughing, sneezing, bending, or changing position. Stress incontinence occurs primarily in women who have had multiple pregnancies or significant weight gain. Additional assessment may reveal the presence of a cystocele, rectocele, uterine prolapse, urethral prolapse, atrophic vaginitis caused by lack of estrogen, obesity, or use of certain antihypertensive medications. The person with stress incontinence is able to completely empty the bladder, and little residual volume remains after voiding.

## Urge Incontinence

Urge incontinence is the involuntary loss of large amounts of urine associated with a strong desire to void. It accounts for 60% to 70% of urinary incontinence in older people. The person complains of losing large amounts of urine day or night and of having a strong desire to void but being unable to hold urine until reaching the bathroom. The person will experience leaking urine 3 to 5 seconds after coughing, rather than with coughing as with stress incontinence. Additional assessment may reveal moderate to high caffeine intake (coffee, tea, cola), atrophic vaginitis, diabetes, infections, degenerative neurologic conditions such as a CVA or Parkinson's disease, alcoholism, or use of certain medications such as sedatives and diuretics. As with stress incontinence, little residual volume remains in the bladder after voiding.

## Overflow Incontinence

Overflow incontinence, the involuntary dribbling of urine caused by an obstruction of the bladder outlet, accounts for 10% to 15% of urinary incontinence in older people. The person complains of dribbling without warning during the day. When voiding, there is a hesitancy and interruption in the stream of urine and the feeling of incomplete emptying of the bladder. If catheterized, there would be more than 100 ml of residual urine present in the bladder. Additional assessment may reveal a fecal impaction, enlarged prostate, diabetes, a spinal cord injury or disc disease, or use of certain drugs such as alcohol, antihistamines, decongestants, phenothiazines, and muscle relaxants.

The person with urinary incontinence requires a thorough evaluation by the health care team. In addition to the causes identified for each type of incontinence, there are multiple environmental factors to assess. Immobility or being unable to get to the bathroom, commode, or bedpan; unfamiliar surroundings; inadequate lighting; dehydration causing concentration of urine, which may irritate the mucosa; and irritation of the bladder wall are all correctable factors that should be considered.

## Voiding Record

There are a variety of methods to record voiding patterns (Wells, 1988). The purpose of the record is to identify the pattern of incontinence in terms of frequency, amount, and conditions surrounding the incontinent episode. It can be kept by the resident, family, or nursing staff. The record requires cooperation by everyone because it encompasses at least one 24-hour period. The resident is observed on an hourly basis to determine whether he or she was incontinent, dry, or voided normally. The amount of urine is documented. If the person was incontinent, the following is noted: the approximate amount of urine, awareness of the urge to eliminate, associated conditions (coughing, sneezing, impaction or urge to defecate, walking, or changing position), and the availability of appropriate facilities. In addition, an accurate record of the amount, type, and time of fluid intake is kept. Analyzing this record will help determine the person's normal patterns of elimination and assist in the development of nursing interventions.

Urinary incontinence is complex. A thorough assessment will help identify the type of urinary incontinence, enabling the health care team to determine appropriate interventions.

## Intervention

Intervention for urinary incontinence depends on the type of urinary incontinence and, whenever possible, the cause. The goal of all treatment is to promote independence and improve function. For stress incontinence, Kegel exercises aim at strengthening the pelvic floor and can be taught by the nurse. The person is taught to find the pelvic floor muscle by trying to stop a stream of urine. The muscle that is pulled is the muscle to be exercised. The person is instructed to tighten the muscle, hold it for a count of 10, and relax for a count of 10. This is repeated 10 to 15 times in the morning, afternoon, and evening. The exercise can be done anytime, anyplace. When teaching the exercise, the nurse needs to emphasize the importance of relaxation as well as tightening. Also, the nurse needs to be sure the person does not use the abdomen, legs (or crossing legs), or buttocks and that the person does not hold his or her breath while exercising. Posting a schedule for the person to mark off when completing the exercise places responsibility on the person and serves as a reminder.

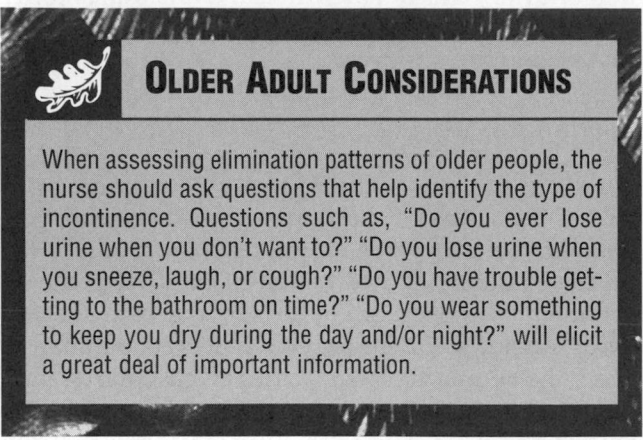

**OLDER ADULT CONSIDERATIONS**

When assessing elimination patterns of older people, the nurse should ask questions that help identify the type of incontinence. Questions such as, "Do you ever lose urine when you don't want to?" "Do you lose urine when you sneeze, laugh, or cough?" "Do you have trouble getting to the bathroom on time?" "Do you wear something to keep you dry during the day and/or night?" will elicit a great deal of important information.

Additional interventions for stress incontinence include oral or topical estrogen for atrophic vaginitis, development of a weight-loss program, wearing loose garments, evaluation of medications (particularly antihypertensive medications), possible use of anticholinergic medications, surgery, and habit training.

The purpose of habit training is to avoid large amounts of urine in the bladder. It begins by examining the voiding record to identify normal frequency patterns. A regular, rigid voiding schedule is then established. The person is taken to the bathroom every 2 hours regardless of whether there is a desire to void and regardless of incontinence.

There are multiple interventions for urge incontinence that can be initiated by the nurse in cooperation with the health care team. First, the nurse assesses the environment to be sure it facilitates normal voiding. This includes ensuring that the bathroom, commode, bedpan, and urinal are accessible and that assistive devices needed for independence are close at hand. Obstacles are removed, and lighting is checked to ensure that it is adequate. It may be necessary to have the resident's eyes examined and vision corrected. The person's mobility may be improved with physical therapy. The occupational therapy department may help design easy-to-open clothing.

Bladder training and habit training for urge incontinence are also useful. The goal of bladder training is to increase the interval between voiding to 4 hours. The person is taught to inhibit the urge to void and increase bladder capacity, thus increasing the interval between voiding. Relaxation exercises often help the person overcome the urge to void. The nurse works with the resident, encouraging slow, deep breathing until the urge disappears. The resident is encouraged to wait 5 minutes and then void. If an accident occurs

before 5 minutes, the waiting time is shortened to 3 minutes. When it becomes easy to wait 3 minutes, the time can be increased to 4 or 5 minutes. The waiting time is gradually increased. To have a successful bladder-training program, the person must maintain adequate intake of fluids, usually between 2000 and 2500 ml/day. Natural diuretics such as coffee, tea, cocoa, cola, and grapefruit juice should be avoided. An evaluation of medications that could cause incontinence should also be performed.

Overflow incontinence is often neurogenic in cause. The resident and family can be taught measures to assist in voiding. The person should sit on the toilet or commode. Deep breathing, blowing through a straw while leaning forward, and the Crede maneuver (manual pressure on the bladder) may help initiate voiding. Each technique may be successful at different times. Because one technique does not work once does not mean that it will not work another time. Successful management depends on patience and a willingness to try various methods.

Another treatment of choice for overflow incontinence is intermittent catheterization. Treatment of incontinence in many health care settings involves the placement of an indwelling catheter, which in turn places the person at risk for infection, decreases independence and mobility, increases the risk of trauma, and increases the need for medical supervision. Sterile intermittent catheterization by a nurse or clean technique taught to a cognitively intact person simulates normal voiding patterns and decreases the risk of infection. In addition, intermittent catheterization promotes independence and functional abilities.

The first intervention for incontinence associated with outlet obstruction is to relieve the obstruction. This may involve removal of the fecal impaction or surgery for an enlarged prostate. Next, medications are evaluated to identify those that tighten sphincters or contribute to urinary retention.

Care of the person with urinary incontinence represents a challenge to the nurse and requires thorough assessment and creative problem solving with the resident, the family, and the health care team.

## Constipation

As with all problems encountered in the long-term care setting, constipation has multiple causative factors. The elderly use more over-the-counter preparations to promote bowel elimination than any other age group. Persistent use of laxatives tends to inhibit normal patterns, thereby creating an impression of constipation that stimulates perpetual use of laxatives. Also, in a misguided attempt to prevent incontinence, the older person may decrease fluid intake, thereby increasing the tendency toward constipation. Diets lacking in roughage and fruit, medications, inhibitory practices (ignoring the bowel reflex as well as using laxatives), and lack of exercise all contribute to constipation. Added to this are cultural beliefs about the importance of regular (often translated as daily) bowel movements.

## Assessment

An accurate assessment of constipation is essential for planning appropriate interventions. The assessment should include the following:

- *Time:* What are the usual days and times of bowel movements?
- *Frequency:* Do bowel movements occur daily, three times a week, twice a week, or weekly?
- *Consistency:* Is the stool formed, hard, soft, or loose?
- *Fluid intake:* What is the amount of daily fluid intake and the type of fluid?
- *Nutrition:* A 24-hour recall is helpful for a variety of assessment areas, including elimination. Ask specific questions regarding foods and amounts consumed at meals, snacks, and bedtime. Note amounts of cereals, fresh fruit, vegetables, and breads.
- *Stimulants:* What does the person use to stimulate bowel movements? This could include coffee, prunes, bran, and other natural laxatives in addition to medications, enemas, suppositories, and digital stimulation.
- *Habits associated with elimination:* What is the usual place for elimination? Are activities such as reading or smoking done during bowel evacuation?
- *Medications:* What medications does the person take? Certain medications cause constipation, such as anticholinergic drugs, aluminum or calcium antacids, and high doses of aspirin.
- *Exercise:* How much and how often does the person exercise? What type of exercise does he or she do?
- *Physical assessment:* A rectal examination to check for impaction, bowel sounds, and skin turgor (dehydration) and a palpation of the abdomen for masses should be performed. Note chronic medical conditions.

## Intervention

If constipation and impaction are present, the bowel must be cleansed before a bowel program can be successful. Laxatives and enemas should be used as needed to clean the bowel. Then the assessment data can be used to identify normal patterns and begin a reeducation of the bowel. When developing a bowel program, it is usually easier to reestablish old patterns than to develop new ones. If the person usually has a bowel movement at bedtime, retraining should begin at this time using the natural cues that the person finds effective. Nutritional stimulants such as bran may be added to the morning or afternoon meals, prunes or other dried fruits may be served, and fresh fruit or bran cereal can be suggested as a snack.

If no bowel movement occurs within the first 48 hours, a gentle stimulant such as a glycerine suppository at the time the person normally has a bowel movement may be needed. Whenever using artificial bowel stimulants, the nurse should start with the most natural and work up to the more irritating.

The person should be encouraged to respond to the urge to evacuate the bowel. The environment should be conducive to having a bowel movement. The nurse can provide privacy and ensure that the bathroom, commode, or bedpan is accessible. No bowel program will work immediately. Each intervention should be given approximately 2 weeks to be effective. The person will usually respond to encouragement and support. Punishing words or actions place an unnecessary barrier to success. For most people it is unnatural to be dependent on others for toileting. Whenever possible, the nurse should facilitate independence.

## Pressure Sores

As a person ages, changes in the skin contribute to the potential for skin breakdown. With aging, there is a decrease in vascularity, subcutaneous fat, elasticity, hair follicles, and temperature and touch receptors. The result is skin that is fragile, easily injured, and slow to heal.

In addition to aging, risk factors for skin breakdown include immobility, diabetes, incontinence, poor nutrition, inadequate fluid intake, and edema. An assessment of the skin of the older person must consider all factors and an accurate description of the altered skin. Pressure sores, in the past called *decubitus ulcers,* are the most common form of alteration in skin integrity and are caused by continued unrelieved pressure. They develop over bony prominences where the pressure causes occlusion of capillaries and local inflammation from inadequate nutrient exchange (Agency for Health Care Policy and Research, 1992a; White et al, 1994). Pressure ulcers are a serious problem that affect approximately 9% of all hospitalized patients and 23% of all nursing home patients. These ulcers are difficult to treat and often result in pain, disfigurement, and prolonged hospitalization. However, prompt and effective treatment can minimize these deleterious effects and speed recovery (Bergstrom et al, 1995).

## Assessment

Pressure sores should be assessed and described using a standard, classification system. Identification of stages helps determine interventions (Figure 18-2 and Box 18-2). Refer to Chapter 40 for further information on pressure sores.

It is extremely useful to photograph pressure sores, including a tape measure in the photograph to indicate size. The photograph serves as both a means to assess the extent of the problem and to evaluate the effectiveness of treatment. Before photographing the pressure sore, permission from the patient or family must be obtained. The picture with the date and location of the wound, along with the treatment plan, are then placed in the record. Pictures should be taken weekly until the lesion is healed. .

## Intervention

A key factor to healing pressure sores is a consistent approach by all who care for the person. The proposed treatment must be given time to work. All long-term care facilities need to develop a skin protocol that fits

their facility and residents. The protocol outlines assessment, identification of the person at risk, preventive measures, and, when pressure sores develop, a protocol for intervention. The treatment protocol requires collaboration with the physician, but the nurse

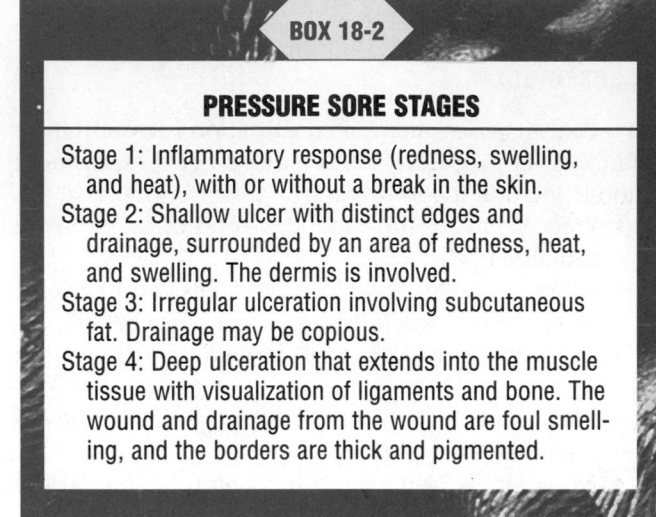

**BOX 18-2**

### PRESSURE SORE STAGES

Stage 1: Inflammatory response (redness, swelling, and heat), with or without a break in the skin.
Stage 2: Shallow ulcer with distinct edges and drainage, surrounded by an area of redness, heat, and swelling. The dermis is involved.
Stage 3: Irregular ulceration involving subcutaneous fat. Drainage may be copious.
Stage 4: Deep ulceration that extends into the muscle tissue with visualization of ligaments and bone. The wound and drainage from the wound are foul smelling, and the borders are thick and pigmented.

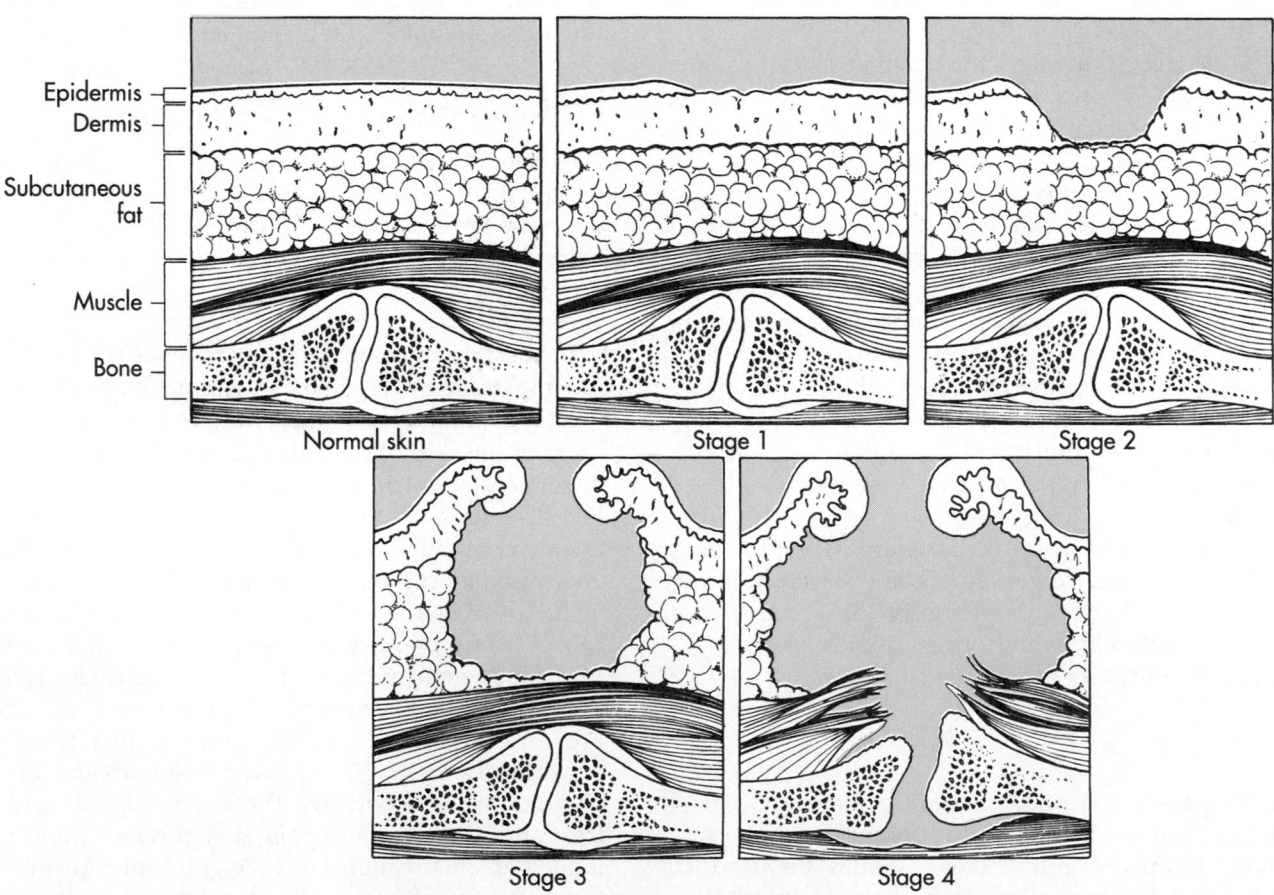

**Figure 18-2**  Normal skin and pressure sore formation.

plays a primary role in the care of pressure sores (Box 18-3).

**NURSE ALERT**

Pressure sores can be prevented by systematic assessment and management as part of the overall plan of care.

Initial interventions aim to identify the person at risk for developing pressure sores as well as to prevent them from ever developing. Once pressure sores begin to develop, interventions are designed according to the extent of the lesions and center around the relief of pressure. Basic nursing interventions include a routine of turning the patient every 2 hours; special mattresses such as a waterbed mattress, a circulating air mattress, or an egg crate mattress; special cushions for the wheelchair; range-of-motion exercises; ambulation; and special skin care. For additional information regarding pressure sores, see Chapter 40.

In addition, residents and families can be taught how to prevent pressure sores and can be encouraged to take part in the treatment plan. Residents who sit in chairs for extended periods should be taught to change position frequently. They can push up on the arms of their chairs to relieve the pressure. Isometric flexion exercises of the buttocks increase circulation and relieve pressure. The nurse may need to remind residents to follow their treatment plans.

There are numerous products for the management of pressure sores. Treatment must begin as soon as redness develops. Once the skin breaks, the wound should be cleansed with an isotonic solution (normal saline). These solutions are not toxic and do not damage healthy skin cells surrounding the ulcer. Wounds that look infected should be cultured. Antiseptics are appropriate for "dirty" wounds only (Bergstrom et al, 1995). Synthetic dressings such as the hydrocolloids (Duoderm; Comfeel), moisture vapor permeable transparent dressings (Opsite; Tegaderm), and absorption dressings (Bard; Debrisar) are useful for Stage-2 and some Stage-3 pressure sores if they are not infected.

**BOX 18-3**    **NURSING PROCESS**

**PRESSURE SORES**

**ASSESSMENT**
- General condition of skin
- Skin over bony prominences
- Awareness of pressure sensation
- Ability to move
- Nutritional status
- Urinary or fecal incontinence
- Amount of shear and friction on skin
- Pressure ulcer staging: color, odor, presence of necrotic tissue, exudate, condition of surrounding skin
- Vital signs and temperature
- Laboratory values: albumin, ferritin, wound culture, white blood cells
- Family's ability to provide associated care

**NURSING DIAGNOSES**
- Impaired skin integrity related to friction, shear, or pressure
- Risk for infection related to open pressure ulcer or poor nutritional status
- Impaired home maintenance management related to long-term therapy
- Risk for caregiver role strain related to long-term therapy

- Altered nutrition: less than body requirements related to chronic illness

**NURSING INTERVENTIONS**
- Maintain preventive measures, including pressure reduction and relief.
- Maintain nutritional needs and management of incontinence.
- Provide aseptic local wound care as ordered.
- Maintain no pressure on pressure ulcer until it has healed.
- Provide perineal hygiene after incontinence.
- Encourage a high-protein, high-caloric diet if not contraindicated.
- Administer antibiotics as prescribed.
- Refer patient to social worker to assist with discharge planning needs.
- Discuss possible need for respite care.

**EVALUATION OF EXPECTED OUTCOMES**
- Pressure ulcer shows evidence of healing
- No evidence of local or systemic infection
- Verbalizes necessary home care measures
- Verbalizes available resources

Deeper wounds and wounds with a great deal of drainage require dressings such as Sorbean. Karaya powder absorbs the exudate without drying the wound.

When necrotic tissue is present, the pressure sore must be debrided. Noninvasive wet-to-dry dressings are often the treatment of choice. However, this debridement process does take time to be effective. Other measures include use of a scalpel and scissors to remove necrotic tissue, followed by enzyme ointments such as Elase to continue debridement. The appearance of pink granulation tissue heralds the end of the debridement process.

Povidone iodine kills bacteria, spores, fungi, and viruses. However, it inhibits the formation of granulation tissue (Thomason, 1989). It is recommended that povidone iodine be used only on dirty wounds and in a dilution of no more than 1%. Hydrogen peroxide helps debride wounds but can damage healthy tissue. It is best used only at the start of wound care for cleansing and debridement. For infected wounds, especially in the presence of diabetes, the physician should be contacted for advice regarding use of systemic antibiotics.

In addition to the physician, other members of the health care team need to be involved in the treatment plan. An in-depth nutritional assessment and treatment plan need to be instituted. When a pressure sore drains, the person loses albumin, a necessary factor in healing. Nutritional interventions include an increase in protein, either at mealtime or by the use of supplements. Periodic albumin levels are needed to monitor nutritional sufficiency. Physical and occupational therapy may help in the development of an activity plan. Special cushions for the wheelchair or assistive devices will help the person move more independently.

Pressure sores severely limit independence and threaten functional ability. Prevention and treatment decisions often rest on the nurse. Resident, family, and staff teaching are important aspects of practice in addition to coordination of care with the interdisciplinary team.

## Decline in Mental Status

A decline in mental status in the elderly is poorly understood and evaluated. Unfortunately, memory loss is often considered a consequence of aging by both the older person and the health care professional. However, a decline in mental status is a symptom rather than a disease and may actually be the symptom of any number of underlying conditions. An important cause of cognitive decline among the elderly is medication. In the nursing home, multiple medications are often used,

doses may be too high, and medications may be given after the underlying problem is resolved, making the medication inappropriate. Periodic reevaluation of all medications should occur on a regular basis.

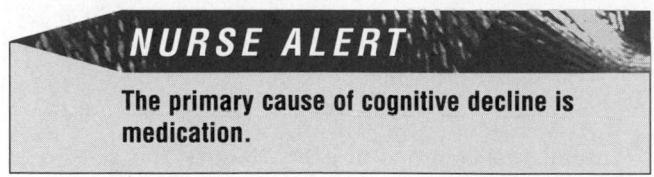

**NURSE ALERT**

**The primary cause of cognitive decline is medication.**

Other causes of cognitive decline include infections (e.g., respiratory or urinary tract infections), metabolic problems (e.g., diabetes or thyroid conditions), poor nutrition, sensory disturbances, tumors, anemia, atherosclerosis, alcohol abuse, trauma, and environmental factors. Confusion is not a simple phenomenon. The person with confusion often requires an extensive evaluation to determine the cause.

There are three D's associated with confusion in the elderly: *d*elirium, *d*epression, and *d*ementia. Although discussed separately, the confused older person commonly has two and often three of the conditions at the same time. See Chapter 6 for a more complete discussion of delirium, depression, and dementia.

## Delirium

**Delirium** is a common, nonspecific presentation of illness in the elderly. It is often the first sign of underlying disease, and it is a symptom in need of evaluation. *Delirium* and *acute confusional state* may be terms used interchangeably to describe the same syndrome. *Delirium* replaces terminology once used to include acute organic brain syndrome, acute dementia, and toxic confusional state. Delirium is a global cognitive impairment of memory and organization of thought. Its onset is sudden and is characterized by uncooperative behavior, drowsiness or hyperactivity, mood swings, inappropriate language, delusions, hallucinations, and confused visual-spatial relationships. Symptoms are more severe at night. The mental status assessment will show an inability to attend to tasks and an altered level of consciousness.

## Depression

Another common cause of confusion is depression. Again, confusion may be the presenting symptom. Depression often goes unrecognized and untreated in the older population, yet the elderly are at highest risk for successful suicides. It is likely that between 30%

and 50% of the residents in long-term care facilities have some type of depression. In addition to confusion, the depressed older person will have a variety of somatic complaints. They are commonly labeled hypochondriacs.

Conditions often associated with or that may trigger depression include thyroid and adrenal abnormalities, Parkinson's disease, and CVAs. The mental status assessment will reveal only mild, if any, impairment. Interviews with the person will be difficult with many "I don't know" answers. The score on the Geriatric Depression Scale (short form) will indicate depression with a score of 5 or higher.

## Dementia

**Dementia,** once called *organic brain syndrome,* is a term used to describe a global cognitive dysfunction with impairment in short- and long-term memory, orientation, abstract thinking, and judgment, as well as personality changes. Disturbances in cortical function that cause aphasia (language disorders), apraxia (inability to carry out motor function), and agnosia (failure to recognize objects and people that are familiar) are also included. The mental status assessment will show a global cognitive impairment, but depending on the stage of the illness, the person may be able to attend to tasks and perform calculations (Besdine et al, 1996). There are many different types of dementia. The most common is dementia of the Alzheimer's type (DAT). Unlike delirium, the onset of DAT is slow and insidious, and the disease is progressive and irreversible. The disease process continues for many years and places considerable burden on the family. Families will report that the person is not the same but may have trouble describing the exact problem. Getting lost while walking or driving or forgetting to turn off the burners on the stove are common behaviors that bring the family to a health care provider.

When assessing the person with dementia, the nurse will note many "near miss" answers to questions and an attempt to conceal problems. The person may also be unsociable, uncooperative, hostile, and confused and disoriented. Because confusion is one of the presenting symptoms and there is no differential diagnosis for dementia, there needs to be a complete evaluation that includes laboratory tests, x-ray examinations, computed tomography scans, magnetic resonance imaging, and psychiatric and neurologic testing.

## Intervention

Caring for the person who has an alteration in thought processes is difficult. The person with delirium needs a consistent, quiet, and calm approach to care. The environment should be organized to avoid extremes and excessive sensory input. The room should be quiet with familiar people nearby to provide care. Changes in personnel and routines should be avoided, and lighting should be decreased at night. Orientation to person, time, and place may be helpful. Once the underlying condition is corrected, the delirium will clear. Mental status will become normal providing there is no other cognitive problem.

Depression should be treated with medication and therapy. There may be a resistance to therapy from the health care workers and the older person. Beneath the resistance is the belief that therapy for the older person is not cost effective and is of little use. The older person, however, will benefit and regain independence and function, as well as have an improved mental status. Reminiscence, life review, and support groups are useful and beneficial interventions that can be initiated by the nurse.

The nursing home resident with dementia needs structure and consistency. Routines are helpful. Because wandering may be a problem, warning devices that let the nurse know that the person is out of bed or opening a door should be used. They allow the person freedom of movement, independence, and functioning ability while maintaining a safe environment. The person can also be seated close to the nurses' station for closer observation.

Of primary importance when caring for the person with dementia is care of the family. Placement of the loved one in a long-term care facility was probably a difficult decision. Watching the slow deterioration and not being recognized are difficult adjustments for any family member. The nurse who reassures the family, offers support, and provides information will help their anticipatory grieving process.

# KEY CONCEPTS

➤ The nursing home is only a part of the long-term continuum of services.

➤ Care of the nursing home resident is challenging and rewarding.

➤ Caring for nursing home residents requires the promotion of autonomy, independence, and improvement of function.

➤ Ethical dilemmas arise when there is tension between promoting autonomy and protecting the safety of the resident.

➤ Providing appropriate care at the end of life requires input and attention from the nursing staff.

➤ A complete assessment of the resident's function, mental status, and level of depression is necessary upon admission to the nursing home and on a routine basis thereafter.

➤ Falls, a significant problem in the nursing home, can be influenced by the resident's gait and balance, muscle strength, sensory changes, and medications.

➤ Physical and chemical restraints in the nursing home may increase injuries and harm the autonomy of the resident.

➤ Behavioral approaches are the best way to deal with troublesome behaviors in the resident with dementia.

➤ Urinary incontinence of the nursing home resident should be carefully assessed and treated.

➤ Constipation can be treated by changes in diet, fluid intake, and exercise, rather than dependence on laxatives.

➤ Pressure sores can usually be prevented by careful attention to position, skin care, hygiene, and nutrition.

# CRITICAL THINKING EXERCISES

1. Describe your personal feelings about the use of life-sustaining methods in the chronically ill.
2. Discuss the risk factors and preventive measures for falls among elderly nursing home residents.
3. Describe your feelings about life as a resident in a nursing home.
4. Discuss the pros and cons of using restraints to prevent falls.

## REFERENCES AND ADDITIONAL READINGS

Agency for Health Care Policy and Research: *Pressure ulcers in adults: prediction and prevention: clinical practice guideline*, Pub No 92-0048, Rockville, Md, 1992a, US Department of Health and Human Services AHCPR.

Agency for Health Care Policy and Research: *Urinary incontinence in adults: clinical practice guideline*, Pub No 92-0038, Rockville, Md, 1992b, US Department of Health and Human Services AHCPR.

Bergstrom N et al: Pressure ulcer treatment: quick reference guide for clinicians, *Adv Wound Care* 8(2):22-44, 1995.

Besdine R et al: *Medical care of the nursing home resident*, Philadelphia, 1996, American College of Physicians.

Cornacchione M, Slusser M: Depression in the long-term-care setting, *Nurs Home Med* 2(2):24-36, 1994.

Ebersole P, Hess P: *Toward healthy aging: human needs and nursing response*, ed 4, St Louis, 1994, Mosby.

Eisenberg MS et al: Cardiopulmonary resuscitation in the elderly, *Ann Intern Med* 113:408-409, 1990.

Evans LK, Strumpf NE: Patterns of restraint: a cross cultural view, *Gerontologist* 12:272, 1987.

Freeman I: Developing systems that promote autonomy: policy considerations. In Kane R, Caplan A, editors: *Everyday ethics: resolving dilemmas in nursing home life*, New York, 1990, Springer.

Mion LC, Strumpf N: Use of physical restraints in the hospital setting: implications for the nurse, *Geriatr Nurs* 15(3):127-132, 1994.

Neugarten B: *Middle age and aging*, Chicago, 1968, University of Chicago Press.

Rader J, Donius M: Leveling off restraints, *Geriatr Nurs* 12(2):71-73, 1991.

Seaver AMH: My world now, *Newsweek*, 123(26):11, 1994.

Semla T et al: Effect of the Omnibus Reconciliation Act 1987 on antipsychotic prescribing in nursing home residents, *J Am Geriatr Soc* 42:648-652, 1994.

Strumpf NE, Evans L: Physical restraints of hospitalized elderly: perceptions of patients and nurses, *Nurs Res* 37:132, 1988.

Tabloski PA et al: Effects of calming music on the level of agitation in cognitively impaired nursing home residents, *Am J Alzheimer Care Res* 10(1):10-15, 1995.

Thomason S: Front-line antiseptics, *Geriatr Nurs* 10(5):235-236, 1989.

Wells T, editor: The rehabilitation management of urinary incontinence, *Top Geriatr Rehabil* 3:1-77, 1988.

White M et al: Skin tears in frail elders: a practical approach to prevention, *Geriatr Nurs* 15(2):95-99, 1994.

# CHAPTER 19

# Home Health Care

## CHAPTER OBJECTIVES

1 Compare and contrast the definitions for home health care and community-focused nursing practice.
2 Identify various types of home care and community-focused providers.
3 List at least six types of services provided by home care agencies.
4 Summarize the historical development of community nursing services and the potential for the future.
5 Discuss the role of the client, family, and informal caregivers.
6 Discuss the roles and activities of team members, especially the nurse.
7 Describe how the nursing process can be used in community-focused practice.
8 Summarize the Omaha System and its use as a tool in community-focused practice.
9 Discuss sources of reimbursement for home care and community-focused services and how reimbursement issues influence nursing practice.

## KEY TERMS

| | |
|---|---|
| assessment | home health care |
| client | nursing process |
| client problem | Omaha System |
| community-focused | quality improvement |
| nursing practice | reimbursement |
| evaluation | team nursing |

"Remember that you are the *guest*." This message is both simple and profound. It should guide the practice of all nursing students and staff who work in the community and provide health-related services to individuals, families, groups, and geographic areas. Although roles and responsibilities vary dramatically, the following all apply to nurses employed in such settings:

1. Need a wide variety of technical and interpersonal skills.
2. Need to be motivated, organized, and honest and must use common sense.
3. Use various terms to describe the recipient of service: client, customer, resident, and patient. *Client* was selected for this chapter to emphasize that the person receiving care needs to be actively involved in health care plans and interventions.
4. Use various terms to describe the specialty. **Community-focused nursing practice,** an umbrella-like term, will be used in this chapter. It refers to the synthesis of nursing practice and public health principles that incorporate a comprehensive, culturally sensitive, and holistic approach to health care and includes services that range from health promotion and disease prevention to sickness care for individuals, families, groups, and communities. Nurses practice in community-focused home care agencies including those that are hospital based, visiting nurse associations, tax supported, and privately or corporately owned. Other settings are tax-supported public health departments, clinics, nursing centers, schools, wellness and occupational health centers, and parish- or church-based nursing programs. Because of the increase in mergers and the seamless approach to health care, more nurses are practicing in the community as employees of large, complex health care systems. As the roles of

nurses blur within these systems, nurses may need to be competent practitioners across the continuum of community, long-term care, and acute care settings.

5. Expect to work with diverse clients (i.e., age, medical and nursing diagnoses, race, religion, income, and values will vary).
6. Enjoy the independence of community-focused practice.
7. Always expect the unexpected!

## BETWEEN PHOEBE AND THE FUTURE

Nursing is the oldest of the arts and the youngest of the professions. Phoebe of Cenchrea (60 AD) is the first visiting nurse identified by name. Community care increased during the early centuries as women in religious orders were allowed by priests to visit homes and provide care outside the convents. St. Vincent de Paul has been credited with introducing the modern principles of visiting nursing and social service. In 1617 he founded the order in France that later became the Sisters of Charity. Over the years, the home continued to be the usual setting for health care; only those who were dying or had no other options were admitted to the "appalling" hospitals (Dolan, Fitzpatrick, Herrmann, 1983; Martin, Scheet, 1992a).

Near the end of the nineteenth century, immigration was at its peak, and thousands of persons arrived from various countries to settle in the United States. Epidemics of influenza, cholera, and other highly contagious diseases were rampant. Physicians were in short supply; it was the nurse who provided needed community-focused services.

In 1877 Francis Root was employed in New York City as the first home visit nurse. In 1893 Lillian Wald and Mary Brewster established the Henry Street Settlement in the same city. Their goal was to offer public health nursing and community-wide programs to population groups of all ages that were at high risk for developing health problems and to clients who had acute and chronic health problems. To accomplish that goal, they initiated a variety of programs at the Settlement and in neighborhood homes after obtaining support from business and political leaders. Collaboration between the Henry Street staff and the New York City Mission home visit staff followed and led to the formation of the Visiting Nurse Service of New York, the largest provider of home health care services in this country. Soon, organized home visit programs were established in populated areas along the East Coast (Figure 19-1). Lillian Wald spread her vision of preventive, curative, and social services for the entire community throughout New York City and the rest of

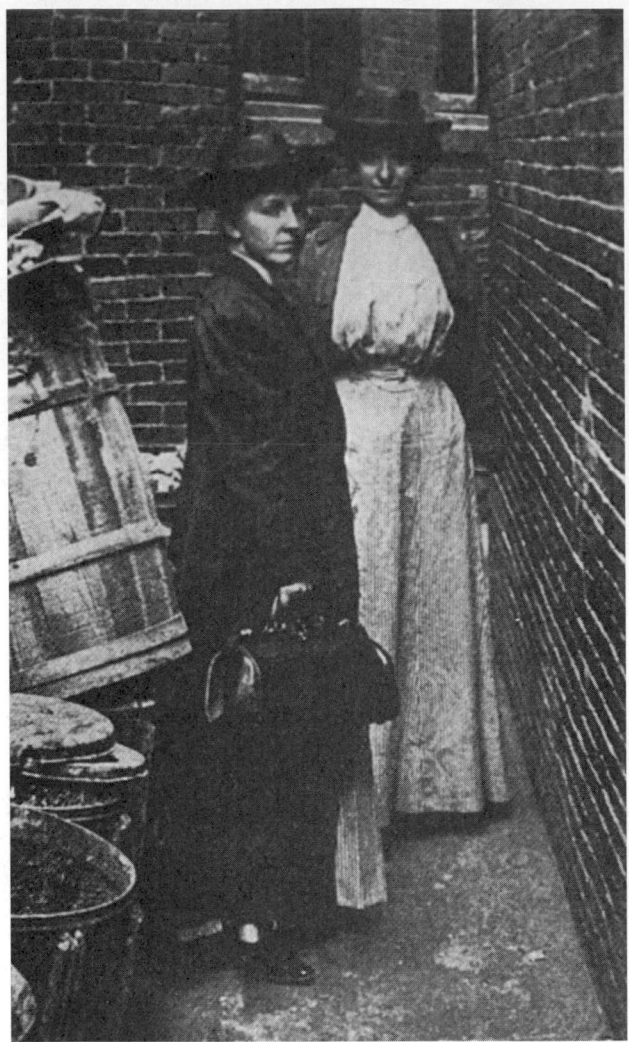

**Figure 19-1**   Two visiting nurses in Boston's North End, 1909. (Courtesy Boston Visiting Nurse Association, Boston. From the Nursing Archives Collection, Department of Special Collections, Boston University.)

the country. In 1912, 2500 nurses were employed by 900 independent visiting nurse associations (Dolan, Fitzpatrick, Herrmann, 1983; Stanhope, Lancaster, 1996).

By 1963 there were 1100 home health and home care aide organizations and hospices in the United States that employed professional registered nurses. The enactment of national Medicare legislation in 1965, the decrease in hospital lengths of stay, and the increase in the elderly population dramatically accelerated the rate of home care agency growth. In 1996, almost 19,000 home care agencies offered services to 7 million clients and accounted for expenditures of more than $36 billion nationally (National Association of Home Care, 1996). Seventeen percent of employed registered nurses (362,648 nurses) were employed by **home health care** and public health agencies. Another 8.5 percent (178,930 nurses) were employed in ambulatory care settings such as physician or nurse solo or group practices and health maintenance organizations (U.S. Department of Health and Human Services, 1996). Approximately 30,000 licensed practical or vocational nurses are employed in home care agencies (National Association of Home Care, 1996). The number of clients receiving Medicare-certified home health services more than doubled between 1991 and 1994. Circulatory system diseases, diabetes, and fractures were the most commonly occurring medical diagnoses for home care clients. These trends and the growth in the home care industry are expected to escalate dramatically as the shift from acute to community-focused care continues (Brown, Barram, Ehrilich, 1994; National Association of Home Care, 1996).

## THE TEAM

The **team** concept is essential for providing effective and economical health care services regardless of the setting. When community-focused services are provided, clients, families, and informal caregivers are the most critical team members. Typically, other team members include a variety of persons who are fulltime, part-time, or contractual employees and include nurses, home health aides and homemakers, therapists, medical social workers, physicians, registered dietitians, and pharmacists. Durable medical equipment is also included in this section; such equipment is important to many of the team members.

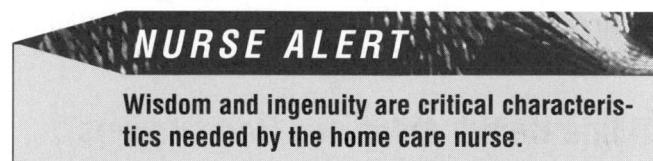

**NURSE ALERT**

Cultural competency is required by all members of the home care team.

### Clients, Families, and Informal Caregivers

**Clients** and their families and informal caregivers are the most powerful members of the team. As the hosts, they decide initially whether to invite the nurse, their guest, into their home. Clients have the power to decide if they will seek care at nursing centers, clinics, and school nurses' offices; they decide if they will return as requested. Clients, not nurses, own their health-related problems. Clients have the power to recognize and deal with their problems and the ability to alter their health status in positive or negative ways (Figure 19-2).

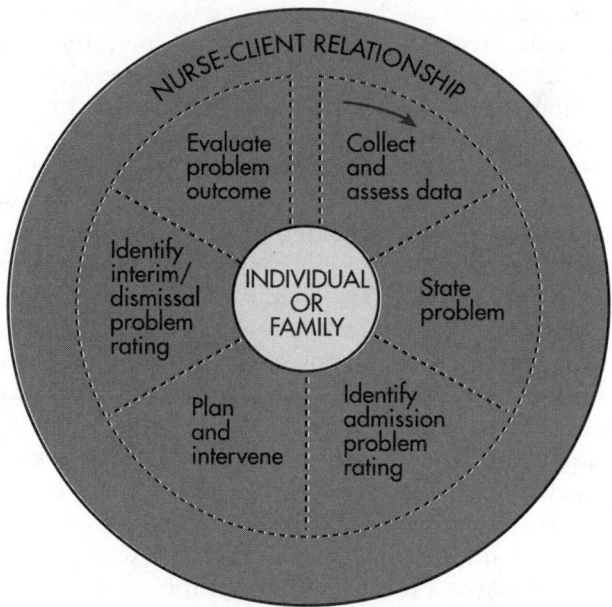

**Figure 19-2**   Conceptualization of the family nursing process. (Redrawn from Martin KS, Scheet NJ: *The Omaha System: applications for community health nursing*, Philadelphia, 1992, Saunders.)

### Nurses

Registered nurses make up the largest group of clinicians employed in community settings; home care agencies employ approximately half of these nurses. Many home care agencies employ associate, diploma, and baccalaureate graduates as well as licensed practical nurses, and some agencies employ advanced practice nurses prepared at the masters level. Some agencies require new staff to have experience in the acute care setting.

**NURSE ALERT**

Wisdom and ingenuity are critical characteristics needed by the home care nurse.

When agencies extended their hours of service to 24 hours a day, 7 days a week, many agencies changed their staffing patterns from a primary nurse or one nurse per geographic area model to a **team nursing** model. Often the baccalaureate-prepared and most experienced nurses serve as the team leaders and case managers, supervising an interdisciplinary team and coordinating the care of a large number of clients in a given geographic area. Typically, teams consist of five to eight members representing nursing, home health aides, therapists, and medical social work. Team members will vary when the team has a specialty focus such as infusion therapy, hospice, pediatric, or enterostomal services. Usually, a team leader or case manager develops a plan of care after obtaining preliminary information from the referral source, client and family, and/or physician. The team leader or case manager may make the admission visit to complete a holistic assessment, provide care, and then assign visits to team members. The team leader or case manager is responsible for all of the following: evaluation of the client's progress, the involvement of the family and informal caregivers, the care provided by the team members, documentation and orders, and the discharge plan. More details about the services frequently provided by nurses will be described later in this chapter.

Many community-focused nurses base their practice on the nursing process, a logical problem-solving or **quality-improvement** approach. The nursing process was suggested in the previous paragraph when the responsibilities of team leaders and case managers were described. For a review of the assessment, problem identification/diagnosis, plan, intervention, and evaluation steps of the nursing process, refer to Chapter 2.

Figure 19-2 depicts the client as the center or hub of the process. It is essential that nurses develop a partnership with clients and work closely with the client's family, significant others, friends, and informal caregivers (Reif, Martin, 1996). Often the nurse is alone when providing care in clients' homes, clinics, schools, or other settings. To practice effectively, efficiently, and safely, nurses need to use the nursing process and care plan, common sense, their nursing bags, and a number of other methods and types of equipment, some of which will be described in this chapter. Before practicing in the community, the professional care provider should become informed about tools that improve communication and safety such as cellular phones, beepers, and computers.

## Home Health Aides and Homemakers

Services provided by home health aides include personal care, assistance with activities of daily living, meal preparation, and bowel and bladder management. Based on educational preparation, agency policy, and other regulations, home health aides may also help with ambulation, perform some exercises, take vital signs, and complete other procedures. Many home health aides attend educational programs sponsored by home care agencies, hospitals, nursing homes, or technical colleges in order to meet employment requirements and become certified and registered. Certification programs usually require 90 to 120 hours of classroom and clinical training. However, because home health agency regulations for certification and registration vary markedly among the states, no basic level of competence can be assumed.

Many larger agencies employ both home health aides and homemakers. Homemakers prepare meals, clean, and take clients to physician and other appointments. They tend to have little or no formal training. The services provided by home health aides and homemakers are determined, scheduled, and supervised by registered nurses.

## Licensed Practical Nurses

The number of licensed practical (vocational) nurses (LPNs) employed by home care agencies varies across the U.S. Many agencies, including some of the largest agencies, do not employ LPNs. However, there is a trend to employ LPNs and bill their services to Medicare as a skilled nursing visit. When LPNs are part of the home care team, they are supervised by and report to registered nurses. Their responsibilities vary; some provide the same services as and are reimbursed as home health aides. In other agencies, LPNs are responsible for procedures such as wound care and dressing changes. For example, if a client requires daily visits, the LPN may visit twice a week and the registered nurse five times a week.

## Therapists

The term *therapists* is often used to describe physical therapists, occupational therapists, and speech and language pathologists. Therapists are educated at the baccalaureate or masters level and must meet registration or licensure regulations. Therapists may be full- or part-time agency employees; however, many provide home care services on a contractual basis.

Although therapy may be the primary reason for referral to home care or other community-focused service, it is usually the second service. Therefore the nurse's admission visit often precedes the therapist's visit. The therapist will complete a limited assessment of the client's status, develop a specialized care plan that becomes part of the total care plan, and provide services. As in other settings, physical therapists focus on range-of-motion exercises, strengthening exercises, and assistance with ambulation and mobility for clients who have fractures, strokes, or other debilitating conditions. Physical and occupational therapists collaborate as they assess the safety of the physical environment and offer suggestions to staff and clients about assistive devices, modifying room arrangements, or making structural changes. The assessment, care plan, and interventions of speech and language pathologists are designed to help the client remain in the home safely. The goal may be to increase speech and language skills through practice and exercises or it may be to obtain and use boards, computers, and assistive devices on the telephone or door.

## Medical Social Workers

Illness and injury are stressful for clients and their families. Social work and counseling services are designed to decrease stress in relation to loss or death, coping skills, moving, budgeting, and financial and other assistance from community resources. Although some agencies employ social workers prepared at the baccalaureate level, most prefer those prepared at the masters level.

## Physicians

Physicians participate in the home care referral process, provide initial medical orders for care, renew orders, and evaluate client progress with agency staff. Physicians often provide direct care and serve as consultants to public health departments. They also serve as consultants to nursing centers and accept referrals from nursing center staff.

## Registered Dietitians

Employment of registered dietitians in community-focused settings is directly related to the increase in clients who have cardiovascular disease and/or diabetes. Some registered dietitians are also providing wellness-oriented services.

## Pharmacists

Accepting a critical number of home visit referrals for intravenous antibiotics and chemotherapy has encouraged many agencies to consider adding a pharmacist and pharmacy department to their staff. The pharmacist may also participate on the hospice team and assist with pain control.

## Durable Medical Equipment

A supply of hospital beds, walkers, dressing supplies, catheters, and other equipment is maintained by the community-focused provider or is available through a contract with another durable medical equipment supplier. As earlier hospital discharges and the use of high technology increase the complexity of home care, the need for new insulin pumps as well as intravenous, ventilator, and ostomy equipment and supplies also

increases. Procedures for obtaining equipment and details related to purchase or lease options vary with the individual supplier and should be included in orientation for students and new employees.

# PROVIDING CARE

Many of the skills and procedures needed in home health care and other community-focused practice settings are similar to those needed in hospitals and residential long-term care facilities. As mergers and the seamless philosophy of health care delivery increase and length of stay decreases, it is even more important for nurses and other health care providers to have the skills needed to function across multiple settings. Details about pathophysiology, technical treatments, procedures, cultural considerations, and interpersonal skills for all settings are well described in other chapters of this book (see Chapters 8 and 9). Nurses who work in the community also share the needs and concerns related to data collection, documentation, and automation with nurses in other areas. The minimum data set for long-term care described in Chapter 18 has some similarities to the Omaha System described in this chapter.

Examples of ways that home care and community-focused practice differ from care in the hospital and other in-patient areas are described in this chapter and many other references (Martin, Scheet, 1992a; Stanhope, Lancaster, 1996). The following description of the Omaha System, the boxes, and the case study offer "how to" information, a beginning foundation for the student or new graduate who wants to provide services in the community setting. The organization of the "how-to" information is based on the **nursing process** and the Omaha System.

## The Omaha System

The **Omaha System** is an assessment care plan that is used by nurses. It is a research-based, comprehensive vocabulary intended to help users describe and measure their practice (Martin, Scheet, 1992a, b). The Omaha System was developed and refined during three Visiting Nurse Association (VNA) of Omaha research projects funded by the Division of Nursing of the U.S. Department of Health and Human Services between 1975 and 1986. Further research focusing on reliability, validity, and usability was funded by the National Institute for Nursing Research of the National Institutes of Health through a 1989 to 1993 RO-1 grant (Martin, Scheet, 1992a; Martin, Scheet, Stegman, 1993). The Omaha System exists in the public domain, so it is equally accessible to students, faculty, and other potential users. The Problem Classification Scheme, the

Intervention Scheme, and the Problem Rating Scale for Outcomes are the three components of the Omaha System.

The System is based on the dynamic, interactive nature of the nursing process, the nurse-client relationship, and related theories of diagnostic reasoning and clinical judgment. It follows principles of taxonomy and consists of terms and codes arranged from general to specific. Terms are intended to be simple, clear, and concise. The System can be used by members of various disciplines in multiple settings to facilitate practice, documentation, and information management.

The Omaha System is one of the four vocabularies recognized and disseminated by the American Nurses Association (Lang, 1995). When implemented in a practice setting, the Omaha System is a model or tool that can be used to introduce new staff to the world of community-focused nursing through a standardized, easily understood system of client problems, nursing interventions, and client outcomes. For experienced staff, it is a series of cues or feedback loops that helps remind the user about possible client problem and intervention options and ways to evaluate the effect of the care provided. Data generated by using the Omaha System in manual or automated client records can provide clinicians, administrators, and researchers with critical information. These clinical data can be converted into trends that can be used to improve practice, facilitate communication, complete reports, meet accreditation

---

**BOX 19-1**

### EXAMPLES FROM THE PROBLEM CLASSIFICATION SCHEME

**11. GRIEF:**
Health promotion
Potential impairment
Impairment
01. Fails to recognize normal grief responses
02. Difficulty coping with grief responses
03. Difficulty expressing grief responses
04. Conflicting stages of grief process among family/individual
05. Other

**29. CIRCULATION:**
Health promotion
Potential impairment
Impairment
01. Edema
02. Cramping/pain of extremities
03. Decreased pulses
04. Discoloration of skin/cyanosis
05. Temperature change in affected area
06. Varicosities
07. Syncopal episodes
08. Abnormal blood pressure reading
09. Pulse deficit
10. Irregular heart rate
11. Excessively rapid heart rate
12. Excessively slow heart rate
13. Anginal pain
14. Abnormal heart sounds/murmurs
15. Other

**27. NEUROMUSCULOSKELETAL FUNCTION:**
Health promotion
Potential impairment
Impairment
01. Limited range of motion
02. Decreased muscle strength
03. Decreased coordination
04. Decreased muscle tone
05. Increased muscle tone
06. Decreased sensation
07. Increased sensation
08. Decreased balance
09. Gait/ambulation disturbance
10. Difficulty managing activities of daily living
11. Tremors/seizures
12. Other

**35. NUTRITION:**
Health promotion
Potential impairment
Impairment
01. Weighs 10% more than average
02. Weighs 10% less than average
03. Lacks established standards for daily caloric/fluid intake
04. Exceeds established standards for daily caloric/fluid intake
05. Unbalanced diet
06. Improper feeding schedule for age
07. Nonadherence to prescribed diet
08. Unexplained/progressive weight loss
09. Hypoglycemia
10. Hyperglycemia
11. Other

requirements, plan new agency programs, and interface with other, non-clinical information within the agency's management information system.

## Problem Classification Scheme

The Problem Classification Scheme is a taxonomy of **client problems** or nursing diagnoses that was developed from actual client data. The Scheme provides a comprehensive method for collecting, sorting, classifying, documenting, and analyzing client concerns and problems. It helps the user separate essential from nonessential data and identify patterns in those data.

The Problem Classification Scheme consists of four levels: domains, problems, modifiers, and signs/symptoms. The domains and problems appear in Box 19-1. The four domains or the first level of the Scheme are general areas that represent community-focused practice and provide organizational groupings for client problems. The domains are Environmental, Psychosocial, Physiological, and Health- Related Behaviors. Client problems, the next level, are the 40 nursing diagnoses that represent matters of difficulty and concern that historically, presently, or potentially adversely affect any aspect of the client's well-being. Modifiers and signs/symptoms appear at the third and fourth levels (Martin, Scheet, 1992a; Martin, Norris, 1996). Grief, neuromusculoskeletal function, circulation, and nutrition are examples of client problems; those problems, their modifiers, and their signs/symptoms are depicted in Box 19-1. In addition, use of the Problem Classification Scheme is illustrated by the case study below and Table 19-1.

## Intervention Scheme

The Intervention Scheme is a systematic arrangement of nursing actions or activities designed to help users identify and document plans and interventions in relation to specific client problems and other concepts of the nursing process. The Scheme represents a research-based effort to link the effectiveness of interventions with diagnoses, an effort not yet accomplished within the nursing profession (Martin, Scheet, 1992a; Martin, Norris, 1996; Bowles, Naylor, 1996).

The first level of the Intervention Scheme comprises four comprehensive categories: Health Teaching,

---

## CASE STUDY

10/20 (Data from referral form): John Smith, age 72, had a mild, left-sided stroke 4 days ago. He now has slight weakness and numbness of right hand and foot. He was newly diagnosed with hypertension and is overweight. He is independent and may be noncompliant. He lives with his wife and is to be discharged from the hospital today.

Orders: Evaluation visit: Assess cardiovascular and neuromuscular status, assess home, assess medication administration. Provide appropriate teaching. Then visit 3 times a week for the first week; 2 times a week for the next 3 weeks to evaluate status, report changes, and continue teaching. See med list.

10/21 (Admission Visit with Julie Jones, RN, BSN): Sarah Smith greets Julie and asks her to come in. As Julie enters, she smells something baking in the oven. Mrs. Smith explains that it is her husband's favorite custard pie. Julie meets John Smith and sits near him. While asking if she may check him over, she opens her bag and takes out her equipment. The couple looks rather annoyed by the entire process. After taking his blood pressure, pulse, and temperature, she measures his ankles and checks him for edema. When Julie asks for their bathroom scale, Mrs. Smith has to search for it. Julie places the scale near another chair and wall. She watches Mr. Smith walk, noticing that his right toe drags and he has other characteristics of a typical hemiplegic gait. Mr. Smith reports that he is 5' 8" tall and weighed 235 pounds in the hospital. Julie talks to the Smiths about his assessment: blood pressure 180/102 and decreased pulses in the lower extremities. She indicates that Mr. Smith is at high risk for having another stroke, noting that this must be difficult for both Mr. and Mrs. Smith. Mrs. Smith raises her voice and says, "If everyone would just leave us alone, John would be okay." Mr. Smith looks surprised and responds to his wife that she knows that is not true, that they both know that he has a serious problem. Mr. Smith admits that he is angry about the lifestyle changes the doctor told him were necessary and the way the doctor talked to him. However, he is beginning to realize the dangers of his present situation and appreciates Julie's genuine concern. During the remainder of the visit, Julie and the Smiths identify initial ways they can work together to decrease Mr. Smith's symptoms, manage his medications, and modify his diet. Julie discusses the teaching guide, *Stroke: Recognizing Symptoms and Risk* (Martin et al, 1998), with the Smiths. The terminology and layout of education materials such as this guide are intended to be client friendly. Julie asks the Smiths to leave the guide on their refrigerator door or in another conspicuous location so they will think about it and make notes when appropriate. Julie plans to discuss the teaching guide during her next visit and use additional guides as appropriate. Mrs. Smith is hesitant but does admit that she had hidden the scale because of her own weight problem, and that she may at high risk for cardiovascular problems.

| TABLE 19-1 | | | | |
| --- | --- | --- | --- | --- |
| **Applying the Nursing Process and the Omaha System** | | | | |
| DOMAIN | CLIENT DATA | PROBLEMS AND SIGNS/SYMPTOMS | RATINGS | INTERVENTIONS |
| Psychosocial | Mrs. Smith raises voice: "If everyone would just leave us alone, John would be okay." Mr. Smith looks surprised; responds to wife that she knows that is not true, they both know that he has a serious problem. Mr. Smith: angry about lifestyle changes doctor told him were necessary and way doctor talked to him. Is beginning to realize the dangers of present situation and appreciates Julie's genuine concern. | 11. Grief: actual/family problem<br>03. Difficulty expressing grief responses<br>04. Conflicting stages of grief process among family/individual | Knowledge = 2<br>Behavior = 2<br>Status = 3 | I. Health teaching, guidance, and counseling<br>10. Communication<br>IV. Surveillance<br>11. Coping skills |
| Physiologic | Mild, left-handed stroke 4 days ago; slight weakness and numbness of right hand and foot. Newly diagnosed hypertension; BP 180/102. Decreased pulses in lower extremities. | 29. Circulation: actual/individual problem<br>03. Decreased pulses<br>08. Abnormal blood pressure reading | Knowledge = 2<br>Behavior = 2<br>Status = 2 | I. Health teaching, guidance, and counseling<br>07. Cardiac care<br>50. Signs/symptoms—physical<br>II. Treatments and procedures<br>50. Signs/symptoms—physical<br>IV. Surveillance<br>50. Signs/symptoms—physical |

Guidance, and Counseling; Treatments and Procedures; Case Management; and Surveillance (Box 19-2). One or more categories are used to develop a plan or document an intervention specific to a client problem. The second level of the Scheme is an alphabetical listing of 62 targets. Targets are defined as objects of nursing intervention or nursing activities that serve to further describe problem-specific intervention categories. For the problem—Grief—and the intervention category—Health Teaching, Guidance, and Counseling—a possible target is communication. For the category Surveillance, a possible target is coping skills. For Circulation and the intervention category Health Teaching, Guidance, and Counseling, possible targets are cardiac care and signs/symptoms—physical. The target signs/symptoms—physical, is also useful for the intervention categories Treatments and Procedures and Surveillance. The third level of the Intervention Scheme is designed for client-specific information. Pertinent, concise words or phrases are generated by

users as they develop plans or document care provided to a specific client. Although not part of the research projects, VNA of Omaha staff organized their suggestions into care planning guides (Martin, Scheet, 1992b). Refer to the case study and Table 19-1 for suggestions about how to use the Intervention Scheme.

## Problem Rating Scale for Outcomes

The Problem Rating Scale for Outcomes is a framework for measuring problem-specific knowledge, behavior, and status relative to a client (see Box 19-1). The Scale is intended to measure client progress and to provide both a guide for practice and a method of documentation. The Scale was designed for use throughout the time of client service. When establishing the initial ratings for client problems, the user creates an independent data baseline, capturing the condition and circumstances of the client at a given point in time.

| BOX 19-2 | NURSING PROCESS |
| --- | --- |

## THE OMAHA SYSTEM

**ASSESSMENT AND NURSING DIAGNOSES**

**Environmental Domain**

- Income
- Sanitation
- Residence
- Neighborhood/workplace safety
- Other

**Psychosocial Domain**

- Communication with community resources
- Social contact
- Role change
- Interpersonal relationship
- Spirituality
- Grief
- Emotional stability
- Human sexuality
- Caretaking/parenting
- Neglected child/adult
- Abused child/adult
- Growth and development
- Other

**Physiologic Domain**

- Hearing
- Vision
- Speech and language
- Dentition
- Cognition
- Pain
- Consciousness
- Integument

- Neuromusculoskeletal function
- Respiration
- Circulation
- Digestion-hydration
- Bowel function
- Genitourinary function
- Antepartum/postpartum
- Other

**Health-Related Behaviors Domain**

- Nutrition
- Sleep and rest patterns
- Physical activity
- Personal hygiene
- Substance use
- Family planning
- Health care supervision
- Prescribed medication regimen
- Technical procedure
- Other

**NURSING INTERVENTIONS**

- Provide health teaching, counseling, and guidance.
- Ensure that patient understands treatments and procedures.
- Provide case management.
- Provide surveillance.

**EVALUATION OF EXPECTED OUTCOMES**

- Knowledge
- Behavior
- Status

This admission baseline is used to compare and contrast the client's condition and circumstances with the ratings completed at later intervals and at client dismissal. The comparison or change in ratings over time can be used to identify client progress in relation to interventions and the effectiveness of the plan of care (Martin, Scheet, 1992a; Martin, Norris, 1996).

The Problem Rating Scale for Outcomes is made up of Knowledge, Behavior, and Status subscales. Knowledge is the ability of the client to remember and interpret information. Behavior is the observable responses, actions, or activities of the client fitting the occasion or purpose. Status is the condition of the client in relation to objective and subjective defining characteristics. The scale for each of the concepts has five categories or degrees for response. For example, for the problems Grief and Circulation, the nurse would identify baseline Knowledge, Behavior, and Status ratings during the first home or clinic visit as illustrated by the case study and Table 19-1.

## Using the Omaha System

The relationships among the nursing process, the Omaha System, and practice in community settings will be described in the following paragraphs.

A community health nurse begins service to a client following an intake or referral process. During a nurse's initial visit and all other visits, the vital importance of establishing and maintaining a positive nurse-client relationship is recognized. Freeman and Heinrich (1981) emphasized that a positive relationship is developed, not discovered. Such a relationship promotes quantity and quality of data and enhances the potential for success and client progress in relation to all components of the nursing process.

A nurse's initial activities include data collection, **assessment,** and analysis (i.e., Problem Classification Scheme). This process involves gathering, clustering, combining, summarizing, and validating diverse subjective and objective information relative to each family member, the family as an interacting unit, and the sociocultural and physical environment. A community health nurse uses principles of epidemiology to enhance systematic data collection and assessment and to identify patterns within client data. The conclusion and logical end product of the data collection and assessment process is problem identification or diagnosis, which involves interpretation of the acquired data.

Planning and intervening are two of the most important concepts of the model to both a client and a nurse (i.e., Intervention Scheme). Campbell (1984) described a broad interpretation of planning and intervention involving nurse and family collaboration to:

- Set priorities
- Identify client status and expected outcomes—outcome criteria or goals relative to specific nursing problems and time frames
- Delineate alternative courses of action
- Choose and take action

Identification of admission, interim, and dismissal ratings quantifies the **evaluation** process (i.e., Problem Rating Scale for Outcomes). Each rating provides a baseline for contrast with later ratings during the period of client service. The evaluation component of the Omaha System allows a nurse to compare a client's health status at different points in time to determine the degree of nursing effectiveness. Through evaluation, a nurse has feedback that can be used to revise and modify plans and interventions with an individual, family, or group. Thus evaluation is both ongoing and terminal (Martin, Scheet, 1992a).

## Nurses' Challenges

The case study and Table 19-1 illustrate challenges experienced by nurses who provide community-focused services. The case study was not intended to depict cultural, safety, documentation, reimbursement, or length-of-stay challenges. However, it does depict examples of typical services home care nurses provide, as well as the benefits of using the nursing

process and the Omaha System. In reviewing the case study, note that the nursing process and Omaha System are used to guide practice and organize documentation.

In the case study, Julie Jones demonstrated the technical, interpersonal, and health education competence of a skilled nurse. Through nonverbal and verbal cues, the Smiths reminded Julie that she was the guest and they were the hosts. Julie was calm and was not offended or judgmental, factors that contributed to her success with the Smiths. She expects less resistance when she returns on the next visit, and she will develop a plan accordingly for that visit. However, just as for the first visit, she always expects the unexpected.

In addition to the time spent during the visit, Julie has responsibilities after the visit. She will document care as well as time, mileage, and other details in accordance with her agency's policies. Table 19-1 is an example of the type of data that will be included in a client record. This information will also be shared with the referral source, the physician, and agency colleagues as appropriate.

## REIMBURSEMENT

The escalating cost of health care is receiving extensive public scrutiny and is changing health care delivery patterns. Refer to Chapter 1 for general information about reimbursement, including private pay and third-party payers such as Medicare, Medicaid, managed care and health maintenance organizations, and private insurance companies.

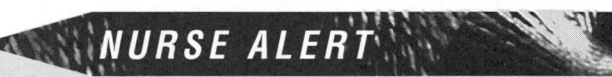

**NURSE ALERT**

For the agency to be reimbursed under Medicare the patient must be homebound and have a physician's approval for the care plan.

Community-focused nurses must be well informed about **reimbursement.** When nursing students or new staff begin providing care in the community, they can expect to learn about reimbursement pertinent to their clients, agency, community, and state. Reimbursement information is an important part of orientation, just as are sessions about technical and interpersonal skills, safety, documentation, durable medical equipment, and community resources.

Helping clients and their families understand their benefits, complete forms, and obtain services and supplies are responsibilities of nurses as well as social workers. At the time of referral, nurses usually collect financial data, discuss options for payment, and ask clients or family members to accept and sign for financial responsibility if third-party payers do not pay their bills. Throughout the period of service, nurses help clients and family members understand complex regulations and their reimbursement status, discuss bills from third-party payers and the agency, and consider alternative sources of reimbursement or service if needed. For example, when clients are no longer eligible for Medicare-reimbursed visits, they may need to arrange for personal care services in order to remain in their homes.

Reimbursement is a critical factor in determining whether clients are eligible for community-focused services. For example, many public health departments, nursing centers, and clinics offer services only to those whose incomes are below a specified guideline. Home care agencies also determine the source of reimbursement before accepting referrals. Increasingly, third-party payers such as managed care and insurance companies require agencies to request prior approval for services and authorize only a specific number or certain types of visits. Thus the nurse, physician, or other health care provider may have limited control over the length of stay. Non-profit home care agencies may receive United Way and other contributions annually, which they can use to provide services to some clients. However, the amount of these funds is usually less than needed for the number of requests for services.

Community-focused services are funded in many ways, and every funding source has specific reimbursement regulations. In addition, variation occurs across geographic areas, especially state lines. Many public health and school health programs are supported primarily by local, state, and/or national taxes and block grants. Persons who have Medicaid benefits receive services from both public health and home care providers. United Way funds, donations from foundations and other groups, fundraising efforts, and private payments have covered a decreasing portion of services over the years.

Beginning with the inception of Medicare in 1966, the home health benefit has been the primary source of reimbursement for services provided by home care agencies. The home health benefit provides for post-hospital services under Part A and services not associated with hospitalization under Part B. The benefits that are available to the recipient of home care services, the charges that recipients must pay, and the reimbursement to home care agencies have varied, with numerous changes in regulations since 1966. Since 1973, agencies have been required to follow the current home health conditions of participation to receive

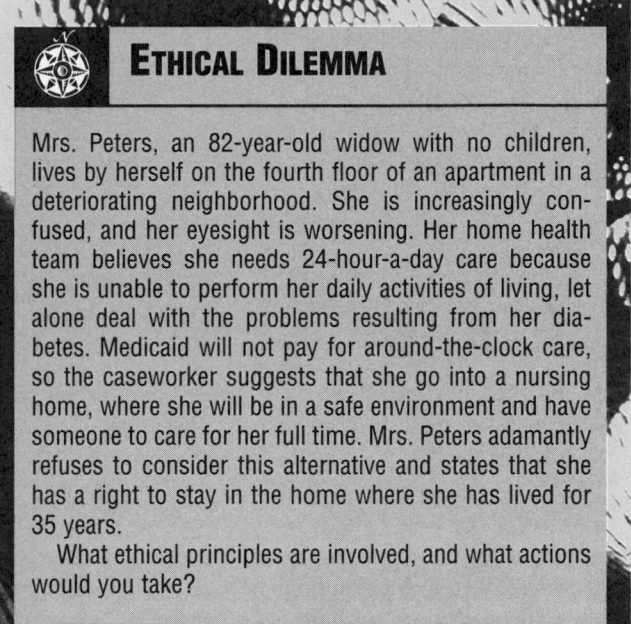

**ETHICAL DILEMMA**

Mrs. Peters, an 82-year-old widow with no children, lives by herself on the fourth floor of an apartment in a deteriorating neighborhood. She is increasingly confused, and her eyesight is worsening. Her home health team believes she needs 24-hour-a-day care because she is unable to perform her daily activities of living, let alone deal with the problems resulting from her diabetes. Medicaid will not pay for around-the-clock care, so the caseworker suggests that she go into a nursing home, where she will be in a safe environment and have someone to care for her full time. Mrs. Peters adamantly refuses to consider this alternative and states that she has a right to stay in the home where she has lived for 35 years.

What ethical principles are involved, and what actions would you take?

reimbursement. For example, the conditions require that a client must require a skilled service, be homebound, and need intermittent services rather than long-term care. During the 1990s concern about escalating health care costs, including home health costs, resulted in significant changes. Managed care enrollment has decreased home care agency's Medicare reimbursement from 90% or 95% to as little as 50% in some states. Currently, the home health conditions of participation are being reviewed; possible revisions focus on patient rights, quality assessment, and performance improvement. Reimbursement for home care may also be changed. Possibilities include a prospective payment system that might be comparable to the diagnostic-related group system developed for hospitals. An alternative is a capitated reimbursement system that would offer agencies a set sum of money for each client; in return, the agency would provide all services needed by that client (Buerhaus, 1997; Garg, Pinsker, Grace, 1997; Martin, Martin, 1997).

Since the onset of the Medicare home care benefit, sickness care has been emphasized and prevention has become the responsibility of public health providers. That distinction is changing as managed care reimbursement increases: managed care companies want their enrollees to improve their health, prevent illness, and limit the amount of expensive sickness care they require. Therefore managed care is changing the type of programs agencies offer, their need for valid and reliable clinical data, and the types of clients they serve (Martin, Martin, 1997).

## THE FUTURE

Without a crystal ball, it is difficult to make predictions about the future of home care and other community-focused services. Many persons believe that the number of agencies, staff, and clients will continue to escalate because of the aging population and the trend toward less institutionalization. They predict this growth despite efforts to curb the total costs of home health care by third-party payers and legislators. Custodial or long-term care remains a dilemma: such services are not covered by Medicare and yet are needed by a growing number of persons.

## KEY CONCEPTS

➤ Nurses and members of other disciplines who provide community-focused services are employed by home care agencies, public health departments, nursing centers, schools, and other agencies.

➤ Home care and public health nursing have a long and distinguished history.

➤ Clients and their families and informal caregivers are the most powerful members of the community-focused team.

➤ Nurses, home health aides, homemakers, therapists, medical social workers, physicians, registered dietitians, and pharmacists are often members of the community-focused delivery team.

➤ Community-focused services should reflect the needs and values of clients and their families.

➤ The steps of the nursing process and the Omaha System offer a logical, comprehensive approach to the delivery of care and the documentation of services in the community.

➤ Reimbursement issues influence the delivery of services in the community.

## CRITICAL THINKING EXERCISES

1. Compare the case study and Table 19-1. Explain the nurse's steps between collecting data and identifying the two problems listed in Table 19-1. Explain why Neuromusculoskeletal and Nutrition are also identified as problems in the chapter.

2. Compare the case study and Table 19-1. Identify what cues in the case study motivated the nurse to provide the specific interventions and to select the PRSO ratings listed in Table 19-1. Discuss why you do or do not agree with those choices.

3. You are a student in a nursing center and will be responsible for Jane Doe's health history, physical assessment, and health education when she comes for her appointment tomorrow. Jane is fourteen years old, pregnant, and has a different cultural background than yours. How will you prepare for this assignment?

4. You are going to change a urinary catheter in the home. Describe what challenges you may face that you probably would not experience in the hospital.

5. How can you know if your client who has diabetes mellitus gives his insulin injections correctly, eats a reasonable diet, and follows your other instructions?

# REFERENCES AND ADDITIONAL READINGS

Bowles KH, Naylor, MD: Nursing intervention classification systems, *Image* 28(4):303-308, 1996.

Brown R, Barram D, Ehrlich E: *Statistical abstract of the United States 1994* (Bureau of the Census, ed 114), Washington, DC, 1994, US Department of Commerce, Economics, and Statistics Administration.

Buerhaus PL: How changes in payment systems are affecting nurses. In McCloskey JC, Grace HK, editors: *Current issues in nursing*, ed 5, St Louis, 1997, Mosby.

Campbell C: *Nursing diagnosis and intervention in nursing practice*, ed 2, New York, 1984, Wiley.

Dolan JA, Fitzpatrick ML, Herrmann EK: *Nursing in society: a historical perspective*, ed 15, Philadelphia, 1983, Saunders.

Freeman R, Heinrich J: *Community health nursing practice*, ed 2, Philadelphia, 1981, Saunders.

Garg ML, Pinsker E, Grace HK: Controlling health care costs: regulation versus competition. In McCloskey JC, Grace HK, editors: *Current issues in nursing*, ed 5, St Louis, 1997, Mosby.

Lang NM, editor: *Nursing data systems: the emerging framework*, Washington, DC, 1995, American Nurses Publishing.

Martin KS, Martin DL: How can the quality of nursing practice be measured? In McCloskey JC, Grace HK, editors: *Current issues in nursing*, ed 5, St Louis, 1997, Mosby.

Martin KS, Norris J: The Omaha System: a model for describing practice, *Holist Nurs Pract* 11(1):75-83, 1996.

Martin KS, Scheet NJ: *The Omaha System: applications for community health nursing*, Philadelphia, 1992a, Saunders.

Martin KS, Scheet NJ: *The Omaha System: a pocket guide for community health nursing*, Philadelphia, 1992b, Saunders.

Martin KS, Scheet NJ, Stegman MR: Home health clients: characteristics, outcomes of care, and nursing interventions, *Am J Public Health* 83(12):1730-1734, 1993.

Martin KS et al: *Mosby's home health client teaching guides: Rx for teaching*, St Louis, 1998, Mosby.

National Association for Home Care: *Basic statistics about home care 1996*, Washington, DC, 1996, The Association.

Reif LJ, Martin KS: *Nurses and consumers: partners in assuring quality in the home*, Washington, DC, 1996, American Nurses Publishing.

Stanhope M, Lancaster J, editors: *Community health nursing: process and practice for promoting health*, ed 4, St Louis, 1996, Mosby.

US Department of Health and Human Services, Bureau of Health Professions, Division of Nursing: *Advance notes II from the National Sample Survey of Registered Nurses*, March, 1996, Rockville, Md (unpublished data).

# CHAPTER 20

# Perioperative Care

## CHAPTER OBJECTIVES

1 Identify four reasons for undergoing surgery.
2 Discuss four negative effects of surgery.
3 Describe the criteria for and the advantages of outpatient surgery.
4 State the major goal of preoperative preparation.
5 Describe the general preoperative preparation of the surgical patient.
6 Identify special considerations for the surgical patient who is obese or older or who has diabetes.
7 Explain surgical asepsis.
8 Describe the roles of the perioperative team.
9 List the common types of anesthesia techniques and their uses.
10 Discuss nursing responsibilities in patient care immediately after surgery.
11 Identify nursing measures that can be used to decrease postoperative discomfort.
12 Explain nursing responsibilities when dealing with the major complications of surgical intervention.
13 Discuss discharge planning for the surgical patient.

## KEY TERMS

| | |
|---|---|
| airway | laparoscopic gastrointestinal |
| ambulation | surgery |
| anesthesia | pain management |
| asepsis | postanesthesia care unit |
| atelectasis | recovery room |
| autoclave | sterilization |
| body image | surgical procedure |
| dehiscence | thrombosis |
| embolism | total parenteral nutrition |
| evisceration | (TPN) |
| hemorrhage | wound healing |
| hypothermia | wound infection |

## THE SURGICAL EXPERIENCE

Modern surgery has alleviated many diseases that in past generations had crippled or killed people. Surgery is performed to arrest or eliminate disease or illness. Surgical procedures are also used for the purposes of examination and reconstruction (Box 20-1). The meaning of surgery varies with each individual, but it is generally a frightening experience to even the most prepared person. Surgery invades one's most intimate privacy. Therefore confidence in the physician, the nurse, and other health care workers is an important aspect of helping the patient cope during this time of need.

**Surgical procedures** may be classified in several ways. A surgical procedure may be done as an emergency or may be scheduled in advance. It may be necessary to save a life, or it may be an optional (elective) procedure that is intended to improve health. Elective surgery can be scheduled in advance, which allows the

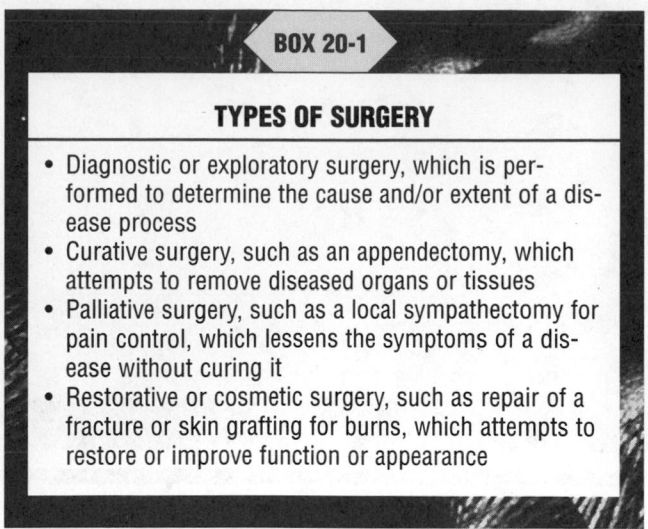

### TYPES OF SURGERY

- Diagnostic or exploratory surgery, which is performed to determine the cause and/or extent of a disease process
- Curative surgery, such as an appendectomy, which attempts to remove diseased organs or tissues
- Palliative surgery, such as a local sympathectomy for pain control, which lessens the symptoms of a disease without curing it
- Restorative or cosmetic surgery, such as repair of a fracture or skin grafting for burns, which attempts to restore or improve function or appearance

individual to prepare for it physically and psychologically. Knowing the purpose and anticipated outcomes of various surgical procedures can help the nurse to educate and support the patient more effectively.

## Negative Effects of Surgery
### Stress

The stress response describes a complex physiologic and psychologic reaction to any external or internal threat to the body's equilibrium. This response can result in profound neurochemical changes in the body. These changes initially help the body cope with the invasive reality of surgery, but if the stress response is too severe or prolonged, the body's defenses become depleted and the immune response is suppressed. Organ failure, infection, and life-threatening electrolyte imbalance can occur. The nurse can minimize the potential for these negative effects of stress by identifying factors (other than the surgical experience) that may be contributing to the patient's concern. Careful preoperative preparation and teaching by the nurse greatly lessen the patient's anxiety. During the preoperative period, the surgeon and the anesthetist carefully evaluate any other physical conditions that may increase the risk related to surgery, such as electrolyte imbalance, diabetes, liver or renal disease, anemia, lung and heart disorders, malnutrition, obesity, or emotional instability.

### Increased Susceptibility to Infection

Intact skin is the body's first line of defense against bacterial invasion. When the skin is surgically incised, the risk of a local infection greatly increases. Suppression of the immune system caused by stress and breaks in skin integrity make infection a real possibility for every surgical patient. Antibiotic therapy may be prescribed prophylactically, but meticulous surgical and postsurgical aseptic techniques are the keys to preventing infection.

## Potential Body Image Changes

**Body image** (subjective feelings about personal appearance) is formed early in life. A surgical procedure may significantly alter this self-perception. Operations that cause a visible change in an individual, such as amputation of a body part, involve not only a physical but also a psychologic loss. The removal of organs that have an emotional and social importance, such as the uterus or testicles, may also profoundly affect a patient despite the fact that there is no visible evidence of change. In some cases, such as cosmetic and reconstructive surgeries, these changes are positive and are desired by the patient. The nurse can help a patient who is undergoing a surgical procedure that may affect body image by encouraging him or her to express any concerns. A number of community support groups exist, such as ostomy clubs and branches of Reach to Recovery for women who have had mastectomies.

## Disruption of Life-Style

Every person who undergoes a major surgical procedure experiences at least a temporary change in lifestyle. A person's career, job security, and social activities may be jeopardized if rehabilitation is prolonged or if normal function has been permanently altered. The nurse can often help the patient identify these potential changes and develop coping strategies and can give referrals to appropriate agencies and resources.

## Spiritual Distress

Spirituality is a uniquely human characteristic. It is a broad concept that represents an individual's search for the meaning of life and death, and it should be considered by nurses when caring for patients who are about to have surgery. Often these issues are not confronted until a patient faces serious illness and the possibility of death. Although some patients may be quite open in expressing their beliefs in a higher power and may find strength and support in this practice, many others exhibit only subtle clues to the state of their spiritual need. Patients may ask the nurse to describe personal beliefs about an afterlife, or they may ask if there is a chaplain in the hospital. It is important to allow patients to discuss these issues and to determine if spiritual support would be useful. To do this comfortably, nurses need to examine their own spirituality. Some nurses may offer to pray with patients or to pray privately for them at a later time. It is very important to support the patient and facilitate personal expressions of spirituality.

## Objectives of Surgical Nursing

The objective of surgical nursing is to prepare the patient mentally and physically for surgery and to assist in full recovery in the shortest time possible and with the least discomfort. The nursing care of surgical patients is a step-by-step process that begins before the patient is admitted to the hospital and ends when recovery is complete and the patient returns to an optimal personal state of health. The nurse who cares for surgical patients needs to have a broad understanding of individual reactions to the surgical procedure. Most surgical patients experience fear and anxiety, and the nurse must be able to recognize the verbal and nonverbal expressions of these emotions and respond in a helping manner. Open communication must be maintained among the nurse, patient, family, and surgeon. The nurse can assist the patient and family by reporting appropriate concerns and questions to the surgeon as they arise or by encouraging the patient to do so. The nurse must possess a wide range of technical skills and keen sense of critical observation. The line between safety and danger in the care of many surgical patients, especially older patients, may be narrow. The alert nurse must recognize early signs of impending complications and report them so that preventive measures may be taken.

## Outpatient Surgery

In the past, a patient needing elective surgery that could not be done in the physician's office was admitted to the hospital for preoperative testing and preparation 1 or more days before the surgery. Many of these surgical procedures are now performed with the patient being admitted, treated, and discharged on the same day. These outpatient (same-day) surgeries have the following advantages:

1. Reduced stress because the patient is not hospitalized and because the atmosphere in these units is generally informal and relaxed
2. Lower costs, which benefit the individual and health care insurers, including industry and government

However, not all surgeries can be done on an outpatient basis (Box 20-2). Although outpatient surgical procedures may not be as extensive as those that take place in the traditional surgical setting, the role and re-

---

**BOX 20-2**

### CRITERIA FOR OUTPATIENT SURGERY

| Patient | Procedure |
|---|---|
| Accepts the idea of outpatient surgery | Is elective and does not produce severe alterations in physiologic status |
| Can follow postoperative discharge instructions | Does not require acute or intensive postoperative care, such as transfusions or intensive monitoring |
| Has a home environment and support system that fosters early postoperative recovery at home | Generally causes only minimal pain that can be managed by oral analgesics |
| Has no other medical conditions that pose a serious risk for home recovery | |

---

sponsibilities of the nurse remain challenging. The nurse still needs to assess and teach the patient and plan for the patient's discharge. All these objectives must be accomplished in a short time. Ideally patient assessment and teaching can occur several days before the procedure when the patient comes to the hospital or freestanding surgical clinic for preoperative diagnostic testing. A telephone interview *and* written assessment and discharge planning forms also help make the outpatient surgical experience safe and satisfactory for the patient.

## ADMISSION OF THE PATIENT

Surgical patients who are admitted to the hospital in emergency situations may be suffering from traumatic injuries received in an accident or from conditions that require immediate surgery, such as acute appendicitis. In these instances, patients may be taken to the operating room with limited preparation. In the absence of an emergency, patients are usually admitted on the morning of surgery according to prearranged plans made by the surgeon. Many patients are admitted for only a few hours to the outpatient unit. The necessary presurgery testing is completed before admission to the hospital. If diagnostic studies or specialized care is required, the patient may be admitted several days before surgery.

The nurse should be ready to receive the patient at the time of admission; a friendly, interested, and unhurried attitude helps the patient feel secure. The physical condition of the patient should be assessed, and the patient should be given a complete orientation to the unit. The nurse should be alert to any fears or apprehensions expressed by the patient and should transmit such information to the surgeon. The patient and family should be encouraged to communicate freely with the physician.

A complete history (including previous illnesses, accidents, and surgeries) and the present illness and its symptoms, duration, and related information are obtained from the patient by both the nurse and the physician (Box 20-3). The nursing assessment includes a psychosocial, spiritual, and educational history of the patient. With children and older adults, members of the patient's family may be helpful in supplying information. Often a number of laboratory examinations may be completed before admission, including urinalysis; a complete blood cell count; and determination of hemoglobin value, bleeding time, clotting time, and hematocrit level. A blood chemistry is ordered, and the nurse should particularly note the preoperative serum potassium level. In some cases a blood glucose test and electrocardiogram may be ordered. Many hospitals automatically require a chest x-ray examination of each patient admitted.

The physician evaluates the patient's nutritional status for dehydration and malnutrition. When severe vomiting and diarrhea have occurred, there may be an electrolyte imbalance and a protein and vitamin deficiency, which can result in decreased resistance to infection and delayed wound healing. To prevent such complications and to improve nutritional status, the patient may be given total parenteral nutrition, also called hyperalimentation, for several days before surgery.

If a **hemorrhage** or slow bleeding has occurred, there may be a decrease in hemoglobin value and red blood cells. It may be necessary to transfuse the patient with whole blood or packed cells or to administer fluids, electrolytes, and vitamins intravenously before surgery. If the patient's blood count is normal and loss of blood during surgery is anticipated, many patients and physicians prefer autologous (self) predonation of blood or the selection of their own donors. Autologous donations must be completed 1 week before surgery, with 1 week allowed between each unit donated. This technique is seen as an additional precaution against exposure to blood-borne diseases, such as acquired immunodeficiency syndrome (AIDS) and hepatitis.

## INFORMED CONSENT

A written statement giving consent to have a surgical procedure performed is required before surgery. This statement is signed by the patient in the presence of an authorized witness. It protects the patient from unsanctioned surgery and protects the surgical team from claims that unauthorized surgery was performed. The statement also implies informed consent, which means that the physician has provided the patient with an explanation of the surgical procedure, the possible consequences of the procedure, and what to expect during the postoperative period.

Patients sign their own operative permits if they are of legal age and mentally capable. A responsible family member may sign the permit if the patient is a minor or if the patient is unconscious or judged to be incapable of understanding his or her actions. Refusal to have the operation is the patient's privilege. The operative permit, when signed, becomes part of the patient's chart.

## PREOPERATIVE PREPARATION

The preparation and care of the patient before surgery have one major goal—to promote the best possible physical and psychologic state of the patient before surgical therapy. To achieve this goal, the patient's individual needs must be ascertained, and his or her strengths and limitations must be evaluated. A plan of care can be developed to help the patient adjust to the surgical experience, both physically and emotionally.

---

**BOX 20-3**

### PATIENT HISTORY

Information collected for the patient history should include the following:

- Past surgical experiences, problems, or complications
- Other illnesses or chronic conditions that the patient has that increase surgical risk, such as diabetes, liver disease, obesity, or cardiorespiratory deficiencies
- The potential for postoperative activity
- All medications the patient is taking, as well as allergies or intolerance to medications because many medications interact with perioperative agents and drugs and can affect recovery
- Habits such as smoking, excessive alcohol use, or a sedentary life-style that could impede recovery
- Support systems available to the patient and any potential problems for recovery in the home environment

## Nursing Assessment

Before any surgery, the nurse must assess the patient for the following:

1. Knowledge and understanding of the surgical procedure and the recovery phase
2. Physiologic status
3. Psychologic status
4. Cultural needs

### Preoperative Patient and Family Teaching

One of the nurse's most important responsibilities during the preoperative period is to teach the patient and family about the upcoming surgery and the postoperative strategies that will speed recovery. The nurse must first find out what the patient already knows, what explanations the physician has already given, and how much the patient needs and wants to know. Excessive and detailed descriptions of the surgical experience may actually increase preoperative anxiety.

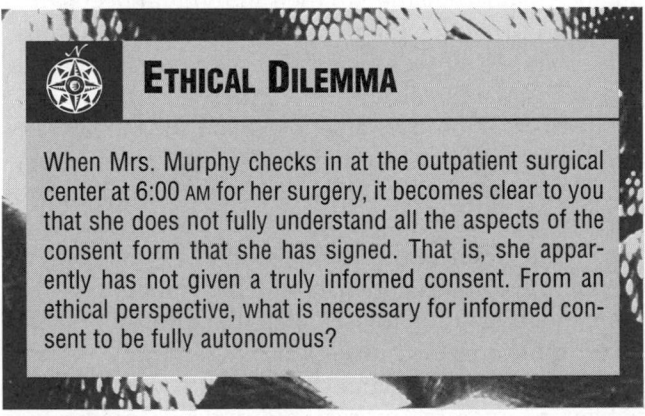

**ETHICAL DILEMMA**

When Mrs. Murphy checks in at the outpatient surgical center at 6:00 AM for her surgery, it becomes clear to you that she does not fully understand all the aspects of the consent form that she has signed. That is, she apparently has not given a truly informed consent. From an ethical perspective, what is necessary for informed consent to be fully autonomous?

### Physiologic Status

The patient's physiologic status is explored by both the physician and the nurse in separate admission histories and examinations. Often the nurse can elicit information that the patient may have neglected to mention to the physician. This information may be important for a successful surgery or may require canceling the surgery.

Individuals vary greatly in physiologic status and needs. Older patients, obese patients, and patients with diabetes require special assessments (Boxes 20-4 and 20-5) (Saltiel-Berzin, 1992; Hogstel, 1994). With shorter and less invasive surgical techniques, many older adults are now considered good surgical candidates if they receive careful preoperative planning and good postoperative care. Ambulatory or outpatient surgery, when possible, is often desirable because it is

less disruptive, is lower in cost, and allows for more contact with family and friends.

### Psychologic Status

An evaluation of the patient's psychologic status and readiness for surgery is also essential. The surgeon

**BOX 20-4**

**Guidelines for Care of the Obese Patient**

| Areas of concern | Assessments and interventions |
|---|---|
| Additional demands on a cardiovascular system that is already overburdened may lead to rapid heart rate and hypertension with exertion. Fatty tissue reduces circulation, so blood clots more easily. | Assess vital signs before and after activity. Pace activities but be sure that the patient is on a consistent schedule of increasing activity, particularly early ambulation. |
| Obese people have more difficulty expanding their chest and moving and walking easily, so respiratory congestion is more likely in the postoperative period. | Assess lung sounds every shift. Ensure that the patient does deep breathing exercises and uses an incentive spirometer, if ordered, every hour when awake. Check the position of abdominal binders often, and position them low on the abdomen to enhance chest expansion. |
| Fatty tissue is less vascular, so wound healing is poor. Wound separation, infection, and incisional hernias are more common. | Assess the incision every shift, and document any redness or drainage. Use sterile technique in giving wound care. Because infections often do not occur until after discharge, teach the patient to assess and care for the incision. |
| Extreme obesity is not acceptable in the U.S. culture, and many people react negatively to the overweight person. | Avoid judgmental behaviors. Anticipate that the patient may need extra assistance with personal hygiene and postoperative activities but may be unwilling to ask. Find gowns, chairs, and other materials that are large enough for the patient's comfort. |

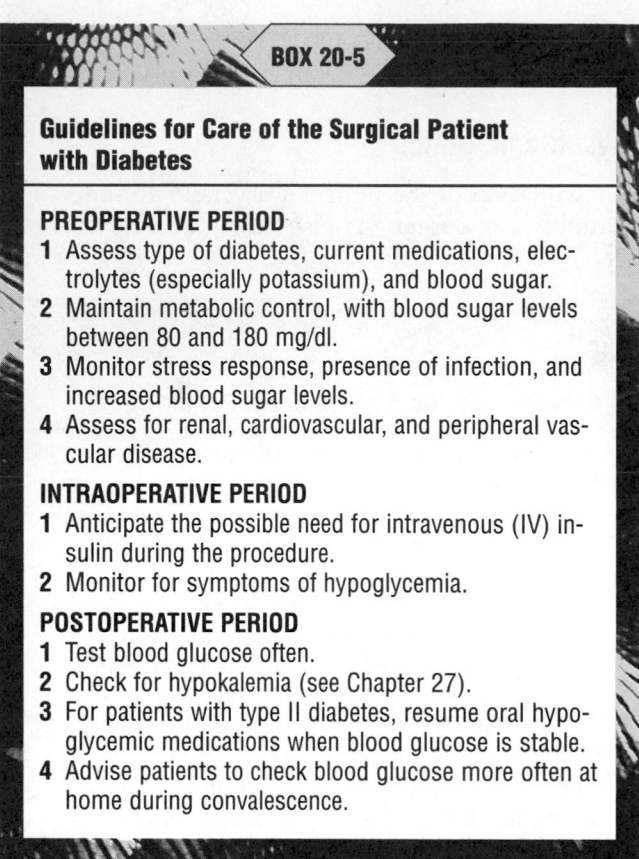

**BOX 20-5**

**Guidelines for Care of the Surgical Patient with Diabetes**

**PREOPERATIVE PERIOD**
1 Assess type of diabetes, current medications, electrolytes (especially potassium), and blood sugar.
2 Maintain metabolic control, with blood sugar levels between 80 and 180 mg/dl.
3 Monitor stress response, presence of infection, and increased blood sugar levels.
4 Assess for renal, cardiovascular, and peripheral vascular disease.

**INTRAOPERATIVE PERIOD**
1 Anticipate the possible need for intravenous (IV) insulin during the procedure.
2 Monitor for symptoms of hypoglycemia.

**POSTOPERATIVE PERIOD**
1 Test blood glucose often.
2 Check for hypokalemia (see Chapter 27).
3 For patients with type II diabetes, resume oral hypoglycemic medications when blood glucose is stable.
4 Advise patients to check blood glucose more often at home during convalescence.

should be informed if the patient is extremely anxious or convinced that the surgery will be fatal. If further explanation by the surgeon does not alleviate excessive anxiety, surgery is often postponed or canceled. The nurse should assess the following:

1. The level of anxiety and specific concerns about surgery
2. Coping patterns of the patient
3. Support systems, which may include family, friends, and religious beliefs and practices
4. Factors that may increase stress levels, such as marital or family discord and financial problems

## Cultural Needs

Cultural sensitivity involves the acceptance of diversity among people. Nurses must examine their own feelings regarding people whose culture differs from theirs, and they must convey respect for the beliefs and customs of all patients. If a patient does not speak English, an interpreter should be called to help with preoperative explanations. The nurse must attempt to find out how the patient feels about surgery, the use of blood transfusions, the disposal of body parts, and personal privacy. Such beliefs are only a few of the many differences among cultures. The status and role

of the nurse also differ among cultures, and the patient's feelings about nurses affect the nurse-patient relationship. Younger members of the patient's family who have been exposed to American culture since childhood are often a great help in language interpretation and cultural clues that help the nurse provide sensitive care to the patient before and after the surgical experience.

## Planning and Interventions
### Preoperative Instruction

Preoperative instructions can help relieve some of the patient's anxiety. Nursing personnel must know what information has been given to the patient and family regarding the surgery. Questioning the patient about what he or she has been told enables the nurse to clarify and reinforce knowledge. The patient's anxieties, needs, and resources must be considered because they vary considerably from patient to patient. The nurse usually informs the patient and family about the hospital routines surrounding the surgical experience in a manner that is sensitive to their individual needs. It is not appropriate for the nurse to discuss the diagnosis and prognosis of the patient. These matters should be referred to the physician.

The nurse should be able to explain the purposes of and the preparation for diagnostic tests, x-ray procedures, laboratory tests, medications, and nursing procedures. The surgical procedure and postoperative expectations often can be discussed with the patient. Preoperative instruction should be planned so that the patient has time to assimilate the information and to ask questions. Various studies regarding preoperative instruction have indicated that a well-prepared patient recuperates more rapidly, needs medication less often, and develops fewer complications after surgery. In addition, the time of hospitalization is often shortened.

Specific patient instructions are often given concerning deep breathing and coughing, turning and moving, medications, and special equipment that may be used postoperatively. Patients should be taught how to take a deep breath and exhale slowly in a sitting position. Such breathing provides good ventilation of the lungs and oxygenation of the blood. After practicing this several times, the patient should take a short breath and cough deeply if congestion is present. Coughing helps remove secretions from the bronchi and the lungs. The patient can be taught to splint an abdominal or thoracic incision by interlacing the fingers and placing the palms over the incision site. A towel or small pillow can also be used. Splinting lessens the muscular strain around the incision when the patient coughs.

## OLDER ADULT CONSIDERATIONS

| Areas of concern | Assessments and interventions |
| --- | --- |
| **PERIOPERATIVE PERIOD** | |
| Aging body systems | Organ systems, including nutritional and hydration status, must be carefully and totally assessed. Preoperative medications are not well absorbed and may have extra side effects. |
| Learning needs | The patient may have hearing or vision problems. Older adults learn well, but more slowly. Ensure that teaching sessions are unhurried and are paced to meet the patient's needs. |
| Evaluation of other health problems | Cardiovascular, renal, and respiratory systems are compromised by age and pose increased surgical risks. Assess, document, and inform the surgeon of any problems. |
| Medical history | In addition to prescription drugs, question the patient carefully about over-the-counter drugs such as aspirin and nonsteroidal antiinflammatory drugs, which can increase bleeding. |
| **INTRAOPERATIVE PERIOD** | |
| Hypothermia | Keep the patient covered as much as possible, and monitor temperature during surgery. |
| Physical trauma | Careful positioning and gentle transfer are needed to prevent bone, joint, and skin injury. |
| **POSTOPERATIVE PERIOD** | |
| Increased danger of aspiration, atelectasis, and airway obstruction because of weakened respiratory muscles | Avoid the supine position. Use narcotics with caution, and evaluate respiratory status often. |
| Increased risk of myocardial infarction, kidney failure, and fluid and electrolyte imbalance as a result of cardiovascular and renal aging | Avoid straining. Careful monitoring of intake and output is needed. Be alert for dehydration, overhydration, congestive heart failure, clotting problems, and urinary retention. Avoid catheterization if possible because of the increased risk of infection. |
| Confusion, sensory deficits | Alert staff if vision or hearing loss exists. Give clear explanations of postoperative events. Provide a safe environment, and assign the same nurses to the patient as often as possible. |
| Pain control | Give the lowest effective dose of analgesics. Use nonchemical pain strategies, such as relaxation techniques, back rubs, and other comfort measures. |
| Slower gastrointestinal motility, constipation | Stool softeners are often needed. Encourage fluids, ambulation, and, if permitted, remedies such as prunes and juices that the patient can take at home to achieve regularity. |

### NURSE ALERT

Vigorous coughing is discouraged after some types of surgeries, such as hernia repair and brain or eye surgery, in which increased intracranial pressure must be avoided.

Postoperative positions should be explained to the patient. Position should be changed often after surgery to improve circulation, increase respiratory function, and prevent venous stasis. Leg exercises are taught if it is anticipated that the patient will not be ambulatory within 1 day after surgery. These exercises include extension and flexion of the knee and hip joints and circular rotation of the foot. Other exercises may be recommended according to the patient's specific surgical procedure.

## Psychologic Preparation

Preparation for surgery should begin as soon as the patient is told that an operation is necessary. The anticipation of any surgical procedure results in an emotional reaction. Much can be done to alleviate fears before and during hospitalization. The patient's reaction depends on many factors, including personality structure and the pattern of reaction to stressful events in the past.

A surgical operation is a stressful situation in which the patient may believe that there is danger of acute pain, serious damage, disability, and death. There is also a fear of the unknown, which can be complicated by fear of anesthesia or fear of separation from activities, family, and friends. Many patients worry about financial problems, family responsibilities, and employment status. Anxiety often increases as the time for surgery draws near.

Reassuring the patient that medications will be available postoperatively to control discomfort helps lower the patient's anxiety. Any special equipment, such as drainage tubes and equipment, intravenous therapy, or an assistive breathing apparatus, should be explained to the patient before surgery. An understanding of this special equipment helps decrease postoperative anxiety. Many patients are placed in intensive care units after extensive surgical procedures. Electronic monitoring equipment may frighten the patient and family if they are not informed of how it contributes to patient care. The patient's family may believe that the patient is in a critical condition when placed in the intensive care unit. The family and the patient should receive the same information. Explanations concerning the patient's care can often be given when the family is present.

The nurse can help the patient, family, and surgical personnel by listening and helping the patient verbalize any fears. Often the patient wants only the opportunity to express fears to a caring, understanding, and accepting person. Members of the patient's family are often not able to listen to or empathize with the patient because of their own feelings and stress.

Patients are more willing to express their feelings if they have established a good relationship with a member of the nursing team. Therefore nurses should try to establish an atmosphere of acceptance and understanding. No attempt should be made to minimize a patient's fears by dismissing them as "normal." A thorough discussion of the patient's concerns and the appropriate explanations or referrals to the physician should be carried out by the nurse. Denial may be one of the major defense mechanisms that the patient uses to deal with stress, and the nurse should not attempt to give detailed descriptions or instructions to a patient who is unable to hear them because he or she has not fully accepted the fact that surgery is needed. The nurse can help dispel any misconceptions and assure the patient that the nurse and physician are available to discuss concerns. Occasionally it is helpful to have the patient talk with other people who have undergone a similar surgery. The patient's family should be included in discussions or explanations whenever possible and should be encouraged to understand the anxiety the patient faces and to visit often.

## Preoperative Orders

The physician writes the preoperative orders for the patient. Hospitals and physicians vary in the type of preoperative preparation desired, but certain routine procedures are fairly common.

### Preoperative Nutritional Care

**Nutrient reserves.** The patient having surgery is at high risk for protein-energy malnutrition. In addition to the fact that food is withheld before surgery and for some time to follow, the patient may already be in a poor nutritional state as a result of the condition requiring surgery. A poor state of nutrition hinders healing and can slow recovery. The surgical process also places physiologic and psychologic stress on patients, which creates added nutritional demands and increases risk of complications. If the surgery is elective and not an emergency, the patient's nutrient body stores should be fortified preoperatively to meet the demands of surgery and the period of limited food intake. Supplemental protein will build tissue and plasma reserves to counteract blood loss during surgery and to prevent tissue breakdown in the immediate postoperative period. Increased carbohydrates will produce stores of glycogen in the liver that will provide energy to support added demands and spare the protein for the work of tissue building. The vitamins and minerals involved in protein and energy metabolism must also be supplied and fluid balance should be ensured to prevent dehydration (Williams, 1995). If the patient is overweight, weight reduction will reduce surgical risk. If the surgery is an emergency, no time is available for building up ideal nutritional reserves and the patient who maintains good nutritional status through a healthy diet is in the best position for meeting the demands and avoiding complications.

**Immediate preoperative period.** Usually nothing by mouth (NPO) is allowed from midnight until surgery the next morning. If the planned surgery is not scheduled until late in the day or will be done using local anesthesia, the patient may be allowed to eat up until 6 to 8 hours before surgery. Withholding food and fluids minimizes the chances of vomiting and of aspirating vomitus into the lungs during or immediately after surgery. Instructions concerning the elimination of food and fluid must be given to the patient before surgery. Accidentally ingesting food or water usually delays surgery, which increases the hospital stay and expense. The nurse is responsible for removing water from the hospitalized patient's room and for communicating the patient's NPO status to everyone involved in his or her care.

## Elimination

For some types of surgery, the physician may request that an indwelling catheter be inserted to keep the bladder empty. A distended bladder can complicate surgical procedures on the lower abdomen and increase the chances of bladder trauma during surgery. The patient who is not catheterized should void before surgery.

Some surgical patients are given a preoperative enema, which may consist of soapsuds, saline, or tap water. Commercially prepared enemas, which are more comfortable for the patient, are being used more often.

Bisacodyl (Dulcolax) suppositories and tablets or other commercially prepared laxative solutions may be ordered instead of enemas. When bowel surgery is to be performed, "enemas until clear" may be ordered, which means that enemas must be given until no fecal matter returns with the solution. The nurse should be sure that all enema solution is returned, and failure to achieve the proper results should be reported to the physician. Solutions such as Go-Lyte are often ordered in place of enemas. To stimulate elimination the day before surgery, the patient drinks one cup of the solution every 15 minutes for 3 hours. A clear liquid diet may be ordered for as many as 3 days preceding the surgery to facilitate bowel cleansing. The administration of enemas or laxatives and the manipulation of the intestines during some surgeries lead to a delay in the return of normal elimination patterns for several days after surgery.

## Skin Preparation

It used to be customary for the nurse to shave the patient on the night before surgery. However, recent research shows that this practice is 10 times more likely to cause wound infection than shaving the incisional area in the operating room just before surgery. The current practice is to avoid shaving the patient if the hair does not interfere with the surgical site. Some institutions use hair removal gels or creams.

If shaving must occur, hair is removed from the area with a sharp, disposable razor. Strokes should be with the grain of the hair shaft to prevent nicking or scraping the skin because such cuts may become sites of infection. If the skin is injured, the surgeon may refuse to perform the surgery. Caution must be used in shaving around moles or warts, and any skin eruptions must be reported. In shaving areas such as the axilla and pubic area, the nurse may clip the long hair first to make shaving easier. Care should be taken not to expose or embarrass the patient, who should be left dry and

comfortable after the procedure. Scrubbing the surgical site with an antiseptic, such as povidone-iodine, may be ordered before the surgery or done in the operating room to decrease wound infection.

## Sedation

The physician usually orders a sedative for the hospitalized patient. The sedative is given at bedtime the evening before surgery to ensure that the patient gets adequate sleep and rest. After administration of the sedative, the patient should be instructed to remain in bed because he or she may experience dizziness or confusion. Side rails should be used with elderly persons, and patients should be observed at frequent intervals. The call light should always be placed within easy reach, and the patient should be taught how to use it properly. Because the majority of patients are not admitted on the morning of surgery, they may not have had adequate rest or may have awakened earlier than usual.

## Day of Surgery
### Visitors

On the day of surgery, the patient should be allowed to rest and should be kept as quiet as possible. Close family members should be advised to arrive at least 1 to 2 hours before the scheduled time of surgery. Time should be allowed for personal hygiene such as bathing, oral care, and shaving. The nurse should allow time in both the inpatient and outpatient settings to make the families and friends of the patients comfortable and to deal with their questions and concerns.

### Assessment

The vital signs (temperature, pulse, respiration, and blood pressure) are checked and recorded. Any temperature elevation must be reported immediately. The skin surface in the surgical area should be assessed for cuts or abrasions if an earlier shave has been done.

The nurse should check the chart carefully to ensure that all data, such as laboratory reports of blood and urine, have been recorded and that a signed operative permit is attached to the chart. Operative permits must be signed before the administration of medications because a patient who has been sedated is not considered legally competent to sign a permit. All preoperative medications and procedures should be accurately charted before the patient goes to the operating room. The nurse documents the preoperative baseline status of the patient, including physical, psychosocial, and spiritual assessments. Charge vouchers and special forms should be included in the patient's chart (Figure 20-1 and Box 20-6).

**NORTHWEST COMMUNITY HOSPITAL**
ARLINGTON HEIGHTS, ILLINOIS 60005
Date: _____
**PREOPERATIVE CHECKLIST**

**PATIENT ASSESSMENT**

☐ ID bracelet attached ☐ Allergy bracelet on

Allergies: _____

_____

Time pt. ate or drank _____ Last menses _____

Time: T_____ P_____ R_____ B/P_____

Height _____ Scaled weight _____

Check for following and remove:
☐ Jewelry/Watch ☐ Hearing aid(s)
☐ Rings taped ☐ Makeup off
☐ Rings removed ☐ Nail polish
☐ Dentures ☐ Wig
☐ Glasses ☐ Prosthesis
☐ Contact lenses ☐ Other_____
Initials: _____

Medication taken at home today: _____

_____

_____

_____

| Preop meds & Dose: | Rte. | Time | Init. |
|---|---|---|---|
| | | | |
| | | | |
| | | | |
| | | | |
| | | | |

**IV start** Time____ Solution _____ Gauge ____

Site _____ Rate _____ By _____

**Preps:**
☐ Enema given ☐ Foley in situ
☐ Douche given ☐ Ted hose on
☐ Hospital gown only ☐ Antiembolism device on
☐ Side rails up ☐ NG tube in situ

Shave prep done by: ____ Site checked by: _____

Voiding time: _____ Time to OR: _____

**CHART** Initial
Consent complete ☐ ____
History & physical complete ☐ ____
Old records on chart ☐ ____

**Test results:**
ECG (age 35 & up – within 1 mo) ☐ ____
Chest x-ray (within 3 mo) ☐ ____
☐ on chart ☐ in x-ray dept. ☐ brought own x-rays

**Labs drawn/on chart:**
CBC ☐ ____ IVY bleeding time ☐ ____
UA ☐ ____ PT/PTT ☐ ____
Chem. pro. (age 14 & up) ☐ __ Coag. pro. ☐ ____
RPR ☐ ____ Preg. test (under 45) ☐ ____

**Additional labs:** _____

| Abnormal labs: | Anes. notified | MD notified | Comments | Init. |
|---|---|---|---|---|
| | | | | |
| | | | | |

**Blood Orders:**
Type and screened ☐ ____
Type and crossmatched ☐ ____
No. units ordered _____
Autologous blood available _____
Directed donor blood available _____
Consent for transfusion signed ☐ ____

**Comments:**
_____
_____
_____
_____

| Initials | Signature | Initials | Signature |
|---|---|---|---|
| | | | |
| | | | |

**Figure 20-1** Preoperative check list. (Courtesy Central Healthcare and Affiliates, October 1994.)

BOX 20-6

# NURSING PROCESS
## PREOPERATIVE PREPARATION

**ASSESSMENT**

- Organ system baselines
- Understanding of and readiness for surgery
- Cultural background and language barriers
- Anxiety, coping ability, and support systems
- Nutritional status, obesity, malnourishment, dehydration
- History of diabetes or cardiac, respiratory, or renal disease
- Medications and allergies
- Laboratory values, particularly serum potassium, complete blood count, clotting time

**NURSING DIAGNOSES**

- Anxiety related to unknown outcomes and unknown environment
- Sleep pattern disturbance related to anxiety and unfamiliar surroundings
- Risk for injury related to premedication sedation
- Knowledge deficit: postoperative exercise and activity, related to lack of exposure to surgery and the hospital environment

**NURSING INTERVENTIONS**
**General**

- Provide a restful environment.
- Explain the operative process.
- Provide patient with the opportunity to verbalize fears.
- Demonstrate and practice deep breathing and coughing.
- Explain postoperative positioning.

- Explain special procedures and equipment and demonstrate when possible.
- Demonstrate and encourage pertinent exercises.
- Explain dietary restrictions, such as nothing by mouth after midnight.
- Prepare skin as ordered.
- Explain and administer medications.
- Provide for spiritual needs.

**Immediate**

- Check that identification band is in place and legible.
- Remove and store hairpins, dentures, jewelry, contact lenses, and prostheses.
- Store valuables.
- Give patient a hospital gown.
- Have patient void; chart time and amount.
- Administer and chart medications.
- Instruct the patient to remain in bed; put the side rails up.
- Complete patient's chart, including the following:
  Operative permit signed
  Laboratory data complete
- Order sheets, progress notes, history, patient status, and response to medication included in chart.

**EVALUATION OF EXPECTED OUTCOMES**

- Demonstrates optimal physical and psychologic status
- Behavior indicates adjustment to the surgical experience
- Postoperative complications avoided

## Prostheses

Just before transportation to surgery, dentures and removable bridges should be removed and placed in a container that is marked with the patient's name. The container should be put in a safe place to prevent loss or damage. Contact lenses and any prostheses (e.g., hearing aids, glasses, and wigs) should be removed and stored or sent to the postoperative recovery unit.

## Makeup

Procedures vary among anesthesiologists, but often they prefer that all makeup be removed before the patient goes to surgery because any reduction of oxygen to the tissues may be observed in the lips, face, and

nail beds or may be detected by the color of the blood at the operative site. Polish must generally be removed from at least one fingernail for the proper use of a pulse oximetry finger monitor, which is a current standard of care during surgery.

## Valuables

Valuables, such as money and jewelry, should be removed and itemized in the patient's presence, sealed in an envelope, and locked up or given to a responsible member of the family. Patients who are being admitted for elective surgery should leave all valuables at home. The nurse should be familiar with hospital policy concerning the care of valuables and should use every precaution to protect the patient's personal property. Often considerable sentiment is attached to a wedding ring, and the patient may be allowed to wear it, but it should be anchored securely with tape to prevent losing it.

## Immediate Preoperative Orders

The patient is given a hospital gown that ties in the back, and all personal articles of clothing are removed. The patient's hair may be covered with a surgical cap. Depending on the type of surgery and the patient's age and condition, the physician may order a retention catheter, which is inserted into the urinary bladder before surgery. The physician may also order intravenous fluids or the insertion of a nasogastric tube before surgery. The surgeon may request that mid-thigh or knee-high elastic stockings be applied or that the patient's legs be wrapped with elastic bandages to help prevent thrombophlebitis. If elastic stockings are ordered, the nurse should follow the manufacturer's directions for measuring and applying them. If elastic bandages are ordered, 4-, 5-, or 6-inch bandages should be used to wrap the patient's legs from the metatarsals to mid-thigh, and the bandages should be fastened securely. Sequential compression devices, if ordered, should be placed correctly on the patient's legs.

Preoperative medications, which are ordered by the anesthesiologist, are usually administered intramuscularly or orally. The purpose of preoperative medications is to reduce the patient's anxiety about anesthesia and to provide a smoother induction. Some medications also reduce secretions, and others reduce postoperative nausea (Table 20-1). Preoperative medications are ordered individually for each patient, and consideration is given to the patient's age and general condition, the presence of other diseases that require medications, and the anesthetizing agent to be administered.

The medication is ordered to be administered on call or at a specific hour, and it is important that the nurse give the medication on time so that its maximum effect is reached during the induction of anesthesia. If for any reason the medication is not administered as directed, the anesthesiologist and/or physician should be notified so that the necessary adjustments may be made. Identification should be attached to the patient's wrist, including such information as the patient's name, room number, hospital number, address, and physician. Some institutions require two identification bands for surgical patients, one on a wrist and one on an ankle.

Just before being medicated, the patient should be requested to void, and the amount and time should be noted. A patient's inability to void should be reported to the physician. Vital signs should be taken and recorded. The nurse should advise the patient to stay in bed after the medication has been given and should put the side rails up.

## Transport

The patient may be transferred to the operating room in his or her own bed or by stretcher, and the patient should be moved carefully and with as little confusion as possible. The nurse should protect the patient from drafts and exposure by applying cotton blankets and should make him or her comfortable with a pillow. The nurse or transport personnel accompany the patient and remain until relieved by a member of the operating room staff. The patient's record is given to the operating room nurse, who is also advised verbally of the patient's name and any significant problem that currently exists. Family members should be told where to wait during the surgery.

# INTRAOPERATIVE CARE

In the past decade, modern surgery has become increasingly sophisticated with the use of new techniques and tools. The common use of endoscopic techniques for surgery has reduced the length of stay and the convalescent period for patients. **Laparoscopic gastrointestinal surgery** (surgery performed through a laparoscope) has become the standard of care for such procedures as appendectomy, cholecystectomy, and bowel resection. Laser surgery, which uses a high-energy beam of light, allows tissue to be cut and destroyed with minimal invasive technique. The conscientious use of aseptic practices remains the primary element of safe surgery. Aseptic surgery began around 1867 with the work of Joseph Lister, an English surgeon. At that time wound infection complicated most surgeries, and puerperal infection was common in obstetric wards. Lister observed the process of wound infection and concluded that it was caused by microbes. On the basis of this belief, Lister began using a solution of carbolic acid in the operating room and also began saturating dressings over wounds. These measures resulted in a remarkable decrease in the incidence of wound infection.

## Surgical Asepsis

Although modern science has progressed since Lister, the basic definition of surgical **asepsis** remains unchanged. Surgical asepsis is a condition in which there is a complete absence of germs. It is absolute. There is no compromise or modification. Many situations on the clinical unit require surgical aseptic techniques, such as catheterization or surgical dressing changes.

**TABLE 20-1**

## Pharmacology of Drugs Used for the Surgical Patient

| DRUG (GENERIC AND TRADE NAME); ROUTE AND DOSAGE | ACTION/INDICATION | COMMON SIDE EFFECTS AND NURSING CONSIDERATIONS |
|---|---|---|
| **Atropine**<br>**Route:** SC<br>**Dosage:** 0.4-0.6 mg | Cholinergic blocker used to reduce secretions before surgery, to calm delirium, and for motion sickness | Dryness of mouth, constipation, and paralytic ileus; contraindicated in glaucoma, myasthenia gravis, and hypersensitivity to belladonna and barbiturates; use with caution in elderly patients and those with benign prostatic hypertrophy, congestive heart failure, hypertension, arrhythmias, and gastric ulcers |
| **Bupivacaine** (Marcaine)<br>**Route:** SC, epidural<br>**Dosage:** Depends on site and length of surgical procedure | Production of local or regional anesthesia | Excitation and/or depression; prolonged loss of sensation at site |
| **Diazepam** (Valium)<br>**Route:** PO, IM, IV<br>**Dosage:** Skeletal muscle relaxation, PO, 2-10 mg 3-4 times daily, 2-2.5 mg in elderly or debilitated patients; IM, IV, 5-10 mg (2-5 mg in debilitated patients) and may repeat in 2-4 hr | Benzodiazepine sedative/hypnotic used to manage anxiety; for preoperative sedation, light anesthesia, and amnesia; as a skeletal muscle relaxant; for status epilepticus; and to manage symptoms of alcohol withdrawal | Dizziness, drowsiness, and lethargy; preexisting CNS depression, uncontrolled severe pain, and glaucoma; use cautiously in hepatic and severe renal disease, suicidal, addicted, elderly, or debilitated patients |
| **Droperidol** (Inapsine)<br>**Route:** IM, IV<br>**Dosage:** Preoperative, IM, 2.5-10 mg ½ hr before surgery; induction, IV, 2.5 mg/20-25 lb given with analgesic or general anesthetic; maintain general anesthesia, IV, 1.25-2.5 mg | Neuroleptic used for premedication for surgery, induction of anesthesia, and maintenance of general anesthesia | Laryngospasm, bronchospasm, dystonia, akathisia, flexion of arms, fine tremors, dizziness, anxiety, drowsiness, restlessness, hallucinations, depression, tachycardia, hypotension, chills, facial swelling, shivering; assess vital signs soon after first dose |
| **Fentanyl Citrate** (Sublimaze)<br>**Route:** IM, IV<br>**Dosage:** Anesthetic, IV, 0.05-0.1 mg q 2-3 min prn; preoperatively, IM, 0.05-0.1 mg q 30-60 min before surgery; postoperatively, IM, 0.05-0.1 mg q 1-2 hr prn | Narcotic analgesic used preoperatively and postoperatively and as an adjunct to general anesthesia when combined with droperidol | Bradycardia, cardiac arrest, respiratory depression, respiratory arrest, and laryngospasm; contraindicated in hypersensitivity to opiates and myasthenia gravis; use with caution in elderly patients and those with respiratory depression, increased intracranial pressure, seizure disorders, and cardiac arrhythmias |
| **Glycopyrrolate** (Robinul)<br>**Route:** PO, IM, IV<br>**Dosage:** Preoperatively, IM, 0.002 mg/lb ½-1 hr before surgery; reversal of neuromuscular blockage, IV, 0.2 mg for each 1 mg of neostigmine or 5 mg IV of pyridostigmine simultaneously; GI disorders, PO, 1-2 mg bid-tid, IM, IV, 0.1-0.2 mg tid-qid, titrated to patient response | Cholinergic blocker used to decrease secretions before surgery and for reversal of neuromuscular blockade, peptic ulcer disease, and irritable bowel syndrome | Dryness of mouth and constipation; contraindicated in glaucoma, myasthenia gravis, gastrointestinal or genitourinary obstruction, tachycardia, hepatic disease, ulcerative colitis, and toxic megacolon |

*Continued*

**TABLE 20-1**

## Pharmacology of Drugs Used for the Surgical Patient—cont'd

| DRUG (GENERIC AND TRADE NAME); ROUTE AND DOSAGE | ACTION/INDICATION | COMMON SIDE EFFECTS AND NURSING CONSIDERATIONS |
|---|---|---|
| **Halothane** (Fluothane, Somnothane) **Route:** Inhaled anesthetic **Dosage:** Minimal alveolar concentration 0.7% in $O_2$ | CNS depressant anesthetic that causes complete anesthesia | Hypotension, cardiovascular depression, lowered body temperature, respiratory depression, malignant hyperthermia, emergence shivering, trembling, confusion, hallucinations, nervousness, and increased excitability; may cause hepatic dysfunction |
| **Isoflurane** (Forane) **Route:** Inhaled anesthetic **Dosage:** Minimal alveolar concentration 1.15% in $O_2$ | CNS depressant anesthetic that causes complete anesthesia | Same as above, except no hepatic complications; exhaled largely unchanged |
| **Ketorolac** (Toradol) **Route:** IV, IM, PO **Dosage:** IV, 15-30 mg q 6 hr; IM, 30-60 mg q6 hr; PO, 10 mg qid | Short-term management of moderately severe pain | Peptic ulceration; renal failure; contraindicated in nursing mothers or patients with active bleeding |
| **Lidocaine** (Xylocaine) **Route:** SC **Dosage:** Usual adult dosage depends on site and length of surgical procedure | Subcutaneously injected local anesthetic with intermediate duration (1-3 hr) | Most common side effects, such as headache, dizziness, convulsions, hypotension, and bradycardia, not present because SC dose is so small; watch for hypersensitivity and persistent loss of sensation at site |
| **Meperidine** (Demerol) **Route:** IM, IV, PO **Dosage:** Preoperatively, IM, 50-100 mg 30-90 min before surgery, IV dose should be reduced; sometimes may be given PO | Narcotic analgesic used preoperatively and for moderate to severe pain | Increased intracranial pressure and respiratory depression; contraindicated if hypersensitive or previously addicted; use with caution in addictive personality, heart disease, respiratory depression, hepatic or renal disease |
| **Midazolam** (Versed) **Route:** IM, IV **Dosage:** Preoperative sedation, IM, 0.07-0.08 mg/kg $\frac{1}{2}$-1 hr before general anesthesia; induction of general anesthesia, 1-10 mg IV | General anesthetic used for preoperative sedation, general anesthesia induction, and other sedation indications | Apnea, bronchospasm, laryngospasm, nausea and vomiting; contraindicated in shock, coma, alcohol intoxication, and glaucoma; use with caution in elderly or debilitated patients or patients with chronic obstructive pulmonary disease, congestive heart failure, chronic renal failure, or chills; has less duration than diazepam; is a better anesthetic |
| **Morphine** (Morhpine) **Route:** PO, IM, IV **Dosage:** IM, 4-15 mg q 4 hr prn; PO, 10-30 mg q 4 hr prn; IV, 4-10 mg diluted in 4-5 ml $H_2O$ for injection over 5 min | Narcotic analgesic used preoperatively and for severe pain | Respiratory depression; contraindicated in addicted patients and patients with hemorrhage, bronchial asthma, and increased intracranial pressure; use with caution in addictive personality, severe heart disease, and hepatic and renal disease |
| **Naloxone** (Narcan) **Route:** IC, SC, IM **Dosage:** Narcotic-induced respiratory depression, IV, SC, IM, 0.4-2 mg, and repeat q 2-3 min if needed; postoperative respiratory depression, IV, 0.1-0.2 mg q 2-3 min prn | Narcotic antagonist used to reverse respiratory depression caused by narcotics, pentazocine, and propoxyphene | Rapid overdosage could predispose to pulmonary edema; almost immediate onset |

| TABLE 20-1 |
|---|

## Pharmacology of Drugs Used for the Surgical Patient—cont'd

| DRUG (GENERIC AND TRADE NAME); ROUTE AND DOSAGE | ACTION/INDICATION | COMMON SIDE EFFECTS AND NURSING CONSIDERATIONS |
|---|---|---|
| **Nitrous oxide** <br> **Route:** Inhaled anesthetic <br> **Dosage:** 50%-70% | Incomplete, "weak" anesthetic | Weak anesthetic with no muscle relaxation; must be administered with 20% oxygen to avoid hypoxia; may cause bowel distention and may contribute to postoperative nausea and vomiting |
| **Pancuronium** (Pavulon) <br> **Route:** IV <br> **Dosage:** 0.1 mg/kg | Nondepolarizing skeletal muscle relaxant (neuromuscular block) | Muscle relaxant anesthetic has a duration of 45-60 min; is reversible with anticholinesterase agents; no histamine release; slow increase in pulse rate initially |
| **Procaine** (Novocain) <br> **Route:** Varies by route of anesthesia <br> **Dosage:** 14 mg/kg at one time | Local anesthetic used for spinal anesthesia, epidural, peripheral nerve block, perineum, lower extremities, and infiltration | Convulsions, decreased level of consciousness, myocardial depression, cardiac arrest, arrhythmias, status asthmaticus, respiratory depression, and anaphylaxis; contraindicated in severe liver disease; use with caution in elderly patients and those with severe drug allergies |
| **Promethazine** (Phenergan) <br> **Route:** PO, IM, IV <br> **Dosage:** Sedation, preoperative/postoperative, PO, IM, IV, 25-50 mg | Antihistamine H₁-receptor antagonist used for motion sickness, rhinitis, allergy symptoms, sedation, nausea, and preoperative and postoperative sedation | Dizziness, drowsiness, respiratory depression, and hypotension; watch for thrombocytopenia with chronic usage; contraindicated in acute asthma attack and lower respiratory disease; use with caution in increased intraocular pressure, renal and cardiac disease, hypertension, bronchial asthma, seizure disorder, peptic ulcers, hyperthryoidism, and benign prostatic hypertrophy |
| **Propofol** (Diprivan) <br> **Route:** IV <br> **Dosage:** Adult dosage depends on length of surgical procedure | Sedative-hypnotic that may be needed for induction and/or maintenance of anesthesia | Cough, airway obstruction, apnea |
| **Succinylcholine** (Anectine, Quelicin, Sucostrin) <br> **Route:** IV, IM <br> **Dosage:** IV, 25-75 mg, then 2.5 mg/min as needed; IM, 2.5 mg/kg, not to exceed 150 mg | Neuromuscular blocker used to facilitate intubation and skeletal muscle relaxation, especially during orthopedic manipulations | Sinus arrest, arrhythmias, prolonged apnea, bronchospasm, cyanosis, respiratory depression, and myoglobulinemia; contraindicated in malignant hyperthermia, penetrating eye injuries, and glaucoma; use with caution in cardiac disease, severe burns, electrolyte imbalances, dehydration, neuromuscular diseases, respiratory diseases, collagen diseases, glaucoma, elderly and debilitated patients |
| **Thiopental Sodium** (Pentothal) <br> **Route:** IV <br> **Dosage:** Induction, 210-280 mg or 3-5 ml/kg; general anesthetic, 50-75 mg given at 20-40 sec intervals; sedation, 12-20 mg/lb | Barbiturate general anesthetic used in short general anesthesia and induction anesthesia before other anesthetics | Respiratory depression, bronchospasm, myocardial depression, arrhythmias, and shivering; contraindicated in status asthmaticus; use with caution in severe cardiac disease, renal disease, liver disease, hypotension, myxedema, myasthenia gravis, asthma, and increased intracranial pressure |

*Continued*

**TABLE 20-1**

## Pharmacology of Drugs Used for the Surgical Patient—cont'd

| DRUG (GENERIC AND TRADE NAME); ROUTE AND DOSAGE | ACTION/INDICATION | COMMON SIDE EFFECTS AND NURSING CONSIDERATIONS |
|---|---|---|
| **Tubocurarine Chloride, Curare** (Tubocurarine) **Route:** IV **Dosage:** IV bolus 0.4-0.5 mg/kg, then 0.08-0.10 mg/kg 20-45 min after first dose if needed for prolonged procedures | Neuromuscular blocker used to facilitate endotracheal intubation, skeletal muscle relaxation during mechanical ventilation, surgery, or general anesthesia | Prolonged apnea, bronchospasm, cyanosis, and respiratory depression; use with caution in cardiac disease, electrolyte imbalances, dehydration, and neuromuscular or respiratory disease |
| **Vecuronium** (Norcuron) **Route:** IV **Dosage:** IV bolus 0.08-0.10 mg/kg, then 0.010-0.015 mg/kg for prolonged procedures | Neuromuscular blocker used to facilitate endotracheal intubation, skeletal muscle relaxation during mechanical ventilation surgery, and general anesthesia | Prolonged apnea and possible respiratory paralysis; use with caution in cardiac disease, electrolyte imbalances, dehydration, and neuromuscular or respiratory disease |

The slightest error may mean prolonged illness or hospitalization for the patient. The nurse should know the methods used to achieve asepsis and the variables that determine the effectiveness or ineffectiveness, whatever method is used.

Surgical asepsis prevents organisms from entering the body. Surgical aseptic techniques are used whenever the skin or mucous membranes are perforated or incised. To prevent contaminants from entering the area of operation or any wound, any object that comes in contact with a wound must be absolutely free of pathogenic organisms. Procedures in operating rooms are carried out under strict surgical asepsis and require preparation of the patient's skin and sterilization of all instruments, linens, dressings, or other materials that come in contact with the wound. Surgical asepsis includes special attire for the surgeon and assistants, properly cleaning and disinfecting all inanimate objects in the room, and maintaining proper temperature and humidity. Laminar airflow systems may be used to reduce the number of airborne organisms. Other terms for surgical asepsis are *sterile technique* and *aseptic technique.*

## Sterilization

**Sterilization** is a process by which all forms of living microorganisms are completely destroyed, including spores and viruses. The sterilization of materials usually occurs in the central processing department of the hospital or surgical area. The method of sterilization is determined by the supplies and equipment that are to be used. In surgical asepsis all supplies and equipment are sterilized before use and are handled only with sterile equipment. Two factors are important in determining the type of sterilization to be used:

1. The type of microorganism, because some pathogens are easily destroyed by ordinary methods of disinfection, whereas others are extremely resistant
2. The degree of contamination, because the greater the amount of contamination, the longer it takes to ensure complete destruction of pathogenic organisms

Heat is one of the most effective and convenient methods of destroying microorganisms. *Boiling,* a form of moist heat, is one of the oldest methods of sterilization. It is commonly used in the home and is adequate under most conditions. Equipment that is to be sterilized by boiling must be completely immersed in the water, and timing begins when the water starts to boil. Most vegetative forms of bacteria are killed if boiled for 10 to 20 minutes.

## Steam Under Pressure

*Steam under pressure* is the most dependable method of sterilizing because it rapidly destroys all forms of microorganisms. This method of sterilizing is called autoclaving. Steam enters the **autoclave** under pressure, which increases the temperature of the steam. During the sterilizing process, the temperature is maintained at approximately 121° C (250° F) and at 15 to 17 pounds of pressure for a specified time. At the completion of the process, the pressure is reduced to zero, and the load is allowed to dry.

## Dry Heat Sterilization

Dry heat sterilization circulates hot air, which is provided by an electric oven sterilizer. This method may be compared to an ordinary baking oven. Dry heat sterilization penetrates many different materials, such as oils and closed containers that are not affected by steam. The type of materials, their packaging, and the loading of the oven determine the time necessary for sterilization. Generally hot air sterilization requires between 1 and 6 hours and in some cases may be longer.

## Ethylene Oxide

Ethylene oxide is a chemical that is found as both a liquid and a vapor. If the liquid form comes into contact with the skin, it causes blisters. Inhaling the gas causes nausea, vomiting, dizziness, and irritation of the mucous membranes. Research has demonstrated that exposure to ethylene oxide gas kills all forms of vegetative bacteria, including spore-forming types, and viruses. Its use has increased in sterilizing equipment that cannot be subjected to other methods of sterilizing, such as instruments with lenses (cystoscope and bronchoscope) and plastic equipment, such as infant incubators and the artificial kidney dialyzer. Polyethylene tubing and some rubber products are usually sterilized with ethylene oxide.

The use of ethylene oxide gas requires special types of sterilizers. The process of sterilization is complex and involves several factors, including temperature, time, moisture, concentration of the gas, and proper packaging of materials. The actual sterilizing time varies from 1 to 4 hours, but all the residual gas must be allowed to dissipate before the supplies or equipment can be used. Therefore materials exposed to ethylene oxide are not used for 24 to 36 hours.

## The Operative Team

Those giving care to the patient during the intraoperative period are generally prepared to be sterile or nonsterile members of the surgical team. Sterile members of the team include the surgeon, who may be assisted by another physician, and the scrub nurse or technician. Nonsterile personnel include the anesthesiologist (a physician) or anesthetist (a nurse), the circulating nurse, and various technicians. To best serve the needs of the patient at a critical time, team members must work efficiently as a unit.

### Scrub Nurse or Technician

As the sterile nursing member of the operative team, the primary role of the scrub nurse or technician is to anticipate the needs of the surgeon and to assist at the operative site. This nurse prepares the instruments

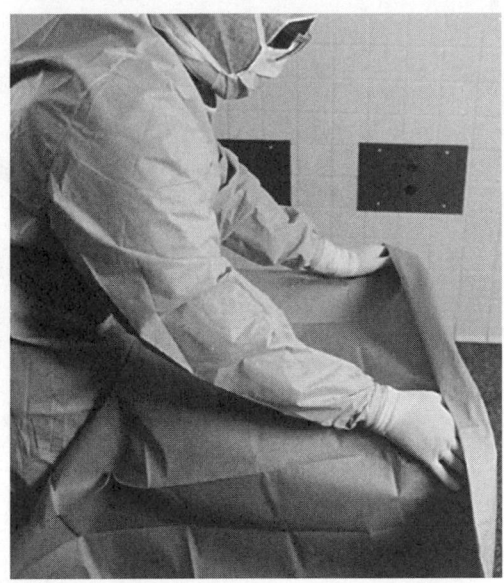

**Figure 20-2**    Scrub nurse protects gloves with cuff of drape when opening inner wrapper of pack, which serves as a sterile table cover. (From Meeker MH, Rothrock JC: *Alexander's care of the patient in surgery*, ed 10, St Louis, 1995, Mosby.)

and materials to be used by the surgeon and may assist with the surgical procedure (Figure 20-2). The scrub nurse or technician must have a thorough knowledge of aseptic technique and the ability and stamina to work efficiently under pressure (Figure 20-3). Manual dexterity and good organizational skills are also important.

### Circulating Nurse

The circulating nurse must be a registered nurse and has a major role in managing the operating room. This nonsterile team member must have an overall picture of the needs of the patient and of the other team members. The duties of the circulating nurse include the following:

1. Maintaining a safe environment for the patient by observing breaks in sterile technique, providing for safe use of complex equipment, and keeping the patient and staff free from hazards
2. Anticipating the need for and obtaining supplies and equipment for the sterile team
3. Communicating information about the patient's status to other members of the health team and to the patient's significant others

### Anesthesia

**Anesthesia** means "the absence of pain." Most patients have some fear of anesthesia. They may worry about going to sleep and not waking up, or they may fear the unknown. Some patients may fear waking

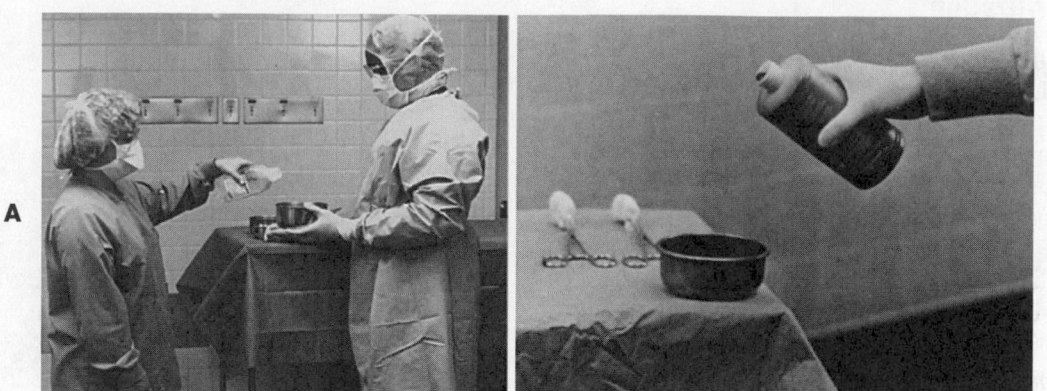

**Figure 20-3** **A,** When pouring solution into receptacle held by scrub nurse, the circulating nurse maintains a safe margin of space to avoid contamination of sterile surfaces. **B,** Care must be used when pouring solution into a receptacle that is on a sterile field to avoid splashing fluids onto sterile field. Placing a receptacle near the edge of the table permits the circulating nurse to pour the solution without reaching over any portion of sterile field. (From Meeker MH, Rothrock JC: *Alexander's care of the patient in surgery,* ed 10, St Louis, 1995, Mosby.)

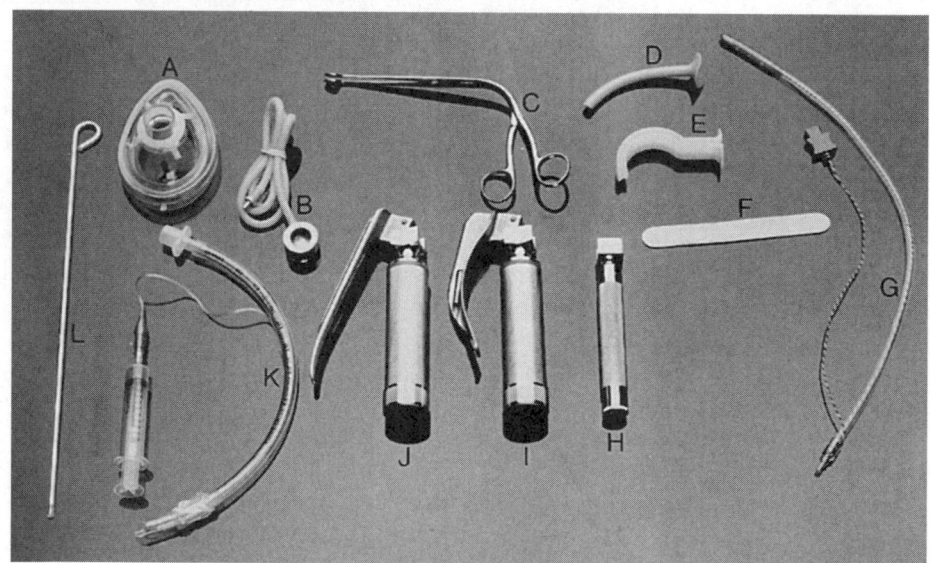

**Figure 20-4** Commonly used anesthesia equipment. *A,* Mask. *B,* Precordial stethoscope. *C,* McGill forceps. *D,* Nasal airway. *E,* Oral airway. *F,* Tongue blade. *G,* Esophageal stethoscope with esophageal temperature monitor. *H,* Pediatric laryngoscope handle. Fiberoptic laryngoscope blades and handles: *I,* MacIntosh. *J,* Miller. *K,* Endotracheal tube. *L,* Intubating stylet for endotracheal tube. (Courtesy Scott and White Memorial Hospital, Temple, Tex. In Meeker MH, Rothrock JC: *Alexander's care of the patient in surgery,* ed 10, St Louis, 1995, Mosby.)

up and experiencing pain during surgery, acting strangely when anesthetized, or experiencing uncomfortable aftereffects, such as nausea and vomiting. Most fears can be allayed if the patient is well informed about the anesthetic chosen and the effects it will produce. The type of anesthetic medication and technique are selected for the individual patient on the basis of his or her physical condition; age; preference; and the type, site, and length of the operation to be performed (Figure 20-4). An anesthesiologist, a physician who specializes in the selection and administration of anesthetics, chooses the anesthetic medication and techniques following a preoperative visit. During the visit, the anesthesiologist assesses the patient's physical and emotional state, discusses individual preferences, explains the procedure of inducing anesthesia, answers questions, and generally promotes confidence and helps relieve anxiety.

**TABLE 20-2**

## Selected General Anesthetics

| DRUG | CHARACTERISTICS | NURSING CONSIDERATIONS |
|---|---|---|
| **Inhalant Agents** | | |
| Isoflurane (Forane) | Volatile liquid; provides good muscle relaxation; rapid induction and recovery; potentiates muscle relaxants significantly | All inhalants depress respirations. Monitor rate and quality of respirations closely. Agent may cause immediate postoperative coughing and laryngospasm. |
| Halothane (Fluothane) | Volatile liquid; rapid induction but poor degree of muscle relaxation; evidence suggests that liver damage may be a side effect; shivering commonly occurs as patient awakens | Anesthesiologist should be informed if patient has any history of liver disease, alcoholism, or gallbladder disease. Keep patient warm postoperatively. Monitor patient closely for cardiac arrhythmias. |
| Enflurane (Ethrane) | Volatile liquid; slow acting but fairly good muscle relaxation and analgesia can be achieved; can cause fatal arrhythmias, particularly in presence of epinephrine-like drugs | Monitor vital signs closely and provide for safety during what is often a prolonged (45-min) wake-up period. Blood pressure may fall, and pulse rate may rise. |
| Nitrous oxide | Gas; very popular, weak agent used in combination with oxygen and other anesthetic agents; nonexplosive; may create hypoxia | Monitor for hypoxia and be prepared to administer oxygen. |
| **Intravenous Agents** | | |
| Short-acting barbiturates: methohexital (Brevital), thiamylal (Surital), thiopental (Pentothal) | Thiopental sodium is most popular of this group; given at onset of surgery to provide rapid and smooth induction; may cause laryngospasm, respiratory depression, and sudden hypotension | Assess postoperative respiratory status closely. Patient may be sedated but may still be in pain and require additional medication. |
| Propofol (Diprivan) | Sedative-hypnotic that may be needed for induction and/or maintenance of anesthesia | Cough, airway obstruction, apnea |
| Narcotic and nonnarcotic analgesics: morphine, meperidine, droperidol (Innovar), fentanyl | Used with other anesthetic agents to provide effective analgesia during surgery; major side effect is respiratory depression | Monitor respirations closely. Keep naloxone (Narcan) on hand to reverse narcotic effect. Use narcotics sparingly or in decreased doses during first 12 hr after surgery. |
| Ketamine (Ketalar, Ketaject) | Dissociative agent used for short procedures; provides analgesia and loss of memory of procedure; often used in pediatric surgery | Protect patients from additional stimuli (noises, touching) during waking period; in adults, may cause confusion and excitement for 24 hr after surgery; assess for hypertension and respiratory depression. |

Anesthesia is induced by a physician anesthesiologist or a certified nurse anesthetist. A nurse anesthetist is a professional nurse who has received postgraduate education in the administration of anesthetics and generally functions under the supervision of an anesthesiologist. The anesthesia team continually monitors the patient's oxygenation vital signs, organ function, and fluid status during the surgery and the immediate post-surgical period. It should be remembered that the patient is sedated and in a strange and sometimes frightening environment. There should be no bright lights or unnecessary noise and talking. Hearing is the last sense to respond to anesthetic agents and the first to return after the effects of the anesthetic wear off. Therefore unnecessary noise, conversation, joking, or inappropriate comments must be avoided by staff members.

The type of anesthetic administered may affect the postoperative condition and the return to consciousness. An understanding of anesthetizing agents helps the nurse assess the patient's condition and anticipate postoperative needs.

## Types

Anesthesia is classified as *general* or *regional*. When the surgeon wishes all sensations in the entire body to be suspended temporarily, the patient is given a general anesthetic. When only a part of the body is involved, the patient may be given a regional anesthetic. General anesthetics include drugs that are administered by inhalation or by injection into the bloodstream (Table 20-2).

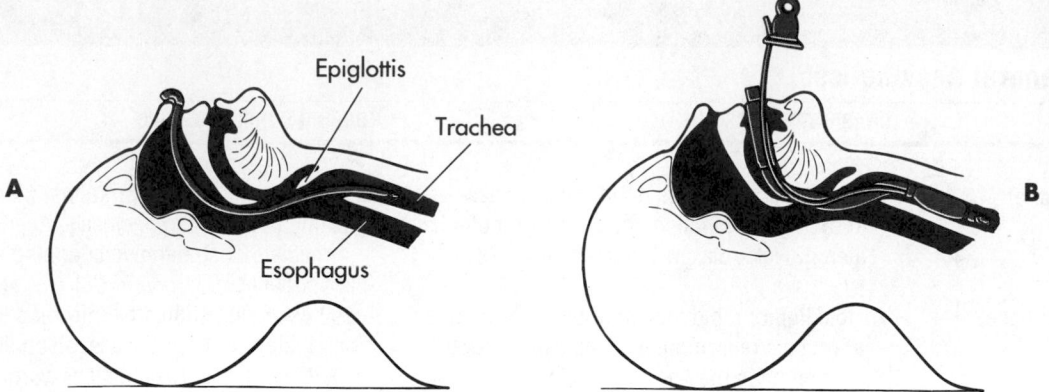

**Figure 20-5** **A,** Intranasal intubation. Note adapter at proximal end of tube that can be used to attach anesthetic equipment. **B,** Oral intubation. Note inflated cuff.

### General anesthesia

***Inhalation anesthesia.*** Drugs used in inhalation anesthesia may be liquids that vaporize, with the patient inhaling the vapor. Examples of such drugs include isoflurane (Forane) and halothane (Fluothane). Inhalation drugs are also in the form of gases, such as nitrous oxide (see Table 20-2). Inhalation anesthetics render the patient unconscious, and therefore awareness of pain and anxiety are eliminated. They also provide muscle relaxation. Inhalation anesthetics are administered in combination with oxygen or air through a mask or through a tube that is inserted into the trachea.

Endotracheal intubation ensures that the airway remains open and that the lungs can be aerated even when the chest wall is entered. The endotracheal tube is held in place by a balloon that is inflated after it is inserted (Figure 20-5). The balloon and the pressure it exerts on the walls of the trachea cause some irritation of the mucosa. Occasionally they can cause postoperative edema in the area, resulting in respiratory difficulty. Therefore when an endotracheal tube has been used, the patient must be watched carefully for symptoms of respiratory obstruction.

***Intravenous drugs.*** Barbiturates, narcotics, and other drugs are administered with inhalation anesthetics and reduce the amount of the inhalation anesthetics required (see Table 20-2). Short-acting barbiturates produce unconsciousness in 30 seconds. The most commonly used intravenous drugs are thiopental (Pentothal) and thiamylal (Surital). When large amounts of these drugs have been given, the patient does not return to consciousness quickly. The patient must be watched carefully for laryngeal spasm, which may be indicated by retraction of the soft tissues around the neck muscles, crowing respirations, air hunger, and restlessness. A pulse oximeter is a simple and essential tool for accurate and ongoing assessment of the patient's blood oxygen levels.

Other intravenous agents, such as morphine, meperidine (Demerol), and fentanyl (Sublimaze), are commonly used to maintain anesthesia throughout the surgical procedure and to provide pain relief in the early postoperative period. These are often used in conjunction with nitrous oxide and are referred to as nitrous-narcotic anesthetics. Ketamine (Ketalar) is a dissociative anesthesia that leaves the patient awake in a trancelike state with no pain or memory of the surgery.

***Muscle relaxants.*** Curare and succinylcholine (Anectine) are powerful depolarizing muscle relaxants that may be administered to increase the relaxation of the abdominal muscles during surgery or to facilitate endotracheal intubation. Pancuronium (Pavulon) is a synthetic neuromuscular blocking agent used primarily to produce skeletal muscle relaxation during surgery after general anesthesia has been induced. It is compatible with all the general anesthetics currently in use. Depolarizing drugs may cause respiratory difficulty by suppressing muscle function. All patients must be monitored carefully.

**Regional anesthetics.** Regional anesthetics use narcotics or local anesthetics to inhibit nerve impulses to various parts of the body (Table 20-3). A local anesthetic drug is injected in and around nerves, which results in anesthesia of the area that is supplied by the particular nerves. Several different drugs may be used, including procaine (Novocain), tetracaine (Pontocaine), and lidocaine (Xylocaine). Regional anesthetics may be divided into the categories of spinal, epidural, nerve block, infiltration, and local.

***Spinal anesthesia.*** To induce spinal anesthesia, a solution of a local anesthetic may be injected into the subarachnoid space, which contains cerebrospinal fluid. The drug anesthetizes nerves as they leave the spinal cord. The method of injection is the same as that for any spinal puncture (Figure 20-6). This type of anesthesia is used for surgery that involves the ab-

**TABLE 20-3**

## Selected Regional Anesthetics

| DRUG | CHARACTERISTICS | NURSING CONSIDERATIONS |
| --- | --- | --- |
| Procaine (Novocain) | Used for infiltration, spinal nerve block; widely used in dentistry; available with or without epinehrine | Observe for allergic reaction. May cause poor local circulation if combined with epinephrine for use on injured fingers or toes. |
| Benzocaine (Solarcaine) | Used topically and available commercially | Avoid use near eyes. May cause skin irritation. |
| Lidocaine (Xylocaine) | Used topically and for infiltration nerve block, such as epidural, caudal, and spinal; rapid action and medium duration; also used to treat cardiac arrhythmias; comes with and without epinephrine | Monitor for changes in vital signs, excitability, and seizures if used systemically. |
| Tetracaine (Pontocaine) | Used topically and for infiltration nerve block, such as spial and caudal; more potent and has more toxicity and longer duration than other agents | Protect patient from injury and burns during the period when no sensation is present. |
| Bupivacaine (Marcaine) | Used for infiltration nerve blocks; spinal; long acting | Observe for allergic or toxic reactions. Monitor and protect patient. |

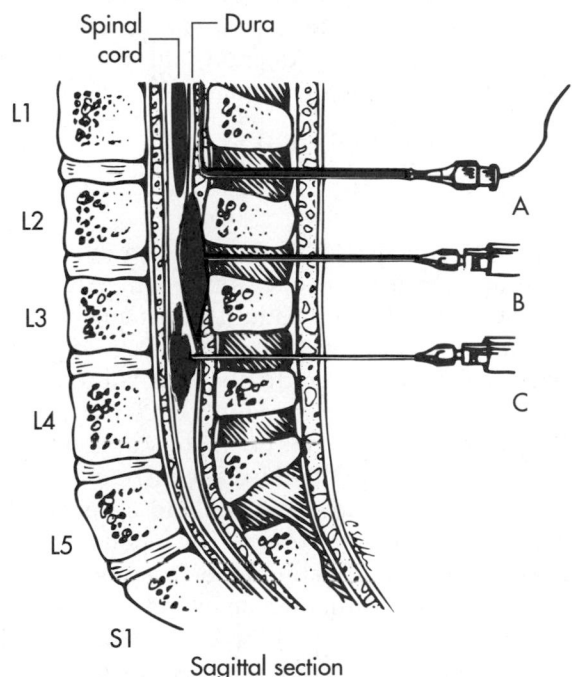

**Figure 20-6**    Location of needle point and injected anesthetic relative to dura. *A*, Epidural catheter. *B*, Single injection epidural. *C*, Spinal anesthesia. (Interspaces most commonly used are L4-5, L3-4, and L2-3.) (From Meeker MH, Rothrock JC: *Alexander's care of the patient in surgery*, ed 10, St Louis, 1995, Mosby.)

domen, perineum, and lower extremities. Use of this method on the upper part of the body or inadvertent migration of medication to the upper spinal canal paralyzes the respiratory muscles and the diaphragm.

The patient may remain awake with spinal anesthesia. Therefore it is necessary that the surgical team avoid any careless conversation that could be misin-terpreted by the patient. During the operation the patient may be aware of pressure or pulling sensations but no pain. After spinal anesthesia, the patient generally is kept flat in bed for several hours. Vital signs, especially blood pressure, should be watched because hypotension may occur. Sensations to the anesthetized part do not return immediately, and careful positioning of the patient is important to prevent later discomfort or pressure injury. The patient may have a severe headache, which is thought to be caused by spinal fluid leaking from the puncture site. The headache often lasts for several days, but analgesics plus an increased oral intake help alleviate the discomfort. Measures taken by the anesthesiologist to reduce the incidence of headache include the use of fine-gauge needles and the placement of a "blood patch" at the insertion site to prevent the leakage of spinal fluid.

*Epidural anesthesia.* Epidural anesthesia involves the injection of a local agent into the extradural space outside the spinal canal. Examples of epidural anesthetics are the sacral and caudal blocks, which are used to anesthetize the perineum during deliveries.

*Peripheral nerve block.* A peripheral nerve block is used to provide anesthesia or freedom from pain in body structures that are innervated by selected nerve systems. Examples include the brachial, femoral, and sciatic nerves.

*Infiltration anesthesia.* Infiltration anesthesia is achieved by injecting a local anesthetic drug directly into the tissues. This type of anesthetic is used for minor operations in which tissue is incised, or it may be used to provide pain control after major operations.

• • •

Because all drugs used for local anesthesia are potentially toxic or may cause an allergic response, the patient should be carefully observed for signs of itching, twitching, convulsions, cyanosis, nausea, and vomiting. The patient's blood pressure, pulse, and respirations should also be carefully checked. The patient is conscious but may be drowsy if a sedative has been administered before the surgical procedure.

**Topical anesthesia.** Drops, sprays, lotions, and ointments are types of topical anesthetics. They are applied directly to the skin or mucosa for temporary anesthesia before a simple procedure or for pain relief. Many of these products are sold over the counter in pharmacies.

## Alternative Forms of Anesthesia

Anesthetic methods such as hypnosis and acupuncture do have the advantage of causing none of the side effects of chemical anesthetics, but these techniques are not widely used or well regarded by many physicians in the United States. Acupuncture is an ancient Oriental method in which fine metal needles are inserted beneath the skin at particular body points to provide anesthesia. There is no clear explanation as to why it is effective, but the technique has been successfully used, particularly for minor procedures. The power of the mind over the body forms the basis for hypnosis as an anesthetic practice. With hypnosis, pain is controlled by the power of suggestion.

## Bloodless Surgery

The risks of accepting a blood transfusion and the refusal of some persons to receive blood on religious and conscientious grounds have motivated caring physicians to develop many alternative ways to treat the patient. In recent years many improvements and developments in techniques, medications, and equipment have facilitated bloodless surgery. These include electrosurgical coagulation, volume expanders, recombinant erythropoietin, hemodilution, intraoperative autologous blood salvage, and predeposit autologous blood.

## Electrosurgical Coagulation

Electrosurgical coagulation is a procedure to limit internal bleeding by coagulating or clotting a patient's own blood during surgery, thus reducing blood loss. Radio frequency (RF) energy is delivered to tissue for the desired clinical effect, such as cutting or coagulation. Benefits of this procedure include reduced blood loss, reduced procedure time, less tissue damage, enhanced healing, and reduced risk of infection.

## Volume Expanders

Volume expanders are intravenous fluids that enhance the circulation of the patient's own blood. The amount of red cells lost is reduced, since each ounce of diluted blood contains a lower concentration of red cells. Examples of volume expanders are crystalloids (Ringer's lactate, normal saline) and colloids (dextran, hetastarch).

## Recombinant Erythropoietin (Epo, Epogen)

Under normal circumstance the kidneys keep track of the oxygen carried by red blood cells in the bloodstream. When the oxygen level is low, the kidneys produce a hormone called erythropoietin that stimulates the bone marrow to make more red blood cells, so that more oxygen can be carried to the body. In the event of a pending surgery, a boost may be given to offset the anticipated decline in red blood cells. Recombinant erythropoietin is then given to stimulate red cell production and accelerate maturation of these cells with surprisingly few, if any, reactions. When given aggressively, in conjunction with iron therapy, it demonstrates a rise in hematocrit levels within 1 week's time.

## Hemodilution

*Hemo* (blood) *dilution* (to dilute or lessen the concentration) takes place in the operating room. After a patient is anesthetized, the anesthesiologist quickly withdraws a large amount of blood by means of gravity drainage. This blood is gradually returned to the patient using equipment arranged in a circuit that is constantly linked to the patient's circulatory system, never being stored. The patient simultaneously receives an equal amount of colloids or crystalloid to replace the volume of the blood withdrawn. The blood is thus diluted, and consequently any blood that is lost in surgery contains very little whole blood but rather a highly diluted mixture of blood and solution. The withdrawn blood is slowly returned to the patient without being stored or having the circuit disconnected. Hemodilution is used primarily when the amount of blood loss is anticipated to be high.

## Intraoperative Autologous Blood Salvage

Intraoperative blood salvage provides the surgical team with a method of maintaining the hemodynamic stability of the patient undergoing surgery by collecting and processing the patient's shed blood and giving it back to the patient without being stored. Cell saver devices continually recirculate the patient's own blood during surgery. Intraoperative blood is salvaged by suctioning, cleaning, and retransfusing back to the patient by means of closed circuit circulation. The cell saver is similar to the heart-lung machine.

### Predeposit Autologous Blood

Predeposit involves the patient's donating his or her own blood before surgery. A patient could donate 1 unit per week and easily accumulate 4 or 5 units by the time of surgery. Autologous predonation not only is safer for the patient by avoiding disease transmission, including human immunodeficiency virus (HIV), but also prevents the consequences of graft versus host blood group incompatibility errors or graft versus host reactions in immunologically suppressed patients. This procedure is not accepted by those who refuse blood on religious grounds.

## Intraoperative Complications

### Malignant Hyperthermia

Malignant hyperthermia is a rapid rise in body temperature that can be triggered by the anesthetic agents or muscle relaxants used during surgery. Its exact pathophysiology is not known, but it is related to a defect in cellular metabolism that results in hypercalcemia. Early warning signs of this potentially fatal complication are tachycardia, muscle rigidity, and a rapid rise in temperature (as much as 1° C every 5 minutes). Treatment consists of cardiopulmonary support during which efforts are made to stabilize vital signs, cool the patient with ice, and reduce muscle spasms with dantrolene (Dantrium). Because this condition is hereditary, the nurse who is preparing the patient for surgery should ask if there has been any family history of this condition or of sudden death during surgery. Patients known to have experienced this complication should be advised to wear a Medic Alert bracelet that identifies this problem.

### Potential Hypothermia

It is not uncommon for patients to experience **hypothermia,** a significant drop in body temperature (95° F or lower), during surgery as a result of low room temperature, incisional exposure of body cavities to the environment, and lowered metabolism. Warm blankets and increased room temperature can limit heat loss.

### Patient Injury

Because patients cannot protect themselves during surgery and anesthesia, the surgical staff must be aware of the potential for harm. Poor positioning may cause skin or nerve damage, as well as respiratory complications. A break in aseptic technique may cause postoperative infection. There are many electrical and equipment hazards because of the increased use of modern equipment. Laser surgery involves special precautions for both patient and staff.

## POSTOPERATIVE ASSESSMENT AND INTERVENTIONS

### Postanesthesia Care

Patients recovering from anesthesia must be closely monitored until their airway reflexes return, their breathing is satisfactory, and their vital signs are stable. Most hospitals maintain facilities for the immediate postoperative care of the patient, and the patient is transferred from the operating room to the postanesthesia recovery unit on a specially designed bed or stretcher. The recovery area, which may be designated as the **postanesthesia care unit** (PACU) or the postanesthesia recovery (PAR), is generally located near the operating room and is equipped with the necessary supplies, drugs, and equipment to care for any emergency that might arise. The **recovery room** is considered a part of the surgical suite and is supervised by the anesthesiologist (Figure 20-7).

The anesthetist or anesthesiologist accompanies the patient from the operating room to the recovery room and advises the nurses of the patient's condition and any special problems that require care or attention. The anesthetist or anesthesiologist ensures that the patient's airway is clear and that his or her vital signs

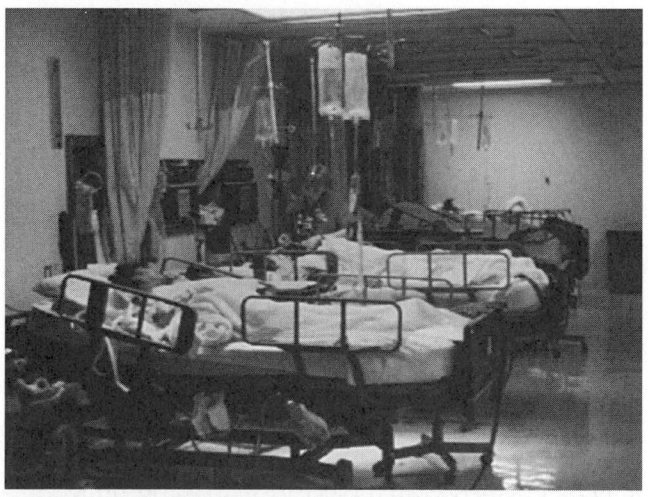

**Figure 20-7** A recovery room or postanesthesia care unit facilitates close observation of the patient during recovery from anesthesia.

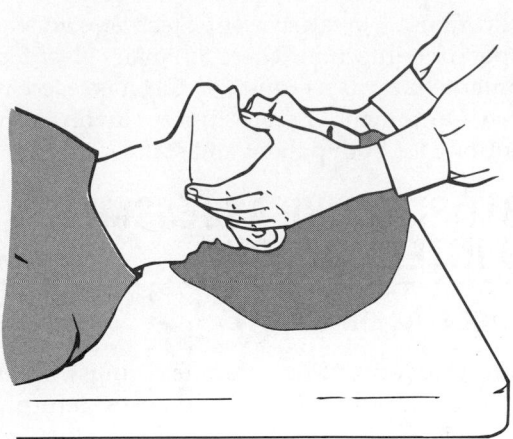

**Figure 20-8** Method of pushing jaw forward to relieve respiratory difficulty.

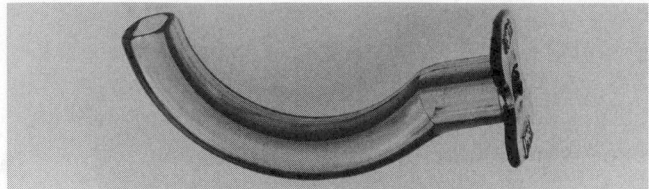

**Figure 20-9** Guedel disposable artificial airway. (Courtesy of Sims Concord Portex, Kean, NH.)

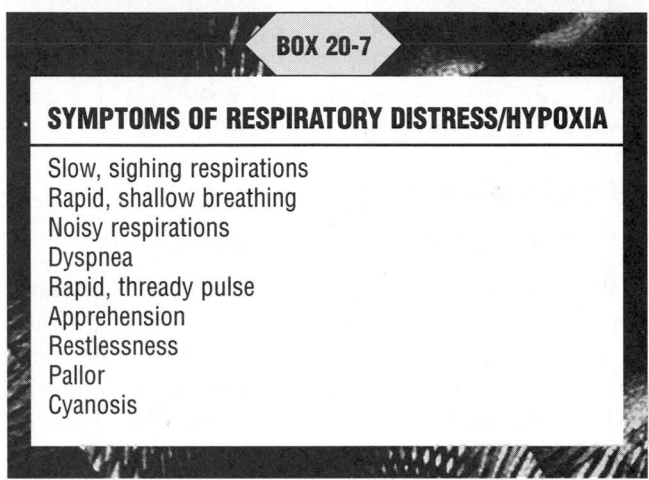

**BOX 20-7**

**SYMPTOMS OF RESPIRATORY DISTRESS/HYPOXIA**

Slow, sighing respirations
Rapid, shallow breathing
Noisy respirations
Dyspnea
Rapid, thready pulse
Apprehension
Restlessness
Pallor
Cyanosis

are satisfactory. Before leaving the patient, the anesthesiologist informs the recovery room nurse of the patient's condition, and the postoperative vital signs are taken. The patient should be protected by side rails on the bed, which may be padded to prevent injury to a particularly restless patient. The patient should be moved as carefully as possible. Anesthetics are stored in the body during surgery, and until they are metabolized, every movement of the patient (e.g., moving from operating table to stretcher or bed, riding in elevators, or wheeling around corners in corridors) may affect vital signs. Regardless of the type of surgery that the patient has undergone, immediate postoperative care should include the maintenance of privacy and warmth, proper body alignment, and **pain management.**

## Airway

The immediate responsibility of the nurse is to ensure that the **airway** is clear and remains clear. If increased secretions obstruct the respiratory passages, they are aspirated with a catheter that has been attached to suction. The catheter must be inserted without suction (suction port open) to prevent damage to the mucous membranes. If secretions have been removed but evidence of respiratory difficulty is still present, the nurse's thumbs and fingers should be placed at the angle of the patient's jaw on both sides, and the jaw should be pushed forward (Figure 20-8). The tongue is the most common cause of airway obstruction and may be grasped with a piece of gauze and pulled forward. If these measures do not open the airway, the nurse may insert an oral or nasal airway or call the anesthesiologist. Often the anesthesiologist leaves an

airway in place until the patient shows signs of regaining consciousness (Figure 20-9).

## Breathing

The patient's respiratory rate should be checked often. Oversedation; shallow, quiet, and slow respirations; noisy respirations; and restlessness may be early signs of respiratory depression. The movement of air into and out of the lungs can be felt by holding a hand near the patient's mouth. Respiratory rates of 30 or above breaths per minute or below 12 breaths per minute should alert the nurse to respiratory difficulty (Box 20-7).

Many anesthetics and anesthetic adjuncts depress the respiratory mechanism. Narcotic anesthetics, sedatives, and neuromuscular blockers all have a negative effect on respiratory activity. The recovery room nurse must be aware of the types of agents used during the surgery and of the time of their administration. The patient who has had a neuromuscular block (curare, succinylcholine) is often requested to lift the head or in some other way demonstrate the return of muscle control before the airway is removed (McConnell, Lawler, 1991).

Patients whose respirations are below 12 breaths per minute as a result of narcotic anesthesia may be medicated with a narcotictagonist such as naloxone (Narcan) or levallorphan (Lorfan). These drugs, given parenterally, work rapidly to reverse narcotic-induced respiratory depression.

## Circulation

The patient's blood pressure and pulse should be taken as ordered or more often as the patient's condition indicates. The patient's preoperative blood pressure should be known so that comparisons can be made. A falling systolic pressure or cardiac arrhythmias should be reported immediately. A critical systolic pressure must be determined for each patient individually and on the basis of preoperative readings. A drop in blood pressure may occur after the administration of certain types of anesthetics, muscle-relaxing drugs, or some tranquilizing drugs. It may also occur as the result of moving the patient or of unrelieved pain. The pulse should be checked for rate, rhythm, and volume. A drop in blood pressure and a weak, rapid, thready pulse with cool, moist skin may indicate severe bleeding or shock, and the physician should be notified immediately. Treatment is based on the cause, and the physician orders the appropriate procedures.

## Drainage

All drainage tubes are connected to the appropriate type of drainage and should be properly connected and patent. Nasogastric tubes are connected to suction, and urinary drainage tubes are connected to the proper drainage container. Dressings should be checked for blood or secretions and constriction, and wound drainage units should be checked for patency. The physician must be notified if bright red bleeding is increasing.

## Intravenous Therapy

The nurse should check and carry out the physician's orders for any procedures or medications, such as administration of intravenous fluids or blood. It is the nurse's responsibility to carefully observe a patient who is receiving intravenous fluids. The rate of flow is ordered, and the number of milliliters per hour must be regulated. The infusion site should be watched for swelling, tenderness, and redness. Blood should appear in the tubing when the nurse aspirates the line with a syringe. If blood does not appear, the intravenous fluid has infiltrated. Infiltration can also be verified by observing continued flow after the vein is compressed with a tourniquet, which is applied above the infusion site. Flow will stop if the needle is still in the vein. The patient's complaint of burning pain at the intravenous site is often the first sign of inflammation or infiltration. When these symptoms occur, the intravenous infusion should be removed and restarted in another area. Nurses should be continuously alert for possible complications, such as respiratory difficulty, circulatory overload, and thrombophlebitis (see Chapter 27).

## Relief of Pain

The awakening patient may complain of pain. Before giving pain-relieving drugs, the nurse should consider the length of time since the preoperative sedatives were administered, the type and action of the anesthetizing agent, the status of vital signs, and the age of the patient. The physician should be consulted whenever any question arises concerning the administration of a narcotic. The patient should be closely monitored for signs of respiratory depression and hypotension. (See Chapter 11 for a complete discussion of pain control.)

## Voiding

The patient may need to void while still in the recovery room and should be encouraged to do so before discharge from an outpatient unit. With the return to full consciousness and the awareness of pain, the patient becomes tense, and voiding may become difficult. The nurse should encourage the patient to void before painful stimuli cause tension or after the pain has been relieved by analgesics. If the patient has an indwelling catheter, the nurse should position the collection unit for optimum drainage. An accurate record of urinary output should be maintained.

## Transfer to Patient's Room or Special Unit

The length of time the patient remains in the recovery room is determined by the immediate postoperative condition. When the vital signs are stabilized and consciousness has been regained, the patient may be transferred from the recovery room. An alert patient can demonstrate orientation to person, place, and time. At the time of transfer the recovery room nurse gives a report about the patient's condition, including any problems that occurred during the immediate postoperative period, to the nurse who will next care for that patient. If the patient needs continued close monitoring, transfer to a special unit may be necessary.

## Intensive Care Unit

The evolution of the intensive care unit (ICU) began in the early 1960s, and almost all units were in large metropolitan hospitals. Now even small rural hospitals have a few beds set aside for the care of critically ill patients. The nurse/patient ratio is low, and the nurses have additional education to provide expert nursing care and to meet any emergency that might arise. The number of beds has increased, and the numbers and types of patients admitted to the ICU have also increased. A patient is admitted to the ICU because of the need for intensive nursing and medical care, which it is assumed cannot be given in the regular clinical units.

The increasing number of patients whose lives may be saved cannot always be cared for adequately in a single unit. Separate ICUs for specific types of patients exist in most large hospitals and include burn units, shock units, coronary care units, respiratory care units, surgical units, neonatal and pediatric care units, and renal care units. Nurses assigned to these units have participated in special courses and are considered experts in intensive care nursing.

## Continuing Postoperative Care

The continued postoperative care of the patient is directed toward the prevention of complications, rehabilitation, and a return to normal living. Family members should be encouraged to see the patient and in some instances may be allowed to remain with the patient beyond visiting hours.

### Comfort and Safety Measures

Postoperative patients should be protected by raising the side rails on the bed. A pillow may be placed under the patient's head, and the head of the bed may be slightly elevated. Because the patient is sensitive to temperature changes, care should be taken to prevent exposure to drafts to avoid chilling. The patient may feel cool to the touch and may complain of being cold because of the cooler temperatures in operating and recovery rooms, as well as the normal circulatory response to stress. The patient may be covered with a blanket until the skin is warm and dry, after which the blanket should be removed to prevent overheating. The patient who becomes too warm becomes restless, and excessive perspiration results in the loss of body fluids and important electrolytes. Oral and back care should be given, and the patient's face and hands should be washed. The patient is turned to the side in Sims' position, with a pillow placed to the back and between the legs to give support. If water intake is not permitted, the lips should be moistened with cool water at intervals. The room should be well ventilated and free from unnecessary noise. The patient should be turned from side to side every 2 hours unless the type of surgery performed limits positioning. Turning is essential to prevent respiratory complications and thrombus formation.

> ### NURSE ALERT
> If the patient's extremities are still cool several hours after surgery, monitor vital signs closely. A failure to "warm up" may be a sign of compensated shock caused by internal bleeding.

### Coughing and Deep Breathing

The purposes of having the patient breathe deeply and cough are to remove mucus and other secretions that accumulate in the respiratory passages during anesthesia and to facilitate expansion of the lungs. Research suggests that forceful expulsive coughing may compromise respiratory recovery by collapsing the alveoli. Coughing exercises therefore are generally done only for patients who have secretions and mucus in the bronchial passageways. When the patient has been taught these exercises before surgery and understands their importance, coughing and deep breathing are accomplished more readily and thoroughly.

Many hospitals use techniques such as encouragement of the patient to yawn, use of the incentive spirometer, and specific respiratory therapies, such as intermittent positive pressure breathing. All these techniques stimulate deep breathing. If coughing is indicated, it is encouraged after deep breathing, should be deep, and should result in expectorating the mass of mucus from the respiratory passages. Better results may be obtained if the patient is placed in a sitting position and if the nurse helps relieve the strain by splinting the incision with a folded towel or pillow. Pain medication that is administered approximately 1 hour before coughing and deep breathing benefits the patient who is experiencing discomfort. If the patient is unable to cough up the mucus and secretions that have accumulated in the respiratory passages, the secretions may need to be removed by suctioning.

Patients who have had surgery of the brain, spinal cord, or eyes should not be permitted to cough because coughing increases intracranial pressure. Lung sounds should be evaluated regularly (i.e., at least once each shift) to assess the lungs for secretions or diminished breath sounds.

## Voiding

Unless an indwelling catheter is in place, the postoperative patient should void within 8 to 10 hours after surgery. The combination of anesthesia, surgery, pain, and apprehension can result in a patient's inability to urinate. A distended bladder can be palpated by examining for fullness above the symphysis pubis. Often the patient is uncomfortable and may void often and only in small amounts.

If the patient's condition permits, the bathroom may be used with the nurse's assistance. Providing adequate hydration through intravenous fluids or taking increased fluids by mouth when permitted facilitates voiding. Running water while the patient is attempting to void, placing the patient's hands in warm water, or pouring warm water over the genital area may also help. The patient should be catheterized only as a last resort and only when the bladder is distended and palpable above the pubis and the patient complains of distress.

If the patient has an indwelling urinary catheter, the nurse should monitor the output every 2 hours for the first 24 hours. Care should be taken to position the collecting unit below the patient to facilitate gravity drainage. Routine catheter care should be followed to minimize the possibility of bladder infection. Records should be maintained of all output.

## Bowel Function

After surgery of the gastrointestinal tract, peristalsis is temporarily absent and usually does not return for approximately 48 hours. The patient's expulsion of flatus or spontaneous movement of the bowels indicates that normal peristalsis has returned. Bowel sounds should be checked once each shift in all four quadrants of the abdomen with a stethoscope, and the nurse should question the patient concerning the passing of gas. Cathartics are not usually administered to surgical patients, and patients should be reassured that usual elimination patterns may not occur for several days. Patients who are accustomed to having a daily bowel movement often become worried. Frequent **ambulation** and extra fluids should be encouraged, and stool softeners may be prescribed.

## Postoperative Nutritional Care

Many surgical patients are not given food until peristalsis returns because eating may result in nausea,

vomiting, and gas formation. They may be allowed sips of cool water or ice chips to moisten the mucous membranes. Before administering oral fluids after surgery, the nurse should check the physician's orders and the patient's ability to swallow. Fluids should initially be given slowly, a few sips at a time.

Intravenous fluids are used routinely to supply hydration and electrolytes. They do not supply energy and nutrients. For example, 5% dextrose in normal saline (0.9% NaCl solution) contains only 200 calories in 1 liter of fluid. Total energy needs postoperatively are about 10 times that amount. Water balance and the prevention of dehydration are constant concerns, and intravenous fluids are used to maintain fluid balance while the patient is NPO or taking limited oral fluids. Patients lose fluids through drainage, vomiting, hemorrhage, fever, and excessive urination so the amount necessary for replacement can be quite high: as much as 7 L per day (Williams, 1995). Oral intake should begin as soon as possible.

A rapid return to nutritious foods should be encouraged to supply the essential amino acids from protein intake that are needed for building tissue. Protein is also essential to maintain adequate albumin levels in the blood. Albumin is necessary for maintaining adequate colloidal osmotic pressure in the blood, which is necessary to draw fluid back into circulation after it leaves the capillaries to nourish the cells. If the fluid leaves the capillaries and does not reenter the blood, volume will diminish and the patient will go into hypovolemic shock (see Chapter 27). This same fluid that cannot return to the blood will remain in the tissues and appear as edema. Generalized edema will affect the function of the heart and lungs, and localized edema will interfere with wound closure and healing. Protein also provides a matrix for the laying down of calcium and phosphorus to form proper bone callus after orthopedic surgery. The major components of the body's immune system that provide defense against infection are protein tissues. Protein is required to carry fat in the bloodstream to tissues to maintain tissue structures and activities and to carry fat to the liver for necessary work in fat metabolism. Protein also combines with fat in the liver and removes it, thus avoiding the fatty infiltration that leads to liver disease. Calories from carbohydrate are necessary in addition to fat and protein to provide the energy needed to spare protein for its essential functions.

**Oral feedings.** Most general surgical patients can and should progress to oral feedings as soon as possible, usually as soon as normal peristalsis in the gastrointestinal tract returns. The nurse checks for bowel sounds to determine the return of peristalsis. The patient usually progresses from clear to full liquids and

**TABLE 20-4**

## Routine Hospital Diets

| FOOD | CLEAR LIQUID | FULL LIQUID | SOFT | REGULAR |
|---|---|---|---|---|
| Soup | Clear fat-free broth, bouillon | Same, plus strained or blended cream soups | Same, plus all cream soups | All |
| Cereal | | Cooked refined cereal | Cooked cereal, corn flakes, rice, noodles, macaroni, sphagetti | |
| Bread | | | White bread, crackers, melba toast, zwieback | All |
| Protein foods | | Milk, cream, milk drinks, yogurt | Same, plus eggs (not fried), mild cheese, cottage and cream cheese, fowl, fish, sweetbreads, tender beef, veal, lamb, liver, bacon, gravy | All |
| Vegetables | | | Potatoes: baked, mashed, creamed, steamed, scalloped; tender cooked whole bland vegetables; fresh lettuce, tomatoes | All |
| Fruit and fruit juices | Fruit juices (as tolerated), flavored fruit drinks | All | Same, plus cooked fruit: peaches, pears, applesauce, peeled apricots, white cherries; ripe peaches, pears, bananas, orange and grapefruit sections without membrane | |
| Desserts and gelatin | Fruit-flavored gelatin, fruit ices and popsicles | Same, plus sherbet, ice cream puddings, custard, frozen yogurt | Same, plus plain sponge cakes, plain cookies, plain cake, puddings, pies made with allowed foods | All |
| Miscellaneous | Soft drinks (as tolerated), coffee and tea, decaffeinated coffee and tea, cereal beverages such as Postum, sugar, honey, salt, hard candy, Polycose, residue-free supplements | Same, plus margarine, pepper, all supplements | Same, plus mild salad dressings | |

From Williams SR: *Basic nutrition and diet therapy,* ed 10, St Louis, 1995, Mosby.

then to a soft or regular diet. Foods allowed in each of these diets are described in Table 20-4.

**Parenteral feeding.** If the patient is unable to eat normally for an extended period of time, protein and other essential nutrients must be supplied intravenously. Solutions containing amino acids, electrolytes, minerals, and vitamins as well as larger amounts of glucose are administered to provide nutritional support. Fat in the form of emulsions is also used to supply needed calories and the essential fatty acid, linoleic acid. The feeding can be supplied through a peripheral vein if a less concentrated solution is being used for smaller nutritional demands over a brief period of time. For larger nutrient demands requiring more concentrated solutions over a long period of time, the feeding catheter must be placed in a large central vein to avoid vein irritation.

The usual site of entry is the subclavian vein, and the catheter is advanced to the superior vena cava (Figure 20-10). This is known as **total parenteral nutrition (TPN).** A basic TPN solution may contain 2.75% crystalline amino acids and 25% dextrose with added electrolytes, vitamins, and trace elements (minerals). The physician and the clinical dietitian determine the needed formula. Nursing responsibilities related to administration of TPN formula are outlined in Box 20-8.

## Tubes

When the patient has a retention catheter in the urinary bladder or a nasogastric tube, the nurse must check it often to ensure that it is draining properly. Irrigations or special procedures that may have been or-

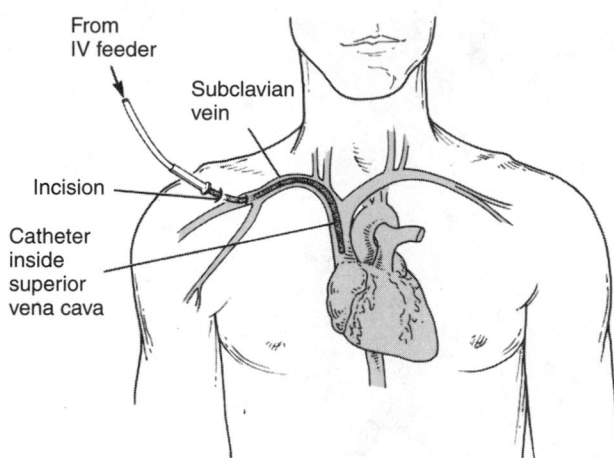

**Figure 20-10** Catheter placement for total parenteral nutrition (TPN) for feeding via subclavian vein to superior vena cava. (From Williams SR: *Basic nutrition and diet therapy,* ed 10, St Louis, 1995, Mosby.)

dered by the physician should be carried out regularly. All drainage should be measured, observed, described, and recorded on the patient's chart.

## Dressings

The nurse must check dressings, wound drainage units, and bed linens beneath the patient often for evidence of excessive drainage or bleeding. If bright red blood appears, the dressing should be observed again within a short period. The surgeon should be notified if there is any increase in bleeding. Dressings should also be checked for constriction of local circulation.

If drainage soaks through the dressing, it may be reinforced with additional dressings until an order has been secured for changing. All wound-dressing changes must be carried out under strict surgical asepsis to promote wound healing. Most hospitals have approved procedures for dressing wounds, and these procedures, including the types of dressings and equipment used, vary among hospitals and surgeons. Some types of dressings, such as those used for severe burns or plastic surgery, may be changed only by the surgeon, and the patient may be given narcotic analgesics and a light anesthetic for the procedure. Abdominal binders may be worn to support the incision while the patient is ambulating. By the time the patient leaves the hospital, no dressing may be required.

Wound drains are commonly used after any surgery in which leakage of fluids around the surgical site is anticipated. Closed drainage systems with the drain exiting the skin through a small stab wound

---

**BOX 20-8**

### ADMINISTRATION OF TOTAL PARENTERAL NUTRITION (TPN) FORMULA

Careful administration of TPN formulas is essential. Specific protocols will vary somewhat. Usually, however, they include the following points:

- *Start slowly.* Give time to adapt to the increased glucose concentration and osmolality of the solution.
- *Schedule carefully.* During the first 24 hours, 1 to 2 L is given by continuous drip, with the slow rate regulated usually by an infusion pump.
- *Monitor closely.* Note metabolic effects of glucose (not to exceed 200 mg/dl) and electrolytes.
- *Increase volume gradually.* After first day, increase by 1 L/day to reach desired daily volume.
- *Make changes cautiously.* Watch the effect of all changes, and proceed slowly.
- *Maintain a constant rate.* Keep the correct hourly infusion rate, with no "catch up" or "slow down" effort to meet original volume order.
- *Discontinue slowly.* Take patient off TPN feeding gradually, reducing rate and daily volume about 1 L/day.

From Williams SR: *Basic nutrition and diet therapy,* ed 10, St Louis, 1995, Mosby.

---

separate from the incision are most common and reduce the risk of incisional disruption and infection (Figure 20-11). These drains empty into a closed reservoir. Open drainage systems, such as the Penrose drain, function through capillary action (Figure 20-12). Fluid from the surgical site is drawn to the body surface and into a dressing. Penrose drains are not used as often now because of the advantages presented by closed drainage systems. If open drainage systems are used, the nurse should change the dressing often, because damp dressings encourage bacterial growth. These dressings are often held in place with Montgomery straps to avoid the repeated use of tape on the skin (Figure 20-13).

## Exercises

Unless contraindicated, exercises should be started as soon after surgery as possible or by the end of the first postoperative day. Starting exercises soon after surgery is especially important if early ambulation is to be delayed. Exercises stimulate circulation; prevent venous stasis, contractures, and loss of function; and facilitate recovery. The patient should be encouraged to

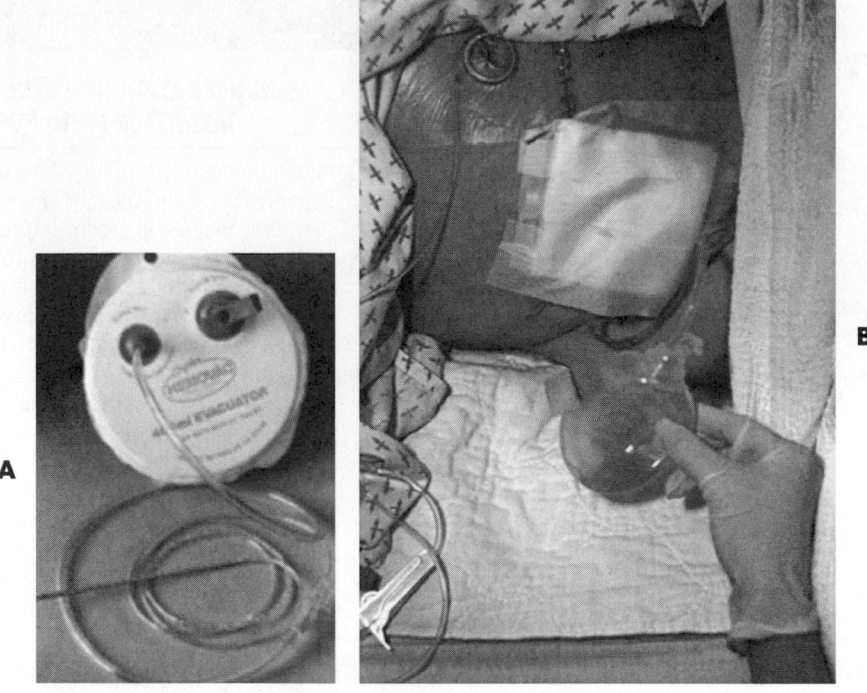

**Figure 20-11**   Closed wound drainage systems. **A,** Portable self-contained. **B,** Jackson-Pratt 100-ml and 400-ml reservoirs with round silicone drains and attached trocars. (**A** from Perry AG, Potter PA: *Clinical nursing skills and techniques,* ed 3, St Louis, 1994, Mosby.)

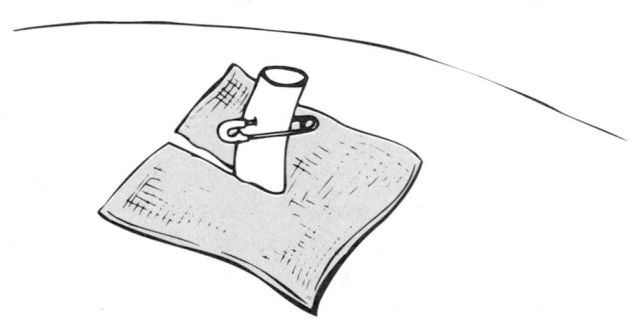

**Figure 20-12**   Penrose drain. (From Perry AG, Potter PA: *Clinical nursing skills and techniques,* ed 3, St Louis 1994, Mosby.)

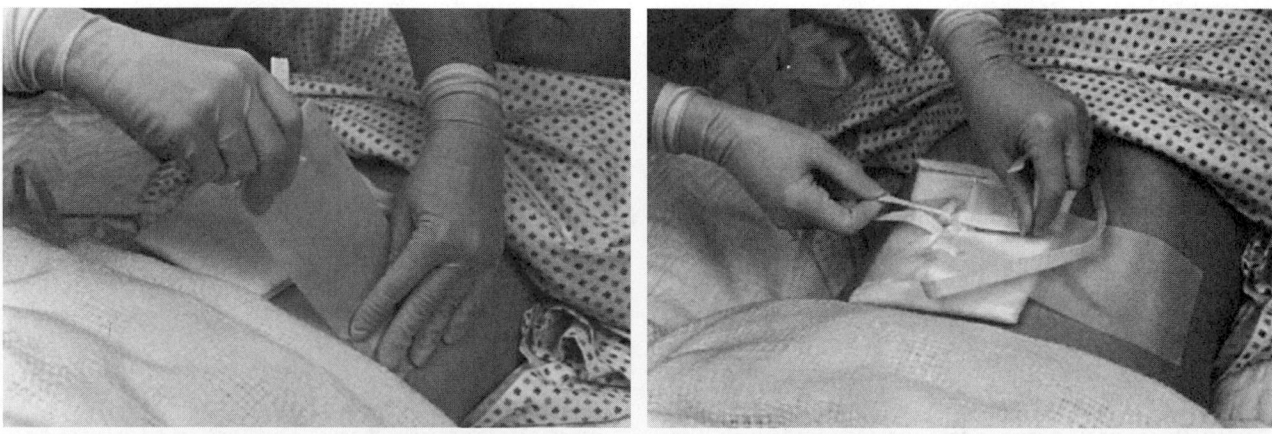

**Figure 20-13**   Montgomery straps may be used when frequent dressing changes are anticipated.

exercise the fingers, hands, arms, feet, and legs. Leg exercises are particularly important to prevent thrombus formation. The patient can alternately flex and extend the legs by bending the knees and straightening the legs while lying in bed. Reminding the patient to perform these exercises encourages the patient to actively participate in recovery.

Pillows should not be placed under the patient's knees, and the knee Gatch of the bed should not be elevated. The patient should not sit on the side of the bed or be up in a chair with the legs dependent for extended periods of time. These positions cause pressure on the veins and engorgement of blood in the lower limbs and contribute to clot formation.

## Wound Healing

**Wound healing** occurs by primary or secondary intention. Most surgical wounds are sutured closely at the time of surgery and heal by primary intention and generally with a minimum of scarring. If a wound is large and has edges that cannot be approximated, it must be allowed to heal by secondary intention, which is the filling of the area from the bottom with scar tissue. Open wounds are far more susceptible to infection. Frequent dressing changes are needed and may include packing these wounds with antiseptic gauze or applying moist dressings. Montgomery straps may be used to avoid tape injuries to the skin when dressings must be changed often.

## Ambulation

Early ambulation facilitates the normal functioning of all body organs and systems and therefore reduces the danger of postoperative complications. Erect posture and activity encourage deep breathing and help prevent lung congestion. Walking stimulates the venous circulation and helps prevent thrombosis. Urinary retention and constipation occur less often in patients who ambulate early in the postoperative period.

Patients are allowed out of bed on the first postoperative day after most major surgeries. Care should be taken while helping a patient get up. If at any time the patient feels faint or nauseous, he or she should return to the last previous comfortable position and remain there for a few minutes before trying to rise again. Getting out of bed and walking soon after a surgical experience may cause apprehension and a fear of pain. The benefits of early ambulation should be well explained before surgery if possible. The type of surgery and the condition of the patient determine when ambulation may be started and the extent of walking permitted.

Ambulation means walking, not sitting in a chair, but it should be a gradual process and should not exhaust the patient. The bed should be elevated to a sitting position before a patient is allowed out of bed. When allowed out of bed, the patient should be assisted by the nurse. A few steps may be sufficient at first. Ambulation permits the patient to be independent, self-sufficient, and able to carry out most self-care activities. It decreases feelings of helplessness, shortens the hospital stay, and enables the patient to regain strength more readily (Box 20-9).

# POSTOPERATIVE CONCERNS

## Pain

Pain is a subjective symptom that indicates physical or emotional distress. The expression of pain varies widely among individuals and cultures. The nurse should remember that pain is always real to the person experiencing it and that efforts should be made toward its relief. The patient may verbally complain of discomfort, or the pain may be manifested in other ways. Facial expressions such as clenched teeth, a wrinkled forehead, widely open or tightly shut eyes, and grimacing are indications of pain but are not always present. Some patients may groan, cry, gasp, or cry out. Body movements, such as muscle tension, immobilization of some or all of the body, kicking, tossing, turning, and rubbing, can also indicate the presence of pain. Observing these symptoms can help the nurse and physician assess the level of pain and provide adequate relief. It is important to remember that some patients in pain will not present a "picture" of pain. The nurse must ask questions to determine the patient's comfort level and offer analgesics. Patients may be unaware that they are permitted to have a pain medication, or they may be reluctant to ask for an analgesic.

The patient's first complaints of pain occur early in the postoperative period. One of the primary responsibilities of the nurse is to evaluate the patient's need for pain medication. When a patient complains of pain, the nurse should note the location of the pain and ask the patient whether it is a constant, intermittent, sharp, dull, or burning sensation. This information should be recorded on the patient's chart. The early administration of a pain-relieving drug, such as morphine or meperidine (Demerol), often provides relief for several hours and permits restful, quiet sleep. Pain resulting from the surgical procedure should diminish after the first 24 to 48 hours, after which new orders are often written for pain management. Pain may be the result of other causes, such as abdominal distention, urinary retention, or casts that are too tight and are pressing on a nerve. A headache sometimes

◁ **BOX 20-9** ▷          **NURSING PROCESS**

## POSTOPERATIVE CARE

### ASSESSMENT
**Immediate**

- Airway and breathing
- Cardiovascular status
- Incision, dressings, drains, intravenous lines
- Level of consciousness, return of voluntary muscle control
- Pain status
- Vital signs
- Skin, nail bed, and lip color

### Continuing

- Ability to cough and breathe deeply
- Respiratory status
- Response to pain interventions
- Incisional healing
- Postoperative complications
- Fluid volume status
- Ability to perform self activities of daily living (ADL)
- Nutrition and elimination patterns
- Support systems after discharge
- Ability to understand follow-up care

### NURSING DIAGNOSES

- Risk for fluid volume deficit/excess related to fluid loss, fluid shift (third spacing), and fluid therapy
- Pain, acute, related to tissue trauma, pressure, or spasms
- Risk for infection related to broken skin and traumatized tissue
- Risk for injury related to electrolyte loss, shock, falling related to surgical intervention
- Impaired physical mobility related to activity restrictions
- Urinary retention related to surgical intervention, anesthesia, analgesia
- Impaired gas exchange related to anesthesia and reduced lung expansion
- Altered nutrition: less than body requirements, related to inadequate nutritional replacement or decreased oral intake

- Activity intolerance related to impaired physical mobility or pain
- Knowledge deficit related to new diagnosis, condition, home care

### NURSING INTERVENTIONS
**Immediate**

- Maintain patent airway.
- Observe for signs of hypoxia.
- Suction secretions from respiratory passageways as necessary.
- Check vital signs often.
- Check dressing often.
- Observe for early signs of shock.
- Maintain proper drainage and/or suction of tubes.
- Provide pain relief.
- Regulate and observe infusion of intravenous fluids.
- Evaluate level of consciousness.

### Continuing

- Encourage deep breathing and coughing.
- Turn and position patient often.
- Evaluate the need for pain medication.
- Position the patient for comfort.
- Encourage voiding.
- Check for flatus or bowel sounds.
- Maintain patency of drainage tubes.
- Measure and record intake and output.
- Care for the wound using aseptic technique.
- Observe for bleeding and drainage.
- Encourage exercises and ambulation.
- Apply antiembolism stockings as ordered; remove for 1 hour every 8 hours.
- Assist with ADL as needed.
- Observe for postoperative complications.

### EVALUATION OF EXPECTED OUTCOMES

- Returns to normal activity and function
- Follows postoperative instructions
- Complications avoided

results from spinal anesthesia, and patients recovering from abdominal surgery experience pain when coughing deeply. The apprehensive and nervous patient may complain of more pain than the calm, passive individual. Older adults may be able to tolerate more pain than younger persons. Obese persons and those who abuse drugs and alcohol often need larger amounts of drugs to relieve pain.

Whatever the cause of pain, the nurse should make every effort to relieve it and to make the patient comfortable. Changing the patient's position, washing his or her face and hands, giving the patient a back rub, applying a cold cloth to his or her forehead, or just sitting with the patient may provide relief and decrease the need for drugs. Drugs such as morphine depress respirations and should not be given when respirations are compromised, when the blood pressure is below what has been established as normal for the patient, or when blood pressure is unstable because shock may result. Narcotics should be given 1 hour before postoperative activities such as ambulation. Nursing care should be given when the patient is receiving the most benefit from the medication. The patient should be told that the medication is for pain. The psychologic effect of knowing that something is being done relieves anxiety and tension, which contributes to the effectiveness of the drug. When a narcotic has been given to an older adult, the nurse must be particularly observant of the patient because the drug may cause restlessness or disorientation.

### Patient-Controlled Analgesia

Pain medication is now commonly administered intravenously with a patient-controlled analgesia (PCA) pump. Morphine or meperidine cartridges are attached to intravenous fluid tubing in a mechanical pump. The patient controls the flow of the medication by pushing a button and is instructed to push the button when any discomfort is present. Overdose is prevented by programming the machine to allow infusion at a predetermined interval. The amount of drug administered is also controlled by settings on the machine. This method gives the patient the ability to control pain and to maintain a consistent level of medication in the blood, which makes pain tolerable. When a PCA pump is used, less medication is required than with the traditional method of allowing pain to return before medication is given.

### Nausea and Vomiting

Postoperative nausea and vomiting result from any one of several causes, including the anesthetic, sensitivity to drugs, surgical manipulation, or serious postoperative complications. Patients who have experienced considerable preoperative vomiting and who fear vomiting postoperatively may be more likely to vomit. A nasogastric tube attached to suction siphonage may be left in place for 24 to 48 hours to keep the stomach empty and to reduce the incidence of nausea and vomiting. Nausea and vomiting that result from anesthesia may last 24 hours or longer. Analgesics may also cause nausea and vomiting. When vomiting appears to be the result of drugs, the physician usually changes the medication order. Most postoperative vomiting is mild and self-limiting and requires little treatment. However, several drugs belonging to the group known as phenothiazines may have an antiemetic effect for some patients and are often ordered by the physician. Some of these include prochlorperazine (Compazine) and promethazine (Phenergan). $H_2$ receptor antagonists, such as cimetidine (Tagamet), ranitidine (Zantac), and famotidine (Pepcid), also reduce postoperative nausea and gastrointestinal distress. If the patient is permitted to have fluids by mouth, sips of ginger ale or cola drinks may be given to relieve nausea. Persistent vomiting results in a loss of body fluids and electrolytes and may be serious.

### Retention of Urine

An overdistended bladder may cause the patient considerable discomfort and actual pain. Patients who have had surgery of the rectum, pelvis, or lower abdomen commonly have difficulty voiding. Catheterization using sterilization technique is indicated when the nurse has exhausted all measures designed to help the patient void. Because a continued inability to void results in overdistention and loss of bladder tone, the physician may order a retention catheter to be inserted until the patient's condition improves (see Chapter 37).

### Abdominal Distention

Abdominal distention occurs when gas accumulates in the stomach and intestines. Many surgical patients have "gas pains" as a result of temporary loss of peristalsis. The cause of gas accumulation in the intestinal tract is not clearly understood. The use of stimulant medications, such as metoclopramide (Reglan), may initiate the return of peristalsis. Severe abdominal distention may interfere with respiratory function. The surgeon may order a nasogastric tube that is inserted through the nose into the stomach and is attached to suction to prevent the stomach from becoming dilated with gas and to prevent further distention (paralytic ileus). Early ambulation can prevent or reduce the amount of distention and can promote the return of peristalsis.

# Complications

The incidence of postoperative complications has been reduced through more careful preoperative preparation for surgery, improved surgical procedures, early postoperative activity, and adequate pain control. However, several postoperative complications continue to occur and probably always will to some extent. The most serious postoperative complications are hemorrhage, surgical shock, respiratory disorders, thrombosis, embolism, wound infection, dehiscence, and evisceration.

## Hemorrhage and Shock

Blood loss may occur during the surgical procedure or after the surgery has been completed and the patient has returned to his or her room. The surgeon evaluates the amount of blood lost during surgery and, if the loss has been large enough, orders a transfusion of appropriate blood products. A secondary hemorrhage may result from an untied blood vessel or from the slipping of a ligature. It may involve a vein or artery and may be external or internal (into a body cavity or organ). All types of hemorrhage create an emergency situation and require immediate steps be taken to control bleeding and to restore blood volume.

Early detection is important to prevent damage to the cells and vital organs and, in some cases, death. The nurse should be conscientious about inspecting the dressings for evidence of bleeding from the wound. When significant bleeding occurs, the patient may require return to the operating room. The nurse should be alert to the symptoms that may indicate internal and external bleeding.

Symptoms of hemorrhage are essentially those of hypovolemic shock. Early signs include cool extremities, restlessness, apprehension, an increasing pulse rate, and oliguria. Later the skin becomes pale, moist, and cool; the respiratory and pulse rates increase; the temperature becomes subnormal; and the blood pressure falls. In addition to blood on dressings, external evidence of hemorrhage may be observed, such as blood in vomitus, in urine, or from the lungs (hemoptysis).

Other causes of postoperative shock are cardiac failure, drug reactions (including anesthetic drugs), transfusion reaction, pulmonary embolism, adrenal failure, and sepsis. Each cause results in a pathologic process that ultimately produces cardiovascular collapse and poor oxygenation of all body tissues. The symptoms of each type of shock are essentially the same as those of hypovolemic shock. Treatment depends on the cause of shock, but oxygen and intravenous solutions are always administered. The patient is kept flat and warm, and vital signs are checked at frequent intervals and recorded (see Chapter 27).

## Respiratory Disorders

Many respiratory complications can be prevented through careful postoperative care. Patients who have a respiratory disease before surgery are most likely to develop complications after surgery. Before surgery, the nurse should observe the patient for congestion, coughing, or sneezing and report such symptoms to the physician. The most common complications are bronchopneumonia, hypostatic pneumonia, bronchitis, pleurisy, and **atelectasis** (see Chapter 22). Maintaining a clear airway, instructing the patient to breathe deeply and to cough, turning the patient regularly, placing the patient in Fowler's position, and encouraging early ambulation are nursing interventions that are designed to prevent respiratory complications.

## Thrombosis and Embolism

Several factors contribute to the formation of a blood clot, or thrombus, in the vein. This complication, called **thrombosis,** is most common in persons who are required to maintain bed rest. Other predisposing factors include tight abdominal binders; injury or pressure to veins, which occurs in the operating room at the time of surgery; decreased respiration and blood pressure; or any condition that results in the decreased flow of blood through the veins. **Embolism** occurs when a blood clot breaks away from a vessel and enters the circulation. Emboli that originate from thrombi in veins usually follow the normal circulatory pathways until the next capillary system is reached, which is that of the lungs. Pulmonary embolism is a serious complication of surgery (see Chapter 22). Postoperative exercises, early ambulation, and frequent position changes are nursing interventions that help prevent these complications. TED hose (elastic support stockings) and pneumatic leg wrappings (sequential compression devices [SCDs]) "squeeze" the legs upward in a sequential manner, which promotes venous blood return. TED hose and SCDs may also be ordered to prevent venous pooling in the legs.

## Wound Infection

Surgical **wound infections** usually are manifest by the fifth postoperative day. The organism most often involved is *Staphylococcus aureus*, but *Escherichia coli*, *Proteus vulgaris*, *Aerobacter aerogenes*, and *Pseudomonas aeruginosa* are also involved. A postoperative wound infection is classified as a hospital-acquired, or nosocomial, infection (see Chapter 15). Factors such as preexisting illness, obesity, advanced age, complicated surgery, and forms of therapy such as radiation and chemotherapy predispose the patient to postoperative infections. A break in surgical asepsis and a

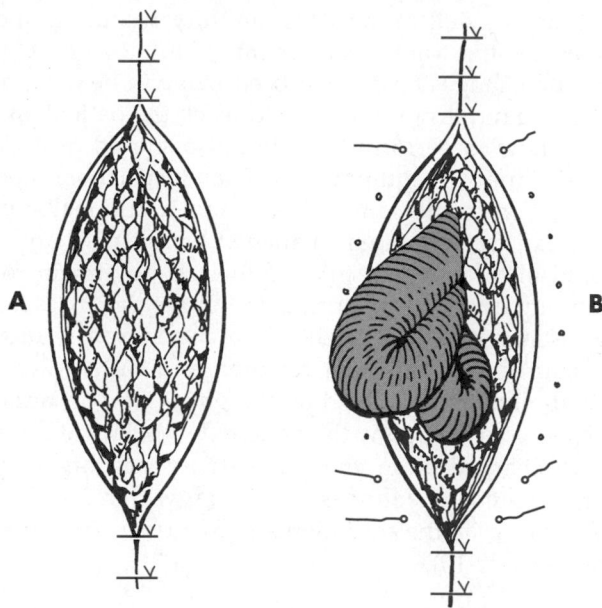

**Figure 20-14** **A,** Wound dehiscence. **B,** Wound evisceration. (From Phipps WJ et al: *Medical-surgical nursing: concepts and clinical practice,* ed 5, St Louis, 1995, Mosby.)

failure to use an aseptic technique during wound care can also result in infection. Infected wounds are cleaned and irrigated by the physician, and often a drain is placed in the incision. The drainage is cultured, and appropriate anti biotic drugs are administered. Clean incised wounds should heal without infection if they are uncontaminated. Infection may also be caused by contaminated intravenous and bladder catheters.

## Dehiscence and Evisceration

**Dehiscence** and **evisceration** may result from infection, abdominal distention, coughing, and poor nutrition. These conditions occur more often in chronically ill or obese patients and usually on the sixth or seventh postoperative day, which is generally when the patient is back home. Both conditions are caused by the sloughing of sutures or staples before healing takes place. In dehiscence some or all of the sutures may give way, which causes the edges of the skin to separate. When evisceration occurs, the incision suddenly opens up and the intestines are released to the outside (Figure 20-14).

Any serosanguineous drainage from the wound of a postoperative patient should be investigated immediately. The wound should be covered with a sterile dressing or a sterile towel held loosely in place. The surgeon should be notified immediately. The nurse should remain calm and should reassure the patient while checking vital signs. The patient should be placed in low Fowler's position, and food or fluids should be withheld until the patient is seen by the physician. Generally the patient is returned to surgery, and the wound is resutured.

---

**BOX 20-10**

### DISCHARGE CRITERIA OR OUTCOMES FOR THE POSTSURGICAL PATIENT

**INPATIENT AND OUTPATIENT**
- The incision is clean and dry and approximated.
- The vital signs are within preoperative normal levels.
- The patient is voiding without difficulty and in adequate amounts.
- The patient has only mild to moderate pain, which is managed by oral analgesics.
- Family or friends are available to transport the patient home and be available.
- The patient has no signs and symptoms of complications, and the patient and family verbalize knowledge of signs and symptoms of postoperative complications.
- The patient is tolerating the prescribed diet and can describe any dietary or activity changes that are necessitated by the surgery.
- The patient or a family member demonstrates an ability to care for the incision, take medications, or do any procedures needed for continuing convalescence.
- The patient can describe the schedule of follow-up care with the physician.
- The patient verbalizes knowledge of community resources and support groups that may be useful in promoting recovery.

**ADDITIONAL INPATIENT CRITERIA**
- The patient is able to carry out activities of daily living without significant increase in pain and fatigue.
- Elimination patterns have been reestablished.
- The patient is able to correctly perform breathing exercises and shows no evidence of respiratory distress.

# PATIENT AND FAMILY TEACHING AND PLANNING FOR DISCHARGE

Careful planning for the transition from the postoperative unit to the home setting or extended care facility is essential for optimum recovery. This planning is done by the patient, family, nurse, and other appropriate members of the health care team. Postoperative hospital stays have decreased in length dramatically in the past decade, which has increased the need for teaching the patient and family numerous procedures and therapies that were once only carried out in the hospital setting. Nowhere is the need more evident than in the outpatient surgery setting. Postoperative patients may be discharged with dressings and urinary and surgical drains still in place and even with ongoing intravenous infusions.

The nurse collaborates with the physician in determining what care the patient and family can provide at home, as well as what community resources and home nursing care agencies may be necessary. If dressing changes or other procedures will be done at home, the nurse not only should teach the patient and family how to perform them but also should provide a small supply of equipment, written instructions, and the location in the community where additional supplies can be obtained. Patients being discharged should also know the time of their appointment for follow-up care with the physician. If the patient is being discharged to an extended care facility, a written summary of the medical regimen and nursing care plan should be completed by the physician and nurse and should accompany the patient. If the patient is being discharged from the day-surgery or outpatient unit, the nurse telephones him or her within 24 hours to follow up on the condition and to answer any questions (Box 20-10).

# KEY CONCEPTS

➤ The nurse can minimize the potential for the negative effects of stress by identifying factors (other than the surgical experience) that may be contributing to the patient's concern.

➤ Stress and breaks in the skin, such as a surgical incision, make infection a real possibility for every surgical patient. Antibiotic therapy may be prescribed prophylactically, but meticulous surgical and postsurgical aseptic techniques are the keys to preventing infection.

➤ The surgical procedure may alter the patient's perception of body image and always causes a temporary or permanent disruption of life-style.

➤ Issues of spirituality (the broad concept that represents an individual's search for the meaning of life and death) are often not confronted until a time of serious illness and the possibility of death. Therefore in preparing the patient for surgery, it is important to support the patient and facilitate his or her personal expressions of spirituality.

➤ The objective of surgical nursing is to prepare the patient mentally and physically for surgery and to assist in full recovery in the shortest time possible and with the least discomfort.

➤ Informed consent means that the physician has provided the patient with an explanation of the surgical procedure, the possible consequences of the surgery, and what to expect during the postoperative period.

➤ The goal of preoperative preparation and care of the patient is to promote the best possible physical and psychologic state of the patient before surgical therapy.

➤ Surgical treatment requires added nutritional support for tissue healing and rapid recovery. Optimal nutritional support involves both oral and venous feeding methods.

➤ Preoperative instruction usually includes deep breathing and coughing, turning and moving, medications, and special equipment that may be used postoperatively. Vigorous coughing is discouraged in cases in which increased intracranial pressure must be avoided.

➤ During the immediate postanesthesia period, the nurse is responsible for ensuring that the airway remains clear, that normal respirations are maintained, and that signs of hemorrhage are treated. The patient's temperature, respiratory rate, blood pressure, and pulse must be monitored; the dressings must be checked; and the drainage tubes and intravenous therapy must be maintained.

➤ Discharge planning must begin before surgery and involves the patient, family, nurse, and other members of the health care team. Resources for the specific needs of each patient must be identified.

# CRITICAL THINKING EXERCISES

1. Mr. Burns is admitted to the hospital for elective surgery. The day before surgery, he is given preoperative care. He is taught how to cough and breathe deeply, turn in bed, and perform leg exercises. In reviewing Mr. Burns's chart, the nurse sees that the consent for surgery has been signed and that all necessary laboratory work is on the chart. However, on the morning of surgery, the nurse enters Mr. Burns's room to assist him with morning care and sees him sitting in his chair fully clothed. When the nurse asks Mr. Burns about this, he states, "I've changed my mind, and I've decided to go home." How would you, as the nurse, respond to this situation? What are some fears that Mr. Burns may have concerning his surgery?

2. Mrs. Hops is admitted to the hospital for removal of her gallbladder. Mrs. Hops is 36 years of age, is 5 feet 4 inches tall, and weighs 194 pounds. She tells the nurse that she has been in the hospital three times, when she delivered her children, but has never had surgery. When she had her last child 4 years ago, she had a blood clot in her leg and had to remain in the hospital for 6 additional days. Why are deep breathing and leg exercises especially important for Mrs. Hops to learn? What complications must the nurse be alert for in caring for Mrs. Hops after her surgery?

## REFERENCES AND ADDITIONAL READINGS

Beare P, Myers J: *Adult health nursing,* ed 3, St Louis, 1998, Mosby.

Black J, Matassarin-Jacobs E: *Luckman and Sorensen's medical-surgical nursing,* ed 4, Philadelphia, 1993, Saunders.

Good M: Relaxation techniques for surgical patients, *Am J Nurs* 95(5):39-43, 1995.

Hogstel M, editor: *Nursing care of the older adult,* ed 3, Albany, NY, 1994, Delmar.

Hulka JF, Reich H: *Textbook of laparoscopy,* ed 2, Philadelphia, 1994, Saunders.

Keep N: Identifying pulmonary embolism, *Am J Nurs* 95(4):52, 1995.

Long B, Phipps W, Cassmeyer V: *Medical-surgical nursing: a nursing process approach,* ed 3, St Louis, 1993, Mosby.

McConnell E, Lawler M: Preventing postop complications, *Nursing* 21(11):33-47, 1991.

McNamara SA: Perioperative nurses' perceptions of caring practices, *AORN J* 61(2):377-387, 1995.

Nicholson C et al: Are you ready for video thoracoscopy, *Am J Nurs* 93(3):54-57, 1993.

Rocuronium Z: A safer fast muscle relaxant? *Am J Nurs* 95(3):56-57, 1995.

Saltiel-Berzin R: Managing a surgical patient who has diabetes, *Nursing* 22(4):34-42, 1992.

Thompson JM et al: *Mosby's clinical nursing,* ed 4, St Louis, 1998, Mosby.

Vernon S, Pfeifer GM: Are you ready for bloodless surgery? *Am J Nurs* 97(9):40-47, 1997.

Williams SR: *Basic nutrition and diet therapy,* ed 10, St Louis, 1995, Mosby.

# CHAPTER 21

## Emergency and Trauma Care

## CHAPTER OBJECTIVES

1 Define the four goals of emergency care.
2 Discuss legislation related to emergency departments.
3 List the characteristics unique to emergency nursing practice.
4 Compare and contrast hospital triage to disaster triage.
5 Describe the steps in cardiopulmonary resuscitation and relief of airway obstruction.
6 Identify the three assessments done on all emergency patients and identify injuries for each assessment area.
7 Identify three life-threatening traumatic injuries affecting airway, breathing, and circulation.
8 Discuss the signs and symptoms of shock and the initial interventions and outcomes.
9 Discuss the precautions to take when administering intravenous conscious sedation.
10 Identify a brief neurologic examination and discuss how it relates to patients with head injuries, environmental emergencies, and psychiatric emergencies.
11 Discuss why violence is a problem in the emergency department.
12 Discuss the four types of maltreatment/abuse and the five areas of maltreatment. Identify the nurse's legal role.
13 Identify three behaviors a psychiatric patient may exhibit during the initial examination in the emergency department.
14 Discuss care of the patient who has overdosed and the patient who is suicidal.
15 Discuss specific selected areas related to emergency care: heat and cold emergencies, head-injured patient, and anaphylaxis.
16 Identify how to help a family who has just experienced sudden death.
17 List the components of critical incidence stress debriefing and discuss what occurs in each component.

## KEY TERMS

against medical advice
agitation
blood alcohol concentration (BAC)
cardiopulmonary resuscitation (CPR)
chain of custody
child maltreatment or abuse
cricothyroidotomy
domestic violence
high-efficiency particulate air respirator/ N95 respirator
hyperthermia
hypothermia
prioritization
resuscitation
sexual assault
stabilization
triage

## EMERGENCY DEPARTMENT

It has been estimated that emergency departments (EDs) are visited by approximately 100 million patients a year. Before 1970 the general public had little awareness of emergency care. The emergency room was seen as the back door to the hospital until legislation was enacted that developed prehospital care, and criteria was set for hospital trauma designation (Table 21-1 and Box 21-1).

**TABLE 21-1**

## Legislation Affecting Prehospital and Emergency Care

| YEAR | LEGISLATION | |
|------|-------------|--|
| 1966 | Highway Safety Act | Federal government established protocols and standards for prehospital care by developing the emergency medical service (EMS). |
| 1973 | Emergency Medical Services Systems Act | Funds allocated to communities for the regionalization of the EMS. These funds provided dollars for the education of EMTs and paramedics. Communities were able to purchase equipment to provide prehospital care such as transport vehicles, telemetry/defibrillation monitors, and medications. |
| 1976 | Trauma System Designation | The American College of Surgeons published an article discussing levels of care for the trauma patient. These recommendations were recognized by the Joint Commission on Accreditation of Healthcare Organizations, and hospitals could voluntarily be classified by these trauma standards. |
| 1986/1990 | Consolidated Omnibus Reconciliation Act (COBRA) | Enacted to prevent "patient dumping," COBRA stated that all hospitals receiving Medicare dollars must perform an initial screening to any person who arrives at an ED to see if a medical emergency exists. Stabilization of the person must occur. If the patient is transferred, a physician at the receiving hospital must accept the person. All medical records including x-ray films must be transferred with the person. This act is constantly under revision (Emergency Nurses Association, 1993). |

**BOX 21-1**

### LEVELS OF TRAUMA CENTER DESIGNATION

**LEVEL I**

Level I trauma centers are regional resource hospitals that provide total care for every aspect of injury. This hospital helps with research and injury prevention. Available resources include 24-hour capability for computed tomography (CT) scans, angiograms, and surgery. Designated specialties can be available within 30 minutes. Patients taken routinely to Level I trauma centers by paramedics are those who do not have spontaneous eye opening; have penetrating injuries to the head, neck, or abdomen; have fallen from a height of greater than 15 feet; or live patients who have been in the same car involving a fatality.

**LEVEL II**

Level II hospitals have the ability to administer 24-hour emergency care by a qualified emergency physician. A surgeon needs to be available on call within 20 to 30

minutes. The hospital needs to have prearranged transfer agreements for critical specialty injuries. Examples of these injuries are burns, spinal cord injuries, acute head trauma, and reimplantation of amputated body parts.

**LEVEL III**

Level III hospitals need to have an emergency physician on call 24 hours a day and available within 30 minutes. They need not have 24-hour capability for CT scans or the ability to perform surgery 24 hours a day. These hospitals are seen in rural settings.

**RURAL HOSPITALS**

Rural hospitals are institutions where life-saving measures may be initiated. The patient is stabilized and transferred to the nearest qualified facility.

From American College of Surgeons: Resources for optimal care of the injured patient, Philadelphia, 1990, The College.

This legislation resulted in the development of improved emergency services and EDs through the establishment of prehospital care and goals for the ED. The ED is now seen as the front door to the hospital, giving patients their first impression of the institution.

## Goals of Emergency Care

The goals of EDs are to stabilize and resuscitate, reduce suffering, provide emotional support, and educate the public on how to care for themselves once they leave the ED. These goals are obtained through the collaborative efforts of the health care team.

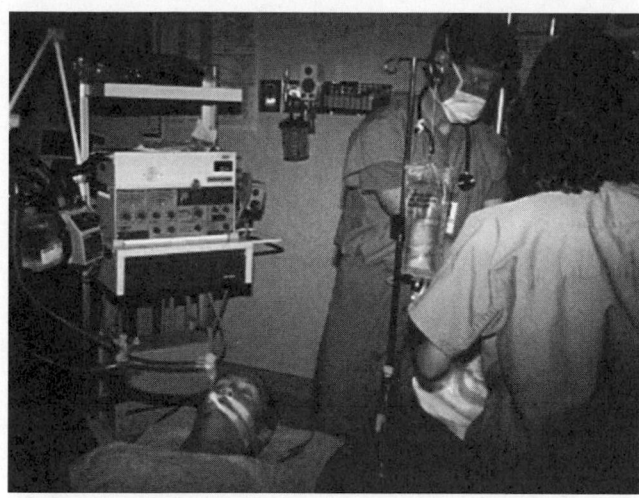

**Figure 21-1** Members of the emergency care team. (Courtesy Michael Clement, MD, Mesa, Ariz.)

## Emergency Care Team

The emergency care team includes many members. The physician, emergency nurse, respiratory therapists, chaplain, social services, patient care representatives, nurses extenders, and x-ray and laboratory technicians all allow the patient coming to the ED to obtain the most complete care (Figure 21-1).

The emergency nurse is a key component of this team. The nurse's responsibilities vary with each situation, the number of emergencies, the available professional personnel, and the policies of the individual institution.

## EMERGENCY NURSING

Emergency nursing as defined by the Emergency Nurses Association (ENA) is the practice of emergency care by a registered professional nurse. Emergency nurses work in a variety of settings: hospitals, urgent-care centers, industrial plants, schools, and nonacute care clinics. The emergency nurse has a role in the prehospital care of patients and in the education of prehospital providers.

Emergency nursing has been recognized as a nursing specialty since 1970, when the Emergency Nurses Association was established. Standards for practice in emergency nursing are established through the ENA. Time is critical when using the nursing processes of assessment and analysis, which include **triage** and **prioritization** and intervention. Emergency nurses manage patients of all ages who require **stabilization** and/or **resuscitation** for life- or limb-saving measures. They also provide crisis intervention. The ED nurse

must provide care in an unpredictable and uncontrolled environment (Dains et al, 1991).

## Characteristics of the Emergency Nurse

Emergency nurses must have the ability to work quickly and efficiently; to continuously prioritize patient care; to be flexible and energetic; and to communicate effectively. The nurse must be able to intervene with families in grief, perform crisis intervention, and diffuse volatile situations. The nurse must teach patients and families expectations of care while being treated in the ED and how to complete the care started in the ED by either providing discharge instructions or facilitating the transition of the patient to another patient care area. Most activities of the nurse include procedures learned in basic and medical-surgical nursing courses. Additional education required includes electrocardiogram interpretation, basics of trauma care, and pediatric care. The nurse may carry out various procedures including administration of medications, catheterization, lavage, and oxygen therapy. The emergency nurse must be able to work as a team member but have the self-confidence to practice autonomously with collaboration of the physician and health care team. The nurse must have good technical skills and be knowledgeable regarding the rapid changes in this highly critical area. Hospitals have developed standards of care and protocols to allow for quicker response to patient illness. The nurse is a patient advocate, who communicates the plan of care and keeps the patient informed as care progresses.

## Role of the Emergency Nurse

The emergency nurse has many roles as the direct caregiver of patients in the emergency department. These roles include triage nurse, primary nurse, and associate primary nurse. Two advanced practice registered nurse roles that are developing for the masters-prepared registered nurse are the clinical nurse specialist and the emergency nurse practitioner. Emergency nurses practicing in the prehospital setting include the emergency communication registered nurse, the prehospital registered nurse, and the flight nurse. Finally, the importance of the ED nurse manager cannot be overlooked.

### Triage Nurse

The triage nurse is the first nurse who assesses all ambulatory patients when they enter the emergency department. For more information about triage, see the triage section.

## Primary Nurse

The primary nurse is the main nursing caregiver for the patient. A complete secondary and focused assessment is performed and the findings communicated to the physician. The primary nurse must be able to give a quick but accurate report to the emergency physician so that a plan of care can be determined. The nurse may order specific tests or x-ray examinations or initiate care according to the policy standards in the ED. The emergency nurse directs professional and ancillary staff while coordinating patient outcomes.

## Associate Primary Nurse

The associate primary nurse may be a licensed practical nurse (LPN), who accepts tasks delegated after the complete assessment of the patient has been completed. The LPN in the ED is becoming a vital team member.

## Emergency Nurse Manager

Because the ED is the front door to the hospital, it is constantly under scrutiny. The nurse manager must be fiscally responsible for the unit, be supportive of the ED staff, and have good public relations and communications skills. The manager must be able to handle patient comments, as well as be proactive in instituting change.

# PATIENT ARRIVAL AND CONSENT

Patients may arrive at the ED in an emergency medical services (EMS) unit (ambulance) from home, work, or an accident scene. They may arrive on their own or be brought by family or friends. They may arrive by helicopter from an accident scene or as a transfer from another facility. No matter how a patient arrives, the care is determined by a systematic approach. All patients receive a screening to see if an emergency exists. The triage nurse usually provides this initial screening. Consent for treatment in the ED must be obtained. This consent is expressed, implied, or involuntary (Box 21-2).

Care should be started or continued immediately when a patient arrives at the ED to prevent complications. However, the nurse's safety should never be jeopardized when administering care.

# INFECTIOUS DISEASE PRECAUTIONS

When preparing to care for any patient, it is imperative that the emergency team is ready to protect itself against infection from the human immunodeficiency

---

**BOX 21-2**

### TYPES OF CONSENT FOR TREATMENT

Expressed—The person comes and asks for care. If the person is under the age of 18, consent should be obtained from the parent or legal guardian. If an emergency does exist, the emergency physician can sign for consent for treatment until formal consent is obtained from the parent or guardian.

Implied—The patient comes in by ambulance and is in need of life-saving measures. It is implied that care is being sought. Consent for care should be obtained from a family member, if possible.

Involuntary—Under the Mental Health Act, treatment can be performed to a patient who refuses treatment if it is determined that the patient is not acting rationally and could potentially harm himself or herself or others. A judge will determine the patient's competence after a court hearing. Patients included may be intoxicated, may have taken an overdose, may be suicidal, or may be psychotic (Klein et al, 1994).

---

virus (HIV), hepatitis B, and tuberculosis (TB) by using Standard Precautions. The emergency team should follow infection-control guidelines as indicated by the Centers for Disease Control and Prevention (CDC). Current federal Occupational Safety and Health Administration published guidelines have been developed to protect the health care worker from contracting TB. The guidelines state that health care workers need to wear a **high-efficiency particulate air respirator** or an **N95 respirator** for high-risk activities such as suctioning and intubation. The N95 respirator is a mask that is to fit the face with a tight seal and filters out inspired air droplet size of 1 to 5 microns (Borton, 1997) (Figure 21-2).

---

**NURSE ALERT**

Hands should always be washed after any contact with a patient, even if gloves were worn. This decreases the chance of transmission of diseases.

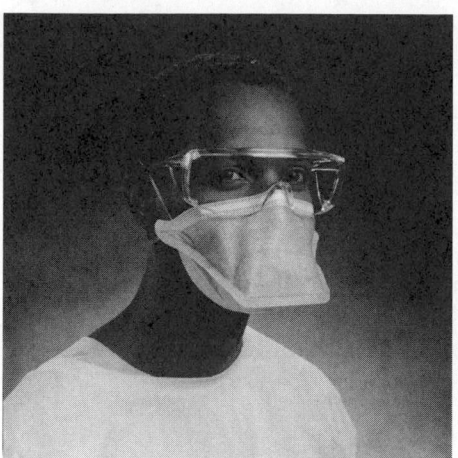

**Figure 21-2**   Health care workers must wear high-efficiency particulate filter respirator when performing high-risk activities such as suctioning and intubation. (Courtesy Kimberly-Clark Corporation, Roswell, Ga.)

# TRIAGE

## Triage Classification

The patient is triaged for determination of treatment. Triage was originally used during World War II to sort out battlefield casualties. The military triage system selected those most likely to live and gave them priority in care and evacuation to medical facilities. This type of triage is still used today during disasters. In contrast, triage used by hospital EDs classifies patients by prioritizing those who are most serious and need the most immediate attention. This is done through the identification of a chief complaint and a brief assessment. The patient is then classified as emergent, urgent, or nonurgent. The classification of expectant or imminent is added during a disaster (Box 21-3).

## Role of Triage during Disaster

The role of triage during a disaster changes to field triage. A temporary satellite health facility is set up at the scene of the disaster. Prehospital triage is initiated by the EMS. Emergency medical technicians (EMTs) are taught to assume the leadership role at the scene of a disaster in deciding the prioritization of patient care and the organized transport of the victims to hospitals. In-hospital triage begins when the patient is received from the ambulance or walks into the ED. Each system depends on the immediate assessment of the patient's status and the identification and immediate treatment of those victims seriously compromised. The Met Tag system is used during a disaster instead of the regular emergency chart because of the great influx of pa-

---

> **BOX 21-3**
>
> ### TRIAGE CLASSIFICATIONS
>
> Emergent refers to a life-threatening problem. If the patient is not seen immediately, he or she will die or lose sight or a limb. Some of these patients are in cardiac arrest, have uncontrolled bleeding, have taken a drug overdose, are experiencing sudden loss of vision, have received chemical or electrical burns, or are in respiratory distress.
>
> Urgent implies that care can be delayed from 20 minutes to 2 hours without significant mortality or increased disability to the patient. These include patients who have open fractures or are experiencing moderate to severe pain. These patients need to be reassessed every 15 minutes to monitor changes in their conditions.
>
> Nonurgent implies that care can be delayed more than 2 hours. These patients have simple rib fractures, sprains, fractures without neurovascular compromise, earaches, or simple lacerations.
>
> Expectant/Imminent is a classification used during a disaster that indicates that the patient will die shortly from his or her injuries. These patients may have experienced an acute head injury with protruding brain matter or extensive burns (Sheehy, 1992).

---

tients. Patients are identified by a color tag system. A red tag means emergent, yellow tag means urgent, green tag means nonurgent, and a black tag means expectant/imminent. The tag, which is securely attached to the patient, includes space for identification of the patient, allergies or current medications, vital signs, medications, treatments, x-ray films, and any significant history. The "expectant" patient who has massive injuries is transported to the hospital after the "emergent" and "urgent" patients have already been treated.

## Telephone Triage

According to ENA's position statement written in conjunction with the position statement by the American College of Emergency Physicians, a diagnosis should never be given over the telephone. The nurse should encourage the caller to come to the ED for care or to see his or her physician. If the patient tells the triage nurse of a situation that could be life-threatening, the nurse should inform the person to call the paramedics and provide whatever information is needed to save the patient's life while waiting for help (Emergency Nurses Association, 1991a).

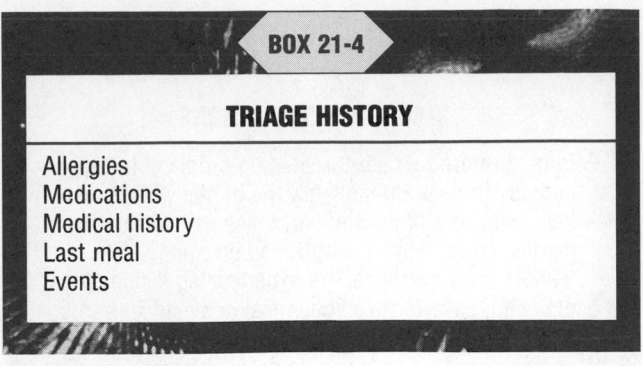

**BOX 21-4**

**TRIAGE HISTORY**

Allergies
Medications
Medical history
Last meal
Events

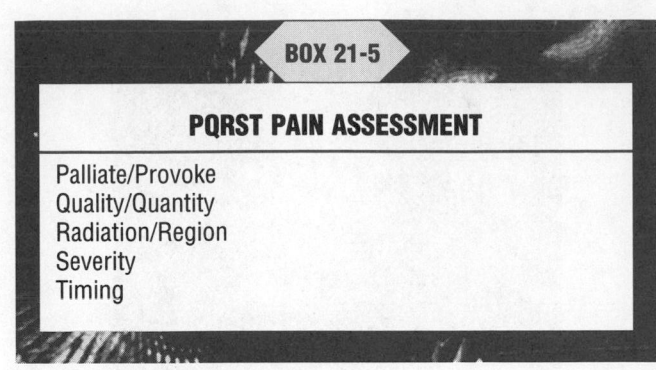

**BOX 21-5**

**PQRST PAIN ASSESSMENT**

Palliate/Provoke
Quality/Quantity
Radiation/Region
Severity
Timing

Telephone triage is performed according to the facility's policies. It is important to understand the Nurse Practice Act regarding who is able to perform this role. In some states it is illegal for an LPN to perform telephone triage.

## Triage Assessment

For stable patients, a brief problem-oriented assessment is conducted to investigate the patient's complaint (Box 21-4). The patient's actual or stated weight is obtained, and, for female patients, the last menstrual cycle is documented.

## EXAMINATION AFTER TRIAGE ASSESSMENT

### History

The patient is assigned to an area where a thorough history and physical examination can be performed. Obtaining a thorough history from a patient allows the health care team to identify problems and determine the degree of concern of the patient's condition. It is imperative to identify and recognize the severity of a patient's condition to allow for an optimal outcome. Some questions to ask are: "What made you seek medical care now? How long have the symptoms existed? Where is the pain? What makes the pain worse or better?" (Box 21-5).

In trauma patients it is important to determine the mechanism of injury or how an injury occurred. Understanding the mechanism of injury allows the health care provider to anticipate potential problems that may arise during the hospital stay. Some sample questions to ask to determine the mechanism of injury include the following:

Was a seat belt worn?
Was a helmet worn?
Was the patient injured at a high or low rate of speed?

How far did the person fall, and what caused the fall?
What instrument was used to cause the injury (gun, knife)?
Who inflicted the injury (male or female, size of assailant)?

This history should augment the history already obtained by the triage nurse or the EMT. The severity of the complaint or condition of the patient will determine who performs the initial examination. The primary nurse conducts the secondary assessment, which is a brief examination to assess and set priorities on all injuries and problems, unless the patient is critically ill or injured. In this case it is not uncommon to have a physician and other members of the health care team work aggressively together to stabilize the patient.

### Physical Assessment

The physical assessment should include inspection, auscultation, and palpation. Percussion may be used during the examination but many times this portion of the physical assessment is deferred because the findings are validated by x-ray or other diagnostic tests. These areas are evaluated during the primary, secondary, and focused assessments (Tables 21-2 and 21-3).

## PRIMARY ASSESSMENT AND INTERVENTIONS

*A*irway, *b*reathing, and *c*irculation (ABCs) are the key components of the first assessment of any patient. The goal of the primary assessment is to identify all life-threatening problems and intervene with resuscitative measures. This is a quick but thorough assessment of the patency of the airway, stability of the cervical spine, ability to breathe, and circulatory status. These are the ABCs of emergency care. In addition, *d*isability (D) is assessed through a brief neurologic examination followed by complete *e*xposure (E) of the patient to allow a more thorough inspection for injuries. Many health care providers are required by the agency they work

## TABLE 21-2

### Emergency Physical Examination

| PRIMARY ASSESSMENT (ABCDE) | ASSESSMENT | INTERVENTION |
|---|---|---|
| Airway/cervical spine | Obstructed | Perform jaw thrust or chin lift. |
| | | Remove debris: teeth, emesis. |
| | | Insert oral/nasal airway. |
| | | Prepare for intubation or a cricothyroidotomy. |
| | Patent | Immobilize cervical spine if this is a trauma patient. |
| Breathing | Absent | Bag/valve/mask at 15 L. |
| | | Prepare for intubation. |
| | | Prepare for positive pressure ventilation. |
| | Present | Administer oxygen if needed (see Figure 21-3). |
| Circulation | Absent | Begin CPR. |
| | Present | Assess location, quality, rate of pulse. |
| | | Assess blood pressure, skin color, temperature, and capillary refill. |
| | | Identify source of bleeding. |
| | | Initiate intravenous access. |
| | | Send type and cross match. |
| Disability (neurologic) | Responsive | Assess level of consciousness. |
| | Unresponsive | Assess response to stimuli (verbal, pain). |
| | | Assess pupils for symmetry and response. |
| | | Prepare to protect patient from harm (secure an endotracheal airway to prevent aspiration; position the patient). |
| Expose | | Completely undress patient. |
| | | Cover patient to prevent heat loss. |

for to have cardiopulmonary resuscitation (CPR) training. This course is offered by the American Red Cross, the American Heart Association, and the National Safety Council. A brief review of clearing an obstructed airway and CPR on an adult patient will be included. Thousands of lives could be saved each year if more people were trained in these rescue maneuvers.

## Airway and Cervical Spine

Is there a patent airway? An airway may be partially or completely obstructed (Figure 21-3). If the airway is partially obstructed, the patient will exchange air. If the air exchange is good, the patient can cough forcefully, dislodging the obstruction. Sometimes the air exchange is good initially but becomes poor. If the air exchange is poor, the patient's cough will be ineffective. There will be a high-pitched noise with inhalations called stridor, a violent respiratory effort using abdominal and intercostal muscles, and even cyanosis. With complete airway obstruction the patient cannot speak, breathe (no air movement), or cough, and he or she may clutch the neck (Figure 21-4). This is the universal choking sign.

## Obstructed Airway

The nurse should ask the patient to speak. If the patient cannot speak, the nurse should attempt to clear the airway. The nurse should stand behind the patient, wrapping the arms around the patient's waist (Figure 21-5). Making a fist with one hand and placing the thumbside against the patient's abdominal midline slightly above the navel and well below the xiphoid process, the nurse should grasp the fist with the other hand. The nurse should then press the patient's abdomen with quick upward thrusts. This process is commonly called the Heimlich maneuver, named for Dr. Harry J. Heimlich, who developed it. Each thrust should be distinct and delivered with the intent of relieving the airway obstruction. The thrusts should be repeated until either the foreign body is expelled or the patient becomes unconscious.

If the patient lapses into unconsciousness, the nurse should position the patient on his or her back and open the airway by performing a chin-lift or jaw-thrust maneuver, which pulls the tongue away from the posterior pharynx. To open the airway using the chin-lift maneuver, the nurse should open the mouth by grasping both the tongue and lower jaw between the thumb

---

**TABLE 21-3**

## Emergency Physical Examination—Secondary Assessment

| AREA OF ASSESSMENT | MODE OF ASSESSMENT |
| --- | --- |
| Head | **Inspect** for any bleeding, depressions of the skull, lacerations, avulsions, embedded foreign bodies, puncture wounds, swelling, and ecchymosis.<br>Look at symmetry of face.<br>**Palpate** for tenderness and bony deformities. |
| Eyes | **Inspect** for bruising around eyes and redness in eyes.<br>Check for contact lenses.<br>Assess gross vision. Is patient able to see from either eye?<br>Assess pupillary response, size of pupils, and symmetry.<br>Assess movement of eyes. |
| Ears | **Inspect** for drainage from ears. Note color of drainage.<br>**Inspect** for bruising behind ears. Check for lacerations. |
| Nose | **Inspect** for drainage from nose. Note color of drainage.<br>**Palpate** for tenderness and bony deformities. |
| Neck | **Inspect** for penetrating objects, tracheal deviation, neck vein distention, swelling, and bruising.<br>**Palpate** for tenderness, tracheal deviation, and subcutaneous emphysema. |
| Chest | **Inspect** for penetrating objects, lacerations, avulsions, embedded foreign bodies, puncture wounds, swelling, and ecchymosis.<br>Look at symmetry and expansion of chest wall.<br>Observe rate of respirations, depth, and use of accessory muscles.<br>**Palpate** for tenderness, bony deformities, and subcutaneous emphysema. |
| Abdomen | **Auscultate** for breath sounds and heart sounds.<br>**Inspect** for penetrating objects, lacerations, avulsions, embedded foreign bodies, puncture wounds, swelling, and ecchymosis.<br>Inspect for protruding abdominal contents and distention.<br>**Palpate** for tenderness or rigidity. |
| Pelvis/genitalia | **Inspect** for deformity of pelvis and blood at the urinary meatus or rectum. Check rectal sphincter tone.<br>Observe for priapism.<br>**Palpate** for tenderness or pain. |
| Extremities | **Inspect** for deformities, lacerations, missing fingers and toes, swelling, and bruising.<br>Assess circulation to area, sensation, and ability to move.<br>**Palpate** for tenderness, pain, and pulses. |
| Back | **Inspect** for deformities, lacerations, and bruising.<br>**Palpate** for tenderness of the spine and costovertebral angle.<br>**Auscultate** for posterior breath sounds. |

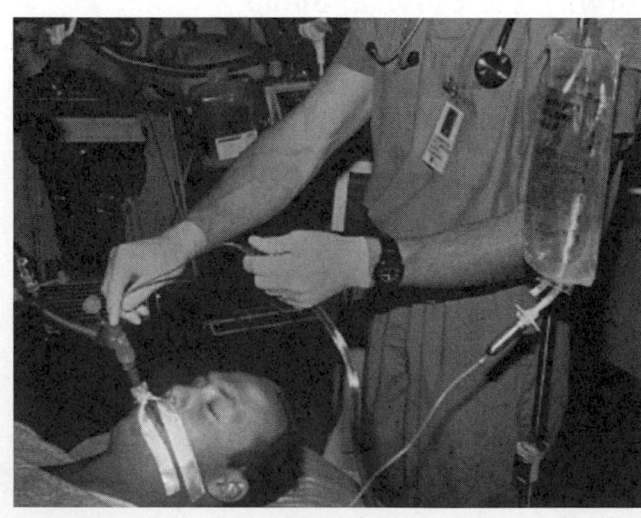

**Figure 21-3**  Patient is intubated to maintain airway. (Courtesy Michael Clement, MD, Mesa, Ariz.)

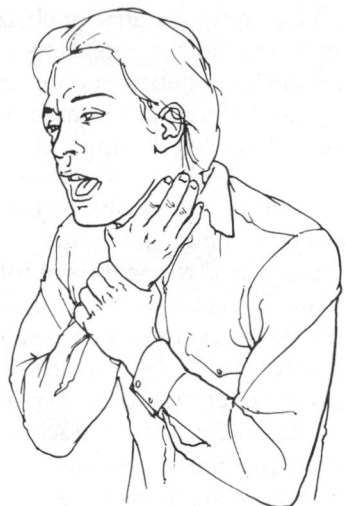

**Figure 21-4**    Universal distress signal for choking. (From Standards and guidelines for cardiopulmonary resuscitation and emergency cardiac care, part 2, *JAMA* 255:2915-2932, 1986.)

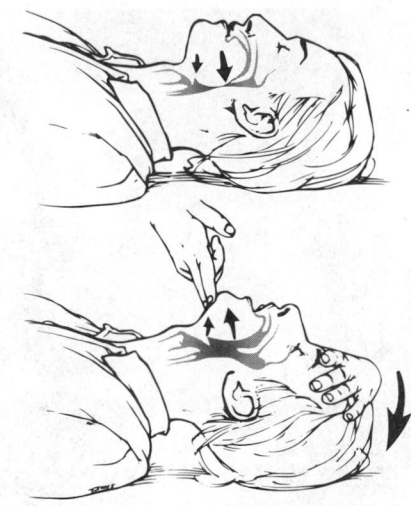

**Figure 21-6**    Head-tilt/chin-lift method of opening airway. (From Standards and guidelines for cardiopulmonary resuscitation and emergency cardiac care, part 2, *JAMA* 255:2915-2932, 1986.)

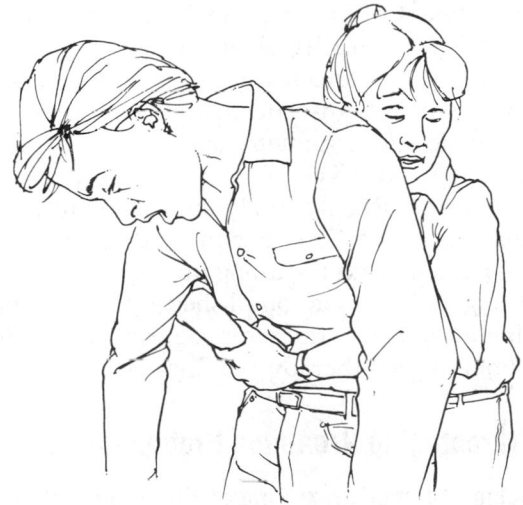

**Figure 21-5**    Heimlich maneuver. Conscious victim with foreign-body airway obstruction. (From Standards and guidelines for cardiopulmonary resuscitation and emergency cardiac care, part 2, *JAMA* 255:2915-2932, 1986.)

---

**BOX 21-6**

### CERVICAL SPINE PRECAUTIONS IN THE TRAUMA VICTIM

The cervical spine should not be hyperextended in a trauma patient because of the potential for a cervical spine injury (JAMA, 1992; Sheehy, 1992). Caution should be taken with all patients with trauma above the clavicles because they may have a cervical spine fracture. The cervical spine should be immobilized until x-ray films have been taken to show that there is no fracture through C7. A trauma patient should be immobilized on a backboard with a cervical collar and paracervical immobilization. If the patient cannot lay flat because of injury and a threatened impairment of breathing, it is necessary to stabilize the cervical spine as best as possible and quickly assess the patient.

---

and fingers, lifting the mandible forward (Figure 21-6). The jaw is supported and this helps tilt the head back. This method should not be used in a suspected cervical spine trauma patient because the neck hyperextends (Box 21-6). In the jaw-thrust maneuver, the nurse should place fingers at the angle of the jaw and push the mandible forward, keeping the patient's head in a neutral position (Figure 21-7).

For adult patients, the nurse should use a finger to sweep the mouth to remove any foreign material such as blood, teeth, or emesis. Sweeping the mouth of a child or infant is not done unless the object is visible. The nurse should then attempt to ventilate the patient by using one of the above methods. If the airway is still obstructed, the nurse should place the heel of one hand against the abdomen, midline above the navel and well below the xiphoid (Figure 21-8). The nurse should place the second hand directly on top of the first hand and press into the abdomen with five quick, upward thrusts. The nurse should check the patient's mouth again for foreign material by sweeping a finger into the mouth, reposition the head, and attempt to

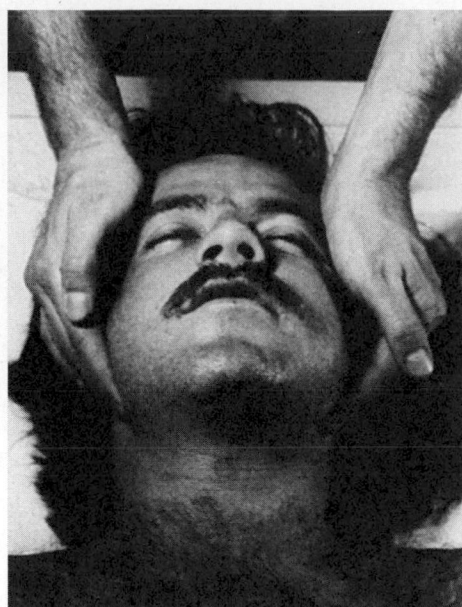

**Figure 21-7**    Jaw-thrust maneuver. (From Sheehy SB et al: *Manual of clinical trauma care: the first hour*, ed 2, St Louis, 1994, Mosby.)

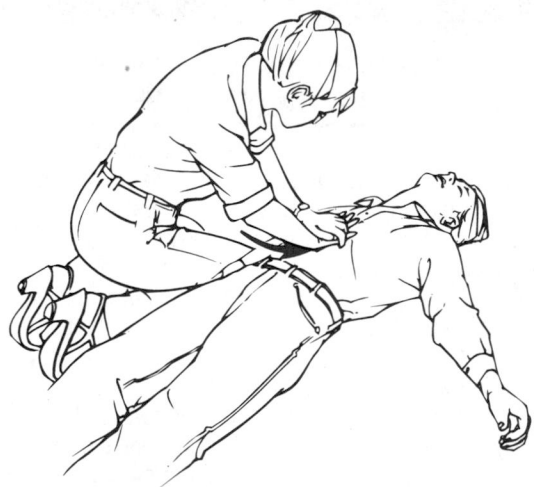

**Figure 21-8**    Heimlich maneuver. Unconscious victim with foreign body airway obstruction. Nurse may be able to perform maneuver more effectively if positioned over patient, straddling patient's thighs. (From Standards and guidelines for cardiopulmonary resuscitation and emergency cardiac care, part 2, *JAMA* 255:2915-2932, 1986.)

ventilate. If the airway is still obstructed, the nurse should repeat the process until the airway is clear. Foreign matter should be removed, and patency of the airway should be determined. If the patient is not breathing, an oral or nasal endotracheal tube should be placed, and rescue breathing should begin.

If a head injury is suspected, a nasotracheal tube should not be used because of a possible basilar skull fracture. A patient with facial fractures or a fractured larynx may have a complete airway obstruction. A laryngeal fracture should be suspected if there are bruises on the neck or if subcutaneous emphysema is observed and palpated in the neck area. Subcutaneous emphysema feels like Rice Krispies crunching. Air is forced into the subcutaneous tissue when the larynx is damaged. The patient may exhibit hoarseness, coughing, or hemoptysis. Emergently, the patient would need a procedure called a **cricothyroidotomy.** This is when an incision is placed in the cricothyroid membrane of the trachea to secure an emergency airway. A tracheostomy will need to be performed later in the operating room to better maintain the patient's airway for a long period. An emergency tracheotomy is usually not performed in the ED because of the potential for uncontrolled bleeding during the procedure.

The abdominal thrust should never be practiced on an individual who is not experiencing airway obstruction.

## Breathing
### Assessment

The assessment of breathing includes rate of respirations, quality of breaths, air movement, use of accessory muscles or intercostal muscles and auscultation of lung sounds. Signs and symptoms of ineffective breathing include asymmetry of chest-wall expansion, cyanosis, altered level of consciousness, distended neck veins, or tracheal shift. If noted, a life-threatening problem exists and intervention needs to be immediate. All patients with breathing impairment need high flow oxygen. This is accomplished by using a nonrebreather mask with a reservoir bag. For more information about oxygen therapy, see Chapter 22.

### Life-Threatening Breathing Problems

**Tension pneumothorax.** One of the easiest life-threatening breathing problems in which to intervene is a tension pneumothorax (Figure 21-9). It is usually caused by blunt chest trauma but can also occur in patients with chronic obstructive lung disease, lung cancer, or patients being positive pressure ventilated with an Ambu bag or a ventilator. A tension pneumothorax is a condition in which air gets in between the parietal and visceral pleurae of the lung but cannot get out. Air gets trapped in this space, compressing the lung tissue. The lung tissue then shifts to the opposite side, compressing the heart and the great vessels. This causes a decrease in cardiac output. If not relieved immediately, the patient will die. Signs and symptoms include severe respiratory distress, tracheal shift to the unaffected side, absent breath sounds on the injured side, distended neck veins, and hyperresonance to percussion. Hyperresonance is a tympanic sound, like the

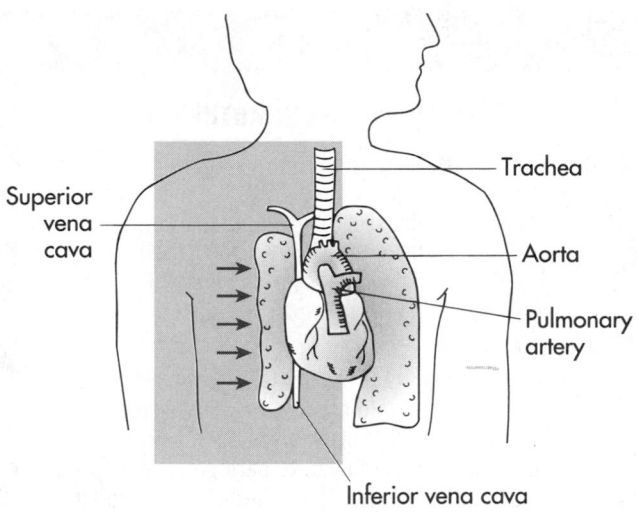

**Figure 21-9**    Tension pneumothorax. (Redrawn from Sheehy SB: *Emergency nursing: principles and practice*, ed 3, St Louis, 1992, Mosby.)

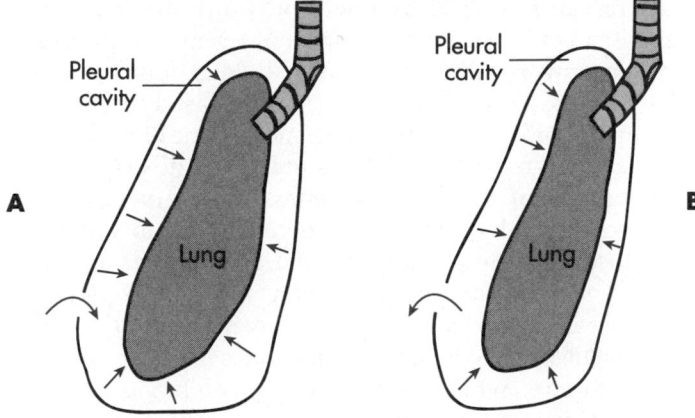

**Figure 21-10**    Open pneumothorax. **A,** Air enters pleural cavity during inspiration. **B,** Air exits pleural cavity during expiration. (Modified from Sheehy SB: *Emergency nursing: principles and practice*, ed 3, St Louis, 1992, Mosby.)

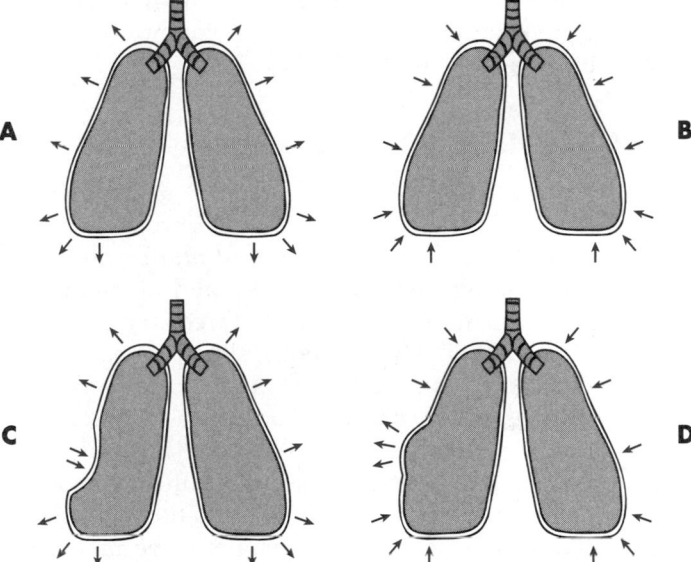

**Figure 21-11**    Flail chest. **A,** Normal lungs during inspiration. **B,** Normal lungs during expiration. **C,** Flail chest during inspiration. **D,** Flail chest during expiration. (Modified from Sheehy SB: *Emergency nursing: principles and practice*, ed 3, St Louis, 1992, Mosby.)

sound of a kettledrum. Immediate treatment is a needle thoracostomy. A hospital policy is written to identify who is able to perform this procedure, and it is usually not an LPN function. A 16-gauge needle is placed in the second-to-third intercostal space at the midclavicular line on the side of the chest that has no breath sounds. Pressure should be relieved, and marked improvement of the patient should be noted. Until a physician can insert a chest tube, intravenous (IV) tubing can be attached to the hub of the catheter and the tubing lowered into a bottle of saline to make a water seal. For more information, see Chapter 22.

**Open pneumothorax.** An open pneumothorax (Figure 21-10) or "sucking chest wound" is usually caused by a penetrating injury such as a gunshot wound or knife injury. The result is that air can enter into the pleural cavity through the chest wall. This especially occurs if the diameter of the hole is greater than two-thirds of the tracheal opening. Signs and symptoms are severe respiratory distress, gurgling, sucking chest sounds, tachypnea, and grunting. Initial treatment includes placing Vaseline gauze over the penetrating injury opening during forceful expiration. The dressing should be taped on three sides to allow air to escape. If air collects in the pleural space after the dressing is applied, a tension pneumothorax could result. The patient will exhibit signs of increasing respiratory distress. The dressing should be loosened or removed to allow the air to escape. The patient will need a chest tube. If the patient has a large, open pneumothorax surgical intervention is needed to repair the defect. The patient will need to be intubated, placed on a ventilator, and prepared for surgery (see Chapter 20).

**Flail chest.** The third condition that poses a life-threatening ventilation problem is a flail chest (Figure 21-11). This is usually caused by a blunt chest trauma such as a fall or a kick to the chest. It also can be the result of compressions during CPR. A flail chest occurs when three or more adjacent ribs are fractured in two or more places, or when the sternum is detached. This allows for a paradoxical (or opposite) movement of that chest segment. On inspiration, when the rest of the rib cage moves outward, the flail segment sinks inward. On expiration, when the rib cage moves inward, the flail segment bulges outward. Because pressure within the chest is decreased as a result of this paradoxical movement, movement of air is decreased. Signs and symptoms are a paradoxical chest movement of the flail segment, respiratory distress, cyanosis, and hypoxia. The patient's respiratory status is closely monitored and arterial blood gases are ordered to monitor the ventilation status. The patient may be intubated and placed on a ventilator.

**Hemothorax.** A final complication of breathing is a hemothorax, which is a collection of blood in the pleural cavity. Enough blood could collect to cause symptoms of shock to develop. Signs and symptoms are difficulty breathing, cyanosis, dyspnea, use of intercostal muscles, dullness with percussion to the area, and signs of shock (tachycardia; hypotension; cool, clammy skin; and decreased urine output). Treatment to improve the patient's breathing is to administer oxygen and prepare for chest-tube insertion. If the patient is bleeding profusely into the hemothorax, autotransfusion may be necessary (Box 21-7).

## Circulation

Circulatory status and the identification of a shock state should be assessed. Ventricular fibrillation is a major cause of loss of cardiac output and cardiac arrest. Determining unresponsiveness and obtaining a defibrillator to terminate this life-threatening emergency is essential. Hypovolemic shock is the most commonly occurring type of shock seen in trauma patients but also can occur in acute gastrointestinal bleeds, and leaking or ruptured aortic aneurysms (see Chapter 27). The objective assessment includes location, quality, and rate of pulse. The location of absent and present pulses gives an estimate of the patient's blood pressure (Table 21-4). If no carotid pulse is palpated, CPR is initiated.

### Basic Cardiac Life Support

Once cardiac function is lost, it must be restored as quickly as possible to avoid cerebral damage. Before starting basic life support, first determine unresponsiveness. This is accomplished by gently tapping the patient's shoulder and asking, "Are you OK?" If the patient does not respond, call for help. This may mean briefly leaving the patient to get additional help. 9-1-1 is the telephone number used in many areas to activate the EMS. Calling for help will allow for access to advanced cardiac life support treatments such as defibrillation, oxygenation, and medications. Next the patient should be assessed for the presence or absence of res-

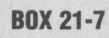

**BOX 21-7**

## TREATMENT FOR HEMOTHORAX

**CHEST TUBE INSERTION SITES**
The chest tube is placed on the affected side, fifth intercostal space, midaxillary line, if fluid is to be relieved. If the tube is to relieve air from the pleural cavity, it is placed in the second intercostal space, midclavicular line (see Chapter 22).

**AUTOTRANSFUSION**
The purpose of autotransfusion is to reinfuse the patient's own blood into the intravascular space. It is performed only from clean areas such as chest trauma from a hemothorax or perioperatively during hip surgery. It is never done from a contaminated area such as the abdomen.

**TABLE 21-4**

## Pulse and Blood Pressure

| PULSE SITE | ESTIMATED BLOOD PRESSURE |
|---|---|
| Carotid only | 60 mm Hg |
| Femoral | 70 mm Hg |
| Radial | 80 mm Hg |

If a radial pulse is present, the systolic blood pressure is at least 80 mm Hg. If a radial pulse is absent but a femoral pulse is present, the estimated systolic blood pressure is 70 mm Hg.

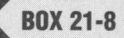

**BOX 21-8**

## ROLE OF FIRST RESPONDER

Many times the nurse will be the first responder to an emergency scene or the first person in a patient's room when an emergency is occurring. The first response has three steps:
1. Check
   The nurse must check the patient and recognize an emergency exists.
2. Call
   Decide to act. Then call for help.
3. Care

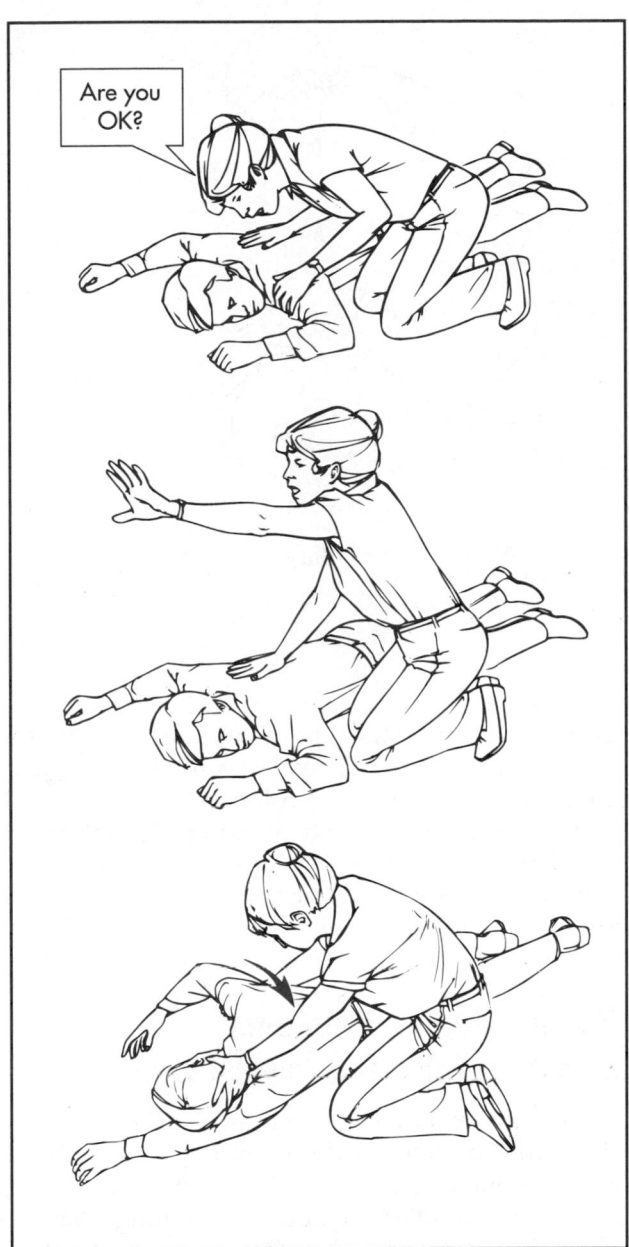

**Figure 21-12** Initial steps in cardiopulmonary resuscitation. *Top,* Determining unresponsiveness. *Center,* Calling for help. *Bottom,* Correct positioning. (From Standards and guidelines for cardiopulmonary resuscitation and emergency cardiac care, part 2, *JAMA* 255:2915-2932, 1986.)

pirations by turning the patient on his or her back (Figure 21-12 and Box 21-8).

**Open the airway.** The airway is opened using the chin lift or jaw thrust (see Figures 21-6 and 21-7). Without muscle tone, the tongue and epiglottis will obstruct the pharynx and larynx.

**Determine breathing.** Breathlessness should be determined by placing an ear over the patient's mouth and nose while maintaining an open airway. The patient's

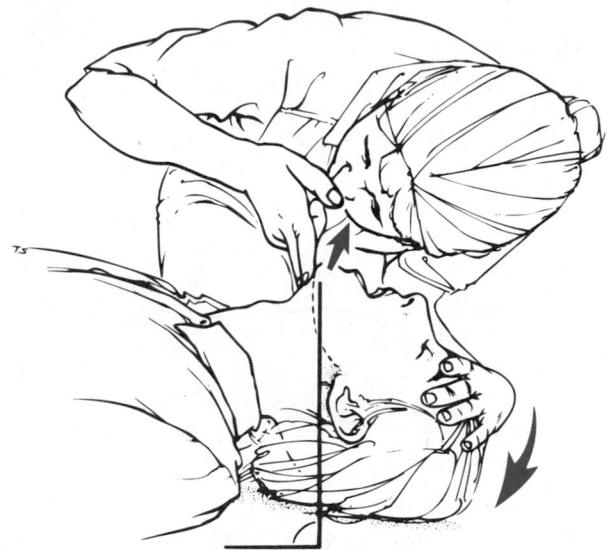

**Figure 21-13** Determination of breathlessness. (From Standards and guidelines for cardiopulmonary resuscitation and emergency cardiac care, part 2, *JAMA* 255:2915-2932, 1986.)

chest should be observed to see if it rises and falls. In addition, air rushing during exhalation should be listened for, and airflow should be felt (Figure 21-13).

**Rescue breathing.** Rescue breathing should begin by sealing the mouth and nose. Two slow breaths of 1½ to 2 seconds each should be delivered. An observation of the chest should be made to see if it rises and falls, and then movement of air should be listened and felt for. If the patient is unable to ventilate, the head should be repositioned and rescue breathing repeated. If the patient cannot be ventilated after repositioning the head, the procedure for airway obstruction previously mentioned should begin.

**Determine circulation.** Circulation should be assessed. The carotid artery should be palpitated for 5 to 10 seconds because it is the strongest palpable pulse. If the pulse is present, rescue breathing should continue at 10 to 12 breaths per minute or 1 breath every 5 to 6 seconds. If the pulse is absent, external compressions should begin. It is important to take time to adequately check for a pulse because external compressions are dangerous to a beating heart.

**Begin external compressions.** External compressions should be performed in the following manner: While kneeling by the patient's shoulders, the palm of a hand should be placed on the sternum, with two fingers above the xiphoid process (Figure 21-14). A second hand should be placed on top of the first. The sternum should be compressed 1½ to 2 inches for adults. Compressions should be equal. Hands should remain on the sternum during upstroke, when the chest should relax completely. The compression rate should be 15

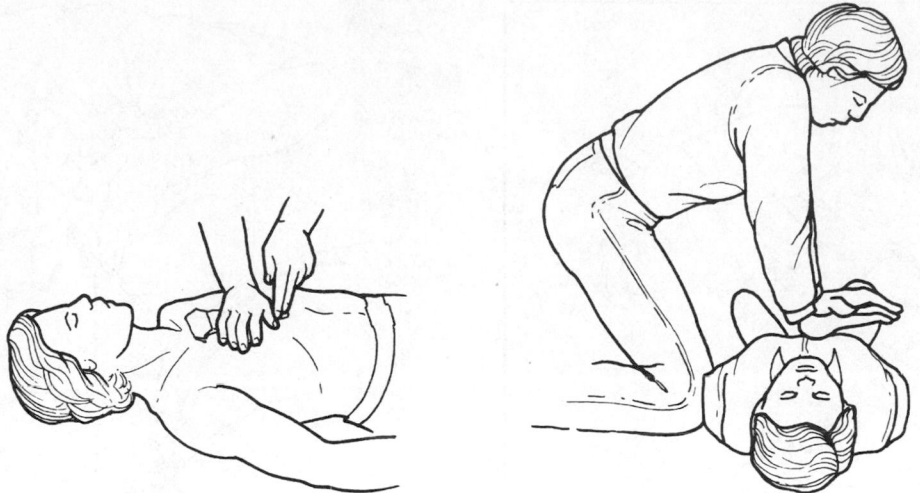

**Figure 21-14**  External chest compression. (From Rund DA et al: *Essentials of emergency medicine,* ed 2, St Louis, 1996, Mosby.)

compressions in 15 seconds to maintain a rate of 80 to 100 beats per minute for an adult. Two breaths should then be administered. Four cycles of 15 compressions and two ventilations should be completed before rechecking the carotid pulse. If the pulse returns, cardiac compressions should be stopped. Once spontaneous respirations begin, the patient will need assessment of the respiratory system. CPR should be performed until the patient regains his or her own pulse or all resuscitative measures have been exhausted (JAMA, 1992).

Any death of a patient in the ED or less than 24 hours after admission to the hospital needs to be reported to the medical examiner. The medical examiner will decide if an autopsy needs to be performed. The Uniform Anatomical Gift Act recognizes the right of a person to donate organs and tissues. The next of kin can make the decision for the deceased if intent is unknown. It is up to the health care professional to address donation with the family. The consent for donation or refusal must be documented in the medical record. This is the law (Emergency Nurses Association, 1992).

All patients with impaired circulatory function should be placed on cardiac monitoring, administered oxygen, and have an IV catheter with a solution of 0.9% normal saline or Ringer's Lactate established. Further cardiac assessment should include capillary refill. However, this may not be an adequate assessment tool if the patient has Raynaud's disease or circulatory problems. Skin color and temperature should be noted, as should any signs of bleeding. The level of consciousness should also be assessed.

Signs and symptoms of hypovolemic shock are decreased level of consciousness; uncontrolled bleeding; tachycardia; hypotension; prolonged capillary refill; and cool, pale skin. The patient in hypovolemic shock has flat neck veins. The patient with a condition that mimics shock, such as cardiac tamponade, would have distended neck veins and distant (more muffled or quieter) heart sounds.

## Life-Threatening Problems
### Uncontrolled External or Internal Bleeding

Uncontrolled external or internal bleeding is a life-threatening condition. External bleeding could be an arterial laceration or venous laceration that has not had pressure applied to stop the bleeding. Ways to control external bleeding are direct pressure, elevation, or use of pressure points. When using pressure points, the nurse should first identify the artery that supplies the area of uncontrolled bleeding. The nurse should compress the artery against the bone that lies behind it to occlude the flow of blood to the bleeding area (Figure 21-15). The nurse must remember that a tourniquet is a last resort and may result in loss of distal limb. Internal bleeding could be from a lacerated spleen or liver or another internal injury such as an acute gastrointestinal bleed. The patient would need a blood sample sent for a type and cross match, and surgery may be required to control the bleeding.

**Military antishock trousers.** Military antishock trousers (MAST) or a pneumatic antishock garment (PASG) may be applied if the patient exhibits signs of shock in the prehospital setting. The effectiveness of these gar-

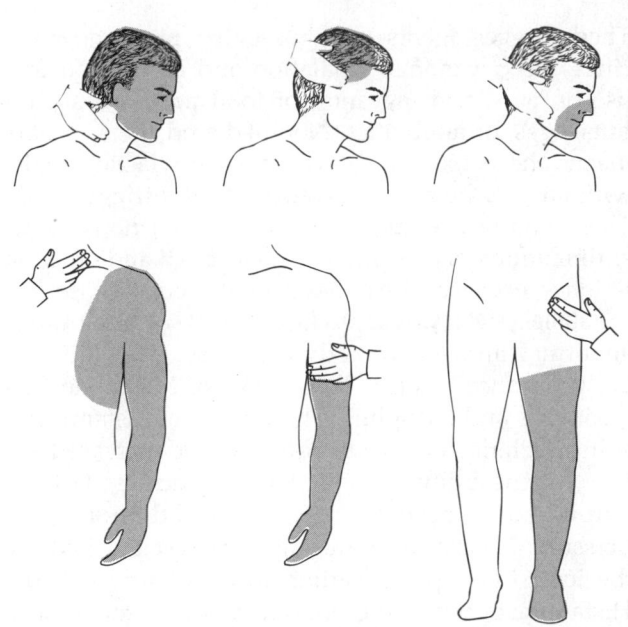

**Figure 21-15** Common pressure point locations to control bleeding. Firm pressure should be applied to the area compressing the artery against the underlying bone. Elevation of the extremity will also help decrease the blood flow to the area to help stop the bleeding.

### NURSE ALERT

**Only red blood cells have hemoglobin, which is necessary to carry oxygen throughout the body.**

ments is presently being evaluated. These garments apply pressure to the lower extremities and abdomen to help increase the blood return to the vital organs and decrease the blood in the lower extremities. They are used to keep the systolic blood pressure greater than 80 mm Hg. They are contraindicated in patients with severe head injury, pulmonary edema, or an intrathoracic bleed. When the garment is inflated, the pulses in the lower extremities must be checked. The garment should never obscure the pulse. Once the blood volume has been restored with blood products and IV fluids, the garment can be removed by deflating the area over the abdomen first and then one leg at a time. If the blood pressure drops more than 5 mm Hg, the deflation is stopped until the blood pressure returns to the previous reading. Many times these garments are removed in the operating room. The operating room staff should be advised not to remove the garment with scissors.

## Cardiac Tamponade

This condition involves the accumulation of blood or fluid in the pericardial sac from blunt chest trauma or from a disease process such as an infection or cancer. Approximately 60 to 100 ml of fluid accumulating in the pericardial sac can impede the heart's ability to pump. Signs and symptoms of cardiac tamponade are distended neck veins, distant heart sounds, and hypotension. Treatment for a pericardial tamponade is a pericardiocentesis. The purpose of this procedure is to remove fluid from the pericardial sac. A needle is placed to the left of the xiphoid process toward the ipsilateral (same side) shoulder. When the needle enters the pericardial sac, fluid is removed. Touching the heart muscle could send the patient into ventricular fibrillation or produce a myocardial laceration.

## Aortic and Great Vessel Injury

If there is trauma to a great vessel such as the aorta or superior/inferior vena cava, the patient is usually dead at the scene of the accident. If the patient makes it to the hospital alive, he or she usually dies within the first 24 hours. A patient may also come to the hospital with excruciating pain from a dissecting aortic or abdominal aneurysm. This is a condition that occurs when there is increased stress on the aorta, causing damage to the middle layer of the blood vessel. This condition is seen in patients with uncontrolled hypertension, arteriosclerosis, and infection. Signs and symptoms include hypovolemic shock, marked variation of blood pressure between the right and left arms, chest wall ecchymosis (if seen in a trauma patient), decreased pedal pulses, widened mediastinum (this is seen on a chest x-ray film and is interpreted by the physician or radiologist), or a bulging pulsatile abdominal mass. The patient needs to go to the operating room to have these extensive injuries repaired (see Chapter 20).

## Lacerated Liver

Traumatic lacerations to the liver are common because of the size of the liver and its location. A ruptured diaphragm may accompany this injury. Fractured ribs on the right side could lacerate the liver. Signs and symptoms of a lacerated liver are hypovolemic shock (caused by hemorrhage), abdominal guarding, right upper-abdominal pain, and positive peritoneal lavage. A positive peritoneal lavage indicates intraabdominal trauma when peritoneal fluid contains a RBC count of greater than 100,000/ml. Many hospitals now do a computed tomography (CT) scan of the abdomen instead of a peritoneal lavage to see if any other abdominal injuries exist. Treatment involves surgery to explore the injury and control the bleeding.

## Ruptured Spleen

The patient with a ruptured spleen initially exhibits blunt abdominal trauma to the left side of the abdomen and may have fractured lower ribs. Signs and symptoms are hypovolemic shock; Kerr's sign, which is pain under the left scapula; guarding of the abdomen; and absent bowel sounds. The shock symptoms are treated as the patient is prepared for surgery.

## Anaphylaxis

Anaphylactic shock is a life-threatening medical emergency. Anaphylactic shock is a systemic response to a type I hypersensitivity reaction. It is potentially fatal and can appear in minutes in people who have been previously sensitized to the allergen.

Immunoglobulin (IgE) antibody formation produces the anaphylactic response after a series of exposures.

These trigger agents are caused by injection of vaccines, insect venoms, inhalation and absorption from use of latex, and ingestion of food products such as nuts, eggs, or antibiotics. Nonmediated IgE formation means the person can have an anaphylactic reaction without ever being presensitized to the trigger agent. These non-IgE reactions can occur from nonsteroidal antiinflammatory drugs, amphotericin B and other antibiotics, exercise, or can have no particular cause.

**Pathophysiology.** Anaphylactic shock results from an abnormal antigen-antibody response. The IgE antibody produced causes the release of histamine from mast cells and basophils. The release of histamine results in arterial and venous dilation and increased capillary permeability. Vasodilation and decreased cardiac output cause a decrease in systolic and diastolic blood pressure. Plasma leaks through the vascular bed into the interstitial space, leading to circulatory collapse. Histamine contracts the smooth muscle of the bronchi, causing bronchospasm, asthma, and panting. The bronchioles constrict and contribute to hypoxemia.

**Assessment.** Initial symptoms of anaphylaxis are edema, itching of the eyes and ears and/or at the site

---

> **BOX 21-9**

## NURSING PROCESS

## EMERGENCY CARE OF INDIVIDUALS IN ANAPHYLACTIC SHOCK

### ASSESSMENT

- Rapid, shallow breathing
- Bronchospasms
- Dyspnea
- Cyanosis
- Restlessness
- "Sense of doom"
- Irritability
- Laryngeal edema
- Hypotension
- Rapid, thready pulse
- Edema and itching at site of injection or insect bite

### NURSING DIAGNOSIS

- Risk for injury related to anaphylactic shock

### NURSING INTERVENTIONS

- Administer oxygen therapy utilizing a non-rebreather mask with a reservoir bag at 15 L.
- Prepare for possible endotracheal intubation or surgical insertion of tracheotomy.
- Initiate two large-bore (size 16- or 18-gauge) angiocaths to infuse copious amounts of 0.9% saline or Ringer's lactate IV solutions.

- Prepare for administration of antihistamines such as Benadryl 50 mg IV over 3 minutes and Tagamet 300 mg IVPB or aminophylline IV drip.
- Administer Solu-Medrol 125 mg IVP or another corticosteroid to decrease inflammation, as ordered.
- Have patient in supine position to increase blood flow to the brain. Administer 0.2-0.5 ml 1:1000 epinephrine solution SC or IM into upper arm and massage site to hasten absorption. Prepare an epinephrine drip for continuous infusion if aggressive IV fluid resuscitation is not adequate. Monitor pulse and blood pressure every 3 to 5 minutes until stable.
- Remove the bee stinger or stop the infusion causing the reaction.
- Place a tourniquet above the site of the antigen. Remove tourniquet every 10 to 15 minutes or until reaction is under control. Apply ice.

### EVALUATION OF EXPECTED OUTCOMES

- Maintains patent airway
- Demonstrates effective breathing pattern
- Maintains hemodynamic stability as evidenced by blood pressure and pulse in normal range
- Reduces systemic absorption of the antigen

of injection, sneezing, and apprehension. In seconds or minutes, edema of the face, hands, and other parts of the body occur. Respiratory distress from bronchospasm, sneezing and coughing, wheezing, dyspnea, and cyanosis follows. Edema of the larynx and laryngospasm may lead to death. Gastrointestinal symptoms such as nausea and vomiting, abdominal pain, and diarrhea may be present. Cardiovascular signs such as arrhythmia, tachycardia, or bradycardia may be followed by circulatory collapse, indicated by a falling blood pressure, pallor, and loss of consciousness. In extreme cases death may occur in 5 to 10 minutes after reaction onset (Box 21-9) (Wyatt, 1996).

Patient teaching should include instructions on how to obtain a Medic Alert bracelet, a warning to avoid the known antigen, a demonstration of procedures to treat an anaphylactic response (use of an Epi pen to self-administer epinephrine), and an explanation of other desensitizing measures (allergy shots).

## Disability

After airway, breathing, and circulation are assessed, an assessment for disability or a brief neurologic examination is performed.

### Neurologic Examination Glasgow Coma Scale

The Glasgow Coma Scale is a reliable tool used to assess levels of consciousness. The coma scale includes a

rank or rating assigned to the patient's best effort at eye opening, verbal response, and motor response. Each is rated, and the total equals from 3 to 15 points. The higher the point value, the better the neurologic examination (Table 21-5). Also included in the brief neurologic examination is an assessment of pupil size and response.

## Exposure

The final step in the primary assessment is to observe the entire body of patient fully exposed. A cover should be placed to prevent hypothermia.

## Primary Interventions

Interventions after the primary examination include inserting an oral/nasogastric tube to decrease abdominal distention, which can impair breathing. An indwelling urinary catheter is inserted to obtain an accurate recording of urine output, which is a valuable indicator of kidney perfusion and hydration. Blood should be drawn for a type and crossmatch, hemoglobin/hematocrit, electrolytes, bleeding studies, and a toxicology screen. Other laboratory examinations ordered would be determined by the nature of the injury.

---

**PATIENT/FAMILY TEACHING**

**ALLERGIC REACTION**

Explain that an allergic reaction is caused by an increased sensitivity to a medication, sting, or food product.
Tell the patient, "You experienced an allergic reaction today," and explain the following:

- Take the medication (Benadryl/Atarax) as prescribed. It will cause sleepiness, so do not drive while on the medication. Take it for at least 3 days. If Tagamet has been ordered, do not drink alcohol with the medication. Tagamet will not cause drowsiness.
- Avoid scratching.
- Avoid hot baths and showers. Tepid or cool compresses may help with itching.
- Return to the ED if experiencing difficulty breathing, lightheadedness, or difficulty swallowing.
- See physician if signs of infection or no resolution of rash occurs.
- Apply for a Medic Alert tag to indicate allergies.
- Avoid the substances that caused the allergic reaction.

---

**TABLE 21-5**

**Glasgow Coma Scale**

| FINDING | SCORE |
|---|---|
| **Eye Opening** | |
| Spontaneous | 4 |
| To voice | 3 |
| To pain | 2 |
| None | 1 |
| | |
| **Best Verbal Response** | |
| Oriented | 5 |
| Confused | 4 |
| Inappropriate words | 3 |
| Incomprehensible sounds | 2 |
| None | 1 |
| | |
| **Best Motor Response** | |
| Obeys commands | 6 |
| Purposeful movement | 5 |
| Withdraw | 4 |
| Flexion | 3 |
| Extension | 2 |
| None | 1 |

Scoring is from 3 to 15. The higher the score the better the neurologic findings. Motor movement is assessed with painful stimuli (pressing on nail bed or sternal rub) (Sheehy, 1992; Klein et al, 1994).

The first hemoglobin and hematocrit are drawn as baseline data because they take hours to show a drop from blood loss. If the mechanism of injury indicates a potential cervical spine injury, cervical spine x-ray films should be obtained before proceeding with further care. **Blood alcohol concentration (BAC)** is routinely obtained if the patient's condition warrants the test. An altered level of consciousness, seizure activity, trauma, or patients who have overdosed are examples of when a BAC would be obtained.

BAC is a test that measures the concentration of alcohol in a person's blood. It is expressed in a BAC percentage. An alcohol blood level of 0.08 to 0.10 is considered legal intoxication. Some mental impairment and physical impairment are noticed at this level (Newell et al, 1993). A patient may be brought to the ED under police custody to obtain a BAC. The patient has the right to refuse the test. If the patient is violent or injury to the patient could occur from the drawing of the sample, someone other than a health care provider should obtain the sample.

> ### NURSE ALERT
> A patient using alcohol or drugs may not respond properly, which could suggest a head injury or an altered response to shock.

## SECONDARY ASSESSMENT

During the secondary assessment all injuries and problems are assessed and prioritized. A full set of vital signs—blood pressure, pulse, respirations, and temperature—is obtained. A complete head-to-toe assessment is performed with a repeat neurologic examination. This assessment is done on an emergency patient to determine what is causing the patient's complaint. Obtaining a thorough history is important to identify and treat the problem. Subjective data (what is said) is as important as objective data (what can be seen and measured). Nurses should look to see if the patient has a Medic Alert tag. If a life-threatening problem occurs during any of the assessments, it must be treated before resuming definitive care. Additional laboratory tests and x-ray examinations are ordered. If the patient is stable, a complete history is obtained.

## FOCUSED ASSESSMENT AND INTERVENTION

Finally a focused assessment is performed. During the focused assessment, interventions may be performed for the specific identified injuries or problem. This is when definitive treatment is completed, which may include interventions such as administering pain medication to make the patient more comfortable or applying a cast to a fracture.

## Immunization

Diphtheria tetanus toxoid (dT) 0.5 ml is administered intramuscularly to all patients who had their last immunization more than 10 years ago and have a break in the skin. This includes fractures, abrasions, animal bites, and burns. For individuals who have never received a dT immunization, they also receive 250 units of tetanus immunoglobulin along with the start of a dT series and repeat injections of dT 1 month and 6 months after receiving the first immunization.

## Removal of Foreign Bodies from the Eye

Many patients come to the ED with complaints of pain in or drainage from the eye. They also may complain of acute vision loss. The emergency caregiver needs to determine the cause of the patient's problem (see Chapter 38). A foreign body in the eye causes pain, often as a result of a corneal abrasion. A corneal abrasion is a scratch to the outer surface of the eye. The objective in removing a foreign body from the eye is to prevent injury to the cornea and conjunctiva (Figure 21-16). If the foreign body is under the lower lid, the lid should be pulled down and the foreign body removed with a cotton swab. If a foreign body is suspected under the upper lid, there are four steps to evert the eyelid to examine the eye. First the patient should close his or her eyelid. Next a cotton swab should be placed at the medial corner of the upper eyelid (eyelashes should be pulled down and back over the swab). Then the eyelid should be everted over the swab. Finally the inside of the eyelid and the eye should be examined to see if any injury is present. Treatment for a corneal abrasion includes applying prescribed antibiotic eye drops to prevent infection and patching the eyelid closed. Patching the eyelid closed allows for decreased movement of the eyelid over the abraded area. This decreased irritation allows the eye to heal. Pain medications are prescribed, and the patient is instructed to rest while the eye is patched. The patient should not drive with the eye patched or open the eye underneath the patch.

## Wound Care

The objectives for the care of a patient with surface trauma are to stop the bleeding, prevent infection, and preserve function. The dT immunization should be administered if needed.

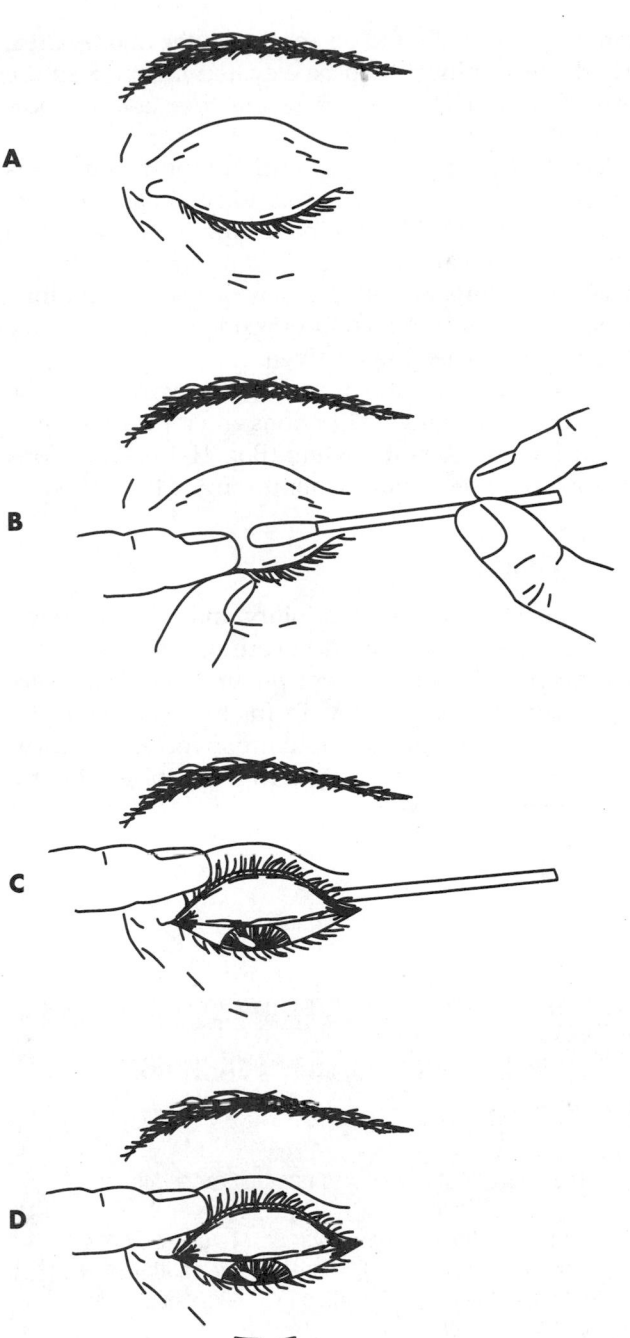

**Figure 21-16** Steps in everting eyelid. **A,** Eyelid. **B,** Placement of cotton swab (eyelashes are pulled down and back over swab). **C,** Eyelid everted over swab. **D,** Examination of inside of eyelid and eye. (From Sheehy SB: *Emergency nursing: principles and practice,* ed 3, St Louis, 1992, Mosby.)

## Abrasions and Lacerations

The first step in treating abrasions and lacerations is to stop the bleeding. This is done either by direct pressure, elevation, or pressure points. The area should be cleaned with soap and water, removing any foreign bodies such as glass or gravel. Definitive treatment for lacerations is to suture if it is a full-thickness wound, or Steri-strip if the wound is partial thickness. An antibiotic ointment such as Bacitracin should be applied, and the wound should be covered with a sterile dressing.

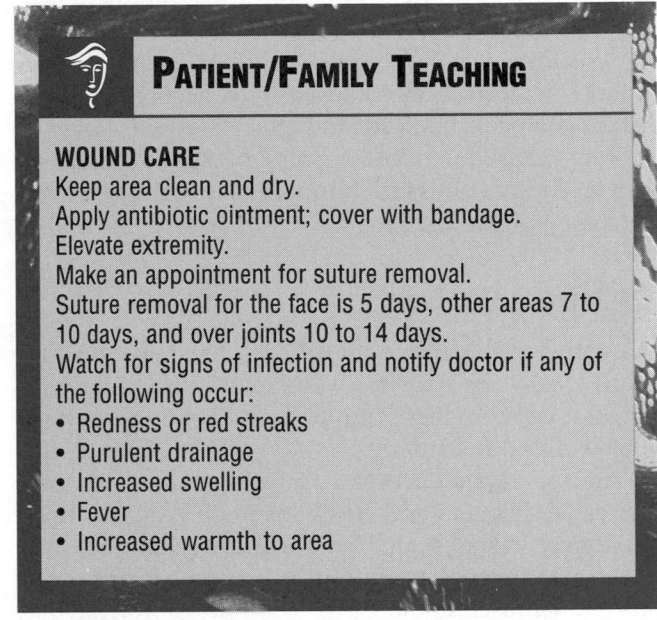

**PATIENT/FAMILY TEACHING**

**WOUND CARE**
Keep area clean and dry.
Apply antibiotic ointment; cover with bandage.
Elevate extremity.
Make an appointment for suture removal.
Suture removal for the face is 5 days, other areas 7 to 10 days, and over joints 10 to 14 days.
Watch for signs of infection and notify doctor if any of the following occur:
• Redness or red streaks
• Purulent drainage
• Increased swelling
• Fever
• Increased warmth to area

## Puncture Wounds

Puncture wounds should be copiously irrigated with 0.9% normal saline, and the physician will determine if a prophylactic antibiotic is needed. An x-ray examination may be ordered depending on the object that caused the injury.

**NURSE ALERT**

Never remove an impaled object. Secure the object. Removal should be done in the operating room.

## Amputation

The ideal treatment for an amputation is to save the amputated part. The amputated part should be placed in a moist but not wet, clean dressing, in a sterile container, and on ice. The amputated tissue should not be frozen. Saline dressings should be placed on the cleansed portion of the remaining body part. Reimplantation may be accomplished, so both parts must be brought for treatment. Both the extremity and the amputated part need x-ray examination. The patient should be prepared for transport to the operating room or a reimplantation center, if appropriate.

## Bites

In the case of a bite the nurse needs to try to determine the type of bite, assess the area of the bite, and determine if the bite affects underlying tissue. A hand bite usually affects the tendon sheath of the hand. The age of the injury should be determined, and the nurse should look for signs of infection. Treatment requires a 10-minute scrub with soap and water. The decision to close the bite is determined by the location and the age of the bite. If the bite is caused by a raccoon or skunk, rabies protocol should be initiated. The area should be loosely dressed. Antibiotics may be started, if appropriate. Animal bites are commonly reported to law-enforcement agencies.

## Contusions (Bruises)

A contusion is a tissue injury that does not break the skin. The injury leads to swelling and discoloration as a result of the release of blood and fluids from damaged cells and capillaries.

The nurse should assess a contusion in the same manner as an abrasion and check for underlying fractures. Treatment includes applying ice and elevating the area. If the area is muscular and if increasing leakage of fluids in the muscle could occur, a compression wrap may be applied with an Ace bandage. Discoloration from a contusion can take 2 to 3 weeks to resolve.

## Crush Injuries

With crush injuries, the nurse should assess patients for neurocompromise, including loss of function, sensation, capillary refill, and pulse. The nurse should also check for compartment syndrome (see Chapter 33). Treatment for crush injuries is ice, elevation, and immobilization.

## Fractures and Dislocations

Initial treatment for a patient with a fracture includes removing jewelry from the extremity and checking the pulse before and after immobilization (splinting) of the fracture. Immobilization can be done with an armboard or many types of splints. Pelvic fractures may be immobilized with the MAST suit. The nurse should always apply the splint above and below the joint to give the maximum immobilization. It is important to check the neurovascular integrity of the extremity. This includes the five Ps: pain, pallor (capillary refill, skin temperature, color), pulses, paresthesia, and paralysis. If a bone has protruded through the skin, a saline or Betadine dressing should be applied to the area. The nurse should never try to relocate the fracture. If no pulse is felt, the physician should be notified immediately. Ice should be applied to the injured area, and the extremity should be elevated higher than the heart. For more information on fractures and dislocations, see Chapter 33.

Administering pain medication to these patients is important. It is sometimes easier to obtain an order for an IV solution of 0.9% normal saline to be started so that pain medications can be given intravenously for an acute fracture. The IV also may be used to administer medications if reduction of a fracture is necessary or if antibiotics need to be given.

Conscious sedation is now being performed in the ED to aid in reducing dislocations and repositioning of closed fractures before casting (Box 21-10). Conscious sedation requires prudent monitoring of the patient.

## Rib Fractures

A rib fracture is a common injury and usually affects one rib. The nurse should encourage the patient to take deep breaths to prevent pneumonia. Analgesics are prescribed for pain. A rib fracture can be a life-threatening problem if the fracture involves the lower ribs, which could lacerate the liver or spleen, or if a flail segment is present.

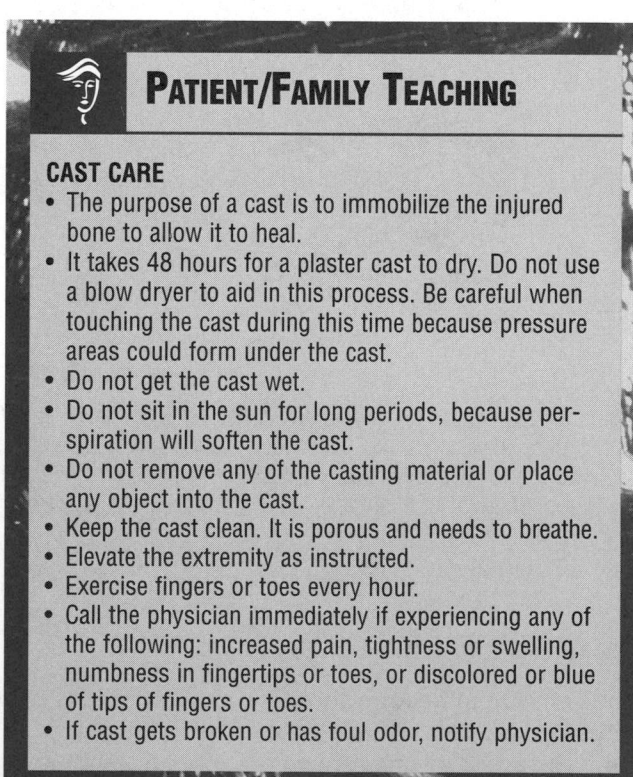

**PATIENT/FAMILY TEACHING**

**CAST CARE**
- The purpose of a cast is to immobilize the injured bone to allow it to heal.
- It takes 48 hours for a plaster cast to dry. Do not use a blow dryer to aid in this process. Be careful when touching the cast during this time because pressure areas could form under the cast.
- Do not get the cast wet.
- Do not sit in the sun for long periods, because perspiration will soften the cast.
- Do not remove any of the casting material or place any object into the cast.
- Keep the cast clean. It is porous and needs to breathe.
- Elevate the extremity as instructed.
- Exercise fingers or toes every hour.
- Call the physician immediately if experiencing any of the following: increased pain, tightness or swelling, numbness in fingertips or toes, or discolored or blue of tips of fingers or toes.
- If cast gets broken or has foul odor, notify physician.

## Guidelines of Conscious Sedation

The purpose of conscious sedation is to depress the level of consciousness but allow the patient to maintain independent airway management and be able to respond with physical and verbal stimulation.

Equipment needed for conscious sedation includes oxygen, suction, Ambu bag/mask, oral/nasal airways and endotracheal tubes, pulse oximeter, sphygmomanometer or noninvasive blood pressure cuff, and cardiac monitoring.

A registered nurse needs to be with the patient during the entire procedure and may not leave to do other tasks. The nurse must be CPR-recognized, have knowledge of the drugs to be given, and be able to monitor arrhythmias and airway. Emergency equipment and personnel should be easily accessible. The steps the nurse should take are as follows:

- Establish an IV.
- Prepare the patient with all the monitoring equipment.
- Receive an order for sedation medication and have the physician in the room while the medication is administered. Commonly used medications for sedation are midazolam or diazepam along with a pain medication such as meperidine, hydromorphone, fentanyl, or morphine sulfate.
- Monitor for signs of hypoventilation (the pulse oximetry reading will drop) continuously and blood pressure and pulse every 15 minutes.
- Observe for arrhythmia on the cardiac monitor.
- Assess arousability and level of consciousness.
- Assess skin condition.
- Document medications given and patient's response. (Berkowitz, 1997; Penn Nurse, 1992).

## Burns

In the case of a burn, the nurse should treat the trauma first—assessing airway, breathing, and circulation—then treat the burn.

The immediate action and intervention of a burn patient is to stop the burning process. This is done before the patient coming to the ED. The area should be cooled with water. Then the extent of the burn, the location, and other possible complications such as smoke inhalation with respiratory involvement should be determined. Debridement of any blistered area that would impede function may be done with a physician's order. The nurse should then cover the burn with a sterile dressing and apply an antibiotic ointment such as bacitracin or Silvadene (see Chapter 41).

## Head Injuries

Head injuries affect a significant number of people each year. They are caused by motor vehicle accidents, sports injuries, assaults, and falls. Patients arriving at the ED with symptoms or a complaint of head injury with a loss of consciousness receive a CT scan of the head to look for any signs of cerebral bleeding (see Chapter 32). It is important for the nurse to instruct the patient and family of symptoms that indicate the need to return to the ED after a head injury.

The goal of treatment of an acutely head injured patient, with a Glasgow Coma Scale of 8 or less, is to prevent hypoxia and hypotension. It is essential to maintain a patent airway and adequate cerebral tissue perfusion. Intubation is necessary to maintain a $PaCO_2$ of 30 to 35 mm Hg. An IV is established to maintain a blood pressure of 100 to 110 systolic (Campbell, 1996; Mattera, 1997). If a change in the neurologic examination indicates increased intracranial pressure (ICP), the physician may decide to place burr holes into the patient's skull to help relieve the pressure until neurosurgery can be performed. Therefore a patient with an altered level of consciousness should be taken, if possible, to a Level I trauma center, where emergency neurosurgery is quickly available. For more information about ICP, see Chapter 32.

### Cerebral Hematomas

There are three types of cerebral hematomas: epidural, subdural, and intracerebral (Figure 21-17). Bleeding causes a hematoma to form. The location of the hematoma determines the symptoms a patient will exhibit.

### Epidural Hematoma

An epidural hematoma involves rapid bleeding between the skull and the dura caused by a laceration of the meningeal artery and vein. The patient has a history of head trauma with a loss of consciousness, followed by a lucid period and a rapid decrease in level of consciousness. The pupils become fixed and dilated on the side of the injury (ipsilateral), and paralysis occurs on the opposite side of the injury (contralateral).

### Subdural Hematoma

A subdural hematoma involves bleeding under the dura. This bleeding can accumulate quickly (acute) within 48 hours or slowly (chronic) within weeks. Patients more prone to chronic subdural hematomas are alcoholics, the elderly, or those on anticoagulants. Symptoms are headache, drowsiness, and confusion. As the symptoms become more severe, ipsilateral

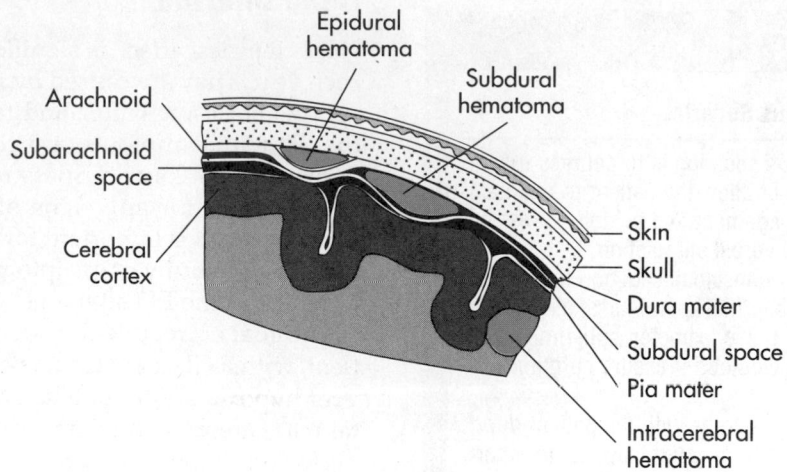

**Figure 21-17** Location of cerebral hematomas.

pupil dilation and contralateral paralysis occur. Symptoms for a chronic subdural hematoma are the same, but symptoms evolve slowly.

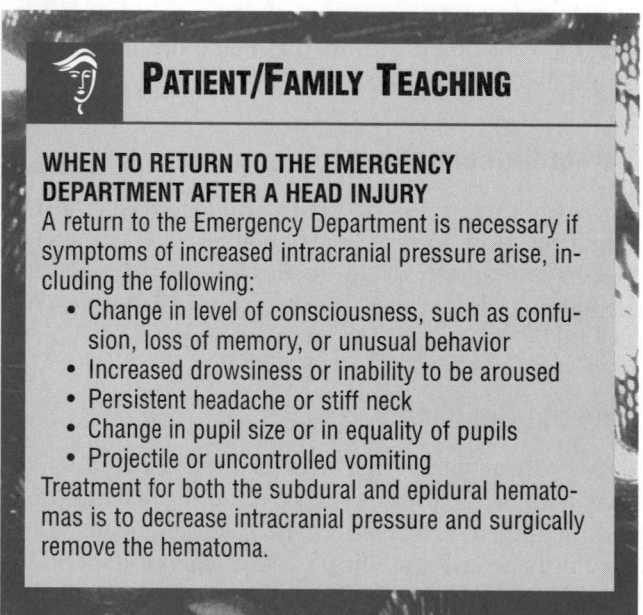

### PATIENT/FAMILY TEACHING

**WHEN TO RETURN TO THE EMERGENCY DEPARTMENT AFTER A HEAD INJURY**
A return to the Emergency Department is necessary if symptoms of increased intracranial pressure arise, including the following:
- Change in level of consciousness, such as confusion, loss of memory, or unusual behavior
- Increased drowsiness or inability to be aroused
- Persistent headache or stiff neck
- Change in pupil size or in equality of pupils
- Projectile or uncontrolled vomiting

Treatment for both the subdural and epidural hematomas is to decrease intracranial pressure and surgically remove the hematoma.

## Intracerebral Hematoma

An intracerebral hematoma is the result of a large contusion to any area of the brain, with small vessel damage. These have high mortality rates because evacuating the hematoma is not as easy as with the two other hematomas. A rapid deterioration occurs.

## VIOLENCE

Recent studies have shown that the fear of violence has replaced economic issues as a national concern.

The CDC has termed violence an epidemic health problem. In 1990 injuries from firearms exceeded injuries from motor vehicle accidents in six states. There have been an increasing number of hospital assaults. The assaults usually occurred in the ED, and the nurse was the person most at risk. The growing number of handguns has led to increased accidental shootings. In the past, a playground disagreement would usually end with a black eye. Now it is not uncommon for it to end with a child being shot. Violence is not only in the streets but in homes as well and includes child and elder maltreatment, spousal abuse, and sexual assault.

Causes of increased violence are poverty, racism, denial of educational opportunities, low self-esteem, disregard for human life, disintegration of the family, and a lack of positive role models.

No family is immune to the effects that violence has on our society. Prevention is the key to solving this problem, and emergency nurses and physicians are trying to intervene. After they continued to see the devastating effects on children, hospitals such as Children's Memorial Hospital in Chicago have developed programs called HELP to educate families about handgun violence. There is also a national organization called STOP. This organization is working to prevent firearm injuries by educating parents and the community about the risks of keeping handguns in the home (Campbell, 1994).

## Emergency Department Violence

The ED is predisposed to violence as a result of its 24-hour accessibility, long waiting times, overcrowding, availability of drugs and hostages, staff shortages, and its utilization by psychiatric patients and patients with drug and alcohol problems. The ENA has a posi-

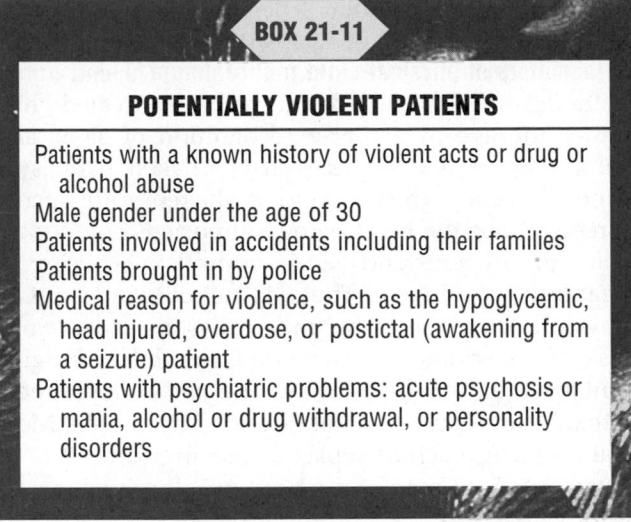

## BOX 21-11

### POTENTIALLY VIOLENT PATIENTS

Patients with a known history of violent acts or drug or alcohol abuse

Male gender under the age of 30

Patients involved in accidents including their families

Patients brought in by police

Medical reason for violence, such as the hypoglycemic, head injured, overdose, or postictal (awakening from a seizure) patient

Patients with psychiatric problems: acute psychosis or mania, alcohol or drug withdrawal, or personality disorders

## BOX 21-12

### TYPES OF MALTREATMENT

Physical abuse involves intentional injury inflicted on the survivor. Some examples are kicking, slapping, biting, shaking, or burning.

Emotional abuse involves behavior is that is degrading, terrorizing, isolating, or rejecting.

Sexual assault/abuse refers to sexual contact to the survivor without consent, by coercion, persuasion, or force.

Neglect includes acts of omission and failure to meet the patient's needs, such as not obtaining medical care when needed or failure to provide food, clothing, and a safe place to live.

Exploitation involves the elderly and includes the improper or illegal use of the patient's resources by a caregiver.

tion statement regarding violence in the emergency setting (ENA, 1991b).

It is important for the emergency nurse to stop violence before it starts. First, potentially violent patients must be identified (Box 21-11). It is imperative that the nurse be aware of signs of increasing aggression so that interventions can occur before the patient or staff gets injured. Signs of increasing verbal aggression are loud talking, rapid speech, increasing verbal threats, or angry tone of voice. Signs of physical agitation or aggression are an inability to stay seated, grinding or clenched teeth, tense posture, or pacing.

Before approaching an angry patient, the nurse needs to ensure that safety measures are taken. Pens in pockets, earrings, and stethoscopes should be removed. The person should be taken to a quiet environment that is safe. Help to control the patient should be readily available. The nurse should not get trapped between the patient and a wall. An exit should always be available.

Communication should be tried first to deescalate the aggression. The nurse should be confident. The patient should be addressed by his or her complete name (Ms. Smith) and allowed to verbalize his or her feelings. The nurse should listen to the patient's response and watch the patient's behavior. Explanations for long delays should be offered.

Second, rapid tranquilization should be tried to control the violent patient. Medications often used are lorazepam (Ativan) combined with thiothixene (Navane) or haloperidol (Haldol).

The nurse should be proactive, restraining the patient if necessary, especially if a painful or uncomfortable procedure is to be performed. It is best to have five people to restrain a violent person. This allows for one person at each extremity and one person at the head.

Nurses need to be involved in the development of security and safety issues in the ED. Panic buttons and panic watches should be available to get help immediately (Dubin, Tardiff, Maier, 1992; Kinkle, 1993).

## Family Violence

Family violence is violence that occurs in a setting where people live together. It includes child and elder maltreatment, spousal abuse, and sexual assault (Box 21-12).

### History

An accurate history and assessment are essential for any patient who comes to the ED as the result of a violent act. The documentation from the emergency visit may be subpoenaed for court. The nurse should approach the survivor in a professional, nonjudgmental, and nonaccusatory manner. The survivor/patient and significant family must be interviewed separately. Open-ended questions and language the patient can understand should be used. The information must be kept confidential. If a child or elder states that a parent/caregiver inflicted the injury, relating this to them could put the patient at risk for further harm. The nurse should listen to responses and compare information for discrepancies. Exact quotes of what the patient stated should be documented, as well as the history of where the injuries happened, the date and time, and whether anyone else was present. The nurse and physician should perform the history and assessment together. If sexual assault is suspected, a person who has special training in this area should do the history and examination. Some nurses have undergone special training to become a sexual assault nurse examiner (SANE). These nurses are called to the ED when a sexual assault survivor is present. This allows for increased accuracy of obtaining evidence and the complete attention of one nurse to the patient's needs.

## Assessment Examination

The patient should fully undress. If it is a child older than 8, consent to perform the physical examination must be granted. Young children may want to stay on a parent's lap for the examination. Other physical signs of injury should be observed. All injuries should be documented using a body map. If bruising is noted, it is important to document the colors of the bruises because this indicates the stage of the healing process. Photographs should be taken of all injuries, and they should be documented. X-ray films should also be obtained for all injuries.

## Child Maltreatment

In 1991 2.7 million cases of child maltreatment were reported to child protection agencies in the United States. This does not reflect all the cases that go unreported. **Child maltreatment or abuse** is any threat to a child's health or welfare. It is required by law in all states that all cases of suspected and actual child maltreatment be reported by emergency personnel to protection agencies. Reporting in good faith and protecting the child from a dangerous situation guarantees immunity from civil or criminal liability. The law does not protect the health care worker who fails to report suspicions.

Persons likely to cause maltreatment can be parents, relatives, close friends, teachers, or babysitters. Maltreatment occurs within every economic class, every religion, and every race.

People who may potentially maltreat a child are those who have drug or alcohol problems, have been maltreated themselves, have a chronic illness, are in crisis and under extreme stress, or have unrealistic expectations of the child. Children who are at risk for potential maltreatment are those with developmental problems or retardation, those of multiple births, or those who were premature.

If the child is in threat of harm or reprisal because emergency treatment has been sought, the ED child protection team should be notified, and the child should be placed in protective custody. This initially means the child will be admitted to the hospital until a

judge can determine what is best for the child (Devlin, Reynolds, 1994; Klein et al, 1994).

**Indicators of physical child maltreatment.** Head injury is the leading cause of death in the maltreated child under the age of 1. Early recognition of signs and symptoms of ICP is necessary. "Shaken baby syndrome" occurs when a child is shaken with intense force without the head being supported. The neck is able to hyperextend and hyperflex, causing a whiplash-type injury. There is no outward sign of physical trauma, but the patient has an unexplained loss of consciousness, increased irritability, bulging fontanels, or seizure activity. The child may appear lethargic and have the inability to suck or feed. Medical problems such as sepsis or meningitis need to be ruled out. A CT scan of the head usually shows a subdural hematoma.

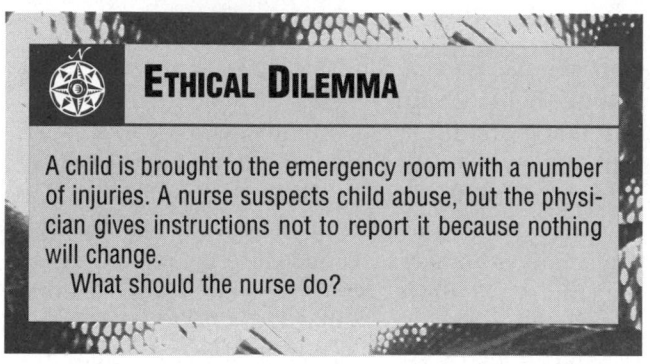

**ETHICAL DILEMMA**

A child is brought to the emergency room with a number of injuries. A nurse suspects child abuse, but the physician gives instructions not to report it because nothing will change.
What should the nurse do?

Other physical indicators of maltreatment are obvious traumas unrelated to the age of the child. Indicators include fractures in multiple stages of healing; ecchymosis or abrasions on wrists or ankles, indicating use of restraints; or bite marks. Burns are of concern if they are circumferential, which indicates immersion injuries, or if they involve the entire buttocks or both hands and wrists. Well-demarcated burned areas suggest the use of a cigarette or a hot instrument, and the shape may identify the instrument used.

The second leading cause of death as a result of child maltreatment is an abdominal injury. Bruising may be minimal or absent as a result of the elasticity of the child's abdomen. When signs of peritonitis or shock occur, it may be too late to help the child.

**Indicators of emotional child maltreatment.** Emotional maltreatment may be harder to identify. Symptoms may include speech disorders, failure to thrive, delayed development, or physical problems such as asthma, headaches, ulcers, or allergies. The nurse should watch how the caregiver interacts with the child. Does he or she push the child away or ignore the child when the child is asking for comfort? It is more difficult for the ED staff to recognize this type of maltreatment because of the short interaction they have with the child and caregiver.

**Indicators of neglect.** Neglect may be suspected if the child is inappropriately dressed, is emaciated, has lice, or has medical needs that go unattended. If the problem is that the caregiver does not have the financial ability to provide these things for the child, the family should be referred to a social agency for assistance.

**Sexual abuse.** Sexual abuse is usually committed by a male family member or male family friend who has gained the child's trust. This person may have been abused as a child.

Certain physical findings may suggest sexual abuse. The nurse should look for bruising or bleeding from the external genitalia, frequent urinary tract infections, pregnancy in adolescents, vaginal or rectal pain or itching, sexually transmitted diseases, or an inability to control urination or defecation in a child who is of an age that control should be obtained. Behavioral findings include sexual promiscuity, age-inappropriate sexual behavior, eating or sleeping disorders, suicide attempts in adolescents, school difficulties, and chronic withdrawal or depression.

## Elder Maltreatment

One million elderly persons are victims of abuse, neglect, or exploitation each year. These numbers have increased because the elderly are living longer and need to turn to their families more for assistance. Many times the family does not know how to respond to the increasing demands placed on them. Individual states have set their own guidelines for reporting elder abuse. Only the states of Wisconsin, Colorado, and New York have voluntary reporting of elder abuse. All other states have mandatory reporting. Protection for reporting suspected abuse is the same as in child abuse.

Victims of elder or geriatric abuse are usually dependent on their abusers. The geriatric patient usually gives up his or her independence to the abuser because of physical health problems such as a cerebral vascular accident or because of a deterioration in mental health. Perpetrators of the abuse are usually dependent on their victims for financial support and may have a problem with mental illness, chronic disease, or drug or alcohol problems. The abuser may be the spouse, child, or grandchild of the victim.

The victim may be in denial that the abuse is occurring because of embarrassment, dependence on the caregiver, and the fear of public scrutiny. The abused also may not want to pursue filing a complaint against the perpetrator because of a fear for his or her life.

Elder abuse is on the rise in the United States. It is up to medical personnel to recognize and report these incidences for the protection of the elderly (Lynch, 1997).

## Battered Patients

Three to four million women are beaten in their homes each year by their husbands or partners. Women make up 94% to 95% of the victims of domestic violence. Domestic violence is sometimes seen by law enforcement agencies as a personal family problem. Domestic violence is the abuse of power in an intimate relationship. **Domestic violence** is also called spousal abuse. There is no mandatory reporting to law enforcement agencies regarding victims of spousal abuse. The ED reports any acts of violence. Domestic violence falls into this category, and these cases are reported to document that an attack has occurred. The victim/survivor has the right to refuse to sign a complaint with the law enforcement agency because the survivors of these attacks are adults and are competent to make their own decisions regarding their care. The current term of survivor is used instead of victim to communicate that the person can take control of these acts of violence.

It is not uncommon for a domestic violence survivor to be seen in an ED many times before he or she is able to decide that this treatment cannot continue. Police officers are sometimes reluctant to pursue complaints in domestic violence cases because many feel it is a family issue. The violence occurs many times before the survivor breaks the cycle. Battering has an effect on the entire family. The person doing the battering to the spouse may also abuse the children in the family. The episodes of violence usually increase in frequency and severity. Of the women murdered in this country, 40% are killed by their husbands or partners. Many women arriving in EDs may have injuries related to being battered (Box 21-13). A police report should be completed

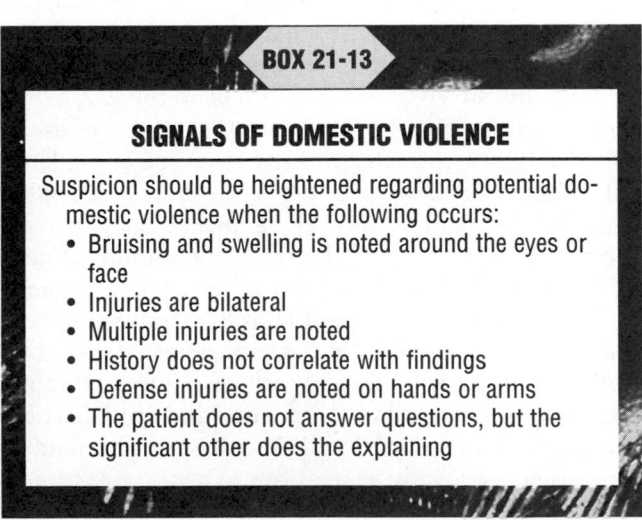

**BOX 21-13**

### SIGNALS OF DOMESTIC VIOLENCE

Suspicion should be heightened regarding potential domestic violence when the following occurs:
- Bruising and swelling is noted around the eyes or face
- Injuries are bilateral
- Multiple injuries are noted
- History does not correlate with findings
- Defense injuries are noted on hands or arms
- The patient does not answer questions, but the significant other does the explaining

even if the patient does not press formal charges of assault and battery.

## Treatment Goals for Survivors of Violent Attacks

The goal of treatment for any survivor of a violent attack is to help the survivor regain control of his or her life. This is done by allowing the survivor to verbalize feelings and make decisions and by supporting those decisions. The person's confidence needs to be regained. The nurse can help by giving the survivor phone numbers of support groups and social agencies. Safety for the survivor and the children should be encouraged. If needed, the nurse can help make arrangements to find a safe place to stay.

All survivors need their physical injuries cared for with follow-up as needed for the specific injuries (Blair, 1992).

## Sexual Assault
### Definition

**Sexual assault** includes all forms of sexual activity performed on another person without that person's consent. Rape is the legal term for sexual assault. It is an act of forced sexual penetration against a man or woman. Sexual assault is a violent crime, and the survivor fears for his or her life. Treatment of sexual assault patients in the ED is usually lengthy, and information obtained through history, physical examination, and gathered evidence will likely be subpoenaed for the criminal court case if the survivor presses charges.

### Treatment Goals for Sexual Assault Survivors

The goal of treatment for the sexual assault patient is to provide medical and psychosocial care in a humane, tactful, and nonjudgmental manner while complying with the law regarding collection of evidence.

When the survivor initially comes to the ED, a one-to-one nurse-patient relationship should be established. Nurses specially trained to assist in evidence collection, counseling, and expert testimony are called *SANEs*. The patient should be placed in a private room, and a sexual assault counselor should be notified. The sexual assault counselor will act as a resource after the patient leaves the ED. It is mandated by law that law enforcement agencies be notified of sexual assaults. The patient should not use the bathroom, change clothes, or eat or drink anything until after the physical examination. The ED staff should attend to the patient as quickly as possible. When a law enforcement officer questions the patient, a counselor or nurse should be in the room. When the physical examination

is performed, the officer should be outside the room, but in some states it may be required that the officer be present during the examination. If this is the case the officer sits at the side of the room parallel to the patient's head or torso so that minimal exposure takes place. Medical information and evidence cannot be released without the patient's consent. The patient is given a choice if he or she wishes to file a police report, but the hospital must notify the police of the attack.

### Documentation

Documentation of sexual assault should reflect a brief subjective account of the survivor's description of the incident. Physical evidence, objective findings, chain of custody of evidence, medications, discharge instructions, pamphlets, and follow-up should also be documented.

All procedures should be explained before the physical examination. The examination entails first treating any life-threatening problems: assessing airway, breathing, and circulation. It is not uncommon for these survivors to have injuries caused by choking. Physical injuries should be documented and photographed, and a pelvic examination of the female patient should be performed.

### Chain of Custody of Evidence

Obtaining evidence and maintaining the chain of custody are very important. **Chain of custody** of evidence is the ability to trace the evidence collected to the point at which it was first obtained. The evidence should stay with the person collecting it until it is sealed and turned over to the next person in the chain. The nurse obtains the samples, seals them, and turns the evidence over to the police only if the patient consents. Specimens should remain unaltered. When collecting evidence for a sexual assault survivor, it is important to have him or her place all clothing in the evidence bags, which are made out of paper. The patient should undress over a sheet so that falling debris can be saved. Evidence kits include equipment necessary to obtain the specimens. Specimens include clothing, pubic hair, head hair, saliva, blood samples, fingernail scrapings, vaginal swabs, and rectal swabs. Laboratory tests obtained are rapid plasma reagin; cultures of affected areas; HIV; urine for sperm, trichomonas, and fungus; and a serum pregnancy test.

### Treatment

Treatment for medical injuries resulting from the sexual assault is then performed. Treatment to prevent sexually transmitted diseases (gonorrhea and Chlamydia) and to prevent pregnancy is initiated in the

ED. A concern today is the risk of contracting HIV. The patient should be counseled regarding this. A patient is tested initially for HIV to make sure he or she did not have the disease before the attack. As a follow-up, patients are tested at 6 months and 1 year to see if they have converted to HIV-positive. It is thought that the likelihood of HIV is rare if conversion has not occurred within the first year.

Medication treatment is ceftriaxone, spectinomycin, or ciprofloxacin, followed by a 7-day dosage of another antibiotic (tetracycline, doxycycline, or erythromycin). Treatment to prevent pregnancy is controversial, but this should be discussed with the survivor. The medication most likely to prevent pregnancy is ethinyl estradiol/norgestrel (Ovral) 12 hours later.

The psychologic effects, referred to as "rape trauma syndrome," can last for a long time. These symptoms include reliving the rape, crying outbursts, fear, anger, inability to sleep, angry outbursts, trouble concentrating, and an inability to remember parts of the event.

The ED should make arrangements for counseling follow-up. Having the sexual assault advocate meet the patient in the ED allows the survivor to develop a rapport with the advocate and gives the survivor a link to help once he or she leaves the ED. Written information regarding all aspects of sexual-assault care should be given to the survivor before leaving the ED (Blair, 1992).

# PSYCHIATRIC EMERGENCIES

The ED is often the clearinghouse for psychiatric patients. It is their first port of entry into a structured health care setting. These patients often arrive in police custody, by paramedics, or by family or friends as a result of a change in the patient's mental status. There are three behaviors the emergency psychiatric patient may exhibit: agitation, confusion, or depression.

## Goal of Psychiatric Care in the Emergency Department

The goal of care for the psychiatric patient in the ED is to keep the patient and staff safe. This is done by providing a safe environment and having the patient observed until definitive care is decided or until the patient is admitted to a psychiatric facility. The patient may need to be chemically sedated with medication or physically restrained to maintain a safe environment. Commonly seen in psychiatric patients are suicidal gestures, acute psychosis, and drug and alcohol problems.

## Agitation

Symptoms of **agitation** are pacing, wringing of hands, tachycardia, hyperactivity, and incessant talking. These patients are at risk of hurting themselves. The symptoms may be caused by drug or alcohol problems, an inability to cope with a crisis, anxiety, or organic brain disease. Interventions need to be performed so the agitated patient does not harm himself or herself. Interventions include talking in a calm, quiet voice. A sedative may be prescribed to calm the behavior. The patient may need to be restrained to avoid injury to the patient or the staff caring for the patient.

## Confusion

Symptoms of confusion are a disheveled appearance, a dazed expression, an inability to follow instructions, and/or an inability to communicate basic needs. Causes of confusion are manic-depressive disease; alcohol or drug withdrawal or intoxication; or a medical problem such as Alzheimer's disease, acute head trauma, seizure disorder, or hypoglycemia. Medical problems need to be ruled out before determining that the cause is psychiatric. Interventions for the confused patient are aimed at protecting the patient because he or she is unable to care for himself or herself. A safe environment should be provided. Stimuli should be decreased by dimming the lights, placing the patient in a quiet room, and speaking softly. The patient should be reoriented to the surroundings. For more information about caring for the patient who is confused, see Chapter 31.

## Depression

Symptoms of depression include being tired all the time, having no appetite, having the inability to sleep, maintaining poor eye contact, and having a loss of interest in life and surroundings. These patients may be a suicide risk. Interventions for the depressed patient include allowing the patient to verbalize feelings. The nurse should try to identify if a suicide attempt is imminent and should protect the patient from harming himself or herself.

## Suicidal Emergencies

Suicidal patients are seen in the ED before receiving psychiatric care. They are often patients who are depressed, have experienced a life crisis, have family problems, or abuse drugs or alcohol. Suicide is the eighth leading cause of death in elderly white males. Adolescent suicide has been increasing. Twenty percent of attempted suicides involve alcohol.

Patients who have a history of suicide attempts usually have an underlying psychiatric problem such as depression or a personality disorder. Suicidal patients who have lost their will to live, have experienced or witnessed a violent attack such as rape, or are under the influence of alcohol or drugs are more likely to follow through with their threats. The nurse should

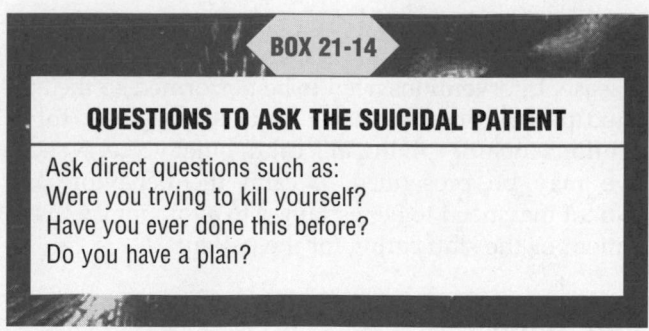

**QUESTIONS TO ASK THE SUICIDAL PATIENT**

Ask direct questions such as:
Were you trying to kill yourself?
Have you ever done this before?
Do you have a plan?

question the patient openly about suicidal thoughts and intentions (Box 21-14). If a plan of how to commit suicide is already thought out, the patient is more likely to attempt suicide again.

Suicidal patients must be kept from harm. A security person or sitter should have direct sight of the patient at all times. The room should be free from anything that the patient could get to harm himself or herself (e.g., instruments, oxygen tubing, and glass). The patient should be completely undressed, and belongings should be stored in a safe place.

Restraints may be necessary to control behavior that could harm the patient or someone else. Once restraints are determined to be necessary, they should be applied. They are not to be used as a threat or a bargaining tool. If restraints are used, the patient should have his or her extremities checked every 15 minutes for circulation, sensation, and mobility. The patient's position should be changed every hour, and the patient should be offered bathroom facilities every 2 hours. Frequent assessments of the patient's psychologic status should be made. If the patient remains violent, chemical sedation should be given. Drugs commonly used are haloperidol (either orally or intramuscularly) or lorazepam intramuscularly until the violent behavior has subsided. Careful monitoring of the respiratory status of suicidal patients is necessary after chemical sedation. The physician, with input from the psychiatric consultant, determines if hospitalization is necessary.

## Overdose Emergency Management

A patient can come to the ED with an accidental or intentional overdose. It is estimated that 5 million overdoses occur annually. An accidental overdose usually involves only one substance. Intentional overdoses usually involve more than one substance. The substances taken should be identified as quickly as possible so that known antidotes can be given. Treatment should never wait until the substance has been identified. Many times the patient arrives with an unknown polydrug ingestion. For any potential emergency patient, the basics must be assessed first. The nurse

should evaluate and intervene on any life-threatening problem affecting the ABCs. Many times these patients need to be intubated because they are unable to protect their airway and their breathing is inadequate. The patient also will need an IV access to be prepared for potential problems and to administer naloxone (Narcan), thiamine, and 50% dextrose. Dextrose is given to patients in case their symptoms are caused by hypoglycemia. A dextrose stick may be obtained before administration of dextrose.

After life-saving measures are instituted, the nurse should obtain a history and complete physical (secondary assessment). The patient should be asked what drugs were taken, when they were taken, how many, and why. If paramedics bring the patient to the ED, they will bring any containers of medications found at the prehospital scene. Measures are then instituted to decrease the absorption of the substance. Definitive measures are performed to help the body eliminate the toxic substances with the least detrimental effects. These procedures are gastric lavage and administering activated charcoal, a cathartic, and any known antidotes for the ingested substances. If the patient does not respond favorably to these treatments, he or she may need to be dialyzed.

**NURSE ALERT**

**Restrain the patient before initiating noxious (painful or uncomfortable) procedures to protect the patient and staff from injury.**

### Gastric Emptying

Ipecac syrup followed by administration of water may be used to help accomplish gastric emptying. Emergency physicians do not like to give this medication because of the effects of retching. If the patient is retching, he or she will be unable to take activated charcoal until the effects of the ipecac have worn off. In addition the patient may be at risk for aspiration if he or she experiences a change in level of consciousness or has seizure activity as a result of the medications ingested before the effects of ipecac end.

Gastric lavage is used to empty any remaining substances from the stomach. An oral or nasal gastric tube is inserted. The patient is then positioned on the left side in Trendelenburg's position. Five liters of tap water are instilled. The amount of water instilled should be the same amount of water returned. A closed gastric lavage system should be used to decrease the chance of exposure to infections. Universal precautions should be followed, including wearing a mask and protective eyewear. Gastric lavage is contraindicated in patients who have ingested hydrocarbons or caustic ingestion. Care should be taken to prevent hypothermia from the administration of the irrigating solution.

## Activated Charcoal

Activated charcoal is used to decrease the absorption rate of the ingested substance. If an oral/nasal gastric tube is in place, the patient should have the charcoal administered through the tube before the tube is removed. The medication also can be taken orally. The usual dose is 1 g/kg, and the total usual adult dose is 50 g. If the patient is to swallow the medication, it can be combined with the cathartic.

## Cathartics

A cathartic such as sorbitol 50 ml or magnesium citrate 4 ml/kg up to 300 ml/kg is given to aid in the elimination of the charcoal. The patient will usually get diarrhea, and the stool will be black. Sorbitol should not be administered to children because studies have shown it can cause retinal hemorrhages.

## Antidotes

The known antidote for the known toxic substance is given after the preceding treatments are completed. A commonly ingested substance is acetaminophen, and the antidote is acetylcysteine (Mucomyst).

## Laboratory Tests

A serum and urine toxicology screen, complete blood count, electrolytes, alcohol level, and arterial blood gases are all laboratory tests that should be ordered for the overdose patient. Specific drug levels will be ordered when the ingested drug is known, such as acetaminophen, aspirin, or digoxin.

## Diagnostic Tests

Cardiac monitoring with an electrocardiogram, pulse oximetry with supplemental oxygen, and a chest x-ray examination are ordered. A CT scan of the head may be ordered for altered mental status.

## Psychiatric Examination

A psychiatric evaluation should be done on all intentional or suspicious accidental toxic ingestions. The patient should be protected from harm and have close observation (Weinman, 1993; Klein et al, 1994).

# POISONINGS

One to two million poisonings occur each year in the United States. Ninety percent of all poisonings take place at home. There are four routes for a poison to enter the body: inhalation, absorption, ingestion, and injection.

## Prevention

Many poisonings can be prevented by educating people about the dangers of products and medications they have at home. Preventing poisonings is the best solution. This is done through patient teaching. Some guidelines to prevent accidental poisonings include the following:
- Keep all medications out of the reach of children. Use containers with childproof covers. Close medications tightly after every use.
- Tell children when they are taking medication and never refer to it as candy.
- Never place dangerous liquids such as paint thinner or gasoline into drinking cups or bottles.
- Read labels before taking any medication.
- Keep all medications and household products in locked cabinets.
- Work in a well-ventilated room when painting or using products that emit fumes.
- Dress appropriately when working outside or hiking. This includes wearing gloves when gardening, and shoes, socks, and long pants when hiking.

## Basic First Aid for Poisoning

For ingestion poisonings the nature of the substance will indicate whether vomiting should be induced. If the substance is a petroleum product such as kerosene, gasoline, or lighter fluid, or if it is a corrosive acid or alkali, vomiting should not be induced because it will further damage the gastrointestinal tract on its return. Toilet bowel cleaners are usually acidic, and drain cleaners and nonphosphate detergents are usually alkaline. Vomiting should never be induced in an unconscious or convulsing patient because of the risk of aspiration. It may be possible to neutralize a corrosive acid or alkali to protect the mucosa of the gastrointestinal tract if the patient is able to swallow. Milk or milk of magnesia will neutralize an acid, and milk, water, or olive oil will neutralize an alkali. Products today have basic first aid instructions on the label. A person involved in a poisoning should contact a poison control center for first aid instructions and the need for follow-up. Many EDs have a poison control index to look up the name of the poison and the advice for first aid. The advice for a triage call is to offer the caller initial first aid instructions and to tell the caller to see a physician or go to an ED for further care. If a patient is unresponsive or is having problems breathing, the EMS should be activated.

For injection poisonings such as bites or stings, the stinger should be removed by scraping it with a credit card. The stinger should never be squeezed, because this can inject more toxins into the bloodstream. Medical help should be sought.

For inhalation poisonings such as chlorine gas or carbon monoxide, the patient should be taken out of the area and given fresh air. Clothing should be loosened to assist with respirations. Help should be called.

For absorption poisonings, the chemical should be brushed off the skin, and the area should be washed with soap and water. Medical help should be sought if there is continued irritation or any sign of respiratory distress (Newell et al, 1993).

## Material Safety Data Sheet

The federal government requires that employees are aware of hazardous chemicals that they could be exposed to in their work area. This law requires employers to educate their staff regarding potential physical and chemical hazards. The government defines what could be considered a hazardous material and mandates that companies supplying these materials have readily available a Material Safety Data Sheet (MSDS). This sheet should be brought with the patient to the emergency department if a chemical exposure has occurred and directs initial emergency and first aid procedures.

# ENVIRONMENTAL EMERGENCIES

Environmental emergencies can be related to extreme heat or cold. They can affect anyone, but the elderly and young, as well as people with chronic conditions such as alcoholism, HIV, or cancer, are extremely vulnerable. The body tries to maintain a core temperature of approximately 37.8° C (100° F).

## Heat Emergencies
### Hyperthermia

**Hyperthermia** is an abnormally high body temperature. As the body temperature rises, the hypothalamus is stimulated and the body tries to compensate for the increase in temperature by first causing peripheral vasodilation. This allows for the heat to dissipate. Then sweat is produced to help the body cool. If the temperature continues to rise, the body will increase heart rate and cardiac output. The kidney will reserve sodium and water. If the temperature is still uncon-

trollable, the patient will begin to exhibit symptoms of heat emergencies: heat stroke, heat cramps, heat syncope, and heat exhaustion.

## Heatstroke

Mortality for heatstroke can be as high as 80%. The body's thermoregulation system is overwhelmed and shuts down. Core body temperature usually goes above 40° C (104° F). Heatstroke is more likely to occur when the temperature and humidity are high. Symptoms include marked confusion, psychotic behavior, and seizures. Skin is hot, dry, and ashen. Heart rate may be very weak and rapid. Signs of dehydration include no urine output, hypotension, tachypnea, and tachycardia. The cells of the brain are injured by the high temperature, and the patient will die if treatment is not initiated to reduce the temperature before the patient is transported to the hospital. The patient should be moved to a cool place, and ice compresses should be applied. Alcohol should never be used to sponge the patient. It can be absorbed through the skin, and the patient can become toxic. An ambulance should be called, and the patient should be transported to the hospital. Interventions begin with the ABCs. Oxygen should be applied, and the patient should be prepped for intubation. Two large-gauge IVs should be established, and vasopressor agents such as Dopamine should be administered if the patient does not respond to IV hydration. A nasogastric tube and Foley catheter should be inserted. The patient should be cooled with a cooling mattress, and the nurse should continuously monitor body temperature. The patient should be on a cardiac monitor so that arrhythmia can be detected. Prevention of shivering is accomplished by administering medications such as chlorpromazine 10 to 50 mg IV.

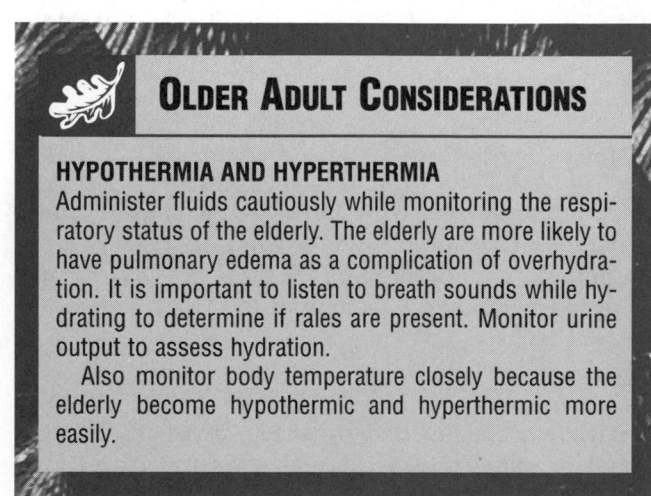

**OLDER ADULT CONSIDERATIONS**

**HYPOTHERMIA AND HYPERTHERMIA**
Administer fluids cautiously while monitoring the respiratory status of the elderly. The elderly are more likely to have pulmonary edema as a complication of overhydration. It is important to listen to breath sounds while hydrating to determine if rales are present. Monitor urine output to assess hydration.

Also monitor body temperature closely because the elderly become hypothermic and hyperthermic more easily.

Seizures are controlled with antineuroleptic medication such as phenytoin (Dilantin) or diazepam.

## Heat Cramps

Heat cramps usually occur in athletes after exercise. The person sweats, and electrolytes become imbalanced. They affect large muscles such as the abdomen, thighs, and calves. The person has lost potassium and sodium through sweat. Electrolytes are further diluted if the person drank water instead of a sports drink containing sodium and potassium.

The treatment for heat cramps begins by getting the patient in a cool environment. Fluids should be replaced with an electrolyte-balanced drink, or IV fluids may be necessary. Salt tablets should not be given, because they irritate the stomach mucosa and cause hypernatremia. When the electrolyte imbalance is corrected, the symptoms resolve.

## Heat Syncope

Heat syncope can occur during exercise. The patient's temperature rises, and the body's blood vessels dilate. This shunt of fluid to the skin can cause symptoms of postural lightheadedness, dizziness, or actual loss of consciousness. Treatment is to get the person into a cool place and rest. The symptoms usually resolve quickly.

## Heat Exhaustion

The patient suffering heat exhaustion exhibits signs of flulike symptoms such as nausea, vomiting, and headache. The skin can be cool and dry, and the patient may have an altered level of consciousness. The body temperature may elevate to 38° C (100.4° F). This person needs IV hydration. The initial IV fluid used is normal saline. The patient should be kept in a cool environment and be given nothing by mouth (Stewart, 1993).

## Cold Emergencies
### Hypothermia

**Hypothermia** is defined as a core temperature less than 35° C (95° F). The body is unable to produce enough heat to maintain its temperature. In mild hypothermia (34° to 35° C [93° F to 95° F]) the patient is conscious and alert and demonstrates tachycardia, tachypnea, cutaneous vasoconstriction, and shivering. With moderate hypothermia (30° to 34° C [86° to 93° F]) symptoms include difficulty speaking, decreased sensorium, and hyperglycemia from decreased utilization of glucose. Shivering has stopped. With severe hypothermia, the nurse will see uncon-

sciousness, deterioration of vital signs, shallow respirations, and cardiac arrhythmias. If no pulse is present, the nurse should begin CPR. The patient should be gradually rewarmed 1 to 2 degrees every hour. The patient should have dry clothes. The worse the hypothermia, the more aggressive the warming techniques. In mild hypothermia the patient's clothes are dry, so warming can be done passively with warm blankets and warmed oral fluids. In severe hypothermia the patient is actively rewarmed with IV fluids, gastric lavage, peritoneal lavage, and oxygen. Pronouncing a patient dead after being hypothermic does not occur until the patient has been rewarmed, which leads to long resuscitative measures.

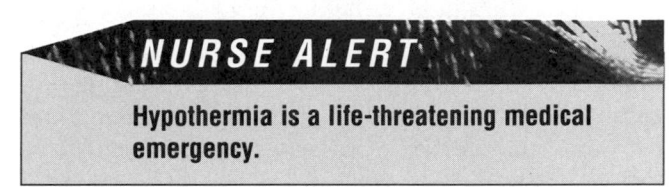

**NURSE ALERT**

Hypothermia is a life-threatening medical emergency.

Patient teaching should include education on layering clothing to stay warm, avoiding alcohol and caffeine when out in the cold, and seeking shelter during a snowstorm or severe weather.

## Frostbite

The skin responds to cold with vasoconstriction, resulting in decreased blood flow and decreased oxygen to the tissue. Severe cold or extended exposure to cold results in damage to vessel walls and leakage of plasma into the interstitial spaces. The blood remaining in the vessel is therefore more concentrated and, together with the narrowed lumen caused by vasoconstriction, results in the formation of small clots that block the small vessels. The pressure from the obstruction causes the arteriovenous shunts to open, and blood bypasses the area. The tissue is essentially without a blood supply. The tissues are cooled to the point that ice crystals form in the extracellular spaces, and the extracellular fluid becomes hypertonic and draws fluid from the cells. If one third of the cells' fluid is lost, dehydration and disruption of enzymatic processes result in injury to the cells. The skin will change to white and will not redden when pressure is applied.

Frostbite most often involves the feet or toes, hands, ears, chin, cheeks, or nose. It is divided into superficial or partial freezing of the skin, or deep, full thickness freezing involving the skin, subcutaneous tissue, and deep tissue.

The frozen tissue looks red and is painful, or it is waxy in appearance, blue or black. The tissue may blister. Treatment involves rapidly rewarming the area. Before starting rewarming, the nurse needs to make sure that there is no chance for refreezing to occur. The temperature of the water for rewarming should be maintained between 37.8° and 40.5° C (100° and 105° F). The tissue should not be rubbed. Rubbing will cause increased cellular damage. The extent of the injury will not be known for at least 24 hours. The frozen area is treated like a burn. Antibiotic ointment should be applied, and the area should be covered with a sterile dressing. The area must be kept from refreezing. If the frostbite is severe and involves tissue beneath the outer layers of the skin, it may permanently remain red and tender, and the affected area will always be very sensitive to cold.

Patient teaching includes information about protecting body parts from further cold injuries, wearing protective clothing, and monitoring the frostbitten areas for signs of infection (Schneider, 1992; Klein et al, 1994).

# DISASTER PREPAREDNESS

Disasters do not occur every day in local communities, but when they do occur, the ED is the unit of the hospital that decides the acuity of the patient and the definitive treatment. A disaster is any situation that causes a large number of victims to seek medical care. It can be caused by natural forces such as hurricane, flood, or tornado. It can be caused by an explosion in an industrial site, or it can be the result of an accident or terrorist and hostage activities. This influx of victims overloads the existing emergency care structure, and an alternative method of deciding treatment for these victims needs to be established. Hospitals now have practice drills to test their disaster plans so that, when a disaster occurs, everyone is familiar with his or her role.

## Types of Injuries

Most casualties from a disaster are surgical in nature, and nursing care is largely the same as that given to any surgical patient. Disaster injuries usually include contusions, lacerations, fractures, crush injuries, burns, and severe hemorrhage from wounds. Many patients suffer from shock, and uninjured persons suffer psychologic stress. In addition, a large group of curious onlookers who feel they must know what is going on is always present.

Disaster nursing differs from emergency nursing only in the number of persons who must be seen. Every effort should be made to protect the individual from further injury and infection, but, in the case of mass casualties, the precise techniques that the nurse has learned may require considerable modification. For more information about triage, see the beginning of this chapter.

## Community Services

Two agencies available to provide services are the Federal Emergency Management Agency (FEMA) and the National Disaster Medical System (NDMS). FEMA activates the government response to secure the disaster area. NDMS coordinates the medical system response.

Community agencies often involved include the fire and police departments, the American Red Cross, Salvation Army, Department of Children and Family Services, Public Health Department, hospitals, clinics, and other agencies. In many disasters the local hospital and medical facilities are adequate for the emergency. However, emergency first-aid centers may be established in schools or churches to care for those with minor injuries and to refer those suffering from more serious injuries to the hospital. If the disaster has caused many deaths, a temporary morgue may need to be set up.

The nurse may assist in various community activities when a disaster occurs. Centers are often set up to immunize large numbers of people when water supplies have been contaminated. Temporary shelters need the assistance of a nurse to help with dealing with families in crisis. The nurse must work with the other disaster team members to help the disaster victims.

## Psychologic Reactions to Disaster

It is normal for the disaster victim to show some signs of disturbance. The victim may tremble or perspire and feel weak and nauseated. After the victim recovers from the first impact of the experience, he or she usually regains composure fairly quickly. Others will panic and seem to lose all ability to make judgments and attempt to escape the situation by fleeing from the site. This reaction can excite others, so it is important to keep a calm manner and reassure persons so they are able to regain control.

It is important that nurses know their own limitations to handle these persons in crisis. Sedatives are usually not prescribed because they can add to the victim's confusion and delay handling of the real problem.

Family and friends can help a disaster victim with support and assistance. The emotional care of the survivor is as important as the physical care. The nurse must convey a feeling of caring if the patient and fam-

## CRITICAL INCIDENCE STRESS DEBRIEFING

Every case of sudden death is different and has a different effect on the health care staff. Critical Incidence Stress Debriefing (CISD) is a support session that occurs after a traumatic event to allow the staff to express feelings. This session usually is best performed 24 to 72 hours after the incident. CISD has shown that if people talk about their feelings, they are better able to resolve them. Unresolved feelings can lead to increased stress.

### COMPONENTS OF DEBRIEFING

The debriefing session is held with the group moderator—a social worker, chaplain, or someone trained in debriefing. The session usually lasts 1 hour, and the group size should be no more than 10 people. There are seven components to the debriefing session: introduction, facts, thoughts, reactions, symptoms, teaching, and closure:

1. Introduction: The group members introduce themselves.
2. Facts: The group starts talking about the facts of the incident. For example: Allen, a local paramedic was brought here by his friends—fellow paramedics—after falling during a routine response drill. He was looking backward and stumbled, hitting his head. He was pronounced brain dead 3 hours after coming to the ED, and life support measures were stopped after organ donation.
3. Thoughts: The group members discuss how they feel, as well as their reactions to the incident. Continuing the ex-

ample, many members state that they feel vulnerable because the accident was so sudden. Discussion also centers on caring for a co-worker in a time of emergency.
4. Reaction: Two questions are answered: How did you feel at the time, and how do you feel now? This is probably the hardest component of the debriefing. Often tears are shed at this point, and physical support with hugs is appreciated by members.
5. Symptoms: The group is asked if it is experiencing any signs or symptoms related to increased stress. It is not uncommon to have nightmares after a traumatic event. Signs of increased stress are physical symptoms: headaches, fatigue, muscle soreness, chest pains, gastrointestinal complaints, inability to concentrate, insomnia, and change of eating habits.
6. Teaching: The group is reminded of the normal response to crisis. It is reeducated regarding the symptoms of increased stress.
7. Closure/Reentry: Finally the group members share how they can help each other better deal with the incident. For example, group members decide to get a plaque for the department honoring the deceased co-worker (Klein et al, 1994).

Not all members of the staff will participate in these sessions. They are voluntary, but the staff who attend the sessions view the response from the session as positive.

ily are to feel comfortable enough to express feelings. It is important to provide a place for family members to express themselves freely.

Psychologic support for the health care team is also important, and critical incidence stress debriefing or management is now an important part of caring for the caregiver after a disaster (Box 21-15).

## SUDDEN DEATH

The ED often deals with sudden death. Sudden death of an infant, a death from a violent attack or car crash, or a natural death from a cardiac arrest or other medical problem all lead to stress for the family of the deceased, as well as for the ED staff.

There is limited time for health care professionals to develop a rapport with families before breaking the news of the death. The grief process begins after the family is told of the death. Each family member's response to the death will vary depending on the person's culture, the closeness of the person to the de-

ceased, the person's learned response to dealing with death, and the circumstances of the death.

On arrival to the ED, the family should be escorted to a quiet room with a phone. It sometimes helps to prepare them by having a health care member (usually the nurse who will be available for the family members while they are in the ED) talk to the family before the actual discussion regarding the death. When addressing the family, the nurse should make introductions and find out who is being addressed. Proper names should be used when speaking to the family of the deceased. The nurse should empathize. The nurse should sit and talk to the family, find out what is already known, and add unknown information. The word dead should be used, so that there is no question regarding the condition of the deceased. The significant others should be encouraged to express themselves. The deceased person can be viewed by the family. This may help to overcome the denial process. It is the family's option to view the deceased. The family should not be rushed into leaving. Some cultures will

NURSING TRANSFER CHECKLIST

Patient Name and ID Number
Address

NOTIFICATION OF RECEIVING FACILITY
Name of agency and unit _____
Name of person notified at receiving facility _____
By whom _____ Date _____ Time _____
Agreed to accept responsibility for care of the patient?  _____ YES _____ NO

TRANSFER INFORMATION
MODE:  _____ Ambulance/ALS  _____ Ambulance/BLS  _____ Helicopter
Other (describe) _____
Name of transfer service or agency _____
Time discharged _____ Time of arrival _____
Required life support equipment _____
Required personnel to accompany patient _____
Physician's Certificate for Transfer completed  _____ YES _____ NO

PATIENT ASSESSMENT/STATUS (within 30 minutes before transfer)

Vital signs:  Time _____ Temp _____ Pulse _____ Resp _____ BP _____

SPECIAL EQUIPMENT OR TREATMENTS
YES     NO
_____  _____    IV Fluids:  Type _____ Rate _____ Site _____
_____  _____    Cardiac monitor
_____  _____    C-spine precautions
_____  _____    Backboard
_____  _____    Cervical collar
_____  _____    Indwelling urinary catheter
_____  _____    Nasogastric tube
_____  _____    Gastric tube
_____  _____    Airway adjuncts
_____  _____        Endotracheal tube
_____  _____        Other _____
_____  _____    Dressings
_____  _____    Splints
_____  _____    Other _____

SENT WITH PATIENT
YES     NO
_____  _____    ED Treatment Record (containing documentation of vital signs on admission and discharge: H & P,
                treatments, medications, physician/nurse signatures, etc.)
_____  _____    Pertinent past medical records
_____  _____    Lab results
_____  _____    EKG
_____  _____    X-rays or reports
_____  _____    Other

Personal belongings: (list all)
_____
_____
_____

**Figure 21-18**   Sample checklist to assure and document via essential information sent with the patient who is transferred to another facility.

bring their entire family to the ED. If this is the case, move the deceased to a room where the family can have some privacy. Before family members leave the ED, it is important for the nurse to give them a name and number to contact if they have any questions. The funeral home is usually the contact that helps once the family has left the ED.

## DISCHARGE TEACHING

After a patient is stabilized and a medical diagnosis has been made or definitive care is complete, the patient is then ready for discharge from the ED. These discharged patients will be admitted to inpatient units, transferred to out of hospital subacute units, or other acute care facilities, or go home. Communication is vital during discharge of the patient. The unit or facility must know what has occurred in the course of the patient's treatment in the ED and the expected outcomes for the patient after they arrive. Many EDs will use a checklist to assure and document the fact that essential information is sent with the patient (Figure 21-18).

If the patient is to be transferred to an out of hospital subacute unit, a copy of the ED chart, a history and physical, and a one-day supply of medications should be sent with the patient. It is essential that the report be given to the accepting facility to identify if any problems would interfere with the safe transfer of the patient. If the patient is being transferred to another acute care facility, a copy of the ED chart, labs, and x-rays must accompany the patient. A physician on staff at the receiving hospital must accept the transfer and the patient must be told of the risks and benefits of the transfer. The transferring physician must certify the benefits that outweigh the risks of transfer. If the patient is going home it is important that they know how to care for themselves to prevent further discomfort.

Patients may leave **against medical advice.** If a patient decides that the care to be rendered is not the care they were seeking, they may decide to leave the hospital. This decision could place them at risk for dying or having their medical condition worsen. It is important that the risks and benefits are stated clearly to the patient and that the patient acknowledges understanding of the information regarding his condition. If the patient still decides to leave it is very important to document the conversation and the patient's response to the information given. Always encourage the patient to return at any time.

The ENA's Standards of Practice emphasize the importance of teaching to help patients and their significant others prevent illness and injury, as well as understand prescribed treatments (Dains et al, 1991). This is accomplished by the constant teaching that

emergency nurses provide. From the moment patients arrive at the ED, teaching is started regarding what care they will receive, the time frame of test results, and the interpretation of test results. This is a collaborative process that is shared by the health care team. Every patient leaving the hospital is given formal discharge instructions that explain how to care for the illness or injury and who to contact later if there is a problem.

Many emergency nurses are involved in educating the public by presenting programs regarding health issues. One organization is ENCARE, Emergency Nurses Cancel Alcohol-Related Emergencies. This organization encourages emergency nurses to speak to high school students regarding the problem of drinking and driving. As stated previously, organizations such as STOP and HELP use nurses to educate the public regarding handgun violence. Nurses also speak at rotary clubs and other meetings about when to use the ED.

Nurses who work in emergency nursing understand that prevention is the key to decreasing accidental injuries.

## TRENDS

Managed care is having an impact on the ED. Since managed-care groups treat patients with minor illnesses in their own offices, the majority of patients admitted to the ED from these groups are acutely ill. The ED physician contacts the managed care physician and they discuss the treatment plan for a patient. If the patient can be transferred to an out of hospital subacute unit to receive IV antibiotics, IV hydration, or rehab this will happen after communication between the managed care case manager and the nurse. The nurse must truly be a patient advocate to ensure that the patient is sent to the proper place to receive appropriate care. This could be to a hospital unit, a rehab or long term care facility, or home with possibly home health.

The ED nurse now is assuming responsibilities for beginning the admission process of the patient. With a decrease in the length of stay of hospital patients, early identification of a patient who may have more complex discharge needs must be identified early in the admission process. Patients who are unable to be admitted to the hospital still may need specialized care at home. The ED nurse or case manager is responsible for making a referral to a home health agency to ensure patient safety on discharge. Sometimes these patients return to the ED in less than 24 hours and need to be readmitted for the same problem as their original admission.

Fast-track systems have been established to separate the critically ill from patients with minor illnesses. Patients who are admitted to observation areas will need the skill of critical care technology. Critical pathways have now been developed to help streamline patient care and facilitate the timely discharge of patients. The ED is the first entry level in these critical pathways.

Because early treatment for illness and injury is known to improve patient outcomes, the ED is becoming more research based. New medications are being tested to improve patients' outcomes from acute ischemic strokes, as well as treatments for acute myocardial infarctions. The ED nurse has a vital role in helping identify patients who meet criteria to participate in the treatment studies. It is the nurse who helps collect the data and administers the medications according to strict guidelines. ED nurses are also conducting research on issues affecting patient care such as assessing patients in pain or evaluating methods of triage.

These are examples of how emergency nursing is constantly changing to meet the needs of the diverse population we care for.

## NURSING CARE PLAN

## PATIENT WITH A HEAT-RELATED EMERGENCY

Marc Stevens is a 26-year-old male who is brought to the emergency department by a friend. The friend states "My friend is barely moving and not acting right." When helping Mr. Stevens out of the car it is noted that he has no breathing impairment, is disoriented, responds to verbal stimuli, and is unable to walk.

The friend reports that they rode bicycles 30 miles before experiencing any problems. The outside temperature is 95° F, but they drank some fluids during the ride. Normally they ride on long trips two to three times per week.

| Medical History | Psychosocial Data | Assessment Data |
|---|---|---|
| No known allergies<br>Takes no medications<br>No significant past<br>  medical history | Unknown | Height 6' 1", weight 176 lbs<br>Well-nourished, muscular appearance<br>Alert and oriented × 2, disoriented to time<br>Answers some questions inappropriately<br>*Vital signs:* Temperature 100° F, pulse 120, respirations 24, BP<br>  100/60, PERRL<br>*Respiratory:* Lungs clear; no dyspnea; respirations deep symmetric<br>*Abdomen:* Soft; nontender; nondistended; hypoactive bowel<br>  sounds.<br>*Skin:* Pale color; cool and dry; no diaphoresis; no surface trauma<br>  head to toe<br>*Cardiovascular:* Apical pulse 124 and regular; orthostatic hypotension; strong peripheral pulses<br>**Laboratory data**<br>Hct 40, Hgb 14.2 g/100 ml, RBC 4.8, BUN 33 mg/100 ml, Cr<br>  1.3 mg/100 ml, Na 130 mg/100 ml, K 3.0 mEq/L, Cl 90 mEq/L<br>**Medications**<br>Normal saline IV wide open rate<br>Oxygen 2 L/min nasal cannula<br>Cardiac monitor<br>Cooling of patient with air conditioner |

# NURSING CARE PLAN

## PATIENT WITH A HEAT-RELATED EMERGENCY—cont'd

**NURSING DIAGNOSIS**
Hyperthermia related to environmental factors

| NURSING INTERVENTIONS | EVALUATION OF EXPECTED OUTCOMES |
| --- | --- |
| Monitor rectal temperature, skin temperature, and overall color. | Rectal temperature 99.6° F |
| Maintain cool environment. | Skin warm and dry |
| Remove excess clothing and covers. | Normal skin color |
| Administer antipyretic medications, if prescribed. | Alert and oriented × 3 |
| Assess for shivering. If it occurs, administer diazepam or lorazepam as ordered. | No agitation |
| Monitor level of consciousness. | Nausea and vomiting subsided |
| Assess for nausea and vomiting. | No shivering |

**NURSING DIAGNOSIS**
Risk for ineffective airway clearance related to decreased level of consciousness

| NURSING INTERVENTIONS | EVALUATION OF EXPECTED OUTCOMES |
| --- | --- |
| Provide airway management as indicated. | Airway remains patent |
| Administer supplemental oxygen. | Pulse oximetry >95% |
| Monitor respiratory status continuously until stable ($O_2$ sat, breath sounds, rate, depth). | Respiratory rate 16 to 20 min |
| Assess for decreased level of consciousness. | Lungs clear bilaterally |
| Position for optimal respiratory effort. | Awake, alert, and oriented × 3 |

**NURSING DIAGNOSIS**
Fluid volume deficit related to peripheral vasodilation, inadequate intake

| NURSING INTERVENTIONS | EVALUATION OF EXPECTED OUTCOMES |
| --- | --- |
| Administer IV fluids as ordered, normal saline at fast rate until stable. | Normal vital signs without orthostatic changes |
| Monitor vital signs, urine output, skin turgor, capillary refill. | Normal sinus rhythm without ectopy |
| Monitor for orthostatic hypotension if indicated. | Urine output 15 to 30 ml/hr |
| Monitor cardiac status with telemetry. | No evidence of dehydration |

**NURSING DIAGNOSIS**
Knowledge deficit related to prevention of subsequent heat illness

| NURSING INTERVENTIONS | EVALUATION OF EXPECTED OUTCOMES |
| --- | --- |
| Assess level of knowledge related to heat illness, discussing early signs and symptoms. | Verbalizes understanding of information |
| Discuss predisposing factors to heat illness (outside temperature, increased activity, lack of hydration). | Identifies early signs of heat illness and measures to prevent heat illness |
| Teach importance of hydration and cooling. | |
| Provide written discharge instructions. | |

# KEY CONCEPTS

➤ The goal of emergency care is to resuscitate and stabilize patients, reduce suffering, provide for emotional needs, and educate regarding discharge instructions and prevention.

➤ Emergency care involves a collaborative approach.

➤ Legislation affecting emergency care includes Consolidated Omnibus Reconciliation Act, mandatory reporting of violent acts, and trauma center designations.

➤ Unique characteristics of emergency practice are assessment, analysis/diagnosis, and treatment of emergent, urgent, and nonurgent individuals of all ages; triage and prioritization; disaster preparedness; stabilization and resuscitation; and crisis intervention.

➤ Priorities differ between daily triage and disaster triage. In daily triage the most critical patient is treated first. In disaster triage the most salvageable patient is treated first. An "expectant" category is added to disaster triage.

➤ Disaster triage starts at the disaster scene. The patients arriving at the hospital have already had their care prioritized at least once.

➤ History, including mechanism of injury, is vital for a thorough assessment and plan of care for the patient.

➤ Primary assessment includes airway, breathing, circulation, and a brief neurologic examination. Intervention is for any life-threatening problem.

➤ Secondary assessment identifies all injuries.

➤ Focused assessment addresses each problem area identified during the secondary assessment. It includes definitive care and patient teaching.

➤ All patients who have impaired skin integrity from an injury receive tetanus (dT) immunization if last booster was given more than 10 years ago and there is no contraindication.

➤ A cervical spine injury should be suspected for any trauma above the level of the clavicle.

➤ When administering IV conscious sedation, resuscitative equipment and medication reversal should be ready.

➤ Changes in the neurologic signs of a head-injured patient indicate the need for immediate intervention.

➤ No family is immune from the effects of violence.

➤ It is mandatory to report any acts of violence to a law enforcement agency.

➤ Safety is the goal for any psychiatric patient.

➤ Anaphylaxis is a life-threatening emergency. After the critical event patients need to be educated on how to avoid a recurrence and measures to take if contact with the allergen occurs.

➤ Eighty percent of all patients who experience heatstroke die.

➤ Frostbitten areas should never be rubbed.

➤ Hypothermic patients are never dead until they are warm and dead. This leads to prolonged resuscitative measures of the hypothermic patient.

➤ The hypothermic patient's temperature should be raised only 1° to 2° an hour.

➤ The emergency nurse needs to be aware of legal and ethical problems that can arise.

➤ If a patient with a head injury has signs of hypovolemic shock, the nurse should look for other injuries that cause bleeding.

➤ The nurse needs to be empathic to families who have just experienced a death. Every family will deal with death differently.

➤ When a traumatic event occurs in the emergency department, a debriefing session should occur between 24 to 72 hours to allow the staff to express feelings and aid in the resolution of those feelings.

# CRITICAL THINKING EXERCISES

1. Contrast the four goals of emergency care with the goals for the general care of any patient.

2. How is triage during a disaster different from daily triage?

3. Compare hypovolemic shock and anaphylaxis. Which symptoms are the same and which are different?

## REFERENCES AND ADDITIONAL READINGS

American College of Surgeons: Resources for optimal care of the injured patient, Philadelphia, 1990, The College.

Berkowitz C: Conscious sedation a primer, *RN* 60(2):32-35, 1997.

Blair TMH, Warner CG: Sexual assault, *Top Emerg Med* 14(4): 58-77, 1992.

Bone LB, Chapman MW: Initial management of the patient with multiple injuries, *Instructional Course Lectures* 39:557-563, 1990.

Borton D: Isolation precautions clearing up the confusion, *Nursing* 27(1):49-51, 1997.

Bukata WR: Thrombolytic therapy for strokes, *Emerg Med Acute Care Essays* 20(11):1-4, 1996.

Cambell J: Policy change in management of head injury patient, *BTLS Bull* (12):1, 1996.

Campbell JC: Violence and our nation's health, *Healthcare Trends Transition* 5(4):10-39, 1994.

Chez N: Helping the victim of domestic violence, *Am J Nurs* 94(7):33-37, 1994.

Dains J et al: *Standards of emergency nursing practice*, ed 2, St Louis, 1991, Mosby.

Devlin BK, Reynolds E: Child abuse: how to recognize it, how to intervene, *Am J Nurs* 94(4):26-32, 1994.

Dubin WR, Tardiff K, Maier G: Overcoming danger with violent patients: guidelines for safe and effective management, *Emerg Med Rep* 13(14):105-112, 1992.

Dwyer B, Weissberg MP, Rund DA: Strategies for recognizing and managing suicidal patients, *Emerg Med Rep* 14(11):91-98, 1993.

Emergency Nurses Association: *Orientation to emergency nursing: diversity in practice*, Chicago, 1993, The Association.

Emergency Nurses Association: *Role of the emergency nurse in tissue and organ procurement: Emergency Nurses Association position statement*, Chicago, 1992, The Association.

Emergency Nurses Association: Telephone advice: *Emergency Nurses Association position statement*, Chicago, 1991a, The Association.

Emergency Nurses Association: *Violence in the emergency setting: Emergency Nurses Association position statement*, Chicago, 1991b, The Association.

Guidelines for cardiopulmonary resuscitation and emergency care, *JAMA* 268(16):2185-2193, 1992.

IV conscious sedation guidelines published, *Penn Nurse* 47(5):7, 1992.

Jackson L: Quick response to hypothermia and frostbite, *Am J Nurs* 95(3):52, 1995.

Kinkle SL: Violence in the ED: how to stop it before it starts, *Am J Nurs* 93(7):22-24, 1993.

Klein AR et al: *Emergency nursing core curriculum*, ed 4, Philadelphia, 1994, Saunders.

Lynch SH: Elder abuse what to look for, how to intervene, *Am J Nurs* 97(1):26-32, 1997.

Malestic S: Fight violence with forensic evidence, *RN* 58(1): 30-33, 1995.

Newell L et al: *Community first aid and safety*, St Louis, 1993, Mosby.

Parker V: Battered, *RN* 58(1):26-29, 1995.

Schneider SM: Hypothermia: from recognition to rewarming, *Emerg Med Rep* 13(1):1-10, 1992.

Sheehy SB: *Emergency nursing: principles and practice*, ed 3, St Louis, 1992, Mosby.

Smith M, Martin F: Domestic violence: recognition, intervention, and prevention, *Med Surg Nurs* 4(1)21-25, 1995.

Somerson S, Justed C, Sicilia M: Insights into conscious sedation, *Am J Nurs* 95(6):26-33, 1995.

Stewart C: Acute hyperthermia: the spectrum of heat emergencies, *Emerg Med Rep* 14(16):133-144, 1993.

Steiner RP, Vansickle K, Lippman SB: Domestic violence: do you know when and how to intervene, *Postgrad Med* 100(1):103-116, 1996.

Trunkey D: Initial treatment of patients with extensive trauma, *N Engl J Med* 324(18):1259-1263, 1991.

Wainscott MP, Morgan DL, Shrestha M: Management of the difficult family in the emergency department, *Top Emerg Med* 14(4):1-11, 1992.

Weinman S: Emergency management of drug overdose, *Crit Care Nurs* 13(6):45-51, 1993.

Wyatt R: Anaphylaxis how to recognize, treat, and prevent potentially fatal attacks, *Postgrad Med* 100(2):87-98, 1996.

# CHAPTER 22

# Respiratory Problems

## CHAPTER OBJECTIVES

1  Describe the normal passage of oxygen and carbon dioxide through the respiratory system.
2  Describe how to obtain relevant subjective information from a patient who is experiencing alterations in respiratory function.
3  Discuss the elements to include when performing a physical examination of the respiratory system.
4  Identify symptoms of respiratory disease.
5  Differentiate age-related changes from pathological changes in the respiratory system.
6  Describe the preparation and care of a patient who is undergoing diagnostic testing to evaluate the respiratory system.
7  Identify at least four nursing interventions that assist patients in reducing retained secretions in the upper airway.
8  Describe nursing responsibilities involved in caring for a patient who is receiving oxygen therapy.
9  Identify threats to patient safety during endotracheal intubation.
10  Describe assessments necessary for a patient after a tracheostomy.
11  List nursing responsibilities when caring for a patient who is mechanically ventilated.
12  Discuss postoperative care of a patient who has had a lobectomy.
13  Describe special considerations for a patient who has closed chest tube drainage.
14  Identify three actions the nurse can use to teach patients how to decrease the spread of respiratory tract infections.
15  Identify symptoms of an upper respiratory tract infection.
16  Differentiate between treatment of viral and bacterial infections in the upper respiratory tract.
17  Discuss interventions that provide symptomatic relief for upper respiratory tract infections.
18  List topics included in patient-family teaching for prevention of upper airway infections.
19  Discuss conditions that may result from trauma or obstruction in the upper airway.
20  Discuss patient education after a total laryngectomy.
21  Describe assessments necessary for a patient after a laryngectomy.
22  List resources available for patients undergoing a total laryngectomy.
23  Describe the pathophysiology and nursing care of patients with chronic obstructive pulmonary disease.
24  Develop a nursing care plan for a patient with pneumonia.
25  Identify risk factors for the development of pulmonary embolism.
26  Discuss ways to prevent the development of atelectasis in a postoperative patient.
27  Describe types of chest trauma and nursing management for each.
28  Identify signs and symptoms of adult respiratory distress syndrome, and discuss patient management.

## KEY TERMS

adventitious sounds
alveoli
atelectasis
bronchiectasis
cilia
cor pulmonale
coryza
crackles
cyanosis
disseminated intravascular
  coagulation
dyspnea
epistaxis
extrinsic asthma
fremitus
hemoptysis
hypoxia
induration
intrinsic asthma

laryngectomy
leukocytosis
lobectomy
orthopnea
parietal pleura
pleural friction rub
pneumonectomy
polyp
pulmonary embolism
sepsis
surfactant
thoracic cage
tonsillectomy
tracheotomy
ventilation
virulence
visceral pleura
wheezes
wheezing

# STRUCTURE AND FUNCTION OF THE RESPIRATORY SYSTEM

## Structure

The primary function of the respiratory system is to provide oxygen that will meet metabolic needs and to remove carbon dioxide, which is an end product of cellular metabolism. The structures of the upper respiratory system include the nose, pharynx, larynx, and trachea (Figure 22-1). The nose serves as a passageway for air to move to and from the lungs. Impurities are trapped by nasal hair and moist mucous membranes, and air is humidified and warmed as it is inhaled into the lungs. The pharynx, or throat, is a tubelike structure with two main functions. It serves as a common pathway for air to enter the trachea and food to enter the esophagus, and it also plays an important role in the formation of sounds, particularly vowel sounds. The pharynx connects the nasal and oral cavities to the larynx, which is commonly referred to as the "voice box." Normally air enters the larynx during breathing and talking. During swallowing, the epiglottis, a flap of cartilage, closes and covers the opening of the lar-

**Figure 22-1**  Anatomy of the thorax and lungs. (From Phipps WJ et al: *Medical-surgical nursing: concepts and clinical practice,* ed 5, St Louis, 1995, Mosby.)

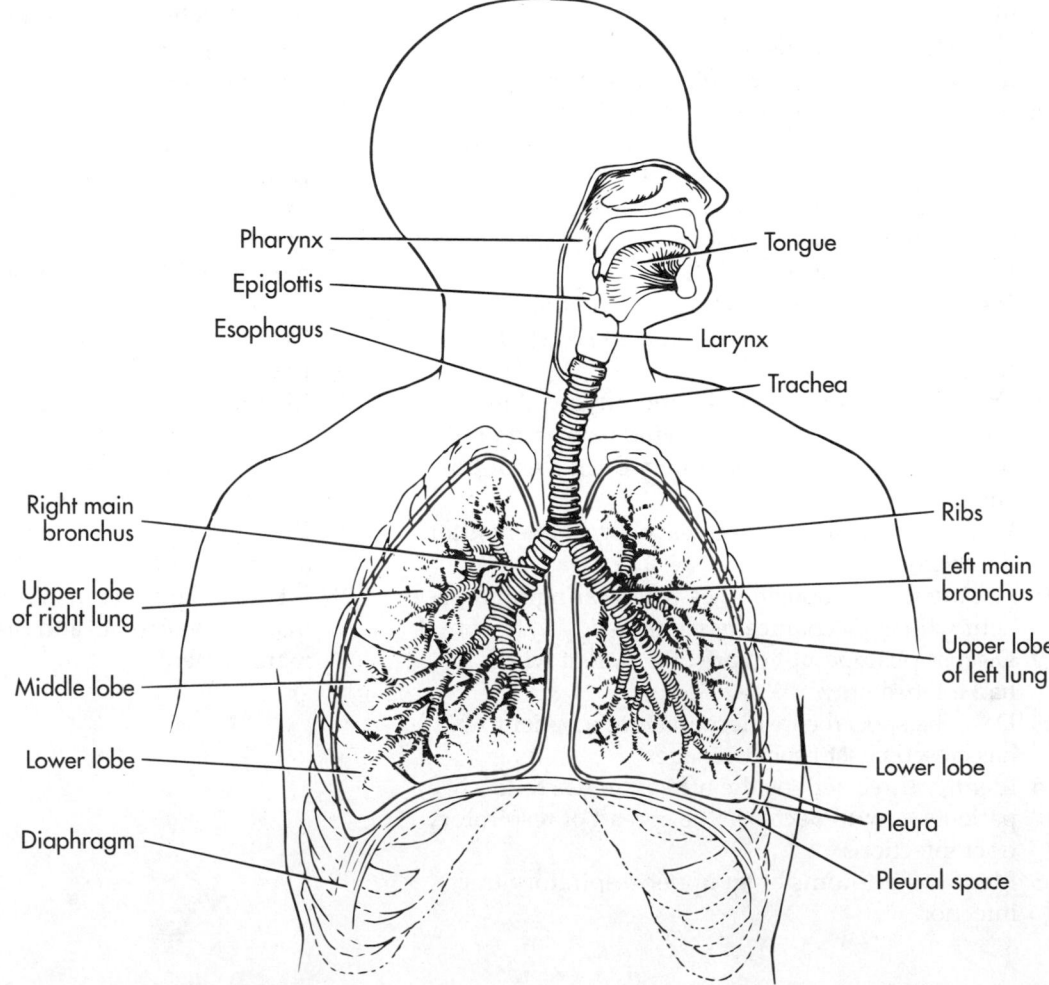

ynx so that food does not enter the larynx and trachea, which is below the larynx. The larynx contains the vocal cords and is located at the upper end of the trachea. The trachea is a 4- to 5-inch-long and 1-inch-wide tube composed of smooth muscle that is supported by regularly spaced rings of cartilage and maintains an open passageway for airflow. At its lower end, (the carina), the trachea divides into the right and left primary bronchi. The right main bronchus is shorter, more vertical, and has a slightly larger diameter than the left bronchus. Because of these characteristics, aspirated foreign bodies often slip down the right mainstem bronchus and lodge in the right lung (Lewis, Collier, Heitkemper, 1996). Mucous membranes line the entire upper respiratory tract, and many of its cells contain fine hairlike projections called **cilia.** Mucus and impurities continually sweep toward the pharynx, where they are expectorated or swallowed.

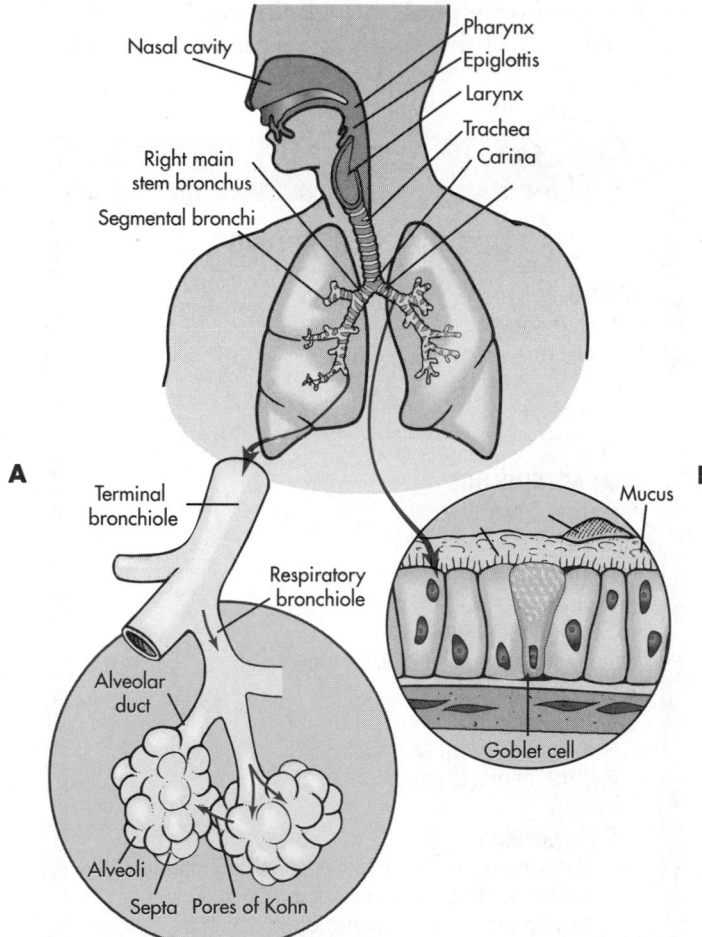

**A**

Labels: Nasal cavity; Right main stem bronchus; Segmental bronchi; Pharynx; Epiglottis; Larynx; Trachea; Carina; Terminal bronchiole; Respiratory bronchiole; Alveolar duct; Alveoli; Septa; Pores of Kohn; Mucus; Goblet cell

**B**

**Figure 22-2** Structures of the respiratory tract. **A,** Pulmonary functional unit. **B,** Ciliated mucous membrane. (Redrawn from Price S, Wilson L: Pathophysiology: clinical concepts of disease processes. In Lewis SM, Collier IC, Heitkemper MM, editors: *Medical-surgical nursing: assessment and management of clinical problems,* ed 4, St Louis, 1996, Mosby.)

The right and left bronchi, their subdivisions, and the lungs form the lower respiratory system (Figure 22-2). The bronchi are similar in structure to the trachea and are lined with ciliated columnar epithelium. Each bronchus enters a lung, where it divides and branches to form bronchioles. The trachea and the bronchi resemble an inverted tree. Further branching of the bronchi produces microscopic alveolar ducts, which end in alveolar sacs called **alveoli** (see Figure 22-2). Inside each lung 300 million alveoli are interlaced in a network of capillaries, where oxygen is transferred to the blood and carbon dioxide is removed from the blood and eliminated from the body. Some of the cells in the alveoli secrete a liquid called **surfactant,** which increases lung compliance (ease of inflation) and keeps alveoli evenly inflated and dry (Lewis, Collier, Heitkemper, 1996).

The lungs are the organs that provide areas for gas exchange. They are separated from each other by the mediastinum. The uppermost portion of the lung, called the apex, extends approximately 1½ inches above the clavicle. The lower part of each lung is called the base. The left lung consists of two lobes, an upper and a lower. The right lung has three lobes: upper, middle, and lower. Each lobe is further divided into two to five segments that are separated by fissures and are extensions of the pleura (see Figure 22-2).

The lower part of the respiratory system and part of the trachea are enclosed in a bony framework known as the **thoracic cage.** The thoracic cage is separated from the abdominal cavity by the diaphragm, which contracts to create a partial vacuum during inspiration and relaxes during expiration, permitting abdominal organs to push upward and help force air from the lungs. The thoracic cavity is lined with a serous membrane, the **parietal pleura,** and each lung is enclosed in a saclike structure of serous membrane, the **visceral pleura.** A potential space exists between the layers of the parietal and visceral pleura. This space is lubricated by a small amount of pleural fluid, which allows the layers of the pleura to glide over each other during breathing. The pleural space can become inflamed and fill with air or fluid, disrupting the negative pressure of the pleural cavity. This loss of normal negative pressure causes the lung to contract and eventually collapse.

## Control of Breathing

Respiration is controlled primarily by the respiratory center in the medulla oblongata of the brain. The phrenic, glossopharyngeal, and vagus nerves innervate the diaphragm, larynx, tracheobronchial tree, and lungs, as well as transmit impulses to and from the respiratory center. Chemoreceptors also play a role in controlling breathing. A central chemoreceptor in the medulla is sensitive to increases in the concentration of carbon dioxide and hydrogen in the cerebrospinal fluid. Additional chemoreceptors in the aortic arch (aortic bodies) and at the carotid bifurcation (carotid bodies) respond to decreases in oxygen and pH and increases in carbon dioxide (Beare, Myers, 1998).

## Ventilation

The function of the respiratory system is to exchange gases, which is accomplished through the process of respiration. Respiration is both external and internal. External respiration **(ventilation)** consists of the movement of oxygen into the lungs (inhalation) and the removal of carbon dioxide from the lungs (exhalation). During the inhalation phase, oxygen from inspired air passes through the permeable membranes of the alveoli and capillaries and reaches the blood. Oxygen combines with hemoglobin in the red blood cells and is transported by the circulatory system to the body cells. Internal respiration is the process by which oxygen is transferred from blood to body cells and carbon dioxide is passed from body cells to blood to be eliminated from the body.

# ASSESSMENT OF SIGNS AND SYMPTOMS OF RESPIRATORY DISEASE

The signs and symptoms most closely associated with respiratory disease are dyspnea, chest pain, cough, sputum production, wheezing hemoptysis, and cyanosis.

## Dyspnea

When breathing becomes difficult or labored and requires considerable exertion, patients are said to have **dyspnea.** Dyspnea is a highly subjective symptom of respiratory difficulty that involves both a physiologic and a cognitive component (Box 22-1) (Gift, 1990). It may result from pain, pulmonary disease, anemia, heart failure, obstruction such as from a pulmonary embolism, or emotional factors. When patients are unable to breathe except in a sitting position, they are said to have **orthopnea.** Orthopnea may occur in individuals with chronic obstructive pulmonary disease

---

## OLDER ADULT CONSIDERATIONS

### PHYSIOLOGIC CHANGES IN THE RESPIRATORY SYSTEM

At all times during the life cycle, the respiratory system is vulnerable to injuries caused by infections, environmental pollutants, and allergic reactions. These are often far more damaging to the system than the decline in function that is a normal component of aging.

Age-related changes include an increased susceptibility to infection because of a decline in the protection normally provided by the intact mucous barrier, a decrease in the effectiveness of the bronchial cilia, and changes in the composition of the connective tissues of the lungs and chest. Elderly persons rely far more on the diaphragm for inspiration, and breathing requires more effort, especially when lying down. Vital capacity declines with age, and it takes longer to inspire or expire air because of the decline in the elastic recoil of the lungs and an increase in the stiffness of the chest wall. Although total lung volume does not change significantly, residual volume increases; and although the alveolar partial pressure of oxygen usually does not change, the alveolar-capillary gradient does increase slightly.

From Beare PG, Myers JL: *Adult health nursing*, ed 3, St Louis, 1998, Mosby.

---

**BOX 22-1**

### DYSPNEA DESCRIPTORS

**TIMING**
Chronic or acute
Episodic or paroxysmal
Onset
Duration
Frequency

**CHARACTERISTICS**
Perceived severity
Phase of respiratory cycle
  Inspiratory
  Expiratory
  Throughout entire cycle
Other symptoms related to dyspnea
Associated factors
  Time of day
  Seasonal or weather changes
  Environmental irritants
  Anxiety
  Body position
    Paroxysmal nocturnal dyspnea (PND): sudden onset while sleeping in recumbent position
    Orthopnea: breathlessness upon assuming recumbent position

From Phipps WJ et al: *Medical-surgical nursing: concepts and clinical practice*, ed 5, St Louis, 1995, Mosby.

(COPD) and heart disease. Dyspnea is one of the most frightening symptoms for patients and their families. Patients often feel their lives are threatened, and, as they become more anxious, their dyspnea may increase. The nurse caring for a patient with dyspnea should be calm, reassuring, and confident and should attempt to determine the underlying cause of the problem. Some relief may be achieved by elevating the head of the bed. The diaphragm descends more easily during inspiration if the upper part of the body is elevated. Supplemental oxygen may be necessary if dyspnea continues or worsens. When dyspnea is assessed, the patient's perception of difficulty is important and can be measured by asking the patient to point to a level of difficulty between 1 and 10, such as demonstrated by the Borg Scale. The nurse can simply ask the patient to rate the shortness of breath from 0 to 10, with 0 signifying no shortness of breath and 10 signifying the worst the patient can imagine.

## Chest Pain

Chest pain of a pulmonary origin may result from a variety of conditions such as pulmonary embolism, pneumonia, pleurisy, and lung cancer (Beare, Myers, 1998). The pain may be described as sharp, stabbing, dull, aching, diffuse, or localized (Table 22-1). Important information includes the location, onset, duration, quality, and quantity of the pain and the setting in which it occurs. The nurse should also be alert to what alleviates the pain and what aggravates it.

## Cough

An irritation of mucous membranes anywhere in the respiratory tract can produce a cough. Coughing protects the lungs against the accumulation of secretions in the bronchi and bronchioles. It is often stimulated by an infectious process or by irritants present in the air, such as smoke, but may be associated with other pulmonary problems (DesJardins, Burton, 1995; Beare, Myers, 1998). The time the cough began (onset) is important to consider. A cough of recent onset is commonly associated with an acute infectious process.

The quality of the cough is also important. Is the cough productive, nonproductive, dry, moist, brassy, barking, hoarse, or hacking? The nurse should ask the patient whether the quality of the cough has changed over time. A severe or changing cough may be associated with bronchogenic carcinoma. The nurse should note at what time of the day the cough occurs and whether it is brought on by specific activities, body positions, or movements.

Coughing at night may be associated with failure of the left side of the heart. Coughing during eating may indicate aspiration of ingested materials into the tracheobronchial tree. Individuals with bronchitis may complain of a productive cough, especially in the morning (Beare, Myers, 1998; Phipps et al, 1998).

## Sputum Production

The goblet cells and mucous glands of the lung secrete mucus that coats the interior lung surface. The lung cilia propel mucus upward toward the pharynx. Sputum production is the reaction of the lungs to any continual irritant. For evaluation and visual inspection of sputum production, the patient should be asked to cough into a white tissue or clean cup. Sputum is evaluated for color, amount, and consistency. The color and consistency of the sputum may point to specific diseases. For example, creamy yellow sputum often occurs with staphylococcal pneumonia, and pink frothy sputum occurs with pulmonary edema. Any change in sputum color, whether from the normal anticipated color or from the patient's baseline color, should be investigated.

## Wheezing

**Wheezing** often occurs in patients who have bronchoconstriction, or airway narrowing. Wheezing is further assessed during the physical examination of the respiratory system when the breath sounds are evaluated.

## TABLE 22-1

### Thoracic-Pulmonary Chest Pain

| ORIGIN | CHARACTERISTICS | POSSIBLE CAUSE |
| --- | --- | --- |
| Chest wall | Well-localized constant ache increasing with movement | Trauma; cough; herpes zoster |
| Pleura | Sharp, abrupt onset increasing with inspiration or with sudden ventilatory effect (cough, sneeze), unilateral | Pleural inflammation (pleurisy); pulmonary infarction; pneumothorax; tumors |
| Lung parenchyma | Dull, constant ache, poorly localized | Benign pulmonary tumors; carcinoma; pneumothorax |

From Phipps WJ et al: *Medical-surgical nursing: concepts and clinical practice*, ed 5, St Louis, 1995, Mosby.

## Hemoptysis

**Hemoptysis** is the coughing up of blood from the respiratory tract. The most common causes of hemoptysis are pulmonary infection, lung cancer, abnormalities of the heart or blood vessels, pulmonary embolism and infarction, and pulmonary artery or vein abnormalities (Beare, Myers, 1998).

A carefully taken history and physical examination are helpful in diagnosing any underlying respiratory disease. Diagnostic evaluation often includes blood testing, chest x-ray examination, and bronchoscopy. Additional studies may be needed to identify the source of the bleeding, which may be the gums, upper respiratory tract, lungs and adjacent structures, or stomach.

True hemoptysis usually contains some frothy portions of bright red blood and is followed by blood-tinged sputum for several days as the site of injury in the lung heals. The pH is alkaline (>7). Hematemesis is the vomiting of blood from the stomach. A patient with hematemesis rather than hemoptysis may have a history of gastric problems, liver disease, or alcoholism (Phipps et al, 1995). Food particles may be evident in the vomitus; the blood is dark red, never frothy; and the pH is acidic (<7).

## Cyanosis

**Cyanosis** is characterized by a bluish discoloration of the skin and mucous membranes. Peripheral cyanosis may be observed in the earlobes, the tip of the nose, or the fingertips. Because peripheral cyanosis may be caused by vasoconstriction as a result of cold or nervousness, it is not a reliable indicator of inadequate oxygenation. Central cyanosis as observed on the mucous membranes of the mouth is noted in severe respiratory disease. Central cyanosis is a certain indicator of inadequate oxygenation and is a late sign of **hypoxia** or decreased oxygen in the blood. For cyanosis to appear, at least 5 g/dl of the normal 15 g of hemoglobin must be deoxygenated. This level approximates the oxygen saturation of venous blood (DesJardins, Burton, 1995). Thus an anemic patient with a hemoglobin level of 8 g/dl would not become cyanotic until in a severely hypoxic condition. Similarly, an individual with a high hemoglobin level of 20 g/dl could be cyanotic if 5 g of hemoglobin were deoxygenated but would not be hypoxic because the hemoglobin level would be normal. Therefore the presence of cyanosis should be identified, but its absence does not guarantee adequate arterial oxygenation. The overall status of the patient must be considered, and the conditions that influence oxygenation must be identified (Carroll, 1996; Beare, Myers, 1998).

# NURSING ASSESSMENT OF THE PATIENT WITH A RESPIRATORY PROBLEM

## History

Individuals with altered respiratory function may seek health care for a variety of complaints, including dys-

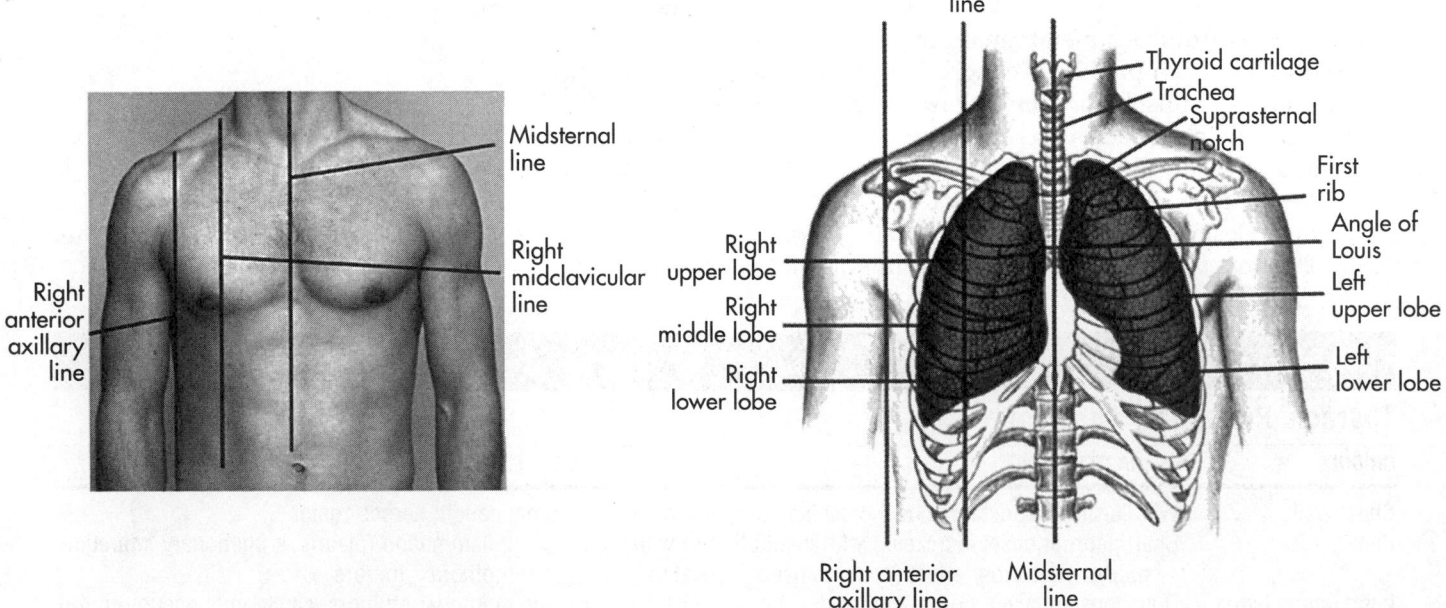

**Figure 22-3** Anterior thorax landmarks. (From Seidel HM et al: *Mosby's guide to physical examination*, ed 3, St Louis, 1995, Mosby.)

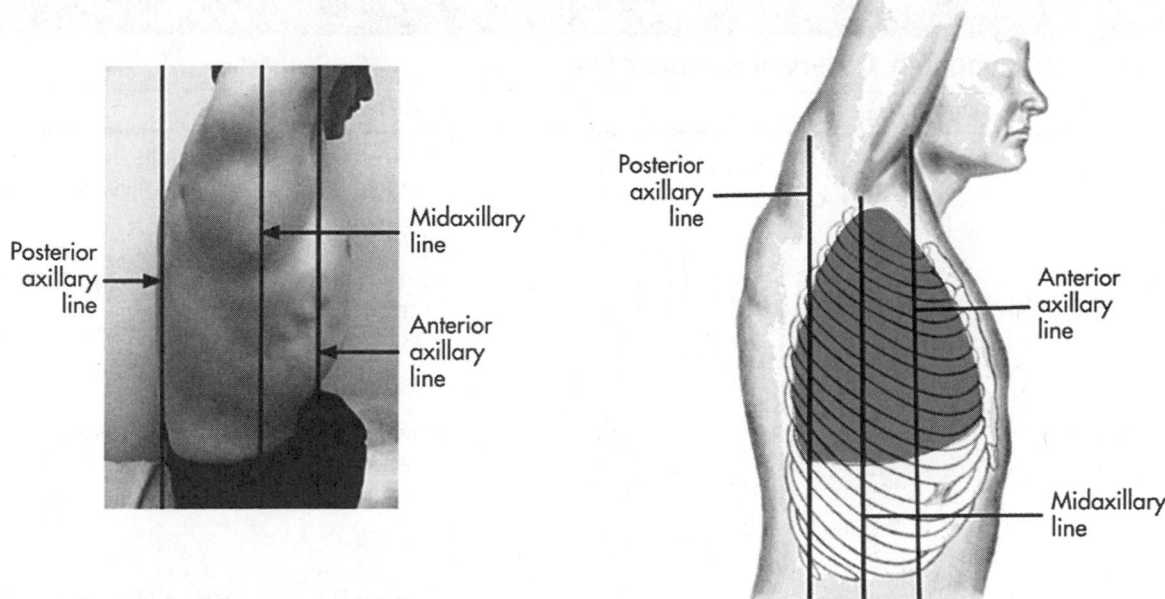

**Figure 22-4** Right lateral thorax landmarks. (From Seidel HM et al: *Mosby's guide to physical examination*, St Louis, 1987, Mosby.)

pnea, chest pain, coughing, sputum production, hemoptysis (blood-tinged sputum), or cyanosis. When a respiratory history is being taken, it is important to determine why the patient is seeking health care. Any complaint should be explored, and the symptom should be evaluated for onset, duration, location, quality, quantity, setting, precipitating factors, aggravating and alleviating factors, and associated signs and symptoms. Other important information includes smoking habits, exercise tolerance, allergens, environmental pollutants, recent respiratory tract infections, exposure to others with respiratory tract infections, medications, and occupational respiratory hazards.

## Physical Examination

After the history is taken, a systematic physical assessment of the patient is performed. Assessment of the lungs and thorax involves the techniques of inspection, palpation, percussion, and auscultation.

### Inspection

The first step in respiratory tract assessment is *inspection*. The entire chest is observed for lesions, scars, skin color, and deformities (Figures 22-3 and 22-4). Normally the ratio of the anterior-posterior diameter to the lateral diameter is 1:2. An increased anteroposterior diameter results in a barrel chest, which is a sign of COPD (Figure 22-5). Other chest deformities associated with respiratory disease that might be evident are

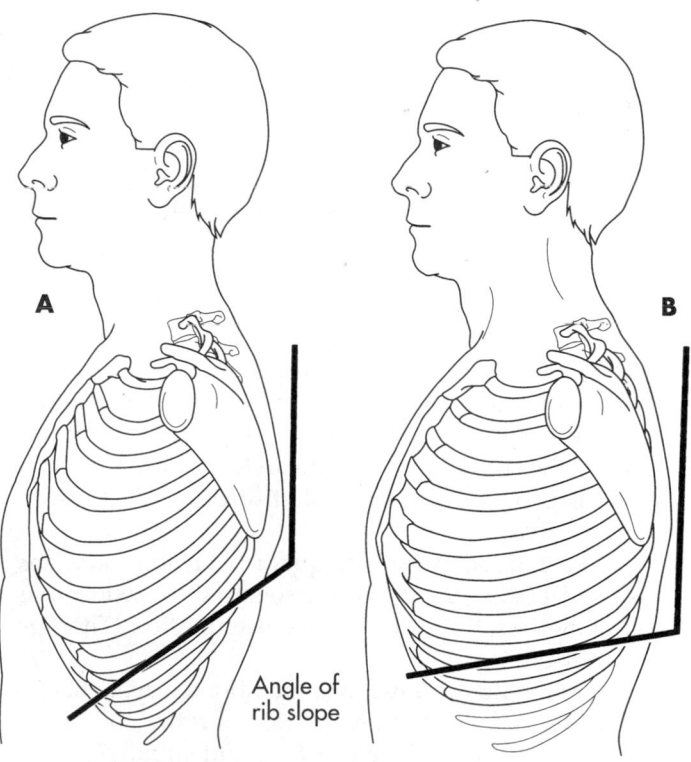

**Figure 22-5** **A,** Patient with normal thoracic configuration. **B,** Patient with increased anteroposterior diameter. Note contrast in the angle of the slope of the ribs. (From Barkauskas VH et al: *Health and physical assessment*, St Louis, 1994, Mosby.)

---

**TABLE 22-2**

## Characteristics of Commonly Observed Respiratory Patterns

| TYPE OF RESPIRATION | DIAGRAM | DISCUSSION |
|---|---|---|
| Normal | | 2-20 respirations/min in adults; regular in rhythm; ratio of respiratory rate to pulse rate is 1:4 |
| Hyperventilation or Kussmaul's respiration | | Increase in both rate and depth; hyperpnea is an increase in depth only |
| Periodic respiration | | Alternating hyperpnea, shallow respiration, and apnea; sometimes called Cheyne-Stokes respiration; often occurs in the severely ill |
| Sighing respiration | | Deep and audible; audible portion sounds like a sigh |
| Air trapping | | Present in obstructive pulmonary diseases; air is trapped in the lungs; respiratory level rises, and breathing becomes shallow |
| Biot's breathing | | Shallow breathing interrupted by apnea; seen in some central nervous system disorders and in healthy persons |

From Barkauskas VH et al: *Health and physical assessment*, St Louis, 1994, Mosby.

---

pigeon chest, funnel chest, and kyphoscoliosis. Kyphoscoliosis is a progressive musculoskeletal deformity characterized by lateral and posterior angulations of the spine, similar to the deformities that occur with osteoporosis or skeletal disorders (Thompson, Wilson, 1996).

The rate, depth, type, and quality of respirations are assessed (Table 22-2). The nurse should consider the following questions during the examination (Thompson, Wilson, 1996):

- Are the lips and mucous membranes cyanotic?
- Does the patient have intercostal retractions?
- Do both sides of the chest expand equally?
- Are the respirations deep or shallow?
- Is the breathing pattern regular or irregular?
- Is the breathing pattern abdominal, thoracic, or paradoxic?

## Palpation

The second step in the physical examination is *palpation*. The patient should be in a sitting position, although a supine position is acceptable if the patient is unable to sit up. The nurse places warmed hands side by side, with the thumbs close together and the fingers spread out over the anterior chest wall. As the patient takes several deep breaths, the nurse compares the respiratory movements of both sides of the chest. The nurse's thumbs should move apart at the same time and be equally distant. The patterns of expansion and contraction are noted, as well as equal or unequal expansion, depression of the chest wall during inspiration, degree of expansion, and diaphragmatic excursion. The nurse palpates the chest for any painful areas, swelling, masses, or crepitation. The trachea is palpated for position. It should be vertical and stretch downward on in-

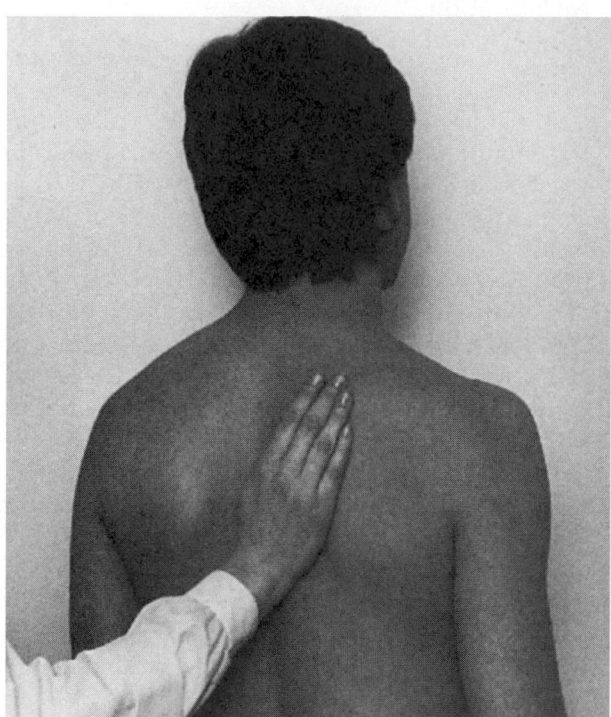 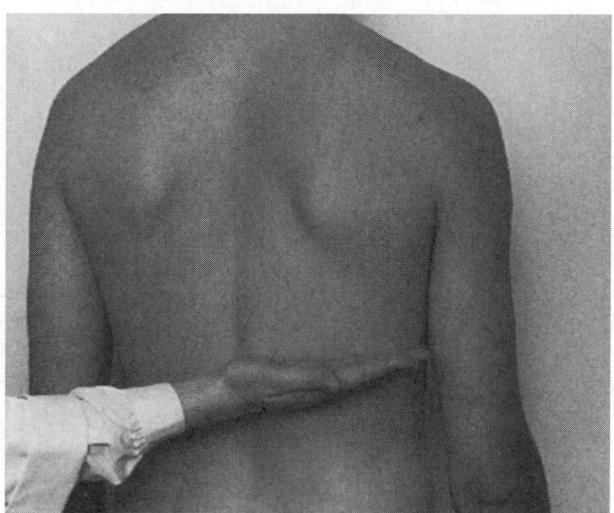

**Figure 22-6** Palpation for assessment of vocal fremitus. (From Malasanos L, Barkauskas V, Stoltenberg-Allen K: *Health assessment,* ed 4, St Louis, 1990, Mosby.)

## TABLE 22-3

### Characteristics of Normal and Abnormal Tactile Fremitus

| TYPE OF FREMITUS | CHARACTERISTICS |
| --- | --- |
| Normal (moderate) fremitus | Varies greatly from person to person and depends on the intensity and pitch of the voice, the position and distance of the bronchi in relation to the chest wall, and the thickness of the chest wall; fremitus is most intense in the second intercostal spaces at the sternal border near the area of bronchial bifurcation |
| Increased tactile fremitus | May occur in pneumonia, compressed lung, lung tumor, or pulmonary fibrosis; a solid medium of uniform structure conducts vibrations with greater intensity than a porous medium |
| Decreased or absent tactile fremitus | Occurs when there is diminished production of sounds, a diminished transmission of sounds, or the addition of a medium through which sounds must pass before reaching the thoracic wall, such as in pleural effusion, pleural thickening, pneumothorax, bronchial obstruction, or emphysema |
| Pleural friction rub | Vibration produced by inflamed pleural surfaces rubbing together; felt as a grating; synchronous with respiratory movements; more commonly felt on inspiration |
| Rhonchial fremitus | Coarse vibrations produced by the passage of air through thick exudates in the large air passages; can be cleared or altered by coughing |

Modified from Barkauskas V et al: *Health and physical assessment,* St Louis, 1994, Mosby.

spiration. The nurse repeats the procedure on the posterior chest wall (Thompson, Wilson, 1996).

**Assessment of fremitus.** Palpation for tactile **fremitus,** or vibrations, is a useful technique. It requires practice but can support other assessment findings. Vocal, or tactile, fremitus is the vibration of the thoracic wall that is produced by the normal spoken word. The nurse places the hand with the palm down on the chest wall, has the patient repeat the phrase "ninety-nine," and compares the transmission of the vibration on both sides of the chest (Figure 22-6). An increased fremitus occurs with secretions or consolidation in the lung, as in pneumonia or atelectasis. Bronchial obstruction or the presence of air or fluid in the pleural space causes a decrease in or absence of fremitus (Table 22-3).

## Percussion

The third step in the respiratory assessment is *percussion* (Figure 22-7). Tapping the surface of the chest wall with the fingers produces sounds that may indicate changes in lung density:

*Resonance* is the normal sound; it is hollow, low pitched, nonmusical, and loudest where the chest is thinnest.

*Dullness* is heard normally over the scapulae and heavy shoulder muscles and over solid organs such as the heart and liver. An area of consolidation, which can occur in pneumonia, produces a dull sound.

A *tympanic* sound may be heard over an area where air is trapped, such as in the hyperinflated lung of a patient with emphysema. The tympanic sound is louder, longer, higher pitched, and drumlike.

### OLDER ADULT CONSIDERATIONS

**RESPIRATORY ASSESSMENT**

**General Approach**
- Allow more time than for a younger adult.
- Articulate clearly; the elderly patient may be hearing impaired.
- Provide clear, concise instructions.

**History Collection**
- Use fewer open-ended questions and provide some choices as needed such as, "Is your chest pain dull, sharp, aching, or stabbing?"
- Repeat questions as needed.
- Be alert for answers that do not appear appropriate. The patient may not have understood the question correctly because of impaired hearing or impaired comprehension.

**Physical Assessment**
- The physical examination itself is not different, but the approach may need to be altered so that the appropriate information is assessed without undue discomfort or embarrassment for the patient.
- Provide an environment with minimal noise, distraction, and interruption.
- Require as few position changes as possible.
- Kyphosis is associated with aging.
- Chest expansion may be decreased.
- Breathing may be more shallow.
- Crackles in the bases in the absence of respiratory or cardiovascular disease may be due to atelectasis or fibrotic lung changes.

Modified from Beare PG, Myers JL: *Adult health nursing*, ed 3, St Louis, 1998, Mosby.

## Auscultation

The final step in the assessment procedure is *auscultation* (Figure 22-7). The patient is instructed to maintain a sitting position and take slow, deep breaths through the mouth. The surroundings should be calm and quiet, and the room temperature should be comfortable. The diaphragm of the stethoscope is placed firmly against the chest wall to decrease the sounds produced by skin or hair rubbing against it. A systematic approach is used, starting at the right scapular area and comparing the sounds heard there with the sounds heard in the left scapular area. The nurse continues down both sides of the posterior side of the chest to the base of the lungs. The procedure is repeated on the anterior side of the chest, and the two sides are compared. The nurse should listen through several respiratory cycles over each area.

Breath sounds reveal important data about a patient's condition. The sounds should be evaluated for location, pitch, quality, intensity, and duration of inspiration and expiration. The nurse should distinguish among three normal types of breath sounds. *Vesicular breath sounds* are heard over most of the normal lung as air passes into the alveoli. They are soft, low-pitched, breezy sounds with an inspiratory phase greater than the expiratory phase. *Bronchial breath sounds* are normally heard over the trachea. If heard elsewhere, they are abnormal and indicate areas of consolidation. Bronchial sounds are loud, high pitched, and hollow with an expiratory phase greater than the inspiratory phase. *Bronchovesicular breath sounds* are heard anteriorly over the mainstem bronchi on either side of the sternum in the first and second intercostal spaces. They are heard posteriorly between the scapulae. If heard elsewhere, they are abnormal. Bronchovesicular sounds are a mixture of vesicular and bronchial sounds and are softer and slightly lower pitched than bronchial sounds, and their inspiratory and expiratory phases are nearly equal (Tables 22-4 and 22-5). Breath sounds may be decreased or absent with shallow breathing, obesity, barrel chest, or fluid in the lung tissue.

Abnormal breath sounds, called **adventitious sounds,** may be superimposed on normal breath sounds and include **crackles, wheezes,** and **pleural friction rubs.** The term "crackles" has replaced "rales," and "wheezes" has replaced "rhonchi"; however, all four terms are used clinically. When describing adventitious breath sounds, the nurse should include the type, location, and timing of the sound (Beare, Myers, 1998).

Crackles (rales) are discontinuous (short, intermittent) fine crackling or bubbling sounds caused by the passage of air through moisture or secretions in the alveoli and small airways and are described as fine, medium, or coarse (Thompson, Wilson, 1996). Crackles

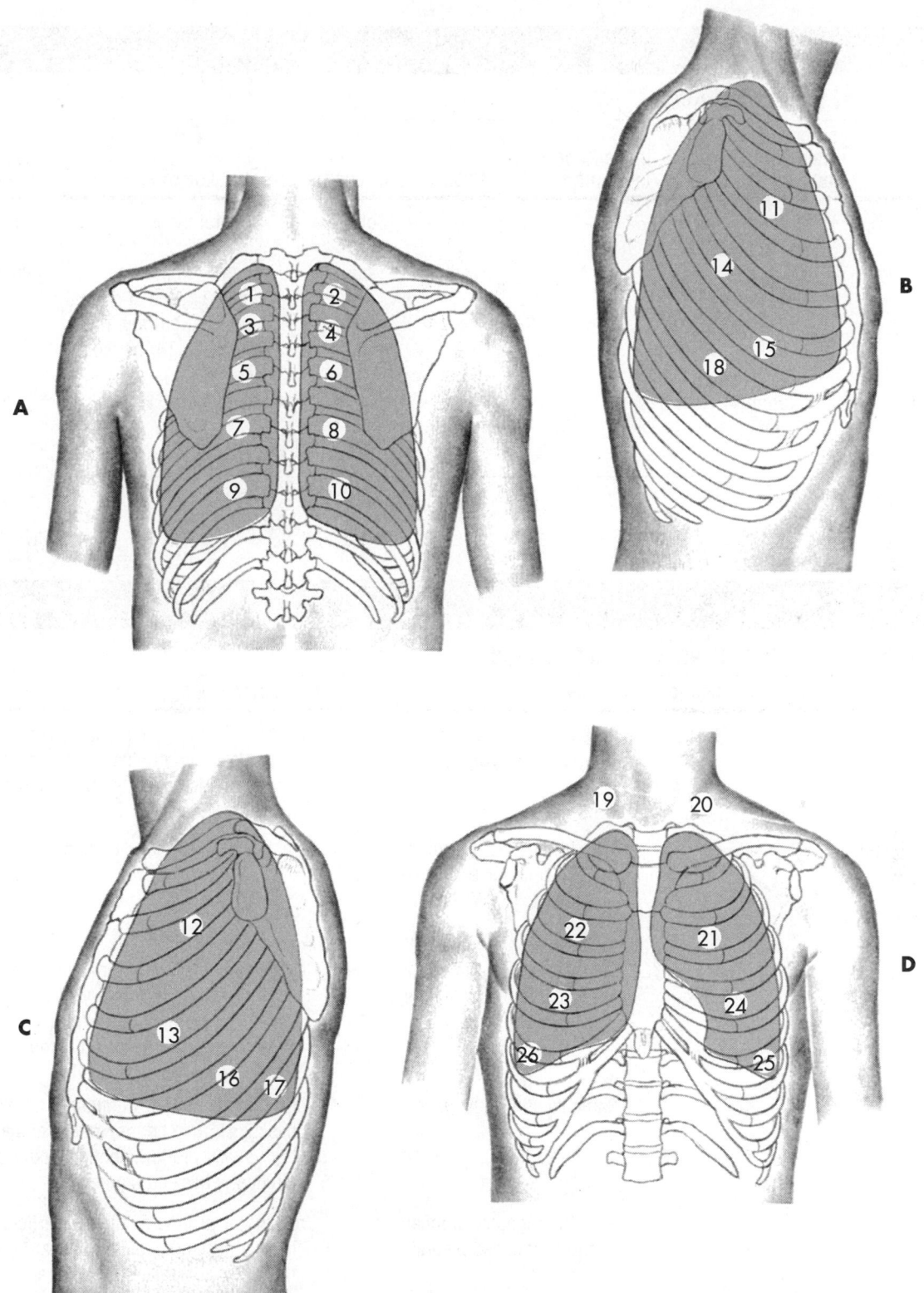

**Figure 22-7** Suggested sequence for systematic percussion and auscultation of the thorax. **A,** Posterior thorax. **B,** Right lateral thorax. **C,** Left lateral thorax. **D,** Anterior thorax. (From Seidel HM et al: *Mosby's guide to physical examination,* ed 3, St Louis, 1995, Mosby.)

---

**TABLE 22-4**

## Characteristics of Breath Sounds

| SOUND | DURATION OF INSPIRATION AND EXPIRATION | DIAGRAM OF OF SOUND | PITCH | INTENSITY | NORMAL LOCATION | ABNORMAL LOCATION |
|---|---|---|---|---|---|---|
| Vesicular | Inspiration > expiration 2.5:1 | | Low | Soft | Peripheral lung | Not applicable |
| Bronchovesicular | Inspiration = expiration 1:1 | | Medium | Medium | First and second intercostal spaces at sternal border anteriorly; posteriorly at T4 medial to scapulae | Peripheral lung |
| Bronchial (tubular) | Inspiration < expiration 1:2 | | High | Loud | Over trachea | Lung area |

From Barkauskas VH et al: *Health and physical assessment,* St Louis, 1994, Mosby.

---

**TABLE 22-5**

## Origin and Characteristics of Adventitous Sounds

| SOUND | DIAGRAM OF SOUND | ORIGIN | CHARACTERISTICS |
|---|---|---|---|
| Crackles*—fine to medium | | Air passing through moisture in small air passages and alveoli | Discrete, discontinuous; inspiratory; have a dry or wet crackling quality; not cleared by coughing; sound is simulated by rolling a lock of hair near the ear |
| Crackles*—medium to coarse | | Air passing through moisture in the bronchioles, bronchi, and trachea | As above; louder than fine crackles |
| Wheezes—sonorous | | Air passing through air passages narrowed by secretions, swelling, tumors, and so on | Continuous sounds; originate in large air passages; may be inspiratory and expiratory but usually predominate in expiration; low-pitched moaning or snoring quality; coughing may alter sounds |
| Wheezes—sibilant | | Same as sonorous wheezes | Continuous sounds; originate in the small air passages; may be inspiratory and expiratory but usually predominantly in expiration; high-pitched, wheezing sounds |
| Friction rubs | | Rubbing together of inflamed and roughened pleural surfaces | Creaking or grating quality; superficial sounding; inspiratory and expiratory; heard most often in the lower anterolateral chest (area of greatest thoracic expansion); coughing has no effect |

From Barkauskas VH et al: *Health and physical assessment,* St Louis, 1994, Mosby.
*Crackles are also called rales or crepitations.

resemble the sound of a cellophane wrapper being gently crinkled and can also be simulated by rubbing locks of hair together between the fingers. They are usually heard on inspiration. Wheezes are caused by air passing through larger airways that have been narrowed by the accumulation of fluids and secretions, by mucosal edema, or by smooth muscle spasms. These continuous sounds are sometimes described as musical and can include an array of pitches from high to low. Wheezes may be expiratory, inspiratory, or both. Pleural friction rubs are caused by rubbing together of the inflamed pleural linings. They produce a grating, squeaking sound, such as that produced when two pieces of leather are rubbed together. The absence of normal breath sounds in their proper locations should also be considered abnormal.

# DIAGNOSTIC TESTS

## Blood Examinations

Routine blood examinations are usually ordered for patients with respiratory disease and may include a red blood cell count, white blood cell count, and hemoglobin determination. Abnormal increases in the number of white blood cells may indicate mobilization of the body's defenses against a respiratory tract infection, whereas significant decreases in red blood cells and hemoglobin level decrease the oxygen-carrying capacity of the blood. Depending on the specific diagnosis of respiratory disease, additional blood studies may be required.

## Arterial Blood Gas Studies

Blood gas analysis provides information necessary in the diagnosis and treatment of patients with acute and chronic lung diseases. The values obtained assess the ability of the lungs to supply adequate oxygen and remove carbon dioxide and the ability of the kidneys to excrete or reabsorb bicarbonate ions for maintenance of normal body pH (Beare, Myers, 1998).

The partial pressure of oxygen in the blood ($PaO_2$) indicates the degree of oxygenation of the blood. The oxygen saturation ($SaO_2$) reflects the percentage of hemoglobin bound with oxygen. The partial pressure of carbon dioxide ($PaCO_2$) indicates the adequacy of alveolar ventilation. The pH and plasma bicarbonate concentration ($HCO_3$) reflect acid-base balance. Normal values for arterial blood gas studies are shown in Table 22-6.

## Sputum Examination

The examination of sputum is performed by persons trained in laboratory methods, but the collection of the specimen is usually a nursing responsibility. Sputum consists of material that is expectorated from the lungs, and it may contain pathogenic and nonpathogenic organisms. Sputum to be used for diagnosis must be collected correctly. Specimens should be collected early in the morning, when sputum production usually is greatest. Before collection, patients should rinse the mouth with clear water, after which they should be encouraged to cough deeply and expectorate into a sterile container. If the specimen obtained is inadequate, sputum may be obtained by inducing coughing with aerosolized mist inhalations or nasotracheal suctioning. If the patient is intubated, tracheal aspiration is accomplished by attaching a mucous trap to the suction source during routine suctioning of sputum. The specimen should be properly labeled and sent immediately to the laboratory.

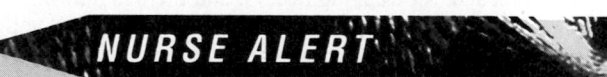

**NURSE ALERT**

The first sputum coughed up in the morning usually contains the most organisms.

---

### TABLE 22-6

### Normal Blood Gas Values of Arterial Blood*

| | |
|---|---|
| $PaCO_2$: Partial pressure of carbon dioxide in arterial blood; gives information about the adequacy of ventilation | 34-45 mm Hg |
| $PaO_2$: Partial pressure of oxygen; the amount of oxygen dissolved in arterial blood | 80-100 mm Hg |
| $SaO_2$: Percent saturation of hemoglobin with oxygen in arterial blood | 97%-100% |
| pH: Hydrogen ion concentration in the blood; acidity/alkalinity of blood sample | 7.35-7.45 |
| $HCO_3$: Plasma bicarbonate concentration; a measurement of the nonrespiratory contribution to acid-base balance | 24-30 mEq/L |

*Arterial blood should be obtained either through a puncture of an artery, such as the femoral or radial, with a small needle or from a catheter previously placed into the artery. All air is expelled after the sample is obtained, and the sample is placed on ice and sent immediately to the laboratory for analysis. If an artery was entered to obtain the sample, direct pressure is applied for at least 5 minutes. If the radial artery is to be used to obtain the arterial sample, Allen's test should be performed to evaluate the patency of the radial and ulnar arteries. In Allen's test the patient is asked to make a fist. The radial and ulnar arteries are then simultaneously compressed, which causes the hand to blanch. The patient is asked to open the fist, and the pressure on the ulnar artery is released while pressure on the radial artery is maintained. The hand turns pink if the ulnar artery is patent (Malasanos, Barkauskas, Stoltenberg-Allen, 1989; Seidel et al, 1995).

Normally sputum is odorless and colorless or white, but in suppurative conditions of the lungs, such as a lung abscess, it may be yellow or green and have a foul odor. Sputum examination using the Papanicolaou (Pap) smear technique may be useful in detecting the presence of cancer cells. The amount, odor, and appearance of sputum should be entered on the patient's record.

## Pulmonary Function Tests

Pulmonary function tests (PFTs) evaluate lung function and may indicate the existence of some impairment or the necessity for additional investigation. They also are used to monitor the patient's respiratory status when disease is present and to evaluate the effectiveness of the therapy instituted. PFTs are useful in evaluating individuals scheduled for upper abdominal or thoracic procedures who have preexisting pulmonary risk factors, including smoking, obesity, dyspnea, cough, or COPD (Beare, Myers, 1998).

The most common pulmonary function tests are performed by spirometry, which measures lung volumes and capacities and flow rates. Lung volumes and capacities are measured to determine the amount of air that can be inhaled and exhaled. Flow-rate measurements are used to evaluate the ability of the individual to move air into and out of the lungs. Flow-rate determinations are helpful in identifying whether altered respiratory muscle strength, lung and chest wall compliance, or airway and lung tissue resistance has affected lung function (Beare, Myers, 1994). Essentially, test values are flow rates during forced breathing maneuvers, usually forced exhalation.

During spirometry the patient sits upright with a noseclip in place. All tight clothing is loosened, and the patient breathes into a mouthpiece connected to a spirometer. A graphic recording (spirogram) is produced. Test results are interpreted on the basis of age, height, weight, and sex. The results are compared with normal values that have been established (Box 22-2).

---

**BOX 22-2**

### VOLUME, CAPACITIES, AND FLOW RATES

Pulmonary function tests that are abnormal and indicate disease are generally classified into three patterns: obstructive, restrictive, or mixed.

*Obstructive disorders* are those that narrow airway passages, which creates an increased resistance to air flow, especially on exhalation. Examples are emphysema, chronic bronchitis, bronchiectasis, and cystic fibrosis. Lung volumes are usually normal or increased. Air trapping occurs, and there is difficulty expelling air via the narrowed airways. Residual volume (RV) is often increased as is functional residual capacity (FRC). Total lung capacity (TLC) may also increase, and vital capacity (VC) may decrease in severe obstruction. Forced expiratory values are usually reduced as a result of air trapping.

In *restrictive disorders* lung expansion is compromised. Therefore volumes and capacities tend to be decreased, but RV and TLC will be normal. Examples of restrictive conditions are pulmonary edema, pneumonia, and kyphoscoliosis. Flow rates may be reduced, normal, or increased.

In patients with more than one disorder, both obstructive and restrictive patterns may be seen. The VC is reduced in *mixed disorders*, and flow rates are reduced out of proportion to the reduced VC (Kersten, 1989; Smeltzer, Bare, 1992).

**LUNG CAPACITIES AND VOLUMES**

Total lung capacity—Total volume of air that lungs can contain when fully inflated

Vital capacity—Maximum amount of air that can be exhaled after maximum inspiration

Inspiratory capacity (IC)—Maximum volume of air inspired after a normal exhalation

Functional residual capacity (FRC)—Volume of air remaining in lungs after a normal expiration

Tidal volume ($V_T$)—Maximum volume of air that can be moved in and out of the lung during quiet breathing (usually 10% of vital capacity)

Inspiratory reserve volume (IRV)—Maximum volume of air that can be inhaled beyond normal inspiration

Expiratory reserve volume (ERV)—Maximum volume of air that can be exhaled beyond normal exhalation

Residual volume (RV)—Amount of air remaining in lungs after maximum expiration

**FLOW RATES**

FVC—Forced vital capacity

$FEV_1$—Forced expiratory volume in 1 second

$FEV_1$/FVC—Ratio of forced expiratory volume in 1 second to the forced vital capacity

FEF 25%-75%—Forced expiratory flow over the midportion of the forced vital capacity

MVV—Maximal voluntary ventilation

Modified from Beare PG, Myers JL: *Adult health nursing*, ed 3, St Louis, 1998, Mosby.

Although nurses usually do not perform the PFT, they should relieve any apprehension that patients may have by explaining the purpose of the procedure. Patient cooperation is important for accurate results. When PFTs are performed preoperatively, the information obtained may allow the nurse to plan preoperative teaching and postoperative interventions, which may include coughing and deep breathing, use of the incentive spirometer, medication education, and information on smoking cessation.

## Radiographic Examination

The chest x-ray examination is one of the most common of all radiographic procedures. It is useful in detecting disease of the chest or in monitoring change over time. Many hospitals require chest x-ray films of all admitted patients.

Because normal pulmonary tissue is radiolucent (allows the x-ray beam to pass through it), densities produced by tumors, foreign bodies, or other conditions may be detected on an x-ray film. A routine chest film consists of posteroanterior (PA) and lateral views. Individuals are usually instructed to take a deep breath and hold it. Once the picture is obtained, they are instructed to exhale.

### Patient Preparation

When chest x-ray examination is prescribed, the nurse should see that the patient wears a hospital gown that is tied in the back. All metal objects above the waist are removed because the presence of metal produces a shadow over the film. Patients are transported to the x-ray department by stretcher or wheelchair and should be accompanied by an attendant. If the patient is too ill to be taken to the x-ray department, a portable x-ray machine may be taken to the patient's bedside. However, the preparation of the patient is the same.

Lung tomography provides clearly focused radiographic images of sections of the lungs at different planes within the thorax. It is useful in further evaluating chest lesions. The nurse should inform the patient that the test takes approximately 30 to 60 minutes and that he or she must remain as still as possible within the x-ray machine. All jewelry and any metal objects should be removed. No restriction of food or fluids is necessary (Lewis, Collier, Heitkemper, 1996).

Computed tomography (CT) is a method in which the lungs are scanned in successive cross sections by a narrow x-ray beam. The test may be performed with or without the injection of a radiopaque contrast medium. The results are subsequently analyzed by computer to identify small nodules, tumors, or other abnormalities that may not be visible on conventional x-ray films. The nurse should inform the patient that the test allows the visualization of structures within the chest, usually takes 45 to 60 minutes to perform, and requires lying very still inside the x-ray machine. The nurse should ensure that jewelry and any metal objects are removed. If scanning will be performed using contrast medium, the patient's sensitivity to iodine-based preparations should be determined. The nurse should inform the patient that because contrast is being used, he or she will be allowed nothing by mouth for at least 4 hours before the test. The patient should be prepared for the sensation of warmth or flushing that may occur with dye injection. If no contrast is being used, food and fluid restrictions are unnecessary.

Pulmonary angiography is a test in which radiopaque dye is injected into the pulmonary circulation, after which a series of x-ray films is taken. This test evaluates the circulation in the pulmonary vasculature and is used to identify thromboembolic disease of the lungs and congenital abnormalities of the pulmonary tree. Ventilation-perfusion lung scans are radiologic tests that are performed to detect pulmonary emboli. Lung scans are used to determine areas of the lung that are being ventilated but not perfused as a result of the presence of an obstruction or clot (pulmonary emboli) in the pulmonary circulation.

## Endoscopy Procedures
### Bronchoscopy

In the past, visualization of the trachea and bronchi was limited by the large, rigid, metal bronchoscope. With the advent of smaller, flexible, fiberoptic bronchoscopes, a more accurate picture of the airway can now be transmitted. The fiberoptic bronchoscope also allows easier passage through the nasal or oral route. After a topical anesthetic has been administered, the bronchoscope is passed through the mouth and into the trachea and major bronchi. The room is darkened, and visualization of the bronchial tree is possible when light is reflected through the instrument. Bronchoscopy is used to remove foreign bodies that have lodged in the bronchi, to suction secretions for laboratory examination, to observe the respiratory passageways for disease, and to obtain biopsy specimens.

**Patient preparation.** The emotional preparation for bronchoscopy is important. The procedure causes a certain amount of discomfort, and an apprehensive, fearful patient may cooperate poorly. Explaining to patients what to expect and teaching them how to breathe and relax during the procedure provides a greater feeling of security and helps relieve their anxiety.

Before a bronchoscopy, no food or fluid by mouth is allowed after midnight. Postural drainage may be ordered in the morning to remove any secretions that may have drained into the trachea or bronchi during the night. Special mouth care should be given after postural drainage, and dentures, bridges, contact lenses, and glasses should be removed. A sedative may be ordered to relieve anxiety. An anticholinergic agent, such as atropine, is also ordered to alleviate symptoms of bradycardia, arrhythmia, and hypotension; to suppress the cough reflex; and to inhibit secretions. If the procedure is performed in the operating room, the usual preoperative nursing measures are required.

**Postprocedure care.** After returning to the hospital room, the patient should be positioned on one side of the body and usually in a semi-Fowler's position for easier removal of secretions. No food or fluids should be given until the gag reflex returns, and vital signs are monitored according to protocol.

Patients should be watched carefully for respiratory difficulties, including bronchospasms and laryngospasms. If a biopsy has been performed, sputum may be tinged with blood for several days. However, the nurse should be alert for any unusual bleeding, and the primary provider should be notified immediately if it occurs. If throat soreness and discomfort are prolonged, a mild analgesic such as aspirin may be ordered. Persistent throat soreness and a hoarse voice should be evaluated because the trachea or larynx can be injured during the procedure.

## Thoracentesis

A thoracentesis is performed to obtain pleural fluid for diagnostic purposes, to obtain a biopsy specimen from the pleura, to remove pleural fluid for therapeutic purposes, or to instill medication (Phipps et al, 1995). The procedure is usually performed in the patient's room. The patient is in a sitting position with head and arms resting on a pillow that has been placed on the overbed table (Figure 22-8). With use of aseptic technique the skin is cleansed, generally in the area of the eighth or ninth rib interspace, and a local anesthetic is injected into the tissues. The patient must be cautioned not to move while the needle is being inserted to prevent damage to the lung or pleura. The pulse and respiration should be checked several times, and the patient should be observed for diaphoresis or any change in skin color (Box 22-3). Chest x-ray examination may be performed after thoracentesis to rule out pneumothorax.

## Pulse Oximetry

Pulse oximetry provides continuous, noninvasive monitoring of arterial oxygen saturation ($SaO_2$), the amount of hemoglobin-carrying oxygen in relation to its total carrying capacity. Pulse oximetry can be used to regulate oxygen therapy in a variety of patients and is useful in evaluating sleep disorders (Patrick et al, 1991; Spyr, Preach, 1990). Oximetry technology allows the nurse to assess minute-to-minute changes in saturation, intervene before hypoxemia produces serious symptoms, and evaluate a patient's response to therapy.

The oximeter consists of two light-emitting diodes (LEDs) and may be applied to any site that has a pulsating vascular bed, such as the finger, toe, or earlobe

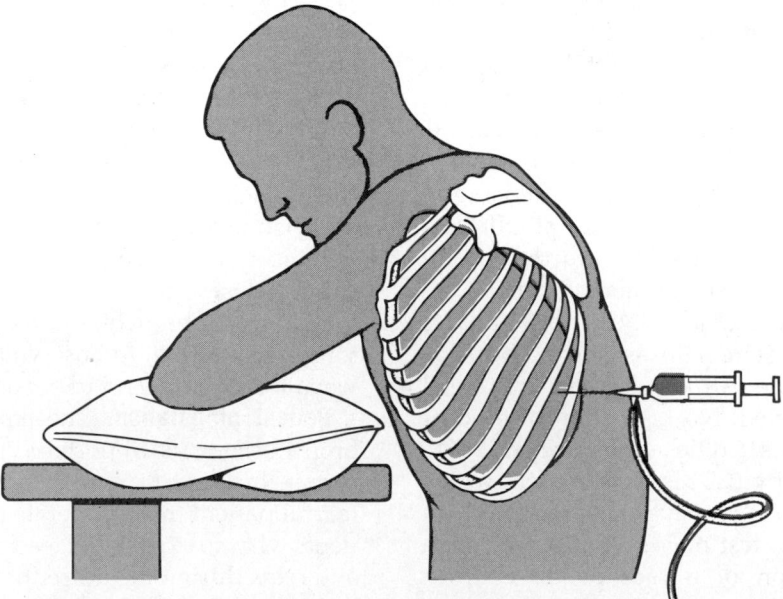

**Figure 22-8** A thoracentesis is performed to obtain a sample of pleural fluid or pleura, to remove accumulated pleural fluid, or to instill medication. (From Beare PG, Myers JL: *Principles and practice of adult health nursing*, ed 2, St Louis, 1994, Mosby.)

(Figure 22-9). The device transmits wavelengths of light through the site and measures infrared and red light absorption through the skin. The signals are returned to the device and displayed on a monitor. A computer within the oximeter calculates oxyhemoglobin saturation on the basis of the fact that red light is more easily transmitted through oxygenated than deoxygenated blood. The value obtained corresponds to the arterial hemoglobin saturation (Carroll, 1997).

The device depends on pulsations from the vascular bed to confirm the presence of a level of blood flow known to be associated with accurate saturation readings. Therefore any condition that alters perfusion (e.g., hypovolemia, hypotension, hypothermia, vaso-

constrictive drugs) may cause no reading to be obtained. Nail polish must be removed to obtain an accurate reading.

Despite its limitations, oximetry is useful. Low values often indicate that a patient needs additional interventions.

## NURSING STRATEGIES FOR COMMON RESPIRATORY PROBLEMS

A variety of treatment modalities are used when caring for a patient who has an alteration in respiratory function. The modalities selected are based on the disorder.

### Coughing

Coughing is used to remove secretions and to provide adequate ventilation in the lungs by maintaining a clear airway. For some patients deep productive coughing may be sufficient. For others the nurse may be responsible for clearing the airway (see "Suctioning"). When possible, before coughing the patient should be placed in a sitting position with the feet supported on the floor. If coughing is painful, the nurse should help the patient by splinting the chest. Some patients need analgesics before coughing to reduce discomfort. Sputum should be collected in tissues and placed in paper bags at the bedside or kept in a sterile container to assess 24-hour sputum production. The patient should be taught to

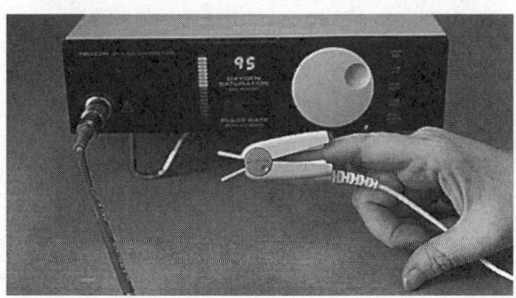

**Figure 22-9**   Oximeter probe that attaches to a finger or an ear. (From Perry AG, Potter PA: *Clinical nursing skills and techniques,* ed 4, St Louis, 1998, Mosby.)

---

**BOX 22-3**

### Guidelines for Care of the Patient Undergoing Thoracentesis

**1** Explain the procedure to the patient. Emphasize the importance of not moving, of breathing quietly, and of not coughing during the procedure to avoid injury to the pleura. Although a local anesthetic is used, the patient may feel some discomfort as the needle enters the pleura.

**2** Obtain baseline vital signs, including blood pressure, heart rate, and respiratory rate. Compare subsequent readings to baseline.

**3** Help the patient obtain the optimal position for performance of the test. If possible, the patient sits on the edge of the bed with the feet supported. Using an elevated overbed table, the patient can maintain a position with the head resting on folded arms (Figure 22-8). Patients who are unable to sit up may be turned onto the unaffected side with the head of the bed elevated approximately 30 degrees.

**4** Provide support and reassurance to the patient as needed.

**5** Monitor vital signs; general appearance; and respiratory rate, depth, and effort throughout the procedure. No more than 1500 ml of pleural fluid should be removed within a 30-minute period because of the risk of intravascular fluid shift with resultant pulmonary edema.

**6** Apply a sterile occlusive dressing over the insertion site after the needle is removed.

**7** After the procedure is completed, position the patient on the unaffected side with the insertion site up. A chest x-ray film is obtained to assess for pneumothorax.

**8** Monitor respiratory status, vital signs, and puncture site after the procedure. Observe for the following complications:
  - Intravascular shift: shortness of breath, hypotension, increased pulse rate
  - Lung trauma: bloody sputum, tracheal deviation, and uncontrollable coughing

take a deep breath, hold it for 1 second, and cough on expiration. Persistent shallow coughing has no value and only tires the patient. Tissues should be folded and placed in the patient's cupped hand. Nurses who handle sputum should wear gloves and wash their hands thoroughly after each encounter.

## Incentive Spirometry and Deep Breathing

The incentive spirometer (IS) is the device most commonly used to promote an individual's ability to take a deep breath (Figure 22-10). The IS is available in several models and consists of one or more small plastic balls on closed chambers that are connected to tubing and a mouthpiece. The patient is instructed to inhale slowly through the tubing, which creates a vacuum and raises the ball(s). An indicator lets the patient know if he or she is breathing deeply enough (Carroll, 1996). Holding the breath at the end of inspiration for 3 to 5 seconds is important to promote air distribution throughout the lung and allow inflation of even the smallest, most distant alveoli. Use of the IS may be taught to patients preoperatively and continued postoperatively. It is especially useful to patients who are undergoing upper abdominal and thoracic surgery.

## Suctioning
### Indications

If a patient is unable to clear secretions with coughing, the secretions may be removed by suctioning. Suctioning is also used to obtain a sputum specimen when the patient is unable to produce a sample by coughing. When a patient is in respiratory distress because of an obstructed airway, the nurse may observe the follow-

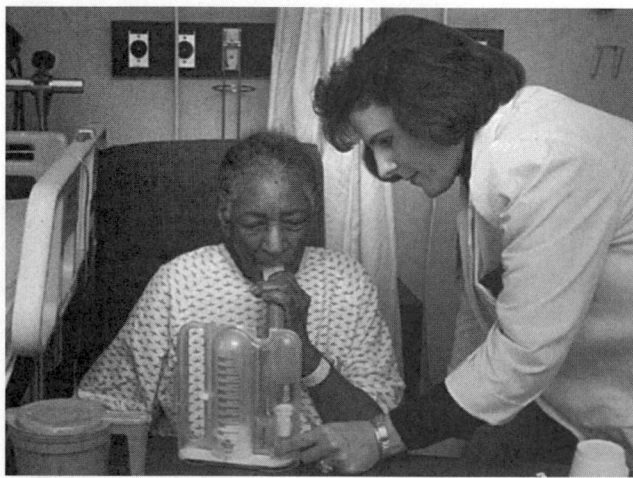

**Figure 22-10**   An incentive spirometer device used by patients to stimulate deep breathing. This procedure facilitates increased expansion of the lungs, which ◆ reduces pulmonary complications.

ing signs: gurgling, increased pulse and respiratory rates, a harsh respiratory sound, restlessness, anxiety, pallor with cyanosis around the mouth, or generalized cyanosis. If the distress is caused by mucus that is obstructing the airway, the patient should be suctioned immediately, carefully, and thoroughly to relieve the symptoms and restore a patent airway. The catheter is inserted through the nose and into the trachea. If a tracheostomy is present, the suction catheter is passed through it.

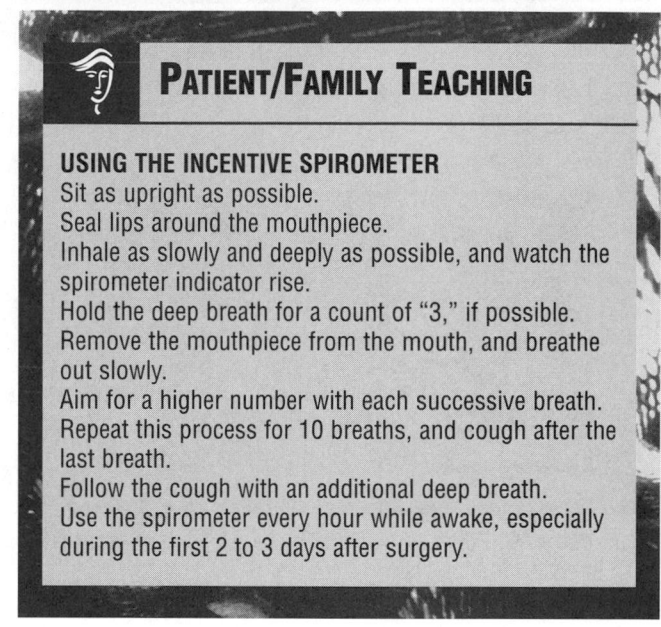

### PATIENT/FAMILY TEACHING

**USING THE INCENTIVE SPIROMETER**
Sit as upright as possible.
Seal lips around the mouthpiece.
Inhale as slowly and deeply as possible, and watch the spirometer indicator rise.
Hold the deep breath for a count of "3," if possible.
Remove the mouthpiece from the mouth, and breathe out slowly.
Aim for a higher number with each successive breath.
Repeat this process for 10 breaths, and cough after the last breath.
Follow the cough with an additional deep breath.
Use the spirometer every hour while awake, especially during the first 2 to 3 days after surgery.

## Equipment

The procedure used to suction a patient's airway involves attaching a whistle-tip catheter to tubing and a continuous suction device. The whistle-tip catheter provides the nurse with fingertip control of the suctioning. During suctioning, sterile gloves are worn and sterile catheters are used to prevent contamination of the respiratory tract. When aspirating secretions, the nurse should maintain strict aseptic technique to prevent serious complications. Separate catheters must be used for nasal and tracheobronchial secretions. The nurse should use caution to avoid injuring the mucous membranes. The procedure should be fully explained to the patient before the procedure is started.

## Procedure

The patient should be hyperventilated and hyperoxygenated before and after suctioning because both air and secretions are removed during suctioning. Several methods may be used to hyperoxygenate patients:

(1) if patients are able, the nurse should instruct them to deep breathe for 1 minute; (2) the nurse should have patients use a face mask and rebreathing bags with oxygen attached; (3) if patients are receiving mechanical ventilation, the oxygen should be increased to 100% for 1 minute and the sigh-cycle button manually depressed two or three times; or (4) patients should be manually ventilated with an Ambu bag that has been adapted to deliver 100% oxygen. Suction should not be applied until after the catheter has been inserted and is being withdrawn. The whistle-tip catheter is rotated while it is being withdrawn, and suction should be made intermittent by removing and replacing the finger to the tube valve during withdrawal of the catheter. If possible, patients should be placed in Fowler's position before the procedure begins. Each suction should not exceed 10 seconds, and an interval of 3 minutes should elapse before the procedure is repeated. During this interval, oxygen is administered and the patient is reconnected to the mechanical ventilator. When suctioning through an airway or an endotracheal or tracheostomy tube, the nurse should insert the tube until resistance is felt (at the carina).

During suctioning, the tip may come into contact with the carina, which stimulates the patient's cough reflex. Although this helps the patient expectorate secretions, the coughing could be violent enough to expel the tracheostomy or endotracheal tube, which is uncomfortable for the patient. Therefore the nurse should ensure that the tube is secured before suctioning. The patient should be informed that suctioning may cause coughing, and the suction catheter tip should be withdrawn from the carina to prevent further cough stimu-

lation. The closed tracheal suctioning catheter system (CTSS) is a new technique for suctioning airway secretions in a patient who is receiving mechanical ventilation. The CTSS is composed of a suction catheter that is enclosed within a plastic sleeve, which can be directed into the endotracheal or tracheostomy tube. The CTSS attaches directly to the ventilator tubing circuit, and ventilator function is not disrupted when it is used. The catheter setup is usually changed once a day.

Saline solution should not be instilled into the endotracheal tube to dilute thick secretions during suctioning. Although this has been a traditional practice, it can lead to a decrease in arterial saturation (the level of oxygen in the arterial blood) and increases the likelihood of pulmonary infection by carrying bacteria into the lower airway (Carroll, 1996).

## Postural Drainage

Postural drainage is used to drain excessive secretions from the lungs (including pus from lung abscesses). Drainage is facilitated by placing the patient in a position that allows gravity to aid in the procedure. The position of the patient should be determined by the area of the lung to be drained. The upper lobes of the lung are best drained in the sitting position, and the lower lobes are best drained in a lying position (Figure 22-11). However, positions vary according to the patient's condition, strength, and respiratory function. Gravity drainage of the lungs can be accomplished in several ways. In most cases younger patients tolerate lowering the head better than older or debilitated patients. If possible, the mouth should be approximately

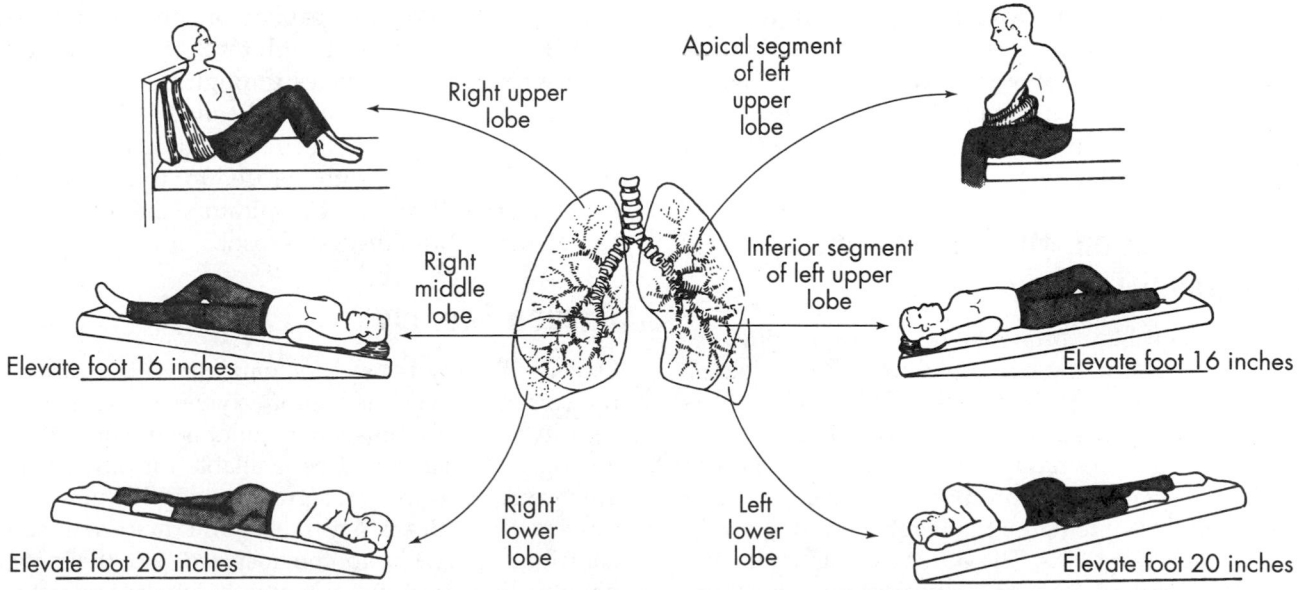

**Figure 22-11**   Postural drainage positions for draining various portions of the lung.

20 inches lower than the base of the lungs. Special beds and tables are available, but the patient's own bed may also be used. During the procedure patients should be encouraged to cough deeply, and after returning to bed they may be expected to cough and expectorate large amounts of sputum.

Older adults with hypertrophic arthritis may be unable to bend their bodies over the bed for postural drainage, but fairly satisfactory results may be obtained by elevating the foot of the bed. Postural drainage often is fatiguing for debilitated patients, and they may be able to remain in the position for only a few minutes. However, with each effort they experience less discomfort. The procedure should be supervised by the nurse and carried out midway between meals to prevent nausea and vomiting. The patient's teeth should be brushed after the procedure, and an antiseptic mouthwash may be used if desired. The patient should be protected from chilling during the procedure and should be allowed to rest after returning to bed. If the drainage is to be measured, it should be collected in a receptacle that is suitable for measuring. The color, amount, and consistency of the drainage should be recorded on the patient's chart.

## Percussion and Vibration

Percussion may be provided during postural drainage. Percussion is performed with the hands cupped so that an air pocket is created within the palm (Figure 22-12). Alternating hands, the caregiver rhythmically claps the chest wall over the involved area to loosen mucous plugs and move them into the bronchi, where they may be drained out or expectorated (Beare, Myers, 1998). Vibration is performed by placing the hands against the chest wall and gently "quivering" them as the patient exhales. Clapping and vibrating are not used when there is a danger of hemorrhage or if the patient complains of pain. The procedure should be performed by a nurse or therapist who has been trained in the technique.

## Throat Irrigation, Humidification, and Aerosol Therapy

Nasopharyngeal and bronchial infections are often relieved with warm throat irrigations. A physiologic saline solution at a temperature of 49° C (120° F) is most commonly used, and irrigations may be performed several times a day. The application of heat to the irritated membranes promotes drainage of secretions; stimulates circulation; and relieves pain, swelling, and muscle spasms. The nurse may assist the patient with the procedure, or the patient may be taught to perform it under professional supervision.

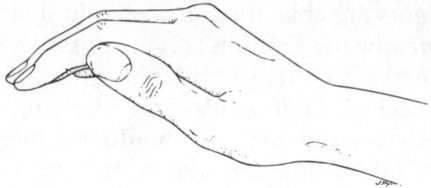

**Figure 22-12** The nurse uses a cupped hand position for chest percussion. (From Beare PG, Myers JL: *Principles and practice of adult health nursing*, ed 2, St Louis, 1994, Mosby.)

Normally air is heated and humidified in the upper airway as it is inhaled. Humidifiers or nebulizers are used when the upper airway is bypassed or when added water vapor is desired to improve patient comfort, mobilize secretions, or deliver inhaled medications (Figure 22-13). Humidifiers add water vapor to inhaled air and are used primarily to moisten dry mucous membranes when a patient receives oxygen therapy. Cool humidifiers provide additional water vapor in the inspired air and are usually adequate if the patient is breathing through the upper airway. However, if the upper airway is bypassed with a tracheostomy, the water vapor must be heated to provide sufficient humidification and to prevent drying of mucous membranes and retention of thick secretions.

Nebulizers produce a fine mist for inhalation therapy. The administration of bronchodilators and mucolytic agents by nebulization is a common part of the therapeutic regimen. A hand-held nebulizer can be used, or the medication can be administered with oxygen under pressure. When oxygen is forced through a nebulizer that contains the medication, it carries fine particles of the medication deep into the respiratory tract. The smaller the particle, the deeper into the lung it can be inhaled. The patient breathes slowly and deeply, holds his or her breath for 3 or 4 seconds after an inspiration, and exhales through pursed lips. The procedure is repeated until all the medication has been inhaled as ordered. The teeth should be brushed and the mouth rinsed after the procedure to prevent soreness. Nearly all forms of respiratory therapy include some form of humidity or aerosol.

## Oxygen Therapy

Oxygen therapy is used for patients with hypoxemia (low arterial oxygen tension). Oxygen is prescribed by the physician, and its management is similar to that of a drug. The many devices available for oxygen therapy are divided into two groups: low-flow and high-flow systems (Beare, Myers, 1998). Low-flow systems contribute partially to the inspired gas the patient breathes (i.e., part of each breath contains room air). Low-flow systems do not provide a constant or known

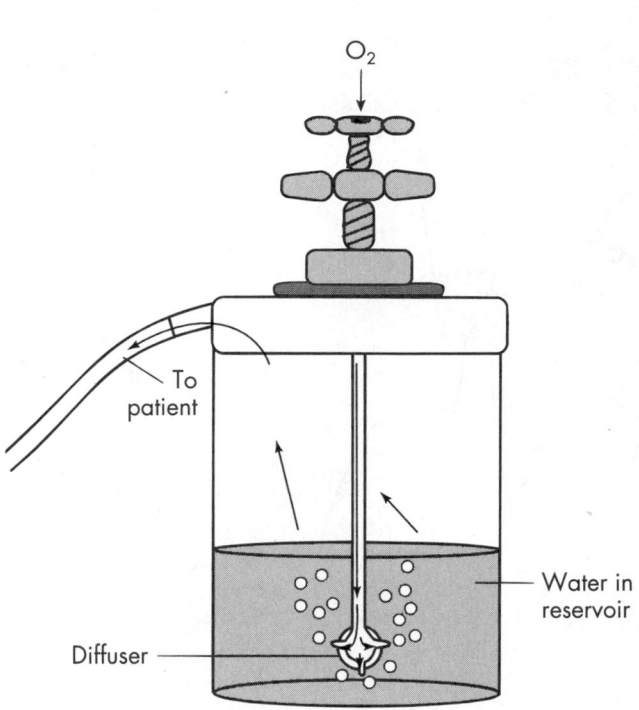

**Figure 22-13**    Bubble humidifier. Gas is directed below the surface of the water and bubbles back to the top. (Modified from McPherson SP: *Respiratory care equipment*, ed 5, St Louis, 1995, Mosby.)

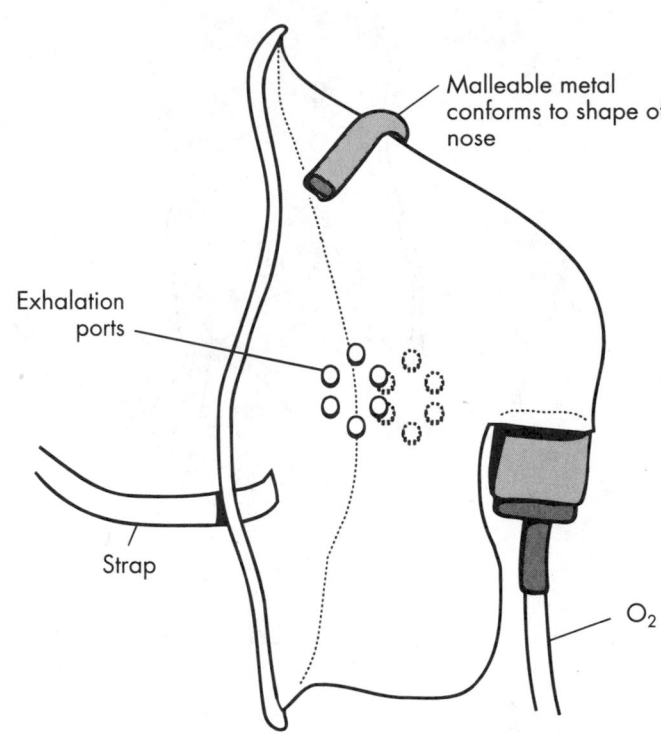

**Figure 22-14**    Simple face mask.

concentration of inspired oxygen. As the patient's breathing patterns change, the amount of oxygen inspired also changes. Examples of low-flow systems include the nasal cannula, simple oxygen mask, partial rebreathing mask, and nonrebreathing mask (Figures 22-14 to 22-16). High-flow systems provide the total amount of inspired gas. A specific percentage of oxygen is delivered independent of the patient's breathing pattern. The Venturi mask is an example of a high-flow system (Figure 22-17).

The decision to administer oxygen, the amount to deliver, and the method to be used depend on the purpose for which it is being administered (Beare, Myers, 1998). The effectiveness of oxygen in the treatment of the patient depends on the pathologic process present. The physician indicates the method by which oxygen is to be given and the number of liters per minute. The nurse responsible for carrying out the directive should act promptly and remember that although oxygen may be beneficial, it may also be dangerous. Therefore the nurse should carefully observe any patient who is receiving oxygen.

## Oxygen by Nasal Cannula

The nasal cannula is useful when an extremely low concentration of oxygen is needed. The oxygen can-

nula is made of plastic and consists of two prongs, which are placed in the nostrils, and either a strap around the head or a plastic bow similar to the bow on glasses, which fits over the ears. The flowmeter should be set at the prescribed number of liters with the oxygen flowing through the cannula before its insertion because the patient may otherwise receive a blast of oxygen that is meant to flush the system. Oxygen concentrations from 24% to 44% may be delivered. At a flow rate of 6 L/min, the nasal cannula delivers a concentration of 44% oxygen. This is the maximum rate a cannula should deliver. The nasal cannula works on the same principle as the Venturi mask, except that the work of mixing oxygen and air is done in the nasopharynx and oropharynx. Therefore whether a patient breathes through the nose or mouth does not matter because oxygen and atmospheric air are mixed before they enter the trachea and lungs. Proper placement of the prongs is important to prevent a direct stream of oxygen against the nasal mucosa. Even with correct positioning of the prongs, a greater degree of nasal drying occurs with this method. When the flow rate is more than 4 L/min, humidification of the oxygen is necessary (Carroll, 1996). If the patient's nasal mucosa becomes dry and irritated, a water-based lubricant may be used to moisten the nostrils.

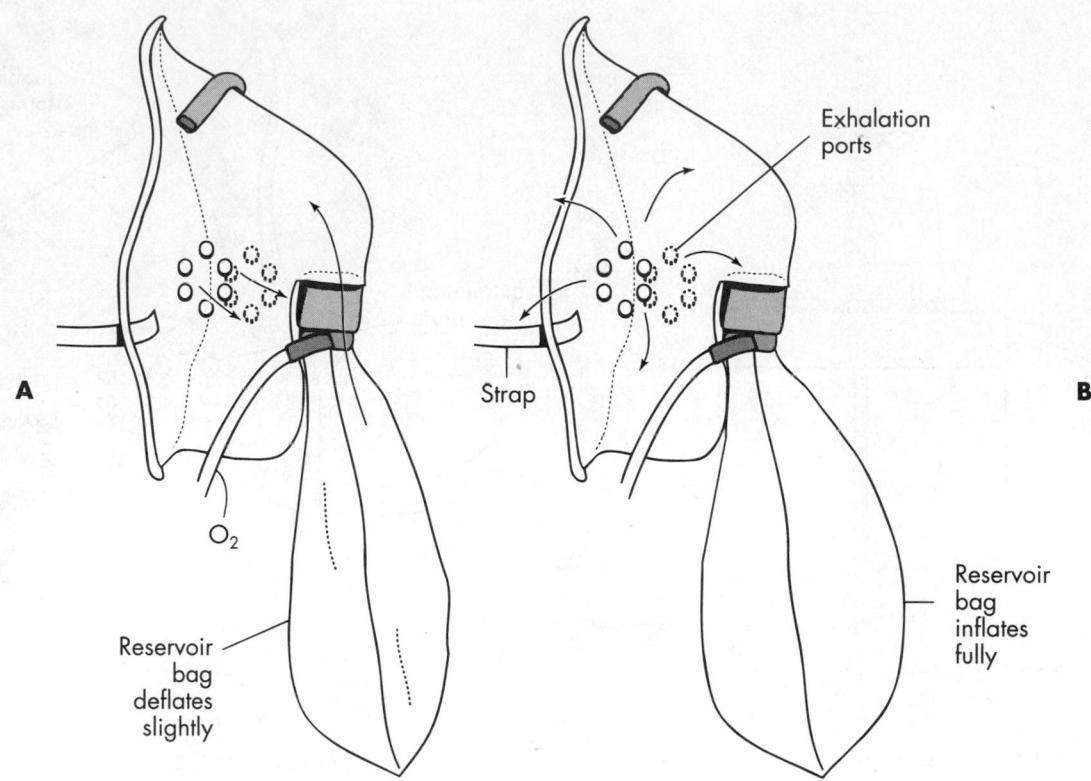

**Figure 22-15**  Partial rebreathing mask. **A,** Inhalation. **B,** Exhalation. Note direction of gas movement indicated by the arrows.

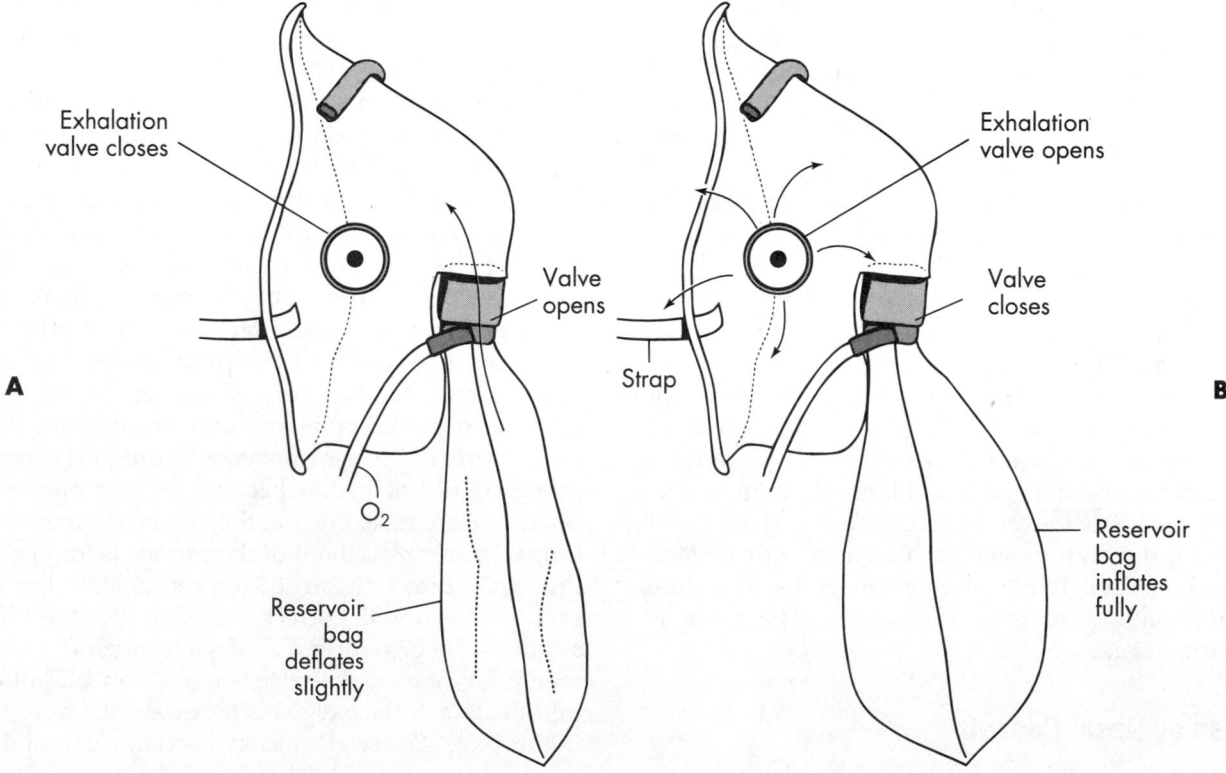

**Figure 22-16**  Nonrebreathing mask. **A,** Inhalation. **B,** Exhalation. Arrows indicate the direction of gas movement.

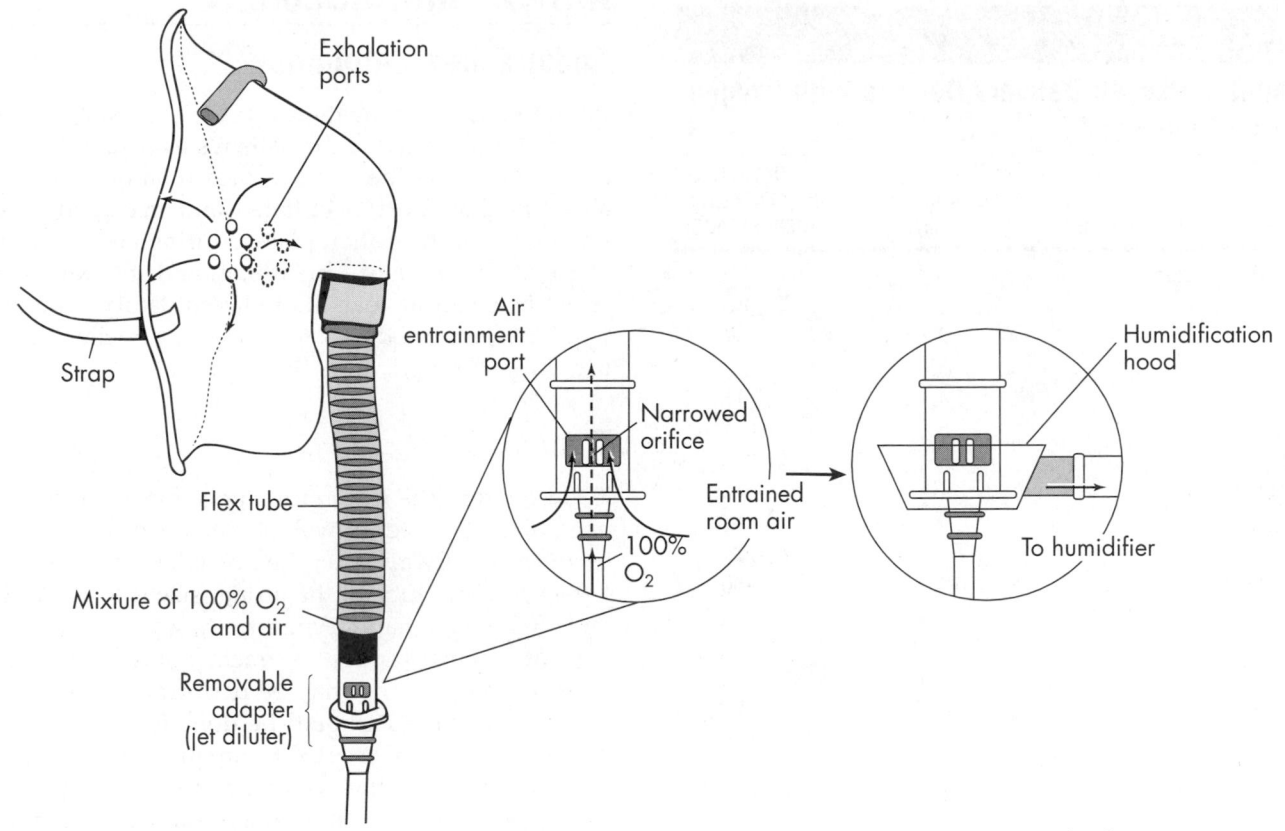

**Figure 22-17**    Venturi mask. A hood has been added to provide humidification and to protect the air ports.

## Oxygen by Mask

Oxygen masks are comfortable and are used when higher concentrations of oxygen than can be delivered by nasal cannula are desired. A simple oxygen mask provides concentrations of oxygen from 40% to 60%, depending on the patient's ventilatory pattern. As the patient inspires, room air is drawn in through the holes in the mask and around the edges and mixes with the oxygen. Flow rates of 5 to 8 L/min are normally required.

Venturi masks, partial rebreather masks, aerosol masks, and nonrebreathing masks are other types of masks that may be used for the patient. Venturi masks are high-flow systems that can deliver oxygen concentrations from 24% to 40%. This system is particularly useful in individuals with COPD at times of infection or exacerbation. They may lose their hypoxic respiratory drive at higher concentrations of oxygen, but because the Venturi mask delivery is well controlled, higher levels can be safely delivered to prevent respiratory failure. Aerosol masks are used with nebulizers and can be adjusted to deliver oxygen concentrations from 22% to 100%. Partial rebreather masks consist of a face mask and a reservoir bag. They can deliver between 35% and 60% oxygen concentration. Nonre-

breather masks have a reservoir that is separated from the mask by a one-way valve to prevent expired air from mixing with supplemental oxygen. Exhaled air is directed out of the mask through exhalation ports. If the mask conforms tightly to the face, 100% oxygen concentration can be delivered (Table 22-7).

Patients vary in their tolerance to oxygen by mask. The head strap should be adjusted to a position that is most comfortable for the patient. A patient who is apprehensive or has acute dyspnea may have a feeling of suffocation. Depending on the patient's condition, the mask should be removed and the face bathed and dried. The mask must be replaced with a nasal cannula during meals. Because moisture tends to collect in the mask, it should be wiped dry regularly. The minimum flow for any type of mask should be 5 L/min.

## Hyperbaric Oxygen

Hyperbaric oxygenation is achieved by exposing the patient to pressure greater than normal atmospheric pressure. As a result, the amount of oxygen dissolved in the plasma is increased, which causes an increase in oxygen levels in the tissues of the body. Therapy is carried out in either small or large

## TABLE 22-7

### Standard Oxygen Delivery Devices With Oxygen Concentration

| OXYGEN DELIVERY DEVICE | FLOW RATE (L/min) | OXYGEN CONCENTRATION (PERCENTAGE) |
|---|---|---|
| **Low-Flow Systems** | | |
| Nasal cannula | 1 | 24 |
| | 2 | 28 |
| | 3 | 32 |
| | 4 | 36 |
| | 5 | 40 |
| | 6 | 44 |
| Simple face mask | 5-6 | 40 |
| | 6-7 | 50 |
| | 7-10 | 60 |
| Partial-rebreather mask | 6-10 | 35-60 |
| Non-rebreather mask | 6-10 | 60-100 |
| **High-Flow Systems** | | |
| Venturi mask | 4 | 24 |
| | 4 | 28 |
| | 6 | 31 |
| | 8 | 35 |
| | 8 | 40 |
| | 10 | 50 |

Modified from Kersten LD: *Comprehensive respiratory nursing: a decision making approach*, Philadelphia, 1989, Saunders.

steel chambers that the patient enters alone or with staff members. All personnel involved undergo rigid physical examination and training. The use of hyperbaric oxygen in the treatment of disease is still in the experimental stage. Although not all authorities agree on its value, most agree that it may serve as an adjunct to other therapies. Researchers also have determined that hyperbaric oxygen may cause severe side effects.

## Oxygen Precautions

Regardless of what method of oxygen administration is used, certain precautions must be taken when a patient is receiving oxygen. Smoking is not permitted because oxygen supports combustion and causes anything that is burning in its presence to burn brighter and faster. When oxygen tanks are being used, they should be secured in such a way that they will not tip over. They should not be placed near lamps, radiators, or other heating devices.

# AIRWAY MANAGEMENT

## Endotracheal Intubation

In endotracheal intubation a tube is passed through the nose or mouth into the patient's trachea. Like a tracheostomy tube, the endotracheal tube has an inflatable cuff that must be inflated and managed in the same manner. It is often placed during an emergency to facilitate a patient's breathing, and the patient receives mechanical ventilation. If ventilatory support is required for more than 2 to 3 weeks, a tracheotomy is usually performed.

## Tracheotomy

A **tracheotomy** is a surgical procedure in which an opening in the anterior wall of the trachea is created to establish an airway. After the procedure is completed, a tracheostomy tube of the proper size is inserted. Patients who have had laryngectomy surgery have permanent tracheostomies. A tracheotomy may be an elective procedure or may be performed in an emergency. If possible it should be done in the operating room under strict aseptic technique. The following signs may indicate the need for a tracheostomy:

- Prolonged intubation—many surgeons consider a tracheotomy after 2 weeks of mechanical ventilation. The tracheotomy permits oral alimentation, verbal communication, and greater patient comfort for ventilation-dependent patients.
- Airway obstruction resulting from a tumor, edema, or infection
- Preliminary tracheotomy in patients who are undergoing head and neck surgery because of anticipated swelling and edema
- Laryngeal dysfunction (e.g., bilateral vocal cord paralysis)
- Trauma with facial fractures, especially mandibular
- Clearance of respiratory secretions in individuals with a depressed cough, neuromuscular disorder, or aspiration

After the surgical procedure a tracheostomy tube is inserted into the opening and tied securely around the patient's neck with cotton tape. Velcro devices are also available to secure the tracheostomy tube. A sterile gauze dressing (unfilled) covers the surgical wound around the tube (Figure 22-18). The tracheostomy tube may consist of two or three pieces: the outer cannula, the inner cannula, and the obturator, or simply a single cannula and an obturator (Figure 22-19). In double-cannula tubes the obturator is used to guide the outer cannula through the surgical opening into the trachea, after which it is removed and the inner cannula inserted into the outer cannula and locked in place. Single-cannula tubes are most com-

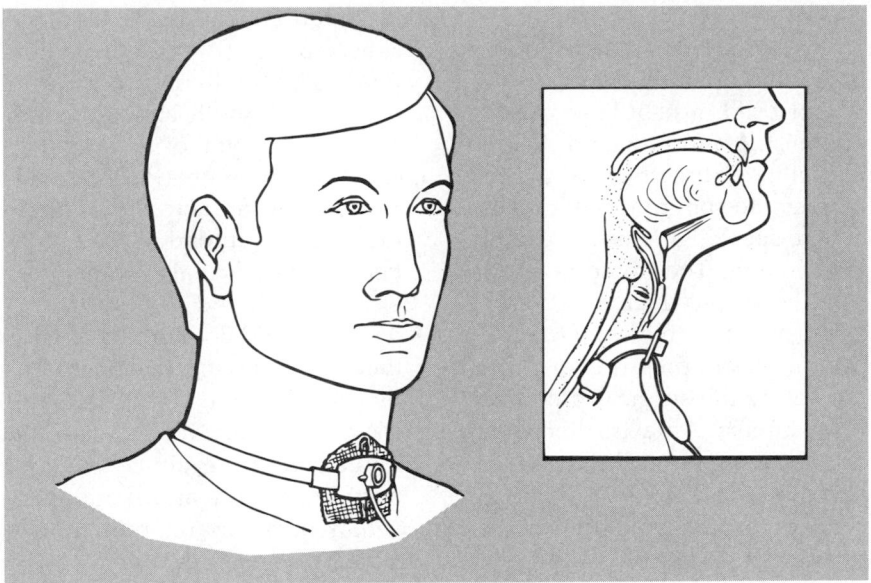

**Figure 22-18**    Cuffed tracheostomy tube is in place and tied around the patient's neck. The wound is protected with a sterile dressing.

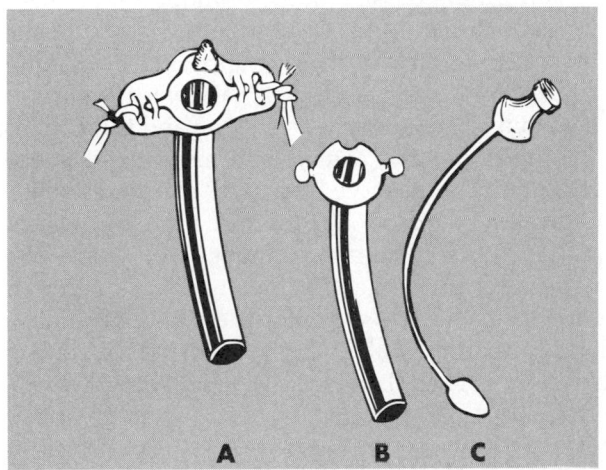

**Figure 22-19**    Tracheostomy tube. **A,** Outer cannula. **B,** Inner cannula. **C,** Obturator.

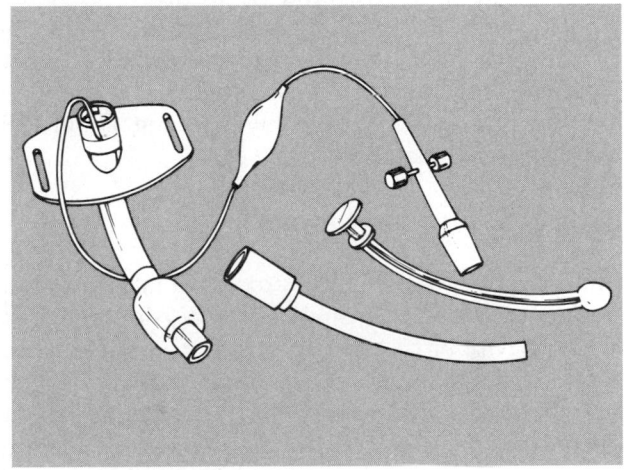

**Figure 22-20**    Cuffed tracheostomy tube.

monly used because newer materials and adequate humidification have eliminated the need for a removable inner cannula.

Generally two types of tracheostomy tubes, cuffed and cuffless, may be used. Cuffed tubes are used when ventilatory support is needed or sometimes to reduce aspiration. These tubes are made of plastic and have an inflatable cuff surrounding the middle portion of the tube (Figure 22-20). The cuff prevents air from leaking around the sides of the tube and holds the tube in place. Although the newer low-pressure, high-volume cuffs minimize irritation to the tracheal mucosa, the cuff pressure should be measured at least every 8 hours. The pressure should be kept at 18 to 21 mm Hg for adequate capillary blood flow. If increased cuff pressures are required, the physician should be notified and the tube changed to a larger size.

The nurse should remember that patients with cuffed tracheostomy tubes in place cannot speak because air does not pass directly through the larynx. These patients should be assured that they will be able to speak normally again when the cuffed tracheostomy tube is removed. Cuffless tubes are used when ventilatory support is not needed and serve to maintain the patency of the tracheotomy tube. These tubes may be plastic or metal.

Maintenance of a patent airway is a primary nursing responsibility. A patient who has a newly created tracheotomy needs suctioning often. If a form of mechanical ventilation is not used, a nebulizer may be used to keep secretions moist. A mid-Fowler's position provides comfort and facilitates breathing. Provision must be made for the patient to communicate because he or she may be unable to speak. Patients are usually apprehensive and fear choking. The nurse must observe the patient for complications, which may include apnea, cyanosis, shortness of breath, bleeding from the wound, and hypotension. Blood pressure measurements should be taken before the surgical procedure and at intervals after the surgery. An extra sterile tracheostomy set of the same size and a tracheostomy insertion tray should be kept at the patient's bedside for emergency use if the tube becomes displaced. Any patient who has undergone a tracheotomy should be closely monitored during the 24 hours after insertion of the tube. Patients who are discharged with a tracheostomy tube must be taught how to care for it (Lewis, Collier, Heitkemper, 1996).

Suction equipment should be available at home. Persons who have a permanent tracheostomy must be instructed not to swim and to use caution when bathing so that water is not aspirated. Scarfs or collars worn around the tracheostomy opening should be made of porous materials.

## Mechanical Ventilation

Pulmonary ventilation is the process of taking oxygen into the lungs and releasing carbon dioxide in the exhaled gas. Under certain conditions the patient is unable to maintain optimum levels of arterial oxygen, carbon dioxide, or both. When this occurs, the patient's survival depends on mechanical ventilation. Several conditions exist for which the patient may need ventilatory assistance. Among these are drug overdoses, respiratory failure, certain neuromuscular disorders, cardiac arrest, and pulmonary edema caused by ventricular failure.

When mechanical ventilation is used, the patient must usually be intubated with an artificial airway and connected to an artificial ventilator. The natural airway is bypassed, which necessitates some form of humidification to prevent drying of mucous membranes and thickening of respiratory secretions. Patients receiving mechanical ventilation therapy require close and careful monitoring. The nurse must be familiar with the ventilator and its connecting tubing. Ventilator settings are prescribed by the physician and should include tidal volume, respiratory rate, frequency of sighs, and percentage of oxygen. Most ventilators can supply several modes or types of ventilatory support. Each requires a different contribution or effort by the patient

to support breathing. These modes include control, assist/control (A/C), intermittent mandatory ventilation (IMV), and continuous positive airway pressure (CPAP). The mode should be ordered according to the severity and type of breathing problem. Positive end-expiratory pressure (PEEP) is often used to improve the oxygen transfer across the lungs of patients receiving mechanical ventilation. The nurse should monitor patients' exhaled tidal volume, respiratory rate, inspired oxygen level, and peak pressure (pressure required to deliver the tidal volume into the patient's lungs) while they are receiving mechanical ventilation. The heart rate and rhythm, blood pressure level, and skin color should be observed carefully. Blood gas studies are performed often to evaluate and optimize ventilatory support. Commonly an arterial catheter is placed to prevent frequent arterial punctures.

The nursing care of patients receiving ventilation therapy includes the following:

- Monitoring all vital signs
- Positioning to provide optimum ventilation
- Frequent turning
- Performing passive range-of-motion exercises
- Recording fluid intake and output
- Assessing airway maintenance and determining the need for suctioning at least every 2 hours
- Maintaining adequate nutrition and fluid balance

If bronchodilating drugs are administered, the patient should be observed for side effects. The nurse should provide emotional support and explain procedures and equipment if the patient is conscious. When conscious, patients may be anxious and require sedation. Before sedatives or narcotics are administered, the blood pressure, pulse, and ventilator parameters should be checked (Lewis, Collier, Heitkemper, 1996).

## THORACIC SURGERY

Surgery of the chest is performed to cure or relieve disease conditions such as bronchiectasis, lung abscesses, lung cancer, cysts, and benign tumors. The type of operative procedure used depends on the purpose. An exploratory thoracotomy is performed to confirm a diagnosis of lung or chest disease. "Thoracotomy" refers to the surgical creation of an opening into the thoracic cavity. Often a biopsy is performed and the chest is closed, with the possibility of future operations to treat the disease process. In some conditions only a small portion or segment of lung tissue may be removed. This procedure is called segmental resection of the lung. Removal of an entire lobe of one lung is a **lobectomy,** whereas removal of an entire lung is a **pneumonectomy** (Figure 22-21). The latter is done most often for treatment of bronchogenic carcinoma. Many patients are cared for in intensive care units or in cardiopulmonary units immediately after surgery. Pneu-

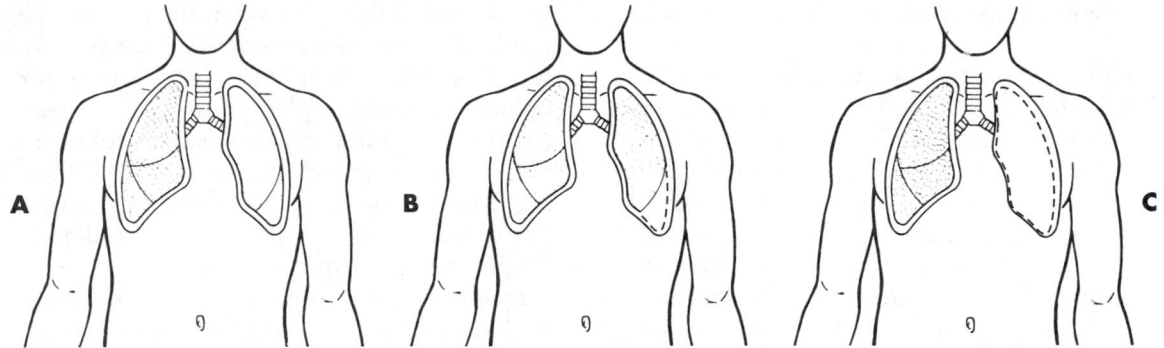

**Figure 22-21**    Lobectomy and pneumonectomy. **A,** Normal lung. **B,** Lobectomy with lower lobe of left lung removed. **C,** Pneumonectomy with entire left lung removed.

monectomy, or lung reduction surgery, is performed to remove hyperinflated portions of the lungs in patients with severe COPD. About one third of one or both lungs may be removed to improve the functioning of the remaining lung tissue.

## Preoperative Assessment and Intervention

The surgeon carefully screens patients being considered for a lobectomy or pneumonectomy because not all patients are eligible for these types of surgery. Many patients are seen in the surgeon's office, and tests and examinations are performed on an outpatient basis. Some patients are admitted to the hospital for their preoperative preparation, which is both psychologic and physical. Patients may have been ill for a long time, and therefore their functional status may have been reduced. Preoperative nutritional evaluation is important because poor nutrition depresses the immune system and impedes wound healing.

Emotional reactions to the proposed surgery may be affected by poor physical status. While efforts are being directed toward improving the physical condition, attempts should also be made to identify and discuss the patient's fears. The nurse should encourage the patient to communicate feelings to the team of caretakers. During this period the team must address any condition that might affect the outcome of surgery.

## Preoperative Preparation

The patient should know that several examinations and tests will be performed. A bronchoscopic examination, electrocardiography (ECG), a chest x-ray examination, and a sputum examination may be performed. Tests of pulmonary function and a number of blood tests may be done. Patients may receive blood transfusions before surgery, and antibiotic drugs are often administered. Drugs by nebulization may also be ordered. Mouth hygiene is extremely important, and

the nurse should ensure that the teeth are brushed in the morning, after each meal, and at bedtime. Postural drainage is performed several times daily, first when the patient is awakened in the morning and last at bedtime. The patient should be encouraged to cough deeply and to expectorate as much mucus as possible during postural drainage. The diet should be nourishing, and the patient should be weighed at specified intervals. Unless contraindicated, the patient should be ambulatory during the preoperative preparation to maintain muscle tone.

The patient should be given an explanation concerning the nursing procedures to be carried out after surgery. Patients should be told that they will be admitted to the intensive care unit for 1 to 2 days postoperatively and that they may have pain because the nerves between the ribs have been cut, necessitating pain medication. In addition, patients should be informed that blood and other fluids may be given, that oxygen will be administered, and that vital signs will be checked often for several hours. If a chest tube will be used after surgery, the patient should be told that it will drain the fluid and air that normally accumulate after chest surgery. Preoperatively the patient should be taught incentive spirometry with coughing and deep breathing techniques and how to do arm and shoulder exercises.

## Postoperative Assessment and Management

After surgery the blood pressure, pulse, and respiration rates are checked frequently according to institutional protocols. Oxygen is administered by a mechanical ventilator, nasal cannula, or mask for as long as necessary. Because a reduction in lung capacity requires a period of physiologic adjustment, fluids may be at a low hourly rate. This prevents overloading the circulation and precipitating pulmonary edema and is especially important in older patients. Fluids by mouth are allowed early in the postoperative period after the patient is fully awake and the gag reflex has returned.

When the patient is conscious and the vital signs have been stabilized, the head of the bed may be elevated to an angle of approximately 30 to 45 degrees. Directions concerning the positioning of the patient should be received. A patient with a pneumonectomy is usually turned every hour from the back to the affected side and should not be completely turned to the unoperated side. This type of turning allows the fluid left in the space to consolidate and prevents the remaining lung and the heart from shifting toward the operative side (mediastinal shift). A patient with a lobectomy may be turned to either side, and a patient with a segmental resection usually is not turned onto the affected side unless the surgeon prescribes this position.

Medication for pain is needed for several days and must be planned for the individual patient. Coughing and incentive spirometry are painful, and better cooperation is secured from the patient if the pain-relieving medication is administered 20 to 30 minutes before he or she is instructed to cough. Coughing must be deep enough to bring up secretions, and the nurse should splint the chest when the patient coughs (Figure 22-22). Both the anterior and the posterior side of the chest must be splinted. The nurse's forearms or palms or a towel is placed around the chest and held tightly, or a pillow may be used to splint the chest. If the mucus is thick and the patient has difficulty bringing it up, respiratory treatments with aerosol may be prescribed. The surgeon should be notified if efforts to cough and bring up mucus fail.

Exercises are begun early in the postoperative period to facilitate lung ventilation and maintain normal muscle tension in the shoulder and trunk. At first the exercises are passive (performed by the nurse), but the patient performs them actively as soon as he or she is ambulatory or able to sit on the side of the bed and stand. The physical therapist assists with the exercises, but, in the absence of the physical therapist, the nurse must be able to teach and to help the patient with the exercises.

The nurse must be constantly on the alert for signs indicating serious complications. Cyanosis, dyspnea, and acute chest pain may indicate atelectasis and should be reported immediately. Increased temperature and pulse may signal the beginning of an infection. Pallor, an increased pulse, and any significant drop in blood pressure may indicate an internal hemorrhage. Dressings should be checked often for the presence of bright red blood, which may indicate an external hemorrhage. Mobilization of the patient with

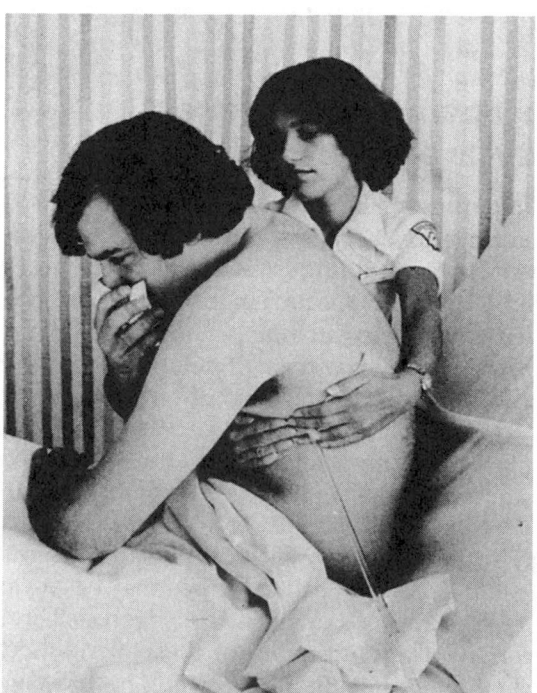

**Figure 22-22** Nurse uses her hands to provide firm support while splinting the patient's incision. This technique lessens muscle stress and reduces discomfort when the patient coughs. Note that the nurse keeps her head behind the patient while he coughs and that the patient is using a tissue to cover his mouth. (From Phipps WJ: *Medical-surgical nursing: concepts and clinical practice*, ed 5, St Louis, 1995, Mosby.)

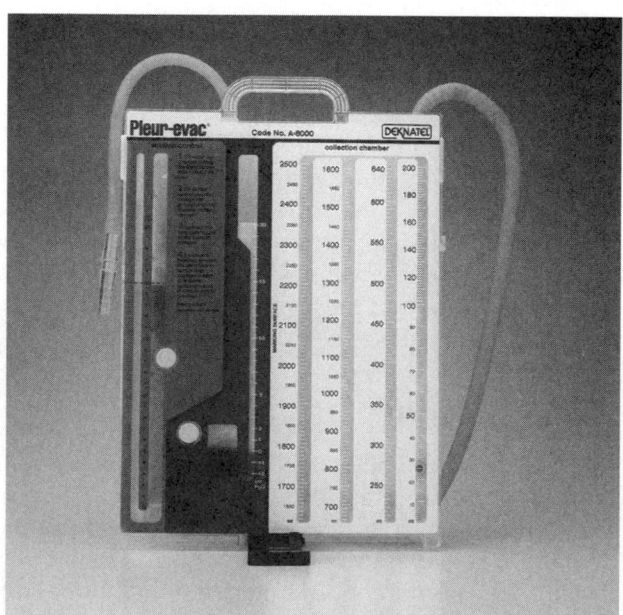

**Figure 22-23** Adult/Pediatric Single Collection Chamber model. (From Genzyme Surgical Products, Fall River, Mass.)

chest surgery may begin on the first or second postoperative day. Initially the patient is allowed to sit on the side of the bed or to stand beside the bed. Ambulation depends on the patient's progress.

## Chest Drainage

When the pleura is entered during surgery, atmospheric air enters the pleural space and the involved lung collapses. Therefore after thoracic surgery the patient usually has one or more chest tubes placed in the pleural cavity, which permit the escape of air so that the lung will expand and allow drainage of fluid from the pleural space. One tube may be placed in the upper chest to remove air, and another tube in a lower position to remove fluids. The chest tubes are then attached to a closed drainage system.

## Systems for Chest Drainage

A chest drainage system must be capable of removing whatever accumulates in the pleural space so that a normal pleural space may be restored and maintained. Self-contained, disposable commercial systems are the most common modalities for water-seal drainage (Figure 22-23), replacing glass bottles. The chest tube is attached to the drainage system. Drainage accumulates in the first chamber or bottle, and water in the second chamber or bottle acts as a seal. It allows air to be removed from the chest but does not allow it to reenter the chest. Suction may be applied to the second chamber to create negative pressure, which facilitates the removal of fluid and air from the pleural cavity. The addition of suction creates constant bubbling in the third chamber.

Figure 22-24 depicts chest tube placement and three types of mechanical drainage systems. The Pleur-Evac

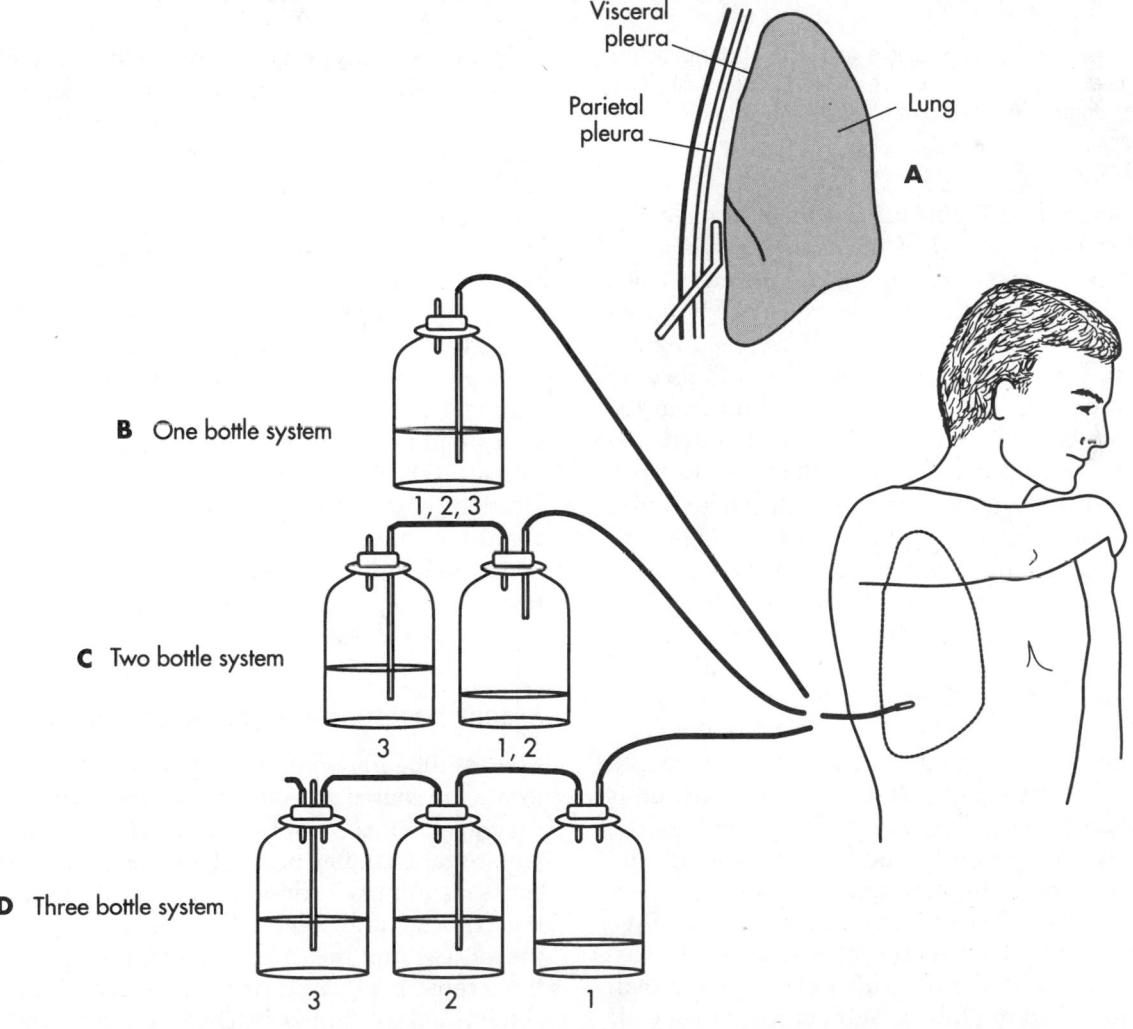

**Figure 22-24**    Chest drainage system. **A,** Chest catheter is placed in the pleural space of the chest cavity. **B,** One-bottle drainage system. **C,** Two-bottle drainage system. **D,** Three-bottle drainage system.

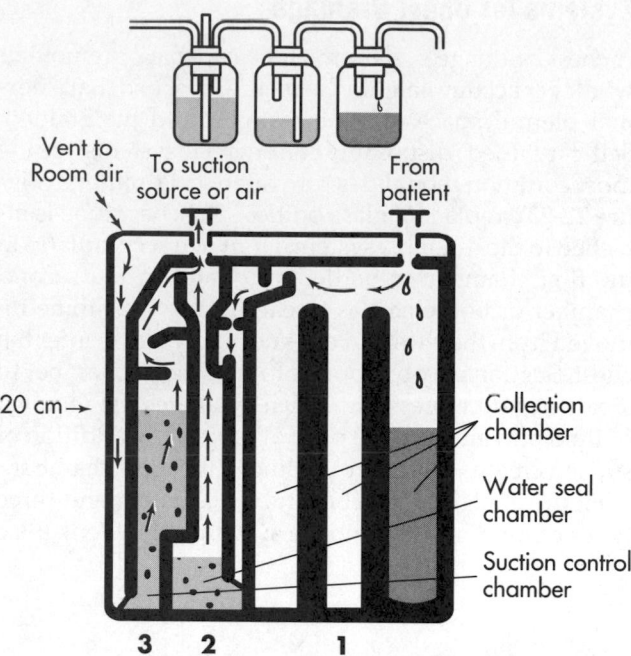

**Figure 22-25**   Pleur-Evac is a single unit with all three bottles identified as chambers. *1*, Collection chamber; *2*, water seal chamber; *3*, suction control chamber. (From Genzyme Surgical Products, Fall River, Mass.)

system is shown in Figure 22-25. In a single-bottle water-seal system the end of the drainage tube from the patient's chest is covered by a layer of water, which allows air and fluid to exit the pleural space but does not allow them to return. Drainage depends on gravity and varies with respirations. As the fluid level in the bottle increases, removing air and fluid from the pleural space becomes more difficult and application of suction may be needed (Lewis, Collier, Heitkemper, 1996). A two-bottle system consists of the same water-seal chamber just described, plus a fluid collection bottle. When fluid drains in this system, the water seal is not affected by the amount of drainage. In a three-bottle system a third bottle is added to the two bottles previously described to control the amount of suction applied (Figure 22-25). The amount of suction is determined by the depth to which the tip of the venting glass tube is submerged in water. The usual depth is 20 cm, which means that 20 cm of water suction is being applied to the chest wall of the patient (Beare, Myers, 1998). In the three-bottle system, drainage depends on gravity or the amount of suction applied. The suction apparatus creates and maintains negative pressure throughout the entire closed drainage system. If the vacuum in the system becomes greater than the depth to which the tube is submerged, outside air can enter the system. The result is constant bubbling in the pressure-regulator bottle, which indicates that the system is functioning properly.

## Assessment

It is important to assess the respiratory status of the patient and to maintain and monitor the chest drainage system. Monitoring the drainage system includes identifying an air leak. An air leak is indicated by constant bubbling in the water-seal chamber (Lewis, Collier, Heitkemper, 1996). Maintaining the drainage system becomes especially important if an air leak is present because as the patient inhales, air is taken into the lungs and small amounts of air may be released from a leak that escapes into the pleural cavity. If no escape route exists for the air (the chest drainage system), a life-threatening tension pneumothorax may develop. Therefore the practice of clamping chest tubes is discouraged. Signs of a tension pneumothorax include an increase in respiratory rate, an increase in heart rate, and cyanosis. The nurse should monitor for a mediastinal shift, which can occur as the lung, heart, and other structures shift away from the pneumothorax (Lewis, Collier, Heitkemper, 1996).

Frequent inspection is necessary to ascertain that the system remains airtight, that it is working correctly, and that the tubing does not become kinked when the patient is lying on his or her side. A small pillow, folded towel, or rubber ring placed under the chest when the patient is in a side-lying position helps prevent obstruction of the tube. If the chest tube accidentally falls out, the nurse should have the patient exhale and should apply an occlusive dressing at the insertion site. The nurse should monitor the patient closely for signs and symptoms of respiratory distress and should notify the physician if they occur. The physician should be notified if drainage is bloodier than expected. If the chest tube comes apart, the nurse should clean the ends with alcohol if it is readily available and should reconnect the tube. If necessary, the nurse should clamp the tube temporarily until the integrity of the system can be restored (Lewis, Collier, Heitkemper, 1996).

## Assessment for Leaks in the System

A chest tube may be clamped for only a brief time to locate the source of leaks in the system and to replace drainage bottles. If continuous bubbling is noted in the water-seal chamber or the Pleur-Evac unit, the nurse starts clamping close to the chest and works down to the drainage unit. When the tube is clamped between the air leak and the drainage unit, the bubbling stops. If the cause is a loose connection, it is reconnected, and if the drainage unit is cracked, it is replaced. If air is leaking into the patient's pleural space, the physician should be notified immediately. The nurse must remember to assess the reasons why the patient has a

---

**BOX 22-4**

## Guidelines for Care of the Patient with Water-Seal Chest Drainage

1 Fill the water-seal chamber with sterile water to the 2-cm water level via the latex suction tubing.
2 If suction is required, fill the suction control chamber with sterile water through the atmospheric vent to the level prescribed. This level is usually 20 cm.
3 Attach the drainage catheter (chest tube) coming from the patient to the latex tubing that is attached to the collection chamber of the Pleur-Evac. Tape this connection securely with adhesive tape.
4 If suction is required, connect the suction control chamber tubing to the suction unit. Turn on the suction unit and increase the pressure until gentle bubbling is produced in the suction control chamber.
5 Ensure that the latex tubing is not looping or kinking.
6 Maintain the tubing and drainage system below the patient's chest at all times to allow gravity drainage and to prevent fluid backup.
7 Monitor the amount of drainage in the collection chamber as ordered. It is calibrated in 2- to 5-ml increments and has a surface on which to mark the time and date of drainage.
8 Help the patient achieve a comfortable position. Use pillows to maintain good body alignment.
9 Medicate the patient with analgesics as needed and document their effectiveness.
10 Encourage movement of the arm and shoulder on the affected side.
11 Gently milk the tubing in the direction of the collection chamber every 2 hours or according to institutional policy.
12 Monitor the water-seal chamber for fluctuations (tidaling), which indicate that the closed-drainage system is patent.
13 Fluctuations in the water-seal chamber stop when (a) the lung has reexpanded, (b) the tubing is obstructed, (c) a dependent loop develops, or (d) the suction control apparatus is not working properly.
14 Monitor the patient for an air leak as indicated by constant bubbling in the water-seal chamber.
15 Use techniques of respiratory assessment and note the patient's respiratory rate, depth, and effort, as well as his or her ease of respirations. Monitor breath sounds and note any adventitious sounds.
16 Encourage the patient to cough and to deep breathe at frequent intervals, and use analgesics as needed to promote comfort.
17 When assisting with chest tube removal, instruct the patient to inhale all the way and perform Valsalva's maneuver as the tube is removed smoothly and quickly.
18 An occlusive dressing with Vaseline gauze is applied immediately to prevent atmospheric air from entering the pleural space. The occlusive dressing may be removed in 24 to 48 hours and changed according to institutional policies.

---

chest tube. If a new air leak develops, it must be investigated immediately.

## Milking and Stripping of Chest Tubes

The nurse should be familiar with the purpose for which the drainage system is being used and the type of drainage to expect. Bloody drainage may form in the tubing and cause an obstruction. To prevent this the physician may prescribe the milking of the tubing. Milking should be done carefully to avoid generating significant amounts of pressure in the chest. Stripping a chest tube is generally avoided because it can generate extreme negative suction pressures. For each patient the physician will determine whether milking and stripping of chest tubes should be done. If this is ordered, it must be done with care, because, with overly vigorous milking or stripping of chest tubes, fragile blood vessels, lung tissue, and fresh sutures can be "sucked" through the holes of the chest tube (Box 22-4).

## Heimlich Chest Drainage Valve

The Heimlich chest drainage valve does not use a water-sealed unit. It is a sterile, disposable flutter valve that is attached between the chest drainage catheter and a drainage collection bag. The flutter valve allows fluid and air to pass through it but prevents any reflux of fluids and air. With the valve in place the patient can be more mobile because it works in any position.

Patient and family education focuses on methods to improve gas exchange, including use of the IS, deep breathing, and coughing. The patient is taught how to splint the incision, and exercises are taught to improve mobility of the shoulder and arm.

## NURSING CARE PLAN
### PATIENT FOLLOWING THORACOTOMY

Mr. Scott is a 71-year-old man who is scheduled for a right lower lobe lobectomy for lung cancer. He has undergone an extensive preoperative evaluation as an outpatient, including routine blood work, an arterial blood gas analysis, a chest x-ray examination, sputum cultures, pulmonary function testing, and a chest CT scan.

| Medical History | Psychosocial Data | Assessment Data |
|---|---|---|
| Denies cardiac disease, hypertension, emphysema, and non-insulin-dependent diabetes mellitus | Widowed; wife died 2 years ago | Alert and oriented × 3 (time, place, and person) |
| | One son, one daughter, six grandchildren | Afebrile, 98.4° F |
| | | *Cardiovascular:* Pulse 84, regular rate without murmurs; skin warm and dry; peripheral pulses palpable bilaterally |
| Has smoked two packs of cigarettes per day for 50 years | Retired engineer | |
| | Practicing Catholic | |
| | Active social life, many friends | *Respiratory:* Respirations 20, not labored, moist cough productive of thin/thick white sputum; scattered rhonchi throughout lung fields; decreased breath sounds right middle and lower lobes; complaining of dyspnea and shortness of breath with exertion |
| Denies alcohol consumption | Owns own home | |
| | *Hobbies:* fishing, chess, crossword puzzles | *Abdominal:* Soft, nontender, nondistended; bowel sounds in all four quadrants; bowel movement morning of admission |
| | | *Skin:* No breakdown noted; no rashes |
| | | Electrolytes within normal limits |
| | | Complete blood count within normal limits |
| | | *Pulmonary function tests:* Ordered |
| | | *Arterial blood gases:* 7.45/35/94/98% |
| | | *Chest x-ray examination:* Consistent with lesion in right lower lobe of lung |
| | | Patient to be NPO after midnight |
| | | IV to be started |
| | | Permit for surgery needs to be signed and witnessed |
| | | Cefazolin (Ancef) on call to the OR |
| | | Anesthesia visit this evening to discuss patient surgical plan |

# CONDITIONS OF THE UPPER RESPIRATORY SYSTEM

## Infectious Respiratory Conditions—Upper Airway Infections

A large number of diseases of the respiratory tract are infectious. Many of these bacterial or viral diseases find their way into the respiratory tract when an individual inhales air that is saturated with the disease organism. Many infections follow a pattern, beginning with what appears to be a common cold but gradually involving all parts of the respiratory tract. A large number of infections of the lower respiratory tract begin as upper respiratory infections.

Invasion of the upper respiratory system by pathogenic microorganisms, usually viral, causes inflammation and edema of the mucous membranes. The mucus-secreting glands become hyperactive and produce large amounts of serous-to-mucopurulent exudate. The cervical lymph nodes enlarge and are tender. Air passages become occluded, which causes impaired pulmonary ventilation. Respiratory rates increase in an effort to get more air to the lungs, and the heart works harder to supply the body's tissues with oxygen. The body mobilizes its forces to combat the invading pathogen, and **leukocytosis,** an increase in white blood cells, occurs. The inflammatory condition of the mucous membranes causes the throat to become red, sore, and dry; the voice becomes hoarse; and a dry painful cough develops. The

## NURSING CARE PLAN
### PATIENT FOLLOWING THORACOTOMY—cont'd

**NURSING DIAGNOSIS**
Ineffective airway clearance related to lung impairment, pain, and general anesthesia as evidenced by secretions, abnormal breath sounds, and increased respiratory rate

| NURSING INTERVENTIONS | EVALUATION OF EXPECTED OUTCOMES |
|---|---|
| Maintain a patent airway. | Airway is patent |
| While patient is on a ventilator, provide endotracheal suctioning to remove secretions until patient able to cough and deep breathe. | Breath sounds clear |
| Teach patient how to use the IS and encourage its use every hour while awake. | Effective cough demonstrated with expectoration of sputum if present |
| Administer humidification and respiratory treatments as indicated. | Splints incision when coughing and seeks analgesic medication before coughing if it has not been given |
| Monitor amount, color, and consistency of sputum. | |
| Assist with postural drainage and chest percussion/vibration as needed. Do not percuss or vibrate over the operative site. | |
| Auscultate breath sounds as ordered or as patient condition warrants. | |
| Teach splinting of incision and medicate before coughing and deep breathing to allow for increased comfort. | |

**NURSING DIAGNOSIS**
Pain related to surgical procedure and resulting thoracotomy incision

| NURSING INTERVENTIONS | EVALUATION OF EXPECTED OUTCOMES |
|---|---|
| Determine location, onset, quality, and quantity of pain. Use pain assessment tools that are available in several textbooks or at health care institutions. | Asks for pain medication when needed |
| Provide analgesics as ordered and determine their effectiveness. | Uses nonpharmacologic modalities to reduce discomfort |
| Attempt to obtain a new or different analgesic order if ineffective pain relief is obtained. | Verbalizes acceptable pain score (usually <3 on 0-10 scale) |
| Instruct patient on nonpharmacologic measures to reduce pain if patient is willing to use them (e.g., relaxation, distraction). | No signs of wound infection |
| Turn and position for comfort at least every 2 hours. | |
| Monitor incision line for healing and identify any signs and symptoms of possible wound infection, including redness, swelling, drainage, and an increase in wound pain. | |

*Continued*

pathogen may invade the contiguous mucous membranes of the sinuses and the ears.

## Acute Coryza (Common Cold)

Acute **coryza** may be caused by one or several viruses. The causative virus is believed to be present constantly in the upper respiratory tract. A person's susceptibility to the virus increases periodically from a wide variety of factors. Symptoms usually appear within 24 to 48 hours after exposure and may be transmitted to others several hours afterward. Symptoms include a chilly sensation and sneezing. The nasal membranes feel hot, dry, and congested. A slight throat irritation may occur, followed by a thin, serous nasal discharge. Nasal congestion causes pressure, which results in headache and tenderness of cervical lymph nodes. If the infection remains uncomplicated, it generally subsides in approximately 1 week. If nasal discharge becomes purulent, it is an indication that the infection is complicated by a bacterial invasion. Symptomatic treatment is appropriate, and the use of

## NURSING CARE PLAN
## PATIENT FOLLOWING THORACOTOMY—cont'd

**NURSING DIAGNOSIS**
Anxiety related to outcomes of surgery, use of many invasive lines/tubes, pain

| NURSING INTERVENTIONS | EVALUATION OF EXPECTED OUTCOMES |
|---|---|
| Explain all procedures in simple terms.<br>If working with patient preoperatively, review preoperative preparation and how patient can help with his or her own recovery.<br>During the postoperative period, limit noise as much as possible and turn down lights to promote rest and sleep.<br>Encourage and support patient and provide opportunities for expression of fears and concerns.<br>Involve family in care and mobilize additional resources (e.g., social work, clinical nurse specialist, clergy) to help patient cope with the diagnosis and outcomes of surgery. | States that anxiety is within a manageable level for him or her<br>Participates in preoperative plan of care<br>Uses appropriate coping skills<br>Uses additional resources if needed |

**NURSING DIAGNOSIS**
Impaired physical mobility of the upper extremities related to thoracic surgery

| NURSING INTERVENTIONS | EVALUATION OF EXPECTED OUTCOMES |
|---|---|
| Assist patient with normal range of motion and function of upper body (arms, shoulder):<br>• Teach breathing exercises to mobilize thorax.<br>• Teach and encourage exercises that promote shoulder abduction.<br>• Help patient to turn and position self in bed, and have patient out of bed to chair and ambulating as condition permits.<br>• Involve physical therapy in care if patient's condition warrants. | Demonstrates arm and shoulder exercises and verbalizes importance of performing them<br>Participates in progressive ambulation program |

**NURSING DIAGNOSIS**
Knowledge deficit related to postoperative recovery and follow-up care needed

| NURSING INTERVENTIONS | EVALUATION OF EXPECTED OUTCOMES |
|---|---|
| Instruct patient in the following regarding home care:<br>• Avoid heavy lifting (greater than 5 lb) until incision is healed.<br>• Take analgesics as prescribed to relieve surgical discomfort, especially before increases in activity.<br>• Use nonpharmacologic measures to promote comfort (e.g., relaxation).<br>• Alternate activities with rest periods; don't try to do too much all at once.<br>• Perform arm exercises and shoulder exercises 3 to 5 times daily.<br>• Practice breathing exercises several times a day.<br>• Avoid bronchial irritants.<br>• Prevent colds or lung infections.<br>• Stop smoking.<br>• Keep follow-up appointment with physician. | Verbalizes the importance of avoiding heavy lifting until incision is well healed, analgesic use to promote comfort, nonpharmacologic measures to relieve discomfort, arm and breathing exercises to regain function, avoidance of bronchial irritants, preventing colds or lung infection, stopping smoking, and keeping follow-up appointments |

antibiotics provides no scientific benefit for viral infections.

## Acute Pharyngitis

Bacteria or viruses from acute coryza may extend to the pharynx, or pharyngitis may occur without prior evidence of a cold. The throat becomes inflamed and red, the tonsils and cervical lymph nodes become tender, and a sensation of rawness and a dry cough may occur. Chronic pharyngitis may result from a chronic infection of the sinuses or nasal mucosa and may not produce any significant symptoms. Acute pharyngitis usually responds to symptomatic treatment, with recovery occurring in approximately 1 week. If the condition is caused by one of several bacteria, such as hemolytic *Streptococcus, Staphylococcus aureus,* or *Haemophilus influenzae,* symptoms may be more serious and complications may occur.

## Acute Laryngitis

Acute laryngitis generally is secondary to other upper respiratory tract infections. The mucous membrane that lines the larynx becomes inflamed, and the vocal cords become swollen. The disease is characterized by hoarseness or loss of voice and a cough. A tracheotomy is required in rare cases. If acute laryngitis remains uncomplicated, it usually clears in a few days.

## Tonsillitis

Acute follicular tonsillitis is an inflammation of the tonsils and is often caused by *Streptococcus* or *Staphylococcus.* The throat is sore and painful; swallowing is difficult; and generalized muscle aches, chills, and a temperature elevation occur. If tonsillitis is caused by hemolytic *Streptococcus,* the symptoms may be more severe, with nausea, vomiting, and an increased leukocyte count. The primary concern is the prevention of complications such as rheumatic fever and nephritis. Repeated attacks of tonsillitis may require surgical removal of the tonsils, or a **tonsillectomy.** Care of a patient who is undergoing a tonsillectomy is discussed later in this chapter.

## Sinusitis

Sinusitis may be acute or chronic and is usually caused by other upper respiratory tract infections. Because mucous membranes of the nasal cavities are contiguous with the sinuses, infection may spread easily to the sinuses. Inflammation of the sinuses may occur from obstructions such as nasal polyps or from a deviated septum that blocks drainage from the sinuses. Sinusitis may also be a complication of influenza or pneumonia and can be caused by allergens. If acute sinusitis is left untreated, it may become chronic or lead to more serious conditions such as meningitis, brain abscess, osteomyelitis, and septicemia.

The primary symptom of sinusitis is pain, which occurs in sites related to the sinus involved. When the maxillary sinus is affected, the pain occurs over the cheeks and may radiate downward to the teeth. A frontal sinus infection causes pain in and above the eyes. The bone over the affected sinus usually is sensitive to slight pressure, and puffiness over the area may be observed (Beare, Myers, 1998). Depending on the extent of the infection and the microorganism involved, the patient may have an elevated temperature, nausea, and loss of appetite. When a continuous postnasal drip into the back of the throat occurs, coughing and soreness of the throat may result. Acute sinusitis can result in lost work time and an inability to perform activities of daily living.

## Influenza

Influenza is an acute disease of the respiratory tract and is accompanied by fever and systemic symptoms. The causative virus is classified as type A, B, or C. Type D is now known as parainfluenza 1, and strains of A are known as A prime, or $A_1$ and $A_2$. In 1968, 1969, and 1974 various parts of the world, including the United States, experienced a fairly mild form of influenza caused by a new strain of the $A_2$ virus, which was called *$A_2$ Hong Kong influenza.*

The first symptoms of influenza develop rapidly. The typical picture is one of chills; a temperature of 39° C to 40° C (102° F to 104° F); severe aching of the back, head, and extremities; sore throat; cough; considerable prostration; sneezing; coated tongue; and weakness. If the infection is uncomplicated, the acute period is usually 3 to 5 days. Some cases do not follow the typical pattern but begin with gastrointestinal symptoms, bronchopneumonia, pleurisy, or sinusitis (Box 22-5). Influenza is especially hazardous for older persons, and the mortality from influenza-pneumonia generally rises sharply during an influenza epidemic.

## Interventions in Upper Airway Infections

The treatment of upper airway infections is directed toward relieving the discomfort of symptoms and preventing complications. Precautionary measures should be taken to prevent the spread of the infection to others. Nasal sprays, moist inhalations, warm saline gargles, throat irrigations, and acetaminophen (Tylenol) provide symptomatic relief and promote comfort. Fluid intake should be increased to provide systemic hydration.

---

BOX 22-5     NURSING PROCESS

## INFLUENZA

**ASSESSMENT**

- Vital signs (fever)
- Cervical lymph nodes
- Respiratory status
- Fluid volume status
- Anorexia, chills, malaise, sore throat

**NURSING DIAGNOSES**

- Ineffective airway clearance related to bronchial secretions
- Risk for fluid volume deficit related to hyperthermia and decreased intake
- Activity intolerance related to weakness

**NURSING INTERVENTIONS**

- Position for optimal breathing (head of bed elevated).
- Encourage bed rest for 2 or 3 days.
- Encourage position changes.
- Provide cool mist humidification, if indicated.
- Administer decongestants, as prescribed.
- Encourage liberal fluid intake (2 L/day) unless contraindicated.
- Plan and encourage rest periods between activities.
- Provide progressive increases in activity as tolerated.
- Encourage high-risk persons to have influenza vaccinations yearly before the "flu" season.

**EVALUATION OF EXPECTED OUTCOMES**

- Clear breath sounds
- No evidence of dehydration
- Able to perform ADLs without fatigue
- Afebrile
- Verbalizes understanding of treatment regimen

---

When pharyngitis or laryngitis accompanies acute coryza, relief may be obtained by cool mist vaporizers, which loosen secretions and reduce inflammation of the mucous membranes. If coughing is disturbing, an analgesic cough mixture or a mild sedative for rest at night may be ordered. When severe pharyngitis is present, the nurse should be alert to the possibility of complications. Temperature, pulse rates, and respiration rates should be checked every 4 hours unless otherwise ordered. A liquid or soft diet and forced fluids may be needed. The patient may be encouraged to drink 2 to 3 L of fluid per day. If the infection is caused by bacteria such as streptococci, the patient should be observed for a skin rash, which might indicate scarlet fever. Blood cultures, a white blood cell count, and a urinalysis may be prescribed. In bacterial infections the white blood cell count may be elevated. When the larynx is involved, the patient should avoid talking. Antibiotic drugs may be ordered when the infection is caused by bacteria.

Most patients with respiratory tract infections are more comfortable when placed in a low (15 degrees) Fowler's position, which allows better drainage of secretions. A cool (20° C to 21° C [68° F to 70° F]), well-ventilated, draft-free, high-humidity room is more comfortable than an overheated room.

### Patient/Family Teaching

The prevention of most upper airway infections is difficult because there are many possible causes. The nurse instructs the patient about the following measures that support the host's defenses and thereby reduce susceptibility to respiratory infections:

- Live healthy; eat a nutritious diet, get adequate rest and sleep, and exercise.
- Avoid excesses in alcohol, smoke, and irritants.
- Ensure adequate home humidification, especially during the cold months.
- Avoid irritants (tobacco, smoke, chemicals) and allergens whenever possible.
- Obtain an influenza vaccination, especially if recommended by a health care provider. (A flu vaccine may be recommended for persons who are over 65 years, have a chronic disease, or are employed in a health care setting.)
- Avoid crowds during the flu season.
- Maintain good dental hygiene.
- Practice good hand washing.

---

**NURSE ALERT**

Flu shots are not recommended during pregnancy or for individuals who are allergic to eggs.
Safety of flu vaccine has not been proved in pregnancy. The vaccine is prepared using egg albumin.

# Obstruction and Trauma of the Upper Airway

## Epistaxis

A nosebleed is rarely fatal or even serious, but it may cause the patient considerable anxiety. A number of causes of **epistaxis** or nosebleed exist. The nasal cavities are supplied by a fine network of blood capillaries, and anything that congests the nasal membrane may rupture a small capillary and result in bleeding. Epistaxis may occur in persons with hypertension, cardiovascular disease, blood dyscrasias, and some communicable diseases. It may also be caused by injury to the nose, nose picking, or forceful nose blowing.

**Assessment.** The cause should be determined by careful examination and assessment. Data to be obtained include history, frequency, and duration of bleeding episodes; precipitating factors; signs of upper respiratory tract infections or allergic conditions; current medications that might influence clotting; history of physical abuse to the face; and measures used to try to stop the bleeding. The patient should also be observed for site, color, and amount of bleeding; signs of respiratory difficulty; and signs of progressing hemorrhage. The primary provider may request laboratory tests to determine the extent and possible cause of the bleeding.

**Intervention.** The patient should be placed in a Fowler's position with the head forward. The patient should be encouraged to let the blood drain from the nose, to breathe through the mouth, and to avoid swallowing the blood because it may cause nausea and vomiting. The nostrils should be compressed tightly below the bone and held for at least 10 minutes. This procedure controls most cases of epistaxis. Ice packs applied to the area may help control bleeding by causing reflex vasoconstriction of the capillaries.

Vasoconstricting agents may be administered topically. These drugs decrease blood supply to the area and control bleeding. A cotton ball or nasal pack is saturated with a 1:1000 solution of phenylephrine and inserted into the nostril. Pressure is applied for several minutes. The cotton ball is removed, and any bleeding is monitored (Beare, Myers, 1998).

If bleeding cannot be controlled, packing the nose may be necessary. Hemostatic agents such as an absorbable gelatin sponge (Gelfoam), packing saturated with a 1:1000 solution of epinephrine, petrolatum gauze, and oxidized cellulose (Oxycel) are often used. A gauze pad can be placed under the nostrils to absorb any drainage or blood. The patient with the nasal packing in place should be monitored for signs and symptoms of infection. Respiratory status should be monitored along with vital signs (Lewis, Collier, Heitkemper, 1996).

Airway patency should be assessed because hypoxemia can occur if the packing slips out of position and obstructs the airway. In rare cases cauterizing the bleeding vessel may be necessary.

**Patient/family teaching.** Patients should be taught proper positioning to facilitate the drainage of blood and the proper application of pressure to the area to control bleeding. Ice packs may also be applied. If bleeding continues, the physician should be notified and the origin of the bleeding determined (Lewis, Collier, Heitkemper, 1996).

## Deviated Septum and Nasal Polyps

The nasal septum divides the two nasal cavities. Most people have some irregularity of the septum but are unaware of the condition unless it is great enough to obstruct breathing. During childhood, injuries to the nose, including fractures, can occur. If not treated, these injuries may result in a bending of the septum to one side or the other. If the deviation is severe, it causes a partial blocking of the respiratory passageway on one side. When obstruction occurs, surgical correction is necessary.

A **polyp** is a small tumor that is attached to the mucous membranes of the nose. It may have been caused by prolonged inflammation of the sinuses, and, because it obstructs free drainage of secretions, the inflammatory condition may be aggravated. Surgical removal may be necessary to relieve the inflammatory condition.

Respiratory obstruction from a deviated septum or nasal polyps may be corrected by a surgical procedure called *submucous resection.* The procedure is performed after administration of preoperative sedation and while the patient is under local anesthesia. After the procedure the nose is packed for approximately 12 to 24 hours. Generally the packing is soaked in liquid petrolatum to facilitate its removal. The patient is placed in a Fowler's position, and analgesics are administered to relieve pain. Because breathing is through the mouth, the patient may be given chipped ice to help keep the mouth moist. Petrolatum jelly may be applied to the lips, and iced compresses may be applied over the nose. The patient should be observed for hemorrhage, which is indicated by expectoration of bright red blood, frequent swallowing, or an increased flow of bright red blood through the packing. After removal of the packing the patient is allowed a diet as desired and bathroom privileges. The patient should be told to expect a loss of the sense of smell for approximately 1 week.

## Enlarged Tonsils and Adenoids

The pharyngeal tonsils (adenoids) are a mass of lymphoid tissue at the back of the nose in the upper pharynx. The palatine tonsils, also composed of lymphoid tissue, are located on each side of the soft palate in the throat. These tissues are normally larger in childhood, and under normal conditions removal is not considered necessary unless they become infected with bacteria and do not respond to conservative treatment. The tonsils also may obstruct the eustachian tube opening in the back of the throat and may cause some loss of hearing. Removing these lymphoid structures surgically may be necessary to restore normal breathing and hearing.

**Intervention.** A tonsillectomy may be performed using a local anesthestic. On return from surgery the patient is placed in a Fowler's position. When a general anesthetic has been given, the patient may be placed on his or her side. Vital signs should be checked, just as for any postoperative patient. An ice collar is applied to the throat to relieve discomfort. The patient should be instructed not to cough or clear the throat, and talking should be discouraged for several hours. The patient should be observed for postoperative hemorrhaging, and care should be directed toward its prevention. The patient should not be allowed to gargle before healing begins because it may dislodge a clot and produce bleeding. If nausea is not present and if no bleeding develops, water or chipped ice may be given. If a temperature elevation occurs, the surgeon should be notified. A trace of blood is to be anticipated, but any unusual amount of bright red blood should be reported immediately. Suction equipment and packing should be available for emergencies.

**Patient/family teaching.** After returning home, patients need to get enough rest, eat soft foods, drink fluids, and gradually resume activity. Because delayed hemorrhaging may occur, bleeding is reported promptly to the physician.

## Foreign Bodies

If foreign materials become lodged in the throat or trachea, emergency treatment must be instituted. If the object cannot be dislodged by the finger, the nurse should stand behind the choking individual, hold the individual below the rib cage, and quickly squeeze (similar to a bear hug). This action, called the Heimlich maneuver, forces residual air and the foreign object out of the respiratory tract.

Aspirated foreign bodies are more likely to enter the right main bronchus, which is larger and in a more vertical position. If the object is small, coughing occurs and slight dyspnea develops. Aspiration of a foreign body often creates an acute emergency and necessitates prompt removal with a laryngoscope or bronchoscope. Occasionally a tracheotomy may be required to establish an airway. The nurse needs to approach the situation with calmness and carry out emergency orders with efficiency. When foreign bodies are removed from the bronchus or lung, steam inhalations may be prescribed along with sedative or analgesic drugs to relieve discomfort.

# TUMORS OF THE RESPIRATORY SYSTEM

## Cancer of the Larynx

Benign or malignant tumors may occur in any part of the respiratory system. Malignant tumors of the upper respiratory system are less common than are tumors in other parts of the body. Cancer of the larynx accounts for a small percentage of neoplasms.

As with malignant tumors in other parts of the body, the cause of carcinoma of the larynx is unknown. However, a strong association exists between cancer of the larynx and both alcohol consumption and tobacco use. When the condition is diagnosed early, a cure is possible. The disease is most common in men over 45 years of age.

### Assessment

The first symptom of laryngeal cancer is hoarseness, which becomes progressively worse without treatment. If this symptom is neglected, metastasis to other structures occurs and pain on swallowing or pain in the vicinity of the "Adam's apple" radiates to the ear. Ultimately the airway becomes obstructed and dyspnea occurs. Carcinoma of the larynx is diagnosed by obtaining a history and by visually examining the larynx with a laryngoscope. Mobility of the vocal cords is assessed. A biopsy is done for laboratory confirmation of the clinical findings. Depending on the location of the tumor and the extent of involvement, a partial or a total laryngectomy is performed.

### Intervention

Treatment varies with the extent of the malignancy and may include radiation therapy, partial laryngectomy, supraglottic laryngectomy, or total **laryngectomy** (removal of voice box) (Table 22-8).

When a total laryngectomy is performed, the larynx, vocal cords, thyroid cartilage, and epiglottis are removed surgically. The trachea is sutured to the anterior surface of the neck as a permanent tracheostomy (Figure 22-26). Because the patient no longer breathes through the nose, he or she has little sense of smell. The patient must be prepared emotionally for the loss of normal speech and the change in normal breathing.

Before the surgery the patient should be given an explanation of the operation, including the way in which

| TABLE 22-8 | | |
| --- | --- | --- |
| **Laryngectomy Surgery for Cancer** | | |
| **TYPE** | **DESCRIPTION** | **VOICE RESULT** |
| Partial laryngectomy; laryngofissure | Opening into larynx through thyroid cartilage with removal of diseased vocal cord | Husky but acceptable |
| Hemilaryngectomy | Same approach as for laryngofissure with removal of diseased false cord, arytenoid, and one side of thyroid cartilage | Hoarse voice |
| Supraglottic partial laryngectomy | Horizontal incision passes above true cords (left intact) with removal of epiglottis and diseased tissue | Normal voice |
| Total laryngectomy | Removal of epiglottis, thyroid cartilage, and three or four tracheal rings; closure of pharynx with trachea; permanent tracheostomy | No voice |

Modified from Phipps WJ et al: *Medical-surgical nursing: concepts and clinical practice,* ed 5, St Louis, 1995, Mosby.

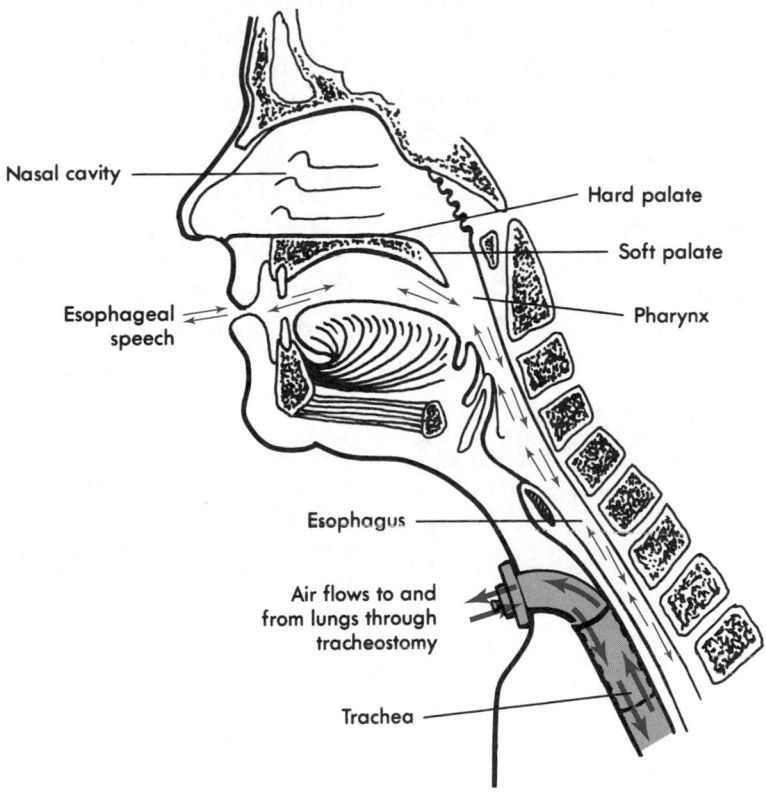

**Figure 22-26**    Permanent tracheostomy. There is no connection between the trachea and esophagus. (From Phipps WJ: *Medical-surgical nursing; concepts and clinical practice,* ed 5, St Louis, 1995, Mosby.)

normal speech is produced and how the operation will affect the production of speech. The patient should also be given information about speech therapy and informed that these resources will be available postoperatively.

After surgery the patient may be placed in the intensive care unit because continuous nursing care should be provided for the first 48 hours, or longer if necessary. If the patient is admitted directly to the surgical unit, it

should be prepared to receive the patient after surgery. Heated nebulizers are used to humidify the air. Equipment for caring for and cleaning a tracheostomy tube should be available, as well as suction, tissues, and a pencil and paper or slate. Some surgeons do not insert a tracheostomy tube because the method of suturing keeps the wound open. If a tube is inserted, it is a laryngeal (laryngectomy) tube, which is slightly larger in diameter and shorter than the ordinary tracheostomy

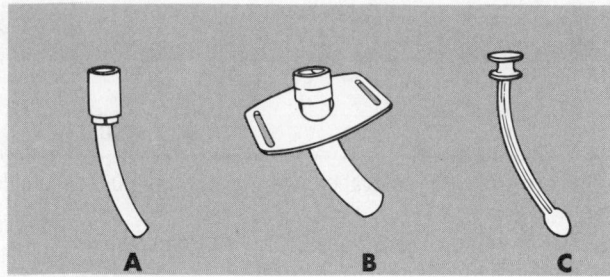

**Figure 22-27** Laryngectomy tube. **A,** Inner cannula. **B,** Outer cannula. **C,** Obturator.

tube (Figure 22-27). If a tube is inserted, a sterile set the same size as the one inserted should be available at the bedside for emergency use if the first tube comes out.

The most important function of the nurse is to keep the airway clear. The nurse must be available to wipe or suction secretions when the patient coughs. In the beginning, suctioning may be necessary as often as every 5 minutes. The suction catheter should not be inserted more than the length of the tube, and the physician should be notified if the secretions cannot be removed. Efforts should be made to prevent wound infection by maintaining aseptic technique. Oxygen may be administered for 1 to 2 days.

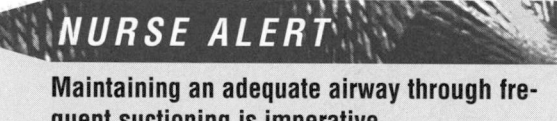

**NURSE ALERT**

**Maintaining an adequate airway through frequent suctioning is imperative.**

The character of respirations must be observed for any rate increase, wheezing, or crowing sounds, which indicate airway obstruction. Secretions may be tinged with blood for 1 or 2 days, but any continued bleeding may be from an internal hemorrhage and should be reported. Meticulous mouth care with an antiseptic mouthwash should be given often. If intravenous fluids are given, they should not be placed in the arm that the patient uses for writing if this can be avoided. The patient may not be allowed anything by mouth for a week. Feedings are given by means of a tube that is passed through the patient's nose. When the patient is allowed food by mouth, the food should be soft until healing is complete. Some surgeons do not order tube feedings but allow patients to eat soft food and drink liquids if they feel well enough. A patient with a laryngectomy usually is most comfortable in a 45-degree Fowler's position, which makes breathing easier. The

lips should be kept moist, and crusts should not be allowed to form around the nares.

As patients improve, they should be taught how to care for their own tracheostomy, and, if they are unable to do so, some member of the family should be taught (Lewis, Collier, Heitkemper, 1996). When a tube is used, it may be left in place for approximately 6 weeks. As soon as the neck wounds have healed, the therapist may begin speech training. Esophageal speech is the means of communication used after a laryngectomy. If esophageal speech cannot be learned, a vibrator or an electronic artificial larynx can be used. Much assistance can be obtained from local chapters of the American Cancer Society, including information on a Lost Cord Club or a New Voice Club. Most patients with total laryngectomies are able to return to normal roles in life, but they should be cautioned about occupational hazards such as dust and fumes and should seek to protect themselves against respiratory tract infections.

## CONDITIONS OF THE CHEST AND LOWER RESPIRATORY SYSTEM

### Chronic Obstructive Pulmonary Disease or Chronic Airflow Limitation

Diseases that interfere with ventilation cause psychologic, physical, and social problems for the patient. Fear, tension, frustration, and panic accompany these diseases. One of the most important aspects of medical and nursing care is the relief of anxiety. Inadequate ventilation disturbs the homeostasis, or equilibrium of the body. Electrolyte balance is affected, changes occur in the extracellular fluid, and serious cardiac complications may occur. The constant shortness of breath, fatigue, and limitation of activity may cause retirement from employment, limitation of social activities, and feelings of social isolation and depression.

Chronic obstructive lung diseases include emphysema, chronic bronchitis, bronchiectasis, and asthma, each of which may result in varying degrees of incapacitation (Box 22-6). Chronic obstructive pulmonary disease accounted for 84,000 deaths in 1989 and is the fifth leading cause of disability in the United States. Unlike heart disease and stroke, COPD has increased in incidence since that time (Higgens, 1993). Emphysema and chronic bronchitis are grouped under the broader terminology of COPD. Clinically it is difficult to quantify the components of the two diseases within one patient. They are discussed separately, but most patients have a mixture of the two obstructive lung diseases.

CHAPTER 22 ♦ Respiratory Problems    **597**

## PATIENT/FAMILY TEACHING

**LARYNGECTOMY AND RADICAL NECK DISSECTION**

**General Hygiene**
- Clean teeth and mouth 3 times daily because the ability to detect mouth odor is lessened; use mouthwash frequently.
- Wear a protective cover over the tracheostomy when taking a shower.
- Wear a protective cover over the stoma while shaving or having a haircut to prevent hair and dust particles from entering.

**Stoma Care**
- Observe the stoma daily for signs of redness, secretions, or swelling; observe also for fever.
- To prevent infection, always wash hands before touching the stoma.
- Clean the stoma twice daily using a clean, damp washcloth; the use of soaps should be avoided because they irritate the skin; tissues may obstruct the airway.
- Apply petrolatum around the exterior of the stoma, if ordered, taking care not to allow any to enter.
- Cover the stoma with a bib (a piece of cotton cloth) to aid in warming and filtering inspired air; a variety of clothing and accessories can be worn by men and women to cover the bib; high-neck sweaters, turtlenecks, and scarfs work well; there should always be easy access to the stoma for inserting a handkerchief or for emergency actions.

**Emergency Care**
- Wear a Medic Alert bracelet or carry a card indicating that a laryngectomy has been done and containing instructions regarding first aid should the stoma become obstructed or a cardiopulmonary arrest occur.
- Swimming may be possible with new commercial covers, but be aware that drowning could easily occur without getting the head wet; other people who have been instructed in first aid measures should be present during swimming.

**Stomal Hydration**
- Additional hydration is needed for the airway; use of commercial humidifiers or a pan of water on the stove or radiator will greatly add to comfort.
- When taking a bath or shower, allow water to accumulate 4 to 6 inches while sitting in the tub or standing in the shower stall on a nonslip mat; a well-wrung towel can be draped around the neck for added moisture and to prevent perspiration from dripping into the stoma.

**Other Healthful Behaviors**
- Moderation is the key rule in all normal activities; move slowly, control emotions, and exercise with moderation to avoid fatigue.
- When coughing, remember to cover the stoma instead of the mouth; moisture and secretions can be expelled onto clothing.
- Report persistent coughing to the primary provider.
- If there is a history of alcohol intake, moderation or abstinence must be practiced; smokers should stop and should seek assistance to do so.
- Use available community resources for support and speech rehabilitation as needed (American Cancer Society, Lost Cord Club).

From Beare PG, Myers JL: *Adult health nursing*, ed 3, St Louis, 1998, Mosby.

## Pulmonary Emphysema

Pulmonary emphysema affects persons of all socioeconomic levels. An estimated 10 million persons in the United States have emphysema. One of every four wage earners over age 45 with emphysema is disabled because of the disease. Emphysema is more common in men than in women, probably because of the higher incidence of smoking in men than women in the earlier part of this century (Beare, Myers, 1998).

Risk factors for pulmonary emphysema include smoking, age, male gender, family history, and hereditary. Smoking is by far the most important risk factor and accounts for 80% to 90% of cases of emphysema. An inherited deficiency of an enzyme, alpha$_1$-antitrypsin, causes emphysema in young adults as well as older people. Air pollution, temperature changes, and humidity appear to exacerbate the disease.

**Pathophysiology.** In pulmonary emphysema the alveolar walls and capillaries are destroyed, which decreases the area available for gas exchange between the bloodstream and the air. Chronic irritation to the bronchi, bronchioles, and alveoli causes inflammation with swelling and secretions. The lumen of the bronchioles narrows, especially during expiration, and air becomes trapped in the alveoli. The alveoli become distended and rupture or become scarred and thickened with a loss of elasticity. Infections hasten the process.

---

BOX 22-6

# NURSING PROCESS

## CHRONIC OBSTRUCTIVE PULMONARY DISEASE

### ASSESSMENT

- Dyspnea
- Hypoxemia
- Productive cough with mucopurulent sputum; barrel-shaped chest
- Use of accessory muscles
- Wheezing; diminished breath sounds with rhonchi and prolonged expiration
- Peripheral cyanosis
- Chronic weight loss
- Anorexia

### NURSING DIAGNOSES

- Impaired gas exchange related to inequality between ventilation and perfusion
- Ineffective airway clearance related to bronchoconstriction, increased mucus production, ineffective cough, and infection
- Ineffective breathing pattern related to shortness of breath, mucus production, bronchoconstriction
- Self-care deficit related to fatigue that is promoted by increase in work of breathing
- Activity intolerance related to hypoxemia and fatigue
- Ineffective individual coping related to effects of illness on life-style
- Anxiety related to respiratory difficulty

### NURSING INTERVENTIONS

- Administer bronchodilators as prescribed.
- Evaluate effectiveness of respiratory treatments.
- Administer oxygen only if ordered and in low concentrations (flow rate of 1 to 2 L/min).
- Teach and demonstrate diaphragmatic breathing and coughing.
- Give patient 6 to 8 glasses of fluids every day unless cor pulmonale is present.
- Provide a diet consisting of several small meals each day.
- Perform postural drainage with percussion and vibration as prescribed.
- Monitor for signs and symptoms of respiratory infections, including change in sputum amount, color, or consistency; shortness of breath; increased coughing.
- Maintain activity level within patient's abilities; encourage alternating activity with rest periods.
- Assist patient in developing a regular activity program to recondition and strengthen muscles; work with other disciplines (e.g., physical therapy) as needed.
- Observe for complications such as cor pulmonale or congestive heart failure.

### EVALUATION OF EXPECTED OUTCOMES

- Verbalizes the need for bronchodilators and for taking them at specified times
- Demonstrates the ability to use and care for the specific respiratory equipment being used
- Uses oxygen when appropriate and verbalizes safe handling of oxygen
- Demonstrates diaphragmatic breathing and coughing
- Verbalizes the need to consume 6 to 8 glasses of fluid each day
- Discusses diet and the need to consume several small meals each day
- Performs postural drainage correctly
- Identifies signs of early infection (e.g., sputum, shortness of breath, increased coughing)
- Verbalizes that pollens, fumes, gases, dusts, and extremes of temperature and humidity are irritants to be avoided
- Verbalizes the importance of maintaining regular activity; understands the need for rest periods and pacing of activities
- Participates in discharge plan
- Explores resources available in the community

---

Expiration of air depends on the elasticity of the lungs, but because of lost elasticity and obstructed bronchioles, not all of the inspired air can be forced out of the lungs. Increased pressure in the alveoli causes them to collapse. Distended air sacs (blebs) occurring on the surface of the lung may rupture and allow air to enter the pleural cavity, causing a spontaneous pneumothorax.

The pathologic changes cause a decrease in vital capacity and an increase in the residual volume of air retained in the lungs. Oxygenation of the arterial blood is decreased, and carbon dioxide tension of the arterial blood is increased in the later stages of disease. The retention of carbon dioxide in the blood may result in respiratory acidosis or carbon dioxide narcosis, stupor, and coma.

**Assessment.** Emphysema has an insidious onset. Dyspnea is the predominant symptom. As the disease progresses, dyspnea is experienced not only on exertion but also at rest. Any emotional upset, exertion, or excitement increases dyspnea and respiratory distress. Other manifestations of the disease include hypoxia, coughing with copious amounts of mucopurulent sputum, a barrel-shaped chest, the use of accessory muscles of respiration, wheezing, grunting on expiration, peripheral cyanosis, digital clubbing, chronic respiratory acidosis, chronic weight loss, anorexia, and malaise. Auscultation of the lung fields reveals diminished breath sounds with rhonchi and prolonged expiration.

**Intervention.** The most important role of the nurse in the treatment of emphysema is prevention. All patients should be encouraged not to start smoking or to quit smoking if they are smokers. Assistance with quitting should be offered with information about smoking cessation programs and aids such a the nicotine patch. Smoking prevention and cessation must be part of the nurse's role both in and out of the hospital. If there is a family history of emphysema, special risk is present and patients should be counseled to consider themselves at high risk for emphysema. When emphysema has been diagnosed, the focus of education should be self-management and avoidance of infection. Patients with emphysema should be encouraged to obtain influenza vaccination in early autumn and should also have pneumonia vaccination.

Patients with emphysema should avoid drafts and abrupt changes of temperature. Windows should be kept closed, and air conditioning is desirable in the hot weather because heat and humidity are usually not well tolerated. Treatment focuses on slowing the advance of the disease, maintaining functional status with moderate exercise, and making breathing as easy as possible. Some patients do better in moderate climates with minimum temperature changes. Severely affected patients should have a bedroom on the first floor of the home if possible. Coughing is the emphysema patient's first defense. Deep breathing, incentive spirometry, and aerosolized bronchodilators loosen secretions and improve ventilation (Haas, Haas, 1990).

Controlled coughing techniques can be used to clear secretions. Low, small, grunting coughs are produced after deep breaths while the abdominal muscles are supported. The patient may be taught to inhale by using the stomach muscles and to exhale by blowing gently through pursed lips. Chest physical therapy such as percussion, vibration, and postural drainage is often effective in removing secretions from affected lungs (Beare, Myers, 1998).

## OLDER ADULT CONSIDERATIONS

### BRONCHODILATOR THERAPY FOR COPD

Age-related changes in pharmacokinetics and the presence of other chronic health problems increase the older adult's risk for side effects associated with bronchodilator drugs used to treat COPD. For theophylline preparations the older adult should have drug level monitored at more frequent intervals than the young adult.

Side effects associated with anticholinergic bronchodilators, such as urinary retention and blurred vision, may be particularly troublesome for the older adult. Ipratropium bromide administered by inhalation will provide therapeutic benefit with fewer systemic side effects. The older adult should exercise caution in using over-the-counter bronchodilators. These drugs usually contain alpha and beta agonists (epinephrine and ephedrine) that can aggravate preexisting health problems such as hypertension or diabetes.

Although metered-dose inhalers may produce fewer side effects, the older adult may have difficulty learning to coordinate drug administration with respiratory activity. Decreased motor function and range of motion in the hands may render the older adult less able to use the device effectively.

From Beare PG, Myers JL: *Adult health nursing*, ed 3, St Louis, 1998, Mosby.

Bronchodilators are prescribed to dilate the airways. Because they relieve muscle spasm in the bronchioles, they improve gas exchange and reduce airway obstruction. Bronchodilators include anticholinergics and beta-adrenergic agonists. Cardiovascular side effects, nervousness, and tremors can be side effects of drugs from both classes. In addition, corticosteroids, mucolytics, expectorants, and, if an infection is present, antibiotics may be prescribed (Table 22-9).

Recent medical research indicates that small doses of an oral corticosteroid, usually prednisone, are beneficial. Usually 5 to 10 mg of prednisone is prescribed as ongoing therapy. During an acute infection or exacerbation, oral antibiotics may be added and corticosteroids increased or given intravenously if there is acute respiratory distress. If steroid therapy is continued, the patient must be monitored for side effects, including gastrointestinal bleeding, loss of bone density, decreased immunity, and increased appetite. When steroids are being discontinued, the dose is gradually reduced and then withdrawn completely.

**TABLE 22-9**

## Pharmacology of Drugs Used in Respiration

| DRUG (GENERIC AND TRADE NAME); ROUTE AND DOSAGE | ACTION/INDICATION | COMMON SIDE EFFECTS AND NURSING CONSIDERATIONS |
|---|---|---|
| **Acetylcysteine** (Mucocil)<br>**Route:** Nebulization via face mask, instillation via tracheostomy tube, or oral<br>**Dosage:** Usual dose is 6-10 ml 10% solution 3-4 times/day | Decreases the viscosity or thickness of mucus and secretions in patients who are debilitated or unable to cough and maintain a patent airway | Nausea, vomiting, rhinorrhea, stomatitis, fever, tracheal and bronchial irritation, chest tightness, and bronchospasm; cautious use in bronchial asthma, debilitated persons with respiratory disease |
| **Codeine** (Used in many cough/cold preparations)<br>**Route:** PO, liquid<br>**Dosage:** Usually 120 mg max over 24 hr; varies with product | Narcotic antitussive used in suppression of nonproductive coughing and relief of mild-to-moderate pain | Lightheadedness, dizziness, sedation, sweating, and nausea; cautious use in asthma or other pulmonary diseases; contraindicated with known or suspected narcotic addiction |
| **Dextromethorphan** (Comtrex, Dimetane-DX, Humidid-DM, Rondec-DM, Tylenol Cold Medication)<br>**Route:** PO, chewable pieces, liquid, lozenges, syrup<br>**Dosage:** 10-20 mg PO q 4 hr or 30 mg q 6-8 hr; controlled-release liquid (60 mg bid) | Nonnarcotic antitussive (cough suppressant), used for nonproductive cough only | Dizziness, GI distress, and drowsiness; contraindicated with MAO inhibitors |
| **Guaifenesin** (Robitussin)<br>**Route:** PO liquid, tablets, capsules.<br>**Dosage:** 100-400 mg q 3-6 hr; max 2.4 g/day | Expectorant used for symptomatic relief of dry, unproductive cough; associated with common respiratory disorders such as colds and bronchitis | Nausea, vomiting, GI distress, and drowsiness; cautious use with persistent cough, high fever, persistent headache, or rash; may decrease platelets and cause bleeding |
| **Ipratropium** (Atrovent)<br>**Route:** Inhaler<br>**Dosage:** Two inhalations 4 times/day, to a max of 12 inhalations within 24 hr | Anticholinergic bronchodilator used in the treatment of bronchospasm associated with asthma, chronic bronchitis, or emphysema | Coughing, dryness of oropharynx, gastric upset, and nervousness; cautious use in glaucoma, prostatic hypertrophy, and bladder obstruction; contraindicated in treatment of acute bronchospastic episodes |
| **Theophylline Ethylenediamine** (aminophylline; closely related to theophylline, Slo-Phyllin, Theo-Dur, Uniphyl, Slo-Bid)<br>**Route:** PO liquids, tablets, capsules, injection, rectal<br>**Dosage:** Highly individualized and adjusted on the basis of serum theophylline levels (optimal range 10-20 g/ml) | Symptomatic relief from or prevention of bronchial asthma and bronchospasm associated with chronic bronchitis, emphysema, and other obstructive pulmonary diseases | GI upset, nausea, nervousness, and urinary frequency; cautious use in elderly with circulatory impairment, renal or hepatic disease, peptic ulcer, hyperthyroidism, and diabetes; contraindicated in hypersensitivity to caffeine, severe gastritis, peptic ulcer disease, and myocardial stimulation |
| **Triamcinolone** (Azmacort)<br>**Route:** Inhaler<br>**Dosage:** 2 inhalations 3-4 times/day; max 16 inhalations/day | An inhaled corticosteroid used in treatment of bronchial asthma | Euphoria, insomnia, and peptic ulcer; bronchodilator inhalers should be taken before corticosteroid inhalers; overuse of inhalers may be harmful; sudden withdrawal of this inhaler could be fatal; corticosteroid inhalers should be terminated gradually if discontinued |

| TABLE 22-9 | | |
|---|---|---|

## Pharmacology of Drugs Used in Respiration—cont'd

| DRUG (GENERIC AND TRADE NAME); ROUTE AND DOSAGE | ACTION/INDICATION | COMMON SIDE EFFECTS AND NURSING CONSIDERATIONS |
|---|---|---|
| **ANTITUBERCULAR AGENTS** | | |
| **Ethambutol** (Myambutol) **Route:** PO **Dosage:** 15-25 mg/kg/day | Antitubercular used in combination with at least one other drug in the treatment of active tuberculosis or other mycobacterial diseases | Optic neuritis; use with caution in renal and severe hepatic impairment |
| **Isoniazid (INH)** (Isoniazid) **Route:** PO, IM **Dosage:** PO, IM, 5-10 mg/kg/day (usually 300 mg) or 15 mg/kg 2-3 times weekly after 2 mo at 300 mg/day | Antitubercular used as a first-line drug in combination with other agents in the treatment of the active disease; also used for prevention of tuberculosis (TB) in patients exposed to active disease | Peripheral neuropathy; contraindicated in acute liver disease and previous hepatitis from INH; use with caution in history of liver damage, chronic alcohol ingestion, severe renal impairment, malnourished patients, and diabetics; possible additive CNS toxicity with other antituberculars; severe reactions may occur with ingestion of foods containing high concentrations of tyramine |
| **Rifabutin** (Mycobutin) **Route:** PO **Dosage:** 300 mg once daily; if GI upset occurs, may give as 150 mg twice daily with food | Antimycobacterial used to prevent disseminated *Mycobacterium avium* complex (MAC) disease in patients with advanced HIV infection and used in the treatment of most strains of *Mycobacterium tuberculosis* | Brown-orange discoloration of tears, saliva, urine, and body fluids; cross-sensitivity with other rifamycins (Rifampin) may occur |
| **Rifampin** (Rifadin, Rimactane) **Route:** PO, IV **Dosage:** PO, IV, 10 mg/kg/day (usual dose 600 mg/day) single dose; may also be given twice weekly | Antitubercular used in combination with other agents in the management of active TB | Nausea, vomiting, heartburn, abdominal pain, flatulence, diarrhea, and red discoloration of all body fluids; use with caution in history of liver disease or concurrent use of other hepatotoxic agents |
| **Streptomycin** (Streptomycin) **Route:** IM **Dosage:** 15 mg/kg/day (not to exceed 1 g) or 25-30 mg/kg (not to exceed 1.5 g) 2-3 times weekly | Antiinfective, antitubercular used in combination therapy for active TB and for streptococcal or enterococcal endocarditis | Ototoxicity and nephrotoxicity; use with caution in renal impairment, neuromuscular diseases, and in the elderly |

Because of the constant high level of carbon dioxide in the blood and tissues of patients with emphysema, the body begins to rely on low levels of oxygen as the main stimulus for respiration. Administering high concentrations of oxygen to such patients may depress their respirations. If prescribed, oxygen should not be administered with a flow rate greater than 2 to 3 L/min unless the patient is in severe respiratory distress. In severe emphysema, oxygen may be administered at least 16 hours a day, with 24 hours often required. Oxygen should be started slowly, and the patient should be observed for restlessness, apprehension, flushed skin, shallow respirations, and stupor. The patient should also be observed for signs of right ventricular failure (**cor pulmonale**). Because the capillaries in the lungs have been destroyed by the disease process, the heart must work harder to pump blood through the diseased lungs. Edema of the feet and legs and distended neck veins may indicate the onset of right ventricular failure. Gastric ulcers also tend to occur in patients with emphysema, although the specific cause is unknown.

Physical therapy should be part of every patient's therapy program. Its purpose is to recondition and strengthen muscles that have become soft and flabby and have lost their tone because of inactivity. Patients should be encouraged to follow a graded program of daily exercise, which may include respiratory muscle training. Patients with emphysema usually breathe most easily when sitting up and find that leaning forward while supporting their upper body with elbows resting on a table will provide some relief of dyspnea (Beare, Myers, 1998). This position is thought to allow greater lung expansion by elevation of the rib cage. Patients may feel less well in the morning because secretions have collected in the lungs and bronchi during the night. A hot drink may loosen tenacious sputum so that it may be coughed up. By the end of the day patients may feel exhausted. They should be encouraged to care for themselves within the limits of their ability. The diet should be nourishing, and gas-forming foods should be eliminated. The appetite may be poor, and several small, attractive meals a day may be better than large meals. Fluids should be encouraged, if appropriate, to avoid the tendency toward dehydration. The nose and mouth should be kept clean, and all nursing care should be adapted to the needs of the individual patient. These needs change as the disease progresses, and the physician, nurse, patient, and family must work together to plan a way of life for the patient.

## Chronic Bronchitis

Chronic bronchitis often occurs with pulmonary emphysema. The diagnosis of chronic bronchitis includes evidence of excessive tracheobronchial secretions on a daily basis for at least 3 months of the year for 2 consecutive years with no other cause. Physiologic findings in obstructive chronic bronchitis are similar to pulmonary emphysema. The incidence of chronic bronchitis is greater among persons who smoke cigarettes, and cigarette smoking is considered the primary etiologic factor. Frequent pulmonary infections and other inhalants may be contributing factors. For example, severe air pollution has been found to aggravate the disorder and cause respiratory failure.

**Pathophysiology.** In chronic bronchitis an abnormal increase in the mucus-secreting cells of the bronchial epithelium and trachea occurs. The goblet cells (so named because of their shape) of the surface epithelium are increased. The bronchi become thickened, and fibrosis of the bronchioles with infiltration by inflammatory cells may occur. Chronic infection of the mucous membranes is usually present, and the sputum may contain a variety of pathogenic microorganisms. The normal function of the cilia is impaired, and they are unable to move secretions upward to be coughed up. Therefore mucous secretions may form pus in small bronchi, where they become a medium for infection.

**Assessment.** The most common physiologic response in chronic bronchitis is a persistent cough with large amounts of sticky but fairly thin liquid mucus. The cough lasts 3 months a year for 2 consecutive years, thus making it chronic. In the presence of shortness of breath the vital capacity is reduced and dyspnea, cyanosis, and wheezing occur. Severely debilitated patients may be unable to cough and clear the respiratory passages, and respiratory function is compromised.

**Intervention.** Treatment of chronic bronchitis includes teaching the patient to adopt a healthy lifestyle. Patients should get adequate sleep and rest, eat a well-balanced diet, and participate in some form of recreational activity. They should be cautioned to avoid exposure to respiratory tract infections, dust, and other irritants. Work that requires being outside during cold or wet weather should be avoided. If a change of employment is necessary, the patient may be referred to the social and rehabilitation service.

The most effective factor in treatment is to encourage the patient to stop smoking. Most methods of treatment, including bronchodilators, nebulized agents, and oral medications, have been shown to have a limited effect on chronic bronchitis. However, some patients may think that they provide some relief. Although antibiotics are often administered to prevent infection, the time to begin such therapy is debatable. When chronic bronchitis with airway obstruction has existed over a long period, respiratory failure and right ventricular failure may develop (Box 22-7).

## Bronchiectasis

**Bronchiectasis** is characterized by a permanent dilation of one or more of the bronchi as a result of repeated infections. A single lobe of one lung or one or more lobes in both lungs may be affected. The left lung tends to be involved more often than the right lung, although both lungs are involved in approximately 50% of patients. The cause of the disease is unknown, and although some cases are believed to be congenital, most appear to result from chronic bronchitis and severe attacks of infectious respiratory disease. Bronchiectasis is primarily a disease of the young and often affects persons 20 years of age or younger.

**Assessment.** In the early stages of bronchiectasis no symptoms may be present, but as the disease progresses, the most characteristic symptom is a productive cough. The cough is worse in the morning, and any change in position may produce paroxysms of coughing. The cough produces large amounts of puru-

| BOX 22-7 | NURSING PROCESS |
| --- | --- |

## CHRONIC BRONCHITIS

### ASSESSMENT

- Vital signs
- Respiratory status (e.g., work of breathing, breath sounds, sputum, cough, cyanosis)
- Restlessness, confusion
- Nutritional status
- Level of anxiety
- Tolerance of activity
- Sputum culture and sensitivity

### NURSING DIAGNOSES

- Ineffective airway clearance related to bronchial secretions
- Impaired gas exchange related to inadequate oxygenation
- Altered nutrition: less than body requirements related to dyspnea and fatigue
- Activity intolerance related to fatigue, work of breathing
- Risk for infection related to decreased pulmonary function, ineffective airway clearance, and stasis of secretions
- Anxiety related to changes in health, hypoxia

### NURSING INTERVENTIONS

- Encourage coughing and deep breathing.
- Position patient for optimal breathing.
- Assist with position changes.
- Provide room and oxygen humidification.
- Administer expectorants, bronchodilators, corticosteroids, and antibiotics as prescribed.
- Encourage fluid intake of 1½ to 2 L/day, unless contraindicated.
- Administer oxygen as prescribed.
- Provide small, frequent feedings.
- Provide a high-protein, low-carbohydrate diet.
- Avoid gas-forming foods.
- Plan rest periods.
- Provide a progressive increase in activity as tolerated.
- Encourage discussion of feelings, fears, concerns.
- Remain with patient during anxious periods.

### EVALUATION OF EXPECTED OUTCOMES

- Clear breath sounds
- No evidence of hypoxia
- $PaO_2$ >60 mm Hg
- Stable weight
- Afebrile
- Acknowledges anxiety
- Demonstrates knowledge of disease process with home care management

lent sputum, which may be tinged with blood. Hemoptysis occurs in a large number of cases, although it usually is not serious. As the disease gradually worsens, fever, chills, fatigue, weight loss, clubbing of the fingers, and a loss of appetite may occur. The diagnosis is made by x-ray examination and bronchoscopy. The only cure is surgical removal of the affected area (lobectomy). However, each patient must be carefully evaluated in relation to pulmonary function and prognosis because not all patients are suitable candidates for such surgery.

**Intervention.** Palliative treatment consists of measures to improve the general health, such as adequate diet, rest, and prevention of respiratory tract infections. Smoking, alcohol, and excessive exercise should be avoided. Irritants from air pollution may contribute to recurrent episodes of acute respiratory tract infections. Sputum cultures often indicate the presence of specific microorganisms, and antibiotic therapy for the

particular pathogen is administered. Postural drainage should be part of the patient's daily routine, and moist inhalations may make it easier to produce thin, tenacious sputum. Many patients are treated on an outpatient basis, but in severe exacerbation the patient is admitted to the hospital. The nurse should encourage and reassure the patient and assist with postural drainage or other chest therapy. Mouth care must be given several times a day, and the use of an antiseptic mouthwash before meals may be desirable. The patient should be constantly on the alert for airway obstruction from large plugs of mucus (Box 22-8).

**Patient/family teaching.** Patients are taught abdominal breathing and postural drainage. They are encouraged to avoid pulmonary irritants such as smoke; to monitor sputum for any changes in amount, color, or consistency; and to obtain an influenza and pneumococcal vaccine if recommended by their health care providers.

BOX 22-8

| | |
|---|---|
| **BOX 22-8** | **NURSING PROCESS** |

## BRONCHIECTASIS

**ASSESSMENT**

- Vital signs
- Respiratory status (breath sounds, cough, sputum)
- Breathing patterns
- Hemoptysis
- Chest x-ray films
- Sputum culture and sensitivity

**NURSING DIAGNOSES**

- Ineffective airway clearance related to bronchial secretions
- Ineffective breathing pattern related to bronchial obstruction and inflammatory process
- Altered nutrition: less than body requirements related to anorexia and dyspnea
- Activity intolerance related to weakness and dyspnea
- Fear related to hemoptysis

**NURSING INTERVENTIONS**

- Position with head of bed elevated.
- Encourage deep breathing and coughing.
- Avoid vigorous coughing.
- Assist with position changes.
- Administer oxygen as prescribed.
- Increase room humidification.
- Administer mucolytic agents, bronchodilators, antibiotics as prescribed.
- Encourage fluid intake to 1½ to 2 L/day, unless contraindicated.
- Provide oral hygiene before meals.
- Provide for small, frequent meals.
- Provide soft or liquid high-protein diet.
- Plan rest periods.
- Encourage adaptive breathing with activity.
- Provide progressive increase in activity.
- Validate sources of fear.
- Encourage discussion of feelings toward illness.

**EVALUATION OF EXPECTED OUTCOMES**

- Breath sounds clear
- Vital capacity optimal for patient
- No evidence of dyspnea
- Tolerating diet without dyspnea
- Stable weight
- Able to express fear

## Asthma

Asthma can be classified as **extrinsic** or **intrinsic.** Extrinsic asthma is caused by substances, or antigens, outside of the body to which the individual is hypersensitive. Approximately half of persons with asthma fall into this category. When it is impossible to determine any extrinsic factor, the disease is considered to be intrinsic asthma, or asthma that results from internal causes. Intrinsic asthma is most often caused by chronic recurrent respiratory tract infections. Attacks may be precipitated by emotional stress, irritating fumes, changes in temperature and humidity, and increased physical activity. Extrinsic or allergic asthma is more common in younger people under 30, while intrinsic asthma is more common in the elderly. However, research indicates that in an older adult, past allergies can continue to be manifested as asthma and in fact a mixed form of the disease may be present (Beare, Myers, 1998).

**Pathophysiology.** In acute attacks of asthma the lumina of the small bronchi become narrow and edematous because of an inflammatory response to various stimuli (Carroll, 1996). The mucus-secreting glands of the bronchi secrete a thick, tenacious mucus, which obstructs the narrowed passages of the bronchi. Inspiration and expiration become difficult, and in an effort to obtain more air the patient uses the accessory muscles of respiration. More air is forced into the lungs than can be expelled, which causes the lungs to increase in size. The vital capacity is decreased, but an increase in the residual volume of air occurs. In a severe attack, cyanosis occurs because of inadequate ventilation. Dyspnea is the primary symptom with wheezing, chest tightening, and rapid shallow breathing. After the acute attack subsides, the narrow lumen widens and the patient is able to cough and produce large amounts of thick, stringy sputum. Although the lungs return to their normal size after an attack, continued episodes lead to permanent impairment and emphysema.

**Assessment.** The characteristic physiologic symptoms of asthma are shortness of breath accompanied by wheezing and coughing. Severe symptoms indicate a severe attack. Pronounced wheezing that progresses to absence of breath sounds in the lungs is an ominous sign and indicates the need for immediate intervention. Results of arterial blood gas studies vary depending on severity and duration of the attack. In asthma, as in chronic bronchitis and emphysema, exhaling is more difficult than inhaling. The patient can reduce dyspnea markedly by sitting up and tilting the head forward during exhalation. After the normal exhalation the patient should gradually contract the abdominal muscles until no more air can be expelled from the lungs and then inhale. This procedure reduces the effort required for exhaling. As a result of the ventilation difficulty the patient may become cyanotic, and asphyxiation and death may occur during prolonged attacks if the patient is not treated with appropriate interventions, including mechanical ventilation. The patient generally perspires freely, may have a weak pulse, and may complain of pain in the chest caused by the respiratory effort. Nausea and diarrhea may occur in children. The cough of persons with asthma is usually tight and dry in the beginning, but, as the attack continues, the thin, mucous secretion becomes copious, thick, and stringy and is expectorated with difficulty.

**Intervention.** Treatment and care of asthma are directed toward three factors: (1) relief of the immediate attack, (2) control of causal factors, and (3) general care of the patient. Adults may be given 0.3 to 0.5 ml of a 1:1000 solution of epinephrine subcutaneously to reverse the inflammatory response, followed by corticosteroids, both parenterally and inhaled, and parenteral aminophylline. Inhaled aerosolized bronchodilators, such as albuterol (see Table 22-9), may be used to supplement therapy in acute exacerbations (Carroll, 1996).

During an acute attack of asthma the patient should be placed in a sitting position with humidified oxygen administered by nasal cannula and be made as comfortable as possible. Humidification of inspired air helps loosen secretions so that they can be expectorated more easily. Dietary orders should be carried out, and the patient should be encouraged to drink adequate amounts of fluid. If the fluid intake is inadequate, intravenous fluids may be ordered. Most attacks subside in 30 to 60 minutes, although they may continue for days or weeks.

Sometimes an asthma attack does not respond to bronchodilator and steroid treatment at home or in the emergency department. When this occurs, the patient is said to have status asthmaticus, a life-threatening complication of asthma. This condition requires hospitalization and intensive therapy with more effective, intravenous medication and respiratory therapy treatments around the clock. Because of increased airway resistance resulting from edema, mucous plugging, and bronchospasm, the symptoms are similar to an asthma attack but more severe and prolonged. Anxiety, fear of suffocation, and panic, which worsen the attack, may result.

The patient with status asthmaticus displays the use of accessory muscles of respiration, hypoxemia, and hypocapnia. Wheezing is usually present but may not be audible if airflow obstruction is severe enough to cause insufficient airflow. Ultimately, respiratory acidosis occurs if the condition does not respond to treatment. If the acidosis is severe, mechanical ventilation may be necessary. In some cases mechanical ventilation may be avoided with oxygen administration, intensive medication therapy, and careful monitoring. This patient requires cardiac monitoring because of the cardiac effects of many of the medications that are given to cause bronchodilation.

The calm reassurance and constant availability that the nurse provides help to relax the patient. Frequent lung assessments are necessary to monitor the effects of therapy. Patients with status asthmaticus must be watched closely because frequent medication adjustments are needed if the patient worsens. Status asthmaticus may continue for days to weeks and may cause death as a result of cardiac or respiratory arrest (Lewis, Collier, Heitkemper, 1996).

The control of asthma depends on finding and eliminating the cause. If the disease is caused by extrinsic factors (allergy), the offending allergen may be identified through skin tests and the patient can be desensitized. If intrinsic factors are suspected, a thorough physical examination should be performed to determine a source of infection, specific organisms, or other physical factors (Box 22-9).

**Patient/family teaching.** Patients with asthma should be advised against smoking and should avoid exposure to cold, wet weather. Sleep, rest, and breathing exercises should be incorporated into activities of daily living.

# RESPIRATORY INFECTIONS

## Acute Bronchitis

Bronchitis is caused by inflammation of the bronchial tree and the trachea. It is caused by infection in the upper respiratory tract but may also result from bronchial irritation caused by exposure to chemical agents or may be a complication of communicable diseases such as measles. Acute bronchitis usually begins with hoarseness and cough, a slight elevation in temperature, muscle aches, and a headache. The cough may be dry and painful but gradually becomes productive. Bed rest is indicated as long as the temperature is elevated. Treatments should be directed toward preventing the extension of the infection. Both plain and medicated cool mist vaporizers soothe irritated respiratory passages. Aerosol therapy may be given, and antibiotics may be ordered. Sedative or

---

BOX 22-9

# NURSING PROCESS

## ASTHMA

### ASSESSMENT

- Personal history of asthma
- Current medications
- Respiratory status (breath sounds, breathing patterns, sputum)
- Evidence of respiratory distress
- Level of anxiety
- Vital signs
- Pulmonary function tests

### NURSING DIAGNOSES

- Ineffective breathing pattern related to anxiety and decreased lung expansion
- Ineffective airway clearance related to secretions and bronchospasm
- Activity intolerance related to imbalance between oxygen supply and demand
- Risk for infection related to steroid therapy and stasis of airway secretions
- Anxiety related to difficulty breathing

### NURSING INTERVENTIONS

- Assist with positions for optimal breathing (head of bed elevated).
- Administer oxygen as prescribed.

- Assist with relaxation techniques.
- Increase room humidification.
- Encourage fluid intake to 1½ to 2 L/day, unless contraindicated.
- Plan rest periods.
- Provide progressive increase in activity as tolerated.
- Assist with nebulizer respiratory therapy and physiotherapy.
- Encourage oral hygiene after aerated corticosteroids.
- Encourage optimal nutrition.
- Assist with identifying coping skills.
- Encourage questions and discussion of feelings.
- Provide accurate information about asthma.
- Provide comfort measures.
- Stay with patient during acute attack.

### EVALUATION OF EXPECTED OUTCOMES

- Vital capacity measurements optimal for patient
- Clear breath sounds
- Able to perform ADLs
- Afebrile
- No evidence of anxiety
- Demonstrates knowledge of disease process and home care management

---

expectorant drugs may be ordered for the cough. If no complications occur, recovery may be expected in a week to 10 days.

# Pneumonia

Pneumonia is a disease of the lungs and is caused by bacteria, viruses, fungi, and mycobacteria. It may occur in comatose or oversedated patients and in those whose pulmonary ventilation is inadequate. It may result from aspiration of infected secretions from the upper respiratory or gastrointestinal tract, may complicate certain viral diseases such as measles or influenza, and may cause complications, including empyema, septicemia, meningitis, and endocarditis. Most community-acquired pneumonia is caused by *Streptococcus pneumoniae* (pneumococcus) and occurs in the very young and in older adults.

Hospital-acquired or nosocomial pneumonias are most often related to bacterial invasion of the lower respiratory tract by *Pseudomonas aeruginosa, Klebsiella pneumoniae,* and *S. aureus* (Figure 22-28). Nosocomial

pneumonias account for 16% of all hospital-acquired infections. Nosocomial pneumonias are often carried from patient to patient by the hands of unknowing hospital personnel. Strict hand-washing protocols before and after patient care and use of universal precautions decreases the incidence of this cause of nosocomial pneumonia. The severity of the infection is related to the number of bacteria invading the patient and the **virulence** of the organisms.

Legionnaires' disease is an acute bacterial bronchopneumonia that is caused by a gram-negative bacillus. Its name is derived from the 1976 American Legion convention in Philadelphia, during which the disease affected 180 people and caused 29 deaths. The bacterium is airborne and has an affinity for stagnant water such as that found in air-conditioning and cooling systems. Therefore it tends to affect people who work together in one building or who come together in large groups, such as at conventions. It tends to occur in epidemics, particularly during the summer, with a severity that ranges from a mild pneumonitis to a multilobar pneumonia with a 10% to 15% mortality.

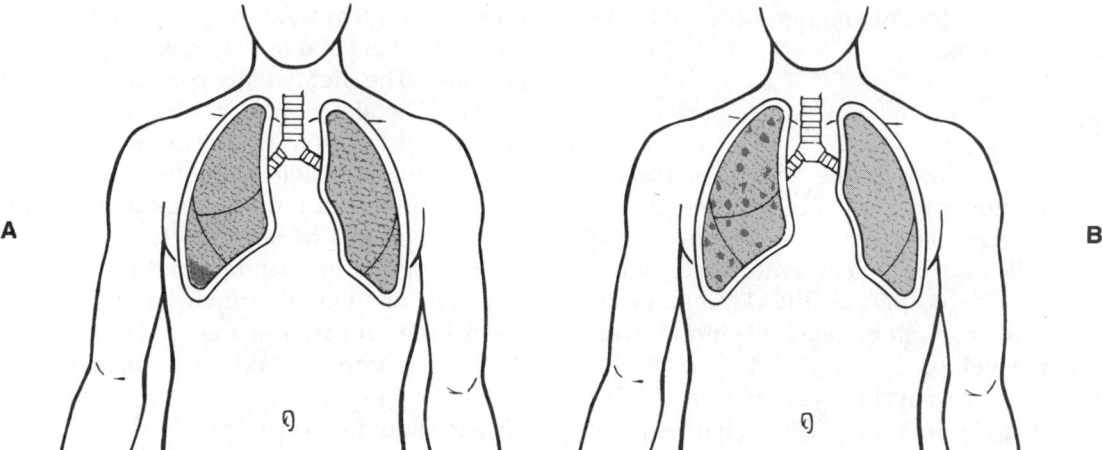

**Figure 22-28** **A,** Bacterial pneumonia may affect one or more lobes of the lung. **B,** Viral pneumonia appears as a patchy distribution throughout the lung.

The symptoms are similar to those of bacterial pneumonia, but the cough may be nonproductive at first and signs of gastrointestinal upset are more likely to be present.

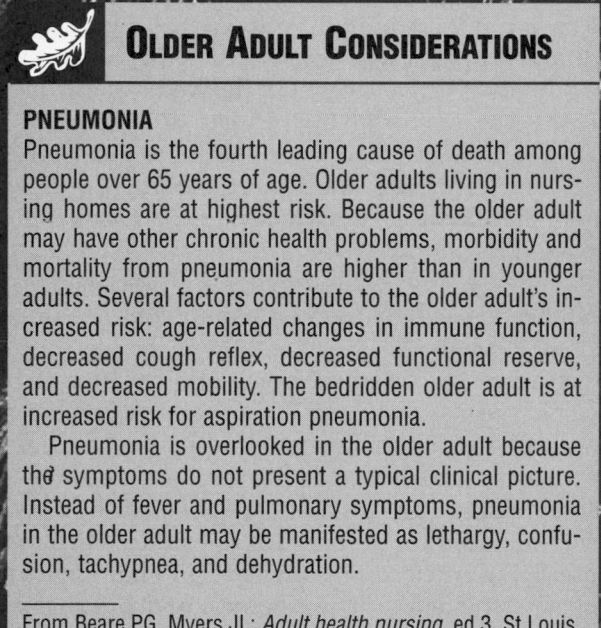

**OLDER ADULT CONSIDERATIONS**

**PNEUMONIA**
Pneumonia is the fourth leading cause of death among people over 65 years of age. Older adults living in nursing homes are at highest risk. Because the older adult may have other chronic health problems, morbidity and mortality from pneumonia are higher than in younger adults. Several factors contribute to the older adult's increased risk: age-related changes in immune function, decreased cough reflex, decreased functional reserve, and decreased mobility. The bedridden older adult is at increased risk for aspiration pneumonia.

Pneumonia is overlooked in the older adult because the symptoms do not present a typical clinical picture. Instead of fever and pulmonary symptoms, pneumonia in the older adult may be manifested as lethargy, confusion, tachypnea, and dehydration.

From Beare PG, Myers JL: *Adult health nursing*, ed 3, St Louis, 1998, Mosby.

Pneumonia caused by a virus usually appears as a patchy infection throughout the lung (Figure 22-28). The onset is slower and is characterized by chills, fever, profuse sweating, aching, and a painful cough.

The sputum is mucopurulent and may contain blood. The temperature elevation generally runs an irregular course, varies even during the day, and may continue for as long as 3 weeks. Viral pneumonia is rarely fatal, and although the patient is extremely uncomfortable, it is less serious than bacterial pneumonia. However, patients with viral pneumonia may require a longer period of convalescence.

Cytomegalovirus is the most common cause of viral pneumonia in immunosuppressed persons. It may occur in patients with organ transplants or acquired immunodeficiency syndrome (AIDS) and in those taking antineoplastic drugs. Cytomegalovirus produces severe pneumonia with high mortality rates. *Pneumocystis carinii* pneumonia has the greatest incidence in patients with AIDS or receiving immunosuppressive therapy.

## Pathophysiology

Infected secretions from the upper respiratory tract drain into the alveoli, where the normal defense mechanisms, such as ciliary action and coughing, are unable to remove them. An inflammatory process begins, and increased amounts of fluid are released in the area. The serous fluid moves easily into additional alveoli and bronchioles. As the process continues, less surface area is available for the absorption of oxygen and the release of carbon dioxide. Leukocytes and a few erythrocytes begin to accumulate in the affected alveoli, and they increase in number until they completely fill each alveolus, which results in consolidation. Phagocytosis begins in the consolidated alveolus, and the area is finally cleared. In the beginning, only one lobe of the lung may be involved, but the infected fluid may spread to the bronchial tree of another lobe and begin another infection process.

## Assessment

Symptoms vary among individuals. However, the onset of bacterial pneumonia is usually sudden and accompanied by severe chills and chest pain. These symptoms are followed by a temperature elevation, which may be as high as 40.5° C (105° F), and an increase in pulse and respiratory rates. A painful, constant cough may develop.

Initially the sputum may be clear or tinged with blood, but within 48 hours it develops a characteristic rusty appearance. The sputum is thick and tenacious and may be expectorated with difficulty. Suction should be available if needed to help clear the airway. Leukocytosis may be present, with the number of white blood cells ranging from 20,000 to 30,000/mm³; the skin is hot and moist; the lips are dry; and the tongue is parched. Nausea, vomiting, diarrhea, and jaundice occasionally appear. Fever blisters (herpes simplex) may appear on the lips and nose, and sores may cover the tongue. Restlessness and delirium may accompany pneumonia.

## Intervention

Nursing care of patients with pneumonia is a major factor in the progress and prognosis of the illness. Pneumonia is debilitating and exhausting. Treatment and care involve keeping the patient as comfortable as possible, planning care to avoid any unnecessary expenditure of energy, and using antibiotic and sulfonamide agents to help the body's defenses overcome the infection. The type of antibiotic used depends on the particular organism present and whether the organism remains sensitive to the drug. Sputum cultures should be obtained before treatment with the antibiotic is started. Analgesics may be used to relieve pain, and nonpharmacologic measures may also be used to promote comfort. The patient may be encouraged to deep breathe and cough if secretions are present. Cough analgesics and increased humidity help to relieve coughing. Oxygen may be prescribed if the patient has cyanosis, dyspnea, or shortness of breath.

The patient's room should be well ventilated, have a temperature between 20° C and 21° C (68° F and 70° F), and be free from drafts. A restful, quiet environment should be provided. The patient should be positioned to allow for the greatest comfort and may be placed in a high (90-degree) Fowler's position or on the affected side. The position should be changed often. The nursing care plan should be made to provide nursing care with periods of uninterrupted rest. Visiting should be limited during the acute phase of the disease. Blood pressure and temperature, pulse, and respiratory rates are checked every 4 hours or as the patient's condition indicates. The diet usually consists of liquids, and the total fluid intake may be increased to 2000 or 3000 ml/day. The patient may need to be encouraged to take food or fluids. If pneumonia occurs in a patient with cardiac disease, the nurse should determine if fluids and sodium are to be restricted. Intake and output records should be maintained. Intravenous fluids designed to maintain electrolyte balance may be ordered. Special mouth care must be given several times each day. A lubricant should be applied to the lips and should be used to soften any crusts on the nares. Fever blisters should be kept dry.

## Tuberculosis

Tuberculosis (TB) continues to be a public health problem in the United States, with over 20,000 cases reported annually. Since 1984, there has not been the decline in TB morbidity that health officials would have expected (see Chapter 14). In fact, there have been substantial increases in TB in areas with a high prevalence of human immunodeficiency virus (HIV) infection (see Chapter 16) and in elderly residents of long-term care facilities, where an estimated 1.5 million infections occur annually (Poker, 1997).

The hazard associated with TB has increased as multiple-drug-resistant strains (MDR-TB) have developed. With effective treatment delayed as health care providers search for an appropriate drug therapy, individuals remain in an infectious state for a longer time, which increases the risk of infecting those with whom they come in contact (Centers for Disease Control and Prevention, 1994).

Pulmonary TB is caused by an acid-fast bacterium, the tubercle bacillus (*Mycobacterium tuberculosis*). It is carried through the air in infectious droplet nuclei, which are produced when the infected person sneezes, coughs, speaks, or sings. When persons breathe air that has been contaminated by an infectious person, they may become infected with the TB organism.

Individuals at greatest risk for TB include those who are immunocompromised, such as with HIV infection; those living in close or crowded conditions, such as homeless shelters, nursing homes, and prisons; and persons who use intravenous drugs and alcohol. The elderly and the malnourished are also at risk.

When the bacillus enters the lung, the body responds by surrounding it with monocytes, which fuse to form giant cells. Fibrous tissue grows around the area, and the central portion of this growth of cells becomes necrotic. The entire inflammatory process is called granulomatous inflammation. If the number of organisms entering the lung is small and the resistance of the body is high, healing occurs by scarring. If a large number of organisms are inhaled into the lung, the inflammation overwhelms the body's defenses and a more extensive destruction of lung tissue occurs, which results in lung cavities. TB can be a primary or secondary disorder. Secondary TB usually occurs late in life or when individuals are immunocompromised.

## Assessment

Symptoms vary from patient to patient depending on the extent of the disease. The most common symptom of pulmonary TB is a cough. Initially the cough is nonproductive, but if left untreated, it becomes productive with mucoid or mucopurulent sputum. Hemoptysis may eventually develop. Patients may complain of pleuritic chest pain and systemic effects, including weight loss, night sweats, fever, malaise, anorexia, and fatigue. TB is detected with skin testing, acid-fast-stained sputum specimens, and chest x-ray examinations.

**TB test—Mantoux.** Tuberculosis is detected by administering a purified protein derivative (PPD) of the tubercle bacillus in an intradermal injection, known as the Mantoux test. The injection is given in the forearm, and the solution is injected into the skin layer, forming a wheal. If the patient is infected with TB, either active or dormant, lymphocytes will recognize the PPD antigen and cause a localized **induration** or hardening of the tissue at the site. The site of the injection is charted and circled and then examined between 48 and 72 hours after injection. Any local induration indicates that the

---

# NURSING CARE PLAN

## PATIENT WITH PNEUMONIA

Mr. Jenkins is a 61-year-old man who comes to the emergency department with a complaint of shortness of breath, chills, fatigue, and "feeling terrible." He states that he has not been well for 1 week, has a loss of appetite, has muscle aches, and feels "very drawn."

| Medical History | Psychosocial Data | Assessment Data |
|---|---|---|
| Denies COPD, cardiac disease, hypertension, and diabetes mellitus | Married 40 years; supportive, caring wife | Alert and oriented × 3 (time, place, and person) |
| Has a history of smoking one pack per day (PPD) of cigarettes since the age of 13 (48 pack years) | Three adult daughters, all with young children, live locally and visit often | Febrile to 101°-103° F; respirations 24 to 26, regular but labored; some use of accessory muscles; painful cough with small amount of sputum (thick, tenacious, yellowish mucoid); oxygen at 3 L |
| Denies alcohol consumption | Full-time truck driver (retired as a limousine driver) | *Respiratory:* Bilateral scattered crackles throughout entire lung fields |
| Has good health behaviors as evidenced by yearly physicals | Practices Catholic religion | *Cardiovascular:* Pulse 86 to 90, regular rate; no murmurs; brachial, radial, femoral, popliteal, and pedal pulses palpable bilaterally |
| Involved in physical sports until 4 years ago; now his activity level is sedentary | Active social life, with many friends | *Abdominal:* Soft, nontender, nondistended, with bowel sounds heard in all four quadrants; bowel movement on day of admission |
| | Owns home | *Skin:* Clean and intact; no broken skin areas, no pressure ulcers or rashes |
| | Insured through private medical insurance | *Laboratory data* |
| | *Hobbies:* Gardening and fixing cars | WBC 18,000, Hgb 12.2, Hct 39, Electrolytes WNL |
| | | Purified protein derivative placed |
| | | Sputum sent for culture and acid-fast bacillus (AFB) |
| | | *Urinalysis:* WNL |
| | | *Chest x-ray:* Consistent with pneumonia bilateral lower lobes |
| | | *Medications* |
| | | IV-D5 ½ N/S at 100 ml/hr cefazolin (Ancef) 1 g in 50 ml D5W over 20 minutes q 6 hr |
| | | Acetaminophen (Tylenol) tabs prn for discomfort |

*Continued*

# NURSING CARE PLAN
## PATIENT WITH PNEUMONIA—cont'd

**NURSING DIAGNOSIS**

Ineffective airway clearance related to tracheobronchial secretions as evidenced by abnormal breath sounds (crackles) and labored breathing

| NURSING INTERVENTIONS | EVALUATION OF EXPECTED OUTCOMES |
|---|---|
| Help the patient cough productively. | Demonstrates effective coughing techniques |
| Teach effective coughing and deep breathing exercises; have patient sit or lie on side with knees flexed. | Verbalizes importance of drinking enough fluid to liquify secretions |
| Splint patient's chest when coughing or straining. | Verbalizes minimal pain and uses measures to reduce pain |
| Administer analgesic before having patient cough. | Airway is free of secretions |
| Use nonpharmacologic measures to reduce pleuritic pain (relaxation, distraction). | Verbalizes need to take antibiotics at prescribed times |
| Humidify air to loosen secretions and promote ventilation. | Maintains oxygen saturation (SaO$_2$) at a predetermined level |
| Encourage fluids 2000-3000 ml daily unless contraindicated. | BP within patient's normal range |
| Perform postural drainage, percussion, and vibration to mobilize secretions. | Temperature normal |
| Administer prescribed antibiotics at correct time intervals. | Pulse and respiratory rate within normal range |
| Provide oxygen as ordered for dyspnea, hypoxemia, or confusion; monitor pulse oximetry to determine effectiveness of oxygen therapy. | Breath sounds clear without evidence of crackles, rhonchi, or decreased breath sounds |
| Monitor patient's response to therapy. | |
| Assess vital signs q 4 hr or as indicated, including blood pressure, pulse, respirations, and temperature. | |
| Auscultate chest q 4 hr or as indicated, identifying crackles (rales) or signs of consolidation (decreased breath sounds, dullness on percussion). | |

**NURSING DIAGNOSIS**

Anxiety related to respiratory difficulties

| NURSING INTERVENTIONS | EVALUATION OF EXPECTED OUTCOMES |
|---|---|
| Teach relaxation techniques. | Demonstrates decreased anxiety through facial expressions and body language |
| Use a caring approach; provide time to listen actively. | Participates in own care |
| Encourage participation in care as tolerated. | Discusses fears and feelings and identifies behaviors of progress |
| Discuss physical feelings and relate them to the compromised lung status. | |
| Help patient compare and contrast behaviors of progress. | |

**NURSING DIAGNOSIS**

Activity intolerance related to imbalance between oxygen supply and demand as evidenced by shortness of breath (SOB) and increased respiratory rate with activity

| NURSING INTERVENTIONS | EVALUATION OF EXPECTED OUTCOMES |
|---|---|
| Provide environment conducive to rest; turn down lights when resting; monitor for noise level. | Lists factors that cause fatigue and shows increasing tolerance with activity level after periods of rest |
| Help patient assume and maintain a comfortable position. | Assumes optimal position for adequate rest and breathing |
| Plan nursing care to include uninterrupted rest periods. | Participates in plans for activities of daily living (ADLs) |
| Encourage patient to help plan activity progression. | |

## NURSING CARE PLAN
### PATIENT WITH PNEUMONIA—cont'd

**NURSING DIAGNOSIS**

Knowledge deficit related to course of illness and health risk behaviors (smoking) as evidenced by verbal questioning

| NURSING INTERVENTIONS | EVALUATION OF EXPECTED OUTCOMES |
| --- | --- |
| Explain the rationale for rest, increased fluids, and activity monitoring because they maintain the body's natural defenses. | States factors that contributed to the illness |
| Discuss behaviors that suggest the need for modification of ADLs; initiate a discussion on smoking. | Identifies behaviors of progress and discusses the rationale for rest, increased fluids, and ADL monitoring |
| Ask if patient is motivated to stop smoking; discuss any previous attempts to quit, and identify the rationale for previous failures; cite statistics related to the risks of smoking, including cardiovascular and pulmonary problems; recommend self-help groups for support. | Identifies the risks involved in smoking, and cites motivational level to quit; plans to attend a self-help smoking cessation group |
| Discuss the importance of obtaining an influenza vaccine and pneumococcal vaccine at specified intervals. | Plans to obtain vaccinations |
| Discuss importance of follow-up examinations after discharge. | Makes an appointment for follow-up care |

patient is positive for tuberculosis infection. The amount of induration is measured in millimeters and recorded (Box 22-10).

**Two-step TB test.** It is common now to use a two-step method, in which a negative reading is followed by another injection of "second-strength" PPD. If this second test is negative, the patient does not have TB.

If the patient is known to have TB, the PPD test is not administered because the local reaction can be severe. Chest x-ray examination is required to determine the presence of disease in the lungs. The PPD test will not cause TB because no live organisms exist in the PPD solution.

## Treatment

Hospitalized patients with active TB should be isolated in negative-pressure rooms until effective medication therapy has been initiated. Usually patients are hospitalized for a short time for diagnostic evaluation and sent home with a prescription for a combination of drugs. Their care and medication compliance are monitored by home care or public health nurses.

Treatment usually requires more than one drug. Triple therapy in the form of streptomycin, isoniazid (INH), and rifampin is prescribed. The Centers for Disease Control and Prevention recommends a minimum of 6 months of therapy with isoniazid, rifampin, and pyrazinamide for the first 2 months, followed by 4 months of isoniazid and rifampin. A 9-month treatment regimen is also acceptable and includes isoniazid and rifampin (see Table 22-9) (Centers for Disease

Control and Prevention, 1994). The best way to measure the effectiveness of therapy for pulmonary TB is to monitor sputum specimens at least every month. In patients with sputum negative for TB before treatment, follow-up treatment focuses on chest x-ray examinations and clinical evaluation of symptoms.

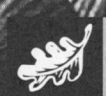

## OLDER ADULT CONSIDERATIONS

**TUBERCULOSIS**

Many factors contribute to the increased incidence of tuberculosis among older adults. Normal age-related changes in immune function and the presence of chronic health problems increase their susceptibility. Many older adults were exposed to tuberculosis when younger because of its former prevalence. The occurrence of tuberculosis in the older adult may represent reactivation of a dormant infection. The decreased immune function limits the usefulness of skin tests in diagnosing the disorder. A chest x-ray film or sputum culture is more accurate.

The classic symptoms may not be present. Instead the older adult may have only weight loss or anorexia as a clinical manifestation. Drug therapy for tuberculosis is effective in the older adult, but more frequent monitoring for side effects is an important part of nursing management.

From Beare PG, Myers JL: *Adult health nursing,* ed 3, St Louis, 1998, Mosby.

---

| BOX 22-10 | NURSING PROCESS |
|---|---|

## ACTIVE TUBERCULOSIS

**ASSESSMENT**

- Respiratory status (breath sounds, cough, breathing pattern)
- Weight loss, anorexia, night sweats, chest pains
- Previous exposure to TB
- Vital signs (temperature q 4 hr)
- Sputum culture (AFB)
- ABGs, if indicated

**NURSING DIAGNOSES**

- Ineffective breathing pattern related to sputum production
- Risk for infection related to active pulmonary TB
- Diversional activity deficit related to isolation
- Ineffective management of therapeutic regimen related to long-term therapy
- Knowledge deficit related to new diagnosis and treatment
- Altered nutrition: less than body requirements related to fatigue, malaise

**NURSING INTERVENTIONS**

- Administer oxygen as prescribed.
- Position for optimal breathing (head of bed elevated).
- Encourage fluids.
- Maintain respiratory isolation.
- Keep tissues at bedside and teach proper disposal of secretions.
- Administer medications as prescribed.
- Encourage expression of feelings.
- Encourage diversional activities.
- Discuss importance of following medical treatment.
- Encourage optimal nutrition.

**EVALUATION OF EXPECTED OUTCOMES**

- Clear breath sounds
- Negative sputum culture
- Stable weight
- Adheres to treatment regimen
- Verbalizes knowledge of TB medications and follow-up therapy

---

## Patient/Family Teaching

Patients and family members need to be aware that not treating TB can have serious consequences. Education should be individualized to meet the needs of the patient and family and should focus on the following objectives:

- Disease process and transmission
- Medication education (understanding of regimen)
- Medication action, dosage, and side effects
- Hand washing
- Use of tissues and proper disposal
- Treatment regimen
- Reporting for sputum monitoring
- Smoking cessation, if indicated
- Encouraging close contacts (family, friends) to report for examination
- Attending follow-up appointments
- Importance of compliance of therapy
- Taking medications as prescribed
- Signs and symptoms of relapse

## Acquired Immunodeficiency Syndrome

Patients with AIDS are at great risk for pulmonary infection, particularly pneumonia caused by *Pneumocystis carinii*. Patients with AIDS also are at risk for TB and Legionnaires' disease (see Chapter 16).

# PLEURAL CONDITIONS

## Pleurisy and Empyema

Pleurisy results from inflammation of any part of the pleura. Several forms of the disease exist, which are referred to as dry pleurisy, wet pleurisy, or pleurisy with effusion. Empyema is characterized by pus formation. Although the disease may occur spontaneously, it is more likely to be a complication of pneumonia or TB. The disease has been less common since the development of antibiotic therapy.

## Assessment

The first symptom may be a severe knifelike pain on inspiration, which may be referred to the shoulder or to the abdomen on the affected side. This pain occurs when the inflamed pleurae rub together during respiration. Coughing, dyspnea, and vomiting may occur, and the patient may hold the abdomen with a boardlike rigidity. Pleurisy with effusion is less dramatic than dry pleurisy, and the first symptom may be dyspnea, which occurs when the accumulation of fluid in the pleural cavity has become large enough to compress the lung. The acuteness of the dyspnea depends on the size of the effusion. Other symptoms are related to the cause and may include a temperature elevation.

If the fluid becomes purulent and empyema develops, the temperature may reach 40.5° C (105° F), with chills, profuse perspiration, and prostration.

## Intervention

The treatment of pleurisy depends on the type and stage of the disease and is directed toward removing the underlying cause through the administration of the appropriate antibiotic to combat the infection. If fluid is present in the pleural cavity, a thoracentesis may be performed and the fluid aspirated, followed by the instillation of an antibiotic. If the pleural fluid has become purulent and empyema has developed, adequate drainage and specific antibiotics must be provided. With antibiotic therapy, the need for an open thoracotomy has been almost eliminated. Patients with pleurisy usually are apprehensive and worried. A quiet environment and a nurse's sympathetic and understanding approach to patients and their conditions help their recovery. Patients are more comfortable if they lie on the affected side and turn toward this side when coughing. Pain should be relieved, and generally the use of acetaminophen is sufficient. Oxygen may be administered if dyspnea is severe. Because pleurisy often follows a debilitating disease, an adequate diet is important. The diet should be high in protein, calories, vitamins, and minerals, and supplemental feedings may be helpful.

## Atelectasis

Atelectasis, or collapse of a part of the lung, is a common postoperative complication that can occur when the patient breathes rapidly and shallowly to prevent pain at the surgical site. The supine position, respiratory depression from narcotics and relaxants, and abdominal distention increase the risk for atelectasis. It may also be seen in smokers, obese individuals who are on prolonged bed rest, and patients with respiratory tract infections or chronic obstructive pulmonary disease (COPD).

## Pathophysiology

Atelectasis occurs from the blockage of air to a portion of the lung. It may result from pressure against the lung as a result of air or fluid in the pleural cavity, tumors, an enlarged heart, or any abdominal condition that pushes the diaphragm upward. It may also result from an obstruction within one of the bronchi. A foreign body or a thick plug of mucus may occlude a bronchus and shut off all air to a portion of the lung. As the air in the isolated part of the lung is absorbed by the capillaries and new air no longer enters, the part involved collapses.

## Assessment

The severity of the symptoms depends on the degree of alveolar tissue involved, the rate at which the obstruction develops, and the presence of a secondary infection. Patients who develop atelectasis usually have dyspnea, anxiety, cyanosis, tachypnea, tachycardia, decreased blood pressure, elevated temperature, and pain on the affected side. Crackles and decreased breath sounds may be auscultated in the affected areas.

## Intervention

The key to the treatment of atelectasis is prevention. Postoperative and other high-risk patients should be taught how to cough and breathe deeply. Mobility should be encouraged, and bedridden patients should be turned and repositioned every 1 to 2 hours. Incentive spirometry may be used to promote deep inspiration and to improve ventilation and bronchial drainage. Chest percussion and postural drainage help with expectoration of bronchial secretions. Suctioning, oxygen, and administration of aerosols and humidity are also used.

## Pulmonary Embolism

A **pulmonary embolism** (PE) is a thrombus (clot) or foreign substance that travels through the systemic circulation and into the pulmonary circulation, which causes a complete or partial obstruction of the pulmonary artery or one of its branches. Generally 90% to 95% of PEs arise from the deep veins of the leg. Other causes of PE include air embolism, fat embolism, septic emboli, tumor emboli, and clots originating from the right atrium or ventricle.

An estimated 50,000 to 100,000 persons die of PE every year (Beare, Myers, 1998). In addition, many cases are thought to go undiagnosed as patients with terminal illnesses die. Most cases of PE result from mobilization of blood clots in the lower extremities (deep vein thrombosis or DVT).

Pulmonary embolism may occur as a postoperative complication of orthopedic surgery certain types of general surgery and gynecologic, obstetric, urologic, or neurosurgical procedures. Patients with various types of disease, usually chronic, are also at high risk for thrombotic events (Beare, Myers, 1998). Risk factors include conditions or events that predispose the individual to venous stasis, vessel wall injury (injury to the innermost lining of the vein), and hypercoagulability (Box 22-11). These three factors are most commonly associated with the development of DVT and subsequent PE. (See Chapter 24 for treatment of DVT.)

Once an embolus lodges, pulmonary blood flow to the area beyond the clot or embolus is interrupted, which results in a ventilation-perfusion mismatch.

Although a portion of the lung is still being ventilated, no blood is flowing to the involved area to pick up oxygen and remove carbon dioxide. To maintain adequate gas exchange, ventilation increases in uninvolved lung areas and bronchoconstriction occurs to reduce wasted ventilation. The airways distal to the embolus constrict, and the alveoli shrink and collapse. Ventilation is shifted away from areas of poor perfusion. Atelectasis may follow.

## Assessment

The symptoms of PE vary with the severity of the condition, but the most common are pleuritic chest pain, tachypnea, dyspnea, and apprehension. Other signs and symptoms include crackles (rales), hemoptysis, tachycardia, cyanosis (in severe cases), and shock. Diagnostic evaluation includes chest x-ray examinations, electrocardiograms (ECG), ventilation-perfusion (V/Q) scanning, and pulmonary angiography. The chest x-ray film may be normal, and the ECG often shows tachycardia. The arterial blood gas measurement shows hypoxemia with a decrease in $PaO_2$. $PaCO_2$ (carbon dioxide) also decreases as a result of tachypnea. With a decrease in $PaO_2$ and $PaCO_2$, the blood becomes more alkaline and the pH increases. The V/Q scan demonstrates areas of ventilation without perfusion. If there is V/Q mismatch, a high probability of PE exists. If a DVT is suspected, evaluation may also include Doppler ultrasonography, duplex scanning, impedance plethysmography, and venography. These tests serve to evaluate lower extremity circulation and determine any obstruction resulting from a thrombus.

## Intervention

The patient must be immediately stabilized, and further assessments must be performed. Continued nursing care focuses on the improvement of gas exchange, the maintenance of optimal cardiac output, the reduction of anxiety, and the relief of pain. When anticoagulation is initiated, the nurse also maintains anticoagulation, monitors for bleeding, and educates the patient regarding the anticoagulant(s) being administered. Nursing measures include the following:

1 Initial stabilization and further assessment
   - Initiate bed rest.
   - Provide oxygen via nasal cannula or face mask.
   - Help patient assume a semi-Fowler's position.
   - Evaluate respirations, noting rate, rhythm, depth, and effort.
   - Arrange for arterial blood gases (ABGs).
   - Obtain intravenous access.
   - Arrange for chest x-ray examinations.
   - Reassess for increased signs of hypoxia, such as pallor, cyanosis, restlessness, nasal flaring, retraction of intercostal spaces, gasping respirations, and use of accessory muscles.
   - Encourage patient to breathe normally.
   - Be prepared to use mechanical ventilation if patient respiratory distress is severe.
2 Improvement of gas exchange
   - Reassess for signs of hypoxemia.
   - Monitor ABGs.
   - Provide oxygen as needed.
   - Position patient to achieve an optimal V/Q relationship.
3 Maintenance of optimal cardiac output
   - Monitor vital signs every 30 minutes to 1 hour.
   - Monitor for cardiac arrhythmias.
   - Maintain IV line patency.
   - Be prepared to administer fluids and medications to maintain cardiac output.

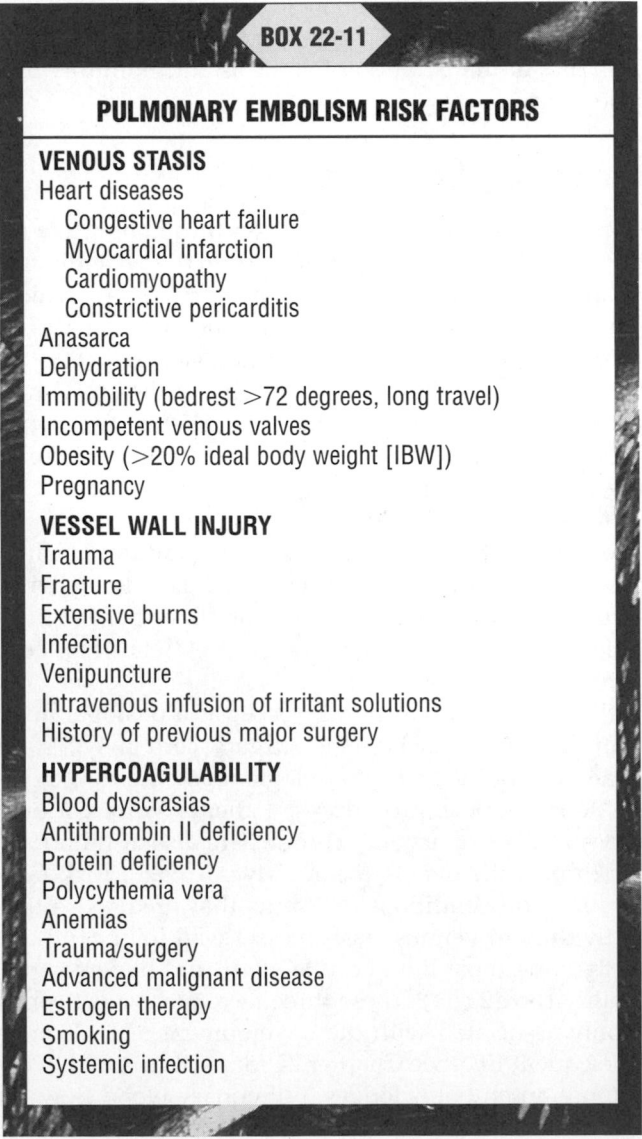

**BOX 22-11**

**PULMONARY EMBOLISM RISK FACTORS**

**VENOUS STASIS**
Heart diseases
    Congestive heart failure
    Myocardial infarction
    Cardiomyopathy
    Constrictive pericarditis
Anasarca
Dehydration
Immobility (bedrest >72 degrees, long travel)
Incompetent venous valves
Obesity (>20% ideal body weight [IBW])
Pregnancy

**VESSEL WALL INJURY**
Trauma
Fracture
Extensive burns
Infection
Venipuncture
Intravenous infusion of irritant solutions
History of previous major surgery

**HYPERCOAGULABILITY**
Blood dyscrasias
Antithrombin II deficiency
Protein deficiency
Polycythemia vera
Anemias
Trauma/surgery
Advanced malignant disease
Estrogen therapy
Smoking
Systemic infection

4 Reduction of anxiety and relief of pain
- Provide pain medication as ordered.
- Provide assurance, approach patient calmly, and maintain as stable (quiet) an environment as possible.
- Position patient for comfort and to optimize V/Q relationship.
5 Maintenance of therapeutic anticoagulation and prevention of bleeding
- Initiate anticoagulation medications as ordered.
- Monitor prothrombin time (PT) and partial thromboplastin time (PTT).
- Monitor for signs and symptoms of bleeding.
- Keep anticoagulant antagonist available.
6 Recognition of the hazards of immobility
7 Patient education

The treatment of PE may include anticoagulation therapy, thrombolytic therapy, or surgery. Intravenous heparin is often the initial treatment. It can begin when the patient is being evaluated and before all diagnostic testing has been completed, especially if there is a strong suspicion of a pulmonary embolus or if the patient's condition is unstable. Heparin is used to prevent the extension and propagation of a thrombus and the development of new thrombi. The patient is usually given a loading bolus of 5000 to 10,000 units, and a continuous infusion is begun. The goal is to maintain the PTT at 1.5 to 2 times normal. Heparin therapy is usually maintained for 7 to 10 days.

Warfarin (Coumadin) administration is usually started while the heparin therapy is being maintained (overlapping of therapies) and continues for 3 to 6 months following a PE. Warfarin works on vitamin K-dependent clotting factors, which are synthesized by the liver (factors II, VII, IX, X). Because the half-lives of these factors range from 6 hours to 90 minutes, it may take 3 to 5 days for the PT to become therapeutic (Box 22-12).

The PT is maintained at approximately 1.5 times the control. Anticoagulation therapy is contraindicated in

---

| BOX 22-12 | NURSING PROCESS |
|---|---|

### PULMONARY EMBOLISM

**ASSESSMENT**
- Respiratory status (breath sounds, breathing patterns)
- Evidence of respiratory distress, apprehension, confusion
- Evidence of thrombophlebitis
- Evidence of bleeding if receiving anticoagulants (skin, stools, urine, sputum)
- Complaints of chest pain
- Skin temperature, peripheral pulses
- Vital signs
- Level of consciousness
- Laboratory studies: ABGs, CBC, PT, PTT

**NURSING DIAGNOSES**
- Impaired gas exchange related to alteration in ventilation/perfusion
- Ineffective breathing pattern related to substernal chest pain, anxiety, hypoxia
- Risk for injury: bleeding related to anticoagulant therapy
- Anxiety related to hypoxia, dyspnea, and sudden change in health
- Risk for decreased cardiac output related to pulmonary hypertension
- Pain related to acute inflammatory process in lungs
- Knowledge deficit related to new medical condition and treatment

**NURSING INTERVENTIONS**
- Administer oxygen as prescribed.
- Anticipate the need for intubation.
- Position for optimal breathing (head of bed elevated).
- Administer anticoagulants as prescribed.
- Monitor IV delivery system.
- Maintain bedrest during acute episode.
- Assist with position changes q 2 hr.
- Administer IV fluids.
- Administer analgesics as prescribed.
- Monitor pulse oximetry continuously during acute episode.
- Provide rest periods.
- Encourage discussion of feelings.
- Provide emotional support.

**EVALUATION OF EXPECTED OUTCOMES**
- ABGs WNL for patient
- Clear breath sounds
- No evidence of respiratory distress
- No pain with respiratory effort
- No evidence of bleeding
- Verbalizes decreased or absent anxiety

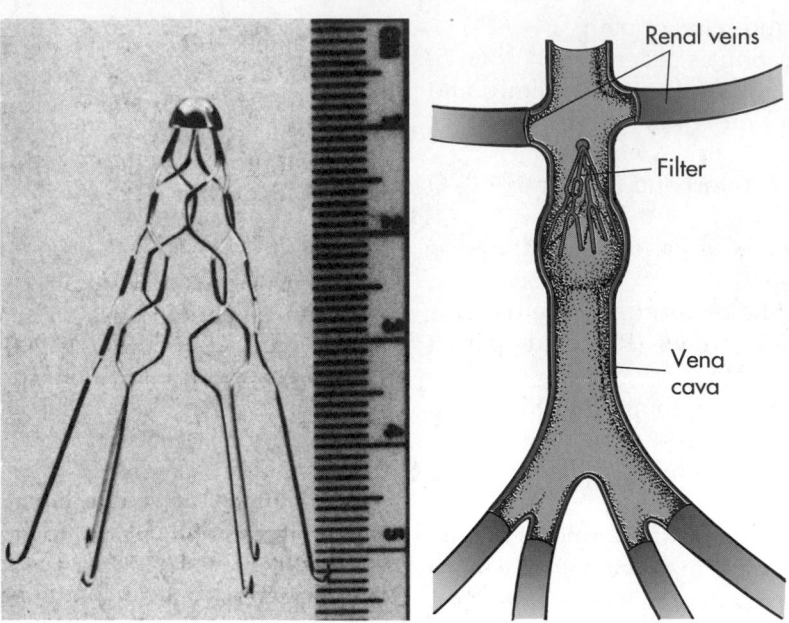

**Figure 22-29** **A,** Greenfield vena cava filter. **B,** Greenfield filter is placed in the inferior vena cava just below the renal veins. (**A** from Davis JH et al: *Surgery: a problem-solving approach*, ed 2, St Louis, 1995, Mosby. **B** from Beare PG, Myers JL: *Adult health nursing*, ed 3, St Louis, 1998, Mosby.)

patients who are at risk for bleeding, and bleeding must be watched for when a patient is receiving heparin or warfarin. Bleeding may be seen in the form of hematemesis, hematuria, or ecchymosis. Before initiation of anticoagulation, a baseline PT/PTT should be obtained, and the hemoglobin level, hematocrit, and platelet count should be monitored at intervals before and during anticoagulation therapy.

Thrombolytic therapy (urokinase, streptokinase, tissue plasminogen activator [t-PA]) may also be used in treatment (White, 1996). These agents result in a more rapid resolution of the thrombi or emboli as they dissolve the existing clot. Because bleeding is a significant side effect, thrombolytics are reserved for those with massive PE or those with severe DVT that affects the thigh or pelvis because the likelihood of the clot embolizing in these patients is greater. Before thrombolytic therapy is initiated, thrombin time (TT), PTT, PT, hematocrit level, and platelet counts are obtained. During therapy all but essential invasive procedures are avoided. If necessary, blood products are used to reverse the bleeding tendency (e.g., fresh frozen plasma). Surgical intervention may be indicated if the patient has persistent hypotension, shock, and respiratory distress. An embolectomy may be performed if the pulmonary artery pressure is greatly elevated and if arteriography shows obstruction in a significant portion of the pulmonary vasculature (Beare, Myers, 1998).

Vena caval interruption is used to prevent recurrent PE by interrupting the venous flow or filtering the venous blood. The use of a Teflon clip to interrupt the flow is rare now, but a variety of filters are inserted to trap clots in the vena cava and prevent their flow to the lungs. The inferior vena cava is entered through the femoral or jugular vein and a filter, such as an umbrella, birdcage, Nitinol, or Venatech, may be inserted. The procedure requires local anesthesia and sedation and is relatively minor (Beare, Myers, 1998). Figure 22-29 illustrates the use of an umbrella filter.

## Patient/Family Teaching

Patient/family education focuses on teaching the patient about the anticoagulant he or she is taking. This information can be provided to patients when Coumadin therapy is instituted. Patients should also be taught how to decrease their risk of DVT or PE (Box 22-13).

## Measures to Prevent Deep Vein Thrombosis and Subsequent Pulmonary Embolism

Nurses have an important responsibility in teaching patients how to prevent DVT and PE (see Box 22-13). Identifying patients at risk for DVT and PE is important, followed by taking action to prevent thrombus formation. These actions include pharmacologic and

## BOX 22-13

### Guidelines for Nursing Care to Prevent Deep Vein Thrombosis and Pulmonary Embolism

1 Prevention is the key.
2 Identify the risk factors that predispose the patient to the development of a DVT.
3 Implement appropriately prescribed prophylactic regimens.
4 Document patient tolerance of prophylactic measures.
5 Assess lower extremities each shift and monitor for signs and symptoms of DVT, including swelling, tenderness, warmth, and redness. Remember to investigate risk factors because the patient may be without symptoms.
6 Encourage early ambulation and leg exercises every hour while the patient is awake.
7 Perform passive range-of-motion exercises if the patient is immobile.
8 Avoid placing pillows directly under the knees.
9 Encourage fluid intake to avoid dehydration and monitor input and output (I&O).
10 Monitor laboratory values as ordered.
11 Educate the patient regarding anticoagulant therapy.

mechanical (nonpharmacologic) modalities. In 1986 the National Heart, Lung, and Blood Institute and the Office of Medical Applications of Research of the National Institutes of Health discussed and agreed on particular prophylactic measures, which take into consideration patient age, health history, risk factors, and the surgery being performed, as well as the efficacy and safety of these measures.

Pharmacologic measures include low-dose subcutaneous heparin usually given as 5000 units two or three times a day until the patient is discharged. It can be used in moderate- or high-risk patients and may also be combined with other mechanical measures. Coumadin may also be used in high-risk patients such as candidates for hip replacement and those with hip fractures. Lovenox (enoxaparin) is a drug that is similar to heparin and is used to prevent blood clots from forming, especially postoperatively in hip replacement patients. It is given by injection into the subcutaneous tissues for about 10 days after surgery. Family members may be taught to give this medication at home and monitor the patient for side effects. Bruising or unexplained bleeding such as nosebleeds, blood in the stool or urine, or bleeding from the gums should be reported to the doctor.

## PATIENT/FAMILY TEACHING

### COUMADIN THERAPY

Coumadin is an anticoagulant and is sometimes called a blood "thinner." Coumadin lengthens the time it takes the blood to clot and helps prevent clots from forming in the bloodstream. You and your health care provider (physician or nurse) are partners in your care.

A blood test must be done to check your body's response to Coumadin. The test is called a "prothrombin time" or "protime." This test is performed every day while you are in the hospital and at scheduled times after you go home. The following guidelines can add to the success of your treatment:

1 Inform your health care provider and dentist that you take Coumadin.
2 Do not take any medicines, especially aspirin, ibuprofen, cold tablets, and vitamin K, without checking with your provider. These medicines can affect your protime.
3 Limit your intake of alcohol.
4 Eat a well-balanced diet. Do not eat large amounts of food that are high in vitamin K, such as liver, dark green leafy vegetables, cauliflower, tomatoes, bananas, fish, cheese, egg yolks, and beef fat.
5 Take your Coumadin at the same time each day according to directions given to you. If you forget to take a pill, call your provider. Do not take another pill to catch up.

6 Obtain your protime blood test as instructed. Your provider will talk with you about where to go (laboratory or hospital) for the test.
7 Notify your provider if you notice any sign of bleeding:
   a Black or bloody bowel movements
   b Blood in the urine
   c Bleeding gums
   d Nosebleeds that do not stop
   e Bad headaches or dizziness
   f Abdominal pain or vomiting of liquid that looks like "coffee grounds"
   g Easy bruising

**Do not** stop taking Coumadin on your own. Instead talk with your health care provider about any concerns or problems you may have.

*Safety measures:*

1 Use a soft toothbrush.
2 Use an electric razor.
3 Do not go barefoot.
4 Talk with your healthcare provider before beginning any contact sports.
5 Carry a card in your wallet or purse to let people know that you take Coumadin.

Mechanical (nonpharmacologic) measures include graduated compression stockings, which may be used in very low-risk patients, and intermittent pneumatic compression (IPC). With IPC, a pair of inflatable sleeves is applied to the patient's lower legs. The sleeves are connected via air tubes to a pump compression unit that rapidly inflates them to a pressure between 40 and 50 mm Hg, maintains the pressure for 10 to 12 seconds, and deflates. IPC is well suited for patients who cannot tolerate anticoagulant therapy because of bleeding risks and can be used in low-, moderate-, and high-risk patients. IPC can also be combined with anticoagulant therapy if indicated.

# TUMORS OF THE LUNG

Tumors of the lung may be benign or malignant. A malignant chest tumor can be primary and arise from within the lung or mediastinum, or it may represent a metastasis from a primary tumor site somewhere else in the body. Because the bloodstream transports free cancer cells from primary cancers elsewhere in the body, metastatic tumors of the lung often occur and may invade the alveoli and the bronchi (Beare, Myers, 1998).

Many tumors of the lung arise from bronchial epithelium. Bronchial adenomas are slow growing and usually benign but are also vascular and therefore produce symptoms of bronchial obstruction and bleeding. Bronchogenic carcinoma is a malignant tumor that arises from the bronchus. Such a tumor is epidermoid and is usually located in the larger bronchi, or it is an adenocarcinoma and arises farther out in the lung. Several intermediate or undifferentiated types of lung cancer also exist and are identified by cell type.

The incidence of malignant tumors (bronchogenic carcinoma) of the lung has been increasing. It is more common in men than in women, but the incidence in women is steadily climbing. It is also more common in smokers than in nonsmokers and is related to the duration and the amount (intensity) of smoking. Additional risk factors include occupational exposure to asbestos, radioactive dusts, arsenic, and particular plastics, either alone or in combination with tobacco smoke.

## Assessment

Depending on the location and size of the tumor, the patient may or may not experience symptoms. Usually a cough and dyspnea are the only signs, and the tumors may have been present for some time before they are detected. The cough may begin as a hacking, nonproductive cough and may later progress to a point at which the sputum becomes thick and purulent. Therefore a cough that changes in character should warrant further investigation. A wheeze may be present if a bronchus becomes partially obstructed, and blood-tinged sputum may also be noted, especially in the morning. Pain is usually a late symptom and may be related to bone metastasis. If the tumor spreads to adjacent structures and lymph nodes, symptoms may occur as a result of obstruction or of pressure on structures. These symptoms include chest pain and tightness, hoarseness, dysphagia, head and neck edema, and pleural or pericardial effusion (Beare, Myers, 1994). Diagnostic evaluation includes many of the tests previously discussed, including a chest x-ray examination, sputum examination, bronchoscopy, and CT scanning. Preoperative evaluation of the patient is important and includes information already presented on p. 582.

## Intervention

Treatment depends on cell type, stage of the disease, and general health status of the patient. It may involve surgery, radiation therapy, and chemotherapy, which may be used alone or in combination. Nursing interventions focus on ways to maintain airway patency, including coughing when indicated, use of the IS, and deep breathing. Oxygen therapy may be used with pulse oximetry and monitored at specified intervals.

The psychologic aspects of caring for the patient with lung cancer are extremely important. The patient may be faced with many decisions and must choose among treatment options. Providing an atmosphere in which the patient can share his or her feelings and concerns is essential. Depending on the particular patient situation, resources to help the individual adjust and cope with the diagnosis are available in the hospital or community and include advanced practice nurses in oncology and mental health, as well as nurses in hospice settings.

# CHEST TRAUMA

Chest trauma accounts for approximately 25% of all trauma-related deaths in the United States. Injuries to the chest are serious surgical emergencies and may involve the thoracic cage, pleura, lungs, heart, diaphragm, and abdominal organs. The care of the patient is determined by the extent of the injury. Patients with chest wounds are often apprehensive, and the nurse should explain procedures that are done to or with the patient (Beare, Myers, 1998). When treating chest trauma, time is of the essence. Patient history focuses on the time the event occurred and on identifying the mechanism of injury. Blood loss is estimated, and, if the patient is responsive, the use of alcohol or drugs is determined.

The physical examination includes assessment of the airway, breathing pattern, vital signs, and skin color. The position of the trachea is assessed, and breath sounds are auscultated. Initial laboratory tests include electrolytes, complete blood cell count (CBC), type and crossmatch, chest x-ray examination, urinalysis, electrocardiography, and arterial blood gases. The patient's level of consciousness is also assessed. Agitation and confusion are signs of decreased blood flow and delivery of oxygen to the brain. Initial management involves maintaining the airway by whatever means possible, including mechanical ventilation. Any pneumothorax or hemothorax is managed, usually via insertion of a chest tube that is connected to water-seal drainage. Hypovolemia is corrected using colloid (e.g., blood products, albumin) and crystalloid, such as dextrose and normal saline or lactated Ringer's solution administered intravenously.

## Rib Fractures

Rib fractures are the most common type of chest trauma. The fifth through the ninth ribs are those most commonly injured. The patient experiences severe pain and muscle spasm at the site of the fracture. Pain is exacerbated by movement, deep breathing, and coughing. Management focuses on pain control. Sedation is used to relieve pain and to allow for deep breathing and coughing. A chest binder may decrease pain on movement. Caution must be taken to relieve pain but not compromise respiratory function. Pain usually shows improvement in 5 to 7 days, at which time nonnarcotic analgesics may be used. Most fractures heal in 3 to 6 weeks.

Multiple adjacent rib fractures can result in a freefloating segment of the rib cage (flail chest). When this occurs, the free segment loses continuity with the rest of the chest wall and moves paradoxically. Therefore, on inspiration, when the rest of the rib cage is moving outward, the flail segment sinks inward. On expiration, when the rib cage is moving inward, the flail segment bulges outward. Because pressure within the chest is decreased as a result of this paradoxical movement, movement of air is decreased. Previously all patients with flail chest were treated with mechanical ventilation, but now mechanical ventilation is avoided unless absolutely necessary. Patients are given analgesics to help decrease pain and to facilitate deep breathing and coughing. The patient should be encouraged to cough and breathe deeply and should be ambulatory as soon as the condition permits.

## Penetrating Wounds

Penetrating wounds may be caused by any foreign object. Knife and bullet wounds may penetrate the lungs and cause an air leak. When this occurs, the air may compress the lung and cause a pneumothorax, or bleeding into the pleural cavity may occur and cause the lung to collapse. Both phenomena are serious because they may lead to cardiac or respiratory arrest unless immediate emergency treatment is given. The patient should be observed for dyspnea, and the blood pressure, pulse, and respiratory rates should be checked at frequent intervals. Oxygen may be administered, and a chest tube may be inserted and connected to closed drainage to remove air and blood. If the injury is such that surgical repair is necessary, a thoracotomy is later performed. An antibiotic and a tetanus toxoid injection generally are administered. A tracheotomy may be required to provide for adequate ventilation in cases in which respiration is severely compromised.

## ADULT RESPIRATORY DISTRESS SYNDROME

Adult respiratory distress syndrome (ARDS) (referred to as shock lung, wet lung, stiff lung, and congestive lung syndrome) is a combination of symptoms that result from direct or indirect injury to the lung. Many factors contribute to the development of ARDS, including viral and bacterial pneumonia, chest trauma, head injury, surgery, any form of shock, oxygen toxicity, smoke inhalation, aspiration of toxic irritants, near drowning, drug overdose, fat or air emboli, **sepsis** (or infection), **disseminated intravascular coagulation,** massive blood transfusions, renal failure, pancreatitis, and radiation injury to the lung.

### Pathophysiology

In ARDS an alteration in the alveolar capillary membrane occurs, and the increased capillary permeability causes fluids to leak into the interstitial spaces, small airways, and eventually the alveoli. The lungs become edematous, and hypoxemia occurs. The fluid affects the activity of surfactant (the lipoprotein that helps maintain the elasticity of the alveolar tissue), and the alveoli collapse, which leads to shunting of blood away from the fluid-filled or collapsed alveoli and interferes with oxygen transport. Plasma and red blood cells escape from the damaged capillaries and cause hemorrhage.

### Assessment

Symptoms of ARDS may occur within hours of the lung injury or may not appear for several days.

Initially the patient experiences rapid, shallow breathing and dyspnea. The dyspnea and tachypnea rapidly become more severe, and hypoxia, intercostal retractions, cyanosis, crackles, rhonchi, and tachycardia appear. Hypoxia and cyanosis respond poorly to oxygen therapy. As the ventilation-perfusion imbalance worsens, the hypoxia becomes overwhelming and results in hypotension and signs and symptoms of respiratory and metabolic acidosis.

## Intervention

Treatment of ARDS is aimed at maintaining adequate alveolar ventilation and tissue oxygenation and at correcting the underlying cause. Many of the respiratory modalities discussed earlier in this chapter are instituted. High concentrations of oxygen are administered through a tightly fitting mask, which allows for the use of continuous positive air pressure. Often the patient requires intubation with mechanical ventilatory support and positive end-expiratory pressure (PEEP). PEEP improves ventilation and perfusion by inflating the alveoli and preventing their collapse. When high positive airway pressures would aggravate lung injury, high-frequency jet ventilation may be required. This type of ventilation delivers small jets of air at a rate of 100 to 900 breaths per minute through a small catheter introduced into the patient's airway. It allows for delivery of high levels of PEEP without raising peak mean airway pressure to the extent required by conventional ventilation (Beare, Myers, 1998). Jet ventilation is used commonly with infants but may be seen rarely with adults.

The newest mode of ventilation used for adults is pressure support. Pressure support provides a small amount of constant positive pressure during the inspiratory effort of the patient. This positive pressure helps overcome the resistance of the endotracheal tube and the demand valve on the ventilator that the patient must trigger to get a breath. Pressure support is useful for weaning when combined with IMV (Esteban et al, 1995).

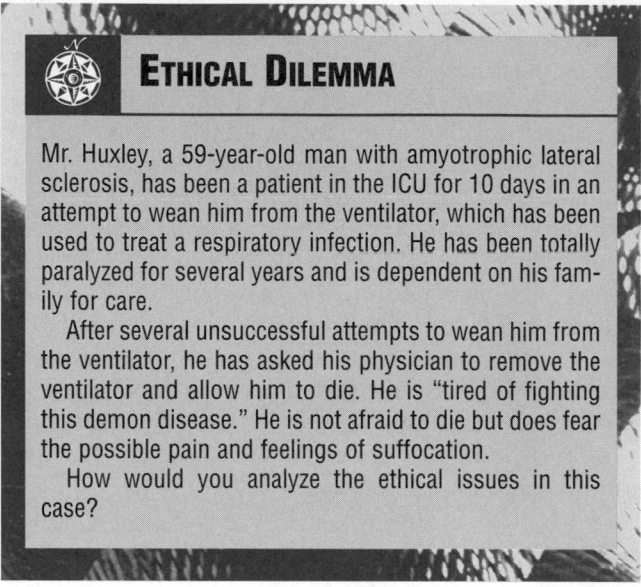

**ETHICAL DILEMMA**

Mr. Huxley, a 59-year-old man with amyotrophic lateral sclerosis, has been a patient in the ICU for 10 days in an attempt to wean him from the ventilator, which has been used to treat a respiratory infection. He has been totally paralyzed for several years and is dependent on his family for care.

After several unsuccessful attempts to wean him from the ventilator, he has asked his physician to remove the ventilator and allow him to die. He is "tired of fighting this demon disease." He is not afraid to die but does fear the possible pain and feelings of suffocation.

How would you analyze the ethical issues in this case?

Nursing care consists of continued support of the patient's respiratory function and of detection and prevention of complications. Vital signs, breath sounds, intake and output, arterial blood gases, and serum electrolytes should be assessed often. Airway patency should be maintained by suctioning using a sterile technique. Ventilator settings are checked often. The patient's position should be changed often, and passive range of motion should be performed. The environment must be quiet and relaxed, and adequate rest periods must be planned. As always, the nurse collaborates with the physician and respiratory therapist and notes respiratory changes promptly (Box 22-14).

# NURSING PROCESS

## ADULT RESPIRATORY DISTRESS SYNDROME

### ASSESSMENT

- Respiratory status (breath sounds, breathing pattern, sputum)
- Vital signs
- Hemodynamic pressures, if indicated (cardiac output)
- Ventilator settings; endotracheal tube (ET) position
- Signs of barotrauma q 1 hr, if on mechanical ventilation
- Urine output
- Skin and nailed color, temperature, quality of peripheral pulses
- Level of consciousness
- ABGs, electrolytes, complete blood count (CBC)
- Chest x-ray examination

### NURSING DIAGNOSES

- Impaired gas exchange related to alveolar-capillary membrane changes
- Ineffective breathing pattern related to decreased lung compliance, fatigue, and decreased energy
- Ineffective airway clearance related to pulmonary and interstitial edema
- Risk for decreased cardiac output related to positive pressure ventilation
- Fear related to difficulty breathing, mechanical ventilation, and inability to communicate
- Risk for infection related to decreased pulmonary function
- Risk for injury: barotrauma related to positive-pressure ventilation and decreased pulmonary compliance
- Risk for impaired skin integrity related to prolonged bed rest/immobility
- Impaired physical mobility related to mechanical ventilation, acute respiratory failure
- Inability to sustain spontaneous ventilation related to acute respiratory failure
- Impaired verbal communication related to endotracheal intubation

### NURSING INTERVENTIONS

- Maintain oxygen delivery system as prescribed, for $O_2$ saturation >90%.
- Provide reassurance.
- Keep health care provider informed of respiratory status.
- Anticipate need for intubation and mechanical ventilation.
- Prevent dislodgment of ET tube with restraints to extremities, as needed.
- Provide nursing care related to ET tube.
- Provide nonverbal means of communication.
- Use pulse oximetry for continuous monitoring of $O_2$ saturation.
- Combine nursing actions to conserve patient energy.
- Turn and position q 2 hr.
- Aseptic suctioning prn, as prescribed.
- Turn and position q 2 hr.
- Administer medications as prescribed.
- Administer IV fluids as prescribed.
- Anticipate need for chest tube placement, if barotrauma occurs.
- Maintain limbs in proper body alignment.
- Perform range-of-motion exercises.
- Initiate activity increases as condition improves.
- Maintain skin integrity.

### EVALUATION OF EXPECTED OUTCOMES

- Maintenance of optimal breathing with assistance as indicated
- $O_2$ saturation >90%
- ABGs WNL for patient
- Breath sounds clear or improved
- Alert mentation
- Urine output >30 ml/hr
- Strong peripheral pulses
- No evidence of barotrauma
- No evidence of skin breakdown

# KEY CONCEPTS

➤ The primary function of the respiratory system is to provide oxygen to meet metabolic needs and to remove carbon dioxide.

➤ The signs and symptoms most closely associated with respiratory disease are dyspnea, chest pain, cough, sputum production, wheezing, hemoptysis, and cyanosis.

➤ Nursing assessment of the patient with respiratory problems begins with the patient history.

➤ Physical assessment of the lungs and thorax includes inspection, palpation, percussion, and auscultation.

➤ Arterial blood gases assess (1) the ability of the lungs to provide adequate oxygen and remove carbon dioxide and (2) the ability of the kidneys to excrete or reabsorb bicarbonate ions to maintain normal body pH.

➤ Pulmonary function tests evaluate lung function. The most common tests are performed by spirometry, which measures lung volumes and capacities and flow rates.

➤ Bronchoscopy allows for visual examination of the lungs.

➤ Thoracentesis is performed to obtain pleural fluid for diagnostic purposes, to remove pleural fluid for therapeutic purposes, to perform biopsy of the pleura, or to instill medication.

➤ Nursing strategies for common respiratory problems include incentive spirometry, coughing and deep breathing, suctioning, postural drainage, percussion, and vibration.

➤ Precautions are important when oxygen is being used because it supports combustion.

➤ The primary nursing responsibility in caring for a patient with a tracheostomy tube is to maintain airway patency. Tracheal suctioning is often required, and secretions should be kept moist. Monitoring for cyanosis, shortness of breath, bleeding from the wound, and hypotension is essential.

➤ The nursing care of patients who are receiving mechanical ventilation includes monitoring vital signs, positioning to provide optimum ventilation, turning, performing active and passive range-of-motion exercises, assessing airway maintenance, determining the need for suctioning, recording intake and output, maintaining adequate nutrition and hydration, and providing emotional support.

➤ Following thoracic surgery, postoperative care focuses on maintaining the closed drainage system;

positioning; encouraging frequent coughing, deep breathing, and use of the incentive spirometer; maintaining patient comfort using medications and techniques such as relaxation; observing for complications; and teaching and reinforcing postoperative arm exercises and activity progression.

➤ Invasion of the upper respiratory system by microorganisms, usually viral, may cause inflammation and edema of the mucous membranes; cervical lymph node enlargement; dryness, redness, and soreness of the mucous membranes of the throat; voice hoarseness with painful cough; and leukocytosis to combat infection. Interventions are directed toward preventing complications, preventing the spread of infection, and relieving discomfort from symptoms.

➤ Hoarseness is often the first symptom of laryngeal cancer. Interventions include radiation therapy and partial, supraglottic, or total laryngectomies. Preoperative preparation, especially psychologic, is important. As the patient improves, the goals are self-care and speech training. Patient teaching focuses on good hygiene, stoma care, emergency care, stomal hydration, and overall healthy behaviors.

➤ COPD causes psychologic, physical, and social problems for the patient. COPDs include emphysema, chronic bronchitis, bronchiectasis, and asthma. Nursing interventions include administration of bronchodilators, evaluation of the effectiveness of respiratory treatments, administration of bronchodilators, evaluation of the effectiveness of respiratory treatments, administration of oxygen, instruction on diaphragmatic breathing, maintenance of adequate hydration and nutrition, performance of postural drainage with percussion and vibration if needed, maintenance of activity level, and development of a regular activity program.

➤ Pneumonia is caused by bacteria, viruses, fungi, and mycobacteria. Most community-acquired pneumonia is caused by *Pneumococcus* and occurs in the very young and in older adults. Interventions are aimed at keeping the patient comfortable, avoiding unnecessary expenditures of energy, and using antibiotic and sulfonamide agents to help the body's defenses overcome the infection.

➤ Tuberculosis is caused by acid-fast bacteria. Signs and symptoms of TB include cough, hemoptysis, pleuritic chest pain, weight loss, night sweats, fever, malaise, anorexia, and fatigue. TB is detected through skin testing, examinations of spu-

## KEY CONCEPTS—cont'd

tum for AFB, and chest x-ray examinations. Treatment requires more than one drug for 6 to 9 months. Patient education includes teaching the patient about the medication regimen and encouraging him or her to remain in close contact with the health care provider so that progress can be monitored.

➤ Atelectasis occurs from the blockage of air to a portion of the lung, which causes collapse. It may be a postoperative complication or may be caused by tumors, an enlarged heart, or obstruction of bronchus by a foreign body or mucous plug. Interventions include deep breathing, incentive spirometry, chest percussion and vibration, and postural drainage. Suctioning, oxygen, administration of aerosols, and humidity are also used.

➤ Pulmonary emboli and infarction are blood clots or other foreign material that originate in the venous system and are carried to the lung. PEs can cause death of lung tissue and infarction. Nursing interventions focus on the initial stabilization of the patient, improvement of gas exchange, maintenance of optimal cardiac function, reduction of anxiety, and relief of pain.

➤ Prevention of deep vein thrombosis is important because 90% to 95% of all pulmonary emboli orig-

inate from the deep veins of the leg. Measures can be pharmacologic, nonpharmacologic, or a combination of the two.

➤ Lung cancer is more common in men than women and is more common in smokers than in nonsmokers. Treatment depends on the cell type, stage of the disease, and general health status of the patient. Treatment may involve surgery, radiation therapy, and chemotherapy, used either alone or in combination.

➤ Chest wounds represent serious medical or surgical emergencies. Patient care is determined by the extent of the injury. Patient history focuses on the time the event occurred, the mechanism of the injury, the estimation of blood loss, and whether alcohol or drugs were used. Physical examination includes the assessment of respiratory and neurologic function.

➤ ARDS has a combination of symptoms that result from direct or indirect injury to lung and changes that occur in the alveolar capillary membrane. Interventions include oxygen therapy, suctioning, percussion, vibration, and postural drainage. Intubation and mechanical ventilation are often required.

## CRITICAL THINKING EXERCISES

1. What are the difficulties in administering oxygen therapy to a patient with emphysema?
2. Explain the dynamics of closed chest drainage for a patient with pneumothorax.
3. Design a plan to prevent the development of a DVT and subsequent PE in a patient with advanced cancer.
4. Outline the preoperative assessment for a patient with a lung tumor who is undergoing a lobectomy.

## REFERENCES AND ADDITIONAL READINGS

Apple S: New trends in thrombolytic therapy, *RN* 59(1):30-35, 1996.

Beare PG, Myers JL: *Adult health nursing,* ed 3, St Louis, 1998, Mosby.

Carroll P: Tradition or science? Spelling the difference in respiratory care, *RN* 59(5):26-30, 1996.

Carroll P: Pulse oximetry—at your fingertips, *RN* 60(2):22-27, 1997.

Centers for Disease Control and Prevention, Division of TB Elimination: *Core curriculum,* ed 3, Atlanta, 1994, US Department of Health and Human Services.

DesJardins T, Burton GG: *Clinical manifestations and assessment of respiratory disease,* St Louis, 1995, Mosby.

Esteban A et al: A comparison of four methods of weaning patients from mechanical ventilation, *N Engl J Med* 332:345-350, 1995.

Gift AG: Dyspnea, *Nurs Clin North Am* 25(4):955-965, 1990.

Haas F, Haas SS: *The chronic bronchitis and emphysema handbook,* New York, 1990, John Wiley & Sons.

Hatfield BO: Cost effective trach teaching, *RN* 60(3):48-49, 1997.

Higgens M: Epidemiology of obstructive pulmonary disease. In Casaburi R, Petty T, editors: *Principles and practice of pulmonary rehabilitation,* Philadelphia, 1993, Saunders.

Kanacki L: How to guide ventilator dependent patients from hospital to home, *Am J Nurs* 97(2):37-39, 1997.

Kersten LD: *Comprehensive respiratory nursing: a decision making approach,* Philadelphia, 1989, Saunders.

Lewis SM, Collier IC, Heitkemper MM: *Medical-surgical nursing: assessment and management of clinical problems,* ed 4, St Louis, 1996, Mosby.

Malasanos L, Barkauskas V, Stoltenberg-Allen K: *Health assessment,* ed 4, St Louis, 1989, Mosby.

Patrick ML et al: *Medical-surgical nursing: pathophysiological concepts,* ed 2, Philadelphia, 1991, Lippincott.

Phipps WJ et al: *Medical-surgical nursing: concepts and clinical practice,* ed 5, St Louis, 1995, Mosby.

Poker AM: Are nursing homes a breeding ground for T.B.? *Nursing Spectrum* 10(3):24, 1997.

Seidel HM et al: *Mosby's guide to physical examination,* ed 3, St Louis, 1995, Mosby.

Smeltzer SC, Bare BG: *Brunner and Suddarth's textbook of medical-surgical nursing,* ed 7, Philadelphia, 1992, Lippincott.

Spyr J, Preach MA: Pulse oximetry: understanding the concept, knowing the limits, *RN* 53(5):38-43, 1990.

Thompson JM, Wilson SF: *Health assessment for nursing practice,* St Louis, 1996, Mosby.

White VM: t-PA for pulmonary embolism, *Am J Nurs* 96(9):34, 1996.

# CHAPTER 23

# Cardiac Problems

## CHAPTER OBJECTIVES

1 Describe the normal flow of blood through the heart and circulatory system.
2 Trace the normal electrical conduction through the heart.
3 Discuss the factors that affect cardiac output and stroke volume.
4 Describe the assessment of a patient with a cardiac disorder.
5 Describe the nursing responsibilities associated with diagnostic testing of patients with cardiac disorders.
6 Identify common cardiac arrhythmias and their effects on cardiac output.
7 List at least three precautions the nurse should teach patients with permanent pacemakers.
8 Describe the major risk factors for coronary artery disease.
9 Identify strategies the nurse should teach patients for reducing their risk of coronary artery disease.
10 Distinguish between the assessment and nursing interventions for angina and myocardial infarction.
11 Describe nursing responsibilities related to the care of patients undergoing invasive therapeutic procedures and cardiac surgery.
12 Describe the nursing assessment and interventions indicated for a patient with acute chronic congestive heart failure.
13 Describe the nursing interventions and patient teaching for a patient with chronic congestive heart failure.

## KEY TERMS

angina pectoris
angioplasty
arrhythmias
arteriosclerosis
atherosclerosis
cardiac output
cardiogenic shock
cardioversion
central venous pressure
cholesterol
congestive heart failure
coronary artery disease

coronary care unit
defibrillation
electrocardiogram
inotropes
isoenzymes
lipoproteins
myocardial infarction
pacemaker
plaques
pulmonary edema
stenosis

## CARDIOVASCULAR STRUCTURE AND FUNCTION

The heart is a fist-sized, hollow, muscular organ that pumps blood through the cardiovascular system. It is behind the sternum, within the mediastinum, between the lungs, and above the diaphragm. The top of the heart, known as the *base,* is just below the second rib. The lower part of the heart, the *apex,* points downward and to the left. The pulsation palpable at the apex, called the *point of maximal impulse (PMI),* is just below the left fifth rib in the midclavicular line. The heart is protected anteriorly by the rib cage and sternum and posteriorly by the rib cage and vertebral column (Figure 23-1).

### Heart Muscle

The heart muscle is made up of three distinct layers. The outer layer, the *epicardium,* is a thin, transparent,

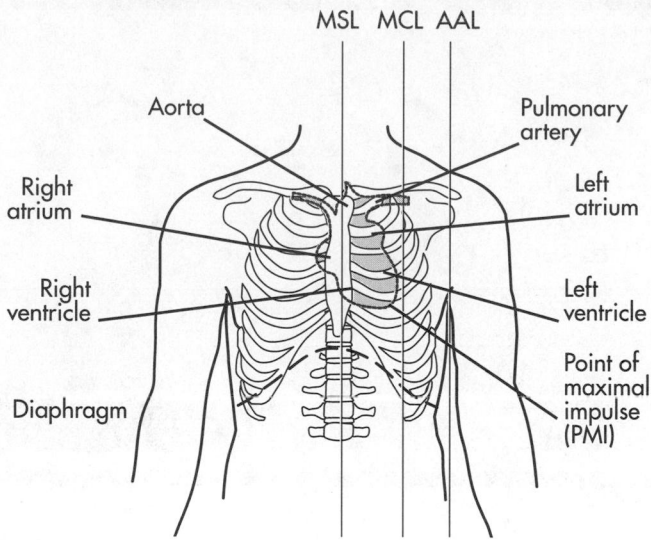

**Figure 23-1** Orientation of the heart within the thorax.

covering layer commonly infiltrated with fat. The middle layer, the *myocardium,* consists of striated cardiac muscle fibers that allow the heart to contract. The inner layer, the *endocardium,* is a thin layer of endothelial tissue that lines the inner cavity of the heart and covers the valves of the heart and the chordae tendineae, the tendons that hold the cardiac valves open. The endocardium is contiguous with the inner lining of the vessels. Inflammation of the endocardium, or *endocarditis,* may be caused by microorganisms such as bacteria, fungi, rickettsiae, and, in rare cases, viruses and parasites.

The heart is surrounded by a fibroserous sac called the *pericardium* or *pericardial sac.* The pericardium consists of an external fibrous layer (the *parietal* layer) and an internal serous layer (the *visceral* layer). The visceral layer adheres to the epicardium. Between the visceral and parietal layers are the ventricular walls. When the ventricles contract, these chordae tendineae prevent the valves from collapsing back into the atrium so that blood does not *regurgitate,* or backflow.

The *pulmonic valve,* between the right ventricle and the pulmonary artery, and the *aortic valve,* between the left ventricle and the aorta, are called *semilunar valves.* These valves prevent blood from regurgitating from the vessels into the ventricles at the end of each contraction.

## Blood Flow through the Chambers and Valves

The movement of blood through the heart requires coordinated functioning of all the chambers, as well as normal opening and closing of all the valves. Contraction of the right and left ventricles, called *systole,* oc-

curs almost simultaneously. As blood flows from the ventricles into the lungs and systemic circulation, the blood in the lungs and circulation returns to fill the right and left atria. When the atria are full and the ventricles are empty, blood flows from the atria into the ventricles. During this filling stage the ventricles are in *diastole* and are not contracting. The atria contract at the end of passive filling to push the remaining blood into the ventricle. This atrial contraction is called the *atrial kick.* When the ventricles are full and the atrial contraction is complete, the ventricles begin their contraction. The differences in pressure in each chamber during systole and diastole regulate the opening and closing of the valves.

If a drop of blood were traced from the right atrium through the cardiovascular system, the flow would progress through each chamber and the valves. The right atrium receives venous blood from all body tissues except the lungs. This blood is returned to the heart through the inferior and superior venae cavae and the coronary sinus. The blood then passes through the tricuspid valve into the right ventricle. During each contraction, the right ventricle pumps venous blood through the pulmonic valve into the pulmonary artery to the lungs, where carbon dioxide is exchanged for oxygen. Oxygenated blood from the lungs returns to the left *pericardial space,* which contains a thin film of pericardial fluid. This serous fluid in the pericardial sac lubricates the two layers to prevent friction during each heartbeat. Inflammation of the pericardium is called *pericarditis.* The cause of pericarditis often is idiopathic, but it may also arise from a viral or bacterial infection. Noninfectious causes of pericarditis include uremia, myocardial infarction, tumors, radiation, and certain pharmaceutical agents (Huether, McCance, 1996).

## Heart Chambers

The heart is made up of four chambers. The thin-walled upper chambers are the *right atrium* and the *left atrium.* The lower chambers, the *right ventricle* and the *left ventricle,* are thick, muscle-walled chambers. The right and left sides of the heart are separated by a *septum.* The myocardium of the left ventricle is thicker than the myocardium of the right ventricle; this difference is related to the pressure the chambers pump against during each contraction. The right ventricle pumps blood into the lower pressure lung circulation, and the left ventricle pumps blood into the higher pressure systemic circulation. Increases in the volume of blood coming into the heart or in the pressure in the pulmonary or systemic circulation increase the work of the heart's chambers and can cause *dilation* or *hypertrophy* of the muscle wall.

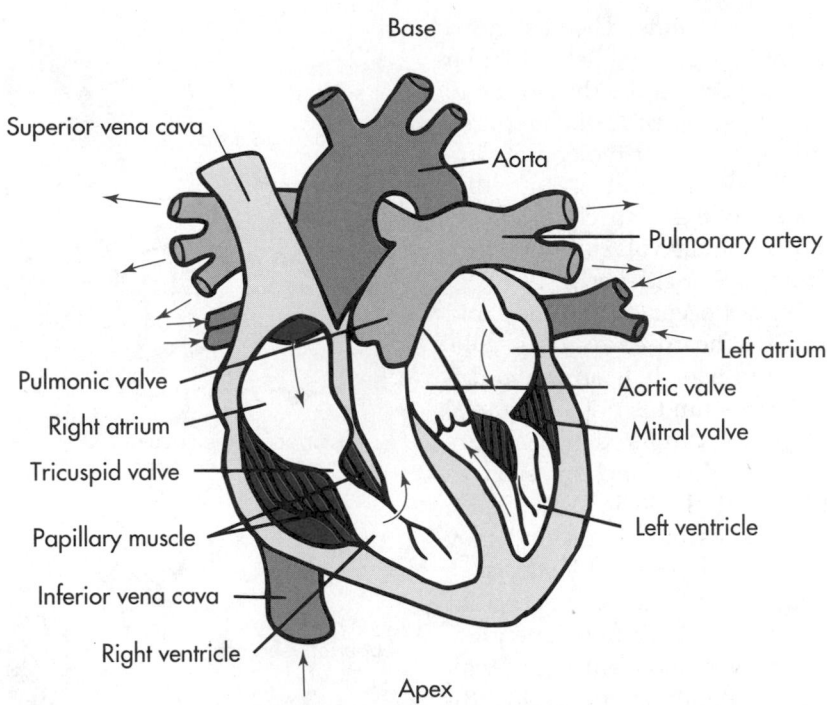

Base

Superior vena cava

Aorta

Pulmonary artery

Left atrium

Pulmonic valve

Aortic valve

Right atrium

Mitral valve

Tricuspid valve

Papillary muscle

Left ventricle

Inferior vena cava

Right ventricle

Apex

**Figure 23-2**   Blood flow through the heart.

**TABLE 23-1**

## Characteristics of the Four Heart Sounds

|  | $S_1$ | $S_2$ | $S_3$ | $S_4$ |
|---|---|---|---|---|
| Sound | Lub | Dub | Ken-tuck-y ($S_1$, $S_2$, $S_3$) | Tenn-ess-ee ($S_1$, $S_2$, $S_4$) |
| Location | Mitral tricuspid valve | Aortic-pulmonic area | Apex | Medial to apex |
| Time | Systolic, longer than $S_2$ | Diastolic, shorter than $S_1$ | Early diastole | Late diastole, presystole |
| Intensity | Louder at apex | Louder at base | Dull | Higher than $S_3$ |
| Pitch | Low | Higher than $S_1$ | Low | Duller than crisp $S_1$ |
| Clinical interpretation | Normal | Normal | Normal in children and young adults or after exercise; in mature adults may be a sign of congestive heart failure or mitral regurgitation | Normally not heard; associated with hypertension, aortic or pulmonic stenosis |

## Heart Valves

The forward flow of blood through the heart is controlled by a series of one-way valves that prevent backflow of blood in the heart during each heartbeat (Figure 23-2). The *tricuspid valve,* between the right atrium and the right ventricle, and the *mitral valve,* between the left atrium and the left ventricle, often are called atrioventricular valves because they direct the blood flow between the atria and the ventricles. These valves have special thin strands of fibrous tissue, called *chordae tendineae,* that anchor the cusps of the valves to the *papillary muscles* on the atrium through the pulmonary

vein. The blood passes through the mitral valve into the left ventricle. During each contraction, the left ventricle pumps blood through the aortic valve into the aorta and on to all parts of the body. Any disruption of the synchrony of the contractions or the functioning of the valves alters the flow of blood through the heart.

## Heart Sounds

The opening and closing of the heart valves causes the blood flow to vibrate, resulting in the heart sounds commonly heard through a stethoscope (Table 23-1). $S_1$

and $S_2$ are the normal heart sounds. The first heart sound, $S_1$, corresponds to the beginning of ventricular contraction (systole) and is produced by the closing of the mitral and tricuspid valves. $S_1$ has a soft *lub* sound. The second heart sound, $S_2$, occurs at the end of ventricular contraction and signals the onset of ventricular diastole (resting). Relaxation of the ventricles results in closing of the aortic and pulmonic valves, which produces the sharp *dub* sound of $S_2$ (Seidel et al, 1995).

A third heart sound, $S_3$, can occur during the rapid early ventricular filling. It is heard early in diastole, just after the $S_2$. The $S_3$ sound usually is quiet and difficult to hear. The third heart sound is not an unusual finding in children and young adults, but in mature adults it suggests altered cardiac function, such as chronic heart failure (Seidel et al, 1995). When $S_1$, $S_2$, and $S_3$ are heard with a stethoscope, the sound they produce has a rhythm similar to the word *Kentucky*.

The fourth heart sound, $S_4$, occurs late in ventricular diastole, after atrial contraction and immediately before $S_1$. Vibration in the valves and ventricular wall creates the $S_4$ sound, but $S_4$ usually is quiet and difficult to hear. A more intense $S_4$ indicates resistance to ventricular filling caused by loss of compliance (stretch) of the ventricular wall; this is common in patients with hypertension (Seidel et al, 1995). When $S_1$, $S_2$, and $S_4$ are heard with a stethoscope, the sound they produce has a rhythm similar to the word *Tennessee*. More information on heart sounds and their auscultation can be found in the Nursing Assessment section of this chapter.

## Coronary Circulation

Like other organ systems the heart has its own blood supply. The two coronary arteries branch from the sinus of Valsalva at the base of the aorta just above the aortic valve. These arteries and their branches surround the heart and provide blood to all portions of the heart muscle and to the heart's electrical conduction system. Blood flow into the coronary arteries occur during ventricular diastole. Coronary veins return deoxygenated blood to the right atrium. Two major coronary arteries provide oxygenated blood to the heart (Figure 23-3).

The right coronary artery and its branches provide blood to the right atrium and ventricle and to the inferior wall of the left ventricle. In most people (90%) the posterior descending coronary artery branches from the right coronary artery; this arrangement is called *right coronary dominant*. In the same percentage of people, the right coronary artery also supplies blood to part of the conduction system called the atrioventricular (AV) node, and in 55% it provides blood flow to the sinoatrial (SA) node (Morton, 1996).

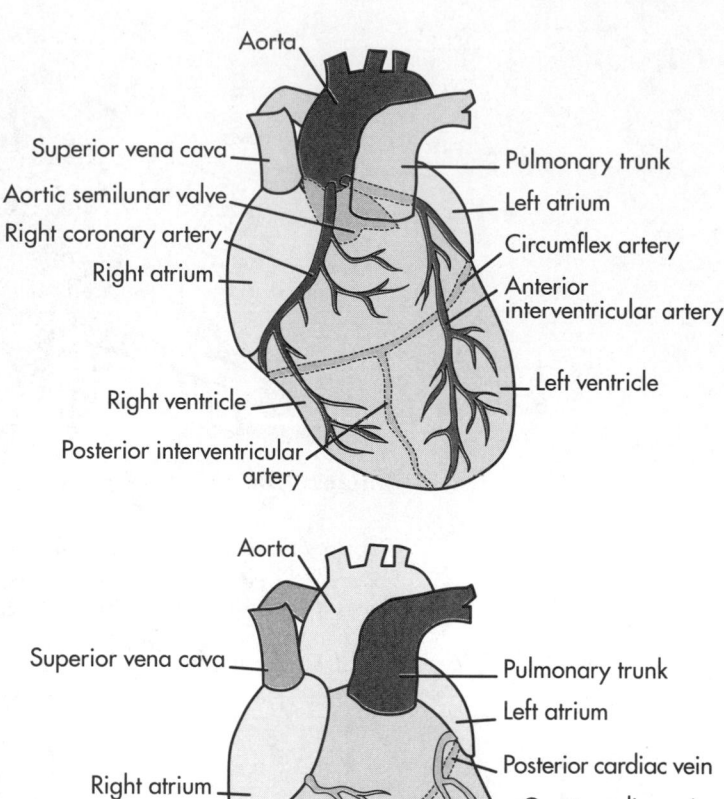

**Figure 23-3**  Coronary arteries and veins.

The left coronary artery begins as one vessel, called the *left main coronary artery,* and then branches into the left anterior descending artery and the left circumflex artery. The left anterior descending artery provides blood flow to the anterior wall of the left ventricle, including the septum and the bundle branches. The left circumflex artery provides blood supply to the left atrium and the lateral wall and to the posterior wall of the left ventricle. In 10% of the population, the posterior descending branch is supplied by the left coronary artery; this is called *left coronary dominant*. The left circumflex artery is the source of blood supply to the SA node in 45% of the left coronary dominant group and to the AV node in 10% (Morton, 1996).

Any disruption of the flow of blood through the coronary arteries reduces the amount of oxygenated blood that arrives at the muscle and conduction system. An imbalance between the supply of oxygen to the heart muscle and the demand for oxygen by the muscle can cause *ischemia,* which is a reversible cellu-

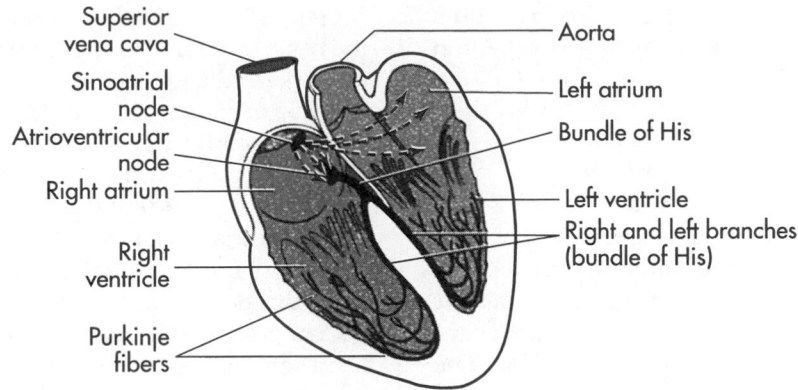

**Figure 23-4**  Conduction system of the heart.

lar injury, or *infarction,* which is tissue death. The effect of ischemia and infarction depends on the area involved and the size of that area. If blood flow is reduced gradually, alternate pathways for blood flow, called *collateral circulation,* may be formed to bypass the narrowed vessel.

## Conduction System

The heart normally beats in an orderly sequence, automatically and regularly. The pattern of systole and diastole is controlled by a specialized electrical conduction system in the myocardial tissue that initiates the cardiac cycle, spreads the excitation over the muscle cells, and maintains the regularity of the cycle (Figure 23-4). The conduction system is composed of the *sinus node, internodal pathways, atrioventricular (AV) junctional tissue,* the *bundle of His,* the *bundle branches,* and the *His-Purkinje system* (Atwood et al, 1996).

The sinus node, also called the *sinoatrial node* or SA node, is located near the junction of the superior vena cava and the right atrium. The SA node initiates the electrical impulse and therefore is known as the heart's normal pacemaker. The impulse spreads over both atria, causing the mechanical contraction of the atrial muscle cells to occur. The impulse is then sent through highly specialized conduction tissue called the *atrioventricular node,* or AV node.

The AV node is situated in the right posterior portion of the interatrial septum, behind the tricuspid valve. The AV node delays transmission of the electrical impulse from the atria to the ventricles to allow time for the atrial kick, which provides maximal filling of the right and left ventricles before the electrical impulse reaches them. After passing through the AV node, the electrical impulse stimulates the bundle of His. The impulse is carried along the bundle of His and its right and left bundle branches.

Because of the size of the left ventricle, the left bundle has two branches, called the anterior and the pos-

terior fascicles. The right and left bundle branches and fascicles subdivide further into the *Purkinje fibers,* which carry the impulse through the walls of both ventricles. The impulse causes the muscle cells in the ventricles to contract.

The wave of electrical current that travels through the conduction system and initiates muscular contraction is the result of rapid changes in the electrolyte concentrations on the inside and outside of the cells. This electrolyte shift, which changes the electrical polarity of the cells, is called *depolarization.* Mechanical contraction follows depolarization of the cell. When the cells return to their normal electrolyte composition, polarity is restored and *repolarization* occurs. This repolarization, or return to normal, prepares the cell to begin the process over again. Transmission of the electrical current and recovery occur very rapidly in order for the heart muscle to contract at the normal rate of 60 to 100 beats per minute. The complete cardiac cycle lasts less than 0.8 seconds. Changes in the serum electrolyte composition can adversely affect the cardiac system (Chapter 27).

The electrical conduction system is extremely complex and highly susceptible to disease, electrolyte imbalances, and lack of blood supply. When the conduction system is damaged, the normal pacemaker function of the SA node may be altered. In this case other components of the conduction system assume the SA node's pacemaker function; this is called an ectopic pacemaker.

The different parts of the conduction system have different rates of initiation of the electrical impulse. The SA node initiates impulses at the normal rate of 60 to 100 times per minute and is the normal pacemaker of the heart. If the AV node is forced to assume pacemaker functions, a rhythmic but slower rate of 40 to 60 beats per minute results (Atwood et al, 1996).

The electrical events that occur within the conduction system of the heart can be detected on the surface of the body by electrocardiograph (ECG) machines, which record the electrical current and display it on a screen or on graph paper. This recording is called an **electrocardiogram** or *ECG*.

## Cardiac Output

The heart normally pumps 4 to 6 L of blood every minute; this is called the **cardiac output.** Cardiac output (CO) is determined by the amount of blood the ventricles eject with each contraction (*stroke volume [SV]*) and the number of times the heart beats every minute, (*heart rate [HR]*), or CO = SV × HR. The amount of cardiac output each person needs varies according to body size, metabolic rate, and activity level. The stroke volume and the heart rate are determined by many factors. Heart rate is controlled by the autonomic nervous system. Stroke volume is affected by preload, afterload, contractility, and heart rate (Darovic, 1995).

According to Starling's Law, the force of the contraction of the heart muscle during systole depends on the amount of stretch placed on the heart's muscle fibers during diastole. The volume of blood in the ventricles at the end of their filling phase (diastole) is called *preload*. This preload stretches the muscle fibers and causes a more forceful contraction. However, if the fibers are stretched too far, the resulting contraction loses its force. Too much preload (overloading the ventricle with blood) overstretches the fibers and diminishes the contraction and thus the stroke volume. Too little preload does not stretch the muscle fibers enough and therefore also causes a weaker contraction and lower stroke volume. The amount of blood volume and the amount of venous return determine preload. Volume overload would cause increased preload, and dehydration would cause decreased preload.

Another factor affecting stroke volume is *afterload*. Afterload is the resistance the ventricle must pump against to eject blood during contraction (systole). The right ventricle pumps its blood through the pulmonic valve into the pulmonary circulation, and the left ventricle pumps its blood through the aortic valve into the aorta and systemic circulation. Any increased resistance from these structures can prevent the ventricle from completely emptying and can reduce the amount of ejected blood (i.e., the stroke volume). To overcome increases in afterload, the heart must work harder. Over time, increased afterload can cause the heart muscle to enlarge, or hypertrophy, or weaken. One example of a condition involving increased afterload is hypertension. Aortic stenosis, or narrowing of the aortic valve, is an example of a structural defect that causes increased resistance to left ventricular ejection. Pulmonary disease may cause increased resistance to right ventricular ejection.

*Contractility* also affects stroke volume. The ability of the heart muscle cells to contract improves the ejection of blood and SV. If some muscle cells cannot contract because of injury, SV is diminished. Contractility can be increased by catecholamines released by the sympathetic nervous system and by many commonly used drugs. The drug digitalis, for example, is used to increase contractility. Contractility can be impaired by ischemia or infarction of the heart muscle cells and by some drugs, such as beta-blockers (e.g., propranolol).

Changes in heart rate also can influence SV. If the heart rate increases, the amount of time the ventricles have to fill decreases and preload decreases, causing less stretch on the muscle fibers and less contractility. The overall effect is a decrease in SV. For most adults, a prolonged heart rate above 150 beats per minute can have detrimental effects on SV. A slow heart rate can alter cardiac output even if SV stays normal. In order to maintain CO, the SV must increase if the HR decreases. A normal response to a decreased SV, as in dehydration, is an increase in HR to maintain overall CO at the normal level.

*Cardiac reserve* is the ability of the heart to respond to the many factors that influence the CO. By adjusting the rate and SV, the heart can increase or decrease its cardiac output as needed to meet the demands of the body. This ability can be diminished in patients with cardiac or other systemic diseases or illnesses, putting them at risk of serious cardiac abnormalities.

## Systemic Vascular Circulation

Blood vessels are a network of arteries, arterioles, capillaries, venules, and veins that circulate blood from and to the heart. The major divisions of this network are the *systemic circulation* and the *pulmonary circulation*. The portal circulation of the liver and the lymphatic circulation are also important components of the body's circulatory status. The systemic arterial system transports nutrients and oxygen to body cells, and the venous system carries waste products to the appropriate organs of the body to be eliminated. All systemic arteries branch from the aorta and subdivide into the arterioles and capillaries. Blood in the venous system of the systemic circulation flows from the venules to the veins and into either the *superior vena cava* or the *inferior vena cava*, both of which flow into the right atrium. Arterial and venous disease can compromise both the cardiac system and other vital organs.

## Pulmonary Vascular Circulation

The pulmonary vascular system carries blood from the right ventricle to the lungs and back to the left atrium. The right and left pulmonary arteries arise from the right ventricle and immediately subdivide into a series of short branches, ending in capillaries that encircle the lungs' air sacs (alveoli), pick up oxygen, and release the waste product, carbon dioxide. The capillaries gradually come together to form pulmonary veins, which carry oxygenated blood from the lungs to the left atrium. Pulmonary disease may cause changes in the pulmonary circulation, increasing the afterload to the right ventricle.

## Blood and Blood Components

Blood volume makes up about 8% of a person's total body weight. This percentage varies with environmental temperature, altitude, individual weight, sex, age, nutrition, and pregnancy. During a normal pregnancy the blood volume increases to about 50% above nonpregnant levels. Approximately 40% of blood is composed of circulating cells, and the other 60% is plasma (Seidel et al, 1995).

Red blood cells transport hemoglobin, which has the unique property of binding and releasing oxygen. The percentage of red blood cells in the whole blood volume is measured as a hematocrit value. White blood cells are the body's first enzymes and are the chemicals needed for the inflammation process and for coagulation of blood. Plasma, which is similar to tissue (interstitial) fluid but contains three times more proteins, contributes to cardiovascular function by maintaining blood volume, blood viscosity, and osmotic pressure.

Each side of the heart, left and right, holds about 4% of the total circulating blood volume. The remaining blood volume is distributed within the vasculature, with approximately 4% in the capillaries, 16% in the arterial vessels and the remainder in the venous vessels (Seidel et al, 1995). Changes in blood volume and blood components disrupt the cardiac system.

## Lymphatic Circulation

Lymphatic fluid is excess tissue (interstitial) fluid that has accumulated around body cells. Lymphatic drainage maintains equilibrium of the fluid surrounding body cells. Lymphatic vessels begin as tiny lymphatic capillaries similar to blood capillaries. These unite and form large vessels (the thoracic duct and the right lymphatic duct) that empty into veins. Lymph moves as a result of skeletal muscle contraction, negative intrathoracic pressure, and the suction effect of blood flow in the veins. The lymphatic fluid flow depends on venous pressure and on the condition of venous vessels. Distributed along the lymphatic vessel system are small, round bodies, called *lymph nodes*, that serve as filters to remove proteins. Lymph node function is related to the immune system. Obstruction of venous vessels or elevated venous pressure can affect the interstitial fluid volume and capillary exchange (Seidel et al, 1995).

## Neurohumoral Controls of the Heart

Many physiologic entities can control the heart. Some of these controls are mediated by the branches of the *autonomic nervous system (ANS)*, the *sympathetic nervous system (SNS)*, and the *parasympathetic nervous system (PNS)* (Seidel et al, 1995). Stimulation of the sympathetic nervous system causes stimulation of the cardiac system through the release of norepinephrine and epinephrine. These catecholamines act on the various receptors to alter cardiac and blood vessel function. Stimulation of *beta$_1$-adrenergic receptors* causes an increase in the heart rate, increased conduction of impulses through the AV node, and increased atrial and ventricular contractility. When *beta$_2$-adrenergic receptors* are stimulated, peripheral vessels dilate and constricted bronchial muscles relax. Stimulation of *alpha-receptors* raises blood pressure by constricting peripheral vascular arterioles.

When the parasympathetic branch of the ANS is stimulated, mediation by the vagus nerve results in an overall inhibition of the cardiac system. In response the SA node slows, lowering the HR, and AV node conduction decreases. Some triggers to ANS stimulation may be exercise, temperature, and emotions. Exogenous catecholamines and other medications can affect the SNS and the PNS.

Baroreceptors are located in the carotid sinuses and aortic arch. They are sensitive to changes in blood pressure and cause temporary changes in HR and blood pressure (BP). For example, a sudden increase in blood pressure stimulates the baroreceptors, causing the vasomotor cardiac control center in the brain to slow the heart rate and lower the blood pressure by vasodilation through inhibition of the SNS and stimulation of the PNS. A decline in blood pressure would result in an increase in the heart rate and vasoconstriction as the body attempts to restore normal pressure.

Chemoreceptors in the carotid arteries and the aorta detect increased levels of carbon dioxide, oxygen deficiencies, or a decrease in pH. When stimulated, these chemoreceptors in turn stimulate the vasomotor center to increase HR and constrict arteriolar and venous reservoirs (Seidel et al, 1995).

Temperature also affects the functioning of the heart. An increase in body temperature increases the metabolic rate, resulting in an increase in SA node discharges and a faster heart rate. Conversely, a drop in body temperature decreases the heart rate by slowing SA node discharge. An extreme change in body temperature (i.e., to below 30° C [86° F]) can precipitate arrhythmias, including ventricular fibrillation and complete cardiac arrest (Cummins, 1994).

# NURSING ASSESSMENT

## History of Current Illness

Nursing assessment begins with a complete history of the patient's current problem. This includes a review of seven aspects of the problem to ensure that no important information is overlooked. These seven dimensions are (1) location, (2) quality (character), (3) quantity (severity), (4) chronology (timetable of events, onset, duration), (5) aggravating or alleviating factors, (6) associated symptoms, and (7) treatment sought and its effect. These seven areas of information are especially important in patients who report chest pain or discomfort. It also is important to ask all patients specific questions that may detect an underlying cardiac problems (Box 23-1).

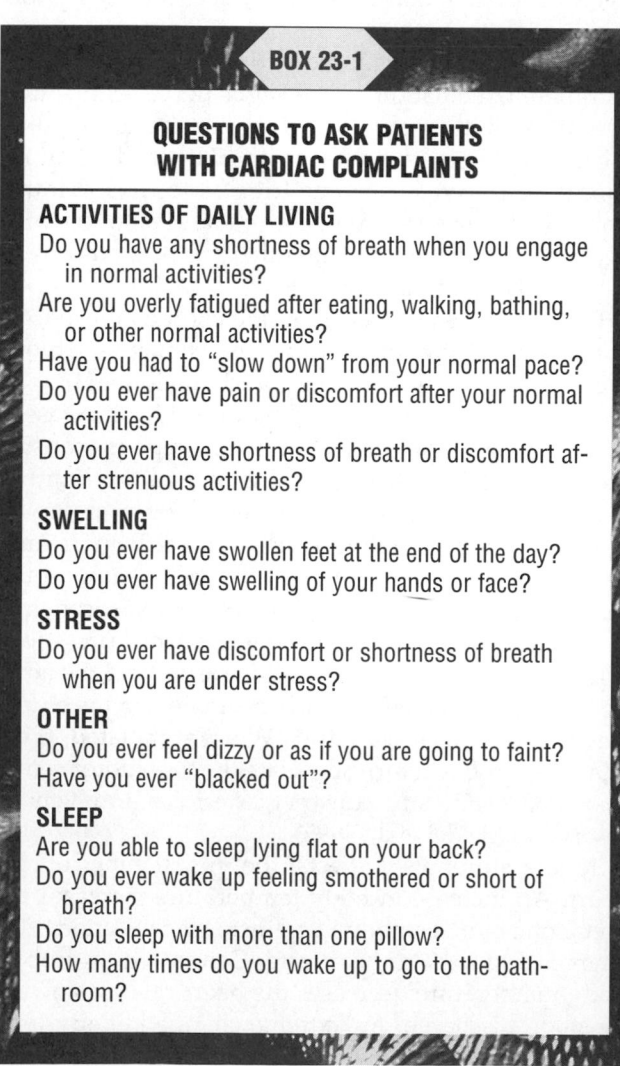

**BOX 23-1**

### QUESTIONS TO ASK PATIENTS WITH CARDIAC COMPLAINTS

**ACTIVITIES OF DAILY LIVING**
Do you have any shortness of breath when you engage in normal activities?
Are you overly fatigued after eating, walking, bathing, or other normal activities?
Have you had to "slow down" from your normal pace?
Do you ever have pain or discomfort after your normal activities?
Do you ever have shortness of breath or discomfort after strenuous activities?

**SWELLING**
Do you ever have swollen feet at the end of the day?
Do you ever have swelling of your hands or face?

**STRESS**
Do you ever have discomfort or shortness of breath when you are under stress?

**OTHER**
Do you ever feel dizzy or as if you are going to faint?
Have you ever "blacked out"?

**SLEEP**
Are you able to sleep lying flat on your back?
Do you ever wake up feeling smothered or short of breath?
Do you sleep with more than one pillow?
How many times do you wake up to go to the bathroom?

## Past Health and Surgical History

Many illnesses can affect the heart either directly or indirectly. The patient should be asked about other illnesses or symptoms that could affect the heart or signal underlying cardiac disease. A complete review of systems may provide much-needed information. For example, the patient may not associate swelling of the feet and ankles or the need for two pillows when sleeping (symptoms suggestive of congestive heart failure) as significant for a cardiac assessment and may not report them unless specifically asked. Past hospitalizations or diagnostic workups for cardiac symptoms need to be explored, and any previous ECGs or chest x-rays should be obtained to serve as a baseline.

## Medications

Many medications, including prescription, over-the-counter, and recreational or abused drugs, can cause cardiac symptoms or problems. A complete list of medications should include the name, strength, and dosage of all medications the patient takes; a note on the patient's understanding of the purpose of the medications; and when the last dose was taken. If the patient cannot give a complete list of medications, family members should be asked to bring the drugs in for evaluation.

## Family History

A complete family history, focusing on cardiac disease or sudden death, should be obtained. Heart attacks

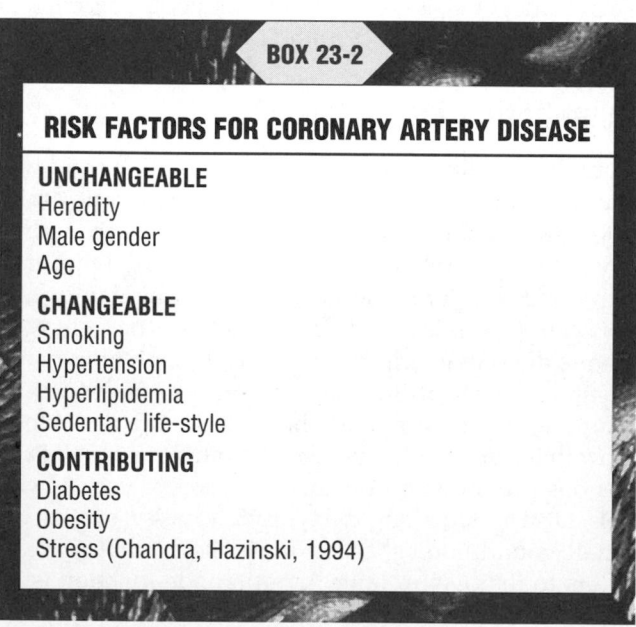

**BOX 23-2**

### RISK FACTORS FOR CORONARY ARTERY DISEASE

**UNCHANGEABLE**
Heredity
Male gender
Age

**CHANGEABLE**
Smoking
Hypertension
Hyperlipidemia
Sedentary life-style

**CONTRIBUTING**
Diabetes
Obesity
Stress (Chandra, Hazinski, 1994)

and sudden death in first-degree family members under 50 years of age are significant risk factors for heart disease.

## Risk Factors

When assessing the cardiac system, it is important to identify risk factors that indicate a higher chance of developing heart disease. The risk factors in Box 23-2 have been identified as contributing to the development of heart disease (Chandra, Hazinski, 1994).

## Physical Examination

After obtaining the patient's cardiac history, the nurse should conduct a systematic physical examination of the heart that includes the four techniques of physical assessment: *inspection, palpation, percussion,* and *auscultation.* The cardiac physical examination is performed with the patient in three positions: sitting, supine, and lying on the left side. Special considerations for assessment of older adults are included in the Older Adult Considerations box.

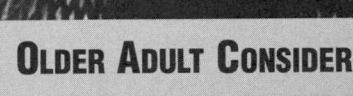

## OLDER ADULT CONSIDERATIONS

- Ventricular walls thicken (S₄ heart sound is common).
- Valves become fibrosed and calcify (more problems occur with stenosis of valves, more murmurs are heard on auscultation).
- Heart rate and cardiac output decline (response to stress is less efficient, return to resting heart rate after activity takes longer).
- Arteries become less elastic (blood pressure rises).
- Heart becomes smaller unless hypertension or heart disease has caused hypertrophy.
- Cellular changes lead to heart block, atrial fibrillation, premature atrial contractions (PACs), and premature ventricular contractions (PVCs) (resulting in more arrhythmias).
- Incidence of coronary artery disease is higher.
- Heart is not as responsive to SNS stimulation (response to stress is blunted, heart rate may not increase as expected).
- Response to myocardial infarction is atypical (shortness of breath is more common than pain).
- Fatigue is a common symptom of heart failure.
- Postural hypotension is more common (vasodilators can aggravate this problem). (Seidel et al, 1995.)

## Inspection

An overall evaluation of the patient should be made during the interview process. Pale or cyanotic skin or nail color, increased work of breathing, prominent vascular patterns, and dependent edema are some of the abnormal objective data related to cardiac function that can be collected during inspection.

Inspection also includes visual assessment of the shape of the patient's chest and observation of the six heart areas for visible pulsations (Figure 23-5). Abnormally shaped thoraces can influence cardiac function. Normally, pulsations are not visible unless the patient is very thin, in which case a slight pulsation may be detected primarily at the PMI. The PMI may be visible in the fifth intercostal space at the midclavicular line. A displaced PMI may be indicative of increased heart size. The finding of an abnormal pulsation in any area requires further assessment via palpation and auscultation (Seidel et al, 1995).

## Palpation

Palpation is used to detect pulsation or vibration (thrills) that may not have been identified with inspection or to further assess pulsations seen during inspection. The same six areas of the chest are assessed. The palmar surfaces of the fingers are used to detect vibrations, and then the pads of the middle and index fingers are used to make finer assessments. Detection of vibrations suggests the presence of a pathologic condition and requires further evaluation through auscultation. Special attention should be given to finding the PMI; this is the most lateral pulsation of the left ventricle, usually detected over the apex of the heart. Normally the PMI, or apical impulse, is an area about 1 cm (about ½ inch) in diameter located in the midclavicular line. A widened or displaced apical impulse or one marked by abnormal vibration indicates cardiovascular disease. An abnormal pulsation is classified as a *lift* if it is a slightly more sustained thrust than normal; a *heave* is an impulse with force that pushes out against the palpating hand. Inability to feel the PMI may be a normal finding in adults because of the thickness of the chest wall (Seidel et al, 1995).

**Heart rate.** Palpation includes determining the heart rate using a peripheral site such as the radial or femoral artery. If the rhythm of the pulse is irregular, it is better to auscultate the heart rate at the apex using the PMI, because early or ectopic beats can be missed when palpating peripherally.

**Arterial pulses.** In addition to determining the heart rate, the nurse should evaluate the quality of the peripheral circulation by examining the pulses. It is important to compare vessels on the right and left sides. The carotid, radial, brachial, femoral, popliteal,

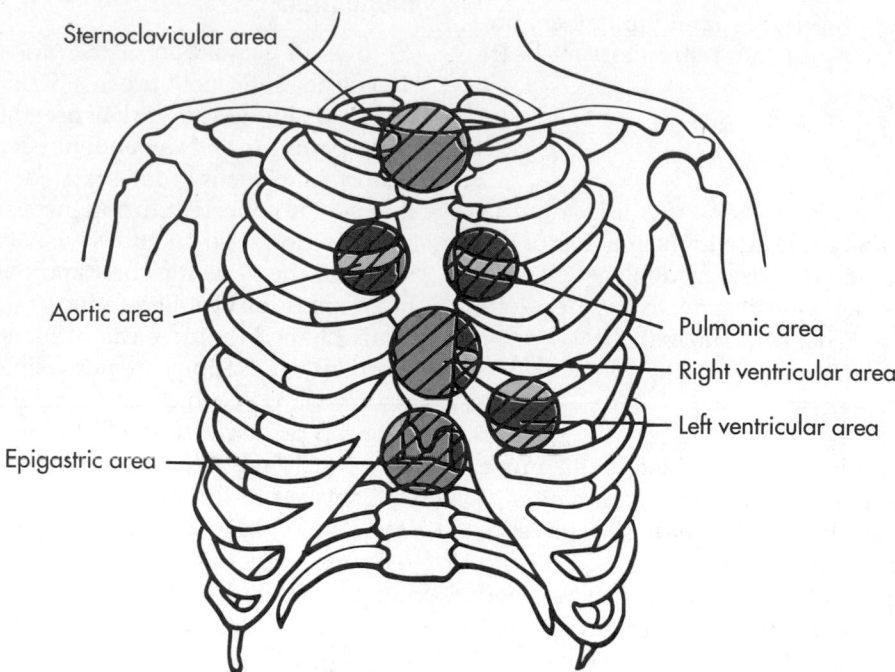

Sternoclavicular area

Aortic area

Pulmonic area

Right ventricular area

Left ventricular area

Epigastric area

**Figure 23-5**     Areas of inspection and palpation for cardiac assessment.

dorsalis pedis, and posterior tibial blood vessels are most commonly assessed. Of these the carotids are easily accessible, but caution is needed; the carotids should be palpated on only one side at a time because excess pressure on this sensitive area may slow the pulse or lower the blood pressure. The most distal vessels usually are palpated in the extremities. Hands and feet that are cool and pale suggest arterial vessel involvement, whereas warm, cyanotic extremities indicate venous problems.

The quality of the pulse is another palpation finding to consider. A weak pulse feels small and may indicate hypovolemia or heart failure. A bounding pulse is caused by increased stroke volume, such as is seen in fever, anemia, or some heart conditions (Bates, 1995). More detailed information on arterial disease and assessment is provided in Chapter 25.

## Percussion

Percussion can be used to determine cardiac borders and overall size, but x-ray examination and fluoroscopy are more accurate diagnostic measures and are more commonly used.

## Auscultation

**Heart sounds.** As described previously, the movement of the heart valves causes turbulent blood flow. Normally the heart has two distinct sounds, $S_1$ and $S_2$. Addi-

tional sounds, $S_3$ and $S_4$, may be present, as may heart murmurs. Using a stethoscope, the nurse listens systematically in five auscultatory areas surrounding the heart (Figure 23-6), first with the diaphragm of the stethoscope and then with the bell. The diaphragm picks up high-pitched sounds, and the bell picks up low-pitched sounds. A quiet environment and concentration are essential for distinguishing normal and abnormal heart sounds. Many nurses close their eyes while listening to avoid distractions. The nurse starts by listening to the heart sounds while palpating the carotid artery. This technique helps identify $S_1$, which is heard simultaneously with the palpation of the carotid pulse.

After listening with the patient in the supine position, the nurse listens with the patient sitting and then lying on the left side. These changes in position can be helpful in identifying abnormal sounds that may be heard in only one position.

Normally no sounds are heard between $S_1$ and $S_2$ or $S_2$ and the next $S_1$. Any extra sound heard may represent an abnormality and should be described and reported. A thorough description includes the timing (during systole or diastole); location (area being auscultated when the sound was heard); patient's position (supine, sitting, or side-lying); and characteristics and intensity (harsh, blowing, soft, loud). The loudness of a murmur is graded on a six-point scale, with the numerator being the loudness of the murmur (from 1 to 6) recorded as a Roman numeral and the denominator recorded as IV.

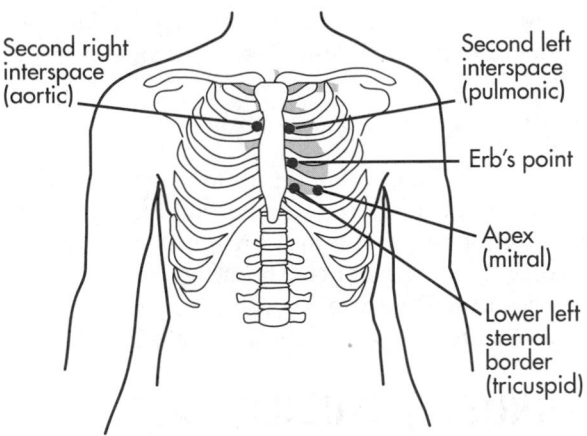

**Figure 23-6**    Areas of cardiac auscultation.

It is vital for the nurse to have confidence in his or her ability to hear and recognize the S₁ and S₂ sounds before expecting to identify S₃, S₄, or *murmurs.* Murmurs are vascular sounds that produce vibrations within the heart or great blood vessels (i.e., aorta and pulmonary vein), and they are most often associated with **stenosis** or regurgitation. Stenosis is the result of thickening of the valvular leaflets, which narrows passages and restricts blood flow. Regurgitation is the backward flow of blood through valve leaflets that have lost their ability to close snugly. Murmurs may be a normal finding, if no other signs or symptoms of cardiovascular disease are found.

Additional heart sounds that may be heard are an *ejection click* (the opening of pulmonic and aortic valves), an *opening snap* (opening of the mitral and tricuspid valves), or the *splitting* of either S₁ or S₂ (a single sound perceived as two sounds). Splitting may be due to a physiologic condition (occurring with respirations) or a pathologic one (related to a cardiovascular problem). Artificial heart valves also may make unusual sounds, depending on the type of material used in their construction.

**Blood pressure.** Auscultation of the cardiovascular system includes measurement of blood pressure (BP). Systolic blood pressure reflects stroke volume and pressure exerted against the interior walls of the aorta; diastolic blood pressure indicates the resistance of the blood vessels. Blood pressure readings vary with age, and the range for adults is 90/60 mm Hg to 140/90 mm Hg. Systolic pressure may vary by 5 to 10 mm Hg between the two arms. The pulse pressure, which is the difference between the systolic and diastolic measurements, usually is 30 to 40 mm Hg. The blood pressure should be taken with the patient in lying, sitting, and standing position if possible. A drop in the systolic blood pressure of more than 15 mm Hg and in the di-

astolic blood pressure of more than 5 mm Hg upon standing is called *postural hypotension,* which may indicate a pathologic condition, such as dehydration, the effects of medication, such as antihypertensives, or prolonged bed rest.

Anxiety can raise blood pressure. The nurse should try to have the patient relax. If the patient is very obese and the standard cuff does not fit well, the nurse can obtain an oversized cuff or use the standard cuff on the forearm and listen over the radial artery. Even scrupulous adherence to good technique for taking the blood pressure can be compromised by conditions such as cardiac arrhythmias, aortic regurgitation, and venous congestion. When cardiac irregularities persist, the nurse may need to take an average of several pressures and record the BP as such. To minimize venous congestion, the nurse should try to avoid repeated, slow inflation of the cuff.

**NURSE ALERT**

Make sure the cuff size is appropriate for the extremity.

## Other Areas of Assessment
### Peripheral Veins

Thrombosis, varicose veins, and edema are signs of venous insufficiency. Tenderness, thickening, or redness over a superficial vein may indicate thrombophlebitis. The nurse should assess all the extremities for these conditions. More detailed information on venous disease and assessment is presented in Chapter 24.

### Venous Measurement

The jugular venous pulse is a good indicator of the hemodynamics (forces resulting in blood circulation) of the right side of the heart and the central venous pressure. Jugular pulsations reflect atrial contractions. The internal jugular veins give a more accurate pressure measurement than do the external jugular veins, which are more visible. When a patient is sitting upright, the jugular veins are not visibly distended. As the patient gradually assumes a supine position, the veins' fill-level should become visible approximately 1 to 2 cm (about ½ to 1 inch) above the level of the manubrium (upper portion of the sternum). When the patient lies flat, the jugular veins pulsate at the top of their length as they transit the neck.

To measure the jugular venous pressure, the head of the bed should be raised to a 45-degree angle and the

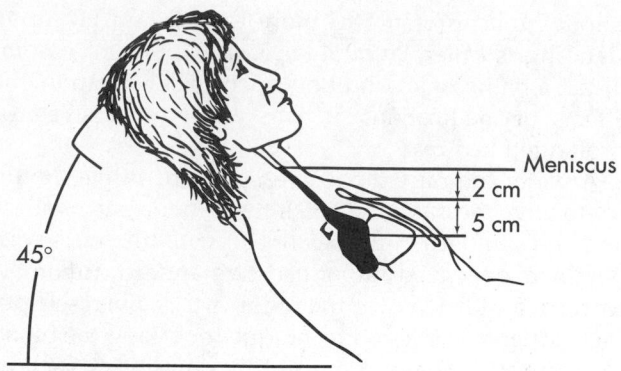

**Figure 23-7** Jugular venous pressure.

nurse should observe the pulsations of the internal jugular vein (Figure 23-7). If these pulsations still cannot be seen, the head of the bed should be lowered until pulsations are visible. The nurse should hold a short ruler on a horizontal plane next to the patient's neck where the jugular pulsations are. The nurse should place another ruler on the sternal angle (the angle of Louis, a bony ridge between the manubrium and the sternum at the level of the second intercostal space) and should extend the ruler vertically. The nurse should measure in centimeters the point where the horizontal ruler crosses the vertical ruler. A change in the jugular venous pressure is most significant when compared with previous readings. An increase suggests hypervolemia, and a decrease suggests hypovolemia. If the patient's pulse is over 90 beats per minute, the value of this assessment is questionable. The nurse should record the height of the venous pressure in centimeters above the sternal angle, as well as the elevation of the patient's head. A measurement of less than 2 cm usually is normal (Seidel et al, 1995).

## Edema

Edema is the accumulation of excess interstitial fluid. Systemic causes include congestive heart failure and kidney disease. Local causes are venous or lymphatic stasis. Edema most commonly is found in dependent parts of the body, that is, the lower extremities in ambulatory patients and the sacral area in patients in the supine position. Edema is not a normal finding and is suggestive of chronic heart failure. It may also be a sign of venous disease, arterial occlusion, or lymphatic obstruction. Edema of one extremity suggests a local cause, whereas bilateral edema indicates a systemic cause. Edema may be described as *pitting edema* if indentation of the edematous area persists after finger pressure is withdrawn. The severity of pitting edema is described by the depth of the indentation, measured

in millimeters. Some practitioners use a four-point scale to grade pitting edema (Seidel et al, 1995).

## Lungs

Assessment of the lungs and pulmonary system also is important in evaluation of the heart. Findings such as crackles, dyspnea, and a rapid respiratory rate can be caused by heart problems. The lungs should be auscultated and the work of breathing and oxygenation level determined as part of the assessment of the heart.

# DIAGNOSTIC STUDIES

## Laboratory Examinations

It usually is important to conduct several laboratory studies to establish an accurate diagnosis or to follow the course of cardiovascular disease.

### Complete Blood Count

The routine laboratory examination comprises a count of red and white blood cells, an estimate of hemoglobin, and a differential count, which includes many different cells that usually are few in number. An increase in the number of white blood cells indicates that an inflammatory condition or tissue destruction is present. Determination of the red blood cell count and the hemoglobin level helps in assessing the oxygen-carrying capacity of the blood. Anemias can adversely affect the amount of blood being carried and the oxygen available to the heart and other organs.

### Acute-Phase Reactants

The erythrocyte sedimentation rate (ESR) and the C-reactive protein (CRP) test are nonspecific tests done to confirm the presence of an inflammatory process. The sedimentation rate is elevated in many conditions, including rheumatic fever and myocardial infarction. It is useful both in diagnosing rheumatic fever and in following the course of the disease.

### Blood Cultures

When *bacterial endocarditis* is suspected, the diagnosis may be established by finding the causative organism in the blood. Often several blood cultures may be necessary before a positive diagnosis can be made.

### Serum Enzyme Tests

Enzymes are proteins that are present in all body cells. Certain enzymes are specific to particular tissues and are present in high concentrations in these tissues, such as the heart, liver, and kidneys. When damage occurs to these tissues, significant amounts of the enzymes are released into the bloodstream.

Cardiac enzymes and **isoenzymes** are specific to heart muscle tissue and are released into the blood during myocardial infarction (MI). Measurement of these enzymes and isoenzymes is useful in diagnosing acute myocardial infarction. Lactate dehydrogenase (LDH) and creatine phosphokinase (CPK) are two enzymes evaluated in the diagnosis of myocardial infarction. The CPK enzyme has three isoenzymes: CPK-MM (found primarily in skeletal muscle), CPK-BB (found in brain tissue), and CPK-MB. The MB isoenzyme is found in cardiac tissue and is not present in significant concentrations in noncardiac tissue, therefore elevations in CPK-MB are specific for cardiac tissue damage. The CPK-MB value can be used to determine both the amount of infarction and the timing of infarction, as well as whether thrombolytic drugs should be given.

The LDH enzyme has five isoenzymes, numbered 1 to 5. Isoenzyme LDH-1 is found in the heart and blood vessels and is compared with LDH-2 to determine if cardiac muscle damage has occurred. Normally LDH-1 is found in lower concentration than LDH-2; the reverse (LDH-1 exceeds LDH-2) is called an LDH "flip" and is indicative of myocardial damage. The total LDH alone is not specific or sensitive for cardiac tissue (Pagana, Pagana, 1996).

Each cardiac enzyme elevates, peaks, and stays in the bloodstream for a different period of time. Table 23-14 contains a list of the enzymes and isoenzymes and their rates of appearance in the serum. The first enzyme to increase is CPK, which increases within 4 to 8 hours after the onset of cellular insult and peaks at 12 to 24 hours. The CPK-MB isoenzyme appears and peaks at the same rate. These enzymes would be detected early in the process of acute myocardial insult. The total LDH does not rise until 24 to 48 hours after MI occurs, and the LDH flip does not occur until 12 to 24 hours later; LDH is used primarily to identify patients who have had a cardiac insult but who did not seek care early in the course. LDH and its isoenzymes are not seen as early after the insult as CPK and thus would not be used for diagnosis in the first 24 hours (Pagana, Pagana, 1996).

Enzyme blood samples are drawn and analyzed at least three times (every 6 to 12 hours) after the onset of symptoms so that the pattern of isoenzyme changes can be established. If an MI has been confirmed by changes in CPK-MB, LDH isoenzymes may not be drawn. A finding of three negative isoenzyme reports, showing no changes in the enzyme levels, rules out myocardial infarction. Recent developments in rapid assays of these isoenzymes have made it possible to rule out an MI within the first 6 hours after the onset of symptoms.

Myoglobin, a protein found in the heart and skeletal muscle, is another value that may be used in the workup for an acute myocardial infarction. Increased levels can be found with cardiac muscle damage. Myoglobin is a very sensitive indicator of muscle damage and rises rapidly. However, it is not a very specific test, and increases also can be seen with trauma, inflammation, and ischemia of other muscle tissues (Pagana, Pagana, 1996).

## Blood Chemistries

The mechanisms that control metabolic balance often are disturbed during serious illness. Assessment of serum electrolytes is important in determining the status of sodium, potassium, chloride, carbon dioxide, bilirubin, calcium, creatinine, glucose, magnesium, phosphorus, alkaline phosphatase, urea nitrogen, and uric acid levels. Changes in serum electrolytes, both elevation and reduction, can have a profound effect on the performance of the heart and can precipitate arrhythmias.

## Cholesterol

**Cholesterol** is one of the major lipid (fatlike) substances in the blood. Increased levels of lipids (hyperlipidemia) have been found to be a major risk factor for vascular disease, including coronary artery disease. It is thought that the lipids accumulate within the inner lining of blood vessels, reducing the diameter of the vessels; this is called **atherosclerosis.** The narrowed blood vessels diminish the circulation efficiency of the blood, which is laden with oxygen and nutrients. Studies show that blood cholesterol levels can be lowered by reducing the dietary intake of food high in saturated fat and cholesterol. Total cholesterol levels are a part of a total lipid profile, which includes lipoproteins and triglycerides. For best results cholesterol levels should be measured after a 12-hour fast and after abstaining from alcohol for 24 hours (Pagana, Pagana, 1996).

## Lipoproteins

**Lipoproteins** carry and help metabolize fat, including cholesterol and triglycerides. Special laboratory tests can be done to identify the levels of the three types of lipoproteins. High-density lipoproteins (HDLs) carry cholesterol away from the arteries and to the liver and prevent cells from taking in lipids. HDL is called the "good" cholesterol, and increased levels can be protective for the arteries and cardiac system. Ideally the ratio of HDL to total cholesterol should be 1:3. Low-density lipoproteins (LDLs) also carry cholesterol, but they carry it to the arteries, and high levels of LDL are associated with an increased risk of heart and vascular disease. This characteristic makes LDL atherogenic (contributing to atherosclerosis). Very-low-density lipoproteins (VLDLs) primarily carry triglycerides. High levels of VLDL also are associated with vascular disease. As with the cholesterol levels, lipoprotein levels should be checked after a 12-hour fast, and they are influenced by dietary intake in the previous 2 weeks (Pagana, Pagana, 1996).

## Triglycerides

Triglycerides are a type of fat in the blood. Like cholesterol and lipoproteins, triglycerides are part of a lipid profile and when elevated can indicate an increased risk of heart and vascular disease. Because alcohol consumption increases the triglyceride level, patients should abstain from alcohol for 24 hours before the test (Pagana, Pagana, 1996).

## Blood Gases

Arterial blood gases help determine the status of the patient's oxygenation and acid-base balance. Hypoxemia (low oxygen) and acidosis (low pH) can have detrimental effects on the functioning of the heart.

## Coagulation Studies

Because many patients with heart problems have had a thrombolic insult, the use of anticoagulation therapies is not unusual. In addition, the current emphasis on reperfusion of the at-risk myocardium with thrombolytic therapies means that many patients will be receiving anticoagulant therapy. Coagulation studies include platelet counts, prothrombin time (PT) counts, partial thromboplastin time (PTT) and activated partial thromboplastin time (APTT) counts, activated clotting time counts, fibrinogen level studies, thrombin time counts, and recalcification time counts. These studies are done before anticoagulants and thrombolytic agents are given to determine the baseline levels; they are repeated frequently to determine the response to and need for adjustments in therapy.

## Monitoring

Patients with heart disease frequently require special monitoring to obtain accurate, objective data that can be used to determine and adjust the plan of care. Two types of monitoring commonly used are ECG monitoring and hemodynamic monitoring. Hemodynamic monitoring typically is done only in an intensive care unit (ICU) or coronary care unit (CCU), where specialized equipment is available and highly trained nurses maintain the monitoring lines, evaluate the effect of treatments on the pressure readings, and adjust the plan of care. ECG monitoring can be done in a variety of settings as long as the needed equipment and personnel trained in the interpretation and intervention for ECG abnormalities are available.

## Electrocardiographic (ECG) Monitoring

The electrical impulses of the heart can be monitored in several ways. One way is to use a portable monitoring system. Portable systems usually are small, can run on batteries for several hours, and can be used during transport of patients from one area to another. They usually have a small screen on which the ECG rhythm can be watched, and they can print out a strip with the waveforms that can be saved in the medical record or used for interpretation. The patient is connected to the machine by adhesive electrodes and lead wires, which are placed in strategic positions over the chest. One type of portable system, called a *defibrillator*, can deliver an electrical shock, called **defibrillation,** to the heart in addition to monitoring the heart's electrical current. Portable systems are useful for monitoring the ECG for short periods and for monitoring patients being moved from one place to another. Portable systems can visualize only 1 or 2 leads (views) at a time. Defibrillators are used in settings where cardiac arrest and the need for emergency measures may occur.

The second type of monitoring system is a nonportable, continuous ECG monitoring system. These systems usually are found in ICUs and are mounted permanently on the wall at the bedside. They run on batteries and usually are not portable, although they may have removable modules that can be used as a portable device. Most of these types of systems can monitor other parameters such as oxygenation (pulse oximetry), heart pressures (hemodynamics), and blood pressure (invasive or noninvasive) in addition to the ECG. As with portable monitoring, the patient is connected to the machines by electrodes and wires, but up to five electrode and lead wire sets can be used to show more than one view of the heart (a lead) at a time. Continuous bedside ECG monitoring usually is found in ICUs and CCUs; a small screen for viewing the ECG waveforms is at the bedside, and a larger screen is at a central monitoring station. The central monitoring station ensures that someone is always watching the ECG rhythm of the patient and can call for help if abnormalities are seen.

The third type of system is telemetry monitoring. In this type of ECG monitoring, the patient is also connected by electrodes and lead wires, but the wires are then connected to a small, lightweight telemetry box that usually is placed in a pouch and worn by the patient like a large necklace. The telemetry unit sends the ECG signal to a central monitoring station via radio waves transmitted to receivers in the ceiling. The telemetry system allows continuous monitoring of the ECG without restricting the patient to the bed or the room. Telemetry ECG monitoring usually is used in intermediate or step-down units.

The 12-lead ECG is another type of ECG monitoring that is done when all 12 views of the heart need to be evaluated. This type of ECG commonly is ordered when patients have chest pain suggestive of myocardial ischemia or injury. The 12-lead technique is also used as a screening tool before surgery and during routine office visits for patients who are over 45 to 50 years of age or who have significant risk factors for cardiac disease. The 12-lead method usually is not a continuous monitoring technique but rather a one-time diagnostic study, with a one-page print out of all the views. In some places 18-lead ECGs are now being used to assess the portions of the heart not visible with a 12-lead ECG method.

## Hemodynamic Monitoring

Hemodynamic monitoring is an invasive method of measuring pressures in the arterial system and heart that provides additional information for the nurse and health care team. Hemodynamic values commonly monitored in the heart are the central venous pressure (CVP), pulmonary artery pressure, pulmonary artery wedge pressure, and cardiac output. Arterial blood pressure also can be monitored invasively through the radial or femoral artery. These pressure measurements can be used along with clinical assessment, diagnostic studies, laboratory values, and calculated hemodynamic indices to obtain a more complete understanding of the patient's physiologic state and response to treatment. Hemodynamic monitoring can provide continuous information on the patient's cardiac functioning and, when completed with technical accuracy, can be a useful tool in managing patient care.

**Central venous pressure.** Central venous pressure (CVP) provides information about the circulating blood volume and right heart function (Figure 23-8). It is a direct reflection of right atrial pressure (RAP) and an indirect reflection of the preload (volume) of the right ventricle. The CVP measurement gives an indication of the patient's volume status and the heart's ability to pump blood. A catheter is introduced into a peripheral or central vein and then threaded into the vena cava or right atrium. The catheter is secured and attached to a pressure monitoring system. This system includes intravenous (IV) fluids and specialized tubing with a transducer (electrical device) that converts the information obtained inside the heart and vascular

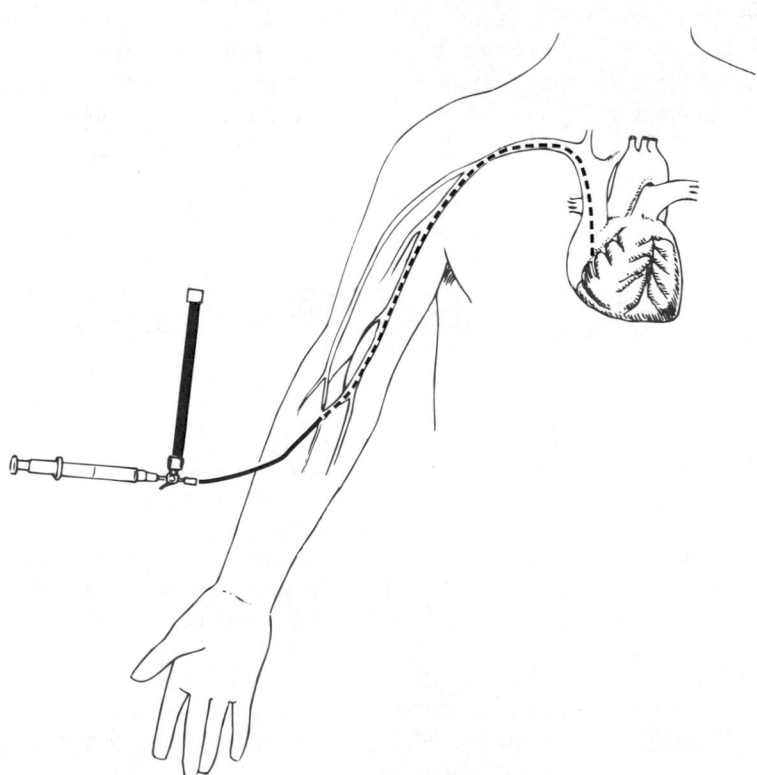

**Figure 23-8** Central venous pressure monitoring. Other sites for insertion can include the femoral vein, basilic vein, internal or external jugular vein, and subclavian vein.

system to a numeral and waveform. Correct placement of the catheter is verified by a chest x-ray. A sterile, occlusive dressing covers the site. In addition to the pressure readings, the CVP line provides a central IV access that can be used for administering fluids and medications and for blood sampling.

The CVP is measured in millimeters of mercury (mm Hg), and the normal range is 2 to 10 mm Hg. An increase in CVP indicates right ventricular failure, or increased circulating blood volume. Conversely, a decrease in CVP suggests hypovolemia. Constriction or dilation of the systemic circulation also can affect the CVP, with constrictions causing an increase and dilation causing a decrease (Darovic, 1995) (Table 23-2).

Complications associated with placement of a CVP catheter include infection, thromboembolism, pulmonary infarction, arrhythmias, and air embolism. The tubing and dressing should be changed according to hospital policy, at which time the site should be observed for any sign of redness, swelling, or drainage. These signs or any complaints of pain from the patient should be documented and reported to the physician.

> ### NURSE ALERT
>
> CVP catheters and any other IV line inserted through a central vein should never be open to air; leaving the end of the catheter open to air may result in an air embolus.

## Pulmonary Artery and Pulmonary Artery Wedge Pressures

Because the CVP alone does not provide an accurate reading of pressure in the left side of the heart, critically ill patients often receive pulmonary artery (PA) catheters (see Figure 23-8). This catheter provides several measurements that are used to determine cardiac performance. The pulmonary artery catheter is placed through a central vein (subclavian or internal jugular) and then advanced through the right atrium and ventricle into the pulmonary artery. The multilumen PA catheter is attached to a pressure transducer and an IV solution source. Placement is verified by a chest x-ray examination. Measurement of the pressures in the heart and pressure waveforms are obtained by means of a continuous electronic monitoring system.

The PA catheter has many lumens, which can be used for fluid and medication administration and pressure monitoring. It also has a balloon on the distal end that, when inflated, can measure the *pulmonary artery wedge pressure (PAWP)*, also called the *pulmonary artery occlusive pressure (PAOP)*, which indicates the functioning of the left side of the heart.

The pulmonary artery pressure is recorded like a blood pressure, with both a systolic pressure and a diastolic pressure. The systolic pressure is recorded during systole of the ventricles, when the mitral valve is closed and the pulmonic valve is open. A column of blood is created between the right ventricle and the left atrium, including the pulmonary vascular system. The systolic pressure, which is an indication of the pressure in the pulmonary vascular system, usually is 15 to 25 mm Hg. Elevation in the PA systolic (PAS) pressure indicates increased pulmonary vascular resis-

### TABLE 23-2

## Hemodynamic Measurements

| PRESSURE MEASUREMENT | NORMAL | CONDITIONS THAT INCREASE PRESSURE | CONDITIONS THAT DECREASE PRESSURE |
|---|---|---|---|
| Central venous pressure | 2-10 mm Hg | Fluid overload, right ventricular failure, left ventricular failure, systemic vasoconstriction | Hypovolemia, systemic vasodilation |
| Pulmonary artery (systolic) | 15-25 mm Hg | Increased pulmonary vascular resistance, pulmonary embolus, hypoxemia, chronic obstructive pulmonary disease (COPD), adult respiratory distress syndrome (ARDS), sepsis | Hypovolemia, systemic vasodilation |
| Pulmonary artery (diastolic) | 6-12 mm Hg | Fluid overload, left heart failure, mitral stenosis/insufficiency, cardiac tamponade, systemic vasoconstriction | Hypovolemia, systemic vasodilation |
| Pulmonary artery wedge | 4-12 mm Hg | Fluid overload, left heart failure, mitral stenosis/insufficiency, cardiac tamponade, systemic vasoconstriction | Hypovolemia, systemic vasoconstriction |

Data from Darovic GO: *Hemodynamic monitoring: invasive and noninvasive clinical application*, ed 2, Philadelphia, 1995, Saunders.

tance; decreases in the PAS suggest hypovolemia (Darovic, 1995).

During diastole of the ventricles, an open column of blood extends from the pulmonary artery through the lungs and into the left side of the heart. Since the mitral valve is open a this time, the electronic "eye" of the catheter can "see" into the left side of the heart. This permits the end of the catheter to measure the pressure, or preload, in the left ventricle. Normally the pulmonary artery diastolic (PAD) pressure is 6 to 12 mm Hg. Increases in the PAD pressure can indicate volume overload or left ventricular failure, whereas decreases usually occur with hypovolemia.

The PAWP obtained during inflation of the PA catheter balloon is 4 to 12 mm Hg and should be nearly the same (within 4 mm Hg) as the PA diastolic pressure (Darovic, 1995). This measurement can be important because the act of inflating the balloon moves the catheter into a portion of the pulmonary artery and out of the pathway of influence that might alter the readings, giving a much better "view" of the left ventricular pressure. See Table 23-2, which lists some conditions that can cause changes in the pressures in the heart.

In addition to providing these measurements, another lumen in the PA catheter ends in a thermistor port (a device for measuring very small changes in temperature) and permits measurement of cardiac output. A small bolus of solution is injected into the catheter, and the thermistor senses the temperature difference. A computer then calculates cardiac output.

PA catheters also have a lumen for measuring the CVP. Some of the newer innovations in PA catheters allow for measurement of the mixed venous oxygen saturation ($SvO_2$), which provides information on oxygen supply and demand in the body and continuous cardiac output readings. Noninvasive monitoring devices also are being used to measure pressures in the heart through recording changes in electrical impedance (electrical resistance) in the chest.

Complications associated with placement of a PA catheter include infection, pulmonary artery rupture, pulmonary thromboembolism and infarction, catheter kinking, arrhythmias, and air embolism. Many of the complications occur during placement or removal of the catheter. The pressure waveforms must be monitored continuously to prevent migration of the catheter into the distal pulmonary circulation, which would cause the catheter to become wedged. When wedging occurs, the blood flow through the pulmonary circulation is halted and a pulmonary infarction can occur.

As with the CVP line, the PA catheter insertion site is covered with an occlusive dressing, and the tubing, dressing, and IV fluids are changed regularly according to hospital policy. In addition, all pressure monitoring lines must be calibrated and adjusted every 8 hours to ensure the accuracy of the readings. Adjustment, calibration, and pressure readings should be done by nurses trained to manage these types of monitoring systems, and patients requiring pressure monitoring usually are in an ICU. These procedures and manipulation of the catheter in place should be done only by a specially trained nurse or by a physician.

# Exercise Tests, Imaging Studies, and Other Tests

## Stress Tests

Stress tests are valuable in diagnosing ischemic heart disease. During a stress test, the patient's ECG, blood pressure, heart rate, and subjective reports of pain are monitored continuously while the patient's heart is subjected to stress. The stress is induced by gradually increasing the level of exercise on a motorized treadmill or bicycle or by administering drugs (e.g., dobutamine or Persantine) that increase the heart rate and increase the workload of the heart without exercise (Pagana, Pagana, 1996). Patients usually are subjected to the stress until they have symptoms, show ECG changes, or reach a calculated heart rate Patients who are unable to exercise because of disability, weakness, or unsteadiness are given a stress test using a drug instead of exercise. Changes in the ECG (e.g., depression or elevation in the ST segment and arrhythmias) and the patient's symptoms are evaluated to determine the likelihood of coronary artery disease.

The stress test is also used to diagnose arrhythmias and to evaluate the patient's cardiac tolerance of exercise before he or she enters an exercise program. The patient needs to understand what the test involves because patient cooperation is necessary. The patient also should know that the test will be stopped if any pain or dyspnea or extreme fatigue occurs. The patient is advised to avoid smoking, to have nothing by mouth except liquids for several hours before the test, and to wear clothing suitable for exercise. Medications that affect the heart, such as beta-blockers, may be withheld before the test.

Stress tests can also be done using radioactive tracers such as thallium and cardiolyte. These tracers, which are injected intravenously before the stress test, collect in regions of the myocardium in direct proportion to the amount of blood flow to that area. The isotopes are then taken up by the myocardial cells and can be visualized during the imaging process. Areas of the myocardium that are not well perfused do not take up the isotopes, producing a "cold spot" on the image (Pagana, Pagana, 1996). The prestress images are compared to the immediate poststress images and the postrecovery images, which allows the effect of stress on the myocardial blood flow to be seen. This procedure can be useful in diagnosing coronary artery disease, determining the progression of previously diagnosed disease, and assessing the effectiveness of various therapies. The imaging study can be done with regular exercise stress tests and with drug-induced stress tests.

Stress tests performed with continuous echocardiograms are done to evaluate structural changes and heart wall dysfunction during stress. These stress echocardiograms are helpful when traditional stress tests are not diagnostic or when the ECG is altered chronically and is not useful in detecting acute ischemia (as with chronic left bundle branch block, which mimics ischemia) (Pagana, Pagana, 1996). Stress echocardiograms are also indicated for women, who have a high false-positive rate with ECG-based stress tests. Stress echocardiogram tests are conducted in a manner similar to that of the traditional exercise stress test, except that the exercise is stopped abruptly and the patient must lie down immediately for the echocardiogram, instead of tapering activity gradually. This change in the procedure is due to the need to get the echocardiogram done before the heart has a chance to return to normal functioning (about 1 minute after exercise stops).

## Ambulatory Electrocardiography

Ambulatory electrocardiography was made possible by a special monitor designed in the 1930s by Dr. Norman J. Holter. Through new technology, it has been redesigned into a compact, battery-operated tape recorder worn by the patient. The Holter monitor records cardiac events that occur as patients carry on in their normal routine of work, sleep, stress, or leisure activity. Three skin electrodes are attached to the patient, and the monitor is worn on the belt or shoulder harness for 24 to 48 hours. A tape recording of all ECG activity is made and then analyzed for any abnormalities. Patients should be instructed to keep the electrodes dry and to record any symptoms, medications taken, or activity in the event diary provided with the monitor. The Holter monitor allows for detection of arrhythmias that may occur intermittently and enables physicians to determine if the events are associated with any special activity by the patient (Pagana, Pagana, 1996).

## Echocardiogram

The echocardiogram is a noninvasive ultrasound of the heart that is used to evaluate the walls and valves of the heart. An echocardiogram uses high-frequency ultrasonic waves, which are bounced off the heart to locate and record the motion of cardiac structures and the flow of blood through the heart. The data are transmitted through an oscilloscope and recorded on photographic paper or film. An echocardiogram is useful in determining the size of the cardiac chamber, the motion of the walls, valvular structure and function, septal motion and thickness, and the thickness of the pericardial sac. It also can indicate the presence of cardiac tumors, pericardial effusion, and congenital heart defects (Pagana, Pagana, 1996).

Before testing the patient should be informed that the procedures are painless and that he or she must lie quietly for approximately 30 minutes. New color Doppler echocardiograms are now available. This technology allows the direction and velocity of blood flow to be recorded and gives the most anatomically correct views of blood flow through the beating heart. With color Doppler echocardiography, valvular leaks, septal defects, and other conditions can be detected with greater ease and accuracy.

An echocardiogram also can be conducted though the esophagus; this is called a *transesophageal echocardiogram (TEE)*. This approach is used when the traditional echocardiogram is not diagnostic, when picture quality is poor (as with obese patients and patients with large lung air spaces), or when the procedure must be done during surgery (TEE does not interfere with the sterile field) (Pagana, Pagana, 1996).

TEE uses an endoscope with an ultrasound transducer on the distal end. The endoscope is advanced through the esophagus into the stomach, where images are recorded from much closer to the heart and without the added interference of the lungs and bony structures of the chest. A TEE can be done as an outpatient procedure, but the patient must have nothing by mouth (be NPO) for 8 hours before the procedure, and sedation is used during the procedure. Complications of TEE are uncommon but can include bradycardia (from vagal stimulation), perforation of the esophagus, bleeding, and hypoxemia. The nurse assisting with the procedure should monitor the heart rate and blood pressure continuously. TEEs are contraindicated in patients with esophageal disorders or diseases or who have difficulty swallowing.

## X-Ray Examination and Fluoroscopy

X-ray examination is a valuable tool for appraising the size and shape of the heart. The heart is easily visualized on a chest x-ray, and its contour can be readily outlined; the thoracic aorta and pulmonary vessels also can be seen. Congestion of the pulmonary circulation suggestive of congestive failure can be evaluated using a chest x-ray. The accuracy of determining the heart's size depends on the type of film (upright or supine) and the position of the x-ray beam (anterior or posterior). Only trained personnel should interpret x-rays.

Fluoroscopic examination allows visualization of the heart in motion and can be a useful tool during insertion of pacemakers and PA catheters when accurate placement of wires and catheters is essential in preventing complications. Fluoroscopy requires the patient and personnel at the bedside to wear protective covering. Because the exposure to radiation is greater with fluoroscopy that with conventional x-rays, the machine is used only intermittently during procedures. No other special preparation is needed.

## Angiography

The chambers of the heart, the valves, and blood vessels are examined by injecting a contrast medium into a vein or artery. X-ray films, called *angiograms,* are then taken. Selective angiography uses a smaller amount of the contrast medium and injects it in or near the area to be studied. This method has proved more satisfactory than injecting the contrast medium into the vein. Selective angiography makes it possible to study any part of the vascular system.

Patients undergoing this procedure should be questioned carefully about allergies, especially to iodine and shellfish, because some people are sensitive to the dye. If the patient has any history of renal failure or renal insufficiency, IV fluid is ordered before and after the procedure to prevent renal failure caused by the contrast dye. Before the examination, food usually is withheld from the patient to prevent nausea and vomiting, and a mild sedative may be given. These patients usually are fearful and apprehensive and need a great deal of education and reassurance.

Potential complications include allergic reactions and bleeding or thrombosis at the site. After the procedure the patient should be monitored for bleeding or hematoma formation at the site of the injection, and vital signs, including blood pressure, should be monitored. Pulses distal to the injection site should be monitored for changes.

## Cardiac Catheterization

Cardiac catheterization requires a team of well-trained physicians and nurses. In the past cardiac catheterization was done only in medical centers that had facilities for open heart surgery, but now portable or freestanding cardiac catheterization laboratories are available for conducting this procedure as an outpatient study. Patients at low risk for complications are candidates for outpatient catheterization.

The purposes of cardiac catheterization are to measure the pressure in the heart chambers and pulmonary arteries, to obtain blood samples from the heart and vessels so that analysis can determine the amount of oxygen and carbon dioxide present, to detect congenital or acquired structural defects, to measure cardiac output, and to evaluate the coronary arteries for narrowing or occlusion.

The catheterization may be done on either the right side or the left side of the heart. In a right heart catheterization the catheter is inserted into the subclavian vein or femoral vein (the brachial vein also can be used) and slowly passed into the heart via the vena cava, the right atrium, and the right ventricle. In a left heart catheterization the catheter is inserted into the brachial or femoral artery and passed via the aorta into the left ventricle.

Dye usually is injected (cardiac angiography) through a catheter in the aorta and into the coronary arteries. The angiography portion of the cardiac catheterization is needed to confirm the presence of coronary artery disease (plaque buildup in the coronary arteries) (Pagana, Pagana, 1996). It also is helpful in evaluating the chambers, valves, and collateral circulation of the heart. Using a fluoroscope, films are taken during the procedure and can be reevaluated after the procedure to make a definitive diagnosis.

Before catheterization the procedure is explained to the patient and a signed consent is obtained. The patient usually is kept NPO for 4 to 8 hours before the test, and an IV line is inserted. In preparation for the procedure the site is shaved and scrubbed, and the peripheral pulses should be assessed and marked with a pen. A baseline assessment of the peripheral pulses assists with the follow-up pulse checks after the procedure. As with other dye studies, the patient should be questioned about sensitivity to iodine, shellfish, and dyes and should be asked about any history of renal failure or renal insufficiency. Extensive teaching must be done, and the patient's questions must be answered. After the catheterization, the nurse should monitor vital signs, examine the insertion site, and assist with activity restrictions during recovery. Possible complications of cardiac catheterization include arrhythmias, perforation of the myocardium, emboli that cause stroke or myocardial infarction, catheter site thrombosis, hematoma, and allergic reactions.

## Electrophysiology Studies

An electrophysiology study (EPS) is an invasive test that assists in the diagnosis and treatment of arrhythmias. With this test the electrical activity of the heart can be evaluated and manipulated. In a technique similar to cardiac catheterization, special electrophysiology catheters are inserted through the femoral vein, into the right heart, and are placed in specific sites along the conduction system. This allows for the electrical activity, SA node function, AV node conduction, and ectopic foci to be evaluated.

During an EPS, the electrophysiologist may stimulate different areas of the myocardium through the catheters, searching for the ectopic site and deliberately provoking arrhythmias under controlled conditions. The arrhythmia is then reversed to normal sinus rhythm by pacing, medication, or cardioversion/defibrillation. Therapy such as medication or catheter-accessed ablation (removal) of the site can then be prescribed or performed. EPS is also done before insertion of implantable cardioverter defibrillator and to evaluate the effectiveness of antiarrhythmic drugs.

## Electrocardiography and Arrhythmias

Heart muscle contraction is the result of an electrochemical process in which electrically charged particles (sodium, calcium, and potassium) on the outer and inner surface of the cell membrane move into and out of the cell. When the myocardial cells are stimulated and change the permeability of their cell membrane (action potential), the surface electrical charges are altered. As discussed previously, the electrical events that occur in the heart can be visualized with an ECG machine. These machines measure the electrical current generated by the heart muscle contraction and display a continuous picture of the electrical current on an oscilloscope.

To obtain an ECG, positive and negative adhesive electrodes are placed on specific areas of the limbs or chest wall (or both) with the heart always between a positive and a negative electrode (Figure 23-9). This procedure provides different views (leads) of the heart's electrical activity. The up or down direction (deflection) of the waveforms on the graph paper depends on whether the electrical wave in the heart is moving toward the positive electrode or the negative electrode or in a line between the two electrodes. The electrodes can be positioned in various places over the chest to record different "views" of the heart. A typical ECG rhythm "strip" is only one view. A 12-lead ECG records the electrical activity of the heart from 12 views.

An ECG recording allows the physician or nurse to review the rate, regularity, and sequence of the electrical currents that travel through the heart; it also can show changes indicative of structural abnormalities, ischemia, infarction of the myocardium, electrolyte imbalances, and drug toxicities. Monitoring of the ECG also is useful for identifying normal and abnormal *heart rhythms* (**arrhythmias**). This can be accomplished by using either a system that continuously displays

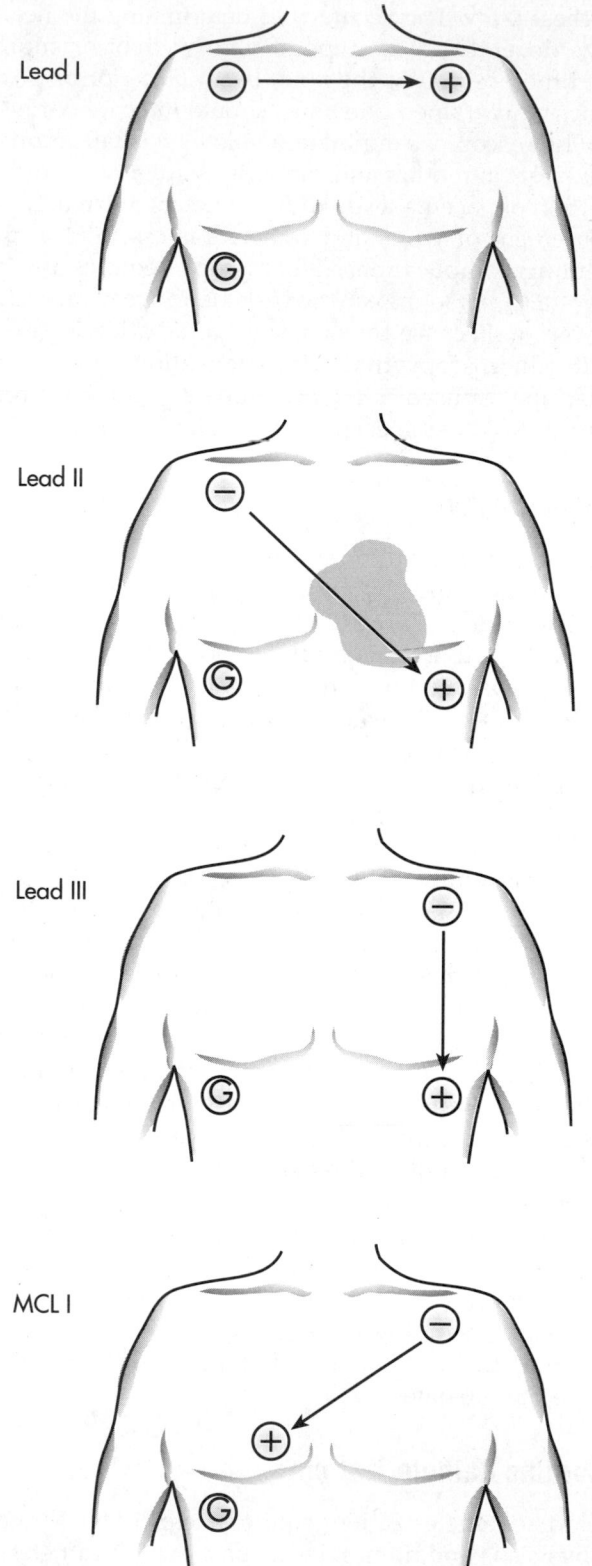

**Figure 23-9** Electrocardiogram electrode placement on the chest. The most common leads monitored are Leads I, II, III, and MCL1. Note that the positive and negative electrodes are positioned differently for each "view" of the heart (lead) but the G (ground) electrode is always on the right lower chest.

the ECG and records a printout when needed, or a system that prepares only a printout. Detection of arrhythmias permits immediate pharmacologic or mechanical (defibrillation/cardioversion) intervention, which can prevent other serious problems.

## Graph Paper

An ECG, the written output of an electrocardiograph machine, appears on graph paper. Time intervals are measured horizontally, and amplitude or force is measured vertically. The graph paper is composed of large and small blocks or squares (Figure 23-10). Each large square contains 25 smaller blocks. Each small block represents 0.04 second of time horizontally and 0.1 mV of amplitude vertically. Each large block containing five small blocks horizontally represents 0.20 second in time (0.4 second × 5 blocks). Each large block vertically represents 0.5 mV in amplitude (0.1 mV × 5 blocks). An understanding of this measurement system is essential to interpretation of an ECG.

## ECG Interpretation

Each contraction of the heart and the electrical forces of depolarization and repolarization that occur during each cardiac cycle should produce a P, Q, R, S, and T wave on the ECG graph paper (Figure 23-11). The first positive deflection above the isoelectric line (baseline) is the *P wave,* which represents the firing of the SA node and depolarization (contraction) of the atria. The *QRS complex* (or waves) is a series of negative-positive-negative deflections that demonstrates the depolarization (contraction) of the ventricles. The positive deflection after the QRS complex is the *T wave,* which represents the repolarization (relaxation) of the ventricle. During this period the heart does not accept an impulse from the SA node, allowing the electrical charges to realign on either side of the cell membrane.

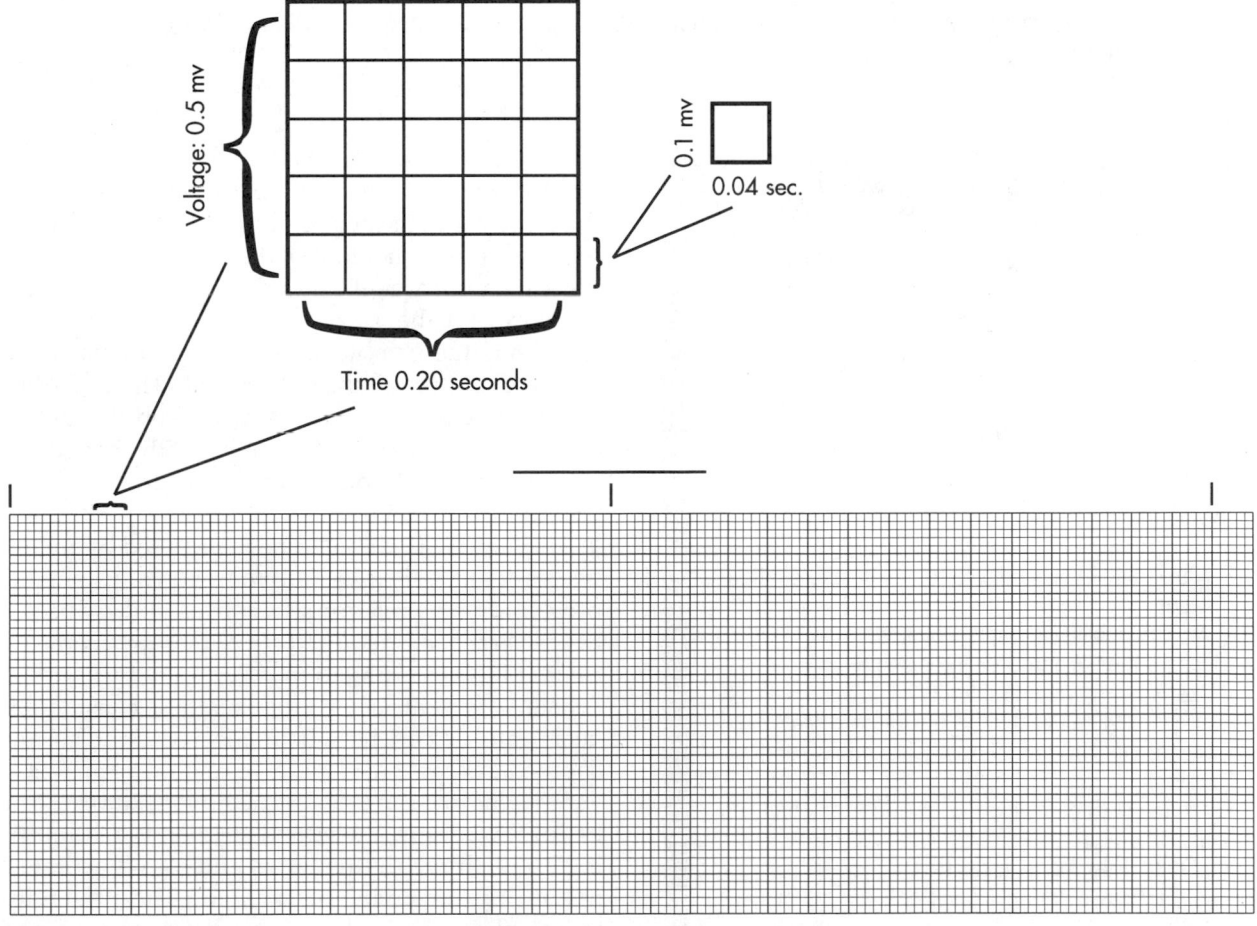

**Figure 23-10**   Electrocardiogram graph paper and measurement.

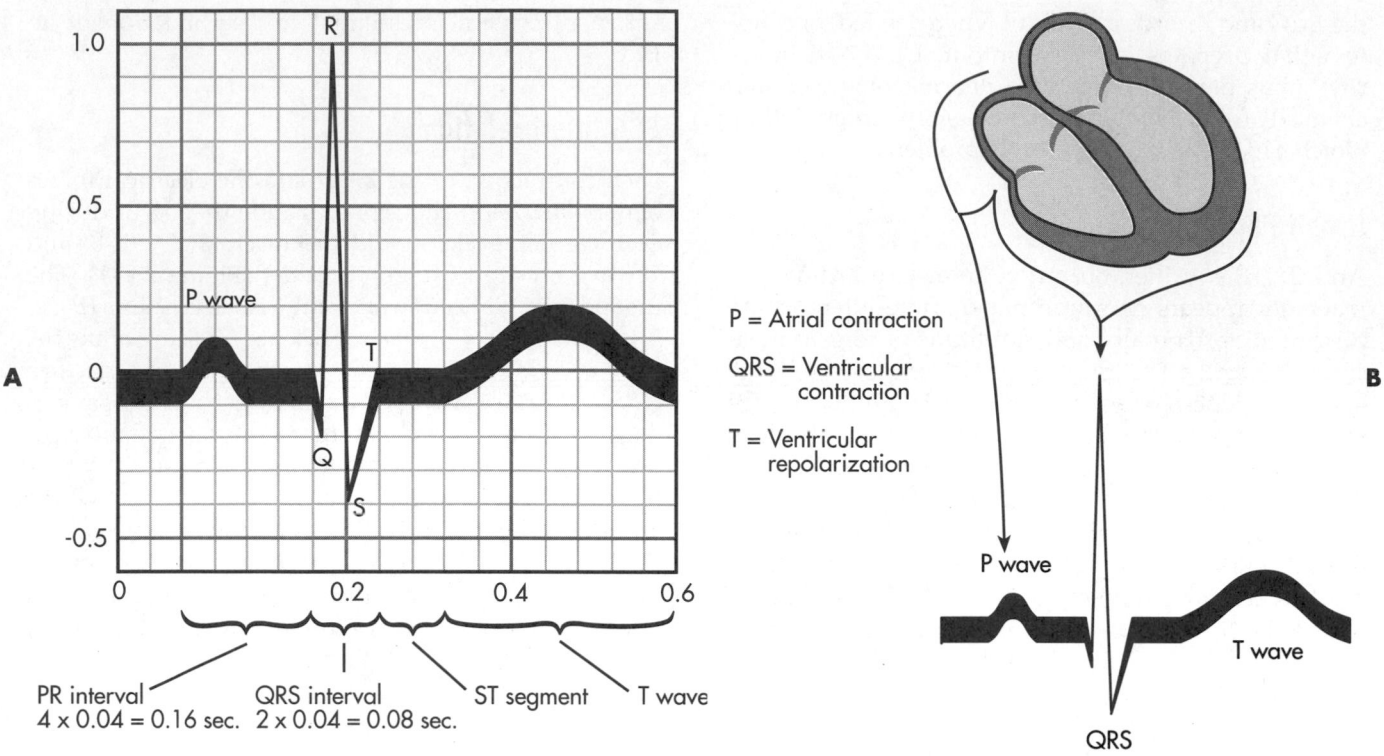

**Figure 23-11**  **A,** Electrocardiogram (ECG) recording of one heartbeat. **B,** ECG waveforms and their relationship to the cardiac cycle.

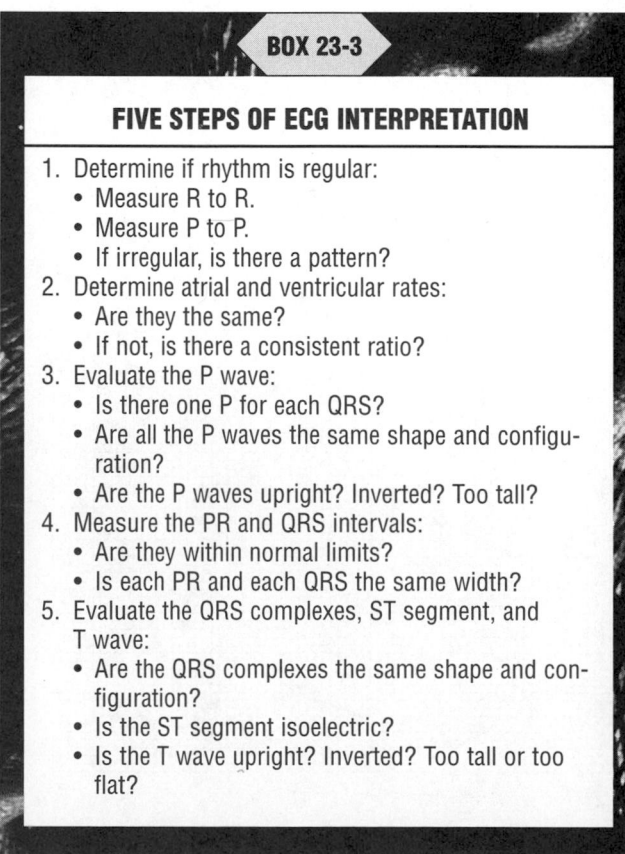

**BOX 23-3**

### FIVE STEPS OF ECG INTERPRETATION

1. Determine if rhythm is regular:
   • Measure R to R.
   • Measure P to P.
   • If irregular, is there a pattern?
2. Determine atrial and ventricular rates:
   • Are they the same?
   • If not, is there a consistent ratio?
3. Evaluate the P wave:
   • Is there one P for each QRS?
   • Are all the P waves the same shape and configuration?
   • Are the P waves upright? Inverted? Too tall?
4. Measure the PR and QRS intervals:
   • Are they within normal limits?
   • Is each PR and each QRS the same width?
5. Evaluate the QRS complexes, ST segment, and T wave:
   • Are the QRS complexes the same shape and configuration?
   • Is the ST segment isoelectric?
   • Is the T wave upright? Inverted? Too tall or too flat?

The spaces between the waves are also important. The *PR interval* is the space between the beginning of the P wave and the beginning of the QRS complex; this represents the time it takes the impulse to travel from the atria and through the AV node. Between the QRS complex and the T wave lies the *ST segment,* which represents the completion of the ventricular contraction and the repolarization period. The angle at the point where the ST segment begins and the QRS complex ends is known as the *J point.* With changes in the ST segment, the J point may deviate from the isoelectric line.

Every ECG strip should be interpreted by following five basic steps (Box 23-3). This creates a systematic approach to interpretation ECG strips and reduces confusion. Practice is required for nurses to become proficient at ECG interpretation.

**Rate.** The ventricular rate usually is considered the heart rate. It can be felt in the radial pulse and is counted in beats per minute. In reviewing an ECG, the ventricular rate can be estimated by counting the number of R waves in a 6-second strip and then multiplying by 10. (If the rhythm is irregular, an exact rate cannot be determined by this method.) The atrial rate can be calculated by counting the P waves in a similar fashion. Usually there is one P wave for each QRS complex, indicating that one atrial contraction occurs for each ventricular contraction. In some arrhythmias the atrial and ventricular rates are different, therefore it is important to determine both.

**Rhythm.** The rhythm reveals whether the patient's heart is beating regularly or irregularly. The atrial and ventricular rhythms should both be evaluated. The atrial rhythm is determined by measuring the distance between two consecutive P waves. Calipers for marking the point on paper at each consecutive P wave often are used to make this measurement but are not necessary. The two caliper points should then be aligned on two P waves (moving left to right) and then used to compare the distance between other P waves. If the distance is equal between all the P waves, the rhythm is regular; if it is unequal, the rhythm is irregular. The ventricular rhythm is determined by the same method, measuring the intervals between the R waves.

**P wave.** The P wave is a result of atrial depolarization. All P waves should point in the same direction. The direction should be appropriate for the lead being recorded. There should be one P wave for every QRS complex, and the distance between them should be regular. All P waves should be similar in shape and size. A difference indicates irritation in the atrial tissue or damage near the SA node.

**PR interval.** The PR interval measures the AV conduction time. It is measured from the onset of the P wave to the beginning of the QRS complex. The normal PR interval is 0.12 to 0.20 second. A shorter PR interval means that the impulse originated in an area other than the SA node. A longer PR interval signifies a delay in the impulse as it passes through the AV node.

**QRS interval.** The width of the QRS complex can reveal important data about the direction of conduction through the ventricles and the length of time it takes the electrical conduction to spread. The QRS complex is measured from the beginning of the QRS to the end of the QRS at the beginning of the ST segment. The normal width is less than 0.02 second. A widened QRS complex may be indicative of conduction delays through the ventricles.

**Configuration and location.** Evaluating the configuration and location of the P, Q, R, S, and T waves on a rhythm strip can bring to light information about the location and extent of myocardial damage and other problems that can disrupt the progression of the electrical current. Each wave should be evaluated systematically. P waves should precede QRS complexes. The QRS complexes should be reviewed for shape, size, direction, and location in relation to the T wave. If the QRS complexes are close to the preceding T wave, the ventricles are contracting prematurely. The T wave represents ventricular relaxation. The closer the QRS is

to the T wave, the greater the risk for serious ventricular arrhythmia. The ST segment can be slightly elevated above the baseline but should not be depressed. It then curves very slightly into the start of the T wave. An abnormality of the ST segment is an early sign of myocardial infarction. T waves should also be observed for size and shape and should deflect in the same direction as the QRS complex. T waves should follow the QRS. Elevated or "tented" T waves can be a sign of elevated potassium levels.

# DISORDERS OF RATE AND RHYTHM OF THE HEART

The pulse (heart rate) is one of the most sensitive indices for assessing cardiac function. Nurses should develop a keen sensitivity to what they feel when obtaining a peripheral pulse. When the heart is functioning normally, the pulse is felt as smooth, regular, equally spaced beats of equal strength and volume that occur 60 to 100 times per minute. Under certain conditions changes occur in the pulse rate and rhythm, indicating a change in the rate and rhythm of the cardiac cycle. These conditions are called cardiac **arrhythmias.**

Cardiac arrhythmias occur both in well people and in those with cardiovascular disease. Any deviation from normal sinus rhythm is defined as an arrhythmia. Arrhythmias may result from an abnormal rate, a site of impulse formation other than the SA node, or abnormal conduction within the system. Arrhythmias can be caused by a number of systemic disorders and diseases. They are categorized by the site of origin, which may be sinus, atrial, nodal (junctional), or ventricular. The nurse may be the first person to detect changes in the patient's pulse and the first to be alerted to the possible presence of arrhythmias. Some arrhythmias can have serious consequences and must be treated immediately to restore a pulse and respirations and to preserve other organ functions. The following sections review the common types of cardiac arrhythmias and their treatment.

## Arrhythmias
### Sinus Arrhythmias

The SA node is the source of all sinus rhythms, but the frequency of its discharge varies. The heart rate increases and decreases as the firing rate of the SA node changes. Figure 23-11 demonstrates a normal sinus rhythm. The SA node normally discharges regularly at a rate of 60 to 100 times per minute.

**Sinus arrhythmia.** If the regularity of the heart rhythm is altered, usually during the inspiratory phase of the respiratory cycle, the change in the sinus rhythm

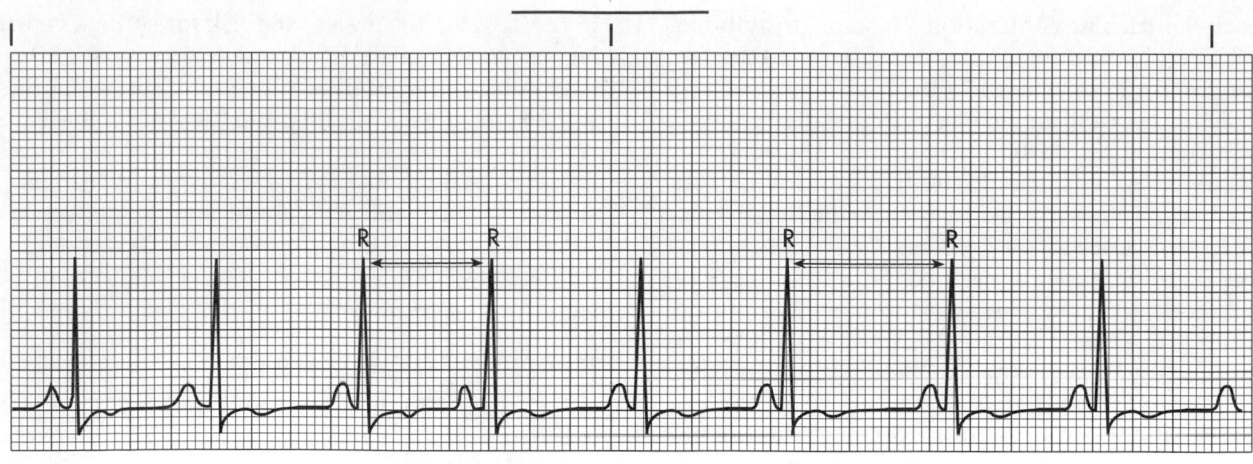

**Figure 23-12**    Sinus arrhythmia.

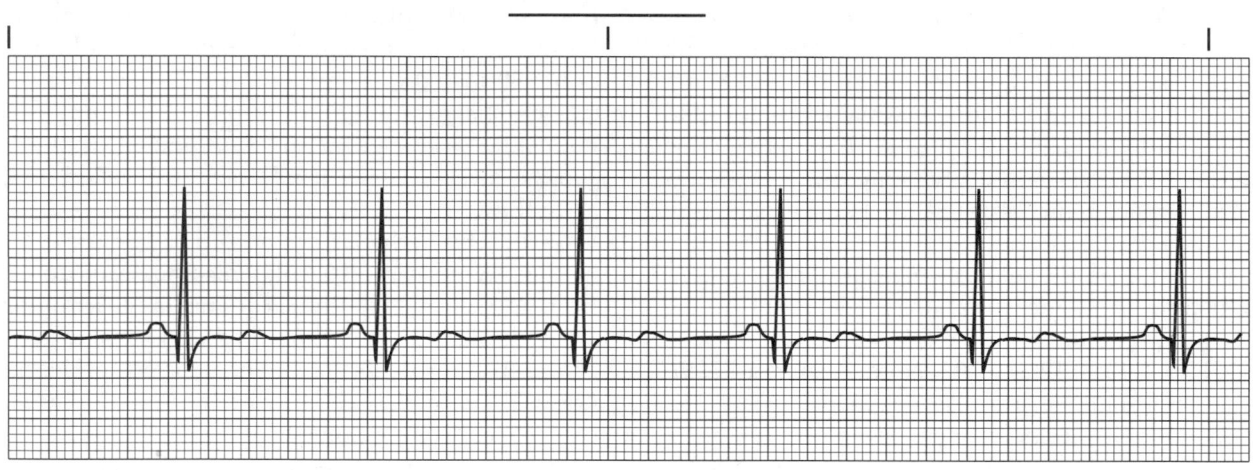

**Figure 23-13**    Sinus bradycardia.

on the ECG is called sinus arrhythmia (Figure 23-12). In healthy young individuals, the rate may vary with respiration asymptomatically. Treatment usually is not needed for sinus arrhythmia.

**Sinus bradycardia.** If the rate falls below 60 times per minute but the complexes and regularity are normal, the arrhythmia is called *sinus bradycardia* (Figure 23-13). Sinus bradycardia may be caused by a defect in the SA node, increased stimulation of the parasympathetic nervous system that slows SA node discharge, or drugs that depress the heart (e.g., beta-blockers, calcium channel blockers, and digitalis). Slowing of the heart rate can cause numerous symptoms indicating a reduction of cardiac output and tissue hypoxia (Box 23-4). If a patient has been found to have a slow heart rate, it is important to determine if the patient has any symptoms such as dizziness and syncope indicating a need for immediate treatment. Possible treatments include administrating atropine to block the parasympathetic nervous system and increase the rate and stimulating the heart with a pacemaker. Drugs that stimulate the sympathetic nervous system (e.g., epinephrine, dopamine and, in rare cases, isoproterenol) also can be used to increase the heart rate (Cummins, 1994).

### NURSE ALERT

**Although bradycardia usually is defined as a heart rate below 60 beats per minute, some patients, such as athletes, have much slower rates that do not require treatment. *Always* evaluate a patient for signs and symptoms before initiating treatment.**

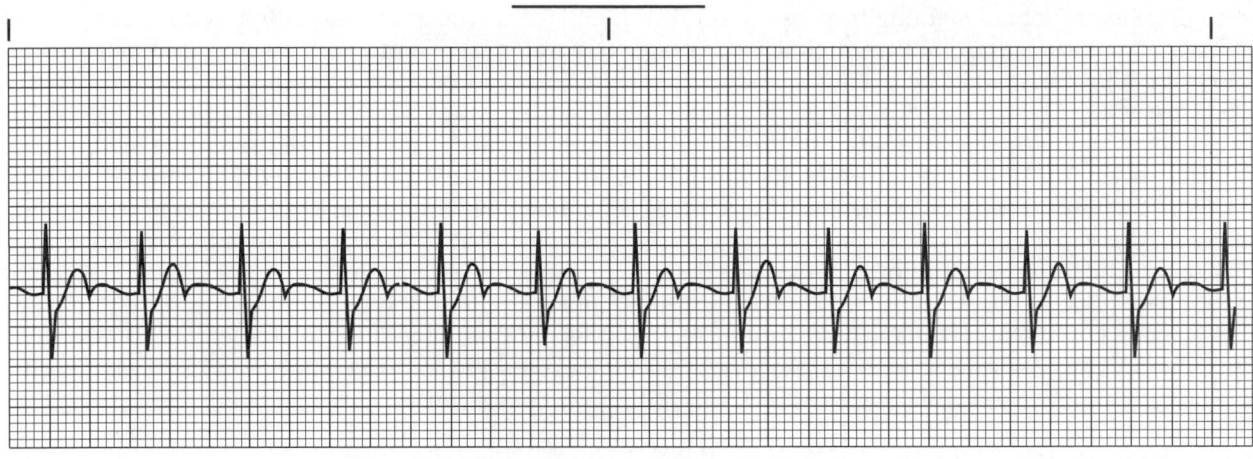

**Figure 23-14**    Sinus tachycardia.

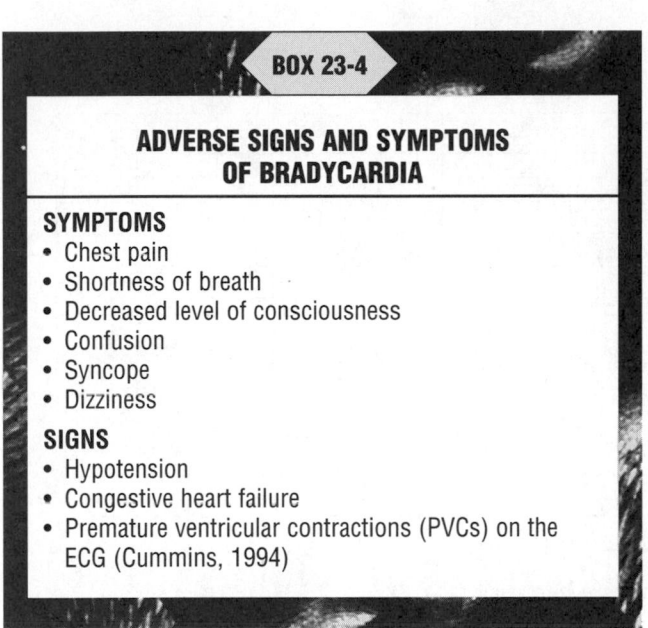

BOX 23-4

### ADVERSE SIGNS AND SYMPTOMS OF BRADYCARDIA

**SYMPTOMS**
- Chest pain
- Shortness of breath
- Decreased level of consciousness
- Confusion
- Syncope
- Dizziness

**SIGNS**
- Hypotension
- Congestive heart failure
- Premature ventricular contractions (PVCs) on the ECG (Cummins, 1994)

**Sinus tachycardia.** A sinus rhythm with normal complexes and regularity but a rate greater than 100 (between 100 and 150) beats/min is called *sinus tachycardia*. (Figure 23-14). Sinus tachycardia is a physiologic response to the need for more cardiac output. Exercise, fever, anxiety, pain, anemia, hypoxemia, hypoglycemia, low fluid volume, and shock are some of the underlying causes of tachycardia. Drugs that stimulate the heart, such as caffeine, nicotine, antihistamines, and epinephrine, also can cause tachycardia. Since an increase in the heart rate increases the workload of the heart, tachycardia can trigger chest pain and myocardial ischemia in patients with underlying cardiac disease. The treatment for sinus tachycardia is aimed at eliminating or treating the precipitating factors.

## Atrial Arrhythmias

Normally the SA node originates the impulse to begin the cardiac cycle. Sometimes, however, an impulse arises from another area of the atrium before the SA node fires. This impulse can stimulate an early contraction of the heart muscle. These ectopic impulses can also take over the pacemaker function from the SA node or can be caught in a pathway along the conduction system and reenter the conduction cycle over and over at a very fast rate. Four of the most common atrial arrhythmia are discussed below.

**Premature atrial contraction.** An early ECG complex that comes from an ectopic focus in the atrium is called a premature atrial contraction (PAC). This impulse usually occurs earlier than expected and is indicated by a P wave with a different configuration from that of P waves of the impulses that begin in the SA node. The QRS complex of the PAC usually is normal, but it may have a different configuration because the normal path of conduction is not followed; this is called aberrancy. A short pause usually is present between the T wave of the PAC and the next P wave (Figure 23-15). PACs are a common arrhythmia. In normal individuals they result from factors such as caffeine, nicotine, or strong emotions (Atwood et al, 1996). In some patients they may be associated with myocardial infarctions, digitalis toxicity, low potassium levels, hypoxia, rheumatic heart disease, or hyperthyroidism (Lilly, 1993). A PAC may be a warning that other atrial arrhythmias are likely to occur. In many patients no treatment is indicated. Eliminating substances or drugs that might be stimulating the ectopic impulses may diminish or stop their occurrence.

If underlying heart disease is thought to be the cause of the PACs, drugs such as quinidine, digitalis, or propranolol may be prescribed.

**Atrial tachycardia.** Atrial tachycardia (Figure 23-16) is an atrial arrhythmia with a very rapid heart rate of 150 to 250 beats per minute. It is caused by an ectopic focus in the atrium that fires repeatedly. When the cause is an underlying drug toxicity, such as digitalis toxicity, the rhythm can be maintained for long periods and is called nonparoxysmal atrial tachycardia. When the cause is a reentry pathway, the tachycardia may start and stop suddenly; these episodes of tachycardia, called paroxysmal supraventricular tachycardia (PSVT), may last for seconds or hours. In a healthy heart they can be brought on by physical exertion, emotional stress, and stimulants like caffeine (Cummins, 1994).

PSVT can also be associated with conditions such as mitral and aortic valve stenosis, Wolff-Parkinson-White syndrome (an accessory pathway disorder), and coronary artery disease. These rapid atrial tachycardias are identified by the excessive rate and a regular rhythm. The P wave frequently is hidden in the preceding T wave and has a different contour than normal P waves. The QRS complex usually is normal.

As with sinus tachycardia, these atrial tachycardias put a strain on the heart muscle and may reduce cardiac output and filling of the coronary arteries. Prolonged rapid heart rates of over 150 beats per minute can compromise cardiac function and cause serious symptoms that require immediate treatment. Box 23-5 presents the signs and symptoms associated with cardiovascular compromise in tachycardias.

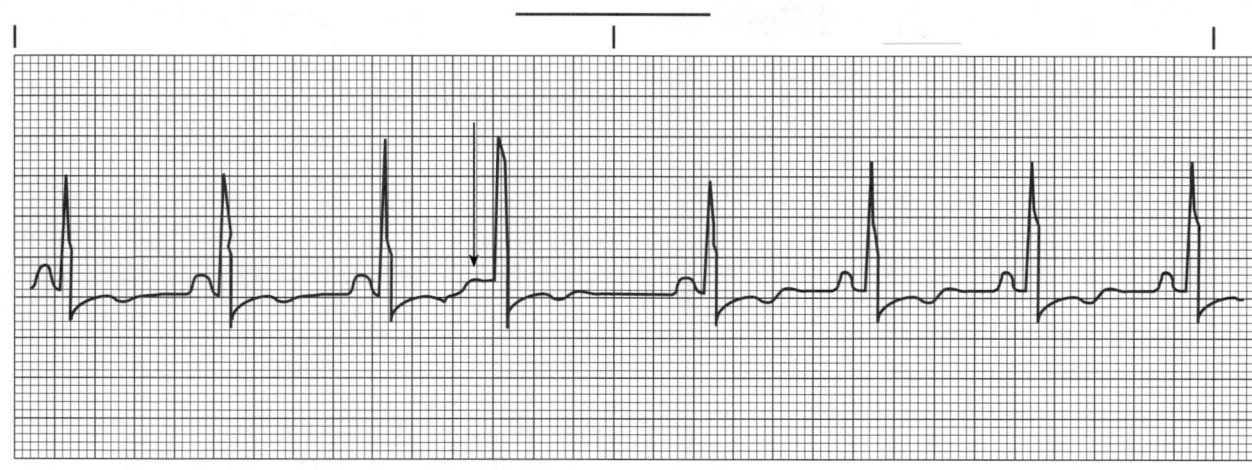

**Figure 23-15**   Premature atrial contraction.

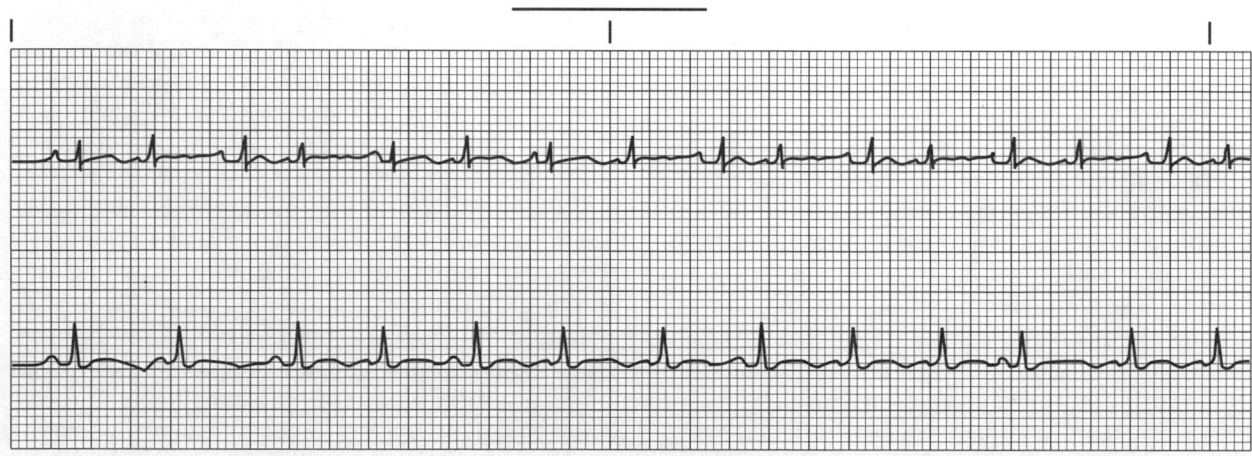

**Figure 23-16**   Atrial tachycardia.

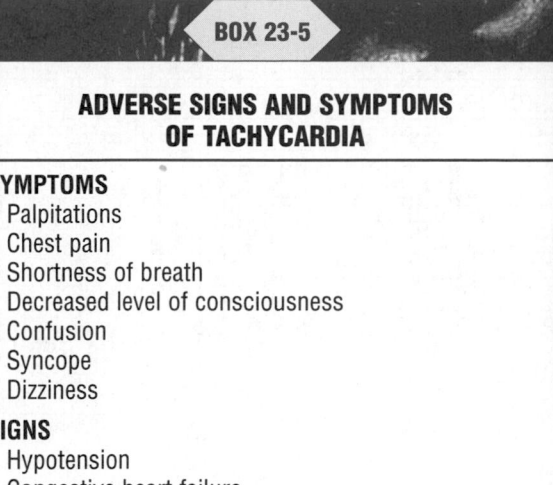

**BOX 23-5**

## ADVERSE SIGNS AND SYMPTOMS OF TACHYCARDIA

**SYMPTOMS**
- Palpitations
- Chest pain
- Shortness of breath
- Decreased level of consciousness
- Confusion
- Syncope
- Dizziness

**SIGNS**
- Hypotension
- Congestive heart failure
- Myocardial infarction (Cummins, 1994)

Treatment of nonparoxysmal atrial tachycardia usually consists of removal of the offending drug. For both paroxysmal and nonparoxysmal atrial tachycardias accompanied by instability and serious signs and symptoms, immediate electrical **cardioversion** is the treatment of choice (Cummins, 1994). Box 23-6 presents information on cardioversion. If the patient is not experiencing serious signs and symptom, the treatment is vagal stimulation and drug therapy. Vagal stimulation may be elicited by carotid massage or the Valsalva maneuver. These interventions increase parasympathetic tone and slow conduction. The current drug of choice for the initial treatment of PSVT is adenosine. This drug has a very short half-life (10 seconds) and causes few long-term side effects. Verapamil may also be used, but it has more prolonged side effects, including hypotension and bradycardia. Patients with recurring atrial tachycardia may be treated with radiofrequency ablation to destroy the accessory pathway and stop the arrhythmia (Cummins, 1994).

**BOX 23-6**

## CARDIOVERSION

Cardioversion is a procedure that gives the heart external electrical stimulation. The external electrical stimulation interrupts the irregular conduction pattern of the heart and restores it to normal sinus rhythm. The patient's heart rhythm is monitored, and the synchronized electrical shock is delivered during ventricular contraction. Delivery of electrical shock at any other time could cause severe, life-threatening arrhythmia. Cardioversion is performed by a physician with the patient's written consent. The nurse monitors the patient's heart rate, rhythm, blood pressure, and respirations throughout the procedure.

**NURSING CONSIDERATIONS AND SAFETY**
- Cardioversion is the process of delivering an electrical shock through paddles placed on the chest at the base and apex of the heart.
- Conductive pads or gel must be used to reduce the resistance and prevent burning of the skin.
- The electrical shock is delivered at the moment a QRS complex is occurring by using a special function of the defibrillator that synchronizes the shock with the heartbeat.
- The shock momentarily stops electrical cardiac activity, allowing a normal pacemaker to take over.
- Cardioversion should be done only by properly trained nurses or physicians after assessment reveals the need for this therapy.

- Cardioversion may be done in an emergency or scheduled as a procedure.
- Unless the patient is unstable and would not tolerate a time delay, sedation should be used.
- If possible the patient should have an IV line, and all emergency equipment should be at the bedside before cardioversion is begun.
- The nurse should be prepared to begin cardiopulmonary resuscitation (CPR) and advanced life support in case asystole occurs after cardioversion.
- The safety measures described in Box 23-7 should be followed.
- The patient can expect to be sore and to have reddened skin where the paddles were placed after cardioversion.
- Vital signs should be taken before the procedure, between shocks, and upon completion of the cardioversion and then every 5 to 10 minutes until the patient is fully alert.
- The patient should have a continuous cardiac monitor for at least 24 hours after cardioversion.
- The preprocedural sedation, all vital signs, the number of cardioversion attempts, the energy used, and the patient's response should be documented in the medical record.
- The patient should be evaluated frequently for respiratory depression, arrhythmias, and any distress after cardioversion. (Cummins, 1994.)

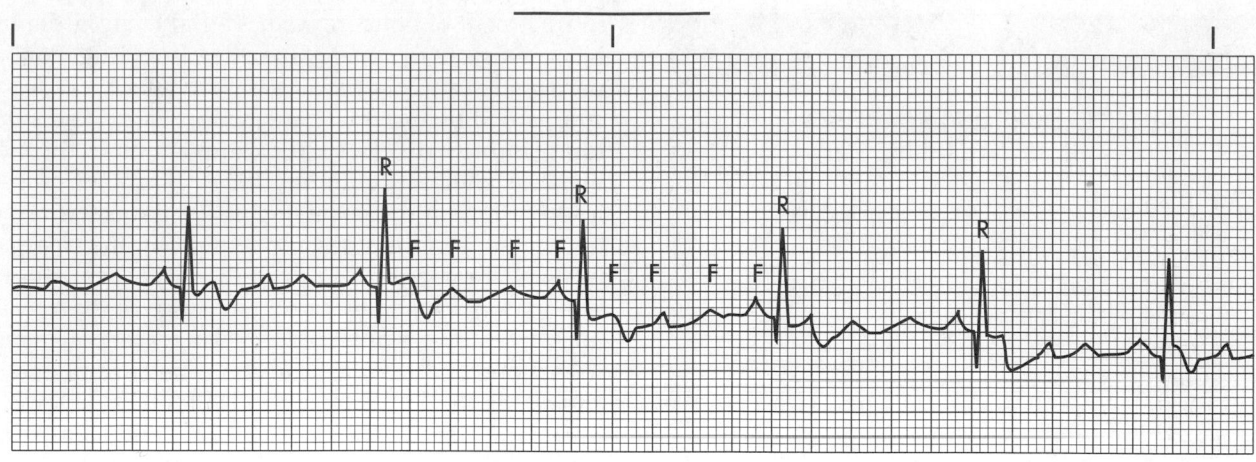

**Figure 23-17**   Atrial flutter.

**Atrial flutter.** *Atrial flutter* is an atrial arrhythmia that occurs at a rate of 250 to 350 beats per minute (Figure 23-17). The impulse originates from an ectopic atrial focus. The regular, rapid atrial rate results in a sawtoothed flutter wave on the ECG tracing. QRS complexes do not follow each flutter wave because the AV node does not transmit each impulse down to the ventricles. Usually a 2:1 ratio of impulses is conducted through the system to the ventricles. This means that the ventricles do respond as quickly as the atria, and the ventricular rate often is half the atrial rate. The QRS complex appears normal unless an aberrant conduction is present.

As are other atrial arrhythmias, atrial flutter usually is the result of a reentry circuit in the atria, and it rarely occurs in the absence of organic heart disease. Cardiovascular problems such as mitral and tricuspid valve disease, coronary artery disease, or cor pulmonale usually are present in patients with atrial flutter (Cummins, 1994).

With atrial flutter, cardiac output remains normal as long as the ventricular rate is within normal limits. If the ventricular rate exceeds 150 beats per minute, signs and symptoms common to other tachycardias may occur. If allowed to persist, atrial flutter can con-vert to atrial fibrillation. Treatment is indicated if the ventricular rate is so rapid that the ventricles cannot fill and the patient becomes symptomatic, or the rhythm persists. The goal of treatment is to slow the ventricular rate or change the rhythm to a sinus node-initiated impulse; this can be accomplished by using electrical cardioversion (a shock to the heart) or drug therapy. If serious signs and symptoms are present, cardioversion is the treatment of choice. If the patient is only mildly symptomatic or has no symptoms, pharmacologic treatment is indicated. The ventricular rate can be slowed with diltiazem, verapamil, digitalis, or beta-blockers (Cummins, 1994).

**Atrial fibrillation.** *Atrial fibrillation* is a chaotic atrial rhythm with a rapid, irregular atrial rate of over 350 beats per minute (Figure 23-18). The ventricular rate can range from as low as 50 beats per minute to as high as 170 beats per minute because the AV node cannot conduct every atrial impulse. Distinct P waves are absent, and the ECG tracing has classic fibrillation waves with an irregular ventricular rhythm. QRS complexes are normal or reflect aberrant (deviant) conduction. PACs usually precede atrial fibrillation.

Atrial fibrillation can be caused by multiple areas of reentry or multiple ectopic areas, and in healthy young people it may be a transient arrhythmia. Continuous atrial fibrillation, however, is associated with heart disease, particularly congestive heart failure. When atrial fibrillation occurs, the atria are not able to complete any organized atrial contraction and thus are not able to contribute their atrial kick. As a result, cardiac output decreases. With atrial fibrillation atrial emptying is incomplete, which can cause pooling of blood around the mitral and tricuspid valves. The pooling can result in the formation of thrombi and an increased risk of

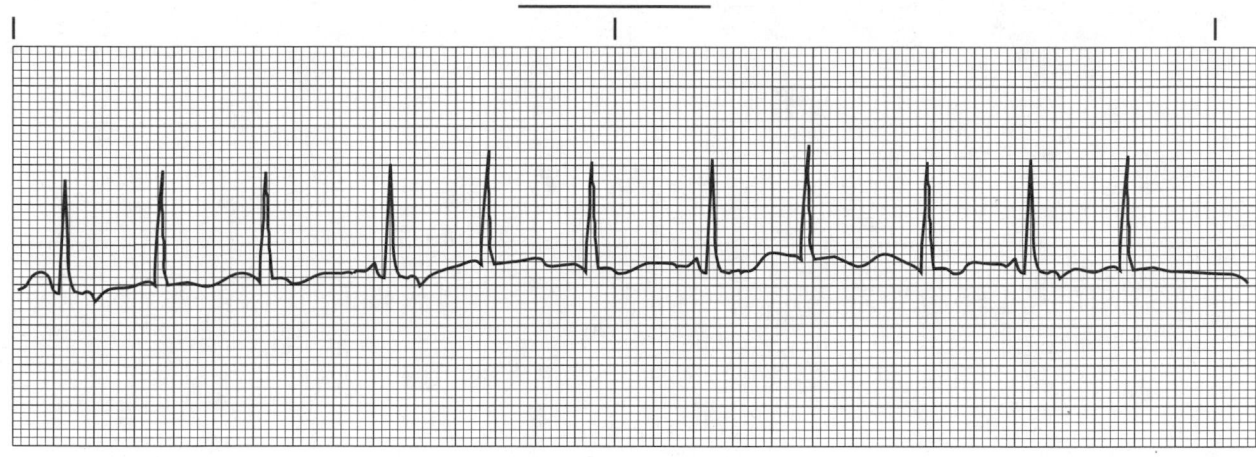

**Figure 23-18**    Atrial fibrillation.

thromboembolization to the brain, lungs, or other organs. The radial pulse is irregular.

Treatment of atrial fibrillation depends on the ventricular rate. If the rate is rapid, rate control can be attempted using pharmacologic agents such as diltiazem, verapamil, beta-blockers, and digitalis. If the patient is having serious signs and symptoms, immediate cardioversion is the treatment of choice. After the rate has been brought under control, cardioversion, either chemical or electrical, is considered (Cummins, 1994).

Chemical cardioversion is the use of drugs to return the rhythm to a sinus node-controlled rhythm. Drugs frequently used for chemical cardioversion are procainamide or quinidine. Electrical cardioversion is an option in unstable situations or when chemical cardioversion has not been successful. The success of cardioversion and prevention of a recurrence of atrial fibrillation depend on the size of the atrium and the length of time the patient has been in atrial fibrillation. Large atria and prolonged atrial fibrillation diminish the likelihood of success. Before cardioversion is attempted, either by chemical or electrical methods, anticoagulation should be initiated unless contraindicated. Anticoagulants prevent formation of thrombi in the atrium (Cummins, 1994).

## Junctional Arrhythmias

The electrical impulse that initiates junctional rhythms originates from areas of the conduction system around or in the AV node. These ectopic junctional beats can occur randomly or can take over the pacemaker function of the heart. The electrical impulse that initiates from the junctional ectopic focus is conducted in a direction opposite that of impulses originating in the SA node. The resulting P wave is upside down and before the QRS, hidden inside the QRS, or after the QRS. The QRS complexes that follow these retrograde P waves usually are normal in configuration. There are several types of junctional arrhythmias, including premature junctional contraction, junctional escape rhythm, accelerated junctional contraction, and junctional tachycardia. This section focuses on junctional escape rhythm.

**Junctional escape rhythm.** When conduction tissue surrounding the AV node takes over the pacing function of the heart, it cannot do so at a rate as high as that of the SA node. Junctional escape rhythms have a rate of 40 to 60 beats per minute (Figure 23-19). Junctional escape rhythms most often occur when the SA node is unable to complete its pacemaker function; they may be seen with acute myocardial infarction that damages the SA node and with disease of the SA node. Because the rate of the junctional escape rhythm is slow, the hemodynamic consequences in the heart and the signs and symptoms are the same as for other types of bradycardia (see Box 23-4). The treatment options, which are the same as for sinus bradycardia, include drug therapy and pacing of the heart to increase the heart rate.

## Heart Blocks

Heart blocks, or atrioventricular (AV) blocks, result from a disturbance in the conduction system at the AV junction. Heart blocks are problematic because of the decrease in conduction of impulses to the ventricles and the reduced ventricular rate. Heart blocks are categorized as first degree, second degree, or third degree.

**First-degree AV block.** First-degree AV block (Figure 23-20) is identified by a PR interval greater than

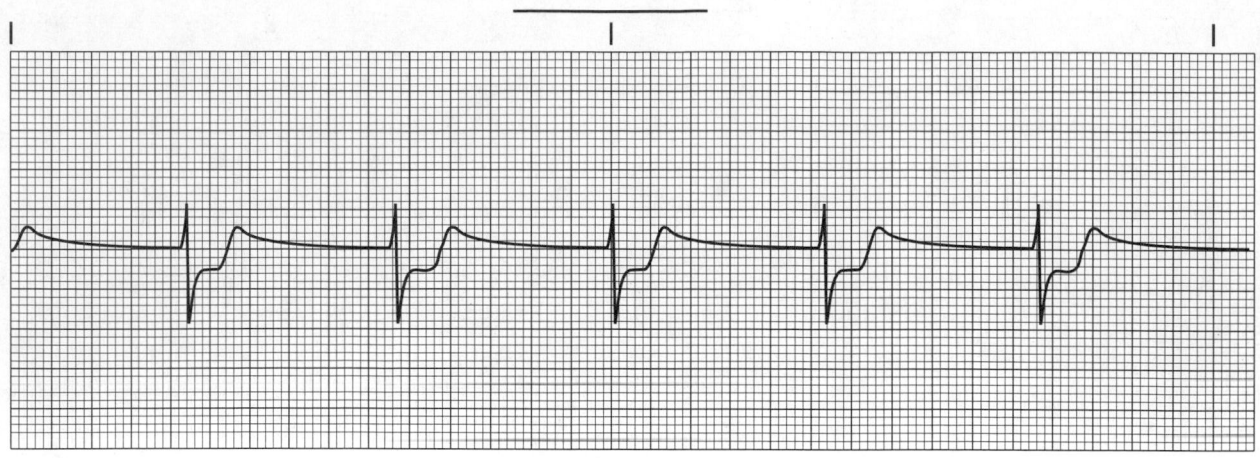

**Figure 23-19** Junctional rhythm.

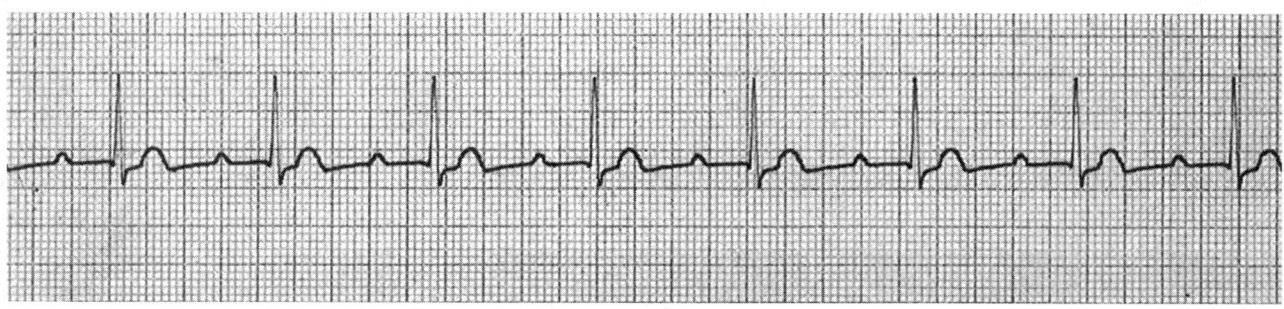

**Figure 23-20** Sinus rhythm with first degree atrioventricular block. (From Smith LF, Fish FH: *Pure practice for ECGs, a practice workbook*, St Louis, 1995, Mosby.)

0.20 second (five small blocks on the graph paper). The impulse originates in the SA node and travels normally through the atria. The conduction is abnormally delayed at the AV junction, but it does pass through, and the ventricles respond normally. Reversible first-degree heart block may result from transient ischemia or from therapy with digitalis, beta-blockers, or calcium channel blockers. Structural causes include myocardial infarction or degenerative changes in the conduction system. Usually no treatment is necessary (Cummins, 1994).

**Second-degree heart block.** Two types of second-degree heart block can be seen. *Mobitz type I* block (sometimes called Wenckebach's block) results from the same conduction defect as first-degree block. However, with each beat the conduction delay through the AV junction increases progressively until the sinus impulse is completely blocked and no QRS complex occurs. On the ECG graph paper, this is seen as a PR interval that gets progressively longer with each beat of the heart until the P wave occurs with no QRS to follow. After the blocked beat, the pattern repeats itself.

This arrhythmia often is seen in patients with inferior myocardial infarction and with the use of drugs that increase parasympathetic tone (e.g., digitalis, propranolol, and verapamil). Treatment involves discontinuing the drug if the condition is drug related. Atropine or other sympathomimetic drugs and pacing also may be used to increase the rate if the bradycardia produces serious signs and symptoms (Cummins, 1994).

*Mobitz type II* heart block is caused by a defect below the level of the AV node, in either the bundle of His or, more commonly, in the bundle branches. On the ECG tracing this rhythm has constant PR intervals, but the atrial impulses are not always conducted down to the ventricles, and more P waves than QRS complexes are seen. Because the SA node is intact, the atrial rate is normal, whereas the ventricular rate is half or less than half the atrial rate. The low rate can cause the same serious decrease in cardiac output and symptoms as in the other bradycardias, sinus bradycardia and junctional escape rhythm. Mobitz type II heart block is a serious arrhythmia usually caused by a lesion in the conduction system, such as an acute anterior myocar-

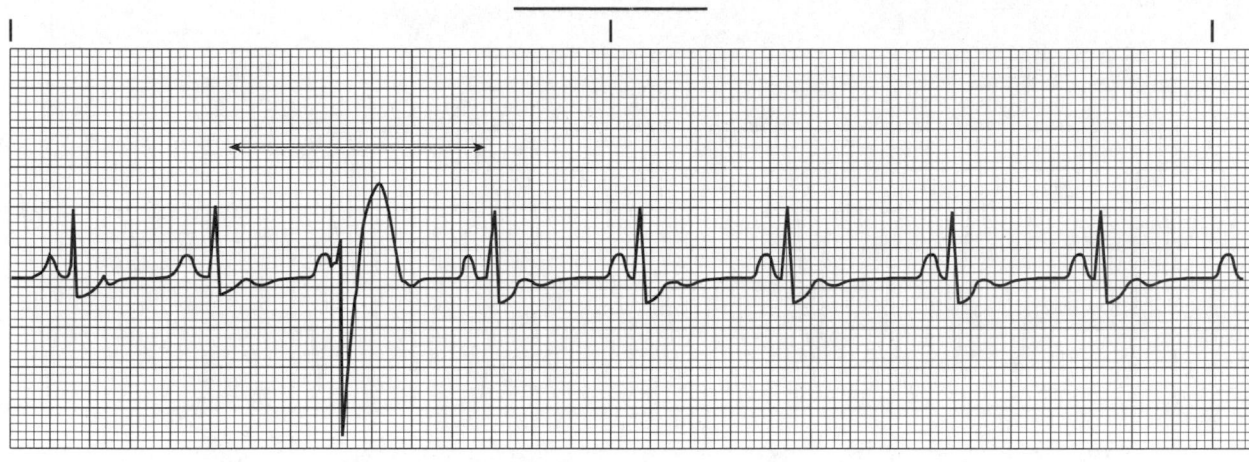

**Figure 23-21**    Premature ventricular contraction.

dial infarction with damage to the ventricular septum. A pacemaker may be required to maintain a normal ventricular rate. If the patient is symptomatic, pharmacologic therapy with atropine, epinephrine, or dopamine can be used until a pacemaker can be obtained (Cummins, 1994).

**Third-degree heart block.** *Third-degree (complete) heart block* occurs when none of the sinus impulses are conducted through the AV junction. The atria and ventricles act independently of one another. The atrial rate usually is regular and of normal frequency. Without stimuli from the SA node, the ventricles use a pacemaker in the ventricular conduction system and beat at a very slow rate, usually 20 to 60 beats per minute. The QRS complex is widened if the ventricular impulse originates in the bundle branch system. Complete heart block may be a result of age, digitalis toxicity, myocarditis, acute myocardial infarction, or cardiac surgery. Because of the ventricular bradycardia, patients with third-degree heart block may experience symptoms of decreased cardiac output. Temporary or permanent cardiac pacing may be needed to maintain the heart rate. Atropine and catecholamine infusions (dopamine or epinephrine) may also be used for temporary therapy (Cummins, 1994).

**Bundle branch block.** *Bundle branch block* is a defect of intraventricular conduction resulting in a conduction delay through the right or left branches of the bundle of His. The PR interval is normal, but the QRS complex is prolonged by at least 0.12 second and may be notched and widened. Myocardial infarction, hypertension, and cardiomyopathy are common causes of bundle branch block. It also can be induced by drugs (e.g., procainamide or quinidine) or caused by hyperkalemia. Treatment focuses on the underlying problem.

## Ventricular Arrhythmias

**Premature ventricular contractions.** *Premature ventricular contractions (PVCs)* are contractions that do not originate from the normal SA node pacemaker (Figure 23-21), but rather arise from an impulse site in the Purkinje fibers. The ventricular contraction occurs earlier than a sinus beat. A P wave does not precede the QRS complex, and the QRS complex is widened, often notched, and may be of greater amplitude (dimension) than normal. The T-wave deflection is in the opposite direction of the QRS complex. Many describe the PVCs as being wide and bizarre-looking compared with normal complexes. A "compensatory" pause usually follows the PVC as the heart waits for another normal SA node impulse. Two PVCs together constitute a couplet, and three consecutive PVCs constitute ventricular tachycardia. When PVCs occur every other beat, the condition is known as *bigeminy;* on every third beat, it is trigeminy. PVCs that occur on or close to the T wave (R on T phenomenon) may start a lethal ventricular arrhythmia.

PVCs may occur in people with or without heart disease and can be expected in patients after a myocardial infarction or cardiac surgery or in patients with myocardial irritability caused by hypoxemia. Because PVCs do not usually create normal ejection from the ventricles, a pulse is not felt when the PVC occurs. The consequences of PVC depend on the number that occurs. Rare PVCs usually are not treated. PVCs that occur in the presence of myocardial ischemia or other causes should be treated by treating the underlying pathologic condition. When pharmacologic therapy is used, most PVCs are treated with antiarrhythmic drugs such as lidocaine or procainamide (Cummins, 1994).

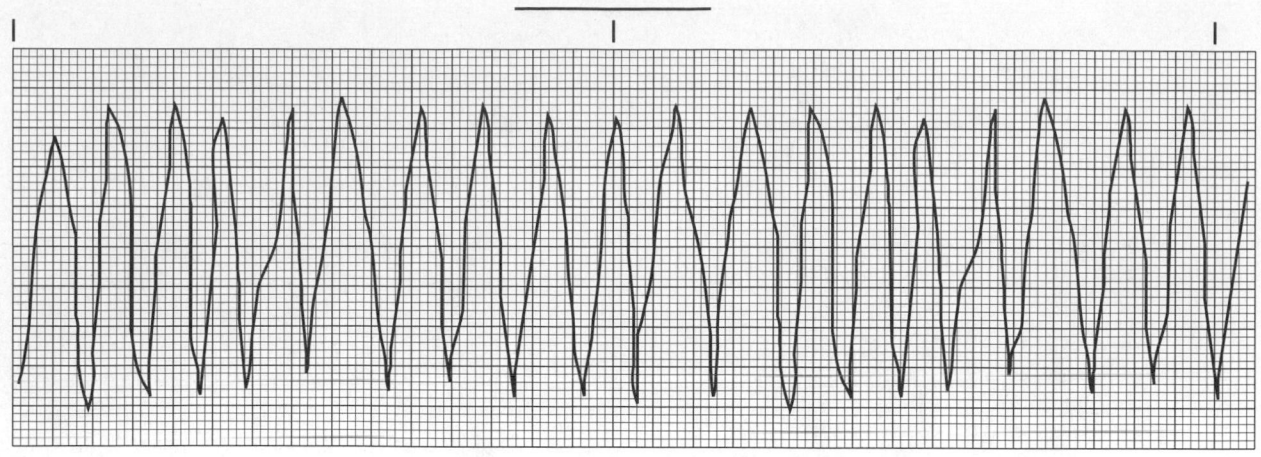

**Figure 23-22**  Ventricular tachycardia.

**Ventricular tachycardia.** *Ventricular tachycardia* is a serious arrhythmia that results from a series of rapid, regular impulses originating in a ventricular ectopic focus (Figure 23-22). The ventricular rate is over 100 beats per minute. P waves are rarely seen. The QRS complex is widened and often notched with greater amplitude. The T wave may be buried in the QRS complex; if visible, it deflects in the direction opposite that of the QRS complex. Ventricular tachycardia can be a complication of digitalis toxicity or myocardial infarction. The consequences of ventricular tachycardia depend on the degree of ventricular dysfunction and the rate of the ventricular contraction.

When ventricular tachycardia is sustained but the patient is stable, treatment consists of drug therapy, such as lidocaine, procainamide, or bretylium. If digitalis toxicity is the cause, the digitalis should be discontinued and potassium levels corrected as necessary. Hypokalemia enhances the toxicity of digitalis by inhibiting the sodium-potassium pump in the cell. When ventricular tachycardia is sustained, a pulse is present, and the patient is suffering symptoms of decreased cardiac output, the treatment of choice is electrical cardioversion (Cummins, 1994).

When the ventricular tachycardia is pulseless, it should be treated with electrical defibrillation (Box 23-7). Defibrillation is similar to cardioversion in that it involves the delivery of an electrical shock for the purpose of depolarizing the myocardium and providing an opportunity for a normal pacemaker to resume functioning. In defibrillation the shock is delivered without synchronizing the delivery with the QRS complex. To be most effective, defibrillation should be delivered quickly after the onset of pulseless ventricular tachycardia (Cummins, 1994).

> ### *NURSE ALERT*
> When defibrillation is being performed, make sure to stay clear of the patient and the bed; contact with the patient or bed can result in an accidental and serious shock.

**Ventricular fibrillation.** *Ventricular fibrillation* is rapid, irregular "quivering" of the ventricles, demonstrated by a wavering baseline and bizarre waveform (Figure 23-23). Ventricular fibrillation often is referred to as "the heart quivering like a bowel of Jello." Ventricular fibrillation may result from myocardial infarction, myocardial ischemia, or chronic disease, such as coronary artery disease or cardiomyopathy. It also can occur with digitalis and quinidine toxicity, a PVC that occurs on a preceding T wave (R on T phenomenon), hypoxemia, hyperkalemia, or accidental electrical shock. During ventricular fibrillation the ventricles cannot deliver blood to the body, and the patient is pulseless.

If the amplitude of the ventricular fibrillation is high, the fibrillation is considered coarse; this usually indicates recent onset of the fibrillation and a better chance for successful recovery with defibrillation. If the amplitude of the fibrillation wave is low, the condition is considered fine ventricular fibrillation; this indicates a more prolonged fibrillation and a diminished chance for recovery. If left untreated, death occurs. The only effective treatment for ventricular fibrillation is electrical defibrillation (Cummins, 1994).

**Asystole.** *Asystole,* also known as ventricular standstill, is the absence of ventricular electrical activity. No

**BOX 23-7**

## DEFIBRILLATION

Defibrillation is the process of delivering an electrical shock to the heart through paddles placed on the chest at the base and the apex of the heart. Conductive pads or gel must be used to reduce resistance and prevent burning of the skin. Defibrillation should be done only by properly trained nurses or physicians after assessment reveals the need for this therapy.

### IMPORTANT SAFETY CONSIDERATIONS

- The patient must be placed in a supine position, on a dry surface, away from pooled water.
- Gel must be applied either to the paddles (or defibrillation pads) or to the surface of the skin where the paddles will be used.
- The defibrillator must be on and the rhythm reevaluated along with the pulse.
- An energy level of 200 joules is recommended for the first shock.
- Paddles must be placed on the chest at the apex and on the right of the upper sternum.

- The paddles must not touch the patient's skin directly and must not touch each other.
- The paddles must not touch any transdermal patches, wires, or tubing.
- No personnel can be in contact with the patient or any tubing and wires connected to the patient.
- No personnel can be in contact directly or indirectly with the patient's bed.
- The person performing the defibrillation must call a signal to clear, such as "I'm clear, you're clear, everyone is clear," checking between to ensure that all are clear.
- All personnel must stay clear until the shock has been delivered.
- After defibrillation the patient's rhythm should be reevaluated, and immediate defibrillation should be attempted again if the rhythm has not changed.
- The number of defibrillations, the energy level used, and the patient's response should be documented in the medical record. (Cummins, 1994.)

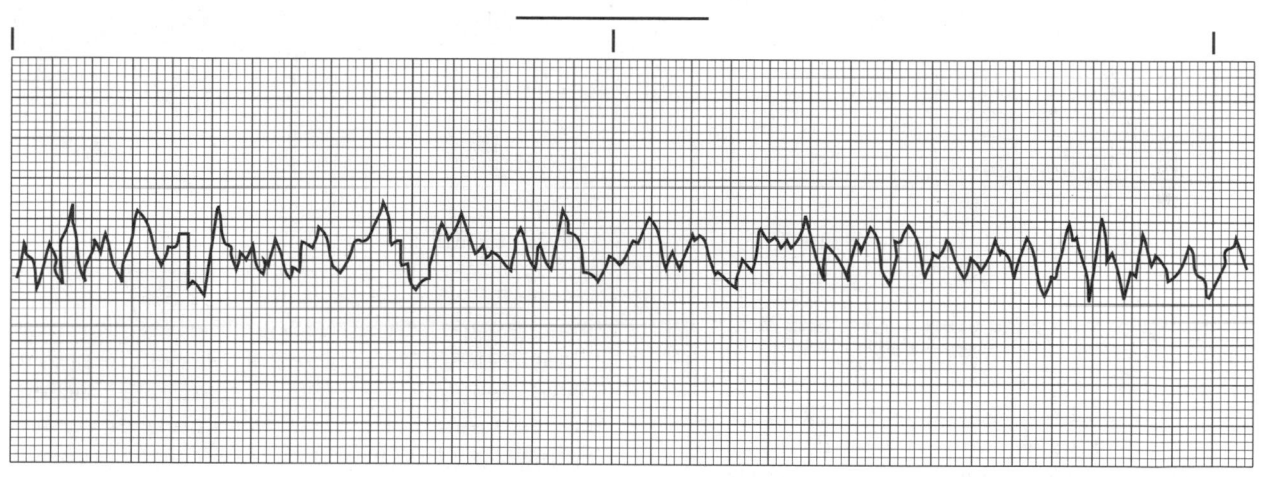

**Figure 23-23**   Ventricular fibrillation.

ventricular contraction occurs, and no pulse is felt. The ECG shows no QRS complexes, although some P waves may be present (asystole) (Figure 23-24). Asystole is a very serious problem that indicates profound myocardial ischemia and a poor prognosis. Underlying causes for asystole include hypoxia, hyperkalemia or hypokalemia, acidosis (low pH), drug overdose, and low body temperature. Asystole also can be the result of advanced cardiac disease or other organ system diseases. In addition to CPR and airway management, asystole should be treated by treating the cause (Cummins, 1994). Other therapy for asystole includes use of drugs such as atropine and epinephrine, and cardiac pacing.

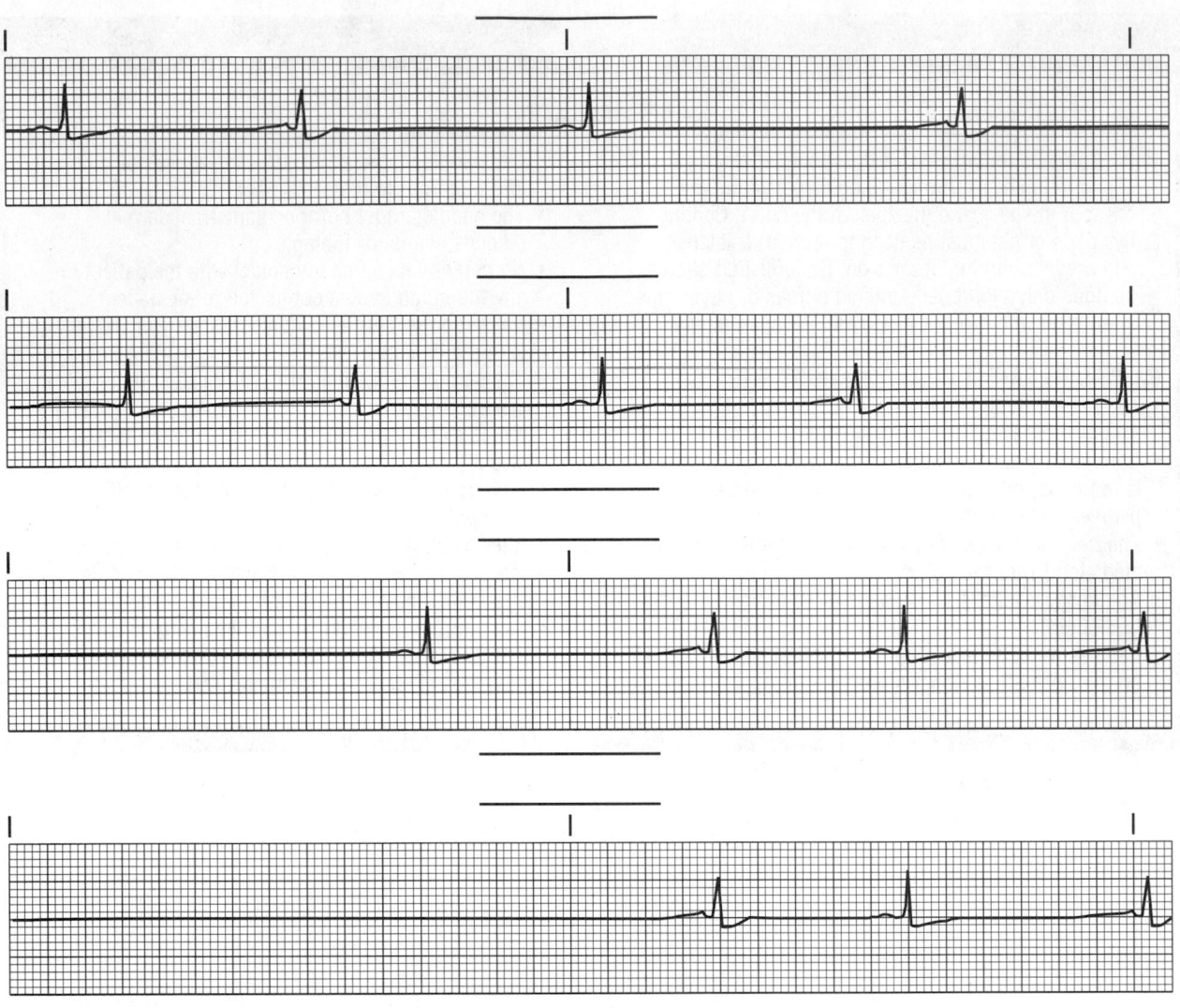

**Figure 23-24** Asystole (ventricular standstill).

## Electrical Therapy for Arrhythmias
### Electronic Cardiac Pacemakers

Electronic cardiac pacing is indicated for any condition in which the heart's SA node fails to initiate the electrical impulse or the impulse is not conducted to the ventricles at the rate needed to obtain good cardiac output. Arrhythmias that may require cardiac pacing include bradycardias (e.g., sinus bradycardia, junctional escape rhythm), heart blocks, and asystole. Pacemakers may also be required when the patient has intermittent periods of slow heart rate. Pacemakers may be internal or external, temporary or permanent, and may provide fixed rate (asynchronous) pacing or demand (synchronous) pacing of the ventricles. The **pacemaker** is a mechanical device that stimulates the heart muscle to contract by creating an electrical current and delivering that current to the muscle via a specialized wire in the heart. Several approaches are possible in initiating use of a pacemaker.

Temporary *transvenous pacemakers* are placed using a wire inserted through the jugular or subclavian vein. The wire is threaded through the right atrium and ventricle and positioned against the inside wall of the right ventricle. Once in place the wire is attached to an external power source. Patients with a temporary blockage of the electrical impulses in the heart, such as after heart surgery or a myocardial infarction, or pa-

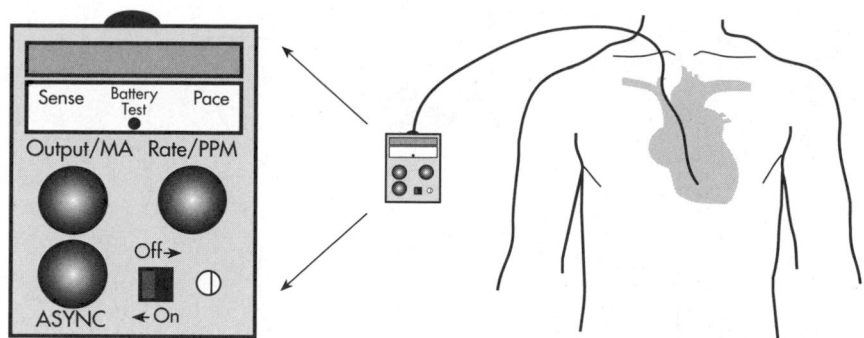

**Figure 23-25**    Temporary transvenous pacemaker.

tients who need a pacemaker during an emergency may receive this temporary type of pacemaker. A transvenous pacemaker can be inserted at the bedside or while the patient is in the operating room or cardiac catheterization laboratory. *Fluoroscopy* (a type of continuous x-ray) commonly is used to guide the pacing wire directly into the right ventricle. The power source of the pacemaker contains numerous controls, which can be set to deliver the appropriate amount of electrical current, the needed rate of delivery of the current, and other specifications (Figure 23-25).

*Permanent pacemakers* are necessary if the patient has irreversible damage to the conductive pathways of the heart. A permanent pacemaker also is inserted through a vein, but the power source is permanently implanted within subcutaneous tissue. The pacemaker's power source usually is inserted into the patient's upper chest, but the abdomen also can be used (Figure 23-26). Permanent pacemakers are implanted in the operating room, with fluoroscopy being used to guide the placement of wires into the cardiac muscle. Permanent pacemakers have become increasingly sophisticated. Newer versions can be placed with both an atrial and a ventricular pacing wire to provide pacing to the atrium and the ventricle (dual chamber) and produce cardiac contractions more like the heart's normal contractions. Some permanent pacemakers can adjust (increase or decrease) the rate of electrical stimulation to meet the patient's needs. The energy source for most permanent pacemakers is a lithium-powered battery that lasts 7 to 10 years.

*External pacemakers* (also known as transcutaneous pacemakers) (Figure 23-27) are used in emergency situations when pacing must be instituted rapidly (Cummins, 1994). These systems use adhesive pads, which are placed on the anterior and posterior walls of the chest over the heart. An external power source delivers the electrical current through the chest wall to the heart. The current needed to create contraction of the heart is much higher than that required by transvenous pacemakers, and it can cause contraction of the chest wall muscles and discomfort for the patient. Sedatives

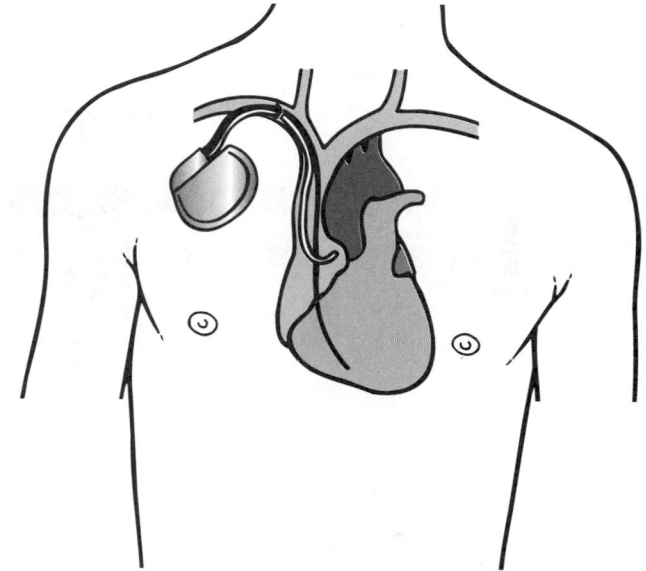

**Figure 23-26**    Permanent pacemaker with pacing wires in both the right atrium and ventricle. (From Lewis SM, Collier IC, Heitkemper MM: *Medical-surgical nursing: assessment and management of clinical problems*, ed 4, St Louis, 1996, Mosby.)

and analgesics frequently are used to provide comfort. Because the electrical current is transmitted through the skin, nursing care for patients receiving transcutaneous pacing includes careful inspection of the skin and repositioning of the electrodes as needed. External pacemakers are used only for a short time, until a transvenous pacemaker can be inserted.

### NURSE ALERT

**Health care providers run no risk of electrical injury during transcutaneous or transvenous pacing. Inadvertent contact with the pacing wire tips or exterior surface of the transcutaneous electrodes will cause only a mild shock, if any.**

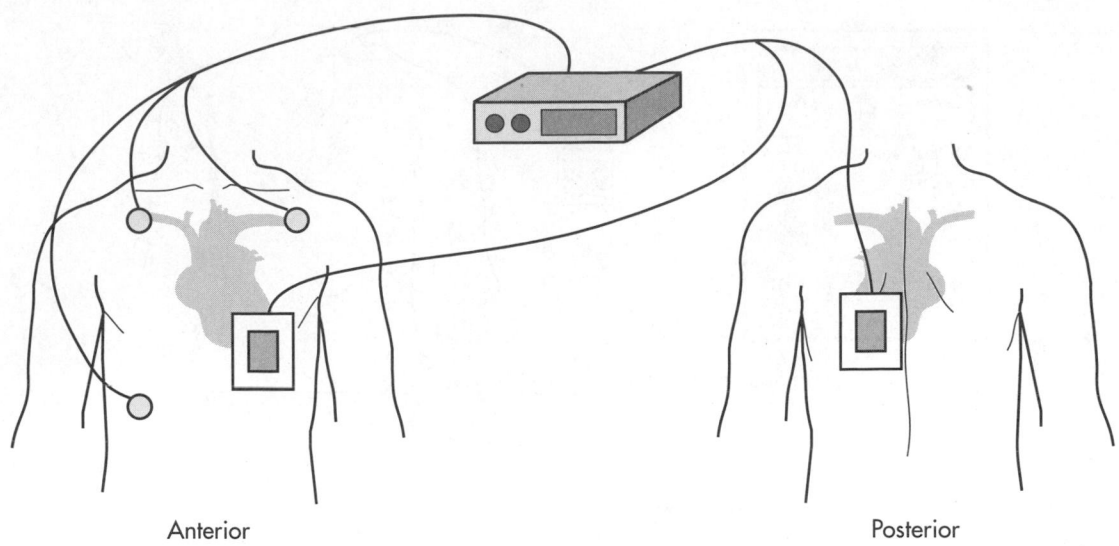

Anterior                                                                 Posterior

**Figure 23-27**   External pacemaker.

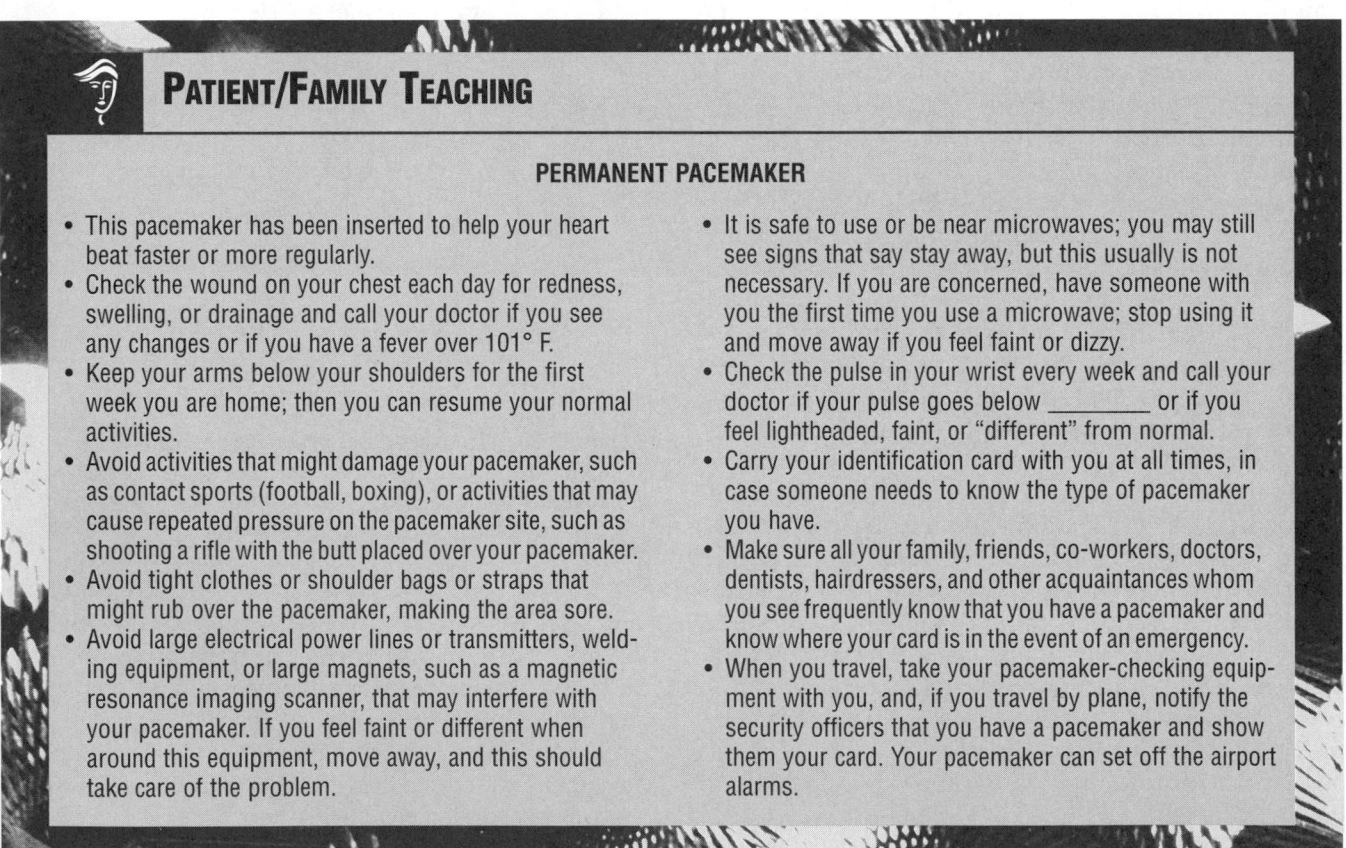

### PATIENT/FAMILY TEACHING

#### PERMANENT PACEMAKER

- This pacemaker has been inserted to help your heart beat faster or more regularly.
- Check the wound on your chest each day for redness, swelling, or drainage and call your doctor if you see any changes or if you have a fever over 101° F.
- Keep your arms below your shoulders for the first week you are home; then you can resume your normal activities.
- Avoid activities that might damage your pacemaker, such as contact sports (football, boxing), or activities that may cause repeated pressure on the pacemaker site, such as shooting a rifle with the butt placed over your pacemaker.
- Avoid tight clothes or shoulder bags or straps that might rub over the pacemaker, making the area sore.
- Avoid large electrical power lines or transmitters, welding equipment, or large magnets, such as a magnetic resonance imaging scanner, that may interfere with your pacemaker. If you feel faint or different when around this equipment, move away, and this should take care of the problem.

- It is safe to use or be near microwaves; you may still see signs that say stay away, but this usually is not necessary. If you are concerned, have someone with you the first time you use a microwave; stop using it and move away if you feel faint or dizzy.
- Check the pulse in your wrist every week and call your doctor if your pulse goes below _____ or if you feel lightheaded, faint, or "different" from normal.
- Carry your identification card with you at all times, in case someone needs to know the type of pacemaker you have.
- Make sure all your family, friends, co-workers, doctors, dentists, hairdressers, and other acquaintances whom you see frequently know that you have a pacemaker and know where your card is in the event of an emergency.
- When you travel, take your pacemaker-checking equipment with you, and, if you travel by plane, notify the security officers that you have a pacemaker and show them your card. Your pacemaker can set off the airport alarms.

**Assessment and intervention.** The nursing care of a patient with a pacemaker is determined by the type of pacemaker and the procedure used for insertion. Complications of transvenous pacemakers are similar for temporary and permanent types; they include pneumothorax (collapsed lung), cardiac tamponade (fluid accumulation in the pericardial sac), infection, pacemaker malfunction, and battery failure. Measures must

be taken to prevent and monitor for complications (Box 23-8), provide for patient comfort, and initiate and complete thorough patient teaching. With any transvenous pacemaker, the patient will have a wound that must be protected from infection. Care must be taken to prevent displacement of the pacing wires and pacemaker malfunction, especially with temporary pacemakers that have exposed wires and an external power source.

<table>
<tr><td colspan="2">

BOX 23-8

## NURSING PROCESS

## PATIENT WITH A PACEMAKER

</td></tr>
<tr><td>

### ASSESSMENT

- Cardiac status (vital signs, cardiac rhythm, edema)
- Neurologic signs (fatigue, syncope, level of consciousness)
- Respiratory status (cyanosis, breathing, crackles)
- Renal status (urinary output, laboratory values)
- Mental status (anxiety, perception of illness, self-concept)
- Pain (location, severity)
- Skin (redness, swelling, drainage at pacemaker insertion site)

### NURSING DIAGNOSES

- Risk for injury related to potential pacemaker malfunction and presence of invasive mechanical device (pacemaker)
- Potential decreased cardiac output related to pacemaker malfunction, postinsertion complications
- Potential infection related to invasive procedure and presence of mechanical device

### NURSING INTERVENTIONS
#### Permanent Pacemaker

- Ensure bed rest for 24 hours.
- Minimize motion of the extremity closest to the insertion site for 48 hours.

#### Temporary Pacemaker

- Ensure bed rest.
- Minimize motion of the extremity closest to the insertion site while the temporary pacemaker is in place.
- Make sure all other electrical equipment is grounded and wear gloves when touching the exposed ends of the pacing wires.
- Tighten the connection on the external power source.
- Keep the external pacemaker box and wires dry, and cover all dials on the face of the box with a plastic shield.

</td><td>

- Check the batteries every 24 hours and replace them when the power is low.

#### Both Types of Pacemaker

- Evaluate the ECG tracing for pacing and sensing; notify the physician if these settings are not appropriate.
- Check the patient's heart rate and compare it with the rate set on the pacemaker; the patient's HR should be the same as or higher than the setting on the pacemaker.
- Monitor vital signs for hypotension, bradycardia, or tachycardia.
- Monitor for urine output over 30 ml/hr and for diminished level of consciousness.
- Keep emergency equipment (drugs, defibrillator, pacemaker adjusting devices) close to bedside.
- Evaluate the patient for shortness of breath, absence of breath sounds on the side of insertion, muffled heart sounds, and distended neck veins.
- Ensure that an x-ray film was obtained after the procedure and that the findings were normal.
- Monitor the insertion site for swelling, redness, and drainage every 8 hours; notify the physician if any signs or symptoms are present.
- Change the dressing over the insertion site as ordered; use aseptic technique.
- Monitor for temperature elevation, and check laboratory data for increased white blood cell (WBC) count.
- Monitor for hyperthermia (temperature over 38.3° C [101° F]).

### EVALUATION OF EXPECTED OUTCOMES

- Normal functioning of pacemaker
- Quick response to potential complications
- Adequate cardiac output
- Wound healing without infection

</td></tr>
</table>

Patients with implanted pacemakers often are apprehensive, fearful, and in pain. The nurse's responsibilities include helping the patient obtain pain relief or control and relieving the patient's fear and apprehension. Adequate teaching about the pacemaker, how it functions, and how it is cared for should be done before insertion, if possible, and then repeated after insertion. Patients with temporary pacemakers may need instruction to prepare them for possible insertion of a permanent pacemaker. Patients with a permanent pacemaker will benefit from knowing that replacing the batteries is a simple procedure required only every 7 to 10 years.

All patients with permanent pacemakers should carry identification or medical alert cards containing information about the manufacturer and the type,

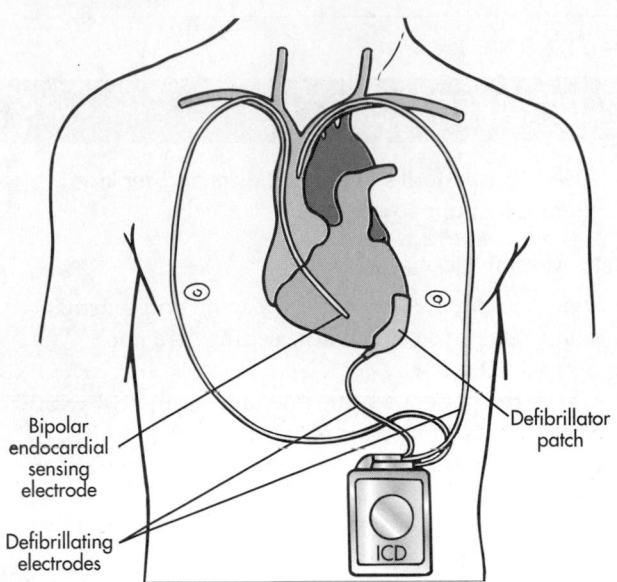

**Figure 23-28**   Implantable cardioverter-defibrillator (ICD). (From Lewis SM, Collier IC, Heitkemper MM: *Medical-surgical nursing: assessment and management of clinical problems*, ed 4, St Louis, 1996, Mosby.)

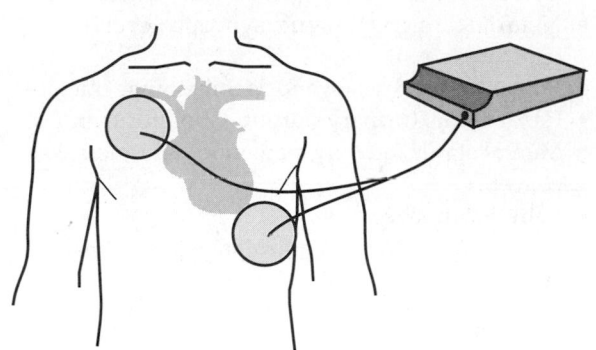

**Figure 23-29**   Automatic external defibrillator.

model, and settings of their pacemaker. Patients with permanent pacemakers also should be taught how to check the radial pulse and count the rate, and how to use any monitoring equipment that comes with the pacemaker. They should check the pulse at least weekly and compare it with the rate for which the pacemaker is set.

In the past patients were taught to avoid many appliances, including microwave ovens. Newer models of pacemakers usually have metal shielding to protect them from external interference (Purcell, Fletcher, 1994b). Most electrical devices can be used safely. Microwave ovens now have special shields and usually will not affect the pacemaker. Arc welding equipment and power transmitters should be avoided. Therapeutic devices such as transcutaneous electrical nerve stimulation (TENS) units and magnetic resonance imagers (MRIs) may create interference. Patients should be taught to inform their therapists about their pacemakers and to use caution near antitheft devices in some stores. Airport metal detectors may be triggered by a pacemaker, therefore the patient may need to provide a pacemaker identification card.

## Automatic Implantable Cardioverter-Defibrillator

Another device available for treating arrhythmias is the *automatic implantable cardioverter-defibrillator* (*AICD* or *ICD*) (Figure 23-28). These devices, which are used in patients who have recurrent ventricular arrhyth-

mias that do not respond to drug therapy, have proven to reduce the risk of sudden cardiac death. This type of arrhythmia-sensing and defibrillation device provides an electrical shock to the heart muscle when a life-threatening arrhythmia occurs, such as ventricular tachycardia or ventricular fibrillation. The power source and "brain" of the device is implanted in the abdomen, similar to a permanent pacemaker, and wires or patches are placed internally on the outside of the heart at the apex. The devices can be programmed to sense an abnormal rhythm and defibrillate the heart. The increasing sophistication of these devices now allows them to analyze the heart's electrical signals and provide pacemaker regulation in addition to defibrillation.

## Automatic External Defibrillator

The *automatic external defibrillator (AED)* (Figure 23-29) is one of the newest electrical devices used to control ventricular arrhythmias. AEDs have arrhythmia-sensing capability and can be used by rescuers who do not have any ECG interpretation experience (Cummins, 1994).

AEDs are connected to the patient by adhesive electrodes, which are placed on the chest in the positions usually used for defibrillation. When placed on a pulseless patient and engaged, the AED analyzes the patient's ECG rhythm and determines if the rhythm is one that requires a shock. With the semiautomatic model, the rescuer initiates the analyze mode by pushing a button, and the AED then, if needed, gives a written or verbal prompt to deliver a shock by pushing the shock button. The fully automated type requires only that the rescuer place the electrodes and turn the device on. If a rhythm requiring a shock is identified, the fully automated AED charges and delivers the shock with no rescuer assistance. With any type of AED, if a rhythm is identified that is not responsive to defibrillation, shocks are not recommended or delivered. These devices are used with increasing frequency in prehospital settings and in remote areas, where a significant time delay is inevitable in the arrival of people trained in advanced cardiac life support (ACLS).

## INTENSIVE CARE UNIT (CORONARY CARE UNIT)

The intensive care unit (ICU) or **coronary care unit** (CCU) is a specially designed unit of the hospital equipped with all the supplies and equipment required, including emergency drugs, to meet the needs of patients who are unstable or critically ill or who require intensive monitoring by the nurse. This type of unit provides continuous monitoring of the patient's cardiac function and other body systems.

The overall objective of the CCU is to save lives. During the early development of these units, emphasis was placed on prompt treatment of patients with cardiac arrest. With the increase in knowledge and understanding of coronary artery disease, the emphasis has come to be placed on preventing cardiac arrest. If not identified, treated, and controlled, minor disorders of rhythm may lead to serious arrhythmias, heart failure, and death. It cannot be expected that all patients admitted to the CCU will survive, but mortality has been reduced significantly.

Large medical centers have specially designed, separate CCUs, but some community hospitals care for cardiac patients in ICUs with other seriously ill patients. Some ICUs and CCUs have wards in which all patients are monitored in one big room with curtain dividers between them, and others have private rooms for each patient. Each system has definite advantages and disadvantages. However, the patient's environmental location is not always the most important factor—the quality of nursing care often is.

Nurses are the key to the success of the CCU. They are the first to provide basic life support and to start treatment of life-threatening arrhythmias. Nurses are with the patient 24 hours a day and are in a position to assess for and detect the first sign of trouble. Their immediate assessment of the problem and appropriate emergency action may be lifesaving. The CCU, with its effective monitoring system and trained personnel,

has effectively reduced deaths from heart attacks in hospitalized patients.

Patients in a CCU may experience extreme emotional and physical stress. They are anxious about loss of function, helplessness, finances, family, and the possibility of death. The CCU environment is foreign and frightening. Coronary care nurses must have the technical proficiency and sensitivity to care for CCU patients and their families in crisis. Much can be done to reassure patients and families by supplying information to relieve anxiety, by listening carefully to the patient, and by treating the patient with respect. The caring and empathy on which nursing was founded is demonstrated during the patient's most serious crises.

Nurses in the CCU often are responsible for keen assessment of the patient's physiologic changes and for taking ECGs, observing and recording cardiac monitor readings, maintaining oxygen therapy, and observing and regulating intravenous fluids. They should also be prepared to provide basic cardiac life support, defibrillation, and intravenous infusions.

## CORONARY ARTERY DISEASE

The leading cause of death in the United States is cardiovascular disease. Since the initiation of a massive campaign to educate people about risk factors, mortality has been declining steadily. Each year complications from cardiovascular disease account for more than 900,000 deaths. More than half of these deaths—about 500,000 people a year—are from acute myocardial infarction. Reducing morbidity and mortality from heart disease is a primary concern of health care providers. The nurse needs to be aware of the risk factors and should help patients modify habits that predispose them to heart disease.

### Arteriosclerosis and Atherosclerosis

**Arteriosclerosis,** commonly called hardening of the arteries, is a process of degeneration and decreasing elasticity of the artery walls caused by chronic inflammation and scarring. This process weakens the vessel walls, predisposing them to hemorrhage, thrombosis, and hypertension. Arteriosclerosis is also related to the aging process. *Atherosclerosis* is a type of arteriosclerosis caused by fatty deposits. It is a generalized disease that involves arteries in different areas, such as the aorta and its major branches, the heart (coronary arteries), and the large arteries of the brain (leading to stroke), and the legs (causing pain during exercise). It is very serious because it is the underlying cause of most heart and brain infarcts and can diminish the functioning of other organs.

## Pathophysiology

Atherosclerosis is a slowly progressive disease characterized by deposits of fat (usually cholesterol and lipids) within the inner lining of the arteries. These deposits initiate a low-grade inflammatory reaction and healing process that eventually results in hard, irregular, multicolored **plaques** (Huether, McCance, 1996). These plaques form fibrous tissue and calcify within the inner lining of the arteries (Figure 23-30). This process weakens and narrows the walls of the major arteries, reducing the blood flow. Both partial and complete obstruction can occur.

If the blood flow is severely reduced by atherosclerosis, the blood trickles and sludges through the vessel and a clot can form, causing complete obstruction. Inadequate blood flow disrupts the oxygen supply and demand balance of the tissues, and the consequences depend on the site being deprived. The process of atherosclerosis begins usually at an early age, and the disease can be considerably advanced in some people before the age of 20.

**Coronary artery disease** (CAD) is the presence of atherosclerosis in the coronary arteries. Whenever obstruction occurs, the tissue beyond the obstruction is deprived of its blood supply, and death of the tissue may result. The term *coronary heart disease (CHD)* is used to describe the presence of CAD accompanied by symptoms such as angina (chest pain) or a history of myocardial infarction. Deprivation of blood to the heart is referred to as *ischemic heart disease*, which may be caused by CAD or other pathologic conditions (Chandra, Hazinski, 1994).

## Assessment

A thorough health history that focuses on risk factors for atherosclerosis is essential in identifying patients with CAD or a high probability of CAD. Many risk factors have been associated with atherosclerosis, but three are considered the most significant: cigarette smoking, hyperlipidemia (elevated serum lipids), and hypertension. As discussed earlier in this chapter, risk factors can be categorized as those that are changeable or modifiable, and those that are not (see Box 23-2). The more risk factors a person has, the greater are his or her chances of developing coronary artery disease compared with a person with fewer or no risk factors (Chandra, Hazinski, 1994). The risk factors for each patient should be evaluated so that interventions can be planned to reduce the risk.

### Unchangeable Risk Factors

Risk factors that cannot be changed include gender, heredity, and increasing age. The death rate from CHD increases with age. Women have a lower incidence of atherosclerosis before menopause, but after menopause the incidence increases steadily, so that at age 75 the morbidity and mortality rates from CAD are almost equal for men and women. Women also have a greater chance of dying after a myocardial infarction than do men (Jensen, King, 1997). A family history of premature CHD in siblings or parents before age 50 or a family history of hyperlipidemia increases the chance of heart disease caused by genetic factors. Race and cultural differences also play a part in increasing risk. It is impor-

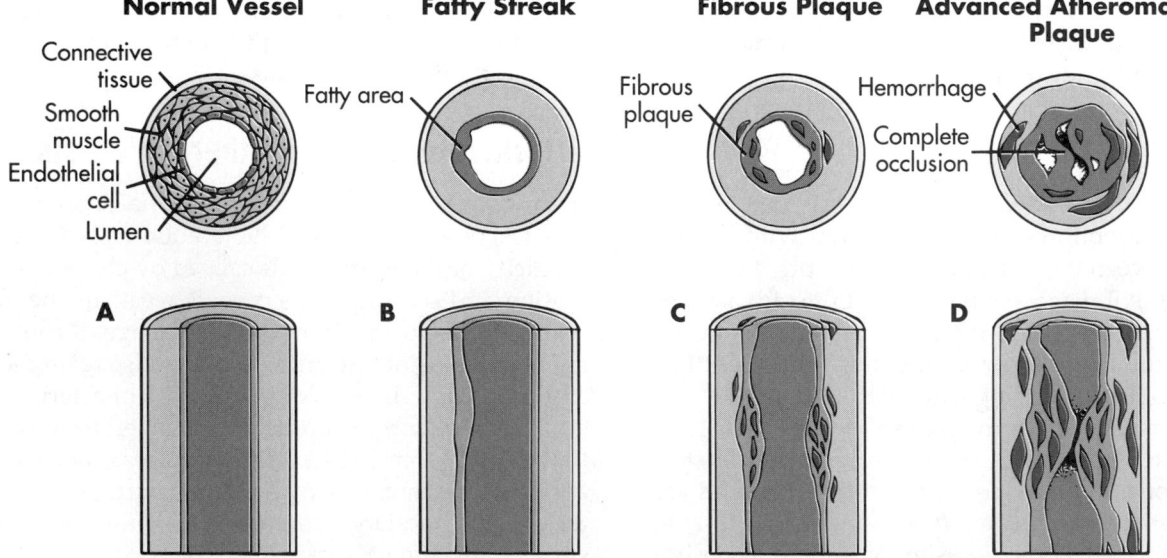

**Figure 23-30**  Progression of atherosclerosis shown in both the longitudinal and the cross-sectional views. **A,** Normal vessel. **B,** First stage, fatty streaks. **C,** Second stage, fibrous plaque development. **D,** Third stage, advanced (complicated) lesions. (From Thelan LA, Davie JK, Urden LD: *Textbook of critical care nursing, diagnosis and management,* ed 2, St Louis, 1994, Mosby.)

tant for the nurse to complete a thorough family history for each patient, identifying the cause of death, if possible, for all deceased family members.

 **ETHNIC/CULTURAL CONSIDERATIONS**

- The risk of myocardial infarction is higher in white middle-aged men.
- African American men have a higher risk of hypertension than white men.
- Hypertension develops earlier and is more severe in African Americans than in whites.
- African Americans with hypertension have a 1½ times higher rate of heart disease than whites.
- African American women have a higher incidence of hypertension and CAD than white women.
- Asians living in America have a lower rate of myocardial infarction than whites, but the rate is higher than that for Asians living in their country of origin.

## Changeable Risk Factors

Some risk factors are changeable or controllable. The American Heart Association has separated the changeable risk factors into two categories, major risk factors and contributing factors. The major changeable risk factors are smoking, hypertension, physical inactivity, and hyperlipidemia. The contributing factors are diabetes, obesity, and stress.

**Smoking.** The death rate from myocardial infarction is significantly higher in smokers. Cigarette smokers have an overall 70% higher rate of CHD. Women who smoke and take oral contraceptives containing estrogen have an increased risk of CAD (Jensen, King, 1997). Smoking plus use of oral contraceptives increases the risk of myocardial infarction to almost 10 times that of women who have neither risk factor.

Exposure to secondhand smoke also has been shown to increase the risk of smoking-related diseases, so that even if the patient does not report being a smoker, determining if other family members or co-workers smoke is important in evaluating risk factors.

The risk of heart disease is related to the number of cigarettes smoked per day and the length of time the patient has smoked. This risk usually is expressed in *pack-years:* the number of cigarettes smoked per day times the number of years as a smoker. A person who smokes 1 pack per day for 30 years is a 30 pack-year smoker. When smoking is eliminated, the death rate falls over time to the level of a nonsmoker.

Smoking and the nicotine in cigarette smoke causes the release of catecholamines that increase the heart rate, causing peripheral vasoconstriction and raising the blood pressure. Inhalation of carbon monoxide in cigarette smoke diminishes the amount of oxygen available for tissues. All the changes caused by smoking put stress on the vascular system and the heart (Huether, McCance, 1996).

**Hypertension.** Hypertension (HTN) increases the incidence of atherosclerosis by putting stress on the arteries and increasing the workload of the heart. Hypertension often is asymptomatic. A history of hypertension (especially hypertension that has not been well controlled) or the presence of high blood pressure on evaluation is a major risk factor for heart disease and stroke (see Chapter 25).

**Sedentary life-style.** Lack of physical activity is another risk factor for heart disease, especially heart attack. The nurse should determine if the patient gets regular, planned exercise that causes perspiration and increases the heart rate (moderate intensity) at least three times a week for 15 to 30 minutes. Many people feel that they have very active lives or jobs, but their activity does not always meet these guidelines. A sedentary life-style increases obesity (a contributing factor in heart disease), lowers the HDL blood levels, and can contribute to stasis of blood and the formation of clots. Activity increases HDL levels, strengthens the heart muscle, and contributes to better weight and diabetes control.

**Hyperlipidemia.** Patients with elevated lipid levels are at increased risk for CAD and CHD. Hypercholesterolemia sometimes is a family trait but most often is due to a diet high in saturated fats (found in red meat, butter, cheese, cream, and whole milk) and cholesterol (found in all animal products). A high serum triglyceride level is associated with obesity, a sedentary life-style, and alcohol ingestion. The risk of heart disease also is increased with changes in the levels of HDL and LDL transport lipoproteins, which were discussed previously. As shown in Table 23-3, an increased risk of heart disease is associated with a specific serum level of cholesterol, triglycerides, and lipoproteins. Reviewing a patient's laboratory values, if available, can be one means of assessing for this risk factor. Another is to review the patient's average diet for excessive intake of fats and cholesterol.

## Contributing Factors

Obesity, diabetes, and stress have been identified as contributing factors in the development of heart disease. Obesity (defined as being 30% over ideal body weight) increases the mortality from CAD because of the higher risk of hypertension, diabetes, a sedentary life-style, and high LDL lipoprotein and triglyceride levels, all of which are common with obesity. The more overweight a person is, the greater is his or her risk.

**TABLE 23-3**

## Cholesterol, Triglyceride, and Lipoprotein Levels Associated with Risk of Coronary Artery Disease

| BLOOD STUDY | NORMAL VALUE | VALUES ASSOCIATED WITH INCREASED RISK |
|---|---|---|
| Total cholesterol | <200 mg/dl | >200 mg/dl |
| High-density lipoprotein (HDL) | >45 mg/dl (men) | Cholesterol:HDL ratio >1:5 |
|  | >55 mg/dl (women) | HDL <35 mg/dl |
| Low-density lipoprotein (LDL) | 60-180 mg/dl | >160 mg/dl in those with known CAD |
|  |  | >190 mg/dl in those with no known CAD |
| Very-low-density lipoprotein (VLDL) | 25%-50% | >25%-50% |
| Triglycerides | 40-160 mg/dl (men) | >150 mg/dl |
|  | 35-135 mg/dl (women) |  |

Diabetes is another contributing factor in CAD, and even when the blood sugar is brought under control, that risk is not eliminated. Diabetes causes acceleration of atherosclerosis partly because of the effects of connective tissue degeneration and elevated lipid levels that are common to even well-controlled diabetics.

Stress produces sympathetic stimulation that puts greater demands on the heart, and this may be the mechanism by which stress increases the risk of CAD. Even in people with no other risk factors and in whom life-style modifications have been made to reduce the risk of CAD, uncontrolled stress appears to affect the development of CAD. The personal response to stress may also play a role in the physical toll on the heart. People who have type A personality traits (e.g., perfectionism, aggression, hostility, and suppressed anger) are more likely to develop CAD. In order to evaluate for these contributing factors, the nurse must get an accurate weight and calculate the ideal versus the actual body weight for each patient. The nurse must also determine the patient's stress level, coping styles, and personality traits. These data are helpful in identifying risks that can be reduced.

### Intervention

There is no effective treatment or cure for arteriosclerosis and atherosclerosis. The process probably begins early in life and develops gradually over the years. Earlier sections of this chapter discussed factors that increase the risk of heart disease and strategies for completing a risk analysis.

Surgical procedures have been developed for removing plaques from certain areas, increasing the circulation, but education, identification, and management of risk factors may prevent or retard the progression of CAD. Each patient seeking care for a cardiac-related event should be evaluated for the risk factors as discussed previously. In addition, nurses should include family members, particularly the children of patients, as appropriate, in discussions about risk factors and reducing risk factors. Many of the changes that will need to be made will affect the family as well as the patient. This can also be a prime opportunity to enhance primary prevention for other members of the family who may be at risk for CAD.

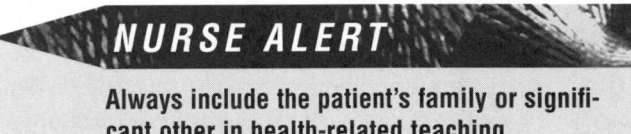

**NURSE ALERT**

Always include the patient's family or significant other in health-related teaching.

### Management of Patients at High Risk

Once the risk factors have been identified, a plan can be made and implemented to assist the patient in making life-style changes. The unchangeable risk factors cannot be altered, but by reducing the changeable factors, the patient can reduce his or her risk for CAD.

The nurse is in an excellent position to teach health-promoting behaviors or to enlist the help of someone who can. However, simply presenting the risks and encouraging patients to make changes may not be enough to convince patients to alter their life-styles. Patients often have a number of risk factors that need to be reduced. Making too many changes at once or excessive pressure from health care providers and family can be overwhelming and can contribute to resistance.

Before beginning health-related teaching, it is very important to understand how patients may view their health habits, their overall health, and the impact making changes will have on their lives. This information, in addition to information on a patient's ability to read, see, hear, and comprehend, is vital in making an appropriate plan. Providing an illiterate patient with a lot of reading material or an elderly patient who has failing eyesight and hearing with a video to watch will

**TABLE 23-4**

## Risk Factor Reduction Strategies

| RISK FACTOR | STRATEGIES FOR REDUCTION | SPECIAL CONSIDERATIONS |
|---|---|---|
| Smoking | Try smoking cessation programs; use gums or patches to reduce withdrawal symptoms; have family member who smokes join in efforts to quit; reduce secondhand smoke exposure. | Some smoking cessation aids are available over the counter, but they are costly. |
| Hypertension | Have BP checked regularly; visit the health care provider regularly; lose weight; exercise regularly; reduce salt intake to 3 g/day; stay on prescribed medications. | The exact amount of salt reduction has not been well established. Limiting added salt and using low-sodium products and salt substitutes reduces sodium intake significantly.<br>A 3 g/day restriction is considered mild restriction; more stringent restrictions may be ordered by the physician or dietitian. |
| Sedentary life-style | Choose an aerobic activity (e.g., walking, cycling, swimming); increase activity gradually to 30 min every other day; remember: any activity is better than no activity. | Patients should consult a health care provider before starting any exercise program, especially if the patient is over 40 years of age or is known to have heart disease. |
| Hyperlipidemia | Lose weight; exercise regularly; reduce intake of saturated fats; reduce cholesterol intake; pay close attention to food labels; avoid fried foods, increase poultry and fish in diet, limit eggs to three a week, bake, broil, or roast food when possible. | Some studies show that plaques can be reduced in size by strict reduction in fat to less than 10 g/day.<br>Goals for cholesterol levels should be:<br>LDL <160 mg/dl with no CHD and fewer than two other risk factors<br>LDL <130 mg/dl with no CHD and two or more risk factors<br>LDL <100 with definite CHD<br>A dietitian can be a great resource for planning diet and cooking changes.<br>Medications to control cholesterol levels may be prescribed if diet does not reduce these levels in 6 mo. With known CHD only 6-12 wk of diet is attempted before drug therapy is initiated. |
| Obesity | Reduce fat and calories; exercise regularly; avoid fad diets and products. | If weight reduction is needed, the advice of a physician or dietitian may be required. |
| Diabetes | Follow prescribed diet; lose weight; check blood sugar regularly; take required medications; visit health care provider regularly. | Many medications for lipid reduction and hypertension affect blood sugar levels. |
| Stress | Identify triggers of stress; try stress reduction seminars, stress reduction tapes, biofeedback, progressive relaxation, yoga; get regular exercise and adequate sleep. | The most effective method of stress reduction varies from person to person. Each individual should use the method that seems to work best. |

not accomplish the goals. Knowing the patient's financial resources also is crucial in selecting cost-effective approaches to care. Table 23-4 presents specific strategies for reducing risk factors.

## Clinical Manifestations

Some people with CAD may not have any signs or symptoms of heart disease, whereas others have numerous manifestations of the underlying coronary artery narrowing. CAD causes three major clinical problems: angina pectoris, myocardial infarction, and sudden cardiac death.

# ANGINA PECTORIS (ANGINAL SYNDROME)

**Angina pectoris** is a condition reflecting a change in the normal balance between myocardial oxygen supply and demand. When myocardial oxygen needs increase (as with exercise, stress, and exertion), normal coronary arteries respond by dilating and the heart responds by increasing the cardiac output. In a person with CAD, atherosclerotic plaques prevent the arteries from improving the blood flow, and the diseased heart is unable to improve its pumping function. These two factors create a deficit in the oxygenated blood that needs to reach the myocardial tissue. This deficit creates reversible ischemia, and the classic transient pain of angina results. At the cellular level, cardiac cells are viable for 20 minutes before irreversible damage or infarction takes place (Huether, McCance, 1996).

Another mechanism of reduced blood flow is coronary artery spasm. The spasms, which commonly occur in the plaque-narrowed, diseased artery, decrease blood flow through the coronary arteries, and the end result is myocardial ischemia.

Angina usually is the result of atherosclerosis in the coronary arteries, but other conditions can predispose a patient to myocardial ischemia and chest pain when no atherosclerosis is present (Table 23-5). In a patient with CAD, myocardial ischemia and angina can be induced by numerous factors. Table 23-6 presents some of the common precipitating factors for the development of angina in patients with CAD. Ischemia also can occur with no symptoms of angina or only minimal discomfort. This is especially true in diabetics and the elderly as a result of neuropathy and alterations in the pain threshold.

## TABLE 23-5

### Nonatherosclerotic Causes of Myocardial Ischemia

| CAUSE | EFFECT |
| --- | --- |
| Low BP and hypovolemia | Cardiac output and blood flow to the coronary arteries decrease. |
| Anemia, chronic lung disease | Oxygen-carrying capacity or the concentration of oxygen on hemoglobin decreases. |
| Valvular disorders, syphilis | Blood flow is obstructed, reducing cardiac output (syphilis can stenose the coronary ostia). |
| Ventricular hypertrophy, hypertension, and release of catecholamines (stimulated by drugs such as cocaine or by stress or shock) | Myocardial oxygen demand increases. |
| Tachycardia, exertion, exercise | Myocardial oxygen demand increases. |
| Bradycardia | Cardiac output decreases. |

## TABLE 23-6

### Precipitating Factors for Angina

| FACTOR | EFFECT |
| --- | --- |
| Exertion: walking; lifting objects or shoveling wet snow; activity done with arms above head, such as hanging out clothes; activities such as sweeping, golfing, or sexual activity | Heart rate increases, diastole (filling of coronary arteries) shortens, and myocardial oxygen demand increases beyond what can be provided. |
| Emotional stress: Anger, fear, excitement; stimulants such as nicotine (cigarette smoking), caffeine, and recreational drugs | Catecholamine release increases heart rate, BP, and workload of the heart; smoking also reduces oxygenation of the blood. |
| Eating a large meal | Blood is diverted from the heart to the gastrointestinal tract, reducing blood flow to the coronary arteries just as the demand on the heart increases to provide more blood flow for digestion. |
| Weather (temperature) changes or moving from inside to outside | Extreme temperature changes increase the demand on the heart and the metabolic rate to carry out the heating or cooling that must occur. |
| Circadian rhythms | The early morning hours, right after wakening, are common times for myocardial ischemia and angina. |

## Assessment

The characteristic symptom of angina is sudden chest pain or discomfort. Some patients describe the discomfort as a pressure, an ache, or a squeezing or uncomfortable feeling (Agency for Health Care Policy and Research, 1994b). Others describe it as a choking, burning, or gassy sensation resembling indigestion. The discomfort most commonly is felt in the substernal region of the chest, but it may radiate to the jaw, neck, shoulders, inside of the arms, or epigastric area or between the shoulder blades (Figure 23-31). The pain can range from minimal to severe enough to completely immobilize the person. Some angina sufferers clutch their chest with an open hand when the pain occurs.

During an acute episode the patient's face may have an ashen appearance, and the patient may be covered with cold, clammy perspiration. These symptoms are due to the sympathetic stimulation that occurs, which causes sweating and vasoconstriction of peripheral vessels. Some patients experience shortness of breath, weakness, or numbness and tingling during the attack. Blood pressure is elevated, as the pulse rate may be. The patient may be extremely apprehensive and have thoughts of death or feelings of impending doom.

Angina usually is transient, lasting only a few minutes to no longer than 20 minutes, and is relieved when the precipitating factor is relieved (Agency for Health Care Policy and Research, 1994b). A complete description of the pain according to the seven characteristics previously discussed is essential in differentiating between the types of angina, a myocardial infarction, and other causes of chest pain or discomfort. Table 23-7 presents a synopsis of the different types of angina. Characteristics that are not commonly seen in patients with cardiac chest pain include changes in the pain with movement, breathing, or positioning, and pain in a specific area of the chest that can be reproduced by palpation. A complete evaluation of the chest should be done to detect any abnormal heart or lung sounds.

## Intervention
### Management of Acute Angina

The nurse must know the acute initial assessment and management of a patient with chest pain (Box 23-9). A rapid "ABC" approach can help in organizing the steps in the process. The initial interventions are

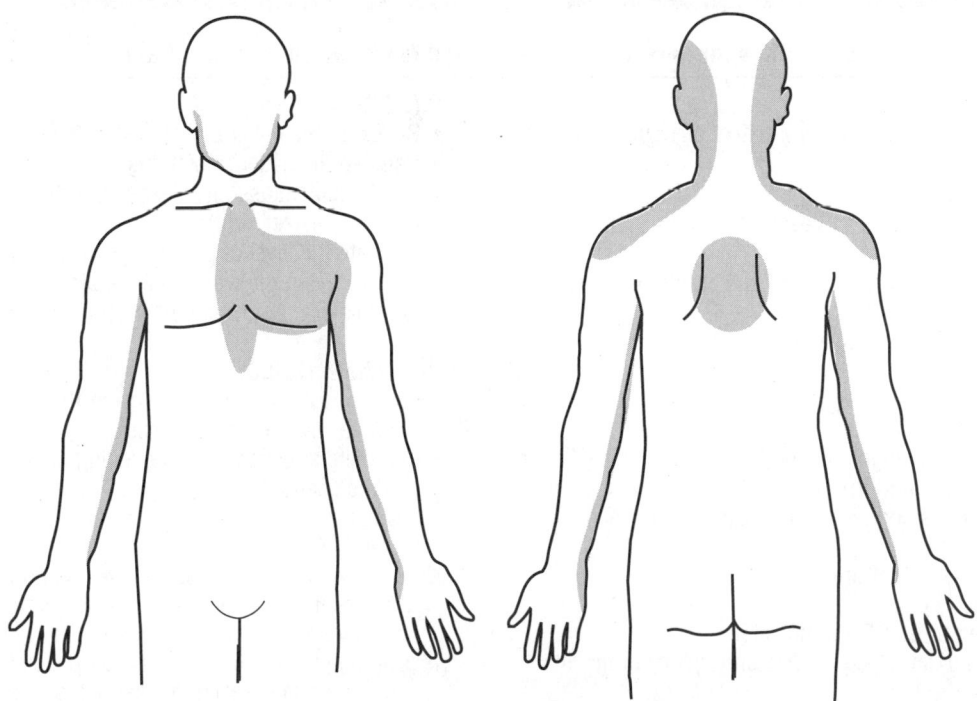

**Figure 23-31**    Areas of pain radiation in angina.

intended to (1) prevent or treat complications that can occur with myocardial ischemia, including arrhythmias (PVCs and ventricular fibrillation), (2) reduce the heart's myocardial oxygen demand, (3) provide for comfort and pain relief, and, as the patient stabilizes, (4) evaluate the extent of the CAD and initiate appropriate therapy.

Angina requires a complete medical workup, which usually includes several laboratory studies and diagnostic tests (Table 23-8) to rule out infarction and determine the extent of the CAD. Once the patient has been evaluated thoroughly, choices for treatment are made, which may include medication alone or an invasive intervention. Invasive interventions, including percutaneous transluminal coronary angioplasty (PTCA), stents, atherectomy, and coronary artery bypass graft (CABG), are discussed in more detail in the section on myocardial infarction.

**TABLE 23-7**

## Types of Angina

| TYPE | CHARACTERISTICS OF PAIN | ETIOLOGY/SPECIAL CONSIDERATION |
|---|---|---|
| Stable angina | Predictable; recurrent pattern of onset, duration and intensity; short duration; exercise induced; can be controlled with medication | Atherosclerotic plaques, coronary artery spasm; can be managed on outpatient basis |
| Unstable angina | Unpredictable; changes in pattern of pain; more frequent episodes; increased intensity; less activity required to provoke an episode; can occur at rest; prolonged duration; medication may not relieve pain | Deterioration or rupture of plaque; spasm or thrombosis of artery; can progress to infarction; can occur in patients with previously stable angina; may be first symptom of CAD; requires hospitalization |
| Prinzmetal's angina | Occurs at rest; not associated with activity | Coronary artery spasm; plaques may or may not be present |

**BOX 23-9**

### Guidelines for Nursing Assessment and Management of Chest Pain

**A (AIRWAY)**
• Determine if the patient has a patent airway.

**B (BREATHING)**
• Assess the rate and effort associated with breathing.
• If the patient is short of breath and respirations are rapid, begin oxygen therapy.
• Have emergency airway equipment at the bedside.

**C (CIRCULATION)**
• Evaluate the vital signs for the hypotension, rapid or slow heart rate, and irregular heart rate, that may signal arrhythmias and need immediate intervention.
• Start an IV line.
• Initiate cardiac monitoring.
• Do a 12-lead ECG.
• Be prepared to do CPR if indicated.
• Have a defibrillator and cardiac emergency drugs at the bedside.

**C (COMFORT)**
• Reassure the patient.
• Remove the patient's clothing.
• Let the patient assume the position that gives him or her the greatest comfort.
• Evaluate the level of pain on a scale from 1 to 10 with 10 being the worst imaginable.
• Administer nitroglycerin or morphine as ordered.

**D (DIFFERENTIALS)**
• Perform a complete evaluation of the patient's pain (use the seven characteristics).
• Complete a focused history, including cardiac history and medication list.
• Evaluate for contraindications of thrombolytic therapy.
Note that many of these assessments and interventions may occur simultaneously. The goal is to stabilize the patient, prevent complications, and initiate appropriate treatment as quickly as possible. Time is muscle in the event of myocardial ischemia.

A patient with stable angina may be evaluated and managed as an outpatient. Patients with unstable angina are admitted to the hospital, usually to the ICU or CCU, if the patient has significant risk factors for CAD or initial studies show a high probability of CAD or a risk of sudden death. In the ICU the patient receives frequent nursing assessments and has continuous ECG monitoring. Patients with unstable angina who are not considered high risk may be admitted to an intermediate care unit where ECG monitoring can be done. Other nursing goals for a patient with angina are reducing anxiety, informing the patient about angina and the treatment plan, and assisting with risk factor modification (Box 23-10).

The most common acute pharmacologic treatment for angina is administration of nitroglycerin, a vasodilator that opens the coronary arteries and increases blood flow to the heart (Agency for Health

---

**TABLE 23-8**

## Diagnostic Studies for Angina

| STUDY | RATIONALE |
| --- | --- |
| Cardiac enzymes and isoenzymes | To detect elevations that would indicate myocardial infarction. |
| Chest x-ray film | To detect any underlying condition, such as pneumonia, pulmonary congestion, enlargement of the heart, or an aortic aneurysm. |
| 12-Lead ECG | To assess for changes that may indicate ischemia or infarction and to evaluate for arrhythmias. |
| Serum lipid levels | To evaluate risk factors. |
| Stress test with or without exercise and with or without nuclear imaging | To determine if exercise induces ischemia. |
| Echocardiogram with or without exercise | To evaluate heart wall and valve functioning. |
| Cardiac catheterization | To evaluate coronary arteries. |

---

**BOX 23-10**    **NURSING PROCESS**

## PATIENT WITH ANGINA

### ASSESSMENT

- Pain (characteristics, severity on 1-10 scale)
- Cardiac status (vital signs, cardiac rhythm, edema, heart sounds)
- Neurologic signs (fatigue, syncope, level of consciousness)
- Respiratory status (rate, rhythm, cyanosis, adventitious sounds)
- Renal status (urinary output, laboratory values)
- Mental status (anxiety, perception of illness, self-concept)
- Knowledge of condition, disease process, medications, risk factors
- Risk factors (presence of changeable risk factors)

### NURSING DIAGNOSES

- Altered tissue perfusion related to myocardial oxygen supply and demand imbalance
- Anxiety related to lack of knowledge of diagnostic procedures, interventions, and illness
- Activity intolerance related to episodes of angina
- Risk for decreased cardiac output related to myocardial ischemia and thrombus formation
- Self-care deficit related to reducing risk for progression of CAD and managing angina

### NURSING INTERVENTIONS

- Instruct the patient to report any symptoms of pain or discomfort.
- Administer nitroglycerin as ordered.
- Administer beta-blockers and calcium channel blockers as ordered.
- Monitor response to drugs.
- Administer oxygen as ordered.
- Make sure the patient gets adequate rest.
- Plan small, frequent meals.
- Orient patient to surroundings and monitoring devices.
- Explain all procedures and diagnostic tests, as well as all medications and their purposes.

*Continued*

BOX 23-10

## NURSING PROCESS

### PATIENT WITH ANGINA—cont'd

- Allow the patient to verbalize his or her feelings and to ask questions.
- Use support personnel and family to help the patient through the initial hospitalization.
- Encourage the patient to participate as much as possible in his or her care and in decision making
- Begin teaching on CAD, risk factors, angina, and the treatment regimen
- Administer sedation as ordered.
- Provide for rest periods; increase activity and participation in care gradually.
- Ensure continuous ECG monitoring.
- Check vital signs frequently.
- Evaluate and treat pain promptly.
- Measure intake and output every 8 hours.
- Assess the patient for edema and for crackles in the lung bases.
- Administer anticoagulants and antiplatelets as ordered.

- Begin expanded patient teaching activities.
- Assist in planning methods of reducing risk factors, and in planning daily activities to reduce episodes of angina.
- Assist in identifying resources to help with lifestyle changes.

### EVALUATION OF EXPECTED OUTCOMES

- Pain or discomfort relieved
- Episodes of angina controlled or minimized
- Anxiety reduced
- Performs activities of daily living without angina
- No complications, or complications treated promptly
- Verbalizes understanding of disease process, procedures, treatment, medications, risk factors, and strategies for preventing angina

Care Policy and Research, 1994). Initially nitroglycerin may be given sublingually (under the tongue) at 5-minute intervals to relieve the acute angina attack. If this does not control the discomfort, nitroglycerin may be given as an IV drip. Both of these routes provide a quick effect of the nitroglycerin (3 minutes for sublingual, immediate for IV). Because of their vasodilating action, all nitrate preparations can cause flushing of the skin, an increase in pulse and respirations, hypotension, and headache (McCormack, 1996). The nurse should monitor for hypotension when administering nitroglycerin. If hypotension occurs, reducing the flow rate of the nitroglycerin (if given IV), elevating the legs, and administering IV fluid usually corrects the problem.

Other drugs that may be used in the acute phase include heparin (an anticoagulant used to prevent thrombus formation), aspirin (to inhibit platelet clumping and prevent the formation of clots), and beta-blockers (to decrease myocardial contractility, the heart rate, and afterload, which reduces the oxygen demand on the heart). Calcium channel blockers also may be given to reduce coronary vasospasm and to depress the myocardium, thereby reducing the oxygen consumption and workload of the heart (Agency for Health Care Policy and Research, 1994b) (Table 23-9). If heparin is used, the patient must be monitored for bleeding complications. Partial thromboplastin time (PTT) values are checked regularly to determine the level of anticoagulation, and the heparin is adjusted accordingly.

## Management of Chronic Angina

The treatment of angina pectoris requires treatment of the whole person, not treatment of the disease only. The patient must understand that he or she can have a full, productive life even with angina. Preventing the angina and reducing risk factors are the primary long-term goals. The patient and family must be educated about the process of CAD and angina, the factors that cause angina and ways to prevent them, medication, and reduction of risk factors. The Patient/Family Teaching box on Angina, p. 673, presents some specific teaching points that should be included in this education.

The patient needs to understand the nature of the pain and what can cause it (see Table 23-6). The nurse can help the patient learn to maintain a daily plan of living that reduces or eliminates the attacks of pain. The patient must get adequate rest, especially after activity and heavy meals. Nitroglycerin can be taken before activities known to cause angina or can be scheduled at times in the day when angina frequently occurs. The patient and family should understand the importance of daily physical activity to strengthen the heart. The nurse should consult with the physician or a rehabilitation exercise specialist to design an appropriate plan of activity progression.

## PATIENT/FAMILY TEACHING

### ANGINA

**Preventing Attacks of Angina**
- Avoid large, heavy meals. If you do eat a heavy meal, you should rest for 1 to 2 hours after eating.
- Avoid going out in extremely hot or cold weather.
  If you must go out in cold weather, wear warm clothing.
  If you must go out in hot weather, avoid strenuous exercise, wear a hat, and rest frequently in the shade.
- Drink decaffeinated tea, coffee, and sodas.
- Don't use tobacco products.
- Get plenty of rest at night.
- Plan exercise, sexual activity, and errands for times when you are well rested and not immediately after eating.
- If you are planning an activity that usually causes an angina attack, taking your nitroglycerin 5 to 10 minutes beforehand may help you avoid angina pain.

**Taking Nitroglycerin for Angina Pain**
- Keep your nitroglycerin tablets with you at all times.
- Store them in the brown bottle they come in and keep the lid on tight.
- Check the date on the bottle every month and get a new bottle when it expires.
- If you feel angina pain:
  Sit down and rest.
  Put one pill under your tongue; you should feel it fizzing or have a warm feeling under your tongue.
  You may feel a normal increase in your pulse, flushing, and a headache as the medicine begins to work. Stay in a resting position and get up slowly after you take the nitroglycerin.
  If the pain is not better in 5 minutes, put another pill under your tongue.
  Wait 5 more minutes and then use one more pill.
  If the pain is not better after three pills 5 minutes apart, **seek medical attention.**

## TABLE 23-9

### Drugs Used for Cardiac Problems

| CLASSIFICATION OF DRUG (GENERIC AND TRADE NAMES); SPECIFIC AGENTS | ACTION/INDICATION | COMMON SIDE EFFECTS AND NURSING CONSIDERATIONS |
|---|---|---|
| **Nitrates** | Vasodilate veins and coronary arteries primarily; provide increased blood flow to the heart muscle and decrease preload; used for treatment of angina and as an adjunct for treating MI and congestive heart failure (CHF) | Can cause hypotension, lightheadedness, dizziness, and tachycardia |
| Nitroglycerin SL (Nitrostat) | Short-acting drug for acute anginal attacks; onset 1-2 min, pain relief 3-5 min. Dissolve under tongue at first sign of attack and q 5 min until relief is obtained; maximum 3 tablets in 15 min. Can be taken before activities that cause chest pain as a preventive measure | Comes in bottle of 100; patient should sit or lie down when taking pill; can cause headache, although tolerance to headache develops within several weeks (use mild analgesic); should be stored in a dry place in a tight container, protected from sun; replace every 6 mo |
| Nitroglycerin translingual (Nitrolingual) | Short-acting drug for acute anginal attacks; lasts longer than nitroglycerin SL. 1-2 sprays (0.4 mg/spray) onto or under tongue for anginal attack, not to exceed 3 sprays in 15 minutes | Costs more that nitroglycerin SL but lasts longer; comes in spray canister with 200 sprays (shelf life is 3 yr) |

*Continued*

**TABLE 23-9**

## Drugs Used for Cardiac Problems—cont'd

| CLASSIFICATION OF DRUG (GENERIC AND TRADE NAMES); SPECIFIC AGENTS | ACTION/INDICATION | COMMON SIDE EFFECTS AND NURSING CONSIDERATIONS |
|---|---|---|
| Isosorbide dinitrate (Isordil,Sorbitrate) Isosorbide mononitrate (ISMO, Imdur) Nitroglycerin (Nitro-Bid) | Long-acting nitrates Oral nitrate; comes in SR (sustained release) strength Longer effects; used for angina and for therapy of MI | Tolerance to nitrates can develop over time; a nitrate-free period of at least 8 hr/day is recommended |
| Nitroglycerin ointment (Nitrol) | Paste; administered in inches on a scaled paper patch; patch is placed with the paste next to the skin and secured as needed | When replacing the paste, old paste is washed off with soap and water; nurse should avoid getting paste on his or her skin and wash it off quickly if this occurs (can cause headache and hypotension); rotate the site of the patch with each new patch; tolerance to nitrates can develop over time; a nitrate-free period of at least 8 hr/day is recommended |
| Transdermal patches (Nitro-Dur, Minitran, Transderm-Nitro) | Medication is released gradually over 24 hr in mg/hr; available in various strengths and rates of release | Use on area of the body free of hair; do not use on distal extremities or in areas of excessive movement; replace patch q 24 hr; rotate sites daily; tolerance to nitrates can develop over time; a nitrate-free period of at least 8 hr/day is recommended |
| Nitroglycerin IV | IV route Used for acute management of angina and MI | Can be absorbed by plastic tubing; glass bottle and special tubing are used in IV system; BP must be monitored carefully during start of infusion and adjustments in rate |
| **Beta-Blockers** Atenolol (Tenormin) Metoprolol (Lopresor) Propanolol (Inderal) | Antihypertensive and antianginal; used to reduce myocardial contractility, heart rate, and BP, reducing oxygen demand; used in angina and MI Can be given IV or PO IV dose is ordered ×3 in acute MI, then oral preparations used | Can cause bradycardia, bronchospasm, and depression Not used with patients who have asthma, COPD, or bradycardia Monitor BP and heart rate during IV administration Should not be reduced or stopped suddenly, can cause MI and sudden death |
| **Calcium Channel Blockers** Nifedipine (Procardia, Procardia XL) Verapamil (Calan, Isoptin) Diltiazem (Cardizem) | Antihypertensive and antianginal; vasodilates coronary arteries and decreases contractility; used for angina and hypertension Can be given IV or PO; comes in sustained release formulas Some physicians order Procardia sublingual; if the drug is given this way, the nurse must make a hole in the capsule and squirt the liquid drug into the patient's mouth | Side effects include hypotension, bradycardia, nervousness, and flushing BP and heart rate must be monitored during IV administration Can also cause constipation and GI upset |
| **Anticoagulants** Heparin | Used to prevent thrombosis in MI Initial bolus is followed by continuous drip | Monitor PTT Can cause prolonged bleeding; nurse must watch for bleeding, hematomas, and petechiae |

## TABLE 23-9

### Drugs Used for Cardiac Problems—cont'd

| CLASSIFICATION OF DRUG (GENERIC AND TRADE NAMES); SPECIFIC AGENTS | ACTION/INDICATION | COMMON SIDE EFFECTS AND NURSING CONSIDERATIONS |
|---|---|---|
| **Antiplatelet Agents**<br>Aspirin | Reduces platelet clumping; used in angina and MI to prevent thrombosis<br>For MI one is given to be chewed and one to be swallowed early in the acute onset, then one daily, one adult, or one baby aspirin may be ordered | Should not be given to patients with a history of GI bleed or hemorrhagic stroke in the past 3 mo or to a patient allergic to aspirin |
| **Angiotensin-Converting Enzyme Inhibitors (ACE Inhibitors)**<br>Enalapril (Vasotec)<br>Captopril (Capoten)<br>Lisinopril (Prinivil)<br>Ramipril (Altace)<br>Benazepril (Lotensin) | Block formation of angiotensin to cause vasodilation; used as antihypertensive; in MI is used to reduce mortality and symptomatic heart failure in patients with left ventricular failure | Can cause high potassium levels in patients taking potassium-sparing diuretics or who have renal failure, and in patients with renal artery stenosis; most common patient complaint is dry cough |
| **Analgesic**<br>Morphine sulfate<br>Given IV in small increments 1-3 mg slowly | Analgesic and vasodilator; reduces myocardial workload and patient anxiety; drug of choice for treating chest pain caused by ischemia | Can cause respiratory depression and hypotension; nurse must watch for decreased respiratory rate and low BP; naloxone can be given to reverse effects |

The patient and family should be educated in the importance of nitroglycerin, the proper way to use it, and the side effects to expect (see the Patient/Family Teaching box on Angina, p. 673). Frequently patients do not take the prn nitroglycerin ordered because of the headache that occurs afterward. Other common medication problems are improper storage, not taking enough tablets during episodes of pain, and taking too many tablets before seeking medical attention. The patient and family also must be taught the steps to take in case rest and nitroglycerin do not relieve the angina. This information should be shared with co-workers and the employee health office if the patient works.

Risk factors are another important teaching focus. The patient and family should be assisted in identifying the risk factors that can be changed and in making a plan to begin this process. Risk factors for CAD and ways to modify them are covered in detail in Table 23-4.

Two major responsibilities of nursing care are to relieve the patient's anxiety and to help the patient and family adjust to the diagnosis of angina, the medical plan of care, and the life-style changes suggested. Helping the family identify community resources and providing counseling, reassurance, and guidance are all important nursing interventions. Outpatient cardiac rehabilitation programs are very helpful in continuing these activities and providing ongoing support for the patient and family, and these programs should be considered as an option.

Medications used in the long-term treatment of angina are the same as those discussed for the acute phase, except that heparin, if used, usually is discontinued after 3 to 5 days, if not sooner. Nitroglycerin normally is continued, as an ointment, a patch, or a long-acting oral agent. However, tolerance to nitroglycerin can develop quickly during long-term therapy. To avoid this, patients usually are given an 8- to 12-hour nitrate "holiday," or nitrate-free time, during the day or night (Agency for Health Care Policy and Research, 1994b). Most patients take their nitrate holiday during the night, when they are not active, but if they have anginal pain during the night, they should take their nitrate-free time during the day. Table 23-9 presents a review of the medications used for anginal pain and the nursing implications for each.

## MYOCARDIAL INFARCTION

**Myocardial infarction**, also called *heart attack*, occurs when one of the coronary arteries or its branches suddenly becomes completely blocked (Figure 23-32). The blockage deprives the myocardial cell of oxygen, and

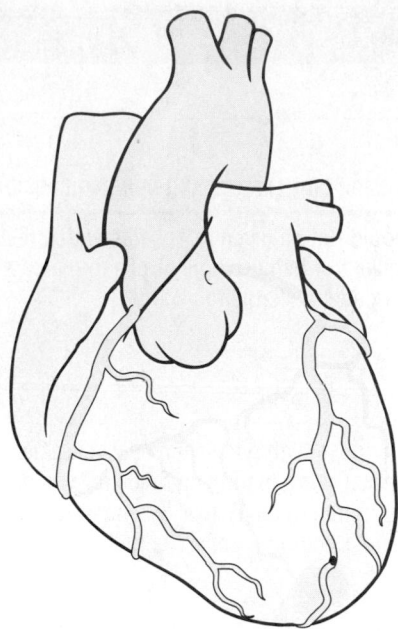

**Figure 23-32** Occlusion of coronary artery, resulting in a myocardial infarction. (By permission of Mayo Clinic, Rochester, Minn.)

ischemia progresses to injury and then infarction (tissue death). There usually is a 20-minute window during which the myocardial cells can survive without permanent damage and death. Unlike with angina, in MI the blockage does not resolve spontaneously, and unless blood flow is reestablished through medical intervention, the myocardial cells suffer irreversible cellular necrosis (death).

MI is most often the end point in the progression of atherosclerotic CAD. Thrombus formation and occlusion of a coronary artery resulting from rupture of plaque are the causative agents in most MIs. This pathologic condition has made the use of thrombolytic (clot buster) agents a standard of practice in the treatment of MI. Other less common causes include coronary emboli, trauma to the heart and coronary arteries, inflammation (vasculitis), and severe imbalances in oxygen supply and demand (cocaine abuse is one possible cause of this) (Urban et al, 1995).

The infarcted tissue loses its ability to contract and conduct electrical impulses. Also, it is surrounded by severely injured and ischemic tissue that either heals or eventually dies. The dead tissue and the varying degrees of injury and ischemia are responsible for the possible complications related to arrhythmias and for the decrease in cardiac output. The degree of impair-

ment and the severity of the MI depend on several factors, including location, size, collateral circulation, and time to presentation.

## Location

Infarctions usually are identified by where they occur; this is described as anterior, posterior, inferior, lateral, or a combination of these. The location of the MI is determined by the coronary artery or branch that becomes blocked. Table 23-10 presents a list of the coronary arteries and the areas of the heart affected during an MI. Most MIs occur in the left ventricle on the anterior wall.

## Size

The size of the myocardial infarction depends on the thickness of muscle involved, the area of the lesions along the coronary artery, the presence or absence of collateral circulation, and the length of time the infarct goes untreated. A *transmural MI* involves the full thickness of the myocardium; a *subendocardial* or *non-Q-wave MI* involves only the inner layer of the muscle.

The location of the blockage along the coronary artery affects the size of the infarction. If the blockage occurs closer to the origin of the coronary artery, more branches are affected and a larger area is damaged. For instance, blockages that occur in the left main coronary artery before it splits into the left anterior descending and circumflex arteries limit blood flow to both branches, creating an extensive area of necrosis.

The presence of *collateral circulation* also influences infarction size. Collateral circulation is arterial branching that occurs when atherosclerotic plaques cause chronic ischemia. These collateral branches divert blood flow around the area of narrowing to keep the muscle cells oxygenated. When CAD occurs slowly over a long period, more collateral vessels are formed, and in the event of complete blockage, heart muscle cells continue to receive blood flow. If the CAD develops quickly or blockage occurs because of spasm or clot formation, adequate collateral circulation may not be present. In this case no alternative route is available for blood flow, and more severe infarction occurs (Urban et al, 1995).

The length of time the infarction goes untreated plays a major role both in the severity of the infarction and in the complications and death rate from MI. The longer the cells are without blood flow, the more damage that occurs. In addition, serious arrhythmias (e.g., ventricular fibrillation) often occur in the first hour af-

**TABLE 23-10**

## Locations of Myocardial Infarctions

| LOCATION | CORONARY ARTERY INVOLVED | COMPLICATIONS/NURSING CONSIDERATIONS |
|---|---|---|
| Inferior | Right | Damage can extend into right ventricle; heart block and bradycardia are common; mitral regurgitation can occur because of papillary muscle rupture; nausea and vomiting can occur; nurse should watch for systolic murmurs and low heart rate. |
| Anterior | Left | Congestive heart failure (CHF), aneurysms, complete heart block can occur; nurse should watch for signs of CHF and low heart rates. |
| Lateral | Circumflex | Usually associated with posterior and anterior MIs; SA node problems and arrhythmias can occur. |
| Posterior | Right or circumflex | Bradycardia, heart block, and CHF can occur; can occur with inferior MI; nurse should watch for signs of CHF and low heart rate. |
| Anteroseptal | Left anterior descending | Considerable muscle damage can occur; ventricular septal defects, CHF, and heart block can occur; nurse should watch for signs of CHF, low heart rate, new onset of systolic murmur. |
| Anterolateral | Left anterior descending | Aneurysm, CHF, and bradycardia can occur; nurse should watch for signs of CHF, low heart rate. |

Data from Morton PG: *Crit Care Nurse* 16(2):85-95, 1996.

ter symptoms begin and are the major reason for sudden cardiac death (Cummins, 1994).

Prompt recognition of the symptoms of MI and aggressive treatment are essential in preventing sudden death.

## Acute Assessment

When evaluating a patient who has chest discomfort, the nurse must complete a rapid evaluation of the patient's airway, breathing, and circulation (the ABCs), the characteristics of the pain, risk factors for CAD, and a physical examination of the heart and lungs, as well as simultaneously beginning initial therapy. The suspicion of MI is based on the patient's symptoms. A concise history and physical examination, done in less than 10 minutes, is the key to fast treatment and improved outcomes (Cummins, 1994).

Because time is critical in limiting damage and preventing complications, a rapid history and physical examination, as well as diagnostic studies and therapeutic interventions, are done in the initial minutes of the patient's presentation. From the time of arrival or the initial complaint of chest pain, the goal is to confirm MI and begin thrombolytic treatment in less than 30 to 60 minutes (Cummins, 1994). The nurse plays an essential role in prompt identification of patients with possible MI and rapid implementation of the therapy.

### NURSE ALERT

Any unusual or prolonged indigestion or discomfort in the chest that persists longer than a few minutes should be evaluated, especially in patients with risk factors for CAD.

## History and Physical Examination

The onset of MI, in contrast to angina, usually occurs when the individual is at rest or engaging in moderate activity. Many patients report being awakened from sleep by the pain and other symptoms. The peak time for the onset of MI is 6 AM to 12 noon, and many occur during the winter months (Cummins, 1994). Severe exertion and emotional stress are other events that can precede the onset of MI.

The typical symptoms of acute MI include a sudden, severe, pressure-like pain in the area of the midsternum and upper abdomen. The pain may increase in severity over time and radiate to the shoulders and down the arms or to the jaw. The left shoulder and the left arm are more often affected. The pain or discomfort may described as crushing, pressure, squeezing, or heavy. Patients often use a closed fist to describe the location and intensity of the pain. In some patients the pain may be mild, or it may be located in the epigastric area and mistaken for indigestion. Women, the elderly, and diabetics may have an atypical presentation of MI, such as vague symptoms or simply shortness of breath (Urban et al, 1995). MI pain is not relieved by rest.

Other cardiovascular symptoms may include a weak, rapid pulse and elevated blood pressure caused by catecholamine release. Sympathetic stimulation can cause sweating (diaphoresis) and vasoconstriction of blood vessels in the skin. The patient may appear pale and ashen and may feel cold and clammy. The blood pressure may drop rapidly if the MI progresses and cardiac output decreases. If cardiac output is affected by the infarction, changes in level of consciousness, as well as pulmonary congestion (crackles heard on auscultation of the chest) and peripheral edema (dependent and jugular vein distension), may occur. Ventric-

ular arrhythmias (e.g., ventricular tachycardia and ventricular fibrillation) are a common complication, and continuous ECG monitoring is a must.

Nausea and vomiting are a common symptom and are due to severe pain or stimulation of vasovagal nerve fibers in the infarcted area. Nausea and vomiting are most common with inferior MI because of the proximity of vasovagal fibers to the inferior border of the heart. In a few hours the patient's temperature rises, but it rarely exceeds 38.3° C (101° F). Most patients are acutely aware of their condition and are extremely apprehensive.

Other data that should be gathered include a list of current medications, and a screen should be done for contraindications to thrombolytic (clot buster) therapy. The criteria for use of thrombolytic agents and the contraindications are presented in Table 23-11.

## TABLE 23-11

### Thrombolytic Drugs

| DRUG | SPECIAL CONSIDERATIONS |
|---|---|
| Alteplase (Activase) | Recombinant tissue plasminogen activator (rt-PA); clot selective, expensive, dosing regimen more time-consuming; heparin given during and after administration |
| Streptokinase | Not clot selective (can cause systemic clot lysis); inexpensive; infusion given over 1 hr; made from *Streptococcus* bacteria—not usually given if patient has had streptococcal infection within the past year; allergic reaction possible; heparin usually given IV after administration |
| Anistreplase (Eminase) | Anisolated plasminogen streptokinase activator complex; not clot selective (can cause systemic clot lysis); expensive; one-time bolus given over 3-5 min; made from *Streptococcus* bacteria—not usually given if patient has had streptococcal infection within the past year; allergic reaction can occur; heparin not usually given |
| Urokinase | Used mostly to treat peripheral thrombi |

**Indications**
History suggestive of MI
ECG evidence of MI
No absolute contraindications
Few or no relative contraindications
Age and length of time to presentation are considered, but no specific guidelines currently are being used.

**Contraindications**
*Absolute*
Active internal bleeding
Possible aortic dissection
Trauma or surgery within past 2 wk
Hypertension that does not resolve with pain control
Recent head trauma or known tumor
Stroke within past 6 mo
Pregnancy
Allergy to drug
*Relative*
Trauma or surgery with past 2 mo
Chronic severe hypertension
Active peptic ulcer disease
History of stroke, tumor, or head injury
Known bleeding problems
Use of anticoagulants
Exposure to agents made from *Streptococcus* bacteria within past 12 mo
Central IV lines

Data from Aragon D, Martin M: *Am J Nurs* 93(9):24-31, 1993.

The nurse also must be vigilant in assessing for possible complications of acute MI. The first 24 hours are critical; however, many life-threatening complications can occur in the following days and weeks. Table 23-12 presents the etiology, assessment findings, and nursing considerations for complications of MI.

## Diagnostic Studies

The initial diagnostic studies for a patient suspected of having an MI are presented in Table 23-13. The 12-lead ECG is the most important study to be done. Because MI is an ongoing process, the 12-lead ECG results may not be abnormal at first, therefore serial ECGs must be done. The 12-lead ECG tracing should be compared to other 12-lead tracings done on the patient if these are available. The 12-lead ECG study will identify the area of infarction. Each area of infarction can produce different side effects, and the nurse must be prepared for possible complications. Cardiac enzyme and isoenzyme levels also are evaluated initially and are reevaluated several times after the first set. A complete review of the enzyme patterns seen with MI can be found earlier in this chapter and in Table 23-14. Several studies, including serum electrolyte and coagulation studies, are done to establish a baseline and to prepare for possible thrombolytic therapy.

## TABLE 23-12

## Complications of Myocardial Infarction

| COMPLICATION | ETIOLOGY | ASSESSMENT FINDINGS/NURSING CONSIDERATIONS |
|---|---|---|
| **First 24 Hours** | | |
| Arrhythmias (See the section Arrhythmias, p. 647, earlier in this chapter.) | Ischemia, sympathetic stimulation, electrolyte imbalances | Most common complication; can be life-threatening; ventricular fibrillation most likely to occur in first few hours after symptoms begin; continuous ECG monitoring must be done. |
| Congestive heart failure (More information can be found in the section Congestive Heart Failure, p. 696.) | Decreased cardiac output because of reduced pumping power | May occur in first 24 hr; can be mild or severe; symptoms include restlessness, rapid respirations, jugular vein distension, dependent edema, decreased urine output, crackles in the lungs, $S_3$ or $S_4$ heart sounds. |
| Cardiogenic shock | Loss of >40% of heart muscle function because of extensive infarction; cardiac output falls significantly | Severe heart failure, hypotension, respiratory compromise, pulmonary edema, and organ failure occur; signs and symptoms can include restlessness, pallor, cool, clammy skin, decreased level of consciousness, tachycardia, decreased urinary output; mortality rate is very high; therapy may include cardiac-stimulating drugs (positive inotropes), vasodilators, vasopressors, and mechanical assist devices, including a ventilator or intraaortic balloon pump. |
| **After 24 Hours** | | |
| Mitral regurgitation | Papillary muscle damage, backflow of blood through mitral valve to left atrium; stresses the left ventricle and decreases cardiac output | Assessment reveals systolic murmur, severe heart failure, shortness of breath; usually requires surgical correction. |
| Septal rupture | Infarction weakens intraventricular septum, hole develops | Assessment reveals harsh systolic murmur, severe heart failure; usually requires surgical correction. |
| Pericarditis | Inflammation of pericardial sac | Usually seen 2-3 days after MI; assessment reveals chest pain aggravated by coughing, breathing, and movement, pericardial rub on auscultation, low-grade temperature; may see changes on ECG; treated with pain medications and antiinflammatory drugs. |
| Ventricular aneurysm | Infarction weakens wall, which bulges with each contraction | Can occur initially or after several days; assessment reveals heart failure, chest pain; may see changes on ECG; ruptured aneurysm is fatal; surgical intervention usually is required. |

Data from Urban N et al: *Guidelines for critical care nursing*, St Louis, 1995, Mosby.

**TABLE 23-13**

## Diagnostic Studies for Acute Evaluation of Myocardial Infarction

| STUDY | RATIONALE | CONSIDERATIONS |
|---|---|---|
| 12-Lead ECG | To assess for ECG criteria for injury and infarction and to locate area of infarction | Should be reviewed by physician within 5 min, ST segment elevations and Q waves are most common findings in acute MI; ECG findings may be normal initially, therefore tracing is repeated at regular intervals. |
| Cardiac enzymes and isoenzymes | To detect elevations consistent with myocardial infarction | Each enzyme has a pattern of elevation and peak; results may not be available rapidly; newer studies are being used to obtain results more quickly. |
| Serum electrolytes | To detect abnormalities that may alter the treatment plan and to establish a baseline | Not useful in determining if MI has occurred. |
| Coagulation studies | To establish a baseline and rule out clotting problems | Thrombolytic agents are contraindicated with coagulation problems; coagulation studies are done frequently after thrombolytic therapy. |
| Chest x-ray film | To rule out underlying pathologic condition that may be causing symptoms and to ensure that no contraindications exist for thrombolytic therapy | |

**TABLE 23-14**

## Cardiac Enzymes and Isoenzymes

| ENZYME | NORMAL VALUES | ELEVATION (hr) | PEAK (hr) | DURATION |
|---|---|---|---|---|
| Creatine phosphokinase (CPK) | *Total CPK:* men: 12-70 U/ml or 55-170 U/L women: 10-55 U/ml or 30-135 U/L | 4-8 | 12-24 | 72-96 hr |
| Lactate dehydrogenase (LDH) | *Total LDH:* 45-90 U/L | 24-48 | 72-144 | 8-14 days |
| Creatine phosphokinase-MB (CPK-MB) | 0% | 4-8 | 12-20 | 48-72 hr |
| LDH-1:LDH-2 ratio | LDH-1:LDH-2 ratio <1 or LDH-1<LDH-2 | 12-24 Abnormal if LDH-1:LDH-2 ratio >1 or LDH-1>LDH-2 | 72-144 | 14 days |

Data from Pagana KD, Pagana TJ: *Mosby's diagnostic and laboratory test reference,* ed 3, St Louis, 1996, Mosby.

## Acute Management and Nursing Interventions

Depending on the situation, many patients who have symptoms of MI are first seen in the Emergency Department, where they are assessed and treated and then transferred to an ICU or CCU. Most patients with MI stay in the ICU or CCU for several days. The goals of intensive therapy are to stabilize the patient's condition, to prevent any increase in the size of the infarct, and to prevent complications. The first 24 hours are extremely important. If aggressive therapy is started within minutes or a few hours after the onset of symptoms, myocardial damage may be reduced or prevented through reperfusion techniques, which include use of thrombolytic agents and invasive procedures for reopening the blocked vessel.

During the acute initial phase of MI, several interventions should be implemented while the diagnosis of MI is confirmed. Initiation of continuous ECG monitoring is crucial to early recognition and treatment of arrhythmias. An IV line must be started to provide a route for medications. If administration of thrombolytic agents is a possibility, two or three large-bore IV lines should be started. Preferred IV sites are those in large peripheral vessels, not central lines. Central IV lines are not compressible and, in the event that thrombolytic drugs are given, can be a site of bleeding.

Pharmacologic management would start on presentation with administration of oxygen, which increases the supply of oxygen to the heart muscle cells (Cummins, 1994). Oxygen usually is started at 4 L/minute using a nasal cannula. Oxygen administration then is adjusted to provide an oxygen saturation over 96%. Oxygen levels need to be lower in patients with chronic obstructive pulmonary disease (COPD) and are started at 1 to 2 L/minute.

> ## NURSE ALERT
>
> **All patients suspected of having MI should be given oxygen. Oxygen—monitoring—IV are the first three interventions for a patient having chest pain.**

Pain relief is of primary importance, and nitroglycerin and morphine sulfate are the drugs of choice for pain control (Cummins, 1994). As a vasodilator, nitroglycerin serves to open the coronary arteries and increase blood flow. Initially nitroglycerin may be given sublingually, but IV nitroglycerin usually is needed to ensure the best control. Care must be taken to prevent large decreases in blood pressure as a result of nitroglycerin administration. Careful titration of the IV dose and frequent BP checks are important nursing interventions. Morphine is the analgesic of choice for the treatment of pain in patients with MI. Morphine provides analgesia and reduces preload and afterload through vasodilation, which reduces the myocardial oxygen demand. The dose of morphine given is 1 to 3 mg IV over 5 minutes, which is repeated at 5-minute intervals until the pain is relieved (Cummins, 1994).

Other drugs commonly given in the initial management of MI are aspirin, heparin, and beta-blockers. Aspirin is recommended because of its antiplatelet-clumping properties. Aspirin has been shown to reduce overall mortality from MI, reinfarction rates, and stroke rates (Cummins, 1994). Unless contraindicated because of ulcer disease or allergy, the patient is given one aspirin to swallow and another to chew (Cummins, 1994). Aspirin is continued daily for life.

With most thrombolytic drugs, heparin is given after the thrombolytic has been administered to prevent recurrence of thrombosis. It also is given to prevent thrombus formation in patients with a large anterior MI, atrial fibrillation, and congestive heart failure (CHF), even without thrombolytic therapy. An initial bolus followed by a continuous drip usually is ordered. Changes in the heparin dose are based on PTT results, with the goal of maintaining the PTT at one and one half to two times the control.

Beta-blockers initially are given intravenously and then orally unless hypotension, bradycardia, heart failure, or asthma are present. Beta-blockers reduce myocardial oxygen utilization and are continued for 1 to 2 years after the MI.

Administration of thrombolytic agents has become standard practice in the treatment of MI. Thrombolytic agents administered early in the course of MI have been shown to reduce mortality (Cummins, 1994). This therapy stops the pathologic thrombotic process that causes most MIs and salvages the muscle cells that are not already dead. To be most effective, thrombolytic drugs must be given as early in the process of MI as possible. Administration within 6 hours of the onset of symptoms gives the most clinical benefit, but administration can improve the outcome of patients who have had symptoms for as long as 24 hours (Cummins, 1994). Currently three drugs are used most often dissolve the thrombus (Urban et al, 1995) (see Table 23-11); they are alteplase, streptokinase, and anistreplase. These agents have different mechanisms of action, pharmacokinetics, and special considerations, but they all function to dissolve the clot causing the MI (Aragon, Martin, 1993). However, drugs that can lyse clots in the coronary arteries also cause clot lysis in other areas of the body. This activity of the thrombolytic agents makes it essential that patients be evaluated for their risk for severe bleeding (see Table 23-11).

Once the patient is determined to be a candidate for thrombolytic therapy, an appropriate agent is chosen based on the patient's characteristics and the institution's and physician's preferences. Each agent has its own protocols for administration, but several common nursing interventions are implemented for patients receiving thrombolytic agents (Box 23-11). Patients receiving thrombolytic agents are monitored closely; continuous ECG monitoring is instituted, and vital signs are checked frequently. As the agent causes lysis of the clot blocking the coronary artery, several events may occur.

The first possible event is restoration of blood flow to the myocardium. The nurse must be able to recognize the indicators of reperfusion, which include ECG changes (ST segments return to normal from their elevated position), resolution of chest pain, and a rapid change in the CPK-MB level (level increases as blood flow washes enzymes into the circulation faster than they normally would have entered it). Reperfusion arrhythmias can occur as blood flow is reestablished. Any number of arrhythmias can be seen, including ventricular tachycardia, ventricular fibrillation, bradycardia, heart block, and short spurts of asystole. Reperfusion arrhythmias may not occur in all patients with

BOX 23-11 | NURSING PROCESS

## PATIENT RECEIVING THROMBOLYTIC AGENTS

### NURSING DIAGNOSES

- Risk for bleeding caused by thrombolytic action of drugs
- Potential decreased cardiac output related to reperfusion arrhythmias
- Potential injury allergic reaction related to drug administration (allergies can occur with streptokinase and anistreplase)
- Potential altered tissue perfusion related to reocclusion of coronary artery

### NURSING INTERVENTIONS
#### Preadministration

- Place two to three large-bore IV lines in peripheral veins; these provide for sites for medication and fluid administration so that other IV lines will not be needed after drug is given.
- Insert any catheters or tubes (e.g., Foley catheter, nasogastric tube); there is less chance of bleeding if these procedures are completed before the drug is given.
- Draw all ordered baseline laboratory studies.

#### Administration

- Monitor infusion accurately; keep ordered rate.

#### Postadministration

- Draw blood needed for laboratory studies from existing IV sites.
- Avoid IM injections; use IV route for medications.
- Avoid arterial punctures.
- Avoid venous sticks; keep IV lines patent and use for drawing blood.
- If venous and arterial sticks are necessary, use compressible sites, because bleeding is more easily stopped when compression can be used.
- Have patient use soft-bristled toothbrush.
- Use an electric razor, not a safety razor, for shaving.
- Avoid trauma (use fall precautions, no precordial thump).
- Apply direct pressure to any arterial or venous sites used for puncture; this limits bleeding and promotes clot formation.
- Take oral temperatures; avoid taking rectal temperature to prevent tissue tears.

- If heparin is given, monitor its administration and maintain desired rate; monitor results of PTT and adjust drip rate as ordered.
- Monitor patient for bleeding:
  Observe guaiac stool, emesis, urine.
  Assess skin, gums, and nose for petechiae, ecchymoses, hematomas.
  Check venipuncture sites for oozing.
  Assess for signs of intracranial bleeding (altered level of consciousness, vomiting, headache).
  Assess for signs of internal bleeding (abdominal pain and tenderness, weakness, distended abdomen).
- Monitor ECG continuously.
- Have emergency drugs and equipment readily available, at bedside is recommended.
- Implement treatment for symptomatic arrhythmias as ordered or according to ACLS guidelines.
- Observe for signs and symptoms of allergic reaction, including itching, rash, swelling of face and tongue, hypotension, and bronchospasm.
- Assess for respiratory distress.
- Prepare to administer IV fluids for hypotension.
- Place patient in modified Trendelenburg position if hypotensive.
- Administer diphenhydramine, epinephrine, and steroids as ordered.
- Observe patient closely for signs of reocclusion, including chest pain and other symptoms seen before thrombolytic agent was given.
- If signs or symptoms are observed:
  Obtain 12-lead ECG tracing.
  Notify physician.
  Administer or adjust nitroglycerin as ordered.
  Administer morphine sulfate as ordered.
  Prepare for invasive procedure or repeat thrombolytic administration.

### EVALUATION OF EXPECTED OUTCOMES

- No major bleeding
- Reperfusion arrhythmias treated quickly
- Allergic reactions recognized and managed
- Reocclusion recognized and treated

restored blood flow, but, if they do occur, the nurse must assess the patient carefully for serious signs and symptoms and treat them as ordered.

Another possible event is failure of reperfusion to occur at all. Persistence of symptoms requires more invasive actions including possible emergency cardiac catheterization. If reperfusion does occur, there is always the risk of reocclusion of the coronary artery. The use of heparin after some thrombolytic agents are administered helps reduce the reocclusion rate. The patient suffering reocclusion initially may seem stable, and reperfusion indicators may have been seen. If another clot forms or a spasm of the coronary artery occurs, the chest pain and other symptoms similar or the ones seen before the thrombolytic agents were given may return. The nurse must be alert to the return of these symptoms and must notify the physician, implement interventions to reduce pain, and prepare for other interventions as ordered by the physician (see Box 23-11).

In some settings patients with confirmed acute MI are taken immediately to the cardiac catheterization laboratory for coronary angiography and invasive treatment. This therapy may be used in patients who are not candidates for thrombolytic therapy, who have clotted grafts from previous coronary bypass surgery, or who have shock or heart failure within 18 hours. The ability to perform invasive treatment depends on the facility. Most patients who have MI receive cardiac catheterization after their condition has been stabilized or after the thrombolytic agents have been administered and the risk of bleeding has been reduced. Treatment options include percutaneous transluminal coronary angioplasty (PTCA), stent placement, atherectomy, and coronary artery bypass graft (CABG). Invasive treatment options are described in a later section.

Patients who experience serious complications such as severe heart failure, **cardiogenic shock,** or life-threatening arrhythmias may require hemodynamic monitoring and respiratory support. They may also require infusions of positive inotropic (stimulating) drugs or mechanical support of heart function with an intraaortic balloon pump. These situations are associated with increased mortality and morbidity and alter the normal progress of an uncomplicated MI.

## Ongoing Assessment and Intervention

As the heart heals, collateral circulation develops and the necrotic tissue in the myocardium is replaced with fibrotic scar formation. With 24 hours many of the inflammatory responses to cellular death have occurred (Huether, McCance, 1996). In 24 to 72 hours, scar tissue formation has begun in the necrotic area. At 2 weeks the scar is still weak. At 6 weeks the infarcted cells

have been replaced with scar tissue. The process of recovery from an MI is slow and gradual, with healing of the injured area occurring at approximately 6 weeks, but convalescence can take several more weeks.

After the initial acute 24 hours, the first 2 weeks after an MI are considered the most dangerous, and the patient's condition is watched closely for 4 weeks. The patient is kept in the ICU or CCU until his or her condition is stable and often until diagnostic and therapeutic interventions have been completed or a medical plan of care has been developed (an average of 2 to 3 days). The patient may be transferred to a step-down unit for continued monitoring and then to a regular nursing unit before discharge. (The entire stay may last 5 to 7 days.)·

The management and care of the patient with MI must be individualized according to the severity of the attack, complications, interventions performed to treat the underlying atherosclerotic plaque, and the patient's progress. Gradually the patient becomes able to return to a normal or nearly normal life. Nursing interventions for patients with MI are designed to (1) reduce pain, (2) monitor for and prevent complications, (3) reduce anxiety, (4) reduce the myocardial oxygen demand, (5) provide education and support to the patient and family, and (6) promote a return to the previous level of functioning (Urban et al, 1995).

Pain reduction, as discussed in the previous section, is an essential nursing function. If IV nitroglycerin is used, it is tapered slowly (called weaning) and discontinued while other nitrates (oral, paste, or patch) are initiated. Most patients begin to receive nitroglycerin sublingually prn (as needed) for pain. As the pain is relieved, the nurse must make sure the patient and family realize that the absence of pain does not mean the injury is any less serious or that permanent damage does not exist. Patients and families often mistake the lack of pain to mean that healing has occurred and that activities can resume at previous levels. They also may think that the lack of pain means no permanent damage has occurred and may deny that they have had an MI. These strong coping mechanisms and misconceptions can jeopardize the recovery process and must be addressed.

Staying alert for complications that can occur after an MI is another important nursing intervention. While the first 24 hours are a very high-risk time for complications such as arrhythmias, other complications may not be seen until later (Urban et al, 1995) (see Table 23-12). Frequent checking of vital signs and continuous ECG monitoring are essential interventions. Fever is a common finding in MI patients; it can increase within the first 24 hours and remain elevated for up to a week. The elevated temperature usually is caused by the inflammatory process, but it also may be due to pericarditis. Intake and output measurements are helpful in detecting the altered fluid volume status that can occur with congestive heart failure. A physical examination every 8 hours, including checking for dependent edema, crackles in the lung bases, and jugular vein distension, also is needed to detect changes early. In addition, the nurse must remember that cardiac monitoring equipment and other monitoring devices have made it possible to detect cardiac disturbances and contribute much to the care of patients, but these machines can increase the patient's fear, anxiety, and apprehension unless their contribution to care is understood. Above all, it should be remembered that machines cannot replace diligent nursing evaluation or provide emotional support and the intelligent, empathetic understanding essential to the patient's progress.

Measures to ease anxiety in the patient and family are needed from the first interaction through the hospital stay and beyond into discharge. It is important for the nurse to be aware of his or her own level of anxiety and to take care to approach the patient calmly and with confidence. Caring for a patient with MI can produce a degree of urgency and concern that can be distressing to the patient. Family and significant others are concerned and scared, and their anxiety may affect the patient. As the patient's anxiety level increases, the systemic effects can lead to increased myocardial oxygen demand, tachycardia, and shortness of breath. The nurse must find out what the patient views as causing the anxiety and intervene as needed. If the patient fears being without loved ones, a change in visiting policies may be needed. If the patient does not understand what is being done, teaching should be done to answer all questions. Orienting the patient and family to the unit, unit routines, what to expect, the monitoring devices being used and why, and how the plan of care will be implemented are interventions that can reduce anxiety. Medication may be ordered to ease the anxiety and help the patient relax.

In addition to anxiety the patient may have other responses to MI, including fear, denial, anger, dependency, and depression. All of these must anticipated and addressed as they occur. Denial can cause the patient to take his or her condition lightly and ignore the restrictions and medical regimen. Fear and dependency may cause the patient to progress more slowly through the recovery and become a "cardiac cripple." Anger may be expressed as acting-out behavior toward the health care team, family, or individual nurse. Depression may not be experienced until discharge, when the patient becomes overwhelmed with life-style changes that must be made. Using many resources, including clergy, counseling services,

patients who have thrived after an MI, and a cardiac rehabilitation program, is helpful in planning specific interventions.

Reduction of myocardial oxygen demand is an essential part of care after an MI. The patient must get maximum rest from the moment of the attack. Procedures should be planned to allow periods of undisturbed rest. Medication may be ordered if the patient is having difficulty sleeping. During the acute phase, visiting may be limited to close members of the patient's family or significant others if these visits stress or tire the patient. Some patients may have increased anxiety with visiting limitations and may do better with a more open visitation policy.

Complete bed rest or limitation of activities is the usual way to provide maximum rest. How long the patient has an activity limitation depends on the extent of the injury. The patient may be allowed up to a bedside commode in the first few hours if activity limitations are causing undue stress. Activity progresses gradually, and the nurse must monitor the patient's response by evaluating the ECG tracing for arrhythmias and observing the patient for shortness of breath, and fatigue during and following activity. Activity should be reduced if the patient experiences pain, arrhythmias, shortness of breath, and extreme fatigue. It is common for patients to tire easily for the first few weeks after an MI. A structured cardiac rehabilitation program with progressive activity and teaching is begun early in the hospital stay and continues in the outpatient setting.

Other interventions to reduce the workload of the heart include diet alterations. The diet usually begins as liquids and progresses to solid as the patient is able to tolerate without nausea and vomiting. A low-sodium, low-fat diet is recommended. Caffeine commonly is restricted to avoid stimulation of the heart. Bowel elimination may be regulated by mild laxatives and stool softeners to prevent constipation and straining, which may induce a vagal response and bradycardia.

Unless contraindicated, pharmacologic interventions are designed to reduce the cardiac workload, prevent complications, and treat specific risk factors such as hyperlipidemia (see Table 23-9). Beta-blockers, described previously, are continued by an oral route. Long-term beta-blocker therapy has been shown to reduce mortality, reinfarction, and sudden death (Cummins, 1994). Aspirin is given daily to reduce the risk of death, reinfarction, and stroke. Oral anticoagulants may be given to patients who have large MIs to prevent thrombus formation and emboli. Angiotensin-converting enzyme (ACE) inhibitors may be ordered because of their role in reducing mortality and heart failure in patients with decreased left ventricular function after MI. Calcium channel blockers may have an

BOX 23-12

## NURSING PROCESS

## MYOCARDIAL INFARCTION

### ASSESSMENT

- Pain: presence, location, quality
- Pulse: quality, rate, rhythm
- Respirations: rate, rhythm, dyspnea
- Skin: color, temperature, moisture
- Mood and mental status
- Knowledge of event and status

### NURSING DIAGNOSES

- Decreased cardiac output related to decreased cardiac perfusion
- Altered tissue perfusion related to interruption of arterial blood flow
- Pain related to poor cardiac perfusion
- Self-care deficit related to weakness
- Anxiety related to inability to control illness
- Impaired physical mobility related to discomfort and activity intolerance
- Risk for fluid volume excess related to cardiac failure
- Risk for ineffective breathing pattern related to discomfort and pulmonary vascular congestion
- Risk for ineffective individual coping related to effect of illness on life-style
- Risk for impaired gas exchange related to pulmonary vascular congestion
- Risk for fear of death related to knowledge of or misperceptions about condition

### NURSING INTERVENTIONS

- Check vital signs often.
- Maintain complete bed rest in the first stage of recovery; transfer the patient to a chair as ordered, and increase activity gradually.
- Observe for signs and symptoms of cardiogenic shock, pulmonary edema, cardiac arrhythmia, and congestive heart failure.
- Allow for long periods of undisturbed rest.
- Restrict visitors, and space visits so they do not interfere with rest periods.
- Administer pain medication as needed.
- Administer oxygen as needed.
- Regulate bowel elimination with laxatives and diet; do not permit straining at defecation.
- Alleviate anxiety or apprehension of the patient and the family.
- Restrict sodium and cholesterol intake; provide a well-balanced diet.
- Orient the patient to his or her surroundings and to any therapeutic devices in use; teach activity restrictions and support the patient's understanding of cardiac rehabilitation principles.

### EVALUATION OF EXPECTED OUTCOMES

- Vital signs within normal limits
- Free of cardiorespiratory complications
- Dietary restrictions on sodium and cholesterol being followed
- Purposes of prescribed medications understood
- Knowledge of what myocardial infarction is and identification of risk factors
- Exercise rehabilitation plan being followed and activity limitations acknowledged
- Adjustments to health problem and any changes necessary in life-style being made

---

adverse effect on outcomes and usually are reserved for patients who cannot take beta-blockers. Diuretics may also be used if the patient has left ventricular failure. Patients need extensive education on the medications ordered, including the action, dosage, and side effects (Box 23-12).

Providing education and support for the patient and family and returning the patient to normal or near normal activities are some of the primary focuses of nursing interventions as the healing process occurs. As with the patient with angina, a patient who has had an MI commonly must make life-style changes to reduce or eliminate the risk factor for CAD (see Table 23-4).

Teaching the patient and family about the anatomy and physiology of CAD and MI, the healing process, risk factor reduction, activity progression and exercise, medications, and common emotions after MI are essential. In addition to these teaching topics, the nurse should be prepared to discuss the signs and symptoms of angina and congestive failure, use of nitroglycerin, and when to seek medical attention (see Patient/Family Teaching box: Angina, p. 673). Many great resources are available for teaching patients who have had an MI. Pointers for teaching are included in the Patient/Family Teaching box: Pointers for Teaching, p. 686.

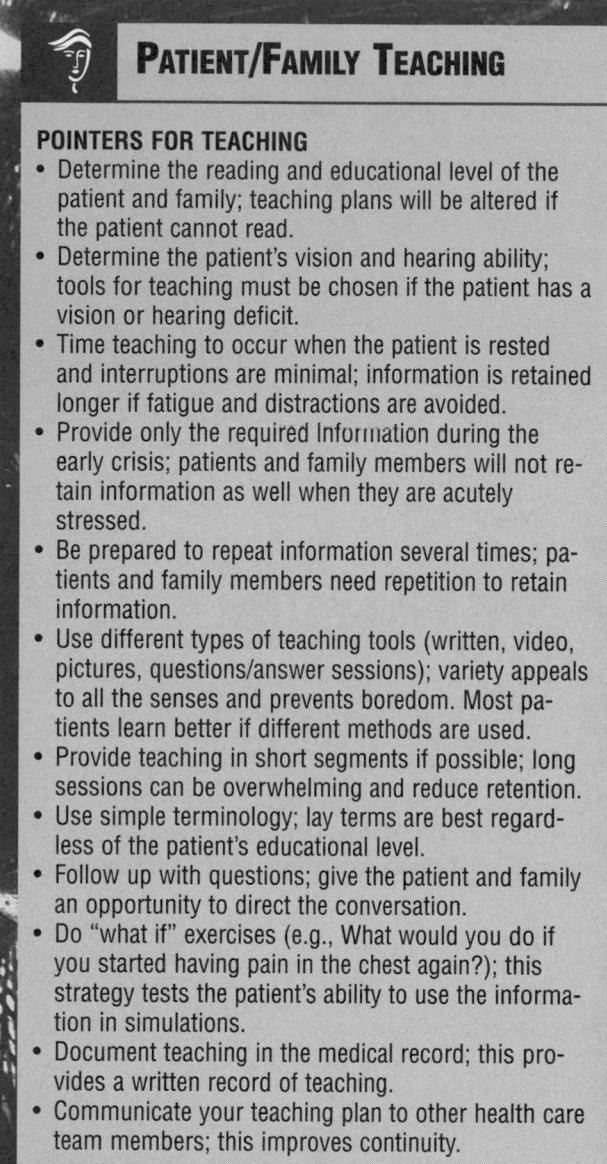

## PATIENT/FAMILY TEACHING

### POINTERS FOR TEACHING

- Determine the reading and educational level of the patient and family; teaching plans will be altered if the patient cannot read.
- Determine the patient's vision and hearing ability; tools for teaching must be chosen if the patient has a vision or hearing deficit.
- Time teaching to occur when the patient is rested and interruptions are minimal; information is retained longer if fatigue and distractions are avoided.
- Provide only the required information during the early crisis; patients and family members will not retain information as well when they are acutely stressed.
- Be prepared to repeat information several times; patients and family members need repetition to retain information.
- Use different types of teaching tools (written, video, pictures, questions/answer sessions); variety appeals to all the senses and prevents boredom. Most patients learn better if different methods are used.
- Provide teaching in short segments if possible; long sessions can be overwhelming and reduce retention.
- Use simple terminology; lay terms are best regardless of the patient's educational level.
- Follow up with questions; give the patient and family an opportunity to direct the conversation.
- Do "what if" exercises (e.g., What would you do if you started having pain in the chest again?); this strategy tests the patient's ability to use the information in simulations.
- Document teaching in the medical record; this provides a written record of teaching.
- Communicate your teaching plan to other health care team members; this improves continuity.

Activity and exercise progression is an important part of the long-term plan of care for a patient after an MI. In many situations the physician orders an exercise stress test during hospitalization to assess the response to exercise and obtain a heart rate goal for the exercise prescription. This is especially true of patients taking beta-blockers, who do not have the normal heart rate increase with exercise. The exercise heart rate may also be calculated by subtracting the patient's age from 220. Patients progress in their activity, as discussed earlier, throughout the hospital stay. Before discharge the patient must be instructed on the activity level to maintain at home, signs of overexertion, when he or she can return to work, usual daily activities, and sexual intercourse. Some guidelines for activity teach-

ing are included in the Patient/Family Teaching box: Acute Myocardial Infarction, p. 687.

Cardiac rehabilitation programs are structured inpatient and outpatient programs designed to help the patient return to optimum functioning through teaching, physical activity, counseling and support, risk factor modification, and use of community resources. These programs use a multidisciplinary approach that involves the services of dietitians, exercise physiologists, vocational rehabilitation counselors, physicians, nurses, and former patients. Cardiac rehabilitation programs have four phases, beginning with the arrival of the patient in the hospital and continuing in the discharge and recovery phase, sometimes for life. Phase 1 and phase 2, which are conducted while the patient is in the hospital, include teaching and activity progression appropriate for each individual and family. Phase 3 involves expanded exercise, teaching, counseling, and connection with community resources during the initial recovery after discharge. Exercise usually is conducted while the patient's ECG, blood pressure, and heart rate are monitored. Phase 4 is the long-term continuation of exercise conditioning and life-style modification.

Cardiac rehabilitation programs can provide support, guidance, and contact with people in similar situations to assist the patient in making the needed life-style changes and continuing them after full physiologic recovery occurs. Cardiac rehabilitation programs are also appropriate for patients with angina, cardiac surgery, and heart failure. It must be stressed that CAD is a chronic disease with no "cure." Lifelong changes are the only way to slow or alter the progression.

## SUDDEN CARDIAC DEATH

Sudden cardiac death is the term used to describe sudden collapse and cardiac arrest. People experiencing sudden cardiac death may have no symptoms before their collapse and may have no history of heart problems. Sudden cardiac death often is the first symptom of heart disease. If symptoms are present before collapse, they are short-lived, lasting less than 2 hours. The arrhythmia that most often causes sudden cardiac death is ventricular fibrillation (Cummins, 1994). The onset of this life-threatening arrhythmia in most cases is extensive CAD; however, MI does not always occur. Of the cases of sudden cardiac death, 75% occur in settings other than the hospital.

### Assessment

Patients with the greatest risk of sudden cardiac death are those who have risk factors for CAD and those who have had a previous MI. Patients with chest pain suggestive of angina or MI must be evaluated quickly

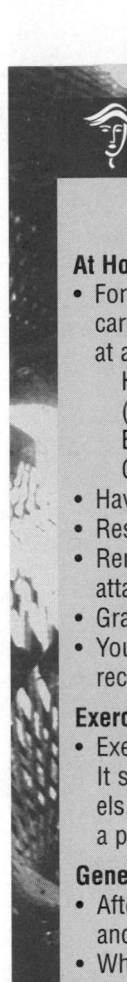

## PATIENT/FAMILY TEACHING

### ACUTE MYOCARDIAL INFARCTION

**At Hospital Discharge**
- For your first week at home, limit your activity to daily care (bathing, shaving, dressing, dining, and walking at a normal pace). Avoid the following:
    Heavy lifting or activities that might make you strain (limit lifting to 5 pounds)
    Extreme hot or cold temperatures
    Getting overtired or doing too much
- Have someone else drive you.
- Rest when you feel the need.
- Remember that it is normal to feel "weak" after a heart attack.
- Gradually add more activities to your daily schedule.
- You can return to work around _____ if your recovery goes smoothly.

**Exercise is Good for You**
- Exercise has many good effects on the heart and body. It strengthens the heart, can lower blood lipid (fat) levels, helps control weight, increases energy, and makes a person feel better.

**General Exercise Guidelines**
- After a heart attack, you need to increase your exercise and activity a little at a time.
- When you exercise, you should check your pulse and slow down if your rate goes above _____.
- Choose an exercise you will enjoy that is rhythmic and uses large muscles. Walking, swimming, and biking are some good choices.
- Do warm up and cool down exercises, such as stretches or slow walking, for 5 minutes before and after exercise. Do not stop or start exercise quickly.

- You should not exercise
    After a meal; wait 2 to 3 hours
    When you are tired
    In extreme cold or hot weather
- You should stop exercising if you have
    Shortness of breath (feeling mildly "winded" is normal with exercise)
    Chest pain
    Dizziness
- If you regularly experience chest pain with activity, your doctor may recommend using nitroglycerin before activity to prevent the pain.

**Sexual Activity**
- Sexual activity is another type of "exercise" or activity that should be resumed gradually.
- The same guidelines for other types of activity apply to intercourse.
- Foreplay is a great warm up exercise.
- Choose the position that is most comfortable for you and your partner.
- Avoid anal intercourse, which can stress the heart.
- Oral stimulation or self-stimulation does not put any added strain on the heart.
- A relaxed, familiar environment with a familiar partner reduces the stress of resuming sexual activity.
- Most people can resume sexual activity when they feel ready and can do moderate activity without chest pain or being short of breath (about two flights of stairs at a brisk pace). Ask your doctor if you are unsure.

and interventions implemented immediately to prevent arrhythmias and arrest. Unconsciousness, pulselessness, and respiratory arrest accompany sudden cardiac death.

## Intervention

Immediate interventions include starting cardiopulmonary resuscitation and calling for help. In the outpatient setting, 911 or the local emergency number should be called immediately upon finding a person who has collapsed. The initiation of defibrillation and advanced cardiac life support (ACLS) measures are the treatments of choice. In the hospital, getting the defibrillator to the bedside and immediate defibrillation of

ventricular fibrillation should be the focus of nursing intervention as cardiopulmonary resuscitation (CPR) is being performed. Defibrillation should not be delayed (Cummins, 1994) (see Box 23-7 and Figure 23-33).

### NURSE ALERT

**All nurses must know and be able to perform cardiopulmonary resuscitation.**

Patients who survive sudden cardiac death receive a complete workup for MI, as described earlier. Diagnostic studies include cardiac catheterization to evaluate the extent of CAD and to help in planning medical

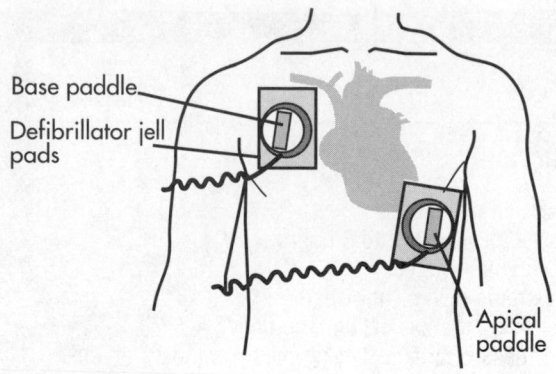

**Figure 23-33**  Placement of paddles in defibrillation.

or surgical intervention. Electrophysiologic studies may also be done to determine the likelihood that sudden cardiac death will reoccur and to evaluate the response to drug therapy. Management choices include pharmacologic agents, such as antiarrhythmic drugs, or insertion of an implantable cardiac defibrillator (ICD).

Nursing interventions should include appropriate teaching and emotional support for the individual patient and family. Sudden death can elicit numerous emotional responses, and the treatment options require major life-style changes. The nurse must be attuned to these needs and plan interventions to address them.

# INVASIVE THERAPEUTIC PROCEDURES AND CARDIAC SURGERY

Invasive interventions and surgery of the heart are some of the most significant accomplishments of medical science in the twentieth century. These procedures saves lives and provide patients with a higher quality of life, free of crippling cardiac conditions. They also require a vast array of equipment and a staff of highly trained, efficient professionals. In no other aspect of medical-surgical care is the team concept of greater importance than in procedures involving the heart. Judgment, technical competence, and skill in observation are demanded of the nurse, and an ability to understand the feelings and emotional responses of the patient is equally important.

The nurse's responsibility begins with diagnosis, continues long after the procedure has been completed, and ends only when convalescence and rehabilitation have returned the patient to his or her optimum condition. Because these interventions must be performed in medical centers with cardiac surgery capability, many patients are away from home and their usual support system. They are in an unfamiliar environment and may be fearful of what is happening to them. The warm, friendly attitude of the nurse contributes to the patient's feeling of security and may lead the patient to talk about his or her fears, anxiety, and other related problems. It is essential that the nurse maintain the focus on the patient and family, even when highly technical procedures with many complications and risks are being performed.

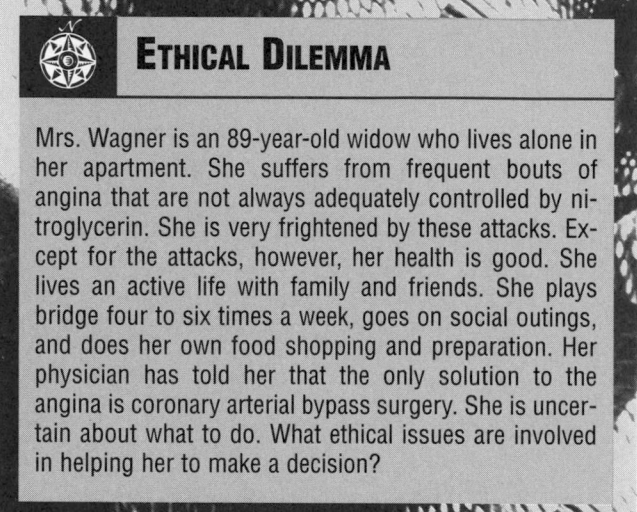

### ETHICAL DILEMMA

Mrs. Wagner is an 89-year-old widow who lives alone in her apartment. She suffers from frequent bouts of angina that are not always adequately controlled by nitroglycerin. She is very frightened by these attacks. Except for the attacks, however, her health is good. She lives an active life with family and friends. She plays bridge four to six times a week, goes on social outings, and does her own food shopping and preparation. Her physician has told her that the only solution to the angina is coronary arterial bypass surgery. She is uncertain about what to do. What ethical issues are involved in helping her to make a decision?

Cardiac surgery may be performed to correct congenital or acquired conditions. It may be performed inside the heart (open heart surgery), or it may be done to relieve or correct some condition outside the heart (closed heart surgery). It may involve the valves of the heart, the heart muscle or its covering, or the great blood vessels of the body. Surgical removal of a patient's diseased heart and replacement with a normal heart (heart transplant) has become fairly routine in some large medical centers. Surgery also is used to treat coronary artery disease, and the coronary artery bypass graft is one of the most commonly performed heart operations in the United States.

The treatment of CAD, angina, and MI may include several types of invasive procedures, cardiac surgery, or a combination of techniques. The option used varies, depending on the patient's overall condition, preexisting chronic diseases, and response to medical therapy and the results of diagnostic studies. The extent of the CAD (the number of vessels involved) and the location and complexity of the atherosclerotic plaque also play a role in the treatment decision. Several treatment options are available, including *percutaneous transluminal coronary angioplasty (PTCA), stent*

*placement, atherectomy,* and *coronary artery bypass grafting (CABG).* Each procedure has indications, advantages and disadvantages, complications and specific
nursing and medical care before and after the procedure. This section provides an overview of the more
common procedures.

## Percutaneous Transluminal Coronary Angioplasty

Percutaneous transluminal coronary **angioplasty**
(PTCA) involves placing a double-lumen, balloon-
tipped catheter into the diseased coronary artery.
When the catheter tip is placed through the lesion, the
balloon is inflated to compress the plaque and dilate
the stenosed area (Figure 23-34). The procedure is performed, using local anesthesia, in the cardiac catheterization laboratory. The catheter usually is inserted
through the femoral vein, but the brachial approach
also can be used.

PTCA is indicated in patients who have plaques that
can be treated with this approach because of the size,
shape, and position of the plaques in the coronary
artery (Pagana, Pagana, 1996). Improved equipment
and techniques have made PTCA easier to do with distal, narrow plaques. PTCA provides an alternative to
bypass surgery, which carries greater risk. With PTCA
the patient is able to be ambulatory in 1 day, has a
shorter hospital stay, can return to work and normal
activity sooner, and does not have to endure an open
procedure and general anesthesia. Shorter stays and
rapid recovery make PTCA a very cost-effective procedure. The major disadvantage is that in 30% of patients, restenosis occurs in the first 6 months (Urban
et al, 1995).

The most serious complication of PTCA is rupture of
the coronary artery during the procedure. If the plaque
is pushed up into the coronary artery instead of being
compressed against the sides, the artery can be severed.
This can cause blood to build up in the pericardial sac,
resulting in cardiac tamponade. Reduced cardiac output and death can occur, and the patient requires immediate bypass surgery. Another complication can occur if a piece of the plaque breaks off and becomes
lodged farther down in the coronary artery. Tissue ischemia and death can result. Other complications possible in the first 24 hours after the procedure are spasm
of the artery and occlusion. Because dye is used in the
procedure, dye-related complications are the same as
those discussed with cardiac catheterization.

Nursing care of patients undergoing angioplasty is
similar to that for a patient undergoing cardiac catheterization. The patient and family need to be taught
about the angioplasty procedure to ease anxiety and to
establish trust and cooperation. The patient must be

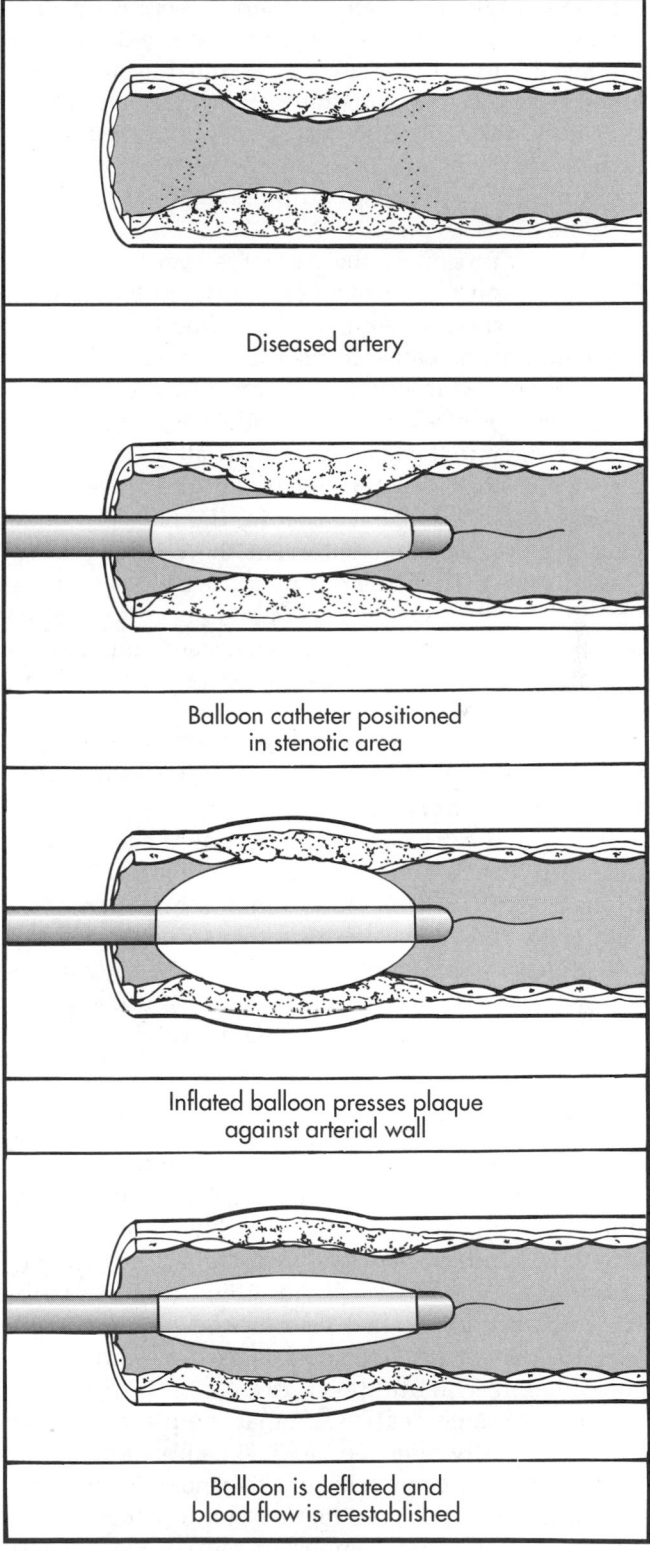

Diseased artery

Balloon catheter positioned
in stenotic area

Inflated balloon presses plaque
against arterial wall

Balloon is deflated and
blood flow is reestablished

**Figure 23-34**   Coronary angioplasty procedure. (From Canobbio M:
*Cardiovascular disorders,* St Louis, 1990, Mosby.)

informed of the risks, and written consent is obtained for bypass surgery in the event it is needed. Identifying sensitivity to dye, as well as renal system problems, is an essential nursing intervention. During the procedure the nurse instructs the patient to report sensations of chest pain. The nurse also continuously monitors the patient's blood pressure, heart rate, and rhythm.

After the procedure the patient is transferred to the CCU or a unit that ensures close monitoring. The patient is watched for excessive bleeding or hematoma formation at the catheter insertion site, chest pain, or arrhythmias, which could indicate that the newly dilated artery is closing. The "sheath" used to introduce the catheter into the femoral vein usually is left in place for several hours after completion of the procedure. It is left in place to make it easier for the physician to repeat the procedure in the event the coronary artery starts to close. The patient is instructed to keep the extremity straight and still for several hours after the procedure is over and the sheath has been removed. The patient normally can ambulate 6 hours after the sheath is removed. The patient can drink immediately after the procedure and should be encouraged to do so to help clear the dye from the body. Eating is resumed after the sheath has been removed.

Patient education after the procedure should focus on modifying risk factors by making needed life-style changes. Restenosis is more common in patients who do not modify their risk factors, especially smokers and those with high blood levels of cholesterol. The hospital stay usually is 3 days or less, and the patient usually can return to work in about 1 week.

## Atherectomy

Coronary atherectomy is another technique for treating the plaques associated with CAD. In this procedure a special catheter with a rotating blade is placed into the occluded artery, and the plaque is cut away by rotations of the blade (Perra, 1995) (Figure 23-35). Atherectomy, also called *percutaneous directional coronary arthrectomy (PTDA)*, often is used instead of or in combination with traditional PTCA.

The advantage of PTDA is that the plaque is completely or partly removed, not just compressed, which reduces the risk of reocclusion. The major limitation is that atherectomy is possible only with plaques in the proximal or middle sections of the coronary artery. Complications and nursing care for atherectomy are similar to those for PTCA.

Another variation of this procedure, called *percutaneous transluminal extraction arthrectomy (PTEA)*, uses a special catheter that cuts away and removes pieces of the plaque. *Percutaneous transluminal rotational coronary*

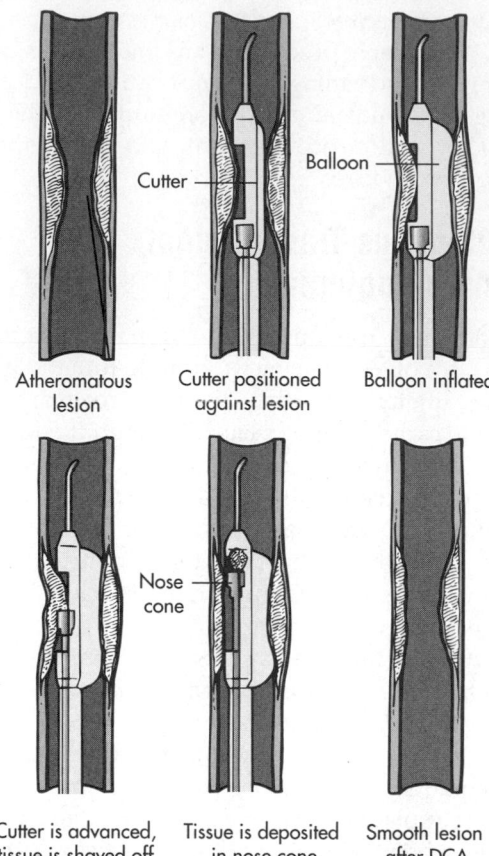

Cutter | Balloon

Atheromatous lesion | Cutter positioned against lesion | Balloon inflated

Nose cone

Cutter is advanced, tissue is shaved off | Tissue is deposited in nose cone | Smooth lesion after DCA

**Figure 23-35** Directional coronary atherectomy (DCA). (From *Heart Dis Stroke* 2:201, 1993, American Heart Association.)

*ablation (PTRCA)* uses a catheter to sand the plaque into fine particles that are absorbed through normal blood processes. Lasers also are used for angioplasty. In laser angioplasty a catheter with a laser on the tip is placed into the coronary artery, and the laser is used to remove the plaque. Lasers are not widely used in all areas, and continued experimentation is needed to refine the procedure.

## Stents

Endovascular stents are small, stainless steel, meshlike tubes placed within the occluded vessel that are expanded over the area of the plaque to hold the vessel open (Figure 23-36). The stent is placed during coronary angioplasty, and the balloon catheter is used to compress the plaque and open the stent. When the catheter is removed, the stent stays in place to support the artery and prevent collapse (Gardner et al, 1996).

The major advantage of the stent is the support it provides to the area of the coronary artery that has undergone angioplasty. This support prevents abrupt closure of the artery. The major disadvantage of stents

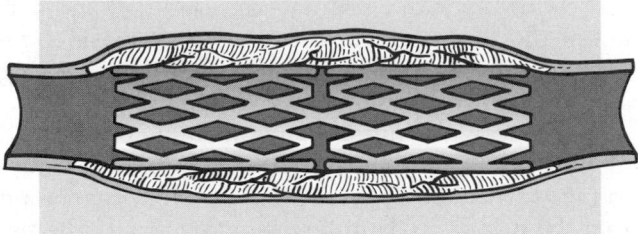

**Figure 23-36**    Endovascular stent. (From *Heart Dis Stroke* 2:199, 1993, American Heart Association.)

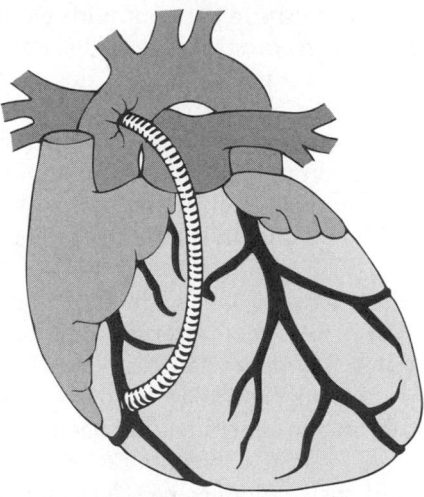

**Figure 23-37**    Aortocoronary artery saphenous vein bypass graft. (From Kinney MR et al: *AACN's clinical reference for critical care nursing,* St Louis, 1993, Mosby.)

is that they are a foreign body and can cause thrombi to form in the coronary artery. Patients must take anticoagulants for at least 3 months after the procedure (Gardner et al, 1996).

The complications of stent placement are bleeding, injury to the vessel, thrombosis of the stent, and coronary artery spasm above or below the stent. If thrombosis or spasm occurs, the patient may suffer a MI. Bypass surgery or stent embolectomy may be required to reopen the coronary artery.

Nursing care of the patient with a stent includes those interventions used for PTCA, in addition to monitoring for signs of stent thrombosis and bleeding. The patient must be educated about the anticoagulant drugs and signs of bleeding. The patient is followed closely after the procedure to monitor PT levels and adjust the anticoagulant dosage.

## Coronary Artery Bypass Graft

A coronary artery bypass graft (CABG) is a surgical procedure performed to create new pathways in the coronary arteries of the heart to "bypass" the blockage caused by CAD. The surgery provides blood flow around the blocked artery to increase the blood and oxygen supply to the heart muscle past the area of stenosis and plaque.

There are two ways to provide new pathways (grafts). In one version, a saphenous vein is removed from the patient's leg and sutured in place to form the bypass. When the vein is removed, it is reversed so that the valves in the vein do not prevent blood flow. One end of the vein is secured in place in the aorta above the junction of the coronary arteries. The other end is connected to the coronary artery beyond the diseased area (Figure 23-37). This method of creating the bypass requires an additional surgical site (the leg). In another version of CABG, either the left or right internal mammary artery (IMA) is used to make the bypass. In this technique the IMA remains attached to its artery of origin (the subclavian artery) at one end, and the other end (disconnected from the chest wall) is at-

tached to the coronary artery past the blockage. These techniques can be used alone or they can be combined to provide bypass for several blocked coronary arteries (triple, quadruple, or more bypasses).

To get to the surface of the heart, CABG most commonly is done using an open chest approach. The sternum is cut down the middle (median sternotomy), and the ribs are spread open to expose the pericardium. Patients often complain of pain in the shoulders, back, and ribs because of this part of the procedure.

Open chest CABG is performed with the use of a complex and highly specialized heart-lung machine, a process called a cardiopulmonary bypass (CPB). Cardiopulmonary bypass is accomplished by using a special machine that diverts the blood from a point before the heart (the right atrium or superior vena cava) past the heart and returns it to the ascending aorta. While the blood is diverted, the machine provides the gas exchange of oxygen and carbon dioxide that normally occurs in the lungs and lowers the temperature of the blood to slow the metabolic processes. The CPB also propels the blood through the circulatory system, filters the blood, and provides a route for delivery of anesthesia.

The heart is stopped during CABG, using a very cold, special electrolyte solution called "cardioplegia," which is infused into the coronary arteries. The asystole that results provides a motionless field for surgery. The combination of CPB, hypothermia, and cardiac arrest allows the surgeon to perform the CABG and reduces some of the complications of the procedure (Urban et al, 1995). However, use of the CPB and the surgery put the patient at risk for numerous complications. Prevention of these complications directs nursing interventions in the first 24 hours after surgery.

CABG is indicated for patients with extensive disease in the left main coronary artery, disease in three or more vessels, disease in two vessels, angina that is not responsive to medical treatment, or hemodynamic compromise after MI or persistent angina (Urban et al, 1995). The decision to perform CABG depends on the findings of diagnostic studies, the patient's coexisting medical problems, and the patient's and physician's preferences.

Major advantages of CABG include longer artery patency than with other interventions (IMA grafts maintain patency longer than saphenous grafts) and better long-term survival than with medical therapy. Major disadvantages include the need to open the chest, with all associated postoperative complications and increased costs, a longer recovery time than with other interventions, and the continuing possibility that the disease will progress and the grafts occlude. CABG does not "cure" the process of atherosclerosis, which is the primary cause of coronary artery disease. Life-style changes to reduce the risk factors that created the CAD must be made to prevent progression of the atherosclerosis and reocclusion of the grafts.

The complications of CABG are similar to those of any surgery of the chest and surgery of the vascular system. Box 23-13 presents an overview of the nursing process for a patient undergoing cardiac surgery.

The care of a patient undergoing CABG is divided into four phases (Urban et al, 1995). The preoperative phase includes cardiac catheterization and other diagnostic studies, which may be done on an outpatient basis, and the immediate preoperative period. The intensive phase includes the day of surgery and the 24-hour period after surgery. The intermediate phase lasts 3 to 5 days and incorporates the transition to discharge. The cardiac rehabilitation phase begins while the patient is in the hospital and continues for several months.

## Preoperative Care

The patient is admitted to the hospital either the day before or the day of surgery or may already have been admitted on an emergency basis after a myocardial infarction. In any event, the patient often is very apprehensive. Before elective surgery, the patient receives detailed examinations, including the laboratory studies and special tests outlined earlier in this chapter. The physician plans for a conference with the patient and family to give them information about the surgery. The nurse should participate in the conference so that information can be repeated and reinforced at a later time.

Before surgery the patient's weight and vital signs are recorded to establish a normal baseline. The patient continues with a sodium-restricted diet and current medication regimen. Unless a reason exists to restrict activity, the patient should be up and walking about to maintain strength and muscle tone.

The surgeon and nurse review with the patient and family the details of the postoperative care, the monitoring that will be done, and the plan for progression from the ICU or CCU to the step-down unit. The patient should be taught how to breathe deeply and cough and how to use a machine to measure the depth of inspiration (an incentive spirometer). He or she should practice this procedure under supervision, because these activities will be essential in preventing respiratory problems after surgery. The patient should be informed that chest tubes, nasogastric tubes, an endotracheal tube (breathing tube), a urinary catheter, hemodynamic monitoring lines, and intravenous lines may be used. The patient also should be assured that vital signs will be monitored frequently and that pain medication will be available. The family should be prepared for the patient's appearance after surgery.

The physical preparation is similar to that for most surgical patients. The skin preparation usually covers a wide area from chin to ankles. A sedative for sleep and rest is recommended the evening before surgery, with fluids and solid foods restricted after midnight. Although the fear is not always verbalized, the patient may expect to die and may have made necessary material preparation. On the day of surgery members of the family and a religious counselor should be permitted to visit the patient.

## Intensive Phase

The first 24 hours after heart surgery are the most critical for the patient. The patient is transferred to an ICU for close assessment and for sophisticated hemodynamic monitoring. Hemodynamic values are very closely monitored. Supporting the patient's recovery from anesthesia and the trauma of CPB and dealing with the autonomic, immune, and stress responses of the body guide the monitoring and nursing interventions.

For the first few hours after surgery, the patient may be given controlled or assisted ventilation and oxygen. This diminishes the possibility of hypoxia and arrhythmias. The nurse must assess the pulmonary system frequently to identify oxygenation or ventilation problems during and after the use of mechanical ventilation.

The potential for volume disorders and coagulopathies is great because of the nature of the surgical insult and the contact the systemic blood has had with the CPB machine (Urban et al, 1995). Close evaluation

BOX 23-13

# NURSING PROCESS

## CARDIAC SURGERY

### ASSESSMENT
#### Preoperative

- Activity tolerance
- Discomfort/chest pain
- Knowledge of procedure and therapeutic plan
- Mental status
- Plans for postdischarge care, including diet and exercise

#### Postoperative

- Cardiac rate, rhythm, and hemodynamic values (early postoperative phase)
- Respiratory rate, volume, adventitious sounds, arterial gas levels
- Fluid volume and electrolyte status (intake output/third spacing)
- Core temperature
- Pain
- Surgical wound drainage
- Activity tolerance
- Level of consciousness, disorientation, and motor/sensory deficits

### NURSING DIAGNOSES

- Ineffective breathing pattern related to discomfort and musculoskeletal impairment related to chest surgery
- Pain related to surgical intervention
- Anxiety related to inability to control illness
- Impaired physical mobility related to discomfort and activity intolerance
- Self-care deficit related to discomfort and activity intolerance
- Fear of death related to knowledge of and perception about condition
- Risk for decreased cardiac output associated with decreased cardiac function
- Risk for altered tissue perfusion related to interruption of arterial blood flow
- Risk for impaired gas exchange associated with possible decrease in cardiac function
- Risk for fluid volume deficit or excess related to altered cardiac function

### NURSING INTERVENTIONS
#### Preoperative phase

- Explain laboratory tests to the patient.
- Monitor apical-radial pulses and blood pressure.
- Weigh the patient daily.
- Continue sodium-restricted diet, diuretics, and digitalis preparations as prescribed.
- Provide activity as tolerated.
- Teach deep-breathing and coughing exercises.
- Explain postoperative care and equipment to the patient.
- Provide emotional support and anticipate the patient's needs.
- Observe for signs and symptoms of cardiorespiratory complications.

#### Immediate postoperative phase

- Check vital signs every 15 minutes until they are stable and then hourly for 24 hours.
- Observe for cardiac arrhythmia.
- Monitor pressures within the heart.
- Report any temperature elevation above 39° C (102° F).
- Administer oxygen and assisted ventilation as ordered.
- Assist patient to cough and breathe deeply every hour.
- Maintain patency of closed chest drainage; observe for excessive drainage.
- Administer intravenous infusions as ordered.
- Maintain the patency of nasogastric tube; give good oral and nasal hygiene.
- Observe for signs of electrolyte imbalance and fluid retention.
- Encourage progressive activity as tolerated and ordered.
- Maintain the patency of the indwelling urethral catheter.
- Measure and record hourly urine output; report if it is less than 30 ml/hour.
- Check and record the specific gravity of the urine every hour.
- Administer pain medication as needed.

*Continued*

| BOX 23-13 | NURSING PROCESS |

## CARDIAC SURGERY—cont'd

- Observe for complications (shock, hemorrhage, pneumothorax, pulmonary edema, cyanosis, and congestive heart failure).
- Check dressings often for amount and type of drainage.
- Observe for disorientation or psychosis.
- Provide frequent rest periods.

**EVALUATION OF EXPECTED OUTCOMES**

- Vital signs within normal ranges
- Deep breathe and cough exercise performed every hour
- Normal fluid and electrolyte balance achieved
- Relief from pain obtained
- Proper rest and sleep obtained
- Postoperative or cardiorespiratory complications absent

of laboratory values, monitoring of all sites for bleeding, and accurate intake and output measurements are important. The stress response can cause an increase in the blood glucose level and may require administration of insulin. Mild systolic hypertension (mean arterial pressure over 95 mm Hg) associated with increased plasma renin and catecholamine levels is not uncommon. Hypovolemia may occur as a result of the bypass procedure itself or as a result of the diuretics given when the procedure is finished.

The myocardium may be irritable, and the potential for arrhythmias is great. Epicardial pacemaker wires permit simple and immediate treatment of bradycardias and heart block, and medication can be used to control atrial fibrillation and ventricular ectopy when indicated. Chest catheters may be used to provide closed drainage for the mediastinum. They are attached to a water-sealed drainage system and must be kept free of clots and kinks. The drainage should be observed for excessive amounts of blood. The amount of drainage in 24 hours depends on the type of surgery and may vary from 400 to 1200 ml in some patients. Absence of drainage must be reported promptly, because fluid may be accumulating in the chest cavity, which results in serious cardiac complication. When turning and positioning the patient, the nurse must prevent disconnection or displacement of the chest catheters.

Antibiotics are given routinely to all patients to prevent infection. X-ray examinations of the chest and ECG studies usually are done within the first 24 hours after surgery. Dressings should be checked often for evidence of any unusual bleeding. Any numbness, tingling, pain, or loss of motion in the extremities should be reported. Assessments for shock, hemorrhage, pneumothorax, pulmonary edema, and congestive heart failure are made at regular intervals.

Providing emotional support for the patient and family after surgery is a crucial nursing intervention. The possibility of death, the many monitoring lines

and machines, the intensive evaluation, and restricted visitation policies of many intensive care areas all combine to create anxiety and crisis in many patients and families. Family dynamics may be strained, and individual role functions may be altered. Assisting the patient and family with coping during the crisis can facilitate recovery. Providing information and frequent updates on the patient's condition, reassuring the patient and family that the things they see, feel, and hear are normal parts of the postoperative phase, and adjusting the plan of care according to the needs of the family and patient are common nursing interventions. Disorientation is common after heart surgery, but it should always be noted and reported.

### Intermediate Phase

When the patient's condition has stabilized, he or she can be transferred to an intermediate care unit, where care continues and the patient is progressed toward discharge. Hemodynamic monitoring lines are removed, the breathing tube (endotracheal tube) is removed (extubation), and the chest tubes and pacemaker wire are removed.

Although the patient's condition is stable, the nurse should continue to assess the vital signs, conduct physical examinations of all body systems, and monitor fluid volume status for any evidence of abnormality. The apical-radial pulse, blood pressure, and respiration are checked and recorded at frequent intervals ranging from 2 to 4 hours. The rhythm, rate, and strength of the pulse should be observed, and the nurse should constantly observe for arrhythmias. The physician should indicate the lowest level of systolic pressure that the patient can tolerate without harmful effects. After surgery involving the coronary arteries, systolic pressure must be watched closely. The incision sites should be assessed for signs of infections. Any elevation of temperature above 39° C (102° F) should be reported because temperature elevation increases the work of the heart and can indicate infection.

Oxygen administration may continue for several days after mechanical ventilation is stopped. Patients may suffer enough discomfort in the surgical sites to prohibit full respiratory excursion. They are encouraged to cough and breathe deeply and to use the incentive spirometer every 1 to 2 hours while awake. Movement of the patient and early mobility also facilitate improved ventilation and prevent venous stasis. Deep breathing and coughing assists in bringing up secretions to maintain a clear airway, but pain is a factor in persuading the patient to comply with this therapy. The nurse should assist the patient by supporting the chest and upper abdomen with a pillow and should give the patient pain medication approximately 30 minutes before pulmonary interventions are performed.

Most patients are allowed fluids by mouth as soon as nausea and vomiting have ceased and the breathing tube has been removed. Intravenous infusions may be maintained for several hours. Occasionally fluid intake is restricted, and an accurate measurement of intake and output must be maintained. A sodium-restricted diet usually is given to the patient as tolerated. Potassium replacement may occasionally be needed. Blood samples are taken on alternating days to monitor serum electrolyte values.

Activity increases as the patient's recovery permits. Patients usually sit in a chair 24 hours after surgery and ambulate short distances 24 to 32 hours after surgery. The patient then begins a prescribed exercise program.

Patients report the most pain during the first 48 hours because of rib retraction during surgery. Meperidine or morphine sulfate may be required for pain relief. However, some patients may require only oral analgesics. It is important for the nurse to assess each patient's pain, requirements for analgesic, and response to medications on an individual basis.

It is not uncommon after a major operation for patients to have a feeling of "let down." Patients often describe it as mild depression. It is important for the nurse to reassure the patient that this is normal and will pass. These patients may also be very emotional about their condition and their survival of the surgery. This show of emotion may be disturbing to the family, and it should be reinforced as normal.

### Cardiac Rehabilitation and Discharge Planning Phase

Patients are leaving the hospital after CABG surgery earlier than ever. It is not unusual for patients who are young and otherwise healthy to be discharged from the hospital as early as postoperative day 5. The length of stay and progression through the stages depends on the patient's overall health before surgery and preexisting chronic diseases.

Because of the decreasing length of stay, it is essential that nurses begin the process of planning for discharge immediately, in some cases even before the day of surgery. Structured cardiac rehabilitation programs with an aggressive inpatient component, care maps or critical paths for postoperative care, and a multidisciplinary approach to all the phases of cardiac surgery are some of the strategies used to progress the patient toward recovery with minimal complications and delays.

Cardiac rehabilitation begins as soon as the patient is stable and includes teaching, activity progression, and risk factor modification. Assessment of the patient's learning abilities and motivation to make needed life-style changes is important in planning for this phase of the recovery.

Patients and families need to know the signs and symptoms that should be reported to the physician. Some of these signs and symptoms are redness or drainage at the incision, decreasing activity tolerance, swelling of the feet, hands, or face, shortness of breath, chest pain, or palpitations. The patient and family should be given a review of follow-up appointments and the plan for outpatient cardiac rehabilitation. They also should be able to perform incision care, as well as respiratory care that may be needed to promote continued recovery.

Other topics that need to be covered are ambulation and activity progression, dietary requirements to help with healing, and life-style modifications specific for the patient. The family needs to be actively involved in this teaching, as well as the day-to-day care of the patient, because they will be the primary caregivers after discharge.

## Minimally Invasive Direct Coronary Artery Bypass (MIDCAB)

The recent introduction of *minimally invasive direct coronary artery bypass (MIDCAB)* has provided a procedure that does not use an open chest approach or CPB. The MIDCAB uses an anterolateral incision just below the nipple to allow access to the chest cavity for bypass of the blocked coronary arteries. Special surgical tools are used to "harvest," or remove, the vessel to be used for the bypass, stabilize the diseased coronary artery for sewing, and complete the bypass procedure (Cardio Thoracic Systems, 1996). The IMA is most often used as the graft vessel in this approach so that only one anastomosis is needed. The heart is not brought to complete cardiac arrest; rather, it is slowed so that grafts can be sewn to the coronary arteries. Although general anesthesia is still used, CPB is not needed. The MIDCAB is still a very new procedure and is not widely available.

Many of the patients currently undergoing this technique are young and healthy, but the MIDCAB is designed for patients requiring CABG surgery who are not good candidates for the traditional approach or who have blockages that can easily be bypassed using this less invasive approach (Cardio Thoracic Systems, 1996).

The major advantages of the MIDCAB are the facts that the chest and sternum are not opened, CPB is not needed, and the heart is not stopped (Cardio Thoracic Systems, 1996). These differences from the traditional approach for CABG result in fewer complications from surgery, CPB use, and trauma to the heart, shorter anesthesia and intubation time, shorter stays in the cardiac recovery area and hospital, reduced need for blood transfusion, and decreased costs. Disadvantages of MIDCAB are that not all bypasses can be done by this approach (anterior vessels are most accessible), and during the procedure complications can require that the chest be opened and the bypass completed by the traditional method.

Complications of MIDCAB are similar to those for CABG with the exception of CPB complications. Some of the more common complications are acute MI, pericarditis, atrial fibrillation, bleeding, pleural effusion, and wound infection (Cardio Thoracic Systems, 1996).

Postprocedural nursing care focuses on early recognition and management of possible complications, activity progression, and preparing the patient for lifestyle changes to reduce risk factors of CAD. In contrast to CABG surgery, after the MIDCAB the mechanical ventilator usually can be stopped and the endotracheal tube removed in the operating room. Oxygen is administered. The patient usually requires only basic hemodynamic monitoring, such as an arterial line to monitor blood pressure and a CVP line for fluid volume status; pacemaker wires are not used. Tubes and drains are minimal and include a chest tube, which usually is removed early in the postoperative recovery. Urine drainage (Foley catheter) is used only in the operating room. Activity begins at the bedside 2 to 3 hours after surgery, with dangling and progresses to being out of bed in a chair as early as 3 to 4 hours after surgery. Ambulation three times a day begins on postoperative day 1, and discharge to home can occur on postoperative day 2. Extensive wound care is not needed because of the small incision (Cardio Thoracic Systems, 1996).

Nursing interventions consist of the usual postoperative care, such as prevention of respiratory complications and pain control. Deep breathing, coughing, and incentive spirometry are done every 1 to 2 hours while awake, and the patient is mobilized early. Incisional pain can be controlled by use of intercostal nerve blocks, an epidural performed by the anesthesiologist during surgery; nerve blocks make the patient more comfortable, and he or she requires less IV pain medication (Cardio Thoracic Systems, 1996). The ECG is monitored continuously, as are vital signs and fluid volume status. Patient teaching and cardiac rehabilitation are the same as for a patient undergoing CABG but must be started and completed earlier because of the more rapid recovery after MIDCAB.

# CONGESTIVE HEART FAILURE

**Congestive heart failure** (CHF) occurs when the cardiac output can no longer meet the needs of the body tissues. CHF is not itself a disease; rather, it is the result of many underlying problems. CHF is a complication of almost all types of heart disease and can be caused by conditions that reduce the heart's ability to pump blood (e.g., arrhythmias and hypervolemia) or those that increase the demand on the heart (e.g., fever and anemia) (Box 23-14).

CHF can be either an acute or a chronic process, depending on the underlying cause and the rate at which the problem develops. Myocardial infarction is the most common cardiac cause of acute congestive heart failure, whereas ischemic heart disease is the most common cause of chronic heart failure.

CHF can be the result of problems with the heart's ability to pump blood out (systolic failure) or problems with the heart's ability to relax and fill with blood (diastolic failure). It also may affect either the right or the left side of the heart or both.

Heart failure is a significant medical problem. Patients with chronic heart failure have high mortality and morbidity, decreased quality of life, and frequent hospital admissions. CHF has become the most frequent and costly hospital discharge diagnosis for patients over the age of 65. Many readmissions are due to patients' lack of understanding failure to follow the treatment regimen. It is important for the nurse to be well prepared to address the needs of patients with acute and chronic CHF.

## Pathophysiology

When the heart fails to pump enough blood to meet the needs of the body, all body organs and tissues are affected. Two types of pumping problems can cause heart failure, systolic failure and diastolic failure.

*Systolic failure*, the more common type of CHF, occurs when the heart muscle is unable to pump forcefully enough to push the blood volume out into the aorta. As a result the cardiac output falls, and the blood that does not go forward and out of the heart puts increased pressure on the ventricular walls and the structures behind the left ventricle. The pulmonary

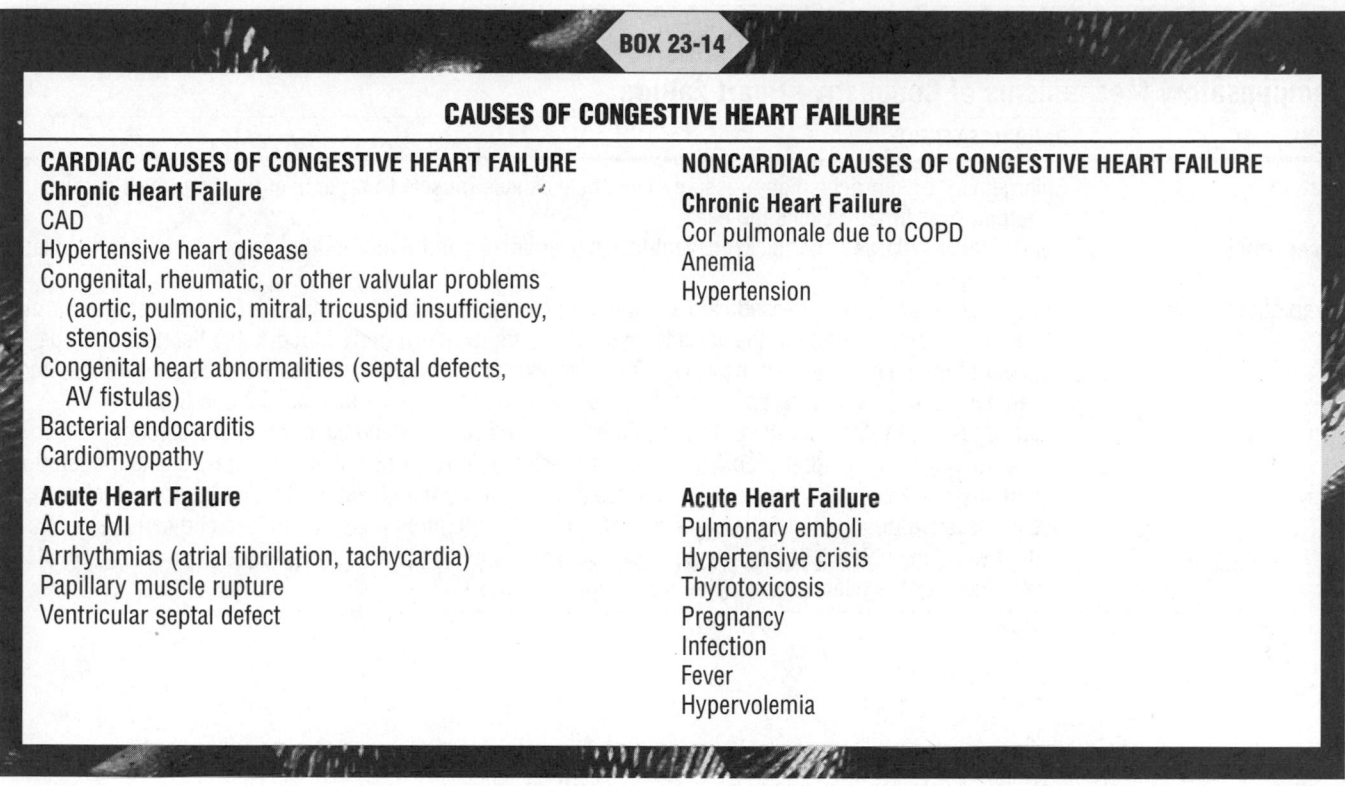

**BOX 23-14**

## CAUSES OF CONGESTIVE HEART FAILURE

| CARDIAC CAUSES OF CONGESTIVE HEART FAILURE | NONCARDIAC CAUSES OF CONGESTIVE HEART FAILURE |
|---|---|
| **Chronic Heart Failure** | **Chronic Heart Failure** |
| CAD | Cor pulmonale due to COPD |
| Hypertensive heart disease | Anemia |
| Congenital, rheumatic, or other valvular problems | Hypertension |
|    (aortic, pulmonic, mitral, tricuspid insufficiency, | |
|    stenosis) | |
| Congenital heart abnormalities (septal defects, | |
|    AV fistulas) | |
| Bacterial endocarditis | |
| Cardiomyopathy | |
| | |
| **Acute Heart Failure** | **Acute Heart Failure** |
| Acute MI | Pulmonary emboli |
| Arrhythmias (atrial fibrillation, tachycardia) | Hypertensive crisis |
| Papillary muscle rupture | Thyrotoxicosis |
| Ventricular septal defect | Pregnancy |
| | Infection |
| | Fever |
| | Hypervolemia |

vascular system becomes congested because it is no longer emptied sufficiently by the left atrium and ventricle. Fluid can leak out of the vessels surrounding the alveoli (air sacs) in the lungs, causing pulmonary edema. As the pressure in the heart chambers increases, the blood begins to back up in the atria and the large veins. Blood returning to the heart cannot be pumped rapidly enough into the congested pulmonary vessels, and the venous system becomes engorged. As the pressure in the venous system rises, other organs of the body, such as the liver, become congested. Because of the increased venous pressure and stasis, fluid is pushed out of the capillaries and venules. The decreased cardiac output also results in a diminished flow of blood to the kidneys, reducing their filtering ability. With reduced renal blood flow, sodium and water are retained in the body, contributing to generalized edema (Beattie, Carrie, 1996).

Systolic failure can be caused by several conditions, including (1) high preload (hypervolemia), which overwhelms the heart's ability to pump; (2) high afterload (hypertension), which restricts the heart's ability to pump blood by causing resistance to the forward flow; and (3) low contractility of the heart muscle (myocardial infarction or ischemia), which reduces the heart muscle's pumping force (Urban et al, 1995). Many times heart failure is the result of a combination of these problems.

In *diastolic failure* the underlying problem is the heart's inability to relax or stretch to let blood come in during the filling phase. In this type of CHF, the heart muscle is stiff or hypertrophied and unable to accept the normal amount of blood. As a result, the heart must work harder to provide the cardiac output needed by the body tissues. The pressures in the heart increase, and pulmonary and venous congestion occur, as in systolic failure. Diastolic failure can be the end result of long-term hypertension, aortic stenosis, and cardiomyopathy that damage the heart muscle and cause hypertrophy of the tissues (Beattie, Carrie, 1996).

The signs and symptoms of CHF depend on whether the process develops acutely or over time. When CHF occurs as a result of a chronic process, the body has time to begin compensating. The compensatory mechanisms help the heart maintain cardiac output so that all body tissues receive the blood supply they need. Dilation, hypertrophy, sympathetic stimulation, and renal changes are the major compensatory mechanisms that occur in CHF (Urban et al, 1995). These mechanisms can have a positive effect on the heart or can worsen the failure. Many of the signs and symptoms and treatment strategies are a result of the compensatory mechanisms (Table 23-15).

The many manifestations of heart failure are related to which ventricle is in failure. Failure of both the right

| TABLE 23-15 |
| --- |

## Compensatory Mechanisms of Congestive Heart Failure

| MECHANISM | RATIONALE/EFFECT |
| --- | --- |
| Dilation | Enlargement of ventricle; high pressure in ventricle causes muscle to stretch; at first improves cardiac output, over time weakens the heart. |
| Hypertrophy | Heart muscle enlarges and thickens; ventricle is overworked and under strain; increases the heart's need for oxygen. |
| Sympathetic stimulation | Occurs in response to decreased cardiac output; heart rate, contractility increase to try to increase cardiac output; vasoconstriction in the vascular system occurs to return more blood to the heart; oxygen demand of the heart increases, heart works harder; vasoconstriction increases afterload (resistance) and can decrease the pumping ability; heart can be overwhelmed by the increased blood flow. |
| Renal changes | Kidneys respond to decreased cardiac output by releasing renin, which causes angiotensinogen conversion to angiotensin; adrenal cortex releases aldosterone in response, and sodium is retained; posterior pituitary releases antidiuretic hormone in response to sodium and water retained; vasoconstriction occurs because of angiotensin release; sodium and water retention increase preload and can overwhelm the heart; vasoconstriction increases afterload, and the heart has more resistance to pumping; Greater workload for the heart results. (Huether, McCance, 1996.) |

and left ventricles is the most common presentation of heart failure, but failure of one ventricle can occur before the other.

The signs and symptoms of right heart failure (Box 23-15) are caused by the congestion of the venous system from the backflow of blood from the right ventricle. Organ congestion in the liver, spleen, and GI tract and systemic venous congestion with peripheral edema and jugular venous distention are common with right-sided failure. Right-sided failure most often occurs because of left ventricular failure but can be the primary type of CHF in patients with chronic obstructive pulmonary disease (COPD), in which case it is called *cor pulmonale*, or heart failure resulting from lung disease, and right ventricular infarctions (Urban et al, 1995). Massive pulmonary emboli also can cause acute right heart failure. Prolonged right heart failure affects the left side of the heart by causing resistance to left ventricular pumping and reduced filling of the left ventricle.

The first area affected by left heart failure is the lungs. Increased congestion and backflow of blood to the lungs can cause **pulmonary edema.** As the left ventricle continues to fail, the right side of the heart is affected by the continued pressure in the heart and the backflow of blood, and symptoms of right heart failure also are seen. Left heart failure usually is the result of heart conditions such as MI and prolonged hypertension, but it also can occur when the demands of the body exceed the heart's ability to pump as in systemic infections, or when the heart is over-

whelmed by rapid increases in preload (volume), as in fluid overload.

## Assessment
### Risk Factors and Precipitating Factors

One of the first assessment skills needed by the nurse is the ability to identify patients at increased risk of CHF and situations that can precipitate heart failure. CHF is a common complication of many types of heart and other body system problems (see Box 23-14). Knowing that CHF can occur after an MI should direct the nurse's assessment focus to the early signs of CHF.

In addition to the more common causes, several other situations or health problems can precipitate CHF, even in patients with healthy hearts (Box 23-16). Anemia, hypervolemia, infection, and fever all increase the demands on the heart, and arrhythmias and hypervolemia can induce CHF by reducing the heart's pumping ability (Urban et al, 1995). A normal, healthy heart may be able to overcome these precipitating factors unless they are severe or prolonged. Hearts that are compromised or at risk may be pushed beyond their ability to compensate. Patients with existing chronic CHF are at increased risk for exacerbations because of their already compromised pumping ability, and they may be affected faster and more severely by the precipitating factors. Early recognition of these causative and precipitating factors can ensure that steps are taken to prevent the development or worsening of heart failure.

BOX 23-15

## SIGNS AND SYMPTOMS OF RIGHT AND LEFT HEART FAILURE

**RIGHT HEART FAILURE**
**Inspection/Palpation**
Heaves
Edema in dependent areas
Ascites
Jugular vein distension
Hepatomegaly
Splenomegaly

**Auscultation**
Murmurs

**History**
Anorexia
Nausea and vomiting
Weight gain
Fatigue
Chest pain

**Other**
Rapid weight gain

**LEFT HEART FAILURE**
**Inspection/Palpation**
Heaves
Increased respirations
Increased heart rate
PMI displaced
Cyanosis
Dry cough
Frothy sputum
Hemoptysis

**Auscultation**
$S_3$ and $S_4$ heart sounds
Crackles in the lung fields
Wheezes in lung fields

**History**
Dyspnea
Exertional dyspnea
Orthopnea
Paroxysmal nocturnal dyspnea
Fatigue
Cough
Nocturia
Palpitations
Chest pain

**Other**
Arrhythmia

Data from Huether SE, McCance KL: *Understanding pathophysiology*, St Louis, 1996, Mosby.

## NURSE ALERT

Acute onset or exacerbations of congestive heart failure usually are caused by underlying problems. The nurse must be a detective in identifying the precipitating cause.

Increasing age, chronic health conditions such as CAD and HTN, and life-style characteristics such as obesity and smoking all increase a person's risk of developing CHF (see Box 23-16). Early in the progression of CHF in this high-risk group, the symptoms may be vague or the patient may be asymptomatic, even though signs indicate that progressive damage to the heart is occurring. Tachycardia at rest, ECG changes indicating hypertrophy of the heart muscle, and x-ray changes indicating an enlarged heart all can be very early signs of CHF that precede the development of symptoms. Recognizing patients at risk for CHF can alert the health care team that screening and health promotion interventions need to be implemented.

Once the process of CHF has begun, it is important for the nurse to pick up on the early signs and symptoms. Intervening early in the process makes CHF much easier to treat. As described in the previous section, the signs and symptoms of CHF depend on whether it is an acute or chronic process and which ventricle (right, left, or both) is involved (see Box 23-15).

### Assessment Findings in Acute CHF

In acute CHF the primary signs and symptoms involve the pulmonary system. *Pulmonary edema,* the leakage of fluid from the pulmonary vascular system into the alveoli, and increased stiffness of the lung tissues cause many pulmonary symptoms. Early in the

---

**BOX 23-16**

### RISK FACTORS AND PRECIPITATING FACTORS IN CONGESTIVE HEART FAILURE

**RISK FACTORS**

**Age**
Incidence increases with age.

**CAD**
All types puts patients at risk, but MI is the most common cause of acute CHF.

**Hypertension (HTN)**
The more severe the hypertension, the higher the risk; HTN can increase the risk to three times that of a person without hypertension.

**Diabetes**
Diabetes is a risk factor even if HTN and CAD are not present.

**Other**
Smoking, obesity, hypercholesterolemia, proteinuria

**PRECIPITATING FACTORS**

**Hypervolemia**
Increased preload can overwhelm the heart's ability to pump.

**Anemia**
Cardiac output must increase to make up for low oxygen-carrying ability of the blood.

**Infection**
The body requires more cardiac output.

**Fever**
Fever increases the body's need for oxygen above what the heart can pump.

**Thyroid Storm**
The body has an extremely high metabolic rate when the thyroid is stimulated, and the heart is overworked.

**Arrhythmias**
Arrhythmias reduce the pumping ability of the heart and may overwork the heart.

**Treatment, Disease, or Life-style Changes in Existing CHF**
With any new illness or sudden onset or problems, such as fever, a normal heart might be able to compensate for the changes, but in CHF compensation cannot occur.
Changes in medication regimen
  Not taking medication
  Changes in dosage (especially decreases)
  Cardiac depressant drugs
  Drugs that cause salt retention
Diet changes
Sodium increases

---

development of CHF, the respiratory rate is increased (tachypnea) and oxygenation of the arterial blood falls (hypoxemia). If the failure continues, hypoxemia worsens, the exchange of carbon dioxide and oxygen decreases, carbon dioxide is retained, (hypercarbia), and a low arterial pH (acidemia) occurs. The patient experiences restlessness and increased shortness of breath and may look pale or cyanotic. As the difficulty breathing continues (dyspnea) and the patient uses accessory muscles for breathing, the respiratory rate increases even more, and the patient may not be able to breathe effectively lying down (orthopnea). The patient coughs, and wheezing and crackles are heard on auscultation of the lungs. The patient may have frothy pink (blood tinged) sputum because of fluid and red blood cells leaking into the alveoli. As cardiac output falls, the patient's heart rate increases because of compensatory mechanisms. BP initially may be slightly increased but then progress to hypotension as compen-satory mechanisms fail. Because of the decrease in cardiac output, the patient may also have the classic look of a patient in shock (i.e., cool, clammy skin) (Huether, McCance, 1996). Acute left ventricular failure is always a serious emergency, and immediate treatment is necessary.

**NURSE ALERT**

Patients in acute congestive heart failure should not be placed in the Trendelenburg position, because it can increase the return of blood to the heart and push the diaphragm up, reducing the pumping ability of the heart and expansion of the lungs. Thus the patient's condition may worsen.

## Assessment Findings in Chronic CHF

When CHF develops as a chronic process, the symptoms usually are a combination of right and left heart failure (see Box 23-15). The most common early symptoms of chronic congestive heart failure are (1) a tendency to become easily fatigued, (2) shortness of breath, usually apparent initially on exertion, such as climbing stairs or walking rapidly, and a slight hacking cough, and (3) swelling of the feet and ankles (Huether, McCance, 1996). The patient may attribute many of these symptoms to the aging process, rather than recognizing them as an indication of a heart problem. He or she may try different home remedies to find relief.

The fatigue associated with CHF is one of the earliest symptoms. In the early stages the fatigue may occur after periods of exercise or activity; it increases in intensity and duration as the failure progresses. The fatigue and activity intolerance that occur with CHF can be one of the most debilitating features of heart failure.

The patient may notice dyspnea only after exertion in the early stages of CHF. As failure progresses, the dyspnea also occurs at rest. As the disease becomes advanced, the dyspnea may be a panting type and may be so severe that the person cannot lie flat in bed at night to sleep (orthopnea) and must remain upright by propping up with pillows or sitting in a chair. Some patients may need several pillows to maintain a partly upright position for sleeping. Increased fluid in the vascular system can cause pulmonary congestion and edema. The patient may be awakened from sleep by severe breathlessness approximately 2 or 3 hours after retiring; this is known as *paroxysmal nocturnal dyspnea (PND)*. The cough may be dry in the early stages but can progress to frothy, and hemoptysis may occur if fluid and blood cells leak into the alveoli.

The swelling of the feet and ankles usually subsides at night when the person is in a supine position and reoccurs during the day when the legs and feet are dependent. The edema, a pitting type, eventually may extend to the face, neck, sacrum, and extremities. Distension of the jugular veins can be seen with increased venous congestion. Patients who are not able to be ambulatory have edema in the most dependent area of their body (the sacral area is a common site for bedridden patients).

The fluid causing the edema in the dependent areas during the daylight hours is reabsorbed when the patient lies down in a more horizontal position. This redistribution of fluid increases blood flow to the kidneys and causes diuresis. The patient may complain of excessive night time voiding (nocturia).

The patient may have excessive weight gain because of the fluid retention. As the venous pressure increases and organs become engorged, the patient complains of pain in the upper abdomen as the liver capsule is stretched and the gastrointestinal tract becomes ede-

matous. The patient is weak and has loss of appetite; malnutrition can be a significant problem in advanced CHF. As CHF progresses, mental status changes because of the decrease in blood flow to the brain.

## Progression and Complications

As CHF worsens, early signs and symptoms give way to symptoms of progression of the failure. The patient becomes more functionally limited. In order to plan interventions, the nurse must take into consideration the effect that CHF has on the patient's ability to complete the normal activities of daily living. CHF often is classified according to the limitations the patient has at each stage (Table 23-16).

The nurse must also assess for complications of CHF, which include organ failure, particularly the liver (see Chapter 36); thrombus formation in the heart and emboli (see Chapter 24); pleural effusions (see Chapter 22); and unstable angina.

## Diagnostic Studies

A patient with new onset CHF, worsening CHF, or acute exacerbations of CHF undergoes a complete diagnostic workup so that any underlying cause can be identified and treated. These studies also assist the health care team in determining the progression of the

---

**TABLE 23-16**

### New York Heart Association Classification of Functional Capacity of Patients with Diseases of the Heart

**Funcational Capacity**

**Class I** Patients with cardiac disease but without resulting limitation of physical activity. Ordinary physical activity does not cause undue fatigue, palpitation, dyspnea, or anginal pain.

**Class II** Patients with cardiac disease resulting in slight limitation of physical activity. They are comfortable at rest. Ordinary physical activity results in fatigue, palpitation, dyspnea, or anginal pain.

**Class III** Patients with cardiac disease resulting in marked limitation of physical activity. They are comfortable at rest. Less than ordinary activity causes fatigue, palpitation, dyspnea, or anginal pain.

**Class IV** Patients with cardiac disease resulting in inability to carry on any physical activity without discomfort. Symptoms of heart failure or the anginal syndrome may be present even at rest. If any physical activity is undertaken, discomfort is increased.

From The Criteria Committee of the New York Heart Association: *Nomenclature and criteria for diagnosis of diseases of the heart and great vessels*, ed 9, Boston, 1994, Little, Brown. See this publication for complete information.

disease and in choosing the best therapy for the patient. The most common diagnostic studies and their use in CHF are presented in Table 23-17. Based on the patient's presentation and the history and physical examination, numerous other studies may be done, such as a ventilation-perfusion scan for suspected pulmonary emboli and measurement of thyroid hormone levels for thyroid storm.

## Intervention

Intervention in patients with CHF has three primary focuses: (1) prevention, (2) treatment of the underlying cause, and (3) management of symptoms (Urban et al, 1995). The nurse can play an important role in all three of these areas.

## Prevention

As mentioned in the assessment section, early recognition of CHF, prevention of CHF, and prompt treatment of precipitating factors in CHF are the nursing goals in patients who have CHF or who are identified as high risk. Some nursing interventions for patients at risk in-

clude monitoring and regulating IV fluids to prevent fluid overload; use of antiembolic stockings and leg exercises to prevent thrombosis, which can lead to pulmonary emboli; teaching patients about their risk for CHF; and life-style changes, such as reducing dietary sodium reduction to reduce fluid retention. The nurse can play a major role in identifying at-risk patients and can contribute to the prevention of acute CHF and CHF exacerbations.

## Treating Underlying Causes

Finding and treating the underlying cause or precipitating factor in congestive heart failure is another focus of management. The assessment and physical examination provide valuable information to direct the diagnostic workup. Diagnostic studies assist in identifying the most appropriate treatment strategy, which may include surgical correction of heart defects such as valvular stenosis and septal, or medical management of acute or chronic conditions such as hypertension, infection, arrhythmias, or MI. Aggressive treatment of underlying causes is needed for both acute and chronic CHF.

### TABLE 23-17

## Diagnostic Studies Used in Congestive Heart Failure

| DIAGNOSTIC STUDY | RATIONALE/USE IN CHF |
|---|---|
| Chest x-ray | Can identify changes in the lung field and pulmonary vascular system caused by pulmonary congestion and edema, and pleural effusion.<br>Can determine the amount of enlargement of the heart; especially helpful when compared with baseline films.<br>Can be used to gauge the response to treatment. |
| Echocardiogram | Used to evaluate valvular function, heart chamber size, ejection fraction, and wall motion abnormalities and to assess for structural changes that can cause CHF.<br>Used to evaluate progression of the disease. |
| Cardiac catheterization | Used to identify abnormalities of coronary arteries. |
| Nuclear imaging studies | Used to identify ischemic heart disease.<br>Can assist in determining the patient's exercise capacity. |
| 12-Lead ECG and continuous ECG monitoring | Used to identify hypertrophy and strain of the ventricles and atrium, arrhythmias, and ischemic changes.<br>Also used to identify changes associated with acute injury or infarction when MI is suspected. |
| Cardiac enzymes and isoenzymes | Used to identify or rule out myocardial infarction as an underlying cause for CHF. |
| Arterial blood gases and pulse oximetry | Used to evaluate oxygenation and ventilation.<br>Used to identify the need for supplemental oxygen or mechanical ventilation.<br>Used to evaluate the patient's response to therapy. |
| Serum chemistries, complete blood cell count, and liver profile | Used to identify underlying electrolyte imbalance, anemia, infection, liver failure, renal insufficiency, and other metabolic causes or complications of CHF. |
| Hemodynamic monitoring | May be initiated in acute CHF and in patients whose condition becomes unstable.<br>Used to monitor the pressures in the heart and arterial system to identify underlying preload, afterload, or contractility problems.<br>Used to monitor the patient's response to treatment. |

## Management of the Symptoms of Acute CHF with Pulmonary Edema

The medical and nursing interventions for patients with acute CHF are directed toward four primary goals: (1) Reducing sodium and water retention, (2) improving the heart's pumping ability, (3) improving oxygenation, and (4) reducing the demands on the heart (Urban et al, 1995). Many of the therapies and pharmacologic agents have an effect on more than one of these goals, and interventions are conducted simultaneously. The patient with acute pulmonary edema often is critically ill and usually is admitted to an intensive care area for continuous monitoring and aggressive treatment.

Reducing sodium and water retention in a patient in acute CHF diminishes the demands on the heart by reducing the amount of blood the heart has to pump; as a result, the effectiveness of pumping increases. Also, since the respiratory symptoms experienced by a patient with acute CHF are due mainly to pulmonary congestion, reducing the volume of fluid in the vessels (preload) improves oxygenation. Volume (preload) is reduced by giving the patient diuretics. The most frequently used diuretics are the loop diuretics, such as furosemide (Lasix) and bumetanide (Bumex) (Agency for Health Care Policy and Research, 1994a). These drugs are given by IV push or infusion to cause rapid diuresis. Vasodilators, such as nitroglycerin and angiotensin-converting enzyme (ACE) inhibitors, also are used in acute CHF (see Table 23-10) to dilate the vessels and displace the volume into the periphery. This displacement reduces the amount of volume (preload) returning to the heart until the kidneys have had a chance to elimi-nate the fluid through diuresis (Agency for Health Care Policy and Research, 1994a). Vasodilators also increase blood flow through the coronary arteries to give the weakened heart more oxygen.

Preload also can be reduced by placing the patient in a sitting position such as high Fowler's position with the legs dependent. This positioning allows gravity to pull the excess volume away from the heart (reducing preload) and can improve lung expansion and oxygenation. When these types of therapies are used, the nurse must monitor intake and output carefully. A urinary drainage (Foley) catheter usually is inserted to drain the bladder and provide a more accurate means of watching the patient's output. The patient also is weighed daily to evaluate the volume status. Physical examinations are needed for evaluation for edema or dehydration.

With excessive diuresis comes the risk of electrolyte imbalances. Potassium may be lost with the administration of diuretics, and the serum potassium level should be checked regularly. Potassium supplements may be given intravenously or orally. The nurse must monitor laboratory values and report any electrolyte imbalances.

The heart's pumping ability is improved by the reduction of preload, as discussed in the previous section. If preload reduction does not improve contractility of the heart, other agents may be needed. The pumping ability of the heart commonly is increased by using drugs to stimulate the heart directly. Drugs that can be used to increase contractility (**inotropes**) include digitalis, dopamine, dobutamine, amrinone, and milrinone (Agency for Health Care Policy and Research, 1994a) (Table 23-18).

---

**TABLE 23-18**

## Inotropes Used in Congestive Heart Failure

| CLASSIFICATION SPECIFIC AGENTS | ACTION/INDICATION/ADMINISTRATION | NURSING CONSIDERATIONS |
|---|---|---|
| **Cardiac Glycosides** Digoxin | Given IV for initial loading, then PO. Increases the force of ventricular contraction and decreases conduction through the AV node to allow more time for ventricular emptying; used in CHF to increase cardiac output. | Can cause toxicity. The nurse must watch for nausea, vomiting, decreased appetite, yellow or blurred vision, and bradycardia; serum levels should be checked regularly; low potassium levels can increase the chances of toxicity, therefore potassium levels should be monitored, especially in patients taking diuretics. |
| **Sympathetic Nervous System Stimulants** | Stimulate the heart, causing increased contractility; given by IV infusion. | Each has its own side effects and considerations; patient should be monitored closely. |

*Continued*

---

**TABLE 23-18**

## Inotropes Used in Congestive Heart Failure—cont'd

| CLASSIFICATION SPECIFIC AGENTS | ACTION/INDICATION/ADMINISTRATION | NURSING CONSIDERATIONS |
|---|---|---|
| **Sympathetic Nervous System Stimulants—cont'd** | | |
| Dopamine (Intropin) | Effects depend on dosage: at low dosage (1-4 $\mu$g/kg/min), increases renal blood flow; at 5-10 $\mu$g/kg/min, increases contractility; at >10 $\mu$g/kg/min, increases contractility and causes vasoconstriction<br><br>Used in acute CHF to increase contractility and improve cardiac output | If infiltration into the subcutaneous tissue occurs, drug can cause tissue necrosis; phentolamine, the antidote for this problem, must be infiltrated into the affected tissue.<br>Can cause increased resistance to ventricular contraction (afterload), myocardial oxygen use, and arrhythmias. |
| Dobutamine (Dubutrex) | Increases contractility through beta-receptor stimulation; used in CHF to increase contractility without increasing vasoconstriction (afterload) | Preferred over dopamine because it does not increase oxygen demand or afterload. |
| **Phosphodiesterase Inhibitors** | Inhibit phosphodiesterase to improve myocardial contractility<br>Increase cardiac output, and cause vasodilation (decreases afterload).<br>Used in CHF to improve the contractility of the heart<br>Given by IV infusion in critical situations and for intermittent use in the home | |
| Amrinone (Inocor) | Increases cardiac output, decreases afterload | Can cause thrombocytopenia (decrease in platelets); platelet count must be monitored; can cause hypotension (nurse must watch BP); can cause ventricular arrhythmias (ECG monitoring required). |
| Milrinone (Primacor) | More potent than amrinone | Side effects similar to those of amrinone; less thrombocytopenia but more hypotension and arrhythmias than with amrinone. |

---

Digitalis can be given intravenously or orally and is used frequently in acute and chronic CHF. Dopamine, dobutamine, amrinone, and milrinone are all potent agents given by IV infusion, and they require close monitoring.

In addition to directly stimulating the heart, it may be necessary to reduce the resistance the heart must pump against (afterload). Afterload is increased by the compensatory mechanisms of CHF. Stimulation of the sympathetic nervous system and the vasoconstriction that results from this stimulation may cause increases in afterload that put extra strain on the weakened heart. Vasodilators reduce afterload, as do some of the inotropes used to improve contractility.

When potent inotropes and vasodilators are used, the nurse must monitor the patient closely for side effects such as hypotension and arrhythmias. Frequent vital sign checks and continuous ECG monitoring are necessary. Hemodynamic monitoring also may be needed if the patient does not respond to initial thera-

pies and cardiac function continues to deteriorate. Hemodynamic monitoring may also be started when these vasodilators and inotropes are used.

Improving oxygenation is a primary initial goal in the care of a patient in acute CHF. The measures discussed previously to reduce volume overload and improve the heart's pumping ability have positive effects on the lungs. While these therapies are implemented, the patient should be given supplemental oxygen and should be monitored closely for improvement or deterioration in pulmonary status. Continuous pulse oximetry should be used to monitor oxygenation, and measurement of arterial blood gases may be ordered to evaluate ventilation and oxygenation.

The patient will be anxious and may be restless and confused because of decreased oxygenation of the brain and air hunger. Intravenous sedation with morphine sulfate can reduce the anxiety and has the additional benefit of reducing preload (Agency for Health Care Policy and Research, 1994a) (see Table 23-9). If the

BOX 23-17

# NURSING PROCESS

## CONGESTIVE HEART FAILURE

### ASSESSMENT

- Respirations: rate, quality, dyspnea, shortness of breath, orthopnea, paroxysmal nocturnal dyspnea, hemoptysis
- Pulse: quality, rate, rhythm, including peripheral pulses
- Weakness, energy level
- Pain (presence, location, quality)
- Skin (edema, color, temperature, moisture)
- Appetite
- Mood and mental status
- Knowledge of condition, diet, medication regimen

### NURSING DIAGNOSES

- Decreased cardiac output related to cardiac failure
- Ineffective breathing pattern related to pulmonary vascular congestion

- Impaired gas exchange related to pulmonary vascular congestion
- Impaired physical mobility related to weakness
- Anxiety related to inability to control illness and ineffective breathing patterns
- Altered nutrition: less than body requirements related to inability to digest large meals and abdominal discomfort
- Self-care deficit related to weakness
- Fluid volume excess related to decreased renal blood flow
- Risk for fear of death related to severity of illness
- Risk for ineffective individual coping mechanisms related to effect of illness on life-style
- Risk for altered thought processes related to poor tissue perfusion

*Continued*

patient has excessive secretions, suctioning may be needed. If the patient does not improve with administration of oxygen and other therapies, placement of a tube in the airway (intubation) and mechanical ventilation may be necessary.

The demands on the heart are reduced through volume reduction and control of preload and afterload (Agency for Health Care Policy and Research, 1994a). Additional measures may be needed if fever, infection, anemia, arrhythmias, or other problems are present that increase the work of the heart. A patient in acute CHF is on bed rest and kept NPO initially. To prevent fatigue and avoid stress on the weakened heart, the nurse should space activities and provide frequent rest periods. As the patient becomes able to take fluid and food orally, small, frequent meals should be offered. Until the patient is able to become more physically active, the nurse should monitor for complications of immobility and implement interventions to prevent them, such as frequent turning and range of motion exercises.

If the weakened heart continues to deteriorate, cardiogenic shock may occur. Mechanical devices, such as intraaortic balloon pump (IABPs), ventricular-assist devices (VADs), and artificial hearts are available in some facilities to reduce ventricular work for short periods (Urban et al, 1995). Dynamic cardiomyoplasty, a surgical procedure that places skeletal muscle around the failing heart, shows promise as a long-term alternative. Once the skeletal muscle has been placed

around the heart, it is stimulated by an electronic pacemaker to contract the ventricle and increase the pumping action (Bove et al, 1995).

The last option for a patient with severe CHF is heart transplantation, but the lack of an adequate number of donor hearts makes this option possible for only a few of those who might need it (Urban et al, 1995).

As with any patient suffering from an acute and possibly critical illness, the nurse must also provide interventions to assist the patient and family with the crisis situation. Support, counseling, information, and teaching are ongoing responsibilities of the nurse. As the patient improves, the nurse may need to prepare the patient and family for dealing with chronic CHF.

## Management of Symptoms in Chronic Congestive Heart Failure

The management of chronic CHF has the same goals as those for acute CHF. Reducing sodium and water retention, improving the heart's pumping ability, improving oxygenation, and reducing the demands on the heart are accomplished by implementing a combination of pharmacologic, dietary, and life-style interventions (Ahrens, 1995). The long-term outcomes sought are to reduce the edema and shortness of breath and increase the patient's activity level. The nurse also must educate the patient and family in ways to manage the treatment regimen and prevent exacerbations of the chronic process (Box 23-17).

---

<BOX 23-17>

## NURSING PROCESS

## CONGESTIVE HEART FAILURE—cont'd

### NURSING INTERVENTIONS

- Position the patient in Fowler's position, with back, arms, and legs supported for optimum respiratory ventilation.
- Observe for signs of fluid excess: pitting edema, dyspnea, cough, pulmonary edema, distended neck veins, and tachycardia.
- Check vital signs often.
- Observe for signs of disorientation or mental confusion.
- Observe for signs of hypokalemia.
- Administer digitalis preparation as ordered and observe for signs of toxicity.
- Administer diuretics as ordered.
- Administer oxygen as needed.
- Turn the patient every 2 hours.

- Provide a quiet, restful environment.
- Allow for periods of rest after activity.
- Provide small, frequent feedings with easily digested items that the patient likes.
- Restrict sodium intake as ordered.
- Weigh the patient daily.
- Explain the therapeutic and side effects of medications, dosing regimen, and diet.

### EVALUATION OF EXPECTED OUTCOMES

- Optimum respiratory ventilation achieved
- Vital signs within normal limits
- Few or no signs of fluid excess exhibited
- Proper rest and sleep achieved
- Purposes of sodium-restricted diet and prescribed medications understood

---

Sodium and water retention and edema are reduced through drug therapy, diet restrictions, and sometimes fluid restrictions. Diuretics are administered to remove excess water the body has retained. When a patient takes diuretics, urinary output increases, edema and ascites are relieved, and breathing is made easier. Because potassium may be lost, potassium supplements may be needed. Potassium may be increased by adding foods rich in potassium to the diet, but the patient should be cautioned about taking supplements and eating potassium-rich food together. Patients should also be taught the symptoms of low potassium levels.

As an adjunct to diuretics, patients with congestive heart failure are placed on a sodium-restricted diet (Ahrens, 1995). The body requires a certain amount of sodium, and any excess normally is excreted by the kidneys. In patients with congestive heart failure, in which water is retained in the tissues, sodium is retained as well. Sodium contributes to water retention, but, when sodium is absent, water is excreted. The sodium-restricted diet often is misunderstood and misinterpreted by the patient to mean no consumption of salt. Selection of foods that are low in natural sodium is most important. The degree of sodium restriction depends on the severity of the heart failure. A normal diet contains up to 7 g of sodium per day. For patients with mild CHF, a sodium restriction of 2 g per day is common. For patients with severe CHF, sodium intake may need to be as low as 500 mg. Fluid restriction may be required for patients with severe CHF.

The patient and family must be taught the role that diuretics and sodium restriction play in the control of the edema. A dietary history and diet preferences will be helpful in planning with the patient and family a diet that limits sodium and provides needed nutrients.

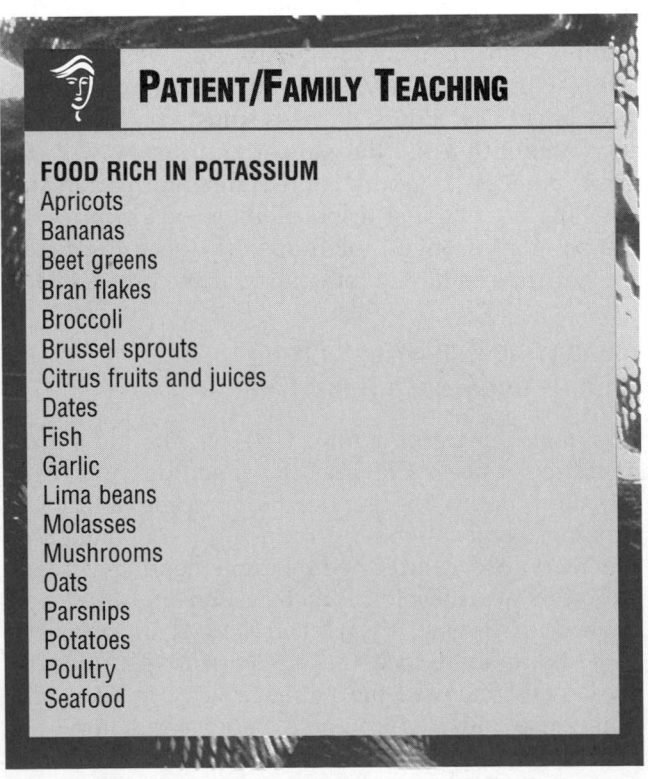

## PATIENT/FAMILY TEACHING

**FOOD RICH IN POTASSIUM**
Apricots
Bananas
Beet greens
Bran flakes
Broccoli
Brussel sprouts
Citrus fruits and juices
Dates
Fish
Garlic
Lima beans
Molasses
Mushrooms
Oats
Parsnips
Potatoes
Poultry
Seafood

Staying on the recommended diet is one of the most difficult parts of the treatment plan for patients with CHF. The dietician or nurse must teach the patient and family foods that are low or high in sodium, and how to read labels to find the sodium content of food. One strategy is to focus teaching on the many foods that are low in sodium, and not on all the food the patient cannot eat (see Patient/Family Teaching box: Low-Sodium Foods). The person who does the shopping and cooking should be actively involved in this teaching. A dietician can also demonstrate or provide recipes for methods of cooking or seasoning that can make food taste better. Low-sodium salt substitutes can be helpful for patients who want to salt their food, but these supplements are high in potassium.

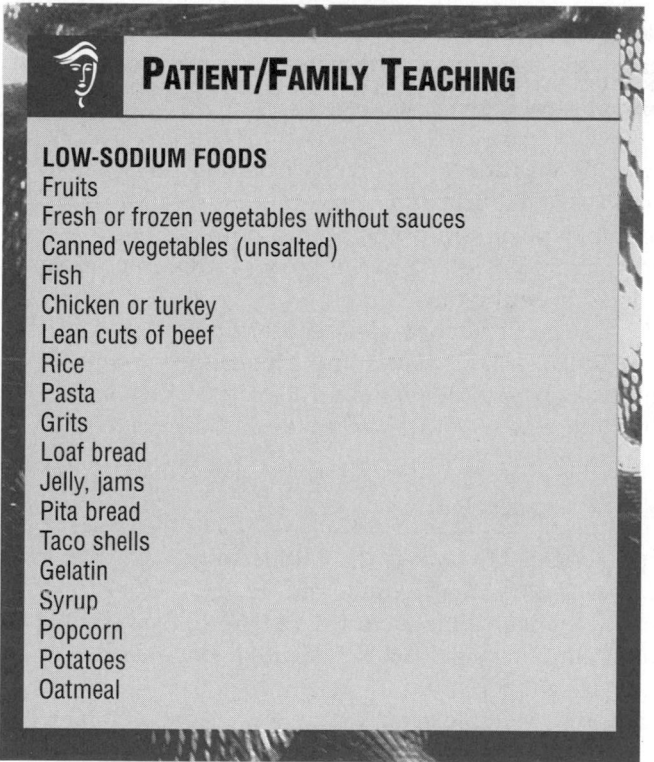

**PATIENT/FAMILY TEACHING**

**LOW-SODIUM FOODS**
Fruits
Fresh or frozen vegetables without sauces
Canned vegetables (unsalted)
Fish
Chicken or turkey
Lean cuts of beef
Rice
Pasta
Grits
Loaf bread
Jelly, jams
Pita bread
Taco shells
Gelatin
Syrup
Popcorn
Potatoes
Oatmeal

Patients should be educated on the type and dosage of diuretics, how to detect edema, and how to weigh themselves daily and track their weight (Purcell, Fletcher, 1994a). One of the most problematic side effects of diuretics for patients is the frequent voiding. Patients may cut back on their diuretics to avoid frequent trips to the bathroom.

As with acute CHF, inotropic agents often are ordered to improve the pumping ability of the heart. Oral agents such as digitalis most often are used for patients with chronic CHF, but if the failure progresses, the patient may receive IV inotropes at home

intermittently. The administration of IV inotropes is conducted and monitored by home health nurses.

The physician often orders an inotropic agent, usually digitalis in some form, to slow the heart rate and increase the force of the beat, thereby improving cardiac output. When digitalis is used, therapeutic levels can be obtained quickly by starting with several large doses. This loading-dose treatment is called *digitalization.* During this time the patient must be carefully monitored for toxic symptoms such as nausea, vomiting, irregular pulse, slow heart rate, diarrhea, anorexia, and visual disturbances. If any of these symptoms occur, the drug should be withheld and the physician notified.

Blood levels of digitalis are usually monitored carefully during the initial doses and during routine administration. As soon as the therapeutic blood level is reached (1 to 2 ng/ml), the patient is put on a daily maintenance dose (McCormack, 1996). It has been the traditional practice of nurses to routinely withhold digitalis preparations from patients with apical pulse rates below 60 beats per minute. Digitalis has only a minor effect on slowing of the SA node. It has a greater affect on the AV node, where it delays conduction and slows the ventricles. Therefore, in patients who have normal sinus rhythm, routinely withholding the dose of digitalis *may* contribute to reduction of the therapeutic level. The appropriate nursing action is to withhold digitalis from patients with symptomatic bradycardia or symptoms of toxicity only until laboratory assessment of therapeutic plasma levels can be done. Hypokalemia predisposes patients to digitalis toxicity. Many patients receiving diuretic therapy are at risk for low potassium levels. Electrolyte values must be checked frequently. The patient and family must be educated about the use of digitalis and the symptoms of toxicity side effects.

Improving oxygenation and reducing the demands on the heart are also important goals for the patient with chronic CHF. Keeping fluid retention and edema down and increasing the pumping effectiveness of the heart are two major interventions previously discussed. Vasodilators such as nitroglycerin and ACE inhibitors are commonly prescribed for chronic CHF to reduce preload, improve ventricular pumping, reduce the heart size, and diminish the detrimental compensatory mechanisms of vasoconstriction (McCormack, 1996). Vasodilators have also been shown to reduce mortality in patients with CHF (Agency for Health Care Policy and Research, 1994a). Providing for a balance of rest and activity, improving nighttime sleep, reducing anxiety and emotional stress, and weight loss are other interventions that should be implemented to reduce the workload on the heart and prevent dyspnea.

The need for rest and for activity restrictions on patients with congestive heart failure must be addressed on an individual basis. Many patients with mild or moderate failure can avoid serious complications such as venous stasis or pulmonary embolism if they are out of bed and leading a relatively normal life. Because the benefits of mobility are well recognized, patients usually are not confined to long periods of bed rest. If the failure is severe, bed rest may be necessary, and the length of rest is determined for the individual patient. The patient and family should be instructed in ways to conserve energy. A physical therapist or exercise specialist may be needed to help the patient review his or her life-style and plan ways to simplify. The patient should be as physically active as the severity of the CHF allows. Unnecessary inactivity can predispose the patient to many complications.

Patients may continue to need to sleep with their heads elevated with pillows or in a chair to avoid nocturnal dyspnea. Sleep may be disrupted, and a mild sedative may help with sleep and rest at night. Patients who experience excessive voiding at night should be taught to schedule their diuretics so that they take effect and cause diuresis during the day. When dyspnea or cyanosis is present, oxygen may be administered, and it may be needed continuously or intermittently at home. Meals should be small to keep the diaphragm low and allow lung expansion. Rest periods taken before and after meals or activities prevent fatigue and dyspnea (Purcell, Fletcher, 1994a).

---

# NURSING CARE PLAN

## PATIENT WITH CONGESTIVE HEART FAILURE AND OLIGURIA

The patient is a 68-year-old woman with morbid obesity who was admitted directly from her physician's office to the Emergency Department with a medical diagnosis of oliguria and congestive heart failure. She has been on continuous oxygen at home because of chronic hypoxia, sleep apnea, and now with increasing dyspnea. She has noticed increasing generalized edema and has a dry, hacking cough that interferes with sleep. She complains of mild abdominal pain unrelated to eating or defecation.

She was cardioverted in the Emergency Department for atrial fibrillation. An echocardiogram done at that time showed a mural thrombus, and she was given anticoagulants. Lasix and Metalazone were administered to increase urinary output. Verapamil (Calan) was given to dilate the coronary arteries and decrease oxygen demand. Procan was given as an antiarrhythmic. She was admitted to the coronary care unit for 5 days and then transferred to a medical unit.

| Medical History | Psychosocial Data | Assessment Data |
|---|---|---|
| Hospitalized as a child for a fractured femur from a bicycle accident<br>Pregnancies complicated by excess weight, preeclampsia, and gestational diabetes<br>C-sectioned 3 times with viable infants; all infants weighed over 4.5 kg (10 lb)<br>Abdominal hysterectomy 12 years ago because of excessive bleeding and fibroid tumors; uterus removed along with both ovaries and tubes<br>Maintained on estrogen therapy until age 60 | Married, supportive husband; three adult children, two live out of state; six grandchildren; one granddaughter in college lives in the home and gives some assistance to her grandmother<br>Jewish religion, husband cantor in temple<br>Retired from lighting supply company as cashier (sedentary activity)<br>Has private health insurance plus Medicare | Oriented to time, place, and person<br>*Vital signs:* T 97 rectally, P 62, R 20, BP 162/78<br>Weight on admission: 162 kg (362 lb) (bed scale)<br>Current weight: 160 kg (351 lb) (6 days later)<br>Height: 5'1"<br>*Skin:* Multiple open, weepy blisters on left thigh and right arm, both draining clear fluid; many open areas on back of thighs and buttocks; evidence of irritation from scratching; blister on right great toe, covered with bandage<br>*Respiratory:* Decreased breath sounds in lower lobes bilaterally; bibasilar crackles (rales) heard; upper lobes clear to auscultation<br>*Cardiovascular:* Apical pulse 68, regular rhythm; neck veins distended<br>*Abdominal:* Pendulous abdomen with many fatty indentations; difficult to hear bowel sounds because of depth of adipose tissue; girth 160-170 cm (64-68 in); abdomen nontender, soft on palpation; midline scars from previous surgeries |

The nurse, patient, and family need to be aware that emotional exertion, like physical exertion, increases metabolic activity and the need for oxygen. The nurse should be alert to signs that indicate anxiety, frustration, and fear. The patient may fear the immediate danger of complications and a prolonged helplessness and loss of independence. The patient may express these feelings verbally or may show them by hostility or failure to cooperate. The patient may feel safe only when someone is nearby, and arrangements may need to be made for a member of the family or others to stay near the patient. Listening to the patient's expressions of concern and explaining procedures and care updates can go a long way toward reducing anxiety. Relaxation therapy, meditation, yoga, music, and many other strategies can be used to assist the patient in controlling anxiety and emotional stress.

Patients with chronic congestive heart failure, like other patients with chronic disease, may have difficulty adapting to the many changes they must make. These patients frequently have to take several medications daily for life, alter their work or leisure activities, and radically change their diet, and they face the prospect of a progressive deterioration in physical ability. Continuous encouragement, frequent reinforcement of teaching, and incremental changes are nursing interventions that can lead to improvement in overall outcomes.

## NURSING CARE PLAN

### PATIENT WITH CONGESTIVE HEART FAILURE AND OLIGURIA—cont'd

| Medical History | Psychosocial Data | Assessment Data |
|---|---|---|
| States she has always been "heavy"<br>Diabetes mellitus type II, (noninsulin dependent), (NIDDM) for 25 years<br>Hypertension for 20 years; has been on various anti-hypertensive drugs with moderately good response; quality compliance to drug therapy<br>COPD-chronic hypoxia and difficulty with ADLs; uses oxygen at home via nasal cannula<br>Biventricular congestive heart failure for past 2 years<br>Sleep apnea, prefers to sleep in recliner<br>Chronic renal failure, requires diuretics daily<br>Atrial fibrillation in past, responded to medications; cardioversion in the Emergency Department—first time needed | Owns home, one level, few stairs; wheelchair ramp being built onto side of house<br>Has never smoked; denies overuse of alcohol or drugs<br>No known food allergies; allergic to sulfa drugs, questionable allergy to some tapes | *Musculoskeletal:* Grossly edematous extremities, 3+ pitting edema; negative pedal, posterior tibial, popliteal pulses; positive femoral pulses felt bilaterally<br>*Urinary:* Foley catheter draining cloudy urine, specific gravity 1.024<br>**Laboratory data**<br>Hgb 9.1, Hct 29, blood sugar 212<br>BUN 63 (normal 5-20)<br>Creatinine clearance 3.7 (normal 0.8-1.4 mg/dl)<br>K 5.2, Na 136<br>$O_2$ sat 94%-97% on oxygen at 2 L, drops to 78%-80% when off oxygen<br>**Medications**<br>40 U NPH insulin daily in morning<br>4 U regular insulin/coverage if blood sugar >160<br>Prednisone 15 mg PO daily<br>Verapamil (Calan) SR 240 mg PO daily<br>Procainamide (Procan) SR 500 mg PO tid<br>Digitalis 0.125 mg PO bid<br>Docusate sodium (Colace) 100 mg PO bid<br>Ducolax 10 mg × 1 prn constipation (rectally)<br>Diet: 1800 calorie ADA diet, with 800 ml fluid restriction |

*Continued*

# NURSING CARE PLAN

## PATIENT WITH CONGESTIVE HEART FAILURE AND OLIGURIA—cont'd

**NURSING DIAGNOSIS**

Decreased cardiac output related to cardiac failure, as evidenced by increasing shortness of breath and inability to perform ADLs

| NURSING INTERVENTIONS | EVALUATION OF EXPECTED OUTCOMES |
|---|---|
| Monitor BP, pulse, cardiac rhythm, temperature, and breath sounds every 4 hours. Record and report changes from baseline. | Less shortness of breath; gradually improvement in ability to perform ADL without undue fatigue |
| Take temperature rectally if dyspnea is present. | BP remains within normal range; signs of hyperkalemia (peaked or elevated T waves, prolonged P-R intervals, widened QRS complexes or depressed ST segments) do not appear on ECG |
| Carefully monitor I&O and specific gravity every 4 hours. Monitor BUN, creatinine, electrolytes, Hgb, and Hct. | |
| Discuss patient's food preferences and plan according to dietary restrictions. Assist her with meal planning. | |
| Provide mouth care every 4 hours. Keep her mucous membranes moist with a water-soluble lubricant. | I&O remain within established limits: intake of no more than 800 ml daily and output no less than 25 ml/hour |
| Keep on oxygen at 2 L via nasal cannula. Explain the rationale for not increasing the oxygen above 2 L at home. | Skin remains free of infection and shows signs of healing, with no new blisters apparent |
| Support patient with positive feedback about adherences to restrictions. | Patient identifies signs and symptoms to report to physician |
| Give skin care every 4 hours. Examine skin daily for signs of breakdown or infection. | Urine specific gravity remains between 1.010 and 1.020 |
| Change patient's position at least every 2 hours. Elevate edematous extremities. | Hct stays above 30 |
| Maintain on bed rest while dyspnea is present. | BUN, creatinine, sodium, and potassium stay within acceptable levels |
| Teach patient to conserve energy. Increase her level of activity as tolerated. Ambulate with assistance until patient's strength improves. Put on antiembolism stockings to increase venous return. Remove for 1 hour every 8 hours. | Participates in passive exercises every 1 to 2 hours when awake |
| Teach patient which foods are rich in potassium (bananas, all citrus fruits and juices, broccoli, bran flakes, raw carrots, prunes). | Demonstrates skill in selecting permitted food |

## NURSING CARE PLAN
### PATIENT WITH CONGESTIVE HEART FAILURE AND OLIGURIA—cont'd

**NURSING DIAGNOSIS**
Fluid volume excess related to congestive heart failure

| NURSING INTERVENTIONS | EVALUATION OF EXPECTED OUTCOMES |
|---|---|
| Weigh daily before breakfast. Check for signs of further dependent edema, such as sacral edema, increasing pitting edema, and increased ascites. | Body weight decreases by 0.9-1.35 kg (2-3 lb) daily; hemodynamic status restored to normal range |
| Monitor fluid restriction of 800 ml; help patient to make a schedule for timed amounts. | Pulmonary status restored to an acceptable range |
| Provide sour hard candy to decrease thirst and improve taste. Explain the reasons for fluid and dietary restrictions. | Reports less dyspnea and experiences more comfort |
| Assess skin turgor for signs of dehydration. Measure abdominal girth daily; compare to previous measurements. Provide sodium-restricted diet; teach patient the foods low in sodium. | Urine specific gravity decreases as urine output increases |
| Administer diuretics as ordered; monitor for increased output as response. | Electrolyte levels, BUN, and creatinine return to as nearly normal a range as possible |
| Assess for peripheral edema; measure girths to check for decreases. Explain the cause for fluid volume excess. | Patient plans 24-hour intake schedule |
| Provide information regarding congestive heart failure, the relationship of diet, medications, activity, and follow-up care. | Patient and family demonstrate adequate knowledge of how excess fluid volume affects congestive heart failure |
| Ask patient to repeat teachings; check for any misinformation. | States the rationales for restricted fluids, medications, and the need for compliance to orders |
| | Complications of excess fluid eliminated |

**NURSING DIAGNOSIS**
Self-care deficit related to shortness of breath, morbid obesity, and fatigue, as evidenced by inability to carry out aspects of self-care such as bathing and personal hygiene

| NURSING INTERVENTIONS | EVALUATION OF EXPECTED OUTCOMES |
|---|---|
| Identify patient's optimum time to attempt self-care (morning, after a period of rest after breakfast). | Grows in ability to perform some self-care needs |
| Provide privacy. Encourage a discussion of feelings related to body size and overall edema. | Demonstrates use of assistive devices |
| Provide dignity to nursing care by showing feelings of acceptance. | Performs some parts of the tasks of bathing and personal hygiene |
| Place all articles of self-care within her reach. | Discusses and shows signs of acceptance of body image |
| Praise patient for any attempts at self-care. | Grows in ability to accept constructive feedback, and plans ways to incorporate new information after discharge |
| Allow ample time to perform tasks. Rewarm bathwater if cold. | |
| Monitor for fatigue. | |
| Encourage her to plan rest periods before moving on to new tasks. | |
| Assist her when necessary. | |
| Check her color and overall adaptations. | |
| Provide constructive feedback. | |

*Continued*

## NURSING CARE PLAN

### PATIENT WITH CONGESTIVE HEART FAILURE AND OLIGURIA—cont'd

**NURSING DIAGNOSIS**

Constipation related to immobility and diet, as evidenced by hard, formed stool and painful defecation

| NURSING INTERVENTIONS | EVALUATION OF EXPECTED OUTCOMES |
|---|---|
| Assess bowel sounds and bowel habits daily.<br>Consult with dietitian for use of prune juice as a fruit exchange.<br>Administer docusate sodium (Colace) or Dulcolax as needed.<br>Encourage as much movement as possible when awake. Progressive ambulation is best once dyspnea decreases.<br>Discuss foods that are high in bulk and roughage.<br>Provide commode at bedside. Maintain privacy. Allow time for evacuation.<br>Keep toilet articles within reach.<br>Instruct patient to avoid straining if possible.<br>Tell patient that abdominal massage may relieve discomfort and promote defecation. | Less pain on defecation<br>Bowel pattern returns to a more normal pattern for patient<br>Identifies the relationship between inactivity, diet, and bowel habits<br>Uses the dietitian as a resource person to discuss food exchanges and foods high in fiber and bulk |

## KEY CONCEPTS

➤ Assessment, palpation, percussion, and auscultation are essential components of a physical examination.

➤ Arrhythmias can be detected by the nurse when taking a radial pulse.

➤ Ventricular tachycardia requires immediate intervention.

➤ When a patient is to receive a mechanical stimulator such as a pacemaker, complete teaching and gentle reassurance by the nurse are essential.

➤ Nonpharmacologic and pharmacologic measures are used to treat hypertension.

➤ Relieving anxiety in the patient who has had a heart attack is a significant responsibility for nurses.

➤ When nurses, physicians, and laypersons perform cardiopulmonary resuscitation and the Heimlich maneuver in emergency situations, countless lives are saved.

# CRITICAL THINKING EXERCISES

1. Mr. Lee was admitted with a myocardial infarction and is now in the telemetry unit in private room. You notice a strong odor of tobacco in his bathroom, and he has had no visitors today. His history includes a 30 pack-year smoking habit. Develop a plan for addressing this problem with Mr. Lee.

2. Mr. Miller is a 47-year-old man who has had a PTCA and is in the telemetry unit. He has been visited by members of the cardiac rehabilitation team, who started teaching him about CAD, and he is now very quiet and teary. When questioned about his change in behavior, he says, "There's no way I can do all the stuff they say I have to do. I am going to die!" What would be your response? What do you think is the underlying problem? What interventions could be implemented to assist Mr. Miller?

3. Mary King, a 61-year-old woman, was admitted with an anterior MI. She has been recovering without complications until this evening, when she began to complain of shortness of breath. On examining her, you note a respiratory rate of 32 and crackles in both lung bases. What other assessment data do you need to gather? What are the possible complications she could be having? What are your nursing priorities?

4. John Colwell is a 52-year-old man who has recently undergone CABG. When his family comes to visit, you notice a strong odor of cigarette smoke, and when they leave, you see empty fried chicken buckets and leftover french fries in the trash can. What problems might you expect with Mr. Colwell's rehabilitation? What interventions could you implement before Mr. Colwell's discharge?

5. Fannie Powell, a 50-year-old woman, originally was admitted for colon surgery. It is postoperative day 2, and she is complaining of a "tight feeling" in her chest. What would your initial assessment include? What interventions would you implement?

## REFERENCES AND ADDITIONAL READINGS

Agency for Health Care Policy and Research: Heart failure: Evaluation and care of patients with left ventricular systolic dysfunction, Clinical Practice Guideline No 11, AHCPR Pub No 94-0612, Rockville, Md, 1994a, US Department of Health and Human Services.

Agency for Health Care Policy and Research: Unstable angina: diagnosis and management, Clinical Practice Guideline No 19, AHCPR Pub No 94-0602, Rockville, Md, 1994b, US Department of Health and Human Services.

Ahrens SG: Managing heart failure: a blueprint for success, *Nursing 95* 25(12):26-31, 1995.

Aragon D, Martin M: What you should know about thrombolytic therapy for acute MI, *Am J Nurs* 93(9):24-31, 1993.

Atwood S et al: *Introduction to basic cardiac dysrhythmias*, ed 2, St Louis, 1996, Mosby.

Bates B: *A guide to physical examination and history taking*, ed 6, Philadelphia, 1995, Lippincott.

Beattie S, Carrie P: Left ventricular diastolic dysfunction: a case report, *Crit Care Nurse* 16(2):37-50, 1996.

Bove LA et al: Nursing care of patients undergoing dynamic cardiomyoplasty, *Crit Care Nurse* 15(3):96-104, 1995.

Cardio Thoracic Systems: Minimally invasive direct coronary artery bypass: the beating heart approach, 1996 (onsite training handout).

Chandra NC, Hazinski MF, editors: *Textbook of basic life support for healthcare providers*, 1994, American Heart Association.

Cummins RO, editor: *Textbook of advanced cardiac life support*, Dallas, 1994, American Heart Association.

Darovic GO: *Hemodynamic monitoring: invasive and noninvasive clinical application*, ed 2, Philadelphia, 1995, Saunders.

Gardner E et al: Intracoronary stent update: focus on patient education, *Crit Care Nurse* 16(2):65-75, 1996.

Huether SE, McCance KL: *Understanding pathophysiology*, St Louis, 1996, Mosby

Jensen L, King KM: Women and heart disease: the issues, *Crit Care Nurse* 17(2):45-52, 1997.

Lewis SM, Collier IC, Heitkemper MM: *Medical surgical nursing: assessment and management of clinical problems*, ed 4, St Louis, 1996, Mosby.

Lilly LS: *Pathophysiology of heart disease*, Malvern, Penn, 1993, Lea & Febiger.

McCormack J, editor: *Drug therapy decision making guide*, Philadelphia, 1996, Saunders.

Morton PG: Using the 12-lead ECG to detect ischemia, injury, and infarction, *Crit Care Nurse* 16(2):85-95, 1996.

Pagana KD, Pagana TJ: *Mosby's diagnostic and laboratory test reference*, ed 3, St Louis, 1996, Mosby.

Perra BM: Managing coronary atherectomy patients in a special procedure unit, *Crit Care Nurse* 15(3):57-68, 1995.

Purcell JA, Fletcher BJ: *A stronger pump: a guide for people with heart failure*, Atlanta, 1994a, Pritchett & Hull.

Purcell JA, Fletcher BJ: *You have a pacemaker*, Atlanta, 1994b, Pritchett & Hull.

Seidel HM et al: *Mosby's guide to physical examination*, ed 3, St Louis, 1995, Mosby.

Smith LF, Fish FH: *Pure practice for ECGs*, St Louis, 1995, Mosby.

Urban N et al: *Guidelines for critical care nursing*, St Louis, 1995, Mosby.

# CHAPTER 24

# Peripheral Vascular Problems

## CHAPTER OBJECTIVES

1 Describe the differences between the structure and function of the arterial and venous vascular systems.
2 Discuss the factors that affect pressure and blood flow in the arterial and venous systems.
3 Describe the assessment of a patient with a disorder of the vascular system.
4 Differentiate between the assessment findings for chronic and acute arterial and venous disorders.
5 Describe the nursing responsibilities associated with diagnostic testing of patients with vascular disorders.
6 Describe the major risk factors for arterial occlusive disease and venous thrombosis.
7 Identify strategies the nurse should teach patients to reduce their risk of arterial and venous vascular disease.
8 Describe nursing responsibilities related to the care of patients undergoing invasive therapeutic procedures and surgery for arterial occlusive disease.
9 Describe the nursing assessment and interventions indicated for a patient who has acute venous thrombosis.
10 Describe the nursing assessment, interventions, and patient teaching for a patient taking oral and intravenous anticoagulants.

## KEY TERMS

| | |
|---|---|
| amputation | emboli |
| aneurysm | intermittent claudication |
| arterial occlusive disease | perfusion |
| arteries | percutaneous translumi- |
| atherosclerosis | nal angioplasty (PTA) |
| bruit | Raynaud's phenomenon |
| Buerger's disease | thrombophlebitis |
| capillaries | varicosed veins |
| capillary refill | veins |
| DVTs | venous stasis |
| Doppler | venous thrombosis |

## STRUCTURE AND FUNCTION

### Blood Vessels

The massive network of blood vessels in the body is collectively called the *circulatory system*. The circulatory system carries the oxygenated arterial blood away from the heart and unoxygenated venous blood back to the heart to be pumped to the lungs. These important functions ensure that oxygen and nutrients are supplied to the organs and tissues and that wastes are directed to the correct removal site. The circulatory system is made up of three major types of vessels: the **arteries, veins**, and **capillaries** (Figure 24-1). Systemic arteries branch from the aorta and divide into the arterioles and then into the smaller capillaries. At the capillary level the blood passes into the venous system via venules that empty into the larger veins for return to the heart. The makeup of the different blood vessels reflects their role in the circulatory system (Huether, McCance, 1996).

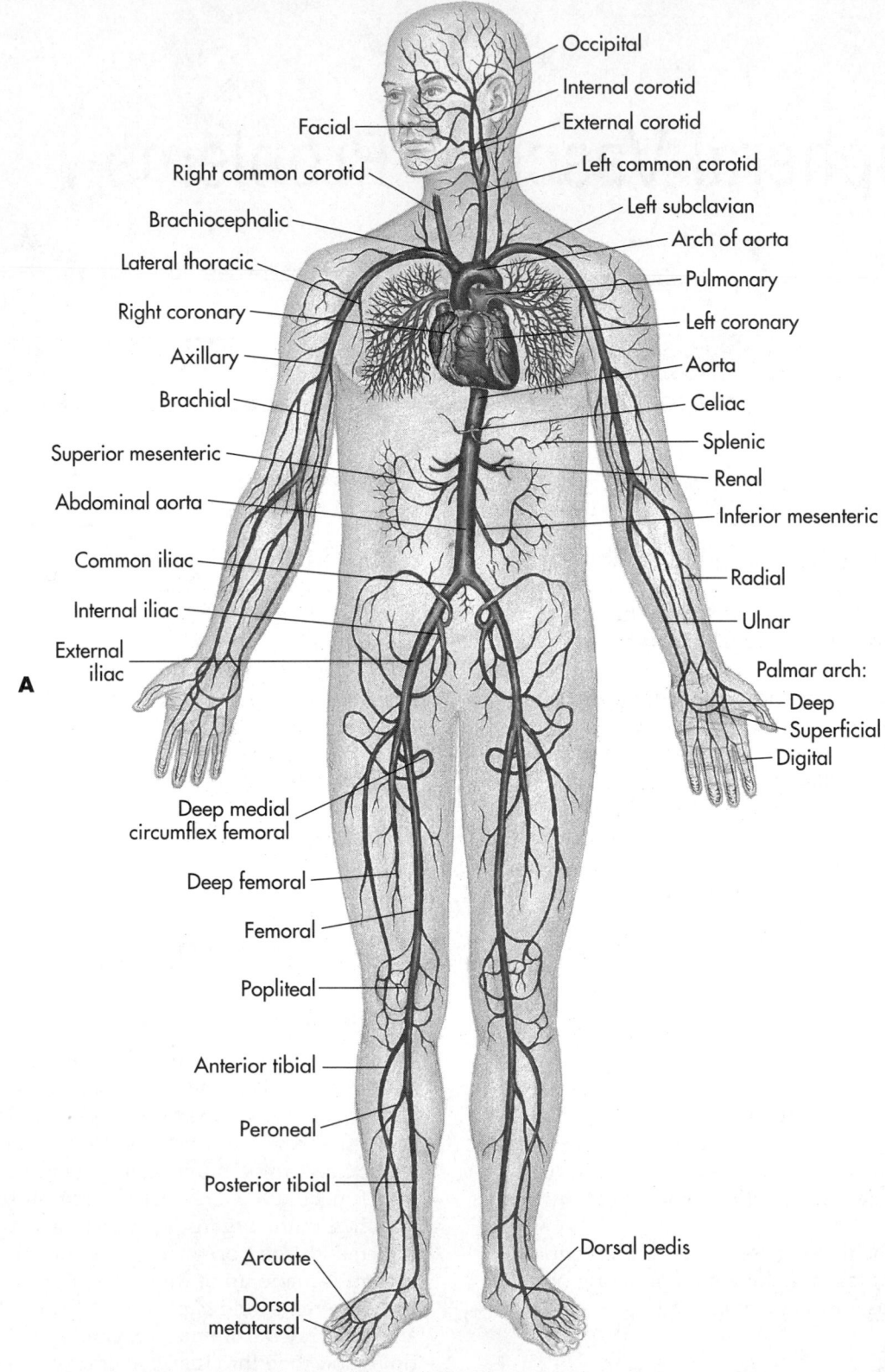

**Figure 24-1** Systemic circulation. **A,** Arteries. **B,** Veins. (From Seidel HM et al: *Mosby's guide to physical examination,* ed 3, St Louis, 1995, Mosby.)

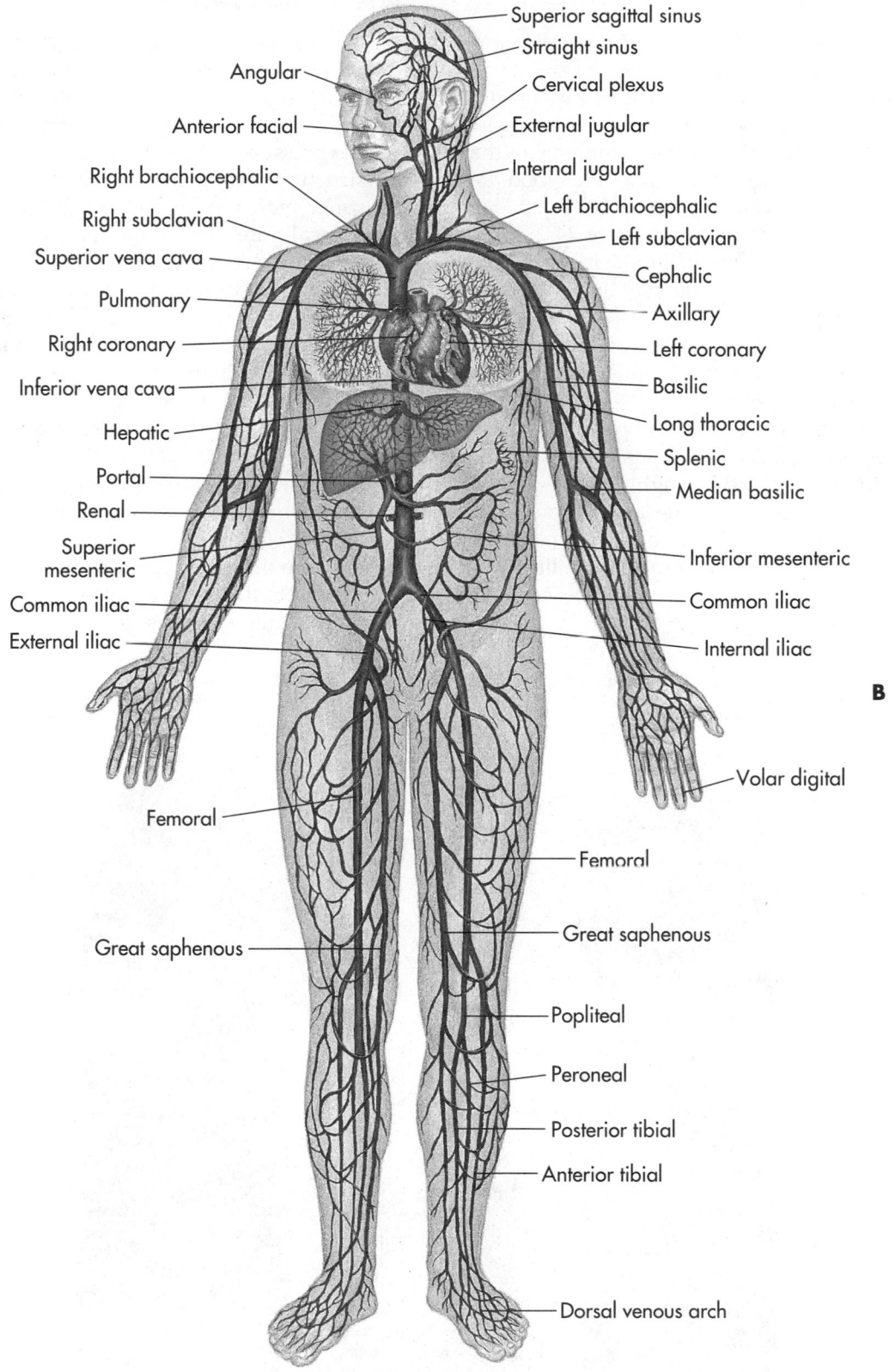

Superior sagittal sinus
Straight sinus
Angular
Cervical plexus
Anterior facial
External jugular
Right brachiocephalic
Internal jugular
Right subclavian
Left brachiocephalic
Superior vena cava
Left subclavian
Pulmonary
Cephalic
Right coronary
Axillary
Inferior vena cava
Left coronary
Hepatic
Basilic
Portal
Long thoracic
Renal
Splenic
Superior mesenteric
Median basilic
Common iliac
Inferior mesenteric
External iliac
Common iliac
Internal iliac
B
Volar digital
Femoral
Femoral
Great saphenous
Great saphenous
Popliteal
Peroneal
Posterior tibial
Anterior tibial
Dorsal venous arch

**Figure 24-1**   For legend, see opposite page.

## Veins and Venules

Veins are large-diameter, thin-walled vessels that return unoxygenated blood from the organs and tissues to the right side of the heart and that direct waste to organs for removal. Veins are more flimsy and better able to distend than arteries. There are also more veins than arteries. Because of the low pressure of the blood flow in the venous system, veins have a series of one-way valves along the internal lumina (Figure 24-2). These valves prevent the backflow of blood in the venous system that would result in pooling of the blood called **venous stasis.** When the valves become damaged or weakened, venous return is compromised and **varicosed veins** (swollen tortuous veins) can develop (Huether, McCance, 1996).

The largest veins are those that empty into the right atrium. The inferior vena cava empties blood from the lower part of the body into the right atrium, whereas the superior vena cava returns the blood from the upper body. The smallest branches of the veins are the venules, which collect blood from the capillary beds and direct it to the larger veins. Figure 24-1 depicts the major veins in the body.

## Arteries and Arterioles

The arterial system begins at the aorta, and branches from the aorta carry oxygenated blood to the organs and tissues. Because it receives blood flow directly from the left ventricle, the arterial system is under greater pressure than the venous system, and therefore the structure of the arterial system is different. Arteries are stiffer, more tensile, and less distensible than veins. Artery walls are thicker and made up of elastic tissue to allow them to stretch during the systolic phase of the heart and spring back during diastole (Huether, McCance, 1996) (see Figure 24-2). Large arteries, such as the aorta, also have some smooth muscle in their lumina. The smooth muscle makes these arteries responsive to autonomic nervous system stimulation.

The branches of the arteries, or arterioles, have lumina made up mostly of smooth muscle with little elastic tissue. Arterioles are very receptive to stimulation of the autonomic nervous system and respond by constricting or dilating. This function of the arterioles makes them the major controller of blood pressure and blood flow to the organs and tissues of the body. Constriction of the arterioles decreases blood flow to tis-

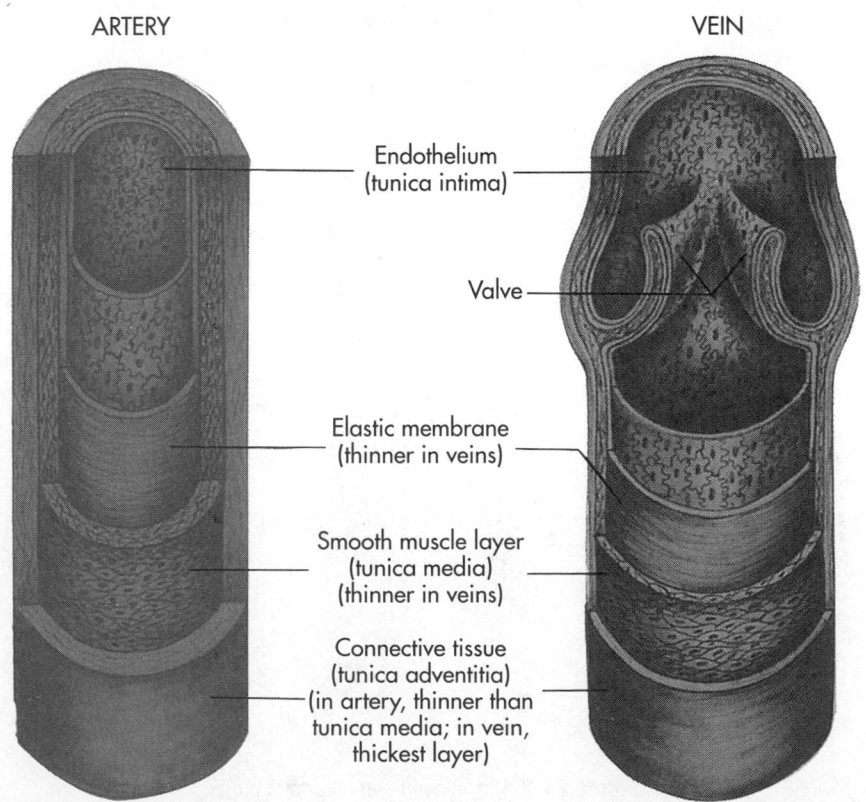

ARTERY                    VEIN

Endothelium
(tunica intima)

Valve

Elastic membrane
(thinner in veins)

Smooth muscle layer
(tunica media)
(thinner in veins)

Connective tissue
(tunica adventitia)
(in artery, thinner than
tunica media; in vein,
thickest layer)

**Figure 24-2** Structure of arteries and veins. (From Thompson JM et al: *Mosby's clinical nursing,* ed 4, St Louis, 1997, Mosby.)

sues, whereas dilation of the arterioles increases blood flow. Constriction of the systemic arterioles can increase the resistance to ventricular ejection and is called *afterload* (Wheeler, Brenner, 1995) (see Chapter 23).

## Capillaries

Capillaries are very thin-walled vessels at the terminal end of the arterial system. Capillaries are made up of endothelial cells with no elastic or smooth muscle tissue like the arterioles and arteries. The capillary bed of the body is very large, with a surface area larger than 100 football fields, and serves to remove waste and provide oxygen and nutrients at the cellular level (Wheeler, Brenner, 1995). Oxygen- and nutrient-rich arterial blood is supplied to the capillary beds by the arteriolar branches of the arteries, and blood containing waste is removed from the capillary system via the venules to be returned to the veins and then to the heart.

## Autonomic Nervous System Control

The sympathetic branch of the autonomic nervous system is the primary regulator of the venous and arterial systems. The parasympathetic nervous system does not play a major role in controlling the vascular system. The sympathetic nervous system has branches that extend into the smooth muscle of the vasculature, and alpha- and beta-receptors in the vessels respond to stimulation. When the alpha-receptors are stimulated, vasoconstriction occurs. When the beta-receptors are stimulated, vasodilation occurs (Huether, McCance, 1996).

## Baroreceptors

Baroreceptors in the aortic arch and the internal carotid artery react to changes in stretch or pressure in the arterial walls. When these receptors are stimulated by increased pressure in the arterial vessels, they signal the vasomotor control center in the brainstem, which suppresses the sympathetic nervous system, causing vasodilation to reduce the pressure. A decreased pressure in the arterial system creates a signal to stimulate the sympathetic nervous system, causing vasoconstriction to raise the pressure.

## Chemoreceptors

Special receptors in the aorta and carotid arteries respond to changes in the amount of oxygen, carbon dioxide, and pH of the blood. When the oxygenation, or pH, of the arterial blood falls, arterioles in the circu-

latory system constrict to increase the blood pressure. When the arterial carbon dioxide level increases, vasodilation occurs, causing a decrease in the blood pressure (Huether, McCance, 1996).

## Pressure and Blood Flow Regulation

The arterial blood pressure is the amount of pressure placed on the arterial wall by the blood as the ventricles contract (systolic pressure) and relax (diastolic pressure). The arterial blood pressure is adjusted constantly to maintain blood flow, or **perfusion,** to the organs and tissues. Changes in body position, muscle activity, and the volume of fluid in the vessels all require changes in blood pressure (Huether, McCance, 1996). The regulation of blood pressure is covered more extensively in Chapter 26. A fall in blood pressure in the arterial system for a prolonged time can reduce the oxygenation of the organs and tissues and cause cellular damage or death.

The amount of blood flow through the arterial system is determined by the amount of blood ejected from the heart (cardiac output), the size of the internal lumen of the artery, the degree of vasoconstriction and vasodilation of the arterioles, and the thickness of the blood. A decreased cardiac output will decrease the flow of blood through the arterial system and thus decreases the amount delivered to the tissues. Plaque buildup in **atherosclerosis** and stiffening of the arteries in arteriosclerosis (see Chapter 23) can alter the lumen size of the artery and reduce blood flow. The stimulation of the autonomic nervous system will create either constriction or dilation of the arterial system and impacts the overall flow of blood.

Arterial pulses are caused by the flow of blood through the arteries during ventricular systole. Pulses are palpable and sometimes visible at specific pulse point locations over the extremities and neck (see "Nursing Assessment"). The characteristics of the pulses in the arterial system can be altered by the amount of blood ejected by the heart with each beat (stroke volume), the dilation or constriction of the artery, and the thickness or viscosity of the blood (Seidel et al, 1995). For example, if the stroke volume is decreased or the artery is very constricted, the pulse will be weaker. If the artery is blocked, the pulse will be absent. Turbulent blood flow through an artery may be caused by partial occlusion of the lumen of the artery, and a **bruit** can be heard with a stethoscope.

The amount of pressure and blood flow in the venous system depends on many factors. The factors include the amount of fluid volume in the body, constriction or dilation of the veins themselves, the flow of blood through the arterial system, the compression of the veins by the skeletal muscles, pressure in the chest and abdominal cavity, and the pressures and flow of blood through the right side of the heart. If the overall blood volume increases, the veins can expand to accommodate the extra volume and provide a storage area for the excess volume. This storage capacity decreases the venous return to the heart and decreases the stress placed on the heart (Seidel et al, 1995). Constriction and dilation of the veins depend on stimulation of the autonomic nervous system. Lack of flow through the arterial system will decrease the blood flow through the venous system and prevent the forward flow of blood back to the heart. Lack of compression on the veins by skeletal muscle will decrease the forward flow of blood, causing venous stasis. Excess pressure in the thoracic cavity or the right side of the heart will also prevent venous return to the heart and will result in engorgement of veins and organs, such as the liver and gastrointestinal system.

## NURSING ASSESSMENT

Nursing assessment always begins with a complete history of the patient's current problem; however, many people with vascular disease are asymptomatic. Identification of patients at risk for either arterial or venous vascular compromise is an important assessment focus for the nurse. Early identification and preventive measures can delay or avert acute or chronic vascular problems. When patients are symptomatic, peripheral vascular diseases can cause a combination of pain, changes in skin temperature and color, changes in pulses, edema, and ulceration. The history and physical examination of a patient with particular complaints will assist in determining if the problem is primarily arterial or venous and if it is acute or chronic so that a plan of care can be developed. Examination of the other vascular systems, including the neurovascular system (carotid arteries, temporal arteries), coronary vascular system (heart valves, jugular veins), and renal vascular system (renal arteries), although usually included in a complete vascular examination, is covered separately in other chapters.

### Patient History
#### History of Current Illness

When a patient presents with a particular complaint, a review of seven aspects of the problem is needed to ensure that no important information is overlooked: (1) location, (2) quality (character), (3) quantity (severity), (4) chronology (the timetable of events, onset, and duration), (5) aggravating or alleviating factors, (6) associated symptoms, and (7) any treatment sought and its ef-

---

**BOX 24-1**

### VASCULAR ASSESSMENT: QUESTIONS TO ASK

Do you ever have swelling of your feet or ankles?
Do you ever have leg cramps or leg pain?
Do the pains or cramps happen when you exercise or when you lie down?
Does elevation of your leg increase or cause pain?
Do cool temperatures increase or cause pain?
How much exercise can you do before the pains start?
Have you noted any changes in the color of your skin?
Have you noted any change in the coolness or warmth of your skin?
Have you noted any sores on your skin, especially in your lower legs and feet?
Have you had any problems moving your arms or legs?
Do your legs ever "give out" or cause you to go limp?
Have you had any recent injury to your legs or arms?
Have you been unable to get up and around?
Have you had trouble with sexual function or ability to have erections?
Have you ever noted any swollen or painful veins in your legs?
Do you wear any special stockings or hose?
Are you required to stand for long periods?

---

fect. This information is especially important in patients who present with complaints of pain or discomfort.

Pain in the legs is a common symptom of lower extremity atherosclerosis and arterial occlusion. Whenever a patient complains of pain in the lower leg, arch of the foot, thigh, hip, or buttocks, disease of the arteries must be considered. Pain in the legs occurring during exercise is called **intermittent claudication.** Male patients who complain of buttock or thigh pain should also be asked about impotence because obstruction in the aortoiliac area (Leriche's syndrome) can cause intermittent buttock and thigh discomfort and sexual dysfunction (Wheeler, Brenner, 1995). In addition, it is important to ask all patients specific questions that may indicate underlying vascular problems (Box 24-1). Arterial disease will be discussed in greater detail in following sections.

### Past Health and Surgical History

Many illnesses can impact the vascular system or put the patient at risk for venous or arterial problems. The patient should be asked about illnesses that could affect the vascular system or increase the risk for underlying vascular disease. Chronic diseases, such as cancer and sickle cell anemia, increase the risk of venous thrombosis, as can recent acute illnesses, such as infections. Diabetes is a major risk factor for arterial disease. A medical history of coronary artery disease or neurovascular disease (e.g., strokes) is an indication of arterial disease that may also affect the peripheral arterial system. A history of hypertension (high blood pressure) or hyperlipidemia (high blood cholesterol levels) is also strongly associated with peripheral vascular disease. A history of clotting problems can also be a risk factor for venous or arterial thrombosis, and more information on this history will be needed. Other risk factors are included in the following section.

A complete review of systems may provide much needed information on symptoms that are signals of vascular disease. For example, the patient may not associate cold feet or leg cramps during walking as symptoms suggestive of arterial disease and may not report them unless specifically asked. Skin changes, presence of wounds, and limitations in activity can all indicate vascular disease and should be investigated further.

It is also important to determine if the patient has had any recent trauma, surgery, or prolonged periods of bed rest that could put him or her at risk for venous stasis or venous or arterial thrombosis. Pregnancy and the 3-month postpartum period is a time of increased risk for venous thrombosis, as is any illness or injury that will keep the patient bedridden for longer than 72 hours. Past hospitalizations or diagnostic workups for vascular disease or symptoms need to be explored, and any previous diagnostic studies should be obtained to serve as a baseline.

## Medications

A complete medication list should include the name, strength, and dosage of all medications taken by the patient, the patient's understanding of the purpose of the medications, and when the last dose was taken. The medication list should include prescription and over-the-counter medications. If the patient cannot give a complete list of medications, family members should be asked to bring the medications in for an evaluation. Medications such as estrogen or progestin replacement or oral birth control pills can increase the risk of deep vein thrombosis (DVT). Patients who are taking aspirin, other antiplatelet agents, or any anticoagulant may have arterial disease in their history or have been identified as high risk. Patients who use cocaine are at risk for aortic dissection.

## Family History

As with cardiac disease, a complete family history should be taken for patients with possible vascular

### TABLE 24-1

### Risk Factors for Peripheral Vascular Disease

| ARTERIAL DISEASE | VARICOSED VEINS | DEEP VENOUS THROMBOSIS |
|---|---|---|
| Major | Gender (female > male) | Damage to vessel |
|   Smoking | |   Trauma |
|   Hyperlipidemia | Family history |   Sugery |
|   Diabetes | Sedentary life-style | Clotting disorders |
| Other | Increasing age |   Sickle cell anemia |
|   Hypertension | Race (whites > African Americans) |   Polycythemia vera |
|   Obesity | |   Hypercoagulable states |
|   Family history | | Venous stasis |
| | |   Bed rest |
| | |   Immobility |
| | |   Sedentary life-style |
| | |   Dehydration |
| | | Cancer |
| | | Obesity |

disease. The focus of the family history for this patient population is to determine if venous disease (varicosed veins, venous clots), hypercoagulable states (thickening of the blood), arterial disease (arterial clots), coronary artery disease (heart attacks, angina), neurovascular disease (strokes), or aortic aneurysms have occurred in the immediate family (parents, grandparents, siblings). All these diseases or problems have a genetic component and increase the risk of vascular problems.

## Risk Factors

When assessing the vascular system, it is important to identify risk factors that, if present, indicate an increased chance of developing peripheral vascular disease or problems (Table 24-1). The risk factors for venous and arterial disease differ, but both should be investigated in a vascular assessment.

The risk factors for disease of the peripheral arteries are the same as those for the atherosclerosis associated with coronary artery disease (see Chapter 23), with smoking, hyperlipidemia, and diabetes as the major contributors. Hypertension, obesity, and familial history of peripheral vascular disease are also risk factors. Peripheral arterial disease increases with advancing age, with the highest risk in men aged 50 to 70 years and postmenopausal women (Cantwell-Gab, 1996). Stress, a risk factor for heart disease, may also be a risk factor for peripheral arterial disease, but it is still not known what the overall impact of stress is.

The risk factors for varicosed veins include female gender, family history, inactivity, obesity, advancing age, and being of white race (see Table 24-1). Females are more than four times more likely to have varicosed veins than males (Seidel et al, 1995). Pregnant women are especially at risk because of the weakening of the walls and failure of the valves caused by higher hormone levels. Women with mothers who have varicosed veins are at increased risk because of the genetic component. With aging the walls of the veins become less elastic and more prone to varicosities. Whites have more varicosed veins than African Americans because of their reduced numbers of valves in the veins of the lower extremities (Seidel et al, 1995). A history of prolonged periods of standing may increase the risk of varicosities. Having varicosed veins can also increase the risk of DVT.

There are three major categories of risk factors for DVT. These categories are known as Virchow's triad and include damage to the vessel, venous stasis, and

## TABLE 24-2

# Characteristics of Arterial and Venous Disease

| | CHRONIC ARTERIAL DISEASE | CHRONIC VENOUS DISEASE | VENOUS THROMBOSIS | ARTERIAL OCCLUSION |
|---|---|---|---|---|
| **Pain** | | | | |
| Location | Calf, foot, thigh, buttock, hip | Lower extremity | Over area of thrombosis | Distal to occlusion |
| Quality | Cramp, ache, sharpness | Aching, heaviness | Localized throbbing | Constant |
| Quantity | Increasing severity as disease progresses | | | Can be excruciating |
| Duration/timing | Claudication Pain at rest as disease progresses | After exercise or when dependent | | Acute onset |
| Aggravating factors | Cold, elevation | Dependency | Touch, movement | |
| Relieving factors | Rest | Rest but takes a while; elevation | Antiinflammatory agents, heat, elevation | |
| **Skin** | Cool, pale, shiny Blackened areas or digits Gangrene in advanced disease Thin, atrophied Ridged, thick nails | Warmer than normal Erythema Increased pigmentation Corona phlebectatia | Inflammation around the vein, with warmth, redness, fever | Discoloration Mottled Cyanotic Cold distal to occlusion |
| **Hair** | Loss over feet, legs | May be thinner on extremity | Not usually lost | Not usually lost unless chronic process preceded acute occlusion |
| **Edema** | Not usually; if edema, it is nonpitting | Dependent, can be pitting | Swelling unilateral >2-cm difference in extremities | Not usually |
| **Pulses** | Decreased or absent | Normal but may be obscured by edema | Normal | Decreased or absent |
| **Ulceration** | Very painful Pain improved with elevation Caused by trauma Irregular shape Covered in crust Around wound, tight, shiny, and itchy Develops rapidly Seen most often on toes Gangrene possible Minimal drainage | Painless unless dependent Ankle or lower leg Reddened, thickened, cobblestone looking Slow to develop Medium to large amounts of drainage No gangrene | Not usually | May occur if occlusion not treated |

clotting abnormalities (Stephen, Feied, 1995). Damage to the vessel can occur following infection, surgery, injury, or trauma. Venous stasis is common in patients on bed rest, who are immobile, or who have a very sedentary life-style. Clotting abnormalities can occur with sickle cell anemia, polycythemia vera, and various clotting protein deficiencies. Cancer can also increase clotting, as can the use of oral contraceptives and hormone replacements. The risk of clotting problems with hormones and birth control pills increases in patients who smoke.

## Physical Examination

Physical examination of the vascular system will include inspection, palpation, and auscultation skills. Percussion is not needed for the examination of the vascular system. Additional examination techniques may be done if the initial examination shows possible disease.

### Inspection

A complete inspection of the arms and legs is needed to identify abnormalities that could indicate problems with arterial blood flow or venous return to the heart. Skin color, texture, and condition; presence and amount of hair; extremity size; and patterns of the veins should be inspection points. Extremities should be compared for symmetric differences since vascular disease may be unilateral (one extremity only). The presence of swollen (varicosed) veins should be assessed with the patient standing (in the supine position varicosities may not be visible), and the whole expanse and both the back and front of the leg should be observed.

Unexpected findings, such as swelling, increased redness (erythema) or blue (cyanotic) color of the skin, pale skin, loss of hair over the lower legs, varicosed veins, and ulcers, can indicate peripheral vascular problems (Table 24-2). These areas of visible changes should be further assessed using palpation, auscultation, or both. If sores (ulcerations) are present, further questioning should be done to assist in determining if the ulcer is related to venous stasis or arterial insufficiency (Box 24-2). Long-term skin changes, such as increased roughness and pigmentation, are signs of prolonged venous insufficiency.

### Palpation

Examination of the vascular system should include palpation of all the peripheral pulses to determine the presence and quality of arterial pulsations. The arterial pulses routinely checked are the radial, femoral, popliteal, dorsalis pedis, and posterior tibial—the ones closest to the surface of the body (Figure 24-3). When palpating pulses, the right and left sides should be palpated at the same time if possible and compared. A scale is frequently used to record the pulse volume (Box 24-3). If repeated pulse checks will be needed, the nurse should use a pen to mark the skin over the area

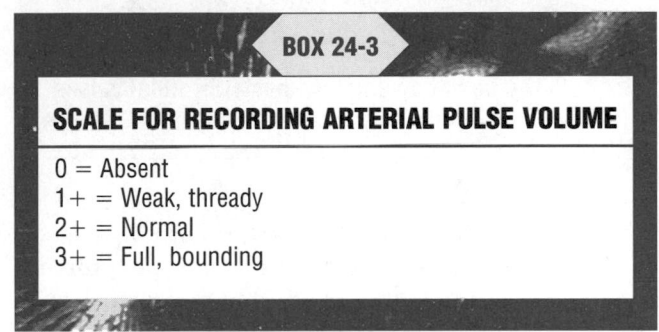

**BOX 24-3**

**SCALE FOR RECORDING ARTERIAL PULSE VOLUME**

0 = Absent
1+ = Weak, thready
2+ = Normal
3+ = Full, bounding

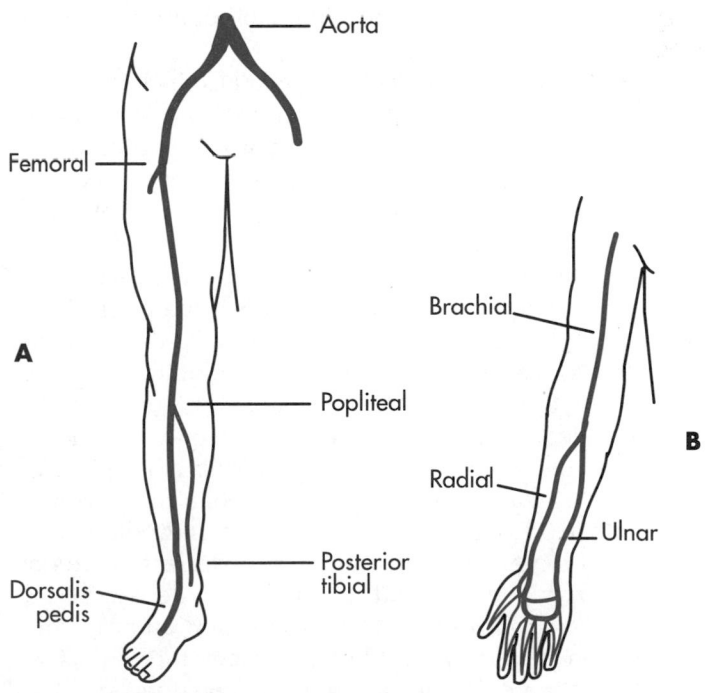

**Figure 24-3  A,** Arterial pulse points in the lower extremity. **B,** Arterial pulse points in the arm. Radial and ulnar pulses connected by vascular arches.

**BOX 24-2**

**QUESTIONS TO ASK ABOUT ULCERS**

What did the sore look like when you first noted it?
What do you think started the sore?
How long did it take for the sore to form?
How painful is the sore?
Have you ever had this type of sore before?

with the strongest pulsation. This mark will allow others to readily find the area for palpation. Weak or thready pulses can indicate low cardiac output, hypovolemia, or decreased flow through the artery because of partial occlusion. Bounding or full pulses can be seen with increased cardiac output, such as after exercise, or with volume overload. Absent pulses can occur with severe decreased cardiac output and with complete arterial occlusion. Absent pulses could signal severe problems and should be more thoroughly evaluated. Assessment of these pulse areas should be done with a Doppler device to determine if any arterial flow is occurring. Any area of decreased or absent pulses should be auscultated with a stethoscope for the presence of a bruit (see below). A determination of the heart rate and regularity can also be accomplished during palpation of the arteries (see Chapter 23).

## NURSE ALERT

**The dorsalis pedis and posterior tibial pulses in the feet may be absent in some well people.**

When palpating pulses, an abnormal palpable vibration (thrill) may be noted. Thrills indicate turbulent blood flow through the artery and can signal arteriosclerosis or atherosclerosis. Any area with a palpable thrill should be auscultated with the bell of the stethoscope to determine if the vibrations are audible (bruits) (Seidel et al, 1995).

Palpation of the vascular system also includes a determination of the **capillary refill** of the extremities. This part of the assessment is important, particularly if the nurse finds any color changes on inspection or pulse abnormalities when the pulses are palpated. Capillary refill can indicate the adequacy of the arterial flow into the extremity. Capillary refill is assessed by elevating the patient's extremity above the level of the heart and pressing on the nail bed or tip of the toe or finger to cause blanching (white coloration) as the blood is forced out of the capillary. When the pressure is relieved, the nurse should watch for and time the return of color to the blanched area. With normal perfusion, the area should return to the preblanching color in less than 3 seconds (Seidel et al, 1995). A capillary refill time of more than 3 seconds signals decreased arterial capillary blood flow and can occur with decreased cardiac output, peripheral arterial occlusion, and vasoconstriction caused by a cold room temperature.

Palpation of the aorta should also be done to determine any enlargement that could indicate bulging of the aorta (aneurysm). The nurse should press deep

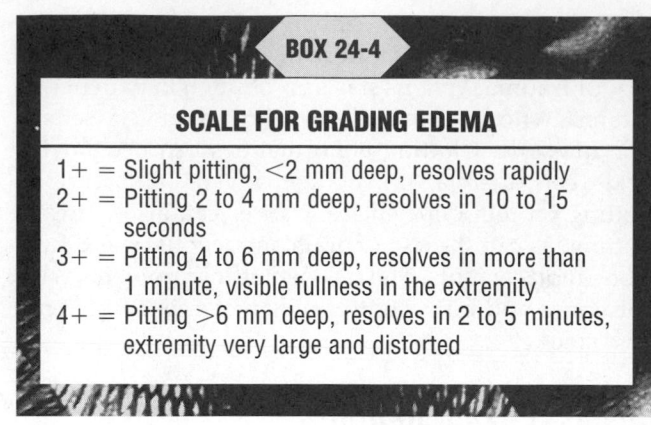

**BOX 24-4**

### SCALE FOR GRADING EDEMA

1+ = Slight pitting, <2 mm deep, resolves rapidly
2+ = Pitting 2 to 4 mm deep, resolves in 10 to 15 seconds
3+ = Pitting 4 to 6 mm deep, resolves in more than 1 minute, visible fullness in the extremity
4+ = Pitting >6 mm deep, resolves in 2 to 5 minutes, extremity very large and distorted

into the middle of the abdomen above the umbilicus with hands on each side of the midline and feel for the aortic pulsation (Seidel et al, 1995). Normally the pulsation may be felt in an anterior direction. If an aortic aneurysm is present, the pulsation will be felt in a lateral direction.

The skin should be palpated for temperature and edema during a vascular examination, particularly in any areas with visible changes in color or pulses. The nurse can check the temperature using the back of the hand and compare side to side. Coolness of an extremity is often felt with arterial disease, and increased warmth can indicate venous insufficiency or inflammation. Any edema noted on inspection should be palpated to determine if the area will indent or pit when pressed for several seconds. The shins and areas below the ankles are common sites for edema in patients with venous insufficiency and should be compressed even if edema is not noted on inspection. Edema may be present with volume overload, malnutrition, heart failure, and lymphatic or venous insufficiency. The edema of vascular insufficiency is usually pitting, as is the edema caused by heart failure (Box 24-4). Any edema associated with arterial disease is normally not pitting, and the edema seen with lymphatic system problems (see Chapter 27) is firm and nonpitting with dimpling and roughness of the overlying skin. DVT can cause swelling of the affected area resulting in unilateral edema (Seidel et al, 1995).

## NURSE ALERT

**If the nurse finds unilateral edema on examination, venous thrombosis of a large vein should be suspected.**

If any varicosities are noted on inspection, they should be evaluated for tenderness or thickness, espe-

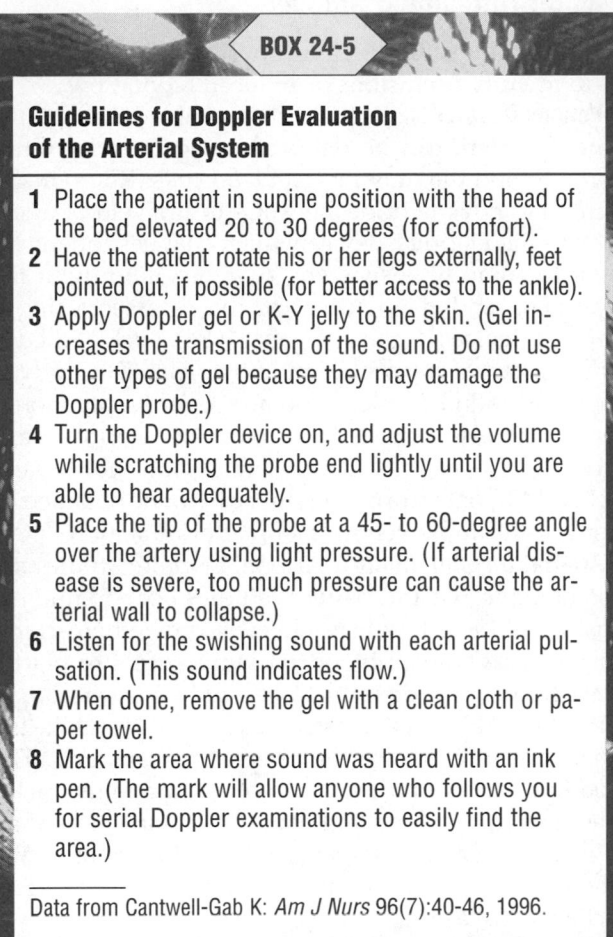

Data from Cantwell-Gab K: *Am J Nurs* 96(7):40-46, 1996.

**BOX 24-5**

**Guidelines for Doppler Evaluation of the Arterial System**

1  Place the patient in supine position with the head of the bed elevated 20 to 30 degrees (for comfort).
2  Have the patient rotate his or her legs externally, feet pointed out, if possible (for better access to the ankle).
3  Apply Doppler gel or K-Y jelly to the skin. (Gel increases the transmission of the sound. Do not use other types of gel because they may damage the Doppler probe.)
4  Turn the Doppler device on, and adjust the volume while scratching the probe end lightly until you are able to hear adequately.
5  Place the tip of the probe at a 45- to 60-degree angle over the artery using light pressure. (If arterial disease is severe, too much pressure can cause the arterial wall to collapse.)
6  Listen for the swishing sound with each arterial pulsation. (This sound indicates flow.)
7  When done, remove the gel with a clean cloth or paper towel.
8  Mark the area where sound was heard with an ink pen. (The mark will allow anyone who follows you for serial Doppler examinations to easily find the area.)

over the middle of the abdomen about 2 cm above the umbilicus (Seidel et al, 1995). Auscultation of other arteries, such as the renal arteries, carotid arteries, and temporal arteries, is discussed in other Chapter 23.

## Doppler Ultrasonography

Using a **Doppler** device to listen for arterial blood flow is another technique that may be required during a vascular evaluation. Dopplers are transcutaneous (through the skin) ultrasound devices that can detect blood flow at various levels. The stronger the Doppler (measured in megahertz—the lower the number, the stronger the Doppler), the deeper it will detect flow. Common bedside Doppler devices are usually 10 MHz and can be used with superficial vessels, such as the radial or dorsalis pedis (Cantwell-Gab, 1996). Doppler use is outlined in Box 24-5.

When using a Doppler device to detect flow of blood, the nurse will hear a swishing sound if flow is present. Sensitive devices can detect flow even in advanced arterial disease. The nurse should remember that the presence of sound using the Doppler device indicates that flow is present; it does not, however, gauge the adequacy of the flow. If flow is heard on one examination and is not heard on following examinations, the nurse should document this finding and notify the physician.

### NURSE ALERT

The presence of sound using a Doppler device for arterial auscultation indicates flow is present. It does not mean the flow is adequate.

cially in any areas with visible redness. Tenderness, thickening, or redness over a superficial vein may indicate **thrombophlebitis** (inflammation and clotting in the vein). Thrombophlebitis can occur in both upper and lower extremities and may be the result of intravenous infusions in upper extremities. Palpation of the veins should be completed while the patient is standing if possible, since veins may become tortuous and more visible when the extremities are dependent.

## Auscultation

Auscultation of the vascular system is focused on using the bell of the stethoscope to listen for humming or swishing sounds (bruits) over the arteries. The presence of bruits can indicate occlusion or narrowing of the artery lumen or bulging of the artery walls (aneurysm). The nurse should listen over all the peripheral arteries and the abdominal aorta and especially closely over those arteries that had diminished pulses, absent pulses, or palpable thrills. Auscultation of the aorta should be done with the stethoscope placed

## Diagnostic Studies
### Laboratory Studies

Many laboratory tests are used for collecting data in patients with vascular disease. These tests may focus on providing baseline data or on monitoring medications such as anticoagulants (heparin or warfarin [Coumadin]) or antiplatelet agents. Specific tests may also be ordered to rule out coagulation abnormalities that lead to hypercoagulable states and increased risk of thrombosis or to identify risk factors that lead to atherosclerosis, such as hyperlipidemia.

### Coagulation Studies

Because many patients with vascular disease are at risk for or have had a thrombotic insult, the use of anticoagulation and antiplatelet therapies is common. Coagulation studies include platelet count, prothrombin time (PT) with international normalized ratio (INR), partial thromboplastin time (PTT), activated partial thromboplastin time (APTT), activated clotting time, fibrinogen level, thrombin time, and recalcification time. The PTT is used to monitor heparin therapy, and the PT with INR is used to monitor Coumadin therapy. These studies are done before the use of anticoagulants and thrombolytic agents to determine the baseline levels and are repeated frequently to determine the response to and need for adjustments in the therapy.

The studies used to identify clotting abnormalities depend on the patient and the individual situation. Some of the most common tests include antithrombin III (AT III), protein C, protein S, and fibrinogen levels. Deficiencies in any of these important clotting system substances can increase the clotting activity of the blood and cause thrombi to form.

## Risk Factor Analysis

Atherosclerosis is the underlying pathologic process in arterial vascular disease, and the patient's risk factors are important to detect in order to plan for reduction. Common laboratory tests for risk factors are serum cholesterol, lipoprotein, and triglyceride levels (see Chapter 23).

## Radiographic Examination

Numerous radiographic tests are available to identify abnormalities of the aorta. These examinations include x-rays, computed tomography (CT) scans, and magnetic resonance imaging (MRI) scans.

**X-ray examination.** Abdominal and chest x-rays can detect enlargement of the aorta in aortic aneurysm, and many aneurysms are detected on routine examinations and with x-ray scans. The chest x-ray scan can show a widened mediastinum or widened thoracic aorta that would be suggestive of thoracic aneurysm. An abdominal film can show calcifications in the abdominal aorta and widening common with abdominal aortic aneurysm. Calcifications can also be seen in the large vessels of the arterial system and would indicate an atherosclerotic process with calcified plaques.

**CT and MRI scans.** The CT and MRI scans are usually used to accurately determine the size of an aneurysm in the aorta. The presence of thrombus formation can also be seen using CT and MRI. These studies may be used following a suspicious x-ray to confirm the presence of the aneurysm and determine the severity. They can also be used to detect thrombi in the vascular system.

## Doppler Ultrasound Studies

Doppler studies can be done on the veins or the arteries to identify occlusions or reduced blood flow.

**Venous Doppler studies.** The flow of blood through the venous system can be detected using Doppler ultrasound to find the moving red blood cells (RBCs) in the vein. The movement of the RBCs in the vein bounces back to the Doppler device, which changes the movement to an audible swishing type of sound. Both the superficial and deep veins can be assessed using a Doppler device (Pagana, Pagana, 1996). Lack of the venous sound means occlusion of the vein. The study is noninvasive and painless, and no special preparation is needed. Duplex Doppler and color flow Doppler variations of the venous Doppler study are newer and yield additional information that cannot be obtained as easily with simple venous Doppler examination.

**Arterial Doppler studies.** Arterial Doppler studies are also noninvasive and painless studies done to find occlusions of the arterial system caused by atherosclerosis. In these studies blood pressure cuffs are placed over the lower extremity to be studied at the thigh, calf, and ankle and inflated and deflated while the blood pressures along the artery are measured. The blood pressures of the legs are compared to the blood pressures in the arms and should not vary more than 20 mm Hg (Pagana, Pagana, 1996). Alterations in the blood pressure measurements below normal indicate occlusive disease.

The arterial Doppler ultrasound is also used to calculate the ankle-brachial index (ABI). The ABI is the ratio of the systolic blood pressure in the ankle to the systolic blood pressure in the arm and is used to measure the degree of arterial disease. In normal people with no arterial disease the ankle blood pressure is the same or a little higher than the arm (brachial) blood pressure, so a calculation of the ratio would be greater than 0.85. In arterial disease the ankle systolic pressure is lower that the arm systolic pressure and the ABI will be less than 1. An ABI of 0.5 to 0.95 indicates mild to moderate arterial insufficiency, and intermittent claudication usually occurs. With an ABI below 0.5 the disease is more severe and pain at rest is common. ABIs below 0.25 usually indicate severe arterial disease and ischemia with possible tissue loss (Cantwell-Gab, 1996). ABIs are usually measured and calculated in the vascular laboratory and do not require any special preparation or poststudy care.

Some patients will have normal ABIs and arterial pressures at rest, and they require ABIs and pressure measurements before and after exercise to identify arterial occlusion (Santilli, Rodnick, Santilli, 1996). In this type of modified Doppler study, the patient has standard resting Doppler pressures taken and then exercises until claudication occurs. Postexercise Doppler pressures and ABIs are taken and compared to the pre-exercise pressures and ABIs.

Duplex Doppler ultrasound is a more extensive Doppler study that can be done on the arterial system. This study gives the Doppler signals to determine the flow patterns of the arteries, and in addition the duplex system produces a two-dimensional image of the artery. Duplex Doppler scanning can locate the level of stenosis more specifically and may be done instead of angiography (Cantwell-Gab, 1996). As with the other Doppler studies, duplex Doppler ultrasonography requires no special preparation or postprocedure care other than patient education.

## Angiography

Angiography is an x-ray study of the arteries using contrast dye. The dye is injected into the artery. This is used to trace the vascular system and determine if blood flow is normal. In angiography of the lower extremities, the dye is injected into a catheter placed in the femoral artery. Timed x-rays are taken frequently after the injection is given to track the flow of the dye through the arterial system. This type of study is important in identifying the exact location of arterial occlusion, the presence of lacerations or tears in the artery, and narrowing or aneurysm in the artery. Angiography is also used to map the arterial system, branches, and collateral circulation before operative revascularization. Angiography can be done electively or as an emergent procedure when complete blockage is suspected (Pagana, Pagana, 1996). Angiography is reserved for patients who are candidates for operative therapy.

Digital subtraction angiography is a more advanced form of computerized angiography that enhances the view of the arterial system using fluoroscopy images taken before and after contrast dye is injected. The preprocedure and postprocedure preparation and care and complications are the same as for standard angiography (Krenzer, 1995; Pagana, Pagana, 1996).

Patients undergoing contrast angiography should be questioned carefully about allergies, especially to iodine and shellfish, because some persons are sensitive to the dye. If the patient has any history of renal failure or renal insufficiency, intravenous fluid will be ordered before and after the procedure to prevent renal failure from the contrast dye. Preceding the examination, food usually is withheld from the patient to avoid nausea and vomiting, and a mild sedative may be given. These patients are usually fearful and apprehensive and need a great deal of education and reassurance. Patients should be informed that they may feel a hot flash during the dye injection and that they will need to keep the extremity straight and still for several hours after the test. The strength of the peripheral pulses should be assessed and documented and the location of the pulses marked on the skin before the procedure to provide a baseline for nursing assessment after the procedure (Pagana, Pagana, 1996).

Potential complications of angiography include allergic reactions and bleeding or thrombosis at the site. After the procedure, the patient should be monitored for bleeding or hematoma formation at the site of the injection, and vital signs, including blood pressure, should be monitored. Pulses distal to the injection site should be monitored for changes. The patient will be required to keep the extremity straight and still for several hours to prevent bleeding at the puncture site. Patients will be encouraged to drink fluids to prevent dehydration and promote diuresis to flush the dye out of the system. Any changes in pulse strength or skin color or temperature, any numbness of the extremity, or any signs of allergic reaction to the dye should be reported to the physician.

# PROBLEMS INVOLVING THE ARTERIES

## Aneurysm

When the wall of an artery becomes weakened from disease or injury, the artery may become distended in the weakened area. This distention is called an **aneurysm**. Aneurysms are usually defined as enlargements in the usual diameter of the artery to more than 1½ times normal (Wheeler, Brenner, 1995). Aneurysms can occur in any arterial system, including the cerebral arteries. This section focuses on aneurysms of the aorta.

The aorta is a very common place for aneurysm formation because of the constant stress on the vessel wall. Aortic aneurysms can be thoracic, thoracoabdominal, or abdominal. Thoracic aneurysms occur in the ascending and transverse portion of the aorta and may involve the aortic valve and the carotid, innominate, and subclavian arteries. Thoracoabdominal aneurysms involve the descending branch of the thoracic aorta from above the diaphragm to the renal arteries. Abdominal aneurysms are usually located below the renal arteries and make up the largest number of aortic aneurysms. Three fourths of all aneurysms involve the abdominal aorta (Wheeler, Brenner, 1995; Huether, McCance, 1996). Other more peripheral sites for aneurysm formation include the popliteal and femoral arteries.

Atherosclerosis is the most common cause of aortic aneurysms. Plaque formation causes erosion of the vessel wall, resulting in loss of elasticity, weakening, and distention. Cigarette smoking and hypertension are also common factors in aortic aneurysm development.

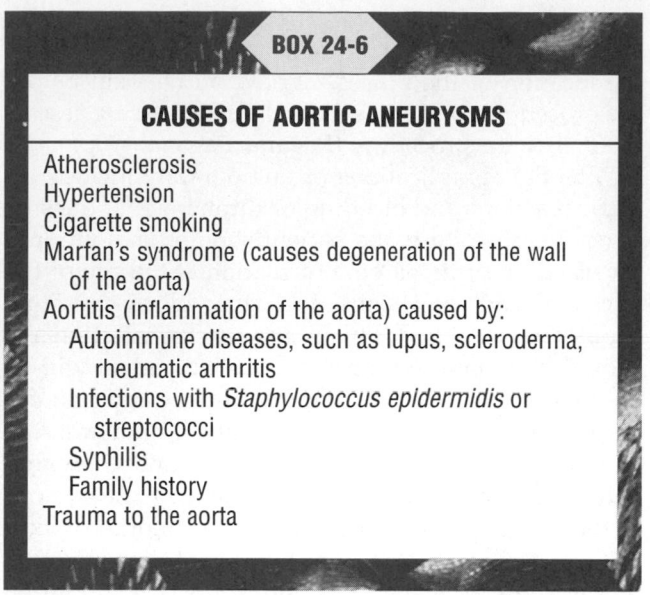

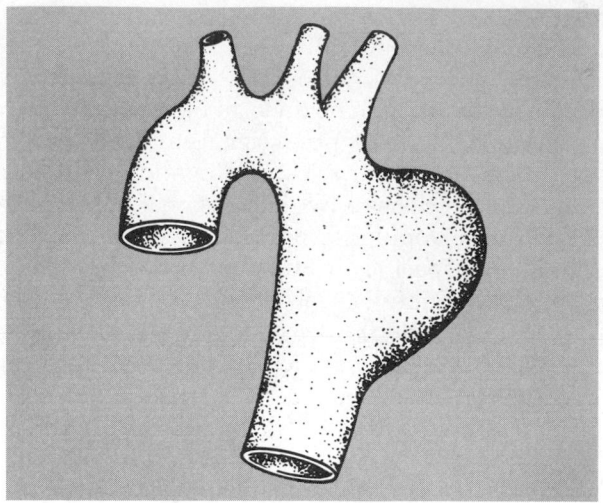

**Figure 24-5**   Saccular aneurysm.

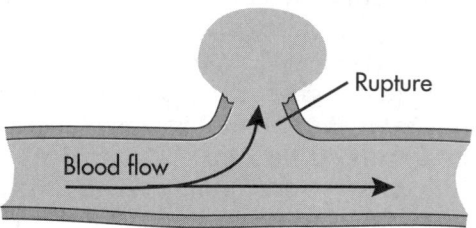

**Figure 24-6**   False aneurysm. (Modified from Lewis SM, Collier IC, Heitkemper MM: *Medical-surgical nursing: assessment and management of clinical problems*, ed 4, St Louis, 1996, Mosby.)

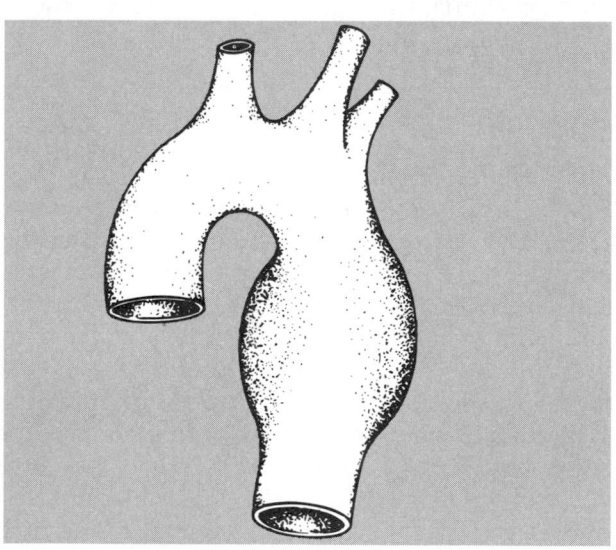

**Figure 24-4**   Fusiform aneurysm.

A family history of abdominal aortic aneurysm has been linked to increased risk for aortic aneurysm development, probably caused by a genetic defect (Dempsey, 1995). Aneurysms also increase with age and are more common in men than in women. Other less common causes of aneurysms include infections (e.g., syphilis), trauma, and autoimmune diseases (Box 24-6).

Aneurysms are classified according to the layers of the arterial wall involved and the shape of the outpouching. A true aneurysm involves weakening of all three layers of the arterial wall and can take on a fusiform shape or saccular shape. A fusiform aneurysm affects the entire circumference of the artery and

is similar to a partially blown up, long balloon (Figure 24-4). A saccular aneurysm involves only a portion of the artery wall and forms an outpouching on one side of the artery (Figure 24-5). Saccular aneurysms are usually the result of trauma. Over time, the distended part of an aneurysm fills with blood and gradually becomes larger and larger, until it has the appearance of a pulsating tumor.

A false aneurysm is not a weakening of the artery wall. It is a complete disruption of the wall with the bleeding contained by surrounding structures or tissues (Figure 24-6). False aneurysms are most frequently caused by trauma or infection and can be complications of surgery or invasive procedures involving the aorta. False aneurysms may appear to resemble a saccular aneurysm on examination.

## Assessment

**History and physical examination.** The symptoms of aneurysm are related to the structures, bones, or nerves that are compressed by the aneurysm, hypoperfusion of an organ, and leakage from the aneurysm. The specific symptoms can vary depending on the location of the aneurysm along the aorta. Most aortic aneurysms are asymptomatic, and their presence is detected through routine x-ray or ultrasound examination.

Thoracic aneurysms are usually not symptomatic. When symptoms are present, they may include diffuse chest hoarseness caused by pressure on the laryngeal nerve or difficulty swallowing because of pressure on the esophagus (Dempsey, 1995). If the aneurysm compresses the vena cava, it can cause distended neck veins and edema of the upper extremities. If the aneurysm presses on the pulmonary structures it can cause coughing and dyspnea (difficulty breathing) (Dempsey, 1995). If dissection of the ascending aorta occurs, the aortic valve may be weakened. The resulting regurgitation of blood back into the heart can cause heart failure. Myocardial infarction can also occur because of decreased blood flow through the coronary arteries.

Thoracoabdominal aneurysms enlarge and cause pressure in the thorax and abdomen. Symptoms include chest pain or shoulder pain. Perfusion to the kidneys, gastrointestinal system, or spinal cord can be decreased, causing renal failure, bowel ischemia, or paraplegia (Dempsey, 1995).

The majority of aneurysms are located below the diaphragm in the abdominal aorta. A common symptom of abdominal aortic aneurysms is back pain. A pulsating mass may be palpated in the upper or middle abdominal area. Bruits may be auscultated in the area around the aneurysm. These aneurysms can also contain emboli that become loosened and migrate to the peripheral arterial system, causing arterial occlusions.

Patients with known or suspected aneurysms should be evaluated for complications. Complications of aneurysms can be life threatening. Rupture of the weakened wall is the most common complication of an aortic aneurysm. If rupture occurs, the outcome and symptoms depend on the extent of the bleeding and the location of the rupture. If the rupture occurs in the posterior section of the aorta, the bleeding will occur in the retroperitoneal space (Dempsey, 1995). The bleeding may be slowed or stopped by surrounding organs. The patient will have severe back pain, and the pooling of blood in the retroperitoneal space may cause a blue discoloration of the back or sides, called *Turner's sign* (Dempsey, 1995). Blood loss causes the classic symptoms of shock, including tachycardia, hypotension, decreased urine output, changes in level of consciousness, and pale, cool, clammy skin.

If the rupture occurs along the front of the aorta, the bleeding progresses more rapidly and blood pools in the abdomen. Massive rapid blood loss occurs, and, frequently with ruptures of this type, the patient

bleeds to death before reaching the hospital. Symptoms of an anterior rupture of the aorta include the signs of shock and a distended tender abdomen.

Patients with known asymptomatic aortic aneurysms will undergo extensive evaluation to determine their readiness for surgery and the extent and size of the aneurysm. It is important for the nurse to thoroughly investigate the patient's past and present health history, including medical and surgical history, review of systems, current medications, risk factors, psychosocial condition, and support system. Assessing the patient's and family's understanding of the diagnostic studies, possible treatment options, and potential complications gives important assessment data needed to plan nursing interventions and teaching activities.

In addition, the nurse should complete a physical examination to detect any abnormalities and establish a baseline for further nursing assessment done after surgery. Determining the quality of peripheral pulses and the functioning of organ systems, such as the kidneys, neurologic system, and gastrointestinal system, provides important baseline data for ongoing nursing evaluations. This information is crucial in preparing the patient and family for major surgery.

**Diagnostic studies.** Aneurysms are diagnosed and evaluated through imaging techniques such as x-ray, CT, or MRI scans, ultrasound examinations, and arteriograms (see previous section on diagnostic studies). Because most aneurysms are asymptomatic, they are usually found during routine studies or during a workup for another problem. Early detection and prompt intervention to prevent complications such as aortic rupture are important.

When a patient presents with pain of the chest and abdomen from an unknown cause, numerous studies may be done to rule out possible causes. These studies include x-rays, a 12-lead electrocardiogram (ECG), abdominal ultrasound, and laboratory tests. The murmur that is heard when aneurysms affect the aortic valve may be evaluated using an echocardiogram. Once an aneurysm is found, further evaluation is done to determine the extent and size.

A known stable aneurysm is evaluated to determine the size of the dilation (measured in centimeters) and whether a thrombus is present in the dilated area (Dempsey, 1995). This is usually accomplished through a CT or MRI scan. The aneurysm is also assessed using an arteriogram to determine how far it extends along the length of the aorta and what other branching vessels are involved. If the aneurysm has ruptured or is leaking and the patient is unstable, these studies are not performed. Emergent or immediate surgery must be done.

Patients who are being considered for surgery to repair the aneurysm undergo numerous laboratory and diagnostic studies to identify other underlying diseases, including arterial disease, pulmonary disease, and cardiac disease. The presence of other problems may increase the risk of surgery and delay or prevent the surgical intervention.

## Medical and Nursing Interventions

The outcome of the diagnostic studies and the evaluation of the size and extent of the aneurysm determine the treatment method. The primary decision is whether the patient will be treated surgically or medically. The overall goal of intervention for an aneurysm is to prevent rupture or leakage of blood.

During the diagnostic workup and decision-making process, the nurse must provide teaching regarding the diagnostic procedures and findings, provide support for the patient, and assist the patient and family in dealing with the anxiety of an uncertain prognosis and treatment plan. The nurse assists with the preparation of the patient for each diagnostic study and the follow-up care after the procedure. Once the treatment decision is made, the nurse focuses on preoperative and postoperative interventions or nonsurgical interventions.

## Surgical Intervention

Decisions regarding surgery are made based on the size and location of the distention, the presence of signs and symptoms, and the risk of surgery for the patient. In patients who are symptomatic or in cases of rupture or leakage, immediate surgery is the treatment of choice. However, controversy exists regarding the indications for surgery in patients who are asymptomatic. In these cases, the size and location of the aneurysm and the patient's risk for surgery are the deciding factors in whether surgery is done.

In general, the larger the aneurysm, the more the risk of rupture, but guidelines vary regarding the size an aneurysm must be before surgery is indicated. Thoracic aneurysms usually require prompt surgical treatment to prevent complications, especially if the aneurysm is enlarging or at risk of rupture. Aneurysms in the distal aorta may be controlled medically before surgical intervention is required (Dempsey, 1995). If surgery is chosen, the studies done during the diagnostic workup will be used to decide the surgical approach to be used and the preoperative preparation needed to get the patient in the best condition for surgery.

**Surgical techniques.** Several surgical procedures for aneurysms are available. Any plaque or thrombus in the aorta is removed, and the weakened area of the aorta is replaced, repaired, or supported. Some aneu-

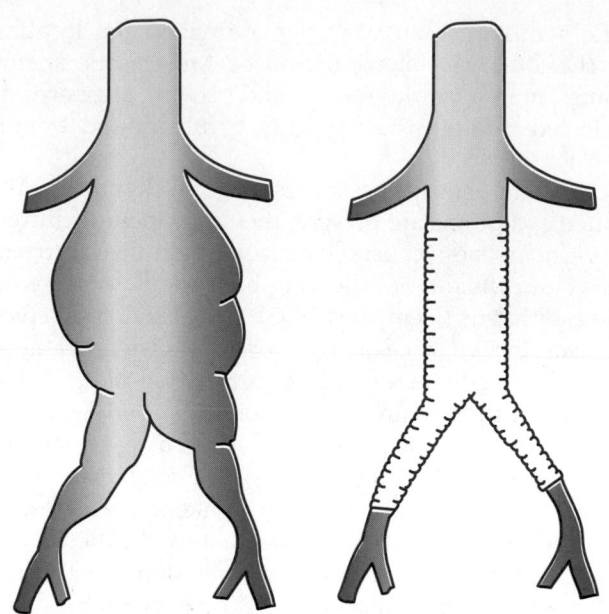

**Figure 24-7** Resection of a fusiform aneurysm with a bifurcated synthetic graft. (Modified from Lewis SM, Collier IC, Heitkemper MM: *Medical-surgical nursing: assessment and management of clinical problems*, ed 4, St Louis, 1996, Mosby.)

rysms can be repaired by removing the distended part of the vessel and either suturing the vessel back together or using a patch graft to cover the area. This technique is most often used with saccular aneurysms. Fusiform aneurysms can be repaired by removing the section of the aorta that is distended and anastomosing the ends of the aorta back together or by using a synthetic graft to replace the weakened section (Figure 24-7). If the aneurysm is in the abdominal aorta and extends into the iliac arteries, a bifurcated graft can be used (see Figure 24-7).

Grafts can also be placed inside or over an incised fusiform aneurysm (Figure 24-8). When grafts are placed over the aneurysm, they provide a stent or extra support for the weakened aortic wall, giving it strength. Grafts are sewn inside the aortic wall when the abdominal aorta is being repaired. This technique prevents the graft from rubbing on adjacent organs and causing erosions.

All these techniques require an open surgical procedure using either a chest (thoracotomy) or an abdominal approach and require clamping of the aorta (called cross clamping) proximal (above) and distal (below) to the aneurysm (Dempsey, 1995). Clamping the aorta increases the risk of clotting so anticoagulation with heparin is usually done. Clamping of the aorta also reduces blood flow to the arterial branches below the clamping site and increases the risk of damage to the

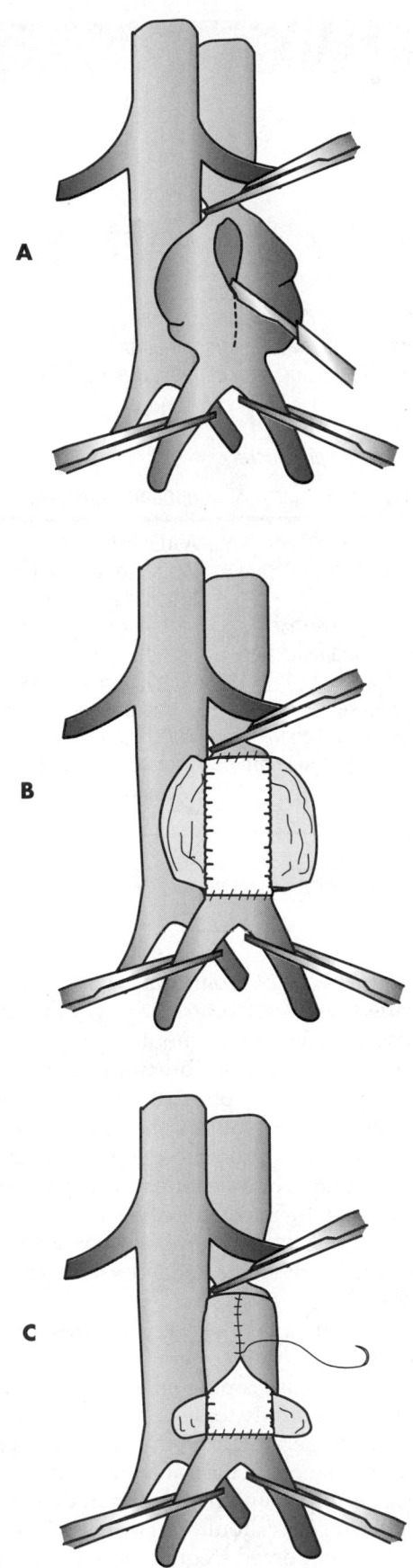

organs distal to the aneurysm. General complications of aortic aneurysm repair are included in Table 24-3.

Specific areas along the aorta require special surgical techniques and postoperative considerations (see Table 24-3). Thoracic aneurysms, especially those in the ascending aorta and aortic arch, can only be repaired if the heart is stopped and cardiopulmonary bypass is used to divert blood around the area being repaired (Dempsey, 1995). Ascending aorta repairs also put the cardiac and brain circulation at risk and can cause complications such as stroke and myocardial infarction. Abdominal aneurysm repairs can compromise perfusion to the gastrointestinal system, kidneys, and spinal cord. When the aorta is clamped above the renal arteries, renal failure is a possible complication. Intraoperative hypothermia allows the aorta to be clamped for longer periods without permanent damage, but hypothermia itself increases the risk for postoperative complications (Dempsey, 1995).

Some aneurysms are now being repaired using an experimental procedure called *endoluminal graft (ELG)*. In this procedure, the patient does not undergo an open resection of the aorta (Hill, 1995). The graft is threaded into the aorta through the femoral artery in the groin. The graft is then placed inside the aneurysm to exclude it and cause the aneurysm to shrink.

All patients undergoing repair of an aortic aneurysm are cared for postoperatively in the intensive care unit (ICU), where close monitoring and specialized equipment are available. General anesthesia is used during the intraoperative period, and nerve blocks may be done or an epidural catheter left in place for pain control in the postoperative period (Hill, 1995). Every effort is made to conserve blood in the patient undergoing aortic aneurysm repair. Cell-saving devices are used during and after surgery to allow autotransfusion of lost blood and prevent the need for donated blood.

**Surgical preparation.** Except in emergent situations requiring immediate surgery, preoperative preparation includes identification and management of any preexisting condition (e.g., pulmonary disease, diabetes, and hypertension) that will increase the patient's risk during and after surgery. Coagulation problems, anemia, malnutrition, and any other

---

**Figure 24-8**  Surgical repair of an abdominal aortic aneurysm. **A,** Incising the aneurysmal sac. **B,** Insertion of synthetic graft. **C,** Suturing native aortic wall over synthetic graft. (Modified from Lewis SM, Collier IC, Heitkemper MM: *Medical-surgical nursing: assessment and management of clinical problems,* ed 4, St Louis, 1996, Mosby.)

---

**TABLE 24-3**

## Surgical Repair of Aortic Aneurysms

**Complications of Aortic Aneurysm Repair**

Disruption in graft patency

Hemorrhage *because of anticoagulation*

Organ ischemia: depends on site; *caused by clamping of the aorta and reduced blood flow to distal organs; hypothermia used to reduce tissue ischemia by decreasing oxygen consumption*

Wound or graft infection, sepsis, poor wound healing

Pulmonary: infection, atelectasis, pneumonia; *caused by general anesthesia and abdominal or thoracic surgical incision*

Gastrointestinal: bleeding, ulceration, ileus, ischemia; *can be caused by stress, general anesthesia, clamping of aorta*

Cardiac: myocardial infarction; *can be caused by emboli from aorta, stress on the heart during and after surgery, preexisting coronary artery disease, aortic clamping*

Renal: acute renal failure; *caused by clamping of aorta above the renal artery, hypotension, emboli*

Neurologic: stroke, paraplegia *caused by clamping of aorta that compromises blood flow to spinal cord*

| ANEURYSM LOCATION | INCISION | USE OF BYPASS | SPECIAL COMPLICATIONS | NURSING CONSIDERATIONS |
|---|---|---|---|---|
| Ascending | Median sternotomy | Yes | Embolization resulting in stroke<br>Myocardial ischemia and infarction | Aortic valve may be replaced<br>Watch for arrhythmias<br>Monitor neurologic status |
| Arch | Median sternotomy | Yes | Embolization resulting in stroke<br>Myocardial ischemia and infarction | Watch for arrhythmias<br>Monitor neurologic status |
| Descending | Lateral chest wall | Maybe | Spinal cord ischemia<br>Pulmonary compromise | Watch peripheral neurologic and pulmonary status |
| Abdominal | Midline abdominal | No | Organ damage involving the kidneys, intestines, and spinal cord<br>Renal failure<br>Ischemic bowel<br>Paraplegia | Watch peripheral neurologic status, urine output, and gastrointestinal system |

Data from Hill EM: *AACN Clin Issues* 6(4):547-561, 1995; Dempsey E: Aortic aneurysms. In Urban N et al, editors: *Guidelines for critical care nursing*, St Louis, 1995, Mosby.

---

correctable problem should be controlled, if at all possible, before surgery. This may require that the surgery be postponed to optimize the patient's health and increase the chances for a good postoperative outcome.

Patients with aneurysms often have other arterial disease as well and may require management of carotid or coronary artery disease before the aortic aneurysm can be repaired. Patients with pulmonary disease or a smoking history may benefit from 2 to 4 weeks of bronchodilators, pulmonary physiotherapy, and smoking cessation (Dempsey, 1995). Patients with diabetes, hypertension, or congestive heart failure may need intensive medical management to optimize cardiac functioning and get chronic conditions well under control. Patients with renal impairment or insufficiency require special consideration and adequate hydration to prevent complications during dye studies and to maintain renal blood flow and perfusion before and following any surgical intervention.

Extensive teaching must be done with the patient and family in the preoperative phase. They should receive instruction regarding the surgical procedure, what to expect in the immediate postoperative phase and the ICU, the types of monitoring that will be done, how the patient will look after surgery, and the postoperative course. The patient should be taught how to complete coughing and deep breathing exercises and how to use a pillow to support the incision site. The patient should also be taught the use of incentive spirometry devices to promote deep inhalation and prevent pulmonary complications. The patient who has been advised to make life-style changes to improve the operative and postoperative risk will need instruction or to be given the needed resources to carry out these changes.

The prospect of major surgery is very stressful for the patient and family. The preoperative phase is an opportune time to discuss coping strategies and encourage the patient and family to develop a plan for the intraoperative, postoperative, and postdischarge phases. The nursing assessment of the patient's support system and resources is important in assisting in this plan. All questions and concerns should be addressed. Teaching may need to be reinforced frequently to ensure retention. Some surgical centers include a tour of the operating area and intensive care area for the patient and fam-

| BOX 24-7 | | NURSING PROCESS |
| --- | --- | --- |

## POSTOPERATIVE CARE: ANEURYSM

### ASSESSMENT

- Pulmonary status, including lung sounds, oxygenation, arterial blood gases (ABGs), pulse oximetry
- Peripheral circulation, pulse quality, color and temperature of extremity
- Vital signs, especially blood pressure
- Cardiac status: electrocardiogram (ECG), hemodynamic pressures, heart sounds, laboratory values
- Renal perfusion: urine output, daily weights, laboratory values
- Gastrointestinal functioning: bowel sounds, flatus, nasogastric tube
- Level of pain and adequacy of pain control method
- Skin: incision and invasive line sites, wound healing, skin breakdown
- Level of anxiety and coping ability

### NURSING DIAGNOSES
#### Actual

- Impaired physical mobility related to pain and presence of invasive lines and drains
- Anxiety related to unfamiliar surroundings, discomfort, and lack of understanding of procedures
- Pain related to tissue trauma during surgery

#### Potential

- Risk for ineffective breathing pattern related to incisional pain and immobility
- Risk for decreased cardiac output related to arrhythmias, heart failure, hemorrhage, and myocardial ischemia
- Risk for altered tissue perfusion related to graft occlusion or failure
- Risk for fluid volume deficit/excess related to blood loss, administration of intravenous fluids, and fluid shifting (third spacing)
- Risk for decreased cerebral perfusion related to intraoperative or postoperative embolism or obstruction of blood flow to the brain
- Risk for decreased renal perfusion related to intraoperative ischemia and hypotension

*Continued*

ily before surgery. Introducing the patient and family to health care workers and letting them see the waiting area, postanesthesia care area, and intensive care room can reduce the anxiety associated with the unknown. Many centers also encourage patients to donate their own blood to be stored for them if a blood transfusion is needed. This is only possible if the surgery is delayed for at least 1 month, to allow time for the body to replace the blood donated.

For the patient undergoing elective aortic aneurysm repair, much of the preoperative preparation may be done on an outpatient basis. The patient may not be admitted to the hospital until the morning of surgery. Important nursing interventions include ensuring all diagnostic studies done during the workup are available, collecting baseline vital signs and physical examination data, completing the preoperative skin preparation and shaving as instructed by the surgeon, and administering preoperative sedation and medications. The nurse should also review and reinforce the teaching that the patient received during outpatient preparation.

Following the procedure, the patient will have intravenous lines and an indwelling urinary catheter in place as well as a nasogastric tube (catheters and nasogastric tubes may be placed after anesthesia is begun). The patient may also require hemodynamic monitoring devices, such as a pulmonary artery catheter and an invasive arterial line for pressure measurement and blood sample collection. The patient may be on a mechanical ventilator for awhile immediately after surgery. If the chest is opened during surgery, the patient will have a chest tube (Hill, 1995). With all these lines and tubes, patients and families must be prepared for the way they will feel and look after surgery. The patient should also be instructed on the type of pain control he or she will be receiving. This can be a combination of nerve blocks, epidural analgesia, and continuous or patient-controlled intravenous analgesia.

**Postoperative care.** As described previously, during the immediate postoperative period patients are cared for in an ICU, with continuous ECG, oxygenation, and hemodynamic monitoring. They usually have numerous tubes and drains, as well as intravenous fluids, medications, and possibly a mechanical ventilator. The care and monitoring of a patient after aortic aneurysm repair can be complex and require continuous nursing vigilance. The nursing plan of care includes interventions to promote normal tissue perfusion to all organs, maintain adequate respiratory system and cardiac functioning, control pain and anxiety, maintain normal fluid balance, and monitor for and prevent complications (Box 24-7).

> BOX 24-7

## NURSING PROCESS

### POSTOPERATIVE CARE: ANEURYSM—cont'd

- Risk for gastrointestinal dysfunction, ischemia, bleeding, ileus
- Risk for infection related to surgical interventions and presence of graft and invasive lines

**NURSING INTERVENTIONS**

- Turn and position patient at least every 2 hours.
- Assist with activities of daily living (ADL) and comfort measures such as mouth care and bathing.
- Monitor for level of pain, and administer pain medications as directed.
- Encourage patient to splint the incision during turning and coughing.
- Administer pain medication 30 minutes before positioning and breathing exercises.
- Orient to environment, explain procedures and activities, and provide information frequently.
- Monitor level of anxiety, and implement strategies to reduce anxiety.
- Provide methods of communication if patient is intubated.
- Observe for signs of hypoxia, adventitious lung sounds, and increased effort or difficulty in breathing.
- Have patient turn, cough, and deep breathe every 2 hours (once mechanical ventilation is discontinued).
- Have patient use incentive spirometry every 2 hours (once mechanical ventilation is discontinued).
- Monitor hemodynamic pressures.
- Monitor vital signs, especially blood pressure.
- Administer fluids or blood products as directed.
- Keep blood pressure within parameters using vasodilators, sedatives, and quiet environment.
- Monitor cardiac rhythm continuously, and observe and treat arrhythmias.

- Evaluate heart sounds for murmurs.
- Monitor laboratory values, especially hemoglobin and hematocrit.
- Measure abdominal girth to detect distention.
- Observe for changes in peripheral pulses or extremity color and temperature.
- Observe for changes in level of consciousness, pupil size and reactivity, and motor and sensory ability.
- Monitor hourly intake and output, daily weight, and blood urea nitrogen (BUN) and creatinine levels.
- Administer fluids, diuretics, and other medications as directed.
- Observe for absence of bowel sounds, abdominal distention, and nausea and vomiting.
- Observe and record amount and color of drainage from nasogastric tube, and report bloody drainage.
- Maintain patency of nasogastric tube, attach to intermittent suction, and irrigate as needed to decompress stomach.
- Monitor for signs of infection: fever, increased white blood cell (WBC) count, and drainage or redness at incision or invasive line insertion site.
- Administer antibiotics as ordered.
- Use aseptic technique when caring for all tubes and drains.

**EVALUATION OF EXPECTED OUTCOMES**

- Progress toward previous level of functioning
- Pain controlled or reduced to tolerable level
- Anxiety reduced
- No complications related to surgical repair
- Normal tissue perfusion and organ function
- Complications identified and managed quickly

Promoting normal tissue perfusion is accomplished first through maintaining patency of the newly grafted or repaired aorta. Hemodynamic monitoring and frequent vital signs are essential nursing assessments in maintaining blood pressure and fluid volume status. Keeping the patient's mean arterial blood pressure within a specific range is an important nursing intervention. An elevated blood pressure can put pressure on the grafted area and cause bleeding or rupture, whereas a low blood pressure will decrease perfusion to vital organs and increase the risk of thrombus formation in the graft. Blood pressure is usually controlled by careful manipulations of vasoactive drugs, sedation, and quiet and rest to keep the blood pressure down. Fluid or blood product administration is used to keep the blood pressure up.

Peripheral perfusion to the extremities is closely watched during the postoperative period. In some cases the pulses in the lower extremities may be decreased or absent immediately following surgery because of spasms in the artery or vasoconstriction from hypothermia (Hill, 1995). As the patient is warmed and recovers from the initial intraoperative trauma, the pulses should return to their preoperative status.

In the preoperative phase all peripheral pulses should be assessed and marked with a pen so that comparisons can be done between the preoperative and the postoperative pulses.

As described in Table 24-3 the specific peripheral areas that can be compromised after aortic aneurysm repair depend on the location of the aneurysm and the position of the clamps during the surgery. The arterial system distal to the surgical site is always at risk, and pulses in all extremities should be checked and documented at regular and frequent intervals (usually every hour for the first 24 hours after surgery). Decreased pulse strength; cool, mottled, blue discoloration; or pain in any extremity should be reported. These changes may indicate an occlusion of the artery from a clot or plaque embolus. Arterial occlusion puts the tissue at extreme risk. Immediate intervention with surgical removal of the clot (called an *embolectomy*) may be needed (Hill, 1995). If the occlusion is not removed, the tissues will be hypoxic and necrosed and amputation may be needed.

Perfusion of the renal, neurologic, and gastrointestinal systems should also be monitored. Renal failure can occur because of clamping of the aorta above the renal arteries during surgery or because of emboli that escape from the aorta and lodge in the arterial blood supply to the kidneys (Hill, 1995). Intraoperative or postoperative hypotension and hypovolemia can also contribute to poor renal perfusion and renal failure. Monitoring of urine output and daily weights to assess for fluid retention or volume loss and careful monitoring of laboratory values, such as the blood urea nitrogen (BUN) and creatinine, are important nursing interventions to detect renal failure in the early stages. A decrease in the hourly urine output below 30 ml/hr for 2 hours with an intact and properly functioning indwelling urinary drainage system should be recorded and reported to the physician (Hill, 1995). Hematuria (blood in the urine) or changes in the color and clarity of the urine should also be reported. These may also indicate ischemic injury to the kidney.

The perfusion to the neurologic system may be decreased during surgical manipulation of the aortic aneurysm and can also occur because of intraoperative or postoperatic emboli, hypotension, and hypovolemia. If this occurs, a stroke or brain infarction may result. Peripheral neurologic deficits, such as paraplegia, can occur if the spinal artery is occluded or clamped during surgery (Hill, 1995). Assessing the neurologic status of the patient, including the level of consciousness, pupil response, and reactivity to light, and the peripheral motor and sensory responses is needed to detect neurologic impairment. Patients may also become confused as a result of pain, lack of sleep, medications, change from their familiar environment,

and preexisting dementia that is exacerbated by acute illness. Any change from the preoperative neurologic functioning should be completely investigated to rule out organic causes.

Bowel ischemia and infarction can result from surgical manipulation of the bowel, reduction in blood flow during aortic cross clamping, and postoperative emboli (Hill, 1995). The nurse must be alert for signs of bowel ischemia, including abdominal pain, tenderness, and distention. Bloody stools or guaiac-positive stools, and, in some cases, diarrhea, can also signal ischemia. If left untreated, bowel ischemia can result in sepsis and death. The treatment of bowel necrosis is resection of the dead areas of bowel.

Promoting adequate respiratory function guides another set of nursing interventions. Initially the patient may be breathing with a mechanical ventilator. As the patient recovers from the anesthesia and regains the ability to breathe without assistance, the tube and mechanical device are removed. As in all patients with thoracic or abdominal incisions, promoting lung expansion and preventing atelectasis, pneumonia, and respiratory failure are important goals. The nursing interventions of coughing, turning, deep breathing, and use of incentive spirometry promote adequate respiratory functioning. The nurse must teach the patient these techniques, along with splinting of the incision, and encourage positioning and early mobility to prevent severe respiratory complications.

Cardiac functioning is also a focus of nursing intervention. The cardiac system may be under great stress following surgery. The surgical techniques used in thoracic aneurysm repair, the use of cardiopulmonary bypass in some procedures, and the possibility of preexisting coronary disease place the patient at risk for myocardial ischemia, myocardial infarction, arrhythmias, and heart failure (Hill, 1995). The patient will have continuous ECG monitoring and hemodynamic lines that can provide valuable data about the heart. The nurse should be alert for arrhythmias, signs of heart failure (elevated hemodynamic pressures, edema, decreased cardiac output), and signs of myocardial ischemia (chest pain and ECG changes).

Alterations in fluid volume can have detrimental consequences for the patient following aortic aneurysm repair. Fluid overload can place stress on the graft and the heart and cause graft failure or heart failure. Hypovolemia can compromise the perfusion of all vital organs. The nurse must monitor volume status using intake and output measurements, daily weights, hemodynamic pressures, vital signs, and physical examination of the patient.

Other postoperative problems can occur. These include intestinal ileus, immobility, pain, anxiety, and infection. The nurse must observe for signs of these problems and implement the needed interventions. Box 24-7 gives specific nursing interventions.

As the patient recovers from the operative procedure, all tubes, lines, and drains are removed, the patient's diet and activity progress, and planning for discharge is started. The patient should receive adequate nutrition as soon as bowel function returns, and the diet usually progresses from clear liquids to a regular diet low in fat and sodium. Nutrition is needed to ensure wound healing and prevent infection, but nausea and vomiting should be avoided because they strain the incision. Pain medications are switched to an oral route when possible, as are other medications. The postoperative course depends on the patient's age, health before surgery, and postoperative complications.

**Discharge planning.** Discharge instructions should include wound care, signs of complications, and activity limitations. As with all major surgery the patient should be able to report any signs of infection, including fever, and redness or drainage of the incision. The patient needs to be instructed to watch the extremities for changes in color, warmth, or strength of the pulses. Pain in the extremities must be reported to the physician. The patient can expect to tire easily and have decreased appetite for the first few weeks after returning home and is advised to avoid heavy lifting and strenuous exercise. Male patients may experience sexual dysfunction following aneurysm repair because of nerve damage and disruption of blood flow to the perianal area (Dempsey, 1995). Impotence should be reported to the physician. The patient may be sent home taking analgesics and other medications, depending on preexisting medical conditions. Complete instructions on the correct dosage, timing, and complications of these medications are necessary before discharge. The patient should also receive teaching to reinforce the life-style changes that are needed to reduce the risk for arterial disease. All patients receiving aortic aneurysm repair are considered to have a chronic disease requiring ongoing management and care. Follow-up appointments should be planned before discharge.

## Nonsurgical Intervention

In some situations, patients may not receive immediate surgical treatment of their aortic aneurysm. These situations may include small aneurysms, patients who are not good surgical candidates because of other medical conditions, and those who refuse surgical intervention.

If medical management of an aneurysm is chosen, the goal is to prevent further enlargement. Control of blood pressure and reduction of the workload of the heart may be accomplished through the use of antihy-

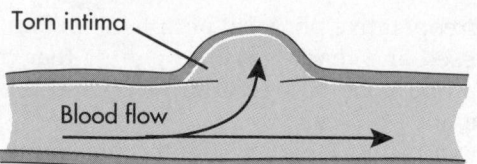

**Figure 24-9** Dissecting aneurysm.(Redrawn from Lewis SM, Collier IC, Heitkemper MM: *Medical-surgical nursing: assessment and management of clinical problems*, ed 4, St Louis, 1996, Mosby.)

pertensive medications and beta-blockers. Treatment also consists of decreased physical activity to reduce the work of the heart and to decrease the arterial pressure. Patients should be instructed to report any symptoms that might indicate enlargement or leakage of the aneurysm and should be told that they will require regular follow-up to detect any problems that would lead to surgery.

For patients who are not suitable candidates for surgery, treatment and nursing care are based on symptoms. If the aneurysm is large and at risk of rupture, the prognosis is poor. Efforts to prepare the family and patient for the possibility of aortic rupture are the focus of nursing interventions in these situations.

## Aortic Dissection

Aortic dissection occurs when the inner lining of the aorta is torn and blood gets between the layers, creating a false lumen (Figure 24-9). The area fills with blood and bulges outward. The dissection of the linings can spread with each pulsation of arterial blood flow, causing disruption to blood flow in the arteries that branch from the aorta (Dempsey, 1995). Aortic dissection is often falsely called a *dissecting aneurysm*. The difference between the two is that in dissecting aortic aneurysm the whole wall of the aorta in a specific area is affected, and in aortic dissection the layers of the wall are separated.

The most likely etiology for aortic dissection is weakening of the lining of the walls of the aorta because of disease or stress. Aortic dissection occurs most often in the thoracic aorta and commonly affects hypertensive men between the ages of 40 and 60 years. Pregnancy, cocaine use, connective tissue diseases, and weightlifting, especially with anabolic steroid use, also increase the risk of aortic dissection (Dempsey, 1995).

Aortic dissection can be life threatening or can stabilize and become a chronic process. A dissection is acute if it has occurred within the last 2 weeks. Most deaths occur in the first 30 days, when the aorta is inflamed and frail (Dempsey, 1995). Aortic dissections are graded using the Stanford classification. Type A dissections involve the ascending aorta, and type B dissections do not involve the ascending aorta. Type A is the most common and has the highest mortality.

## TABLE 24-4

### Complications and Clinical Manifestations of Aortic Dissection

| LOCATION | COMPLICATIONS | CLINICAL MANIFESTATIONS |
|---|---|---|
| Ascending aorta | Cardiac tamponade | Hypotension, distended neck veins, muffled heart sounds, paradoxical pulse (blood pressure drop during inspiration) |
| | Aortic valve dysfunction | Murmur |
| | | Left ventricular failure: shortness of breath, pulmonary edema |
| Aortic arch | Decreased arterial flow to brain | Decreased or absent carotid and temporal pulses |
| | | Decreased level of consciousness |
| | | Dizziness, syncope |
| | | Strokelike symptoms |
| Descending | Subclavian artery involvement | Decreased pulse and blood pressure on affected side |
| | Hemothorax | Dyspnea, tachypnea, hypoxemia, decreased breath sounds on affected side |
| Abdominal | Spinal cord ischemia | Weakness, paralysis, numbness in lower extremities |
| | Renal ischemia | Decreased urinary output, renal failure |
| | Bowel ischemia | Abdominal pain and tenderness, distention, decreased bowel sounds |
| | Lower extremity arterial occlusion | Pain, pallor, pulselessness in lower extremities |

Data from Hill EM: *AACN Clin Issues* 6(4):547-561, 1995; Dempsey E: Aortic aneurysms. In Urban N et al, editors: *Guidelines for critical care nursing*, St Louis, 1995, Mosby.

The problems and complications associated with aortic dissection depend on the location of the dissection along the aorta (Table 24-4). The most common complication of aortic dissection is rupture. If rupture occurs, the pericardial sac or the pleural space will fill with blood. If the hemorrhage occurs into the pericardial sac, cardiac tamponade and death may occur. If the hemorrhage occurs into the pleural space, a massive hemothorax and respiratory failure can occur (Dempsey, 1995).

## Assessment

**History and physical examination.** The pain of aortic dissection is usually described as a "tearing" or "burning" type of pain that occurs after vigorous movement (Dempsey, 1995). The pain becomes less severe over time and is replaced by a deep aching. If the ascending aorta is dissecting, the pain will be focused in the anterior part of the chest. Neck pain is common with dissection of the aortic arch, and back and abdominal pain occurs with dissection of the descending aorta. The pain can start in one area, particularly the chest, and migrate to other areas above and below the diaphragm and to the back or shoulder. The pain mimics that of a myocardial infarction for many patients.

The area of dissection determines the specific symptoms (see Table 24-4). Other symptoms include pulse deficits and discrepancies in the blood pressure between the arms and the legs (arms being lower than legs). The pressure occurring during dissection may cause stimulation of baroreceptors and the release of catecholamines causing tachycardia and

an increase in blood pressure. It is important to determine if the patient is a cocaine user because use of beta-blockers, common as a treatment for dissection, may cause paradoxic hypertension in cocaine intoxication.

**Diagnostic studies.** The diagnostic studies conducted for suspected aortic dissections are similar to those done for aortic aneurysm. An ECG will be done to rule out myocardial infarction as the cause of the chest pain. A chest x-ray can identify many dissections but cannot determine the exact extent or the patency of the aortic valve. Options for stable patients include a CT or MRI scan and angiography of the aorta (aortography). Unstable patients may be evaluated using transthoracic ultrasonography.

The priority laboratory study for suspected aortic dissection is the type and crossmatch needed to prepare blood for transfusion. If rupture occurs, the patient will lose massive amounts of blood rapidly.

## Medical and Nursing Interventions

In the patient who is stable, control of blood pressure and control of heart rate are the major management strategies to reduce the risk of rupture of the dissection. The myocardial workload and force of myocardial ejection are also decreased to keep the pulsation in the aorta low and avoid rupture of the weakening aortic wall. Intravenous beta-blockers, such as propanolol and esmolol (see Chapter 23), are used to decrease contractility of the heart, and intravenous vasodilators, such as nitroprusside are used to rapidly lower blood pressure. The goal for blood pressure is usually 100 to 120 mm Hg (on the higher end of the range for patients with hypertension), and for heart rate the goal is 60 to 80 bpm (Dempsey, 1995).

> ### NURSE ALERT
>
> **Monitor blood pressure closely in patients receiving intravenous vasodilators. Hypertensive patients who normally have a higher blood pressure may have changes in level of consciousness resulting from decreased cerebral perfusion if the blood pressure is reduced too low or too quickly.**

If the patient does not have any complications, type B dissections may be treated using nonsurgical intervention. Supportive care is given, including pain control, control of blood pressure and heart rate, and monitoring for complications. If the patient has lost significant amounts of blood into the false lumen, blood transfusions may be needed. Type A dissections with or without complications usually need thoracic surgery. Patients who are unstable are referred immediately for surgery. Any life-threatening complications are managed as needed until surgery can be performed.

Nursing interventions for the patient who is unstable include starting at least three large-bore intravenous lines, assessing and managing the ABCs (airway, breathing, and circulation), and obtaining the necessary laboratory work to begin rapid transfusion of blood. If a hemothorax is present, the nurse should prepare to assist with a chest tube insertion. If pericardial tamponade is present, a pericardiocentesis is performed. Preparation of the patient and family for surgery is the next priority. In this type of crisis, the family needs much support.

In the patient who is stable, nursing interventions include starting large-bore intravenous lines in case of emergency, monitoring pain and providing pain relief, monitoring intravenous drug infusions, observing for signs and symptoms of complications, and providing support and information to the patient and family. The level of pain and adequacy of pain control methods are used to gauge the stability of the dissection and thus are critical nursing interventions. The nurse should also observe for signs of blood loss (e.g., tachycardia, increased anxiety and restlessness) and for signs of end-organ ischemia (e.g., decreased urinary output). Peripheral pulse checks and vital signs are done frequently.

The use of potent intravenous antihypertensive and vasoactive drugs requires close nursing supervision. These drugs are usually titrated to maintain vital signs within strict parameters. Continuous ECG and blood pressure monitoring is done (Dempsey, 1995). Usually an indwelling arterial monitoring line is used to provide continuous blood pressure readings. The patient who is receiving this type of intervention will be admitted to an ICU.

Other nursing interventions for aortic dissection involve keeping the patient calm, quiet, and in bed. These interventions reduce the heart rate and blood pressure and prevent extension of the dissection. Sedatives and analgesics are commonly administered to control pain and anxiety.

If surgery is performed, the postoperative care is the same as with patients who have an aortic aneurysm repair. The postoperative course varies from patient to patient, and discharge planning priorities are the same as those for a patient after aneurysm repair. If surgery is not performed, the patient will most likely be sent home taking oral antihypertensives and beta-blockers. The patient and family will need teaching regarding the importance of continuing these medications and the dosage and timing of administration. The patient will also need instruction on signs and symptoms that indicate complications (e.g., return of the pain; changes in level of consciousness, pulses, or urine output).

## Arterial Occlusions

Occlusion of the arterial system can be an acute or a chronic process. Acute arterial occlusions occur suddenly and may be (1) the result of chronic arterial disease with arterial narrowing, (2) caused by emboli that obstruct the artery, or (3) the result of trauma to the artery (Table 24-5). Blood flow to the areas supplied by the artery is suddenly stopped, and tissue ischemia, injury, and infarction can occur.

Chronic arterial disease has been directly linked to atherosclerosis (see Table 24-5). The buildup of plaques in the intimal layer of the arteries leads to narrowing and obstructions, which decrease the blood flow in the artery. In chronic occlusions, pain, disability, and loss of limb can occur.

Any major arteries may be affected by occlusive disorders, and the assessment findings, medical or surgical management, nursing interventions, and prognosis depend on the location and severity of the occlusion. The following section focuses on arterial occlusion in the extremities. Occlusions in the arterial systems of the brain, heart, and kidneys are discussed in Chapters 30 and 32.

### Acute Arterial Occlusion

Regardless of the cause, acute arterial occlusions are considered surgical emergencies since the obstruction puts the tissues beyond the occlusion at grave risk. As discussed previously, emboli, thrombi, and trauma are

## TABLE 24-5

### Causes of Arterial Occlusion

| ACUTE ARTERIAL OCCLUSION | CHRONIC ARTERIAL OCCLUSION |
|---|---|
| **Emboli from:** | **Atherosclerosis** |
| Heart: endocarditis, myocardial infarction, mitral valve disease, atrial fibrillation, cardiomyopathies, artificial heart valves | **Risk factors** |
| Thrombosed aortic aneurysm | Smoking* |
| Arterial system after surgery or invasive procedures | Hyperlipidemia* |
| | Hypertension* |
| **Thrombosis of existing plaque in artery** | Diabetes |
| | Obesity |
| | Family history |
| **Trauma to artery** | Sedentary life-style |
| Trauma to extremity | |
| Indwelling arterial lines | |
| Arterial blood collection | |
| Invasive procedures with arterial entry sites | |

*Major risk factors.

the most common causes. **Emboli** from cardiac sources are frequent causes of arterial occlusions. Many cardiac conditions increase the risk of thrombus formation (see Table 24-5). Pieces of these thrombi can become dislodged, travel to the arterial system, and become clogged in an artery at a branching point or get caught in an area of atherosclerotic narrowing. Embolic sources for arterial occlusion can also include blood clots or plaque particles that break free from thrombosed aortic aneurysms or that break free during surgery or procedures involving the arterial system (Howland-Gradman, 1995). Chronic arterial disease and the resulting plaque can also serve as a source for arterial occlusion. If the plaque ruptures and a thrombus forms, it can severely or totally occlude the artery. Thrombi, spasm, or compression of the artery can also occur from direct accidental trauma to the artery (crushing injury, knife wounds, gunshot wounds), trauma during invasive tests (arteriography, arterial blood drawing for arterial blood gases), and trauma during surgical procedures (arterial bypasses, aortic aneurysm repairs) (Howland-Gradman, 1995).

The severity of the signs and symptoms and the degree of tissue loss depend on the amount of obstruction (partial or complete), whether particles of the embolus lodge in smaller vessels, the underlying condition of the arterial system, and the location of the obstruction. If the obstruction is complete, tissue damage progresses more rapidly and symptoms are more severe. If small particles of emboli "spray" throughout the arterial system, the tissue damage is greater and more widespread (Howland-Gradman, 1995). If chronic arterial disease is present, collateral circulation develops and may provide an alternative route for blood flow to

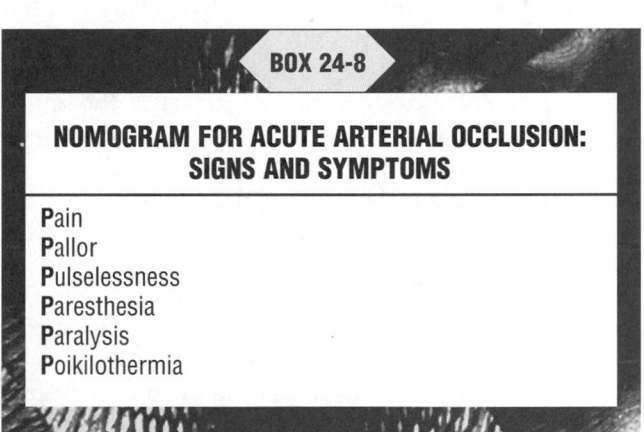

**BOX 24-8**

**NOMOGRAM FOR ACUTE ARTERIAL OCCLUSION: SIGNS AND SYMPTOMS**

**P**ain
**P**allor
**P**ulselessness
**P**aresthesia
**P**aralysis
**P**oikilothermia

the affected extremity. The collateral flow can prevent the degree of tissue damage that would occur in an extremity that does not have these additional pathways. Arterial occlusions located in the proximal portion of the artery will reduce or halt blood flow to a much greater amount of tissue. The more distal the obstruction, the more limited the damage.

### Assessment

***History and physical examination.*** The signs and symptoms of acute arterial occlusion are commonly described as the five "Ps": pain, pallor, pulselessness, and possibly paresthesia and paralysis (Seidel et al, 1995) (Box 24-8). The pain, pallor, and pulselessness of the extremity occur early after the onset of the occlusion as a result of the disruption of the arterial blood flow that causes tissue ischemia and injury. The pain may be excruciating in the early stages and decrease as the occlusion continues. The pain may be replaced by numbness as tissues die and sensation decreases. The pain is usually felt in areas distal to the area of occlusion. Pallor may be present initially and will progress to cyanosis if the occlusion is not removed. The paresthesia (altered sensation) and paralysis occur because of damage to nerve tissue and may not appear until late in the progression of the arterial occlusion (Krenzer, 1995). If interventions occur quickly, the patient may not ever report or exhibit changes in sensation and movement. If paresthesias or paralysis does occur before intervention, it may not be corrected by removal of the blockage and restoration of the blood flow because permanent damage may have occurred. Changes in skin temperature of the affected extremity are also common and are known as *poikilothermia* (Seidel et al, 1995). When arterial flow is reduced, the skin loses its warmth and is cool or cold to the touch depending on the room temperature. This sign of arterial obstruction is often used as the sixth "P" in the nomogram (see Box 24-8).

In arterial systems that are not affected by chronic disease, these signs and symptoms have a very sudden onset. In the patient with chronic arterial disease, the signs and symptoms may not appear suddenly but may be more of a progression or increase in the severity of the symptoms that the patient already experiences on an ongoing basis.

Other assessment data that should be collected include a quick review of the patient's history to determine underlying causes, evaluation of the extremity to detect any areas of obvious trauma, and evaluation of the artery using a Doppler device to detect the presence of any blood flow. Since the interventions for acute arterial occlusion may include the use of anticoagulants and thrombolytic agents, the patient should be questioned about bleeding or clotting abnormalities and sensitivity to any drugs.

***Diagnostic studies.*** Diagnostic studies done on patients with acute arterial occlusion may be limited to baseline laboratory studies, such as PT, APTT, and complete blood count (CBC). These are used to guide the administration of anticoagulants and thrombolytic agents. The need for immediate intervention to remove the occlusion dictates the type of diagnostic studies that are conducted. Studies to evaluate the arterial system and locate the occlusion, such as arteriography, are not performed unless therapeutic interventions will be done in conjunction.

Once the patient is stabilized, it may be necessary to conduct a complete evaluation of the arterial system and initiate tests to determine the site of origin of the embolus. Because the cardiac system is a common source for emboli resulting in arterial occlusion, numerous tests may be needed to rule out each of the possible cardiac etiologies.

**Medical and nursing interventions.** Several treatment options are available for the patient with acute arterial

occlusion. In severe limb-threatening occlusion, an embolectomy or thrombectomy may be performed to remove the occlusive material. In these procedures a balloon-tipped catheter is placed into the affected artery and advanced beyond the occlusion (Hill, 1995). The balloon is then inflated and the catheter slowly removed. The balloon will capture the clot, and it will be pulled out of the artery as the catheter is removed. Once this is accomplished, the artery is clamped below the area of occlusion and irrigated to remove debris (Hill, 1995). Immediately after the procedure is performed, the circulation is assessed, and if the circulation is not restored the procedure is repeated until the occlusive material is completely removed and blood flow resumed. Intravenous anticoagulants (heparin) are administered by continuous drip following the procedure to prevent further clot formation. Since embolectomy does not remove the arterial plaque, the patient may require further intervention, such as angioplasty or stent placement (discussed in the next section) to maintain adequate blood flow.

Another treatment option is the use of thrombolytic agents, such as urokinase or streptokinase, to dissolve the occluding clot (Howland-Gradman, 1995). These agents are administered directly into the affected artery at the site of the clot using a catheter inserted into the artery. Arteriography with contrast dye is used to locate the clot and evaluate the effectiveness of the lysis of the clot during and following the procedure. The patient is usually given short-term continuous intravenous heparin after the administration of thrombolytic agents. Thrombolytic therapy does not remove the plaque from the arterial wall. Following thrombolysis, the patient still requires additional interventions to remove the plaque or bypass the narrowed artery to restore blood flow.

Long-term management after the acute episode is directed at identifying and treating the cause. If the cause of the occlusion is a chronic condition, the patient is given oral anticoagulants, such as warfarin (Coumadin). If chronic arterial disease precipitated the acute occlusion, bypass surgery or other invasive procedures and risk factor reduction (described in the following section) are the focus of management strategies.

The nursing interventions for acute arterial occlusion should focus on identification of those at risk, early recognition, patient support and education, close observation of the affected limb, and monitoring of medications. Identification of those patients at risk for arterial occlusion is an essential nursing role. As described in the previous section, patients who have undergone invasive procedures or surgery involving the arterial system are at high risk for limb-threatening occlusion. Frequent assessment of the circulation is critical in identifying the signs and symptoms of reduced blood flow so that rapid intervention can be done. Assessment strategies (e.g., establishing baseline pulses, skin color, and temperature; marking pulses; use of consistent pulse strength evaluation scales) should be implemented. Documentation of findings and prompt physician notification of deviations from baseline should be done.

Patients who are experiencing acute arterial occlusion will be understandably anxious. They are experiencing severe discomfort and are at risk of losing their limb. The nurse must provide the patient and family with information regarding the procedures, medications, and plan of care as appropriate throughout the crisis. After the crisis has past, the nurse plays an important role in preparing the patient for discharge. The patient will require teaching on follow-up care and visits, risk factor reduction, medication regimen, and the signs of recurrent occlusion. If the revascularization procedure is unsuccessful, the nurse is in a vital position to assist the patient and family in dealing with preparations for and rehabilitation after amputation.

Other nursing management consists of observing the affected limb for signs of reocclusion and monitoring the anticoagulant administration. The affected extremity should be protected from further injury and watched for the development of wounds or ulcers. Because the patient will be on bed rest initially, the nurse must take action to prevent pressure areas. Anticoagulant administration and the use of thrombolytic agents put the patient at risk for bleeding complications. Frequent laboratory studies will be ordered to assess the adequacy of the anticoagulants, and the nurse should monitor the patient for any signs of abnormal or increased bleeding. Guidelines for nursing care of patients receiving anticoagulants are included in Box 24-9. Additional nursing interventions, such as risk factor modification, long-term drug therapy, and progressive exercise, will be the same as for patients with chronic arterial disease (see the following section).

## Chronic Arterial Occlusion

Chronic arterial occlusion, also called *peripheral arterial disease, arteriosclerosis obliterans,* or **arterial occlusive disease,** is a progressive process occurring most often in the lower extremities (Howland-Gradman, 1995). Arterial occlusive disease has been directly linked to atherosclerosis, with buildup of plaques in the intimal layer of the arteries that leads to narrowing of the lumen and obstruction of blood flow.

Although smoking, hyperlipidemia, and hypertension are the three major risk factors for peripheral arterial disease (see Table 24-5), obesity, sedentary lifestyle, family history of occlusive disease, and diabetes are all considered predisposing factors (Howland-Gradman, 1995). The disease is more common in men than women and increases with advancing age.

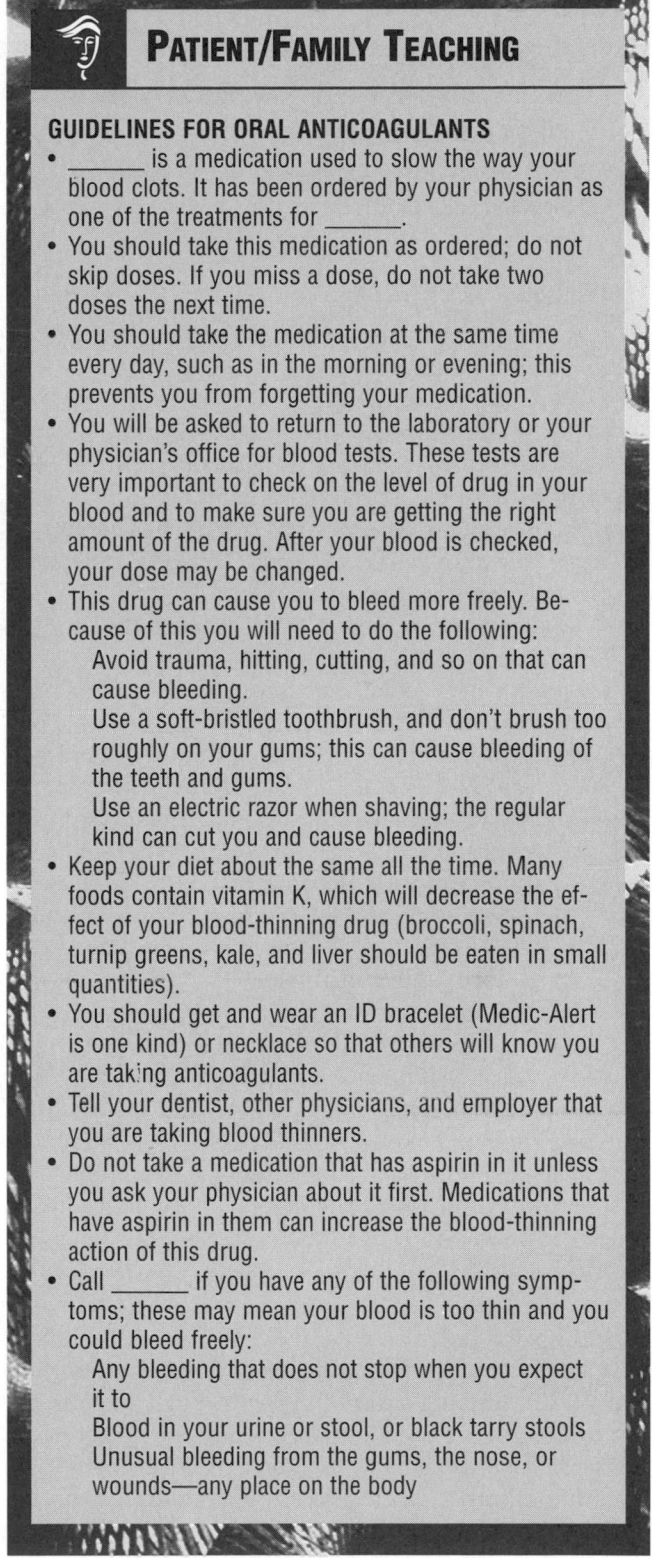

### PATIENT/FAMILY TEACHING

#### GUIDELINES FOR ORAL ANTICOAGULANTS

• _____ is a medication used to slow the way your blood clots. It has been ordered by your physician as one of the treatments for _____.
• You should take this medication as ordered; do not skip doses. If you miss a dose, do not take two doses the next time.
• You should take the medication at the same time every day, such as in the morning or evening; this prevents you from forgetting your medication.
• You will be asked to return to the laboratory or your physician's office for blood tests. These tests are very important to check on the level of drug in your blood and to make sure you are getting the right amount of the drug. After your blood is checked, your dose may be changed.
• This drug can cause you to bleed more freely. Because of this you will need to do the following:
  Avoid trauma, hitting, cutting, and so on that can cause bleeding.
  Use a soft-bristled toothbrush, and don't brush too roughly on your gums; this can cause bleeding of the teeth and gums.
  Use an electric razor when shaving; the regular kind can cut you and cause bleeding.
• Keep your diet about the same all the time. Many foods contain vitamin K, which will decrease the effect of your blood-thinning drug (broccoli, spinach, turnip greens, kale, and liver should be eaten in small quantities).
• You should get and wear an ID bracelet (Medic-Alert is one kind) or necklace so that others will know you are taking anticoagulants.
• Tell your dentist, other physicians, and employer that you are taking blood thinners.
• Do not take a medication that has aspirin in it unless you ask your physician about it first. Medications that have aspirin in them can increase the blood-thinning action of this drug.
• Call _____ if you have any of the following symptoms; these may mean your blood is too thin and you could bleed freely:
  Any bleeding that does not stop when you expect it to
  Blood in your urine or stool, or black tarry stools
  Unusual bleeding from the gums, the nose, or wounds—any place on the body

Arterial occlusive disease is a systemic problem, and most patients who have disease in one arterial bed have disease in other systems as well, especially the heart. All arterial systems can be affected, but the atherosclerotic process most often occurs in main arteries,

BOX 24-9

# NURSING PROCESS

## PATIENTS RECEIVING ANTICOAGULANTS

### NURSING DIAGNOSES

- Risk for bleeding related to anticoagulation
- Knowledge deficit related to new pharmacologic regimen

### NURSING INTERVENTIONS

- Avoid intramuscular injections; use intravenous route for medications.
- Avoid arterial punctures.
- Have patient use soft-bristled toothbrush.
- Use electric razor for shaving (no razor with blade).
- Avoid trauma; use fall precautions.
- Apply direct pressure to any arterial or venous sites used for puncture to limit bleeding and promote clot formation.
- Take oral temperatures; avoid rectal temperatures because they can tear tissue.
- Monitor intravenous rate frequently.
- Monitor results of blood levels; adjust drip rate or dosage as ordered: activated partial thromboplastin time (APPT) monitored for intravenous heparin therapy, prothrombin time and international normalized ratio monitored for warfarin therapy.
- Monitor patient for bleeding:
    Observe stool, emesis, and urine; test for blood.
    Assess skin, gums, and nose for petechiae, ecchymosis, and hematoma.
    Check venipuncture sites for oozing.
    Assess for signs of intracranial bleeding: altered level of consciousness, vomiting, headache.
    Assess for signs of internal bleeding: abdominal pain and tenderness, weakness.
- Instruct patient on action, dosing, and complications of prescribed drug and when to call health care provider.

### EVALUATION OF EXPECTED OUTCOMES

- No major bleeding complications
- Any bleeding identified promptly and interventions implemented
- Patient able to verbalize the actions, dosing, and complications of the prescribed drug and situations requiring notification of the health care provider or immediate attention
- Special considerations for heparin
    Monitor activated partial thromboplastin time, and adjust intravenous rate as ordered
    Subcutaneous heparin requires no special blood monitoring
    Dosages may be based on weight, so an accurate patient weight is essential
    Can cause thrombocytopenia: monitor platelet counts
    Protamine sulfate: antidote for warfarin (Coumadin)
    See also discussion of deep vein thrombosis in this chapter
- Special considerations for warfarin
    Given orally
    Initial doses may overlap intravenous heparin use by several days
    Drugs that increase effects of warfarin: metronidazole, phenytoin, aspirin
    Drugs that decrease effects of warfarin: barbiturates, rifampin, cholestyramine
    Foods high in vitamin K can decrease effects of warfarin (green leafy vegetables, onions, liver)
    Vitamin K: antidote for warfarin

including the aorta and its lower extremity branches, as well as the carotid and subclavian arteries (Figure 24-10). Smaller arterial systems, such as those in the lower part of the leg and foot, are the target of arterial disease in diabetic persons. With diabetic persons the atherosclerotic process is accelerated, occurring at a younger age than in the person without diabetes (Howland-Gradman, 1995).

Patients with chronic arterial occlusive disease can have isolated areas of narrowing, but in advanced cases multiple areas may be present. Blood flow distal to the area of narrowing will be decreased, and collateral circulation may develop to provide the ischemic area with alternative routes for blood flow. In the early

stages, the chronic arterial disease may produce no symptoms. As the disease advances, symptoms (e.g., claudication) become more severe and tissue necrosis occurs. Complications of arterial occlusive disease include tissue atrophy, chronic ischemic ulcers, acute arterial occlusion, gangrene, and infection. If blood flow is not increased, amputation of the extremity may be necessary.

### Assessment

***History and physical examination.*** A health history should include collection of information on risk factors, health habits, past history of arterial disease in any system, and use of medications. Screening of pa-

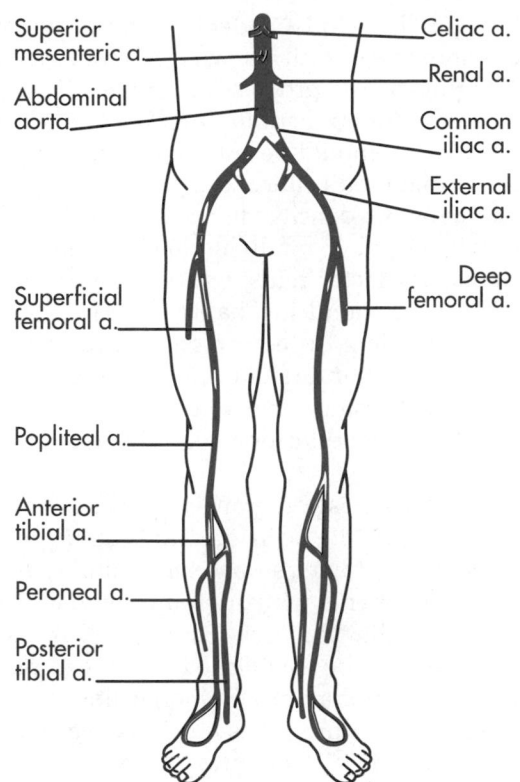

**Figure 24-10** Common anatomic locations of atherosclerotic plaques in the aorta and lower extremities. (Modified from Lewis SM, Collier IC, Heitkemper MM: *Medical-surgical nursing: assessment and management of clinical problems,* ed 4, St Louis, 1996, Mosby.)

tients for the major risk factors of arterial disease is important in identifying those at high risk so that risk reduction strategies can be implemented before arterial disease progresses. Specific health history questions arc included in the assessment portion of this chapter.

In the early stages of arterial disease the patient may not be symptomatic. Patients may not have any significant pain or changes in the pulses or skin on the affected extremity until a large lesion is present. The degree and presentation of symptoms depend on the area affected and the amount of occlusion.

As arterial narrowing progresses, the resulting tissue ischemia produces pain beyond the lesion when the patient exercises. This intermittent claudication is reproducible with the same amount of activity each time and is relieved with rest. If the patient is sedentary and does not have regular physical activity, intermittent claudication may not occur because the patient does not walk long enough to produce ischemia (Cantwell-Gab, 1996). In addition, patients may adjust their activity level to avoid pain and thus will not have the classic claudication symptoms. When interviewing patients with suspected arterial disease or risk factors for arterial disease, it is important to find out as much detail as possible about their level of activity.

Claudication usually occurs in the muscle groups one joint below the area of disease (Cantwell-Gab, 1996). Lesions in the femoral or popliteal arteries produce pain in the calf. Lesions in the aortoiliac arteries may produce pain in the buttocks and thighs (Santilli, Rodnick, Santilli, 1996). Disease that involves the internal iliac artery may cause impotence in male patients. If the patient has disease in more than one area, pain may be experienced in more than one location. Patients may describe their claudication pain in several ways. The quality of the pain may vary depending on the site. Claudication in the calf may be described as a sharp cramping pain, whereas claudication in the hip and thigh may be more of an aching discomfort associated with weakness in the extremity (Cantwell-Gab, 1996).

As the arterial occlusion becomes more advanced, pain occurs at rest. This presentation of pain indicates the ischemia has progressed to a critical level. Rest pain is usually most troublesome at night (with the extremity elevated, ischemia worsens) and may be relieved by lowering the extremity into a dependent position (gravity improves blood flow). The patient may need to sleep in a chair to obtain adequate rest. In very severe cases, the pain may be so severe that even narcotic analgesics will not provide relief (Cantwell-Gab, 1996).

Paresthesia (numbness, tingling, burning) may also occur in patients with arterial disease. These altered sensations are the result of nerve ischemia and occur most often in the feet. With progression of the disease the paresthesias can worsen to loss of sensation and inability to feel deep pain. Once the arterial disease progresses to this point, injuries and trauma to the extremity can occur because the patient cannot detect the insult.

Other signs that arterial disease is present include atrophy of the skin (causing it to appear shiny and tight) and loss of hair on the lower leg. Reduced blood flow will also cause the extremity to appear pale or become pale when elevated. In addition, the extremity will take on a red (hyperemic) or blue (cyanotic) coloration when placed in the dependent position. As described in the assessment section of this chapter, pulses distal to the area of disease will be diminished or absent. Using a Doppler device to evaluate the pulses may produce the swishing sound that indicates blood flow, but flow may not be adequate. The presence of pulses by Doppler examination does not rule out arterial disease. Capillary refill in the affected extremity will be prolonged as a result of poor perfusion, and the extremity may be cooler than normal below the level of the lesion.

Chronic arterial occlusion also predisposes the patient to ischemic ulcers. These ulcers typically occur over bony areas on the ankle and on the toes and will heal slowly because of poor blood flow. Ischemic ulcers are very painful and do not bleed much when manipulated. Gangrene and infection are also common skin manifestations of chronic arterial disease.

***Diagnostic studies.*** Diagnostic studies to evaluate a patient with suspected chronic arterial disease include coagulation studies to provide a baseline and identify hypercoagulable states, cholesterol screening to identify hyperlipidemia, and arterial Doppler studies to determine the exact location and extent of the disease. (See the previous section on diagnostic studies for a more complete description.) A Doppler study with calculation of the ABI is the most important study currently used for the evaluation of patients with chronic arterial disease (Santilli, Rodnick, Santilli, 1996). The ABI provides a noninvasive method of determining the extent of the occlusion and is used to observe the progression of the disease process, determine if and when surgical intervention is needed, and observe patients postoperatively after revascularization surgery. Exercise Doppler studies can be used to detect changes in blood flow following exercise. Duplex Doppler imaging and arteriography are used to more specifically locate and assess the arterial disease. Arteriograms, which are invasive, are usually reserved for patients who are going to undergo surgery or angioplasty (Santilli, Rodnick, Santilli, 1996).

**Medical and nursing interventions.** Arterial occlusive disease is progressive with no cure, but the disease can be slowed through risk factor modification. Treatment is aimed at improving circulation, relieving pain, improving the quality of life, preventing complications such as injury and infection, slowing the progression of the disease, and preventing ischemia (Cantwell-Gab, 1996). The type of therapy implemented depends on the location, cause, and size of the obstruction. Options for conservative, noninvasive management of chronic arterial occlusive disease include risk factor modification, a progressive exercise program, drug therapy, and injury prevention. In severe cases where conservative management is not helpful, pain becomes incapacitating or occurs at rest, or studies indicate a critical reduction in blood flow, operative or endovascular procedures may be used (Santilli, Rodnick, Santilli, 1996).

**Nonsurgical interventions.** Risk factor modification should be part of the treatment plan for all patients with chronic arterial disease regardless of the use of invasive procedures. Patients should be assessed for risk factors such as hypertension, diabetes, hyperlipidemia, and smoking. Hypertension and diabetes should be brought or kept under tight control. Patients who smoke cigarettes should be strongly encouraged and given adequate resources to facilitate smoking cessa-

tion. Smoking is an independent risk factor for arterial disease, and those patients who continue to smoke are at high risk for progression of the disease and eventual amputation (Santilli, Rodnick, Santilli, 1996). Hyperlipidemia should be controlled through a combination of diet modification and possibly medications to maintain low-density lipoprotein (LDL) levels below 100 mg/dl (Santilli, Rodnick, Santilli, 1996). Additional risk factor reduction strategies for atherosclerosis can be found in Chapter 23. The nurse will be key in providing the education needed to promote risk factor reduction and in assisting the patient in identifying and using other resources that can facilitate risk factor modification and changes in health behavior.

Progressive exercise programs improve exercise performance, relieve the pain of claudication, improve functional ability, increase overall wellness, and decrease risk in patients with arterial disease (Cantwell-Gab, 1996; Santilli, Rodnick, Santilli, 1996). Exercise guidelines should be established by an exercise specialist or physical therapist. Some facilities have vascular rehabilitation programs much like cardiac rehabilitation programs that provide equipment and monitoring of exercise progression.

The goals of drug therapy for chronic arterial disease are to decrease metabolic activity or increase blood flow to the affected muscle groups (Santilli, Rodnick, Santilli, 1996). Choices for drug therapy include agents to decrease the viscosity of the blood (e.g., pentoxifylline [Trental]) and antiplatelet agents (e.g., dipyridamole [Persantine], ticlopidine [Ticlid], and aspirin). With the exception of pentoxifylline, no drug has been specifically shown to be effective (Santilli, Rodnick, Santilli, 1996). Patients who have operative procedures that involve grafting may be given anticoagulants (e.g., warfarin [Coumadin]) (Table 24-6). The nursing role in pharmacologic management includes monitoring anticoagulant and other drug therapy and providing patient teaching for those who will continue medication in an outpatient setting (see the box on p. 742). For more information on anticoagulant therapy see the section on DVT in this chapter.

Nursing intervention plays a crucial role in preventing complications and injury. The feet and lower extremities should be inspected regularly for broken areas and interventions implemented to prevent skin breakdown. The lower extremities should be kept clean and lubricated to prevent dryness and cracking of the skin, but the feet should not be soaked in water for extended periods of time. Prolonged wetness, such as from soaking or sweating, can cause the skin to become weakened and will increase the chances of infection. If ulcers are present they should be kept clean

## PATIENT/FAMILY TEACHING

### GUIDELINES FOR ARTERIAL DISEASE
#### Exercise Guidelines
- Regular exercise, particularly walking, can increase the distance that patients can walk and improve functional ability.
- Patients who are cleared by their physician to begin walking should follow the following guidelines:
  Walk two to four times daily to the point when pain occurs.
  Walk for 30 to 60 minutes each time.
  Use a treadmill or bicycle exercise as a good alternative to walking.
  Record your walking time and distance for each exercise session.
  After the pain begins, sit down and rest until the pain subsides; then begin walking again.
  Wear shoes that fit well and are wide toed to avoid pressure sores.
  Always wear cotton stockings or hose.
  Never walk barefoot.
  Treat cuts or blisters promptly.
- It may take 3 to 6 months for walking times and distances to improve.

#### Foot and Skin Care
- Wear comfortable, wide-toed shoes with cotton socks or hose.
- Look at your feet daily, and treat any cuts, blisters, or sores promptly.
- Avoid trauma to the feet; always wear shoes or slippers when walking.
- Have any ingrown toenails or calluses removed by a health care professional.
- Report any redness or swelling of open areas to your health care provider promptly.

- Keep toenails trimmed straight across the top of your toes to avoid ingrown toenails.
- Avoid hot water bottles or heating pads; they can injure your feet.
- Keep your feet clean and dry.
- Do not soak your feet; this can weaken the skin and cause cracks and sores.
- Use a mild lotion to prevent dry skin.
- Check the water in your bath with your fingers, not your toes; you may have less feeling in your toes and may not be able to tell temperature as well with your toes.
- Avoid cold temperatures; cold slows blood flow.
- Use sunscreen to protect against sunburn.
- Avoid wearing garters or stockings that are tight and put pressure on your legs; this can decrease blood flow.
- Avoid sitting or standing for long periods; this can decrease circulation.
- Do not cross legs when sitting or lying down; this can also decrease circulation.

#### Changing Risk Factors
- Even if you have had surgery for your arterial disease, you need to work to reduce your risk factors.
- Health problems, such as diabetes, high blood pressure, and high cholesterol levels, can make your disease worse.
- Cigarette smoking greatly increases the problems of arterial disease.
- Stopping smoking, eating a low-fat and low-cholesterol diet, and taking your medications for diabetes and high blood pressure are important things for you to do to slow your arterial disease. Your health care provider can help you make the needed changes to improve your health.

Data from Santilli JD, Rodnick JE, Santilli SM: *Am Fam Physician* 53(4):1245-1255, 1996.

---

and dry, and pressure over and around the ulcer should be avoided. A skin care consultation may be needed to determine the best skin care product to use. Ulcerations are a common complication of arterial disease. These ulcers are very slow to heal without adequate blood flow. Any increased redness, warmth, or drainage from the ulcer should be reported promptly so that therapy to prevent the spread of infection can be initiated. Any position that causes legs to be crossed or hips and knees to be flexed for long periods should be discouraged. Restrictive clothing, such as garters or tight shoes, should be avoided. The patient should also be instructed to avoid chilling and cold environ-

ments. The nurse must teach the patient how to properly evaluate the extremities and maintain meticulous foot care.

**Surgical interventions.** Surgery or invasive interventions may be necessary to restore circulation. Surgery is indicated when the disease causes pain at rest, claudication severely restricts activity, or ischemia is severe. Many procedures are now available to restore blood flow in arterial occlusive disease. The type of procedure chosen depends on the degree and location of the lesion and the patient's overall health status. Commonly used procedures for arterial occlusive disease include **percutaneous transluminal angioplasty**

## TABLE 24-6

## Drugs Used to Treat Arterial Occlusive Disease

| DRUG | ACTION/INDICATION | SIDE EFFECTS/NURSING INDICATIONS |
|---|---|---|
| **Anticoagulants** | | Abnormal bleeding can occur with both |
| Warfarin (Coumadin) | Inhibits vitamin K–dependent clotting factors<br>Taken orally on a daily basis for long-term anticoagulation | Risk of excessive bleeding; may have other effects when used with certain drugs; contraindicated in pregnancy<br>Vitamin K in large doses reverses action<br>Teach patient signs of bleeding and who to contact in an emergency |
| Heparin | Enhances antithrombin III to inhibit clotting<br>Given intravenously by infusion pump to slow clot progression or prevent clotting<br>Can be given subcutaneously for prophylaxis | Same as for Warfarin; patient should have frequent platelet counts done |
| **Antiplatelet Agents** | Reduce platelet clumping<br>Used for medical management of arterial occlusive disease to decrease incidence of clot formation | |
| Aspirin | Usually ordered one per day | Over-the-counter medication; can cause gastrointestinal distress and abnormal bleeding |
| Dipyridamole (Persantine) | | Prescription drug; taken on empty stomach; side effects: hypotension, prolonged bleeding times, nausea, vomiting, diarrhea; nurse should monitor blood pressure and observe for signs of abnormal bleeding |
| Ticlopidine (Ticlid) | | Prescription drug; can cause neutropenia and thrombocytopenia: monitor white blood cell (WBC) and platelet counts; can increase bleeding times: monitor for abnormal bleeding; other side effects: diarrhea, vomiting, flatulence, dyspepsia |
| **Drug to Decrease Blood Viscosity** | | |
| Pentoxifylline (Trental) | Increases red blood cell flexibility, decreases plasma viscosity, decreases platelet aggregation, increases blood flow to extremity<br>Used to treat claudication | Side effects: dyspepsia, nausea, vomiting, dizziness, agitation; should be taken with food; do not crush pills<br>Usually given to patients for 1-3 mo to gauge response; if no response, drug is discontinued |
| **Thrombolytic Agent** | | |
| Urokinase (Abbokinase) | Used to lyse clot causing occlusion; will not have an effect on plaque in the arterial wall; once clot is removed and blood flow restored, plaque may be treated with angioplasty or removed through surgical intervention<br>Agent of choice infused through a catheter placed in clot; procedure usually done in the radiology department | Can cause systemic bleeding complications; patients should be evaluated for contraindications to thrombolytic administration<br>After infusion, nurse should monitor for increased bleeding and maintain bleeding precautions |

**(PTA),** stent placement, and bypass grafting. Atherectomy and laser procedures are also possible alternatives but are not widely used. In severe cases, when other revascularization attempts have failed, amputation of the extremity may be necessary.

The PTA is an invasive procedure usually done in the radiology department using fluoroscopy. During a PTA, a balloon-tipped catheter is inserted into the artery and guided into the area of narrowing or occlusion (Howland-Gradman, 1995). Once the catheter is placed into and past the atherosclerotic plaque, the balloon is inflated to push and flatten the plaque against the arterial wall. As the plaque is flattened the lumen of the artery is widened and blood flow will increase. This procedure is similar to the PTCA done for coronary artery disease (see Chapter 23). The advantage to PTA is that it is less invasive and less expensive than traditional surgical interventions, can be done with local anesthetic and sedation, and has fewer complications than bypass surgery (Hill, 1995; Cantwell-Gab, 1996; Dempsey, 1996). The disadvantages include the risk of restenosis of the artery and the need for administration of antiplatelets and anticoagulants before and after the procedure.

Complications of PTA are similar to those of arteriography (see the section of this chapter on diagnostic studies). In addition to bleeding and clot formation, angioplasty can cause dissection of the artery. Complete occlusion and tissue ischemia can occur if a piece of the plaque breaks off and becomes lodged further down in the artery. Other complications possible in the first 24 hours after the procedure include spasm of the artery and occlusion. Because dye is used in the procedure, dye-related complications are the same as those with angiography.

Nursing care of patients undergoing angioplasty is similar to that of a patient undergoing angiography. The patient and the family need to be knowledgeable about the angioplasty procedure to reduce anxiety and establish trust and cooperation. The patient must be informed of the risks, and a consent will be obtained for bypass surgery in the event it is needed emergently. Identification of sensitivity to dye and renal system problems is an essential nursing intervention. During the procedure, the nurse instructs the patient to report sensations of pain. The nurse will also continuously monitor the patient's blood pressure and heart rate and rhythm.

After the angioplasty procedure, the patient is transferred to a unit that ensures close monitoring. The patient is then watched for excessive bleeding or hematoma formation at the catheter insertion site. Limb pain or changes in color, warmth, or pulses in the extremity indicate that the newly dilated artery is closing. Close monitoring of the affected extremity is an important nursing intervention, and inspection of skin color, palpation of skin temperature and pulses, and assessment of the arterial pulses with a Doppler device are done at frequent intervals—usually every 15 minutes for the first hour, every 30 minutes for the second hour, and every shift thereafter (Cantwell-Gab, 1996). Any change from the baseline should be reported immediately. The patient is instructed to keep the extremity straight and still for 6 to 8 hours after the procedure is completed and the femoral sheath removed, and he or she is usually placed on bed rest for the first 24 hours. A pressure dressing is usually applied to the catheter insertion site. The head of the bed should be kept flat or raised no higher than 30 degrees. The patient can usually drink immediately after the procedure and should be encouraged to do so to help clear the dye used in the procedure from the body. Patients are also usually given anticoagulant therapy (e.g., heparin). The nurse must monitor APTT levels and observe for signs of bleeding. Patient education after the procedure should focus on modifying risk factors by making needed life-style changes.

To reduce the risk of restenosis of the artery following PTA, many surgeons are placing intravascular stents instead of or in addition to the PTA procedure. Stents are small, stainless steel, meshlike tubes placed within the occluded vessel and expanded over the area of the plaque to hold the vessel open. The stent is placed during angioplasty, and the balloon catheter is used to compress the plaque and open the stent. When the catheter is removed, the stent stays in place to support the artery and prevent collapse (Hill, 1995; Cantwell-Gab, 1996; Dempsey, 1996).

The major advantage of the stent is the support it provides to the area of the artery that has undergone angioplasty. This support prevents abrupt closure of the artery. The major disadvantage of stents is that they are a foreign body and can cause thrombi to form in the coronary artery. Patients must be given anticoagulants for at least several months following the procedure.

The complications of stent placement are bleeding, injury to the vessel, thrombosis of the stent, and artery spasm above or below the stent. If thrombosis or spasm occurs, the patient may suffer acute arterial occlusion. Bypass surgery or stent embolectomy may be required to reopen the artery.

Nursing care of the patient with a stent includes those interventions used for PTA in addition to monitoring for signs of stent thrombosis and stent dislodgement. The patient must be educated about the anticoagulant drugs that he or she is taking and signs of bleeding. The patient will be observed closely after the procedure to monitor PT levels and adjust the anticoagulant dosage. Life-style modifications are also a focus of the follow-up care after stent placement.

Bypass grafts to provide an alternative route for blood flow around areas of narrowing or occlusion are considered when other treatments have failed or are impossible because of the location and size of the atherosclerotic plaque. The approach and type of graft depend on the location of the occlusion. Common types of bypass grafts are included in Table 24-7. The greater saphenous vein is most often used to create the bypass in the arterial system. If the veins of the lower extremities are varicosed or have already been used for other bypass surgery, an upper extremity vein can be used

---

**NURSE ALERT**

If an upper extremity vein is to be used for the arterial bypass, the vein should not be used for intravenous therapy or venipuncture for laboratory studies. These procedures can cause infection or damage to the vein and make it unusable as the graft.

---

(Cantwell-Gab, 1996). Synthetic grafts may also be used if no other vein is available, and these grafts are also used frequently in bypasses involving the aorta and iliac arteries. Veins are the preferred graft material because they have a lower rate of infection and a higher rate of remaining patent.

Because of the more invasive nature of the surgical procedure, arterial bypass graft surgery is associated with numerous complications, including graft infection, graft failure (occlusion), wound infections, pulmonary complications, and other common complications of major surgery. Bypass surgery also requires longer hospitalization and is associated with higher mortalities than less invasive interventions (Howland-Gradman, 1995). The common surgical approaches are included in Table 24-7.

For all bypass procedures, routine preoperative care includes an in-depth assessment of the patient's risk for surgery. The cardiac, renal, and pulmonary systems are evaluated to determine any impairment that could cause increased intraoperative and postoperative complications. Of particular concern is a history of

---

**TABLE 24-7**

## Common Bypass Graft Procedures

| TYPE | PICTURE | NURSING CONSIDERATIONS | TYPE | PICTURE | NURSING CONSIDERATIONS |
|------|---------|------------------------|------|---------|------------------------|
| Femorofemoral bypass | | Used for unilateral claudication or ischemia | Aortoiliac bypass | | Usually uses synthetic graft |
| Femoropopliteal bypass | | Usually uses vein graft | Aortobifemoral bypass | | Usually uses synthetic graft |

carotid artery or coronary artery disease. Arterial disease in the neurologic or cardiac system may need to be addressed before peripheral arterial disease can be treated.

The nursing role in the preoperative phase includes collection of data regarding the patient's health history and current physical state. Of greatest importance is the establishment of a baseline vascular assessment. Preoperative vascular parameters (e.g., color, temperature, and pulse quality) are compared with the findings postoperatively. In addition, the nurse is integral in providing patient and family teaching and support and in preparing the patient and family for the postoperative phase. Because the patient may not be admitted until the day of surgery, preoperative teaching and evaluation are often done on an outpatient basis.

Postoperatively, the patient may be monitored in an ICU or may be placed on a general surgical unit. The level of monitoring required determines where the patient will be cared for. Numerous complications can develop following bypass grafting, and the major nursing interventions in the immediate and ongoing postoperative phase should be to monitor for and prevent these complications (Boxes 24-10 and 24-11).

Close monitoring of the affected extremity and the operative site is essential in the immediate postoperative period. Because graft failure and graft infection often result in limb amputation, any alteration from normal should be reported and treated immediately. The

---

**BOX 24-10**

### COMPLICATIONS FOLLOWING BYPASS GRAFT SURGERY

**OPERATIVE SITE OR GRAFT RELATED**
Graft failure or occlusion
Graft infection
Aneurysms at the anastomosis
Bleeding
Hematoma formation
Compartment syndrome (swelling in the tissues) compresses the graft
Wound infection

**OTHER**
Renal failure from use of dyes, hypovolemia, or surgery involving renal arteries
Spinal cord ischemia from surgical manipulation of spinal artery
Bowel ischemia from anesthesia or bowel manipulation
Pulmonary infections from postoperative immobility, pain, or anesthesia
Skin breakdown from immobility
Sexual dysfunction from disruption of pelvic autonomic nerves

Data from Hill EM: *AACN Clin Issues* 6(4):547-561, 1995.

---

**BOX 24-11**

## NURSING PROCESS

## POSTOPERATIVE BYPASS GRAFT SURGERY

**ASSESSMENT**
- Pulmonary status including lung sounds, oxygenation, arterial blood gases (ABGs), pulse oximetry
- Peripheral circulation: pulse quality, color, temperature, and capillary refill of extremity; Doppler pulses
- Vital signs, especially blood pressure
- Cardiac status: heart rate and rhythm, electrocardiogram (ECG) if indicated, heart sounds, laboratory values
- Renal perfusion: urine output, weights, laboratory values
- Gastrointestinal functioning: bowel sounds, flatus, nasogastric tube if indicated
- Level of pain, and adequacy of pain control method

- Skin: incision and invasive line sites, wound healing, skin breakdown
- Level of anxiety and coping ability

**NURSING DIAGNOSES**
**Actual**
- Pain related to decreased peripheral perfusion and incision site
- Impaired mobility related to pain and recent intervention

**Potential**
- Risk for acute decreased tissue perfusion related to hematoma formation, graft failure, or occlusion
- Risk for alteration in skin integrity

*Continued*

BOX 24-11

# NURSING PROCESS

## POSTOPERATIVE BYPASS GRAFT SURGERY—cont'd

### NURSING INTERVENTIONS

- Assess level of discomfort or pain, and medicate as ordered.
- Evaluate effectiveness after each dose of analgesic.
- Notify the surgeon of any excruciating pain.
- Assess pulses, sensory and motor function, skin temperature and color, capillary refill, and swelling of extremities.
- Notify the surgeon of paresthesias, loss or decrease in peripheral pulses, coldness or discoloration of feet, prolonged capillary refill, and excessive swelling.
- Assess incisional site for bleeding, hematoma, or swelling.
- Assess vital signs, and administer medication to control blood pressure.
- Keep head of bed flat or elevated as ordered.
- Avoid bending at knees and use of knee Gatch on hospital bed.

- Keep operative site free of binding bandages or bed linens; use a bed cradle if needed.
- Avoid prolonged dependent position of extremity.
- Avoid trauma to lower extremity: keep heels protected from pressure, avoid the use of tape, avoid bumping feet.
- Reposition patient frequently.
- Elevate extremity above the level of the heart if swelling occurs.

### EVALUATION OF EXPECTED OUTCOMES

- Patient pain free or pain controlled adequately to allow for activity progression and rest
- Extremity warm and pink with good pulses
- No hematoma, infection, swelling, or skin breakdown
- Mobility increased to presurgical level

nurse must evaluate the color, temperature, capillary refill, and arterial pulses distal to the operative site. These evaluations may be done as often as every 15 minutes during the first few hours after surgery, and any alterations from baseline should be reported immediately. In addition, the patient must be monitored for the development of excessive bleeding, hematoma formation, infection, and pulmonary or cardiac complications. Severe pain, loss of pulses, changes in sensation, or discoloration or coolness of the extremity may indicate occlusion of the bypass graft and should be reported immediately. Swelling or hematoma formation on the suture line can impair blood flow through the graft and must be reported and treated quickly. Symptoms of graft infection include swelling, redness, pain, fever, and bleeding.

### NURSE ALERT

**Remember that the presence of pulses by Doppler assessment does not mean flow is adequate. Loss of a peripheral pulse that has previously been present must be reported immediately.**

The nurse is also responsible for preventing injury to the operative extremity and avoiding any pressure

that could occlude the new graft. The operative site should be kept free of binding bandages and should be cushioned from pressure. Although elastic bandages or support stockings may be used in the postoperative phase, they should not create excessive pressure that could block the new grafts. Knee or hip flexed positions should be avoided. The patient should be repositioned often to prevent pressure on bony prominences. When the patient is allowed to sit or stand, the extremity should not be left dependent for prolonged periods to avoid edema and pressure on the graft sites. If swelling occurs, the extremity should be elevated above the level of the heart. The pulmonary system, gastrointestinal system, and renal system are assessed regularly to avoid complications such as pulmonary infections, ileus, and renal failure. The patient is usually given intravenous heparin and monitored for bleeding complications.

The patient's diet and activity gradually progress during the postoperative period. Patient teaching before discharge includes all the risk factor modifications previously discussed, wound and incision care, the use and complications of anticoagulant therapy, and signs of decreased circulation. General patient teaching guidelines for chronic arterial disease are also appropriate for patients following bypass surgery or other invasive treatments (see Box 24-11).

**Amputation** of the ischemic extremity will be needed if revascularization attempts fail. Amputations are usually accomplished in stages, only removing the portion of the extremity that is necessary to prevent progression of gangrene and necrosis. Amputations are done as distally as possible to maintain a functional limb. More distal amputations also decrease the dependency of the patient on prosthetic devices. Unfortunately, because circulation is compromised, the rate of healing for amputations for arterial occlusive disease is poor (Hill, 1995).

Before amputation, nursing interventions should focus on providing support and education to the patient and family. The need for amputation means failure of other treatment attempts and permanent loss of part or all of a body part. Emotional responses of patients can range from anger, denial, guilt, or overwhelming grief to relief that persistent pain will be removed. Anger, depression, and anxiety are common patient responses. The nurse must evaluate the meaning of the amputation for each individual patient and plan interventions that will assist with the grieving or emotional process. Cultural and religious beliefs, particularly regarding the disposition of the amputated limb, should also be taken into consideration and accommodated as appropriate when planning care. The patient and family should be educated on the postoperative course, the possibility of phantom pain, and the resources for prostheses and rehabilitation. The overall goal is to restore the patient to the highest level of functional ability possible.

In the postoperative period, care of the stump should be one of the major nursing functions. The dressing and care of the remaining limb (the stump) are integral parts of the rehabilitation process. Complications following amputation include contractures, misfit of the prosthesis, and infection and vascular insufficiency in the distal part of the stump (Hill, 1995). The nurse should closely monitor the incision site for bleeding, infection, and circulation. The new distal pulses in the stump should be palpated frequently to ensure blood flow is adequate. The stump should be dressed according to the surgeon's orders to prepare it for prosthesis fitting.

The rehabilitation process should begin soon after surgery with consultation from physical therapy and occupational rehabilitation experts. These professionals can assist with activity progression and teach the patient to transfer or ambulate. They will also measure, fit, and show the patient how to use the prosthesis. Some patients may benefit from counseling or a short stay in a rehabilitation facility.

Nursing knowledge of the patient's beliefs, fears, and responses to the amputation is essential in the discharge planning process. In addition, a thorough assessment of the patient's occupation, social environment, and support systems is needed to plan a smooth transition to home. Patients with limited family support, with other physical limitations (e.g., visual or physical impairment), or who are elderly may require additional resources to return to independent living. High-risk patients may be unable to resume independent living and may require home health or long-term care placement.

## Other Arterial Diseases
### Raynaud's Phenomenon

**Raynaud's phenomenon,** also called *arteriospastic disease,* is a chronic peripheral vascular disorder that often affects young women. Raynaud's phenomenon is characterized by episodes of vasospasm of the small skin arteries, primarily of the fingers, but vasospasm can also occur in the earlobes and toes (Krenzer, 1995). The cause is unknown, but Raynaud's phenomenon is often seen in conjunction with collagen diseases, such as lupus, scleroderma, and rheumatoid arthritis (Huether, McCance, 1996). Other predisposing factors include occupations that require repeated pressure on the fingertips, such as typing and the use of vibrating equipment. Attacks are often triggered by cold, emotional stress, or vasoconstricting agents (e.g., caffeine and nicotine). The vasospasm of the arteries of the hands or feet leads to blanching or white discoloration of the fingers or toes. This white color change is followed by cyanosis, or blue discoloration, and then by rubor, or red coloration. The rubor of Raynaud's is caused by hyperemia following the spasm. Because the process is caused by spasm and not complete occlusion, the pulses of the affected extremity are not affected. The changes in color are usually accompanied by a sensation of coldness and numbness followed by throbbing pain, tingling, and swelling (Huether, McCance, 1996). Attacks usually last only a few minutes but can last for several hours. A complication of Raynaud's phenomenon includes skin breakdown of the digit progressing to gangrenous ulcers (Wheeler, Brenner, 1995).

Because symptoms spontaneously subside in most cases, treatment may not be required. In severe cases the patient may be given vasodilators or beta-blockers to prevent spasms. Sympathectomy or severing of the nervous tissue that causes the vasoconstriction is reserved for severe cases (Huether, McCance, 1996).

Nursing interventions for patients with Raynaud's phenomenon include counseling and patient education. The patient should be reassured that the disease is unlikely to lead to serious disability and that the symptoms can be controlled and prevented. The patient should keep the extremities warm and avoid contact with cold objects. Stressful situations that precipitate the attacks should be identified and dealt with accordingly. Care should be taken to prevent injury or infection to the affected extremities. Smoking and caffeine use should be discouraged. Some patients find that soaking the hands or feet briefly in warm water can decrease the spasms and provide relief of symptoms during an attack (Krenzer, 1995).

### Buerger's Disease

**Buerger's disease,** also called *thromboangiitis obliterans,* is an acute inflammation of the arteries and veins of the upper or lower extremities (Huether, McCance, 1996). The inflammation leads to development of lesions that eventually cause thrombus formation. This results in decreased blood flow to the legs and feet. Leg ulcers and gangrene are frequent complications. Although the underlying cause is unknown, the disease only occurs in smokers, with the highest incidence in young men who are heavy smokers (Huether, McCance, 1996). A family tendency toward Buerger's disease has been found.

Symptoms include asymmetric intermittent claudication similar to that of arterial occlusive disease. Peripheral pulses may be absent or diminished, and the extremities may be cold, numb, tingly, red, or cyanotic (Huether, McCance, 1996). Sensitivity to cold, paresthesia, ulcers, and gangrene can also occur. In severe cases the arterial occlusion may require amputation.

The primary treatment for Buerger's disease is to have the patient stop smoking (Wheeler, Brenner, 1995). The patient should be referred to aggressive smoking cessation programs and should be counseled on the progressive course of the disease, including amputation, if smoking is not stopped. Anticoagulants and vasodilators may be used, but these pharmacologic agents are not frequently successful. Skin and foot care to prevent infections is vital, and exposure to cold and trauma should be avoided.

## PROBLEMS INVOLVING THE VEINS

Problems involving the veins and venous systems are frequently encountered by nurses. Because of the vital role that nurses play in the implementation and main-

tenance of intravenous therapy and in prevention of complications of prolonged bed rest in hospitalized patients, nurses are in a prime role for identification of risk factors for venous problems, prevention, and early identification and treatment.

Varicosed veins, venous thrombosis with superficial thrombophlebitis or DVT, and chronic venous insufficiency with venous stasis ulcers are the most common peripheral venous problems. Pulmonary embolus formation can be a serious, even deadly, venous problem (see Chapter 23).

## Varicosed Veins

Varicosed veins, also called *varicosities,* are dilated veins most commonly found in the superficial saphenous venous system of the legs (Wheeler, Brenner, 1995) (Figure 24-11). Varicosed veins can range from small to large and tortuous, and they most often affect women. There are two types of varicosed veins. Primary varicosed veins are the most common and are caused by dysfunction of the valves, vein wall dilation, or both (Olivencia, 1996). Primary varicosed veins have a familial tendency with congenital weakness of the wall of the vein as the underlying disease.

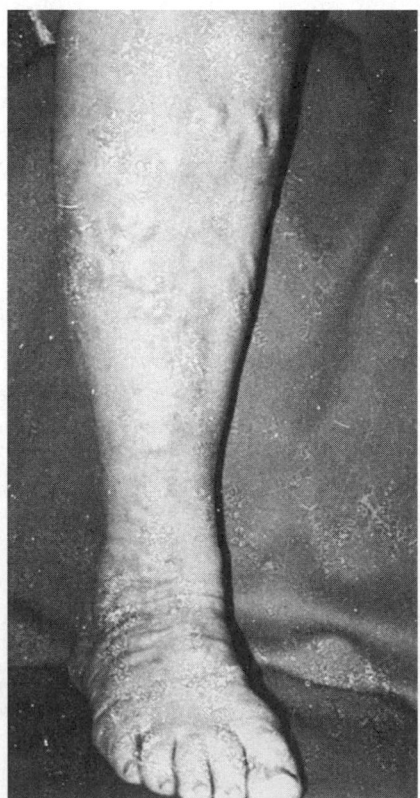

**Figure 24-11** Varicosed veins on lower leg with nodular bulges. (From Bowers AC, Thompson JM: *Clinical manual of health assessment,* ed 4, St Louis, 1992, Mosby.)

Secondary varicosed veins develop in patients who have previous inflammation of the vein (phlebitis), obstruction in the venous system, venous malformations, or arteriovenous fistulas. Secondary varicosed veins can occur in the lower extremities, esophagus (called *varices*), or the anorectal area (called *hemorrhoids*).

Anything that increases the pressure in the veins or structural weakness of the vein wall can cause varicosed veins. Box 24-12 gives common predisposing factors to varicosed veins. In patients with existing varicosed veins numerous environmental and lifestyle variables can worsen varicosed veins (Box 24-13).

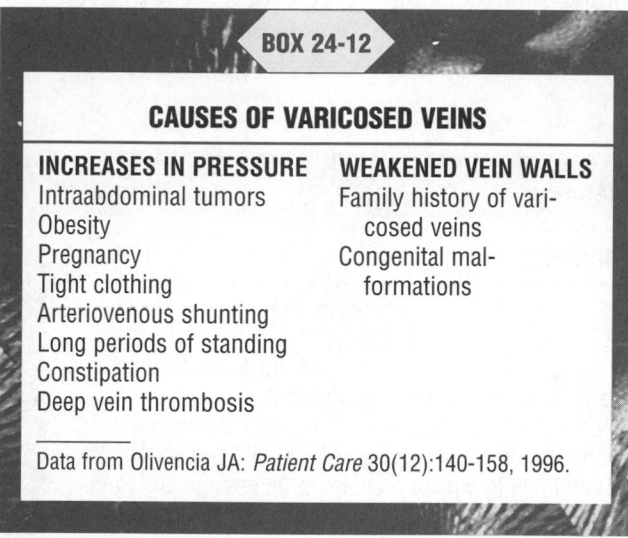

**BOX 24-12**

### CAUSES OF VARICOSED VEINS

| INCREASES IN PRESSURE | WEAKENED VEIN WALLS |
|---|---|
| Intraabdominal tumors | Family history of varicosed veins |
| Obesity | Congenital malformations |
| Pregnancy | |
| Tight clothing | |
| Arteriovenous shunting | |
| Long periods of standing | |
| Constipation | |
| Deep vein thrombosis | |

Data from Olivencia JA: *Patient Care* 30(12):140-158, 1996.

**BOX 24-13**

### FACTORS THAT WORSEN VARICOSED VEINS

Overexposure to the sun: damages the elastic layer of the vein

Use of hot tubs: causes pooling of blood in the legs and veins; dilates the veins

Heating via floor vents: dilates veins and causes venous pooling

Tight clothing: increases pressure

High-heeled shoes: keep the calf muscles from pumping venous blood back to the heart

Lack of exercise: weakens muscles that promote venous return

Weightlifting or heavy lifting: increases pressure on the venous system

Exercises that involve jumping: damage valves

Excessive sitting or standing: decreases venous return

Data from Olivencia JA: *Patient Care* 30(12):140-158, 1996.

As superficial veins suffer weakening or increased pressure, the veins enlarge and the valves become stretched and no longer close correctly to prevent backflow of blood. As the backflow of blood continues, blood is no longer effectively pumped back toward the heart. This continued backflow increases the pressure in the vein even further, and edema develops.

## Assessment

**History and physical examination.** The clinical manifestations of varicosed veins vary among patients and can include swollen tortuous bulging veins, skin thickening and pigmentation changes, and venous stasis ulcers. Symptoms include aches or pains, particularly after prolonged standing or before and during menstruation. The pain of varicosed veins may improve with walking or elevation of the legs. Cramplike pain may occur at night. Swelling of the lower extremity may also occur. Corona phlebectatica is an area with tiny veins concentrated around the ankles and feet that is seen with chronic venous insufficiency (Olivencia, 1996).

The nurse should assess all patients for the presence of risk factors and evidence of varicosed veins. Evaluation of the extremities should be done with the patient in a standing position. Because thrombophlebitis and venous stasis ulcers are common complications of varicosed veins, the nurse should also assess for redness, tenderness, and skin lesions over the lower extremities.

**Diagnostic studies.** A duplex Doppler study is recommended in patients who have bulging varicosities of the distal or middle thigh, the anterior medial aspect of the calf, or extending distally from the popliteal fossa (Olivencia, 1996). This study can determine the competence of the veins, the extent of dilation, and whether a blood clot is present. Duplex Doppler studies are most often used before invasive intervention for severe varicosities. Veins that are dilated but not varicosed can be reversed through conservative treatment. Varicosed veins are irreversible and may require invasive therapy.

## Medical and Nursing Interventions

Medical and nursing interventions for varicosed veins should begin with early identification and prevention of varicosed veins. Patients with familial history or risk factors for varicosed veins should be counseled to avoid sitting or standing for prolonged periods, to maintain ideal body weight, to avoid constrictive clothing, and to wear supportive stockings to prevent excessive pressure on the venous system. These measures assist with reducing pressure in the venous system and can prevent progression of varicosities.

Once varicosed veins are present, treatment usually starts with conservative therapy and progresses to invasive therapy for cosmetic and symptom control. The goals for chronic varicosed veins are to improve venous return to the heart, prevent complications, relieve discomfort, and improve the appearance. Therapy depends on whether the varicosed veins are secondary or primary in nature. For secondary varicosed veins, the underlying cause must be treated first if possible. If chronic obstruction as a result of a tumor is the underlying cause, the tumor must be removed for improvement in the varicosities to be seen. Primary varicosities are progressive and will not resolve without treatment (Olivencia, 1996).

Conservative therapy for varicosed veins, including compression stockings, exercise, weight loss, and regular periods of leg elevation, is usually implemented before invasive treatments are considered (Olivencia, 1996). The nurse can serve in a crucial role by providing education and resources for patients to facilitate compliance with this initial management.

The first-line conservative treatment for varicosed veins is the regular use of compression stockings. In patients with potential for varicosed veins or in the early stages of varicosed veins, compression stockings can be obtained over the counter from medical supply stores. If varicosed veins are already present or the condition worsens, the patient should wear graduated compression stockings. The nurse should instruct patients on the proper use and care of compression stockings (Box 24-14). Men and young women may resist wearing compression stockings because of a concern over their appearance and cost. Obese and pregnant patients should have their stocking individually fitted by a

---

**BOX 24-14**

## COMPRESSION STOCKINGS

**WHO NEEDS COMPRESSION STOCKINGS?**
People who work in professions that require standing: teachers, nurses, factory workers
People with varicosed veins or chronic venous insufficiency
People with thrombophlebitis or lymphedema
People with risk factors for varicosed veins

**WHAT TYPE OF STOCKINGS SHOULD BE WORN?**
Over-the-counter stockings can be worn initially; purchased at medical supply stores or via mail
Graduated compression stockings should be worn by those with worsening varicosed veins; purchased in medical supply stores with a prescription from the physician

**WHEN ARE COMPRESSION STOCKINGS CONTRAINDICATED?**
Arterial occlusive disease
Uncontrolled congestive heart failure
Open leg ulcers

**WHAT TYPES OF GRADUATED COMPRESSION STOCKINGS ARE AVAILABLE?**
Graduated compression stockings come in different classifications depending on the amount of pressure
  Class 1: 18-25 mm Hg pressure for mild varicosed veins with minimal symptoms
  Class 2: 26-35 mm Hg pressure for large varicosed veins with increasing symptoms

  Class 3: 36-49 mm Hg pressure for severe varicosed veins with complications
  Class 4: >50 mm Hg pressure; infrequently used
Many colors and styles now available
Special stockings for pregnant women available
Compression stockings should be individually measured and fitted to ensure they are large enough and long enough for the person wearing them; some people may require custom fitting

**HOW SHOULD STOCKINGS BE USED?**
Put on in the morning before getting out of bed and kept on all day until bedtime
Put on before venous pooling has occurred, and if possible should be put on with the legs elevated above the level of the heart
Should not bind at the waist, groin, or knees
May come with special gloves to assist with putting them on
Care taken to keep the toes from being compressed and bent when stockings are applied

**HOW SHOULD STOCKINGS BE CARED FOR?**
Follow manufacturer's guidelines for washing and drying: use mild soap and let air dry; commercial dryers can damage the elastic fibers and make the stockings loose
Replace after 4-6 months before they lose their elasticity
Have two pairs at least so that one pair can be washed and dried while the other pair is being worn

Data from Olivencia JA: *Patient Care* 30(12):140-158, 1996.

trained professional. It is important for the nurse to strongly encourage the use of compression stockings and reemphasize the complications that can occur from progressive venous insufficiency, such as clot formation, bleeding, and increased discomfort and disfigurement.

Regular exercise, such as walking, and control of weight are also important treatments for varicosed veins. Patients who are overweight should be assisted with weight reduction. Patients who are ambulatory should be instructed to walk daily to promote venous return. Patients who are bedridden or have problems with ambulation need to be taught leg exercises, such as pumping of the feet to exercise the calf muscles and improve venous return. Patients who are required to stand or sit for long periods must be taught to change positions frequently and take breaks to walk or do leg exercises, such as standing up on tiptoes or pumping the feet (Olivencia, 1996).

Patients with varicosed veins, especially those with swelling of the lower extremities, should be instructed to elevate their feet above the level of the heart two or three times per day for 15 to 20 minutes to promote venous return and decrease edema (Olivencia, 1996). Patients should also be advised to avoid wearing high-heeled shoes and restrictive clothing and sitting in hot tubs, all of which can worsen varicosed veins (Olivencia, 1996).

Varicosed veins can be unsightly, and many patients will express concern over the appearance of their legs. Many products can be used to cover the blue discoloration of the veins and improve the appearance of the legs. Patients should be discouraged from overexposure to the sun because this can damage the vein walls and worsen the varicosities.

Invasive procedures can also be used to treat varicosed veins for cosmetic reasons. Invasive therapy for varicosed veins includes injection sclerotherapy, ambulatory phlebectomy, and surgery, including vein stripping, vein ligation, and segmental resection. These therapies may be indicated for patients with moderate to severe varicosed veins not responsive to conservative treatment, for cosmetic treatment, or for those patients who have complications from varicosed veins.

Sclerotherapy involves using a sclerosing agent, such as hypertonic saline or sodium tetradecyl sulfate, injected into the varicosed vein to cause irritation, inflammation, and eventual thrombosis of the vein (Olivencia, 1996). It is most often used for small or medium-sized varicosed veins, but it can be used for larger veins in patients who are not good surgical candidates. Sclerotherapy is usually done in an outpatient setting and causes mild discomfort during and after the injection. Complications include swelling, pain, superficial phlebitis, DVT, and rare allergic reactions

to the sclerosing agent (Olivencia, 1996). Following sclerotherapy the extremity is usually wrapped with an elastic bandage for 24 to 48 hours to compress the vein and promote fusion of the vein walls. The results of sclerotherapy are not immediate, and improvement may take as long as 4 weeks to be seen. Patients who have undergone sclerotherapy should continue with conservative therapy to prevent recurrence.

Ambulatory phlebectomy is the removal of the varicosed vein through numerous small 1- to 3-mm incisions made down the extremity (Olivencia, 1996). Through these incisions the vein is ligated and removed in sections. The procedure is commonly completed on an outpatient basis with the patient under local anesthesia.

Vein stripping, ligations, and segmental resections, which are also methods to remove the vein, are used for more severe cases of varicosed veins (Olivencia, 1996). These procedures can be done on an outpatient basis, but complicated cases are commonly performed in the hospital. The physician usually sees the patient before surgery to mark the route of the veins that are to be removed. The long saphenous vein, which branches from the groin and extends to the ankle, is often the one removed. One or both extremities may be involved. Recuperation depends on the complexity of the procedure and can range from 1 day to 3 to 4 weeks.

Hospitalization may be required. If the patient is hospitalized, it is usually limited to 24 to 48 hours for observation and pain control. Most vein surgery can be done using spinal or epidural anesthesia, but some procedures may require general anesthesia. Complications of surgical intervention to remove varicosed veins include hematomas, infection, and injuries to the arteries and nerves that run next to the veins.

Hospitalized patients who have had surgery for varicosed veins must be monitored for complications. The extremity is wrapped firmly with elastic bandages following the procedure to prevent swelling and pressure on the ligated vein ends. The knee Gatch section of the bed should not be raised, but the foot of the bed may be elevated about 8 inches to facilitate the return of venous blood. The foot and toes should be observed for skin color and edema, and the patient should be encouraged to move them as soon as possible. The patient may have some pain for several days after surgery. Patients should be encouraged to walk as soon as allowed and discouraged from sitting and standing. An elastic stocking is worn for several weeks. Patients should also be taught to avoid scratching and bruising the legs. The patient should not sit with the legs crossed and should be advised to avoid wearing clothing that may compress veins in the groin and thighs or irritate the incisions. The staples or sutures used for closure of the skin will be removed during the follow-up visit with the physician, and the patient should be taught the signs of infection and incision care before discharge.

## Venous Thrombosis

**Venous thrombosis** is one of the most common problems associated with the venous system. Abnormal clots can occur anywhere in the venous system, and the severity, complications, and treatment depend on the location and extent of the thrombus. *Thrombophlebitis* is the term usually used to describe inflammation accompanied by a blood clot in the vein. Thrombi or thrombophlebitis in the venous system can be either in the superficial venous system or the deep venous system. Thrombi in the deep venous system are also called DVTs.

A classic triad of factors (Virchow's triad) is responsible for thrombus formation in the venous system. These factors are stasis of venous circulation, hypercoagulability of the blood, and damage to the vessel wall (Huether, McCance, 1996). Patients who have conditions that slow venous blood flow, thicken the blood or increase clotting of the blood, or damage the blood vessels are at risk for developing venous thrombi and thrombophlebitis. Prophylactic interventions for DVT are given in Box 24-15. Box 24-16 includes some of the underlying conditions that affect Virchow's triad. Patients with multiple risk factors have an even higher possibility of venous thrombosis.

Superficial thrombophlebitis is most often caused by vessel damage—in the arms the culprit is usually intravenous catheters, and in the legs it is usually related to varicosed veins (Stephen, Feied, 1995). DVT can form in any area, including the pelvis or arms, but lower extremity DVT is the most common. Lower extremity DVTs are categorized as distal or proximal. Distal DVTs are those that form in the deep veins of the calf, and proximal DVTs are those that form in the popliteal, femoral, or iliac veins (Stephen, Feied, 1995).

---

**BOX 24-15**

### PROPHYLACTIC INTERVENTIONS FOR DEEP VEIN THROMBOSIS

**INTERVENTIONS THAT PROMOTE VENOUS RETURN/PREVENT VENOUS STASIS**
Early ambulation
Range of motion (active or passive)
Leg exercises and dorsiflexion of feet to use calf muscles
Pneumatic compression stockings or boots

**INTERVENTIONS THAT PREVENT HYPERCOAGULABILITY**
Adequate oral intake or use of intravenous fluids to prevent dehydration
Avoidance of drugs that increase hypercoagulability if possible
Low-dose anticoagulant therapy using subcutaneous route of administration

---

**BOX 24-16**

### RISK FACTORS FOR THROMBOPHLEBITIS

**VENOUS STASIS**
Varicosed veins
Obesity
Sedentary life-style
Immobility: postoperative, paraplegic/quadriplegic, or bedridden patient or one who sits for long periods
Pregnancy
Postpartum state
Congestive heart failure
Atrial fibrillation: blood pools in atrium
Drugs: steroids

**HYPERCOAGULABLE STATES**
Polycythemia vera
Anemias
Dehydration
Malnutrition
Cancer
Protein C, protein S, or antithrombin III deficiency
Systemic lupus erythematosus
Systemic infections
Oral drugs: oral contraceptives, estrogen replacements
Cigarette smoking
Smoking + oral contraceptives = double risk factor

**VESSEL DAMAGE**
Venipuncture
Intravenous therapy, especially prolonged
Intravenous drugs: high-dose antibiotics, potassium, chemotherapy, hypertonic saline
Intravenous drug abuse
Diabetes
Upper extremity risks: cervical rib, clavicular, rib fractures; pacemaker leads; central lines; dialysis catheters; repetitive motion, such as pitching, scrubbing, or lifting heavy loads overhead
Trauma to vessels secondary to surgery or fractures

**OTHER**
History of thrombophlebitis
Advanced age: can impact all risk factors

Proximal DVTs are considered more serious because of increased risk of complications such as pulmonary emboli and severe local symptoms caused by venous occlusion. Upper extremity DVT can occur in patients with trauma to the shoulder or clavicle, indwelling central venous lines, or repetitive motion injuries, such as can occur with pitching or scrubbing, in addition to hypercoagulable states and slow venous flow (Kurgan, Nunnelee, 1995).

The development of venous thrombi occurs when one or more factors of Virchow's triad are present (Wheeler, Brenner, 1995). Blood cells adhere to form a thrombus that grows until the lumen of the vessel is partially or totally occluded. If the thrombus detaches, it becomes an embolus that flows through the venous system. If the embolus does not become lodged in the smaller venous system, it can be carried back to the right side of the heart and to the pulmonary circulation (Stephen, Feied, 1995). If the thrombus remains attached to the walls of the vessel, it will either become more organized and adhere to the wall or be lysed.

When the venous system is occluded, the skin discoloration ranges from red to deep purple or blue. Pressure in the venous system causes leakage of fluid into the interstitial spaces and results in edema. Compression on the local nerves and edema leads to pain. The activation of the clotting cascade that occurs in venous thrombosis also initiates the inflammatory response and contributes to the tenderness, swelling, and redness in the area of the thrombus (Huether, McCance, 1996). If venous occlusion and edema are severe, arterial blood flow can be compromised, resulting in signs and symptoms of decreased arterial perfusion (see Box 24-8).

## Superficial Venous Thrombophlebitis

### Assessment

**History and physical examination.** Palpable firm or hard veins with tenderness, warmth, and redness along the length of the vein are the most common signs and symptoms of superficial thrombophlebitis. The patient may also have a mild temperature and an elevated white blood cell count because of the inflammatory response. In severe cases the whole extremity may be swollen and tender to touch. Either the legs or the arms may be affected depending on the cause. Patients with intravenous lines and varicosed veins should be regularly assessed for the development of thrombophlebitis, and preventive and therapeutic interventions should be implemented.

**Diagnostic studies.** Patients with superficial thrombophlebitis may have noninvasive duplex or color flow Doppler studies to rule out a thrombosis in the deep venous system (Stephen, Feied, 1995). If a causative DVT is identified, it must be treated.

### Medical and Nursing Interventions

For patients at risk for superficial thrombophlebitis, the major nursing management focuses on prevention (see Box 24-16). Regular evaluation of intravenous sites for redness or swelling, rotation of intravenous sites every 48 to 72 hours, prompt removal of intravenous catheters when they become tender, swollen, or red, and slow or diluted administration of drugs and fluids known to cause vein irritation are preventive measures that can be implemented by the nurse. Patients with varicosed veins should be taught the factors that worsen varicosed veins. Compression stockings and leg exercises can promote venous return and prevent venous stasis. Care should also be taken to avoid the use of leg veins for intravenous therapy and to prevent other trauma to the legs.

The patient who develops superficial thrombophlebitis is usually treated with elevation of the extremity, moist heat application, and nonsteroidal antiinflammatory agents (Stephen, Feied, 1995). Any source of irritation, such as intravenous lines, must be discontinued. If the legs are affected, compression stockings with a >30 mm Hg pressure gradient should be used to prevent progression of the thrombosis (Stephen, Feied, 1995).

Placing patients with superficial thrombophlebitis on bed rest, a common intervention in the past, is now deemed unnecessary and risky since bed rest increases the risk of venous stasis and thus increases the risk of further thrombosis (Stephen, Feied, 1995). Patients should remain ambulatory using compression stockings unless severe swelling or pain prevents mobility. In this case patients should be assisted to complete range of motion and foot-pumping exercises at least every 2 hours. Mobility should resume as soon as possible as the swelling and pain subside.

Mild analgesics and nonsteroidal antiinflammatory drugs (e.g., aspirin and ibuprofen) are usually given to control the discomfort and decrease the inflammatory process. In severe thrombophlebitis, codeine may be needed to control the pain. Care must be taken to prevent further tissue irritation and trauma. The patient with severe thrombophlebitis may also be tender to any touch or pressure over the site. In this case the nurse should leave the area uncovered or provide a cradle for linens so that they do not touch the extremity. If thrombophlebitis of the lower extremities is recurrent, invasive interventions such as those described in the section on varicosed veins may be needed.

# Deep Vein Thrombosis
## Assessment

**History and physical examination.** Because many **DVTs** can be prevented, a crucial nursing assessment function is to evaluate patients for risk factors that would contribute to the development of venous thrombosis (see Box 24-16). Implementation of preventive measures is important for patients who have multiple risk factors for the development of DVT but should be implemented for all patients with even one risk factor, particularly decreased mobility. In patients with existing DVT, nursing assessment should focus on assessment of complications of DVT, namely, pulmonary emboli and chronic venous insufficiency.

Patients with lower extremity DVT may present with classic symptoms of unilateral leg pain, edema, and warm, reddened skin over the site of the thrombus. Other patients with DVT may have no symptoms at all. Patients with DVT may have a temperature or may be afebrile. Homan's sign (pain when the foot is dorsiflexed [pushed back toward the lower part of the leg]) can also be seen, but absence of Homan's sign (no pain on dorsiflexion) does not rule out DVT. A positive Homan's sign can be elicited in patients who have tight calf muscles and no DVT. If the venous occlusion and edema impair arterial circulation, the limb can become cool and pale, with diminished pulses. Other symptoms of DVT include tenderness of the extremity, a feeling of tightness, heaviness, or a dull ache that worsens when walking. Since clinical assessment data can be varied and misleading, any patient suspected of having lower extremity DVT will usually undergo diagnostic testing.

Patients who have thrombosis in larger venous systems, such as the inferior vena cava, will have poor venous return in both legs and may have bilateral edema and cyanosis. If the superior vena cava is involved, the patient may have edema and cyanosis of the upper extremities, trunk, and face. Thrombosis in the upper extremities, although rare, will cause unilateral edema and cyanosis of the arm (Kurgan, Nunnelee, 1995). The discomfort of upper extremity thrombosis is commonly described as a dull or achy feeling in the arm or shoulder. Other manifestations include prominent veins in the upper chest or shoulder, dependent redness, and tenderness over the vein (Kurgan, Nunnelee, 1995). Patients with indwelling central venous or dialysis catheters, fracture of the ribs or clavicle, or thoracic or breast surgery should be monitored for upper extremity DVT (Kurgan, Nunnelee, 1995).

**Diagnostic studies.** The noninvasive diagnostic tests most often used for DVT include venous Doppler, duplex Doppler, and MRI, with the duplex Doppler test being the most widely used (Stephen, Feied, 1995). Invasive tests using contrast dye, such as contrast venograms, ventilation-perfusion scans (VQ scans), and pulmonary arteriograms, are reserved for situations in which ultrasound tests fail to yield the needed information (venograms are done in that case) or the patient is also suspected to have a pulmonary embolus (VQ scans or pulmonary arteriograms are done in that situation). In addition, the patient will usually have coagulation studies, such as PT, APTT, platelet count, and bleeding times, to establish a baseline before the administration of anticoagulants. If a hypercoagulable or a malignant cause of the DVT is suspected, other laboratory and diagnostic studies will be needed.

## Medical and Nursing Interventions

Prophylactic interventions are extremely important for the prevention of DVT. Box 24-17 includes common measures used for preventing venous thrombosis and DVT. Prophylactic interventions can include activity, pharmacologic agents, or mechanical devices. The most appropriate interventions should be implemented for all patients who have risk factors for DVT.

Promotion of venous return and prevention of venous stasis can be accomplished through early ambulation and leg exercises, especially in patients who are bedridden during illness or after surgery. In patients who are unable to ambulate or actively complete leg exercises, passive range of motion or continuous passive range of motion devices can be used. Compression stockings or pneumatic compression stockings are also used to promote venous return and are recommended for all at-risk patients unless contraindicated. Ensuring adequate oral intake, accurate intake and output measurements, and noting trends in intake and output volumes can prevent dehydration and hypercoagulability. Patients at risk for DVT should not take or be given drugs that increase hypercoagulability unless medically necessary. The most common pharmacologic intervention to prevent DVT is the administration of subcutaneous heparin (usually 5000 units given subcutaneously every 8 hours). Intravenous heparin or oral anticoagulants will not be needed for prevention unless the patient has a history of DVT or a hypercoagulable state that requires aggressive anticoagulant therapy. Long-term prevention for patients with continuous risk includes smoking cessation, avoiding long periods of standing or sitting, exercise, and use of compression stockings.

Once a diagnosis of DVT is made, the patient is usually admitted to the hospital (if not already hospitalized) so that intravenous heparin therapy can be started. The overall goals of care for the patient with DVT are prevention of progression of the clot and prevention of complications such as pulmonary embolus (see Box 24-17).

> **BOX 24-17**

# NURSING PROCESS
## DEEP VEIN THROMBOSIS

### ASSESSMENT

- Pulmonary status, including lung sounds, oxygenation, arterial blood gases (ABGs), and pulse oximetry if shortness of breath, tachypnea, or chest pain occurs
- Peripheral circulation: pulse quality, color, temperature, and capillary refill of extremity; Doppler pulses; presence of edema; compare sides
- Vital signs, especially temperature
- Cardiac status: heart rate and rhythm, electrocardiogram (ECG) if indicated, heart sounds, laboratory values
- Fluid volume status: urine output, weight, laboratory values, intake
- Level of pain and adequacy of pain control method
- Skin: color and texture changes, breakdown
- Gastrointestinal: color of stool, stool guaiac test
- Renal: color of urine, presence of hematuria
- Neurologic: mental status, level of consciousness, signs of intracranial bleeding
- Level of anxiety and coping ability
- Risk factors for venous thrombosis

### NURSING DIAGNOSES
**Actual**

- Pain related to edema and impaired venous return
- Knowledge deficit related to new diagnosis, medical regimen

**Potential**

- Risk for impaired skin integrity related to altered tissue perfusion, edema
- Risk for potential complication—pulmonary embolus

### NURSING INTERVENTIONS

- Keep affected extremity elevated above the level of the heart.
- Apply compression hose or compression devices as ordered.
- Administer analgesics as ordered.
- Monitor level of discomfort and effect of analgesics.
- Administer antiinflammatory agents.
- Monitor edema, and compare sides daily; measure circumference of extremity.
- Apply warm moist heat as ordered.
- Instruct patient to avoid crossing legs.
- Do not use knee Gatch or pillows under knees.
- Maintain bed rest or activity level as ordered.
- Instruct patient to perform leg and foot exercises.
- Provide patient/family education regarding disease process, procedures, medications, life-style modifications, compression stockings, exercise progression, and preventive measures to reduce risks.
- Assess skin for signs of breakdown or ulceration.
- Assist patient to reposition every 2 hours.
- Avoid trauma to extremity.
- Provide skin and wound care as needed.
- Monitor for signs and symptoms of pulmonary embolus.
- Notify physician immediately of changes in pulmonary status.

### EVALUATION OF EXPECTED OUTCOMES

- Patient pain free or pain controlled adequately to allow activity progression and rest
- Patient and family able to verbalize understanding of disease process, medical regimen, use of medications, use of compression stockings, preventive measures, life-style modifications, and follow-up care needed
- No skin breakdown
- No complications from deep vein thrombosis

Continuous intravenous heparin therapy is the treatment of choice for all patients with DVT regardless of the site (Stephen, Feied, 1995). Intermittent or subcutaneous administration of heparin is insufficient to produce adequate systemic anticoagulation and is used for prevention only (Stephen, Feied, 1995). Newer low-molecular–weight heparin and other types of heparin are showing promise and may replace intravenous heparin but are not widely used at present.

The action of heparin for DVT is not to dissolve the clot but to slow or prevent progression of the clot. For this reason it is critical that the heparin is begun quickly and in appropriate amounts with frequent monitoring of serum laboratory values so that the dosage can be titrated.

In preparing for beginning an intravenous heparin infusion, the nurse should obtain an accurate patient weight. Newer formulas for calculating intravenous heparin loading dosages and continuous infusion rates are based on body weight, and an accurate weight is essential in providing the correct dosage of heparin to achieve effective blood levels within a short time (Stephen, Feied, 1995). The nurse should also arrange for baseline laboratory values, including APTT, PT, INR, platelet count, hemoglobin, and hematocrit, to be obtained before initiating heparin therapy. The most current procedure for beginning intravenous heparin therapy is to give a loading dose and then begin a continuous drip (Stephen, Feied, 1995). Close monitoring of the APTT levels is essential in providing the most effective anticoagulation. Initially the APPT is obtained 6 hours after the start of the heparin and every 6 hours for the first 24 hours (Stephen, Feied, 1995). The rate of the heparin infusion will be adjusted based on the APTT until a therapeutic level is achieved. Once a therapeutic level is obtained, the APTT will usually be monitored daily. Therapeutic APTT levels of 1.5 to 2 times the control value should be achieved in 48 hours for prevention of clot progression to be most effective (Stephen, Feied, 1995). It is essential that the nurse track the APTT level and notify the physician of levels above or below the therapeutic range. If the APTT level goes above the therapeutic range, the patient is at risk for bleeding complications and the infusion may be stopped temporarily or reduced. If the APTT level is below the therapeutic range, the heparin infusion is increased and rechecked in 6 hours.

The patient's platelet level should also be watched during heparin infusions because of the risk of heparin-induced thrombocytopenia (HITT) (Malyuk, 1996). Platelet levels that drop below 10,000 are an indication of HITT. HITT may not occur until 2 days after heparin is begun, and the platelet level will usually return to normal in 2 to 4 days after the infusion is discontinued (*Physician's drug handbook,* 1995; Malyuk, 1996). If HITT develops, heparin is stopped and other anticoagulants are begun.

Once heparin therapy is begun and the blood anticoagulant levels are stable, the patient will be given an oral anticoagulant, such as warfarin (Coumadin). Because warfarin takes several days to achieve full anticoagulant levels, heparin and warfarin are continued together for 4 to 6 days (*Physician's drug handbook,* 1995). Warfarin levels are monitored using the PTT and INR. Typical therapeutic levels are PTT 1.3 to 2 times control and INR 2.0 to 3.0 times control. Warfarin will usually be continued for 6 weeks to 3 months after clinical evidence of thrombosis has subsided (*Physician's drug handbook,* 1995).

If venous occlusion is severe, the DVT is extensive, or arterial circulation is impaired, an invasive procedure, such as a thrombectomy, or pharmacologic agents, such as thrombolytics ("clot busters"), may be used. For thrombolytics to be most effective, they should be administered within 48 hours of the onset of the DVT (Stephen, Feied, 1995).

Patients receiving heparin or warfarin should be monitored for abnormal bleeding. Nosebleeds, bleeding gums, or oozing of intravenous sites or the surgical incision site may occur if anticoagulant levels are too high. Bleeding into the gastrointestinal and urinary systems can occur, and stools and urine should be examined for evidence of blood. Stool guaiac and urine tests for hematuria should be done daily or when blood is suspected. Changes in mental status may indicate cerebral bleeding and are a cause for concern. Bleeding prevention measures should be initiated for all patients taking anticoagulants (see Box 24-9). Whether to place the patient with DVT on bed rest, as has been done in the past, is still controversial. Because venous stasis and progression of the clot can be increased significantly by bed rest, patients who have distal DVT (below the knee in the calf area) are usually not placed on bed rest (Stephen, Feied, 1995). These patients should ambulate if possible. Patients who have more proximal DVTs may continue to be placed on bed rest to prevent any detachment and embolization of the venous clot. Compression stockings with >30 mm Hg pressure should be used for patients with lower extremity DVT (Stephen, Feied, 1995). Pressure on the affected extremity, such as the use of the knee Gatch and crossing of the legs, should be avoided.

Fear of the possibility of blood clots in the lungs, prolonged hospitalization, and the need for long-term drug therapy and life-style changes will understandably create anxiety in patients with DVT. The nurse must provide interventions to assist the patient and family in dealing with the short-term and long-term medical regimen, the hospitalization and follow-up care, and the impact that all of this will have on their lives. Discharge instructions should stress risk factor reduction and medication use.

Patients receiving warfarin require extensive teaching regarding the dosage, timing of the dose, and complications of anticoagulant therapy. Because many drugs and foods can interact with warfarin, the nurse should educate the patient about drugs that can increase or decrease the anticoagulant effects of the drug and the foods (especially those containing vitamin K) that can decrease the effects (see Box 24-9). Patients who are discharged taking oral warfarin will also need to have their PT and INR levels drawn and monitored frequently and should be knowledgeable of the follow-up visit schedule that will be required.

# Venous Stasis Ulcers

DVT and varicosed veins can lead to chronic venous insufficiency and venous stasis ulcers (Olivencia, 1996). When the venous system has been disrupted and valves become incompetent, chronic venous stasis and edema can occur, producing permanent skin changes and predisposing the skin and tissues to breakdown. Chronic skin changes include increased red-brown coloration of the skin on the lower leg, leathery, dry skin texture, and the development of dermatitis (Huether, McCance, 1996). Chronic venous congestion and edema prevent tissue from receiving adequate nutrients and oxygen, leading to skin breakdown and ulceration, particularly over the medial ankle area. Depending on the amount of venous stasis, the ulcerations can range from small and superficial to large and extensive (Huether, McCance, 1996).

In evaluating the patient with chronic venous insufficiency and venous ulcers, the nurse must examine the lower extremities for chronic skin changes and evidence of scarring from previous ulcers or the presence of new ulcerations. Any ulceration should be assessed for color, size, shape, depth, the presence of odor or drainage, and the degree of pain.

The classic venous ulcer is painless unless dependent and has a moist pink wound base with moderate to large amounts of drainage and irregular wound edges (Krenzer, 1995). If the ulcer has gone without treatment, the wound may be large and deep with scar tissue on the wound edges. Infected wounds will have purulent drainage and an odor.

## Medical and Nursing Interventions

For patients with chronic venous insufficiency and skin changes without ulceration, prevention of trauma and ulceration and reducing venous stasis and edema are the primary goals. The patient should be instructed to elevate the extremity as much as possible and avoid trauma or irritation of the delicate tissues. Foot care guidelines described in previous sections are important teaching points for these patients. The use of compression stockings and elastic bandages and regular exercise will also reduce venous stasis and help prevent breakdown. The patient will also require teaching regarding wound care if ulcerations do occur and the signs of infection that should be reported.

Once ulcerations occur, the goal is to promote healing and prevent infection. Elevation of the affected extremity is essential to reduce edema and venous stasis. Compression stockings should not be used until the open wound is healed. Elastic bandages and special casing systems, such as Unna boots, may be ordered to provide compression (Olivencia, 1996). Wound dressing systems can range from a simple sterile gauze to more advanced hydrocolloidal dressings. The nurse should change and dress the wound as ordered and apply the prescribed compression device. If elastic bandages are used, they should be wrapped firmly from the toes to the knees with the leg elevated above the level of the heart. Antibiotic therapy may be used if signs of infection, such as increased pain and drainage or fever, are observed. Ulcers that fail to heal may require surgical debridement to remove infected or necrotic tissue or skin grafting. Patients with venous ulcerations should be instructed on proper wound care, use of elastic wrapping, the need for elevation, and signs of infection. Patients should also be instructed on the need for adequate diet and rest to promote healing and prevent infection.

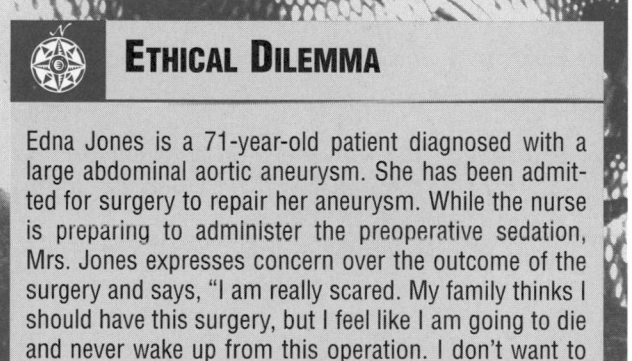

### ETHICAL DILEMMA

Edna Jones is a 71-year-old patient diagnosed with a large abdominal aortic aneurysm. She has been admitted for surgery to repair her aneurysm. While the nurse is preparing to administer the preoperative sedation, Mrs. Jones expresses concern over the outcome of the surgery and says, "I am really scared. My family thinks I should have this surgery, but I feel like I am going to die and never wake up from this operation. I don't want to go through with this." The operating room team is already set up for the surgery and waiting for the nurse to bring Mrs. Jones down. What actions should the nurse take? How would you advocate for this patient's rights?

## NURSING CARE PLAN

### ANXIETY

Mr. Cox is a 54-year-old man who has been diagnosed with deep vein thrombosis (DVT) of the deep venous system in his right calf. He has just been admitted to your unit for the initiation of intravenous heparin. He is nervous, jittery, and tearful. When questioned about how he is coping, he says, "I am so worried about how I am going to pay for all of this. I don't have medical insurance, and now that I have to be in this hospital bed I can't work. The doctor says I could get a clot in my lung. I don't understand how this happened to me and how I am going to get along. What if I get really sick and can't drive anymore?"

| Medical History | Psychosocial Data | Assessment Data |
|---|---|---|
| No previous hospitalizations | Married with three children 14, 12, and 10 years old, all living at home | Oriented, anxious, tearful, jittery |
| No chronic illnesses | | Vital signs: blood pressure 140/72, heart rate 103 bpm, respirations 24/min and unlabored |
| No current medications | Drives a truck for a shipping company 6 days per week | |
| | Wife is stay-at-home mother | Right leg swollen, painful, and reddened on anterior aspect of calf, pulses +4 bilaterally |
| | Can read and write; has completed high school and technical training | |
| | No visual or hearing impairment | |

**NURSING DIAGNOSIS**

Anxiety related to hospitalization, alteration in provider role, lack of understanding of disease process and medical regimen, fear of complications

| NURSING INTERVENTIONS | EVALUATION OF EXPECTED OUTCOMES |
|---|---|
| Take time to sit with the patient and listen to his concerns. | Vital signs |
| Begin patient teaching, focusing on the current concerns: | Subjective data |
|   Explain the process of DVT development, the medical regimen, and the plan of care. |   Patients report of anxiety |
|   Explain the low risk of emboli with distal DVT and the precautions that will be taken to prevent pulmonary embolus. |   Verbal report of understanding |
|   Explain the use of heparin, heat, and elevation in preventing worsening of the DVT. | Objective data |
|   Describe the normal hospital course and plans for discharge. |   Level of anxiety |
|   Use simple terminology, and allow time for questions. |   Episodes of tearfulness |
| Obtain written information for the patient to review. |   Level of participation in plan of care and plan for adjusting to hospitalization and medical regimen |
| Have the patient begin to write down questions so they can be addressed in future teaching sessions. | Vital signs stable with reduced pulse and respiratory rate |
| Obtain a social services consultation to assess financial status and obtain needed resources. | Patient verbalizes understanding of teaching points |
| Determine diversional activities and comfort measures that would appeal to the patient, and provide them if possible. | Patient expresses concerns and feelings |
| Help the patient with relaxation techniques. | Patient reports reduced feelings of anxiousness and fear |
| Determine the spiritual or social resources that would comfort the patient and contact clergy or significant others for the patient. | Patient used relaxation techniques and diversional activities |
| | Patient has reduction in fearful episodes |
| | Patient participates in planning strategies to cope with hospitalization and medical regimen |

## KEY CONCEPTS

➤ Early detection and preventive measures may delay or avert acute or chronic vascular problems.

➤ Treatment for patients at risk of arterial occlusive disease includes improving circulation, relieving pain, improving the quality of life, and preventing infection and ischemia.

➤ The major risk factors for developing vascular problems include smoking, hyperlipidemia, and diabetes.

➤ Complications following amputation include contractures, poor fit of prosthesis, infection, and vas- cular insufficiency. Nursing care is directed toward these potential problems.

➤ Patients with known or suspected aneurysms should be evaluated and monitored for complications.

➤ For patients with chronic venous insufficiency, further trauma, ulceration, and reduction of stasis and edema are primary goals.

➤ Patients with arterial occlusions are considered to be surgical emergencies.

## CRITICAL THINKING EXERCISES

1. You are completing a vascular assessment on a patient 2 days after a right femoral popliteal bypass for arterial occlusive disease. You begin with a Doppler assessment of the pedal pulses and are unable to auscultate arterial flow. What are the possible reasons for this finding? What other assessment data should you gather to confirm or rule out your suspicion? What interventions should you implement?

2. During your rounds on the surgical ward, you find that the intravenous pump for one of your patients has been accidentally turned off. The medication running was heparin. This patient has been admitted for deep vein thrombosis in the right calf. What steps should you take to resume the therapy safely?

3. Mary Quattlebaum is a 92-year-old patient admitted from the nursing home with congestive heart failure and pulmonary edema. She has a peripheral intravenous line in the right forearm with maintenance fluids infusing. She is also receiving potassium supplements through the intravenous site because of a low serum potassium level. She begins to complain that the site is sore. What assessment data do you need to gather regarding the condition of the site? What are the potential complications that could occur from the intravenous line? What are indications that the line should be removed or restarted in another location? If you are unable to restart the intravenous line, how would you problem solve this situation?

## REFERENCES AND ADDITIONAL READINGS

Cantwell-Gab K: Identifying chronic peripheral arterial disease, *Am J Nurs* 96(7):40-46, 1996.

Dempsey E: Aortic aneurysms. In Urban N et al, editors: *Guidelines for critical care nursing*, St Louis, 1995, Mosby.

Hill EM: Perioperative management of patients with vascular disease, *AACN Clin Issues* 6(4):547-561, 1995.

Howland-Gradman J: Peripheral vascular disease. In Urban N et al, editors: *Guidelines for critical care nursing*, St Louis, 1995, Mosby.

Huether SE, McCance KL: *Understanding pathophysiology*, St Louis, 1996, Mosby.

Krenzer ME: Peripheral vascular assessment: finding your way through the arteries and veins, *AACN Clin Issues* 6(4):631-644, 1995.

Krikorian RK, Vacek JL: Peripheral arterial disease: when to consider percutaneous revascularization, *Postgrad Med* 97(6):109-117, 1995.

Kurgan A, Nunnelee JD: Upper extremity venous thrombosis, *J Vasc Nurs* 13(1):21-23, 1995.

Lewis SM, Collier IC, Heitkemper MM: *Medical-surgical nursing: assessment & management of clinical problems*, ed 4, St Louis, 1996, Mosby.

Malyuk DL: Drug therapy for pulmonary embolism or deep vein thrombosis. In McCormack J, editor: *Drug therapy: decision making guide*, Philadelphia, 1996, Saunders.

*Nurse Practitioner Prescription Reference* New York, 1998, Prescription Reference.

Olivencia JA: Varicosed veins: not just a cosmetic problem, *Patient Care* 30(12):140-158, 1996.

Pagana KD, Pagana TJ: *Mosby's diagnostic and laboratory test reference*, ed 3, St Louis, 1996, Mosby.

Santilli JD, Rodnick JE, Santilli SM: Claudication: diagnosis and treatment, *Am Fam Physician* 53(4):1245-1255, 1996.

Seidel HM et al: *Mosby's guide to physical examination*, ed 3, St Louis, 1995, Mosby.

Skidmore-Roth L: *Mosby's 1997 nursing drug reference*, ed 10, St Louis, 1996, Mosby.

Stephen JM, Feied CF: Venous thrombosis: lifting the clouds of misunderstanding, *Postgrad Med* 97(1):36-46, 1995.

Wheeler EC, Brenner ZR: Peripheral vascular anatomy, physiology, and pathophysiology, *AACN Clin Issues* 6(4):505-514, 1995.

# CHAPTER 25

# Hypertension

## CHAPTER OBJECTIVES

1 Describe the mechanisms involved with the regulation of blood pressure.
2 Differentiate between primary and secondary hypertension.
3 Discuss the risk factors related to the development of primary hypertension.
4 Discuss the clinical manifestations and complications related to target-organ damage.
5 Describe the nonpharmacologic treatment therapies for the prevention and control of hypertension.
6 Describe the different antihypertensive medication classifications and name two medications in each group.
7 Discuss the nursing management of the hypertensive patient, with a focus on patient education.
8 Discuss the management of the older patient with hypertension.
9 Describe the etiology, clinical manifestations, and treatment of the patient in hypertensive crisis.

## KEY TERMS

adrenergic receptors
angiotensin II
arterial blood pressure
baroreceptors
benign hypertension
cardiac output
chemoreceptors
diastolic blood pressure
hypertension

hypertensive crisis
malignant hypertension
peripheral vascular
  resistance
primary hypertension
receptors
secondary hypertension
systolic blood pressure

## REGULATION OF BLOOD PRESSURE

The regulation of blood pressure (BP) is primarily determined by two factors: cardiac output (CO) and peripheral vascular resistance (PVR).

$$BP = CO \times PVR$$

**Cardiac output** is defined as the volume of blood pumped out by the left ventricle with each heartbeat (stroke volume) multiplied by the heart rate (HR) for 1 minute:

$$CO = SV \times HR$$

**Peripheral vascular resistance** is the sum of all the resistive forces that oppose the movement of blood flow in the circulatory system. This is determined by the vasomotor tone and the diameter of the blood vessels, mainly the small arteries and arterioles, in the peripheral vascular system. **Arterial blood pressure** is the force blood exerts on the wall of a blood vessel as it flows through. The **systolic blood pressure** (the peak pressure the within the vessels immediately following ventricular contraction) is primarily affected by CO. The **diastolic blood pressure** (the pressure in the blood vessels during ventricular relaxation) is mainly affected by PVR. Any change, either up or down, in CO or PVR will cause a corresponding change in the BP.

The regulation of BP is accomplished through both short-term and long-term mechanisms aimed at keeping the mean arterial pressure within a range that is adequate for tissue perfusion. Short-term adjustments of BP (those occurring over seconds to hours) involve the neural system, including baroreceptors and autonomic nervous system, and hormonal mechanisms. Long-term regulation of BP is accomplished primarily through renal regulation (sodium and water) and hormonal influences.

## Neural Regulation

### Baroreceptors

**Baroreceptors** (pressoreceptors) are pressure-sensitive nerve cells located in the walls of the large arteries and in the arch of the aorta. The carotid and aortic baroreceptors are the main baroreceptors responsible for the control of blood pressure. They react to changes in the stretch of the vessel wall and when stimulated send impulses to the sympathetic vasomotor center in the brain stem to bring about changes in heart rate or vascular smooth muscle tone. Baroreceptors are capable of only short-term BP regulation because they become adjusted to prolonged changes in BP and recognize the new BP as "normal."

### Chemoreceptors

**Chemoreceptors** are located in small structures called carotid and aortic bodies, which lie in close proximity to the baroreceptors in the aortic arch and carotid sinus. Although primarily responsible for the regulation of respirations, chemoreceptors also transmit impulses to the vasomotor center when there is a decrease in the oxygen or hydrogen ion content of the blood or a decrease in the carbon dioxide content. The result is an increase in sympathetic stimulation with resulting vasoconstriction and an increase in BP.

## Autonomic Nervous System

The heart is innervated by both the sympathetic and parasympathetic divisions of the autonomic nervous system (ANS). The ANS affects BP regulation by influencing heart rate, contractility, and PVR. Parasympathetic control of BP is via the vagus nerve. Vagal stimulation results in a slowing of the heart rate, thereby decreasing CO and lowering BP.

The neural control center for the sympathetic nervous system, called the vasomotor center, is located in the medulla of the brain stem. Stimulation of the sympathetic nervous system produces an increase in heart rate and contractility that results in an increase in CO and perfusion of blood to the vital organs. Sympathetic stimulation also causes vasoconstriction of the peripheral blood vessels, which increases PVR. Even a small change in the diameter of the arterioles will cause a large change in PVR.

The actions of the sympathetic nervous system are mediated by the chemical neurotransmitter norepinephrine. Sympathetic neurons also respond to epinephrine and dopamine. The membrane proteins that enable the neurotransmitters to exert their effects are called **receptors.** The receptors of the sympathetic nervous system are called **adrenergic receptors.** There are two different types of adrenergic receptors:

alpha and beta, which are further classified as alpha-1 and alpha-2 receptors, and beta-1 and beta-2 receptors. Alpha-1 receptors are mainly located in vascular smooth muscle and respond to sympathetic stimulation with vasoconstriction. Alpha-2 receptors are found throughout the central nervous system and are part of a negative feedback loop. They respond to stimulation by inhibiting sympathetic outflow from the brain. Beta-1 receptors are located primarily in the heart, with some also in the vascular smooth muscle. Beta-2 receptors are primarily in the bronchioles. When stimulated, beta-1 receptors act to increase heart rate, speed of conduction, and force of muscle contraction.

## Renal Regulation

The renin-angiotensin-aldosterone system plays a key role in the regulation of BP. Renin is an enzyme secreted from the juxtaglomerular apparatus in the kidney and is released in response to decreased renal blood flow and renal artery pressure. Stimulation of the sympathetic nervous system also causes the release of renin. When released, renin combines with angiotensinogen to form angiotensin I. Angiotensin I travels in the blood to the lungs where it is converted to angiotensin II, a potent vasoconstrictor, by the angiotensin-converting enzyme. Angiotensin II influences the regulation of BP actively through vasoconstriction of blood vessels and indirectly by stimulating the release of aldosterone from the adrenal cortex. Aldosterone causes the kidneys to reabsorb sodium and water, thereby increasing blood volume and CO. The renin-angiotensin-aldosterone system functions via a negative feedback loop. With the resultant increase in blood volume and CO, there is an increase in renal blood flow, which in turn stops the sympathetic stimulation and therefore the release of renin (Figure 25-1).

## Hormonal and Chemical Regulation

Many different hormones and chemicals play a role in the regulation of blood pressure. They exert their affects by either changing the diameter of the blood vessels or adjusting the total blood volume.

Epinepherine and norepinephrine are released in response to sympathetic nervous stimulation by the adrenal medulla. When released, they cause an increase in CO and vasoconstriction of the abdominal and cutaneous arterioles and veins, resulting in an increase in PVR. Vasodilation of the arterioles in the cardiac and skeletal muscles also occurs.

**Angiotensin II** is a potent vasoconstrictor. It stimulates the adrenal cortex to release aldosterone, which

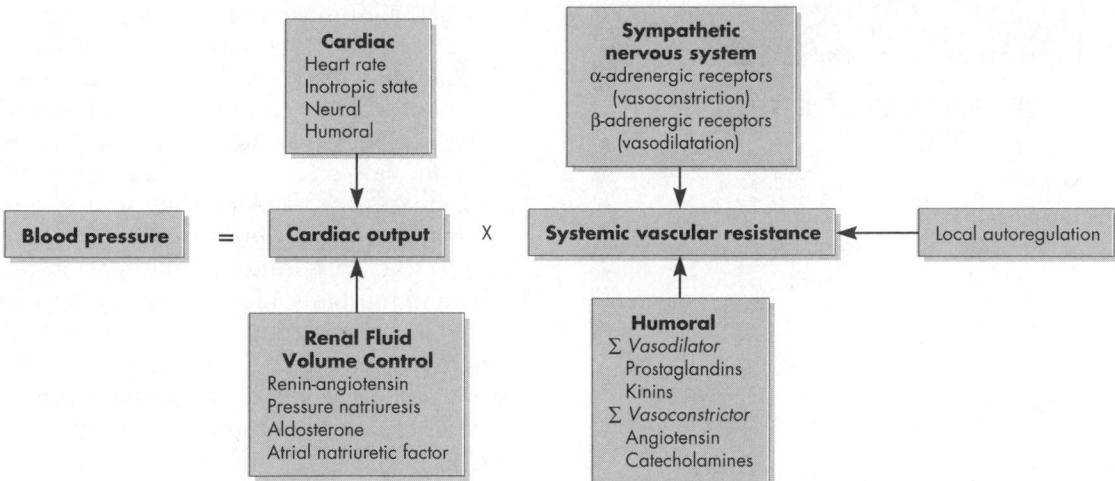

**Figure 25-1**    Factors influencing blood pressure. (Redrawn from West JB: *Physiological basis of medical practice*, ed 12, Baltimore, 1991, Williams & Wilkins. In Lewis SM, Collier IC, Heitkemper MM: *Medical-surgical nursing: assessment and management of clinical problems*, ed 4, St Louis, 1996, Mosby.)

stimulates the kidneys to retain sodium and water, thereby increasing CO.

Antidiuretic hormone (ADH) is produced by the hypothalamus and released by the posterior pituitary gland in response to decreases in blood volume and blood pressure. ADH stimulates the kidneys to retain water, thereby increasing blood volume and CO. ADH also has potent vasoconstrictive properties.

Histamine and kinins, when released from mast cells, cause vasodilation during the inflammatory response. They also cause an increase in capillary permeability, enhancing fluid loss from the intravascular space.

# HYPERTENSION

**Hypertension** is defined as a persistent elevation of systolic blood pressure (SBP) ≥140 mm Hg and/or diastolic blood pressure (DBP) ≥90 mm Hg. Guidelines from the Fifth Report of the Joint National Committee on the Detection, Evaluation, and Treatment of High Blood Pressure (JNC-V) recommend that the diagnosis of hypertension be made only after the initial elevated BP reading is confirmed on at least two subsequent visits, one to several weeks apart (unless SBP is ≥210 and/or DBP ≥140). To ensure blood pressure values are representative of the patient's normal level, the blood pressure measurement should be obtained after the patient has had an opportunity to rest for 5 minutes and has neither smoked nor ingested caffeine within 30 minutes of the measurement.

Hypertension is classified as either primary (essential) hypertension or secondary. **Primary hypertension** accounts for approximately 90% to 95% of all hyper-

tension and has no identifiable cause. It typically occurs between the ages of 25 and 55 years and affects men and women equally. Primary hypertension may be further classified as benign or malignant. **Benign hypertension** is a term used to describe uncomplicated hypertension. **Malignant** (or accelerated) **hypertension** refers to a rapidly progressive elevation of blood pressure associated with acute end-organ damage (e.g., left ventricular hypertrophy, retinitis, and papilledema). A characteristic finding is inflammation of the arterioles in the eyes. The prevalence of malignant hypertension is greatest in African American males younger than 40. In the absence of medical treatment, malignant hypertension is often fatal.

**Secondary hypertension** develops as the result of an identifiable cause and accounts for less than 5% of newly diagnosed hypertension in adults. It is often associated with problems within the renal or endocrine system. Secondary hypertension is often reversible when the underlying problem is treated or controlled (Box 25-1 and Table 25-1).

The JNC-V classifies the severity of hypertension according to four stages plus a high-normal category (Table 25-2). Hypertension is a major risk factor for both cardiovascular and cerebrovascular disease. Those patients with high-normal BPs are at a greater risk for the development of hypertension than those with normal BPs and should be monitored frequently (JNC-V, 1993).

## Epidemiology

Approximately 60 million people in the United States have high blood pressure. It is estimated that only 50%

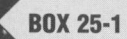

## CAUSES OF SECONDARY HYPERTENSION

**RENAL**
Chronic nephritis
Acute glomerulonephritis
Diabetic nephropathy
Primary sodium retention
Polycystic kidney disease
Renin-producing tumors

**VASCULAR**
Coarctation of aorta

**ENDOCRINE**
Acromegaly
Hypothyroidism
Hyperthyroidism
Hyperparathyroidism
Hypercalcemia
Cushing's syndrome
Primary aldosteronism
Pheochromocytoma

**MEDICATIONS**
Estrogen-containing oral contraceptives
Nonsteroidal antiinflammatory drugs
Mineralocorticoids
Glucocorticoids
Tricyclic antidepressants
Nasal decongestants
Monoamine oxidase inhibitors
Cold preparations
Erythropoietin
Appetite suppressants
Caffeine excess
Alcohol excess
Nicotine

**OTHER**
Pregnancy-induced hypertension
Increased intracranial pressure
Brain tumor
Encephalitis
Lead poisoning
Guillain-Barré syndrome
Acute stress

of the actual number of people with hypertension are diagnosed as such because many are asymptomatic and go undiagnosed until complications develop. Hypertension is more common in African Americans than in Anglo Americans and in both races is more prevalent in the less educated. The incidence of hypertension increases with age for all groups and is higher in men than in women until middle age, when the reverse is true. In addition, hypertension-related morbidity and mortality rates are higher for men than for women in all age-groups and higher in African Americans as compared to Anglo Americans. Residents of the Southeastern United States have a higher incidence of hypertension than those in the rest of the country (JNC-V, 1993).

## ETHNIC/CULTURAL CONSIDERATIONS

- Incidence of hypertension is higher in African Americans than in Anglo Americans.
- More prevalent in less educated vs. educated in all groups.
- Incidence increases with aging in all groups.
- Incidence is higher in males than females until age 55; then the reverse is true.
- Men have higher morbidity and mortality rates than women in all age groups, and African Americans have higher rates than anyone else.
- People who live in the Southeastern United States have higher incidence of hypertension than those living in the rest of the country.

## Risk Factors and Pathophysiology

There are many factors associated with a patient's relative risk of developing primary hypertension. The identification of nonmodifiable risk factors and management of modifiable risk factors are the primary objectives in the prevention of hypertension (Box 25-2).

## TABLE 25-1

### Assessment Findings Suggestive of Secondary Hypertension

| FINDING | CAUSE |
| --- | --- |
| Tachycardia, pallor, headache, palpitations, excessive sweating | Pheochromocytoma |
| Truncal obesity, moon face, pigmented striae | Cushing's disease |
| Diminished or absent lower extremity pulses, leg claudication, delayed or absent femoral pulsations | Aortic coarctation |
| Abdominal bruit | Renovascular hypertension |
| Fatigue, polyuria, muscle cramps, weakness | Hyperaldosteronism |

**TABLE 25-2**

## Classifications for Blood Pressure for Adults Age 18 Years and Older* and Recommendations for Follow-up Based on Initial Set of Blood Pressure Measurements for Adults

**INITIAL SCREENING BLOOD PRESSURE†**

| CATEGORY | SYSTOLIC (mm Hg) | DIASTOLIC (mm Hg) | FOLLOW-UP RECOMMENDED‡ |
|---|---|---|---|
| Normal§ | <130 | <85 | Recheck in 2 years |
| High Normal | 130-139 | 85-89 | Recheck in 1 year‖ |
| Hypertension¶ | | | |
|    Stage I (mild) | 140-159 | 90-99 | Confirm within 2 months |
|    Stage II (moderate) | 160-179 | 100-109 | Evaluate or refer to source of care within 1 month |
|    Stage III (severe) | 180-209 | 110-119 | Evaluate or refer to source of care within 1 week |
|    Stage IV (very severe) | ≥210 | ≥120 | Evaluate or refer to source of care immediately |

Modified from Joint National Committee on Detection, Evaluation, and Treatment of High Blood Pressure, *Arch Intern Med* 153:154-188, 1993.

*Not taking antihypertensive drugs and not acutely ill. When systolic and diastolic pressures fall into different categories, the higher category should be selected to classify the individual's blood pressure status. For instance, 160/92 mm Hg should be classified as stage 2, and 180/120 mm Hg should be classified as stage 4. Isolated systolic hypertension is defined as systolic blood pressure of 140 mm Hg or more and a diastolic blood pressure of less than 90 mm Hg and staged appropriately (e.g., 170/85 mm Hg is defined as stage 2 isolated systolic hypertension). In addition to classifying stages of hypertension on the basis of average blood pressure levels, the clinician should specify presence or absence of target organ disease and additional risk factors. For example, a patient with diabetes and a blood pressure of 142/94 mm Hg, plus left ventricular hypertrophy, should be classified as having stage 1 hypertension with target organ disease (left ventricular hypertrophy) and with another major risk factor (diabetes). This specificity is important for risk classification and management.

†If the systolic and diastolic categories are different, follow recommendations for the shorter-time follow-up (e.g., 160/85 mm Hg should be evaluated or referred to source of care within 1 month).

‡The scheduling of follow-up should be modified by reliable information about past blood pressure measurements, other cardiovascular risk factors, or target-organ disease.

§Optimal blood pressure with respect to cardiovascular risk is less than 120 mm Hg systolic and less than 80 mm Hg diastolic. However, unusually low readings should be evaluated for clinical significance.

‖Consider providing advice about life-style modifications.

¶Based on the average of two or more readings taken at each of two or more visits after an initial screening.

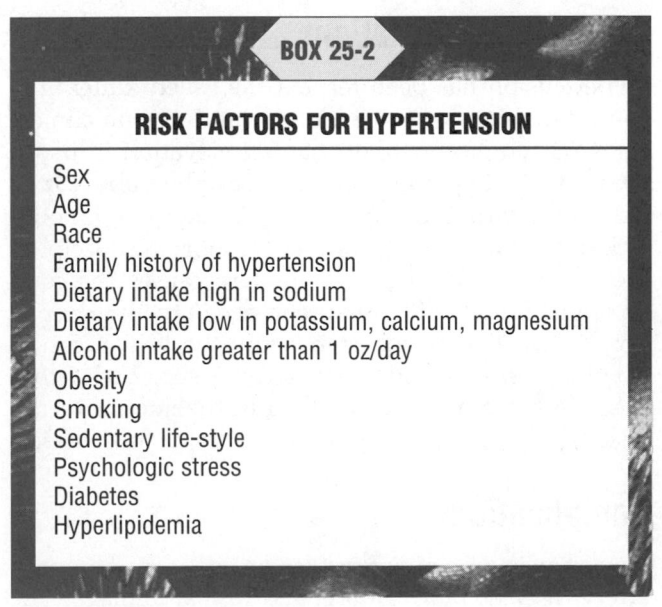

**BOX 25-2**

### RISK FACTORS FOR HYPERTENSION

Sex
Age
Race
Family history of hypertension
Dietary intake high in sodium
Dietary intake low in potassium, calcium, magnesium
Alcohol intake greater than 1 oz/day
Obesity
Smoking
Sedentary life-style
Psychologic stress
Diabetes
Hyperlipidemia

## Family History

Although the exact roles family history and heredity play in the development of hypertension are not known, studies have shown that patients with a family history of hypertension are twice as likely to develop hypertension than those with none (Porth, 1990). Many experts believe that environmental factors combine with genetic factors to produce abnormally high blood pressures.

## Age

More than 50% of persons over the age of 65 are estimated to be hypertensive. With increasing age, the baroreceptor reflexes probably become less sensitive to changes in the fluid volumes within the arteries, and the arteries become less compliant to changes in the amount of blood. The arteries become increasingly rigid, contributing to higher pressure being exerted by the blood against the vessel walls.

## Sex

Males are affected by hypertension earlier than females until the age of 55, and thereafter, women are affected more often. Men also experience hypertension at higher rates and have a greater risk of morbidity and mortality associated with cardiovascular complications.

### Race

In the United States, African Americans have a greater incidence of hypertension than Anglo Americans and at any given blood pressure have greater morbidity and mortality rates. The reason for this is unclear, but it is thought to be related to dietary factors, heredity, and environmental stresses.

### Obesity

For years it has been recognized that there is a close correlation between excess body weight and hypertension. Recent studies have suggested that the distribution of body fat is a more accurate indicator of risk for hypertension. Central obesity (truncal or abdominal as evidenced by a waist-to-hip ratio above 0.85 in women and 0.95 in men) is associated with hypertension. The goal is to attain and maintain body weight within 15% of the ideal (JNC-V, 1993).

The majority of obese patients with hypertension will benefit significantly from weight reduction. Weight reduction also enhances the effects of most pharmacologic therapies. A reduction of 2.2 pounds (1 kg) usually results in a 1 mm Hg decrease in BP (Beilin, 1994).

### Dietary Factors

The effect of dietary sodium intake on hypertension has been studied for years. Certain groups may be "salt sensitive" and tend to be more affected by sodium intake. Those groups include African Americans, the elderly, and those with a family history of hypertension. In some patients there may be an underlying inherited pathologic abnormality in sodium transport in the renal tubules, resulting in the retention of sodium and water (Zellner, Sudhir, 1996).

Other epidemiologic studies have implicated an inverse relationship between low dietary intake of potassium, calcium, and magnesium and the development of hypertension. Excessive intake of caffeine has been weakly linked as a risk factor. A recent study showed a significant reduction in systolic and diastolic ambulatory pressures in normotensive patients who omitted the intake of caffeinated coffee (Superko et al, 1994).

Although hyperlipidemia is not a direct risk factor for the development of hypertension, it is a major risk factor for coronary artery disease, as is hypertension.

### Excessive Alcohol Intake

Alcohol promotes vasodilation, causing a decrease in BP. It acts by inhibiting the release of ADH from the hypothalamus and inhibits the vasomotor center in the medulla.

### Smoking

The nicotine in tobacco mimics the effects of catecholamines and causes vasoconstriction by directly stimulating the postganglionic synaptic neurons. Nicotine also stimulates the release of increased amounts of norepinephrine and epinephrine.

### Sedentary Life-Style

A sedentary life-style has been linked to the development of hypertension and is strongly associated with increased mortality from coronary artery disease (Zellner, Sudhir, 1996). Regular aerobic exercise can aid in weight reduction, raise levels of high-density lipoproteins in relation to total blood cholesterol, and facilitate cardiovascular conditioning, and it may reduce BP.

### Stress

Emotional stress has been found to increase the production of plasma catecholamines and stimulate the sympathetic nervous system to raise BP. Job stress was identified as a risk factor for the development of hypertension in a 1990 study by Schnall and co-workers (Schnall, 1990).

## Clinical Manifestations

Hypertension has been termed the "silent killer" because in the early stages it often produces no clinical signs or symptoms other than an elevation in blood pressure. As hypertension advances, the patient may develop a variety of symptoms. The most commonly reported symptom is an early morning occipital headache. Increased blood pressure causes the cerebrospinal fluid (CSF) pressure to rise in the lying position. When the person stands up, the CSF pressure slowly decreases and the headache subsides. Other possible symptoms include fatigue, dizziness, blurred vision, palpitations, angina, and epistaxis (nosebleed).

## Complications

Hypertension is a major risk factor for stroke, coronary artery disease, renal failure, and retinal damage. The chance of developing complications associated with hypertension increases with the severity of the hyper-

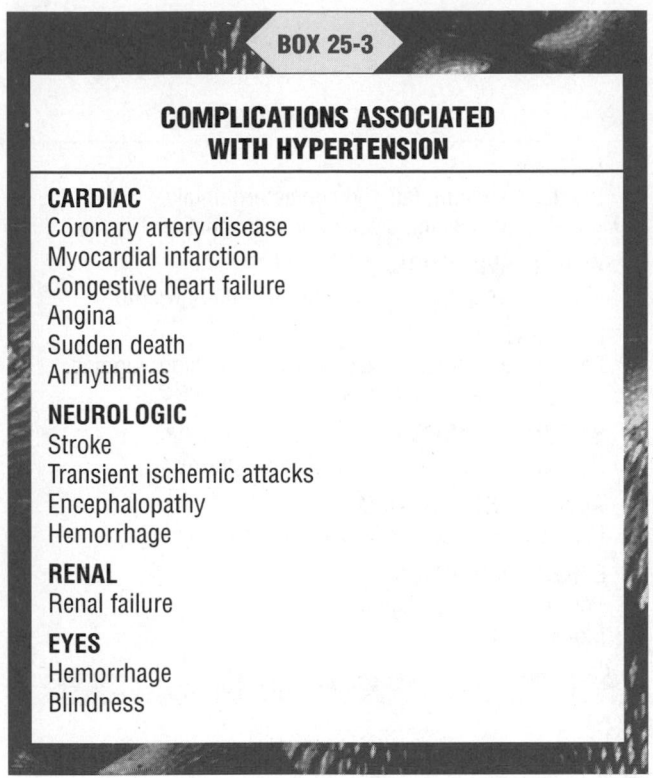

**COMPLICATIONS ASSOCIATED
WITH HYPERTENSION**

**CARDIAC**
Coronary artery disease
Myocardial infarction
Congestive heart failure
Angina
Sudden death
Arrhythmias

**NEUROLOGIC**
Stroke
Transient ischemic attacks
Encephalopathy
Hemorrhage

**RENAL**
Renal failure

**EYES**
Hemorrhage
Blindness

tension and the length of time without treatment. The primary sites of hypertension-related organ damage are the heart, brain, kidneys, and eyes, although any system may be involved (Box 25-3).

# Prevention
## Primary Prevention

The goal of primary prevention is to identify nonmodifiable risk factors and identify and manage the modifiable risk factors associated with hypertension. Education is a key component in primary prevention. Health programs have focused on teaching the public the following aspects of the effects and prevention of hypertension:

- Hypertension's serious negative effects on the eyes, heart, kidneys, and brain
- Dietary modifications, such as low sodium intake and a decrease in saturated fat intake
- Smoking cessation
- Moderate consumption of alcohol (less than 2 ounces/day)
- Maintenance of optimal body weight
- Stress reduction techniques

## Secondary Prevention

Secondary prevention is focused on screening clients for hypertension. Hypertension screening should be

an automatic part of office visits. Patients identified at high risk, such as African Americans (especially men), the elderly, obese persons, and those with a family history, should be followed more closely.

## Tertiary Prevention

Tertiary prevention is aimed at controlling high BP and preventing or minimizing the associated potential complications. Hypertension is a chronic disease, and patients need ongoing medical follow-up for the rest of their lives. With proper medical management, the complications associated with hypertension can be prevented or reduced.

# Medical Management
## Diagnosis

Hypertension is diagnosed when the average of two blood pressure measurements obtained on separate occasions, at least one or several weeks apart after the initial elevated measurement, produce a systolic reading of ≥140 mm Hg and/or a diastolic reading of ≥90 mm Hg. Because blood pressure measurements may be affected by many variables, it is important that consistent measurement techniques be followed.

A complete history and physical examination should be performed on all patients diagnosed with high blood pressure before therapy is initiated. The medical history includes questions about any previous diagnosis of hypertension and treatments, current medications, dietary history, family history of hypertension or other cardiovascular disorders, job and emotional stress level, information about possible target organ damage (CHF, coronary artery disease, stroke, renal disease, retinopathy), and other cardiovascular risk factors (smoking, sedentary life-style, obesity, alcohol consumption, dyslipidemia, diabetes mellitus) (Box 25-4).

The physical examination focuses on identifying evidence of target organ damage and secondary causes of hypertension that may be reversible. All patients with high blood pressure need to have their height and weight measured. A funduscopic examination of the eyes is performed, with an emphasis on spotting arteriovenous nicking, retinal exudates, hemorrhages, and papilledema. The patient's neck is assessed for jugular venous distention and carotid bruits, and the thyroid is palpated for enlargement. Auscultation of the heart is performed for rate and rhythm, murmurs, clicks, rubs, enlargement, and S3 and S4 heart sounds. Breath sounds are auscultated for signs of congestive heart failure (CHF). The abdomen is assessed for hepatosplenomegaly and bruits. The extremities are examined for diminished, absent, or unequal peripheral

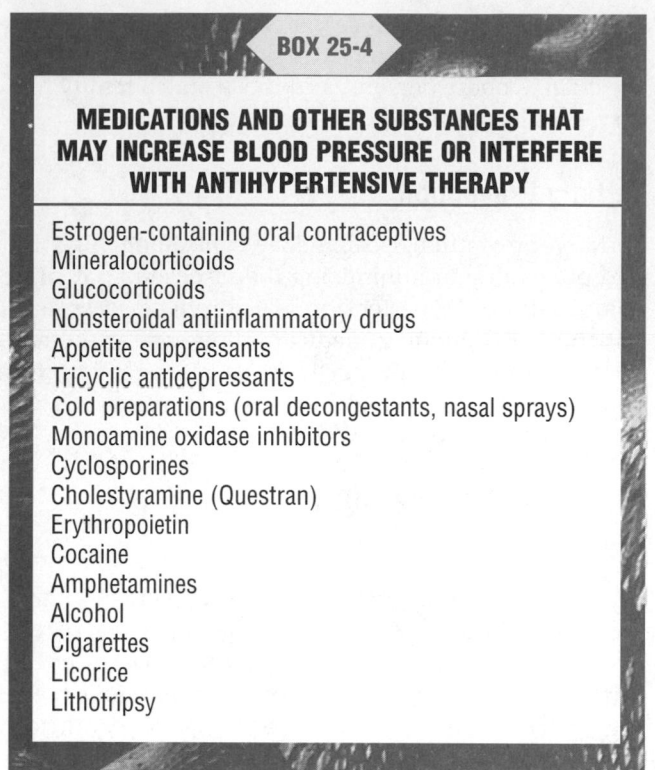

BOX 25-4

### MEDICATIONS AND OTHER SUBSTANCES THAT MAY INCREASE BLOOD PRESSURE OR INTERFERE WITH ANTIHYPERTENSIVE THERAPY

Estrogen-containing oral contraceptives
Mineralocorticoids
Glucocorticoids
Nonsteroidal antiinflammatory drugs
Appetite suppressants
Tricyclic antidepressants
Cold preparations (oral decongestants, nasal sprays)
Monoamine oxidase inhibitors
Cyclosporines
Cholestyramine (Questran)
Erythropoietin
Cocaine
Amphetamines
Alcohol
Cigarettes
Licorice
Lithotripsy

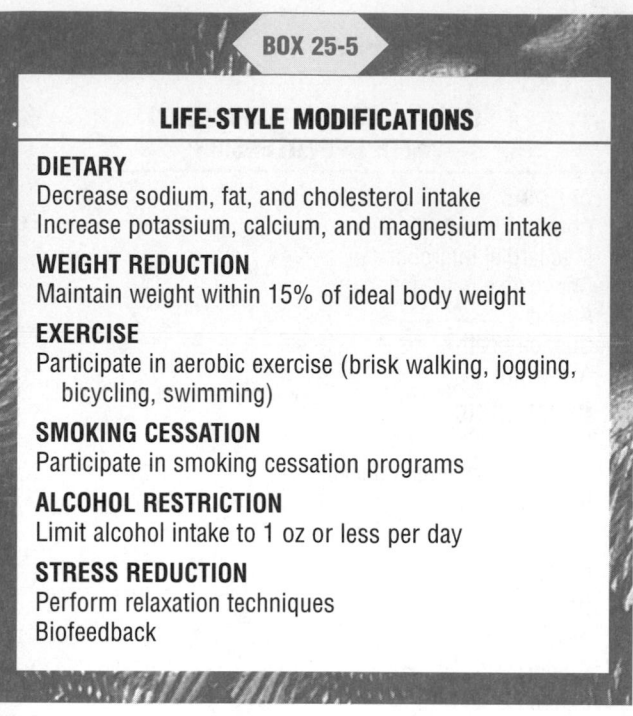

BOX 25-5

### LIFE-STYLE MODIFICATIONS

**DIETARY**
Decrease sodium, fat, and cholesterol intake
Increase potassium, calcium, and magnesium intake

**WEIGHT REDUCTION**
Maintain weight within 15% of ideal body weight

**EXERCISE**
Participate in aerobic exercise (brisk walking, jogging, bicycling, swimming)

**SMOKING CESSATION**
Participate in smoking cessation programs

**ALCOHOL RESTRICTION**
Limit alcohol intake to 1 oz or less per day

**STRESS REDUCTION**
Perform relaxation techniques
Biofeedback

pulses, decreased capillary refill, and edema. A neurologic examination is also important for all patients with high blood pressure.

Routine laboratory tests usually performed before therapy is begun include a complete blood cell count, fasting blood sugar, BUN, serum creatinine, electrolytes, calcium, a lipid profile, and urinalysis. A 12-lead ECG is obtained to monitor for dysrhythmias, left ventricular hypertrophy, and signs of myocardial damage. A chest x-ray may also be done. More extensive studies may be done for the patient with suspected secondary causes of hypertension.

## Treatment

The goal of medical management is to control the hypertension and prevent target organ damage. Treatment is aimed at keeping the SBP below 140 mm Hg and the DBP below 90 mm Hg (except in the elderly). Many factors influence the type of medical treatment initiated: the degree of pressure elevation, presence of risk factors, and the presence and extent of target organ damage (Box 25-5). Figure 25-2 depicts the stepped-care approach to the treatment of hypertension.

Step-down therapy may be tried after a year of good blood pressure control. The dose and number of medications are slowly reduced to the lowest amount that keeps the BP within the desired range. Close follow-up is essential to monitor for any elevation requiring further treatment (JNC-V, 1993).

**Nonpharmacologic therapy.** Life-style modification for at least 3 to 6 months after the initial diagnosis of hypertension is recommended as the initial therapy to be used with patients with stage I and II hypertension. Strategies include weight reduction, sodium restriction, limited alcohol intake, exercise, smoking cessation, and stress reduction. Life-style modifications are especially beneficial for patients who have additional cardiovascular risk factors (e.g., diabetes, hyperlipidemia). Management of hypertension through life-style modification has many benefits at minimal cost or risk to the patient (JNC-V, 1993) (see Box 25-5).

***Diet.*** Dietary management of hypertension can be accomplished through moderation of dietary sodium; adequate intake of potassium, calcium, and magnesium; reduction of dietary saturated fats and cholesterol; and a reduction in caloric intake for those who are overweight.

The association between blood pressure and sodium intake has been supported in epidemiologic observations and clinical trials. In short-term trials, hypertensive individuals have shown a reduction in SBP by an average of 4.9 mm Hg and DBP by 2.6 mm Hg with a moderate sodium restriction. Not all individuals benefit from sodium restriction. Patients with low renin activity (African Americans and the elderly) appear to be more "salt-sensitive" and are more likely to respond to a reduction in sodium intake (JNC-V, 1993).

The average American consumes in excess of 9 g of sodium chloride (NaCl) per day. The Joint National

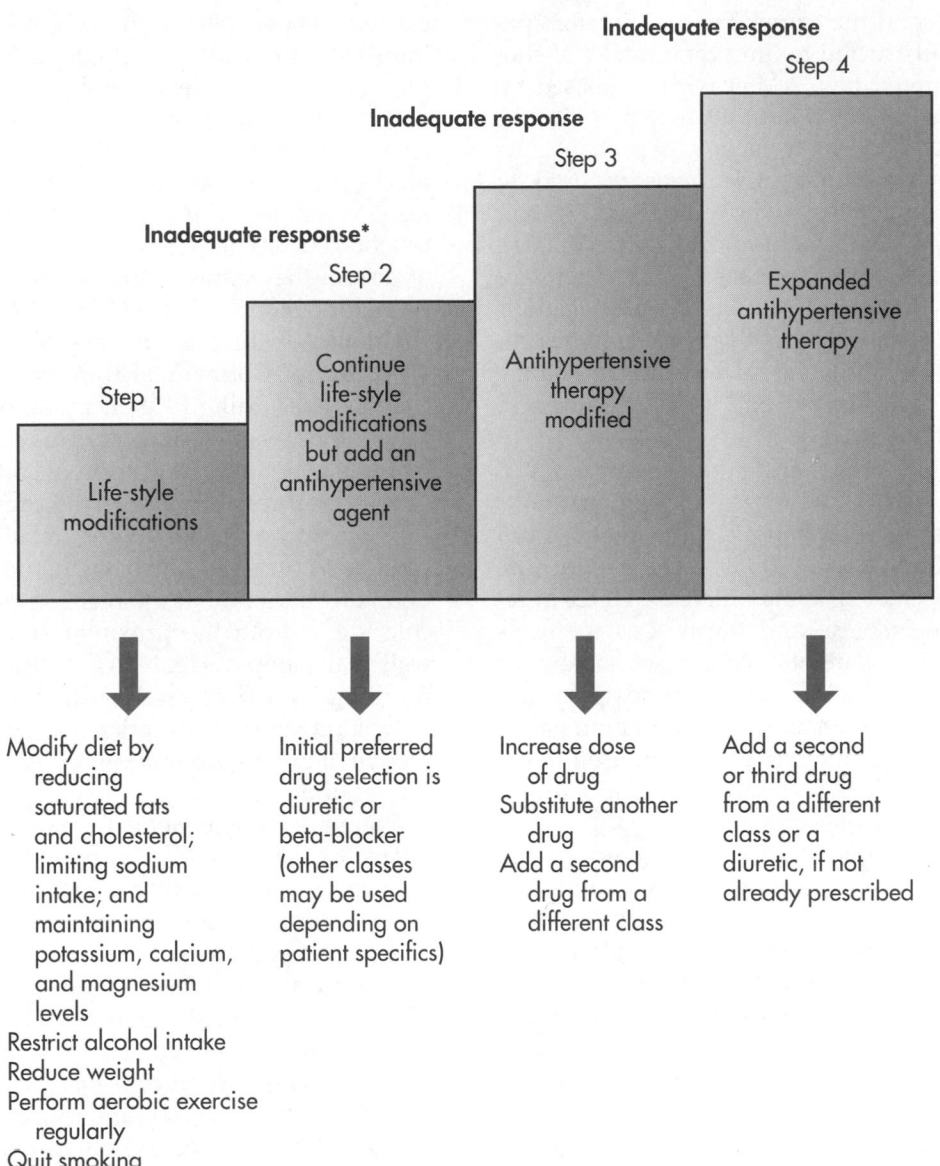

**Figure 25-2**    Stepped-care approach for treating hypertension. (Modified from The Joint National Committee on Detection, Evaluation, and Treatment of High Blood Pressure: *Arch Intern Med* 153:164, 1993.)

Committee recommends that sodium intake be limited to less than 6 g of sodium chloride (<2.3 g of sodium) per day. Most individuals can achieve this by not adding salt during food preparation or at the table and by avoiding processed foods preserved in salt.

A diet with substantial potassium intake may augment the antihypertensive effects of weight reduction, sodium restriction, and antihypertensive medications. Increased BP may be caused by a lowered potassium; therefore it is recommended that patients with hypertension maintain an adequate daily potassium intake (about 100 mEq/day).

Some studies have shown an inverse relationship between both the intake of calcium and the intake of magnesium and blood pressure. Although some patients have shown a reduction in BP with an increased calcium intake, the overall effect is small. To date, there is not enough evidence to support increasing calcium intake in excess of the recommended allowance of 800 to 1200 mg/day. There is also no evidence that increasing magnesium intake will reduce BP.

Although hyperlipidemia has not been shown to cause hypertension, it is the primary risk factor in the development of coronary artery disease. Hypertension follows as the second major risk factor. Therefore patients should be instructed to limit their intake of cholesterol and saturated fats. A diet with decreased fat intake will also help with weight reduction.

***Weight reduction.*** Weight reduction is probably the most effective nonpharmacologic measure used to treat hypertension in patients who are 10% above their ideal body weight. Even moderate weight reduction has been associated with decreases in BP. Therefore weight reduction to within 15% of ideal body weight is recommended for all obese patients with hypertension. Weight loss can independently reduce BP and the risk of cardiovascular disease, and it tends to improve self-esteem and body image.

***Exercise.*** A regular program of aerobic exercise (such as brisk walking, biking, swimming, or jogging) yields a modest decrease in BP in patients with stage I and II hypertension. Exercise also aids in weight reduction, reduces cardiovascular risk, may increase HDLs in relation to total cholesterol, and improves a person's sense of well-being. Patients with heart disease or other health problems should be advised to have a complete physical examination before beginning an exercise program. They should also be advised to begin their exercise program slowly and gradually increase the intensity as tolerance allows.

***Alcohol intake.*** Multiple studies have demonstrated an association between consumption of more than 1 to 2 ounces of alcohol per day and the development of hypertension. Therefore alcohol intake should be limited to 1 ounce of alcohol per day—the equivalent of the amount of alcohol in 2 ounces of 100-proof whisky, 8 ounces of wine, or 24 ounces of beer. Alcohol intake should be avoided by patients with additional disease processes such as diabetes mellitus and liver disease.

***Smoking cessation.*** The nicotine in cigarettes increases heart rate and produces peripheral vasoconstriction. Although there is no direct relationship between smoking and the development of hypertension, all persons who smoke should be encouraged to enroll in a smoking cessation program. Patients who smoke may not receive the same effect from antihypertensive medications as nonsmokers. For those who continue to smoke, they should be advised not to smoke within 30 minutes of having their BP checked.

***Stress reduction.*** Although studies have shown that stress can acutely raise BP, the role of stress-management techniques (relaxation therapies, biofeedback, etc.) in the treatment of hypertension is still controversial. To date there are not enough data to justify the use of stress-management techniques as a definitive therapy for the treatment or prevention of hypertension (JNC-V, 1993).

**Pharmacologic therapy.** Pharmacologic therapy should be initiated in patients with sustained blood pressure readings above 140/90 mm Hg who have shown no improvement in BP control after 3 to 6 months of nonpharmacologic therapy. Antihypertensives are classified as diuretics, beta-blockers, angiotensin-converting enzyme inhibitors (ACE inhibitors), calcium channel blockers, alpha-1 agonists, central-acting alpha agonists, combined alpha- and beta-blockers, and vasodilators. Antihypertensives have two primary modes of action: they either decrease the PVR or reduce the circulating blood volume (Table 25-3 and Box 25-6).

***Diuretics.*** Diuretics are one of the first-line drugs used in the treatment of hypertension. Diuretics are classified according to their mode of action: thiazide, loop, or potassium sparing. Thiazide diuretics work by inhibiting the reabsorption of sodium and chloride in the distal renal tubules. This causes an increase in the excretion of urine. The net result is a reduction in plasma volume, cardiac output, and renal blood flow. Loop diuretics inhibit the reabsorption of sodium and chloride in both the proximal and distal tubules as well as the loop of Henle. Again, this causes a diuresis resulting in a decreased cardiac output. The use of potassium-sparing diuretics avoids the potential depletion of potassium that can occur with the other two classes of diuretics.

There are many benefits to using thiazide and other related diuretics for the control of hypertension. These are inexpensive, can be prescribed in once-daily dosing, enhance the efficacy of other antihypertensives, and are especially effective in the elderly, African American, and low-renin hypertensive patients.

Unwanted metabolic effects of thiazides include hypokalemia, hyperuricemia, hypomagnesemia, and impaired glucose tolerance. Most can also elevate total cholesterol, triglycerides, and low-density lipoproteins (LDLs) and may decrease high-density lipoproteins (HDLs). Many of these effects can be minimized by using low dosages. Other potential side effects include precipitation of an acute gout attack, rash, photosensitivity, impotence, and fatigue. Diuretics may be ineffective for patients in renal failure.

***Beta-blockers.*** Beta-blockers work to reduce BP by inhibiting the production of renin. Beta-blockers also inhibit the beta-1 alpha adrenergic receptors, thereby decreasing CO and reducing the HR, force of contractions, and speed of impulse conduction. These effects make beta-blockers a good choice of antihypertensive therapy for patients with angina or who have had a myocardial infarction.

Potential side effects include orthostatic hypotension, bradycardia, bronchospasm, exacerbation of CHF, increased insulin resistance, sexual dysfunction, aggravation of arterial insufficiency, increased serum triglycerides, and reduced HDL levels. Beta-blockers are contraindicated for patients with asthma, CHF, peripheral

*Text continued on p. 779.*

**TABLE 25-3**

## Pharmacology of Drugs Used in Hypertension

| DRUG (GENERIC AND TRADE NAME); ROUTE AND DOSAGE | ACTION/INDICATION | COMMON SIDE EFFECTS AND NURSING CONSIDERATIONS |
|---|---|---|
| **DIURETICS (THIAZIDE AND RELATED DIURETICS)** | | |
| **Chlorothiazide** (Diuril) Route: PO Dosage: Initially 0.5-1 g once or twice daily, qod, or 3-5 days/wk | Promotes renal excretion of sodium, water, and potassium. Initially blood volume and cardiac output are decreased, but with continued therapy levels rise to normal. | Increased BUN, uric acid, blood glucose, calcium, cholesterol, LDLs, and triglycerides Decreased potassium GI upset, dry mouth, thirst, polyuria, fatigue, muscle weakness, tachycardia, gout, leukopenia, agranulocytosis |
| **Hydrochlorothiazide** (Esidrix, Hydro-Diuril, Oretic) Route: PO Dosage: 25-200 mg/day, max: 200 mg/day | Higher than normal doses rarely enhance effect on BP and can worsen adverse effects. | Sexual dysfunction may occur Advise patient that orthostatic hypotension may be potentiated by alcohol, narcotics, and barbiturates Monitor electrolytes Advise patient to supplement diet with foods high in potassium |
| **Methyclothiazide** (Enduron) Route: PO Dosage: 2.5-10 mg/day | | Thiazides may potentiate cardiotoxicity of digitalis and NSAIDs may decrease effects |
| **LOOP DIURETICS** | Comparable to thiazides | Same as thiazides, including reversible hearing loss, metabolic alkalosis |
| **Bumetanide** (Bumex) Route: PO Dosage: 0.5-2 mg/day, max, 10 mg/day | Act on ascending loop of Henle to minimize reabsorption of sodium and water Drug of choice in patients with renal failure | Monitor for electrolyte imbalances Effects of drug increase with dose Monitor patient weight Avoid administering before bedtime to prevent frequent urination and loss of sleep |
| **Ethacrynic acid** (Edecrin) Route: PO Dosage: 50-200 mg/day | | |
| **Furosemide** (Lasix) Route: PO Dosage: Initially 20-80 mg/day, max 600 mg/day | | |
| **POTASSIUM-SPARING DIURETICS** | Promotes excretion of sodium and water and retention of potassium by blocking action of aldosterone in distal loop | Increased BUN, potassium Decreased sodium GI disturbances, rash, hirsutism, gynecomastia in men, photosensitivity, irregular menses, drowsiness, confusion, headache, vertigo, dry mouth, blood dyscrasias |
| **Amiloride** (Midamor) Route: PO Dosage: 5-10 mg/day | Amiloride and Triamterene act on distal tubule to block potassium excretion independently of aldosterone | Monitor for hyperkalemia, especially in patients with renal insufficiency |
| **Spironolactone** (Aldactone) Route: PO Dosage: 25-200 mg/day | Weak diuretic when used alone, potentiates actions of other antihypertensive drugs | Administer after meals to reduce nausea Do not use potassium supplements |
| **Triamterene** (Dyrenium) Route: PO Dosage: Initially 100 mg twice daily, max. 300 mg/day | | |

All dosages are for PO administration unless otherwise stated.

*Continued*

**TABLE 25-3**

## Pharmacology of Drugs Used in Hypertension—cont'd

| DRUG (GENERIC AND TRADE NAME); ROUTE AND DOSAGE | ACTION/INDICATION | COMMON SIDE EFFECTS AND NURSING CONSIDERATIONS |
|---|---|---|
| **BETA BLOCKERS** | | |
| **Acebutolol** (Sectral)<br>**Route:** PO<br>**Dosage:** 200-800 mg/day, max 1.2 g/day in 2 divided doses<br><br>**Atenolol** (Tenormin)<br>**Route:** PO, IV<br>**Dosage:** 50-100 mg/day, max 100 mg/day<br><br>**Metoprolol** (Lopressor)<br>**Route:** PO, IV<br>**Dosage:** 100-450 mg/day in 1-2 divided doses<br><br>**Nadolol** (Corgard)<br>**Route:** PO<br>**Dosage:** 40-80 mg/day, max. 320 mg/day<br><br>**Propranolol** (Inderal)<br>**Route:** PO<br>**Dosage:** Initially 40 mg bid, maintenance 120-240 mg/day, max 640 mg/day | Blocks beta-adrenergic receptors in the heart and peripheral vessels to decrease cardiac output, sympathetic stimulation and renin secretion by kidney | Avoid concomitant use with calcium channel blockers<br>Bronchospasm, bradycardia, CHF, hypoglycemia, fatigue, nightmares, insomnia, palpitations, hypotension, weakness, impaired peripheral circulation, GI disturbances, decreased exercise tolerance, orthostatic hypotension, thrombocytopenia, impotence (rarely)<br>Assess patient for signs of heart failure<br>Instruct patient to take own pulse daily to monitor for bradycardia or irregularity<br>Advise patients with diabetes that these medications may mask signs of hypoglycemia<br>Advise patients with heart disease that sudden withdrawal may be dangerous<br>Contraindicated in patients with asthma, COPD, CHF, and heart block. Use with caution in diabetes and peripheral vascular disease |
| **ANGIOTENSIN-CONVERTING-ENZYME (ACE) INHIBITORS** | | |
| **Benazepril** (Lotensin)<br>**Route:** PO<br>**Dosage:** Initially 10 mg/day, may increase to 20-40 mg/day in 1-2 divided doses, max 80 mg/day<br><br>**Captopril** (Capoten)<br>**Route:** PO<br>**Dosage:** Initially 25 mg 2-3 times daily, after 1-2 wk may increase to 50 mg 2-3 times daily, max. 450 mg/day<br><br>**Enalapril** (Vasotec)<br>**Route:** PO, IV<br>**Dosage:** Initially 2.5 mg/day, max. 40 mg/day in 1-2 divided doses | Inhibits conversion of angiotensin I to angiotensin II blocking release of aldosterone thus reducing sodium and water retention<br>Reduces peripheral vascular resistance without affecting cardiac output | Increased potassium<br>Loss of taste, fever, rash, cough, bone marrow depression, orthostatic hypotension, tachycardia, hemolytic anemia, granulocytosis<br>May cause renal damage with proteinuria<br>Advise patient to use aspirin substitute as aspirin may decrease drug's effectiveness<br>Loss of taste may decrease patient's desire to eat |

**TABLE 25-3**

## Pharmacology of Drugs Used in Hypertension—cont'd

| DRUG (GENERIC AND TRADE NAME); ROUTE AND DOSAGE | ACTION/INDICATION | COMMON SIDE EFFECTS AND NURSING CONSIDERATIONS |
|---|---|---|
| **Fosinopril** (Monopril)<br>**Route:** PO<br>**Dosage:** 20-40 mg/day in single or 2 divided doses, max. 80 mg/day | | |
| **Lisinopril** (Prinivil, Zestril)<br>**Route:** PO<br>**Dosage:** 20-40 mg/day | | |
| **Quinapril** (Accupril)<br>**Route:** PO<br>**Dosage:** Initially 10 mg/day, maintenance 20-80 mg/day in 1-2 divided doses | | |
| **Ramipril** (Altace)<br>**Route:** PO<br>**Dosage:** 2.5-20 mg/day in single or 2 divided doses | | |
| **CALCIUM CHANNEL BLOCKERS** | | |
| **Amlodipine** (Norvasc)<br>**Route:** PO<br>**Dosage:** 5 mg/day, max. 10 mg/day | Inhibits the influx of calcium into smooth muscle cells (primarily arteries) causing arteriolar vasodilation and decreased peripheral vascular resistance | Headache, nausea, dizziness, hypotension, peripheral edema, weakness, flushing, arrhythmia, GI disturbances, constipation<br>Use with caution in patients with CHF<br>Be aware may exacerbate asthma, diabetes, and peripheral vascular disease<br>Verapamil may cause bradycardia |
| **Diltiazem** (Cardizem)<br>**Route:** PO<br>**Dosage:** Initially 180-240 mg/day, usual range 240-360 mg/day, max. 480 mg/day | | |
| **Nifedipine** (Procardia)<br>**Route:** PO<br>**Dosage:** 30-60 mg/day, max. 120 mg/day | | |
| **Verapamil** (Calan, Isoptin)<br>**Route:** PO<br>**Dosage:** 80 mg tid, max. 360 mg/day in 3 divided doses, elderly or small patients Initially 40 mg tid | | |

*Continued*

**TABLE 25-3**

## Pharmacology of Drugs Used in Hypertension—cont'd

| DRUG (GENERIC AND TRADE NAME); ROUTE AND DOSAGE | ACTION/INDICATION | COMMON SIDE EFFECTS AND NURSING CONSIDERATIONS |
|---|---|---|
| **ALPHA-1 ADRENERGIC BLOCKERS** | | |
| **Doxazosin** (Cardura) <br> **Route:** PO <br> **Dosage:** Initially 1 mg/day, monitor BP for 2-6 wk and slowly increase q 2 wk if needed to max 16 mg/day | | Prevent hypotension and syncope by giving small first dose at bedtime and advising patient not to get up for three hours <br> Cautious use in elderly because of orthostatic hypotension |
| **Phentolamine** (Regitine) <br> **Route:** IM, IV injection <br> **Dosage:** 5 mg IV or IM 1-2 hours before surgery | Blocks alpha-adrenergic receptors thus reducing peripheral vascular resistance by dilating arterioles and venules | Cardiac dysrhythmias, acute prolonged hypotension, orthostatic hypotension, tachycardia, weakness, flushing, lightheadedness, first dose syncope, palpitations |
| **Prazosin** (Minipress) <br> **Route:** PO <br> **Dosage:** Initially 1 mg 2-3 times daily, usual range 6-15 mg/day in divided doses, max. 20-40 mg/day | | |
| **Terazosin** (Hytrin) <br> **Route:** PO <br> **Dosage:** 1-5 mg/day in am, max, 20 mg/day | | |
| **CENTRAL-ACTING ALPHA-AGONISTS** | | |
| **Clonidine** (Catapres) <br> **Route:** PO, transdermal <br> **Dosage:** Initially 0.1 mg bid, usual range 0.2-0.6 mg/day in divided doses; max. 2.4 mg/day | Inhibits central vasomotor centers, thus decreasing sympathetic outflow to the heart, kidneys, and peripheral vasculature. Causes decrease in BP, peripheral vascular resistance, and heart rate | Dry mouth, sedation, dizziness, constipation, fatigue, orthostatic hypotension, headache, bradycardia, fluid retention, rebound hypertension if drug abruptly withdrawn, impotence <br> Chewing gum or hard candies help to relieve dry mouth <br> Advise patient that alcohol and sedatives can increase central nervous system depression <br> Patients with diabetes may need increased insulin doses <br> Advise patient not to abruptly stop taking drug as rebound hypertension may occur |
| **Guanabenz** (Wytensin) <br> **Route:** PO <br> **Dosage:** Initially 4 mg bid, may increase by 4-8 mg/day q 1-2 wk, max. 32 mg bid | | |
| **Methyldopa** (Aldomet) <br> **Route:** PO, IV <br> **Dosage:** Initially 250 mg 2-3 times daily, maintenance 500 mg-2g/day in 2-4 divided doses, max. 3 g/day | | |

**TABLE 25-3**

## Pharmacology of Drugs Used in Hypertension—cont'd

| DRUG (GENERIC AND TRADE NAME); ROUTE AND DOSAGE | ACTION/INDICATION | COMMON SIDE EFFECTS AND NURSING CONSIDERATIONS |
|---|---|---|
| **VASODILATORS** | | |
| **Hydralazine** (Apresoline) Route: PO, IV Dosage: Initially 10 mg 4 times a day, max. 300 mg/day in 4 divided doses | Dilates peripheral blood vessels by relaxing vascular smooth muscle | Headache, tachycardia, palpitations, flushing, angina, dyspnea, GI disturbances, weakness, hypotension Monitor for reflex tachycardia Usually used in conjunction with other antihypertensives as they tend to increase sodium and water retention |
| **Minoxidil** (Loniten) Route: PO Dosage: Initially 5 mg once daily, usual range 10-40 mg/day, max. 100 mg/day | | |
| **Sodium nitroprusside** (Nipride) Route: IV Dosage: Average dose is 3 $\mu$g/kg/min, max. is 10 $\mu$g/kg/min | | |

---

**BOX 25-6**

### POTENTIAL CAUSES OF POOR RESPONSE TO PHARMACOLOGIC THERAPY

Noncompliance with plan (see Box 25-8)
Drug related
  Drug dose too low
  Inappropriate combination of drugs
  Inappropriate selection of drugs based on individual profile
  Drug interactions
    Adrenal corticosteroids
    Nonsteroidal antiinflammatory drugs
    Cyclosporine
    Oral contraceptives
    Nasal decongestants
    Antidepressants
    Sympathomimetics

Licorice-containing substances
  Cocaine
  Amphetamines
Associated conditions
  Smoking
  Excessive alcohol intake
  Obesity
  Secondary causes of hypertension (see Box 25-1)
  Malignant hypertension
Volume overload
  Inadequate diuretic
  Excessive sodium intake
  Renal failure
  Fluid retention related to decreased blood pressure

Modified from Joint National Committee on Detection, Evaluation, and Treatment of High Blood Pressure, *Arch Intern Med* 153:154-188, 1993.

---

vascular disease, heart block greater than first degree, and type I diabetes mellitus. African Americans and the elderly tend to respond poorly to beta-blockers in comparison to other classifications of antihypertensive medications.

***Angiotensin converting enzyme inhibitors.*** Angiotensin converting enzyme (ACE) inhibitors act by interfering with the renin-angiotensin-aldosterone system by blocking the formation of angiotensin II (a potent vasoconstrictor that also stimulates the release of aldosterone). ACE inhibitors also increase the levels of bradykinins, thereby causing vasodilation of arterial and venous vessels.

ACE inhibitors are generally well tolerated. The most common side effect is a dry chronic cough, particularly common at night. Adults with diabetes and hypertension benefit from ACE inhibitors because they decrease proteinuria and stabilize renal function in diabetic nephropathy. ACE inhibitors are contraindicated in patients with renal artery stenosis because of the risk for acute renal failure. Patients taking ACE inhibitors should have their renal function monitored.

***Calcium channel blockers.*** Calcium channel blockers inhibit the influx of extracellular calcium ions across the cell membranes of the vascular and cardiac cells. The resultant vasodilation causes a relaxation of the arteriolar smooth muscle and a decrease in peripheral vascular resistance. Calcium channel blockers are useful with or as an alternative to beta-blockers. They frequently require titration up to the most effective dosage.

The major side effects associated with the use of calcium channel blockers are related to their vasodilatory effects: headache, flushing, palpitations, and ankle edema. Because there are no adverse effects on plasma lipids, glucose metabolism, or renal function, they are suitable for use in patients with asthma, diabetes, renal failure, and claudication.

***Alpha-1-adrenergic blockers.*** Alpha-1-adrenergic blockers work to lower the BP by blocking the alpha-1-adrenergic receptors in arteriolar smooth muscle. This causes vasodilation of the arterioles and veins, thereby reducing PVR.

First dose orthostatic hypotension is a potential problem that can be minimized by taking an initial low dose and by using alpha-1-adrenergic blockers at bedtime. Other reported side effects include weakness, fatigue, headache, palpitations, and nasal congestion. Alpha-1-adrenergic blockers have a positive effect on plasma lipids, decreasing total cholesterol and triglycerides and increasing HDLs. In addition to their antihypertensive effects, they also have been shown to increase urinary flow in men with benign prostatic hypertrophy.

***Central-acting alpha agonists.*** Central-acting alpha agonists are alpha-2 receptor agonists. They act by inhibiting the sympathetic vasomotor center in the brain, resulting in decreased PVR and heart rate.

The most common side effects are dry mouth, sedation, and orthostatic hypotension. They should be used cautiously in the elderly. Patients are advised that abrupt discontinuation, especially of clonidine, may cause a severe rebound hypertension characterized by headache, nausea, vomiting, anxiety, and increased BP. Central-acting alpha agonists have no significant effects on serum lipids, renal function, or glucose metabolism.

***Vasodilators.*** Vasodilators act by producing relaxation of vascular smooth muscle, resulting in vasodilation and decreased PVR. Potential adverse effects include tachycardia, fluid retention, headache, palpitations, and nasal congestion; angina may be precipitated in patients with coronary heart disease.

## Nursing Management
### Assessment

A complete assessment, including history and physical examination, should be performed on all patients diagnosed with hypertension. The focus should be on identifying signs and symptoms that indicate target organ involvement, identifying symptoms associated with secondary causes of hypertension, and identifying the presence of other cardiovascular risk factors. Assessment of the patient's BP includes measurements taken while lying, sitting, and standing. Measurements should be taken in both arms to determine baseline data and document any bilateral pressure differences. It is important to follow the guidelines for BP measurements presented in Box 25-7. Also see Box 25-8.

---

**BOX 25-7**

**Guidelines for Accurate Blood Pressure Measurement**

1 Seated with arm supported and at heart level.
2 Blood pressure cuff should be of appropriate size (the rubber bladder should encircle at least two thirds of the arm) and applied to the patient's bare arm to ensure accurate measurement.
3 The patient should not have consumed coffee or smoked for 30 minutes before the measurement.
4 The patient should rest for 5 minutes before the measurement is taken.
5 A mercury sphygmomanometer, recently calibrated aneroid manometer, or validated electronic device should be used to take the blood pressure readings.
6 Initially blood pressure measurements should be taken in both arms.
7 Record both the systolic and diastolic pressures.
8 Assessment is based on the average of two or more readings, taken at least 2 minutes apart. If there is more than a 5 mm Hg difference between the first two readings, additional readings should be obtained.
9 Inform the patient of the numeric blood pressure measurement and advise about the need for periodic remeasurement.

---

Modified from US Department of Health and Human Services: The fifth report of the Joint National Committee on Detection, Evaluation, and Treatment of High Blood Pressure (JNC-V), Washington, DC, 1993, National Institutes of Health.

<| BOX 25-8 |>    **NURSING PROCESS**

## HYPERTENSION

### ASSESSMENT
### Subjective Data

- Past medical history including any disease entities putting patient at risk for target organ damage or hypertension (CHF, diabetes, stroke, CAD, PVD, kidney disease)
- Assessment of risk factors (smoking, alcohol intake, obesity, sedentary life-style, hyperlipidemia, age, sex, ethnicity)
- Family history of hypertension, cardiovascular disease, diabetes
- History of any previously diagnosed hypertension age of onset, treatment, compliance, any side effects from antihypertensive therapy
- Presence of early morning headache, blurred vision, spontaneous epistaxis, angina, dizziness, confusion, dyspnea on exertion
- Knowledge of hypertension: definition, risk factors, effects on the heart, brain, and kidneys
- Current prescribed and over the counter medications (see Table 25-9)
- Emotional, financial, or job-related stress
- Dietary preferences and pattern

### Objective Data

- Two or more blood pressure measurements taken on both arms at least 2 minutes apart with the patient in supine and standing positions
- Height and weight
- Funduscopic examination of the eyes assessing for arteriovenous nicking, papilledema, hemorrhage, cotton wool patches
- Examination of the neck for bruits, jugular venous distention, thyroid enlargement
- Auscultation of the heart for heart rate, murmurs, rubs, clicks, S3, S4, evidence of left ventricular enlargement, arrhythmias
- Examination of the abdomen for organomegaly, aortic/renal bruits
- Palpitation of pulses (carotid, brachial, radial, femoral, popliteal, posterior tibial, dorsalis pedis): quality, symmetry, rate, amplitude
- Auscultate lungs: for crackles, wheezes
- Palpate extremities for edema
- Neurologic examination for signs of stroke, TIA, hemorrhage
- Evaluation of lab tests: possible findings include abnormal potassium, elevated BUN, creatinine, glucose, LDLs, triglycerides, total cholesterol, low

HDLs, proteinuria, glucosuria, EKG demonstrating left ventricular hypertrophy, CXR revealing cardiomegaly, aortic dilation

### NURSING DIAGNOSES

- Altered health maintenance related to knowledge deficit about disease process, complications, and management of hypertension
- Altered health maintenance related to lack of exercise
- Altered nutrition: more than body requirements related to high caloric, fat, and sodium intake
- Altered sexuality patterns related to side-effects of antihypertensive medications
- Anxiety related to ability to adhere to plan of care, possible complications, life-style modifications needed to control disease, and need for life-long follow-up
- Body image disturbance related to having an identified disease
- Knowledge deficit related to disease process, potential complications, life-style modifications needed to reduce risks, nutritional requirements, treatments, and medications
- Decreased cardiac output related to increased workload of the heart and vasoconstriction
- Noncompliance with the treatment regimen related to asymptomatic characteristic of disease, financial constraints, inability to adhere to life-style modifications, side-effects of antihypertensive drugs, and lack of understanding about seriousness of disease and potential complications

### NURSING INTERVENTIONS

- Monitor BP in left and right arms in lying, sitting, and standing positions
- Inform patient of numerical blood pressure measurement
- Monitor weight
- Monitor visual acuity, note any visual changes
- Monitor for signs and symptoms of target-organ damage (eyes, brain, kidney, heart, etc.)
- Involve patient and family in education
- Provide all education in both verbal and written form in language appropriate to the individual's level of understanding
- Provide time for the patient to verbalize fears and concerns, or to ask questions
- Discuss disease process, risk factors, complications

*Continued*

BOX 25-8

## NURSING PROCESS

### HYPERTENSION—cont'd

- Educate about signs and symptoms of target organ damage
- Encourage life-style changes (dietary modifications, smoking cessation, alcohol intake, stress reduction, exercise, and weight reduction)
- Educate about antihypertensive agents (purpose, dosing, side-effects, ways to minimize side-effects)
- Stress importance of continuing therapy even if BP is WNL
- Teach home BP monitoring techniques
- Encourage patient to keep a diary of BP measurements and related important information
- Encourage verbalization of fears and concerns
- Involve patient/family in plan of care
- Set realistic goals with the patient
- Educate about stress reduction techniques and biofeedback
- Provide reassurance that BP can be controlled with appropriate therapy
- Reinforce education and clarify misunderstandings at follow-up visits
- Provide positive feedback for behavioral modification and blood pressure reduction
- Make appointment for next follow-up visit and send appointment reminders
- Monitor laboratory results: CBC, electrolytes (especially K+), BUN, creatinine, FBS, cholesterol, urinalysis, EKG and CXR results

**EVALUATION OF EXPECTED OUTCOMES**

- BP reduction to within goal range
- No evidence of target organ damage
- Patient verbalizes fears and concerns
- Patient demonstrates knowledge about disease process, risk factors, and complications associated with hypertension
- Patient demonstrates knowledge about treatment modalities including diet modifications, weight reduction, exercise, smoking cessation, alcohol limitation, stress reduction, and medications (name, rationale for use, dosing, frequency, side effects and ways to minimize them)
- Evidence of adherence to plan of care
- Patient keeps follow-up appointments
- Patient/family demonstrate proper BP measurement technique and documentation
- Able to verbalize understanding of need for life-long follow-up care
- Patient demonstrates ability to accurately take pulse rate and determine target heart rate
- Weight is reduced/maintained in goal range

---

**NURSE ALERT**

Not following proper procedure for blood pressure measurement can affect the accuracy of the measurement.

## Interventions

The goal of hypertension management is to lower the BP to as close to normal levels as possible. The usual treatment for hypertension is a plan for life-style modifications for 3 to 6 months for patients with a hypertension classification of stage 2 or less and life-style modifications plus antihypertensive therapy for all others. Life-style modifications are based on individual risk factors but may include dietary restrictions of sodium and fat, weight loss, exercise, smoking cessation, moderation of alcohol intake, stress reduction, and the need for follow-up health care. Because the patient or significant other is ultimately responsible for following the therapeutic plan, counseling and education on an ongoing basis are essential. The patient needs to be instructed about the disease process, potential complications, risk factors, dietary restrictions, weight control, exercise, smoking cessation, alcohol intake, stress reduction, and any pharmacologic therapies initiated (medication, dosing, side-effect profile, etc.).

**Patient/family education.** The patient needs to fully understand what hypertension means and how this disease may affect the body. The effects of hypertension on the heart, brain, kidneys, and eyes need to be clearly understood to facilitate compliance to the therapeutic plan. Refer to the Patient/Family Teaching Box.

**Dietary modifications.** Food habits are often very difficult to change. Restriction of sodium intake to less than 6 grams of sodium chloride per day is appropriate. Patients should be advised to avoid adding salt to their food during cooking or at the table, to replace

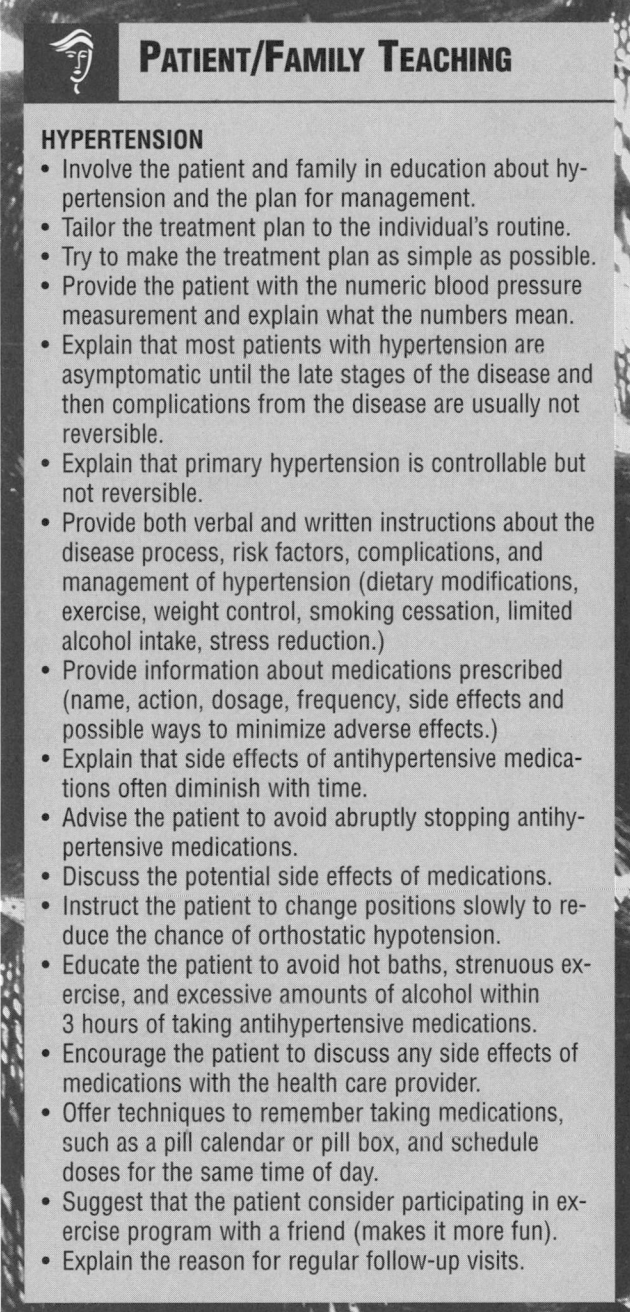

**PATIENT/FAMILY TEACHING**

**HYPERTENSION**

- Involve the patient and family in education about hypertension and the plan for management.
- Tailor the treatment plan to the individual's routine.
- Try to make the treatment plan as simple as possible.
- Provide the patient with the numeric blood pressure measurement and explain what the numbers mean.
- Explain that most patients with hypertension are asymptomatic until the late stages of the disease and then complications from the disease are usually not reversible.
- Explain that primary hypertension is controllable but not reversible.
- Provide both verbal and written instructions about the disease process, risk factors, complications, and management of hypertension (dietary modifications, exercise, weight control, smoking cessation, limited alcohol intake, stress reduction.)
- Provide information about medications prescribed (name, action, dosage, frequency, side effects and possible ways to minimize adverse effects.)
- Explain that side effects of antihypertensive medications often diminish with time.
- Advise the patient to avoid abruptly stopping antihypertensive medications.
- Discuss the potential side effects of medications.
- Instruct the patient to change positions slowly to reduce the chance of orthostatic hypotension.
- Educate the patient to avoid hot baths, strenuous exercise, and excessive amounts of alcohol within 3 hours of taking antihypertensive medications.
- Encourage the patient to discuss any side effects of medications with the health care provider.
- Offer techniques to remember taking medications, such as a pill calendar or pill box, and schedule doses for the same time of day.
- Suggest that the patient consider participating in exercise program with a friend (makes it more fun).
- Explain the reason for regular follow-up visits.

foods with a high salt content (e.g., canned fruits and vegetables, processed foods, carbonated beverages, and fast foods) with potassium-rich foods (e.g., oranges, bananas, asparagus, green leafy vegetables, freshly cooked meats, and whole grains). The use of herbs and spices to flavor food instead of salt should be encouraged. Over time, most individuals will adapt to the decrease in sodium.

Patients are advised to lower their daily intake of saturated fats and cholesterol. Although hyperlipidemia has no direct effect on BP, it is a major risk factor for cardiovascular disease. A low-fat diet will also aid in weight reduction.

**Weight reduction.** For those who are overweight, instructions should include weight loss through diet and exercise. An individualized, monitored weight reduction program should be established, taking into consideration the individual's food preferences, financial status, and life-style. The overall goal is to reduce and then maintain weight within 15% of the patient's ideal body weight. If pharmacologic therapy is required, a weight loss program should still be encouraged.

**Exercise.** Regular aerobic exercise can reduce BP, aid in weight reduction, and improve overall cardiovascular health. The patient should be encouraged to find some form of aerobic exercise that is enjoyable (brisk walking, swimming, jogging, bicycling) and should gradually build up to 30 to 45 minutes 3 to 5 times a week. Patients with known cardiovascular disease or other serious health problems should have a thorough physical examination before beginning an exercise program.

**Alcohol and smoking restrictions.** Patients should be advised to limit their intake of alcohol to one ounce or less of alcohol per day. This is the equivalent of 24 ounces of beer, 8 ounces of wine, or 2 ounces of 100-proof whisky. For those who smoke, smoking cessation programs should be strongly encouraged.

**Stress reduction.** Although relaxation techniques and biofeedback are not recommended for the definitive treatment of hypertension, some patients do find them beneficial.

**Drug therapy.** As with any medication, education about the purpose, dosage and schedule, possible drug interactions, potential side effects, and ways to minimize the unpleasant side effects of the medication is essential. After the initiation of any pharmacologic antihypertensive therapy, it is imperative to plan for scheduled blood pressure checks to determine if the therapy is effective and if any adjustments are needed in the dosing or type of medications. Table 25-3 describes the major classifications of antihypertensive medications.

**Patient noncompliance.** In patients with hypertension, noncompliance can be a major problem. If patients are active members in the design of the treatment plan there is greater likelihood of its success. A good primary care provider works closely with the patient to develop a therapeutic regimen that is acceptable. Box 25-9 identifies possible reasons for a patient's lack of adherence to the plan.

**Home monitoring.** Home blood pressure monitoring, using a reliable instrument, needs to be taught to all patients and significant others who are capable of accurately taking a BP reading. Home BP monitoring is a very useful adjunct to office readings, especially for suspected "office" or "white coat" hypertension (office BP measurements are consistently elevated but repeatedly normal when taken elsewhere), evaluation of

---

BOX 25-9

## FACTORS CONTRIBUTING TO NONCOMPLIANCE

- Financial constraints (cost of medications can be high)
- Instructions not clear
- No written instructions
- Unpleasant side-effects of medications
- Memory deficits (forget to take medication, forget to make or keep follow-up appointments)
- Inconvenient dosing schedule
- Inadequate or no patient education
- Sexual dysfunction related to medications
- Lack of patient involvement in development of plan
- Patient feels well so does not understand need to continue taking medication
- Abrupt withdrawal of antihypertensive medications
- Lack of trust between patient and caregiver

---

drug resistance, evaluation of nocturnal BP changes, monitoring of episodic hypertension, or evaluation of symptoms associated with antihypertension therapies. Fine tuning of dosages and timing of antihypertensive medications is facilitated through the use of home monitoring. Blood pressure measurements should be done a minimum of once a week after the readings have become stable (unless otherwise directed). Patients should be instructed to keep a written diary of all BP measurements and any pertinent information related to elevated or lowered readings, and they should bring the diary to office visits. Home BP monitoring often gives patients an added incentive to follow the prescribed plan of care. They are actively involved in the day-to-day management of their BP.

## Gerontologic Considerations

Approximately 50% of all persons over the age of 65 in the United States have an elevated systolic or diastolic blood pressure. With advancing age, specific structural and functional changes occur in the peripheral vascular system that place the elderly at increased risk for the development of hypertension. The following changes in the peripheral vascular system are responsible for the changes in blood pressure that occur in the elderly:

- Loss of connective tissue elasticity
- Decreased compliance of vessel walls caused by atherosclerosis
- Decreased baroreceptor response
- Reduced renal function
- Increased peripheral vascular resistance

Hypertension management is essentially the same in the elderly as it is in younger patients, although the elderly are often more prone to have adverse effects related to therapy. The goal of therapy is to reduce the blood pressure, identify and reduce risk factors, prevent complications related to hypertension (CAD, stroke), and minimize adverse affects of therapy.

The elderly often have decreased appetites and taste sensations, making them more prone to nutritional deficiencies related to dietary restrictions. Many are on fixed incomes, which makes the purchase of medications and healthful foods difficult. Pharmacologic management of hypertension is more difficult in the elderly. Because baroreceptor reflexes are blunted, there is greater risk for orthostatic hypotension, and they should be instructed to rise slowly from sitting or lying positions. Dosages of antihypertensive agents should be started low and advanced slowly to reduce the risk of hypotension related to decreased metabolism and excretion of drugs. The elderly should be started with low-dose antihypertensives and the dosages increased slowly to reduce the risk of adverse effects. If possible, sustained-release agents should be used to enhance compliance. Reminding patients to swallow the medication whole, without breaking it in half or chewing it, will enhance the effect of the medication.

---

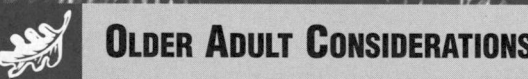

## OLDER ADULT CONSIDERATIONS

- Start with low dosages of antihypertensive medication and advance slowly to reduce potential side effects (especially orthostatic hypotension and dizziness).
- The elderly are especially sensitive to volume depletion; be careful with the administration of diuretics.
- Teach elderly patients to change positions slowly to reduce dizziness and orthostatic hypotension.
- With decreased taste sensation and appetite, the elderly may be prone to nutritional deficiencies.
- Be aware of potential interactions with other medications the patient may be taking.
- Carefully monitor the therapeutic effects of medical management in the older patient.

---

## Hypertensive Crisis

A hypertensive *emergency* is an acute rise in blood pressure, usually to a systolic pressure greater than 200 mm Hg or a diastolic pressure greater than 120 to 130 mm Hg, accompanied by severe symptoms and potential target organ complications. Signs and symptoms may include severe headache, nausea, vomiting, confusion, stupor, lethargy, chest pain, shortness of breath, visual loss, papilledema, focal deficits, seizures, coma, CHF, and renal insufficiency. Target organ damage is evidenced by signs and symptoms of encephalopathy, acute myocardial ischemia, pulmonary edema, CVA, renal failure, or aortic dissection. A hypertensive crisis may be precipitated by a number of causes, including but not limited to exacerbation of chronic hypertension, sudden withdrawal of antihypertensive medications, acute or chronic renal failure, renal artery disease, pheochromocytoma, CVA, eclampsia, preeclampsia, acute myocardial infarction, unstable angina, intracranial hemorrhage, dissecting aortic aneurysm, and primary aldosteronism (Porsche, 1995).

Hypertensive *urgencies* include accelerated or malignant hypertension without the associated symptoms or evidence of target organ damage.

A **hypertensive crisis** is a life-threatening medical emergency. It is imperative that the patient receive immediate treatment. Treatment is aimed at rapidly reducing the BP with the use of intravenous antihypertensive medications to prevent or limit target organ damage.

## ETHICAL DILEMMA

Mrs. Santos is a 45-year-old, obese, Hispanic female who was diagnosed with severe hypertension 1 year ago. She is married and has three young children. Despite repeated education related to the management of hypertension and to the seriousness of complications related to hypertension, Mrs. Santos does not adhere to the medical plan. She verbalizes understanding about the medical plan and the potential complications but states that she feels good and would rather not take any medications. She says she has a hard time trying to stick to a "diet" because she loves to eat and is too busy taking care of her children to find time to exercise. Despite appointment reminder calls, she often misses scheduled follow-up appointments. What is your ethical responsibility to this patient in relation to the control of her hypertension?

## NURSING CARE PLAN

## HYPERTENSION

Mr. Leonard is a 35-year-old obese Anglo American male who has come to the office for a physical and hypertensive work-up. Two weeks ago at a hypertension screening clinic held at his local YMCA, Mr. Leonard was found to have an average blood pressure of 168/102. Mr. Leonard states that he is rarely sick and has not been to his doctor in 3 years. He does admit to being under a lot of stress lately.

| Medical History | Psychosocial Data | Assessment Data |
|---|---|---|
| Hospitalizations: appendectomy age 12. | Married with three children ages 3, 7, and 9. Wife is pregnant with twins (unplanned but both are happy about it); is due in 2 months and is on bed rest. Describes marriage as strong and supportive. Wife is unemployed. | Height 6' 0", Weight 240 lbs |
| Medical history: Hiatus hernia diagnosed 5 years ago. | | B/P |
| Health risk behavior: | | Lying: left 174/98; right 168/100 |
| Smokes 1 pack cigarettes per day × 15 years | | Sitting: left 170/96; right 164/96 |
| Drinks 5-6 beers on weekends | Works as an assistant vice president for a local insurance company; is worried about losing his job because company is in process of downsizing. | Standing: left 166/92; right 164/94 |
| Gets minimal exercise | | Heart: regular rate and rhythm, apical rate 92, no murmurs, rubs |
| Family history: | | Respiratory: bilateral breath sounds clear to bases, rate 18 |
| Father: age 67, uncontrolled HTN, stroke 6 months ago | Religion: Roman Catholic; occasionally goes to church | Abdomen: large, round, soft, positive bowel sounds, no bruits |
| Mother: age 65, breast cancer, depression | Hobbies: surfing the Internet, golf (but does not get to play as often as would like), watching sports on TV | Neurologic: WNL |
| Older brother: HTN under control with medication | | Musculoskeletal: full ROM |
| Younger sister: alive and well | | Circulation: strong palpable pulses bilaterally, good capillary refill |
| Medications: Pepcid 20 mg PO hs, PRN | | Eyes: WNL, vision R 20/20 L 20/20 |

*Continued*

# NURSING CARE PLAN

## HYPERTENSION—cont'd

**NURSING DIAGNOSIS**

Altered health maintenance related to knowledge deficit about disease process, complications, and management of hypertension.

| NURSING INTERVENTIONS | EVALUATION OF EXPECTED OUTCOMES |
|---|---|
| Educate patient (verbal and written) about disease process, risk factors, and complications associated with hypertension. | Patient describes disease process, risk factors, and potential complications associated with hypertension. |
| Describe possible signs and symptoms associated with target organ disease. | Patient lists signs and symptoms to report to health care provider. |
| Teach the patient/family how to do home BP monitoring. | Patient verbalizes understanding of and agreement with plan of care to treat hypertension (including pertinent information about diet modifications, weight control, exercise, smoking cessation, alcohol limitation, stress reduction, and medications). |
| Discuss applicable life-style modifications (dietary changes: sodium restriction, adequate potassium, calcium, and magnesium intake, low fat and cholesterol intake; weight control; exercise; smoking cessation; limited alcohol intake; and stress-reduction techniques). | |
| Devise diet plan, in collaboration with patient, for weight reduction, and initiate counseling with dietitian as needed. | Patient verbalizes understanding of need for follow-up care. |
| Allow time for patient to ask questions and express concerns. | Patient/family member demonstrates appropriate method of taking BP. |
| Teach about any antihypertensive medications prescribed (name, purpose, dosage, route, time, frequency, side effect profile, and ways to minimize side effects) | Patient verbalizes fears and concerns. |
| Include family in teaching whenever possible. | Patient understands and adheres to therapeutic plan. |

**NURSING DIAGNOSIS**

Altered nutrition: more than body requirements related to high calorie, fat, and sodium intake

| NURSING INTERVENTIONS | EVALUATION OF EXPECTED OUTCOMES |
|---|---|
| Instruct patient in dietary modifications necessary to reduce weight. | Patient verbalizes accurate information about dietary modifications necessary to reduce weight. |
| Develop individualized diet plan, taking into considering life-style, food preferences, cultural considerations, and financial status. | Patient can identify ways to decrease intake of sodium, identify foods high in potassium and calcium and those low in cholesterol and saturated fats. |
| Provide nutritional information about food content (fat, caloric, cholesterol, and sodium content). | |
| Initiate dietary consultation as needed. | Patient adheres to the plan, evidenced by reduction in BP and weight. |
| Develop exercise program with patient (find something he would like to do). Encourage patient to exercise with a friend. | |

## NURSING CARE PLAN
## HYPERTENSION—cont'd

**NURSING DIAGNOSIS**
Altered health maintenance related to lack of exercise.

| NURSING INTERVENTIONS | EVALUATION OF EXPECTED OUTCOMES |
|---|---|
| Develop in collaboration with the patient an aerobic exercise program. | Patient verbalizes accurate information about benefits of exercise. |
| Encourage patient to do something that gives enjoyment. | Patient is able to demonstrate how to take pulse and calculate target heart rate. |
| Instruct patient to start slow and progress as tolerated. | Patient demonstrates compliance with the plan. |
| Instruct patient on warm-up and cool-down periods. | Patient's BP decreases. |
| Teach patient how to take pulse and how to calculate target heart rate range for maximal aerobic benefit. | |
| Encourage patient to exercise with a family member or friend. | |

# KEY CONCEPTS

**REGULATION OF BLOOD PRESSURE**
➤ Arterial BP is the force blood exerts on the wall of a blood vessel as it flows through.
➤ Systolic BP is the peak pressure within vessels immediately following ventricular contraction.
➤ Diastolic BP is the pressure in blood vessels during ventricular relaxation.
➤ Regulation of BP is calculated by cardiac output $\times$ peripheral vascular resistance.
➤ Cardiac output (CO) is the volume of blood pumped out the left ventricle with each heart beat.
➤ Peripheral vascular resistance (PVR) is the sum of all resistive forces that oppose movement of blood flow in the circulatory system.
➤ Any change in CO or PVR will cause a corresponding change in BP.
➤ Short-term adjustments of BP are made by baroreceptors and the autonomic nervous system and hormonal influences.
➤ Long-term regulation of BP is under renal and hormonal influences.

**NEURAL REGULATION**
➤ Baroreceptors are pressure-sensitive nerve cells in large arteries and the arch of the aorta that react to changes in stretch of vessel walls.

➤ Chemoreceptors transmit impulses to the vasomotor center to increase sympathetic stimulation with resulting vasoconstriction in response to a decrease in $O_2$ or hydrogen ion content or a decrease in $CO_2$ content.
➤ The autonomic nervous system influences heart rate, contractility, and PVR. The parasympathetic division (vagus nerve) slows heart rate. The sympathetic nervous system (SNS) is located in the medulla, and stimulation increases heart rate and contractility and causes vasoconstriction of peripheral blood vessels.
➤ The SNS has two types of membrane protein receptors (called alpha- and beta-adrenergic receptors) that allow neurotransmitters to work.
➤ Alpha-1 receptors in vascular smooth muscle are responsible for vasoconstriction.
➤ Alpha-2 receptors are located throughout the CNS and inhibit sympathetic outflow from the brain as part of the negative feedback loop.
➤ Beta-1 receptors are located in the heart; they increase heart rate, speed of conduction, and force of muscle contractions.

**RENAL REGULATION**
➤ Regulation is provided by the renin-angiotensin-aldosterone system.

*Continued*

## KEY CONCEPTS—cont'd

### HORMONAL AND CHEMICAL REGULATION

➤ Regulation is by epinephrine, norepinephrine, angiotensin II, antidiuretic hormone, atrial natriuretic factor, histamine and kinins, endothelin, nitric oxide.

### HYPERTENSION

➤ Definition: persistent elevation of SBP ≥140 mm Hg and/or DBP ≥90 mm Hg confirmed by minimum of two subsequent elevated readings taken at least 1 week apart, after the initial elevation.
➤ Classifications:
   Primary: no identifiable cause, accounts for 90%-95% of all cases
   Secondary: hypertension resulting from identifiable cause, 5% of cases
   Benign: uncomplicated
   Malignant: rapidly progressive elevation of BP associated with target organ damage and requiring immediate treatment
➤ Joint National Committee classifies severity of HTN according to four stages I = mild, II = moderate, III = severe, and IV = very severe.

### EPIDEMIOLOGY

➤ Approximately 60 million people in the United States are hypertensive, and as many as 50% go undiagnosed because of the asymptomatic nature of the disease
➤ Hypertension is most prevalent in African Americans
➤ Incidence of hypertension increases with age
➤ Hypertension morbidity and mortality rates are higher for men than women and higher in African Americans than Anglo Americans.

### RISK FACTORS FOR DEVELOPMENT OF HYPERTENSION

➤ Non-modifiable (family history, age, race, sex)
➤ Modifiable (obesity; high salt intake; low potassium, magnesium, and calcium intake; excessive alcohol intake; smoking; sedentary life-style; stress)

### CLINICAL MANIFESTATIONS

➤ Patients are often asymptomatic until late in disease process.
➤ The most common symptom is early morning occipital headache.

### COMPLICATIONS

➤ Hypertension is a major risk factor for stroke, coronary artery disease, renal failure, and retinal damage.
➤ Complication potential increases with severity of hypertension and length of time without treatment

### PREVENTION

➤ Primary: identify nonmodifiable risk factors and identify and control modifiable risk factors. Patient education is the key component
➤ Secondary: screening for hypertension, especially for those at increased risk
➤ Tertiary: management of hypertension and prevention and/or control of complications

### MEDICAL MANAGEMENT

➤ Diagnosis of hypertension is by complete history and physical, routine laboratory tests
➤ Treatment should be by the stepped care approach to therapy.
➤ Life-style modifications include dietary modifications, weight reduction, exercise, smoking cessation, alcohol limitation, stress reduction.
➤ Pharmacologic therapy is with diuretics, beta-blockers, angiotensin converting enzyme (ACE) inhibitors, calcium channel blockers, alpha-1 adrenergic blockers, central-acting alpha-agonists, and vasodilators.

### NURSING MANAGEMENT

➤ A complete history and physical examination should be performed.
➤ The goal is to lower the BP to as close to normal as possible while preventing complications associated with hypertension.
➤ Patient/family education: the most important intervention is an understanding of the disease process, the risk factors, and the treatment plan.
➤ Dietary modifications include the following:
   Limit salt intake to less than 6 grams of NaCl per day
      Increase intake of potassium, calcium, and magnesium
      Decrease daily intake of saturated fats and cholesterol

## KEY CONCEPTS—cont'd

➤ Weight reduction is undertaken to reduce and maintain weight within 15% of ideal body weight.

➤ Exercise: regular aerobic exercise should be performed three to five times a week.

➤ Alcohol restriction: the patient should drink no more than one ounce of alcohol/day.

➤ A smoking cessation program should be encouraged.

➤ Education about stress reduction techniques and biofeedback is provided.

➤ The patient must be educated about the drug name, purpose, dosage, frequency, timing, potential side effects, and ways to minimize side effects.

➤ Patient noncompliance is multifactorial: the practitioner needs to investigate reasons why the individual is noncompliant with the plan of care.

➤ Home BP monitoring should be performed using the proper technique and a diary used for recording measurements.

### GERONTOLOGIC CONSIDERATIONS

➤ Half of the persons in the United States over age 65 are hypertensive.

➤ The physiologic changes responsible for changes in BP in elderly include loss of connective tissue elasticity, decrease in compliance of vessel walls, decreased baroreceptor response, reduced renal function, and increased peripheral vascular resistance.

➤ Management is essentially the same as with younger persons.

➤ Special considerations for the elderly include the following: decreased appetite and taste sensations may make the elderly more prone to nutritional deficiencies when on special diets, fixed incomes make purchasing healthful foods and medications difficult, a greater risk for orthostatic hypotension exists, and metabolism and excretion of drugs are decreased in the elderly.

### HYPERTENSIVE CRISIS

➤ Hypertensive crisis is defined as an acute rise in blood pressure, usually to systolic BP >200 mm Hg and/or diastolic BP >120 mm Hg, with associated signs and symptoms indicative of target organ damage. This is a medical emergency requiring immediate pharmacologic intervention to rapidly lower BP.

## CRITICAL THINKING EXERCISES

1. You work in a medical clinic in a low-income housing project and are caring for a middle-aged woman who is noncompliant with the prescribed medication regimen. Describe your assessment to identify those factors that might be interfering with her ability to follow the prescribed plan of care.

2. How would you assess for target organ damage in an elderly patient?

3. Why is screening for high blood pressure so important?

4. A 48-year-old African American male has the following blood pressure readings over the past 4 weeks: 162/90, 174/88, and 166/94. He is 20% over his ideal body weight, frequently eats at fast food restaurants, and does minimal exercise. What interventions should be initiated by the provider?

### REFERENCES AND ADDITIONAL READINGS

Barker L: Hypertension. In Barker L, Burton J, Zieve P, editors: *Principles of ambulatory medicine,* Baltimore, 1995, Williams & Wilkins.

Barron H, Amidon T: Options in antihypertensive drug therapy, *Postgrad Med* 100(4):89-94, 1996.

Beilin L: Non-pharmacological management of hypertension: optimal strategies for reducing cardiovascular risk, *J Hypertens Suppl* 12(10):S71-S81, 1994.

Futterman L, Lemberg L: Hypertension, stroke, and noncompliance: an avoidable triad, *Am J Crit Care* 5(3):227-233, 1996.

Ganda O, Simonson D: Controlling lipids and blood pressure, *Patient Care* February 15:61-64, 66-67, 70-72, 1995.

Griffith C: Hypertension: evaluation and management, *Physician Assist* September: 25-28, 31-34, 36-40, 42, 44-45, 1995.

Hamdy R, Hudgins L, Compton R: Management of hypertension in older patients, *South Med J* 86(10):2S1-2S6, 1993.

Hanes D, Weir M, Sowers A: Gender considerations in hypertension pathophysiology and treatment, *Am J Med* 101(3A):10S-21S, 1996.

Henshaw C: Alteration in blood pressure. In Copstead L, editor: *Perspectives on pathophysiology*, Philadelphia, 1995, Saunders.

Joint National Committee on Detection, Evaluation, and Treatment of High Blood Pressure: Fifth Report of the Joint National Committee on Detection, Evaluation, and Treatment of High Blood Pressure, *Arch Intern Med* 153:154-188, 1993.

Kaplan N: Resistant hypertension: what to do after trying "the usual," *Geriatrics* 50(5):24-25, 29-30, 33, 38, 1995.

Marieb E: *Human anatomy and physiology*, ed 3, Redwood City, Calif, 1995, Benjamin/Cummings.

Mattson C: *Pathophysiology: concepts of altered health status*, ed 5, Philadelphia, 1998, Lippincott.

Murphy J: *Nurse practitioners' prescribing reference*, New York, 1998, Prescribing Reference.

Phipps W et al: *Medical-surgical nursing: concepts and clinical practice*, ed 5, St Louis, 1995, Mosby.

Porche R: Hypertension: diagnosis, acute antihypertension therapy, and long-term management, *AACN Clin Issues* (6)4:515-525, 1995.

Porth C: *Pathophysiology: concepts of altered health states*, ed 3, Philadelphia, 1990, Lippincott.

Reynolds E, Baron R: Hypertension in women and the elderly, *Postgrad Med* 100(4):58, 60-63, 67-69, 1996.

Rubenstein E, Federman D: High blood pressure. In Rubenstein E, Federman D, editors: *Scientific American medicine*, New York, 1993, Scientific American.

Sadowski A, Redeker N: The hypertensive elder: a review for the primary care provider, *Nurse Pract* 21(5):99-100, 102, 105-112, 118, 1996.

Sanson-Fisher R, Clover K: Compliance in the treatment of hypertension: a need for action, *Am J Hypertens* 8:82S-88S, 1995.

Schnall P et al: The relationship between "job strain," workplace diastolic pressure, and left ventricular mass index, *J Am Med Assoc* 263:1929-1935, 1990.

Schotte D, Stunkard A: The effects of weight reduction on blood pressure in 301 obese patients, *Arch Intern Med* 150(8):1701-1704, 1990.

Skidmore-Roth L: *Mosby's nursing drug reference*, St Louis, 1997, Mosby.

Stein P, Black H: The role of diet in the genesis and treatment of hypertension, *Med Clin North Am* 77:831-847, 1993.

Superko N et al: Effects of cessation of caffeinated-coffee consumption on ambulatory and resting blood pressure in men, *Am J Cardiol* 73:780-784, 1994.

Trottier D: Hypertension. In Lewis SM, Collier IC, Heitkemper MM, editors: *Medical-surgical nursing: assessment and management of clinical problems*, ed 4, St Louis, 1996, Mosby.

Tucker S et al: *Patient care standards: collaborative practice planning guidelines*, ed 6, St Louis, 1996, Mosby.

Zellner C, Sudhir K: Lifestyle modifications for hypertension, *Postgrad Med* 100(4):75-79, 1996.

# Hematologic and Lymphatic Problems

## CHAPTER OBJECTIVES

1 Discuss the importance of the blood components as a measure of health and illness.
2 Describe the common diagnostic tests for blood disorders.
3 Differentiate among hemorrhagic, iron-deficiency, pernicious, sickle cell, and aplastic anemias according to their pathophysiologic features and nursing assessment and intervention.
4 Discuss the significance of leukocytosis and leukopenia as indicators of illness.
5 Discuss the nursing care plan for the patient with leukemia and anemia.
6 Discuss the pathophysiology, assessment, and nursing interventions in caring for patients with hemorrhagic disorders.
7 Differentiate among leukemia, Hodgkin's disease, non-Hodgkin's lymphoma, and multiple myeloma.

## KEY TERMS

| | |
|---|---|
| anemia | leukopenia |
| blood dyscrasias | lymphangitis |
| ecchymoses | lymphedema |
| erythrocytes | lymphoma |
| erythropoietin | multiple myeloma |
| hemophilia | petechiae |
| Hodgkin's disease | polycythemia |
| leukemia | reticulocyte |
| leukocytes | sickle cell anemia |
| leukocytosis | thrombocytes |

## FUNCTION OF BLOOD

The circulatory system is the transportation system of the body. Through its vast network of vessels, blood carries oxygen to the cells and returns carbon dioxide to the lungs to be eliminated. It transports food to nourish the cells so that they may carry on their normal functions and carries away waste products of cell metabolism. Water, electrolytes, hormones, and enzymes, all of which have important functions in keeping the body in a state of equilibrium (homeostasis), are transported by the blood. Heat is carried by the blood, thereby regulating body temperature. Immune cells and antibodies that help prevent disease are also important parts of the blood. Through a complex system, the blood provides clotting factors and prevents serious loss of fluids in case of injury. It also prevents clot formation in blood vessels, which would seriously interfere with the oxygen supply to the cells. Any disease or condition that affects the blood or its transport system may pose a serious threat to the individual.

## STRUCTURE OF BLOOD

The blood is slightly sticky and has a characteristic odor and a faint salty taste. It is bright red in the arteries because it is carrying oxygen; it is dark red in the veins because the cells have taken up the oxygen and the blood is carrying carbon dioxide to be eliminated by the respiratory system. The blood is comprised of two parts: the liquid part, called *plasma*, which constitutes slightly more than half of the total volume; and the formed or solid elements. The formed elements have been divided into several groups: (1) **erythrocytes**, or red blood cells; (2) **leukocytes**, or white blood cells; and (3) **thrombocytes**, or platelets. Platelets are not considered cells, but cell fragments.

Blood volume remains fairly constant in one person, but there are variations among individuals. Factors such as age, sex, size of the body frame, and the amount of adipose tissue may affect the volume of circulating blood. Adults generally have 5 to 7 L of circulating blood volume.

## Plasma

Plasma contains no cells and is estimated to be approximately 90% water. It is a clear, straw-colored fluid with a large number of substances dissolved in it. Among the most important of these substances are the plasma proteins, which include serum albumin, serum globulin, and *fibrinogen* (Figure 26-1). The proteins have some individual functions, but all of them are important in nutrition and regulation of blood volume through osmotic pressure. Serum albumin, in particular, influences blood volume because it comprises more than half of the total proteins. Serum globulins are divided into α-, β-, and γ-globulins. The γ-globulins are significant in the immune response because they are the body's antibodies. Fibrinogen contributes to blood coagulation through its role in the formation of fibrin. Other substances dissolved in plasma include urea, uric acid, glucose, respiratory gases, hormones, and electrolytes. Minute amounts of other substances essential to the body are also found in plasma. Plasma can be separated from the formed elements, and because it contains the proteins that assist in the clotting of blood, it may be administered for several bleeding disorders.

## Erythrocytes
### Formation

Erythrocytes are formed in the red bone marrow, which develops in the pelvis, vertebrae, ribs, skull, and proximal ends of the femur and humerus. Before birth the red blood cell production is carried on by the liver and the spleen. The production of erythrocytes (erythropoiesis) is a continuous process, and in the absence of disease, the number of erythrocytes remains relatively constant.

### Number

The number of erythrocytes is usually slightly higher in men (4.5 to 6 million/mm³ of blood) than in women (4.3 to 5.5 million/mm³ of blood). In the newborn infant the number may be increased (5 to 7 million/mm³ blood), but it gradually decreases to adult levels by 15 years of age. A **reticulocyte** is an immature red blood cell (Pagana, Pagana, 1997). Recent discovery of substances called hematopoietic growth factors has contributed to an understanding of erythrocyte homeostasis. **Erythropoietin** is one of the growth factors that stimulates marrow production of red blood cells. It is thought that the kidney produces erythropoietin in response to low tissue oxygen levels. In addition to

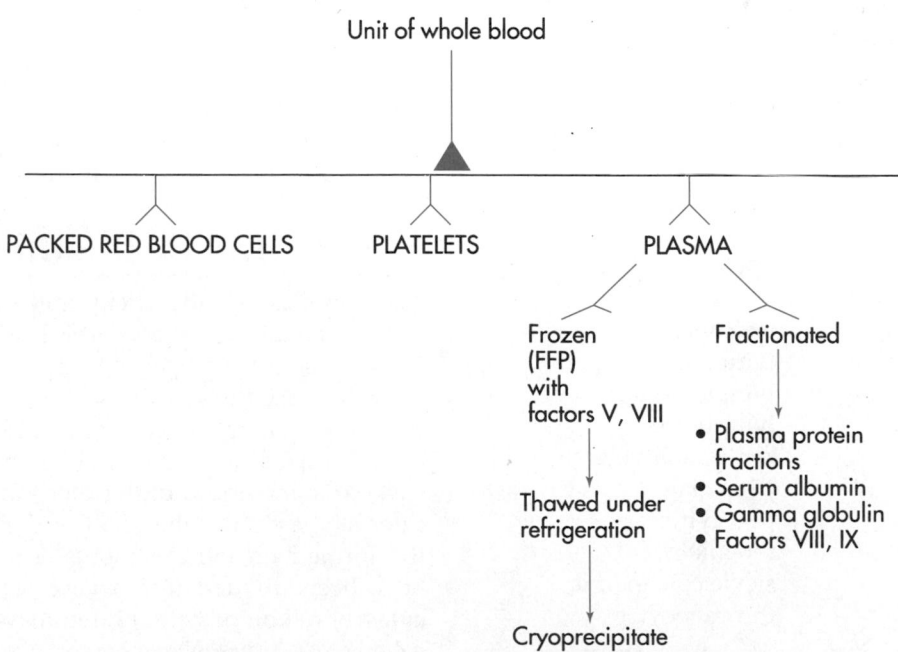

**Figure 26-1**   Reduction of unit of whole blood into fractions.

the growth factors, effective erythropoiesis requires healthy bone marrow with normal stem cell populations and adequate supplies of folic acid, vitamin $B_{12}$, and iron.

## Hemoglobin

The main ingredient of the erythrocyte is hemoglobin. Within each red blood cell there are millions of molecules of hemoglobin. The amount of hemoglobin in the red blood cell depends on adequate iron storage, which is essential for the synthesis of hemoglobin and for the oxygen-carrying ability of the hemoglobin molecule. Hemoglobin carries oxygen to the cells of the body, and thus the amount of oxygen available to the cells depends on the amount of hemoglobin in the blood. Hemoglobin is measured in grams per deciliter of blood, whereas red blood cells are measured in millions per cubic millimeter of blood.

## Effects of Blood Loss

Loss of blood through hemorrhage causes a decrease in the amount of circulating fluid, the number of red blood cells, the amount of hemoglobin, and, in turn, the amount of iron. Because the oxygen-carrying power of the blood has been decreased, the heart must work harder to supply the cells with oxygen. Thus a person suffering from loss of blood may be expected to have an increased pulse rate. There will also be an increase in the respiration rate as the body attempts to provide more oxygen for circulation. Chronic blood loss also causes anemia, although, in this case, the blood volume in the vascular system is stabilized more readily.

## Response to Disease

Certain diseases of the blood and blood-forming organs may affect the production of erythrocytes so that the number is decreased or their structure is immature. In some genetic diseases the erythrocytes may have an abnormal shape. In contrast to the disease states mentioned that cause anemia, some disorders cause an overproduction of erythrocytes. Having too many red blood cells in the circulation is undesirable and may at times be life threatening.

## Leukocytes
### Formation

Leukocytes, in a manner similar to that of erythrocytes and thrombocytes, arise from stem cells in bone marrow. Disorders of white blood cells can result from overproduction, underproduction, or abnormal maturation of any one or all leukocyte cell lines.

### Number

Leukocytes, or white blood cells, are not as numerous as the erythrocytes, or red blood cells. The number of white blood cells in 1 $mm^3$ of blood varies between 5000 and 10,000. The number is essentially the same for men and women. When there is an increase of more than 10,000 white blood cells, it may indicate the presence of some pathologic condition. Such an increase is called **leukocytosis**. Under some conditions there may be a decrease in the number of leukocytes, which is called **leukopenia**. *Granulocytopenia* is a term that is used interchangeably with leukopenia but refers specifically to a low number of circulating granulocytes or neutrophils.

### Classification

Leukocytes are classified as granular or nongranular, depending on the color of their cytoplasm and the shape of their nuclei. Granular leukocytes are called *granulocytes*, and approximately 50% to 75% of leukocytes are granulocytes. Approximately 50% of the mature granulocytes released from the bone marrow into the circulation adhere to the walls of small blood vessels. The remainder pass from the circulation into the tissues to perform their specific functions. The granulocytes are divided into three types: *neutrophils, basophils,* and *eosinophils.* The nongranular leukocytes, or *agranulocytes,* comprise less than one third of the cells and include the *lymphocytes* and *monocytes.*

**Granulocytes.** The primary function of the *neutrophils* is *phagocytosis,* the ingestion and digestion of debris and foreign material throughout the body. They are the first cells to arrive at the scene when an inflammatory reaction is stimulated. Neutrophils are attracted to the foreign substance in response to chemicals that are released from inflamed tissue. Neutrophils are also referred to as *myelocytes, polys,* and *granulocytes.*

The basophils do not phagocytize material but contain powerful chemicals such as histamine and heparin that can be released locally. They are important during the inflammatory process in modulating the formation of clots and their growth. The specific function of these cells is not completely understood.

The eosinophils appear to play a role in allergic or foreign protein reactions and are elevated in number in patients with allergies or parasitic infestations.

**Agranulocytes.** The monocytes become larger phagocytic cells when stimulated and play an important role in the inflammatory process. Lymphocytes are the primary cells concerned with the development of immunity. Although they arise from stem cells in the bone marrow, maturation occurs in the lymphatic or reticuloendothelial systems.

The leukocytes have many functions in the body, and their mobility allows them to protect the body from infection and to repair damaged tissue. A differential count of white blood cells is often an important aid to the physician in establishing a diagnosis. For example, in suspected acute appendicitis, an increase in the number of white blood cells, together with clinical symptoms, may indicate to the physician the need for an appendectomy (Lewis, Collier, Heitkemper, 1996).

## Differential Count

A differential count is a measure of the total number of white blood cells or leukocytes and the percentage of each of the five classes. For many patients, one drop of blood obtained from a fingertip is sufficient for this test. After the specimen is placed on a slide, it is examined under a microscope, and each type of leukocyte is identified and counted. Each type of cell is reported as a percentage of all classes of white blood cells. In various diseases certain kinds of cells may be increased; for example, in some bacterial infections the number of lymphocytes may increase.

## Thrombocytes
### Formation

Thrombocytes, or platelets, are tiny, fragile elements in the blood. They are formed in red bone marrow and are thought to be minute fragments of larger cells called *megakaryocytes.*

### Number

The exact number of platelets is unknown, but various estimates have placed the number from 150,000 to 500,000/mm³ of blood. In the hemorrhagic disorder called *thrombocytopenia,* a decrease in the number of platelets may cause serious bleeding, whereas in other diseases there may be an abnormally high number of platelets, called *thrombocytosis.*

### Function

The primary function of platelets is to control bleeding. When an injury to a blood vessel occurs, the platelets concentrate at the site of the injury and control bleeding by forming thrombotic plugs and by releasing a substance, factor III, that is necessary for coagulation and the formation of fibrin. Platelets continue their activity in helping to shrink the clots and bring together the margins of the damaged vessel.

# THERAPEUTIC BLOOD FRACTIONS

Blood may be broken down into its component parts so that patients with certain conditions may be given specific blood fractions to meet their individual needs (Table 26-1; see Figure 26-1).

## Blood Plasma

Plasma may be separated from whole blood that has been stored, or it may be separated from fresh blood taken from a donor and immediately frozen. The primary use of plasma is to treat conditions in which clotting of the blood is defective. When fresh blood plasma is used, it contains all of the factors essential for clotting, including the antihemophilic factor.

## Platelets

Platelets may be separated from whole blood and administered to patients with severe hematologic disorders, open-heart surgery, and postoperative bleeding. The demand for platelets has increased, and it is now believed that patients who are bleeding from any site, internal or external, and whose platelet count is below 20,000/mm³ of blood should receive platelets. The administration of platelets has been a lifesaving measure for many patients who are receiving chemotherapy for malignant disorders.

Platelets are administered most often in the form of a concentrate that has been separated from one or more units of whole blood. The advantage of the platelet concentrate is that it may be infused in only 50 ml of fluid. When long-term administration is required, it avoids overloading the circulatory system.

## Pheresis

In platelet pheresis, whole blood is removed from a donor through a needle in one arm. The blood is then circulated through a cell separator where platelets are removed. All the other blood components are returned to the donor through a needle inserted into the opposite arm (Lewis, Collier, Hietkemper, 1996). Pheresed platelets, also called *single-donor platelets,* decrease the antigens to which a patient is exposed. For patients who are at risk for developing antibodies to donor platelets, platelets matched for human lymphocyte antigen (HLA) are preferred over pooled or random donor platelets and single donor pheresed platelets. The life span and functional capacities of platelets are diminished when these antibodies develop. This also interferes with successful bone marrow transplantation. With the exception of hemolytic reactions, the patient receiving platelets may have reactions similar to

TABLE 26-1

## Pharmacology of Drugs, Blood, and Blood By-Products

| DRUG (GENERIC AND TRADE NAME); ROUTE AND DOSAGE | ACTION/INDICATION | COMMON SIDE EFFECTS AND NURSING CONSIDERATIONS |
|---|---|---|
| **Albumin**<br>**Route:** IV in 5% solution<br>**Dosage:** 250 ml and 500 ml; 25% solution: 50 ml and 100 ml: 5% solution infuse 1 to 10 ml/min, or more rapidly if patient in shock; 25% solution infuse 0.2 to 0.4 ml/min | Blood by-product used for acute liver failure, burns, hemolytic disease of newborn, as well as volume expansion when crystalloid solutions are not adequate; shock and massive hemorrhage | Cross match unnecessary; cannot be used as plasma substitute because albumin contains no clotting factors; watch for circulatory overload hypertension |
| **Cryoprecipitate and factor VIII**<br>**Route:** IV<br>**Dosage:** 5 to 20 ml depending on preparation method; rapidly 1 to 2 ml/min | Both are blood by-products; Cryo used to treat von Willebrand's disease, hypofibrinogenemia, or factor XIII deficiency; factor VIII used for deficiencies, including hemophilia type A | ABO compatibility preferred; contraindicated in undefined coagulation deficiency; watch for infectious diseases and allergic reactions |
| **Epoetin alfa** (Epogen)<br>**Route:** IV, SQ<br>**Dosage:** IV or SQ 50-100 units/kg 3 times a wk, then adjust dosage by increments of 25 U/kg to maintain hematocrit | Treatment of anemia associated with chronic renal failure, for anemia secondary to AZT in HIV infection | Hypertension or seizures; use may increase need for heparin in dialysis |
| **Factor II, VII, IX, and X complexes**<br>**Route:** IV<br>**Dosage:** Infuse 2 to 3 ml/min | Freeze-dried prepared blood by-product made from pooled plasma; used for hemophilia type B, congenital factor VII or X deficiency | Cross matching unnecessary; use only with specific factor deficiency; watch for allergic reactions and infectious diseases |
| **Folic acid** (folate, vitamin B)<br>**Route:** PO, IM, SQ<br>**Dosage:** 0.25 to 1.0 mg/day for anemia. 0.1 to 1.0 mg/day as dietary supplement | Used in treatment of anemia, given during pregnancy to promote normal fetal development | Use with caution in uncorrected pernicious anemia |
| **Granulocyte colony stimulating factor** (Filgrastim, Neupogen)<br>**Route:** SQ, IV<br>**Dosage:** 5 $\mu$g/kg/day | Stimulates the production and function of neutrophils; used for the prevention and treatment of neutropenia | Bone pain may occur |
| **Granulocyte macrophage colony stimulating factor** (Sargramostim, Leukine, Prokine)<br>**Route:** IV<br>**Dosage:** 250 $\mu$m²/day over 4 hr | Stimulates the production and function of granulocytes, monocytes, macrophages; used for patients receiving chemotherapy or who have had a bone marrow transplant | Bone pain, lethargy, fever, myalgia, rash may occur. Use caution in patients with history of cardiac disease. |

*Continued*

**TABLE 26-1**

## Pharmacology of Drugs, Blood, and Blood By-Products—cont'd

| DRUG (GENERIC AND TRADE NAME); ROUTE AND DOSAGE | ACTION/INDICATION | COMMON SIDE EFFECTS AND NURSING CONSIDERATIONS |
|---|---|---|
| **Iron** (ferrous) salts<br>**Route:** PO, IV, IM<br>**Dosage:** PO 200 mg/day; IM, IV total dose = 0.0476 kg (14.8 − patient hemoglobin) + 1 ml/5 kg up to 14 ml for iron stores | Treatment and prevention of iron-deficiency anemias | Hypotension, staining at IM site, constipation, diarrhea, nausea, dark stools, epigastric pain, staining of teeth in liquid preparations; use cautiously with peptic ulcer and inflammatory bowel disease |
| **Phytonadione** (AquaMEPHYTON, Vitamin K₁)<br>**Route:** PO, IM, SQ<br>**Dosage:** 2.5 to 10 mg, repeat PO in 12-48 hr if necessary; SQ or IM in neonates 0.5 to 1.0 mg within 1 hr of birth | Prevention and treatment of anemias; antidote for overdose of salicylates and oral anticoagulants; nutritional deficiencies and prolonged total parenteral nutrition; prevention of hemorrhagic disease in the newborn | Large doses counter the effects of oral anticoagulants; use caution in use with liver disease |
| **Plasma**<br>**Route:** IV<br>**Dosage:** 185 to 225 ml/bag; may be infused rapidly 10-20 ml over 3 min or slowly if potential for circulatory overload exists | Blood by-product separated from RBC and frozen within 6 hr after collection; contains plasma proteins, fibrinogen, and factors V, VIII, and IX, as well as water, electrolytes, sugars, proteins, vitamins, minerals, hormones, antibodies, used to increase levels of clotting factors when there is a deficiency | Cross matching unnecessary, must be ABO compatible; not for nutritional supplementation or volume expansion; watch for infectious diseases, allergic reactions, circulatory overload, hemolytic reactions |
| **Platelets** (Platelet concentrate)<br>**Route:** IV<br>**Dosage:** 50 to 70 ml; may be infused rapidly 1 unit in 10 min or less; must be infused within 4 hr | Platelets are blood by-products centrifuged from plasma; used for bleeding as a result of deficiency in platelet function or number | Cross matching unnecessary, but ABO compatibility preferred; watch for infectious diseases and septic, toxic, allergic, or febrile reactions |
| **Red blood cells** (packed RBCs)<br>**Route:** IV<br>**Dosage:** 250-350 ml, depending on specific bag volume; infuse up to 4 hr only | Blood by-product prepared by removing up to 90% of the plasma; used for blood loss and anemia | Cross matching and ABO compatibility necessary; watch for all hemolytic, febrile, allergic reactions (including urticaria up to anaphylactic shock); also circulatory overload, hyperkalemia as a result of potassium release, hepatitis, HIV, CMV, and other infectious diseases; watch for reactions; especially with massive transfusion |
| **Whole blood**<br>**Route:** IV<br>**Dosage:** 400-500 ml; infuse over no more than 4 hr | Whole blood consists of RBC, platelets, plasma, anticoagulant, preservative; when stored, it loses clotting factors and releases potassium; used to treat acute, massive blood loss, but is not often given; instead crystalloid and colloid solutions, RBC, or other blood components are given | Cross matching and ABO compatibility is necessary; watch for all reactions as mentioned for RBC transfusion |

those from whole blood transfusions. Therefore close observation of the patient is essential.

## Plasma Protein Fractions

Plasma proteins may also be given as individual blood components.

### Gamma Globulin

The primary use of gamma globulin is in the prevention or modification of infectious disease. Immune human gamma globulins are fractions of blood obtained from persons with circulating antibodies against a specific disease. Such persons may have antibodies as a result of having had the disease or having been immunized against it. When administered to nonimmune persons, immune human gamma globulin prevents disease or complications of diseases such as tetanus, mumps, pertussis, or rubella.

### Serum Albumin

Purified human serum albumin may be administered to maintain osmotic pressure of the plasma. It is useful in any condition in which the albumin/globulin ratio has been lowered. It may be administered to burn patients as well as to treat hypovolemic shock and liver disease.

### Fibrinogen

Fibrinogen is an essential factor for clotting blood. Fibrinogen is converted into fibrin, an essential part of a blood clot, by thrombin in the presence of calcium ions. A deficiency of fibrinogen may exist as a congenital disorder or an acquired condition resulting from massive hemorrhage, prolonged active bleeding, or other hematologic conditions dependent on the clotting mechanism.

### Cryoprecipitate

Cryoprecipitate, prepared by the thawing of fresh frozen plasma, contains an average of 150 mg of fibrinogen and is used to restore a patient's clotting factors to normal ranges (American Red Cross, 1994). Cryoprecipitate also contains factor VIII (the antihemophilic factor), factor XIII, and von Willebrand's factor. A deficiency in any one of these coagulation factors can result in severe bleeding. Cryoprecipitate may be used to correct the deficit. However, replacing the specific factor concentrate that is deficient is usually preferred (American Red Cross, 1994).

## Packed Red Blood Cells

Packed red blood cells are red blood cells without the plasma. The cells and the plasma are separated by centrifugation of whole blood. In conditions in which the blood volume is normal but the number of red blood cells and amount of hemoglobin are decreased, packed red blood cells may be given to the patient. Because packed red blood cells are placed in only a small amount of fluid, the danger of overloading the circulatory system is avoided. The removal of plasma containing white blood cells and antibodies reduces the risk of allergic reaction. To provide safer transfusions to recipients, whole blood is rarely administered except when specifically indicated, as in the case of massive hemorrhage or total blood transfusions to newborns.

## Leukocytes

Leukocytes may be obtained through a special process called *leukapheresis*, or *granulocytapheresis*. Because leukocytes cannot be obtained in sufficient amounts from a single unit of blood, it is necessary to obtain them from a single compatible donor by removing the leukocytes and replacing the blood. The procedure yields leukocytes that are predominantly granulocytes. Recipients of this component are those with life-threatening, low white blood cell counts who have infections that are unresponsive to antibiotic therapy; those with leukemia or immunosuppressive disorders; and those undergoing extensive field radiation therapy or intensive chemotherapy. Granulocytes have a short survival time and must be infused as soon as possible after collection—in less than 24 hours. The infusion must be given slowly, and the recipient should be observed closely for negative reactions. The long-term therapeutic benefit of granulocyte transfusion is still questionable and continues to be evaluated. Leukocyte transfusions are not usually administered in community hospitals.

## COLLECTION OF BLOOD

The collection and storage of blood began during World War II. Because of the progress of medical science, whole blood, plasma, and blood fractions have become essential to the practice of modern medicine. Along with the increased demand have come improved methods of collection, storage, and distribution. At present there are three main collection systems: the American Red Cross, hospitals, and commercial centers. The American Red Cross maintains regional centers for the collection of blood and mobile units that may be taken to communities, industrial plants, or college campuses. The arrival of the mobile unit is usually the culmination of drives for donors sponsored by local citizens. Some hospitals collect blood to meet their individual needs. Commercial blood centers have recently begun to flourish in the community. These centers collect and process blood components. Donors often are members of the patient's family, friends of the patient, or other persons interested in the patient. In an emergency, when large amounts of blood may be needed, the hospital may call on citizens of the community or the American Red Cross to help meet its needs.

## Testing

Although all prospective donors are examined and interviewed, donors may be unwilling or unable to provide an accurate history about exposure to and incidence of blood-transmitted diseases, including acquired immunodeficiency syndrome (AIDS), hepatitis, syphilis, malaria, cytomegalovirus, or Epstein-Barr virus. Therefore the Food and Drug Administration requires that all donated blood be tested for antibodies to human immunodeficiency virus (anti-HIV); hepatitis B surface antigen (HB$_s$Ag); antibody to hepatitis B core antigen (anti-HB$_c$); antibody to hepatitis C virus (anti-HCV); antibody to human T-cell lymphotropic virus, type I (anti-HTLV-I); and syphilis. However, such donor screening and testing does not totally eliminate the risk of transmitting disease by transfusion (American Red Cross, 1994).

## Autologous Blood

In many areas blood collection agencies can store autologous (one's own) blood for use in elective surgery. Recent technologic developments also allow the reinfusion of a patient's blood shed during and after surgical procedures. These developments contribute to the safer use of blood products but have limited application in high blood use groups.

## NURSING RESPONSIBILITIES FOR DIAGNOSTIC TESTS

A large number of blood tests are done for diagnostic purposes, but some are useful in guiding the physician in the course and treatment of disease. Some tests are performed on capillary blood and require only a few drops, which are usually secured by pricking the finger or the earlobe. Blood for other tests requiring a larger amount of blood is secured from a vein with a needle and syringe. Some of the more common tests are reviewed here, and others are found in different sections of this book, according to their relation to specific diseases. Table 26-2 lists normal hematologic values for various diagnostic tests.

## Complete Blood Cell Count

The complete blood cell count (CBC) is the most common of all tests made on the blood. It consists of a count of the erythrocytes and leukocytes, a measurement of hemoglobin and hematocrit, and a differential count of the leukocytes. A platelet count is often included. The physician orders the examination, which is made by persons trained in laboratory methods. However, it is often the responsibility of the nurse to execute the proper forms and notify the laboratory of the physician's request. Many hospitals require that routine blood counts be completed for all patients on admission, and some hospitals route the patient from the admission office to the laboratory for the examination before the patient is admitted to the clinical unit. Elevated red blood cell counts may indicate polycythemia or dehydration; lowered counts may suggest anemia. Elevated white blood cell counts may result from infection or leukemia, whereas decreased counts may suggest bone marrow depression from various causes.

## Hemoglobin

Hemoglobin (Hgb) is the oxygen-carrying pigment of the red blood cells that gives blood its red color. Its primary function is to transport oxygen from the lungs to the tissues of the body. Measurements of the total amount of hemoglobin in the peripheral blood are important in diagnosing different types of anemias. Hemoglobin electrophoresis is used to identify various abnormal hemoglobins in the blood. The most common abnormal hemoglobin is seen in sickle cell anemia.

## Hematocrit

The hematocrit is a measure of the percentage of red blood cells in the total blood volume. In anemia, after hemorrhage and in extracellular fluid excess, the hematocrit value is lowered; in dehydration it is increased. A microhematocrit test may be performed on capillary blood, which is secured by pricking the finger.

## Coagulation Tests

Tests for coagulation measure the ability of the blood to clot, which may be affected by many factors. The criteria most commonly used to measure the clotting ability of blood are bleeding time, prothrombin time, and partial thromboplastin time (PTT) (Phipps et al, 1995).

### Bleeding Time

The bleeding time test measures the amount of time it takes for platelets to interact with the wall of the blood

TABLE 26-2

## Normal Values for Complete Blood Cell Count Tests

| TEST | NORMAL RANGES | RELATIVE VALUES (% OF TOTAL WHITE BLOOD CELLS) |
|---|---|---|
| **Differential White Blood Cell Count** | | |
| *Granulocytes* | | |
| Neutrophils | 3000-7000 | 60%-70% |
| Eosinophils | 50-400 | 1%-4% |
| Basophils | 25-100 | 0.5%-1% |
| *Agranulocytes* | | |
| Lymphocytes | 1000-4000 | 20%-40% |
| Monocytes | 100-600 | 2%-6% |
| | | |
| **Red Blood Cell Count** | | |
| Men | 4.5-5.4 million | |
| Women | 3.6-5 million | |
| **Red Blood Cell Indices** | | |
| Mean corpuscular volume | 84-99 $\mu^3$/red blood cell | |
| Mean corpuscular hemoglobin | 26-32 $\mu^3$/red blood cell | |
| Mean corpuscular hemoglobin concentration | 30%-36% | |
| | | |
| **Hematocrit Values** | | |
| Men | 40%-50% | |
| Women | 37%-47% | |
| | | |
| **Hemoglobin Values** | | |
| Men | 14-16.5 g/dl | |
| Women | 12-15 g/dl | |
| | | |
| **Platelet Count** | 150,000-400,000 mm³ | |
| | | |
| **Normal Values for Coagulation Tests** | | |
| Bleeding time | | |
| Earlobe method | 1-6 min | |
| Forearm method | 1-9 min | |
| Prothrombin time | 11-16 sec | |
| Partial thromboplastin time | 30-45 sec | |
| Fibrinogen level | 160-415 mg/dl | |
| Lee-White clotting time | 5-10 min | |
| | | |
| **Reticulocyte Count** | 0.5%-2% | |

vessel to form a clot or hemostatic plug. A small stab wound is made in either the earlobe or forearm, and the time it takes for a clot to form is measured and recorded. The bleeding time test is most useful in detecting vascular abnormalities and has some value in detecting platelet abnormalities or deficiencies. Its principal use is in the diagnosis of von Willebrand's disease, a hereditary defect involving factor VII that causes excessive bleeding.

## Prothrombin Time

Prothrombin is converted to thrombin in the clotting process. When prothrombin time is increased, it indicates a longer time for clotting to occur. When greatly increased, the prothrombin time warns of a person at risk for bleeding or hemorrhage. The time may increase in the presence of some diseases or when the patient is receiving coumarin therapy. All patients receiving coumarin therapy should be tested often. A decreased prothrombin time may indicate intravascular clotting and suggest a patient at risk for thrombus formation.

## Partial Thromboplastin Time

A more sensitive test than the prothrombin time is the PTT. The PTT is affected by the reduction of even one of the clotting factors. Heparin dosage is often regulated by monitoring the PTT to maintain specific levels of therapy. When the PTT is greatly increased, the possibility of bleeding is also increased. Patients should be assessed for any sign of bleeding, such as ecchymoses, bleeding from gums or any body surface, tarry stools, or bloody urine. A low PTT may indicate a patient at risk for clot formation.

## Reticulocyte Count

A **reticulocyte** is an immature red blood cell that still contains a nucleus. The reticulocyte count gives an indication as to the function of the bone marrow in relation to red blood cell production (Pagana, Pagana, 1997). A normal reticulocyte count is 0.5% to 2.0%. An increased reticulocyte count in a patient with anemia shows that the bone marrow is attempting to compensate for the low red blood cell count by producing more cells. A low reticulocyte count in a patient with anemia indicates inadequate red blood cell production possibly because the bone marrow is missing a component necessary for the production of the cells.

## Sedimentation Rate

The test for sedimentation rate measures the time required for the red blood cells to settle to the bottom of a test tube, usually based on a duration of 1 hour. The test is most often used to observe the course of some diseases, such as rheumatic fever and rheumatoid arthritis.

## Blood Gas Analysis

A blood gas analysis is used to measure the oxygen and carbon dioxide content of the blood and to determine the functional ability of the lungs to maintain adequate gas levels in the blood. Blood is secured from the radial or femoral artery. The test is used primarily in respiratory diseases and disorders and guides the physician in the administration of oxygen or medications (see Chapter 22).

## Schilling Test

Intrinsic factor secreted by the gastric mucosa is necessary for the absorption of vitamin $B_{12}$. The Shilling test is used to diagnose pernicious anemia in which the intrinsic factor is deficient and in which a reduction of vitamin $B_{12}$ absorption results. Normally a person ingests and absorbs more vitamin $B_{12}$ than needed, with the excess excreted in the urine. However, when vitamin $B_{12}$ cannot be absorbed, it passes on through the gastrointestinal system without appearing in the urine. To perform the Schilling test, an injection of vitamin $B_{12}$ is given to meet body needs, with subsequent administration of oral radioactive vitamin $B_{12}$. If absorption is unimpeded, the excess vitamin $B_{12}$ should be found in the urine. All urine is collected for 24 hours, and the amount of radioactive vitamin $B_{12}$ is measured. Little or no radioactive vitamin $B_{12}$ in the urine indicates an absorption problem. The next step is to determine whether the malabsorption results from intrinsic factor deficiency or some other cause, such as intestinal disease. The Schilling test is repeated, and oral intrinsic factor is added. If the radioactive vitamin $B_{12}$ in the urine now rises, it is clear that an intrinsic factor deficiency is the problem, which establishes a diagnosis of pernicious anemia. If radioactive vitamin $B_{12}$ remains low, other malabsorption causes are implicated.

## Bone Marrow Biopsy and Aspiration

Bone marrow is aspirated to obtain a specimen of cells for biopsy. A bone marrow biopsy involves removing a core of marrow (Figure 26-2). Examination of the cells gives an indication of their reproductive ability and is useful in the diagnosis of certain blood dyscrasias. A local anesthetic is injected into the area surrounding the biopsy site. The most common site in adults and children over 18 months of age is the posterior iliac crest (Figure 26-3). The nurse's role is to reinforce the explanation of the procedure with the patient and to assist with positioning. Guided imagery techniques can be used to elicit patient cooperation and to minimize the pain associated with the procedure. Because of the risk of bleeding, pressure should be applied to the site for 5 minutes, and the patient should be closely observed (Lewis, Collier, Heitkemper, 1996). If the patient has a problem with prolonged bleeding, the puncture site should be assessed often for oozing or frank bleeding; pressure should be applied if this occurs.

## Blood Chemistry

The chemical analysis of blood involves a large number of tests, some of which are carried out on whole blood, a few on plasma, and others on blood serum. Many of these tests are related to the diagnosis of specific diseases and are discussed elsewhere. Blood for chemical analysis is usually collected early in the

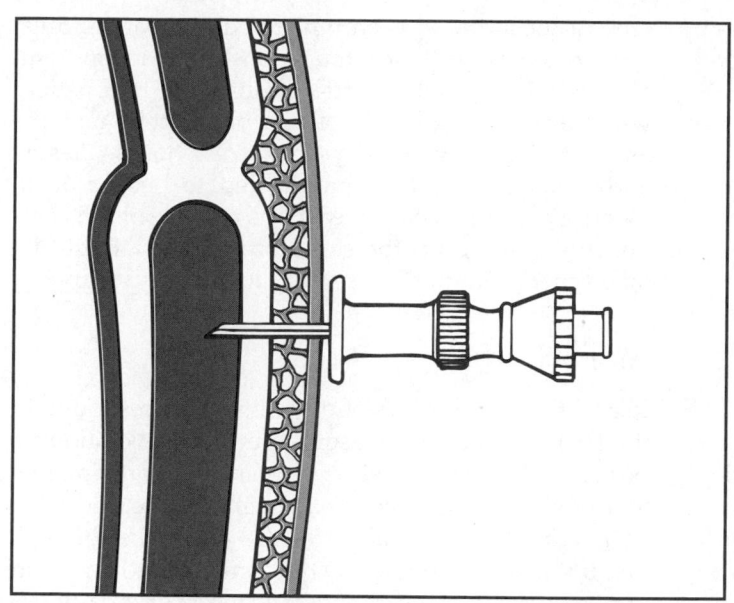

**Figure 26-2** Bone marrow aspiration: penetration into marrow cavity. (From Powers LW: *Diagnostic hematology,* St Louis, 1989, Mosby.)

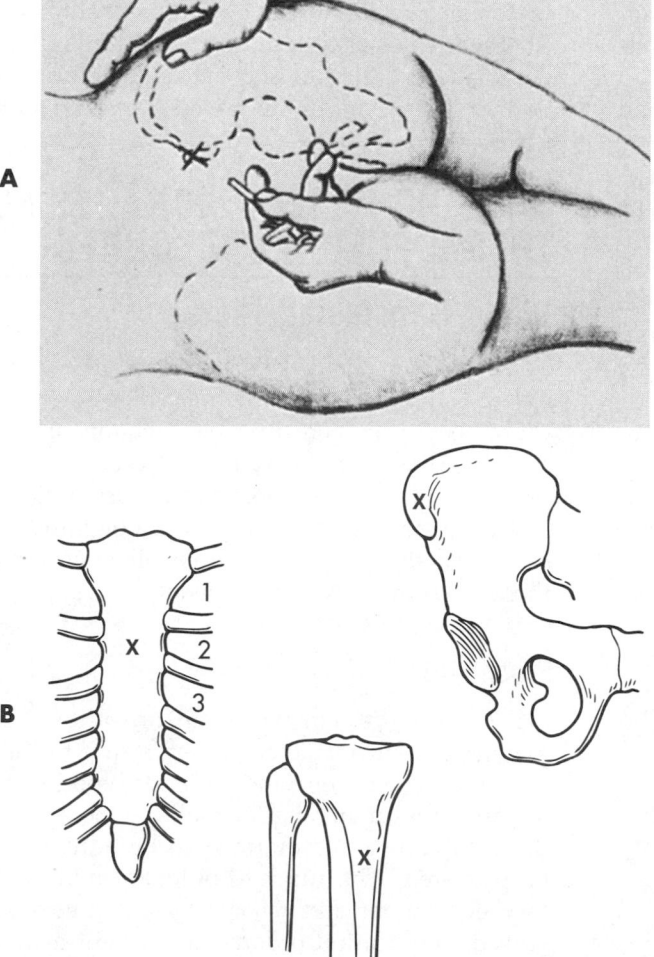

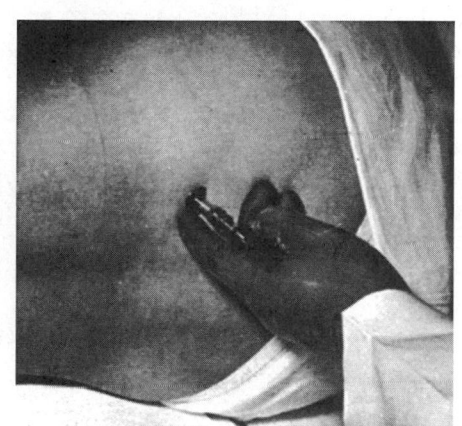

**Figure 26-3** **A,** Bone marrow aspiration; posterior iliac crest. *Left,* Drawing of anatomic site. *Right,* Photograph of aspiration technique. **B,** Sites for bone marrow aspiration; sternum, iliac crest (most common), and tibia. (**A,** *right* from Miale JB: *Laboratory medicine hematology,* ed 6, St Louis, 1982, Mosby; *left,* from Bauer JD: *Clinical laboratory methods,* ed 9, St Louis, 1982, Mosby; **B,** from Phipps WJ et al: *Medical-surgical nursing: concepts and clinical practice,* ed 5, St Louis, 1995, Mosby.)

morning, while the patient is in a fasting state. The patient may not be allowed anything by mouth after midnight, and breakfast may be withheld.

## Blood Typing and Cross-Matching

It is important for the blood of the donor and the blood of the recipient to be compatible. If they are not, the patient may suffer a severe or fatal reaction. There are many different systems for matching blood, and more than 100 different blood factors are known. However, the most familiar system classifies blood types as A, B, AB, and O (Table 26-3). A and B antigens are located on the membranes of red blood cells. The presence or absence of one or both of these antigens is the basis for the type of blood in each individual (Lewis, Collier, Heitkemper, 1996). If an individual has type A blood, he or she has A antigens; an individual with type B blood has B antigens. An individual with type AB blood has both A and B antigens; an individual with type O blood has neither antigen. If an individual does not have a specific antigen, that individual has antibodies to the antigen. An individual with type A blood has anti-B antibodies. An individual with type O blood has anti-A and anti-B antibodies. An individual with type AB blood has neither anti-A nor anti-B antibodies.

It is always best to transfuse the patient with blood of his or her own type whenever possible. For example, a patient with type A blood should receive type A blood. A patient with type AB blood can receive type AB blood, type A blood, type B blood, or type O blood because AB blood does not contain antigens against either A or B blood. For this reason, individuals with type AB, Rh-positive blood are considered universal recipients because they can technically receive any type blood.

If the same blood type cannot be secured for a transfusion or if there is a delay in typing and crossmatching, the type O, Rh-negative, may be used in an emergency because type O blood has neither A nor B antigens. Individuals with type O, Rh-negative blood are considered universal donors. However, when non-crossmatched blood is administered, the patient must be watched carefully for indications of a reaction. Usually 500 ml of whole blood administered to a patient will elevate the number of red blood cells and the amount of hemoglobin by 15% in 24 hours. Plasma and platelets may be administered to people of all blood types, but because reactions to these blood components may occur, the same precautions should be taken as for blood.

## Rh Factor

In addition to the kinds of protein substances found in the four types of blood, some persons have an extra protein substance called the *Rh factor.* Approximately 85% of all persons have this protein and are said to be *Rh positive;* the remaining 15% are said to be *Rh negative.* It is just as important to determine the Rh factor in cross-matching blood for transfusion as it is to determine the blood type. If an Rh-negative person is transfused with Rh-positive blood, he or she may develop antibodies against the Rh-positive factor. If given further transfusions with Rh-positive blood, he or she may develop severe reactions. An Rh-positive fetus in utero may precipitate the formation of antibodies in an Rh-negative mother. If any of these antibodies reaches the fetal circulation, it may cause the infant to be stillborn or may result in the disease called *erythroblastosis fetalis.*

# NURSING RESPONSIBILITIES FOR THERAPEUTIC PROCEDURES

## Blood Transfusion Therapy

There are three primary reasons for administering blood: (1) to replace or maintain blood volume, (2) to preserve the oxygen-carrying function of the blood, and (3) to increase or maintain the coagulation abilities of the blood. A transfusion introduces whole blood, or any of its components, from a donor into the bloodstream of the recipient. Whole blood is rarely used these days, even in an emergency.

### Procedures

When the physician writes an order for a blood or platelet transfusion, the request is sent to the laboratory with a sample of the patient's blood so that typing and cross-matching for that specific patient can be done and the pints or units to be administered can be prepared. The nurse should assemble the necessary equipment and record the patient's vital signs. Any premedication ordered to prevent a transfusion reaction, such as acetaminophen and diphenhydra-

---

**TABLE 26-3**

## ABO Blood Types

| RECIPIENT'S BLOOD TYPE | COMPATIBLE DONOR TYPE |
| --- | --- |
| A | A, O |
| B | B, O |
| AB | A, B, AB, O |
| O | O |

mine (Benadryl), should be administered. A registered nurse is responsible for the administration and handling of the blood product once it arrives on the unit. Most institutions require that two licensed nurses check the blood product before administration. The blood or platelets should be checked for expiration date, and the label indicating the patient's name, room number, and identification number should be compared with the patient's identification band. The patient's blood group and Rh status should be compared with the donor's blood group and Rh status for all blood transfusions. If any discrepancy is found, the blood is not given. Blood products brought to the unit should be used immediately or returned to the blood bank. The transfusion is administered through an infusion set with a filter in the drip chamber that will remove any precipitates or clots that may form (Figure 26-4). The physician may order an additional leukocyte removal filter for patients who may need many transfusions over a course of time. This filter traps white blood cells and helps prevent the patient from developing antibodies to future donated blood products (Higgins, 1996; Shuey, 1996). The infusion line is primed and rinsed with saline because other solutions, especially those containing glucose or dextrose, can cause hemolysis of the cells. The blood filter should not be used for more than 4 hours, and a unit of blood should not be transfused for more than 4 hours.

After the transfusion has begun, the nurse should carefully observe the patient while the first 50 ml is infused. Symptoms of severe reaction are usually seen during the first 50 ml of blood or platelet infusion. The infusion should be started slowly—at 5 ml/min or less for the first 15 minutes (Flynn, Bruce, 1993). Vital signs should be taken according to the institution's policy, but usually before and 15 minutes after the transfusion is started and frequently during the transfusion. The patient should be observed for symptoms of potential complications. After the transfusion is completed, the empty blood bag should be returned to the laboratory.

## Transfusion Reactions

Transfusion reactions from contaminated blood, the presence of antibodies to donor cells, and allergic reactions can occur after only a small amount of blood has been given. If symptoms of a reaction occur (Table 26-4), the transfusion should be discontinued, the intravenous tubing should be changed, and the vein should be kept open with a slow saline solution drip. The blood should not be destroyed but should be sent back to the laboratory for examination to determine the cause of the reaction.

## Circulation Overload

Circulation overload is a complication that can result from too rapid fluid infusion. Cough, increasing pulse rate, dyspnea, and edema are symptoms of this complication. Packed cells rather than whole blood are indicated for patients who are susceptible to circulatory overload. This includes people with cardiac and renal impairment, as well as the elderly. Furosemide (Lasix)

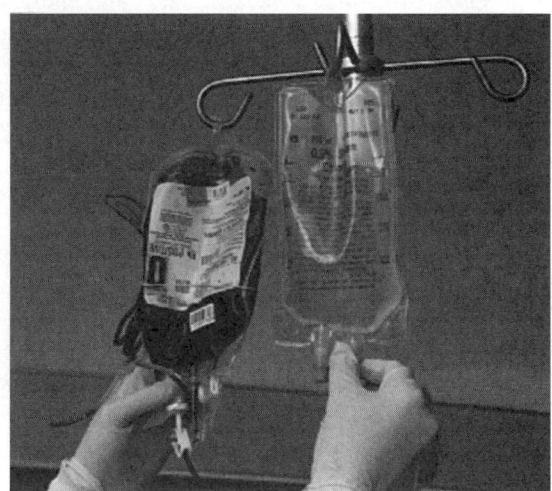

**Figure 26-4** Blood is transfused through tubing that has a special filter. The tubing is flushed with normal saline before and after the blood is administered.

---

**TABLE 26-4**

## Blood Transfusion Reactions

| TYPE OF REACTION | CAUSE | SYMPTOMS |
|---|---|---|
| Allergic | Hypersensitivity to antibodies in donor's blood | Urticaria, pruritus, fever, anaphylactic shock |
| Hemolytic | Incompatibility | Nausea, vomiting, pain in lower back, hypotension, increase in pulse rate, decrease in urinary output, hematuria |
| Pyogenic febrile (most common) | Antibodies to donor platelets or leukocytes or contamination of blood | Fever, chills, nausea, headache, flushing, tachycardia, palpitations |

is frequently ordered for patients at risk for circulation overload who are receiving more than one unit of blood.

## Air Embolism

Air embolism is a rare but often fatal complication from a blood transfusion and is caused by air being allowed to enter the circulation. This is most likely to occur when blood is being given under pressure. Symptoms that indicate an air embolus include chest pain, acute shortness of breath, and shock. The patient should be turned immediately onto his or her left side, and his or her head should be lowered below the level of the heart. Air embolism is a rare complication but requires immediate action if it occurs.

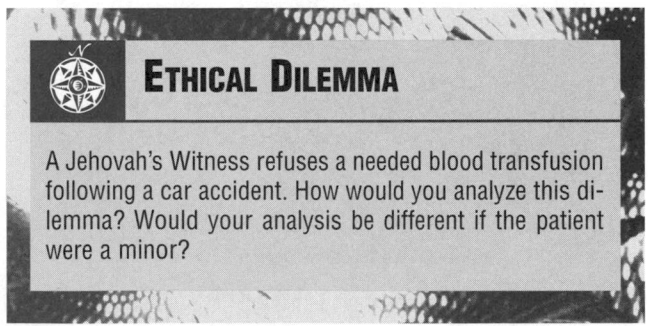

**NURSE ALERT**

When the patient is receiving blood, notify the physician of a drop in blood pressure, a rise in pulse, chills, or fever. Chest pain, shortness of breath, and shock indicate air embolism. Turn the patient to his or her left side, stop the infusion, call for life support, and notify the physician.

**ETHICAL DILEMMA**

A Jehovah's Witness refuses a needed blood transfusion following a car accident. How would you analyze this dilemma? Would your analysis be different if the patient were a minor?

## Interventions

Policies and procedures related to transfusion of blood or its components vary between institutions, but the care of the patient should always include strict adherence to universal precautions and measures to prevent transfusion reactions through proper identification of blood donor and recipient compatibility and careful handling of the blood product to prevent contamination and hemolysis. The specific action the nurse takes varies with the type of reaction that is suspected. In general, vital signs should be monitored throughout the transfusion, and the patient should be assessed for

signs and symptoms that indicate a reaction. When assessments indicate circulatory overload, the nurse slows the transfusion rate and raises the head of the bed. When a hemolytic reaction is suspected, the nurse monitors the patient for shock, taking frequent blood pressure and pulse measurements, recording accurate intake and output, and obtaining a first-voided urine specimen. If the patient complains of itching and wheezes within the first few minutes of the transfusion, an allergic reaction should be suspected. Chills and fever occurring about 1 hour after the start of a transfusion indicate a pyogenic reaction. If the physician determines that these symptoms are not a result of hemolytic reaction or contaminated blood, the patient may be treated with antipyretics and steroids to alleviate the symptoms; the transfusion is then continued.

# THE PATIENT WITH BLOOD DYSCRASIAS

**Blood dyscrasias** are diseases or disorders of the blood and blood-forming organs. These include a wide range of conditions with varying prognoses. Life-style may predispose persons to certain disorders, whereas heredity may account for others. Often the cause is unknown. Similarly, treatment may cause a dramatic response or simply be palliative. Some diseases may be controlled, but a lifetime of compliance to treatment is required. Box 26-1 is a partial classification of diseases and disorders of the blood and the blood-forming organs. These include red blood cell, white blood cell, and hemorrhagic disorders.

## Disorders of Erythrocytes

**Anemia** is not a disease but a condition resulting from one or a combination of causes. It is defined as a lower than normal number of red blood cells and quantity of hemoglobin. The major manifestations of anemia, including pallor, decreased activity tolerance, and orthostatic hypotension, result from the body's attempts to provide adequate levels of oxygen to the brain and other vital organs. Vasoconstriction of peripheral blood vessels in the skin and blood vessels in the kidneys are the mechanisms that are responsible for the symptoms of anemia. Anemia accompanies several diseases, and its development may be so insidious that an individual is unaware of the condition until symptoms appear. Anemia may develop slowly when there is a slow bleeding from the intestinal tract, or it may develop quickly if there is a massive hemorrhage. Anemia is usually present in diseases in which there is destruction of red blood cells or when there is immature development of the red blood cells. Any condition that

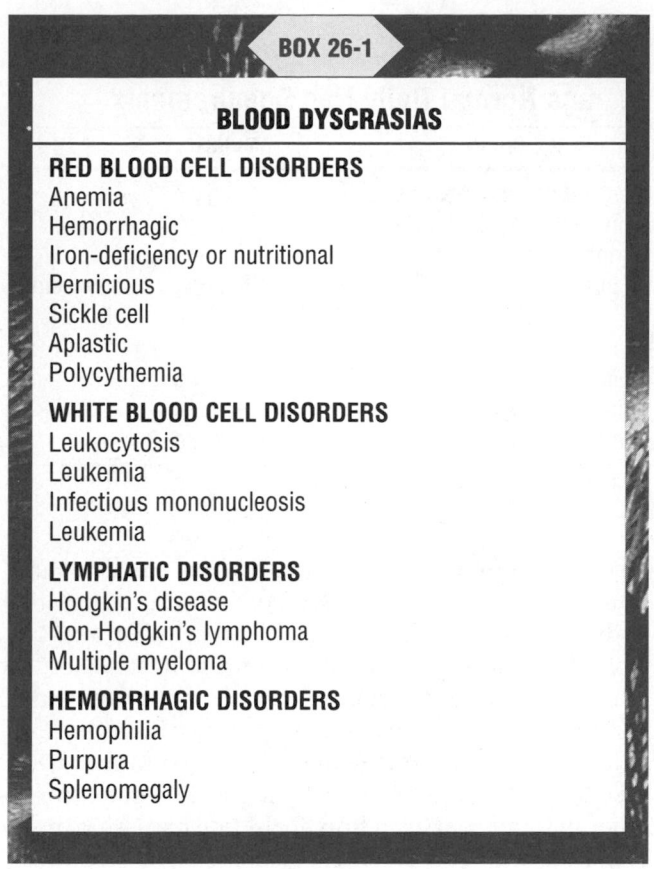

causes a decrease in red blood cells, in hemoglobin, and in iron will cause varying degrees of anemia.

## Assessment of the Patient with Anemia

The nurse should examine the patient's skin for the texture and level of hydration and for the presence of any ulcerated areas. The nurse should also assess the eyes for pallor of the conjunctiva or a yellowish tinge to the sclera and for brightness or luster. The oral cavity is assessed for color, and the tongue is assessed for any evidence of sores or swelling. The patient should be asked about the presence of such symptoms as headaches, ringing in the ears, dizziness with position changes, difficulty concentrating, or difficulty swallowing. Other areas included in the assessment are the diet history and a past or present history of blood loss from the rectum, hemorrhoids, urine, vomitus, and prolonged or frequent menstrual bleeding. The nurse should inquire about a history of gastric ulcer, gastric or colon surgery, anemia, or a family history of anemia or blood disease.

## Hemorrhagic Anemia

Anemia resulting from loss of blood may be acute or chronic. Acute anemia or hypovolemic shock occurs when there has been a sudden loss of a large amount of blood. This may be caused by traumatic injury, hemoptysis, hemorrhage at childbirth, ulcerative lesions, and disorders of coagulation. Anemia may result from lesser degrees of hemorrhage or slow bleeding, such as that from a bleeding gastric ulcer or bleeding hemorrhoids.

**Pathophysiology.** The loss of blood decreases the amount of circulating fluid and hemoglobin and the amount of oxygen carried to the tissues of the body, which must have oxygen to survive. Blood loss may be classified as severe, moderate, or mild. The degree and rapidity of the blood loss are related to the severity and number of symptoms observed in the patient.

Severe blood loss may be caused by trauma if large blood vessels are ruptured or severed. Massive uterine hemorrhage may accompany childbirth or may result from cancer. A ruptured tubal pregnancy may release large amounts of blood into the peritoneal cavity. Severe blood loss can also occur when the number of platelets in the blood is low or when the coagulation process is abnormal.

Less severe blood loss occurs in many conditions, including prolonged or frequent menstrual periods, a bleeding gastric ulcer, or bleeding hemorrhoids.

**Assessment.** When blood loss is severe, the patient may experience hematogenic or hypovolemic shock. Symptoms include prostration, thirst, a rapid pulse rate, pallor, hypotension, clammy skin, or mental confusion because of decreased oxygen supply to the brain. When anemia is caused by slow bleeding, the symptoms are less dramatic. Fatigue is a primary symptom. The volume and rate of the pulse are normal. On exertion, the blood pressure may drop and tachycardia may occur. There is a tendency toward fainting and dizziness because of orthostatic hypotension. If bleeding continues for a prolonged period, pallor will develop and shortness of breath on exertion, headache, drowsiness, and menstrual disturbances may occur.

**Intervention.** In the case of massive hemorrhage, measures are taken to control the bleeding, treat for shock, and replace the volume of circulating fluid (see Chapter 27). Patients should be observed for evidence of further bleeding. They should lie flat and be kept warm, and vital signs should be taken at frequent intervals. Care should be taken to prevent injury to a restless or confused patient.

The immediate concern in chronic bleeding is to locate and remove the cause. This requires a carefully taken history and physical examination. Laboratory examination and x-ray studies may be required. Depending on the degree of anemia, blood transfusions may be given and iron therapy instituted.

The patient may or may not be given iron preparations. If any disorder of the intestinal tract makes the

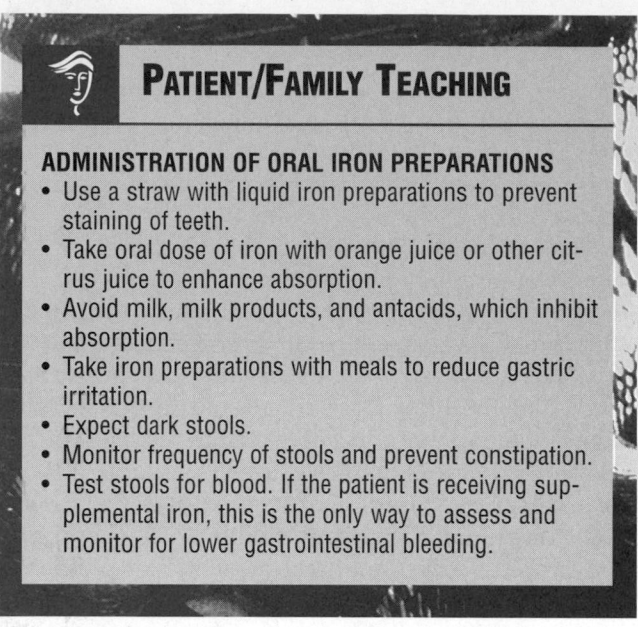

**PATIENT/FAMILY TEACHING**

**ADMINISTRATION OF ORAL IRON PREPARATIONS**
- Use a straw with liquid iron preparations to prevent staining of teeth.
- Take oral dose of iron with orange juice or other citrus juice to enhance absorption.
- Avoid milk, milk products, and antacids, which inhibit absorption.
- Take iron preparations with meals to reduce gastric irritation.
- Expect dark stools.
- Monitor frequency of stools and prevent constipation.
- Test stools for blood. If the patient is receiving supplemental iron, this is the only way to assess and monitor for lower gastrointestinal bleeding.

| TABLE 26-5 |
| --- |

**Average Normal Daily Iron Requirements**

| SEX AND AGE-GROUP | AMOUNT |
| --- | --- |
| Men and postmenopausal women | 10 mg |
| Women during childbearing period | 18 mg |
| During pregnancy | 15-35 mg |
| Infants | 1.5 mg/kg of body weight (approximately 5-15 mg) |
| Children | 10-18 mg |
| Adolescent boys | 10-15 mg |
| Adolescent girls | 10-25 mg |

oral administration of iron undesirable, it may be given intramuscularly in the form of iron dextran (Imferon). It is given in the gluteal muscle in 1- to 5-ml injections daily or less often, and it may be continued until the hemoglobin returns to normal. Deep injection using the Z-tract method is necessary to avoid leakage into subcutaneous tissue, which stains skin.

*NURSE ALERT*

**When administering liquid iron preparations, have the patient use a straw to prevent staining of teeth. Take iron in citrus juice with meals, but not with milk products, for best absorption.**

## Iron-Deficiency (Hypochromic) Anemia

Anemia caused by iron deficiency is the most common type of anemia. It is estimated that 90% of the iron-deficiency anemia in adults is found in women. It is the most common cause of anemia in infancy and childhood. The iron stored by the fetus in utero is depleted during the first 6 months after birth. Iron deficiency occurring after the infant is 6 months old is usually the result of inadequate iron in the diet. Average normal daily iron requirements are found in Table 26-5.

Approximately two thirds of all iron in the body is in the hemoglobin of the blood. For the most part this iron is used over and over, with essentially no excretion, and small reserves are available if needed. Re-

serves are stored in the bone marrow, spleen, liver, and muscle; in menstruating women almost all of the body's iron is stored in the red blood cells. Sources for storage include iron recycled from the destruction of old blood cells and dietary intake. Because iron is not lost through normal excretion, anemia caused by loss of iron must result from some other cause. In the adult, diet is a factor only if iron is being lost by some route other than normal excretion, including excessive menstrual bleeding, repeated pregnancies with blood loss and transfer of iron to the fetus in utero, and blood loss from the gastrointestinal tract, as might occur from carcinoma (Erickson, 1996). In some cases the body fails to assimilate and use iron.

**Pathophysiology.** Loss of blood is the most common cause of iron-deficiency anemia, which is characterized by a decrease in hemoglobin in the red blood cells. Although the red blood cell count may be within a normal range, the cells are microcytic and poorly shaped and therefore are unable to carry their normal amount of hemoglobin. The body gradually exhausts its supply of stored iron, and the blood develops an abnormally low color index (hypochromia). Iron is an essential constituent of enzymes within the cells, and without it, the metabolism of the cell is affected. Eventually the entire body suffers.

**Assessment.** Iron-deficiency anemia develops gradually, and the individual may consult a physician because of fatigue and weakness. Sometimes during the early stages, the anemia may be found on a routine physical examination. Symptoms include pallor, dyspnea, palpitation, and loss of appetite. The nails become brittle and poorly shaped, the tongue is sore, and in some instances there may be difficulty in swallowing. The hemoglobin level will be found to be as low as 10 mg/dl of blood, and if the condition is severe it may be lower. The most reliable test for the diagnosis of iron-deficiency anemia is a bone marrow biopsy.

**TABLE 26-6**

## Commonly Used Iron Preparations

| DRUG | NURSING CONSIDERATIONS |
|---|---|
| **Oral Administration** | |
| Ferrous sulfate (Feosol) 300 mg (most common and least expensive) | Do not administer with tetracyclines, antacids, eggs, milk, coffee, or tea, which inhibit absorption. |
| Ferrous gluconate (Fergon) 900 mg | Give with meals to reduce gastric irritation. |
| Ferrous fumarate (Ircon) 600-800 mg | Black and tarry or dark green stools or constipation may occur. |
| | Encourage foods high in iron. |
| **Intramuscular Injection** | |
| Iron dextran (Imferon) | Use Z-track method for IM injection. |
| IM not to exceed 250 mg/day | Monitor blood pressure and heart rate. |
| IV 100 mg/day as a bolus or dilute total dose and infuse over 1 to 6 hr | Assess for signs and symptoms of anaphylaxis (rash, pruritus, edema, and wheezing) |
| | Monitor hemoglobin, hematocrit, and reticulocyte values |

**Intervention.** In the absence of observed bleeding, a thorough examination should be made to locate any internal source of bleeding. Treatment for iron-deficiency anemia is the administration of iron and the identification and treatment of the cause. Commonly used iron preparations are found in Table 26-6. Iron is absorbed much more slowly when administered orally than it is when injected, and administration may have to be continued for several months. For varying reasons some patients cannot be given iron orally and must receive it intramuscularly. When iron is injected, the results are faster and the duration of therapy is shortened. However, it does carry some risk—fatal reactions have been reported but are rare.

Most patients with iron-deficiency anemia are cared for in the physician's office or the outpatient clinic. Patients should be evaluated for compliance with iron replacement regimens because of the drug's tendency to cause gastrointestinal problems. If the patient is experiencing side effects that prevent compliance, there are actions that can be taken to minimize the discomfort. When the problem is constipation, reducing the daily dose is helpful; for gastric distress the patient can be instructed to take the drug with meals. Another reason for noncompliance may be the cost of the drug. The nurse should consult the pharmacist for a less expensive preparation or should contact a social worker who may be able to identify sources of financial assistance (Spratto, Woods, 1994). Replacement iron is usually given orally, 90 to 300 mg/day. Therapy continues for 2 to 4 months after the hemoglobin, hematocrit, and reticulocyte levels return to normal, indicating that the anemia is reversed. This could be a total of 6 months or more (Spratto, Woods, 1994).

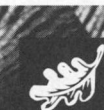 **OLDER ADULT CONSIDERATIONS**

Anemia is not a normal consequence of the aging process but is primarily a result of deficiencies commonly found in older populations. The elderly often lack the money or mobility to purchase and prepare foods. Others may lack interest in cooking or eating as a result of decreased sense of smell and taste or from loneliness. Dentures, alcoholism, and chronic illness can also affect nutritional intake.

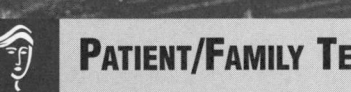 **PATIENT/FAMILY TEACHING**

**IRON DEFICIENCY ANEMIA**
- Patient education regarding iron therapy and proper diet is vital.
- Foods high in iron should be identified: eggs, organ meats, red kidney beans, dried raisins, apricots, yellow vegetables such as carrots and turnips, spinach, and whole wheat bread. (The addition of eggs and organ meats may need to be evaluated and modified if the patient needs to decrease his or her cholesterol intake.)
- Teenagers in particular need help with diet modification.

# Pernicious Anemia (Vitamin B₁₂-Deficiency Anemia)

Until 1928 pernicious anemia was considered incurable, and the patient was subject to remissions, relapses, and ultimately death. Although the disease remains incurable, modern treatment has made it possible for the patient to have a normal life span. Patients with pernicious anemia who die usually do so from some other cause. The disease primarily affects middle-aged and older persons. Individuals who have had a total or partial gastrectomy will inevitably develop the disease because the gastric fundus (the source of the intrinsic factor) has been removed. Persons who are strict vegetarians and persons with a history of surgery or disease of the ileum are at risk for vitamin B₁₂-deficiency anemia. Pernicious anemia is not the same as iron-deficiency anemia; however, it is believed that iron-deficiency anemia of long duration may predispose an individual to pernicious anemia.

**Pathophysiology.** An intrinsic factor secreted by the fundus of the stomach is necessary for the absorption of vitamin B₁₂ by the intestinal mucosa. Persons who have pernicious anemia lack this intrinsic factor and thus develop vitamin B₁₂ deficiency. Vitamin B₁₂ is a necessary element in the production of erythrocytes and nervous system function. In pernicious anemia red blood cells in the bone marrow fail to mature and are abnormally large (Hawley, 1996). Their rate of destruction exceeds their rate of production. The erythrocytes that do reach the bloodstream may be few in number and abnormally large or megaloblastic. The red blood cell count may be low, and the hemoglobin is decreased. The skin may have a pale lemon-yellow color (mild jaundice) because of the excessive death rate of the red blood cells, which causes the bile pigments to be increased in the blood serum. There is little or no secretion of hydrochloric acid in the stomach.

**Assessment.** The onset of pernicious anemia is usually insidious, with symptoms of a slowly developing anemia. Pallor develops gradually, and there is a yellowish tint to the skin. There may be palpitation, nausea, vomiting, flatulence, indigestion, constipation, and often diarrhea. There is soreness and burning of the tongue, which appears smooth and red, with infection around the teeth and gums. Fever, weakness, anorexia, and difficulty in swallowing may also occur. Neurologic symptoms may develop, including tingling of the hands and feet and loss of sense of body position. Cerebral symptoms include loss of memory, mental confusion, and depression. Personality changes and behavior problems can also occur.

Severe neurologic impairments can result from inappropriate treatment and inadequate diagnostic evaluation of vitamin B₁₂-deficiency anemia. These impairments include partial or total paralysis, which results from destruction of the nerve fibers of the spinal cord. Peripheral nerve damage causes the paresthesia and lack of position sense seen in this disorder.

**Intervention.** Once the diagnosis has been established, the treatment consists of injections of hydroxocobalamin (vitamin B₁₂). If the anemia is severe, the patient may be transfused with packed red blood cells. The patient may also require treatment for coexisting conditions such as cardiovascular disorders. Injections of vitamin B₁₂ must be continued throughout the person's lifetime. Treatment is individualized, but one injection every 2 months may keep the patient free of symptoms. The nursing care of the patient depends to some extent on the stage the disease had reached when it was discovered. While the patient is confined to the hospital, his or her vital signs should be checked daily and recorded. An increase in pulse and respiration is to be expected, especially with exertion, but any great change should be reported immediately. The patient should clean his or her mouth several times a day using a solution that is non-irritating to the mucous membranes. Commercial mouthwash containing alcohol should be avoided.

Meals should be carefully planned to provide a diet high in protein, vitamins, and minerals. It is better to use complete proteins of a high order, such as meat, milk, eggs, and shellfish. Because the patient may have a poor appetite, considerable encouragement to eat may be needed. The attractive preparation and serving of food will often stimulate the patient's appetite. Unusually hot, acid, salty, and spicy foods should be avoided because of the soreness of the mouth. Constipation may be treated with mild laxatives prescribed by the physician.

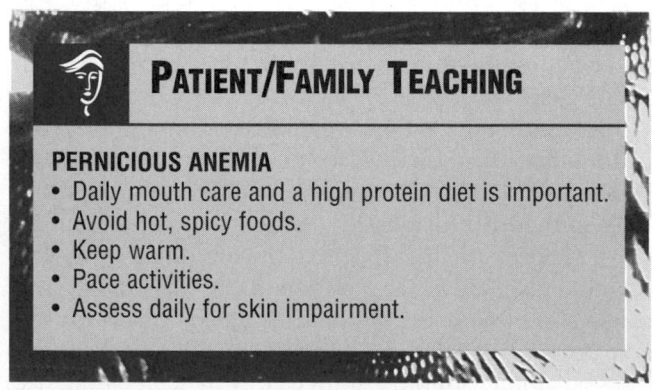

**PATIENT/FAMILY TEACHING**

**PERNICIOUS ANEMIA**
- Daily mouth care and a high protein diet is important.
- Avoid hot, spicy foods.
- Keep warm.
- Pace activities.
- Assess daily for skin impairment.

Patients with pernicious anemia are especially sensitive to cold, and extra lightweight, warm blankets may be needed. Cotton flannel nightclothes, a warm bed jacket, and bed socks will make the patient more comfortable. Hot-water bottles and electric heating pads should be avoided because of the danger of burning the patient.

Nursing care of the patient with a vitamin B$_{12}$-deficiency anemia also includes evaluation of patient problems such as self-care deficits, fatigue, weakness, activity intolerance, and potential for injury. The goals of care are to conserve energy and prevent injury. Energy can be conserved by assisting the patient with physical care and balancing activities with rest periods. Passive exercises maintain bone and muscle mass that would otherwise be depleted during prolonged inactivity. As soon as they can be tolerated, active exercises such as progressive ambulation should be instituted. Loss of independence and altered self-image are common problems and must be considered in the plan of care. Maintenance of skin integrity is managed by frequent skin inspections, position changes, and the use of protective devices. Intensive and comprehensive rehabilitation programs are appropriate for individuals with severe neurologic deficits and can be instituted when the anemia is corrected.

Most patients with pernicious anemia are older than 40 years of age, and lifetime patterns have been established. Learning that they have an incurable disease may cause considerable emotional shock for some patients. The patient may reject the diagnosis and lose valuable time needed for therapy. The nurse may help the patient by stressing how regular treatment will help the patient feel well, be well, and live a happy, normal life. Persons who are economically depressed may need assistance from a community social agency and Medicaid, and elderly persons may be provided for through the Medicare program.

## Sickle Cell Anemia

**Sickle cell anemia** is found primarily among blacks, and its distribution is worldwide. The disease is a genetic hemolytic blood disorder affecting both men and women. Approximately 1 of every 10 black Americans carries the gene for the abnormal sickle hemoglobin and therefore has the sickle cell trait, an asymptomatic condition. A child whose parents each carry the gene trait inherits sickle cell anemia (Marchiondo, Thompson, 1996). Sickle cell anemia is diagnosed most often in children, often in infancy, and the mortality rate is high. Only half of the patients with sickle cell anemia live beyond 20 years of age, although survival rates are increasing with improved care.

Screening clinics have been established in many areas of the United States to identify persons with the trait. Although there is no preventive treatment or cure for the disease, counseling helps the person avoid the

factors that may predispose him or her to a serious exacerbation. Furthermore, couples who either have the trait or have sickle cell disease should be advised of the risks involved so they can make informed decisions about becoming parents. The risk of having a child with sickle cell anemia depends on the genetic characteristics of the prospective parents.

**Pathophysiology.** Sickle cell anemia is caused by an abnormal hemoglobin molecule (hemoglobin S). When the molecule is present in the red blood cell, it causes the cell to acquire a sickle or crescent shape when the oxygen supply is decreased (Blaylock, 1996). This crisis can be precipitated by fever, infection, and dehydration (Chiocca, 1996). The sickle-shaped cell cannot move normally through the blood vessels and tends to block or clog small vessels. As tissue hypoxia worsens and as more oxygen is given up to the tissues, further sickling occurs, blood viscosity increases, hemolysis increases, and more clots form in the microcirculation. A sickle cell crisis ensues.

**Assessment.** The life of the sickled cell is short, and the production of new cells is not fast enough to keep oxygen supplied to the tissues of the body. The person may experience attacks of severe pain in various organs and in the bones. There may be fever, anemia, and thrombi in the lungs and spleen, and the spleen may be enlarged. Leg ulcers may occur. Because of red blood cell destruction, jaundice is often seen. Children develop abnormal growth patterns, and infections account for the high mortality in very young children. These persons are especially susceptible to osteomyelitis and to pneumonia caused by the pneumococcus bacterium. The rate of maternal complications in pregnancy, such as hemorrhage and eclamptic conditions, is reported to be high.

**Intervention.** Treatment is preventive and supportive. Children should be immunized against preventable diseases. Any activity that causes stress or requires strenuous exercise and would limit oxygen supply should be avoided. Good health habits including rest, proper diet, avoidance of respiratory tract infections, and regular medical supervision should be encouraged. If an acute exacerbation (crisis) occurs, the patient is admitted to the hospital and placed on a regimen of bed rest. The patient may experience fever; severe pain in the chest, joints, and abdomen; edema; and leukocytosis. Routine administration of analgesics is indicated for pain during a crisis, as is assistance with activities of daily living and frequent rest periods. Because dehydration contributes to sickling, oral or intravenous administration of fluids is important. Local applications of heat may be used to relieve pain, but cold applications should not be used because cold promotes sickling. Bacterial infection is a serious complication of sickle cell anemia, and immunization to prevent pneumococcal pneumonia in these patients is recommended. Death from sickle cell anemia usually results from the long-term effects of repeated tissue damage in major organs such as the heart, kidneys, and liver.

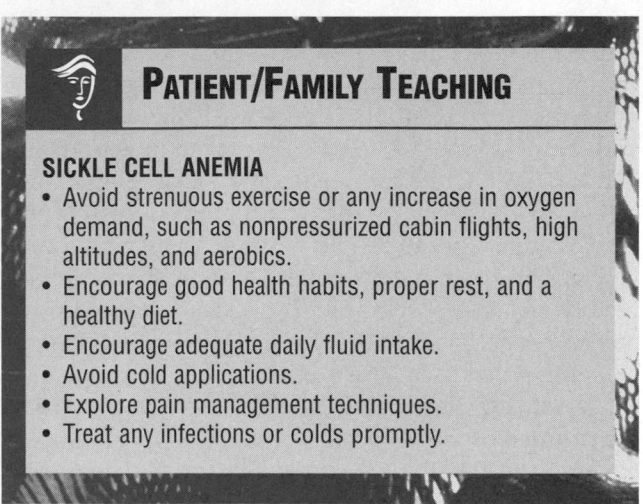

**PATIENT/FAMILY TEACHING**

**SICKLE CELL ANEMIA**
- Avoid strenuous exercise or any increase in oxygen demand, such as nonpressurized cabin flights, high altitudes, and aerobics.
- Encourage good health habits, proper rest, and a healthy diet.
- Encourage adequate daily fluid intake.
- Avoid cold applications.
- Explore pain management techniques.
- Treat any infections or colds promptly.

**NURSE ALERT**

Do not use cold applications for pain relief with sickle cell anemia because cold promotes sickling.

The patient with sickle cell anemia and his or her parents need a great deal of encouragement and emotional support during the long course of chronic illness. Repeated hospitalizations that begin in early childhood often cause ineffective family and patient coping. The loss of independence can lead to depression and to noncompliance with crisis prevention approaches. The adolescent is particularly vulnerable to ineffective coping because many activities such as vigorous athletics must be avoided, as must situations where exposure to infection is a risk. It is difficult to achieve the developmental tasks of childhood and adolescence while having to cope with a chronic and life-threatening illness. Early referral to resources such as the Sickle Cell Foundation can provide the patient and family with support.

The nurse needs to maintain a sensitive awareness of the needs of each age group afflicted with sickle cell anemia. A common need is the presence of a trusting relationship with health care providers. An area of po-

tential conflict in this relationship is that of pain management (Pasero, 1996). In a sickle cell crisis, pain is severe. However, it is often ineffectively managed because of caregiver attitudes and lack of knowledge. When the patient seeks pain relief but cannot obtain it because of these problems, trust is threatened and the patient experiences alienation from the staff. If the patient uses strategies that exacerbate the alienation, a vicious cycle begins and the patient suffers needlessly. The nurse is in the best position to prevent this escalation of events through early recognition and appropriate management of symptoms.

## Aplastic Anemia

Aplastic anemia results from bone marrow failure that is congenital or acquired. It may be induced by radiation, chemicals, or drug therapy, especially with antineoplastic drugs and chloramphenicol. This is a severe, life-threatening anemia with a poor prognosis and requires careful medical management and excellent nursing care.

**Pathophysiology.** In aplastic anemia, insufficient blood cells are produced as a result of an interference with the stem cells in the bone marrow. In rare instances, only the red blood cells are affected, but usually there is depression of all the cells originating in the bone marrow. This depression of red blood cells (erythrocytes), white blood cells (leukocytes), and platelets (thrombocytes) is referred to as *pancytopenia.*

**Assessment.** The reduction of erythrocytes produces classic signs and symptoms of anemia: pallor, weakness, dyspnea, and hypoxia. The patient may be tired, lethargic, or confused because of the lack of oxygen to the brain. Infection poses a real threat because of decreased white blood cells (leukopenia). Thrombocytopenia (reduced thrombocytes or platelets) increases the risk of bleeding. Even an intramuscular injection may produce a site for fatal bleeding.

**Intervention.** The cause of aplastic anemia must be identified promptly and removed or discontinued if possible. Bone marrow suppression is expected with certain antineoplastic drugs or radiation therapy, and therefore laboratory values should be monitored often to maintain control. The margin for therapeutic treatment in such cases is exceedingly narrow. Supportive treatment includes transfusions of packed red blood cells and platelets as indicated.

Blood transfusions are avoided to prevent iron overloading and the development of antibodies to tissue antigens. However, if frequent, multiple blood transfusions are administered, the drug deferoxamine mesylate (Desferal) may be ordered to promote iron excretion and prevent iron overload. Platelet transfusions that are HLA matched are used to treat serious bleeding in the thrombocytopenic patient. Cautious use of blood transfusion is necessary to minimize the risk of rejection for the bone marrow transplant candidate.

A splenectomy may be required in patients with hypersplenism when it is responsible for destruction of normal platelets or for marrow suppression of platelet production. Steroids and androgens are sometimes used in an attempt to stimulate the bone marrow.

Bone marrow transplantation is the treatment of choice in patients under the age of 50 who have a compatible donor. Bone marrow transplantation involves several processes: immunosuppression of the recipient with or without total lymph node irradiation and high-dose chemotherapy (see Chapter 12). Bone marrow or stem cells are collected from a compatible donor. Stem cells can be aspirated directly from bone marrow in the pelvis sternum or ribs. Stem cells can also be obtained through a procedure that separates them from circulating blood. The donor bone marrow cells are then infused intravenously into the recipient and migrate to the bone marrow cavities. Establishment of the graft (engraftment), if it takes place, occurs in 10 to 30 days. During that period the patient is at enormous risk for severe and irreversible bleeding and infection.

The patient receives immunosuppressive therapy for approximately 6 months to prevent rejection and graft-vs-host disease. In 30% to 70% of patients, graft-vs-host disease occurs with varying degrees of severity. The long-term physical problems include skin changes that cause contractures and muscular wasting, fluid and electrolyte abnormalities caused by chronic diarrhea, fatigue, and jaundice and pruritus caused by inflammation of the liver. Patients and families are confronted with numerous stressors, including prolonged hospitalization and isolation from friends and support systems, an altered patient self-concept as a result of physical changes and the inability to carry out role responsibilities, and the need to learn complex care regimens after discharge from the hospital.

Patients with aplastic anemia are highly susceptible to infection, thus nursing care should be directed toward prevention. Strict aseptic technique must be used for dressing changes and administration of intravenous fluids or medications. Meticulous care to prevent impaired skin and mucous membrane integrity includes avoiding intramuscular injections, rectal medications, and the use of rectal thermometers. When bed rest is prescribed, the patient should be helped to change position often to prevent the development of decubitus ulcers caused by tissue hypoxia. Protective devices such as egg crate or water mattresses are indicated. Patients should be encouraged to cough and deep breath every 2 hours while awake to prevent pulmonary complications such as pneumonia.

Bowel movements must be kept soft and regular to prevent irritation to the mucous membrane, which could act as a site for infection. Rest periods and assistance will help alleviate shortness of breath and conserve energy. Thrombocytopenia should alert the nurse to assess the patient for signs of bleeding, and even the slightest trauma must be prevented. The patient's urine and stool should be monitored for occult or gross bleeding. Assessment of the oral cavity includes noting the presence of bleeding gums or bleeding from mucosal areas. Medications should be given orally whenever possible. Although the prognosis is poor, careful medical and nursing management improves the chance of survival (Box 26-2).

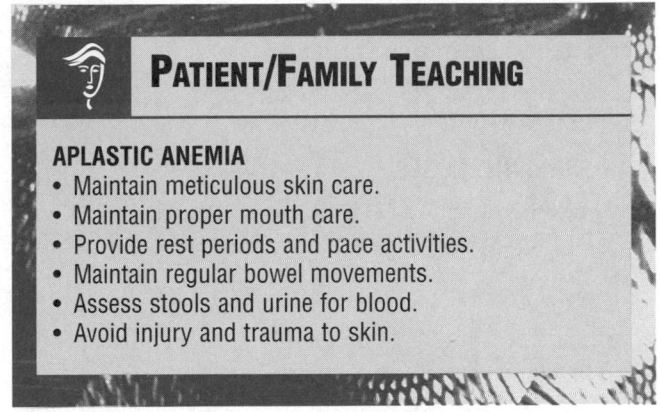

**PATIENT/FAMILY TEACHING**

**APLASTIC ANEMIA**
• Maintain meticulous skin care.
• Maintain proper mouth care.
• Provide rest periods and pace activities.
• Maintain regular bowel movements.
• Assess stools and urine for blood.
• Avoid injury and trauma to skin.

## Polycythemia

**Pathophysiology.** **Polycythemia** is a chronic disease caused by a proliferation of erythrocytes in the bone marrow. It occurs most commonly in middle-aged men of Jewish ancestry. The red blood cell count may range from 7000 to 10 million/mm³ of blood. The disease occurs in two forms: primary (true) and secondary (relative). The cause of primary polycythemia is unknown. In the absence of cardiorespiratory disease, the oxygen content of the blood is normal but the rate of flow is decreased and the viscosity is increased. The decreased rate of flow and increased viscosity may lead to thrombosis in small blood vessels. The leukocyte count is increased in primary polycythemia and may reach 25,000 to 50,000/mm³. Increased numbers of platelets predispose the patient to intravascular thrombosis. The spleen and liver are enlarged, and bleeding in the form of ecchymosis occurs in mucous membranes and skin. The secondary form of the disease accompanies several other chronic disorders, including cardiac and pulmonary disease. This form has been associated with benign and malignant tumors, particularly malignant tumors of the kidney. In the absence of infection the leukocyte count is near normal.

◁ **BOX 26-2** ▷　　　　　　　　**NURSING PROCESS**

## ANEMIA

### ASSESSMENT

- Nutritional status and appetite
- Oral mucosa and skin
- Gastrointestinal system for nausea, abdominal distention, diarrhea, constipation, and enlarged spleen or liver
- Tolerance to activity
- Dyspnea at rest or with exertion, weakness, or fatigue
- Vital signs
- Bleeding tendency or active bleeding
- Signs and symptoms of heart failure
- Laboratory studies (hemoglobin, hematocrit, red blood cell indices, reticulocyte count, folate, vitamin $B_{12}$)

### NURSING DIAGNOSES

- Altered nutrition: less than body requirements related to anorexia
- Pain related to decreased oral mucous membrane integrity
- Activity intolerance related to an imbalance between oxygen supply and demand
- Risk for impaired skin integrity related to immobility
- Risk for injury related to decreased hemoglobin
- Risk for impaired gas exchange related to inadequate oxygen-carrying capacity
- Risk for trauma (falling) related to weakness
- Anxiety related to prescribed treatment plan
- Altered family processes related to hospitalization
- Knowledge deficit related to prescribed diet and medication therapy

### NURSING INTERVENTIONS

- Encourage small, frequent meals.
- Provide a pleasant dining environment.

- Provide oral hygiene before meals and as needed.
- Provide cool, bland foods if indicated.
- Provide frequent rest periods.
- Encourage patient to request assistance with activities.
- Increase activity as tolerated.
- Elevate head of bed as tolerated.
- Prevent unnecessary exertion.
- Prevent skin breakdown.
- Provide an atmosphere of acceptance.
- Provide positive reinforcement.
- Encourage family to visit.
- Prevent falls.
- Keep environment free of clutter.

### EVALUATION OF EXPECTED OUTCOMES

- Tolerates prescribed diet
- Describes foods high in specific dietary need (iron, vitamin $B_{12}$, folate)
- Mucous membranes remain intact
- Verbalizes pain relief
- Participates in required activity
- Verbalizes need for assistance
- No evidence of respiratory distress
- Maintains vital signs within normal limits for patient
- Maintains complete blood cell count within normal range for patient
- Verbalizes sources of anxiety
- Participation of family members in patient's care
- Maintains intact skin
- Verbalizes signs and symptoms of anemia and reportable conditions

---

The causative factor in secondary polycythemia is decreased oxygen in the blood.

**Assessment.** Symptoms of polycythemia are caused by the effects of massive numbers of red blood cells, which result in hyperviscosity of the blood and hypervolemia. The patient may complain of headache, fatigue, night sweats, pruritus, paraesthesia, and dyspnea. The spleen and liver will be enlarged, and bruises may be seen on the skin and mucous membranes. These persons appear to be predisposed to gout and peptic ulcers.

**Intervention.** The objective of treatment of polycythemia is to suppress the bone marrow, reduce the blood cell mass, maintain the hematocrit value at or below 50%, and reduce the leukocyte and platelet count. Phlebotomy and the removal of up to 500 ml of blood at intervals may accomplish the objectives for some patients. Chemotherapeutic drugs may also be used, including melphalan (Alkeran), chlorambucil (Leukeran), and busulfan (Myleran). Radioactive phosphorus ($P^{32}$) may be administered intravenously. Combinations of phlebotomy with chemotherapy or radioactive phos-

CHAPTER 26 ◆ Hematologic and Lymphatic Problems

phorus are used to provide sustained control of this disease. Persons who survive for 10 years or longer often develop leukemia. The role of the nurse is supportive and directed at minimizing the symptoms. The patient should be encouraged to maintain good health habits and regular medical supervision.

## Disorders of White Blood Cells

### Leukocytosis

Leukocytosis is an increase in the number of white blood cells. It is both a protective and a destructive mechanism. In many diseases that are potentially dangerous, leukocytes are increased and play an important role in helping the body overcome an infection. In some forms of leukemia, large numbers of immature leukocytes are produced, causing changes in the spleen, liver, and lymph nodes. Although the number of leukocytes is increased, the cells are immature and do not offer protection against infection.

### Leukopenia

Leukopenia is a condition in which the number of leukocytes is greatly reduced. When the granulocytes are reduced, serious bacterial infection may occur. There are numerous conditions causing leukopenia, including chemical agents known to be toxic to the body. Among these are the antineoplastic drugs. Whenever leukopenia occurs, the patient should be protected from infection. Because the protective mechanism offered by the leukocytes has decreased, the patient's life could be in danger if infection should develop.

### Infectious Mononucleosis

Infectious mononucleosis is an acute infectious disease involving the white blood cells. The number of leukocytes may be increased from 10,000 to 25,000/mm³. The lymphocytes are also increased, some of which will be immature, although most will be mature. The clinical manifestations of the disease involve the lymphoid tissues of the body, particularly the lymph nodes and the spleen (see Chapter 14). The Paul-Bunnell (heterophil antibody) test is used to determine the presence or absence of antibodies to the Epstein-Barr virus, which causes infectious mononucleosis.

### Leukemia

**Leukemia** is a group of neoplastic disorders resulting in widespread proliferation of white blood cells and their precursors throughout the body. It is a disease of the bone marrow, which is where leukocytes are formed. There is excessive production of nonfunction-

ing leukocytes, which crowd the bone marrow and slow the production of red blood cells and platelets (Shelton, Baker, Stekler, 1996). Specific causes of leukemia are unknown, but ionizing radiation, viruses, certain antineoplastic drugs, and genetic abnormalities have been linked to the disease.

Leukemia may be acute or chronic and is classified according to the type of cells involved, such as granulocytes, monocytes, and lymphocytes.

Acute lymphoblastic leukemia is the form most common in children, but chronic forms may also occur. Chronic leukemia is more common in persons older than 45 years of age, but acute leukemia may occur in adult persons of any age. Approximately 50% to 60% of all leukemia in the United States is classified as acute leukemia.

### Acute Leukemia

The acute leukemias are divided into lymphocytic leukemia (ALL), which originates from lymphocytes, and myelocytic leukemia (AML), which originates from granulocytes. ALL occurs primarily in children, and AML occurs primarily in adults. In children the disease usually affects those 2 to 4 years of age, with most deaths occurring in children under 2 years of age. Regardless of the type of the cells involved, whether in children or adults, the characteristics and progress of the disease are similar.

**Pathophysiology.** Abnormal growth of immature cells, or blasts, will occur. AML is diagnosed when bone marrow aspiration and biopsy show an overgrowth of immature cells of the myeloblast. ALL is characterized by lymphoblasts, which are cells that are precursors of lymphocytes.

Early in the course of acute lymphoblastic leukemia, lymphatic tissues are involved, including lymph nodes and the spleen. The enlarged lymph nodes may be the first signs of the disease in some persons. In all forms of acute leukemia, the leukemic cells multiply in the bone marrow. Their proliferation causes a decrease in the production of red blood cells and shortens their life. With the reduction of erythrocytes, anemia may develop. The platelets are also reduced, possibly interfering with the blood clotting mechanism resulting in bleeding. During the course of the disease almost all organs of the body become involved. With treatment, remissions may occur, during which blood cell production may return to nearly normal levels.

**Assessment.** The onset of the disease in children often begins with a slight cold or tonsillitis. The temperature may range from low to high grade. The child may complain of headache and abdominal pain; in the very young child, pain may be evidenced by crying, restlessness, and reluctance to move or be moved. The onset of the disease in adults may be traced to a cold from which recovery was slow. This is followed by prostration, weakness, anemia, and anorexia. If the anemia is severe, there may be pallor. Ulcerations may occur around the mouth, skin, and rectum. Bleeding varies from ecchymosis and petechiae to purpura, which may become necrotic and ulcerative. Bone pain results from the rapid proliferation of cells in the mar-

row. Symptoms will vary widely because various organs or parts of the body are involved.

**Intervention.** Tremendous progress in the treatment of leukemia has been made during the last decade by using a complex combination of drug and radiation therapy (see Chapter 12). The survival of children with ALL has increased from an average of 3 months before modern therapy to the point where the majority of

---

◁ **BOX 26-3** ▷          **NURSING PROCESS**

## LEUKEMIA

### ASSESSMENT

- Vital signs
- Body sites for evidence of infection (oral cavity, skin, perineum, rectum)
- Respiratory system for evidence of congestion
- IV sites and bone marrow biopsy sites for evidence of bleeding
- Signs and symptoms of bleeding (skin, urine, stool, emesis, sputum, nose, gums)
- Dizziness with position changes and orthostatic hypotension
- Tolerance to activity
- Mental status for signs of restlessness, agitation, confusion
- Lymphadenopathy, pallor, or fatigue
- Laboratory studies (whole blood cell count, platelet count, hemoglobin, hematocrit)

### NURSING DIAGNOSES

- Risk for infection related to leukopenia
- Risk for injury related to thrombocytopenia
- Activity intolerance related to weakness and fatigue
- Risk for ineffective coping related to loss of health and associated stress
- Knowledge deficit related to diagnosis and treatment
- Anticipatory grieving related to potential loss of life

### NURSING INTERVENTIONS

- Report abnormalities in vital signs.
- Encourage optimal personal hygiene.
- Provide frequent oral hygiene.
- Wash hands before patient contact.
- Reduce number of visitors.
- Prevent patient contact with persons with respiratory infections, flu, etc.
- Administer antibiotic and antifungal medications on time, as ordered.

- Encourage deep breathing and coughing.
- Use protective devices (e.g., egg crate mattress) to prevent skin breakdown.
- Assist with frequent position changes; provide skin care.
- Report any bleeding or evidence of infection.
- Avoid IM injections, indwelling catheters, rectal thermometers, suppositories.
- Apply pressure to venipuncture sites and bone marrow biopsy sites for 5 minutes.
- Provide patient with soft toothbrush.
- Instruct patient to use an electric razor.
- Provide patient with shoes or slippers when ambulating.
- Have patient change position slowly and wait for assistance with ambulation.
- Keep siderails up.
- Provide frequent rest periods.
- Assist with self-care activities.
- Establish communication.
- Assist patient and family with coping.
- Provide referral for home care as needed.

### EVALUATION OF EXPECTED OUTCOMES

- Describes signs and symptoms of infection and preventive measures
- Maintains adequate nutrition
- Demonstrates no evidence of active bleeding
- Laboratory values within normal range for patient
- Avoids physician trauma
- Verbalizes a need for assistance
- Spaces activity throughout the day
- Demonstrates progression with activity and endurance
- Strives toward independence
- Begins coping with life-style changes

those treated have no evidence of the disease after 5 years. AML (nonlymphocytic) has shown less response to treatment.

Bone marrow transplantation may be selected as the treatment of choice if initial remission of the acute leukemia has been induced. Before transplantation, the patient's bone marrow cells and leukemic cells must be killed by massive chemotherapy with or without total body irradiation (Belcher, 1993). The patient may succumb to infection or hemorrhage. Graft-vs-host disease, a condition that occurs if the donor bone marrow cells recognize the patient's cells as foreign and attack them, can also be fatal.

Many of the symptoms concurrent with leukemia are the result of treatment rather than the disease. Side effects of the chemotherapeutic drugs and reactions to radiation therapy should be noted (see Chapter 12). If the person receives blood transfusions, packed red blood cells, or platelets, he or she must be observed for transfusion reaction. When numerous transfusions are given, the danger of reaction is increased. Hematomas or hemorrhage may occur from any trauma to the skin. Infections and hemorrhage account for many complications of leukemia, and the nurse must be constantly alert to protect the patient from infection and to report immediately any severe bleeding or indication of infection (Box 26-3).

The patient with acute leukemia may come into the hospital several times during the course of the disease. Examinations and treatment may be painful experiences especially for a child, and he or she may be fearful. The nurse should do everything possible to relieve the anxiety of both the patient and family members. Parents of a child with leukemia need tender, loving care at this time as much as the child. A referral to the Leukemia Society of America will offer an additional source of information and support.

## Chronic Leukemia

Chronic leukemia is confined almost entirely to adults and generally develops slowly. The major classes of chronic leukemias are divided into lymphocytic (CLL) and myelogenous (CML) leukemia. The individual may be completely asymptomatic when the disorder is discovered by routine physical examination.

**Pathophysiology.** CLL may progress slowly, or it may progress rapidly to a fatal termination. The leukocyte count is increased, and lymph nodes throughout the body are enlarged but are not painful. There is an increased incidence of infection. CML is characterized by the presence of a chromosomal marker, the Philadelphia chromosome. In CML the spleen becomes enlarged. Without treatment, CML will progress to an acute stage (blast crisis). Death usually occurs within a few months after blast crisis occurs (Lewis, Collier, Heitkemper, 1996).

**Assessment.** All forms of chronic leukemia are characterized by similar symptoms, including weakness, fever, bone pain, loss of appetite, loss of weight, anemia, enlargement of body organs, and hemorrhage.

**Intervention.** The objectives of treatment in chronic leukemia partially depend on the kind of cells that are involved. In CML the purpose of treatment is to bring about a reduction in the number of leukocytes and thrombocytes and in the size of the spleen. When the white blood cell count is kept at or near normal, other symptoms are modified. In CLL the primary consideration is directed toward relief of the conditions that arise from the increased production of lymphocytes, such as enlarged and painful lymph nodes and spleen, anemia, and a decrease in the number of platelets. Drugs commonly used in chronic leukemia include chlorambucil (Leukeran), hydroxyurea, corticosteroids, and cyclophosphamide (Cytoxan). Irradiation of lymph nodes is often used, and blood transfusions may be given if the anemia is severe. Although drugs are not curative, they help prolong life expectancy for patients with chronic leukemia. The median survival time for patients with CML is $3\frac{1}{2}$ to 4 years, whereas that for patients with CLL is 6 years (Beare, Myers, 1994). The nursing care required during severe relapses is the same as that for patients with acute leukemia. When the patient is ambulatory in the hospital or in the home, regular daily rest periods should be observed to minimize fatigue and weakness.

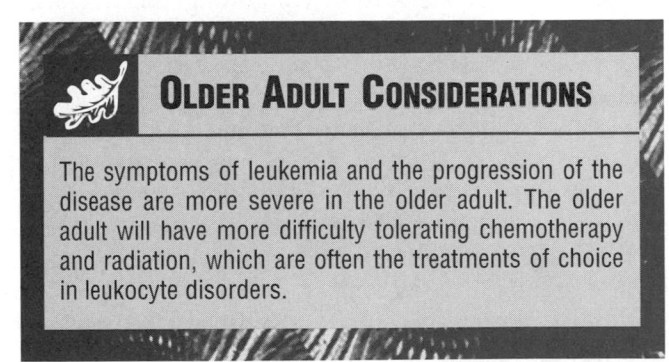

### OLDER ADULT CONSIDERATIONS

The symptoms of leukemia and the progression of the disease are more severe in the older adult. The older adult will have more difficulty tolerating chemotherapy and radiation, which are often the treatments of choice in leukocyte disorders.

## Hemorrhagic Disorders
### Hemophilia

**Hemophilia** is a general term that is applied to a group of diseases that have certain things in common. They are all hereditary diseases characterized by prolonged bleeding time. They all exhibit a deficiency in one or more of the factors essential for coagulation of the blood.

**Pathophysiology.** The most common form of hemophilia is classic hemophilia A, a deficiency of factor VIII. This form appears only in males and is transmitted by the female. Christmas disease (hemophilia B) occurs in the same manner as hemophilia A but is a result of a deficiency of factor IX. A third form of the disease is von Willebrand's disease (hemophilia C, vascular hemophilia), which occurs in both men and women. von Willebrand's disease involves a deficiency of the von Willebrand coagulation protein (Lewis, Collier, Heitkemper, 1996).

**Assessment.** Severe bleeding may occur in any part of the body. Repeated hemorrhages into joints (hemarthrosis) such as ankles, knees, and elbows may damage them to the extent that mobility is difficult. Hemorrhage into muscles may lead to contractures. Bleeding occurs into soft tissues and throughout the gastrointestinal tract, and minor injuries such as cuts, lacerations, or bruises may lead to fatal bleeding. There may be hematomas and hematuria, and anemia is often present.

**Intervention.** Treatment of hemophilia is first preventive. The individual with hemophilia in any form must be guarded against injuries. Contact sports are contraindicated. Parents should receive instruction concerning activities for young children and should know when an injury is serious enough to call the physician. Genetic counseling should be available to the family. If there has been a severe hemorrhage, fresh whole blood may be given. At the present time cryoprecipitates or commercial concentrates of factor VIII are the treatment of choice for persons with hemophilia A. In hemophilia B, concentrates containing the deficient factor IX may be administered. In hemophilia C, cryoprecipitate is given. Mild to moderate hemophilia A and von Willebrand's type I may be treated with a synthetic analog of vasopressin. This has been shown to increase factor VIII levels and can reduce the risk of AIDS and hepatitis transmitted by blood transfusions. The nurse needs to monitor the patient for side effects of the drug, which include fluid retention, tachycardia, hyponatremia, and hypokalemia. The blood pressure and pulse rate are measured often during the infusion, and fluids are usually restricted. Patients experiencing pain from joint or muscle complications may need analgesics to relieve pain. Analgesics containing aspirin or narcotics are usually avoided.

When injections are unavoidable, the nurse should use a small needle and apply firm pressure to the injection site for some time after the injection. The patient should be helped to remain quiet by the use of a recommended sedative, if necessary. The diet should be high in iron, vitamin C, and protein, and include high-protein drinks between meals. The application of cold compresses and pressure sometimes lessens the amount of bleeding into the tissues. Persons with hemophilia should inform physicians and dentists of this condition. Identification, which indicates that the person has hemophilia and names the type, should be worn or carried.

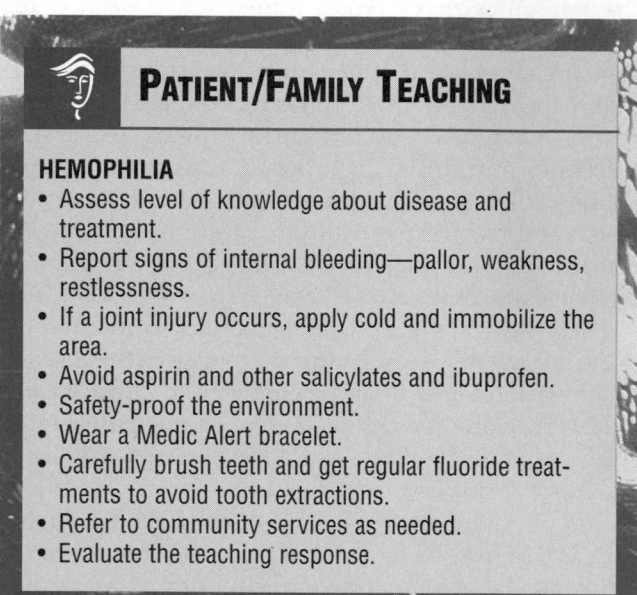

**NURSE ALERT**

When giving medication by injection to patients with leukemia or hemophilia, use the smallest gauge needle possible and apply firm pressure to the site for at least 1 minute after the injection. Do not massage the injection site.

**PATIENT/FAMILY TEACHING**

**HEMOPHILIA**
- Assess level of knowledge about disease and treatment.
- Report signs of internal bleeding—pallor, weakness, restlessness.
- If a joint injury occurs, apply cold and immobilize the area.
- Avoid aspirin and other salicylates and ibuprofen.
- Safety-proof the environment.
- Wear a Medic Alert bracelet.
- Carefully brush teeth and get regular fluoride treatments to avoid tooth extractions.
- Refer to community services as needed.
- Evaluate the teaching response.

Some psychosocial concerns are common to the hemophiliac and family and must be addressed. In hemophilia A and B, the gene is transmitted by the mother, who may experience guilt feelings and thus compensate by overprotecting the child. As in sickle cell anemia or in any chronic condition that requires extra attention for the affected child, sibling rivalry and jealousy may be exaggerated. The hemophilic child learns early that trauma is associated with bleeding and may use defense mechanisms such as denial to cope. In adolescence and young adulthood this can be manifested in risk-taking behavior. Other adaptations include stress-related spontaneous bleeding and passive reliance on others, neither of which is an effective coping response. The nurse can assist the patient and family by recognizing these responses and confronting them. Referral to the National Hemophilia Foundation may be helpful.

## Vascular Purpuras

**Pathophysiology.** Purpura may be divided into two categories: those associated with the destruction of platelets and those caused by failure of the bone marrow to produce platelets. Idiopathic or autoimmune thrombocytopenic purpura (ITP) is caused by the destruction of the platelets in the blood (Shuey, 1996). The destruction results in a greatly reduced number of platelets and leads to bleeding. The disorder occurs in an acute form in children and may progress to a chronic disorder. It also occurs as a chronic disorder, most commonly in young, adult females. Destruction of the platelets is caused by an antiplatelet factor in the plasma. In the chronic form, it may occur as a complication of a primary disease or after the ingestion of certain drugs. In some forms the platelets are deposited in large numbers in the spleen, causing splenomegaly. The second form of the disease, thrombocytopenic purpura, is caused by a failure in the production of platelets, which may be the result of damage to the bone marrow. Drugs and chemicals or conditions that require massive blood transfusions may result in purpura.

**Assessment.** Purpura is a condition in which there are small, spontaneous hemorrhages into the skin or mucous membrane. Tiny hemorrhages appearing as pinpoint purplish spots are called **petechiae;** larger hemorrhages are called **ecchymoses.**

**Intervention.** Treatment and care depend on discovering and eliminating the cause. If purpura is caused by the destruction of platelets, both the acute and chronic stages of the disorder are treated with steroids. In some situations removal of the spleen may be indicated. If purpura is caused by a drug, withdrawing the drug usually corrects the condition.

## Splenomegaly

The spleen is located in the upper part of the abdominal cavity under the lower part of the rib cage. It has four major functions: removal of microorganisms from the blood, formation of red blood cells under abnormal conditions, removal of old red blood cells and platelets from the circulation, and storage of blood. In blood dyscrasias, in which blood cell production in the marrow is compromised, the spleen may assume the function of producing all the blood cells. Not all of the functions of the spleen are understood. Enlargement of the spleen occurs in several diseases and is called *splenomegaly.*

**Pathophysiology.** Chronic congestive splenomegaly is commonly associated with certain blood dyscrasias in which removal of the spleen, splenectomy, may be indicated. Various disorders affecting the spleen may also require its removal. Injury to the organ, especially a crushing type, is always a surgical emergency. Splenectomy is done only as a reluctant, final intervention in children.

**Postoperative nursing intervention.** The nursing care of the patient after a splenectomy is essentially the same as that for other patients after abdominal surgery (see Chapter 20). Because the spleen has a rich blood supply and the patient may have a blood dyscrasia, it is important that the patient be carefully observed for postoperative hemorrhage. The patient should be carefully monitored for the development of a subphrenic abscess in the dead space created by removal of the spleen.

# FUNCTION OF THE LYMPHATIC SYSTEM

The lymphatic system has many functions including transport of lymph, production of lymphocytes and antibodies, phagocytosis, and absorption of fats and fat-soluble matter from the intestine (Belcher, 1993). Lymph nodes are located near the vessels of the lymphatic system. These vessels collect fluid from the interstitial spaces and transport the fluid back into the general circulation.

# STRUCTURE OF THE LYMPHATIC SYSTEM

The organs of the lymphatic system include the thymus, bone marrow, spleen, lymph nodes, tonsils, and Peyer's patches in the small intestine (Schindler, 1991).

## Disorders of the Lymphatic System

**Lymphoma** is a general term applied to any neoplastic disorder of the lymphoid tissue, including Hodgkin's disease. Benign lymphoma is rare. Malignant lymphomas are classified by predominant cell type and pattern of cell arrangement.

## Hodgkin's Disease

**Pathophysiology. Hodgkin's disease** is classified as a malignant lymphoma and involves the maturation of T-lymphocytes (Reed-Sternberg cells), the lymph nodes, and lymphatic tissues (Shelton, Baker, Stecker, 1996). The disease occurs more often in men than in women and in those 15 to 34 and over 50 years of age. In the past, Hodgkin's disease was always fatal, but now many persons can be cured. Early diagnosis in stage I and treatment with radiation can offer a 90% to 100% cure. The cause of Hodgkin's disease is unknown, although environmental, genetic, infectious, and immunologic causes have been studied.

**Assessment.** The first sign of the disease in two thirds of all cases is an asymptomatic enlargement of a lymph node in the neck (Shelton, Baker, Stecker, 1996). As the disease progresses, the deep lymph nodes in the mediastinum and the retroperitoneal cavity and adjacent tissues become involved.

When systemic symptoms such as loss of 10% of body weight, fever, and night sweats are present, the prognosis is less favorable, regardless of the stage of disease at diagnosis; this is denoted as "B" in the staging system (i.e., stage IIB Hodgkin's disease). The spleen and liver become enlarged, and in about one fifth of cases the bone marrow is affected. Symptoms are associated with the extent of lymph node and organ involvement. Mediastinal lymph node involvement can compress the trachea and underlying lung tissue, causing dyspnea and difficulty in swallowing. Retroperitoneal involvement is associated with edema of the lower extremities and back pain. Jaundice and fatigue are symptoms of liver involvement. The diagnosis is usually established by biopsy of a lymph node and identification of large atypical cells called Reed-Sternberg cells.

Intervention. Hodgkin's disease is classified into stages according to pathologic findings and the probable prognosis. From stage I, each subsequent stage represents increased activity and progression of the disease. Depending on the stage, treatment may be curative or only palliative. In stages I and II, treatment consists of radiotherapy of the involved lymph nodes and the contiguous tissues with a view toward cure. In later stages a combination of radiotherapy and chemotherapy is used. When the disease becomes widespread, radiotherapy has little benefit and chemotherapeutic drugs and steroids are administered in cycles. Although a cure may not be achieved in the late stage of the disease, remission extending over several years may occur. Nursing management of the patient with Hodgkin's disease includes intervention to reduce the effects of problems such as dyspnea, pain, fatigue, pruritus, and impaired skin and mucous membrane integrity. The patient is especially susceptible to infection and should be protected against respiratory tract infections and skin infections, which may result from scratching. Treatment of Hodgkin's disease contributes to the severity of the patient's problems.

## Non-Hodgkin's Lymphomas

**Pathophysiology.** Non-Hodgkin's lymphomas are a group of malignant neoplasms which are characterized by immature lymphocytes. The cause of non-Hodgkin's lymphomas is unknown. Because each of the non-Hodgkin's lymphomas is a different entity, the symptoms and course of each disease vary. Some lymphomas are slow growing (low grade), whereas others progress more rapidly (high grade).

**Assessment.** The main symptom of the non-Hodgkin's lymphomas is a painless enlarged lymph node. Other symptoms may include fever, night sweats, and weight loss. Lymph node biopsy is the method used to diagnose the specific type of lymphoma present. Staging for non-Hodgkin's lymphoma is similar to staging for Hodgkin's disease.

**Intervention.** Treatment for non-Hodgkin's lymphomas includes radiation therapy or chemotherapy depending on the specific type of lymphoma and the stage of the disease. Stem cell transplantation, using the patient's own stem cells or those of a compatible donor, is also used as a treatment (Lewis, Collier, Heitkemper, 1996). The prognosis for non-Hodgkin's lymphomas is usually less favorable than that of Hodgkin's disease.

Nursing care is aimed at patient teaching to prevent infection and recognize early symptoms of infection. Lymphoma is often a chronic illness with an unpredictable course. The nurse needs to offer support to the hospitalized patient by listening to concerns about the uncertain future (Wells et al, 1995).

## Multiple Myeloma

**Pathophysiology. Multiple myeloma** is a cancer of plasma cells which results in abnormal production of immunoglobulins. Immunoglobulins are plasma proteins produced by lymphocytes in lymph nodes and other lymphatic tissues (Belcher, 1993). These abnormal plasma cells no longer function to protect the patient. As the disease progresses, these plasma cells destroy bone and invade lymph nodes, the liver, the spleen, and the kidneys (Lewis, Collier, Heitkemper, 1996). The exact cause of multiple myeloma is unknown.

**Assessment.** No symptoms are usually present early in multiple myeloma, often not occurring until the kidneys are damaged or an infection occurs (Shelton, Baker, Stecker, 1996). Skeletal pain develops with bone destruction, and pathologic fractures are common. When the destroyed bone releases calcium, the increased levels of calcium in the blood can cause kidney damage, gastrointestinal symptoms, or changes in neurologic status.

**Intervention.** Chemotherapy is administered to destroy the abnormal plasma cells. Radiation therapy to specific bones involved can decrease pain at that site and aid in healing. Decreasing the elevated blood level of calcium by hydration and medication helps alleviate the neurologic and gastrointestinal symptoms and may prevent renal damage. Nursing care is focused on pain management and prevention of injury. Extra care should be taken when moving the patient to prevent pathologic fractures. The patient with an elevated calcium level needs to be protected from injury relating to confusion.

## Lymphedema

**Pathophysiology. Lymphedema** is a condition in which the lymphatic structures become obstructed. This condition is considered primary if the lymph channels are malformed or absent, as after dissection during surgery for cancer. Secondary lymphedema is a result of damage to the lymph vessels from infection, direct trauma, or obstruction.

**Assessment.** When lymph channels cannot drain the interstitial fluid adequately, the fluid accumulates within the tissues. The resulting swelling may be pitting edema. If it is painful, there is an inflammatory process present as well. It may be debilitating to patients who suffer cosmetic and functional losses. Progressive attacks of lymphedema with fibrosis of the subcutaneous tissues are known as *elephantiasis.*

**Intervention.** Conservative management of lymphedema involves applying increased pressure on the affected extremity in an attempt to move the fluids in the tissues (Humble, 1995). One method to encourage fluid to move from tissues to lymph vessels is positioning the affected limb at the level of the heart. Exercise also promotes drainage of fluid through muscle contraction. Another effective method is the use of a physician-prescribed elastic compression device to be worn on the extremity involved (Humble, 1995).

## Lymphangitis

**Pathophysiology. Lymphangitis** is an acute inflammation of the lymph vessels caused by the invasion of bacteria such as the streptococcus organism. It is characterized by red streaks that follow the course of the vessel involved.

**Assessment.** The patient with lymphangitis may experience an elevated temperature and chills. In some patients, the lymph nodes along the course of the vessel may be swollen and tender. Usually, however, the inflammatory condition terminates at the first lymph node. The condition may be serious if the causative organism reaches the bloodstream because septicemia may occur.

**Intervention.** Treatment of lymphangitis is based on controlling the underlying cause. Warm, moist dressings may need to be applied over the affected vessels. Skin care should be scrupulous, and all abrasions should be given immediate attention. The affected part is elevated, and antibiotic therapy is prescribed. The condition usually responds quickly to therapy. Any abscesses that form may require incision and drainage.

# NURSING CARE PLAN

## PATIENT WITH APLASTIC ANEMIA

Mr. Edwards is a 40-year-old male on the medical unit with a diagnosis of aplastic anemia. He saw his private physician 2 weeks earlier with complaints of fatigue, epistaxis, easy bruising, and hematuria. Since admission, he has undergone multiple diagnostic studies and is currently being prepared to transfer to an oncology regional center as a potential candidate for a bone marrow transplant. Various members of his extended family are being considered as potential donors, but no one has been identified as a tissue match as yet.

Mr. Edwards states that he lost 20 lbs before admission, but he has regained 5 lbs since admission. He received 10 units of cryoprecipitate the second day of his hospital stay, 1 unit of fresh frozen plasma the third day, and 2 units of packed red blood cells the fourth day. Implantation of a porta-cath into the right subclavian region was performed under local anesthetic.

Mr. Edwards has no known food or drug allergies. Aspirin and nonsteroidal antiinflammatory drugs are contraindicated because of his pathologic condition.

| Medical History | Psychosocial Data | Assessment Data |
|---|---|---|
| No previous hospitalizations, history of occasional premature ventricular contractions (PVCs), noted on recent in-office ECGs; has hypertension (HTN), which is under control with atenolol (Tenormin), 50 mg/day<br><br>Spontaneous passing of a kidney stone (nephrolithiasis), 1 year before current illness<br><br>As a Vietnam veteran was exposed to Agent Orange while on ground patrol in that country (prolonged exposure)<br><br>*Health risk behaviors:* Smoked 3 to 4 packs of cigarettes per day × 21 years; drinks 2 to 3 cans of beer per day × 15 years<br><br>*Health strengths:* Has yearly physical examinations; eats a low fat diet, exercises at least twice per week (plays tennis); works out at the gym when he feels that his weight is climbing<br><br>*Family History*<br>Father died at age 67 from myocardial infarction (MI)<br><br>Mother alive and well, age 65, only health problem is hypertension, which is under control with medication<br><br>Older brother Sam died 3 months ago from a motor vehicle accident<br><br>Younger brother Joe, age 38; excellent health; lives in Europe<br><br>Two sisters, ages 33 and 34, both in good health; supportive relationships; all said to be willing to be tested as a candidate for bone marrow transplant | Married for 16 years; periods of separation × 2; states that the last visits to the marriage counselor have strengthened their communication skills and now they have a quality "understanding" relationship; one daughter Sally, age 14, who is currently being shielded from the knowledge of the gravity of her father's illness; large extended family on wife's side<br><br>Has worked at automotive factory for 22 years; has HMO-oriented health insurance plan<br><br>*Religion:* Protestant; goes to church sporadically<br><br>*Hobbies:* Bowling, fishing, some contact sports; likes TV, but dislikes reading | Appears chronically ill; oriented × 3 (time, place, and person)<br><br>Height 6', weight 195 lb<br><br>*Skin:* Pale, with evidence of multiple bruises in various stages of healing; bruises mostly on trunk and upper arms; no rashes, no evidence of skin breakdown<br><br>Anterior chest wall has two intact, sutured incisions with no dressings; very slight serosanguineous drainage from lower incision; no redness or edema present in either incision<br><br>Hematoma 5 × 6 cm noted to the right of incisions; patient keeping ice over the swelling<br><br>*Respiratory:* Rate 16-20; regular depth and rhythm; clear to percussion and auscultation<br><br>*Abdominal:* Soft, nondistended; positive bowel sounds heard in all four quadrants<br><br>*Cardiovascular:* Apical pulse of 78; best heard over apex<br><br>*Musculoskeletal:* Full range of motion all joints<br><br>***Laboratory data***<br>WBC 6000<br>RBC 2.69<br>Hgb 7.3<br>Hct 23.4   } All low = pancytopenia<br>Platelets 114,000<br>Oxygen saturation level = 79-81 without additional oxygen; improves up to 95 with 4 L oxygen continuously |

## NURSING CARE PLAN

## PATIENT WITH APLASTIC ANEMIA—cont'd

| Medical History | Psychosocial Data | Assessment Data |
|---|---|---|
| *Medications*<br>atenolol (Tenormin) 50 mg PO daily<br>allopurinol 300 mg PO bid<br>phytonadione (aqua METHYTON)<br>   15 mg PO bid<br>methylprednisolone (Solu-medrol)<br>   20 mg PO q 6 hr | | BUN, creatinine, chloride, and potassium within normal limits<br>Calcium high at 11.2 (nl = 8.5-10.4)<br>Sodium (Na) high at 148 (nl = 135-145)<br>Albumin low at 3.2 (nl = 3.3-5.0)<br>PT high at 14.0<br>PTT high at 42.5<br>IV 1000 ml normal saline at 100 ml/hr; may discontinue if PO intake adequate; convert to a heparin lock |

### NURSING DIAGNOSIS
Risk for infection related to pancytopenia and surgical incision

| NURSING INTERVENTIONS | EVALUATION OF EXPECTED OUTCOMES |
|---|---|
| Monitor vital signs at least every 4 hours and report any deviations from the baseline.<br>Minimize the risk of infection by careful handwashing. All personnel, family, visitors, and staff need to comply.<br>Use strict aseptic technique when inserting IV lines, changing dressings, and providing wound care.<br>Have patient cough and deep breathe every 4 hours to help remove secretions and prevent pulmonary complications.<br>Help patient turn q 2 hr; provide skin care, especially to bony prominences to prevent venous stasis and skin breakdown.<br>Ensure adequate nutritional intake. Patient needs 2000 calories daily. Offer high protein supplemental snacks; patient likes milkshakes if cold.<br>Arrange for reverse isolation if WBC count falls low. Monitor flow and number of visitors. Explain rationale to patient and family.<br>Educate patient and family about good handwashing techniques and/or any other factors that increase infection risks. | Temperature and vital signs remain within the normal range<br>WBC and differential count remain within a normal range<br>Cultures do not grow pathogens<br>Demonstrates appropriate personal/oral hygiene<br>Incision site (port-a-cath) remains clear and pink and free of purulent drainage<br>IV sites do not show signs of inflammation; skin does not exhibit signs of breakdown<br>Lists risk factors that contribute to infection; remains free of infection |

### NURSING DIAGNOSIS
Risk for injury or fatigue related to altered hemodynamics

| NURSING INTERVENTIONS | EVALUATION OF EXPECTED OUTCOMES |
|---|---|
| Monitor daily laboratory values and document findings; report any abnormal values immediately to the physician.<br>Assess for excessive bleeding, fatigue, or new bruising; inspect skin daily during bath.<br>Guaiac all stools. | Laboratory values improve after the infusion of platelets and packed RBCs<br>Fatigue will be lessened, and patient identifies ways to conserve energy; bruising diminishes |

*Continued*

# NURSING CARE PLAN

## PATIENT WITH APLASTIC ANEMIA—cont'd

### NURSING INTERVENTIONS

Monitor neurovital signs. Monitor for changes in level of consciousness (LOC) or any signs of confusion. Keep on oxygen at 4 L. Check oxygen saturation levels q 4 hr. Monitor for a fall of $O_2$ saturation level if off oxygen.

Assess for hematuria, epistaxis, blood in the stool, or dyspnea.

Maintain IV hydration as ordered. Monitor intake and output.

Force fluids (at least 1000 ml per shift) while on the allopurinol.

Maintain patient safety measures such as no aspirin or nonsteroidal antiinflammatory drug (NSAID) products.

No intramuscular injections when platelet count is so low. Put pressure on any venipuncture sticks for 5 minutes.

Assist patient in and out of bed; monitor for safety.

Monitor administration of blood and blood products. Assess baseline vital signs before and during any procedure according to hospital protocol.

Check laboratory values before and after treatments, and watch for adverse reactions during the administration of any blood or blood products (assess for rash, hives, fever, or generalized urticaria).

Teach patient ways to conserve energy (e.g., alternate periods of rest).

Inform patient of the adverse effects of smoking, and encourage him to stop.

### EVALUATION OF EXPECTED OUTCOMES

No signs of covert or overt bleeding

Has no untoward reaction during transfusion therapy

Clotting profile returns to normal limits

Patient improves in his ability to carry out ADLs

### NURSING DIAGNOSIS

Risk for anxiety related to diagnosis as evidenced by restlessness, insomnia, aggression toward staff and family, changes in communication patterns, and verbalization of inability to cope and meet role expectations

### NURSING INTERVENTIONS

Spend 10 minutes with patient twice each shift; convey a willingness to listen.

Give patient concise explanation of anything that is about to occur.

Avoid information overload, because an anxious patient cannot assimilate many details. Make no demands on patient. Identify and reduce as many environmental stressors as possible.

Have patient state what types of activities promote feelings of comfort, and encourage him to perform them. Remain with patient during severe anxiety. Include him in decisions related to care when feasible.

Support the family in coping with patient's anxious behavior. Allow extra visiting periods with his family if this seems to allay anxiety.

Teach patient relaxation techniques to be performed at least every 4 hours, such as guided imagery, progressive muscle relaxation, and meditation.

Praise patient for initiating discussion with daughter; encourage daughter to share feelings.

Refer patient to community or professional mental health resources as needed

### EVALUATION OF EXPECTED OUTCOMES

Patient reports decreased restlessness and anxiety; has longer periods of uninterrupted sleep

Patient and family have quality discussions on the projected effects of the illness and life-style changes that might be necessary

Daughter is included in the family discussions, and the exclusion behaviors are eradicated

Patient and wife identify their usual patterns of coping and relate these to the perceived illness threat; draw strength from one another

Patient practices relaxation techniques on an ongoing basis

## NURSING CARE PLAN
## PATIENT WITH APLASTIC ANEMIA—cont'd

**NURSING DIAGNOSIS**

Knowledge deficit related to lack of information regarding treatment protocol as evidenced by questioning drugs, side effects, and infusion therapies

| NURSING INTERVENTIONS | EVALUATION OF EXPECTED OUTCOMES |
|---|---|
| Establish an environment of mutual trust and respect to enhance learning. | Expresses a desire for new knowledge related to his treatment protocol |
| Ascertain what patient already knows; clarify any misinformation; negotiate with patient to develop goals for learning. | Demonstrates newly learned skills and health-related behaviors |
| Select teaching strategies, such as discussion of visual materials and demonstration. | Develops realistic learning goals |
| Answer patient's questions honestly. Refer him to physician on matters related to medical protocol. | Can state each drug he is taking, the correct dosage, the rationale for use, and some common side effects |
| Give clear explanations on the drugs that the patient is taking. Explain the dose, time, and need for compliance. | Writes down any questions related to his medical regimen to further enhance his knowledge about his illness |
| Teach the patient the skills that he must incorporate into his daily lifestyle (dressing changes). Have patient give a return demonstration. | Indicates an openness to discuss the potential of bone marrow transplantation and the availability of a matched donor |
| Provide emotional support if patient questions the overall prognosis. | |
| Discuss bone marrow transplantation after the concept is introduced to him. Encourage the patient to ask further questions. Reinforce the prevention of infection. | |

## KEY CONCEPTS

➤ Blood, through its network of vessels, carries oxygen to cells and returns carbon dioxide to the lungs to be eliminated.

➤ Blood is comprised of a liquid component called plasma and formed solid elements.

➤ Cells are divided into (1) erythrocytes, or red blood cells; (2) leukocytes, or white blood cells; and (3) thrombocytes, or platelets.

➤ Types of diagnostic tests for blood disorders include complete blood cell count, coagulation tests, blood gas analysis, Schilling test, bone marrow aspiration, reticulocyte count, blood typing and cross-matching, and Rh factor.

➤ Blood transfusion reactions include allergic, hemolytic, pyogenic, circulation overload, and air embolism.

➤ Hemorrhagic anemia results from a loss of blood, which decreases the amount of circulating fluid and hemoglobin and the amount of oxygen delivered to the tissues.

➤ Symptoms of acute hemorrhagic anemia include thirst, rapid pulse rate, pallor, hypotension, and clammy skin.

➤ Interventions for massive hemorrhage include controlling the bleeding, treating for shock, and replacing circulating volume.

➤ Anemia caused by iron deficiency is the most common type of anemia.

➤ Loss of blood is the most common cause of iron-deficiency anemia.

➤ Symptoms of iron-deficiency anemia include pallor, dyspnea, palpitations, and loss of appetite.

➤ Pernicious anemia results from the lack of an intrinsic factor and the subsequent development of vitamin $B_{12}$ deficiency.

➤ Symptoms of pernicious anemia include pallor, nausea, vomiting, indigestion, constipation, diarrhea, and anorexia.

*Continued*

# KEY CONCEPTS—cont'd

➤ Treatment of pernicious anemia includes injections of vitamin B$_{12}$, a high-protein diet, warm comfortable clothing, and rest periods.

➤ Sickle cell anemia is caused by an abnormal hemoglobin molecule (hemoglobin S).

➤ Symptoms of sickle cell anemia include fever, anemia, enlarged spleen and lungs, and jaundice.

➤ Treatment of sickle cell anemia includes avoidance of stress and strenuous exercise, analgesics for pain, fluid therapy, avoidance of respiratory tract infections, and rest periods.

➤ In aplastic anemia, insufficient red blood cells are produced as a result of an interference with the stem cells in the bone marrow.

➤ Symptoms of aplastic anemia include pallor, weakness, dyspnea, hypoxia, lethargy, and fatigue.

➤ Treatment of aplastic anemia includes antineoplastic drugs and radiation or bone marrow transplantation.

➤ Polycythemia is caused by a proliferation of erythrocytes in the bone marrow.

➤ Symptoms of polycythemia include complaints of headache, fatigue, night sweats, pruritus, and dyspnea.

➤ The main treatment of polycythemia is to suppress the bone marrow, reduce blood cell mass, maintain the hematocrit at or below 50%, and reduce the leukocyte and platelet count.

➤ Leukocytosis is an increase in the number of white blood cells. In some forms of leukemia, the number of leukocytes is increased; however, the cells are immature.

➤ Leukopenia is a condition in which the number of leukocytes is greatly reduced. Patients with leukopenia need to be protected against infection.

➤ Leukemia is a neoplastic disorder resulting in widespread proliferation of white blood cells and their precursors throughout the body.

➤ Leukemia may be acute or chronic and is classified according to the type of cells involved.

➤ Nursing care for the patient with leukemia includes monitoring vital signs, inspecting for skin impairment, conserving the patient's energy, performing frequent oral hygiene, preventing infection, and monitoring white blood cell counts.

➤ Hemophilia refers to hereditary bleeding diseases that have prolonged bleeding times. The forms are classic hemophilia A, Christmas disease (hemophilia B), and von Willebrand's disease (hemophilia C).

➤ Symptoms of hemophilia include repeated hemorrhages into joints, ankles, knees, and elbows; hematomas; hematuria; and anemia.

➤ Intervention for hemophilia includes prevention of injury, genetic counseling, transfusion therapy, avoidance of injections and aspirin, a high-iron and high-protein diet, and analgesics for pain.

➤ Symptoms of Hodgkin's disease include enlarged lymph nodes in the neck, weight loss, fever, and night sweats.

➤ Hodgkin's disease is classified into stages according to pathologic findings and probable prognosis.

➤ Non-Hodgkin's lymphoma is a classification of malignant diseases involving painless enlargement of lymph nodes.

➤ Multiple myeloma is cancer of the plasma cells and can cause renal disease and pathologic fractures.

# CRITICAL THINKING EXERCISES

1. Mr. Atkins, 38 years of age, has been admitted to the hospital with a tentative diagnosis of bleeding gastric ulcer. A significant symptom is dark, tarry stools, fairly frequent in number and of a very fetid odor. Physical and laboratory examinations indicate that blood loss has caused a dangerously low hemoglobin and marked reduction in the number of red blood cells. The physician has ordered immediate typing and cross matching for 3 units of blood. However, Mr. Atkins' religious beliefs forbid him to receive blood, and he steadfastly refuses the blood transfusion.

   Although there is a medical problem involved, what nursing interventions can assist the patient?

2. Janice, 25 years of age, has been admitted to the hospital with terminal acute leukemia. There are numerous ulcerated areas around her gums, lips, and nares. Any effort to clean these areas causes additional bleeding. As a result, they remain encrusted with dried blood.

   What is the patient's problem? What are the possible solutions? Have you ever encountered this problem before? How did you deal with it?

3. Mr. Smith, age 20, is newly diagnosed with Hodgkin's disease. Consider the following:
   a. Psychologic impact of the disease
   b. How you would support the coping abilities of the patient
   c. The major teaching points to discuss with the patient
   d. Possible community resources and support groups

4. Mrs. Johnson, a 42-year-old mother, is admitted to the hospital for treatment of multiple myeloma. Knowing pathologic fractures are common in patients with multiple myeloma, what safety measures would you suggest both for her hospital stay and for her home?

## REFERENCES AND ADDITIONAL READINGS

American Red Cross: *Circular of information for the use of human blood and blood components,* Washington, DC, 1994, The American Red Cross.

Beare P, Myers J: *Principles and practice of adult health nursing,* ed 2, St Louis, 1994, Mosby.

Belcher AE: *Blood disorders,* St Louis, 1993, Mosby.

Blaylock B: Sickle cell leg ulcers, *Medsurg Nurs* 5(1):41-43, 1996.

Chiocca EM: Sickle cell crisis, *Am J Nurs* 96(9):49, 1996.

Erickson JM: Anemia, *Semin Oncol Nurs* 12(1):2-14, 1996.

Flynn JBM, Bruce NP: *Introduction to critical care skills,* St Louis, 1993, Mosby.

Hawley K: Pernicious anemia, *Am J Nurs* 96(11):52-53, 1996.

Higgins VL: Leukocyte-reduced blood components: patient benefits and practical applications, *Oncol Nurs Forum* 23(4):659-667, 1996.

Humble, CA: Lymphedema: incidence, pathophysiology, management, and nursing care, *Oncol Nurs Forum* 22(10):1503-1509, 1995.

Lewis SM, Collier IC, Heitkemper MM: *Medical-surgical nursing: assessment and management of clinical problems,* ed 4, St Louis, 1996, Mosby.

Marchiondo K, Thompson A: Pain management in sickle cell disease, *Medsurg Nurs* 5(1):29-33, 1996.

Pagana K, Pagana T: *Mosby's diagnostic and laboratory test reference,* ed 3, St Louis, 1997, Mosby.

Pasero CL: Pain control, *Am J Nurs* 96(1):59-60, 1996.

Phipps WJ et al: *Medical-surgical nursing: concepts and clinical practice,* ed 5, St Louis, 1995, Mosby.

Schindler LW: *Understanding the immune system,* Pub No 92-529, Washington, DC, 1991, National Institutes of Health.

Shelton BK, Baker L, Stecker S: Critical care of the patient with hematologic malignancy, *AACN Clin Issues* 7(1):65-78, 1996.

Shuey KM: Platelet-associated bleeding disorders, *Semin Oncol Nurs* 12(1):15-27, 1996.

Spratto G, Woods A: *RN magazine's nurse's drug reference,* Albany, NY, 1994, Delmar.

Wells ME et al: Reducing anxiety in newly diagnosed cancer patients: a pilot program, *Cancer Pract* 3(2):100-104, 1995.

## CHAPTER 27

# Fluids and Electrolytes

## CHAPTER OBJECTIVES

1 Identify the compartments of body fluid.
2 Differentiate between intracellular and extracellular fluid.
3 Identify the major ways fluids are gained and lost from the body.
4 Explain the processes involved in fluid and electrolyte exchange throughout the body.
5 Identify the signs and symptoms of primary fluid and electrolyte imbalances.
6 Explain the role of body systems in controlling acid-base balance.
7 Discuss the causes of acid-base imbalance.
8 Describe the symptoms of acidosis and alkalosis.
9 Interpret blood gas values to determine the types of acid base imbalance.
10 State the primary nursing responsibilities in maintaining intravenous therapy.
11 Compare and contrast the types of solutions used for fluid and electrolyte therapy.
12 Differentiate among the major types of shock according to cause.
13 Identify the goals of drug therapy in the major types of shock.
14 Outline the nursing management of the patient in shock.

## KEY TERMS

acidosis
alkalosis
anion
cardiogenic shock
cation
electrolytes
extracellular fluid
hypercalcemia
hyperchloremia
hyperkalemia
hypernatremia
hyperphosphatemia
hypertonic (hyperosmolar)
hypervolemia
hypocalcemia
hypochloremia
hypokalemia

hypomagnesemia
hyponatremia
hypophosphatemia
hypotonic (hypo-osmolar)
hypovolemia
hypovolemic shock
interstitial fluid
intracellular fluid
intravascular fluid
ions
isotonic (isoosmolar)
neurogenic shock
osmolality
osmolarity
third spacing
vasogenic shock

## BODY FLUIDS

Body fluids are essential to each of the billions of cells that make up the body. Body cells receive nutrients and discharge wastes into the environment, but the fluid is trapped beneath the skin, and volume and chemical composition are regulated precisely by intricate and complicated homeostatic mechanisms.

### Water Content of the Body

Water is the solvent of the body, the liquid in which other substances such as **electrolytes** are dissolved. Although the human body appears solid, approximately two thirds of it is liquid. Approximately 75% of an infant's body weight is water, whereas average adult men have approximately 60% and women approximately 50% water in their bodies. The percentage of body weight that is water decreases with age. Obese individuals have a smaller percentage of body weight in water because fat contains little water. Therefore the obese and the aged are at greater risk in situations that involve fluid loss because they have reduced fluid reserves. Infants and very young children are also at great risk because they have a higher ratio of body surface to body weight, immature kidneys that are less able to reabsorb water when necessary, and a higher percentage of fluid in the interstitial space, where water is more readily lost from the body (Figure 27-1).

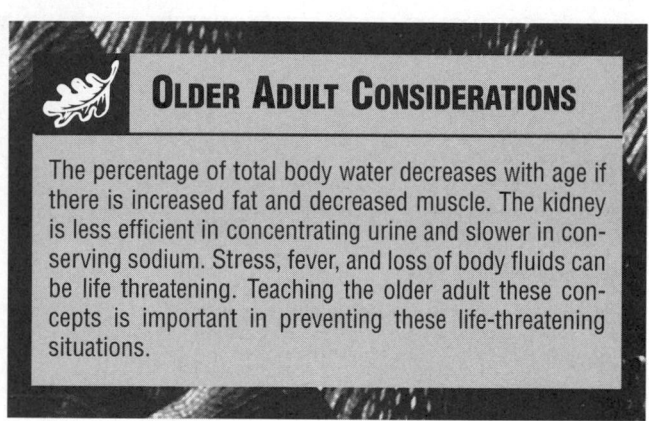

### OLDER ADULT CONSIDERATIONS

The percentage of total body water decreases with age if there is increased fat and decreased muscle. The kidney is less efficient in concentrating urine and slower in conserving sodium. Stress, fever, and loss of body fluids can be life threatening. Teaching the older adult these concepts is important in preventing these life-threatening situations.

## Body Fluid Compartments

Three fourths of the total amount of body fluid is located within the body cells as **intracellular fluid** (ICF). The remainder of the fluid is located outside the body cells as **extracellular fluid** (ECF). Approximately one fourth of the ECF is plasma of **intravascular fluid,** and three fourths is interstitial fluid. **Interstitial fluid** is found between the cells and in the lymph system. Intraocular fluid, cerebrospinal fluid, gastrointestinal tract fluids, and fluids within body organs are considered transcellular and are part of the interstitial portion of the ECF. The ECF maintains the proper environment for cellular life. It supplies food, oxygen, water, vitamins, and electrolytes, and it carries away wastes. The ECF must be constantly monitored and controlled by sensitive homeostatic mechanisms to maintain appropriate volume and chemical composition and to keep the body healthy (Figure 27-2).

## Fluid Spacing

The distribution of body water is also classified by the space it occupies. First spacing means that there is a normal distribution of fluid in both the extracellular and intracellular compartments. Second spacing refers to an excess accumulation of interstitial fluid (edema). **Third spacing** is fluid accumulation in areas that nor-

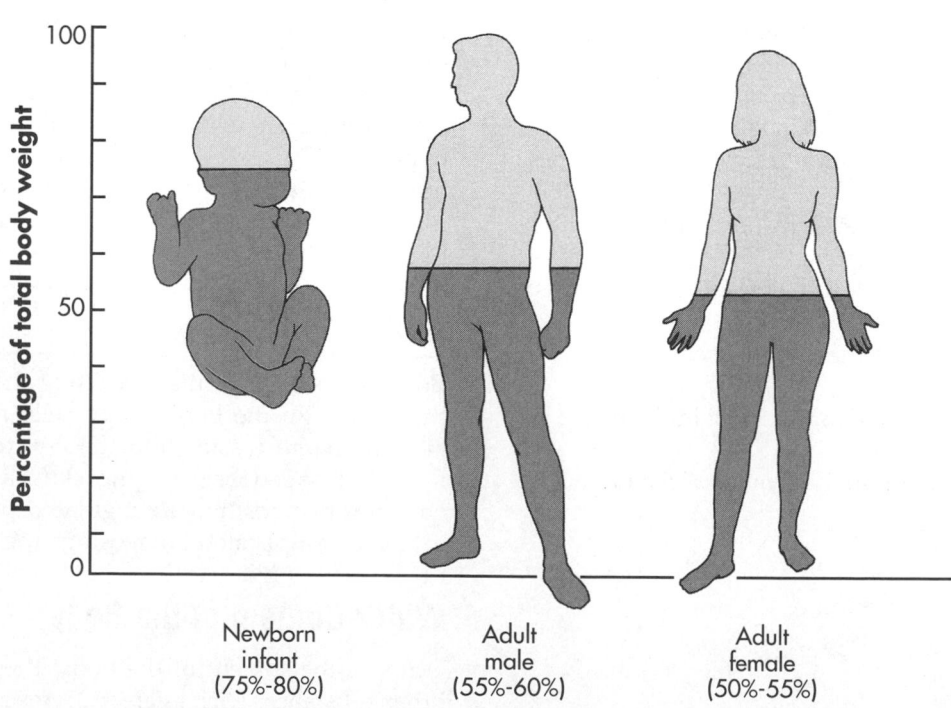

**Figure 27-1** Proportion of body weight represented by fluid. (Courtesy Rolin Graphics. From Thibodeau GA, Patton KT: *Structure and function of the body*, ed 10, St Louis, 1997.)

mally have no fluid or a minimal amount of fluid. Examples of third spacing include ascites, edema associated with burns, and the accumulation of fluid in bowel tissue that occurs with peritonitis. Third spacing can take fluid away from the normal fluid compartments and produce **hypovolemia.**

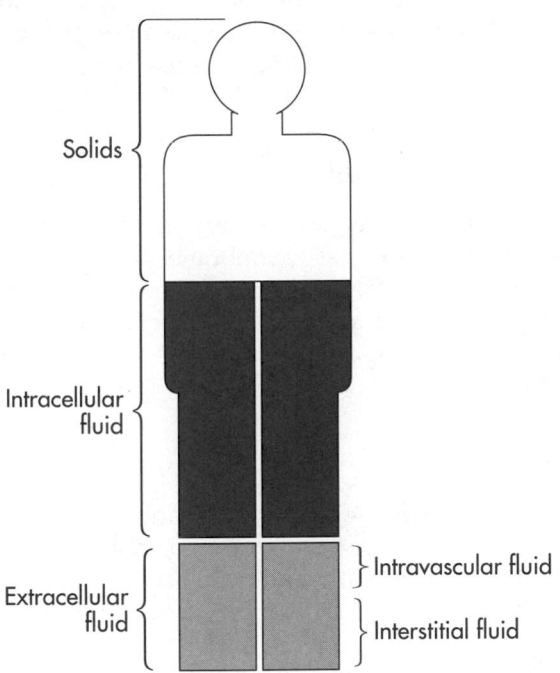

**Figure 27-2**   Comparison of intracellular fluid to extracellular fluid. (Modified from Horne MM, Heitz UE, Swearingen P: *Pocket guide to fluid, electrolyte, and acid-base balance*, ed 3, St Louis, 1997, Mosby.)

## Electrolytes

Substances that are dissolved in body fluids are called *solutes.* Solutes are nonelectrolytes and electrolytes. Nonelectrolytes are compounds that do not separate into charged particles when dissolved in water. Glucose is a nonelectrolyte. **Electrolytes** separate into particles, called ions, that develop an electric charge when placed in water. For example, salt (NaCl) breaks up, or ionizes, into sodium ($Na^+$) and chloride ($Cl^-$). **Cations** are positively charged ions, and **anions** are negatively charged ions. The principal ions in the body are listed in Table 27-1. Oppositely charged ions attract each other, and like charges repel each other. All electrolytes are found inside and outside the cell. However, ECF contains large amounts of sodium, chloride, and bicarbonate ions. Sodium is the major cation, and chloride is the major anion. ICF contains large amounts of potassium, sulfate, and phosphate. Potassium is the major cation, and phosphate is the major anion. Protein is more concentrated in the plasma. Normally the total number of positive and negative charges is equal on both sides of the cell membrane.

To anticipate and prevent their depletion, it is helpful to know what electrolytes are found in which body fluids. For example, gastric secretions have a high concentration of hydrogen ions, and pancreatic secretions contain high bicarbonate concentrations. Sodium is abundant in bile and in gastric and pancreatic secretions.

## Gains and Losses

Fluid and solutes, including electrolytes, are gained primarily through the intake of food and water. A small

## TABLE 27-1

### Normal Electrolyte Content of Body Fluids

| ELECTROLYTES (ANIONS AND CATIONS) | EXTRACELLULAR* | | INTRACELLULAR (mEq/L) |
|---|---|---|---|
| | INTRAVASCULAR (mEq/L) | INTERSTITIAL (mEq/L) | |
| Sodium ($Na^+$) | 138.0-145.0 | 146.0 | 15.0-20.0 |
| Potassium ($K^+$) | 3.5-5.0 | 5.0 | 150.0-155.0 |
| Calcium ($Ca^{++}$) | 4.5-5.5 | 3.0 | 1.0-2.0 |
| Magnesium ($Mg^{++}$) | 1.5-2.5 | 1.0 | 27.0-29.0 |
| Chloride ($Cl^-$) | 96.0-106.0 | 114.0 | 1.0-4.0 |
| Bicarbonate ($HCO_3^-$) | 22.0-26.0 | 30.0 | 10.0-12.0 |
| Protein ($Prot^-$) | 16.0 | 1.0 | 63.0 |
| Phosphate ($HPO_4^{--}$) | 1.7-4.6 | 2.0 | 100.0-104.0 |
| Sulfate ($SO_4^{--}$) | 1.0 | 1.0 | 20.0 |
| Organic acids | 5.0 | 8.0 | 0.0 |

Modified from Phipps WJ, Long BC: *Medical-surgical nursing: concepts and clinical practice*, ed 5, St Louis, 1995, Mosby.
*Note that the electrolyte level of the intravascular and interstitial (extracellular) fluids is approximately the same and that sodium and chloride contents are markedly higher in these fluids, whereas potassium, phosphate, and protein contents are markedly higher in intracellular fluid.

amount of water is also gained as a by-product of the metabolism of carbohydrates, fats, and proteins. This process is known as *oxidation*. Under normal circumstances, fluid gains will approximately equal fluid losses. For example, the daily urinary output is approximately equal to intake of fluids. The difference can be ±300 cc and still be considered "equal" and normal. The water derived from solid foods and through the metabolism of nutrients (oxidation) will approximately equal the water lost via the lungs, stool, and skin, the insensible loss. This difference can be ±600 to ±1000 cc per day and still be considered normal. Patients can gain water and solutes from the use of nasogastric tubes, rectal tubes, and intravenous therapy. In renal failure, fluid loss does not compensate for fluid gain.

Fluid and electrolyte deficits are common because of the many abnormal states that contribute to fluid loss. Water and electrolyte loss occurs normally through respiration, urination, perspiration, lacrimation (crying), and defecation. Abnormal conditions that result in a loss of fluid and electrolytes include burns, wound drainage, hemorrhage, vomiting, and diarrhea. Therefore during an illness, gains and losses are not always equal. Abnormal losses accumulate during the illness and may cause serious problems.

## Calculation of Fluid Gain or Loss

A sudden weight change is the best indicator of a fluid gain or loss. One liter of water weighs 1 kg, or 2.2 pounds. Drinking 1 cup of water (240 ml) results in a weight gain of about ½ pound. Large weight gains or losses (2 to 4 kg) over a short period (12 to 24 hours) can be accounted for by fluid gain or loss. Diuretic therapy can cause the fluid loss, whereas acute heart failure can cause fluid retention.

## Measurement of Electrolytes

Electrolytes are measured both by weight and by combining power (the ability of the electrolyte to combine with other electrolytes). Electrolyte weight is expressed in milligrams per deciliter (mg/dl). Combining power is expressed in milliequivalents per liter (mEq/L).

# FLUID AND ELECTROLYTE EXCHANGE

## Passive Transport

Fluids and electrolytes move through the body by passive and active transport systems. Passive transport of fluid and electrolytes occurs through diffusion (con-

centration differences), filtration (pressure differences), and osmosis (diffusion of water molecules).

## Diffusion

Diffusion is based on the principle that molecules and ions flow through a semipermeable membrane from an area of higher concentration to an area of lower concentration (from where there is more of the substance to where there is less). Diffusion moves molecules (solutes, particles) into and out of cells.

## Facilitated Diffusion

Some molecules require a carrier to move more rapidly across the cell membrane. This process is called *facilitated diffusion*. Molecules move from higher to lower concentration as in simple diffusion. For example, in the transportation of glucose into the cell, insulin acts as the carrier molecule.

## Filtration

Filtration is the movement of fluid and electrolytes by the pressure or force that is exerted as a result of the weight of the solution. Movement occurs from an area of higher pressure to an area of lower pressure.

## Osmosis

Osmosis is the diffusion of water through a semipermeable membrane, which is a membrane that allows only particles of a certain size to pass through. A cell membrane is a semipermeable membrane. When solutions of different concentrations exist, one on each side of the semipermeable membrane, water passes through the semipermeable membrane from the weaker solution to the more concentrated solution in an attempt to equalize the strength of the solutions on each side of the membrane (Figure 27-3).

Diffusion, filtration, and osmosis are passive transport systems. Water and electrolytes continually move between the intravascular fluid, interstitial fluid, and intracellular fluid by all of these processes. Any change in the composition of one fluid is quickly reflected in changes in the others.

## Active Transport

Some substances can also be moved through semipermeable membranes by an active transport system. In this process energy is needed to move ions from an area of low concentration to an area of high concentration. The sodium-potassium pump is an example of

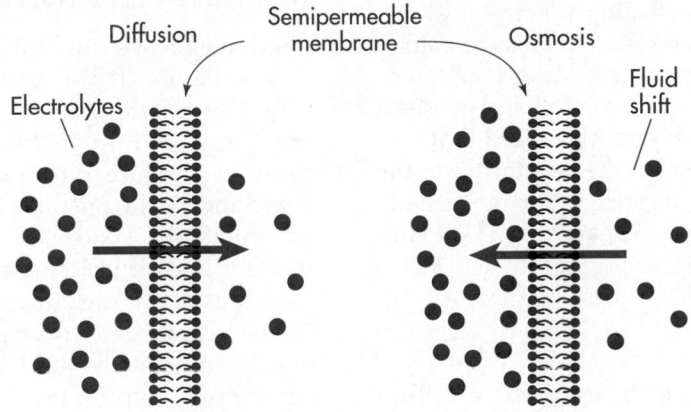

**Figure 27-3**     Osmosis and diffusion through a semipermeable membrane.

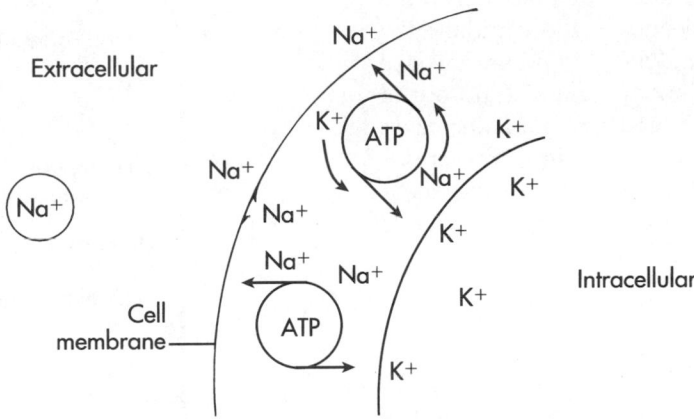

**Figure 27-4**     Sodium-potassium pump. As sodium diffuses into the cell and potassium out of the cell, an active transport system supplied with energy delivers sodium back to the extracellular compartment and potassium to the intracellular compartment.

active transport. During neuromuscular function, sodium diffuses into the cell and potassium diffuses out of the cell. Each is returned to its original place with the aid of the energy source, adenosine triphosphate (ATP). This process maintains the majority of sodium outside the cell and potassium inside the cell (Figure 27-4).

## Osmotic Pressure

Osmotic pressure or force is a term used to describe the "pulling" of water in the process of osmosis. Osmotic force is measured in units of milliosmoles (mOsm). **Osmolarity** and **osmolality** are both measurements of osmotic pressure. Osmolality measures the total milliosmoles of solute per unit weight of solvent (mOsm/kg). Osmolarity measures the total milliosmoles of solute per unit of total volume of solution (mOsm/L). Osmolality is the more acceptable term for

body fluids because it allows for a comparison of body fluids that do not have the same weight for equal volume, such as plasma and urine. Osmolarity is used to compare solutions of equal weight and volume, such as plasma and intravenous (IV) solutions. Normal body fluid osmolality is between 275 and 295 mOsm/kg. A patient's body osmolality tells if he or she is adequately hydrated, overhydrated, or dehydrated.

## Osmotic Movement of Fluids

Fluids added to the body that have the same osmolality as the fluid inside the cell are called **isotonic**, or **iso-osmolar.** Solutions that contain more water (are more diluted) than the ICF are hypotonic, or hypoosmolar. Solutions with less water (more concentrated) than the cell are **hypertonic** or **hyperosmolar.** Normally the ECF and ICF are isotonic to one another, and no movement of water occurs. Although there is a constant exchange of substances (including electrolytes) between the compartments, there is no net loss or gain of water. If a hypotonic fluid is introduced and surrounds the cell, water moves into the cell and causes it to swell and possibly burst. Hypertonic fluid that surrounds a cell draws water from the cell to dilute the ECF, which causes the cell to shrink and eventually die. IV fluids and their osmolarity are discussed later in this chapter (Figure 27-5).

## Hydrostatic Pressure

Hydrostatic pressure is the force exerted by a fluid against the walls of its container. Pressure in the vascular system is generated primarily by the force of the pumping heart. The hydrostatic pressure in the vascular system is higher on the arterial side than it is on the venous side. At the arterial end of the capillary the pressure measures approximately 32 mm Hg. The size of the capillary bed and the movement of fluid out of the capillary and into the interstitial fluid decreases the pressure to approximately 15 mm Hg at the venous end of the capillary. Hydrostatic pressure is the major force in the movement of water out of the capillaries and into the interstitial fluid (Figure 27-6).

## Oncotic Pressure/ Colloid Osmotic Pressure

Oncotic pressure, also called *colloid osmotic pressure,* is the pressure caused by colloids in solution. Colloids are particles that are too large to pass through a semipermeable membrane. Proteins are an example of a colloid. More protein is found in the plasma than in the interstitial space, so they create an osmotic force that pulls fluid from the interstitial space.

## Capillary Fluid Movement

Fluid must leave the capillary to enter the interstitium (interstitial fluid) and bathe the cells. It must also return. The amount and the direction of fluid movement are determined by the interaction between (1) the hydrostatic pressure in the capillary and in the interstitial space and (2) the oncotic pressure in the plasma and in the interstitial space. Hydrostatic pressure is higher than the oncotic pressure at the arterial end of the capillary and therefore forces fluid into the interstitium. At the venous end, hydrostatic pressure is lower than oncotic pressure, so fluid is drawn back into the capillary by plasma proteins (see Figure 27-6).

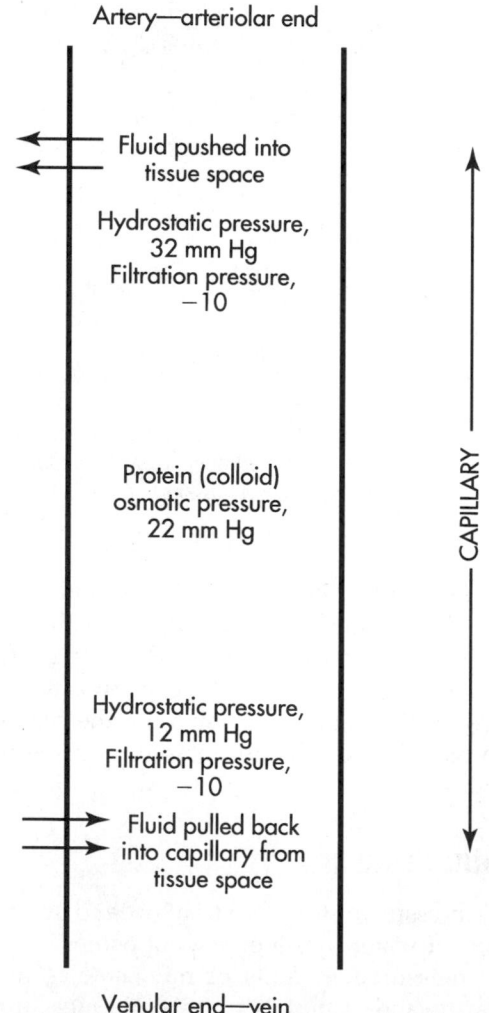

**Figure 27-6** Control of fluid movement from intravascular to interstitial space and return to intravascular space. HP, Hydrostatic pressure: pressure of blood against blood vessel walls; COP, colloid osmotic pressure: osmotic pressure exerted by plasma proteins, mainly albumin; FP, filtration pressure: HP minus COP (FP may be positive or negative).

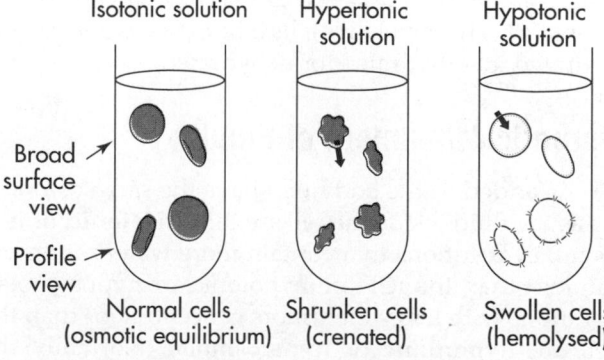

**Figure 27-5** Effect of osmotic pressure on the cells. (From Horne MM, Heitz UE, Swearingen P: *Pocket guide to fluid, electrolyte, and acid-base balance,* ed 3, St Louis, 1997, Mosby.)

## Fluid Shifts

An alteration in capillary and/or interstitial pressure causes an abnormal shift of fluid from one compartment to another. Edema is caused by a shift of fluid from the plasma to the interstitial space. Dehydration occurs when fluid shifts from the interstitial space to the plasma.

### Shifts of Plasma to Interstitial Fluid (Edema)

Plasma shifts to the interstitial fluid if the hydrostatic pressure rises in the vascular system. It also shifts if colloidal osmotic pressure is decreased in the plasma, because an adequate "pull" is not exerted to keep fluid in the capillary or to draw it back from the interstitial space. If oncotic pressure rises in the interstitial space, fluid is pulled and remains there. All of these shifts result in edema.

### Increase in Venous Hydrostatic Pressure

If the pressure is higher than normal at the venous end of the capillary, the movement of fluid back into the capillary is inhibited. The high pressure can be caused by anything that obstructs venous return of blood to the heart, such as congestive heart failure, tourniquets, thrombi in the venous system, fluid overload, or poor venous return resulting from varicose veins.

### Decrease in Plasma Oncotic Pressure

If the plasma oncotic pressure is too low, fluid is not drawn back to the capillary from the interstitium. Oncotic pressure decreases in several cases: (1) when protein is lost from the plasma, as seen in some kidney diseases; (2) when protein is not synthesized, as seen in liver disease; and (3) when insufficient protein is ingested, such as in malnutrition. Edema occurs in all of these cases.

### Increase in Interstitial Oncotic Pressure

Damage to capillary walls from trauma, burns, or inflammation allows plasma proteins to escape into the interstitial space. This shift results in an increase in interstitial oncotic pressure, which draws fluid into the interstitial space and retains it. This phenomenon explains the edema that occurs with tissue damage or inflammation.

## Shifts of Interstitial Fluid to Plasma

An increase in the oncotic (osmotic) pressure of the plasma draws fluid from the interstitium. The administration of colloids (albumin), dextran, mannitol (an osmotic diuretic), or hypertonic solutions may be ordered to achieve this result and relieve some patients of edema.

Hyperglycemia, as seen in uncontrolled diabetes mellitus, also pulls fluid from the interstitium. An increase in the hydrostatic pressure of the tissues shifts fluid into the plasma, as is seen when elastic bandages or hose are worn to decrease peripheral edema.

# REGULATION OF FLUID AND ELECTROLYTES

## Hypothalamus

The thirst mechanism is located in the hypothalamus and regulates the ingestion of water in the conscious person. The thirst mechanism is stimulated by hypotension and increased serum osmolality. A dry mouth causes the patient to drink.

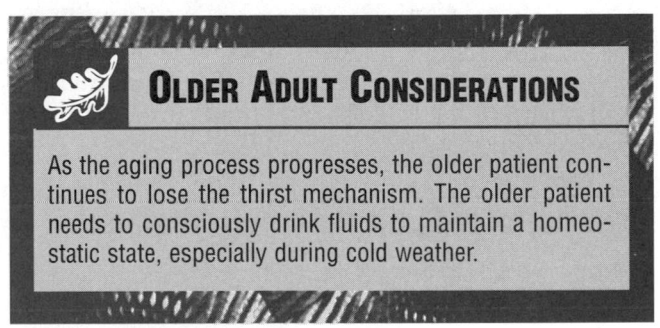

**OLDER ADULT CONSIDERATIONS**

As the aging process progresses, the older patient continues to lose the thirst mechanism. The older patient needs to consciously drink fluids to maintain a homeostatic state, especially during cold weather.

## Hormonal Regulation

Fluid and electrolyte balance is also maintained by three hormones: the antidiuretic hormone (ADH), aldosterone, and parathormone. ADH is produced in the hypothalamus and is stored and released from the posterior pituitary gland. It acts on the renal tubules to retain water and decrease urinary output. Aldosterone is produced by and secreted from the adrenal cortex. It increases sodium and water reabsorption while increasing potassium excretion in the renal tubules. The reabsorption of water and sodium results in increased circulatory volume (McCance, Huether, 1994).

Both ADH and aldosterone act in the kidney, which normally reabsorbs 99% of the fluid that is filtered in the glomerulus. Parathormone is produced by the parathyroidal glands. It promotes the absorption of calcium from the intestine, the release of calcium from the bones (bone resorption), and the excretion of phosphate ions by the kidneys.

# FLUID AND ELECTROLYTE IMBALANCES

Fluid and electrolyte imbalances occur when the homeostatic mechanisms that normally control volume and concentration are ineffective. Disturbances are primary when they are directly related to the amount of fluid or electrolyte. For example, a large amount of salt intake over a short time can result in sodium excess. Disturbances can also be of a secondary nature when other pathologic processes in the body contribute to fluid and electrolyte imbalances. Body fluid disturbances accompany many illnesses. Therefore every patient is a potential victim. The very young and the very old are at high risk.

To provide a basis for the understanding of these processes, the most important and most common imbalances are presented separately. However, because of the intricate and interacting nature of the mechanisms that control the body fluid composition, several types of imbalances usually occur at one time. Because ICF is inaccessible for analysis, fluid and electrolyte imbalances are determined by examining the ECF. The effects of a change in one fluid compartment are rapidly transmitted to the others. Therefore the ECF accurately reflects the state of all fluids throughout the body.

## Extracellular Fluid Volume Imbalances

Volume disturbances of the ECF (the plasma and interstitial fluid) can be classified as a volume deficit or a volume excess.

### Isotonic Extracellular Fluid Deficit

Isotonic extracellular fluid deficit, or hypovolemia, occurs when both water and electrolytes have either been lost from the body or trapped in an area of the body in such a way that they are unavailable to the circulation, which occurs in second and third spacing. Examples of third spacing include fluid accumulation at the site of burns or massive soft tissue injury, the collection of fluid in the peritoneal cavity (ascites), and shifts of fluid from the intravascular space to the interstitial and intracellular spaces after abdominal and chest surgery.

Third spacing with tissue injury results from increased capillary membrane permeability, which allows fluid and albumin to leave the capillary and enter the interstitial space. This shift reduces colloid osmotic pressure in the plasma and increases colloid osmotic pressure in the interstitial space, which pulls greater amounts of fluid into the interstitial space and depletes the circulating volume. The patient requires fluid replacement and may need albumin to restore the plasma colloid osmotic pressure. In the patient with burns a normal reabsorption occurs in 48 to 72 hours. The capillaries begin to heal, and plasma proteins are replaced or reabsorbed through the lymphatic system. Therefore fluid is drawn back into the plasma, and **hypervolemia** can result if the return is too rapid or too much IV fluid is administered. Diuretics are administered if fluid volume becomes excessive (see Chapter 23).

Hypovolemia occurs with any abrupt decrease in fluid intake, an acute loss of secretions or excretions, or a sudden shift of fluid to the interstitial space. It often results from a combination of these forces. The most common cause of isotonic extracellular fluid deficit is loss of fluids through the gastrointestinal tract by vomiting and diarrhea. Other conditions that lead to hypovolemia include intestinal obstruction, peritonitis, and acute pancreatitis. All of these involve inflammation, which diverts fluid from the intravascular space to the inflamed tissues. Fistulas (abnormal channels between organs or parts) can cause fluid loss.

No specific laboratory tests can indicate when a fluid deficit is occurring. However, the patient's signs and symptoms plus results from other more nonspecific laboratory tests can indicate that the condition is developing. The isotonic extracellular fluid deficit can result in an acute weight loss, often in excess of 5% of body weight; decreased body temperature; low blood pressure; increased respiratory rate; delayed vein filling; anorexia; nausea; vomiting; and shock. Oliguria, a urinary output below 30 ml (0.5/kg/hr) in 1 hour, can occur in severe cases. Treatment involves correcting the cause of the deficit and replacing the fluid with oral or parenteral solutions that have a normal balance of water and electrolytes, such as lactated Ringer's solution (Box 27-1).

In either type of extracellular fluid deficit, the components of the blood are more concentrated as a result of the fluid loss. The increased concentration elevates the hematocrit and hemoglobin values and red blood cell count.

### Extracellular Fluid Excess

When there is an excess of water and electrolytes in the ECF, a state of hypervolemia exists. Hypervolemia commonly occurs when the kidneys are not functioning properly or when isotonic intravenous solutions are being administered too rapidly. Congestive heart failure and malnutrition can also result in retention of water and electrolytes.

There are no specific tests to indicate excess ECF. However, the hematocrit and hemoglobin values and red blood cell count may decrease as a result of the di-

## FLUID VOLUME DEFICIT: HYPOVOLEMIA (ISOTONIC FLUID DEFICIT)

**ASSESSMENT**

- Decreased temperature
- Low blood pressure
- Tachycardia
- Weak pulse
- Increased respiration
- Delayed vein filling
- Cold extremities
- Weakness
- Restlessness
- Weight loss
- Nausea and vomiting
- Anorexia
- Decreased urinary output
- Shock
- Increased hematocrit and hemoglobin values and red blood cell count

**NURSING DIAGNOSIS**

- Risk for injury related to hypovolemia

**NURSING INTERVENTIONS**

- Monitor administration of oral and IV fluids.
- Monitor vital signs.
- Observe for signs of shock.
- Record body weight daily.
- Observe skin turgor.
- Maintain accurate intake and output (I&O) records.
- Observe for oliguria.
- Monitor and communicate laboratory results.
- Observe fluid accumulation in "third spaces."

**EVALUATION OF EXPECTED OUTCOMES**

- Fluid deficit corrected
- Hydration increased
- Shock prevented
- Progressive weight loss prevented
- Skin elastic
- Renal function maintained; output 30 ml/hr
- Therapy modified accordingly
- Fluid remobilized

lution effect of the excess fluid. Patients most commonly display symptoms of pitting edema, dyspnea, hoarseness, a bounding pulse, acute weight gain, puffy eyelids, and engorgement of peripheral veins. All symptoms are caused by the accumulation of excess fluid throughout the body. The treatment for isotonic extracellular fluid excess involves correcting the underlying cause, withholding fluids, restricting sodium intake, and administering diuretics (Box 27-2).

## Hypertonic Extracellular Fluid Deficit

When body water loss exceeds electrolyte loss or when excess electrolytes are ingested or administered, the remaining fluid is hypertonic. Water moves out of the cell to dilute the ECF. Cell dehydration results, and this condition is referred to as dehydration (Box 27-3). The thirst response is triggered by the hypertonic ECF. The skin is flushed, the skin and mucous membranes are dry, and body temperature increases. Skin turgor is poor, and the skin produces a "tenting" effect when grasped between two fingers. Normal skin turgor prompts the skin to quickly return to its former position when released and can be described as "elastic." The best place to check skin turgor is directly below the clavicles (Figure 27-7).

A common cause of dehydration is the administration of concentrated tube feedings to an unconscious patient, who is unable to respond to the thirst mechanism. Hyperglycemia that occurs with uncontrolled diabetes mellitus also produces dehydration. A deficiency of ADH or a diseased kidney that does not respond to ADH results in profound diuresis, which leads to dehydration. Dehydration also results from excessive pulmonary water loss with high fever and diarrhea in infants, as well as excessive sweating without water replacement.

## Primary Water Excess

An excess of body water that occurs without excess electrolyte accumulation is called *primary water excess* (formerly termed *water intoxication*). The ECF is hypotonic, and water moves into the cells, causing them to swell. Cerebral edema occurs, which causes confusion, weakness, and lethargy. Seizures may also result. Increased volume results in increased central venous pressure (CVP) and jugular vein distention. The patient experiences a sudden weight gain. Skin will be warm and moist.

Water excess with hypotonicity is seen in patients with renal failure who have taken too much fluid by

---

BOX 27-2

## NURSING PROCESS

## FLUID VOLUME EXCESS: HYPERVOLEMIA (ISOTONIC FLUID EXCESS)

### ASSESSMENT

- Acute weight gain
- Decreased hemoglobin and hematocrit values and red blood cell count
- Skin warm, moist
- Pitting edema
- Puffy eyelids
- Bounding pulse
- Engorged peripheral veins
- Dyspnea, increased respiratory rate
- Hoarseness
- Moist crackles in lungs
- Cyanosis
- Cardiac enlargement

### NURSING DIAGNOSIS

- Risk for injury related to hypervolemia

### NURSING INTERVENTIONS

- Record body weight daily.
- Maintain accurate I&O records.

- Monitor and communicate laboratory results.
- Observe and document skin integrity.
- Monitor vital signs.
- Assess neck veins.
- Observe for pulmonary edema.
- Restrict fluids and sodium as ordered.
- Administer medications as ordered.
- Check lung sounds.
- Elevate head of bed 45 degrees.

### EVALUATION OF EXPECTED OUTCOMES

- Fluid accumulation prevented; normal weight maintained
- Laboratory values normal
- Vital signs within normal limits
- Neck veins flat
- Oxygenation adequate

---

BOX 27-3

## NURSING PROCESS

## FLUID VOLUME DEFICIT: DEHYDRATION (HYPERTONIC FLUID DEFICIT)

### ASSESSMENT

- Thirst
- Flushed skin
- Dry skin and mucous membranes
- Decreased skin turgor; nonelastic (tenting)
- Increased body temperature
- Increased hematocrit and hemoglobin values and red blood cell count
- Weight loss
- Decreased urinary output

### NURSING DIAGNOSIS

- Risk for injury related to dehydration

### NURSING INTERVENTIONS

- Ask patient if he or she is thirsty.
- Observe skin and mucous membranes.

- Apply moisturizing creams.
- Monitor vital signs (frequency determined by condition).

### EVALUATION OF EXPECTED OUTCOMES

- Fluid deficit corrected
- Hydration increased
- Shock prevented
- Progressive weight loss prevented
- Skin elastic
- Renal function maintained; output 30 ml/hr
- IV therapy modified accordingly
- Fluid remobilized

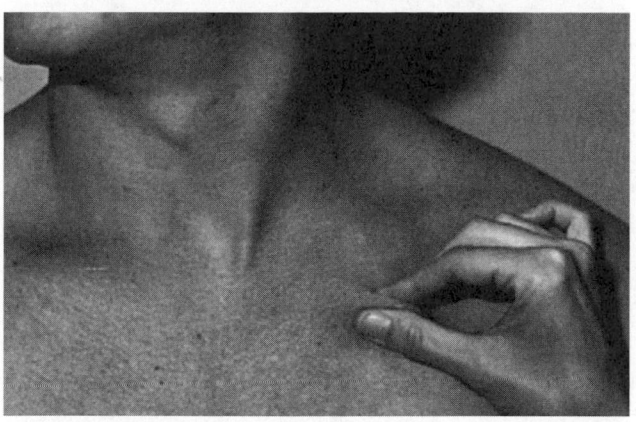

**Figure 27-7** Assesment of skin turgor. When normal skin is pinched, it resumes shape within seconds. If the skin remains in a "tent" shape for 20 to 30 seconds, the patient has poor skin turgor (tenting). (From Seidel HM et al: *Mosby's guide to physical examination,* ed 3, St Louis, 1995, Mosby.)

---

| BOX 27-4 | NURSING PROCESS |
| --- | --- |

## FLUID VOLUME EXCESS: OVERHYDRATION (HYPOTONIC FLUID EXCESS) (WATER INTOXICATION–PRIMARY WATER IMBALANCE)

### ASSESSMENT

- Acute weight gain
- Decreased serum sodium
- Decreased hemoglobin, hematocrit
- Skin warm, moist
- Edema
- Full, bounding pulse
- Increased blood pressure, jugular distention
- Increased CVP
- Confusion
- Lethargy
- Seizures
- Moist crackles
- Urine specific gravity below 1.003

### NURSING DIAGNOSIS

- Risk for injury related to overhydration

### NURSING INTERVENTIONS

- Weigh daily.
- Obtain accurate I&O.
- Restrict fluid intake as ordered.
- Monitor laboratory results.
- Observe and document skin integrity; protect from heat, cold, pressure.
- Monitor vital signs.
- Note central venous pressure.
- Assess orientation.
- Establish seizure precautions.
- Monitor lung sounds.
- Check urine specific gravity.

### EVALUATION OF EXPECTED OUTCOMES

- Weight loss; return to previous weight
- Laboratory values normal
- Skin warm, dry, elastic
- Neck veins flat
- Vital signs and CVP within normal limits
- Oriented to time, place, person
- Injury avoided
- Lungs clear
- Specific gravity within normal limits

---

mouth or have been given excessive IV fluids. Administration of 5% dextrose in water after surgery or trauma can result in overhydration because the water is hypotonic after the glucose is metabolized. The water "dilutes" the plasma, and the hypotonic plasma enters the cells and overhydrates them. Balanced solutions are usually given and include dextrose to provide calories and isotonic fluids to maintain fluid volume after surgery (Box 27-4).

**NURSE ALERT**

Expect to administer balanced IV solutions to patients after surgery or trauma. Avoid dextrose in water if cerebral edema is present or probable because dextrose will metabolize and water will enter the brain cells and increase cerebral edema.

## Electrolytes in Body Fluids

Electrolytes are measured in milliequivalents per liter (mEq/L), which indicates their chemical combining activity. For example, 1 mEq of a sodium cation can combine with 1 mEq of an anion such as chloride or bicarbonate. Cations and anions are found in equal milliequivalents in the plasma. The normal levels are usually given on laboratory reports, and normal ranges may vary slightly from one laboratory to the next, depending on the equipment. The normal ranges cited in this text are commonly accepted but may vary slightly when compared to a specific laboratory.

Electrolytes function as a group to promote neuromuscular irritability, maintain body fluid volume and osmolality, distribute body water between fluid compartments, and regulate acid-base balance (Phipps, Long, 1995). Each electrolyte has specific functions, which are affected when there is a deficit or a surplus. There are two basic ways by which changes in electrolyte concentration can be produced: (1) by altering the total quantity of the electrolyte in the body and (2) by altering the total quantity of water in the ECF in which the electrolyte is dissolved. For example, an excess of sodium can be caused by an increased intake of sodium, decreased output of sodium, decreased intake of water, or increased output of water. Generally a combination of these factors produces the imbalance. This principle applies to all of the extracellular electrolytes.

## Sodium

Sodium is the chief cation of the ECF and accounts for 90% of all the extracellular positive ions. It is largely responsible for maintaining the proper relationships of body fluids by regulating fluid balance and osmotic pressure. Sodium has several functions:

- Plays a vital role in numerous chemical reactions
- Participates in the generation and transmission of nerve impulses
- Assists in maintaining acid-base balance
- Is necessary for the regulation of water reabsorption and excretion in the kidney tubule

A normal serum sodium level of 138 to 145 mEq/L and intracellular sodium concentrations of 10 mEq/L are necessary to balance body fluids. If there is too much sodium outside the cell (**hypernatremia**) or too little inside, water leaves the cell and causes it to shrink. If intracellular sodium increases or extracellular sodium decreases (**hyponatremia**), water moves into the cell and causes it to swell. Both shrinking and swelling disturb normal cellular activity in the central nervous system. The major role of sodium in neuromuscular transmission is demonstrated by the changes in muscle tone that are seen as early signs of abnormalities. Shrinking or swelling in cerebral cells results in dysfunction.

---

**NURSE ALERT**

Use normal saline to irrigate nasogastric tubes. To minimize loss of electrolytes from stomach tissues. In some agencies, tap water is considered acceptable.

---

Sodium levels are controlled by the hormone aldosterone, which is secreted by the adrenal cortex when sodium levels are low. Aldosterone stimulates the renal tubules to reabsorb more of the sodium, which could otherwise pass out of the body in the urine. In doing so, potassium is excreted to replace the reabsorbed sodium. Thus aldosterone directly affects sodium and indirectly affects potassium. Once normal levels of sodium are reached, aldosterone secretion decreases. In this way, the concentration of sodium is maintained in normal limits. A daily intake of 2 to 4 g sodium is needed to replenish stores. Because the body stores sodium well, a decreased intake does not immediately result in a deficit.

**Sodium deficit.** A sodium deficit, or hyponatremia, can be caused by loss of sodium or by an excess of water. It is usually caused by excessive perspiration associated with the drinking of plain water; losses from the gastrointestinal tract because of (or related to) vomiting, diarrhea, or nasogastric suction; or administration of a potent diuretic. Too much salt is lost, or the intake of water is excessive.

A sodium deficit can also be caused by adrenal insufficiency. The adrenals secrete aldosterone, and without sufficient aldosterone, the patient fails to retain sodium. Dilutional hyponatremia can occur with a fluid overload that is caused by congestive heart failure, cirrhosis of the liver, or by the administration of excessive hypotonic IV solutions.

In a sodium deficit there are too few particles in relation to the amount of water present. The ECF is therefore hypoosmolar, or hypotonic. In an attempt to create equilibrium, the water moves into the interstitial spaces and the cells by osmosis. The cells become swollen and cause symptoms of anorexia, headache, nausea, vomiting, mental disturbances, and confusion followed by disorientation, convulsions, and coma. The deficit affects transmission of nerve impulses, which causes abdominal cramps and muscle weakness. Treatment usually includes the administration of normal saline or, with a severe deficit, 3% or 5% hypertonic saline solution if the kidneys are healthy. Hypertonic solutions must be administered slowly to prevent pulmonary edema. If too much water is the cause of the sodium deficit, fluids are restricted while sodium is gradually added (Box 27-5).

| BOX 27-5 | NURSING PROCESS |
|---|---|

## SODIUM DEFICIT: HYPONATREMIA

**ASSESSMENT**

- Plasma sodium <133 mEq/L
- Low urine specific gravity
- Anorexia, nausea, vomiting
- Weakness
- Headache
- Muscle cramps
- Abdominal cramps
- Confusion
- Disorientation
- Convulsions
- Coma with severe deficit

**NURSING DIAGNOSIS**

- Risk for injury related to hyponatremia

**NURSING INTERVENTIONS**

- Encourage diet high in sodium if ordered.
- Weigh daily.
- Check specific gravity q8h.

- Monitor neurologic status.
- Monitor vital signs.
- Monitor administration of IV fluids.
- Monitor serum electrolyte levels as ordered q2-4h.
- Maintain accurate intake and output records.
- Observe for a change in status.
- Pad side rails of bed.
- Place head in lateral position if seizure occurs.
- Restrict fluids if deficit is caused by excess water.

**EVALUATION OF EXPECTED OUTCOMES**

- Serum sodium level increased; within normal limits
- Specific gravity within normal limits
- Early symptoms observed
- More severe symptoms prevented
- Renal compensation for low serum sodium level determined
- Volume overload prevented
- Patient safety maintained
- Airway maintained

---

If sodium is lost in equal proportions with water, the ECF remains isotonic but its volume is decreased. Serum sodium levels are normal, and the patient's symptoms are related to circulatory collapse caused by decreased ECF volume. Isotonic fluids are administered to replace fluid and electrolytes.

> ### NURSE ALERT
> Because sodium regulates fluid balance, a patient with a sodium imbalance also can be expected to have a fluid imbalance.

**Sodium excess.** A sodium excess, or hypernatremia, can occur in any condition in which fluids that contain little sodium are lost in excess, such as the losses that accompany profuse watery diarrhea. When the water in the plasma is decreased, the electrolyte readings increase even though the total amount of the electrolyte in the body has not changed. Because sodium is the most abundant electrolyte, it is the first to show changes.

When a large amount of salt is ingested over a short time, acute sodium excess can occur. Following the laws of osmosis, water from the cells flows into the more concentrated ECF. This helps dilute the ECF but leaves the cells in need of water.

The high levels of sodium in the ECF draw fluid from the cells and result in cellular dehydration. Therefore the symptoms of hypernatremia are those of dehydration: dry, sticky mucous membranes; dry tongue; fever; thirst; flushed appearance; weakness; and irritability. Shallow, rapid breathing; fluttering eyelids; and muscle spasms that lead to stupor, seizures, and coma can occur. Laboratory data indicate increased levels of plasma sodium and chloride, and the specific gravity of the urine is elevated.

> ### NURSE ALERT
> Sodium and potassium imbalances often occur inversely. If sodium is high, potassium may be low, and vice versa.

Hypernatremia occurs in victims of salt-water drowning; renal disease; and hyperaldosteronism, which results in reabsorption of too much sodium by the kidney. Normal sodium levels are restored by infusion of hypotonic saline solutions, administration of furosemide (Lasix) or hydrochlorothiazide

(HydroDiuril) to promote sodium excretion, and dietary restriction of sodium (Box 27-6).

When sodium is gained over a longer period of time, water is also retained. Sodium and water increase together in similar proportions, so serum sodium levels are within normal limits. Because the ECF remains isotonic, the cells of the body do not swell or shrink and there are no symptoms of cerebral irritability or depression. The result of this isotonic imbalance is increased volume of ECF, which causes edema and circulatory overload. Patients who are retaining sodium and fluid are placed on a low-sodium diet (2 g/day or less). Processed foods, dairy products, and salty foods are high in sodium.

## Potassium

Potassium ($K^+$) is the major intracellular cation. It is responsible for ICF balance, a regular heart rhythm, conduction of neuromuscular impulses, conversion of glucose to energy in the cell, protein synthesis, and regulation of acid-base balance. The normal potassium range is 3.5 to 5 mEq/L. This is the amount in the ECF that can be measured by diagnostic testing. It is an indirect measurement of the level of potassium found in the cell, where it is much more abundant.

> ### NURSE ALERT
>
> **The body does not store potassium well, so a deficit can occur quickly if potassium intake is poor or the loss excessive.**

Potassium affects acid-base balance because it acts as part of the body's buffer system. If the body becomes acidotic **(acidosis),** hydrogen ions move into the cell to reduce their number in the ECF. As hydrogen enters the cell, potassium exits in exchange for hydrogen ions, which raises the serum level of potassium. This elevated serum potassium level is called a false positive because actual levels of potassium in the body have not changed. In **alkalosis** the plasma is low in hydrogen ions, so hydrogen leaves the cell and enters the plasma to compensate. Potassium then leaves the plasma and enters the cell, and **hypokalemia** results. In these cases, the potassium imbalance is treated by correcting the acid or base imbalance.

Plasma potassium falls about 0.6 mEq/L for each 0.1 unit rise in blood pH. A level below 3 mEq/L is toxic. Plasma potassium increases about 0.6 mEq/L for each 0.1 unit fall in blood pH. Regardless of the cause,

---

| BOX 27-6 | NURSING PROCESS |
| --- | --- |

## SODIUM EXCESS: HYPERNATREMIA

**ASSESSMENT**

- Plasma sodium >150 mEq/L
- Dry, sticky mucous membranes
- Dry tongue
- Flushed appearance
- Thirst
- Oliguria
- Increased BP
- Elevated temperature
- Weakness
- Irritability, excitability
- Disorientation
- Shallow, rapid breathing
- Fluttering eyelids
- Muscular spasm
- Seizures
- Stupor
- Coma

**NURSING DIAGNOSIS**

- Risk for injury related to hypernatremia

**NURSING INTERVENTIONS**

- Encourage low-sodium diet if ordered.
- Observe skin and mucous membranes.
- Maintain accurate I&O records.
- Monitor administration of IV fluids.
- Monitor vital signs.
- Administer muscle relaxants and/or diuretics as ordered.
- Observe seizure precautions.
- Maintain life support systems during therapy.

**EVALUATION OF EXPECTED OUTCOMES**

- Serum sodium levels decreased
- Deficit of water corrected
- Rapid correction avoided
- Efficacy of treatment determined
- Temperature and BP within normal limits
- Muscle spasms controlled

a serum potassium level below 3 mEq/L or above 5.5 mEq/L can produce toxic effects.

The role of potassium in neuromuscular function is to excite or irritate nerve cells, resulting in muscular contraction. Smooth, skeletal, and cardiac muscle depend on potassium for proper contraction and function. Heart muscle is particularly sensitive to an imbalance.

Large amounts of potassium are found in secretions and excretions of the body such as sweat, saliva, gastric juice, and stool. Unlike with sodium, the body has no effective mechanism for conserving potassium and continues to excrete potassium in the urine even when the levels are already low. Because 90% of the potassium is excreted in the urine, levels increase if kidney function is impaired. To replenish potassium stores, 40 to 60 mEq of potassium are needed daily.

**Potassium deficit.** Probably the most common cause of potassium deficit, or hypokalemia, in the United States is the use of diuretics without potassium supplementation. Loop diuretics, like furosemide (Lasix), and thiazide diuretics, like chlorothiazide (Diuril), increase potassium excretion. Loop diuretics are drugs that act by inhibiting the active reabsorption of chloride ions in the ascending limb of Henle's loop. Because chloride draws sodium with it, sodium reabsorption is also prevented. Therefore sodium chloride is retained in the tubule and excreted in urine, carrying water with it. Thiazide diuretics block sodium and chloride reabsorption in the distal convoluted tubule, which results in increased excretion of sodium, chloride, and water. With both loop and thiazide diuretics, the high concentration of sodium in the distal convoluted tubule causes an increased exchange of sodium and potassium, which in turn causes additional potassium to be pulled in and excreted.

Some diuretics spare potassium because they act in ways that do not cause potassium excretion. An example is spironolactone (Aldactone), which inhibits the action of aldosterone in the distal tubule. Aldosterone normally causes more sodium to be reabsorbed in the distal tubule, and potassium is excreted. When its action is inhibited by Aldactone, less sodium is reabsorbed. It is excreted and at the same time potassium is "spared."

Other factors that contribute to potassium loss are insufficient potassium intake; inefficient gastrointestinal absorption; and abnormal gastrointestinal losses as a result of diarrhea, vomiting, and ileostomy drainage. Metabolic alkalosis causes potassium to move into the cell in exchange for hydrogen ions, which reduces extracellular potassium levels. This condition is corrected by treating the alkalosis rather than by administering potassium.

## OLDER ADULT CONSIDERATIONS

A high percentage of older adults take diuretics to treat hypertension. This places them at high risk for a potassium deficit. Potassium supplements are prescribed to offset the potassium loss. Teach the importance of taking both medications at all times and never to stop one without stopping both. Many older adults also take digitalis to strengthen heart function, which can produce toxic effects if potassium is low. Watch for signs of potassium deficit and digitalis toxicity. Anorexia may be the first sign for both.

## NURSE ALERT

The following are characteristics of patients at risk for potassium deficit:
- Taking loop or thiazide diuretics
- Unable to intake anything by mouth
- Severe anorexia (chemotherapy)
- Unable to chew or swallow
- Gastric suction applied
- Severe diarrhea
- Stress

*Effects of stress on serum potassium levels.* Stress stimulates the pituitary gland, which causes the release of ADH from the posterior pituitary. ADH causes the body to retain water and sodium and to reduce urine output. This action maintains blood volume, which may be needed if one is threatened physiologically or psychologically. Stress also causes the adrenal cortex to secrete aldosterone, which results in the retention of sodium, chloride, and water and in the loss of potassium. Therefore stress can be a factor in hypokalemia.

## NURSE ALERT

If a patient states that he or she is too worn out to do anything, or feels "washed out," suspect a potassium deficiency. Ask about other symptoms.

***Assessment.*** Many of the signs and symptoms of potassium deficit result from its effect on the nervous and muscular systems. As a result of the deficit, the nerve cells are not as "excited" as they need to be to produce good muscle function. Skeletal muscle weakness and fatigue are common early complaints. The decreasing tone of the smooth muscle of the gastrointestinal tract can produce symptoms of anorexia, vomiting, distention, and possible paralytic ileus. Decreasing blood pressure, a weak pulse, faint heart sounds, and paralysis of the respiratory muscles are later signs. Cardiac arrhythmias are common, and the electrocardiogram may show a flattened T wave and the presence of a U wave (Figure 27-8). Ventricular tachycardia and cardiac arrest may occur when the levels are very low. Hypokalemia reduces the ability of the renal tubules to concentrate waste, which results in an increased fluid loss in urinary output. Laboratory data show low potassium levels in plasma.

***Intervention.*** Hypokalemia is treated with oral or IV supplements of potassium chloride (KCl). KCl should not be given if urine output is less than 30 ml per hour because excretion of potassium will be inadequate, which quickly results in **hyperkalemia.** Because of the effect of potassium on the cardiac muscle, a deficit should not be corrected rapidly. Correcting the deficit too rapidly can also cause tetany. KCl supplements added to IV solutions should never exceed 60 mEq/L, and 40 mEq/L is preferred. The rate of IV administration of KCl should not exceed 20 to 40 mEq/hr to prevent hyperkalemia and cardiac arrest. KCl is always diluted when administered intravenously. It is never given as a bolus IV push because the concentrated solution can cause cardiac arrest. Even in solution, KCl can be very irritating to the vein at the site of entry. Central venous lines inserted in the subclavian or a peripheral vein are preferred. Any underlying disease that is causing the potassium deficit must be identified and treated.

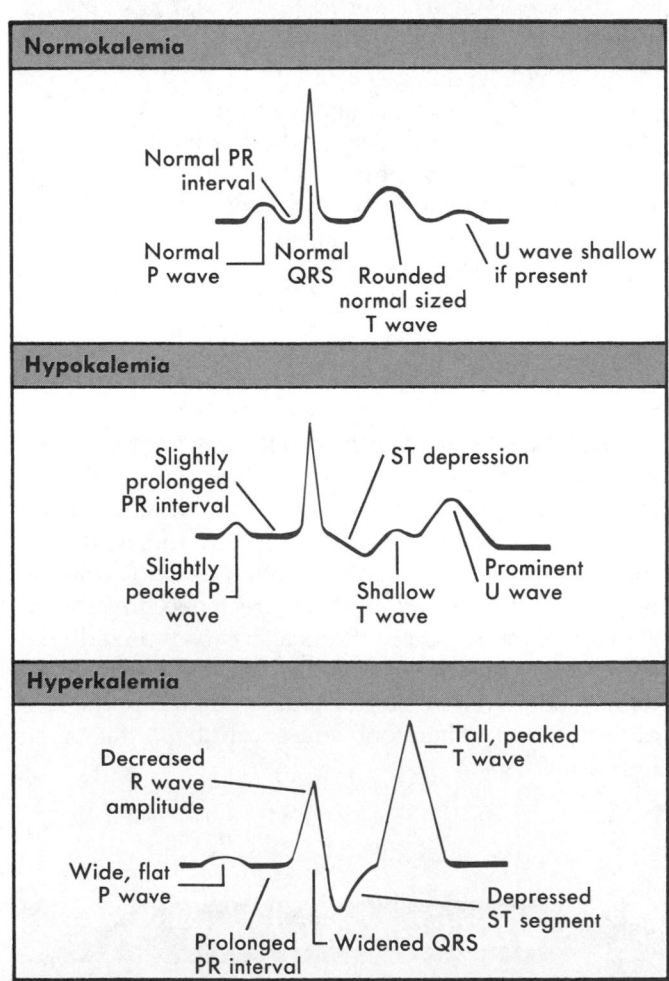

**Figure 27-8** ECG changes with potassium imbalance. (From McCance KL, Huether SE: *Pathophysiology: the biologic basis for disease in adults and children,* ed 2, St Louis, 1994, Mosby.)

## NURSE ALERT

**When KCl is administered intravenously, it is always mixed in solution. Give slowly and never exceed 20 to 40 mEq/hr.**

Mild deficits can be treated with a dietary intake of potassium. Preventing and treating deficits requires a knowledge of dietary sources of potassium (Box 27-7). Individuals who are taking diuretics that cause potassium loss, especially thiazide and loop diuretics, need to increase their dietary intake of potassium and need to know the signs and symptoms of a deficit. At the earliest sign they should increase intake and report their symptoms to their health care provider (Box 27-8).

***Hypokalemia and the patient taking digitalis.*** Digitalis is a cardiotonic drug that is used to slow conduction from the sinoatrial node to the atrioventricular node and strengthen the heartbeat. It is given to a patient with a failing heart to increase the heart's capability as a pump, a positive inotropic effect. Inotropic drugs increase the force of contraction of the heart, which improves its efficiency. Frequently the same patient is taking diuretics, which act to reduce ECF volume and reduce the workload of the pumping heart. Loop and thiazide diuretics cause a loss of potassium, so the patient taking drugs of this type is at a greater risk of potassium deficiency. When the potassium level falls

BOX 27-7

## SOURCES OF POTASSIUM (in mg)

| | |
|---|---|
| Butternut squash, 1 cup baked, 1200 | Prune juice, 1 cup, 600 |
| Lima beans, dry, 1 cup cooked, 1200 | Parsnips, 1 cup cooked, 590 |
| Spinach, 1 cup cooked, 1160 | Split peas, 1 cup cooked, 590 |
| Black beans, 1 cup cooked, 1000 | Blackstrap molasses, 1 tablespoon, 580 |
| Soybeans, 1 cup cooked, 970 | Dates, 10 medium, 520 |
| Pinto beans, 1 cup cooked, 940 | Potato, 1 medium, cooked, 500 |
| Navy beans, 1 cup cooked, 790 | Orange juice, 1 cup, 500 |
| Acorn squash, ¼, baked, 750 | Skim milk powder, ¼ cup, 490 |
| Green lima beans, 1 cup cooked, 720 | Beet greens, 1 cup, 480 |
| Papaya, 1 medium, 710 | Banana, 1 medium, 440 |
| Cantaloupe, ½ medium, 680 | Low-fat milk, 1 cup, 430 |
| Avocado, ½ medium, 650 | Kohlrabi, 1 cup cooked, 430 |
| Raisins, ½ cup, 650 | Peas, fresh, 1 cup, 420 |
| Kidney beans, 1 cup cooked, 630 | Brussels sprouts, 1 cup cooked, 420 |
| Chard, 1 cup cooked, 600 | Nectarine, 1 medium, 410 |

BOX 27-8

# NURSING PROCESS

## POTASSIUM DEFICIT: HYPOKALEMIA

### ASSESSMENT

- Plasma potassium <3.5 mEq/L
- Muscular weakness
- Fatigue
- Vertigo
- Electrocardiographic changes
- T wave flattened
- U wave present/prominent
- Anorexia
- Vomiting
- Distention
- Paralytic ileus
- Decreasing blood pressure
- Weak pulse
- Faint heart sounds
- Respiratory muscle paralysis

### NURSING DIAGNOSIS

- Risk for injury related to hypokalemia

### NURSING INTERVENTIONS

- Note serum potassium level.
- Encourage diet high in potassium if indicated.

- Monitor administration of replacement solutions.
- Assist if ambulating to prevent injury.
- Monitor ECG results.
- Monitor bowel sounds and palpate and measure abdomen for distention.
- Maintain accurate I&O records.
- Observe for metabolic alkalosis (secondary to hypokalemia causing shift of hydrogen to the cell so needed $K^+$ can move from cell to plasma; metabolic alkalosis can also cause hypokalemia).
- Monitor vital signs.

### EVALUATION OF EXPECTED OUTCOMES

- Potassium level slowly returns to normal
- No falls
- Safety maintained
- Changes in heart rhythm secondary to decreased potassium detected at onset; cardiac arrest prevented
- Absence of tingling and twitching; pH normal
- Bowel sounds present, all quadrants
- Shock and respiratory arrest prevented

below normal, a patient who is taking digitalis is more likely to develop a toxic reaction to the drug.

Digitalis toxicity can be mild and can cause anorexia, nausea, and visual disturbances in which the visual field appears to have a yellow cast. Symptoms can also be severe and lead to fatal arrhythmias (irregular heart rhythms). Most patients receiving digitalis and diuretics have diseased hearts that may be more likely to have irregular rhythms.

> ## NURSE ALERT
>
> A patient who develops hypokalemia while taking digitalis is likely to develop a toxic reaction, which could be fatal. The nurse must observe the patient for symptoms of potassium deficit and teach the patient to do the same. The nurse must also teach patients that these drugs, as well as all drugs, should be taken as prescribed and that the patient should not change medication dosages without first consulting a physician.

**Potassium excess.** Hyperkalemia occurs most often when the kidneys are unable to excrete potassium adequately (renal failure). It can also occur soon after massive injury, such as burns and crushing injuries. Cellular destruction releases large amounts of intracellular potassium into the ECF. Severe infections and chemotherapy with cytotoxic drugs can also cause cellular destruction (catabolism). The destroyed cells release their intracellular potassium into the interstitial fluid. Administering blood that is near its expiration date may also cause an excess of potassium as a result of the breakdown of old red blood cells. Metabolic acidosis causes potassium to leave the cell and enter the ECF in exchange for hydrogen ions, which results in an elevated serum potassium. Adrenal insufficiency leads to retention of potassium in the serum because aldosterone is deficient and sodium is not reabsorbed. Therefore the potassium that is normally excreted in exchange for sodium remains in the body. Administering IV potassium solutions too rapidly may also lead to a potassium excess.

Many of the early symptoms of potassium excess are nonspecific. Electrocardiogram (ECG) changes usually occur early, but often the patient is not monitored for these changes. Because potassium plays a major role in neuromuscular activity, muscle twitching is an early sign. Facial and respiratory muscles may become involved, and paresthesias (numbness, tingling) of the face and tongue may develop. Gastroin-

testinal symptoms of nausea, diarrhea, and intestinal colic are also related to neuromuscular overexcitability. Flaccid paralysis may develop. The most serious effect of a high potassium level is on the cardiac muscles. Cell excitability is increased, but cardiac contractions are weaker, which can result in a dilated, flaccid heart. Tachycardia is seen and is followed by bradycardia and dysrhythmia, which may lead to cardiac arrest. The conduction system of the heart is disturbed, and ectopic beats appear on the ECG. Changes include tall, peaked T waves; a shortened Q-T interval; a prolonged PR interval followed by a disappearance of the P wave; and a widening of the QRS complex (see Figure 27-8). Laboratory data indicate levels of potassium in the plasma in excess of 5.5 mEq/L. ECG changes become more severe at higher levels.

> ## NURSE ALERT
>
> Monitor cardiac function closely in hyperkalemia. Cardiac cell overstimulation leads to life-threatening changes in heart rate and rhythm. Tachycardia is followed by bradycardia. ECG monitoring is necessary.

The treatment of potassium excess varies according to the type and severity of the underlying problem. In mild cases, potassium intake is avoided and any IV solutions should omit potassium. An ion-exchange resin, sodium polystyrene sulfonate (Kayexalate), can be used orally, rectally, or by nasogastric tube to treat hyperkalemia. It binds with potassium in the gastrointestinal tract and is eliminated. When given rectally, it is administered as a retention enema and retained for 30 to 60 minutes. A potassium-wasting diuretic such as furosemide also brings down potassium levels by causing potassium to be excreted.

If the condition is acute, 10 or 20 U of regular insulin is administered along with intravenous hypertonic dextrose solution (25% to 50%). As the dextrose accompanied by insulin enters the cell, potassium is carried along (facilitated diffusion) and lowers potassium levels in the ECF. The effects are temporary but provide time for the other measures to restore balance.

Sodium bicarbonate may also be added to alkalinize the plasma. Sodium bicarbonate causes hydrogen to enter the plasma from the cells in an attempt to restore acidity. Potassium leaves the plasma and enters the cell in exchange for hydrogen, thus lowering serum potassium. Sodium bicarbonate also provides sodium, which antagonizes the effects of potassium on the myocardium. This effect also is only temporary. Peri-

| BOX 27-9 | NURSING PROCESS |
| --- | --- |

## POTASSIUM EXCESS: HYPERKALEMIA

**ASSESSMENT**

- Plasma potassium >5.0 mEq/L
- Electrocardiographic changes: tall, peaked T waves, shortened Q-T interval, prolonged PR interval followed by disappearance of the P wave, widened QRS complex; bradycardia, arrhythmias leading to cardiac arrest
- Tachycardia followed by bradycardia
- Muscle twitching and weakness
- Hyperactive deep-tendon reflexes
- Nausea, diarrhea, intestinal colic (abdominal cramps)
- Paresthesias of the face, tongue, and extremities
- Ascending paralysis in severe cases; could result in respiratory arrest

**NURSING DIAGNOSIS**

- Risk for injury related to hyperkalemia

**NURSING INTERVENTIONS**

- Note serum potassium results; encourage diet low in potassium if taking food.

- Monitor ECG results, vital signs.
- Administer calcium solutions to neutralize potassium; use with caution if patient is receiving digitalis preparations.
- Monitor muscle tone.
- Monitor deep-tendon reflexes.
- Check bowel sounds; observe level of hydration.
- Observe and report paresthesias.
- Check respirations q15min to qh.

**EVALUATION OF EXPECTED OUTCOMES**

- Potassium level slowly returns to normal
- Abnormal electrical conductions detected and treated at onset; normal sinus rhythm resumed
- Muscle activity normotonic
- Bowel sounds present, all quadrants; no report of nausea or diarrhea; well hydrated
- No report of numbness
- Respirations 14/min or more

---

toneal dialysis and hemodialysis can also be used in emergencies.

IV administration of calcium may be ordered to stimulate heart contraction by antagonizing the effects of excess potassium on heart muscle. However, calcium solutions should be used cautiously with patients who are receiving digitalis preparations. Calcium sensitizes the heart to digitalis, and digitalis toxicity can result and cause severe visual, gastrointestinal, neuropsychologic, and cardiac disturbances (Box 27-9).

## Calcium

Calcium (Ca) is absorbed through the small intestine. Vitamin D is essential for the absorption of calcium. The majority of calcium in the body is stored in the teeth and bones. It is absorbed by the bones from the ECF during bone formation. It also flows out of the bone and back to the ECF, a process called *bone resorption*. Although normal levels of serum calcium are low, it is an important ion for the transmission of nerve impulses. Intracellular calcium is essential for the contraction of muscle tissue. Extracellular calcium is necessary for blood clotting (factor IV of the coagulation cascade) and for tooth and bone formation. It is needed for the absorption and use of vitamin $B_{12}$ and is essential for maintaining a normal heart rhythm. Extracellular calcium stabilizes the cell membrane and blocks sodium transport into the cell, thus decreasing the excitability of the cell. A decreased serum calcium level causes increased nerve and muscle cell excitability. Many enzyme systems are activated by calcium.

Calcium levels are regulated by the parathyroid hormone and by calcitonin. When serum calcium levels drop, the parathyroid gland increases secretion of the parathyroid hormone, which draws calcium from the bones to the circulating serum (bone resorption). Parathyroid hormone also increases gastrointestinal absorption of calcium and increases renal tubule reabsorption of calcium.

Calcitonin is the other hormone that regulates calcium balance. It is produced by the thyroid and is stimulated by high serum calcium levels. It opposes the action of parathyroid hormone and thus lowers the serum calcium level by decreasing gastrointestinal absorption, by increasing bone mineralization (preventing bone resorption), and by promoting renal excretion.

Laboratory tests can measure ionized serum calcium or total serum calcium. It is more difficult to measure ionized calcium, so the routine test measures total calcium. Total calcium is measured in milligrams, and the normal level is 8.6 to 10.6 mg/dl. Ionized calcium is measured in milliequivalents, and the normal range is 4.5 to 5.5 mEq/L. Total calcium includes the calcium bound to albumin and other proteins, which is about 44% of the circulating calcium in the body. The remainder is ionized and is the portion that is biologically active and can cause problems by being too high or too low. The amount of bound calcium decreases when serum albumin drops, which causes a decrease in total serum calcium. Therefore a normal serum calcium level accompanied by low serum albumin is actually indicative of **hypercalcemia** because the ionized calcium now represents a higher percentage of the serum calcium. Conversely, a high albumin level causes bound calcium to increase. Therefore a normal total calcium level accompanied by hyperalbuminemia actually indicates an ionized calcium deficit, or **hypocalcemia.** Serum pH also affects calcium binding to albumin. Acidosis decreases calcium binding, which leads to more ionized calcium. Alkalosis increases calcium binding. Box 27-10 describes a method used to determine a "correct" total calcium reading in the presence of high or low albumin levels. It is provided to illustrate the relationship between albumin and calcium.

**Calcium deficit.** A calcium deficit, or hypocalcemia, is often associated with excessive gastrointestinal losses. Because calcium levels in the serum are regulated by the parathyroid glands, hypoactive or absent glands can also lead to a calcium deficit. When a thyroidectomy is performed, the parathyroid glands can be removed inadvertently, or postoperative edema can temporarily restrict the flow of parathyroid hormone and cause a calcium deficit. Pancreatic diseases (e.g., acute pancreatitis), massive subcutaneous infections, and peritonitis may lead to extraction of calcium from the ECF and cause a calcium deficit. Multiple blood transfusions can cause hypocalcemia because the citrate used to anticoagulate the blood binds with calcium.

**Assessment.** The signs and symptoms of calcium deficit result from neuromuscular irritability because there is not enough calcium to decrease the excitability of the nerve and muscle cells. Tetany occurs, which is characterized by tingling of the extremities, muscle cramps and twitching, carpopedal spasms (sharp flexion of the wrist and ankle joints), and convulsions. Tetany is a state of increased neuroexcitability and sustained muscle contraction. Because the peripheral nerves are affected first, carpopedal spasm is one of the first signs of tetany (Figure 27-9, A). Early signs of tetany are evident if carpal spasm occurs when the brachial artery is occluded by constriction, such as when a blood pressure cuff is applied to the upper arm

**BOX 27-10**

**FORMULA TO CORRECT CALCIUM READINGS DISTORTED BY ABNORMAL ALBUMIN LEVELS**

**HYPOALBUMINEMIA**
1 Subtract patient's serum albumin level from the normal level (4.0 mg/dl).
2 Multiply that remainder by a correction factor of 0.8.
3 Add that product to the total calcium level found in the laboratory results.

**Example:**
1 4.0 mg/dl (normal serum albumin)
−1.7 mg/dl (patient's albumin level)
2.3 mg/dl (remainder)
2 2.3 mg/dl (remainder)
×0.8 (correction factor)
1.84 mg/dl (product)
3 1.84
+10.1 mg/dl (patient's total calcium level)
11.94 mg/dl adjusted total calcium level, which indicates hypercalcemia

**HYPERALBUMINEMIA**
1 Subtract normal albumin (4.0 mg/dl) from the patient's albumin level.
2 Multiply the remainder by a correction factor of 0.8.
3 Subtract that product from the total calcium level found in the laboratory results.

**Example:**
1 6.4 mg/dl (patient's albumin)
−4.0 mg/dl (normal albumin)
2.4 mg/dl (remainder)
2 2.4 mg/dl (remainder)
×0.8 (correction factor)
1.92 mg/dl (product)
3 8.6 mg/dl (patient's total calcium level)
−1.92
6.68 mg/dl adjusted total calcium level, which indicates hypocalcemia

and inflated. Carpal spasm is evident within 3 minutes if hypocalcemia is present. This phenomenon is called *Trousseau's sign.* Patients can also be checked for Chvostek's sign, which involves tapping the face over the facial nerve in front of the ear (Figure 27-9, B and C). If the face twitches, the results are positive and indicate a calcium deficit. Laryngeal stridor, dysphagia, dysarthria, cardiac dysrhythmia, and convulsions are also seen with tetany. ECG changes and x-ray films of bones are helpful in establishing a diagnosis. Changes in the blood clotting process can also be observed. Laboratory data indicate low calcium levels in the urine and plasma.

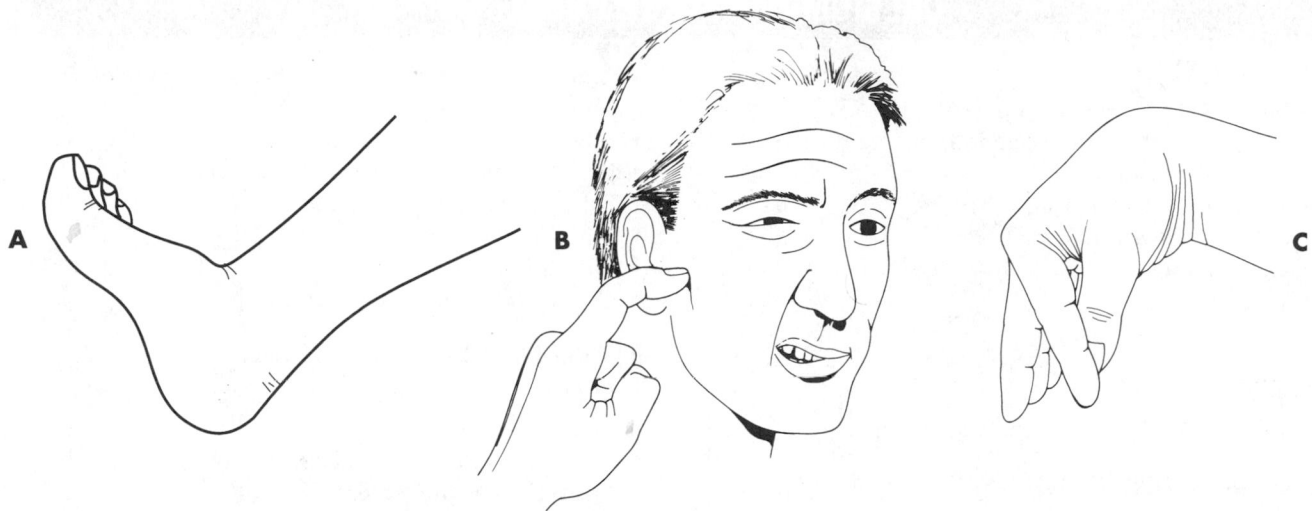

**Figure 27-9** **A,** Carpopedal spasm—hyperflexion of the wrist and ankle. **B,** Chvostek's sign—a contraction of the facial muscle elicited in response to a light tap over the facial nerve in front of the ear. **C,** Trousseau's sign—a carpal spasm (hyperflexion at the wrist) induced by inflating a blood pressure cuff beyond the systolic pressure.

*Intervention.* Symptoms of calcium deficit must be treated immediately. Any patient who has had thyroid surgery must be watched closely for signs and symptoms of calcium deficit. Calcium levels must be returned to normal while the cause is being identified and treated. Calcium carbonate can be given orally if symptoms are less severe. IV calcium gluconate is administered if symptoms are life threatening. The IV infusion site must be checked frequently because calcium infiltration can cause sloughing of the tissue. Calcium is not given intramuscularly because it precipitates (separates out of solution) in the muscle. Calcium-rich foods are prescribed along with vitamin D supplements to help absorb calcium from the gastrointestinal tract. Synthetic parathyroid hormone (parathormone) can also be given (Box 27-11).

---

**NURSE ALERT**

Observe the patient after a thyroidectomy for calcium deficit. Ask the patient about tingling of the fingertips, and look for Trousseau's sign when taking blood pressure readings.

---

**Calcium excess.** Hypercalcemia is a state of excess calcium in the serum. It most often occurs as a result of a tumor of the parathyroid glands. However, it is also associated with excessive administration of vitamin D,

multiple fractures, multiple myeloma, and prolonged immobilization. Renal diseases may prevent calcium excretion and result in abnormally high calcium levels in the body fluids.

Calcium excess produces depression of neuromuscular activity. Signs and symptoms include lethargy and decreased muscle tone. The patient demonstrates decreased memory span, confusion, disorientation, and fatigue. Nausea, vomiting, and constipation may occur, and cardiac dysrhythmias are evident. Deep bone pain may be present if the excess serum calcium is caused by bone resorption. High levels of serum calcium can result in kidney stones, which cause flank pain. As calcium levels continue to rise, psychoses and coma may develop. Laboratory data indicate high levels of calcium in the urine and plasma.

*Intervention.* Treatment of hypercalcemia is aimed at increasing urinary excretion of calcium. This can be accomplished by administering a loop diuretic. If the patient can take fluids by mouth, he or she must drink 3000 to 4000 ml of fluid daily to promote renal excretion of calcium and decrease the possibility of renal calculus formation. Synthetic calcitonin may be given to reduce gastrointestinal absorption, increase return of calcium to the bone, and promote renal excretion. Mithramycin, a cytotoxic antibiotic, inhibits bone resorption and thus lowers serum calcium. Corticosteroids may be used to decrease bone turnover and reabsorption in the kidney tubules. Weight-bearing exercise is encouraged to enhance bone mineralization. The underlying cause must be identified and treated (Box 27-12).

BOX 27-11

## NURSING PROCESS

# CALCIUM DEFICIT: HYPOCALCEMIA

### ASSESSMENT

- Serum calcium level <8 mg/dl
- Tingling of extremities; abdominal cramps; carpopedal spasm
- Positive Chvostek's sign
- Positive Trousseau's sign
- Convulsions
- ECG changes
- Delayed blood clotting

### NURSING DIAGNOSIS

- Risk for injury related to hypocalcemia

### NURSING INTERVENTIONS

- Encourage increased dietary intake of calcium.
- Monitor administration of IV solutions containing calcium; monitor serum calcium.
- Instruct patient regarding expected symptoms.
- Establish and maintain communication with patient, encouraging symptom report.
- Check for Chvostek's sign.
- Compress brachial artery to check for Trousseau's sign.
- Monitor neurologic status.
- Maintain quiet environment, subdued lighting.
- Establish seizure precautions.
- Monitor vital signs.
- Monitor clotting times.
- Observe for hemorrhagic areas.

### EVALUATION OF EXPECTED OUTCOMES

- Mild calcium deficit corrected through dietary measures
- Bradycardia, which is caused by giving too much IV calcium, is prevented
- Patient reports altered neuromuscular sensations
- Absence of facial twitch
- Absence of carpal spasm
- Absence of seizure activity
- Injury prevented
- Arrhythmias controlled
- Bleeding avoided

BOX 27-12

## NURSING PROCESS

# CALCIUM EXCESS: HYPERCALCEMIA

### ASSESSMENT

- Serum calcium >11 mg/dl
- Lethargy
- Decreased muscle tone
- Deep bone pain
- Flank pain
- Kidney stones (renal calculi)
- Hypertension
- Nausea and vomiting
- Thirst
- Anorexia
- Constipation
- Psychoses
- Coma, cardiac arrest

### NURSING DIAGNOSIS

- Risk for injury related to hypercalcemia

### NURSING INTERVENTIONS

- Eliminate calcium from diet.
- Use caution if patient is receiving digitalis.
- Monitor neurologic status.
- Encourage patient to communicate symptoms.
- Medicate for pain as ordered.
- Observe for passage of calculi.
- Strain urine.
- Monitor vital signs.
- Provide IV isotonic saline as ordered or PO fluids if tolerated (3000-4000 ml daily).
- Provide small, frequent meals.
- Encourage mobility as patient condition permit.
- Reorient patient to reality.
- Maintain life support systems.
- Support family members.

### EVALUATION OF EXPECTED OUTCOMES

- Calcium level within normal limits
- Myocardial response to digitalis monitored; arrhythmias prevented
- Able to perform activities of daily living
- Stones sent to laboratory if passed
- Blood pressure within normal limits
- Output equals intake
- Hydrated and able to take diet
- Optimal nutritional status maintained
- Constipation decreased
- Patient feels more secure, less fearful
- System integrity maintained throughout hypercalcemic period
- Family members able to voice their concerns

## Magnesium

Magnesium (Mg) is the second most abundant intracellular cation. Approximately half of the magnesium in the body is contained in the bone, and 40% to 50% is found in the cells of the heart, liver, and skeletal muscle. Approximately 1% is found in the ECF. Normal serum magnesium is 1.8 to 2.4 mEq/L. Magnesium depletion may be present even if levels are normal because such a small percentage is in the ECF sample that is analyzed. Magnesium activates many enzymes that are needed for carbohydrate and protein metabolism. Without magnesium, potassium is excreted to excess. Magnesium also influences the use of calcium and protein. It is involved in the sodium-potassium pump, which moves sodium out of and potassium into the cells. Therefore it plays a crucial role in maintaining normal muscle and nerve activity. Neuromuscular excitability is profoundly affected by alterations in serum magnesium. Recent studies indicate that magnesium protects the heart from damage by influencing cardiac enzyme activity and calcium and potassium levels in myocardial and vascular muscle tissue.

**Magnesium deficit.** A magnesium deficit (**hypomagnesemia**) is rarely the result of diet but does occur in cases of severe malnutrition, chronic alcoholism, prolonged diarrhea, intestinal malabsorption, prolonged nasogastric suction, and prolonged IV therapy that lacks magnesium. It is believed that chronic alcoholism accompanied by liver disease leads to a lack of digestive enzymes, which reduces magnesium absorption and causes a deficit. Hypoparathyroidism, prolonged diuretic therapy as with congestive heart failure, and the diuresing phase of renal failure can also produce a magnesium deficit. Patients with gastrointestinal cancer who are receiving chemotherapy are also at increased risk. The cancer interferes with absorption, and the patient is often anorexic, which further reduces magnesium intake.

Increased neuromuscular and central nervous system irritability result from a magnesium deficit and produce symptoms similar to those of a calcium deficit, such as agitation, paresthesias, hyperreflexia, tremors, leg cramps, muscle twitching, jerking, tetany, and convulsions. Cardiac arrhythmias occur in severe cases. Serum calcium and magnesium levels can provide an accurate diagnosis (Box 27-13).

The patient with a magnesium deficit has discomfort as a result of neuromuscular excitability. The nurse should move the patient and handle the patient's extremities gently. The nurse should also keep the room quiet and the lighting subdued to reduce stimulation. A linen cradle should be used to reduce the weight of bed linens, which could provoke spasms. If an oral diet is allowed, soft foods will prevent choking and aspiration from laryngeal or esophageal spasms.

Treatment of a mild deficit requires oral supplements and an increased intake of magnesium-rich foods such as nuts, bananas, peanut butter, whole grains, and green vegetables. Diet can be supplemented with magnesium-based antacids such as Mylanta, Gelusil, Maalox, or Milk of Magnesia. A more

---

**BOX 27-13**

**NURSING PROCESS**

## MAGNESIUM DEFICIT: HYPOMAGNESEMIA

**ASSESSMENT**
- Serum Mg 1.0 mEq/L or less
- Leg cramps, agitation
- Esophageal and laryngeal spasm
- Muscle twitching, hyperreflexia, jerking (tetany)
- Convulsions

**NURSING DIAGNOSIS**
- Risk for injury related to hypomagnesemia

**NURSING INTERVENTIONS**
- Monitor serum Mg levels daily or after each 16 mEq supplement of Mg is administered.
- Provide a bed cradle for linens, a quiet room, and subdued lighting.
- Provide a soft diet if PO food allowed.
- Check deep-tendon reflexes.
- Administer Mg as ordered.
- Monitor urine output and vital signs.

**EVALUATION OF EXPECTED OUTCOMES**
- Serum Mg between 1.0 and 3.0 mEq/L
- Agitation reduced; cramps not evident
- Swallows without choking or aspirating food
- Muscle activity normotonic
- Urine output >30 ml/hr or physician notified
- Respiratory rate >12 or physician notified
- BP within normal limits

severe deficit requires IV or intramuscular administration of magnesium sulfate. Oral replacement can be used to prevent a deficit in individuals who are predisposed to a deficit.

Magnesium given intravenously must be given slowly to prevent cardiac or respiratory arrest. The patient receiving magnesium sulfate intravenously or intramuscularly must be observed closely to avoid excess. Renal function must be observed and the physician notified if output falls below 30 ml per hour. Without adequate renal function, an excess can develop easily because magnesium is excreted by the kidneys. Vital signs and deep-tendon reflexes must be checked hourly. A decrease in blood pressure, weak or absent deep tendon reflexes, or a decrease in respirations below 12 per minute indicate toxicity. In addition, symptoms of flushing, generalized warmth, thirst, sweating, anxiety followed by lethargy, and decreased motor function should be reported immediately and the drug discontinued. Toxicity can produce coma. In the event that toxicity develops, calcium gluconate should be administered because it antagonizes the action of magnesium and reverses the symptoms of toxicity. If calcium gluconate is administered via the same IV line used for the magnesium, the line must be flushed thoroughly before the calcium gluconate is added because the calcium will precipitate with the sulfates of the magnesium preparation and stop the infusion.

> ## NURSE ALERT
>
> **Magnesium given intravenously must be administered slowly to prevent cardiac or respiratory arrest.**

**Magnesium excess.** A magnesium excess (hypermagnesemia) is less common. It is found in patients with renal insufficiency who are unable to excrete magnesium adequately. It is also found in severely dehydrated patients who develop oliguria and magnesium retention. Patients with renal failure must avoid antacids that contain magnesium, such as Gelusil. A magnesium excess depresses neuromuscular and central nervous system functions. Symptoms include a generalized sense of warmth; decreased deep-tendon reflexes, which leads to flaccid paralysis; low blood pressure; depressed respirations; and drowsiness and lethargy, which lead to coma and respiratory arrest (Box 27-14). The ECG reveals arrhythmias, and cardiac arrest may result. Treatment must be aimed at correcting the underlying cause. Dialysis may be necessary to eliminate the excess and prevent life-threatening symptoms.

---

◁ **BOX 27-14** ▷       **NURSING PROCESS**

## MAGNESIUM EXCESS: HYPERMAGNESEMIA

**ASSESSMENT**

- Serum Mg 3.0 mEq/L or more
- Nausea and vomiting
- Generalized sense of warmth
- Decreased deep-tendon reflexes
- Flaccid paralysis may develop
- Low blood pressure
- Depressed respirations
- Respiratory arrest
- Drowsiness and lethargy
- Coma
- Arrhythmias and cardiac arrest

**NURSING DIAGNOSIS**

- Risk for injury related to hypermagnesemia

**NURSING INTERVENTIONS**

- Monitor serum Mg levels.
- Prepare patient for dialysis if ordered.

- Observe and report sense of warmth.
- Observe deep-tendon reflexes qh or as ordered.
- Check movement of extremities.
- Check BP qh or as ordered.
- Monitor respirations; report drop to <14/min.
- Monitor level of consciousness qh or as ordered.
- Monitor cardiac rhythm.
- Maintain life support systems.

**EVALUATION OF EXPECTED OUTCOMES**

- Serum Mg between 1.0 and 3.0 mEq/L
- Tolerating normal diet
- No report of sense of warmth
- Normotensive
- Movement of extremities is retained
- BP within normal limits
- Respirations 14/min or above
- Alert, oriented
- Normal sinus rhythm

## Chloride

**Chloride deficit.** Chloride is the major extracellular anion. It is a component of hydrochloric acid in the stomach and plays a role in the transport of carbon dioxide by red blood cells. Chloride is excreted by the kidney and is affected by aldosterone secretion. When aldosterone is released to cause sodium reabsorption, chloride is also reabsorbed. Chloride is secreted into the gastrointestinal tract, and **hypochloremia** can occur if there is a loss of gastrointestinal secretions as seen in vomiting, diarrhea, and nasogastric suctioning. Plasma chloride levels change with and resemble sodium levels. Chloride is lost along with sodium in patients who are receiving diuretic therapy, but urinary loss of chloride may be greater than the loss of sodium. Gastric fluids contain a higher proportion of chloride, so a loss of gastrointestinal fluids causes more chloride than sodium to be lost. When chloride is depleted and unavailable for reabsorption with sodium, the bicarbonate ion is reabsorbed to maintain the cation-anion balance. The increase in bicarbonate may cause metabolic alkalosis. The normal chloride level is 96 to 106 mEq/L. Hypochloremia occurs at levels below 95 mEq/L. The symptoms of hypochloremia are the same as those of hyponatremia and metabolic alkalosis.

**Chloride excess. Hyperchloremia** occurs with hypernatremia because chloride ions move with sodium ions. Such movement occurs in a severely burned patient when fluid is remobilized from the edematous burned areas to the vascular compartments, usually a few days after the burn is sustained.

Hyperchloremia can also result from hyperaldosteronism or renal failure. Excessive aspirin ingestion and sodium polystyrene (Kayexalate), the drug used to treat hyperkalemia, can cause chloride excess. Excess chloride interferes with bicarbonate reabsorption and results in metabolic acidosis. Symptoms of hyperchloremia are those of acidosis: lethargy, confusion, weakness, and stupor. The patient's breathing becomes deep and labored as the lungs attempt to correct the problem by blowing off carbon dioxide to reduce carbonic acid. IV sodium bicarbonate is administered to return the pH to normal. The kidneys retain the bicarbonate and eliminate chloride. A change to slow, shallow breathing indicates that the patient has too much bicarbonate and is trying to conserve carbon dioxide to restore normal acidity. Frequent assessment is necessary.

## Phosphates

Phosphate levels vary inversely with calcium levels. A high calcium level usually means a low phosphate level and vice versa. The parathyroid hormone that promotes calcium uptake also inhibits absorption of phosphate. Both electrolytes are deficient when the imbalance is caused by malnutrition or malabsorption.

**Hypophosphatemia** results from inadequate intake, poor absorption (e.g., shortening of the gastrointestinal tract), loss caused by thiazide diuretics, hyperparathyroidism, and lead poisoning. Alkalosis reduces serum phosphate levels. Hypophosphatemia is treated with supplements of oral sodium and potassium phosphates. (NeutraPhos K). Severe cases require IV administration of sodium phosphate or potassium phosphate.

**Hyperphosphatemia** occurs most often in patients with renal failure. They also have hypocalcemia, and those symptoms are the most obvious. Patients with renal failure often take aluminum hydroxide or aluminum carbonate to bind phosphate in the gastrointestinal tract and prevent its absorption into the bloodstream.

## PROTEIN IMBALANCES

Plasma proteins attract water and act as colloids, which creates colloidal osmotic pressure within the vascular system.

Hyperproteinemia (protein excess) is rare but can occur with dehydration, which causes the blood to be more concentrated. Hypoproteinemia (protein deficit) can occur over a long period of time when intake is reduced, such as in anorexia, malnutrition, starvation, fad dieting, and true vegetarian diets. Gastrointestinal diseases involving poor absorption can result in a protein deficit. Surgery and severe burns require cell growth and repair, which increases the use of protein by the body. Inflammation can cause cell membrane changes that allow protein to shift out of the ECF to a "third space," as is seen with ascites. The breakdown of protein increases with increased metabolic and catabolic states such as fever, infection, and certain malignancies. Hemorrhages can cause a protein deficit, and large amounts of protein, especially albumin, are lost through the kidneys in nephrotic syndrome.

Major abdominal or chest surgery (e.g., coronary bypass surgery) involves massive tissue trauma, inflammation, increased catabolism, and damage to red blood cells. This combination of factors may result in protein loss, and fluids may shift to tissues because of the reduction in colloidal osmotic pressure. Generalized edema develops (second spacing), and the blood pressure drops because of reduced intravascular volume. Urine output is low.

Symptoms of protein deficit include edema (from decreased colloidal osmotic pressure), slow healing, anorexia, fatigue, and anemia. The body eventually breaks down tissue to obtain needed protein, which results in muscle loss. Infusion of IV fluids most likely increases the edema rather than raises intravascular volume. Administration of albumin restores colloidal osmotic pressure, draws the fluids back from the tissues, raises blood volume and blood pressure, and increases urinary output. The nurse should be alert to the development of and increase in edema in a postsurgical patient. A high-carbohydrate, high-protein diet with protein supplements is required to treat a protein deficit. Hyperalimentation may be necessary if the patient is unable to eat a normal diet or if the gastrointestinal system is not functioning.

# ACID-BASE IMBALANCES

## Hydrogen Ion Concentration

The normal composition of body fluids depends not only on the volume of fluid and concentration of various electrolytes but also on the concentration of the acids and bases, or alkalies, in the body. Acids are substances that can release hydrogen ions ($H^+$), and bases are substances that can accept hydrogen ions. It is the concentration of hydrogen ions that determines whether a solution is acidic, basic, or neutral. The pH scale measures the amount of acidity or alkalinity of fluids. On a scale of 1 to 14, a pH of 7 is neutral. Anything below 7 is considered acidic, and anything above 7 is considered alkaline. The normal pH of ECF ranges from 7.35 to 7.45 and therefore is slightly alkaline. The range required to support life is from 6.8 to 7.8.

## Acid-Base Regulation

The body controls pH with buffer systems, the lungs, and the kidneys. The buffers react immediately. The respiratory system responds almost instantaneously and begins to lose effectiveness in a few hours. The kidneys may need 6 to 10 hours to achieve acid-base balance in a younger adult, but in the elderly person it may take 18 to 48 hours (Weldy, 1996). Unlike the lungs, the kidney can reach and maintain a balance for a long period. If a problem exists with respiratory or kidney function, the body may not be able to successfully regulate acid-base balance.

## Buffer Systems

The buffer system is the primary regulator of acid-base balance. Buffers react with an acid or base to prevent a large change in pH. They act chemically to change strong acids into weaker acids or to bind with acids to neutralize their effect.

The primary buffer is the carbonic acid/bicarbonate system. Bicarbonate neutralizes hydrochloric acid (HCl) by combining with it and changing it to a weaker acid (carbonic acid) ($H_2CO_3$) and a salt (NaCl). A ratio of 20 parts of bicarbonate to 1 part carbonic acid maintains an adequate supply of bicarbonate to combine with and neutralize acids. The carbonic acid that is formed is broken down to water and carbon dioxide ($CO_2$). $CO_2$ is excreted by the lungs, and water is excreted by the lungs and kidneys. This action maintains the 20:1 ratio and the normal pH. A second buffer, the phosphate buffer system, works in a similar way.

The intracellular and extracellular proteins are also buffers. Their amino acids include free acid radicals, which can contribute hydrogen ions, and free basic radicals, which can dissociate and combine with hydrogen to form water. Hemoglobin is also a buffer. It regulates pH by shifting chloride in and out of red blood cells in exchange for bicarbonate. The level of oxygen in the blood triggers this chloride shift, which is capable of raising or lowering bicarbonate levels as needed. The cell acts as a buffer by shifting hydrogen into and out of the cell. If hydrogen is increased in the ECF, the cell accepts hydrogen in exchange for another cation, usually potassium because it is abundant in the cell.

## Pulmonary System

The lungs help maintain acid-base balance by controlling the amount of carbon dioxide that is released into the air during respiration. Carbonic acid in the ECF of the pulmonary capillaries dissociates into $CO_2$ and water. When respiration is suppressed, carbonic acid accumulates in the body fluids because less $CO_2$ is excreted. When respirations are stimulated, the levels of carbonic acid within the body fall. The rate and depth of respiration and thus excretion is regulated by the respiratory center in the medulla in the brain, which is triggered by the level of $CO_2$ and hydrogen ions.

## Renal System

The kidneys selectively excrete or resorb bicarbonate and excrete hydrogen ions as needed by the body.

## Alterations in Acid-Base Balance

Two general types of disturbances in the body result in an upset of the balance between the base bicarbonate and the carbonic acid. Body metabolic processes add base bicarbonate to or subtract it from the ECF. The respiratory process adds carbonic acid to or subtracts it from the ECF. Metabolic processes can also produce acid. Therefore a state of acidosis can be caused by lowering the amount of base bicarbonate or by increasing the amount of carbonic acid or metabolic acids. A state of alkalosis can be caused by increasing the amount of base bicarbonate or decreasing the amount of carbonic acid. Each of these conditions alters the ratio of base bicarbonate to carbonic acid. Acid-base imbalances can take one or a combination of these forms, each of which alters the ratio of base bicarbonate to carbonic acid.

## Metabolic Acidosis

A base bicarbonate deficit, or metabolic acidosis, can result either from the accumulation of too many acid by-products of metabolism or from the loss of bicarbonate. Abnormal metabolic processes such as diabetes, renal insufficiency or failure, and shock produce metabolic acidosis by the accumulation of acids within the body. Anaerobic metabolism produces lactic acidosis, and fasting or starvation can produce ketosis, caused by increased fat metabolism for energy. Excessive bicarbonate is lost in renal insufficiency and severe diarrhea; via ileostomy, ureterosigmoidostomy, intestinal or biliary fistula, and intestinal suction; and as a result of increased chloride levels.

The laboratory test used to differentiate between the two types of metabolic acidosis is the anion gap (or R factor). The anion gap is the difference between the concentration of the cations (sodium and potassium) and the sum of the chloride and bicarbonate anions. This difference reflects the concentration of anions in the ECF. When metabolic acidosis is caused by a loss of bicarbonate, the anion gap is normal at 13 mEq/L or below. When the cause is an excess of metabolic acids, the gap is increased above 13 mEq/L. Acidosis resulting from bicarbonate loss is called *normal anion gap acidosis;* acidosis resulting from excess metabolic acid is called *high anion gap acidosis* (Table 27-2).

Signs of metabolic acidosis include deep, rapid respirations; weakness; disorientation; diarrhea; and drowsiness leading to stupor and coma. Any state of acidosis depresses the central nervous system. The lungs attempt to compensate for the state of acidosis by increasing the rate and depth of respirations, which reduces the amount of carbonic acid in the system. This type of breathing is known as *Kussmaul's respiration.* The serum pH level is below 7.35, the pH of the urine is lower than normal, and the serum bicarbonate level is decreased or normal, depending on the cause. Serum potassium levels are elevated when acidosis occurs as a result of the exchange of intracellular potassium for hydrogen ions.

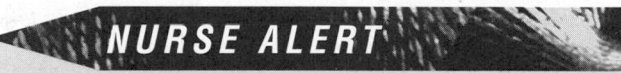

**NURSE ALERT**

**A patient using an increased rate and depth of respirations (Kussmaul's respiration) is trying to correct metabolic acidosis by eliminating $CO_2$.**

Appropriate therapy for metabolic acidosis is treatment of the underlying cause. Bicarbonate can be given intravenously to counteract the excessive acids in the blood. Often sodium lactate is given because the liver metabolizes sodium lactate into bicarbonate. In renal failure, dialysis may be the treatment of choice (Box 27-15).

## Metabolic Alkalosis

A base bicarbonate excess, or metabolic alkalosis, can result from either the loss of acid in the body or from the accumulation of bases in the blood. Loss of acid can occur with excessive vomiting or from gastric suction, which removes the upper gastrointestinal secretions that are high in hydrochloric acid. Administration of potent diuretics can cause a loss of hydrogen and chloride ions and result in a relative increase of bicarbonate in the blood. Ingestion of an excessive amount of sodium bicarbonate or antacids causes accumulation of base in the ECF.

---

**TABLE 27-2**

## Anion Gap

| ANION GAP TYPE | VALUES | CAUSES |
|---|---|---|
| Normal anion gap | 12 ($\pm$2) mEq/L | Diarrhea, renal tubular acidosis, or pancreatic fistula causing a direct loss of $HCO_3^-$; addition of chloride-containing acids |
| Increased anion gap | >14 mEq/L | Lactic acidosis, uremia, diabetic ketoacidosis, or salicylate and methanol toxicity, resulting in accumulation of nonvolatile acids with decrease in $HCO_3^-$ |

From Horne M, Heitz U, Swearingen P: *Fluid, electrolyte, and acid-base balance,* ed 3, St Louis, 1997, Mosby.
Anion gap $= Na^+ - (Cl^- + HCO_3^-)$

## NURSING PROCESS

## METABOLIC ACIDOSIS: BASE BICARBONATE DEFICIT OR METABOLIC ACID EXCESS

### ASSESSMENT

- Serum pH <7.35
- Low urine pH
- Decreased serum bicarbonate
- Increased serum potassium
- Decreased blood $CO_2$
- Diarrhea
- Increased rate and depth of respirations
- Weakness, drowsiness
- Disorientation
- Shock
- Stupor
- Coma

### NURSING DIAGNOSIS

- Risk for injury related to metabolic acidosis

### NURSING INTERVENTIONS

- Monitor pH and potassium values.
- Keep bicarbonate readily available.
- Monitor laboratory results.
- Monitor heart rhythm.

- Maintain accurate I&O records.
- Monitor vital signs.
- Monitor neurologic status and level of consciousness.
- Observe orientation.
- Observe for decreased BP and/or increased pulse.
- Administer medications as ordered to correct metabolic acidosis.
- Maintain life support systems.

### EVALUATION OF EXPECTED OUTCOMES

- Patient's response monitored
- pH within normal limits
- Serum potassium within normal limits
- IV fluids administered at prescribed rate
- ECF volume deficit avoided
- Respiratory compensation for metabolic imbalances observed
- Alert and oriented
- Safety maintained
- Shock prevented
- Integrity of body systems maintained

---

The major signs and symptoms of metabolic alkalosis include nausea, vomiting, and diarrhea. Muscles cramp and have increased tone, and symptoms similar to tetany may appear. Often patients are confused and irritable, and convulsions can occur. The lungs attempt to compensate by decreasing the rate and depth of respirations to conserve carbonic acid. Plasma bicarbonate levels, serum pH, and urine pH are increased. Plasma potassium levels are lowered in alkalosis, as hydrogen moves out of the cell and forces potassium into the cell.

The underlying cause of metabolic alkalosis must be determined and treated. Excessive losses should be replaced, and acidifying solutions can be given orally or intravenously. The specific treatment depends on the cause (Box 27-16).

### NURSE ALERT

Hyperventilation results in respiratory alkalosis. Have the patient use a paper bag to rebreathe $CO_2$ and restore carbonic acid.

### Respiratory Alkalosis

A carbonic acid deficit, or respiratory alkalosis, is caused primarily by hyperventilation, which can result from anxiety, fever, or lack of oxygen. Some drugs can stimulate the respiratory center and cause hyperventilation. Too much $CO_2$ is excreted during hyperventilation, so carbonic acid levels decrease. Common symptoms of respiratory alkalosis are related to increased neuromuscular irritability and include headache, dizziness, paresthesias, tingling of the fingertips and around the mouth, and tetany. The blood pH is above normal, the blood gas $CO_2$ level is low, and the urine pH increased. The bicarbonate level of the plasma may be normal or slightly lowered. Serum potassium levels are usually lowered in alkalosis. Treatment consists of sedation, emotional support, and the use of a bag to rebreathe exhaled $CO_2$ (Box 27-17).

### Respiratory Acidosis

A carbonic acid excess, or respiratory acidosis, is caused by any condition that interferes with the normal release of $CO_2$ from the lungs. Emphysema, bronchitis, pneumonia, and asthma are conditions that in-

> BOX 27-16

# NURSING PROCESS

## METABOLIC ALKALOSIS: BASE BICARBONATE EXCESS

### ASSESSMENT

- Serum pH >7.45
- Increased urine pH
- Increased serum bicarbonate
- Decreased serum potassium (<4 mEq/L)
- Blood $CO_2$ tension increased
- Nausea and vomiting
- Diarrhea
- Decreased rate and depth of respirations
- Confusion
- Irritability
- Increased muscular tone and cramps
- Twitching
- Tingling, numbness (tetany)
- Convulsions

### NURSING DIAGNOSIS

- Risk for injury related to metabolic alkalosis

### NURSING INTERVENTIONS

- Monitor laboratory values.
- Observe for signs of hypokalemia.
- Monitor administration of IV fluids.
- Maintain accurate I&O records.
- Monitor vital signs.
- Monitor neurologic status.
- Orient patient to reality.
- Observe change in level of consciousness.
- Maintain quiet environment.
- Administer muscle relaxants as ordered.
- Observe for signs of increased muscle tone and cramps, indicating tetany.
- Establish seizure precautions.

### EVALUATION OF EXPECTED OUTCOMES

- Patient's response monitored
- Abnormal laboratory results communicated
- Serum potassium within normal limits
- Fluid balance maintained
- Respiratory compensation for metabolic imbalance observed
- Patient more assured, less fearful
- Decreased need for psychotropic agents
- Decreased oxygen need; conservation of patient's energy
- Injury prevented

> BOX 27-17

# NURSING PROCESS

## RESPIRATORY ALKALOSIS: CARBONIC ACID DEFICIT

### ASSESSMENT

- Elevated blood pH
- Decreased serum $CO_2$
- Increased urine pH
- Plasma bicarbonate normal or slightly decreased
- Serum potassium lowered
- Headache
- Dizziness
- Paresthesias
- Tingling, numbness (tetany)

### NURSING DIAGNOSIS

- Risk for injury related to respiratory alkalosis

### NURSING INTERVENTIONS

- Monitor laboratory values.
- Observe patient for signs and symptoms of primary disease process that could contribute to respiratory alkalosis.
- Administer pain medication as ordered.
- Reassure patient.
- Educate patient concerning breathing techniques.
- Monitor sensorium.
- Observe for signs of tetany.

### EVALUATION OF EXPECTED OUTCOMES

- Patient's response monitored
- Primary disease treated with correction of carbonic acid deficit
- Headache controlled
- Hyperventilation decreased
- Oxygenation improved
- Patient alert and oriented
- Injury prevented

terfere with the normal transport of gases across the pulmonary membrane. In addition, sedatives, narcotics (morphine), and brain trauma may affect the respiratory center in the medulla and depress respirations. Carbonic acid levels increase. Patients become weak, restless, drowsy, and disoriented, and may lose consciousness. Headache and muscle twitching may lead to convulsions. The pulse rate increases, and arrhythmias may occur. Cyanosis is usually a late sign. The plasma pH is low, and the blood gas $CO_2$ level is elevated. The bicarbonate level is normal or elevated in an attempt to compensate. Serum potassium is usually elevated during acidotic states.

Severe respiratory acidosis can be an emergency. Treatment measures should first involve improvement of ventilation; mechanical ventilation may be necessary (Box 27-18).

### NURSE ALERT

**Hypoventilation results in respiratory acidosis. If the patient demonstrates slow, weak respirations or signs of hypoxia, look for signs of respiratory acidosis.**

## Interpretation of Blood Gas Values

When evaluating laboratory reports of blood gas values, the nurse should first determine if the pH level is normal or indicates acidosis (below 7.35) or alkalosis (above 7.45). The nurse should next evaluate the bicarbonate and carbonic acid levels. Normal bicarbonate is 22 to 26 mEq/L. Carbonic acid is measured by the $Paco_2$, and its normal range is 35 to 45. If the pH indicates acidosis and the bicarbonate level is low and the carbonic acid or $Paco_2$ level is normal, the patient has a base bicarbonate deficit, or metabolic acidosis. If the pH indicates acidosis and both bicarbonate and carbonic acid are normal, the cause is excess metabolic acid, or metabolic acidosis. If the pH level indicates acidosis and the carbonic acid level is high while the bicarbonate is normal, the patient has a carbonic acid excess, or respiratory acidosis. With an alkaline pH level, a high bicarbonate level indicates metabolic alkalosis, and a low carbonic acid level indicates respiratory alkalosis (Box 27-19).

## Compensation

The "normal" value in each of these situations gradually becomes abnormal in the body's attempt to compensate by balancing carbonic acid and base bicarbon-

---

**BOX 27-18** | **NURSING PROCESS**

### RESPIRATORY ACIDOSIS: CARBONIC ACID EXCESS

**ASSESSMENT**

- Decreased blood pH
- Increased serum $CO_2$
- Plasma bicarbonate normal or increased
- Serum potassium increased
- Weakness
- Restlessness
- Disorientation, drowsy
- Headache
- Muscle twitching
- Convulsions
- Increased pulse
- Arrhythmias
- Cyanosis

**NURSING DIAGNOSIS**

- Risk for injury related to respiratory acidosis

**NURSING INTERVENTIONS**

- Monitor laboratory values.
- Maintain patent airway.
- Provide suction as necessary.
- Monitor administration of IV fluids.

- Assist with transfer.
- Provide oxygen as ordered.
- Provide emotional support.
- Monitor neurologic status.
- Provide reorientation.
- Establish seizure precautions.
- Monitor vital signs.
- Administer medications as ordered.
- Perform chest percussion and postural drainage as ordered.
- Place patient in semi-Fowler's position if indicated.

**EVALUATION OF EXPECTED OUTCOMES**

- Arterial blood gases within normal limits
- Serum potassium decreased via the dilutional effect of IV fluids
- Injury prevented
- Oxygen level increased
- Patient verbalizes increased awareness of environment
- Arrhythmias avoided
- Transport of gases across the pulmonary membrane facilitated

ate levels. This compensation causes the pH to move toward normal. Because balance is being attempted but has not yet been achieved (pH is still abnormal), this state is termed partially compensated. Once the pH has returned to normal, the state is referred to as being compensated because even though the bicarbonate and carbonic acid levels may be abnormal, they have achieved a proper balance. With continued treatment, these levels are returned to normal while a normal pH is maintained.

## INTRAVENOUS THERAPY

IV therapy is a primary therapeutic technique that is used to treat patients with fluid and electrolyte imbalances or to prevent their occurrence. The three types of solutions commonly used are categorized according to the strength of their composition, or their osmolarity (Box 27-20).

---

**BOX 27-19**

### BLOOD GAS INTERPRETATION*

1 Is pH acid or alkaline? (normal range: 7.35-7.45) Give it a name: acidosis or alkalosis

2 Look for the cause: acidosis results from ↑ acid or ↓ base; alkalosis results from ↓ acid or ↑ base. Therefore check the levels of bicarbonate and carbonic acid.

3 Is bicarbonate ($HCO_3^-$) level normal? (22-26 mEq/L). If yes, go on. If no, is it high or low? Does it explain the condition named in step 1? (Example: If acidosis, a low bicarbonate level could explain the cause; a high bicarbonate level would not cause acidosis)

4 Is carbonic acid ($Paco_2$) normal (35-45 mm Hg)? If yes, go back to bicarbonate level. If no, is it high or low? Does it explain the condition? (Example: If acidosis, a high carbonic acid level could explain the cause; a low carbonic acid level would not cause acidosis)

5 Give it another name related to the possible cause. If it is caused by a change in bicarbonate level, it is a metabolic imbalance. If it is caused by a change in carbonic acid level, it is a respiratory imbalance. Acidosis with bicarbonate level ↓ = metabolic acidosis. Acidosis with carbonic acid level ↑ = respiratory acidosis. Alkalosis with bicarbonate level ↑ = metabolic alkalosis. Alkalosis with carbonic acid level ↓ = respiratory alkalosis. The second name comes from the possible cause.

6 Look for compensation. Metabolic acidosis, carbonic acid level ↓ (to compensate). Metabolic alkalosis, carbonic acid level ↑. Respiratory acidosis, bicarbonate level ↑. Respiratory alkalosis, bicarbonate level ↓. If pH is abnormal, it is uncompensated. If pH is normal and carbonic acid or bicarbonate levels are abnormal, it is compensated.

7 There are now three names:

| | |
|---|---|
| Compensated or Uncompensated | choose this name last |
| Respiratory or Metabolic | choose one of these names second |
| Acidosis or Alkalosis | choose one of these names first |

### EXERCISES: ASSIGN THREE NAMES TO THE FOLLOWING:

| pH | $HCO_3^-$ | $CO_2$ |
|---|---|---|
| 7.23 | 14 | 32 |
| 7.10 | 28 | 63 |
| 7.51 | 25 | 26 |
| 7.55 | 34 | 43 |
| 7.36 | 34 | 56 |

---

*Answers are in Instructor's Resource Manual.

---

**BOX 27-20**

### PARENTERAL SOLUTIONS

**HYPOTONIC SOLUTIONS (0.45% SALINE, D5%/0.45% SALINE, 2.5% DEXTROSE, 0.33% SALINE, D5%/W*)**
Decrease intravascular osmolarity
Result in intracellular hydration
Used for cellular dehydration
Complications: shock and increased intracranial pressure
Contraindications: anasarca (total body edema), cerebral edema, hypotension

**HYPERTONIC SOLUTIONS (D10%/NS, D5%/NS, D5%/RL, 8% AMINO ACIDS)**
Increase intravascular osmolarity
Result in intracellular and interstitial dehydration
Used for intravascular expansion by shifting intracellular and interstitial fluids
Complications: circulatory overload
Contraindications: intracellular dehydration, hyperosmolar states

**ISOTONIC SOLUTIONS (NS, RINGER'S SOLUTION, RL, 10% DEXTRAN 40 IN 0.9% SODIUM CHLORIDE)**
Do not change osmolarity
Result in total body water expansion
Complications: circulatory overload
Contraindications: circulatory overload; alkalosis

---

*D5%/W is isotonic as a solution before infusion, but because the glucose is rapidly metabolized, leaving plain water, it has the effect of a hypotonic solution in the blood.

## Types of Solutions

Isotonic, or isoosmolar, solutions have the same tonicity as plasma. No osmosis occurs between two isotonic solutions when they are separated by a membrane, such as a cell membrane. These solutions are similar to normal blood plasma. They provide water, electrolytes, and carbohydrates and do not change body osmolarity.

Hypertonic, or hyperosmolar, solutions are stronger than isotonic solutions because they have more solutes dissolved in them per unit of volume. When introduced into the plasma they send electrolytes into the cell via diffusion and draw water from the interstitial space and from the cells via osmosis, thus expanding plasma volume even more.

**Hypotonic,** or **hypoosmolar,** solutions are weaker than isotonic and hypertonic solutions. Osmosis causes the fluid to enter the cell in an attempt to equalize the concentration of solutes on either side of the cell membrane. Therefore these fluids cause cellular hydration and stimulate kidney function. These solutions usually contain carbohydrates in water or hypotonic saline. The carbohydrate is metabolized, and the water is free to be absorbed by the cells or is eliminated.

> ### NURSE ALERT
>
> **Do not administer 5% dextrose in water or other hypotonic intravenous solutions to patients with stroke or head injury. Such solutions enter the cell and increase cerebral edema and intracranial pressure.**

When administering IV fluids, it is important to provide adequate fluids for hydration while preventing fluid overload. Too much fluid (fluid overload) decreases the normal body osmolality. A high body osmolality indicates dehydration. A patient's osmolality can be determined by a formula that is based on sodium, blood urea nitrogen (BUN), and blood glucose levels (Box 27-21). A shortcut calculation is based on the sodium level only (sodium level × 2 = approximate body osmolality). Normal body osmolality is between 275 and 295 mOsm/L.

## Techniques and Equipment

Fluids are introduced into veins through metal needles or through plastic cannulas that are inserted by sliding them over a metal needle. An IV infusion tubing set and a bottle or plastic bag filled with the appropriate solution are prepared before the procedure is started

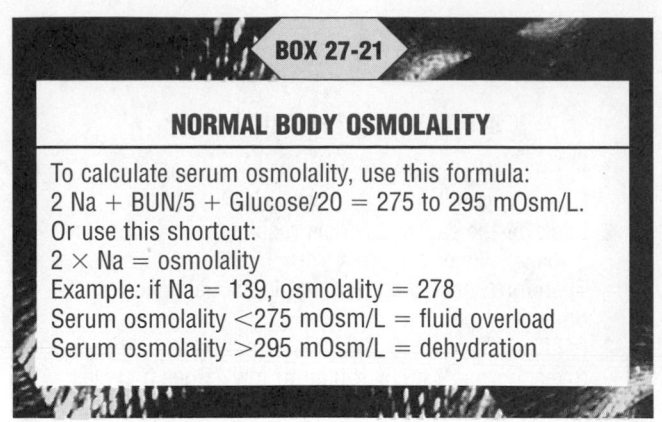

**BOX 27-21**

### NORMAL BODY OSMOLALITY

To calculate serum osmolality, use this formula:
2 Na + BUN/5 + Glucose/20 = 275 to 295 mOsm/L.
Or use this shortcut:
2 × Na = osmolality
Example: if Na = 139, osmolality = 278
Serum osmolality <275 mOsm/L = fluid overload
Serum osmolality >295 mOsm/L = dehydration

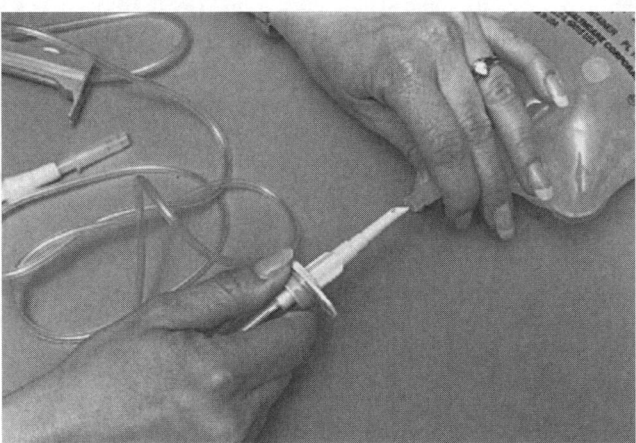

**Figure 27-10** Tubing insertion site is inserted into bag. Tubing clamp is opened slowly. Tubing is filled with IV fluid in preparation for attachment of the needle adapter of the infusion set to the hub of the cannula that is inserted in the vein. (From Potter PA, Perry AG: *Basic nursing: theory and practice,* ed 3, St Louis, 1995, Mosby.)

(Figure 27-10). The clamp on the tubing is closed, the tubing is connected to the bag, and the clamp is opened to fill the tubing with fluid. A vein is selected and the site is cleansed. Any long hairs in the area are cut. Figure 27-11 illustrates the sites commonly used for intravenous infusion. The needle is inserted, and the over-the-needle cannula, if present, is advanced into the vein. The needle adapter of the infusion set is connected to the hub of the catheter. The fluid is started, and a proper flow rate is established. The catheter is secured, usually with narrow tape, and may be covered with a transparent layer of gauze dressing, depending on the procedure accepted in each agency.

In the rare case that a vein cannot be accessed, a cutdown may be necessary. A cutdown requires a small incision through the skin and into the vein to insert a catheter. The catheter is sutured in place and the wound is dressed to prevent infection.

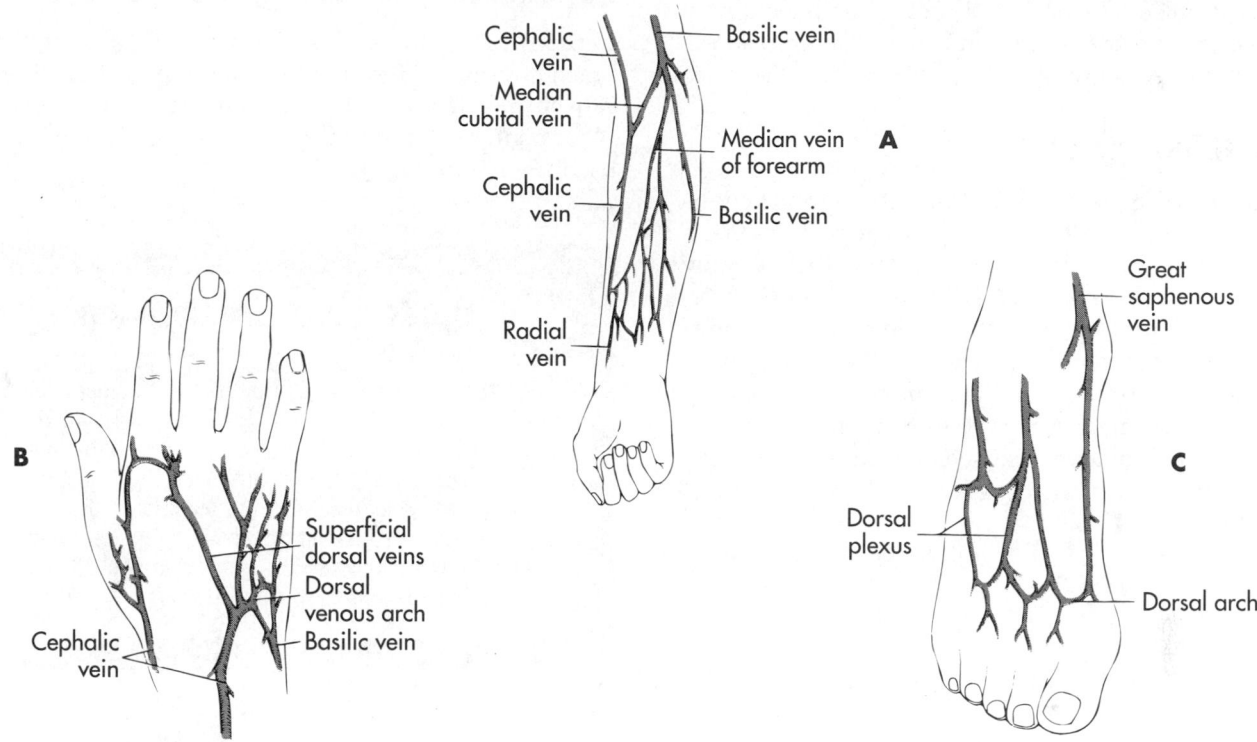

**Figure 27-11**    Common intravenous sites. **A,** Inner arm. **B,** Dorsal surface of hand. **C,** Dorsal surface of foot (used primarily for pediatric patients). (From Potter PA, Perry AG: *Basic nursing: theory and practice,* ed 3, St Louis, 1995, Mosby.)

## Complications
### Local

The nurse observes and monitors the patient's IV fluids. The prescribed flow rate must be regulated. The IV site is watched for infiltration, which is caused by displacement of the IV needle from the vein into the surrounding tissue. Infiltration is characterized by swelling of the affected tissue. The patient may experience a burning sensation at the needle site. The infiltrated site is pale, cool, edematous, and is firm or hard to the touch. To confirm infiltration, a tourniquet can be applied above the infusion site. The solution continues to flow if the solution is infiltrating the surrounding tissues but will stop flowing if the needle is still in the vein. If infiltration is confirmed, the IV line must be discontinued and restarted at another site. Warm compresses can be applied to the infiltrated site to promote reabsorption of the IV fluid.

Thrombophlebitis is a more common complication in which the vein becomes inflamed and a clot forms. Redness, warmth, and edema occur at the injection site, and the patient complains of pain along the vein. When thrombophlebitis occurs, the IV infusion should be discontinued, and warm, moist compresses should be applied to reduce pain and stimulate healing.

### Systemic

Systemic complications that may occur from IV infusions include fluid overload (circulatory overload), embolism, and infection. Nurses should be continuously alert for symptoms of circulatory overload, which include respiratory distress and increased venous pressure. Shortness of breath, increased respirations, coughing, increased blood pressure, bounding pulse, and distended veins can also signal circulatory overload. If infusion continues, pulmonary edema can result.

Air embolism occasionally occurs when substantial amounts of air enter the blood through an improperly running infusion. The apparatus should be checked often, and the infusion should be stopped or the solution changed before the bottle and tubing are empty. Such actions prevent air from entering the vein. Sudden vascular collapse can occur from air embolism, with the patient showing signs of shock and loss of consciousness.

A pulmonary embolism results if the clot that forms in the process of thrombophlebitis breaks loose and travels to the lungs. Sudden and severe respiratory distress is an indication of pulmonary embolism and requires emergency treatment. If nausea, vomiting, an increased pulse rate, and chills occur, the patient may be experiencing a systemic infection. The infusion is stopped immediately, and the physician is called.

## Central Venous Lines

Fluids can also be infused through central venous lines. In the operating room the doctor inserts a catheter into the right atrium of the heart, usually through the subclavian vein. These catheters can remain in place for long periods, which reduces the need for frequent venipuncture. These catheters can have more than one lumen to allow infusion of multiple solutions and/or medications. Using strict aseptic technique, the site must be cleansed and dressed regularly and observed for signs of infection (Figures 27-12, *A* and 27-13).

## Peripherally Inserted Central Catheter

Central lines can also be introduced in a peripheral brachial vein and inserted into the right atrium. These can be inserted by the registered nurse, but correct placement must be verified by x-ray before the line is used (Figure 27-12, *B*).

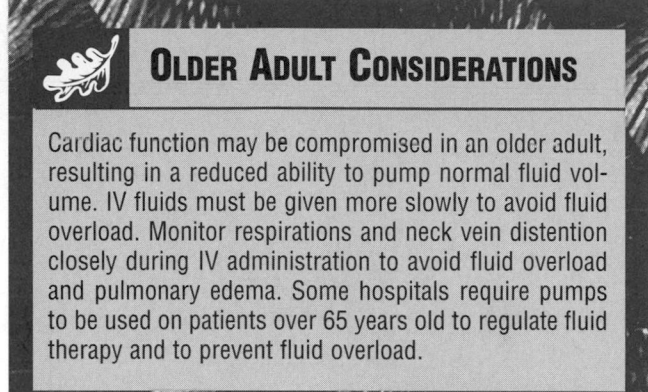

### OLDER ADULT CONSIDERATIONS

Cardiac function may be compromised in an older adult, resulting in a reduced ability to pump normal fluid volume. IV fluids must be given more slowly to avoid fluid overload. Monitor respirations and neck vein distention closely during IV administration to avoid fluid overload and pulmonary edema. Some hospitals require pumps to be used on patients over 65 years old to regulate fluid therapy and to prevent fluid overload.

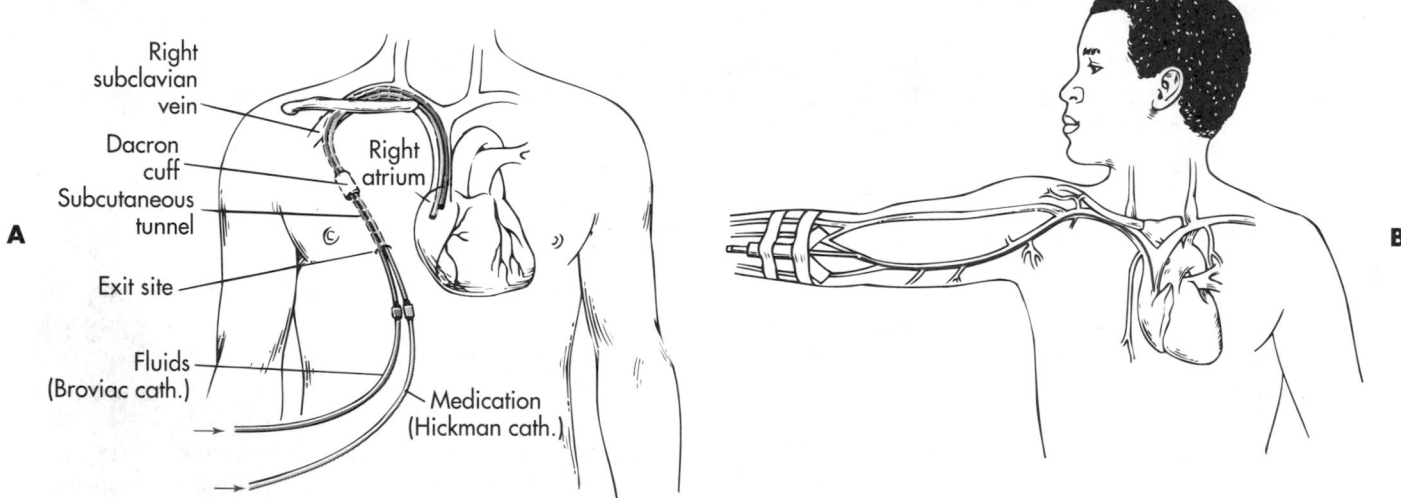

**Figure 27-12** **A,** Central venous catheter with double lumen. **B,** Peripherally inserted central catheter.

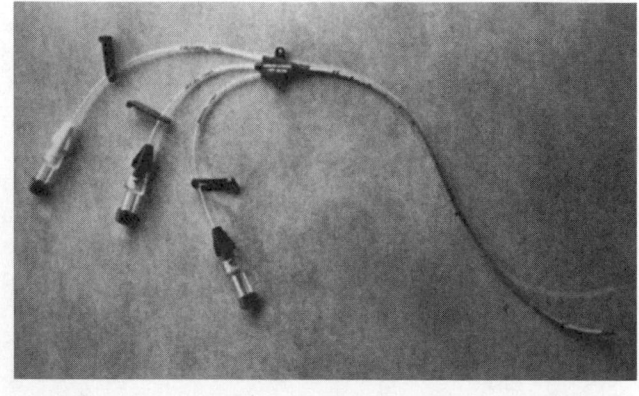

**Figure 27-13** ARROWg+arg Blue Antiseptic Surface Triple Lumen Catheter. (From Arrow International.)

# SHOCK

The basic abnormality that occurs when a state of shock develops is an imbalance between the tissue needs and its supply of adequately oxygenated blood. Contributing to this is a disproportion between the volume of blood and the vascular space in which it is circulating. Lack of oxygen results and leads to altered chemical activity within all the cells of the body. Normal metabolic processes that produce the energy needed for work within the cell are interrupted. Lactic acid is produced, which diffuses out of the cells into the ECF, causing a state of acidosis.

## Body Response to Shock

Although the causes of various forms of shock differ, many of the compensatory mechanisms that counteract the effects of shock are the same. Loss of fluid volume or a disproportion between fluid volume and the size of the vascular space causes the blood pressure regulatory mechanisms to react.

Decreasing blood pressure excites the vasoconstrictor center of the brain (medulla oblongata), and epinephrine and norepinephrine are released from the adrenal medulla. The effect is vasoconstriction of the peripheral blood vessels and an increased heart rate and strength of the contraction. These mechanisms may be successful in elevating the blood pressure and increasing the cardiac output in mild shock. The kidneys secrete the hormone renin when the blood pressure falls. Renin produces angiotensin, which is a powerful vasoconstrictor. To return the blood volume to normal, the body releases aldosterone from the adrenal cortex, which causes sodium reabsorption and water retention by the kidney tubules. This increases ECF and blood volume and decreases urinary output.

## Assessment of Shock

The signs and symptoms of shock are similar, regardless of the cause. The basic property of shock is decreased blood flow and therefore decreased delivery of oxygen, nutrients, hormones, and electrolytes to the cells. There is also a decreased removal of metabolic wastes. Signs of shock are a direct result of the body's attempt to counteract the effects of decreasing cardiac output.

Subtle, early signs of shock include an increased pulse rate, increased respirations, a mild drop in blood pressure, oliguria, and restlessness. Weakness; lethargy; pallor; cool, moist skin; rapid, shallow respirations; decreasing body temperature; a rapid, thready pulse; and progressively decreasing blood pressure with a narrowing pulse pressure occur later. Pulse pressure is the difference between the systolic and di-

astolic blood pressures. A normal pulse pressure is 40 mm Hg. For example, a blood pressure of 128/88 would produce a pulse pressure of 40. Pulse pressure narrows in early shock because of a decreased systolic blood pressure.

## Types of Shock
### Hypovolemic Shock

Shock can be classified in several ways. **Hypovolemic shock** results from a loss of fluid available to the circulation. It is caused most often by hemorrhage but can also result from the loss of body fluids such as in dehydration caused by diabetic ketoacidosis; severe, extended vomiting; or diarrhea. Burns and other trauma can trap fluid at the site of the injury and decrease the volume of the bloodstream. Tissue injury that occurs during trauma or surgery can increase the permeability of capillary membranes and allow albumin to leave the circulating blood. This disturbs plasma colloid osmotic pressure and allows fluid to shift from the circulation to the tissues (see Figure 27-6). Hypovolemia results, and shock is a potential danger.

Hypovolemic shock is an extension of fluid volume deficit. Loss of plasma results in hemoconcentration. Loss of fluid volume results in less venous blood returning to the right side of the heart. Therefore less blood is pumped out of the heart into the vascular system. Insufficient oxygen is provided to the body cells and abnormal metabolic processes result, which leads to metabolic acidosis.

**Assessment.** An objective assessment includes location, quality, and rate of pulse. The location of a pulse that can be palpated can give an estimate of the patient's blood pressure (Box 27-22).

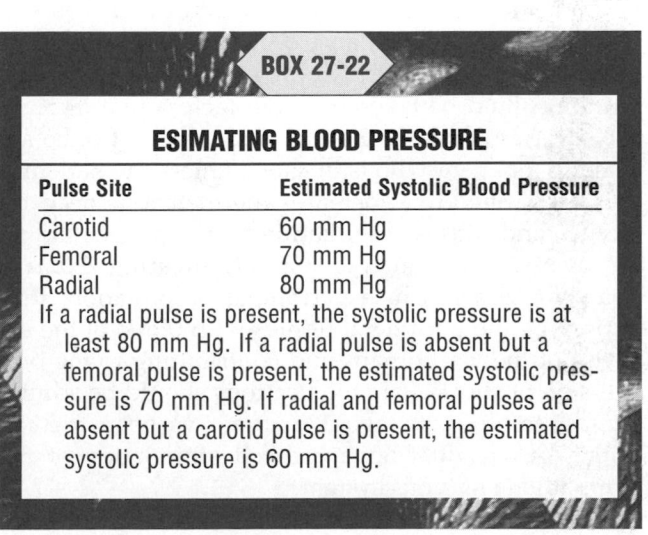

**BOX 27-22**

### ESIMATING BLOOD PRESSURE

| Pulse Site | Estimated Systolic Blood Pressure |
| --- | --- |
| Carotid | 60 mm Hg |
| Femoral | 70 mm Hg |
| Radial | 80 mm Hg |

If a radial pulse is present, the systolic pressure is at least 80 mm Hg. If a radial pulse is absent but a femoral pulse is present, the estimated systolic pressure is 70 mm Hg. If radial and femoral pulses are absent but a carotid pulse is present, the estimated systolic pressure is 60 mm Hg.

Signs and symptoms of hypovolemic shock are decreased level of consciousness; uncontrolled bleeding; tachycardia; hypotension; prolonged capillary refill; and cool, pale skin. A person in hypovolemic shock has flat neck veins. Cardiac tamponade, a condition that mimics shock, results in distended neck veins and distant (muffled or quieter) heart sounds.

**Intervention.** Prevention of shock is the best possible treatment. Shock must be anticipated as a possible complication after surgery or in any condition that involves significant blood loss. Early signs of shock should be observed and treatment instituted before the condition becomes life threatening.

The primary objective in treatment is to restore adequate tissue perfusion of oxygenated blood. The blood volume must be restored and the hemorrhage controlled. If uncontrolled bleeding is the cause of hypovolemic shock, bleeding must be controlled or stopped. Applying pressure to the artery that supplies the area of uncontrolled bleeding reduces blood flow (see Chapter 21). The hand or an additional firm object (a sand bag) is held on the artery to compress it against the bone that lies behind it. A tourniquet is a last resort because it is likely to result in loss of the extremity. The patient is given oxygen at a rate of at least 6 L/min. A large-bore IV catheter, 18 g or greater, is used to initiate an IV line. Ringer's lactate or normal saline is the usual fluid ordered.

Patients should be kept supine, and those who do not have head injuries may have their lower extremities slightly elevated. Trendelenburg's position is avoided because gravity pushes the abdominal organs up against the chest, which interferes with diaphragmatic excursion and cardiac contractions. Position changes should be made slowly and gently. Observations should be made systematically and recorded in written form. Pertinent observations include blood pressure, pulse, respirations, skin color, temperature, IV and oral fluid intake, urinary and other forms of fluid loss, a running balance of I & O, and level of consciousness.

Care should be taken to avoid factors that increase the severity of shock. External heat should not be applied to a patient who is in shock unless the patient is shivering. Shivering increases the metabolic need for oxygen and causes vasodilation, so the patient should be covered just enough to stop the shivering. External heat would also cause peripheral vasodilation, thus supplying the peripheral tissues with blood at the expense of the vital organs and contributing to the progression of shock. Pain medications should be administered carefully to avoid extreme vasoconstriction, which can result from increased stimulation of the sympathetic nervous system.

A central venous catheter is inserted. Frequent monitoring of central venous pressure is done to prevent the danger of overhydrating the patient. Overloading the patient's circulatory system can lead to pulmonary edema, which further impedes the amount of oxygenation and $CO_2$ removal that can occur in the lungs. Patients receiving high-humidity oxygen can absorb some of the humidity through their lungs. Daily chest x-ray films are beneficial in monitoring the development of pulmonary edema. Diuretics such as furosemide may help prevent fluid accumulation in the pulmonary bed. Arterial blood-gas determinations indicate the patient's oxygen and $CO_2$ levels, as well as acid-base balance.

Military antishock trousers (MASTs) or pneumatic antishock garments (PASGs) may be applied. These garments apply pressure to the lower extremities and abdomen to help increase the blood return to the vital organs and decrease the blood volume in the lower extremities. They are used to keep the systolic blood pressure above 80 mm Hg. MASTs and PASGs are contraindicated in patients with severe head injury, congestive heart failure, or an intrathoracic bleed. When the garment is inflated, the pulse must be checked in the lower extremities. The garment should never obscure the pulse. Once the blood volume has been restored with fluids and blood products, the garment can be removed by first deflating the area over the abdomen and then over one leg at a time. If the blood pressure drops more than 5 mm Hg, the deflation is stopped until the blood pressure returns to the previous reading. If the patient requires surgery to control bleeding, these garments may be left in place and removed in the operating room after the surgery is complete.

## Normovolemic Shock

Shock that results from causes other than fluid loss is termed normovolemic shock. **Cardiogenic shock** results from a failure of the heart to pump adequate amounts of blood into the systemic circulation to fully perfuse and therefore oxygenate the body tissues. Cardiogenic shock is easiest to treat in its early stages but is not easily identified. It is not easily reversed if it is not identified early. The seriousness of the precipitating factors tends to shadow the impending shock. Precipitating factors include arrhythmias, myocardial infarction, or congestive heart failure. Decreased blood pressure, a decreased level of alertness, and decreased renal function are all present in cardiogenic shock and reflect the failure of the heart as a pump.

**Neurogenic shock** and **vasogenic shock** both result from vasodilation, or an increase in the size of the vascular bed with a normal blood volume. Blood pressure decreases, and therefore venous blood returned to the heart is decreased, which contributes to decreased cardiac output. In both types of shock, venous pooling results, and tissue hypoxia and cell death occur.

Although vasodilation occurs in both neurogenic and vasogenic shock, the causative factors of each differ. The cause of neurogenic shock is nerve stimulation or nerve blocks, such as those arising from deep general anesthesia, spinal anesthesia, postural hypotension, drug reactions, brain damage, or insulin shock. Vasogenic shock occurs as a result of factors that directly affect the blood vessels. Vasodilation in vasogenic shock is followed by a decrease in venous return, cardiac output, blood pressure, and volume of blood to the tissues. Cellular anoxia and destruction occur. Anaphylactic shock and septic shock are examples of vasogenic shock.

Anaphylactic shock results from an abnormal antigen-antibody response. The IgE antibody produced causes the release of histamine from mast cells and basophils (see Chapter 7). The release of histamine results in arterial and venous dilation and increased capillary permeability. Vasodilation and decreased cardiac output cause a decrease in systolic and diastolic blood pressure. Plasma leaks through the vascular bed into the interstitial space, which leads to circulatory collapse. Histamine contracts the smooth muscle of the bronchi and causes bronchospasms, asthma, and panting. The bronchioles constrict and contribute to hypoxemia. The patient initially complains of dizziness, drowsiness, and itching of the eyes and ears. Confusion; diaphoresis; edema of the hands, lips, and eyelids and tongue; and laryngospasm quickly appear. The reaction rapidly progresses to complete respiratory obstruction and distress and circulatory collapse.

Treatment requires immediate elimination of the antigen, such as removing a bee stinger or stopping an infusion that caused the reaction. The patient should be placed in a supine position to increase blood flow to the brain. An open airway must be maintained, and oxygen is given at 5 to 10 L/min. IV fluids should be started, and the patient is placed on a cardiac monitor. Epinephrine is given to block the release of histamine, counteract bronchospasms, and prevent circulatory collapse. Antihistamines, corticosteroids, and aminophylline are given to supplement the effects of epinephrine. After recovering from the acute episode, the patient must be fully informed of the allergy to avoid future exposure (Box 27-23).

Septic shock is caused by the metabolic end-products of bacteria. During the early phase of septic shock, the vessels are dilated and the patient may have a fever. There is still adequate blood flow to the brain, as indicated by the patient's alertness. Urinary output, which reflects renal perfusion, is adequate. The pulse may be moderately elevated, but the increase in heart rate does not support an adequate cardiac output, and

---

> **BOX 27-23**

## NURSING PROCESS

## EMERGENCY CARE OF INDIVIDUALS IN ANAPHYLACTIC SHOCK

**ASSESSMENT**
- Rapid, shallow breathing
- Bronchospasms; dyspnea
- Cyanosis
- Restlessness, sense of doom; irritability
- Laryngeal edema
- Hypotension
- Rapid, thready pulse
- Edema and itching at site of injection or insect bite

**NURSING DIAGNOSIS**
- Risk for injury related to anaphylactic shock

**NURSING INTERVENTIONS**
- Prepare for oropharyngeal intubation or surgical insertion of tracheotomy.
- Provide oxygen therapy per order.
- Prepare for administration of antihistamines such as Benadryl 50-100 mg IM, aminophylline IV drip. Administer corticosteroids to decrease inflammation as ordered.

- Administer 0.1-0.5 ml 1:1000 epinephrine solution SC or IM into upper arm and massage site to hasten absorption.
- Prepare to administer vasopressor drugs such as levarterenol bitartrate (Levophed) and high-dose dopamine (Intropin).
- Monitor pulse and blood pressure q3-5min until stable.
- Place a tourniquet above the site of the injected antigen; remove tourniquet q10-15min or until reaction is under control; apply ice.

**EVALUATION OF EXPECTED OUTCOMES**
- Patent airway maintained
- Effective breathing pattern demonstrated
- Hemodynamic stability maintained as evidenced by blood pressure and pulse in normal range
- Systemic absorption of the antigen reduced

systolic blood pressure slowly falls. Hyperventilation results in metabolic alkalosis.

The late phase of septic shock is marked by decreased mentation, which may lead to confusion and stupor. The sluggish blood is prone to clot, especially within the smaller vessels. This condition is known as *disseminated intravascular coagulation*. The clotted vessels are unable to deliver oxygen and nutrients to the affected tissues. The widespread clotting depletes blood clotting factors, and the patient begins to hemorrhage. Metabolic acidosis results from cellular hypoxia and the inability of the clotted vessels to carry cellular waste products from the affected areas. Arterial and venous constriction contribute to cold, pale, and clammy skin with a below-normal body temperature. Constriction of the renal arteries leads to decreased perfusion of the kidneys, and little urine is produced. Acute or chronic renal failure is the second most common cause of death in septic shock.

## Drug Therapy for Shock

Various types of drug therapy are ordered according to the cause of shock. Vasoactive drugs, which affect vascular tone, can be categorized into various groups according to the following actions: constriction/dilation of arterioles, constriction/dilation of veins, or increasing myocardial contractility. Vasoactive drugs include norepinephrine, nitroprusside, and dopamine. Inotropic agents are also used. For example, dobutamine is used because it improves cardiac performance without increasing myocardial oxygen demand. This would be important if the patient was in cardiogenic shock because the heart itself is the primary cause of the shock state. But if the cause was vascular collapse secondary to hemorrhage, norepinephrine could be given for the inotropic effect on the heart and its properties as a potent vasoconstrictor. Management is actually more complex than this. The patient's condition must be closely monitored to avoid increasing myocardial contractility at the expense of myocardial oxygen demand.

Noninotropic drugs, such as nitroprusside, that equally dilate arterioles and veins also decrease cardiac oxygen demand and increase perfusion of peripheral vessels. However, perfusion of the vital organs is decreased. Other drugs used to treat shock include antiarrhythmics (lidocaine, procainamide), antibiotics (tobramycin, gentamicin), and diuretics (ethacrynic acid).

## PSYCHOSOCIAL SUPPORT

This chapter has considered the biologic alterations in a patient who has fluid and electrolyte imbalances or one who is in a state of shock. However, the patient leads a biopsychosocial existence. Therefore biologic alterations are likely to affect both psychologic and social spheres.

Many of the conditions previously discussed affect mentation to various degrees. Progressive lethargy and weakness or intermittent confusion may frighten one patient, cause another to withdraw, and inspire anger and hostility in yet another. Various family members also have diverse responses. Responding to patients and their families in a calm, reassuring manner is often all that is needed to decrease fears, encourage communication, and lessen anger.

Patients and family members will have many questions, both verbalized and nonverbalized: Why does he twitch so uncontrollably? He was normally so active, why is he so sleepy all the time? Why doesn't my wife recognize me? Why are all those needles in her arm? What is that machine for? Often the only answer required is factual information that is communicated in words that are understood by the patient or family member. However, sometimes it is not information that is sought, but rather someone to listen attentively. Emotional support is not necessarily exclusively verbal. It can be a gentle touch on the shoulder or maintained eye contact when someone trusts the nurse enough to ask a question or share his or her anxieties.

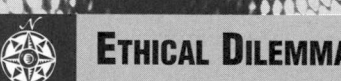

### ETHICAL DILEMMA

Mrs. Smith is an 88-year-old woman who has been admitted for dehydration, anemia, and a deteriorated cognitive state. She has a long history of depression and has expressed over many years her apparent wish to die. She is also nearly deaf. According to her daughter, Mrs. Smith has lost approximately 25 pounds over the past year. The patient had a mastectomy for breast cancer 25 years ago. Before admission, Mrs. Smith was living in her own apartment. Family members visited often and provided cooked meals and other necessities.

One problem in treating Mrs. Smith is that she refuses to eat with any regularity. During rehydration she had to be restrained because of combativeness. She has also refused intravenous (IV) and nasogastric (NG) tube feedings. Her family is concerned about her lack of nutrition and hydration, but they do not want to see her physically restrained and fed against her wishes. There is also the problem of placement. Mrs. Smith's apartment has been relinquished by her family, and family members state that they are not in a position to provide the necessary care to their mother within their homes.

What are the ethical questions related to the care of Mrs. Smith? Should she be fed via an IV and/or an NG tube?

## NURSING CARE PLAN

## PATIENT WITH HYPOKALEMIA

**NURSING DIAGNOSIS**

Mr. Baxter is a 73-year-old male who has been admitted from the emergency room with a diagnosis of dehydration, abdominal pain, and hypokalemia. He had been well at home until the past week, when he began experiencing nausea, vomiting, and abdominal discomfort. He attributed this to a flu until 6 days had passed and the abdominal pain increased in severity. He has not moved his bowels in 3 days. Abdominal x-ray examinations reveal a small bowel obstruction.

| Medical History | Psychosocial Data | Assessment Data |
|---|---|---|
| Myocardial infarction × 2, most recent 2 years ago; has participated in cardiac rehabilitation and is able to continue moderate activities around the house | Lives independently in own single-level home with wife of 52 years | Height 5'10", weight 155 lb<br>Vital signs: T 99.2, P 100, R 18, BP 102/64<br>Alert and oriented × 3<br>In moderate distress; pleasant and personable |
| | Active lifestyle; is avid gardener | *Skin:* intact, pink, warm, and dry; poor skin turgor |
| Congestive heart failure, which is under control with medications; very compliant with taking his cardiac medications and has continued to take them despite nausea this past week | Very involved with extended family; has 4 children, 10 grandchildren, and 6 great-grandchildren | *Eye-ear-nose-throat (EENT):* mucous membranes dry; lips dry and cracked<br>*Respiratory:* lungs clear to auscultation; diminished breath sounds; bilateral bases; respirations nonlabored, shallow, and symmetrical<br>*Cardiovascular:* apical pulse 100, slightly irregular; no jugular vein distention or edema; weak peripheral pulses bilaterally |
| Hypertension for 20 years | Religious affiliation is Baptist; he and his wife attend church every week and are involved in activities of the church | *Abdomen:* firm, distended abdomen; bowel sounds absent; NG tube inserted in the ER is draining a moderate amount of bile-colored fluid |
| Colectomy 3 years ago for adenocarcinoma | | *Musculoskeletal:* full, active range-of-motion (ROM) in all extremities. Soft, slightly flabby muscles; gait even, slow, and steady |
| No known allergies | Nonsmoker; minimal alcohol usage | *Urinary:* decreased urine output; indwelling urinary catheter inserted in the ER is draining 30 ml/hr; urine is clear, dark amber color |
| Wife has severe osteoarthritis but has remained active; no cardiopulmonary disease | | **Laboratory data**<br>Hemoglobin 12.2, Hematocrit (HCT) 38.3, BUN 31, Chromium (Cr) 1.3, WBC 12,000 |
| Children are healthy | | Na, 134 K 2.3, Cl 92 |
| Father died of heart disease | | *Chest x-ray:* Clear, no evidence of infiltration, atelectasis, or vascular congestion |
| Mother had diabetes | | *ECG:* Normal sinus rhythm; occasional unifocal premature ventricular contraction (PVC); flattened T wave; U wave present |
| | | **Medications**<br>*Home:* Lasix 40 mg qd<br>NitroDur 0.4 mg patch qd<br>Digoxin 0.25 mg qd<br>Cardizem 30 mg qid<br>*Hospital:* Demerol 50-75 mg IM q 3 hr prn<br>Compazine 10 mg IM q 6 hr prn<br>D5/0.45 saline with 40 mEq KCl at 125 ml/hr<br>Nasogastric tube to low intermittent suction |

# NURSING CARE PLAN

## PATIENT WITH HYPOKALEMIA—cont'd

### NURSING DIAGNOSIS

Fluid volume deficit related to nausea, vomiting, diuretic therapy, NG tube as evidenced by poor skin turgor, dry mucous membranes, decreased urine output, concentrated urine, decreased blood pressure

| NURSING INTERVENTIONS | EVALUATION OF EXPECTED OUTCOMES |
|---|---|
| Assess skin turgor, mucous membranes, vital signs, and level of consciousness. | Vital signs stable and within normal limits for patient |
| Maintain accurate I&O. Monitor urine output q2h during acute illness. | Urine output >30 ml/hr and urine yellow |
| Maintain IV fluids at prescribed rate. | Supple (elastic) skin turgor |
| Observe for signs of orthostatic hypotension. | Moist mucous membranes |
| Monitor serum electrolytes, primarily K, and report abnormal values. | Tolerating diet and fluids without nausea or vomiting |
| Explain all treatments and procedures to patient and family. | |

### NURSING DIAGNOSIS

Risk for decreased cardiac output related to hypokalemia and potential effect on cardiac conduction system

| NURSING INTERVENTIONS | EVALUATION OF EXPECTED OUTCOMES |
|---|---|
| Monitor vital signs, level of consciousness, and peripheral pulses. | BP and pulse within normal limits for patient |
| Monitor heart rhythm for arrhythmia, and report irregularities immediately. | Regular cardiac rhythm |
| Administer potassium as prescribed. | Strong and equal peripheral pulses |
| Provide rest to reduce oxygen demands. | Serum potassium within normal limits |
| Monitor for signs and symptoms of digitalis toxicity because hypokalemia enhances action of digitalis. | |

### NURSING DIAGNOSIS

Pain related to gastric distention, decreased GI motility, vomiting as evidenced by verbal complaints and nonverbal pain behavior

| NURSING INTERVENTIONS | EVALUATION OF EXPECTED OUTCOMES |
|---|---|
| Assess pain for severity, location, duration, and quality q2-4h. | Abdominal distention and pain decreased |
| Assess abdominal distention and bowel sounds q8h. | Reports tolerable level of pain |
| Medicate as needed with analgesic. | NG tube patent and functioning while in place |
| Respond immediately to complaint of pain, and monitor effectiveness of analgesic. | Nausea and vomiting resolved |
| Help patient assume a comfortable position. Maintain elevation of head of bed. | |
| Medicate as needed with antiemetic. | |
| Maintain patency of NG tube, and irrigate prn with 30 ml normal saline. | |
| Provide comfort measures (massage, relaxation). | |

## NURSING CARE PLAN
## PATIENT WITH HYPOKALEMIA—cont'd

**NURSING DIAGNOSIS**
Knowledge deficit related to complication of diuretic therapy and acute illness

| NURSING INTERVENTIONS | EVALUATION OF EXPECTED OUTCOMES |
|---|---|
| Assess patient and family level of understanding of illness. Review the correlation between diuretic use, vomiting, and hypokalemia. Review other conditions that may lead to hypokalemia. Instruct on medication action, dosage, and side effects. Teach the importance of ingesting potassium-rich foods (oranges, bananas, tomatoes, dark green leafy vegetables, milk). Review signs and symptoms to report to primary physician. | Verbalizes causes of hypokalemia Identifies potassium-rich foods Verbalizes understanding of medication administration |

## KEY CONCEPTS

➤ Infants, the aged, and the obese are at higher risk in situations that involve fluid loss.

➤ A 5-pound weight gain represents 2 L of fluid retained.

➤ A solution that is equal in concentration to fluid in the cell is hypotonic. A solution that is higher in concentration is hypertonic, and a solution that is lower in concentration is hypotonic.

➤ Shifts of plasma to interstitial fluid (edema) result from elevation of venous hydrostatic pressure, a decrease in plasma oncotic pressure, or an elevation of interstitial oncotic pressure.

➤ Shifts of interstitial fluid to plasma result from an increase in oncotic pressure of plasma or an increase in hydrostatic pressure of the tissues.

➤ An isotonic ECF deficit (hypovolemia) occurs when fluids and electrolytes are lost equally.

➤ Symptoms are low blood pressure, a weak pulse, weight loss, and shock.

➤ A hypertonic ECF deficit (dehydration) occurs when more water is lost than electrolytes, which causes water to leave the cell to dilute the ECF.

➤ Symptoms are tenting and dry mucous membranes.

➤ An isotonic ECF excess occurs when water and electrolytes are retained. Symptoms are edema, a bounding pulse, and dyspnea.

➤ A hypotonic ECF excess (primary water excess) occurs when water intake exceeds electrolyte intake. Symptoms of confusion, lethargy, and seizures result from cerebral edema.

➤ The following is a list of symptoms of electrolyte imbalances:

Hyponatremia: anorexia, nausea, vomiting, diarrhea, muscle cramps, abdominal cramps

Hypernatremia: same as dehydration (dry and sticky mucous membranes, flushed appearance, thirst, oliguria, irritability, excitability, disorientation, muscle spasms)

Hypokalemia: weakness, anorexia, nausea, vomiting, abdominal distention, prominent U wave on ECG

Hyperkalemia: muscle twitching, paresthesias of the face and tongue, tachycardia followed by bradycardia, peaked T waves on ECG

Hypocalcemia: tingling, twitching, tetany, carpopedal spasm, positive Chvostek's sign and positive Trousseau's sign as a result of increased nerve and muscle cell excitability

Hypercalcemia: lethargy and decreased muscle tone as a result of depressed neuromuscular activity

Hypomagnesemia: similar to hypocalcemia (tingling, twitching, tetany)

Hypermagnesemia: lethargy, decreased tendon reflexes, depressed respiratory rate, low blood pressure

Hypochloremia: same as hyponatremia and metabolic alkalosis (anorexia, nausea, vomiting, diarrhea, muscle cramps, abdominal cramps, twitching, tetany)

## KEY CONCEPTS—cont'd

Hyperchloremia: same as acidosis (lethargy, confusion, weakness, stupor)

➤ Phosphate levels vary inversely with calcium levels. If calcium is high, phosphate is low and vice versa.

➤ Hypoproteinemia results in reduced colloidal osmotic pressure in the plasma, which causes edema.

➤ Acid-base balance is regulated by the buffer systems, the lungs, and the kidneys. The primary buffer system is carbonic acid/bicarbonate. The cells are buffers. The lungs control $CO_2$. The kidneys excrete or reabsorb bicarbonate and excrete hydrogen ions as needed.

➤ Metabolic acidosis is caused by a deficit of base bicarbonate or an excess of acid byproducts from metabolism. Symptoms of metabolic acidosis are Kussmaul's respiration, weakness, disorientation, drowsiness, stupor, and coma.

➤ Metabolic alkalosis is caused by an excess in base bicarbonate. Symptoms of metabolic alkalosis are nausea, vomiting, diarrhea, muscle cramps, twitching, and tetany.

➤ Respiratory alkalosis is caused by a carbonic acid deficit. Symptoms of respiratory alkalosis are paresthesias, numbness, headache, tingling, and tetany.

➤ Respiratory acidosis is caused by an excess in carbonic acid. Symptoms of respiratory acidosis are weakness, restlessness, drowsiness, disorientation, headache, muscle twitching, and convulsions.

➤ Interpreting blood gas values requires three steps:
Step 1. Name the pH level (acidosis or alkalosis).
Step 2. Look at bicarbonate and carbonic acid levels. Identify the abnormality that can cause what was found in Step 1. Add either "respiratory" or "metabolic" to the name.
Step 3. Look for compensation. Add "compensated" or "uncompensated" to the name.

➤ A quick formula to determine body serum osmolarity is $2 \times$ sodium level.

➤ The following is a list of types of shock:
Hypovolemic shock: caused by a loss of fluid available to circulation
Cardiogenic shock: caused by pump failure (heart is the pump)
Neurogenic shock: caused by vasodilation following nerve stimulation or nerve block
Vasogenic shock: involves vasodilation resulting from factors affecting blood vessels
Anaphylactic shock: results from an abnormal antigen-antibody response
Septic shock: results when the metabolic end-products of bacteria cause vasodilation; can result in disseminated intravascular coagulation

➤ To treat shock, remove or treat the cause, replace blood volume, provide oxygen, and position patient supine or with feet elevated if cerebral edema is not present or likely

## CRITICAL THINKING EXERCISES

1. Describe the differences between the processes of osmosis and diffusion.
2. Explain the fact that a severe burn will result in extracellular fluid volume deficit.
3. Describe the effects of aldosterone on sodium and potassium levels in the bloodstream.
4. Explain the fact that patients who are taking thiazide or loop diuretics are likely to develop hypokalemia.
5. Develop a list of discharge instructions for the patient receiving thiazide diuretics.

## REFERENCES AND ADDITIONAL READINGS

Ahern J: A guide to blood gases, *Nurs Stand* 10(49):50-52, 1995.

Batory-Griffith GA: Learning the ins and outs of IV therapy, *Nursing* 26(8):58-59, 1996.

Bove LA: Restoring electrolyte balance: calcium and phosphorus, *RN* 59(3):47-52, 1996.

Braxmeyer DL, Keyes JL: The pathophysiology of potassium balance, *Crit Care Nurse* 16(5):59-73, 1996.

Cirolia B: Understanding edema, *Nursing* 26(2):66-69, 1996.

Cornock MA: Making sense of arterial blood gases and their interpretation, *Nurs Times* 92(6):30-31, 1996.

Held JL: Cancer care: correcting fluid and electrolyte imbalances, *Nursing* 25(4):25-28, 1995.

Horne MM, Heitz UE, Swearingen PL: *Pocket guide to fluid, electrolyte, and acid-base balance,* ed 3, St Louis, 1997, Mosby.

Hunter E et al: Relationship of local IV complications and the method of intermittent IV access, *J Intravenous Nurs* 18(4):202-206, 1995.

Lamb J: Peripheral IV therapy, *Nurs Stand* 9(30):32-35, 1995.

Levine TT: Central intravenous lines: your role, *Nursing* 26(4):48-49, 1996.

Lilley LL: Revisiting digoxin toxicity, *Am J Nurs* 96(8):14, 16, 1996.

Lilley LL, Guanci R: Persistent potassium problems, *Am J Nurs* 97(6):14, 1997.

Masoorli S: Home IV therapy comes of age, *RN* 59(10):22-25, 1996.

Mays DA: Turn ABG's into child's play, *RN* 58(1):36-40, 1995.

McCance KL, Huether SE: *Pathophysiology: the biologic basis for disease in adults and children,* ed 2, St Louis, 1994 Mosby.

O'Donnell L: Complications of MI: beyond the acute stage, *Am J Nurs* 96(9):24-31, 1996.

Perez A: Electrolytes: restoring the balance, *RN* 58(11):32-37, 1995.

Perez A: Restoring electrolyte balance: hypokalemia, *RN* 58(12):33-36, 1995.

Phipps WJ, Long BC: *Medical-surgical nursing: concepts and clinical practice,* ed 5, St Louis, 1995, Mosby.

Potter PA, Perry AG: *Basic nursing: theory and practice,* ed 3, St Louis, 1995, Mosby.

Seidel HM et al: *Mosby's guide to physical examination,* ed 3, St Louis, 1995, Mosby.

Venfrolio LG: Would you hang these IV solutions? *Am J Nurs* 95(6):37-39, 1995.

Weldy NJ: *Body fluids and electrolytes: a programmed presentation,* ed 7, St Louis, 1996, Mosby.

White VM: Hyperkalemia, *Am J Nurs* 97(6):35, 1997.

Wilkinson R: Nurses' concerns about IV therapy and devices, *Nurs Stand* 10(35):35-37, 1996.

Williamson JC: Acid-base disorders: classification and management strategies, *Am Fam Physician* 52(2):584-590, 1995.

Wolpert N: An orderly look at calcium metabolism disorders, *Nursing* 20(7):60-64, 1990.

# CHAPTER 28

# Endocrine Problems

## CHAPTER OBJECTIVES

1 Identify patient responses that may indicate potential problems of the endocrine system.
2 Describe the pathophysiology, course, prognosis, and treatment of endocrine gland disorders.
3 Describe nursing management of patient responses to hypersecretion or hyposecretion of specific endocrine glands.
4 Outline the actions that patients and providers take to prevent, detect, and treat complications from changes in endocrine function.

## KEY TERMS

| | |
|---|---|
| acromegaly | goiter |
| aldosterone | goitrogens |
| androgens | homeostasis |
| atrophy | idiopathic |
| catecholamines | mineralocorticoids |
| Chvostek's sign | myxedema |
| endogenous | polyendocrine deficiency |
| exogenous | syndrome |
| giantism | tetany |
| glucocorticoids | Trousseau's phenomenon |

## ENDOCRINE ORGAN FUNCTION

The endocrine organs are ductless, highly vascularized glands composed of specialized cells that synthesize hormones. These hormones pass directly into the tissue fluid, are absorbed into the blood, and are carried by the blood to other sites in the body. Hormones are chemical messengers that ultimately influence the activity of various body organs.

Endocrine glands produce minute amounts of hormones, which are secreted at predictable intervals. Hormones bind to specific cellular receptors in various sites in the body and regulate intracellular metabolism. Each hormone reacts with receptor sites (hormone-binding sites) on specific cells in target organs. For example, the thyroid gland synthesizes thyroxine, which acts at several cellular sites, including the cell membrane, mitochondria, and nucleus. Thyroxine acts to increase the production of energy for metabolism in all body tissues.

Other important hormones affect reproduction, responses to injury and stress, fluid and electrolyte balance, growth and maturation, and energy production. Exocrine glands, in contrast, secrete substances through ducts that empty into specific parts of the body. Sweat glands are exocrine glands that discharge substances directly onto the skin. The pancreas produces enzymes that are secreted into the pancreatic duct and carried into the gastrointestinal (GI) tract.

The endocrine glands are interrelated and interdependent. They play an essential role in maintaining homeostasis and in regulating blood pressure and neuromuscular contraction. Overproduction or underproduction of hormones can cause serious and sometimes life-threatening illness. Figure 28-1 shows the location of the endocrine glands.

The *thyroid gland* is the largest of the endocrine glands. It consists of two lobes and is located in the neck below the pharynx and anterior to the trachea, with a lobe on either side of the trachea. The two lobes are connected by a strip of thyroid tissue called the *isthmus.* The thyroid gland stores iodine and secretes three hormones: thyroxine ($T_4$), triiodothyronine ($T_3$),

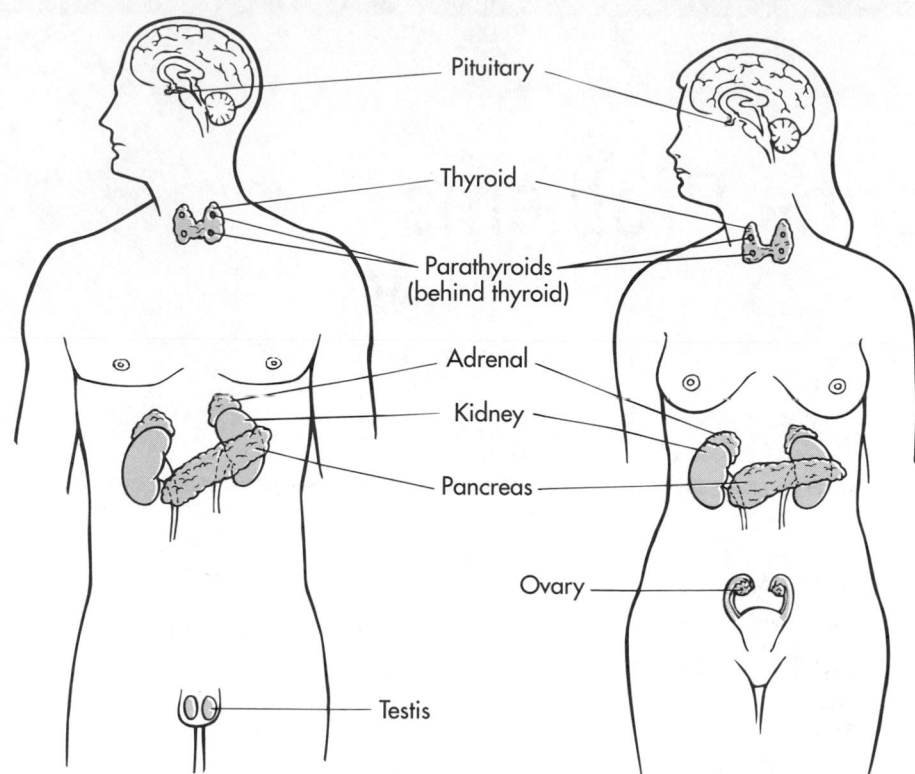

**Figure 28-1** Location of the endocrine glands.

and thyrocalcitonin (calcitonin). The primary function of the thyroid gland is regulation of metabolism, the rate at which nutrients are oxidized to provide energy for the body. $T_4$ and $T_3$ produce similar effects; $T_4$, however, acts more slowly and is longer lasting than $T_3$. Any disturbance in the secretion of $T_4$ may result in hyperthyroidism or hypothyroidism. A congenital absence of the thyroid gland causes cretinism in the infant, a deficiency of secretion may result in **myxedema** in the adult, and increased secretion may result in Graves' disease. Calcitonin acts to reduce the level of calcium in the blood by increasing the movement of calcium from the blood into the bones.

The *parathyroids* are usually four small glands, but there may be more or fewer. They are arranged in pairs and embedded in the posterior lateral lobe of the thyroid gland. The parathyroids release parathormone, which helps to maintain the **homeostasis,** or relative consistency, of the calcium levels in the blood and body fluids. The presence of this hormone tends to increase the level of calcium in the blood and the excretion of phosphates.

The two *adrenal glands* are located immediately above the kidneys. Each adrenal gland consists of two parts, which function as separate glands. The outer section, the adrenal cortex, produces several different hormones that are essential to life, such as the **glucocorticoids,** the **mineralocorticoids,** and the sex hor-

mones. The glucocorticoids cortisone and hydrocortisone regulate much of the cell activity of the body and maintain an optimum internal environment for the cells. They also regulate the body's ability to adapt to constant changes in the external environment. The mineralocorticoids help regulate electrolyte metabolism. **Aldosterone** is the most important mineralocorticoid, and its primary function is to maintain homeostasis of the sodium concentration in the blood. Small amounts of the male hormone androgen and the female hormone estrogen are also secreted by the adrenal cortex. The inner section of the adrenal gland, the adrenal medulla, secretes the **catecholamines** epinephrine and norepinephrine, two hormones that tend to increase and prolong the effects of the sympathetic nervous system. Epinephrine and norepinephrine primarily affect smooth muscle, cardiac muscle, and glandular activity and are responsible for the "fight or flight" response to stress.

The hypothalamus and the pituitary gland, which are located at the base of the brain, integrate the functions of the endocrine system and the nervous system. Hypothalamic hormones are secreted into the local venous circulation, where they immediately react with receptors and either stimulate or inhibit the synthesis and release of anterior pituitary hormones. The pituitary gland (hypophysis) consists of an anterior lobe (adenohypophysis) and a posterior lobe (neurohy-

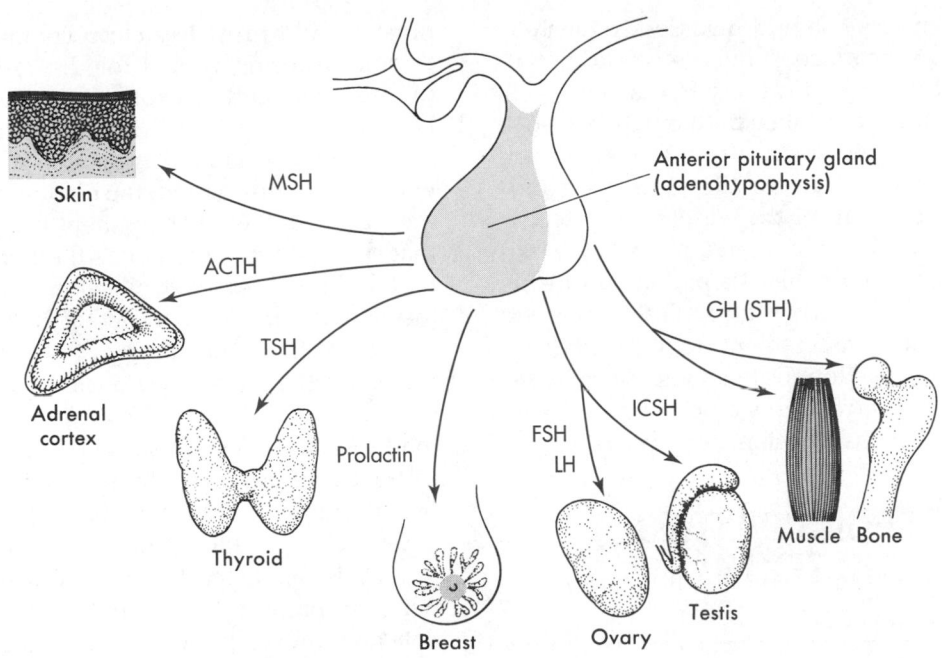

**Figure 28-2**    Target organs of hormones released by the anterior lobe of the pituitary gland. (From Beare P, Myers J: *Adult health nursing,* ed 3, St Louis, 1998, Mosby.)

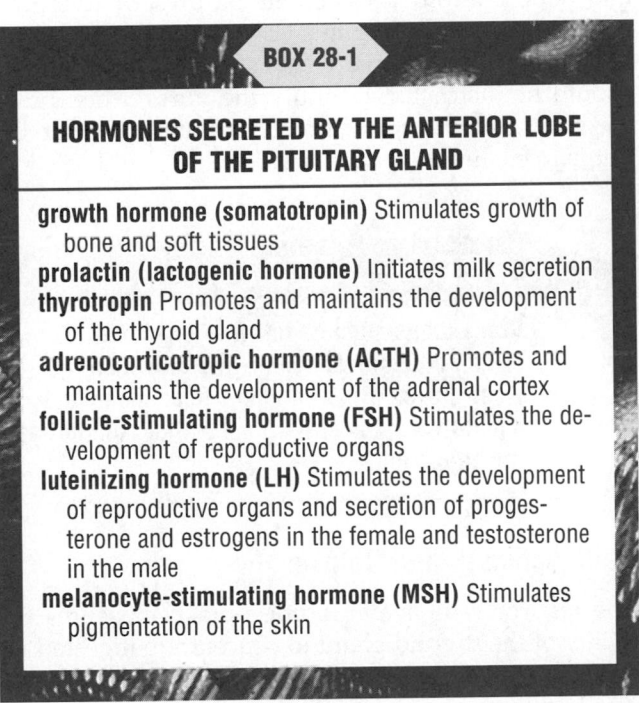

### BOX 28-1

## HORMONES SECRETED BY THE ANTERIOR LOBE OF THE PITUITARY GLAND

**growth hormone (somatotropin)** Stimulates growth of bone and soft tissues

**prolactin (lactogenic hormone)** Initiates milk secretion

**thyrotropin** Promotes and maintains the development of the thyroid gland

**adrenocorticotropic hormone (ACTH)** Promotes and maintains the development of the adrenal cortex

**follicle-stimulating hormone (FSH)** Stimulates the development of reproductive organs

**luteinizing hormone (LH)** Stimulates the development of reproductive organs and secretion of progesterone and estrogens in the female and testosterone in the male

**melanocyte-stimulating hormone (MSH)** Stimulates pigmentation of the skin

pophysis). The anterior lobe secretes growth hormone, thyroid-stimulating hormone (TSH), adrenocorticotropic hormone (ACTH), prolactin, gonadotropic hormones, and beta-lipotropin (Box 28-1). The target organs for these hormones are shown in Figure 28-2. The posterior lobe of the pituitary is a continuation of the hypothalamus. The hormones secreted by the posterior pituitary originate in the hypothalamus; they in-

clude antidiuretic hormone (ADH), or vasopressin, and oxytocin. Antidiuretic hormone regulates the fluid volume in the body by facilitating water reabsorption in the renal tubules. It also is a potent vasoconstrictor. Oxytocin affects uterine contractions and lactation, stimulating breast tissue to secrete milk into the mammary ducts.

In females, the gonads, or sex glands, are the ovaries, which secrete estrogen, progesterone, and small amounts of **androgens.** The male sex glands are the testes, which secrete testosterone and androsterone. These hormones are important in the development of sex characteristics and in the reproductive process. The male and female reproductive systems are discussed in Chapters 42 and 43. The pancreas has both exocrine and endocrine functions and is discussed in Chapter 29.

## NURSING ASSESSMENT

Endocrine problems often are difficult to assess because of the various effects of each hormone on body function. A health history is the first approach to assessment of the patient. Problems of the cardiovascular, pulmonary, renal, or neurologic systems or of other body systems should be identified. Previous endocrine disorders and the presence of hypertension should be noted. The signs and symptoms of endocrine disorders vary and can be subtle. Symptoms that should be assessed include changes in smell, taste, speech, skin, personality, and energy level. Possible signs of endocrine problems also should be assessed, such as visual disturbances, headaches, muscle weakness, excessive hunger or thirst, and urinary frequency.

A history of medications taken by the patient also is important. Many medications affect the endocrine glands and could contribute to the patient's symptoms. Physical assessment of the endocrine system is difficult because the thyroid gland is the only endocrine gland that is palpable. Palpation can determine if the gland is enlarged or if nodules are present. The primary physical assessment tool for the endocrine system is inspection. Data should be collected on the individual's general appearance, apparent age, facial expression, hair distribution, and stature.

# NURSING RESPONSIBILITIES FOR DIAGNOSTIC TESTS AND PROCEDURES

Many of the tests used to diagnose a possible endocrine disorder, to follow its course, and to evaluate the results of therapy are performed on blood and urine. The amount and type of specific hormones can be estimated through chemical analysis of these body fluids. When an excess or deficiency is suggested, further tests and procedures may be done to determine the effect on the whole body. Many of these tests require nursing interventions to ensure that specimens are collected properly. Some procedures require withholding of food and fluids and collection of urine specimens. To ensure that the test results provide reliable information about the patient's endocrine status, procedures must be followed accurately.

> **NURSE ALERT**
>
> A history of allergy should be determined and clearly noted before any tests are done.

## Procedures
### Blood Chemistry

Analysis of endocrine gland functions often is done by hormone assay. Serum levels of hormones such as $T_3$ or $T_4$ indicate whether appropriate amounts of hormones are being secreted. However, not all hormone levels can be easily determined by blood level.

### Urinalysis

A 24-hour urine collection may be necessary for hormone analysis. Collection may start at any hour. The nurse should provide a clean container large enough to hold all urine voided for the 24-hour period. The procedure should be explained to the patient, and the hour at which collection is started should be carefully noted. Because the test measures substances *produced* within a 24-hour period, the bladder must be empty at the start of the test. The patient is asked to void, and that specimen is discarded. All other urine voided after that hour is saved. Collection is stopped at exactly the same hour the next day; at that hour the patient voids, and the urine becomes the last part of the specimen. It is the nurse's responsibility to see that the patient voids the last specimen exactly 24 hours from the time the collection started. For ease of collection, 24-hour urine tests usually are conducted from 7:00 AM one morning to 7:00 AM the next morning.

Several precautions must be taken in conducting urinalysis. First, the bottle should be clearly labeled with the patient's name and room number and the date and time collection began. Second, all urine must be collected and saved. Finally, the container holding the urine must be maintained as specified for the diagnostic test. A preservative or refrigeration may be required. Patients should be taught to collect their urine and pour it into bottles containing preservatives and never to void directly into a bottle containing a chemical. If the preservative used is an acid, the patient should be instructed to notify the nurse when he or she voids, and the nurse should pour the urine into the bottle to ensure the patient's safety.

> **NURSE ALERT**
>
> Precautions must be taken when collecting urine and blood samples. The nurse should wear gloves while obtaining specimens and should wash his or her hands after completing the collection.

### Radioactive Iodine Uptake

The test for radioactive iodine uptake measures the ability of the thyroid gland to concentrate ingested iodine. A small amount of radioactive iodine is administered orally to the patient, either in capsule form or in a colorless, odorless drink. The amount is called a *tracer dose.* After 24 hours the amount of radioactive iodine stored in the thyroid gland is measured by a Geiger counter—a type of instrument called a *scintillator,* which is held near the thyroid gland. Patients with overactive glands are found to store a high percentage of the iodine, whereas those with underactive glands take up a small amount of the iodine.

## Thyroid Ultrasonogram

The patient is brought to the x-ray area for radiologic visualization of the tissue structure. In an ultrasonogram, ultrasonic waves reflect off the organ, and a picture of the findings appears on an oscilloscope and paper printout.

## Thyroid Scan

The patient is given radioactive iodine-131 ($^{131}$I), and the uptake is quantitatively measured by the external passing of the scintillator over the throat. The scintillator is connected to a recording device that provides a record of the activity. The scan is used in connection with other tests and is used to differentiate between a nonmalignant condition and a possible malignancy of the thyroid gland.

## Triiodothyronine (T$_3$) Resin Uptake Test

In the T$_3$ resin uptake test, a blood specimen is taken from the patient, and $^{131}$I is added to the blood in the laboratory. Normally the red blood cells take up 11% to 19% of the iodine. In hypofunction of the gland, less is taken up, whereas in hyperfunction, more is taken up. The advantage of the test is that the patient does not have to be given the $^{131}$I.

## Nursing Responsibilities

Several thyroid function tests use $^{131}$I. Nursing responsibilities include reassuring the patient and encouraging cooperation. Patients should realize that the test will not make them radioactive. Care must be taken to ensure that the patient does not receive iodine before the test. Drugs that contain various iodine preparations, contrast mediums used in x-ray examinations, iodine used as a skin antiseptic (Betadine), and iodized salt are all forms of iodine that should be avoided. The nurse should question the patient about any hypersensitivity to iodine before any testing with this drug is done.

Other diagnostic tests performed to detect or monitor the course of endocrine disturbances require some patient education. The two noninvasive tests are computed tomography magnetic resonance imaging. For computed tomography (CT scan), patients should be told that a picture of the gland will be taken by a machine that moves around them. *Magnetic resonance imaging* (MRI) involves the use of a magnet, radiowaves, and computers to make an image of the entire body. It is a painless scanning procedure that requires no special preparation. The presence of any metal inside the patient's body, such as pacemakers, heart valves, or clips, must be determined before the test.

For invasive tests, such as arteriography, a contrast medium is injected into a vein, and the medium travels to the organ to be examined. X-ray pictures of the gland are taken once it can be visualized on the screen. Some people may feel a warm sensation when the medium is injected, which is normal.

# NURSING RESPONSIBILITIES FOR THERAPEUTIC PROCEDURES

The treatment for endocrine disorders varies greatly, depending on the type of disorder. However, some nursing responsibilities are the same regardless of the problem. The fluid and electrolyte balance should be monitored as necessary by recording fluid intake and urinary output and by weighing the patient daily. Vital signs should be assessed, and the patient's neurologic status should be monitored when indicated.

Endocrine disorders are often traumatic, both physically and emotionally, and support should be given to the patient and family. Many endocrine disorders, such as diabetes and Addison's disease, require lifelong treatment that may be costly and inconvenient to the patient. Feelings of frustration are common, and the nurse should help the patient and family deal with these feelings by encouraging them to talk openly about the disorder and about the changes that need to occur in their life-styles.

Endocrine disorders are chronic and cause changes in a patient's self-image, behavior, and life-style. For these reasons, patient preparation, as well as support and encouragement in developing new coping strategies, are essential components of the management of endocrine disorders. Both patient and family must understand the disorder and be prepared to deal with the life-style changes it may necessitate.

Teaching the patient about long-term drug therapy for maintaining his or her health is important because replacement therapy often is required for life. The nurse's instructions should be precise, and demonstrations may help both the patient and significant others understand the information. Because stress may interfere with the response to medication, the nurse should explore with the patient potential stressors and the most appropriate methods of dealing with them. The nurse also should emphasize that the medication must be taken consistently, even if the person feels normal. The expected results, possible side effects, and methods of minimizing side effects should be discussed. It is particularly important that the patient understand the signs and symptoms of possible complications, so that he or she will know when to call the primary care provider. Consistent adherence to a daily regimen can help prevent acute episodes. Patients should be encouraged to carry an identification card with pertinent medical information or to wear a medical alert device at all times. They also should be guided to local support groups for help in coping with the disorder.

# THE PATIENT WITH DISEASES AND DISORDERS OF THE ENDOCRINE SYSTEM

## Disorders of the Thyroid Gland

### Simple (Endemic) Goiter

Any enlargement of the thyroid gland is called a **goiter.** *Endemic,* or *simple,* goiter results when dietary iodine is insufficient for the synthesis of thyroxine. To compensate for the insufficiency, the pituitary gland secretes excessive amounts of thyroid-stimulating hormone (TSH), causing the gland to hypertrophy. Iodine deficiencies in food and water can be found in certain areas of the United States, and it is in those areas that the occurrence of endemic goiter has been greatest. The marketing and use of iodized salt has reduced the incidence of this type of goiter.

Some foods and drugs act as **goitrogens,** which inhibit the synthesis of thyroid hormone. Turnips, rutabagas, soybean products, and peanuts are potent goitrogens. Seafood, green, leafy vegetables, peaches, peas, strawberries, and radishes are less potent goitrogens. Thyroid-inhibiting drugs, sulfonamides, and salicylates also can reduce the synthesis of thyroid hormone. However, goitrogens usually cause goiters only in individuals who have a low iodine intake (Lewis, Collier, Heitkemper, 1996).

An increase in physiologic demands, such as pregnancy, lactation, puberty, infections, and other body changes, also can result in an inadequate iodine supply. For instance, endemic goiter is more common in girls and usually occurs just before puberty, after which it may disappear completely. These types of goiter usually produce no symptoms unless they become large and exert pressure on adjacent structures, such as the trachea. When this occurs, the patient may experience mild neck discomfort, a chronic cough, difficulty swallowing, and respiratory difficulty (Lammon, Hart, 1993).

The best treatment for goiters is prevention, achieved through adequate amounts of dietary iodine. However, once goiters have developed, treatment is aimed at reducing the size of the gland with iodine and thyroid preparations. Large goiters may be removed surgically to relieve pressure or to improve appearance. A subtotal thyroidectomy usually is performed. Individuals living in areas with a known deficiency of iodine in the water and soil should be encouraged to use iodized salt and to eat foods rich in natural iodine, such as leafy vegetables and seafood.

## Hyperthyroidism

Hyperthyroidism occurs when the circulating levels of thyroid hormones ($T_4$, $T_3$, or both) are elevated. The incidence is six times higher in women, and the condition often occurs between 30 and 50 years of age. A previous iodine deficiency is believed to predispose people to hyperthyroidism. The condition may be **idiopathic** or may be caused by thyroid gland hypertrophy, neoplasms, inflammatory processes, or autoimmune disorders. Hyperthyroidism often follows infection or emotional stress. The increase in hormone production speeds up all the body's metabolic processes and gives rise to characteristic signs and symptoms. The most common form of hyperthyroidism is Graves' disease, followed by multinodular goiter.

**Graves' disease.** Graves' disease is an autoimmune disorder of unknown origin that occurs primarily in genetically susceptible individuals. The patient's immune system produces thyroid-stimulating antibodies, which circulate in the bloodstream and attack thyroid tissue. The ensuing damage stimulates thyroid tissue to multiply (hyperplasia), and the thyroid gland enlarges, resulting in increased levels of thyroid hormones. Exacerbations and remissions are common despite ongoing treatment.

**Multinodular goiter.** Multinodular goiter is characterized by the formation of small, discrete nodules that secrete thyroid hormone. The signs and symptoms of this condition are slower to develop and are less severe than those of Graves' disease. Often the patient has a history of simple goiter for a period of years before diagnosis. Multinodular goiter is more common in women in their sixth or seventh decade (Lewis, Collier, Heitkemper, 1996).

Diagnostic tests for hyperthyroidism indicate that serum $T_4$ and $T_3$ are elevated. $T_3$ resin uptake ($T_3RU$) also is elevated. Thyroid-stimulating hormone (TSH) is subnormal and occasionally undetectable. A radioactive iodine uptake (RAIU) test may be done, especially to differentiate Graves' disease from other forms of thyroid disorders. A patient with Graves' disease shows a diffuse uptake of the radioactive iodine of 25% to 95%, compared with other conditions that show an uptake of 5% or less. Electrocardiographic (ECG) tracings may indicate tachycardia, atrial fibrillation, and changes in the P and T waves.

**Assessment.** Excess production of thyroid hormones increases the metabolism, resulting in an increase in all physiologic processes. It also increases the effects resulting from stimulation of the sympathetic division of the autonomic nervous system. The appetite increases, but the person loses weight and is thin. The systolic blood pressure rises, and the pulse rate is much faster, even while the individual is at rest. The thyroid gland may be enlarged. The skin is warm, and the patient perspires freely and is sensitive to heat. Palpitations tachycardia, and atrial fibrillation may occur. When the fingers are extended, a fine tremor may be seen. The patient may also experience fatigue, weakness, a disruption in menstruation, a disturbance in sleep, and constipation or diarrhea. Profound personality changes may occur, marked by episodes of irritability, excitability, and crying that may occur spontaneously. Such personality changes often are difficult for friends and family members to understand. Therefore it is important that nurses provide emotional support for the family and the patient, to help them understand that the patient's emotional state is related to hormonal changes and should subside as the hormone levels decline. The patient may have a bulging of the eyeballs, known as *exophthalmos*, which gives the person a startled expression. This is a result of retraction of the upper eyelid, which is caused by fluid retention in extraocular muscles and impaired venous drainage from the orbit of the eye. The patient may have excessive tearing, blurred vision, and a feeling of pressure behind the eyes. Treatment may or may not relieve symptoms (Figure 28-3). It should be noted that women over age 50 often do not manifest the standard symptoms of hyperthyroidism but show instead the cardiovascular symptoms, which could include shortness of breath, palpitations, or chest pain.

**Intervention.** The treatment of patients with hyperthyroidism is directed toward reducing the activity of the thyroid gland and the excessive production of thyroxine (Box 28-2). The disease may be treated with antithyroid drugs, surgical removal of the gland, or therapeutic doses of radioactive iodine.

Iodine preparations, propylthiouracil, and saturated solutions of potassium iodide (SSKI) may be given to alleviate the symptoms of hyperthyroidism. These preparations prevent the release of thyroxine but are only temporarily effective. Liquids usually are diluted with fruit juice, water, or milk and are administered through a straw to prevent staining of the teeth. Side effects include a metallic taste, epigastric discomfort, nausea, and vomiting. Iodine preparations are most useful before thyroid surgery or in emergency situations but are rarely used for long-term therapy.

Propranolol (Inderal) relieves many of the symptoms of hyperthyroidism, tachycardia, and hypertension. The beta-adrenergic blockers help prevent critical complications from thyroid hormone excess. Because of their effectiveness, beta-blockers often are used in conjunction with antithyroid drugs.

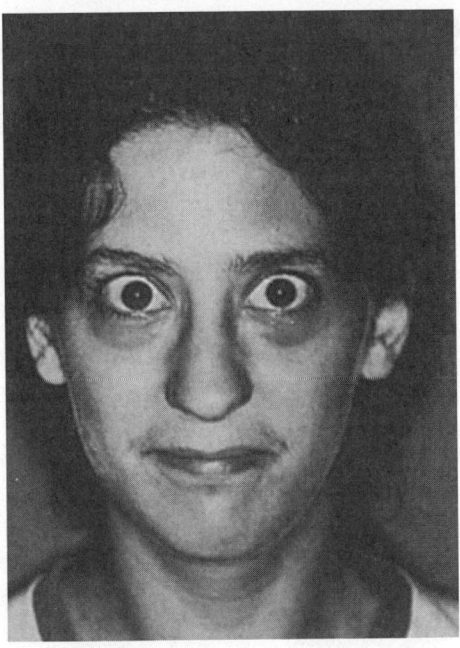

**Figure 28-3** Exophthalmos in hyperthyroidism. Note severe retraction of upper and lower lids. (From Rose LF, Kaye D: *Internal medicine for dentistry*, St Louis, 1983, Mosby.)

Radioactive iodine also may be given for hyperthyroidism. The drug acts the same as nonradioactive iodine. After an oral dose it enters the bloodstream and becomes concentrated in the thyroid gland, where it destroys the cells. This treatment is inexpensive and easily administered. Those involved with patient care should wear gloves when giving radioactive iodine and when disposing of the patient's excreta. The major side effect is hypothyroidism.

Each patient must be considered as an individual, and patience and tact may be required in meeting nursing needs. If exophthalmos is present, the eyes must be protected from irritation. The environment should ensure rest and quiet and should be be free of annoying distractions. Because the patient is sensitive to heat, the room should be private, well ventilated, and cool. Visitors should be limited to family and significant others, and efforts should be made to interpret the patient's erratic behavior as a part of the disease. The patient needs emotional as well as physical quiet and should be protected from situations that increase emotional tension and anxiety. Psychotherapy may be beneficial.

The diet should be high in calories and vitamins, with carbohydrate supplements. Extra servings should be available, and between-meal opportunities to eat may be given if sufficient calories are not taken in with

<table>
<tr><td colspan="2">

| BOX 28-2 | NURSING PROCESS |
</td></tr>
</table>

## BOX 28-2 ▷ NURSING PROCESS

# HYPERTHYROIDISM

### ASSESSMENT

- Mental status (diminished attention span, emotional lability)
- Cardiovascular (increased systolic blood pressure; decreased diastolic blood pressure; tachycardia at rest; arrhythmia; complaints of palpitation, chest discomfort, and dyspnea)
- Skin (flushed, warm)
- Hair (fine, thinning)
- Eye (lid retraction, decreased visual acuity, complaints of eyes tiring easily)
- Metabolic changes (decreased weight; increased food intake; decreased serum cholesterol and triglycerides; complaints of intolerance of heat, fatigue, sleep disturbance, and change in libido)
- Musculoskeletal (muscle weakness, decreased muscle tone, tremors)

### NURSING DIAGNOSES

- Altered nutrition: less than body requirements related to increased metabolism
- Altered thought processes related to personality changes
- Sleep pattern disturbance related to increased metabolism
- Ineffective thermoregulation associated with increased metabolism
- Knowledge deficit related to altered metabolism
- Anxiety related to inability to control illness
- Ineffective individual and family coping related to personality changes

### NURSING INTERVENTIONS

- Keep environment quiet and calm.
- Limit visitors.
- Monitor vital signs and temperature.

- Promote diet high in protein, vitamins, calories, and fluids.
- Discourage intake of caffeinated foods (coffee, cocoa, chocolate, cola, tea).
- Monitor for potential adverse effects of medications (rash, fever, conjunctivitis, generalized discomfort).
- Protect eyes from trauma, especially with exophthalmos.
- Weigh patient daily.
- Observe for respiratory problems, tetany, or voice changes after thyroidectomy.
- Observe for signs of complications of hyperthyroidism (thyrotoxicosis, thyroid crisis, or thyroid storm), including elevated temperature, rapid pulse and respirations, pain, dyspnea, confusion, restlessness, and alteration in level of consciousness.
- Provide emotional support to patient, significant others, and family.
- Educate patient, significant others, and family to watch for adverse effects of medications and for signs of thyroid crisis.

### EVALUATION OF EXPECTED OUTCOMES

- Verbalizes the rationale for reducing environmental stimuli
- Follows a diet high in protein, vitamins, calories, and fluids
- Avoids intake of caffeine
- Describes the medication regimen and potential side effects of medications
- Discusses the need for protecting eyes from trauma
- Weighs self daily
- Recognizes signs of complications of hyperthyroidism

the regular meals. Patients should be permitted to choose food, especially if the appetite is poor, and a visit from the dietitian may be helpful in ascertaining the patient's likes and dislikes. If the patient is to be cared for at home, the visiting nurse may visit the home and help plan the patient's care.

## Thyroidectomy

Part or all of the thyroid gland may be surgically removed because of malignancy, exophthalmic goiter, or any other severe condition affecting the gland and adjacent structures. A thyroidectomy is not an emergency procedure, and the patient must have normal thyroid function before surgery is done; this may require 2 to 3 months of drug therapy. Surgery usually is done only in cases involving a carcinoma or large goiter. Nursing care after thyroid surgery requires more than routine postoperative care because of the location of the incision. Swelling around the incision can cause airway obstruction, and a tracheotomy tray should be available for emergency intervention. The patient

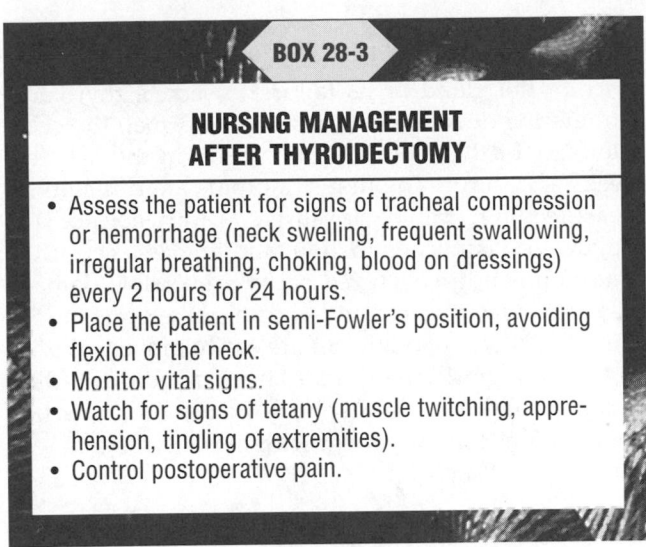

**BOX 28-3**

## NURSING MANAGEMENT AFTER THYROIDECTOMY

- Assess the patient for signs of tracheal compression or hemorrhage (neck swelling, frequent swallowing, irregular breathing, choking, blood on dressings) every 2 hours for 24 hours.
- Place the patient in semi-Fowler's position, avoiding flexion of the neck.
- Monitor vital signs.
- Watch for signs of tetany (muscle twitching, apprehension, tingling of extremities).
- Control postoperative pain.

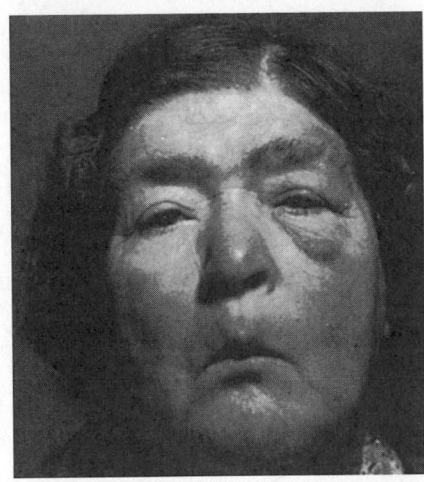

**Figure 28-4**    Adult with severe hypothyroidism, showing typical puffiness around the eyes. (From Schottelius BA, Schottelius DD: *Textbook of physiology,* ed 18, St Louis, 1978, Mosby.)

should be observed for **tetany** arising from problems with calcium metabolism related to injury to the parathyroid gland and also for voice changes resulting from injury of the vocal cords (Box 28-3).

Thyroid crisis (storm) is a rare complication that can occur before surgery or in the early postoperative period. It may also occur after severe physical or emotional stress. In thyroid storm, increased amounts of thyroid hormones are released into the bloodstream, resulting in a sudden increase in metabolism. The heart rate, pulse rate, and temperature rise, and the patient becomes apprehensive and restless and finally may become comatose and die. The patient is given oxygen, intravenous fluids, and sedatives and is placed on a hypothermia blanket to control his or her temperature. Administration of cardiac drugs may be indicated if heart failure is imminent. This serious complication is the reason why the patient's condition must be stabilized with antithyroid drugs before surgery.

### NURSE ALERT

**Marked tachycardia, a fever over 38.7° C (100° F), flushing, sweating, agitation, and restlessness are symptoms of a thyroid storm (thyrotoxic crisis). Delirium and coma can occur within 24 hours.**

## Hypothyroidism

Hypothyroidism is the result of undersecretion of thyroxine by the thyroid gland or, in some cases, of complete lack of secretion. It may occur after surgical re-

moval of the gland if too much thyroid tissue is removed. When production of thyroid hormones is diminished, the symptoms are almost the reverse of those that characterize hyperthyroidism. All metabolic processes of the body are diminished. Three conditions are recognized as resulting from hypothyroidism: myxedema, juvenile myxedema, and cretinism, all of which are actually forms of the same deficiency occurring at different ages.

*Myxedema* is the term applied to hypothyroidism in adults. The symptoms usually occur gradually and include sensitivity to cold, dryness of the skin and hair, weight gain despite a loss of appetite, and a gradually appearing dull facial expression with thickening of the lips and puffiness around the lips and eyes (Figure 28-4). The individual becomes lethargic and may fall asleep at intervals; the speech is slurred, and response is slow. Impaired memory, personality changes, and depression may also occur. The pulse is slow, and the patient complains of severe fatigue.

The treatment is replacement of the deficient hormone by administering synthetic triiodothyronine ($T_3$), levothyroxine, or desiccated thyroid. Replacement therapy is instituted gradually, and it may require 2 weeks or longer for effects to become noticeable. Complete subsidence of symptoms may require up to 2 months or more of therapy, and once therapy is begun, it must be continued for life. Because thyroid hormone increases the metabolism, the patient's cardiovascular status must be monitored, especially during the initial weeks of therapy.

*Juvenile myxedema* is similar to adult myxedema and varies in degree of severity. Moderately severe disease delays both physical and mental growth. Puberty also is delayed, and the child tends to be lethargic. The treatment is administration of levothyroxine or desiccated thyroid, which is well tolerated by children. The dose administered is sufficient to relieve the symptoms but not large enough to cause hyperthyroidism. The dosage needs to be adjusted periodically as metabolic needs increase.

Emotional support is particularly important for these children. In addition to the normal changes of adolescence, they must deal with the changes caused by hypothyroidism and its treatment. Adolescence often is associated with feelings of rebellion; therefore teaching the importance of management of hypothyroidism and compliance with therapy is essential.

*Cretinism* is the result of a complete absence of thyroid secretion from birth, which may be caused by absence of the gland or its failure to secrete thyroxine. Intrauterine development usually is normal; the characteristics of the condition may begin in the first few weeks after birth. The first symptoms are difficulty in breast-feeding, failure to thrive, protrusion of the tongue, dry skin, constipation, and a hoarse cry. If the condition is not recognized early, irreversible damage may occur in physical and mental development. Because the effects of cretinism are easily prevented with an early diagnosis, many states have mandated testing of thyroxine ($T_4$) levels after birth. Box 28-4 summarizes interventions for the patient with hypothyroidism.

---

**BOX 28-4**

## NURSING PROCESS

## HYPOTHYROIDISM

### ASSESSMENT
- Mental status (slowing of intellectual functions, altered memory somnolence, lethargy or confusion)
- Cardiovascular (peripheral edema, bradycardia, possibly cardiorespiratory complications)
- Skin (cool, pale, may become dry and thickened)
- Hair (thin)
- Metabolic (weight gain, decreased appetite, tiredness, weakness, intolerance to cold, constipation, increased serum triglycerides and cholesterol)
- Neurologic (slowed speech, deepened voice, lethargy progressing to coma, slow reflexes, paresthesia)
- Reproductive (decreased libido, change in menses)

### NURSING DIAGNOSES
- Altered nutrition: more than body requirements related to decreased metabolism
- Altered thought processes related to personality changes
- Ineffective thermoregulation related to decreased metabolism
- Chronic low self-esteem related to depression
- Knowledge deficit related to altered metabolism
- Ineffective individual and family coping related to personality changes

### NURSING INTERVENTIONS
- Keep environment warm.
- Promote care of skin with lotions.
- Monitor effects of medications, especially those that depress the depress central nervous system;

drugs may be potentiated because of decreased metabolism.
- Assess carefully for signs of infection because resistance to infection may be decreased.
- Prevent constipation by encouraging good bowel habits (exercise and eat diet high in fiber, fruits, and fluids).
- Prevent hypoxia by encouraging deep breathing and moving.
- Promote good nutritional status by reducing caloric intake if necessary to promote weight loss.
- Support patient and family emotionally during treatment, which usually leads to dramatic reversal of symptoms.
- Educate patient and family to watch for side effects of therapy, such as tachycardia, sleeplessness, palpitations, and anxiety.

### EVALUATION OF EXPECTED OUTCOMES
- Verbalizes principles of good skin care and demonstrates ability to perform this care
- Describes the medication regimen and potential side effects of medications (tachycardia, sleeplessness, palpitations, anxiety)
- Discusses signs of infection (redness, warmth, fever)
- Practices good bowel habits by exercising and eating a diet high in fruits, fiber, and fluids
- Follows a well-balanced diet and monitors weight
- Performs deep-breathing and moving exercises every 1 to 2 hours

## Thyroiditis

Thyroiditis is an inflammation of the thyroid gland. Acute thyroiditis results from a bacterial or fungal infection of thyroid tissue. Subacute granulomatous thyroiditis is thought to be caused by a viral infection. $T_4$ and $T_3$ are elevated in acute and subacute thyroiditis, and TSH is low. If the inflammation continues, $T_4$ and $T_3$ become depressed, and TSH becomes elevated. Autoimmune thyroiditis (Hashimoto's thyroiditis) is an insidious, chronic inflammation of the thyroid gland that results in destruction of thyroid tissue and consequent hypothyroidism. Thyroid hormone levels usually are reduced in Hashimoto's thyroiditis and TSH is high.

Infections usually have an abrupt onset and often are self-limiting, with complete recovery within a few weeks. Specific antibiotics are used for bacterial infections. Nonsteroidal antiinflammatory drugs (NSAIDs) or salicylates are used to reduce inflammation and discomfort. Corticosteroids may be given if the inflammation remains after 24 hours of drug therapy. Thyroid hormone is given if the patient is hypothyroid. Nursing management includes educating the patient about the specific thyroid disorder and symptoms requiring further treatment. Encouragement and reassurance are important in helping the patient accept the long-term aspects of the illness.

## Tumors of the Thyroid Gland

Tumors of the thyroid gland may be benign or malignant and may be associated with hyperthyroidism. Some tumors secrete thyroxine, because they are composed of the same type of cells as that found in normal thyroid tissue. If the tumor secretes appreciable amounts of the hormone, hyperthyroidism develops, and the symptoms are the same as those generally associated with hyperthyroidism. Surgical removal generally is indicated for nodular-type tumors.

Carcinoma of the thyroid may be any of several types. Some types grow slowly and metastasize first to the lymph nodes, then to the lungs and bones. Other types progress rapidly, and some may be fatal within a few weeks. Surgery has proven to be the most satisfactory method of treatment, although radioactive iodine and x-ray therapy may be used in conjunction with surgery for some types. The nurse may care for patients for whom treatment is only palliative. The same physical care and emotional support are necessary as for all patients with terminal cancer.

## Disorders of the Parathyroid Glands

Hyperparathyroidism is one of the more common endocrine disorders. It is characterized by excessive secretion of parathormone (PTH), a hormone that assists in the regulation of calcium and phosphate, two minerals particularly important for bone metabolism. PTH stimulates bone resorption, resorption of calcium by the renal tubules, and activation of vitamin D. The most common cause of hyperparathyroidism is an adenoma or a benign neoplasm, although it can be associated with other diseases such as chronic renal failure, malabsorption, and vitamin D deficiencies.

An excess of parathyroid hormone causes a calcium imbalance by allowing the calcium in the bones to be removed and migrate into the bloodstream. The bones become weak, tender, and painful, and spontaneous fractures may occur. The appetite may become poor, constipation may be present, and the patient may have fatigue, depression, weight loss, and loss of muscle tone, which makes walking difficult. The blood calcium level increases, and renal calculi, composed chiefly of calcium salts, may form in the kidneys. Small tumors, which are detected by x-ray examination, may form in the bones. The treatment is surgical removal of the tumor or removal of the overactive gland. After surgery all symptoms should disappear, and the bones gradually strengthen.

The goals of nursing care are to help the patient remain active and maintain a high fluid intake and to prevent complications. As with thyroid disorders, reassurance and support are necessary for adjustment to the long-term effects of the disorder.

Hypoparathyroidism results from inadequate production of PTH. When too little parathormone is secreted, the level of calcium in the blood declines and phosphorus increases. The deficiency of the hormone may result from injury to the glands or removal of too much parathyroid tissue during a thyroidectomy or radical neck surgery. The primary symptom is tetany caused by suddenly diminished levels of blood calcium. Tetany is characterized by tingling of the lips, fingers, and toes, increased muscle tension, and spasms of smooth and skeletal muscles. The patient may have tightness in the throat and difficulty swallowing and usually is anxious. **Chvostek's sign,** a muscle spasm that occurs when the face is tapped below the temple, may be seen, as may **Trousseau's phenomenon,** a carpopedal spasm that occurs when a blood pressure cuff is used to interrupt arterial circulation for 3 minutes. The combination of muscle spasm and laryngeal spasm can lead to airway obstruction.

Tetany is treated with calcium gluconate, given either intravenously or by slow push over 10 minutes. This may be accompanied by parathormone solution and vitamin D. Intervention for acute episodes includes maintenance of the airway. Convulsions may occur. If the patient is able to cooperate, rebreathing lowers the body pH. ECG monitoring is indicated. Oral calcium supplements may be prescribed for long-term management. Hormone replacement of PTH is not indicated because of its potent side effects.

Patients need instruction in nutrition and in the importance of consistent drug therapy and a high fluid intake. Meals high in calcium are encouraged, and foods containing oxalic acid, which reduces calcium absorption (e.g., spinach, rhubarb, bran and whole grains), should be avoided. Written materials help emphasize important points. Information about signs and symptoms of hyperparathyroidism and hypoparathyroidism can help patients recognize the need to call their physician.

## Cushing's Syndrome

Hyperfunction of the adrenal cortex produces a spectrum of clinical abnormalities known as Cushing's syndrome. The adrenal hormones are divided into three primary classifications: glucocorticoids, which regulate metabolism; mineralocorticoids, which regulate sodium and potassium levels; and androgens, which contribute to growth, development, and sexual activity. Prolonged administration of high doses of corticosteroids is the most common **exogenous** cause (originating outside the body) of Cushing's syndrome. A tumor in the anterior pituitary gland or a tumor of the adrenal cortex is the most common **endogenous** cause (originating inside the body) of Cushing's syndrome.

The characteristic symptoms of Cushing's syndrome reflect exaggeration of the normal functions of adrenal hormones (Figure 28-5). An excess of glucocorticoid can result in observable changes in personal appearance that are stressful to the patient. Weight gain results from the accumulation of adipose tissue in the face, neck, trunk, and cervical area, creating a "humpback" appearance. Sodium and water retention may also be a problem. Increased metabolism results in protein wasting, and muscle weakness occurs, especially in the extremities. Loss of protein in the bone leads to osteoporosis and eventually pathologic fractures, compression fractures of the vertebrae, and bone and neck pain. Protein deficit results in thin, weak, easily bruised skin, and wound healing may be delayed. Glucose intolerance can arise from glucocorticoid-induced insulin resistance. The excess of mineralocorticoids may cause hypertension. Excess androgens may result in changes in secondary sex characteristics in both genders, including menstrual irregularities in women and an increase in body hair and acne. Mood swings, irritability, anxiety, and insomnia are among the many other effects of Cushing's syndrome.

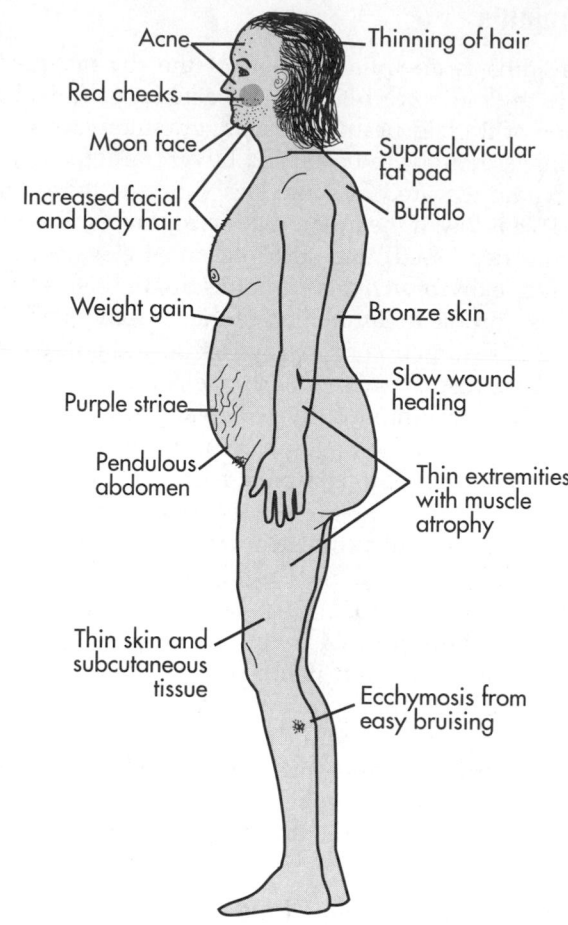

**Figure 28-5**  Common characteristics of Cushing's syndrome. (Redrawn from Lewis SM, Collier IC, Heitkemper MM: *Medical-surgical nursing: assessment and management of clinical problems*, ed 4, St Louis, 1996, Mosby.)

A variety of chronic diseases are treated with adrenal steroids, even when no adrenal disease is present. Such diseases include rheumatoid arthritis, leukemia, emphysema, and ulcerative colitis. Drugs such as prednisone have potent antiinflammatory effects, which can be of great therapeutic value. However, most patients treated with adrenal steroids develop Cushing's syndrome to a variable degree, and serious complications and side effects can occur. Careful observation is important. If Cushing's syndrome is a result of prolonged administration of steroids, gradual discontinuation of the drug, reduction of the dosage, or administration on alternate days may be tried.

The treatment for endogenous conditions usually involves surgery. If the pituitary gland is involved, hypophysectomy (removal of the gland) or irradiation of the pituitary gland may be performed. Good neurosurgical nursing skills are required (see Chapter 30). Before surgery, any underlying conditions such as hypertension, hyperglycemia, or fluid electrolyte imbalance must be controlled. Because glands are highly vascularized, hemorrhage may occur. Manipulation of glandular tissue during surgery may result in release of excessive amounts of hormones, which may destabilize the patient's condition. After surgery, the blood pressure and fluid and electrolytes must be monitored carefully. The 24 to 48 hours after surgery is a critical period, during which instability is mostly likely to occur.

In inoperable cases or when residual glandular tissue is present, powerful drugs are available that suppress hormone production (mitotane). However, side effects are common, including anorexia, GI bleeding, nausea, vomiting, dizziness, skin rashes, double vision, and depression.

The primary nursing goal is to assist the patient to participate actively in the therapeutic plan. This includes adjusting the life-style to accommodate the disorder, preventing complications such as fractures and infections, and maintaining an appropriate body weight and a positive self-image.

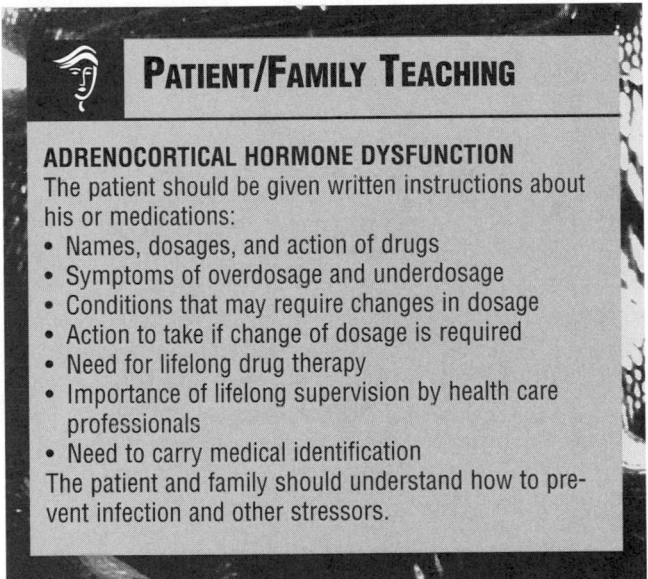

## PATIENT/FAMILY TEACHING

**ADRENOCORTICAL HORMONE DYSFUNCTION**
The patient should be given written instructions about his or medications:
- Names, dosages, and action of drugs
- Symptoms of overdosage and underdosage
- Conditions that may require changes in dosage
- Action to take if change of dosage is required
- Need for lifelong drug therapy
- Importance of lifelong supervision by health care professionals
- Need to carry medical identification
The patient and family should understand how to prevent infection and other stressors.

## Addison's Disease

Hypofunction of the adrenal cortex, resulting in insufficient secretion of glucocorticoids and mineralocorticoids, results in Addison's disease. It is a relatively rare condition, usually autoimmune in origin. In Addison's disease the body forms antibodies against its own adrenal cortex, causing **atrophy** and destruction of tissue. When Addison's disease is accompanied by other endocrine dysfunctions, **polyendocrine deficiency syndrome** may be present. Infectious conditions such as tuberculosis, fungal infections, or infec-

tion with the human immunodeficiency virus (HIV) can cause Addison's disease, as can noninfectious conditions such as hemorrhage, infarction, or metastatic cancer. Occasionally the disease arises secondary to chemotherapy.

Symptoms result from the inadequate amounts of adrenocortical hormones in the blood and body fluids. Progressive weakness, fatigue, anorexia, and weight loss are common. Other GI symptoms are nausea, vomiting, diarrhea, and abdominal pain. The patient may show signs of hypoglycemia, such as nervousness, increased perspiration (diaphoresis), headache, and trembling. These symptoms result from the inadequate amount of circulating cortisone and hydrocortisone. The normal fluid and electrolyte balance is disrupted, and the patient may have a deficiency of sodium and chloride and an excess of potassium because of insufficient aldosterone. Hyperpigmentation of the skin in areas of the body exposed to the sun can result in a bronze coloring resembling a tan.

Hypotension is the most dangerous symptom of Addison's disease. During stress from infection, surgery, trauma, hemorrhage, or emotional states or as a result of abrupt withdrawal of adrenocortical hormone replacement therapy, the patient may go into shock. The circulatory collapse that occurs does not respond well to vasopressors and fluid replacement; glucocorticoids must be administered to reverse the condition. An addisonian crisis (acute adrenal insufficiency) is a serious exacerbation of the disease that may be a life-threatening emergency. Along with a sudden drop in blood pressure, tachycardia, fever, weakness, confusion, and fluid and electrolyte imbalances, including dehydration, may occur. Treatment involves management of shock and immediate glucocorticoid replacement.

Addison's disease is treated by reestablishing a state of normal hydration and then replacing hydrocortisone and fludrocortisone (Florinef) (Table 28-1). Glucocorticoids usually are prescribed in divided doses in the morning and afternoon. Mineralocorticoids are taken daily, usually in the evening. This schedule approximates normal circadian rhythm and reduces the side effects. Both these medications should be taken after meals because they may cause gastrointestinal upset. Once therapy has begun, it is essential that the patient understand that Addison's disease is a lifelong disorder and medications should not be adjusted or stopped except under the guidance of a health care professional.

When any illness or stress occurs, even if it is mild, patients may be advised to increase the dosage of glucocorticoids to prevent adrenal crisis. Patients should carry a MedicAlert tag or card identifying them as having Addison's disease and listing emergency measures

**TABLE 28-1**

## Pharmacology of Drugs Used for Endocrine Disorders

| DRUG (GENERIC AND TRADE NAME); ROUTE AND DOSAGE | ACTION/INDICATION | COMMON SIDE EFFECTS AND NURSING CONSIDERATIONS |
|---|---|---|
| **Calcitriol** Route: PO Dosage: 0.25 mg q day initially | Used for patients with hypocalcemia and those in chronic renal failure | Monitor calcium levels; discontinue if hypercalcemia occurs |
| **Fludrocortisone Acetate** (Florinef) Route: PO Dosage: 0.1-0.2 mg daily | Used to promote increased reabsorption of sodium and loss of potassium from the renal tubules, used in adrenal insufficiency | Flushing, sweating, hypertension; contraindicated with acute glomerulonephritis; use with caution in patients with congestive heart failure and osteoporosis |
| **Levothyroxine** (Synthroid, Levothroid, $T_4$) Route: PO, IV Dosage: PO, 12.5-50 $\mu$g as a single daily dose initially; may be increased q 2-4 wk; usual maintenance dosage is 75-125 $\mu$g/day | Used for replacement or substitution therapy in diminished or absent thyroid function of many causes | Irritability, insomnia, nervousness, tachycardia, arrhythmias, and weight loss; contraindicated in recent myocardial infarction or thyroidtoxicosis; use with caution in patients with cardiac disease, severe renal insufficiency, and uncorrected adrenocortical disorders, and in the elderly; can be safely used in pregnancy |
| **Methimazole** (Tapazole) Route: PO Dosage: 15 mg q day initially | Used to treat hyperthyroidism; inhibits synthesis of thyroid hormone; may be used preoperatively for thyroidectomy | Observe patient for hyperthyroid symptoms |
| **Prednisone** Route: PO Dosage: 5-60 mg/day single dose or divided doses; maintenance dose may be given daily or every other day | Used systematically and locally in a wide variety of chronic diseases, including inflammations, allergic, hematologic, neoplastic, and autoimmune conditions; also used for replacement therapy in adrenal insufficiency | Depression, euphoria, hypertension, nausea, anorexia, diminished wound healing, petechiae, ecchymoses, fragility, hirsutism, acne, adrenal suppression, muscle wasting, osteoporosis, increased susceptibility to infection, moon face or buffalo hump appearance; chronic treatment leads to adrenal suppression; never abruptly discontinue drug; use of the drug may mask presence of infections, and it should be administered at the lowest possible dose for the shortest period of time |
| **Propylthiouracic** (PTO) Route: PO Dosage: 15 mg q day initially | Used to treat hyperthyroidism; inhibits synthesis of thyroid hormone; may be used preoperatively for thyroidectomy | Observe patient for hyperthyroid symptoms |
| **Strong Iodine Solution, Lugol's Solution** Route: PO Dosage: Strong iodine solution 0.1-0.3 ml (3-5 drops) tid | Used as an adjunct with other antithyroid drugs in preparation for thyroidectomy | Hypothyroidism, diarrhea, and hypersensitivity; use with caution in patients with tuberculosis, bronchitis, hyperkalemia, and impaired renal function |
| **Vasopressin** (Pitressin) Route: IM, SC, nasal spray Dosage: Diabetes insipidus IM, SC 5-10 U bid to qid as needed; abdominal distention, IM 5 U, then q 3-4 hr, increasing to 10 U if needed; nasal spray as ordered | Antidiuretic hormone used for diabetes insipidus, abdominal distention postoperatively, and bleeding esophageal varices | Contraindicated in patients with chronic nephritis |

to be taken. The patient should carry an emergency kit at all times consisting of 100 mg of intramuscular hydrocortisone, syringes, and instructions. Patients and families must know the signs and symptoms of inadequate or excessive steroid levels and must understand the need to report symptoms promptly.

The goals of nursing care are to assist the patient in adapting to and managing the illness and in avoiding addisonian crisis. Given appropriate guidelines, the patient and family can learn to adjust the medications according to life situations. With careful attention to all aspects of the disease, people with Addison's disease have a normal life expectancy.

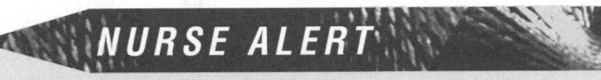

### NURSE ALERT

**A severe drop in blood pressure heralds an addisonian crisis.**

## Secondary Hypoadrenalism

Steroid (hydrocortisone) therapy is commonly used in the treatment of asthma and ulcerative colitis. Long-term treatment with steroids leads to atrophy of the adrenal glands. If steroid therapy is withdrawn too suddenly, symptoms similar to those of Addison's disease occur. The patient feels lethargic and weak and may become hypotensive. The response to stress such as surgery may be severe depression; therefore it is important to know if a patient scheduled for surgery has been undergoing steroid therapy. Withdrawal from steroid therapy must be done very slowly to allow the adrenal glands to recover.

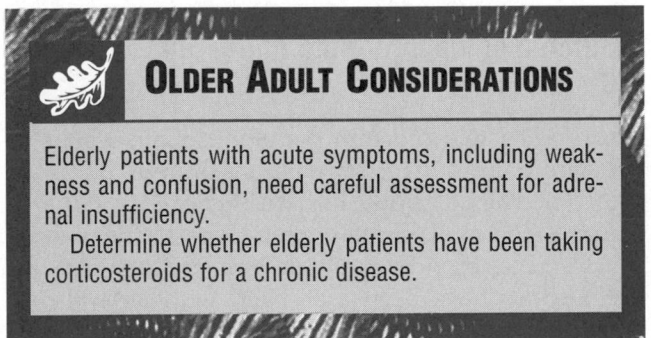

### OLDER ADULT CONSIDERATIONS

Elderly patients with acute symptoms, including weakness and confusion, need careful assessment for adrenal insufficiency.

Determine whether elderly patients have been taking corticosteroids for a chronic disease.

## Pheochromocytoma

Pheochromocytoma is a catecholamine-producing tumor of the adrenal medulla. These tumors are generally small and benign; and only a tiny number are malignant. Pheochromocytoma is believed to be associated with neurofibromatosis and tumors of the thyroid gland and may be hereditary.

Symptoms arise from the hypersecretion of epinephrine and norepinephrine. The characteristic symptom is hypertension. However, the hypertension may be variable, being persistent and chronic or occurring in intermittent attacks. Because of the elevated blood pressure, pheochromocytoma often is confused with essential hypertension. Other symptoms may include severe headache, excessive sweating, nausea, vomiting, palpitation, and nervousness with acute anxiety. During an acute attack, tachycardia, hyperglycemia, and polyuria may occur.

The diagnosis of pheochromocytoma may be made by testing the urine for elevated levels of metanephrine (a byproduct of epinephrine metabolism), using a 24-hour urine collection. When collecting the specimen, the urine should be kept on ice in a dark container with a preservative (hydrochloric acid). Pheochromocytoma may also be diagnosed by urine levels of vanillylmandelic acid (VMA), by intravenous pyelography, or by aortography. A CT, MRI, or ultrasound scan also may be useful for diagnosis. The treatment is removal of the tumor.

## Adrenalectomy

Adrenalectomy is the surgical removal of the adrenal gland. The preoperative preparation of the patient is the same as that for other abdominal surgery. Postoperative care may require administration of hydrocortisone if the adrenal cortex has been removed. When surgery has been done because of pheochromocytoma, the patient's condition may be critical for the first 48 hours. Shock may occur because of the abrupt fall in blood pressure. Blood pressure must be monitored continuously and the patient must be observed for hemorrhage, which may be external or internal. Urinary output must be observed for signs of oliguria. Vasopressor drugs are administered intravenously. Caution should be used when administering narcotic drugs for pain because some of these drugs have a tendency to cause hypotension. After the critical period the recovery progresses normally. If both adrenal glands are removed, the patient requires lifelong hormone replacement therapy.

## Disorders of the Pituitary Gland
### Hypersecretion of the Anterior Pituitary Gland

**Growth hormone excess.** Hypersecretion of the anterior lobe of the pituitary gland results in overproduction of growth hormone. This condition usually is the result of a benign pituitary tumor. The overgrowth of soft tissue and bones causes either **giantism** or

**acromegaly,** depending on the time of onset. If the overproduction of growth hormone occurs before growth is complete and before the epiphyses of the long bones have closed, giantism occurs. Growth usually is proportional, and children may grow to 2.4 m (about 8 feet) tall and weigh more than 135 kg (300 pounds). Other growth disorders also may occur, and these children may have a shortened life span. Fortunately, the condition is rare.

Acromegaly occurs in adults, and although it is more common than giantism, it also is rare. The onset, which is insidious, often occurs in the third or fourth decade of life. The bones increase in thickness and width, the hands and feet become enlarged, and deformities of the spine and mandible develop (Figure 28-6). The paranasal and frontal sinuses also enlarge, resulting in coarse facial features. At the same time, the soft tissue throughout the body enlarges. The tongue may enlarge, causing speech difficulties and hoarseness. Other systemic effects may include hypertension, enlargement of the heart, neuropathy, gastrointestinal distention, muscle weakness, and joint pain. Headaches and visual disturbances also can occur. Since growth hormone is an antagonist to insulin, hyperglycemia can occur, with associated diabetic complications.

Treatment for growth hormone excess may involve surgery, radiation, drug therapy, or combinations of therapies. Drug therapy usually is not completely effective and more often is used as an adjunct to other therapy. The goal is to return production of growth hormones to normal levels. The prognosis depends on the patient's age at onset, when treatment is initiated, and the underlying pathologic condition. Good neurosurgical preoperative and postoperative care is necessary for patients treated surgically (Chapter 30).

**Other anterior pituitary hormone excess.** Excess secretion of other trophic hormones also can occur. This usually results in signs and symptoms related to hormone excess from the target organ. For example, if levels of TSH are high, hyperthyroidism develops; if levels of ACTH are increased, Cushing's disease results.

## Anterior Pituitary Gland Deficit

Hypofunction of the anterior pituitary gland is a rare condition that often stems from an infection, vascular disease, tumor, or autoimmune disorder. Growth hormone deficit is most common, although deficiencies of TSH, ACTH, prolactin, and gonadotropins can occur. Signs and symptoms associated with hypofunction of the pituitary gland vary with the degree of pathology and the particular hormones in deficit. Symptoms often are nonspecific, such as weakness, fatigue, headache, sexual dysfunction, dry skin, and increased susceptibility to infection. The underlying problem that causes the hypofunction should be treated, and appropriate replacement therapy should be initiated.

Low levels of growth hormone during childhood result in slow but proportional growth (dwarfism). Except for their small size, these individuals appear normal. Replacement drug therapy is available, although expensive. The best results are obtained if treatment is begun early, before growth is complete.

Sheehan's syndrome is a relatively rare condition that can occur after postpartum hemorrhage. Deficiencies of prolactin, FSH, and LH may occur as a result of slow degeneration and necrosis of the pituitary gland that occurs because of damage caused by lack of oxygen during the acute hemorrhage. Failure to lactate, amenorrhea, and infertility may occur, followed by hypothyroidism and a change in secondary sex characteristics. If hormone replacement therapy is begun early, the condition often is reversible.

## Syndrome of Inappropriate Antiduretic Hormone (ADH Excess)

Excess ADH released into the bloodstream results in the syndrome of inappropriate antidiuretic hormone (SIADH). The condition has various causes. Often it occurs secondary to malignant tumors that release ADH, such as bronchogenic carcinoma. Pulmonary infections also have been associated with SIADH. Release of excessive ADH may be associated with head trauma, meningitis, delirium tremens, Addison's disease, stress, and medications.

Excess ADH increases reabsorption of water into the circulation from the renal tubules. The extracellular fluid expands, and sodium deficit occurs from dilution of the plasma. Fluid retention, concentrated urine, muscle cramps, weakness, and weight gain without

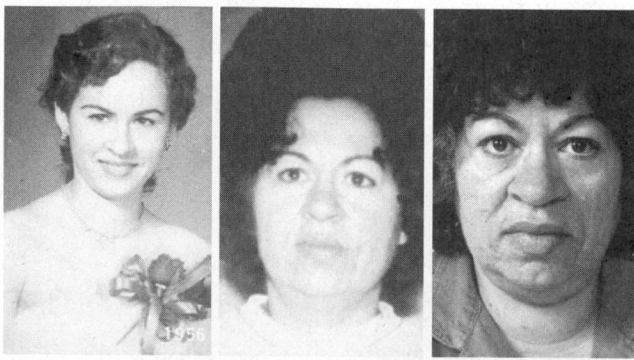

**Figure 28-6** Progressive development of facial features of acromegaly. (Courtesy Linda Haas, Seattle. From Lewis SM, Collier IC, Heitkemper MM: *Medical-surgical nursing: assessment and management of clinical problems*, ed 4, St Louis, 1996, Mosby.)

edema occur. Urinary output is low, and urine specific gravity is high. As the condition progresses, confusion, lethargy, anorexia, headache, convulsions, and coma can occur as a result of cerebral edema. Cardiac symptoms also may be present.

The goal of treatment is to return the fluid volume to normal. Restriction of fluid intake may result in a gradual return to normal. Diuretics may be necessary. The condition often is self-limiting when caused by trauma, infection, or drug therapy but may become chronic if malignancy or metabolic diseases are the underlying cause. Patients susceptible to the syndrome (i.e., those with malignant neoplasms, pulmonary infections, or central nervous system trauma or infection) should be carefully monitored for SIADH. Low but highly concentrated urinary output with a low specific gravity, signs of sodium deficit, a sudden weight gain, and alteration of consciousness often signal the onset of SIADH. When the condition is chronic, patients must be assisted in developing strategies for self-management. The discomfort caused by a restricted fluid intake can be moderated by sucking on ice chips or hard candy.

## Diabetes Insipidus (ADH Deficit)

Any condition that interferes with the synthesis of ADH production or release results in diabetes insipidus (DI). Such conditions include head trauma, brain tumors, infection of the central nervous system, and cranial surgery, although some cases are idiopathic in origin. The onset of DI can be sudden, as in a complication after surgery. ADH functions to increase the amount of water reabsorbed from the kidney tubules, and in its absence large amounts of urine are excreted, as much as 10 L daily. Therefore, the main characteristic of DI is excretion of a large amount of urine that has a low specific gravity. A severe fluid volume deficit can occur if the patient cannot compensate for the condition by drinking large amounts of fluid. Extreme thirst, weight loss, poor skin turgor, hypotension, and tachycardia are indications of a fluid volume

deficit (Chapter 27). Central nervous system manifestations and shock can result if treatment is delayed.

Identification and treatment of the underlying cause of the condition are essential. Maintenance of a normal fluid and electrolyte balance is the treatment goal. Treatment includes parenteral fluids and ADH replacement therapy either parenterally or by nasal spray. Nursing management requires monitoring of fluid intake and output and appropriate intervention for complications. Adequate fluids should be kept readily available. Nurses should assist patients with long-term management of replacement therapy and with management of their symptoms.

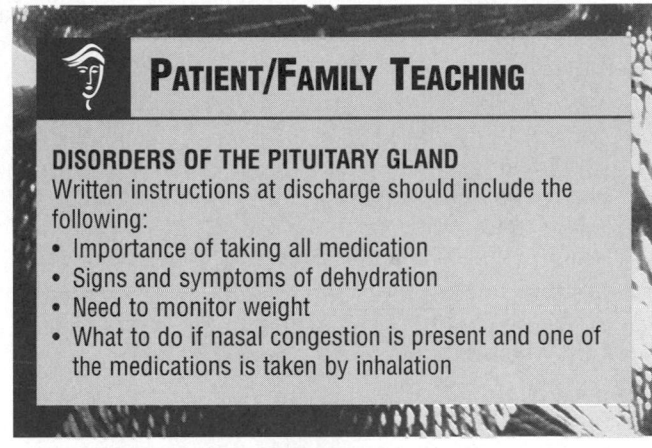

**PATIENT/FAMILY TEACHING**

**DISORDERS OF THE PITUITARY GLAND**
Written instructions at discharge should include the following:
- Importance of taking all medication
- Signs and symptoms of dehydration
- Need to monitor weight
- What to do if nasal congestion is present and one of the medications is taken by inhalation

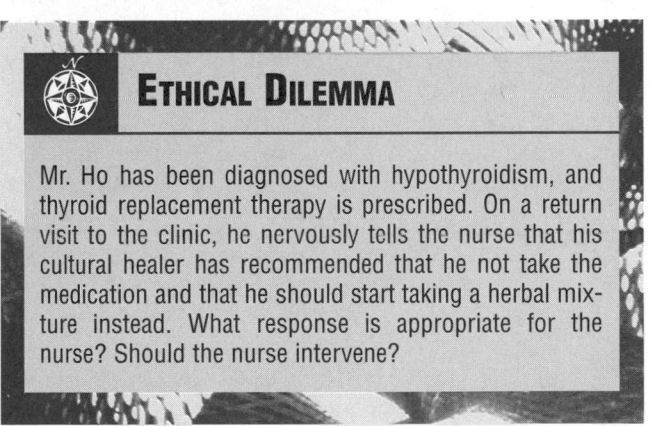

**ETHICAL DILEMMA**

Mr. Ho has been diagnosed with hypothyroidism, and thyroid replacement therapy is prescribed. On a return visit to the clinic, he nervously tells the nurse that his cultural healer has recommended that he not take the medication and that he should start taking a herbal mixture instead. What response is appropriate for the nurse? Should the nurse intervene?

# NURSING CARE PLAN

## PATIENT WITH HYPERTHYROIDISM

Mrs. Reynolds is a 34-year-old female who is admitted to the medical unit for a diagnostic workup after having palpitations, tachycardia, and an enlarged thyroid gland that was identified on a routine health visit to her private medical doctor (PMD).

Significant in her history is the fact that she has lost 20 pounds within the past 2 months without exercising or dieting. Her menstrual cycle has been erratic for the past 6 months, with no menses for the past 3 months. She denies being pregnant. She states she is currently stressed over her husband's projected employment transfer to the west coast and away from her extended family. She complains of heat intolerance and frequent episodes of "sweating." She states she is easily fatigued and has had periods of insomnia and constipation. She describes herself as feeling irritable and having crying outbursts without warning.

| Medical History | Psychosocial Data | Assessment Data |
|---|---|---|
| Tonsillectomy and adenoidectomy, age 10 yr | Married 12 yr; quality relationship with husband; dated 6 yr while in college and after; only stressor due to husband's frequent traveling with his work (consultancy business and sales) | Thin, frail-appearing woman with obvious exophthalmos; height 5'8"; weight 53.1 kg (118 lb) |
| Appendectomy at 14 yr old; no other surgeries | | *Skin:* Warm with evidence of recent diaphoresis; no rashes, lesions, or bruises |
| Hospitalized three times for childbirth; all routine vaginal deliveries without complications | | *Musculoskeletal:* Steady gait; full range of motion all joints |
| Immunizations up to date | | Fine tremors noted when fingers extended |
| No known food or drug allergies; has received antibiotics in past without problems | Own home; has cleaning lady once per week | *Neck:* Diffuse swelling of anterior portion of neck; isthmus of gland palpable; no specific nodules palpable |
| Both parents alive and in good health; both employed full time and supportive to their children | Works part-time as librarian in media center at grammar school | *Respiratory:* Lungs clear to percussion and auscultation; RR 24-26; regular rate and rhythm |
| Two brothers in good health; both lawyers | Has three children: Steve, age 9; Melissa, age 6; and Adam, age 5; all in excellent health | *Cardiovascular:* BP 146/84 (normal baseline 118/72); apical pulse 96-100; no bruits; all peripheral pulses symmetric; atrial flutter documented on ECG |
| Identical twin sister recently diagnosed with Graves' disease | | |
| Family history of hypertension in maternal grandmother, age 79 | Jewish faith; children attend Hebrew school | *Abdominal:* Bowel sounds heard all four quadrants; slight distension |
| Adult onset diabetes in paternal uncle, age 70; good management | Has private health insurance | *Laboratory data* |
| Cancer of the breast in maternal aunt, decreased age 52 | *Hobbies:* Avid reader, gardening, some traveling; is a gourmet cook | Hgb 12.1, Hct 37.8, WBC 8000, platelets 320,000, BUN 16, electrolytes WNL |
| Excellent health behaviors: yearly physical, Pap smear, mammogram | | Thyroid ultrasonogram reveals marked diffuse swelling bilaterally |
| Has never smoked; denies use of alcohol and drugs; some use of over-the-counter (OTC) cold remedies/analgesics (aspirin, Tylenol) | | Thyroid scan reveals a nonmalignancy condition |
| | | $T_3$ triiodothyronine ($T_3$) resin uptake test shows 24% of iodine uptake |
| | | *Medications* |
| | | SSKI 300 mg PO every 4 hours; dilute in 4 oz orange juice |
| | | Inderal 20 mg PO qid |
| | | Colace 100 mg PO daily |
| | | Multivitamin tab 1 PO daily |
| | | Tylenol 300 mg PO prn headache |

## NURSING CARE PLAN

## PATIENT WITH HYPERTHYROIDISM—cont'd

**NURSING DIAGNOSIS**

Altered nutrition: less than body requirements related to increased metabolism, as evidenced by rapid weight loss and chronic fatigue

| NURSING INTERVENTIONS | EVALUATION OF EXPECTED OUTCOMES |
|---|---|
| Weigh patient daily (same time, same scale) and record results. | Remains at or above specified weight (156.7 kg [125 lb]) and shows a steady increase of (0.9 kg [2 lb]) bimonthly |
| Monitor fluid I & O (likes milkshakes as between-meal snack). | Consumes at least 90% of meals served and all of between-meal snacks |
| Provide high-calorie, high-carbohydrate diet. Assist her with menu choices and discuss rationale for choices. She likes pasta, some creamed soups, and fresh fruits. Patient hates broccoli. | Plans appropriate diet for discharge for 1 wk postdischarge; can explain the rationale for her choices |
| Refer to dietitian for teaching related to incorporating special dietary needs into gourmet cooking. | |
| Monitor bowel sounds once per shift. Check for episodes of constipation. Hold Colace if stools are loose. Teach same to patient. | |
| Provide oral hygiene at least twice per day. | |
| Remind patient to try to eat at least 90% of each meal tray. Record results on calorie count sheet. | |

**NURSING DIAGNOSIS**

Body image disturbance related to exophthalmic appearance as evidenced by statements of anxiety and wearing dark glasses

| NURSING INTERVENTIONS | EVALUATION OF EXPECTED OUTCOMES |
|---|---|
| Assess patient's usual coping patterns. | Discusses the change in her body image |
| Encourage discussion of feelings by initiating comments related to self-esteem and self-worth. Cite behaviors of progress. | Takes an active role in planning hygiene and self-care |
| Introduce patient to available personnel (by mutual consent) who have had similar condition (it is not a rare condition). | Expresses at least two positive feelings about herself daily |
| Praise efforts to participate in self-care. | Identifies coping strategies that aid situations |
| Discuss hairstyle changes that might enhance self-image. | |
| Actively listen for expressions of anxiety. | |
| Guide thinking along positive channels. | |
| Protect eyes from trauma. | |
| Monitor for complete closure while asleep to prevent corneal drying. | |

*Continued*

# NURSING CARE PLAN

## PATIENT WITH HYPERTHYROIDISM—cont'd

### NURSING DIAGNOSIS

Sleep pattern disturbance related to increased metabolism

| NURSING INTERVENTIONS | EVALUATION OF EXPECTED OUTCOMES |
|---|---|
| Ask patient what factors are conducive to sleep. Discourage intake of caffeinated foods such as coffee, cocoa, tea, chocolate, and cola drinks. Keep environment restful and calm. Plan to provide period for uninterrupted sleep. Provide patient with normal sleep aids such as back rubs, pillow, food, drinks, and personal hygiene measures. Ask patient to discuss sleep pattern from previous night. Teach patient relaxation techniques such as meditation, guided imagery, and muscle relaxation exercises. Plan medication schedule to allow for maximum rest. Limit visitors to those specified by patient. Reduce environmental stimuli at bedtime (dim lights, soft music, closed doors). | Sleeps at least 6 hr without interruption and expresses a feeling of being well rested Does not exhibit signs and symptoms of sleep deprivation Discusses life-style changes to induce sleep after discharge to home Performs relaxation techniques at bedtime |

### NURSING DIAGNOSIS

Knowledge deficit related to physical status as evidenced by statements of "immediate recovery"

| NURSING INTERVENTIONS | EVALUATION OF EXPECTED OUTCOMES |
|---|---|
| Ascertain what patient already knows about Graves' disease. Urge her to ask questions. Suggest she write down major concerns. Determine if she enjoys learning through media (is a librarian) such as videotapes, audiotapes, or books. Begin negotiating learning objectives with her. Plan mutual establishment of goals. Set times for discussion and include her husband if needed. Discuss possible adverse side effects of medications. Answer any questions pertaining to the possibility of surgery. | Discusses newly acquired knowledge Develops realistic learning goals Identifies specific changes in her life-style needed to promote optimal health Discusses a reasonable time frame for condition to subside Feels free to question the possibility of surgery if necessary |

# KEY CONCEPTS

➤ Endocrine glands secrete hormones that act as chemical messengers, ultimately altering the activity of a variety of body organs.

➤ Endocrine glands include the thyroid gland, the parathyroid glands, the adrenal glands, the pituitary body, the gonads, and the pancreas.

➤ All patients requiring therapeutic procedures for endocrine disorders require maintenance of a patent airway, monitoring of fluid and electrolyte balance, assessment of vital signs and neurologic status, emotional support, and education about their condition.

➤ A simple goiter is an enlargement of the thyroid gland that occurs when dietary iodine is insufficient for synthesis of thyroxine. Iodized salt has reduced the incidence of this condition.

➤ Hyperthyroidism, or Graves' disease, is caused by an overactive thyroid gland that produces an excess of thyroid hormone.

➤ The symptoms of hyperthyroidism are a result of an accelerated metabolic rate, which causes increases in all physiologic processes. Common symptoms include increased appetite, weight loss, increased systolic blood pressure and pulse rate, sensitivity to heat, arrhythmias, palpitation, tremors, weakness, and bulging of the eyeballs as a result of lid retraction.

➤ Treatment of patients with hyperthyroidism is directed toward reducing the activity of the gland by antithyroid drugs, surgical removal of the gland, or therapeutic doses of radioactive iodine.

➤ Hypothyroidism is the result of an undersecretion of thyroxine by the thyroid gland. Myxedema, juvenile myxedema, and cretinism are alternate forms of this deficiency that occur at different ages.

➤ In adults, symptoms of hypothyroidism occur gradually and include sensitivity to cold, dryness of the skin and hair, weight gain, and a dull facial expression with puffiness around the lips and eyes.

➤ Treatment of hypothyroidism replaces the deficient hormone.

➤ Disorders of the parathyroid glands interfere with the calcium balance in the blood.

➤ Tetany results from a decreased level of blood calcium.

➤ Surgery for hyperthyroidism or replacement of deficient parathormone extract, calcium salts, and vitamin D for hypothyroidism controls the conditions.

➤ The adrenal cortex produces several different hormones that are essential to life. Cortisone and hydrocortisone regulate cell activity and the internal environment of the body. Aldosterone is a mineralocorticoid that maintains homeostasis of the sodium concentration in the blood. The catecholamines, epinephrine and norepinephrine, increase and prolong the effects of the sympathetic nervous system.

➤ Addison's disease is hypofunction of the adrenal cortex. It is a lifelong disease requiring consistent hormone replacement. Addisonian crisis is a serious exacerbation of the disease.

➤ Hyperfunction of the adrenal cortex results in Cushing's syndrome. Fat accumulation in the face, neck, and trunk; weakness; muscle wasting; fluid and electrolyte imbalance; irritability; and other symptoms are common. Adrenalectomy may be performed.

➤ Disorders of the pituitary gland are uncommon. However, hypersecretion of the anterior lobe of the pituitary gland can result in conditions such as acromegaly in adults and diabetes insipidus.

# CRITICAL THINKING EXERCISES

1. Compare the pathophysiology and resulting signs and symptoms of hypothyroidism and hyperthyroidism.

2. Design a patient teaching plan for a patient with diabetes insipidus.

## REFERENCES AND ADDITIONAL READINGS

Anonymous: Pharmacology update: know the disease, understand the treatment, *J Pract Nurs* 46(2):22, 1996.

Davis-Martin S: Pearls for practice: disorders of the adrenal glands, *J Am Acad Nurse Pract* 8(7):323-326, 1996.

Finding JW: Cushing's syndrome: an etiologic workup, *Hosp Pract* 27(10):107-112, 114-118, 121-122, 1992.

Ford AR: Healthy adrenal glands: support for menopause A Friend Indeed: for Women in the Prime of Life . . . 13(2): 1-3, 1996.

Handerhan B: Recognizing adrenal crisis: how to respond to severe steroid withdrawal, *Nursing* 22(4):33, 1992.

Healy PF: Self-test: caring for patients with endocrine disorders, *Nursing* 25:22, 1995.

Hershamn JM et al: A savvy approach to thyroid testing, *Patient Care* 26(3):134-137, 140-142, 144-145, 1992.

Johnson D: Pathophysiology of thyroid storm: nursing implications, *Crit Care Nurse* 3(6):80-86, 1993.

Johnson JL, Felicerta JV: Hyperthyroidism: a comprehensive review, *J Am Acad Nurse Pract* 4(1):8-14, 1992.

Lammon C, Hart G: Recognizing thyroid crisis, *Nursing 93* 23(4):33, 1993.

Lewis SM, Collier JC, Heitkemper MM: *Medical-surgical nursing: assessment and management of clinical problems,* ed 4, St Louis, 1996, Mosby.

Mundy GR: Evaluation and treatment of hyperkalemia, *Hosp Pract* 29(6):79-84, 1994.

Ober PR, editor: Endocrine crisis, *Endocrinol Metab Clin North Am* 22(2):181-453, 1993.

O'Donnell M: Emergency! Addisonian crisis, *Am J Nurs* 97(3):41, 1997.

Roberts A: The adrenal glands, *Nurs Times* 91(45):34-36, 1995a.

Roberts A: The adrenal gland. Part 2, *Nurs Times* 91(45): 31-33, 1995b.

Roberts A: The adrenal gland. Part 3, *Nurs Times* 92(2):31-33, 1996.

Romeo JH: Hyperfunction and hypofunction in the anterior pituitary, *Nurs Clin North Am* 31(4):769-778, 1996.

Rusterholtz A: Interpretation of diagnostic laboratory tests in selected endocrine disorders, *Nurs Clin North Am* 31(4):715-724, 1996.

Spittle L: Diagnoses in opposition: thyroid storm and myxedema coma, *AACN Clin Issues Crit Care Nurs* 3(2): 300-308, 1992.

Streff MM, Pachucki-Hyde LC: Management of the patient with thyroid disease, *Nurs Clin North Am* 31(4):779-796, 1996.

Trivalle C et al: Differences in the signs and symptoms of hyperthyroidism in older and younger patients, *J Am Geriatr Soc* 44(1):50-53, 1996.

# CHAPTER 29

# Diabetes

## CHAPTER OBJECTIVES

1 Discuss the nursing responsibilities to identify potential problems of the endocrine system.
2 Describe the nursing interventions to manage patient responses to hypersecretion or hyposecretion of specific endocrine glands.
3 Describe the pathophysiology, course, prognosis, and treatment of diabetes mellitus.
4 Compare and contrast the risk factors, onset, and course of the acute complications of diabetes mellitus.
5 Outline the actions that patients and providers take to prevent, detect, and treat diabetic complications.
6 Discuss the palliative treatment goal of diabetes to reduce symptoms, control hyperglycemia, and prevent complications.
7 Describe some examples of patients' responses to diabetes mellitus that indicate the uniqueness of this disease.
8 Describe nursing interventions that foster self-care of patients with diabetes to perform activities of daily living.
9 Describe some special educational needs of the elderly patient with diabetes.

## KEY TERMS

acetone
diabetes mellitus
glucagon
glycohemoglobin
homeostasis
hormone
hyperglycemia
hyperglycemic, hyperosmolar, nonketotic coma
hypoglycemia
insulin reaction
ketoacidosis
ketone
ketonuria
ketosis
metabolism
type I diabetes mellitus
type II diabetes mellitus

## DIABETES MELLITUS

**Diabetes mellitus** is the most common endocrine disorder in the United States. The American Diabetes Association estimates that there are 16 million people in the United States with diabetes. More than 625,000 new cases are diagnosed each year. Nearly 11% of the population older than 65 years old have diabetes. Approximately 1 in every 20 Americans is or will be affected by this metabolic problem. Diabetes mellitus is a chronic, currently incurable health problem that results from defects in insulin action or secretion or usage. It represents a heterogeneous group of anatomic and chemical problems characterized by high blood glucose levels. In addition to the initially observed problem with carbohydrate metabolism, individuals who have diabetes mellitus also have a deficit in their conversion of proteins and fats.

Although the cause of diabetes mellitus is currently unknown, there are probably diverse causes. Known risk factors for developing diabetes mellitus are heredity, environment, and life-style. Blood relatives of people who have diabetes, especially type II diabetes mellitus, are more likely to develop diabetes than are individuals not related to anyone with the disease. Overweight individuals and those who lead a sedentary life-style are more prone to develop type II diabetes mellitus. Certain viruses and autoimmune factors have been associated with the development of the disease and are thought to play a role in its cause. Chickenpox-type viruses have been associated with the development of type I diabetes mellitus. The present thinking is that diabetes develops as a result of a combination of risk factors.

Diabetes is the leading cause of blindness, heart attack, stroke, and gangrene. Improvements in therapeutic techniques have increased the average life span of the individual who has diabetes, but prevention through health education of the complications of the disease is appropriate.

## Pathophysiology

An adequate supply of insulin in the body is necessary for the body cells to combine oxygen and glucose to produce the energy necessary for body functions. In the absence of insulin several metabolic changes occur. Glucose accumulates in the blood and is excreted in the urine. The body is then required to use proteins and fat for energy, which under certain conditions will lead to metabolic acidosis.

The symptoms of diabetes mellitus result from insulin deficiency. Insulin is secreted by the beta cells in the islets of Langerhans in the pancreas. The deficiency may result because of diminished or absolute lack of insulin or as a result of resistance to insulin action at the cell level. Lack of enough usable insulin causes **hyperglycemia,** a high blood glucose level.

Diabetes mellitus is classified as either insulin-dependent (IDDM), **type I diabetes mellitus,** or as noninsulin-dependent (NIDDM), **type II diabetes mellitus** (Table 29-1). Formerly IDDM individuals were classified as having juvenile-onset, or brittle, diabetes. NIDDM individuals previously were described as having stable, or adult-onset, diabetes. Clinically many patients lie between the two extremes, and nursing interventions are directed toward individual responses to diabetes and its treatment, regardless of classification. However, because the pathogenesis, treatment, and possible complications of the types differ, the two classes are discussed separately.

Diabetes is a complex phenomenon. The analogy of insulin helping to unlock the cell wall so that circulating glucose can enter into the cell has been used as a learning device for patients. The absorption of glucose into the cell, the resultant circulating glucose level, and its potential spill into urine are different, depending on the presence or absence of available insulin.

## Assessment

The two classifications differ in respect to insulin dependency, onset and symptoms, and intensity of treatment. Type I diabetes mellitus commonly has a sudden onset marked by an excessive concentration of

---

**TABLE 29-1**

## Comparison of Type I and Type II Diabetes Mellitus

| TYPE I (IDDM) | TYPE II (NIDDM) |
| --- | --- |
| Less than 10% of known cases of diabetes mellitus | 90%-95% of all known cases of diabetes mellitus |
| Any age; peaks at ages 5 and 11 | Over age 30 |
| Usually thin | Obese |
| Abrupt symptoms | Few symptoms |
| Ketosis prone | Nonketosis prone |
| Severe insulinopenia | Insulin levels normal, depressed, or elevated |
| Dependent on insulin for life | Not dependent on insulin for life |
| Autoimmune disease | Autosomal-dominant inheritance |
| At risk for complications of retinopathy, neuropathy, and nephropathy | At risk for microvascular and macrovascular complications |

*IDDM,* Insulin-dependent diabetes mellitus; *NIDDM,* noninsulin-dependent diabetes mellitus.

glucose in the blood and the presence of the three polys associated with diabetes: polyuria, polydipsia, and polyphagia accompanied by weight loss.

Lack of insulin initiates a chain of events that accounts for the initial symptoms of type I diabetes mellitus. With an insulin deficiency, glucose cannot enter the cell and accumulates in the bloodstream. This is evidenced by hyperglycemia. Because the body cannot use this glucose for food or energy, it keeps piling up until the kidneys excrete it. Glucose is dissolved in fluid in the bloodstream, so when it is excreted by the kidneys (glycosuria), not only is it wasted but so is the water in which it is dissolved. This accounts for the polyuria, or excessive urination. The increase in the amount of fluid lost makes the individual thirsty, polydipsia, so the patient drinks extra liquids to maintain fluid balance. Instead of being absorbed into the cell, glucose is lost in urine. Because those calories were not used, the appetite mechanism is stimulated and the individual becomes hungry and eats an excessive amount of food (polyphagia). There is no weight gain because calories are wasted when the glucose is excreted into the urine.

Individuals who develop type I diabetes mellitus are usually young, of normal weight or have recently experienced weight loss, and often show signs of polyuria, polydipsia, polyphagia, and **ketosis** (an accumulation of ketone bodies in the blood and tissues). When left untreated, other symptoms that result include dry skin and mucous membranes, constipation, and signs of fluid and electrolyte losses. These undiagnosed individuals may develop diabetic ketoacidosis (DKA) and die unless this process is stopped by exogenous insulin (insulin that is produced outside the body). Most people who have type I diabetes mellitus require insulin to manage their diabetes.

Type II diabetes mellitus symptoms are usually so mild that the condition may exist undetected and untreated for a considerable period. Often individuals are middle-aged and overweight. They have some endogenous (produced within the body) insulin, but its secretion may be slow or subnormal or a problem with its use at the cellular level may exist. When this diabetes exists for a long time and is untreated, symptoms of varied severity may occur. These symptoms include skin infections such as boils and carbuncles and arteriosclerotic conditions, particularly of the eyes, kidneys, lower extremities, and coronary and cerebral blood vessels. Some people who have type II diabetes are able to control the disease with diet and exercise alone; others require the addition of an oral antidiabetic agent, and a third group requires insulin. Type II diabetes mellitus is characterized by a slow, insidious onset and may go undetected for years.

## Treatment Goal

The therapeutic goal of diabetes management is to maintain a blood glucose level that is as close to normal as possible while allowing the patient to maintain a normal life-style. Treatment includes maintaining normal blood glucose level, exercise, nutrition, medication, and patient education. Diabetes cannot be cured, but its symptoms can be controlled and its pathologic course may be kept in check. The therapeutic management of diabetes mellitus is palliative. The goals of hyperglycemia reduction, prevention of acute complications (insulin reaction; DKA; and **hyperglycemic, hyperosmolar, nonketotic coma**), and forestalling chronic complications (microvascular and macrovascular angiopathies) guide clinicians as they plan the diabetic regimen with the individual. The acute complications of diabetes are discussed later in this chapter.

Priorities of nursing care are first concerned with immediate patient needs and then with long-range needs because diabetes at the present time is a lifetime disease. Patients must assume a great deal of responsibility for their self-care management and become partners with clinicians who provide needed health care. Because individuals who have diabetes become managers of their chronic illness on a day-to-day basis, they are not always in a patient role. Therefore instead of always labeling people who have diabetes as patients, they should be referred to as persons or individuals. The word *diabetic* should only be used as an adjective to describe a component of the regimen, such as diabetic meal plan. The label *diabetic* should never be used to refer to a person, rather they are people with diabetes.

## Diagnostic Tests

The initial diagnosis of diabetes mellitus is accomplished by analyzing the patient's blood glucose level. Neither glucose nor ketones are normally present in urine. Their presence indicates the possibility of diabetes mellitus and the need for additional diagnostic tests. Glucose in urine means that the blood glucose level has exceeded the renal threshold, which is the blood glucose level for an individual that must be reached before circulating glucose is removed from the blood by the kidneys. The presence of **acetone,** one of the ketone bodies produced in abnormally large amounts in uncontrolled diabetes mellitus, in the urine means the body has rapidly broken down fats to use as energy and that some of the breakdown product has been removed from the bloodstream and is present in the urine. Severe dieting or a high-fat diet can also cause **ketonuria,** an excess of ketone bodies in the urine.

Consistency in the diagnosis of diabetes is being achieved by the use of criteria recommended by the National Diabetes Data Group of the National Institutes of Health (Sperling, 1988). The diagnosis of diabetes can be made for nonpregnant adults when one of the following signs is present: (1) classic symptoms of diabetes and hyperglycemia with a random plasma glucose level of 200 mg/dl or greater; (2) a fasting venous plasma glucose level at least equal to 140 mg/dl on two occasions; or (3) an elevated venous plasma glucose level once after drinking glucose and before the 2-hour point *and* at the 2-hour point in an oral glucose tolerance test. A fasting plasma glucose level over 130 mg/dl should be an indication for further testing in children. DKA can occur rapidly in young children, so early diagnosis and treatment is especially important.

An oral glucose-tolerance test is done after an individual has eaten a high carbohydrate diet for 3 days. The person fasts from the evening before the test until the last specimen has been obtained. On the day of the test an initial fasting blood sample is drawn and is sent to the laboratory. The patient is given a pure glucose drink. Consuming the very sweet-tasting drink on an empty stomach may make the person feel a little nauseous. Because the test is terminated if vomiting occurs, the nurse should instruct the patient to assume a comfortable position during the test. Blood samples are collected at various specified intervals of 30 minutes until the test is complete. An elevated glucose level at the 2-hour point usually indicates some disorder of carbohydrate metabolism.

Another common test is a 2-hour postprandial blood sugar test that is drawn exactly 2 hours after the patient finishes the specified meal. Individuals who do not have diabetes mellitus would have a 2-hour postprandial blood glucose level that had returned to the normal premeal range.

> ### NURSE ALERT
>
> **The patient who has a fasting blood glucose level taken in the morning should be told that breakfast will not be served until after the blood specimen has been taken.**

Immediately after the diagnosis is made, health care providers monitor the status of the individual's diabetes and responses to treatment. Patients are taught to self-monitor their own blood glucose as soon as possible. Patients learn the rationale for and techniques to correctly obtain the desired specimen and test it for the amount of glucose.

Urine testing provides an approximation of the individual's blood glucose level. An individual's renal threshold determines when blood glucose spills over into urine. For adults with no renal problems, this threshold is approximately 170 to 200 mg, which means the blood glucose level must be least 170 mg before any glucose could be wasted into the urine. Individuals determine their own renal threshold by recording their blood glucose values and comparing them with their urine glucose values. The lowest blood glucose value at which glucose spills into the urine is an estimate of the renal threshold. Urine testing remains valuable for the detection of acetone **(ketones)** which can identify people at risk for developing ketoacidosis.

When insulin is being used, the frequency and timing of the testing of the blood sugar (glucose) varies. The variety is caused by the number of insulin injections the patient is using, the peak action of that insulin, and the goals for therapy. Individuals who control their disease by diet alone or with an oral antidiabetic agent may occasionally be asked to test a blood sugar after a meal (postprandial) to identify how the pancreas is handling the challenge of food. Only in rare cases, such as a newly diagnosed elderly patient being managed by diet only, would testing for glucose in the urine be considered after meals.

Urine testing is the only method patients can use to test for ketones. The patient should be instructed to test urine for ketones if there is a large amount of glycosuria, if there is a blood glucose level over 240 mg/dl, or if there are symptoms of illness. When acetone is present in the urine, the body has metabolized fatty acids. This can occur during a usual overnight fast, and a trace amount may be expected every morning. Conversely, larger amounts of ketone bodies can be a sign that the person requires more insulin.

## Monitoring

Self-monitoring of blood glucose levels may be done with the use of commercial products such as visual strips or with meters. A finger stick is done, and capillary blood is placed on the test strip. After a certain amount of time, the reagent strip turns to a color indicating the amount of glucose in the blood. A color comparison of the strip to the chart indicates the amount of glucose present. Meters can automate the calculation and give a readout of the glucose level. Home measurement of blood glucose is recommended for all individuals on insulin therapy and oral antidiabetic medication.

In 1994 the American Diabetes Association issued a policy statement strongly recommending that certain classes of patients self-monitor their blood glucose levels (American Diabetes Association, 1994a). Some patients require frequent insulin dose adjustments on the basis of blood glucose levels. These patients include those who are (1) receiving intensive insulin therapy by insulin pump or multiple daily injections, (2) pregnant or plan to be, or (3) prone to hypoglycemia but who may not experience warning signs of hypoglycemia. In another policy statement the American Diabetes Association stressed the importance of blood glucose self-monitoring to meet treatment goals. They stated that patients must be taught blood glucose self-monitoring if their treatment goals included maintenance of specific blood sugar levels, prevention of severe hyperglycemia, prevention of frequent hypoglycemia, and insulin adjustment to meet life-style changes (American Diabetes Association, 1994b).

Individuals who are taught to monitor their diabetes at home need to follow the same precautions that nurses in health care facilities take with similar diagnostic products. The most important precaution is the most basic: read and carefully follow the manufacturer's directions! The individual should wait the exact number of seconds required before examining the strip or solution for color change or result. He or she should be sure to use the specific color chart or automatic device designed for the test, if applicable. The individual should observe the reagents and color strips to be sure they have not discolored or gone bad, which would make them inaccurate. The individual should test the calibration of instruments used to ensure their accuracy and should clean them regularly according to package directions. He or she should store all testing materials in a place safe for both the product and the people who live in the same environment. There are many glucose meters on the market today. Most are extremely easy to use, and the nurse can assist the patient by following package or video instructions. Patient technique should be observed before discharge to ensure proper home use. All blood glucose monitoring requires patients to puncture the skin to obtain blood samples. Companies are working on noninvasive blood glucose testing using near-infrared light that can see through the skin. Although the new technology could be expensive, it would reduce many problems with technique and compliance (National Diabetes Information Clearinghouse, 1993).

**Glycohemoglobin** levels are another diagnostic test used in diabetes. Glycosylated hemoglobin forms when glucose in the blood attaches to the hemoglobin in the red blood cells. The higher the blood glucose level, the more glucose is attached and the higher the result. Because blood glucose levels reflect the present, they are easily influenced by recent events and are useful in determining daily insulin or dietary requirements. The glycohemoglobin level represents the degree of glucose control achieved during the previous 2 to 3 months and is a general indicator of long-term metabolic control. Glycohemoglobin production increases in the presence of hyperglycemia. An elevated glycohemoglobin level means that the patient's blood

glucose levels were consistently high for 6 to 8 weeks previously. Because the palliative goal of diabetes therapy is to achieve good metabolic control without complications, glycohemoglobin levels are assessed periodically, between 1 and 4 times per year.

Providers and patients must exercise some general precautions regarding the use and interpretations of the glycohemoglobin diabetic diagnostic tests. This specific test and range of normal may differ from setting to setting. The important consideration is not to memorize lists of laboratory values but to know what the normal ranges of values are in the laboratory that is being used.

> ### NURSE ALERT
>
> The normal ranges of the glycohemoglobin (HgALc) may vary according to the laboratory used.

## Meal Plan

There is no standard diabetic diet. Meal plans are developed for the individual patient on the basis of caloric needs, nutritional requirements, and usual eating habits. Many patients with type II mild diabetes mellitus are maintained by controlling their food intake and exercise. Some meal plans control calories and are commonly prescribed for older, obese patients who do not require insulin therapy. The metabolic picture of obese patients with type II diabetes mellitus often improves after they reduce their weight.

For patients who have unstable type I diabetes mellitus, the meal plan is first calculated and then the amount of insulin necessary to metabolize it is established. A meal plan controls the amount of carbohydrate, protein, fat, cholesterol, fiber, and calories. The amount of food is divided into specific amounts to be eaten at meals and for snacks at predetermined times.

Usually the food-exchange lists prepared jointly by the American Diabetes Association, the American Dietetic Association, and the United States Public Health Service are used in planning the patient's therapeutic meal plan. Seven lists of exchangeable foods have been defined: (1) foods with a minimum caloric content that are allowed as desired ("free food"); (2) vegetables; (3) fruits; (4) bread; (5) meat; (6) fats; and (7) milk. Each item on a specific list is equal in nutritional value, and similar amounts are interchangeable with one another (Figure 29-1). A specified number of exchanges is allowed for each meal and snack according to the caloric needs of the patient and the prescribed plan (Table 29-2).

The individual's usual life-style, preferences, use of insulin or oral hypoglycemic agents, and cultural differences are considered when the meal plan is established. Because the discipline of dietary restrictions and the need to eat at prescribed time intervals are so demanding, it is crucial that the meal plan be accommodated into the patient's routine as much as possible. Creativity of health care providers exercised within therapeutic guidelines can help minimize the tedium of following the same plan day after day. Individuals can be taught how to eat at fast-food chains and to correctly "augment" their diet. For instance, a person who craves a large glass of orange juice in the morning but is allowed only 4 ounces can be taught to add 4 ounces of sugar-free orange tonic to their juice. Eight ounces of frosty, cold, orange-juice-tasting liquid can be had for one fruit exchange.

In 1994 the American Diabetes Association released new dietary guidelines for people with diabetes. Sugars and starches are now one food category and can be exchanged. However, food containing carbohydrates must still be measured. If a high-sugar food is selected, one gets a smaller amount than with a low-sugar counterpart. For example, $\frac{1}{3}$ cup of frosted flakes would be equal to $\frac{3}{4}$ cup of corn flakes. Many high-sugar foods contain fat and should be avoided (American Diabetes Association, 1994b).

Counting carbohydrates has become the cornerstone to dietary management in patients desiring "tight" control on intensive insulin therapy, normally someone with type I diabetes mellitus. Basically, the amount of insulin to be taken premeal is determined

## TABLE 29-2

### 1200 Calorie Meal Plan

|  | BREAKFAST | LUNCH | AFTERNOON SNACK | DINNER | EVENING SNACK |
|---|---|---|---|---|---|
| Time | 7 AM | 12 PM |  | 6 PM |  |
| Number of choices |  |  |  |  |  |
| Lowfat milk | $\frac{1}{2}$ cup | $\frac{1}{2}$ cup |  |  | $\frac{1}{2}$ cup |
| Vegetable |  | 1 |  | 2 |  |
| Fruit | 1 | 1 |  | 1 |  |
| Bread | 1 | 1 | 1 | 1 | 1 |
| Meat |  | 1 | 1 | 2 |  |
| Fat | 1 | 1 |  | 1 |  |

Cholesterol 153 g, protein 61 g, fat 41 g.

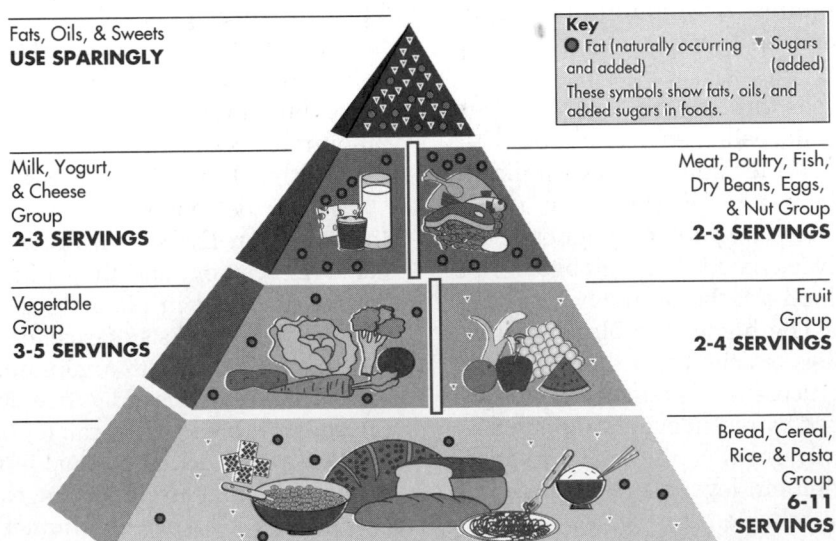

**Figure 29-1** The food guide pyramid, a guide to daily food choices. Each food group provides some, but not all, required nutrients. (From US Department of Agriculture, Human Nutrition Information Service, 1992.)

by the amount of carbohydrate to be consumed at the meal plus a correctional factor if the glucose is out of range.

Diet therapy for people who have type I diabetes mellitus follows a specific time frame. When the action of insulin is at its peak, patients must have enough circulating glucose in their bloodstream to move into the cells. A specific amount of carbohydrate, protein, and fat in the form of food exchanges is calculated. The time frame for eating the exchanges is specified. Thus a package of peanut butter crackers eaten 3 hours after lunch, instead of being a casual snack, is an important component of an individual's diabetes therapy. A bedtime snack also prevents reactions during the night. Patients can be taught to exchange meals and snacks to accommodate special events in their lives.

## Insulin

Many individuals who have diabetes require insulin. In the United States insulin is commercially derived from the pancreas of a pig or cow or synthesized in a laboratory. The new synthetic human insulins (Humulin, Novolin) are the purest forms of insulin. Patients should not switch to synthetic insulin without close monitoring of dosage by the health care provider. The amount of insulin needed depends on the individual and varies at different times for the same person. The type of insulin needed also varies. The purpose of administering insulin is to replace a deficiency. Its action is to enable the body to metabolize food, absorb glucose into the cell, and thus lower the blood glucose level. Many types of insulin are in current use. Each insulin has three expected time frames: (1) *onset* is the time between the injection of insulin and when it starts to be effective in the body, (2) *peak* is the time when the insulin action is at its highest, and (3) *duration* is the length of time the insulin effect is expected to last in the body. Insulins are classified according to their time frame of action and duration of effect as one of three types: (1) fast acting or short duration, (2) intermediate acting or medium duration, and (3) slow acting or long lasting (Table 29-3).

Product information circulars and current drug books provide precise data about the composition of specific insulins and their action. Health care professionals examine patients' blood glucose records and relate the values to food eaten, exercise, and symptoms of possible insulin reactions. They learn the approximate times after an injection that the insulin has its onset, peak, and duration for that individual. Adjustments in dose are then made until the best dose and type of insulin is found to achieve the individual's goal of blood glucose levels. Insulin used on a daily basis may be stored at room temperature for 1 month, as long as it is not exposed to direct sunlight or kept near a heat source. Unopened insulin can be stored safely in the refrigerator until the expiration date on the bottle.

## TABLE 29-3

### Insulins Sold in the United States

| PRODUCT | MFG | STRENGTH | PRODUCT | MFG | STRENGTH |
|---|---|---|---|---|---|
| **Rapid-acting (onset <15 min; usual duration 3-5 h)** | | | Novolin L (lente) | Novo Noridks | U-100 |
| *Human analog* | | | Novolin N (NPH)*† | Novo Nordisk | U-100 |
| Humalog (insulin lispro)* | Lilly | U-100 | *Pork* | | |
| | | | Iletin II L (lente) | Lilly | U-100 |
| **Short-acting (usual onset 0.5-2.0 h; usual duration 4-6 h)** | | | Iletin II N (NPH) | Lilly | U-100 |
| *Human* | | | Purified pork L (lente) | Novo Nordisk | U-100 |
| Humulin R (regular)* | Lilly | U-100 | Purified pork N (NPH) | Novo Nordisk | U-100 |
| Novolin R (regular)*† | Novo Nordisk | U-100 | | | |
| Velosulin human (regular, buffered) | Novo Nordisk | U-100 | **Long-acting (usual onset 4-6 h; usual duration 18-24 h)** | | |
| *Pork* | | | *Human* | | |
| Iletin II R (regular) | Lilly | U-100, U-500 | Humulin U (ultralente) | Lilly | U-100 |
| Purified pork R (regular) | Novo Nordisk | U-100 | | | |
| | | | **Premixed combinations** | | |
| **Intermediate-acting (usual onset 3-6 h; usual duration 12-20 h)** | | | *Human* | | |
| *Human* | | | Humulin 50/50 (50% NPH, 50% regular) | Lilly | U-100 |
| Humulin L (lente) | Lilly | U-100 | Humulin 70/30 (70% NPH, 30% regular)* | Lilly | U-100 |
| Humulin N (NPH)* | Lilly | U-100 | Novolin 70/30 (70% NPH, 30% regular)*† | Novo Nordisk | U-100 |

Modified from Skyler JS: *Medical management of type 1 diabetes*, ed 3, Alexandria, Va, 1998, American Diabetes Association.
*Indicates availability in cartridges for pens, in addition to vials.
†Indicates availability in "prefilled" disposable pens, in addition to cartridges and vials.
*Mfg*, Manufacturer.

Insulin is administered in units that have been standardized so that it is the same no matter where it is purchased or from which pharmaceutical manufacturer it comes. Insulin is available in concentration of 100 units/ml (U-100) and in a 10-ml vial in the United States. Insulin syringes are calibrated in units of 100 to correspond to that concentration of insulin (100 units/ml). Small-gauge (28-29), short (½-inch) needles are used. There is also a 1-inch needle for use by pediatric patients or very thin adults. One-milliliter (U-100) syringes are suitable for patients with higher dosages. Low-dose syringes that hold 50 units of U-100 concentrated insulin are available for those who require minimum amounts of insulin. U-30 and U-25 insulin syringes are available, especially for use by children or those with impaired vision or on small doses of insulin. The most important consideration is that the patient understands that each line on the U-100 syringe equals 2 units, whereas on all other syringes each line equals 1 unit.

The skills required to inject insulin are less complex than the skills of drawing insulin into a syringe. The patient may be fearful of the first self-administered injection. Teaching the patient to inject should always be the first teaching done because this is the source of the most anxiety.

Before teaching the mechanical skills for drawing insulin, the patient should be assessed for ability to see the syringe markings and manual dexterity to handle the equipment. The patient should be taught to always check the label on the bottle. Intermediate- and long-acting insulin should be gently rolled to ensure that all sediment is mixed into the liquid (Figure 29-2). The insulin vial should be placed on a firm surface, and its top should be cleaned with alcohol. The syringe should be handled carefully so as not to stress the small needle, and sterile technique should be used. The patient should then remove the needle cover and draw in the amount of air equal to the amount of insulin to be removed from the vial. The air is injected into the vial, and the vial is inverted in the patient's hand so that the tip of the needle is covered by insulin and the bottle is not resting on the needle. The plunger is pulled halfway down the syringe, and air bubbles are eliminated. Then the correct amount of insulin is withdrawn from the vial.

If the patient is receiving two insulins that can be mixed in the same syringe, some modifications are made to the procedure. Additionally, careful reading of each bottle label is imperative. To ensure patient consistency and to avoid contamination, the shorter-acting insulin should be drawn first. Both insulin vials are cleansed and placed on a firm surface. The amount of air to be injected into the longer-acting insulin is drawn and injected into the vial, and the needle is removed. Then the correct amount of air for the shorter-acting insulin is injected into that bottle, the vial is inverted, the bubbles are removed, and the insulin is removed. Without letting any of the shorter-acting insulin leave the syringe, the longer-acting bottle is entered, the needle tip is covered, and the correct amount of insulin is withdrawn.

Patients are given careful instructions so that dose errors are avoided. If the patient's dose is 10 units of Regular insulin and 20 units of NPH insulin, the following instructions would be given so that the patient would correctly draw up a total dose of 30 units:

1. Draw up 20 units of air, inject it into NPH vial, and remove the syringe.
2. Draw up 10 units of air, inject it into the Regular vial, invert the bottle, cover the needle with insulin, fill the syringe halfway, remove the air bubbles, push or pull the plunger until there are exactly 10 units of insulin and no air in the syringe, and remove the syringe from the vial.
3. Without losing any of the Regular insulin in the syringe, inject the needle into the NPH vial, cover the tip of the needle with NPH insulin, and slowly pull the plunger back until it reaches 30 units on the syringe.
4. Remove the needle from the NPH bottle and proceed with the injection.

A total dose of 30 units (10 Regular and 20 NPH) was drawn into the same syringe.

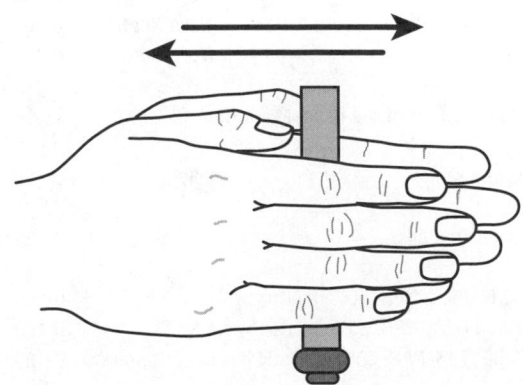

**Figure 29-2** Method for rolling NPH insulin. Vial is rolled between the palms.

**NURSE ALERT**

If too much insulin is pulled from the NPH bottle, it may not be pushed back into either bottle. The syringe is discarded, and the patient must begin the process again.

Because mixing insulin may be a problem for some patients, taking two separate injections may be one safe solution. Premixed insulins may be purchased (Novolin or Humulin 70/30) when the required dose is 30% Regular insulin and 70% NPH insulin (see Table 29-3). Sample instructions for measuring insulin are found in Figure 29-3.

The method currently used for injecting insulin is to inject the insulin into the subcutaneous tissue. Once the correct dose is prepared, the patient is taught to clean the skin and to pinch up a large fold of skin and fat. Holding the syringe like a pencil, the needle is injected into the skin at a 90-degree angle all the way to the hub. The insulin should be injected through the subcutaneous tissue into the loose space made by the

pinch. Once all the insulin has been injected, the pinch of skin is released before the needle is withdrawn to avoid loss of insulin. The first time the patient self-injects insulin, the nurse should select a site that is easily reached, such as the thigh or abdomen. The patient should be guided through the procedure and assisted as needed.

The sites for injection should be rotated to prevent lipodystrophy, which may interfere with absorption and lead to the formation of scar tissue. Possible injection sites should be chosen on the basis of the condition of the skin, patient preferences, manual dexterity, and the sensitivity of the individual to site changes. Preferred sites are the lateral surface of the upper arms, the abdominal tissue just below the rib cage, the anterolateral surfaces of the thigh, and the upper buttock (Figure 29-4). Any atrophied or hypertrophied area should be avoided, including scar tissue, nevi, or moles. If insulin is given in the same site for a time, scar tissue may form, which leads to erratic absorption of the insulin. The site chosen for the insulin injections affects the rate of absorption. The most rapid absorption is from the abdomen, and the arm site is second.

---

DOSE  *10 Reg.*
       *20 NPH*

INSTRUCTIONS FOR MEASURING INSULIN

### Mixed Dose

1. Turn cloudy bottle upside down and roll between hands.

2. Wipe off tops of bottles with cotton and alcohol.

3. Pull plunger to . . *20* . Put needle through top of cloudy bottle and push plunger down, putting air into bottle. Take needle out empty.

4. Pull plunger to . . *10* . . . . Put needle through top of clear bottle and push plunger down. Leave needle in bottle.

5. Turn bottle upside down and pull plunger halfway down syringe. Push all insulin back in bottle;

6. Pull plunger halfway down syringe and check for bubbles.* If no bubbles present, push plunger to . *10* . units of regular insulin and take out needle.

   *If bubbles present, repeat step 5 before completing step 6.

7. Turn cloudy bottle upside down and stick needle through rubber top.

8. Pull plunger slowly to . *30* . . units.
   ( . *10* . + *20* . ). Take out needle.

9. Wipe skin with alcohol and cotton and pinch.

10. Pick up syringe like a pencil and push needle straight into skin. Push plunger down.

11. Release pinch, press alcohol next to needle and pull out.

**Figure 29-3**   Instructions for measuring a mixed dose of insulin.

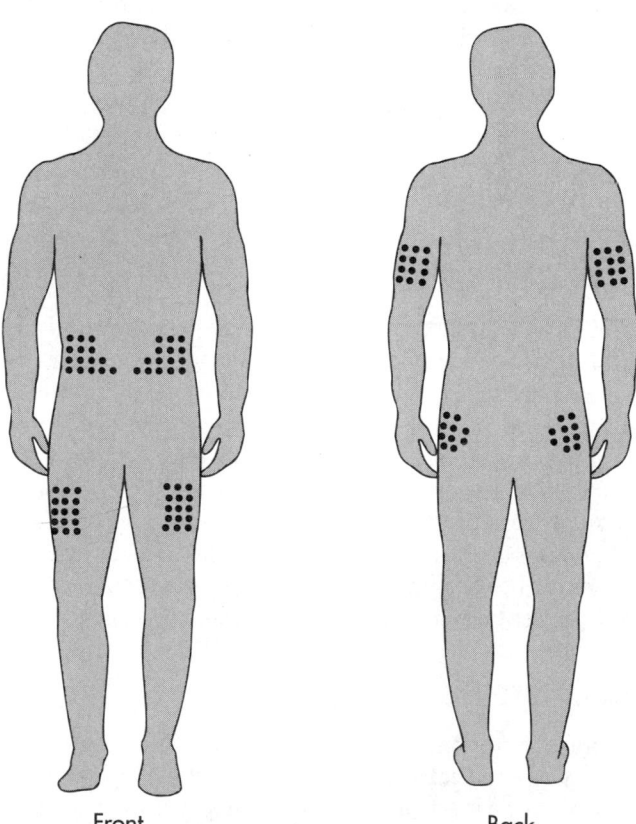

Front          Back

**Figure 29-4**   Rotation sites for insulin injections. (Modified from Potter PA, Perry AG: *Basic nursing: theory and practice*, ed 3, St Louis, 1995, Mosby.)

Patients should be instructed to use these sites if blood glucose levels are elevated.

Once the prescribed dose of insulin has been injected, the patient should record the amount and site in a record book. The used syringe and needle should be placed in a covered container (e.g., coffee can) before disposal.

A family member or significant other should be taught the insulin administration technique for times when assistance is needed. For patients who have problems meeting acceptable skill levels in any component of the insulin administration process, problem solving should be done so that individuals are as independent as possible. For instance, if a patient cannot see well enough in the morning to accurately draw up insulin but can manipulate injecting insulin, there are several alternatives. A visiting nurse can draw up a week's supply and leave them, a family member or a neighbor could be asked for daily assistance, or a magnifier could be used on the syringe. If the person can see better at the end of the day, which is not uncommon, the insulin for the next day can be drawn up the night before and stored in the refrigerator. Proper lighting is essential.

There are also several devices on the market to aid patients with injections. Some patients with unstable diabetes and changing life-styles may be candidates for intensive treatment. The first is multiple injections of insulin, and the second is the use of the insulin pump. Both of these treatments require motivation and special education but do allow for greater flexibility in meal scheduling and exercise programs.

## Risk for Infection

People who have diabetes are believed to have a lowered resistance to infection, and their abrasions or wounds may heal more slowly than those of individuals who do not have diabetes. These observed phenomena may be secondary to an etiologic factor of immunologic suppression of white blood cells or may exist because of the effect of high blood glucose levels when diabetes is uncontrolled. General skin care to prevent the accumulation of pathogenic organisms and prevent drying should be carried out daily.

## Foot Care

Because many patients are at risk for foot problems because of potential vascular complications and peripheral neuropathy from their diabetes, the most important aspect of hygiene is proper care of the feet. Feet should be washed daily with warm water (avoid hot water) and mild soap and dried well. The area between the toes should be especially dry, and no lotion or lanolin should be applied to this area. Nails should be filed slightly longer than the shape of the toe. Corns and calluses should be smoothed with a pumice stone or emery board. Patients should be told to avoid bathroom surgery and to consult a podiatrist for very tough toenails or corns that require cutting. Feet should be examined daily, and any problem should be reported to the health care provider.

Even a trivial injury should be reported early because care for a minor problem can prevent its escalation into a major one. Other aspects of foot care include wearing properly fitting shoes, not going barefoot, and avoiding anything constricting (e.g., round garters or tightly fitting knee-high hose) that could decrease circulation to the feet. Shoes should be broken in gradually. The best time to purchase shoes is at the end of the day to ensure proper fitting. Heating devices for the feet (e.g., hot water bottles) should never be used, and feet should never be soaked.

## Exercise

One of the American pioneers in diabetes treatment, Dr. Elliot Joslin, viewed diet, exercise, and insulin as three "frisky ponies" that together control diabetes. After insulin became readily available as a therapy, the Joslin Clinic noted that patients who returned to farm work or other active jobs were in better metabolic control than their patients who had a more sedentary lifestyle. Exercise is believed to exert its physiologic benefit by changing the cell wall permeability so that movement of glucose into the cell is increased, by directly lowering blood glucose levels because glucose is used for energy, and by increasing the uptake of free fatty acids. Exercise also increases the level of high-density lipoproteins and lowers cholesterol and triglyceride levels. This is important because individuals who have diabetes are at a greater risk for cardiovascular diseases.

Just as diet and insulin therapies are individualized, so too are exercise regimens. Health care professionals are aware of potential complications from exercise and characteristics of those individuals for whom exercise would be considered dangerous. Therefore the specific exercise plan should be mutually decided upon by the patient (to fit into daily activities) and the provider (to prescribe the proper amount and adjust the diet and insulin as necessary). Exercise may be contraindicated for some individuals. Others may need cardiovascular screening before an exercise prescription is given.

Weight control, lower insulin requirements, and a sense of well being are positive outcomes of an ongoing exercise program. Integrating regular exercise into a daily routine can be difficult. For those who integrate the activities required of diabetes management into their routine, the addition of an exercise plan may be especially difficult. This underscores the importance of the patient and provider collaborating in the development of activities of daily living that are acceptable to the individual who has diabetes.

## Insulin Reaction

The goal of diabetes therapy is to prevent or delay the onset of chronic complications without precipitating acute complications. Achieving a near-normal blood glucose level at all times is ideal but is difficult to achieve in actuality. Shifts in blood glucose levels are inevitable, and these may result in one of the acute complications of diabetes. An insulin reaction, or hypoglycemic (low blood glucose) reaction, is the most common acute complication of diabetes, especially in patients who use insulin. Individuals who use insulin should be taught to expect some insulin reactions, to learn what are the most likely causes for a hypoglycemic event, and to recognize their own early warning signs. Both patients and providers must incorporate prevention, detection, and management of reactions into the overall treatment plan.

An insulin reaction results from either a drop in blood glucose level to an amount not tolerated by the individual (usually under 70 ml/dl of blood). This drop in blood glucose is caused by too much insulin or diabetes medication, too much exercise, or delayed or omitted food intake. In the first case, a blood test would reveal a "normal" blood glucose level, but the individual would still experience and exhibit the symptoms of a reaction. Once individuals recognize their reaction patterns, their opinion of whether or not they are in reaction is what determines if treatment is required. When in doubt, treat!

Hypoglycemic reactions are caused by too little circulating glucose. The reaction may be caused by too much insulin or exercise and not enough food. An increased amount of insulin, not enough food at the time insulin is peaking, alcohol consumption, or strenuous exercise without an insulin decrease or food increase may precipitate a reaction. Reactions come on rapidly. They can be mild or extremely severe. The most common symptoms are a trembling sensation, profuse perspiration, irritability, and dizziness. Additional signs may be generalized muscle weakness, headache, tingling sensations of the lips or tongue, blurred or double vision, an unsteady gait, palpitations, pallor, and hunger (Table 29-4). Without immediate treatment, the patient may become confused, lose consciousness, and develop seizure activity.

The immediate treatment is to raise the blood glucose level. Simple carbohydrates such as juice, glucose tablets, or regular soda should be ingested. Some pa-

tients monitor their blood glucose level before treating to make an appraisal of how much carbohydrate they need. Such monitoring allows patients to gain a closer approximation of what symptoms they experience at various levels. Treatment must never be delayed because symptoms rapidly progress. If a suspected reaction is treated with 4 ounces of ginger ale and later on it is discovered that the patient was in error when the diagnosis was made, there is no harm done. Extra calories from the ginger ale are better than the risk of not treating a possible reaction or waiting too long.

Patients should be taught to carry a simple carbohydrate with them at all times so they can immediately treat suspected reactions and prevent serious ones. In a hospital setting, a conscious patient who experiences an insulin reaction is treated with fruit juice, regular soda, honey, jelly, or milk. If a patient is unconscious, nothing is given by mouth. One of two methods is used to quickly raise the blood glucose level. The length of time the patient has been unconscious and the setting in which the patient was found determine which to use. If the patient is unconscious at home or if it is known that the patient just became unconscious, then glucagon would be the first treatment to use. Endogenous glucagon is a hormone secreted by the alpha cells of the islets of Langerhans. In the presence of low blood glucose levels, glucagon is secreted and stimulates the liver to break down glycogen, which in turn releases glucose into the bloodstream and raises the blood glucose level. An exogenous glucagon preparation would be given subcutaneously or intramuscularly to stimulate a glucose release from stored glycogen.

Once conscious, the patient should ingest some easily absorbed carbohydrate and then some more complex food. Family members are taught to administer glucagon by using a glucagon emergency kit. A side effect of glucagon is nausea, so the patient and families should be told of this during the teaching session. After the initial treatment of an unconscious reaction, the patient and family should be instructed to investigate the cause of the low blood sugar. Repeated unconscious reactions should be reported to the physician.

If the patient does not immediately respond to the glucagon or if the patient has been unconscious for awhile, intravenous glucose is required. Approximately 20 to 30 ml of a concentrated glucose solution (50%) is given, and patients usually respond rapidly. Additional complex carbohydrates, protein, and fat are provided as soon as the patient can tolerate them because the intravenous glucose rapidly passes from the bloodstream into the cells. Insulin reactions should not be overtreated. The day after a reaction, the patient may normally experience rebound hyperglycemia. The ideal treatment for an insulin reaction is to give enough but not too much extra carbohydrate. One

TABLE 29-4

## Characteristics of Hyperglycemia and Hypoglycemia (Insulin Reaction)

|  | HYPERGLYCEMIA | HYPOGLYCEMIA (INSULIN REACTION) |
|---|---|---|
| Cause | Dietary excesses<br>Too little insulin<br>Infection<br>Decreased exercise with same dietary intake<br>Another disease or condition that taxes available insulin<br>Emotional stress | Dietary deficit (too little food or delayed meals)<br>Too much insulin<br><br>Increased exercise without dietary supplement or insulin reduction |
| Symptoms | Early<br>    Gradual loss of appetite<br>    Increased thirst<br>    Nausea and vomiting<br>    Dry skin, flushed face<br>    Headache<br>    Weakness<br>Late<br>    Diabetic acidosis<br>    Kussmaul's respirations<br>    Sweet, fruity odor to breath<br>    Decreased blood pressure<br>    Increased pulse | Early<br>    Lassitude<br>    Lethargy<br>    Inability to concentrate<br>    Hunger<br><br>Late<br>    Trembling sensation<br>    Profuse perspiration<br>    Irritability<br>    Generalized muscle weakness<br>    Blurred or double vision<br>    Headache<br>    Tingling sensation of lips or tongue |
| Blood glucose | Greater than 240 mg/dl | Less than 60 mg/dl |
| Urinary glucose | Positive | Negative |
| Urinary ketones | Positive |  |
| Progression | Gradual | Rapid |
| Intervention | Regular insulin<br>Fluid and electrolyte replacement<br>Mannitol if cerebral edema is present | Simple carbohydrates by mouth (orange juice, sugar)<br>20-30 ml of 50% glucose intravenously<br>1-2 mg of glucagon subcutaneously or intramuscularly |

suggestion is to wait 10 to 20 minutes after giving carbohydrates; if the symptoms have not disappeared in that time, the carbohydrate should be repeated.

When patients begin taking insulin, they may experience a reaction while their dose is being adjusted. Experiencing a reaction at this time may help them recognize what a reaction feels like and give them confidence in treating future reactions. As individuals gain more experience with their illness, they should be able to detect initial warning signs and learn their particular signs of impending reaction. For example, a growling stomach may indicate an impending insulin reaction.

Patients need to be taught when to expect reactions and how to prevent them. Once they learn when their insulin peaks, they should be instructed to eat an appropriate snack a little in advance to prevent hypoglycemia. If strenuous weekend-only exercise is planned, then, depending on body size and whether one wishes to gain or lose weight, either less insulin is used that day or more food is taken. Regularity in times of insulin administration, eating, and exercise is the best way to prevent insulin reactions. Personal identification (e.g., a Medic Alert bracelet) should be worn. These alerts indicate the disease and the possibility of a hypoglycemia reaction.

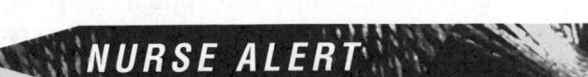

**NURSE ALERT**

When a patient is taking Precose or a sulfonylurea, treatment for hypoglycemia includes glucose gel, glucose tablets, or skim milk.

# COMPLICATIONS

## Diabetic Acidosis (Ketoacidosis)

Diabetic acidosis, also known as *ketoacidosis* or *DKA*, is a serious acute complication of diabetes that leads to death if untreated and is always considered an emergency. Ketoacidosis may occur in an undiagnosed individual, and it may be the first indication of the disease. Ketoacidosis is more prevalent in individuals who have type I diabetes mellitus. Although it is unusual, it may occur in individuals who do not require insulin to manage their diabetes.

The immediate cause of DKA is always lack of insulin and the subsequent accumulation of glucose and waste products from increased fat and protein metabolism. The onset is gradual and can be caused by any events that result in decreased available insulin or increased insulin requirements. Too little insulin, the flu, infection, or stress are some possible causes of DKA. Because the pathophysiology of DKA is similar to untreated type I, uncontrolled diabetes, early DKA symptoms are similar to the classic signs of new-onset, type I diabetes mellitus. Initial symptoms are polyuria, polydipsia, and polyphagia, which may go unnoticed until some other symptoms such as nausea, vomiting, appetite loss, weakness, headache, dry skin, and flushed face occur (see Table 29-3). Often patients think they have these symptoms because they have a virus. This is why all sick days are treated as if they might mean an impending DKA.

Unchecked DKA can lead to complex metabolic processes that result in fluid and electrolyte loss, dehydration, starvation, and reduction in the acid-base buffering system. Late symptoms of DKA are related to these metabolic sequelae and include sweet, fruity breath, decreased blood pressure, increased pulse, and Kussmaul's respirations. Kussmaul's respirations, characteristic of late DKA, are a rhythmic cycle that includes a pattern of loud, deep, and rapid respirations followed by apnea. Body chemistries reflect this picture of metabolic acidosis. Patients exhibit high blood glucose levels, low pH and carbon dioxide, and altered electrolytes and have fatty acid breakdown products (ketones) in the urine. A blood glucose level may be well over 1000 mg/dl. This complication is the exact opposite of an insulin reaction. Usually the classic signs and symptoms of DKA allow the diagnosis to be made quickly. If symptoms are unusual and there is doubt as to which acute complication has occurred, the patient should be treated for an insulin reaction. If the patient has DKA that is incorrectly diagnosed as an insulin reaction and glucose is given, the only harm done is the waiting for a few minutes to see if the glucose is effective.

Patients with DKA look and feel seriously ill. They may become comatose if treatment is delayed. Emergency treatment is necessary to reverse the hyperglycemia, dehydration, acidosis, and electrolyte imbalance. Quick-acting insulin is given intravenously and is followed by subcutaneous or intravenous infusion of insulin. Rapid infusion of intravenous fluids is used to reverse the dehydration. Electrolytes are closely monitored, and supplements are given as required. These seriously ill patients require intensive nursing care, focusing mainly on the observation and management of symptoms. The treatment goal for DKA is to reverse the metabolic imbalance without causing fluid overload or hypoglycemia.

Once the patient's condition has been stabilized, the cause of the DKA must be discovered. Alterations in diabetes management and education of the patient and others should be tailored to prevent future occurrences.

## Hyperglycemic, Hyperosmolar, Nonketotic Coma

A severe but less commonly seen acute complication of diabetes is hyperglycemic, hyperosmolar, nonketotic coma (HHNC). Individuals who do not require insulin to manage their diabetes are susceptible to this problem. It is more common among elderly patients and may occasionally be the first indication that the individual has type II diabetes mellitus. The syndrome was named from its observed clinical signs and symptoms. There is no ketoacidosis, but the other defining characteristics of the problem, hyperglycemia and hyperosmolality, are very intense. Extreme dehydration is treated with massive amounts of fluid replacement, and very small amounts of insulin are used to reverse the hyperglycemia. These patients are critically ill and require intense monitoring as their metabolic problems are reversed.

Once the critical phase has passed, the cause of the HHNC must be discovered. Often it is secondary to an infection or another illness. This explains a general rule of thumb in diabetes management. No matter what other disease process may be present, metabolic control of diabetes must be concurrent with other disease management.

## Chronic Complications

Macrovascular and microvascular changes, functional disturbances in the nervous system, and infection are the major categories of impairment of long-term or uncontrolled diabetes mellitus. A syndrome called diabetic *triopathy* results when severe pathologic changes have occurred in the peripheral nerves (neuropathy), eyes (retinopathy), and kidneys (nephropathy). The primary focus of the treatment of the complications of diabetes is early detection and initiation of treatment to delay or minimize progression.

According to the American Diabetes Association, diabetes and its complications are the fourth leading cause of death by disease in the United States. Diabetes is a major health problem because approximately 2.3 million hospital days are attributed to it. A clinical study was started in 1985 to examine the relationship between efforts to lower blood glucose and the long-term complications of diabetes. This clinical research was conducted in 29 centers across the United States, and the results were released by the American Diabetes Association in 1993. The results of the Diabetes Control and Complication Study showed that improved blood glucose control reduced the risk of clinically meaningful retinopathy by 76%, nephropathy by 54%, and neuropathy by 60%. This study clearly demonstrates that near-normal glucose levels are the best means of preventing diabetic complications (McCarren, 1993).

Individuals who have diabetes often develop macrovascular changes caused by atherosclerosis. These changes usually occur earlier and are more severe than in individuals without diabetes. Some specialists estimate the anatomic changes of a patient's cardiovascular system to be consistent with that expected according to their chronologic age plus the number of years they have had diabetes. These patients are in high-risk groups for problems with their peripheral vascular system, such as intermittent claudication or gangrene. Stroke and coronary artery disease also result from macrovascular changes.

Microvascular problems are caused by changes in the capillary basement membrane. High levels of circulating glucose in uncontrolled diabetes are believed to cause thickening and damage to these small vessels. Capillaries in the eye and kidney can be affected and can cause retinal problems that may lead to blindness. Other vision changes may occur from cataracts secondary to prolonged hyperglycemia. Also, glomerulosclerosis may cause renal failure.

High blood glucose levels probably account for the increased susceptibility that individuals with diabetes have for infections. Metabolic imbalances also contribute to problems that are evidenced in the central or peripheral nervous systems. Sensory and motor fibers can be affected and contribute to the "at-risk" foot. The ease with which individuals who have diabetes can acquire infection; poor circulation, which impedes healing; and diminished sensation to lower extremities guide patient teaching regarding foot care. Patients are taught to observe their feet daily because an abrasion or infection may be present but not felt.

## Other Complications

Surgery for any reason causes physiologic stress regardless of whether one has diabetes or not. The individual who has type II diabetes mellitus that is under metabolic control by diet alone may require insulin for several days when hospitalized for major surgery. Patients who previously required insulin have increased insulin requirements. One half of the anticipated insulin dose is usually given preoperatively and the remainder in the recovery room. An intravenous glucose

solution runs during the perioperative period. Blood glucose levels are monitored closely, and supplemental insulin or glucose is administered as required.

Routine tests that require the patient to take nothing by mouth can complicate the hospitalization of those who have diabetes. The length of the procedure and sensitivity of the patient to periods of fasting or withholding insulin determine what is ordered for each individual. Some patients may tolerate half of their usual insulin dose (including rapidly acting insulin), whereas others may need to receive an intravenous glucose infusion.

When "sick days" occur, more tailoring of the therapeutic plan may need to be made. Sick days refer to a period of physiologic stress that can be caused by injury, emotional trauma, surgery, drugs, or infection. Sick days should be treated as days of impending DKA or HHNC. Blood glucose levels and urine ketones need to be monitored every 4 hours, and patients must be in contact with their health care provider during the duration of the illness. Extra insulin may be needed even if only fluids such as ginger ale instead of a full diet are all that can be tolerated. Patients should be reminded that they must always take their insulin dose even if they are unable to eat because of nausea and vomiting.

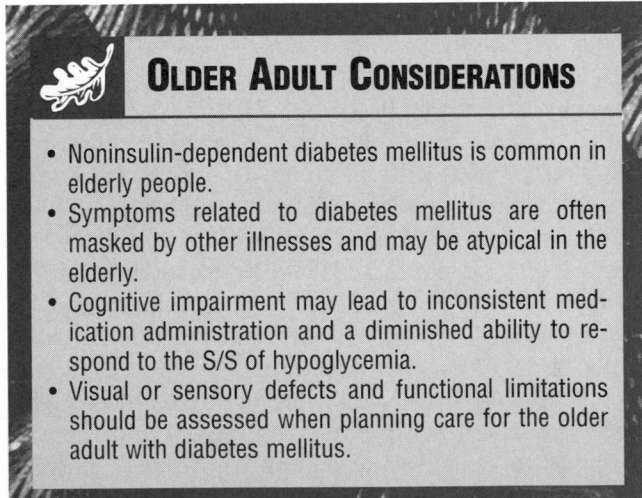

### OLDER ADULT CONSIDERATIONS

- Noninsulin-dependent diabetes mellitus is common in elderly people.
- Symptoms related to diabetes mellitus are often masked by other illnesses and may be atypical in the elderly.
- Cognitive impairment may lead to inconsistent medication administration and a diminished ability to respond to the S/S of hypoglycemia.
- Visual or sensory defects and functional limitations should be assessed when planning care for the older adult with diabetes mellitus.

## PATIENT AND FAMILY TEACHING

The American Association of Diabetes Educators has issued a position statement that recommends a careful adjustment of diet, exercise, and medications and suggests that individualized education be based on the person's intellect, motivation, physical ability, and social and personal resources. Individual cultures must be acknowledged and incorporated into the development of the entire plan of care.

One patient may be taught how to eat at a fast-food restaurant chain by following a specific list of what to order. Another individual may have the ability to exchange foods quite accurately and, by following a few suggestions, could eat within the diet at almost any restaurant. This same patient might be taught a sophisticated algorithm to increase the usual insulin dose by 10% to 20% during a sick day. Conversely another individual might be told, "Call your provider to find out what to do whenever you have the flu."

The most important feature of patient teaching is that its success depends on both the ability and willingness of individuals to incorporate their therapeutic plan into their daily routine. In collaboration with their health care provider, individuals' plans of care must be stylized to their beliefs, values, and attitudes. If a plan does not work, a new one must be developed jointly. A patient should not be labeled *noncompliant,* but rather an effort must be made to establish a joint alliance of patient and provider.

Nursing interventions for people who have diabetes are directed toward the diagnosis and treatment of their actual and potential responses. The steps of the nursing process are the organizing framework to summarize general nursing interventions for people with diabetes, regardless of setting (Box 29-1).

The type of diabetes, general health status, personal ability, regimen complexity, and individual differences are some of the factors that determine expected outcomes for specific patients. Outcome criteria determine when patients are prepared to be the self-care manager of their disease, require additional assistance, or require a change in their therapeutic plan.

Patients need to have adequate knowledge about their diabetes. They should have an understanding of the rationale that determines their individual care plan and should possess the requisite skills to manage their therapeutic regimen. An integration of patients' cognitive and behavioral skills should be demonstrated as they monitor, make decisions, and carry out their diabetes activities of daily living. Good metabolic control without acute complications is the expected therapeutic outcome.

Patients should understand the rationale for their treatment on the basis of the pathophysiologic condition that exists. This includes specific components of their therapy, such as monitoring glucose level, giving medications, acting on the basis of blood and urine testing, and eating the correct foods. Blood and urine chemistry levels should be as close to normal range as possible. Desirable near-normal ranges for someone with diabetes include a fasting venous plasma glucose level of 70 to 150 mg/dl, no sugar or acetone in preprandial urine specimens, a glycohemoglobin level less than 1.5 times normal (acceptable range for an individual with diabetes would be approximately 4.5% to 9%), and a 2-hour postprandial blood glucose level close to

fasting range. Nurses are responsible for ensuring that patients demonstrate knowledge of the prevention, detection, and treatment of complications such as hypoglycemia and hyperglycemia (see Box 29-1).

Because there is no known cure for or prevention of diabetes mellitus, early detection and careful treatment are the current therapeutic interventions. Individuals who develop diabetes become managers of their chronic illness and become partners with health care providers who prescribe therapy. Interventions must be guided to assist patients to successfully live with this disorder so that its catastrophic complications are prevented. Nurses with creativity and ingenuity can make the difference between a regimen that is impossible for the patient to accept and one that accommodates culture and life-style. The pharmaceutical companies that make insulin and the companies that manufacture diabetes equipment (meters and syringes) are wonderful resources for educational materials. These materials are available free of charge and can be obtained in several languages to meet the needs of a culturally diverse population.

## HYPOGLYCEMIA

An abnormally low level of blood glucose may also occur in the absence of diabetes. It may be caused by disease of the liver or pancreas or disease of the pituitary or adrenal gland. The symptoms include hunger, weakness, anxiety, pallor, headache, sweating, and rapid pulse. One type, known as *functional hypoglycemia,* has an unknown cause. The symptoms are variable and often occur several hours after meals or exercise. The attacks may last from minutes to days. Treatment is based on relieving the immediate attack, followed by removing the cause when it is known. In mild attacks orange juice or hard candy may relieve the symptoms, whereas for patients with severe cases glucose may be administered intravenously. Patients may be given low-carbohydrate, high-protein intake with restriction of simple sugars; frequent, small meals are usually prescribed. This type of meal plan should help prevent hypoglycemic episodes.

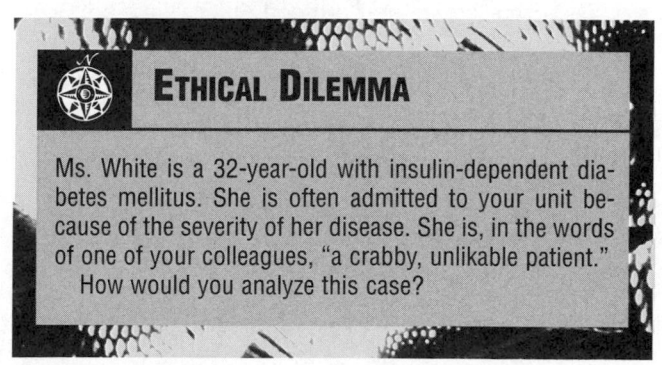

### ETHICAL DILEMMA

Ms. White is a 32-year-old with insulin-dependent diabetes mellitus. She is often admitted to your unit because of the severity of her disease. She is, in the words of one of your colleagues, "a crabby, unlikable patient." How would you analyze this case?

BOX 29-1 > **NURSING PROCESS**

## DIABETES MELLITUS

### ASSESSMENT

- Mental status: anxiety and fear
- Cardiovascular: dizziness, palpitations, and changes in blood pressure and pulse
- Respiratory: changes in respiratory rate and depth, breath odor
- Skin: changes in skin turgor, temperature, and color
- Gastrointestinal: polyphagia, nausea, vomiting, polydipsia (excessive thirst), and abdominal pain or bloating
- Metabolic: changes in blood glucose levels, blood pH
- Urinary: glycosuria, polyuria, and ketonuria
- Neuromuscular: tiredness; lethargy; weakness; tremors; headache; visual changes; changes in level of consciousness; change in reflexes, muscle mass, and strength
- Fluid status: intake and output, tongue appearance, moisture of mucous membranes, and firmness of eyeballs

### NURSING DIAGNOSES

- Altered nutrition: less than body requirements related to insulin deficiency
- Anxiety related to inability to control illness
- Risk for fluid volume deficit related to polyuria
- Chronic low self-esteem related to chronicity of illness
- Knowledge deficit related to complex management of illness
- Ineffective individual and family coping related to chronicity of illness
- Risk for infection related to metabolic changes
- Impaired tissue integrity related to metabolic change

### NURSING INTERVENTIONS

- Monitor blood glucose levels (normal fasting level: 70-150 mg/dl).
- Promote nutritional status by planned meal plan.
- Monitor vital signs.
- Weigh patient daily.
- Encourage moderate levels of activity, which lower blood sugar levels.
- Test urine for ketones if blood glucose is more than 240 mg/dl.
- If patient is taking oral agents, observe for adverse effects such as nausea, vomiting, rash, photosensitivity, and alcohol intolerance.
- Monitor for signs of insulin reaction, such as diaphoresis (excessive perspiration), shaking, tachycardia, and anxiety.
- Observe for signs of diabetic ketoacidosis, such as nausea, vomiting, facial flushing, weight loss, polydipsia, and positive urine tests for ketone.

- Provide emotional support for patient and family.
- Educate patient and family regarding basic pathophysiology and management of diabetes.
- Foster independence in self-care management.
- Assess patient's health status, psychosocial functioning, and social support.
- Assess patient's and significant others' ability to comprehend and integrate diabetes activities of daily living into their usual life-style pattern.
- Observe condition of feet and skin.
- Collaborate with patient, family, and diabetes clinicians to identify a therapeutic plan that provides the best metabolic control possible within the limitations of patient ability and acceptability.
- Decide how best to implement the plan so that patient becomes independent in self-management techniques as soon as possible without becoming overwhelmed.
- Incorporate the therapeutic plan of the patient care setting into the patient's individualized care plan. For example, use laboratory results of blood glucose values so patient can relate how he or she feels in relation to varying blood glucose levels; if the patient takes urine tests, he or she can learn renal threshold.
- Promote patient confidence and independence in carrying out diabetes activities of daily living. For example, under decreasing supervision, patient should draw up and inject own insulin, perform urine or blood test, and select foods for meals and snacks.
- Evaluate patient's skill level and coping ability so refinements can be made in care plan.
- Collaboratively determine patient outcome expectations regarding the degree of metabolic control to be achieved, specific patient and significant other responsibilities in the home setting, and mechanisms to evaluate diabetes control, regimen ease and difficulty, and adherence to the therapeutic plan.

### EVALUATION OF EXPECTED OUTCOMES

- Blood and urine chemistries close to normal range
- Basic pathologic condition of diabetes explained
- Rationale for treatment regimen explained
- Prevents, detects, and treats hypoglycemia and hyperglycemia
- Foods exchanged properly
- Manages self-care on a sick day
- Health care provider called appropriately
- Complications prevented

## KEY CONCEPTS

➤ The most common endocrine disorder is diabetes mellitus, a disorder resulting from insulin deficiency. Diabetes mellitus is classified as either insulin-dependent (type I) diabetes mellitus or as noninsulin-dependent (type II) diabetes mellitus. Insulin is necessary for the body cells to combine oxygen and glucose to produce the energy necessary for body functions.

➤ The therapeutic goal for diabetes management is to maintain as close to normal a blood glucose level as possible while allowing the patient to maintain a normal life-style. This is done through administration of insulin or oral hypoglycemic agents, control of diet, and prevention of complications.

➤ Hyperglycemia and hypoglycemia are serious acute complications and should be avoided. Over time, poorly controlled diabetes mellitus can result in changes throughout the body.

## CRITICAL THINKING EXERCISES

1. Explain the characteristics of type I and type II diabetes mellitus.
2. State two reasons for patients with diabetes to maintain good blood sugar control.
3. State the four categories of oral antidiabetic agents and their action on glucose control.
4. Discuss four special teaching strategies in teaching the elderly patient with diabetes.

## REFERENCES AND ADDITIONAL READINGS

American Diabetes Association: Position statement: nutrition recommendations and principles for people with diabetes mellitus, *Diabetes Care* 11:1517-1520, 1993.

American Diabetes Association: Census statement: self-monitoring of blood glucose, *Diabetes Care* 18(1):81-85, 1994a.

American Diabetes Association: Position statement: nutrition recommendations and principles for people with diabetes mellitus, *Diabetes Care* 17(5):519-522, 1994b.

American Diabetes Association: Clinical practice recommendations 1996, *Diabetes Care* 19(suppl 1):S1-S118, 1996.

American Diabetes Association: Diabetes 1996 vital statistics.

Beaser RS: *The Joslin guide,* New York, 1995, Simon & Shuster.

Burch WM: *Endocrinology for the house officer,* ed 2, Baltimore, 1990, Williams & Wilkins.

Christensen MH et al: How to care for the diabetic foot, *Am J Nurs* 91(3):50-58, 1991.

Clement S: Diabetes self-management education, *Diabetes Care* 18(8):1204-1214, 1995.

Collier JH, Brodbeck CA: Assessing the diabetic foot: plantar callus and pressure sensation, *Diabetes Educ* 19(6):503-508, 1993.

Cradock S: Diabetes mellitus at diagnosis, *Nurs Stand* 10(30):47-48, 1996.

Deakens DA: Teaching elderly patients about diabetes, *Am J Nurs* 94(4):38-42, 1994.

DeWit SC: *Kean's essentials of medical surgical nursing,* ed 3, Philadelphia, 1992, Saunders.

Epstein CD: Fluid volume deficit for the adrenal crisis patient, *Dimens Crit Care Nurs* 10(4):210-217, 1991.

Eye KL, Janney L: Identification of need for education in self-monitoring of blood glucose, *Am J Health Syst Pharm* 53(12):1456-1457, 1996.

Franz MJ et al: Nutrition principles for the management of diabetes and related complications, *Diabetes Care* 17(5):490-518, 1994.

Harris MI, Cowie CC, Howie LJ: Self-monitoring of blood glucose by adults with diabetes in the United States population, *Diabetes Care* 16(8):1116-1122, 1993.

Herman W, editor: *The prevention and treatment of complications of diabetes,* ed 2, Atlanta, 1991, National Center for Chronic Disease Prevention and Health Promotion.

Keegan A, editor: 1994 Buyer's guide to diabetes supplies, *Diabetes Forecast* 46(10):49-78, 1993.

Kistel F: Using blood glucose meters—part I, *Nursing 93* 23(3):34-42, 1993a.

Kistel F: Using blood glucose meters—part II, *Nursing 93* 23(4):50-53, 1993b.

Kistel F: Using blood glucose meters—part III, *Nursing 93* 23(5):51-54, 1993c.

Lammon C, Hart G: Recognizing thyroid crisis, *Nursing 93* 23(4):33, 1993.

Lebovits HE, editor: *Therapy for diabetes mellitus and related disorders*, Alexandria, Va, 1991, American Diabetes Association.

Lewis SM, Collier IC, Heitkemper MM: *Medical-surgical nursing: assessment and management of clinical problems*, ed 4, St Louis, 1996, Mosby.

Lundman B, Norberg S: Coping strategies in people with insulin-dependent diabetes mellitus, *Diabetes Educ* 19(3): 198-204, 1993.

McCarren M: DCCT—the results, *Diabetes Forecast* 46(9):48-51, 1993.

McCarren M: A new faster insulin? It's here! *Diabetes Forecast* 49(8):24-34, 1996.

Mundy GR: Evaluation and treatment of hypercalcemia, *Hosp Pract* 29(6):79-84, 1994.

National Diabetes Information Clearinghouse: Noninvasive blood glucose monitoring, *Diabetes Dateline* Spring 1993, Clearinghouse.

Ober PR, editor: Endocrine crisis, *Endocrinol Metab Clin North Am* 22(2):181-453, 1993.

Peragallo-Dittko V, Godley K, Meyer J: *A core curriculum for diabetes education*, ed 2, Chicago, 1993, American Association of Diabetes Educators.

Policoff SP: Diseases your doctor may miss, *Ladies Home J* 107(6):104, 106-109, 1990.

Scherer JC: *Introductory medical surgical nursing*, ed 5, Philadelphia, 1991, Lippincott.

Schmidt LE et al: The relationship between eating patterns and metabolic control in patients with non-insulin-dependent diabetes mellitus (NIDDM), *Diabetes Educ* 20(4):317-321, 1994.

Sherwin R: Pill time, *Diabetes Forecast* 49(3):36-45, 1996.

Sinclair AJ, Turnball CJ, Croxson SC: Document of care for older people with diabetes, *Postgrad Med J* 72(848):334-338, 1996.

Steuer R: The light at the end of the meter, *Diabetes Self-Manage* 10(3):42-44, 1993.

Stolar MW: Clinical management of the NIDDM patient: impact of the American Diabetes Association practice guidelines, *Diabetes Care* 18(5):701-707, 1995.

Tucker SM: *Patient care standards: collaborative practice planning guides*, ed 6, St Louis, 1995, Mosby.

Zehrer CL, Gross CR: Patient perceptions of benefits and concerns following pancreas transplantation, *Diabetes Educ* 20(3):217-219, 1994.

# CHAPTER 30

# Neurologic Problems

## KEY TERMS

| | |
|---|---|
| acetylcholine | dysarthria |
| aura | dysphagia |
| automatism | Glasgow Coma Scale |
| autonomic nervous system | hemiparesis |
| bradykinesia | herniation |
| cell body | intracranial pressure |
| cerebrospinal fluid | Monro-Kellie doctrine |
| cholinergic crisis | myasthenic crisis |
| coma | nuchal rigidity |
| consciousness | orthostasis |
| craniotomy | papilledema |
| dementia | paresthesia |
| dopamine | proprioception |
| ptosis | reticular formation |
| reflex | seizure |
| reticular activating system | tentorium |
| | tremor |

## STRUCTURE AND FUNCTION OF THE NERVOUS SYSTEM

The nervous system is the body's most highly organized and complex system. It controls the motor, sensory, and autonomic ("automatic") functions of the body. The nervous system receives sensory information from within and outside the body, interprets information sent to the brain, and determines the body's responses to these messages. In this way, the nervous system controls and coordinates all systems of the body so that it can function as an integrated whole.

The nervous system is divided into the central nervous system and peripheral nervous system. The central nervous system is composed of the brain and spinal cord (Figure 30-1). The peripheral nervous system is made up of 12 pairs of cranial nerves, 31 pairs of spinal nerves, and the cell bodies, ganglia, and fibers of the autonomic nervous system.

### Central Nervous System

The brain is divided into three major areas: the cerebrum, the brain stem, and cerebellum (Figure 30-2). The cerebrum is divided into two cerebral hemispheres, which are connected by the corpus callosum. The left hemisphere provides motor and sensory control to the right side of the body, and the right hemisphere controls the left. The hemispheres are composed of pairs of frontal, parietal, temporal, and occipital lobes, which

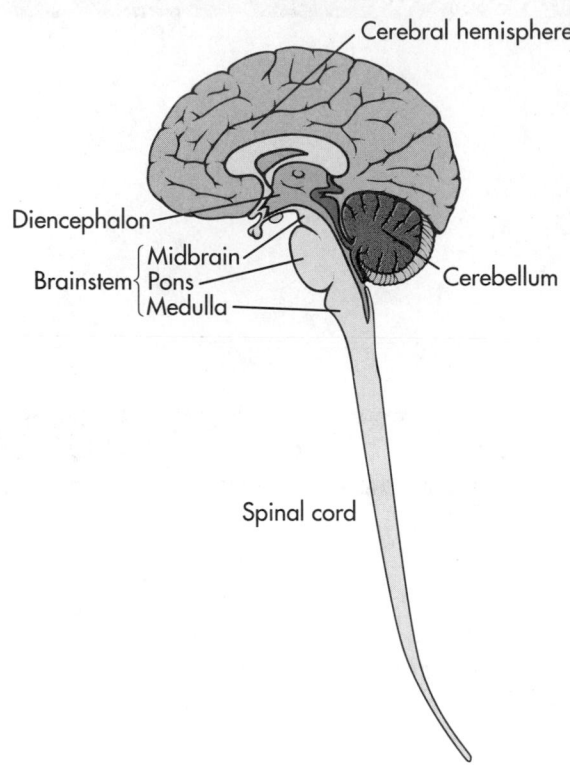

**Figure 30-1**    Major divisions of the central nervous system. (From Lewis SM, Collier IC, Heitkemper MM: *Medical-surgical nursing: assessment and management of clinical problems* ed 4, St Louis, 1996, Mosby.)

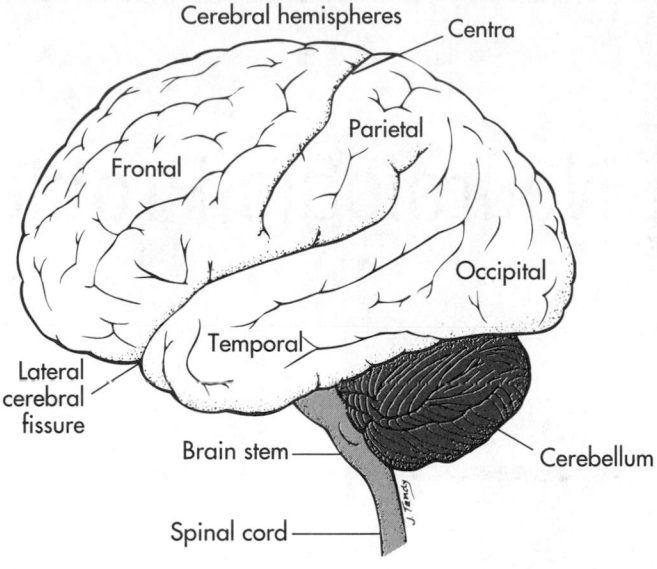

**Figure 30-2**    Major parts of the brain.

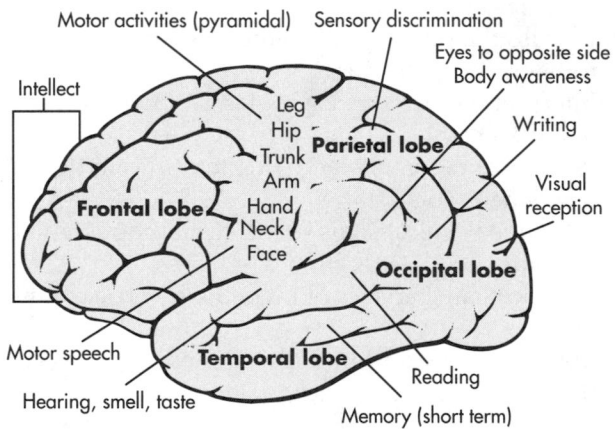

**Figure 30-3**    Each area of the brain controls a particular activity. (From Lewis SM, Collier IC, Heitkemper MM: *Medical-surgical nursing: assessment and management of clinical problems*, ed 4, St Louis, 1996, Mosby.)

provide specific functions for receiving, analyzing, and storing information for future use and for controlling conscious voluntary movements (Figure 30-3). The cerebellum, located under the occipital lobe of the cerebrum and behind the brain stem, contains nerve connections to and from the cerebrum and brain stem. It assists in the coordination of movement, maintenance of muscle tone, and equilibrium. The brain stem, composed of the midbrain, pons, and medulla, is the pathway for impulses between the brain and spinal cord, with some fibers going through the cerebellum. The vital centers for control of respiration, cardiac function, and vasoconstriction of blood vessels are located in the brain stem. All the sensory and motor pathways pass through the brain stem, and many fibers cross over to the other side of the brain stem, which explains why injury to one side of the brain may result in loss of function on the opposite side of the body (Figure 30-4).

The spinal cord is a slender cylinder of nerve tissue extending from the brain stem to the approximate level of just above the waist (first lumbar vertebra) (Figure 30-5). Spinal nerve roots extend beyond the tapered end of the spinal cord, forming the cauda equina ("horse's tail"). Ascending (sensory) and descending (motor) nerve fibers within the spinal cord form pathways to carry impulses to and from the brain and the spinal nerves that communicate with muscles and glands in the periphery of the body. The spinal cord also contains pathways responsible for involuntary responses to a stimulus, such as response to pain, maintenance of muscle tone essential for body posture, and the deep tendon reflexes (Figure 30-6).

The brain and spinal cord are protected from injury by the skull, the meninges, and cerebrospinal fluid.

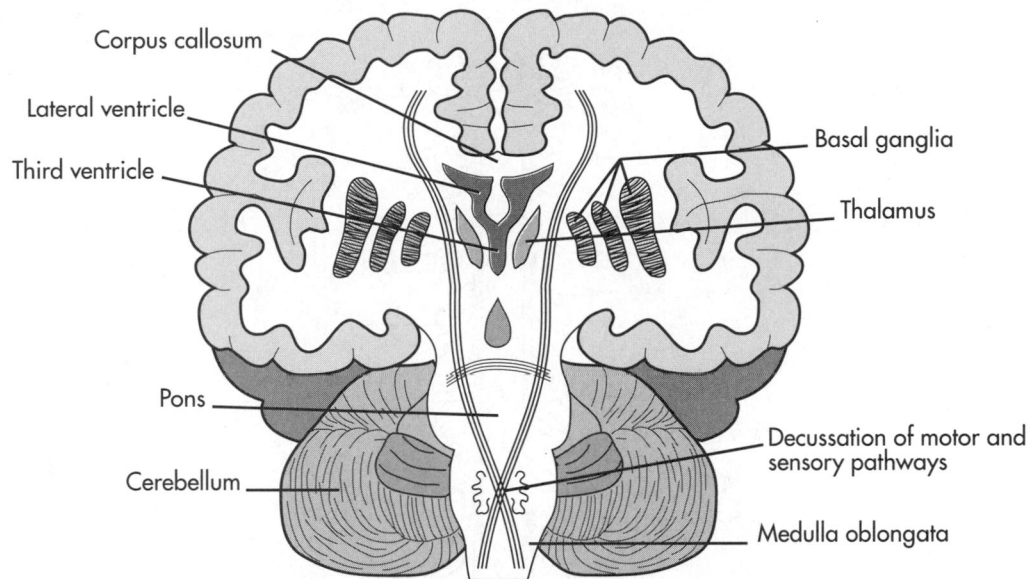

**Figure 30-4**    Oblique coronal section through the cerebrum and brain stem.

The skull, or cranium, is the bony covering of the brain; the spinal cord is encased within the vertebral column. The meninges are three layers of connective tissue that completely enclose the brain and spinal cord in a continuous covering (Figures 30-7 and 30-8). In addition to providing protection, the meninges contain the blood vessels that supply the brain and spinal cord. **Cerebrospinal fluid** (CSF) is a clear, watery liquid that fills the ventricular system (Figure 30-9) of the brain and the subarachnoid space of the meninges and completely encases the brain and spinal cord. The CSF provides nutrients, moisture, lubrication, and an effective liquid cushion for the brain and spinal cord.

## Peripheral Nervous System

Cranial nerves provide specialized motor and sensory functions, including the specialized senses of sight, hearing, taste, smell, and other functions. Each cranial nerve, like all other nerve cells (also called neurons), has a **cell body** as its metabolic center and contains the nucleus and cytoplasm of the nerve. Cell bodies of the cranial nerves originate from or near the brain stem (Figure 30-10). The spinal nerves arise from the spinal cord and transmit information from and to the brain so that movement and sensation can be provided to the periphery of the body. The **autonomic nervous system** carries information to smooth muscle (heart, lungs, intestines, bladder) and glands (salivary, adrenal, pancreas). It has long been

thought that these functions could not be voluntarily controlled; however, recent research indicates that it may be possible to control these "autonomic" functions.

Further divisions of the autonomic nervous system are the sympathetic and parasympathetic systems, which function together to maintain a relatively balanced internal environment for the body. Sympathetic nervous system fibers arise from cell bodies lying in the spinal cord at the chest and waist levels (thoracic 1 to lumbar 2 levels). Extending from the cell bodies are ganglia (collections of neurons) that lie close to the spinal column (Figure 30-11). The chemicals norepinephrine and **acetylcholine** are produced by the sympathetic nervous system and are responsible for the generalized physiologic responses that prepare the individual for "fight or flight." Increased heart rate and blood pressure, an increased blood supply to skeletal muscles and heart, and vasoconstriction of the blood vessels of the skin are examples of these responses. The parasympathetic nervous system is composed of cell bodies that lie in the brain stem and in the sacral spinal segments (sacral 2 to sacral 4 levels). Ganglia of the parasympathetic nervous system are located in or near the structures they affect, such as the heart, lungs, digestive tract, and other organs. The parasympathetic nervous system produces only acetylcholine, which allows the body to maintain a state of equilibrium by conserving and restoring the body's energy stores. Functions of the parasympathetic nervous system include slowing the heart rate,

*Text continued on p. 918.*

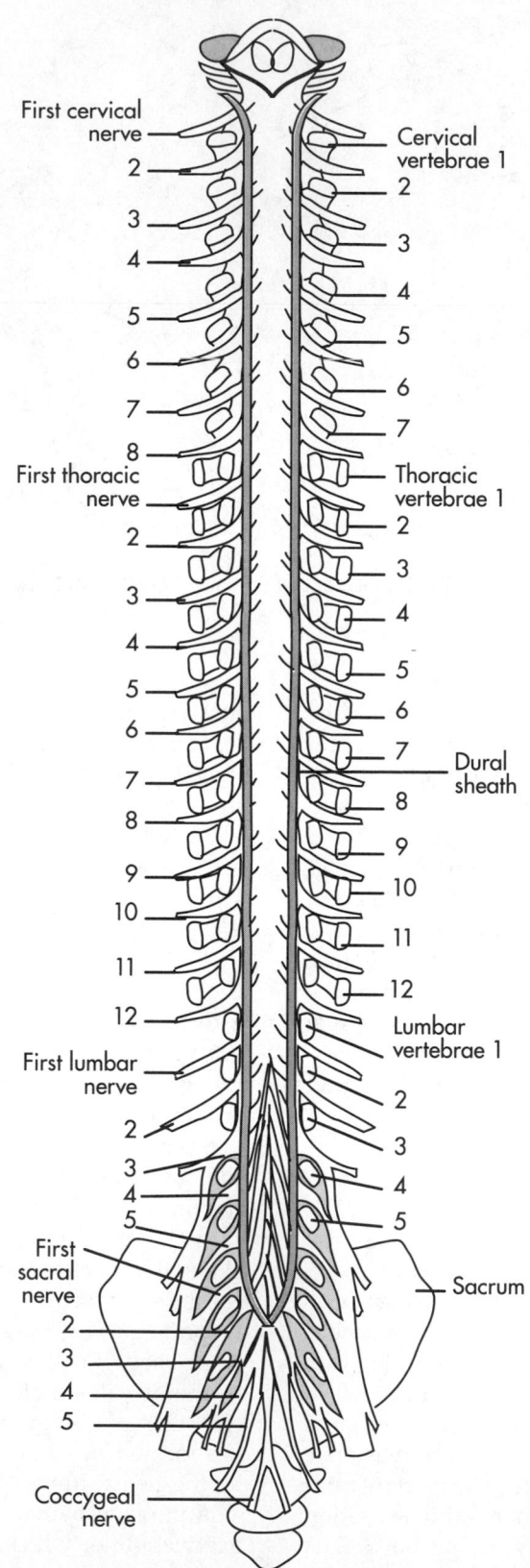

First cervical nerve

2

3

4

5

6

7

8

First thoracic nerve

2

3

4

5

6

7

8

9

10

11

12

First lumbar nerve

2

3

4

5

First sacral nerve

2

3

4

5

Coccygeal nerve

Cervical vertebrae 1

2

3

4

5

6

7

Thoracic vertebrae 1

2

3

4

5

6

7

8

9

10

11

12

Lumbar vertebrae 1

2

3

4

5

Dural sheath

Sacrum

**Figure 30-5** Spinal cord lying within the vertebral canal. Spinal nerves are numbered on the left side, and the vertebrae are numbered on the right side.

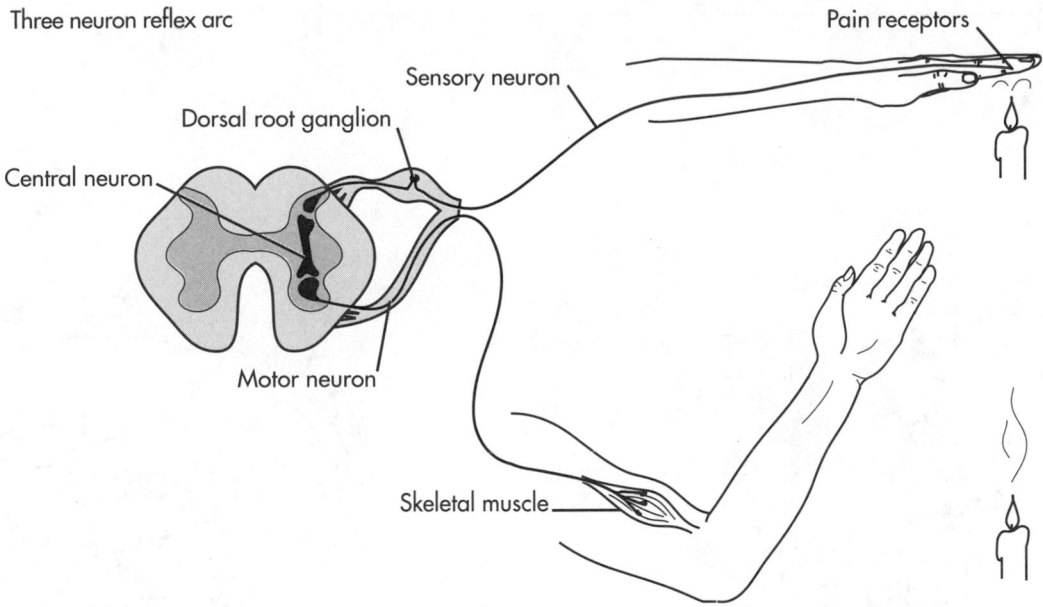

Three neuron reflex arc

Pain receptors

Sensory neuron

Dorsal root ganglion

Central neuron

Motor neuron

Skeletal muscle

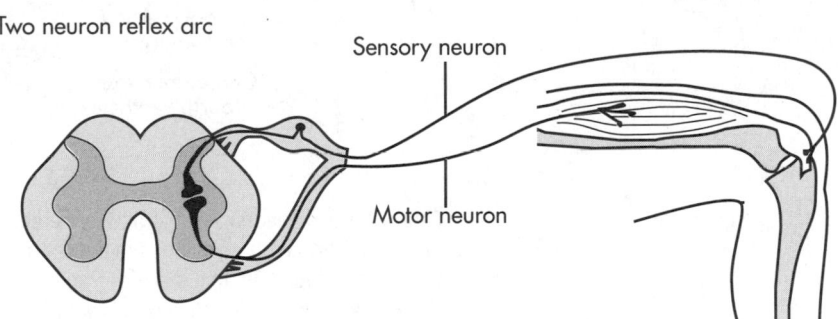

Two neuron reflex arc

Sensory neuron

Motor neuron

**Figure 30-6**  Diagram of a flexor reflex *(top)* and a stretch reflex *(bottom).*

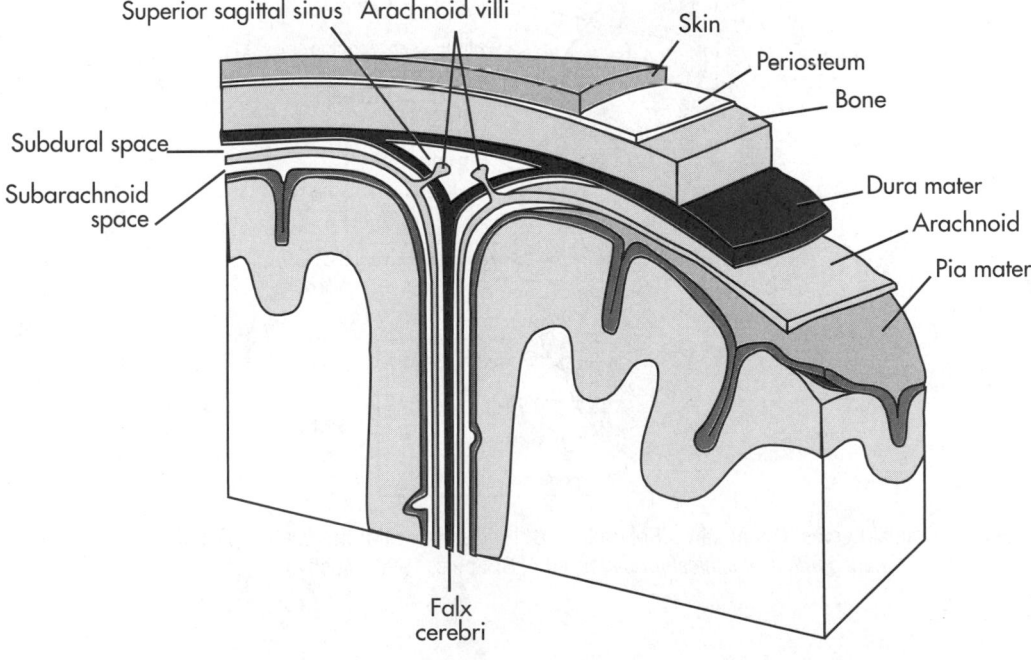

Superior sagittal sinus   Arachnoid villi

Skin

Periosteum

Bone

Subdural space

Subarachnoid space

Dura mater

Arachnoid

Pia mater

Falx cerebri

**Figure 30-7**  The cranial meninges.

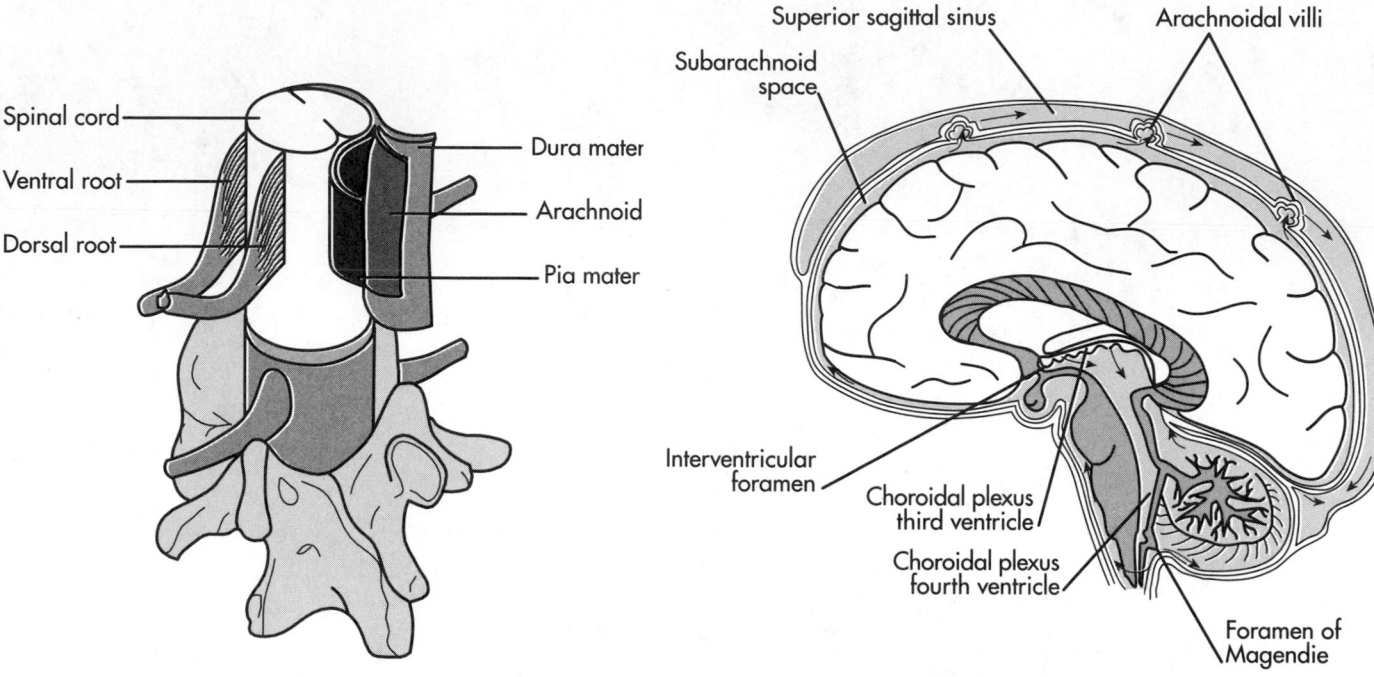

Spinal cord
Ventral root
Dorsal root

Dura mater
Arachnoid
Pia mater

**Figure 30-8** Spinal cord and meninges.

Superior sagittal sinus
Arachnoidal villi
Subarachnoid space

Interventricular foramen
Choroidal plexus third ventricle
Choroidal plexus fourth ventricle
Foramen of Magendie

**Figure 30-9** Diagram of the flow of cerebrospinal fluid from the time of its formation from blood in the choroid plexuses until its return to the blood in the superior sagittal sinus. (Redrawn from Hickey JV: *The clinical practice of neurological and neurosurgical nursing,* ed 4, Philadelphia, 1997, Lippincott.)

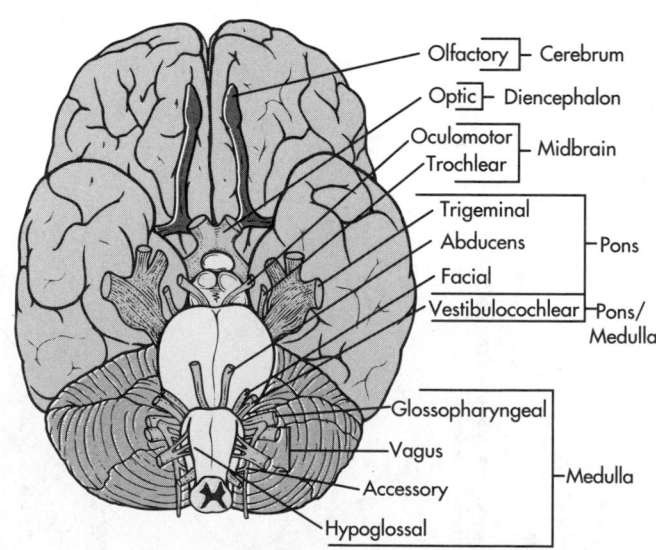

Olfactory — Cerebrum
Optic — Diencephalon
Oculomotor
Trochlear — Midbrain
Trigeminal
Abducens — Pons
Facial
Vestibulocochlear — Pons/Medulla
Glossopharyngeal
Vagus
Accessory — Medulla
Hypoglossal

**Figure 30-10** Cranial nerves. (From Lewis SM, Collier IC, Heitkemper MM: *Medical-surgical nursing: assessment and management of clinical problems,* ed 4, St Louis, 1996, Mosby.)

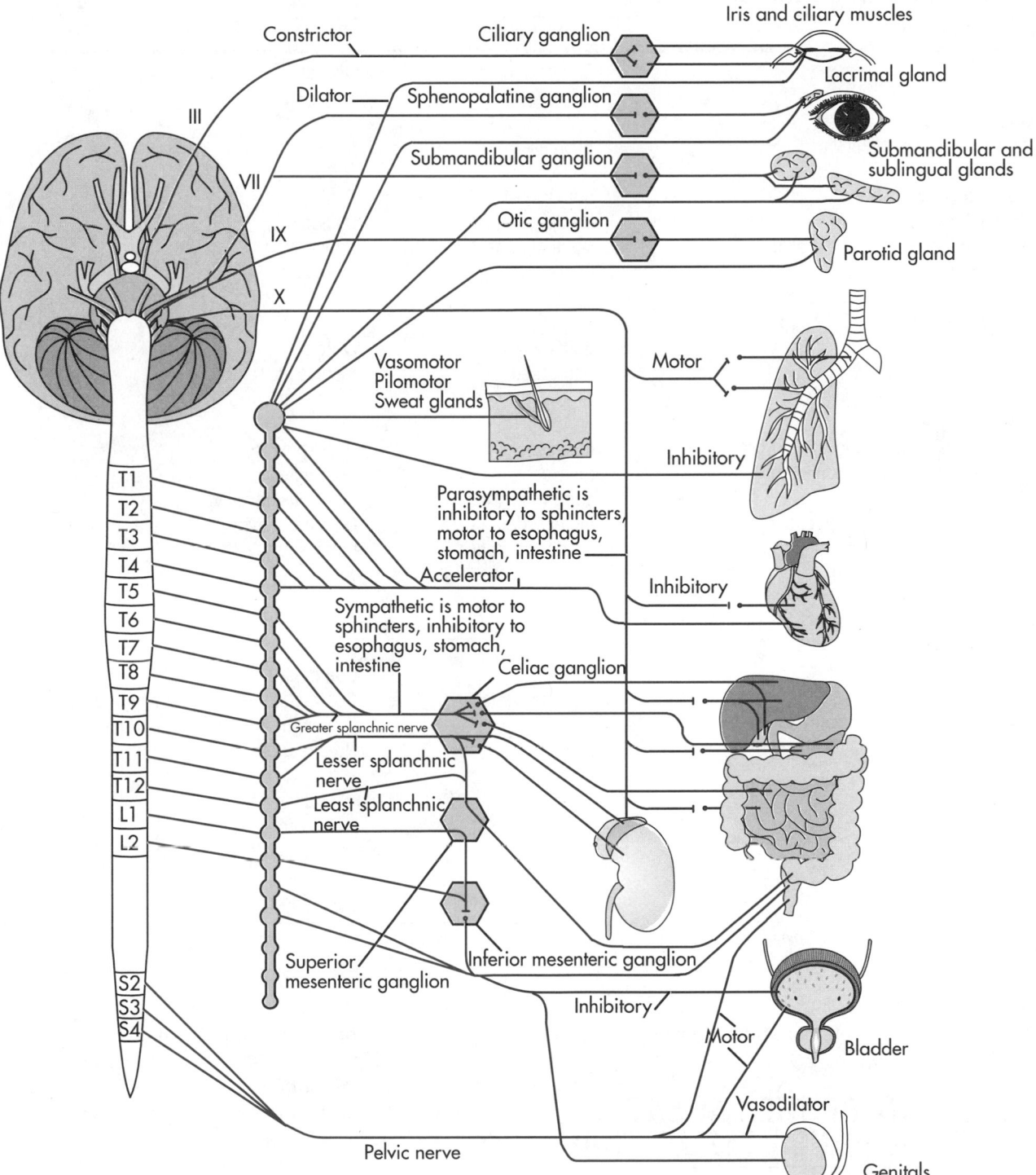

**Figure 30-11**    Diagram of the autonomic nervous system, including the parasympathetic, or craniosacral, fibers and the sympathetic, or thoracolumbar, fibers. Note that most organs have a double nerve supply.

**TABLE 30-1**

## Autonomic Effects of the Nervous System

| STRUCTURE OR ACTIVITY | PARASYMPATHETIC EFFECTS | SYMPATHETIC EFFECTS |
|---|---|---|
| **Pupil** | Constricted | Dilated |
| **Circulatory System** | | |
| Rate and force of heartbeat | Decreased | Increased |
| Blood vessels | | |
| In heart muscle | Constricted | Dilated |
| In skeletal muscle | No direct effect | Dilated |
| In abdominal viscera and the skin | No direct effect | Constricted |
| Blood pressure | Decreased | Increased |
| **Respiratory System** | | |
| Bronchioles | Constricted | Dilated |
| Rate of breathing | Decreased | Increased |
| **Digestive System** | | |
| Peristaltic movements of digestive tube | Increased | Decreased |
| Muscular sphincters of digestive tube | Relaxed | Contracted |
| Secretion of salivary glands | Thin, watery saliva | Thick, viscid saliva |
| Secretions of stomach, intestine, and pancreas | Increased | No direct effect |
| Conversion of liver glycogen to glucose | No direct effect | Increased |
| **Genitourinary System** | | |
| Urinary bladder | | |
| Muscular walls | Contracted | Relaxed |
| Sphincters | Relaxed | Contracted |
| Muscles of the uterus | Relaxed; variable | Contracted under some conditions; varies with menstrual cycle and pregnancy |
| Blood vessels of external genitalia | Dilated | No direct effect |
| **Integument** | | |
| Secretion of sweat | No direct effect | Increased |
| Pilomotor muscles | No direct effect | Contracted (gooseflesh) |
| **Medullae of Adrenal Glands** | No direct effect | Secretion of epinephrine and norepinephrine |

From Chaffee EE, Lytle IM: *Basic physiology and anatomy*, ed 3, Philadelphia, 1980, Lippincott.

increasing gastric secretions, and increasing peristalsis (Table 30-1).

## ASSESSMENT OF THE PATIENT WITH NEUROLOGIC DYSFUNCTION

### The Neurologic Examination

The neurologic examination is performed to determine the presence of neurologic dysfunction, to localize dysfunction within the nervous system, and to aid in the diagnosis of disorders within the nervous system. The neurologic examination is also used to monitor known neurologic deficits for worsening or improvement. It can be performed by a physician or advanced practice nurse. The staff nurse's ability to interpret data obtained by the neurologic examination is helpful in identifying specific areas of concern and focus, as well as in providing valuable information for use in neurologic nursing assessment. For example, a patient with a middle cerebral artery distribution stroke is likely to have **hemiparesis,** or weakness of one side of the body. This patient is likely to need assistance with many activities of daily living, including mobilization, nutritional intake, and hygiene.

The neurologic examination involves the systematic evaluation of the patient's mental status, cranial nerve function, motor function, sensory function, cerebellar function, and reflexes. The mental status portion of the examination consists of assessing level of consciousness and observing the patient's behavior, speech, emotional status, affect, and mood. In addition, testing of orientation, memory, and higher level cognitive function (e.g., spelling or serial arithmetic, judgment, and abstract thinking) is performed. Assessing level of consciousness is also an important nursing responsibility for patients with suspected or known neurologic dysfunction. Change in alertness, agitation, confusion, or any other decrease in the level of consciousness is often the first sign of increased intracranial pressure and should be recognized and reported immediately.

The cranial nerve examination provides information regarding the functioning of the 12 pairs of cranial nerves, which also reflects the function of their points of origin, primarily the brain stem (Table 30-2). Evaluation of the pupils is a part of the cranial nerve examination and also an important component of the nursing assessment of patients with neurologic dysfunction. When evaluating pupils, it is important for the nurse to note the pupil size, shape, movement, reaction to light, and symmetry (left compared to right in size, shape, reaction). Normal pupils are round, dilate in dim light, react briskly to light, and are symmetric. Variation is normal, however, with one pupil being slightly larger than the other, which is known as anisocoria. Deviation from these normal findings may indicate an increase in intracranial pressure and should be reported immediately. Change in normal pupillary function is especially emergent if accompanied by any change in the patient's level of consciousness.

Examination of the motor system is conducted systematically, beginning with the upper extremities and trunk, then the lower extremities. Muscle size, tone, range of motion, and strength and the presence of involuntary movements such as **tremor** are assessed. A standard five-point scale is commonly used to assess strength, with 5/5 being normal and 0/5 representing no movement or contraction. The sensory examination evaluates the patient's ability to perceive various types of stimuli and is conducted in the same systematic manner as the motor examination. Perception of pain, temperature, light touch, vibration, and position sense **(proprioception)** are commonly part of the sensory examination.

The assessment of cerebellar function includes observation of gait for detection of balance and evaluation of the patient's ability to perform coordinated tasks with the upper and lower extremities for assessment of coordination. The **reflex** examination provides important information about nervous system function. A deep tendon reflex is elicited when the tendon is stretched, as when tapped by a reflex hammer (see Figure 30-6). Reflexes usually assessed include the biceps,

**TABLE 30-2**

## Cranial Nerves and their Functions

| CRANIAL NERVE | FUNCTION |
|---|---|
| Olfactory | Smell |
| Optic | Visual acuity, visual fields |
| Oculomotor | Pupil constriction, lens shape, eyelid opening, extraocular movements |
| Trochlear | Downward and inner eye movement |
| Trigeminal | Jaw opening and chewing, sensation in eye, face, and mouth |
| Abducens | Lateral eye movement |
| Facial | Facial movement, anterior taste, saliva secretion |
| Acoustic | Hearing and equilibrium |
| Glossopharyngeal | Swallowing and phonation, gag reflex, posterior taste, saliva secretion, nose sensation, carotid reflex |
| Vagus | Phonation, sensation of nose gag, and tongue, secretion of digestive enzymes |
| Spinal accessory | Motor; turn head, shrug, speech |
| Hypoglossal | Tongue for speech and swallowing |

Modified from Malasanos L, Barkauskas V, Stoltenberg-Allen K: *Health assessment*, ed 4, St Louis, 1990, Mosby.

triceps, and brachioradialis in the upper extremities and patellar and Achilles reflexes in the lower extremities. The plantar response is a superficial reflex that is included in this portion of the examination. An extensor plantar response (upward movement of the great toe with fanning of remaining toes) is also known as the Babinski sign and is normal in the newborn. After infancy, the Babinski sign indicates a disruption of nerve fibers in the spinal cord, brain stem, or brain. Other reflexes normal in the newborn, but abnormal after maturation of the nervous system, include the sucking, rooting, and snout reflexes.

The findings of the neurologic examination may indicate the need for further assessment, with the help of diagnostic tests.

## Neurodiagnostic Studies
### Lumbar Puncture

A lumbar puncture (LP) consists of using a needle and stopcock apparatus to withdraw approximately 8 to 10 ml of cerebrospinal fluid (CSF) from the lumbar subarachnoid space. The procedure is carried out for diagnostic and assessment purposes and usually is performed in a treatment room or the patient's hospital room. The nurse should explain the procedure to the patient, emphasizing the need to remain in the

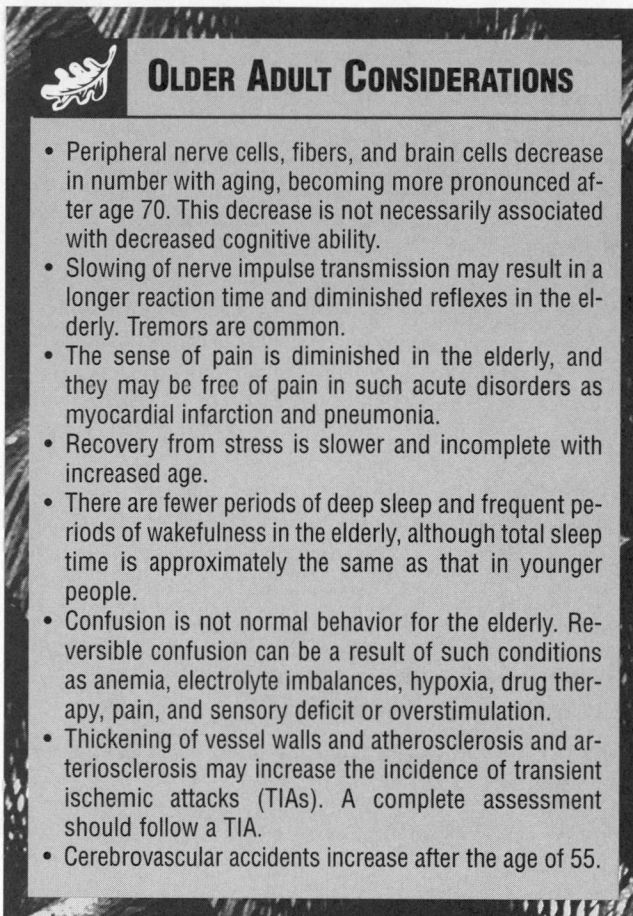

## OLDER ADULT CONSIDERATIONS

- Peripheral nerve cells, fibers, and brain cells decrease in number with aging, becoming more pronounced after age 70. This decrease is not necessarily associated with decreased cognitive ability.
- Slowing of nerve impulse transmission may result in a longer reaction time and diminished reflexes in the elderly. Tremors are common.
- The sense of pain is diminished in the elderly, and they may be free of pain in such acute disorders as myocardial infarction and pneumonia.
- Recovery from stress is slower and incomplete with increased age.
- There are fewer periods of deep sleep and frequent periods of wakefulness in the elderly, although total sleep time is approximately the same as that in younger people.
- Confusion is not normal behavior for the elderly. Reversible confusion can be a result of such conditions as anemia, electrolyte imbalances, hypoxia, drug therapy, pain, and sensory deficit or overstimulation.
- Thickening of vessel walls and atherosclerosis and arteriosclerosis may increase the incidence of transient ischemic attacks (TIAs). A complete assessment should follow a TIA.
- Cerebrovascular accidents increase after the age of 55.

preferred position and to remain very still. Questions should be encouraged, and any myths or erroneous information should be corrected. Lumbar puncture is a routine procedure performed on many patients with suspected or diagnosed neurologic dysfunction and very rarely causes severe pain or untoward effects. During the procedure, the patient is placed in a side-lying position near the edge of the examination table with the head flat and neck flexed, knees flexed, and back bowed (Figure 30-12). Occasionally, the patient may need to be in the sitting position, leaning forward with head down and back bowed. A local anesthetic is used to minimize discomfort caused by the needle puncture, but the patient usually feels pressure as the needle with stylet is inserted. Strict aseptic technique is followed while the needle is placed between the L3 and L4 or L4 and L5 disc space. This is below the approximate level of the end of the spinal cord, which for most individuals is at the L1 level. As the needle is inserted, the patient may feel some pain extending down one leg. When the needle reaches the subarachnoid space, CSF pressure is measured using a stopcock and manometer. Specimens of CSF are collected in three or more test tubes and sent for diagnostic studies. Typical laboratory studies done on CSF include measurement of glucose, cell count, protein, gram stain, culture and sensitivity, and other tests specific for the suspected diagnosis, such as Lyme titer or HIV studies.

Throughout the procedure, the nurse should provide support and encouragement and assist the patient to relax and lie or sit very still. The patient's response to the procedure, including level of anxiety, and any changes that occurred in pulse, respiratory rate, or skin color should be observed, reported, and recorded.

Following LP, the patient may be advised to lie or semi-recline for a few hours and is encouraged to drink fluids to hasten the body's replacement of the removed CSF. Continuous loss of fluid occasionally occurs from leakage at the puncture site, usually beneath the skin, which may cause headache. To relieve headache, patients are given a mild analgesic such as acetaminophen and are encouraged to continue fluid intake and remain in a flat position.

## Computed Tomography Scan

Computed tomography (CT) scanning is a diagnostic technique used in patients with neurologic dysfunction to study structures of the brain or spinal cord. An intravenous radiopaque material (contrast) can be used to better delineate and visualize certain structures or abnormalities by depicting tissue of different densities, for example, to distinguish stroke and certain tumors. Scans are taken at several different levels of the brain or spinal cord and compiled by a computer to produce a series of pictures showing "slices" of the tissue being studied. CT scans pose little risk to the patient and have taken the place of or reduced the need for several older, invasive diagnostic tests, such as myelogram.

The nurse should explain the procedure to the patient, emphasizing the need to lie very still throughout the scan. Normal activities can be assumed as soon as the procedure is completed.

## Magnetic Resonance Imaging and Angiography

Magnetic resonance imaging (MRI) is similar to CT scanning, except that radio waves and magnetism rather than x-rays are used to obtain the picture "slices" of the brain or spinal cord. As with CT scans, an intravenous radiopaque (contrast) material can be used to show greater contrast between tissues of different densities, such as blood and brain tissue. Magnetic resonance angiography (MRA), which is the same procedure as MRI with intravenous contrast and is often done at the time of MRI, is used to specifically visualize the carotid and cerebral arteries. Before MRI

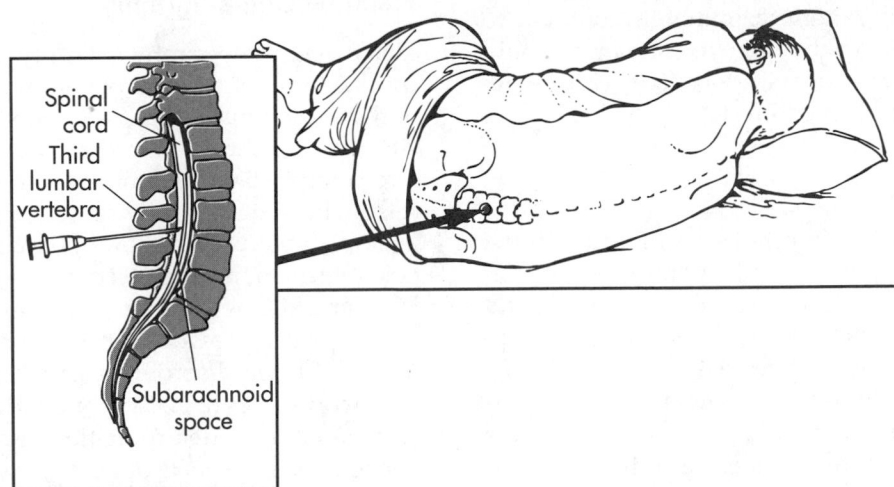

**Figure 30-12**    Patient position for lumbar puncture. An imaginary line can be drawn from the iliac crests, above L4 and L5. (From Beare PB, Myers JL: *Principles and practice of adult health nursing,* ed 2, St Louis, 1994, Mosby.)

and MRA, the nurse should explain the procedure to the patient, including the necessity to lie without moving in a small, closed cylinder (Figure 30-13). If the patient is claustrophobic, a mild sedative such as diazepam or lorazepam can be prescribed. The magnetic field of the MRI machine causes malfunction of pacemakers, and, depending on proximity to the body part being imaged, can cause damage to tissue surrounding the metal. All suspected metal within the body, such as metal sutures and artificial joints, residual shrapnel, and even metal fragments in the eye should therefore be reported to the imaging center. External metal and jewelry must be removed before MRI. After MRI and MRA, patients can resume usual activities, with standard precautions following sedation use if such medication was used.

MRI produces images with sharpness and detail not obtainable with any other study currently available. It is used in evaluating brain and spinal cord edema, tumors, hemorrhage, stroke, and other abnormalities. MRA can be used to evaluate carotid and cerebral artery stenosis and other abnormalities of the arterial system.

## Cerebral Angiography

A cerebral angiogram consists of injecting a radiopaque contrast material into an artery for visualization of the cerebral arterial system, frequently including the vessels leading to the brain from the aorta. As the contrast fluid circulates, a series of x-rays is taken and abnormalities such as aneurysms, tumors, and stenosis of the carotid artery can be defined. The puncture site of the catheter for cerebral angiography (usually the femoral or, less often, the brachial artery)

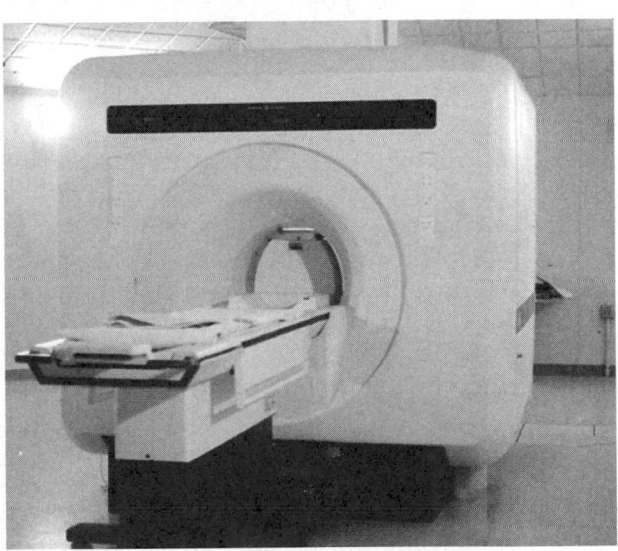

**Figure 30-13**    Clinical setting for magnetic resonance imaging (MRI). (From Lewis SM, Collier IC, Heitkemper MM: *Medical-surgical nursing: assessment and management of clinical problems,* ed 4, St Louis, 1996, Mosby.)

is cleaned with antiseptic, and local anesthetic is injected. A catheter is inserted and advanced to the aorta and base of the carotid or vertebral artery, and radiopaque dye is injected. Patients with sensitivity to the radiopaque material may have nausea, vomiting, or an allergic reaction that requires medication. After the procedure, direct pressure is applied to the puncture site for 10 or more minutes, followed by pressure dressing and close observation for signs of bleeding or hematoma. Vital signs and neurologic status are monitored frequently. The patient must remain on bed rest with the punctured extremity immobilized for 4 to 8 hours. Pulses distal to the puncture site also should be monitored. Normal activities usually can be resumed after the period of bed rest.

## Myelography

A myelogram involves taking a series of x-rays of the spinal cord and surrounding subarachnoid space following injection of radiopaque contrast fluid through a lumbar puncture. Myelography is used to locate an abnormality, such as a tumor, within the spinal canal that is blocking the flow of CSF. A water-soluble contrast material usually is used because it is self-absorbing and nonirritative. As with all diagnostic tests, the nurse needs to explain the procedure to the patient and family when appropriate. Questioning about past allergic reactions, especially those associated with contrast material used in other tests, is important in preventing possible anaphylactic shock.

The patient's vital signs and neurologic status are monitored after the myelogram. The head of the patient's bed should be elevated at a 30-degree angle for several hours after the myelogram to decrease the likelihood of contrast material pooling in the brain. Contrast material that is allowed to accumulate in the brain unimpeded increases the incidence of headache, nausea, vomiting, and possible seizure. The patient's increased intake of clear fluids enhances the body's normal circulation and replacement of CSF, thereby speeding the elimination of contrast material from the body.

The use of myelography has declined significantly since the advent and accessibility of newer, less-invasive imaging techniques such as MRI and CT, which are frequently performed with no contrast material and require no postprocedural monitoring.

## Carotid Doppler and Ultrasound Studies

A carotid duplex study combines ultrasound and Doppler techniques to detect the blood cells of circulating blood as they move through the common, internal, and external carotid arteries. The frequency of transmission of the ultrasound signal is registered as sound and recorded on a graph as blood velocity. Increased blood flow velocity can result from stenosis of a blood vessel, indicating carotid artery occlusive disease. If the ultrasound duplex indicates severe carotid stenosis or occlusion, a carotid angiogram or MRA may be indicated to show more exact information. Carotid duplex scanning is painless and does not require preparation or monitoring. After the test, the patient can resume normal activities.

## Electroencephalography

Electroencephalography (EEG) typically records electrical activity of the neurons in the outer area (cortex) of the brain. Small metal electrodes are placed on specific areas of the scalp and are connected by wires to a recording machine similar to an electrocardiograph (ECG). In some specialty centers, EEG electrodes may be implanted deep into brain tissue for obtaining specific information about electrical activity of the brain. Standard EEG is painless, and, though not as specific as ECG, it can provide helpful information in the evaluation of brain disorders such as epilepsy, the effects of other diseases (e.g., liver and kidney disease) on the brain, and in the determination of brain death. EEG is performed in a quiet, darkened room and takes 1 to 2 hours to complete. The patient having an EEG is advised to avoid stimulants such as coffee and cola and may be asked to stay awake for a specified period of time before the EEG to induce a drowsy state or sleep during the procedure. There is no preparation for the test unless specific orders are given. The patient can assume regular activities after EEG.

## Electromyography and Nerve Conduction Velocity Studies

Electromyography (EMG) is a diagnostic test that measures and records the electrical activity associated with skeletal muscles being innervated by motor neurons. Needle electrodes are inserted into the muscle and connected by wires to the electromyograph machine for graphic recording of the electrical activity. Nerve conduction velocity (NCV) involves applying electrodes to the skin, usually an extremity, and recording the length of time between onset of a brief electrical impulse and its resulting wave of depolarization in the nerve nearer the center of the body (proximal). For example, a stimulus may be applied to the thumb with depolarization measured in the median nerve at the wrist. If the nerve is damaged or compressed, slower or absent nerve conduction velocity is depicted on the graph. Before EMG and NCV, the nurse should explain the procedure to the patient, specifically, that there is mild to moderate discomfort but no severe electrical shock or pain. The patient can assume normal activities after EMG and NCV.

## Evoked Potentials

Evoked potential (EP) testing is the recording of electrical activity in a specific sensory nerve pathway as the pathway is stimulated. For example, the patient is given a stimulus such as a blinking light (visual EPs), a clicking noise (auditory EPs), or a mild electrical impulse on a finger or wrist (somatosensory EPs). Electrodes placed on specific areas of the scalp and appropriate area of the skin record the electrical activity as the nerve is stimulated. The length of time for a stimulus to travel from its source to the brain (conduction time) is recorded and then compared to normal ranges. If the conduction time is longer than normal, damage somewhere along the involved nerves is indicated. EPs can help in the diagnosis of such conditions as tumor of the auditory cranial nerve (acoustic neuroma) and multiple sclerosis. No pain is associated with this test, and no preparation or aftercare is necessary.

# GENERAL CONSIDERATIONS IN NEUROLOGIC NURSING

## Altered States of Cerebral Functioning

**Consciousness** can be thought of as a continuum, ranging from a state of complete arousal or wakefulness to that of sleep (normal function of the nervous system) or coma (abnormal manifestation of the nervous system). The **reticular formation,** a group of nerve cells within the brain stem, contains the **reticular activating system,** which is the regulating system for arousal. Unconsciousness, or a state in which the individual is unresponsive to sensory stimuli and lacks self-awareness, is a symptom of many conditions. It may mean neurologic tissue has been injured as a result of trauma or disease or that another body system is affecting the central nervous system. In **coma,** the cerebral hemispheres, the brain stem, or both are not functioning normally, and the patient is unresponsive to all stimuli (Box 30-1).

The cerebral cortex is the outer layer of the cerebral hemispheres and contains neurons that provide complex functions. In addition to controlling motor function and sensation throughout the body, the cortex is essential for highly complex and sophisticated aspects of mental functioning, such as language, memory, and thought processes. These functions can be disrupted and even permanently disturbed after head injury or disease affecting the brain.

It is the nurse's responsibility to assess and accurately record any changes in the patient's neurologic status. Level of consciousness is often the first sign of deteriorating cerebral function. Even a subtle change in behavior, which may be an early sign of decreased level of consciousness, could be important to the patient's treatment and outcome and should be promptly reported and documented.

One tool available for accurate, objective monitoring of level of consciousness is the **Glasgow Coma Scale** (GCS). Developed in 1974, it is still considered

the standard for assessing and monitoring level of consciousness (Juarez, Lyons, 1995). The GCS evaluates three aspects of cerebral functioning: eye opening, verbal response, and motor response. Each of these three areas is scored according to the patient's best response to verbal command or painful stimulus (Box 30-2). Pressure applied to the fingernail bed by a blunt object such as a pencil or pen is the preferred stimulus, since the patient can be injured by other methods such as pinching, pin prick, and sternal pressure. Scores from the three GCS sections are added to determine the total level of consciousness score. The total GSC score and individual section scores are sufficiently specific to discriminate between different or changing states of consciousness (Kerr, Walleck, 1996). Other vital components of neurologic nursing assessment include evaluation of pupillary movement and response to light and extremity strength testing. These parameters are often included with the GSC on an assessment form for monitoring patients with impaired consciousness.

Many subjective terms have been used to describe the various degrees of consciousness between total alertness and orientation to coma. However, no agreement has been reached on the manifestations of these states, and confusion often exists when subjective terms are used. When used appropriately, the GCS score eliminates the subjectivity associated with levels of consciousness, and descriptions such as "obtunded" and "stupor" may be avoided.

### NURSE ALERT

Deterioration in level of consciousness is frequently the *first* sign of increased intracranial pressure. Changes in pupillary response, weakness, headache, seizures, or vomiting may indicate *continued* increasing intracranial pressure.

### ETHICAL DILEMMA

What ethical issues, questions, and dilemmas can you identify that may affect patients with a diagnosis of dementia? How are their families affected? How can the nurse assist the patient and family in dealing with these issues and situations?

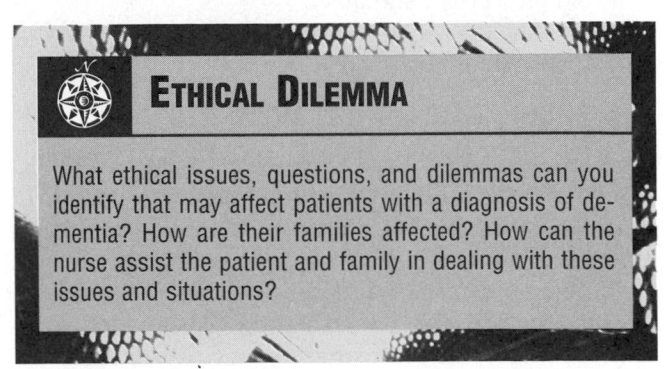

◀ BOX 30-1 ▶      NURSING PROCESS

## THE UNCONSCIOUS PATIENT

**ASSESSMENT**

- LOC
- Neurologic status
- Vital signs
- Respiratory characteristics
- Laboratory studies: ABGs, pulse oximetry, electrolytes
- Fluid volume status
- Nutritional status

**NURSING DIAGNOSES**

- Ineffective airway clearance related to neurologic deficit
- Total incontinence related to unconsciousness
- Ineffective breathing pattern related to unconsciousness
- Impaired swallowing related to unconsciousness
- Risk for injury related to unconsciousness
- Impaired physical mobility related to unconsciousness
- Altered nutrition: less than body requirements related to altered intake pattern
- Altered oral mucous membranes related to unconsciousness
- Self-care deficit related to unconsciousness
- Risk for impaired skin integrity related to decreased mobility

**NURSING INTERVENTIONS**

- Ensure open airway; insertion of oral airway or placement of endotracheal or tracheostomy tube may be necessary.
- Position patient in lateral or semiprone position to facilitate drainage of oral secretions.

**EVALUATION OF EXPECTED OUTCOMES**

- Maximum pulmonary function maintained
- Aspiration prevented
- Skin integrity maintained

- Adequate nutrition status maintained
- Tracheal and oral secretions aspirated by suctioning patient as necessary
- Vital signs and neurologic signs (level of consciousness, motor function, pupillary response) checked every 15 minutes for first few hours, then every 4 hours or as ordered
- Patient turned every 2 hours
- Proper body alignment maintained by positioning patient to allow patent airway and prevention of foot drop, wrist drop, joint contractures, and pressure sores
- Antipressure mattresses and devices used as available to prevent pressure to bony surfaces and all pressure points
- Eyes protected from irritation and corneal ulceration with use of eye shields, eye irrigations with physiologic saline, and eye lubricants and ointments as ordered
- Intravenous fluids or tube feedings monitored closely; do not give unconscious patients oral fluids
- Oral hygiene provided frequently, including emollients for lips to prevent cracking
- Urinary output closely monitored; if indwelling catheter is in place, traction prevented and closed system maintained
- Bowel care, such as suppositories, provided as needed and ordered to maintain bowel elimination
- Patient treated with care and dignity, explaining all procedures and your actions
- Emotional support and reassurance provided to family; family members allowed to assist in care when feasible
- Remember that, depending on the cause of brain dysfunction, level of consciousness may vacillate, and the patient may be able to hear some or all of your words

## Increased Intracranial Pressure

An understanding of the concept of increased **intracranial pressure** (IICP) is fundamental to the care of patients with neurologic problems. Uncontrolled and untreated IICP can lead to irreversible neurologic pathology and cardiopulmonary arrest.

The **Monro-Kellie doctrine** describes normal intracranial pressure as the maintenance of constant volumes of the major components within the skull: brain tissue, blood, and cerebrospinal fluid. If a small increase occurs in one of these components, the body can compensate by making changes in the remaining two components (Geraci, Geraci, 1996). However, this compensatory response is limited because the skull is an inflexible vault, and continued or increased total volume will result in IICP. If the increased pressure is

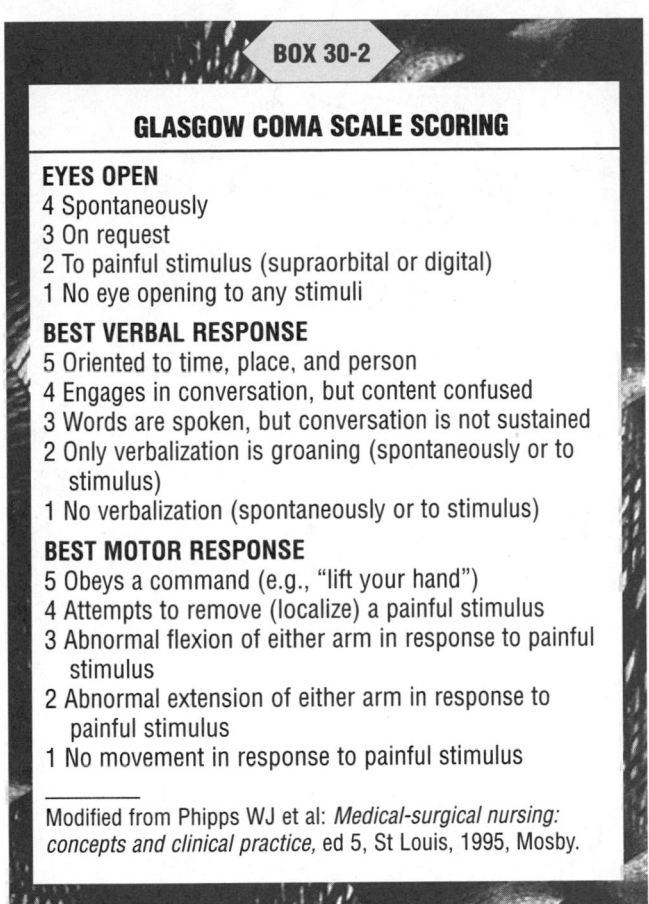

BOX 30-2

## GLASGOW COMA SCALE SCORING

**EYES OPEN**
4 Spontaneously
3 On request
2 To painful stimulus (supraorbital or digital)
1 No eye opening to any stimuli

**BEST VERBAL RESPONSE**
5 Oriented to time, place, and person
4 Engages in conversation, but content confused
3 Words are spoken, but conversation is not sustained
2 Only verbalization is groaning (spontaneously or to stimulus)
1 No verbalization (spontaneously or to stimulus)

**BEST MOTOR RESPONSE**
5 Obeys a command (e.g., "lift your hand")
4 Attempts to remove (localize) a painful stimulus
3 Abnormal flexion of either arm in response to painful stimulus
2 Abnormal extension of either arm in response to painful stimulus
1 No movement in response to painful stimulus

Modified from Phipps WJ et al: *Medical-surgical nursing: concepts and clinical practice*, ed 5, St Louis, 1995, Mosby.

ally, any condition that causes generalized edema of the brain (cerebral edema) can cause IICP. Cerebral edema maybe the result of organ disease or dysfunction (e.g., hepatic or renal encephalopathy) and lead toxicity. The rate of increase in intracranial pressure due to such generalized dysfunction may be gradual, and therefore tolerated by the patient without causing abrupt symptoms such as **papilledema.** When intracranial pressure rises gradually, there are fewer obvious signs, especially in the early stages of the situation or disease (Guyton, 1992). Confusion, agitation, and drowsiness are typical early signs in the alert patient with slowly progressing IICP (Hickey, 1997) (Box 30-3).

Establishment of a baseline nursing assessment for all patients at risk for IICP is imperative, since detection of even subtle changes can be crucial in the prevention of irreversible brain damage. Rising intracranial pressure is a true emergency and a primary consideration in the care of patients with neurologic dysfunction. Early signs and symptoms of IICP may include a deterioration in the level of consciousness, changes in pupillary response (Figure 30-15), weakness on one side of the body (hemiparesis), headache, seizures, and vomiting. If IICP is untreated and continues to rise, level of consciousness continues to decline, pupillary dilation of one pupil may occur, and vital sign changes of slow pulse, widened pulse pressure, and respiratory irregularities occur. These late signs of IICP are indicative of impending brain herniation.

**Herniation** of the brain is the protrusion of a portion of the brain through an opening or a defect in the skull. The most common site of brain herniation is at the opening of the tentorium, called the *tentorial notch* (Evans, 1995) (Figure 30-16). The **tentorium** is the tough layer of dura mater that lies between the cerebrum—which is above the tentorium in the supratentorial space—and the cerebellum and brain stem, which are below the tentorium, in the infratentorial space. Herniation in this area is called *uncal* herniation because it is the uncus of the temporal lobe that is forced through the opening of the tentorial notch. During this process, the third cranial nerve (oculomotor nerve) is compressed as it exits through the tentorial notch, causing dilation of the pupil on the same (ipsilateral) side as the herniation. If this condition is not relieved almost immediately (usually by emergency placement of subarachnoid catheter or screw or by **craniotomy**), pressure to vital structures in the brain stem results in irreversible changes and death.

Medical treatment of patients with IICP focuses on rapid detection, support of body systems (e.g., respiratory and cardiovascular), and methods to decrease intracranial pressure. Osmotic diuretics (e.g., mannitol), loop diuretics (e.g., furosemide and ethacrynic acid), and corticosteroids (e.g., dexamethasone) are the most

not alleviated, damage to brain structures and ultimate total decompensation occurs, leading to death (Evans, 1995). Other factors that influence intracranial pressure are changes in the pressures of arterial and venous circulation, abdominal and thoracic cavity pressure increases, posture (i.e., flexion of neck, head lower than body), and increase in body temperature.

Intracranial pressure can be measured during lumbar puncture by measuring the cerebrospinal fluid (CSF) pressure as it drains through a manometer, by inserting a catheter into one of the ventricles of the brain, or by inserting a screw or bolt into the subarachnoid space within the meninges (Figure 30-14). Normal CSF pressure with the head of the patient's bed elevated 30 degrees is 80 to 180 cm of water (by LP manometer) and 0 to 15 mm of mercury (by catheter pressure transducer). Elevation of the head at 30 degrees is usually best for patients with the potential for IICP because it facilitates normal gravity of CSF away from the cerebral structures.

A variety of conditions can cause IICP, such as cerebral tumor, hematoma, abscess, and malabsorption of CSF caused by obstructive hydrocephalus (occlusion of normal CSF flow and reabsorption, leading to enlargement of cerebral ventricles and IICP). Addition-

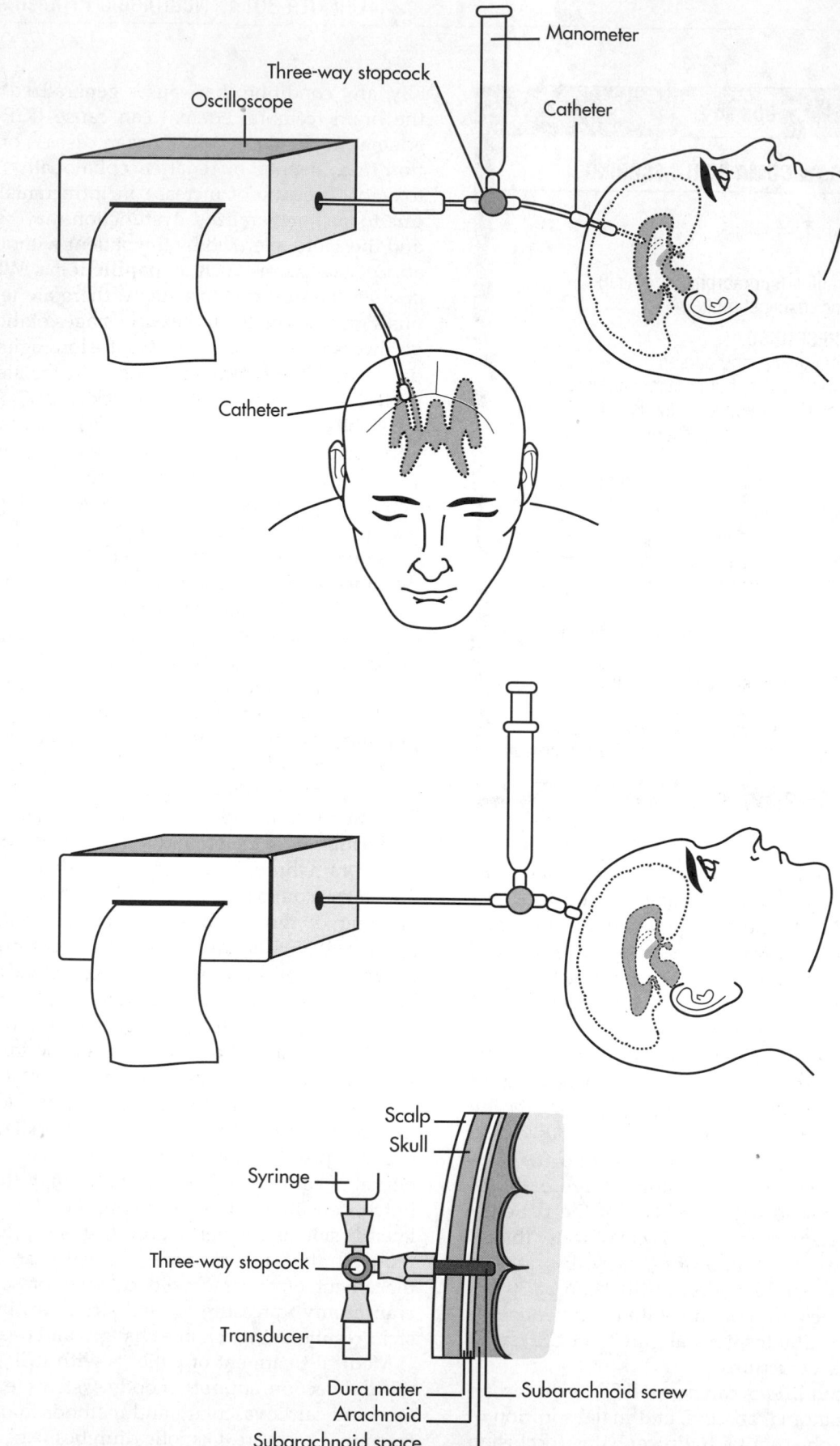

**Figure 30-14** Major intracranial pressure monitoring devices. **A,** Ventricular catheter monitor. **B,** Subarachnoid screw or bolt monitor. (Redrawn from Smeltzer S, Bare B: *Brunner and Suddarth's textbook of medical-surgical nursing,* ed 8, Philadelphia, 1996, Lippincott-Raven.)

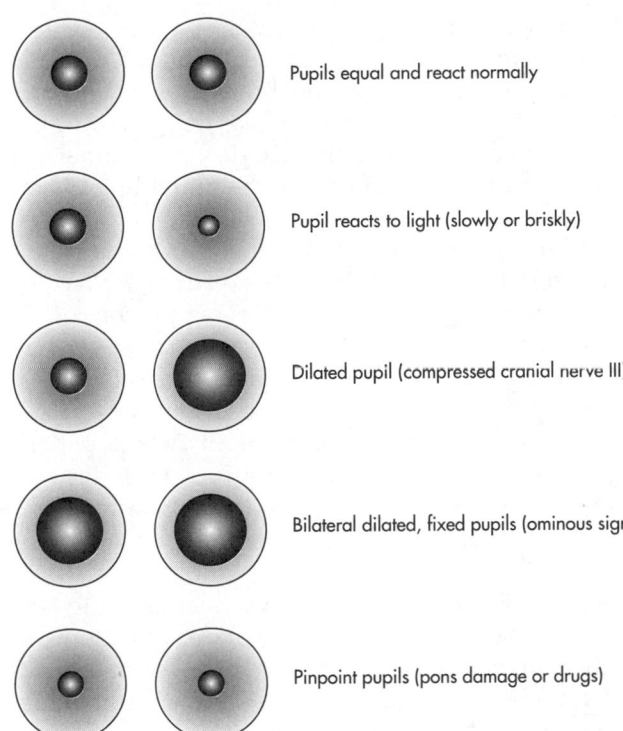

Pupils equal and react normally

Pupil reacts to light (slowly or briskly)

Dilated pupil (compressed cranial nerve III)

Bilateral dilated, fixed pupils (ominous sign)

Pinpoint pupils (pons damage or drugs)

**Figure 30-15**   Pupillary check for size and response. (From Lewis SM, Collier IC, Heitkemper MM: *Medical-surgical nursing: assessment and management of clinical problems,* ed 4, St Louis, 1996, Mosby.)

---

**BOX 30-3**

### EARLY AND LATE SIGNS AND SYMPTOMS OF INCREASED INTRACRANIAL PRESSURE

**EARLY SIGNS AND SYMPTOMS**

LOC: restlessness, irritability, mild confusion, personality changes, or agitation; lower Glasgow Coma Scale (GCS) score

Pupils: drooping of eyelid (ptosis), ovoid pupil, delayed or sluggish reaction, unilateral change in pupil size

Vision: blurred; diplopia; decreased visual acuity

Motor: pronator drift (weakness and pronation of outstretched arm); decreased grasp strength; weakness, especially on one side

Sensory: decreased response to touch or pinprick

Headache: early morning headache; possible vomiting with or without nausea

Speech: slow or slurred

Memory: may be impaired

Appearance of cranial incision: postoperative bulging or edema

Vital signs: no change

Cranial nerves: II (early papilledema), III (ptosis, abnormal pupillary responses) may be seen

Seizure activity: may or may not occur

**LATE SIGNS AND SYMPTOMS**

LOC: difficult to arouse; requires more stimulus for response; low GCS score; coma

Pupils: unilateral enlarging pupil, progressing to fixed and dilated; papilledema; progressing to bilateral fixed and dilated

Motor: dense weakness, decorticate or decerebrate posturing, flaccid muscles

Sensory: only response may be decorticate or decerebrate posturing

Headache: worsening, with projectile vomiting

Speech: may only groan to stimulus

Respiratory: irregular rate; Cheyne-Stokes progressing to central neurogenic hyperventilation or other pathologic patterns; arrest if IICP not relieved

Vital signs: rising systolic BP with widening pulse pressure, bradycardia; tachycardia, fall in BP, temperature changes if IICP not relieved

Cardiac (in varying sequence): Q-waves with ST depression, elevated T waves, supraventricular tachycardia, sinus bradycardia, A-V block, PVCs, agonal rhythm, cardiac arrest if IICP not relieved

Cranial nerves: II (papilledema, decreased visual acuity), III, IV, VI (pupillary and eye movement dysfunction); all if IICP not relieved

Abnormal reflexes: Babinski sign; oculocephalic reflex abnormalities (e.g., doll's eyes)

---

widely used medications for treatment of IICP and play an important part in its management (Ozuna, 1996a). Control of fluid intake, fever, blood pressure, and respiratory rate are also crucial while seeking the cause and a definitive treatment of IICP. Patients are monitored continuously in the intensive care unit (ICU) and need mechanical ventilation. Mild hyperventilation for IICP caused by trauma and selected encephalopathies is a standard intervention in many centers (Bond, 1996). The mechanism of reduced IICP by hyperventilation is believed to be an increase in the expiration of carbon dioxide that causes blood vessels in the high blood flow areas of the brain to be constricted, which causes blood to be shunted to areas with reduced blood flow (Geraci, Geraci, 1996). Continuous intracranial pressure monitoring can be accomplished in the ICU by using a transducer connected to a catheter that is inserted into one of the lateral ventricles, or to a screw or bolt that is placed in the subarachnoid space. CSF can be drained through either of these devices, which may be done to further reduce intracranial pressure. Surgery to remove any causative, resectable lesion, such as subdural hematoma, abscess, or other expanding lesion, further assists in reducing intracranial hypertension (Hickey, 1997).

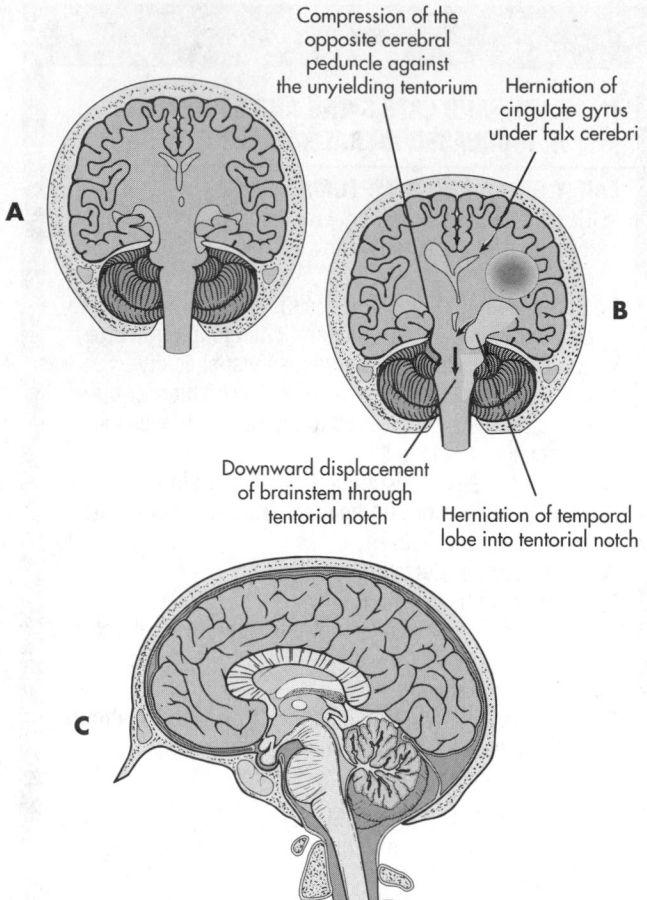

Compression of the opposite cerebral peduncle against the unyielding tentorium

Herniation of cingulate gyrus under falx cerebri

Downward displacement of brainstem through tentorial notch

Herniation of temporal lobe into tentorial notch

**Figure 30-16**  Herniation. **A,** The normal relationship of intracranial structures. **B,** Shift of intracranial structures. **C,** Downward herniation of the cerebellar tonsils into the foramen magnum. (Redrawn from McCance KL, Huether SE: *Pathophysiology: biological basis for disease in adults and children,* ed 2, St Louis, 1994, Mosby.)

Nursing goals for patients with increased intracranial pressure are to detect and control any factors that may further increase the pressure (see Box 30-3).

## Care of the Patient with Seizure Disorder

A **seizure** is a sudden, excessive discharge of electrical impulses from nerve cells in the brain that usually produces a brief disturbance in brain function. Changes in behavior and body function can occur, although actual signs and symptoms of a seizure depend on the location, duration, and pattern of abnormal discharge (Faught, 1995). Seizures can occur at any age and can be associated with previous trauma and a variety of diseases and disorders, or they can occur spontaneously with no apparent cause. Seiz-

ures may not follow a particular pattern, even in the same individual. The characteristics of a seizure depend on the area of the brain from which the seizure activity originates, called the seizure *focus.* Everyone has a seizure threshold, which under certain circumstances could cause the individual to have a seizure.

*Seizure disorder* and *epilepsy* are interchangeable terms used to denote seizures that recur over time. Approximately 0.5% to 2% of the population of the United States have some form of seizure disorder, with 80% having the first seizure before the age of 20 years. About 5% of persons report the occurrence of a seizure at some time in their lives. In about 70% of patients with seizures, no identifiable neurologic or systemic disorder is found. Because there is no known cause of the seizures, this condition is known as idiopathic epilepsy.

Seizure disorders or the increased tendency to have seizures may be inherited. Other causes of seizures are birth injury, congenital malformations, head trauma, and lesions in the brain such as stroke and tumor. Single seizures that may occur as the result of hypoglycemia or other reversible metabolic state and febrile convulsions associated with high fever during infancy or early childhood are not considered seizure disorders (epilepsy). Treatment with an antiepileptic medication is usually begun if more than one provoked seizure occurs within a year.

The International Classification of Epileptic Seizures uses standardized terminology in describing different seizure types to improve communication and study of epilepsy. This classification of seizures is based on the clinical manifestations of seizures and their corresponding electroencephalograms (EEG) (Faught, 1995). The previously used terms *grand mal, petit mal,* and *temporal lobe* have been replaced by nomenclature described in the following paragraphs.

**NURSE ALERT**

When caring for the patient with a seizure disorder:
- Do not leave the patient unattended during a seizure.
- Prevent injury due to falls.
- Place the patient's head in a lateral position.
- Place patient on the floor or bed.
- A plastic airway or padded tongue blade should be inserted between the patient's back teeth *only* if the patient's jaw is relaxed.
- Observe and record all aspects of the seizure.

Seizures are divided into the two broad categories: *generalized* and *partial*. Generalized seizures are caused by abnormal (epileptic) discharges over the entire cerebral cortex, with no apparent focus of abnormality. Partial (focal) seizures begin in a specific area of the cortex, and the abnormal discharges of electrical activity may remain the area of the focus or may spread to other areas or the entire brain.

## Generalized Seizures

*Generalized tonic-clonic seizures,* historically called "grand mal" seizures, are characterized by loss of consciousness and stiffening of the entire body (tonic phase), followed by alternating flexion and extension of the body, neck, and extremities (clonic phase). Initially, there may be a high-pitched cry that is caused by spasm of the respiratory muscles forcing air from the lungs and through the constricted vocal cords. This may be followed by a period of cyanosis during the tonic phase, due to inhibition of the respirations by muscle rigidity. The clonic phase begins within a few seconds, with convulsive jerking of all muscles. Bowel and bladder incontinence, tongue-biting, and excessive salivation with frothy drooling may occur. This is the *ictal* phase of the seizure and is followed by a period of unresponsiveness for several minutes to several hours. This is the *postictal* period, and may be followed by normal sleep. If any of the different types of seizures occur without full recovery between them, *status epilepticus* exists. Although there are many types of status epilepticus, tonic-clonic status epilepticus constitutes a medical emergency associated with substantial morbidity and mortality (Hickey, 1997). If the continuous seizure activity of tonic-clonic status cannot be interrupted and controlled, brain damage, ventilatory and circulatory insufficiency, cardiac dysrhythmias, and damage to virtually all body systems can occur, leading to death (Blissitt, 1996).

Typical *absence* (petit mal) *seizures* consist of a brief period of loss of consciousness and staring. No preictal or postictal change occurs in the individual's activity, and the entire episode may go unnoticed by the patient or observers. These seizures occur almost exclusively in children and rarely progress past adolescence. An atypical form of absence seizure is not as rare among adults and consists of brief staring that may be preceded by a warning, followed by unusual and nonpurposeful activity. The individual usually is confused for a short period postictally. Typical and atypical absence seizures are characterized by the same unique EEG pattern, which is a 3-Hz per second spike and wave pattern. This pattern has both a lower amplitude and slower rhythm than the pattern of tonic-clonic seizures (Ozuna, 1996a).

## Partial Seizures

Partial seizures, although of many types, all begin in a focal area of the brain. *Simple partial seizures* are brief and do not cause loss of consciousness. The individual may experience an unusual sensation or uncontrollable movement of an extremity. The seizure activity may spread to other parts of the entire brain, which would result in a generalized tonic-clonic seizure. This generalization of the seizure focus was previously known as a *jacksonian seizure. Complex partial seizures* usually begin with an abnormal focus of epileptic activity in the temporal lobe, which explains the older term, "temporal lobe epilepsy." With complex partial seizures, consciousness is altered, and movement and nonpurposeful activity may be involved, explaining the descriptor "psychomotor seizure," popular for many years. Complex partial seizures may be characterized by repetitive and nonpurposeful movements or by inappropriate activity, such as picking at objects or clothing or simply walking about. These motions are called **automatisms.** The patient often has an **aura** at the beginning of a complex partial seizure, which may consist of an unusual smell, visual image, or other sensation, such as the feeling that an event has occurred before *(déjà vu).* Although the aura is part of the seizure, it serves as a warning for many individuals (Evans, 1995). Patients may have no recollection of a complex partial seizure, although they may be disoriented or confused for a few seconds and then able to resume usual activities.

## Intervention

The goal of treatment for patients with seizure disorders is prevention. This is best accomplished when the affected individual is knowledgeable and accepting of this chronic condition, since the primary treatment—medication—is often required throughout life. Health maintenance through diet, exercise, adequate rest, stress reduction, and other aspects of a healthy lifestyle are as important as medication for overall quality of life. Alcohol is strongly contraindicated for individuals with seizures because of its interactions with antiepileptic drugs and its propensity for lowering seizure threshold. Psychologic aspects of having a seizure disorder are extremely important, especially among children of school age and teenagers. Common fears of these patients are ridicule by peers, embarrassment, and limitations concerning ability to drive, participate in recreation and sports, and seek or maintain employment. Counseling is often part of the initial treatment plan, and psychologic assessment and support should be ongoing in most cases. As in other chronic conditions, the individual's psychologic state affects his or her quality of life and the ability and willingness to follow the therapeutic plan of care (Ozuna, 1996b).

Antiepileptic medications act by either raising the brain's threshold for seizure activity or preventing spread of the seizure focus in the brain. Commonly used antiepileptic medications are phenytoin (Dilantin), carbamazepine (Tegretol), divalproex (Depakene, Depakote), phenobarbital, and primidone (Mysoline). Ethosuximide (Zarontin) is used almost exclusively in children for the treatment of typical absence seizures. Gabapentin (Neurontin) and lamotrigine (Lamictal) are newer medications, recently approved for use with another antiepileptic medication. Felbamate (Felbatol) is restricted to individuals not responsive to other antiepileptic medications. The effective dosage of antiepileptic medications to prevent seizures varies with each individual. As with all medications, patients should be taught signs and symptoms of side effects and effects of toxic levels of antiepileptic medications. of Blood cell count and liver function should be monitored regularly, and other tests should be done to detect possible adverse effects. In a small percentage of individuals not responsive to antiepileptic medications, surgical resection of the area of abnormal EEG electrical discharge is indicated.

The nurse should be aware of all patients who are admitted to the hospital and have a history of seizures and be alert for possible seizure activity in those individuals. Change in routine, especially in a stressful environment or circumstances, can cause seizures. Hospitalized patients also may be affected by conditions that can lower seizure threshold or may have started taking medications that will complicate their current antiseizure regimen. If a seizure occurs, the patient should be protected from injury, and activity before, during, and after the seizure should be observed and documented as accurately as possible (Box 30-4). Aspiration of saliva is a risk during the postictal period of a tonic-clonic seizure if the patient is not positioned to allow drainage of oral secretions. Observation and documentation of the individual's seizure should include the following:

- Time of onset, duration, and cessation of motor activity (ictus)
- Presence or absence of preseizure symptoms or activity (aura)

---

| BOX 30-4 | NURSING PROCESS |
| --- | --- |

## SEIZURES

### ASSESSMENT

- Frequency, duration, and type of seizure activity
- Aura before alteration in consciousness
- Sequence of events: preseizure activity, part of body first affected, and progression
- Respiratory rate and character during and after seizure activity
- Alteration or loss of consciousness, orientation, memory, speech and pupillary response postictally

### NURSING DIAGNOSES

- Risk for injury related to seizure activity and postictal change in consciousness
- Ineffective airway clearance related to seizure activity and postictal decrease in consciousness
- Ineffective breathing pattern related to seizure activity and postictal decrease in consciousness
- Risk for incontinence related to seizure activity
- Impaired swallowing related to change in consciousness
- Impaired physical mobility related to change in consciousness
- Self-care deficit related to change in consciousness
- Impaired verbal communication related to change in consciousness
- Knowledge deficit related to condition and prognosis

### NURSING INTERVENTIONS

- If patient is standing, assist to floor and place pillow or other padding under head.
- Do not leave patient unattended; do not attempt to move patient.
- Remove nearby furniture and objects away from patient if possible.
- Ensure privacy as much as possible; instruct nonmedical and unnecessary staff to vacate area.
- Insert folded gauze pad or other soft, flat material between patient's back teeth only if patient's jaw is relaxed. Do not attempt to force open patient's mouth if jaw is rigid.
- Maintain patent airway and adequate ventilation postictally; suctioning and oxygen may be needed.
- Accurately record all aspects of seizure and activities, body movement, behavior before, during, and after seizure.
- Padded side rails; keep bed in low position at all times.
- Accompany patients with frequent seizures when necessary for them to leave nursing unit.
- Administer anticonvulsant medication as ordered; notify physician if patient unable to take medication for any reason.

- Level of consciousness before, during, and after seizure activity
- Type and location of body movements
- Presence of respiratory difficulty or cyanosis
- Presence of tongue-biting or urinary or fecal incontinence
- Position or movement of eyes
- Behavior or activity after the seizure (postictal)
- Any injury occurring as a result of the seizure

**Patient and family teaching.** Education of individuals and their appropriate family members is an integral part of the nursing care of patients with seizure disorders. Understanding the nature of the condition and the individualized treatment plan is especially important. Side effects, interactions with other medications, and the necessity of taking antiepileptic medications as prescribed should be stressed. Omitting even one or two doses of antiepileptic medication can result in a seizure in some individuals. Adequate rest, exercise, balanced diet, and avoidance of strenuous and stressful activities are thought to contribute to the control of seizures and to a better quality of life. General guidelines for the safety of individuals who have not been seizure free for at least 1 year include avoiding heights, refraining from operating heavy or intricate machinery with moving parts, and avoiding any other situation that could place the individual or others at risk if a seizure occurs. State laws vary, but most states allow individuals with a history of seizures to drive if they have been seizure free for 1 year. The Epilepsy Foundation of America can provide information and support regarding the many issues of living with seizure disorder to the affected individual and his or her family.

---

### NURSE ALERT

**During a generalized tonic-clonic seizure:**
- **Do not leave the patient unattended during the seizure.**
- **Prevent injury.**
- **Place the individual on a bed if possible. If he or she is sitting or falling, assist them to the floor and place a pillow or other protection under the head.**
- **Remove objects that could cause injury. Do not restrain.**
- **Keep bystanders at a distance and provide privacy for the patient when possible.**
- **Observe and record activity before, during, and after the seizure.**
- **Following the seizure, turn the individual to his or her side to provide an open airway and drainage of oral secretions.**

---

## Care of the Patient with Central Nervous System Infection
### Meningitis

Meningitis is an acute inflammation of the inner layers of the meningeal covering of the brain and spinal cord. The causative bacteria or virus invades the cerebrospinal fluid (CSF), resulting in purulent rather than clear, watery fluid. The CSF may increase and subsequently cause increased intracranial pressure, especially if the infection spreads to the brain and causes encephalitis. The most common organism causing meningitis is *Streptococcus pneumoniae*, which is the cause of many upper respiratory tract infections. However, many different organisms can cause meningitis, which also may occur after an upper respiratory tract infection or other systemic infection, from a direct wound into the skull, and less frequently from extension of an adjacent infected area (e.g., otitis, mastoiditis). Sporadic epidemics occur, especially in crowded living conditions. Children under the age of 6 years, older adults, and debilitated persons are more at risk for meningitis. It usually causes acute, serious illness and can result in permanent disability and even death.

**Assessment.** The onset of symptoms of meningitis varies according to the causative organism. Clinical symptoms usually develop with 48 hours but may have a more rapid onset of 8 to 12 hours. Diagnosis is based on symptoms, clinical evaluation, and examination of the CSF, including cultures to determine the organism. Symptoms include severe headache, **nuchal rigidity** (stiff neck that is painful with movement), fever, lethargy, and confusion. A skin rash is common in meningitis caused by meningococcal bacteria. Symptoms of meningitis caused by syphilis, which is rare except among HIV-infected patients, may range from mild photophobia and headache to severe headache, nuchal rigidity, seizures, and cranial nerve abnormalities causing pupillary, facial, and auditory problems (Hook, 1995). If the meningitis progresses, regardless of the causative organism, the patient can develop severe symptoms, including seizures and decreased level of consciousness leading to coma.

**Intervention.** Treatment of meningitis begins with prompt administration of and ongoing treatment with intravenous antibiotics. Analgesics such as codeine may be necessary for headache and severe neck pain. A quiet, darkened room should be provided to diminish photophobia and headache, and seizure precautions should be taken. Isolation precautions usually are unnecessary beyond the judicious hand washing and standard precautionary care given to every patient. For meningococcal meningitis, however, strict isolation precautions are necessary to prevent disease transmission.

Supportive measures necessary for any acutely ill patient are likewise necessary for patients with meningitis, including neurologic assessment (GCS, pupillary responses, motor function), vital signs, turning at regular intervals, maintaining good body alignment with head of bed elevated 30 degrees and neck straight or in extension for comfort, and accurate monitoring of fluid intake and urinary output. Control of fever and prevention or control of seizures are necessary. The patient must be observed for evidence of increasing intracranial pressure (see Box 30-3).

Residual disability and even death can occur in patients with meningitis. Sequelae may include visual impairment, deafness, cognitive impairment, and seizure disorder.

## Encephalitis

Encephalitis is an acute, febrile illness caused by inflammation of the brain. It is more often caused by a virus than by bacteria or other organism, and it can be a complication of measles, chickenpox, or mumps. Epidemics of encephalitis have been caused by a virus harbored by wild birds and horses and transmitted by ticks and mosquitoes (e.g., equine encephalitis). The fatality rate of encephalitis is 5% to 20%, with the highest rates occurring among those with herpes simplex virus and equine viruses (Kerr, Walleck, 1996).

**Assessment.** The initial symptoms of encephalitis are similar to those of meningitis but are more gradual. Headache, high fever, seizures, confusion, and drowsiness are usually seen. Cerebral edema is a result of generalized infection and damage to the brain and requires urgent treatment to prevent irreversible brain damage or death due to increasing intracranial pressure (IICP). Assessment for early signs of IICP and ongoing monitoring for changes in status are crucial (see Box 30-3).

**Intervention.** Corticosteroids and hypertonic intravenous solutions such as mannitol are used to control cerebral edema. Vidarabine and acyclovir are specific agents shown to reduce mortality in herpes simplex encephalitis (Kerr, Walleck, 1996). Nursing care requires careful observation and detection of changes, especially those denoting IICP. The patient is usually critically ill, and supportive nursing care is based on condition and symptoms. Respiratory distress, seizures, and immobility are common nursing considerations. A nasogastric tube or hyperalimentation nutrition may be needed to provide nutrition. In those patients who survive, many have residual neurologic disability requiring rehabilitation.

## Care of the Patient with a Chronic Neurologic Disorder

Many neurologic diseases are not well understood and have no known cure, despite ongoing research in many areas of the country and world. Devastating, progressive physical and mental deterioration can result, from neurologic chronic disease, changing and challenging many aspects of life for the patient, family, and caregivers. Conditions may develop quickly, as in Guillain-Barré syndrome, or over a period of months or years, as may be seen with Alzheimer's disease and multiple sclerosis. The degree of disability varies, and some disorders, such as amyotrophic lateral sclerosis, lead to death. Diagnosis of many neurologic disorders is difficult to determine, adding to the anxiety and uncertainty of the patient and family. The primary goals of nursing care for patients with chronic neurologic disorders are preventing complications, facilitating self-care and independence when possible, and providing supportive care as needed. Psychosocial support and education throughout all phases of diagnosis, treatment, and care are vital to accomplishing the nursing care goals.

## Multiple Sclerosis

Multiple sclerosis (MS) is a chronic, progressive disease of the myelin sheath, the protective covering of the many nerve cells (neurons) in the central nervous system. It affects women more often than men, and the usual age of onset is between 15 and 50 years. Approximately 250,000 to 350,000 people in the United States are known to have MS (Schapiro, 1997). In multiple sclerosis, myelin is broken down and replaced by plaque. The severity of this degenerative sclerosis varies in severity and location in the brain and spinal cord, which explains the wide range and severity of symptoms among patients. Many experts believe MS is caused by an inflammatory response caused by the individual's immune system, perhaps triggered by a virus in genetically susceptible individuals (McGuinness, 1996). The disease usually begins with periods of exacerbations and remissions of days' or weeks' duration (exacerbating/remitting form), but may begin—or rapidly progress—to more static, though progressive (chronic/progressive) MS. When the myelin sheath is first damaged, symptoms may be mild, or barely noticeable by the affected individual. Myelin is capable of regenerating in the very early stage of most cases of MS, but, as the disease progresses, the loss of myelin allows the underlying neurons to be permanently damaged. Symptoms (exacerbations) are then more pronounced. Recovery (remission) following each exacerbation is increasingly less complete over time, and, depending on the amount of damage to neurons, permanent loss of function eventually occurs. The degree of disability also varies widely, and some patients with MS are able to maintain independent or assisted living throughout a normal lifespan. Others may be severely limited in activities or become bedridden in a few years. In most cases the onset of MS at a young age indicates a more severe form of the disease with increased disability.

**Assessment.** Because of the variable and sometimes insidious onset of MS, the diagnosis may not be made until long after the first symptoms appear. Diagnosis is based on clinical examination, symptoms, and laboratory examination of CSF. MRI enhancements typically contributed to MS plaque are frequently seen in the brain or spinal cord but may not be visible in the early stages of the disease. Early symptoms vary widely and may be manifested as eye pain (optic neuritis), vague or pronounced numbness, bladder retention or urgency, problems with balance, or other problems. Attention deficits and other changes in cognition have been observed and reported in some patients with MS, even in mild or early stages (Jansen, Cimprich, 1994). The disease may progress slowly, with long remissions or plateaus of stability; or it may progress rapidly, with brief or no apparent remissions. Severe, advanced MS can cause paralysis, spasticity, tremor, incontinence, slurred speech, and changes in mental status. Although MS is not fatal, it can lead to chronic complications of immobility such as pressure sores, pneumonia, and bladder and kidney infections that can hasten death.

**Intervention.** There is no current cure for MS; however, intravenous corticosteroid drugs have been effective in reducing the severity of exacerbations in many patients. It is thought that steroids act by reducing inflammation and edema at the site of demyelination in the neuron. According to recent studies, intravenous steroids have been found to be more effective and to have fewer side effects than oral steroids (Ozuna, 1996b). Immunosuppressive drugs such as azathioprine (Imuran) have also been used, but neither steroids nor immunosuppressive drugs have been shown to affect the ultimate outcome and progression of MS. Two forms of beta-interferon (Betaseron; Avonex) are approved for the treatment of MS patients with exacerbating/remitting forms of MS. Research studies have shown that these drugs reduce the number and severity of MS exacerbations (Kelley, 1996). It is hoped that this will affect the speed of disease progression and thereby lessen the severity of disability. Although intravenous steroids are sometimes used for worsening symptoms, currently nomedication has been approved for treatment of chronic/progressive MS.

The nurse can contribute to the achievement of maximum independence, prevention of complications,

and psychosocial well-being of individuals with MS by providing symptomatic and supportive care. Physical and occupational therapists can help patients maximize and conserve strength and assist them in modifying their homes and work environments as necessary. Very warm, humid temperatures can increase weakness and fatigue, so hot baths and showers should be avoided. Many MS patients stay indoors with air-conditioning as much as possible in hot weather. Safety measures should be considered in all activities of daily living, especially if patients have motor and sensory deficits that could lead to falls, burns, or other injuries. A well-balanced diet and regular exercise are necessary to maintain function and mobility and consequently contribute to independence. Education and support of the patient and family are major components of care, especially since there is no specific individual prognosis. As in other chronic illnesses, the entire family unit is affected. The National Multiple Sclerosis Society is an excellent source of information and support for individuals affected by MS, and there are local chapters in many communities.

## Amyotrophic Lateral Sclerosis

Amyotrophic lateral sclerosis (ALS, Lou Gehrig's disease) is a fairly rapidly progressive disease caused by degeneration of motor neurons in the brain stem and spinal cord. The cause of ALS is unknown, and the disease usually leads to death in 2 to 6 years. Suspected, but not as yet proven, causes of ALS include endotoxins and immunologic disturbances (Eisen, 1995). Muscle weakness or slurred speech (**dysarthria**) and difficulty swallowing (**dysphagia**) are the usual presenting symptoms and are the result of the injured motor neurons being unable to produce or transmit signals from the brain to the muscles. The onset of ALS usually is between 40 and 70 years of age and affects men twice as frequently as women.

Goals for nursing care of patients with ALS include maximizing function and preventing complications while supporting the patient and his family. Cognition remains intact, so the patient can have input into the decisions regarding his or her care. Ethical issues involving end-of-life decisions can be major considerations, as respiratory failure may occur weeks to months before death occurs, usually as result of a complicating infection. Although many patients oppose living out their lives with ventilatory support and without the ability to move or speak, others have lived seemingly comfortably with 24-hour nursing care. Electronic communication devices that are activated with minimal pressure, such as a very soft finger touch, allow the patient to print words and sentences. Each decision about end-of-life events is a personal one, and the patient and family should be provided as much information and support as possible, as early as possible, and feasibly. Discussion and decisions pertinent to ventilatory support, nutrition, and other issues before the late stages of the disease are therefore of utmost importance. The ALS Foundation is an excellent resource for information and support to patients and their families.

## Parkinson's Disease

Parkinson's disease (PD) is a chronic, progressive disease of the basal ganglia, which are a group of nerve cell bodies (nuclei) located deep within the brain. Typical symptoms of PD are resting tremor, **bradykinesia** (slow movements), muscular rigidity, and problems with balance and vital signs related to changes in position **(orthostasis)** (Dowling, 1995). The pathophysiology of PD is an imbalance between dopamine and acetylcholine, chemicals released by neurons in the basal ganglia that function to influence control of body movement. **Dopamine** regulates or inhibits the nerve cells that release acetylcholine, the substance that excites nerve cells to function. In the imbalance caused by PD, dopamine is depleted, allowing acetylcholine to be released unopposed. This causes uninhibited excitation of acetylcholine, which results in movement disorders. The cause of the decrease in dopamine is unknown, although some forms of parkinsonism are caused by chemicals, drugs, and a type of encephalitis prevalent in the 1920s. Most individuals, however, have the primary (idiopathic) form of PD, for which no cause has yet been discovered. Considered to be one of the most common neurologic disorders of the elderly, symptoms of PD typically become apparent between the ages of 50 and 70 years. Dementia occurs in 30% to 70% of patients with PD (Koller et al, 1994), and depression may be as high as 50% (Reich, 1995).

**Assessment.** The onset of PD is gradual, with tremor, or stiffness of the trunk or neck, slight change in gait, or other subtle signs. The three classic signs of PD are tremor, described as a "pill-rolling" movement of one or both hands when at rest; rigidity or stiffness of the body or extremities resulting in difficulty initiating and sustaining movement, and bradykinesia, which is the loss of automatic movements such as blinking, swallowing, and swinging the arms when walking. No specific test has been developed for PD, but the diagnosis can be made with the presence of two of the three classic signs listed above and a positive response to anti-Parkinson's medication.

Limitations of function in the patient with PD caused by tremor, rigidity, or bradykinesia can be significant, especially as the disease progresses. Initiation of movement is delayed, and even turning in bed,

walking, and rising from a chair are agonizingly slow or impossible for patients with severe symptoms. A shuffling gait, with little or no arm swing, and a stooped posture are common (Figure 30-17). As the disease progresses, symptoms can become quite severe, with an absence of blinking and facial expression, giving the face a masklike appearance; a decrease in spontaneous swallowing, causing drooling; a soft, low, and monotonous voice; and a lack of posture adjustment, giving the patient a statuelike appearance.

**Intervention.** Treatment of PD is symptomatic, supportive, and palliative. Medication, exercise, psychosocial interventions when necessary, and safety measures to prevent injury are the primary methods of treatment (Box 30-5).

**Medications.** Levodopa with carbidopa (Sinemet), a combination drug, is the most widely used medication for Parkinson's disease. It is particularly effective for the treatment of rigidity and bradykinesia. Levodopa is given to replenish the basal ganglia with dopamine, with carbidopa contributing to the amount of levodopa that reaches the basal ganglia. Only about 1% of ingested levodopa reaches the brain for initial conversion into dopamine in the basal ganglia, as most of the levodopa is converted by chemicals in the liver and intestine to dopamine outside the brain in the periphery

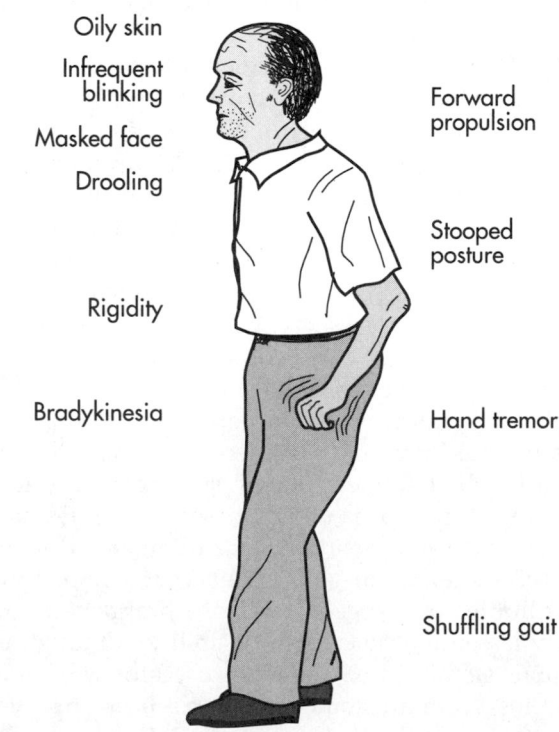

**Figure 30-17** This patient displays several outward characteristics of Parkinson's disease.

of the body. Carbidopa, which has no therapeutic effects of its own, suppresses this breakdown of dopamine by the liver and intestines to allow more dopamine to reach the brain. Excessive amounts of levodopa and carbidopa cause involuntary movements of the neck, body, and extremities (dyskinesias) and can even cause worsening of PD symptoms ("end of dose symptoms"). The smallest dose of levodopa/carbidopa that will relieve symptoms is therefore desired. Side effects include nausea, agitation, confusion, hallucinations, and the dyskinesias mentioned above. The drug is contraindicated in patients with glaucoma. A diet high in protein is thought to reduce the therapeutic effects of levodopa/carbidopa; therefore pa-

tients may be advised to take the medication 30 to 60 minutes before eating.

Selegiline (Eldepryl) was introduced as a neuroprotective medication that would slow down progression of the effects of PD. Although no studies of selegiline have demonstrated its effectiveness in halting the progression of PD (Silverstein, 1996), its use improves the effectiveness of lower doses of levodopa/carbidopa.

Bromocriptine (Parlodel) and pergolide (Permax) are medications used in Parkinson's disease to activate dopamine receptors in the basal ganglia. They prolong the therapeutic response to levodopa/carbidopa and can reduce drug-induced dyskinesias. There is a 30%

---

| BOX 30-5 | NURSING PROCESS |
| --- | --- |

## PARKINSON'S DISEASE

### ASSESSMENT

- Motor system, functional ability, activities of daily living, mental status, and emotional state
- Rigidity and slowness of body movement
- Patterns of mobility
- Communication patterns
- Medication information
- Nutrition status and swallowing ability
- Home environment

### NURSING DIAGNOSES

- Impaired physical mobility related to coordinated movements
- Self-care deficit related to altered movement patterns
- Anxiety related to inability to control illness
- Risk for injury related to altered movement patterns
- Constipation related to altered movement pattern
- Ineffective individual and family coping related to chronicity of illness
- Hopelessness
- Knowledge deficit related to drug therapy regimen
- Body image disturbance related to change in body movement

### NURSING INTERVENTIONS

- Observe for L-dopa side effects—check pulse rate and rhythm four times a day; take blood pressure in lying and standing position.
- Administer L-dopa with meals to decrease nausea.

- Reduce stress- and anxiety-producing situations—allow patient plenty of time to perform such activities as eating and dressing.
- Encourage patient to exercise and use all muscles and joints—range-of-motion exercises should be done several times a day.
- Carry out regular daily exercise program to maintain function.
- Practice writing and singing aloud.
- Use march music and lines placed at intervals on the floor to encourage larger steps.
- Encourage exercises to improve balance.
- Use stool softeners and suppositories as necessary to prevent constipation.
- Involve family and patient in all aspects of planning and giving care.
- Provide emotional support to patient and family—be calm and reassuring.

### EVALUATION OF EXPECTED OUTCOMES

- Takes appropriate precautions to prevent injury
- Sets realistic goals
- Participates in self-care as appropriate
- Reports satisfaction with self-care despite limitations
- Relates rationale for interventions
- Describes own anxiety and coping patterns; uses coping mechanisms effectively
- Demonstrates ability to understand and express self
- Demonstrates initiative and autonomy in making decisions
- Describes methods to prevent constipation

to 50% adverse effect rate of nausea, confusion, nightmares, agitation, hallucinations, paranoia, dyskinesias, and/or postural hypotension with these drugs.

Anticholinergic drugs such as trihexyphenidyl (Artane) and diphenhydramine (Benadryl) are less effective than levodopa/carbidopa in relieving symptoms of PD but generally produce fewer side effects (Lehne, 1994). These drugs are often helpful in relieving symptoms of PD, especially tremor. Anticholinergic drugs act by blocking the access of acetylcholine, an excitatory neurotransmitter, to the cholinergic receptors that contribute to the symptoms of PD. They may cause dry mouth, blurred vision, urinary retention, constipation, and tachycardia, especially in the elderly.

Amantadine (Symmetrel) promotes the release of dopamine from terminals in the basal ganglia but with less profound responses. Side effects are similar to those of the anticholinergic drugs (Table 30-3).

Other than medications, stereotaxic surgery to correct severe tremor or refractory dyskinesias is currently the only treatment for symptoms of PD. Performed in centers specializing in these procedures, stereotaxic surgery is limited to patients with medication-refractory PD. The procedure is usually effective for a few years and carries a moderate risk of stroke.

Nursing care of the patient with Parkinson's disease is symptomatic and supportive, with emphasis on safety and facilitation of the patient's maximum independence. Because PD, as well as many of the medications used for its treatment, can cause orthostatic hypotension, the patient is at particular risk for falls. Education of the patient, family, and caregivers of this and other risks is of major importance. Understanding by the patient and family of the medication regimen, including possible side effects, is crucial. Scheduling medications around meals and activities throughout the day can make a great deal of difference in the patient's level of function. For maximum effect, medications usually are carefully balanced and monitored and adjusted as indicated by symptoms. Diet, elimination, and exercise are important in the program of care. As for all patients with chronic disease, psychosocial support and information about community resources can make a positive difference in the quality of life for PD patients, and for all involved, especially as the disease progresses. The American Parkinson Disease Association, Inc., and the National Parkinson Foundation, Inc., are national organizations that can provide valuable information and have local chapters throughout the United States.

## Alzheimer's Disease

Alzheimer's disease (AD) is a chronic, degenerative disease that causes gradual, progressive decline in cognition (**dementia**) and other functions of the brain. Women are affected more often than men, and onset is usually after the age of 45 years. It is the major cause of dementia in the elderly, but the familial form of AD may strike younger adults as well. Although the etiology of this disease remains unknown, brain tissue of patients with AD has shown degenerative changes caused by neurofibrillary tangles, which are thought to occur because of accumulation of a protein (Duara, 1996). Major research is under way to investigate this theory further, as well as to study other possible causes and treatments for AD. Research has already suggested that risk factors may be associated with AD, such as prior head injury and history of malaria (Kawas et al, 1996). Abnormal immune function, viral infection, and genetics are among widely considered etiologies. Decline in short-term memory is one of the most common initial signs of AD, with changes in speech, judgment, and behavior being other possible early manifestations. As the disease progresses, attentiveness, long-term memory, personal hygiene, and even recognition of familiar surroundings and family members are impaired. Eventually, the individual is unable to communicate or perform any voluntary motor function, such as stand, walk, or swallow. Progression of symptoms leading to major disability and total dependence varies over time but can span as long as 20 years. Death usually is caused by a complication of immobility, such as aspiration pneumonia. There is no known treatment.

Nursing care of the AD patient is supportive, with patient comfort and family support being major objectives. Patients with AD respond more readily to tone of voice and gestures than to the content of conversation. A calm, slow manner will usually project a feeling of comfort and acceptance to the patient (Stolley, 1994). Prevention of injury, nutrition support, and maximum quality of life for patient and family require education and resources for all involved. Depression, a common consequence of the responsibility of being caregiver for a family member with AD, often surfaces within the first year (Burns et al, 1996). The nurse needs to recognize the needs of caregivers and provide or facilitate support whenever possible. National, state, and local associations for the support of patients with AD and their caregivers are excellent resources for materials, information, and as support groups.

## Guillain-Barré Syndrome

Guillain-Barré syndrome (GBS) is an acute, potentially fatal inflammation of the peripheral nerves that can involve the entire body. Symptoms most often begin in the lower extremities but can also first occur in the

**TABLE 30-3**

## Pharmacology of Drugs for Neurologic Disorders

| DRUG (GENERIC AND TRADE NAME); ROUTE AND DOSAGE | ACTION/INDICATION | COMMON SIDE EFFECTS AND NURSING CONSIDERATIONS |
|---|---|---|
| **Amantadine** (Symmetrel)<br>**Route:** PO<br>**Dosage:** 100 mg 1-2 times qd | Antiviral agent also used for the initial or adjunct treatment of Parkinson's disease | Dizziness, ataxia, insomnia, hypotension, skin mottling; use with caution in seizure disorders, liver, cardiac, and renal disease, and in elderly |
| **Bromocriptine** (Parlodel)<br>**Route:** PO<br>**Dosage:** 1.25 mg tablet bid with meals initially; increase gradually according to symptoms | An adjunct drug for Parkinson's disease used to reduce motor fluctuations; may prolong action of carbidopa/levodopa | Nausea; psychiatric reactions such as confusion, agitation, nightmares, hallucinations, and paranoid delusions; dyskinesias; orthostatic hypotension |
| **Carbamazepine** (Tegretol)<br>**Route:** PO<br>**Dosage:** Begin with 200 mg at bedtime and increase by 200 mg q 1-3 days until therapeutic range achieved; usual dose is 800-1200 mg daily in divided doses 3-4 times qd. Newer, sustained-release form can be given twice daily | Antiepileptic drug for prophylaxis of generalized tonic-clonic and partial seizures<br>Also used for neuropathic pain disorders, such as trigeminal neuralgia | Diplopia, drowsiness, ataxia, malaise, headache if advanced too rapidly; bone depression is rare; however, drug is contraindicated in patients with history of blood disorders; use with caution in hepatic and cardiac disease |
| **Carbidopa/Levodopa** (Sinemet)<br>**Route:** PO<br>**Dosage:** 10/100, 25/100, 25/250 tablets: 2-6 or more daily in frequent, divided doses; 50/300 sustained-release tablets (CR): 2 or more qd. Strength and frequency according to symptoms | Used for relief of the symptoms of Parkinson's disease, especially bradykinesia and rigidity | Involuntary movements, nausea and vomiting, cardiac dysrhythmias, orthostatic hypotension, hallucinations, psychiatric disturbances; foods high in protein are thought to inhibit action, therefore, administer 30 min before or 1 hr after eating |
| **Selegiline** (Eldepryl)<br>**Route:** PO<br>**Dosage:** 5-mg tablet at breakfast and lunch | First 1-2 yr: may retard progression of Parkinson's disease and prolong effects of carbidopa/levodopa | Insomnia; dosage may need to be decreased if there are increased side effects of carbidopa/levodopa |
| **Trihexyphenidyl** (Artane)<br>**Route:** PO<br>**Dosage:** 1-2 mg/day initially; increase gradually by 2 mg 3-5 days; maintenance dose 3-15 mg/day in 3-4 divided doses | Used in the management of Parkinson's disease, primarily for tremor | Dry mouth, blurred vision, urinary retention, constipation, tachycardia (may be dose-related); confusion, depression, hallucinations; use with caution in elderly; do not discontinue abruptly |
| **Valproic acid** (Depakene, Depakote)<br>**Route:** PO<br>**Dosage:** 750-1500 mg/day in 2-3 divided doses | Antiepileptic drug used to prevent generalized and partial seizures; also used for treatment of headache and in psychiatric disorders | Give with food to prevent nausea and indigestion; uncommon: weight gain, weight loss, hair loss, tremor (may be dose related); liver damage, blood disorder; contraindicated in pregnancy |

hands or cranial nerves. Usual symptoms are numbness, tingling **(paresthesia)**, weakness, and pain in the feet (less commonly the hands) that spreads over all extremities toward the body. This process may take hours or days and may affect the peripheral nerves of the entire body and brain stem. Symptoms can vary in intensity, and pain can be severe. The autonomic nervous system may be affected in severe cases of GBS, which can cause such problems as orthostatic hypotension, hypertension, bradycardia, and heart block.

Progression of GBS to the lower brain stem affects the cranial nerves, which can cause paresthesia and weakness of the face, weakening of the eye muscles, and dysphagia. The most serious complication of GBS is respiratory failure, and approximately 20% of patients require ventilatory support. The cause of GBS is unknown, but it is believed to be an immune response in susceptible individuals with trauma, viral infection, surgery, viral immunization, or neoplasm affecting the lymphatic system. Between 5% and 10% of patients with GBS do not survive because of respiratory failure or cardiac dysrhythmias (Michalek, Walleck, 1996). Survivors of GBS usually have a complete recovery, although rehabilitation over weeks and months is usually necessary. In the chronic form of GBS, paralysis evolves more slowly and the cranial nerves are not affected. Full recovery does not usually occur, and, although patients may gradually improve over 1 to 2 years, they may be left with varying degrees of paresthesia and weakness. Men and women are affected with GBS equally, and it usually occurs between the ages of 20 and 50 years.

The diagnosis of GBS is based on symptoms, neurologic examination, CSF examination, and electromyogram (EMG) results. Primary treatment is with plasmapheresis or intravenous immunoglobulin, and corticosteroids can be used as an additional medication. Nursing care plays a vital role in the management of GBS. The nursing focus is assessment of baseline neurologic and respiratory functions and careful monitoring for changes from the patient's baseline. Respiratory insufficiency is the major complication of GBS, and early detection and treatment with mechanical support to provide adequate ventilation may be lifesaving. Pneumonia, deep vein thrombus (DVT), pulmonary embolism (PE), and skin breakdown are also potential, serious complications, along with other problems of impaired mobility. Education and psychosocial support of the patient and family are required on an ongoing basis, during both the acute and rehabilitation phase of GBS.

## Myasthenia Gravis

Myasthenia gravis (MG) is a chronic neuromuscular disease characterized by fluctuating weakness. The weakness results from an interruption in the action of acetylcholine, the neurotransmitter substance that carries the nerve impulse from the nerve fiber to receptor sites that stimulate the muscle to contract. After it is stimulated, the muscle produces cholinesterase, an enzyme that inactivates acetylcholine, thus allowing the muscle to relax after use. This process occurs at the neuromuscular junction. In MG, an autoimmune response is thought to produce antibodies that act at the neuromuscular junction to reduce the number of attachment sites available for acetylcholine. This reduction results in insufficient muscle contraction and weakness. The etiology of the autoimmune process is not known, although a viral infection is suspected as a precipitant of the disease (Ozuna, 1996a). Tumor of the thymus gland (thymoma) is found in approximately 15% of persons with MG, and 85% of these improve with removal of the thymus gland (thymoma). The course and prognosis of MG are variable. There may be short-term remissions, a stable, chronic condition, or severe, progressive disease.

Myasthenia gravis occurs most often between 20 and 30 years of age, with women being affected slightly more than men. In patients with thymoma and MG, the majority are men over the age of 50 years.

**Assessment.** The primary symptom of MG is muscle weakness or fatigue, which occurs after activity and improves with rest. The muscles most often involved are those used for moving the eyes and eyelids, chewing, swallowing, speaking, and breathing. When these muscles are affected, **ptosis** (drooping of eyelids), dysarthria, dysphagia, nasal speech, and shortness of breath may occur. The muscles of the trunk and extremities also can be affected, with the neck and hip muscles typically weaker than those of the distal extremities. The muscles affected by MG are generally strongest in the morning and become exhausted with continued activity. Sensation and all other neurologic function, including cognition, are normal in MG, and the muscles themselves are not affected.

The diagnosis of MG is made on the basis of history, physical examination, and electromyography (EMG). Intravenous administration of a test dose of edrophonium chloride (Tensilon, Enlon), a short-acting cholinesterase inhibitor that slows the breakdown of the neurotransmitter acetylcholine, results in brief improvement in the strength of the affected muscles in the individual with MG. This test can be done at the patient's bedside or in the office or outpatient area; however, bradycardia, bronchial constriction, and other effects of uninhibited action of acetylcholine may occur. Therefore the patient should be monitored closely during and immediately after the test, and atropine should available if needed to reverse bradycardia and other effects of Tensilon (Lehne, 1994).

**Intervention.** Oral anticholinesterase drugs are the mainstay of treatment. Neostigmine (Prostigmin) and pyridostigmine (Mestinon) are two of the most successful in this group of drugs. One if these is given as ordered to prolong the action of acetylcholine by inhibiting cholinesterase at the neuromuscular junction. The action is the same as Tensilon, but with longer, more gradual action. Dosage must be tailored for each individual, as too little medication can cause an exacerbation of symptoms, called **myasthenic crisis,** and overmedication can produce **cholinergic crisis**, which causes generalized weakness. Either of these situations can cause severe respiratory distress and the need for ventilatory assistance. Corticosteroids also can be used to suppress the immune response in MG, and less often, cytotoxic drugs such as azathioprine (Imuran) and cyclophosphamide (Cytoxan). Many drugs are contraindicated or should be used with extreme caution in patients with MG. Among classes of drugs that should be evaluated before use include anesthetics, antibiotics, dysrhythmics, antipsychotics, barbiturates, diuretics, narcotics, muscle relaxants, thyroid preparations, and tranquilizers (Ozuna, 1996b). Thymectomy is indicated in patients with thymoma and in certain other cases.

Plasmapheresis, the process of washing acetylcholine-receptor antibodies from the plasma, is a short-term treatment indicated for patients in crisis or when corticosteroids are contraindicated (e.g., in preparation for surgery). Education of the patient and family should include measures for conserving strength, medication action and side effects, and the recognition of symptoms that indicate a pending emergency (myasthenic crisis, anticholinergic crisis). The nurse should always include psychosocial support and information about community and national associations, such as the Myasthenia Gravis Foundation, Inc., in the plan of care.

# REHABILITATION FOR NEUROLOGIC DISORDERS

Rehabilitation of the patient with a neurologic disorder is integrated in all aspects of care and begins on admission. Self-care—a basic tenet of rehabilitation—should be encouraged, with the patient performing as many activities of daily living as possible and reasonable, with assistance as needed. The patient should not be rushed in these endeavors and should be praised and encouraged in all efforts and progress, no matter how small. Timing of activities is important, and new learning experiences should be attempted only when the patient is well rested.

Independence in mobility, either walking or by using a wheelchair, helps to diminish the patient's feelings of helplessness. The nurse is involved in teaching the patient to transfer from bed to wheelchair and wheelchair to toilet, by leading with the nonpara-lyzed side of the hemiparetic patient, or by assisting the patient with generalized weakness according to individual needs. In assisting the hemiparetic patient, the nurse should assist the patient to dress the weak side first and support the patient's weak side when walking. A belt placed around the patient's waist and held in back for support helps to maintain balance and offers the patient a feeling of security. A sling or other individualized upper extremity support of the affected arm and hand following stroke can prevent separation of the shoulder joint (subluxation). The apparatus should be applied so that the hand is fully supported and aligned so that the hand is positioned higher than the wrist and the wrist higher than the elbow to prevent edema. A forearm splint to maintain functional positioning of the hand and wrist is often used to prevent wrist drop and flexion contractures.

The patient who has suffered a severe neurologic insult has experienced changes that may be overwhelming. Although intellect may be intact, the body may no longer respond as desired and expected. The patient may be unable to speak intelligibly, move at will, or control even basic bodily functions. Self-perception may be altered drastically, and emotional reactions are to be anticipated. There may be outbursts of anger, tears, or depression in response to the fear, anxiety, and frustration the patient may be experiencing. By remaining calm, supportive, and reassuring, the nurse can provide opportunities for the patient to express his or her feelings and to experience positive feedback during the crucial early stages of recovery and rehabilitation.

The nurse shares with other team members the responsibility of preparing the patient for discharge. Team members may include physical therapist, occupational therapist, speech therapist, neuropsychologist, dietitian, and social worker. Both the patient and family should be involved in planning for care after discharge. If the patient is to return home, the environment should be assessed for safety, with any necessary assistive devices installed before discharge.- Extensive teaching, depending on the degree of neurologic deficit, may be needed to provide the patient and family with the knowledge, skill, and confidence to maintain the patient at home. Home health assistance, such as visiting nurses and aids, may be needed, especially until the family is comfortable providing care at home. Physical therapy and speech therapy also can be provided in the home, depending on availability and resources of the patient. The family should be encouraged to maintain as normal a home environment as possible, with consideration for the patient's capabilities.

## NURSING CARE PLAN

## PATIENT WHO IS CONFUSED

Mr. Wilson is a 19-year-old male who was brought into the trauma center by the police after having been found wandering aimlessly along a dirt road by a passing motorist. Details of the patient's accident are still not complete, but the police found an overturned, smashed motorcycle approximately 500 feet from where the patient was discovered. On arrival, it was noted that the patient was not wearing a helmet and had a strong odor of alcohol on his breath. A blood-alcohol level was drawn, as well as other drug toxicology studies, but the results are being kept confidential on the advice of his lawyer. Identification was confirmed through a wallet found near the cycle. His vital signs have been stable but difficult to obtain because he has been combative since his arrival. Physical examination also has been difficult to perform because of his altering states of cooperation.

He has a large facial laceration extending from just above the right eyebrow to the center midhair line (approximately 8 cm). Frontal swelling is noted along his forehead. Skull x-ray examinations are negative for a fracture, and he has had a cranial CT scan. The laceration was sutured with 6-0 nylon sutures and xylocaine.

He is moving all extremities without evidence of pain or tenderness. Abdominal trauma is being questioned because he has guarding and wincing on palpation of the left upper quadrant. Serial hematocrits have been stable, ruling out a ruptured spleen. Vital signs are stable, and his pupils are equal and reactive to light. He has been uncooperative in testing his hand grasp. His condition is felt to be stable, but he is being admitted for observation because of the ingestion of unknown substance(s) and possible loss of consciousness at the scene of the accident. His score on the Glasgow Coma Scale is 12, with orientation only to self.

| Medical History | Psychosocial Data | Assessment Data |
|---|---|---|
| Provided by anxious parents, who were notified once identification had been established | Lives with parents and three younger brothers | Well-developed, well-nourished male who is oriented to self only; cannot state orientation to time, place, or persons |
| Generally good health; recently passed Army physical examination and was awaiting orders to attend basic training; had plans to join the Reserves to obtain its college assistance program | Second year of college; business major | Does not appear to recognize parents |
| | Reported to be in scholastic jeopardy due to low grades | Vital signs stable: T 99, P 84, R 22, BP 126/78 |
| | | *Skin:* Color good; multiple abrasions on right forehead; sutures dry and intact; no evidence of infection |
| | Active in sports, likes basketball best | Abrasions also on right chest wall; no drainage |
| | Has part-time job at local McDonald's | No rashes, no edema |
| | | *Head:* Patent nares; no discharge |
| | Has had driver's license since age 16 | Cut on upper lip; central upper incisor loose |
| Immunizations up-to-date; last tetanus booster 2 years ago because of a foot laceration with sutures | One conviction of driving while intoxicated (DWI), age 18 | *EENT:* Full extraocular movements (EOMs); pupils round, equal, and react to light accommodation; visual acuity intact |
| | | No complaints of dizziness or diplopia |
| No known food or drug allergies. No history of hospitalization/surgeries | Has attended mandatory DWI classes; license just renewed | *Respiratory:* Regular rate and rhythm; no use of accessory muscles |
| | | Chest movements symmetric; clear to percussion and auscultation; no rales, rhonchi, or rubs |
| | Covered by parents' health insurance | *Abdominal:* Soft; slight tenderness in upper left quadrant, with some guarding on palpation; nondistended; bowel sounds present all quadrants |
| | Protestant religion; no active church involvement | *Musculoskeletal:* Moving all extremities well; full range of motion |
| | | Equal grasps and sensations; DTRs intact, 2+, and symmetric |
| | | Babinski sign negative; unable to test for Romberg's sign |

## NURSING CARE PLAN
## PATIENT WHO IS CONFUSED—cont'd

| Medical History | Psychosocial Data | Assessment Data |
|---|---|---|
| | Said to have many girlfriends, recently depressed over loss of special girlfriend | Is right-handed |

*Neuro:* Follows commands inconsistently; speech rambling; some echolalia

No memory of events before accident

Cannot name president of United States or identify basic colors

Will count to 10 only; no ability to add or subtract

Periods of increased agitation and crying

Unable to test all cranial nerves owing to lack of cooperation

Will shrug shoulders, blink, raise eyebrows, smile, frown, and yawn

*Cardiovascular:* Apical pulse 82 and regular; no diaphoresis

**Laboratory data**

Hct stable at 34-36; checked every 3 hours for first 24 hours

Hgb 12.2; oxygen saturations stable at 96-98

Platelets, electrolytes, liver function tests (LFTs), BUN, FBS all within normal limits (WNL)

Urinalysis WNL; no gross or microscopic hematuria

Chest x-ray and flat plate of abdomen all negative

**Medications**

No medications

IV 1000 ml D5W in Ringer's lactate at 80 ml per hour

IV removed by patient; decision to restart pending tolerance of PO fluids

Clear liquid diet; advance as tolerated; nursing judgment

### NURSING DIAGNOSIS

Sensory/perceptual alterations related to head trauma and question of drug ingestion as evidenced by confusion, anxiety, and apprehension

### NURSING INTERVENTIONS

Assess patient for signs and symptoms of decreased cerebral tissue perfusion: dizziness, syncope, blurred or dimmed vision, diplopia, or any change in his visual field.

Monitor for a decreased level of consciousness, seizures, paresthesia, motor weakness, paralysis, and unequal pupils (late sign), or an absent pupillary reaction to light.

Monitor vital signs every 2 hours until stable. Report any deviations from the baseline.

Orient patient to reality: call him by name. Tell him your name and why you are with him.

Give background information (time, place, and date) often throughout the day.

Orient him to his environment, including sights and sounds. (Example: "This is a hospital. I am a nurse caring for you. You are hearing the food cart go down the hall.")

Have parents bring in photos and personal articles from home.

### EVALUATION OF EXPECTED OUTCOMES

Does not show signs of altered tissue perfusion related to an interruption in cerebral blood flow

Level of consciousness does not deteriorate

Communicates in a lucid manner

Reestablishes a sleep-wake cycle

Shows an interest in external environment

Demonstrates an increased ability to react to reality

At discharge, oriented to self, person, place, and time

Periods of agitation, anxiety, and confusion diminished or absent

*Continued*

# NURSING CARE PLAN

## PATIENT WHO IS CONFUSED—cont'd

| NURSING INTERVENTIONS | EVALUATION OF EXPECTED OUTCOMES |
|---|---|
| Talk to patient while providing care. Encourage the family to discuss past and present events with him.<br>Arrange to be with him at predetermined times to avoid feelings of isolation.<br>Turn on the TV and radio for short periods of time, based on his interests, to help him orient to reality.<br>Hold his hand while talking to soothe him.<br>Monitor his response.<br>Continually monitor neurologic signs and report changes immediately.<br>Always approach in a calm, gentle manner to avoid startling him.<br>Encourage regular sleep patterns and routines.<br>Encourage the family to visit often. Provide reassurances and explanations to aid their understanding of his condition.<br>Suggest that friends send cards rather than visit or call during the acute stage. | |

**NURSING DIAGNOSIS**

Risk for injury related to the question of drug ingestion and cerebral trauma

| NURSING INTERVENTIONS | EVALUATION OF EXPECTED OUTCOMES |
|---|---|
| While orienting patient to the environment, state his boundaries.<br>Assess his ability to use the call bell.<br>Keep the side rails up at all times, with the bed in the low position and the wheels locked.<br>Keep a light on at night to prevent falls.<br>Conduct a close watch on him, especially when he is agitated.<br>Teach the family about the need for safe illumination, especially if he has distorted images.<br>Monitor his gait when he ambulates. Have two people ready if he is unsteady.<br>Have a system in place to call for assistance if he is extremely agitated.<br>Assist patient when eating.<br>Monitor for safe use of utensils.<br>Have him do as much self-care as possible (e.g., brushing teeth). Praise him for any attempts.<br>Discuss the need for nonskid slippers or sneakers when ambulating.<br>Assess his visual acuity before ambulation.<br>Discuss safety after returning home with his parents. Inquire into their ability to remain home with him until he feels safe.<br>Discuss the effect of patient's confusion on his younger siblings. | Remains safe and free of injury while in a confused state<br>Identifies factors that could increase potential for injury<br>Cooperates in keeping himself free from harm<br>Parents incorporate safety teachings into discharge plans<br>Cooperates in applying safety measures to prevent injury<br>Family develops strategies to maintain safety upon discharge to home<br>Optimizes ADL within sensorimotor limitations |

# NURSING CARE PLAN
## PATIENT WHO IS CONFUSED—cont'd

**NURSING DIAGNOSIS**

Impaired verbal communication related to the questionable history of drug ingestion and the cerebral trauma, as evidenced by periods of crying, echolalia, and garbled speech

| NURSING INTERVENTIONS | EVALUATION OF EXPECTED OUTCOMES |
|---|---|
| Speak slowly and distinctly when addressing patient. | Needs are met consistently |
| Stand where he can see and hear you. | Patient and family communicate at a |
| Reorient him to reality. Use a large calendar and reality orientation boards. | satisfactory level |
| | Correctly answers two direct questions |
| Use short, simple phrases and yes-or-no questions, especially when his frustration level is high. | By the time of discharge, echolalia is gone and speech is no longer garbled |
| Be prepared to repeat the words or directions. | Communicates basic needs (e.g., use |
| Monitor for signs of understanding (nodding his head, frowning). | of the urinal, need for privacy) to staff and his family through ges- |
| Encourage his attempts at communication. | tures and sign language before re- |
| Listen carefully for identifiable words. Provide reinforcement when he is lucid. | gaining oral ability |
| Allow ample time for a response. | |
| Do not answer questions for him. Teach his family the same. | |
| Do not pretend to understand if you do not. This only adds to his confusion. | |
| Remove distractions from environment during his attempts to communicate (e.g., lower the sound on the TV). | |
| Adjust his care plan as progress develops. | |

**NURSING DIAGNOSIS**

Pain: headache related to cerebral trauma as evidenced by crying and wincing with head movement and swelling in the frontal area of his head

| NURSING INTERVENTIONS | EVALUATION OF EXPECTED OUTCOMES |
|---|---|
| Determine how patient usually responds to pain. | By body language, indicates that ag- |
| Assess for nonverbal signs of headache (wrinkled brow, clenched fists, squinting, rubbing head, avoidance of bright lights and noises). | gravating factors have been de- creased or eliminated |
| Assess for any verbal attempts at communication of pain. | Cooperates more fully in his neuro- logic assessments and participates |
| Assess for factors that seem to aggravate head pain. | in nursing care activities |
| Implement measures to relieve the pain (quiet environment, dim lights, avoidance of any sudden movements). | Obtains relief from headache as evi- denced by verbalization of head- |
| Provide nonpharmacologic measures for headache relief (e.g., cool cloth to forehead, back rub, distraction). | ache relief, relaxed facial expression, and body posturing |
| Involve family to assist in soothing pain by gentle touch. | Shows increased participation in activities |
| Administer nonnarcotic analgesics if ordered. | |
| Monitor results. Consult physician if above action fails to relieve headache. | |

# KEY CONCEPTS

➤ The purpose of the neurologic examination is to determine the presence or absence of neurologic dysfunction and to localize the site of a pathologic condition.

➤ Common diagnostic studies include lumbar puncture, electroencephalogram, electromyogram, computed tomography, and magnetic resonance imaging.

➤ Care of patients with altered states of cerebral functioning is a primary function of the neurologic nurse. Any changes in a patient's neurologic status should be assessed, reported, and documented immediately.

➤ The Glasgow Coma Scale is a tool developed for standardized, accurate reporting of a patient's level of consciousness.

➤ Deterioration in the level of consciousness is often the *first* sign of increasing intracranial pressure and should be recognized, reported, and documented at the first sign of change.

➤ Changes in pupillary response to light, vital signs, and motor weakness are *late* signs of intracranial pressure and constitute an extreme emergency. Any changes in these parameters should be reported and documented immediately.

➤ Nursing responsibilities while the patient is having a seizure are to protect from injury and accurately observe and record behavior before, during, and after the episode.

➤ Appropriate antibiotic therapy, supportive measures, and rehabilitation are interventions for infections of the nervous system.

➤ Chronic disorders affecting the nervous system may develop over a period of days or years and can cause some degree of chronic disability. Nursing care is supportive and is based on actual or potential problems of the patient and family.

# CRITICAL THINKING EXERCISES

1. What are important nursing considerations in caring for a patient during a seizure? What behaviors should you observe and record during the seizure?
2. Discuss some ways that the patient with multiple sclerosis might conserve energy and avoid becoming overly fatigued.

3. What is the difference between a cholinergic and a myasthenic crisis? Discuss some important nursing considerations to prevent these situations from occurring.

## REFERENCES AND ADDITIONAL READINGS

Blissitt PA: Physiologic responses to generalized convulsive status epilepticus, *J Neurosci Nurs* 28(6):396, 1996.

Bond EF: Critical care. In Lewis SM, Collier IC, Heitkemper MM, editors: *Medical-surgical nursing: assessment and management of clinical problems,* ed 4, St Louis, 1996, Mosby.

Brodie MD, Dichter MA: Antiepileptic drugs, *N Engl J Med* 334(3):168-174, 1996.

Burns R et al: Caring for the caregiver, *Patient Care* 30(18): 108-112, 1996.

Cason CL, Sample JG: Preparatory information for myelogram, *J Neurosci Nurs* 27(3):182-187, 1995.

Dowling GA: Sleep in older women with Parkinson's disease, *J Neurosci Nurs* 27(6):355-362, 1995.

Drugs for epilepsy, *The Medical Letter* 37(947):37-40, 1995.

Duara R, Douglas G, Gerard S: Unlocking the mysteries of Alzheimer's disease, *Patient Care* 30(18):44-56, 1996.

Eisen A: Amyotrophic lateral sclerosis, *Intern Med* 34(9): 824-832, 1995.

Evans MJ: *Neurologic-neurosurgical nursing,* Springhouse, Penn, 1995, Springhouse.

Faught RE: Diagnosis and classification of epileptic seizures, *Fed Prac* (suppl) 7-8, 1995.

Foreman MD: Nursing strategies for acute confusion in elders, *Am J Nurs* 96(4):44-49, 1996.

Geary SM: Nursing management of cranial nerve dysfunction, *J Neurosci Nurs* 27(2):102-108, 1995.

Geraci EB, Geraci T: A look at recent hyperventilation studies: outcomes and recommendations for early use in the head-injured patient, *J Neurosci Nurs* 28(4):222-233, 1996.

Guyton AC: *Human physiology and mechanisms of disease,* ed 5, Philadelphia, 1992, Saunders.

Hickey JV: *The clinical practice of neurological and neurosurgical nursing,* ed 4, Philadelphia, 1997, Lippincott.

Hook EW, Ennis DM: Selected spirochetal infections: syphilis and Lyme disease. In Barker LR et al, editors: *Principles of ambulatory medicine,* ed 4, Baltimore, 1995, Williams & Wilkins.

Howser RL: Corticosteroid therapy, *Am J Nurs* 95(8):44-48, 1995.

Jansen DA, Cimprich B: Attentional impairment in persons with multiple sclerosis, *J Neurosci Nurs* 26(2):95-102, 1994.

Johnson CC: Clearing up the confusion, *Nursing 95* 25(11):39-45, 1995.

Juarez VJ, Lyons M: Interrater reliability of the Glasgow Coma Scale, *J Neurosci Nurs* 27(5):283-286, 1995.

Kawas C, Schneider LS, Whitehouse PJ: Treating Alzheimer's disease: today and tomorrow, *Patient Care* 30(18): 62-83, 1996.

Kelley CL: The role of interferons in the treatment of multiple sclerosis, *J Neurosci Nurs* 28(2):114-120, 1996.

Kernich CA, Kaminski HJ: Myasthenia gravis: pathophysiology, diagnosis and collaborative care, *J Neurosci Nurs* 27(4):207-215, 1995.

Kerr, ME, Walleck, CA: Intracranial problems. In Lewis SM, Collier IC, Heitkemper MM, editors: *Medical-surgical nursing: assessment and management of clinical problems,* ed 4, St Louis, 1996, Mosby.

Koller WC, Silver DE, Lieberman A: An algorithm for the management of Parkinson's disease, *Neurology* 44(12 [suppl 10]):S1-S52, 1994.

Lehne RA: *Pharmacology for nursing care,* ed 2, Philadelphia, 1994, Saunders.

Leppik IE: Current management of status epilepticus, *Pharmacol Ther* 21(suppl 5):6-20, 1996.

Lewis SM, Collier IC, Heitkemper MM: *Medical-surgical nursing: assessment and management of clinical problems,* ed 4, St Louis, 1996, Mosby.

McGuinness S: Learned helplessness in the multiple sclerosis population, *J Neurosci Nurs* 28(3): 163-170, 1996.

Michalek DH, Walleck CA: Peripheral nerve and spinal cord problems. In Lewis SM, Collier IC, Heitkemper MM, editors: *Medical-surgical nursing: assessment and management of clinical problems,* ed 4, St Louis, 1996, Mosby.

O'Hanlon-Nichols T: Intracranial tumors, *Am J Nurs* 96(4): 38-39, 1996.

Ozuna JM: Nervous system. In Lewis SM, Collier IC, Heitkemper MM, editors: *Medical-surgical nursing: assessment and management of clinical problems,* ed 4, St Louis, 1996a, Mosby.

Ozuna JM: Chronic neurologic problems. In Lewis SM, Collier IC, Heitkemper MM, editors: *Medical-surgical nursing: assessment and management of clinical problems,* ed 4, St Louis, 1996b, Mosby.

Parker CD: Emergency! Fast action for subarachnoid hemorrhage, *Am J Nurs* 95(1):47, 1995.

Reich SG: Common disorders of movement: tremor and Parkinson's disease. In Barker LR, Burton JR, Zieve PD, editors: *Principles of ambulatory medicine,* ed 4, Baltimore, 1995, Williams & Wilkins.

Schapiro RT et al: Living with multiple sclerosis: the outlook improves, *Patient Care* 31(1):87-92, 1997.

Silverstein PM: Moderate Parkinson's disease, *Postgrad Med* 99(1):52-68, 1996.

Specht DM: Cerebral edema, *Nursing 95* 25(11):34-38, 1995.

Stolley JM: Alzheimer's disease, *Am J Nurs* 94(8):34-40, 1994.

Testani-Dufour L, Morrison CAM: Brain attack: correlative anatomy, *J Neurosci Nurs* 29(4):213-222, 1997.

Vernon GM, Jenkins M: Health maintenance behaviors in advanced Parkinson's disease, *J Neurosci Nurs* 27(4):229-235, 1995.

# CHAPTER 31

# Cerebrovascular Accidents

## CHAPTER OBJECTIVES

1 Identify two major categories of stroke.
2 Describe the signs and symptoms of stroke.
3 Explain the goal of acute stroke management.
4 Describe nursing interventions for a patient with decreased mobility.
5 Discuss nursing assessment for a patient with the stroke effect of neglect.
6 Explain which side of the brain is affected in patients with communication disorders.
7 List the stroke-related impairments that might affect a patient's nutritional status.
8 Describe stroke-related factors that might contribute to changes in elimination.
9 Explain altered sleep patterns in stroke.
10 Discuss the effect of poor family coping on stroke patients.
11 List the signs and symptoms of cerebral edema.
12 Identify factors affecting a patient's risk for pneumonia.
13 Discuss circulatory complications of stroke.
14 Describe the most frequent cause of injury in hospitalized stroke patients.
15 Describe a major complication of depression that follows a stroke.

## KEY TERMS

agnosia
aphasia
apraxia
ataxia
deep vein thrombosis (DVT)
dysarthria
dysphagia
embolus
hemianopsia
hemiplegia
hemorrhagic stroke
ischemic stroke
neglect
spasticity
thrombosis
transient ischemic attack (TIA)

Cerebrovascular disease is the third most common cause of death in the United States and the most common cause of permanent neurologic disability in adults. However, the death rate from this disease has declined since the 1970s, largely as a result of improved health habits (e.g., a decrease in cigarette smoking and improved exercise habits) and improved medical management of diseases such as hypertension and hypercholesteremia. Current mortality data show a greater frequency of stroke among men than women and a greater frequency among nonwhites than whites (Gillum, 1988). The stroke rate is 50% higher in African American men than in Caucasian men and 130% higher in African American women than in Caucasian women. The incidence of hypertension and atherosclerosis bears a direct relationship to the incidence of cerebrovascular disease.

## PATHOPHYSIOLOGY

Strokes can be classified into two major categories, **ischemic stroke** and **hemorrhagic stroke** (Figure 31-1). An ischemic stroke has either a thrombotic or an embolic mechanism. A thrombotic stroke results from the

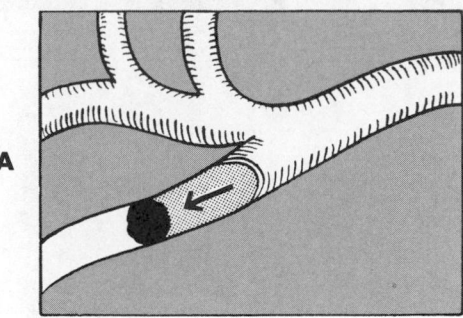

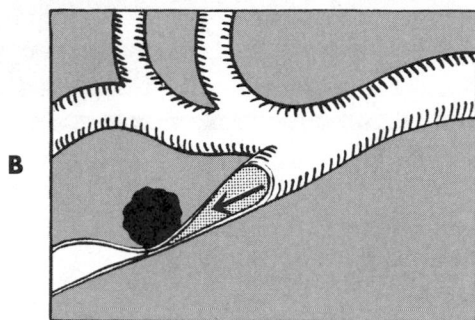

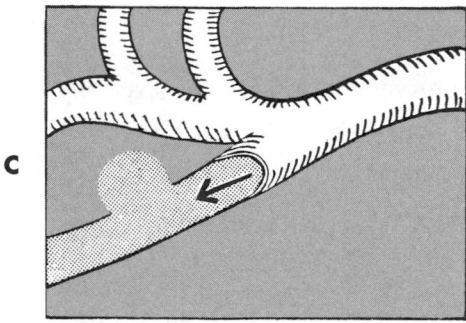

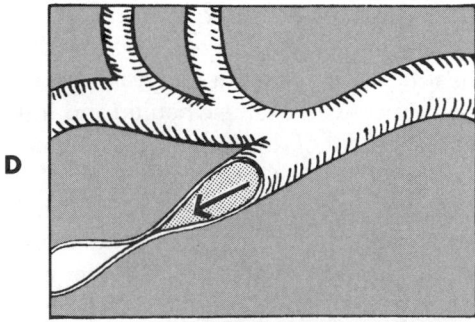

**Figure 31-1** Causes of cerebrovascular accident. **A,** Blood clot formation in the blood vessel, resulting in occlusion and ischemia. **B,** Pressure on the blood vessel from a blood clot, tumor, or anything that compresses the blood vessel, resulting in ischemia. **C,** Rupture of the blood vessel with hemorrhage into adjacent tissue. **D,** Closing of the blood vessel caused by spasm or contraction, resulting in blockage of blood flow and ischemia.

narrowing and ultimate occlusion of a vessel by an atherosclerotic plaque **(thrombosis).** Before an actual thrombotic stroke occurs, many patients experience a **transient ischemic attack (TIA).** A TIA is characterized by the sudden onset of a neurologic deficit that lasts less than 24 hours and that leaves the patient at his or her neurologic baseline. It is a warning sign of a stroke, and, if intervention is taken, the patient often is spared a significant neurologic event.

An embolic stroke is caused by blockage of a cerebral blood vessel by a small clot **(embolus);** these clots most often are tiny emboli that are carried to the brain as a result of atrial fibrillation. The onset and progression of symptoms usually are rapid because of the sudden ischemia in the brain.

A hemorrhagic stroke occurs as either an intracerebral or a subarachnoid hemorrhage. Intracerebral hemorrhage involves bleeding into the brain tissue caused by the rupture of a small blood vessel, often as a result of hypertension. The site of hemorrhage usually is deep within the brain tissue. A major hemorrhage can cause herniation and death. Subarachnoid hemorrhage occurs as a result of bleeding into the subarachnoid space; it often is a result of a ruptured aneurysm or an arteriovenous malformation.

## ASSESSMENT

### Acute Stroke

Stroke is considered an emergency. As soon as symptoms of stroke are apparent, it is important to recognize these symptoms and act on them immediately. The early signs and symptoms of stroke depend on the cause, location, and extent of the insult. TIAs precede many thrombotic events. Symptoms may include difficulty with speech, visual changes, dizziness, headache, confusion, or motor weakness. If left untreated, these symptoms may progress to more permanent deficits. Hemorrhagic events occur more suddenly and without warning. Headache, seizures, and rapid deterioration in level of consciousness may occur.

When a new stroke first comes to medical attention, the patient's respiratory, cardiac, and neurologic status must be evaluated rapidly. A large stroke or hemorrhage can cause cerebral edema, which could lead to a threat to respiratory status. Stroke is sometimes caused by cardiac arrhythmias or myocardial infarction. It is important to evaluate for these possibilities immediately. The patient's initial neurologic examination should include an assessment of level of consciousness, limb movement, and language. Obtaining an accurate history of the event also is important. It is essential to determine the time of onset of the symptoms because this information might affect treatment decisions. If the patient cannot provide this information, a family member or witness to the event might be a good source of information.

## Effects of Stroke

Once the patient's condition is stable, the effects of the stroke can be evaluated in more detail. A patient with a stroke involving the right side of the brain has **hemiplegia** (paralysis) involving the left side of the body, because the motor nerve pathways cross from one side of the brain to the other in the brainstem (Figure 31-2). If the left side of the brain is involved, the patient has hemiplegia on the right side. Because the speech center (Wernicke's and Broca's area) is located in the left hemisphere, the patient may also have difficulty speaking or understanding the spoken word **(apha-**

**sia).** The patient with involvement of the right hemisphere tends to have perceptual problems. He or she may not recognize the hemiplegic part and may ignore it altogether **(neglect).** In addition, the patient may be impulsive and often presents a safety risk. Other problems include difficulty swallowing **(dysphagia),** bladder and bowel incontinence, and loss of vision toward the hemiplegic side **(hemianopsia).** A patient with a stroke in the brainstem tends to have problems with coordination **(ataxia),** swallowing, eye movements, and sometimes paralysis. Some patients with brainstem strokes have a change in level of consciousness because the reticular activating system is located in the brainstem. A patient who suffers a stroke in the cerebellum may have problems with coordination, balance, and eye movement (Box 31-1).

## Risk Factors

Identification of stroke risk factors sometimes can help in determining the cause of the stroke and can identify possible treatment for reducing the risk of another stroke. Of the primary risk factors, some can be controlled (e.g., hypertension) and some cannot (e.g., age) (Wolf et al, 1991). Other primary risk factors include diabetes, heart disease, cigarette smoking, sex, race, previous stroke, heredity, and atrial fibrillation.

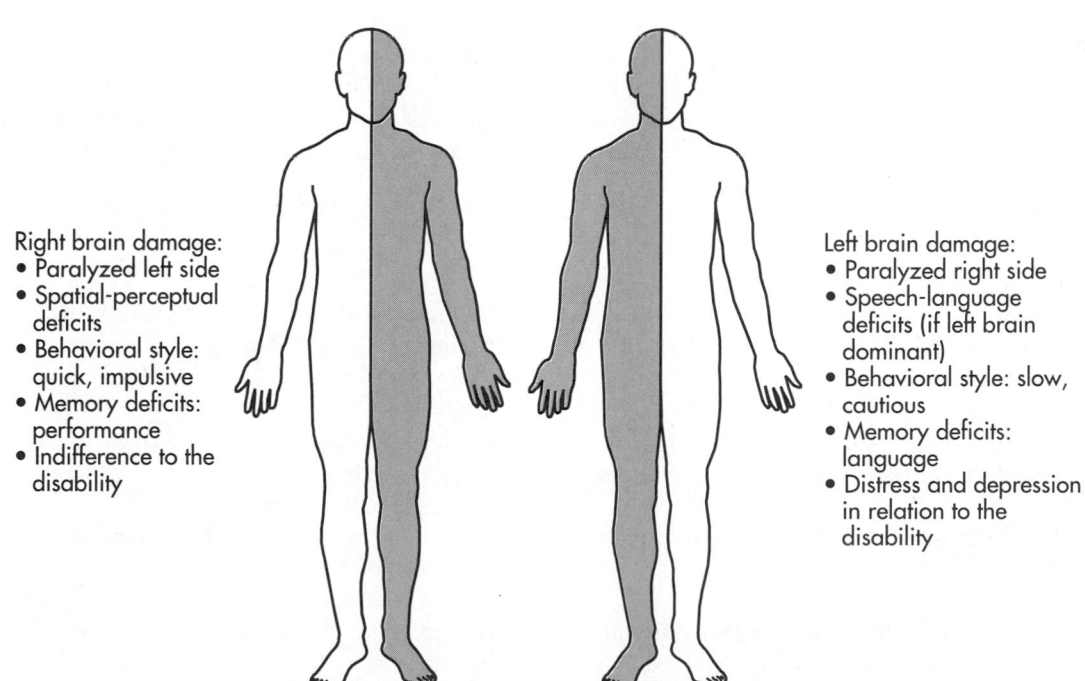

Right brain damage:
• Paralyzed left side
• Spatial-perceptual deficits
• Behavioral style: quick, impulsive
• Memory deficits: performance
• Indifference to the disability

Left brain damage:
• Paralyzed right side
• Speech-language deficits (if left brain dominant)
• Behavioral style: slow, cautious
• Memory deficits: language
• Distress and depression in relation to the disability

**Figure 31-2**   Manifestations of right-sided and left-sided stroke. (Redrawn from Lewis SM, Collier IC, Heitkemper MM: *Medical-surgical nursing: assessment and management of clinical problems*, ed 4, St Louis, 1996, Mosby.)

| BOX 31-1 | NURSING PROCESS |
|---|---|

## PROBLEMS ASSOCIATED WITH LEFT HEMISPHERE INFARCTION

### ASSESSMENT

- Neurologic status
- Speech and language ability
- Motor function of upper and lower extremities
- Sensory and perceptual deficits
- Nutritional status
- Swallowing ability
- Bowel and bladder elimination

### NURSING DIAGNOSES

- Impaired verbal communication
- Impaired physical mobility
- Risk for injury
- Bathing/hygiene self-care deficit
- Dressing/grooming self-care deficit
- Risk for impaired skin integrity
- Sensory/perceptual alterations: tactile and visual
- Altered nutrition: less than body requirements
- Feeding self-care deficit
- Impaired swallowing
- Risk for aspiration
- Risk for fluid volume deficit
- Altered urinary elimination
- Constipation
- Toileting self-care deficit
- Body image disturbance
- Ineffective individual coping

### NURSING INTERVENTIONS
#### Aphasia

- Talk slowly in a normal tone of voice.
- Allow uninterrupted time when communicating with the patient.
- Do not rush the patient.
- Eliminate extra stimulation in the environment.
- Use simple words and phrases and short sentences.
- Use gestures, along with words, to convey an idea.
- Listen carefully to the patient's attempts to speak.
- Do not try to force the patient to talk if he or she is unable to do so.
- Teach family members methods of communication.

#### Mobility

- Increase activity level as soon as the patient is stable.
- Encourage the patient to participate in all ADL.
- Perform regular range of motion exercises for paralyzed limbs.
- Properly position the patient in the bed or chair.

#### Hemianopsia

- Position the patient so that activity is toward the nonparalyzed side.
- Approach the patient from the nonparalyzed side.
- Place objects within the patient's visual field.
- Encourage the patient to turn his or her head toward the paralyzed side to increase the viewing area.

#### Nutrition and Hydration

- Assess the patient's ability to swallow.
- Maintain accurate intake and output records.
- Perform calorie counts if intake seems to be decreased or weight is decreasing.
- Assess the patient's ability to feed himself or herself.
- Provide a pleasant, encouraging environment at mealtimes.
- Supervise patients at risk for aspiration.
- Place the patient in an upright position with the head flexed for meals.
- Provide foods with an appealing taste.

#### Urinary Incontinence

- Determine the patient's previous urinary pattern.
- Maintain a urinary incontinence record.
- Monitor intake and output.
- Assess for problems with mobility, communication, and level of consciousness, which might affect the patient's ability to ask to void or to use the toilet.
- Establish a toileting schedule.

### EVALUATION OF EXPECTED OUTCOMES

- Demonstrates improved ability to understand and express self
- Reports less frustration with communication
- Participates in self-care as appropriate
- Demonstrates satisfaction in self-care despite limitations
- Achieves or improves control of own body
- Achieves urinary continence
- Participates in toileting
- Shares feelings about changes in perception of self
- Describes own anxiety and coping patterns; uses coping mechanisms effectively
- Adequate nutrition status maintained
- Injuries prevented
- Skin integrity maintained

Secondary risk factors (e.g., high cholesterol, physical inactivity, and obesity) contribute to the risk of heart disease and stroke.

## Diagnostic Tests

If a stroke is suspected, the diagnostic test most commonly done is the computed tomography (CT) scan. CT scanning is highly sensitive to blood and can be critical in identifying patients with intracerebral or subarachnoid hemorrhage. If the stroke is the ischemic type, it may not be detected by the CT scan if the scan is done within 24 hours of onset. Magnetic resonance imaging (MRI) can detect an acute ischemic stroke earlier than CT scanning, although it is not as readily available as the CT scan in many places. Overall, MRI is becoming more popular as it becomes more available and as its development improves in detecting hemorrhages (Fisher, 1995).

A number of techniques are available for examining the arteries that supply the brain to determine if vascular disease might have been the cause of a stroke. Carotid ultrasound scans often are done to assess the external carotid arteries to determine if a critical stenosis of one of the arteries might have caused the stroke. Cerebral angiography is another method of examination. Although it is more invasive than ultrasonography, it provides a good picture not only of the external carotid arteries but also of the arteries in the brain. It is used to identify aneurysms or arteriovenous malformations in the brain that might be responsible for a hemorrhagic stroke. Magnetic resonance angiography is used to examine the intracerebral vasculature. This method is less invasive than cerebral angiography because it does not require a contrast agent or any intervention. Transcranial Doppler imaging can be done to assess the flow of blood in the intracerebral vasculature.

Additional tests might be performed to help in determining the etiology of the stroke. An echocardiogram might be performed to look at the structure and function of the heart. This would help determine if the heart muscle is weak or if a structural defect could have been responsible for generating a clot. An electrocardiogram and cardiac telemetry can help identify any arrhythmias, such as atrial fibrillation, that might have contributed to the formation of a clot. Although it is not done frequently, an electroencephalogram might be done to help locate the area of damage or to identify the possibly of epileptic activity from the area of the stroke.

## STROKE INTERVENTION

### Acute Intervention

In the acute phase, medical management and nursing care are directed toward maintaining cerebral circula-

tion to prevent ischemia of cerebral tissue. Managing blood pressure and fluid volume and maintaining head position are essential elements of ensuring adequate cerebral perfusion pressure (Shepard, Fox, 1995). It has been hypothesized that an increase in blood pressure is a protective mechanism in ischemic stroke, therefore high blood pressure often is left untreated. The American Heart Association (AHA) has recommended treatment of systolic blood pressure over 220 mm Hg and mean arterial pressure over 130 mm Hg (Adams et al, 1994). The National Stroke Association recommends treatment of diastolic pressure over 120 mm Hg (McDowell et al, 1993). These parameters would be modified for patients with coexisting diseases such as acute myocardial infarction (MI) and congestive heart failure and for patients with hemorrhagic stroke.

It is important to remember that when blood pressure must be lowered in an acute stroke patient, care must be taken to do so slowly. In the initial hours after a stroke, the patient is kept on bed rest with the head of the bed down; this is done to help ensure that the ischemic area receives adequate circulation. The head of the bed is elevated if the patient has a large ischemic or hemorrhagic infarct; this helps reduce intracranial pressure from edema. The patient receives intravenous fluid to help maintain circulating volume and adequate blood pressure. Fluid may be restricted in cases involving a large hemorrhage or cerebral edema. Careful monitoring of the patient's neurologic status is important during the acute phase of stroke.

### Drug Therapy

Several drugs are under investigation for use in the treatment of acute ischemic stroke (Whitney, 1994). Currently, however, only one drug, alteplase (Activase), is available for this purpose. Alteplase is a thrombolytic drug that works by dissolving the clot that caused the stroke and restoring circulation to the area. However, it must be given within 3 hours of the onset of stroke symptoms. For a number of reasons, most stroke victims do not arrive at the hospital in time to receive this drug. Patients often do not recognize symptoms of stroke, or they may deny that they are having stroke symptoms. The need to educate the public about stroke and stroke symptoms is great. Alteplase has been used for a number of years in victims of acute MI.

Patients must meet several criteria to be eligible to receive alteplase. The stroke symptoms cannot be either too severe or too mild, as determined by a neurologist. A CT scan should be obtained before administration of the drug to assess for any intracranial or subarachnoid bleeding, because such bleeding or a history of it is a contraindication for alteplase. Other

**TABLE 31-1**

## Pharmacology of Drugs Used in Stroke Prevention

| DRUG (GENERIC AND TRADE NAME); ROUTE AND DOSAGE | ACTION/INDICATION | COMMON SIDE EFFECTS AND NURSING CONSIDERATIONS |
|---|---|---|
| **Acetylsalicylic Acid** (Aspirin, ASA) **Route:** PO, tablet **Dosage:** 81-325 mg qid | Reduces the formation of blood clots by inhibiting platelet aggregation | GI bleeding, nausea, vomiting, stomach upset, ulcers, easy bruising, black, tarry stools, ringing in the ears |
| **Heparin** (Heparin) **Route:** IV **Dosage:** Titrated based on partial thromboplastin time (PTT) | Reduces the coagulability of the blood by inhibiting the formation of fibrin clots | Easy bruising, nosebleeds, dark, tarry stools, blood in urine, hemorrhage, thrombocytopenia (rare); regular monitoring required for PTT, platelet count, hematocrit, and occult blood in stool |
| **Ticlopidine** (Ticlid) **Route:** PO, tablet **Dosage:** 250 mg bid | Reduces the formation of blood clots by inhibiting platelet aggregation | Diarrhea, nausea, vomiting, stomach upset, abdominal cramping, flatulence, decreased appetite, neutropenia; contraindicated in patients with hematopoietic disorders such as neutropenia and thrombocytopenia |
| **Warfarin** (Coumadin) **Route:** PO, tablet **Dosage:** Titrated based on prothrombin time (PT) or the International Normalized Ratio (INR); average dosage is 2-5 mg once a day at bedtime | Reduces the clotting ability of the blood by inhibiting the synthesis of vitamin K–dependent clotting factors | Easy bruising, prolonged bleeding from cuts, dark, tarry stools, blood in urine, nosebleeds, bleeding gums; contraindicated in pregnant patients and those at risk for falls; regular visits required for monitoring of PT; patient should avoid alcohol, foods high in vitamin K, aspirin, and nonsteroidal antiinflammatory drugs (NSAIDs) |

contraindications are evidence of an intracranial neoplasm, arteriovenous malformation, or aneurysm; recent intracranial surgery or head injury; uncontrolled hypertension; and active internal bleeding or possible bleeding diathesis, including the use of anticoagulants.

Once a patient has been given alteplase, blood pressure and neurologic status should be closely monitored for 24 hours. Bleeding precautions should be observed, and the patient should not receive any anticoagulant or antiplatelet therapy for 24 hours after administration of alteplase.

Several drugs are used to prevent a subsequent stroke (Table 31-1). Anticoagulation often is started if an embolic stroke is suspected, as in the case of atrial fibrillation. Intravenous heparin is used initially because it has an immediate effect. If the physician determines that the patient will continue anticoagulation therapy after discharge, the patient is started on the oral anticoagulant warfarin (Coumadin). While the patient is undergoing anticoagulation therapy, the prothrombin time or International Normalized Ratio or partial thromboplastin time must be closely monitored. A patient who is discharged with a prescription

for warfarin must be taught the potential risks of the drug and the need for follow-up with the physician for routine drawing of blood.

Aspirin and ticlopidine (Ticlid) also are used to prevent stroke. Both drugs act on platelet adherence to reduce the occurrence of thrombosis and clot formation. Some consider ticlopidine a greater risk than aspirin because it can cause thrombocytopenia (Blissitt, 1992).

## STROKE REHABILITATION

The rehabilitation of a stroke patient requires the participation of several members of the health care team. It is essential that team members collaborate and set goals together with the patient and family. Members of the health team caring for a stroke patient can include the physical therapist, occupational therapist, social worker, nurse, physician, speech-language pathologist, swallowing therapist, and psychologist. Many of the issues concerning rehabilitation are discussed in greater detail in Chapter 17. This chapter highlights rehabilitation issues specifically related to stroke.

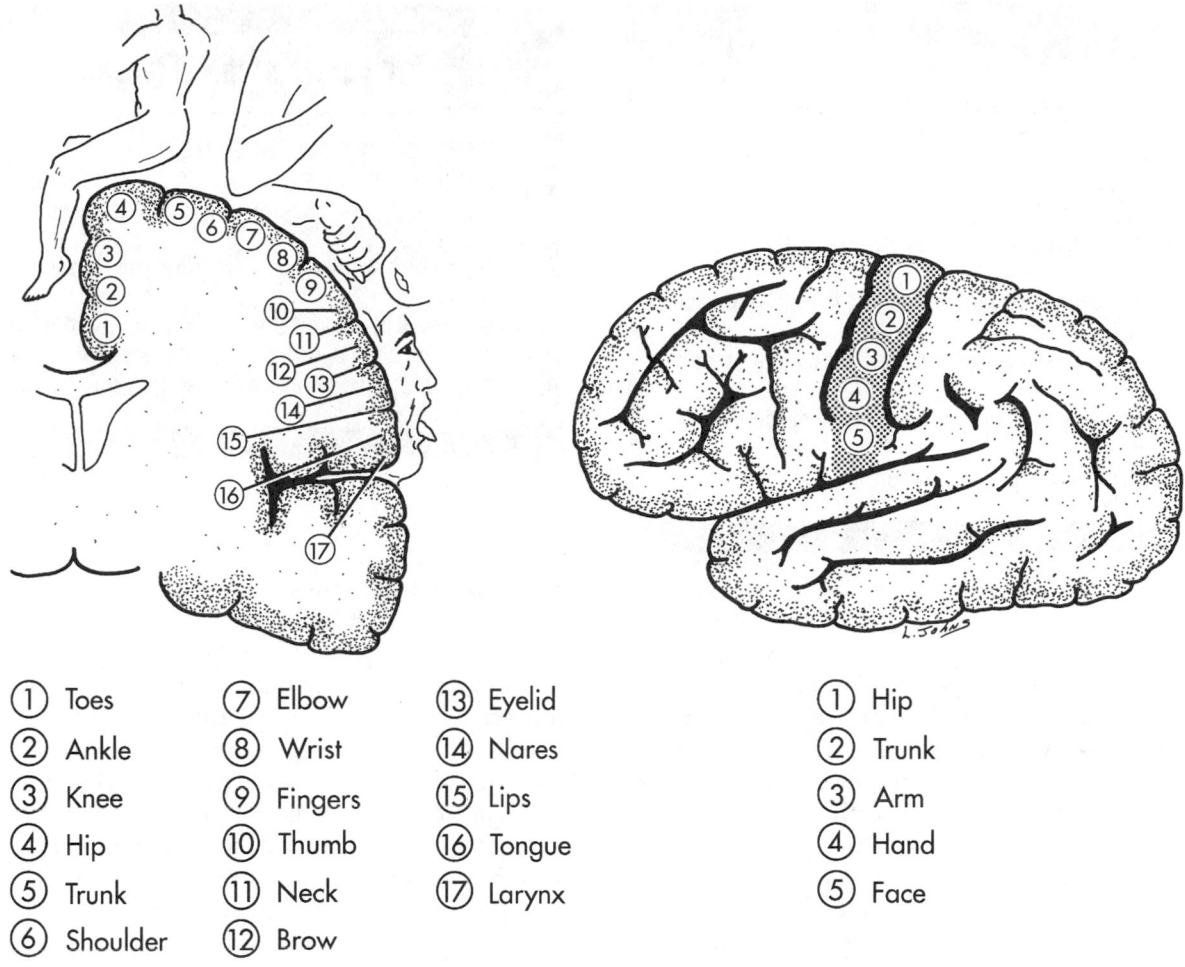

| ① Toes | ⑦ Elbow | ⑬ Eyelid | ① Hip |
|--------|---------|----------|-------|
| ② Ankle | ⑧ Wrist | ⑭ Nares | ② Trunk |
| ③ Knee | ⑨ Fingers | ⑮ Lips | ③ Arm |
| ④ Hip | ⑩ Thumb | ⑯ Tongue | ④ Hand |
| ⑤ Trunk | ⑪ Neck | ⑰ Larynx | ⑤ Face |
| ⑥ Shoulder | ⑫ Brow | | |

**Figure 31-3**  Motor strip of the cerebral cortex. (From Bronstein KS, Popovich JM, Stewart-Amidei C: *Promoting stroke recovery: a research-based approach for nurses*, St Louis, 1991, Mosby.)

## Mobility

Stroke can cause varying levels of impairment in functional mobility. Weakness can range from very mild to very severe. Typically, the weakness is unilateral and is referred to as hemiplegia. The area of the brain primarily responsible for motor movement is located in the frontal lobe of the cortex and is called the motor strip (Figure 31-3). Stroke can also affect a person's ability to coordinate movements, which can be referred to as ataxia. The cerebellum is responsible for motor coordination. A number of other pathways and areas of the brain contribute to motor movement and coordination, but further discussion of these is beyond the scope of this chapter.

A patient who is hemiplegic and relatively immobile is at risk for developing contractures, pressure ulcers, pneumonia, thrombosis, and constipation. Proper positioning, range of motion of the joints, and early mobilization can help prevent complications of immobil-

ity. The patient's level of activity should be increased as soon as his or her condition is medically and neurologically stable. Early mobilization not only reduces complications from stroke but also can increase the patient's overall feeling of well-being.

Assessment of mobility involves evaluation of the patient's strength, muscle tone, and coordination of movement. Guidelines for assessing limb strength are presented in Box 31-2; although this method may be subjective, it is useful in tracking the patient's motor strength in the acute phase of the stroke. Diminishing strength can be an indication of worsening of the stroke. With muscle tone, the weak limb or limbs initially are flaccid. Over time the affected limb begins to develop increased tone and **spasticity**, which is increased resistance to stretching of the limb.

The patient's ability to coordinate movement also can affect his or her level of mobility. The nurse can assess for evidence of poor coordination while the

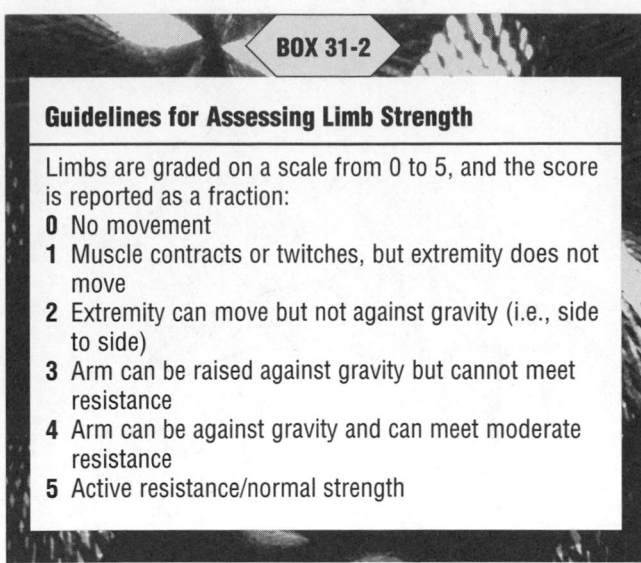

**BOX 31-2**

**Guidelines for Assessing Limb Strength**

Limbs are graded on a scale from 0 to 5, and the score is reported as a fraction:

**0** No movement
**1** Muscle contracts or twitches, but extremity does not move
**2** Extremity can move but not against gravity (i.e., side to side)
**3** Arm can be raised against gravity but cannot meet resistance
**4** Arm can be against gravity and can meet moderate resistance
**5** Active resistance/normal strength

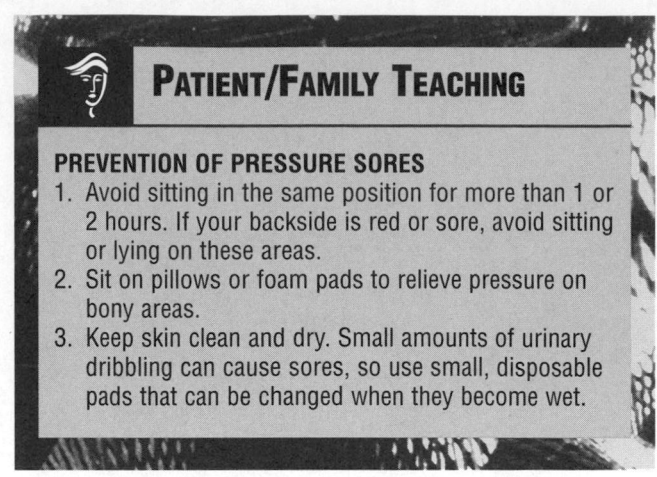

**PATIENT/FAMILY TEACHING**

**PREVENTION OF PRESSURE SORES**
1. Avoid sitting in the same position for more than 1 or 2 hours. If your backside is red or sore, avoid sitting or lying on these areas.
2. Sit on pillows or foam pads to relieve pressure on bony areas.
3. Keep skin clean and dry. Small amounts of urinary dribbling can cause sores, so use small, disposable pads that can be changed when they become wet.

patient attempts to participate in activities of daily living (ADL). Once the patient's activity level has increased, tools are available for assessing the ability to function in ADL that involve motor components. Examples of these tools are the Barthel Index and the Functional Independence Measure.

The overall goal in treating a stroke patient with deficits in mobility is to increase the patient's level of independence and ability to participate in activities of daily living. The stroke patient should be encouraged to participate in all activities right from the beginning. Patients unable to change position themselves must be repositioned on a regular schedule. Both positioning and range of motion exercises can be initiated in the acute phase of the stroke. Once the patient's condition is medically and neurologically stable, the patient's ability to move within his or her environment can be determined.

Working with the therapists, the nurse can evaluate the stroke patient's level of mobility. Initially, it may be possible only to assess the patient's ability to turn from side to side and to move up in bed. If the patient can tolerate having the head of the bed up (as indicated by a stable neurologic and hemodynamic status), the activity level can be slowly increased. The patient's ability to come to a sitting position on the edge of the bed and to maintain balance should be the first step in assessing tolerance to increased activity. Assessing the patient's ability to come to a standing position, to bear weight, and to transfer from the bed to a chair should be the next step. Finally, the patient's gait and ability to ambulate should be evaluated. Throughout this assessment process it is essential that the nurse work with the therapists. The nurse also must make sure

that proper techniques are used for transferring and ambulating the patient.

The stroke patient and family members should be instructed in the potential risks of immobility and the importance of encouraging functional independence. Family members and patients can be taught range of motion exercises, which encourage early involvement and contribute to prevention of contracture formation. The patient and family can be taught measures for preventing skin breakdown. Tips on skin care and relieving pressure are presented in the Patient/Family Teaching box above.

## Sensory and Perceptual Deficits

A stroke patient often is left with sensory and perceptual defects. Changes in sensation and the ability to perceive their environment put stroke patients at risk for injury. Sensory deficits can include diminished or lost sensation in affected parts of the body, diminished or lost vision, and diminished or lost joint position sense (the patient's sense of position of self in space). Visual field deficits often are present on the same side of the body as the hemiparesis (Figure 31-4). Changes in perception can include **apraxia**, which is the inability to carry out previously learned motor skills with no weakness or sensory, cognitive, or coordination impairment. **Agnosia**, the inability to recognize familiar objects, also is an impairment in perception. Stroke patients with right hemisphere lesions also can suffer from **neglect**, or failure by the patient to pay attention to the affected side of the body. Often times a patient has a combination of sensory and perceptual difficulties. For example, in a classic right hemisphere stroke, the patient could have a visual field deficit (hemianopsia), diminished sensation on the left side, and neglect of the left side.

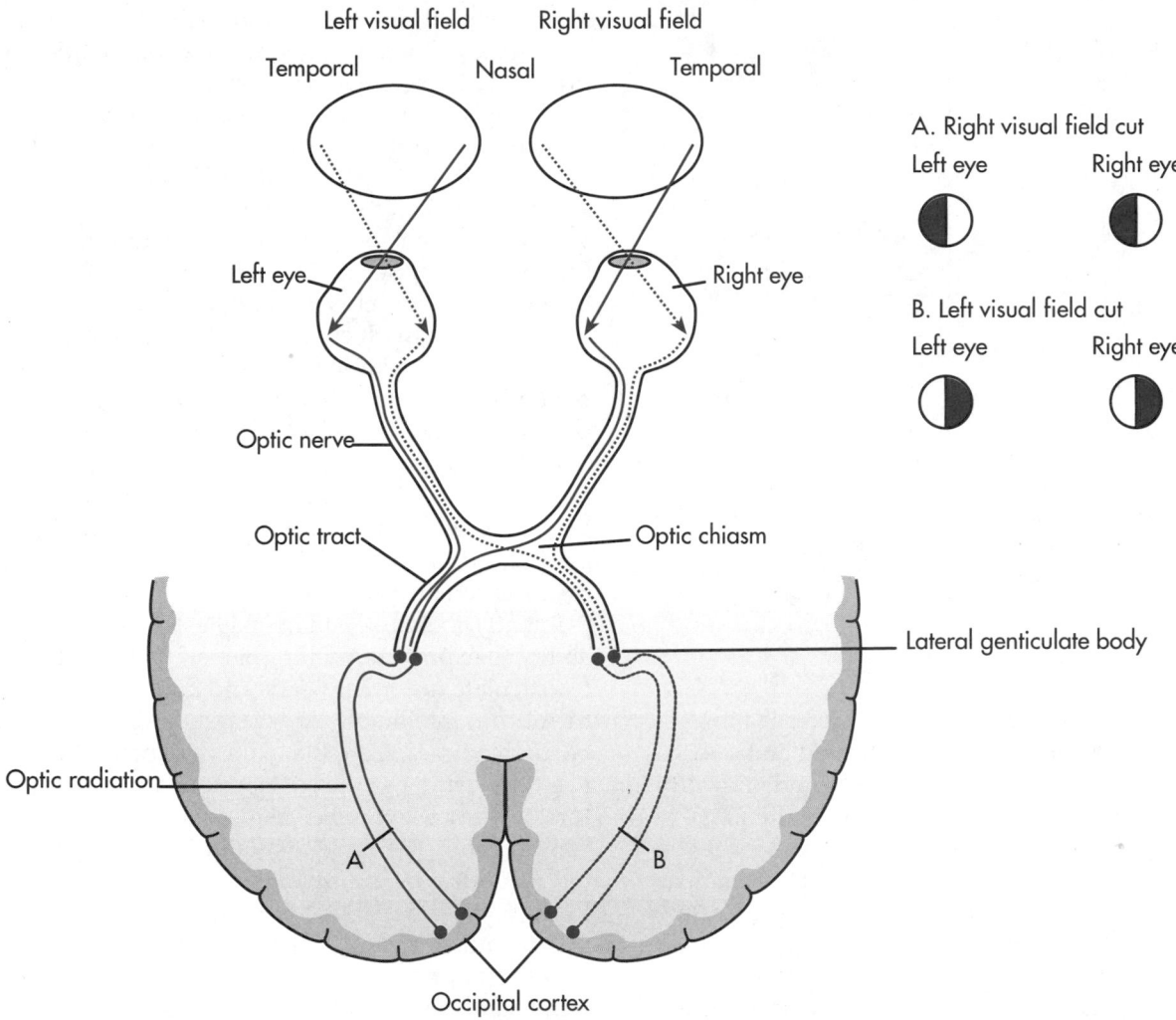

**Figure 31-4**   If a stroke affects the visual pathway as indicated in *A* and *B*, the patient experiences visual field deficits corresponding with the interruption of the pathway. (Redrawn from Bronstein KS, Popovich JM, Stewart-Amidei C: *Promoting stroke recovery: a research-based approach for nurses*, St Louis, 1991, Mosby.)

In conjunction with the occupational therapist, the nurse can assess the patient's sensory and perceptual deficits. Because the nurse is with the patient for most of the day and assists the patient with ADL, he or she is in the unique position to assess for these deficits during routine care. For example, the nurse might make the assessment that the patient is not washing the left side of the body or not eating the food on the left side of the plate. The patient may tend to look only to the right side of the room and despite requests may not turn his or her head to the left side (Baggerly, 1991) (Figure 31-5). These signs indicate that the patient is experiencing the syndrome of neglect. Apraxia might be suspected if the patient seems puzzled about what to do when handed a toothbrush. Sensation to touch can be assessed simply by touching the patient, when the eyes are closed, on each side of the body and assessing for a response. Patients often can report a decrease in sensation. The nurse can make a gross assessment of the patient's visual fields by sitting in front of the patient, having the patient look straight at the nurse, and presenting a stimulus (e.g., the nurse's finger), starting from the outer aspect of the field of vision. Each eye can be tested separately by having the patient cover one eye. The patient should indicate when the stimulus is detected.

When sensory-perceptual deficits are present, the patient's safety is the primary concern. If a loss of sensation on one side of the body is assessed, the patient is at risk for pressure sores and soft tissue damage on that side. In conjunction with the therapists, the nurse must begin teaching the patient the importance of

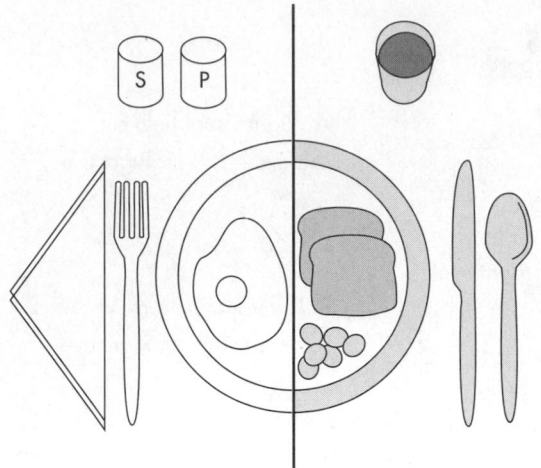

**Figure 31-5**   Spatial-perceptual deficits in stroke: a patient with homonymous hemianopsia cannot see the food on the left side. (Redrawn from Lewis SM, Collier IC: *Medical-surgical nursing: assessment and management of clinical problems*, ed 4, St Louis, 1996, Mosby.)

changing position and of having an increased awareness of the lack of sensation of the affected limbs. A patient with neglect syndrome poses some difficulty with education if he or she is not easily attending to the affected side; it is difficult to educate someone who is unaware that something is wrong with them. The nurse must make sure that the patient remains safe and that the patient's family is educated appropriately about the patient's problem with neglect. A patient with hemianopsia must be taught how to scan the environment. For example, if the patient has a visual field deficit on the right side, he or she must be instructed to turn the head to the right to obtain visual information about the right side of the environment. This is especially important to ambulatory patients, to prevent them from walking into objects.

## Communication Deficits

Deficits in communication occur in up to 40% of stroke survivors (Gresham et al, 1995). Communication disorders most commonly occur in patients who have had a left hemisphere stroke. In order to understand problems with communication, it is helpful to understand what is normal when we communicate. Language and speech are part of normal communication. Language is the use of written and spoken words and expressions to communicate ideas. Speech is the "articulatory and phonetic aspect of verbal expression" (Victor, Adams, 1993). Changes in language often are referred to as the aphasias. Aphasia is the inability to understand or articulate language. Aphasia can manifest as an inability to understand what is being said to a person (a problem with reception) or as difficulty in

saying what the person wants to say (a problem with expression). Often the patient has a combination of expressive and receptive problems.

Changes in speech include **dysarthria** and speech apraxia. Dysarthria is caused by an impairment in the motor aspect of speech, often described as slurred speech. Apraxia of speech is loss of the ability to convert what the person intends to say into spoken words (Bronstein, Popovich, Stewart-Amidei, 1991). These disorders in speech and language often coexist in stroke patients with communication difficulties.

A nurse can take several steps to assess the stroke patient's ability to communicate. When possible, the person's baseline level of communication should be assessed. For example, did the person have difficulty hearing before the stroke? Was he or she able to read and write? Once a prior level of functioning has been established, the current level of speech and language function can be assessed.

Initially, the nurse can quickly establish the person's ability to express himself or herself. Is the patient able to articulate his or her needs and answer questions? Is the output intelligible, or is it jargon or too slurred to be understood? Can the person express his or her needs by using gestures or pointing at objects and pictures? The nurse can then assess the patient's ability to comprehend. The patient should be given short, simple requests. For example, the patient could be asked to show the nurse his or her right hand. When doing this, the nurse should make sure not to provide any visual prompting (e.g., should not show his or her own right hand when making the request). If the patient can comply with a simple request, the request is made a little more complex by adding a few steps. If the patient appears not to understand the spoken word, the nurse should move on to using gestures to see if the patient can understand visual cues.

The patient's ability to understand the written word and to write should be assessed as well. The nurse should have the patient read a brief paragraph or a few sentences. If the patient's speech is unintelligible, the nurse should write a brief request on a piece of paper and see if the patient can read it and follow the request. The nurse then should have the patient attempt to write a sentence, which is assessed for logicalness and glaring grammatical errors.

Caring for a patient with communication problems involves collaboration among all members of the health care team, the patient, and the family. A speech and language pathologist can perform a detailed assessment and suggest many helpful methods for communicating with the individual patient.

In devising a plan of care for a patient with a communication disorder, the nurse must take into account several possible considerations. The nurse must attempt to allow uninterrupted time with the patient when communicating. The patient should not be rushed through an exchange, and the nurse should try not to finish sentences for a patient unless he or she clearly is becoming frustrated and is looking for assistance. The nurse should attempt to reduce extra stimulation in the environment. Background noise, such as a television or radio, can be distracting and can make it difficult for the patient to filter information. The nurse should give instructions in slow, simple sentences and should use gestures along with words to convey an idea. Pictures or props can be used if the patient appears to understand visual messages.

The nurse also should be aware of his or her tone of voice, because it can convey a message. The patient should be encouraged to speak slowly and to speak louder if the speech is slurred, because this makes it easier for others to understand. The nurse should let the patient know when he or she does not understand what the patient is saying. The nurse also should acknowledge the patient's frustration and sadness over the loss of the former ability to communicate. The patient should be given positive feedback when improvements have been made in attempts to communicate. The family must be educated about the change in the patient's ability to communicate and must be taught ways of communicating with the patient.

---

### CASE STUDY

Mr. Henry is a 74-year-old man with a newly diagnosed left hemisphere stroke. He recently was admitted to a rehabilitation unit and is adjusting to his new environment. The nurse has noticed that Mr. Henry periodically becomes agitated. He bangs on his bedside table and pulls at his clothing. By obtaining an incontinence record, the nurse observes that his periods of agitation frequently coincide with episodes of incontinence. The nurse implements a toileting schedule, and the speech pathologist gives Mr. Henry communication cards. As a result, the episodes of agitation and incontinence have decreased dramatically.

---

## Nutrition

Many stroke-related impairments can make meeting nutritional needs difficult for stroke patients. Such impairments include newly acquired physical disabilities, the increased energy demands of rehabilitation, and increased metabolic requirements after a stroke (Buelow, Jamieson, 1990). Meeting these extra nutritional demands can be complicated by motor impairments, sensory-perceptual impairments, changes in attention level and level of consciousness, impaired communication, and impaired ability to swallow. Malnutrition can put the patient at increased risk of infec-

tion, diminished wound healing, and diminished ability to participate in rehabilitation.

Detecting dysphagia (a change in the ability to swallow) and identifying the potential risk for aspiration are primary concerns in stroke patients. Dysphagia has been documented in 25% to 47% of stroke patients (Holas, DePippo, Reding, 1994; Smithard et al, 1996). Of stroke patients determined to be dysphagic, 51% to 73% aspirate, although not all of those develop pneumonia (Holas, DePippo, Reding, 1994). Patients are more likely to have dysphagia if they have had a stroke in the brainstem or a large hemispheric stroke (Horner et al, 1991). Many of the cranial nerves involved in the complex process of swallowing originate in the brainstem. Large hemispheric strokes usually cause severe motor impairment that affects the muscles in the face and neck, impairing the ability to swallow.

---

### NURSE ALERT

**Patients who have had a brainstem stroke or a large hemispheric stroke are at higher risk for dysphagia.**

---

It is not uncommon for an elderly stroke patient to arrive at the hospital in an already compromised nutritional state. This accentuates the importance of first addressing the patient's baseline nutritional status. Obtaining the patient's height and weight is part of the baseline assessment and of the continual nutritional assessment. Maintaining an accurate record of intake and output, along with caloric counts, can alert the nurse to problems the patient might have in meeting nutritional needs. A serum albumin level above 3 g/dl indicates that protein needs are being met.

Nursing assessment of stroke-related deficits includes identification of dysphagia. Some indications that a patient is dysphagic are choking or coughing while attempting to eat, dysphonia or a "wet"-sounding voice, facial weakness that leads to pocketing of food in the cheek, delay in the swallowing reflex, and difficulty handling oral secretions. If the nurse suspects that the patient has dysphagia, the health care team should discuss the possibility of aspiration and measures to be taken to prevent the patient from aspirating. The physician or swallowing therapist might suggest videofluoroscopy to help determine the patient's risk of aspiration. Care of the dysphagic patient should be a collaborative effort.

The patient also should be observed for difficulty with self-feeding caused by motor weakness. For example, this condition might affect the patient's ability to cut food and feed himself or herself, and it could affect the ability to sit in an upright position. Sensory-perceptual deficits could interfere with mealtimes as well. A patient with a severe neglect syndrome or visual field deficit might not see or be aware of food on one half of the plate. The patient's level of attention and level of consciousness also can affect the ability to participate in mealtimes.

Mealtimes for a stroke patient should be pleasant and positive experiences. The patient should be seated in an upright position with proper support for the hemiparetic limbs. The patient's day should be planned so that he or she is well rested at mealtimes. A patient with a diminished level of consciousness is at risk for aspirating, and oral feeding should not be attempted. The nurse should ask the patient or family what the patient likes and dislikes. The nurse also should make sure that the patient has proper dentition. If the patient is known to have sensory or perceptual problems, he or she should be cued to attend to the "ignored" side of the plate. Nursing supervision and assistance should be provided until it is determined that the patient can feed himself or herself safely and independently. If it has been determined that the patient is at risk for aspirating, specific interventions for that patient should be decided upon by the team members caring for the patient. For example, the patient's diet could be modified to consist of foods and textures he or she can tolerate. It is important for the nurse to educate the patient and family about any special needs associated with meals.

If nutritional needs are not being met orally, a decision must be made on ways the patient can meet those needs. In the acute phase of stroke, this often is accomplished by means of a nasogastric (NG) tube, which is a temporary means of providing enteral nutrition. Stroke patients who cannot swallow initially often improve to the point that they can safely swallow some or all foods. If the patient's ability to swallow does not return, a more permanent tube, such as a gastrostomy tube, needs to be placed. If the patient cannot speak for himself or herself, placing or removing any sort of feeding tube can present a dilemma for the patient's family or proxy. An NG tube should be assessed every shift to ensure that it is in place. Techniques for assessing the position of an NG tube are presented in Box 31-3.

A chest x-ray film might be done initially to assess proper positioning of the feeding tube by the physician, but the nurse can use other methods as part of the daily patient assessment. Residual gastric contents can be withdrawn and tested for an acidic pH, because gastric contents should be acidic. The nurse can inject a small amount of air into the NG tube and auscultate the stomach with a stethoscope. The injected air should make a gurgling sound, indicating that the tube is in the stomach. Respiratory difficulties or difficulty speaking could be indications that the NG tube has become dislodged and is not in the stomach. If it is suspected that the tube is in the patient's lungs, the end of the tube can be submerged in water and assessed for bubbling, which would indicate that it is in the lungs. However, this method is not completely reliable, because bubbling does not occur if the tube is pressed against the pleural tissue (Metheny, 1993).

Another nursing intervention for patients with an NG tube is monitoring of residual gastric volumes to prevent regurgitation and possible aspiration. This should be done more frequently once tube feeding has been started. After it has been established that the patient is tolerating the rate and volume of tube feeding,

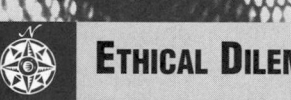

## ETHICAL DILEMMA

Mrs. Williams is an 84-year-old, previously independent woman admitted to the hospital for management of a large left frontal stroke. Several days after her stroke, Mrs. Williams is awake and alert and follows people with her eyes but is not able to speak or obey requests. She does not have the initiative to feed herself and so is being fed with a nasogastric tube. The health care team has recommended that she be placed in a nursing home. Mrs. Williams' children have said that she had expressed her desire not to live in a debilitated state. The family met with the medical team and voiced concerns about their mother's wishes. Mrs. Williams' primary care physician has determined that she has no chance for further recovery and has agreed with the family to discontinue tube feedings, medications, and any other treatments. Should this patient's tube feeding and medications be discontinued? Who determines an individual's quality of life?

---

**BOX 31-3**

### Guidelines for Determining Proper Position of Nasogastric Tube

1 Chest x-ray
2 pH of residuals
3 Observe for respiratory changes and difficulty speaking
4 Auscultation for gurgling in the stomach
5 Bubbling under water

monitoring can be done less often. If the residual volume is high, the tube feeding should be withheld for about 1 hour, the residual rechecked at the end of the hour, and the tube feeding restarted. The nurse should work in collaboration with the nutritionist and the physician in determining the maximum allowable residual volume for an individual patient and the rate the tube feeding should run.

Positioning is another important factor in caring for a patient with an NG tube. The head of the patient's bed should always be elevated 30 to 45 degrees during tube feeding and for 30 minutes after tube feeding has stopped. This is important to keep in mind when planning the patient's day. For example, if the patient must lie flat for a chest physical therapy session, the nurse must make sure that the tube feeding has been shut off and the patient has remained upright for 30 minutes before the treatment is given.

## Bowel and Bladder Elimination

Urinary incontinence is fairly common in the early stages of stroke, although it resolves in a large number of patients (Brocklehurst et al, 1985). Several areas of the brain are involved in regulating bladder function. If these areas are affected by a stroke, this might contribute to changes in bladder control. Changes most often experienced by stroke patients are urinary frequency, dysuria, urge incontinence, and urinary retention (Bronstein, Popovich, Stewart-Amidei, 1991). Constipation and fecal impaction are the most common complications of bowel elimination in stroke. Fecal incontinence is less common.

It is not clear how the brain contributes to bowel elimination, although it is thought that the brain influences bowel function through cortical inhibition (Bronstein, Popovich, Stewart-Amidei, 1991). Factors other than the location of the stroke that might contribute to elimination problems are changes in mobility, sensation and perception, cognition, nutrition, hydration, and communication. Complications that can arise as a result of alterations in urination include skin breakdown and urinary tract infections. Fecal impaction is the main complication of altered bowel elimination. Urinary and bowel incontinence can both contribute to depression, social embarrassment, and possible need for institutionalization.

Because most stroke patients are older, it is important to consider elimination problems that might have been present before the stroke. The prevalence of urinary incontinence in people over 60 years of age living in the community ranges from 15% to 30%. Women have twice the prevalence of urinary incontinence of men (Agency for Health Care Policy and Research, 1992). This could be related to loss of pelvic floor mus-

cle tone because of multiple births, a higher incidence of infection, a prolapsed uterus, and reduced bladder capacity. Older men are at increased risk of urinary incontinence because of enlargement of the prostate, increased bladder neck tone, and reduced bladder capacity. Older men and women also are at higher risk of having a history of constipation and possible chronic use of laxatives.

Once a baseline assessment of elimination has been done, stroke-related deficits that might interfere with elimination can be identified. For example, the patient might have difficulty communicating the need to void because of aphasia. Altered mental status and cognition might interfere with the stroke patient's ability to identify and communicate the need to use the toilet, resulting in urinary or fecal incontinence. Diminished mobility caused by the stroke might prevent the patient from reaching a toilet or commode in time. Immobility, poor hydration, and a decrease in oral intake can contribute to constipation.

Other assessments that can be made include a urinary incontinence record, monitoring of intake and output, assessing for a postvoid residual, and assessing for bowel elimination. These assessments and interventions for both urinary and fecal impairment are described in further detail in Chapter 37.

## Rest and Sleep

Sleep and rest can be affected by stroke. An inversion of sleep-wake cycles, with agitation in the night and lethargy in the daytime hours, has been identified in large hemispheric strokes. Patients who have had a hemispheric stroke have been shown to have a reduction in sleep efficiency and altered rapid eye movement (REM) sleep compared with healthy volunteers (Korner et al, 1986; Mohsenin, Valor, 1995). Patients with stroke can also have an increase in the incidence of sleep apnea (Dyken et al, 1996). Pain, incontinence, inability to move in bed, muscle spasms, and hospital disruptions also can interfere with the stroke patient's ability to sleep (Agency for Health Care Policy and Research, 1992).

It is essential that stroke patients get the proper sleep and rest so that they can participate in rehabilitation. A history of sleeping patterns should be assessed to determine the patient's baseline. Consideration should be given to sleep problems in the elderly. As people age, they report more frequent waking and feeling less rested after sleep. The patient's sleeping pattern should be observed, and possible environmental disruptions should be identified. Problems with muscle spasms and discomfort should be identified as possible sources of sleep disruption.

When developing a plan of care for the stroke patient, sleep and rest periods need to be an integral part of the plan. Limiting naps during the day can help encourage sleep throughout the night, although a patient undergoing rehabilitation should be given adequate periods of rest between therapies. Toileting before bed and discouraging the use of products that might interfere with sleep (e.g., alcohol and caffeine) can help encourage sleep. A quiet, peaceful environment with limited disruptions should be encouraged. Assisting the patient with position changes and using nonnarcotic medications for pain and discomfort can reduce pain and muscle spasm during sleep. Use of pharmacologic interventions for sleep should be limited; they should be used only when other attempts to help the patient sleep have failed.

## Patient and Family Education

Stroke patients and their families require continual support throughout recovery. A stroke is a crisis situation for the victim and the family. The family's immediate concerns are the patient's medical condition and whether their loved one will survive. The roles and relationships in the family may be threatened by the stroke patient's cognitive and physical disabilities. Patients and their families require education and support throughout acute hospitalization, rehabilitation, and return to the community.

Education of the stroke victim and family varies, depending on the time of recovery, the knowledge deficits identified by the health care provider, the family members' and patient's perceived educational needs, and the current level of family functioning. A stroke can devastate interpersonal relationships and require reassignment of roles in the family. The family members' ability to cope with these changes can affect their ability to learn. Family members often are the ones to assist with the education and compliance of the stroke patient and frequently are responsible for coordinating the patient's care. If families are coping poorly, it is difficult to expect compliance with education provided by health care providers (Evans et al, 1992). Early identification of a family that is having difficulty with coping can create the opportunity to offer the family counseling. Clear and open communication between the health care team and family members can be the key to identifying educational needs.

Education of the stroke patient and family can cover many factors. Teaching the patient and family about modifying risk factors and preventive measures almost always is needed (see Patient/Family Teaching box).

Evans and others (1992) outline concepts that are most important in the education of the stroke patient and the family. These include educating and counseling the patient and family on the effects of physical loss, cognitive and perceptual disorders, and language impairment. These researchers also stress the impor-

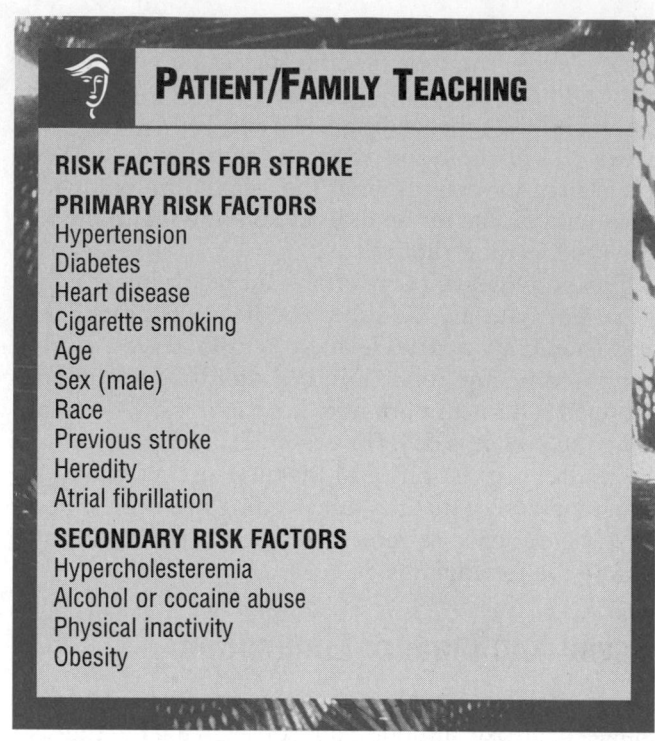

tance of including the effects of stroke on sexuality. The effect of the stroke on family roles and relationships also is a potential educational need. Robinson-Smith and Mahoney (1995) explored the effect of stroke on older couples' relationships 6 months and 12 months after the stroke. They found that these couples were redefining the balance in their marriage, were experiencing changes in social function and physical changes, and were feeling concern about their future. Vanetzian and Corrigan (1995) explored the educational needs of family caregivers 1 month and 6 months after a stroke. They found that most caregivers put the most importance on wanting to learn how to assist a disabled family member and learn more about gaining access to health and human services. The findings of both of these studies can guide education and support later in recovery.

## COMPLICATIONS OF STROKE

### Acute Neurologic Complications

Acute neurologic complications that occur after a stroke include cerebral edema, increased intracranial pressure, seizures, and stroke recurrence or hemorrhage. During daily assessments of the acute stroke patient, the nurse can assess for signs or symptoms of these complications.

Death in the first week after a stroke commonly is caused by edema and increased intracranial pressure (Silver et al, 1984). Although cerebral edema occurs within hours of a stroke, the signs and symptoms might not be clinically evident until 1 to 4 days later. The main symptom of cerebral edema is a decreased level of consciousness. Other signs and symptoms are pupillary asymmetry, fixed pupils, periodic breathing patterns, headache, or vomiting. It is important to prevent conditions that would increase intracranial pressure. Fever, overhydration, hypoxia, hypercapnia, and head position all can contribute to increasing intracranial pressure. Interventions include mildly restricting fluid intake and possibly administering diuretics such as furosemide or mannitol. Hyperventilation might be attempted to increase the amount of oxygen and decrease the amount of carbon dioxide, which will decrease intracranial pressure. Fevers should be treated, because cerebral blood flow increases with elevation in temperature. An increase in cerebral blood flow can contribute to increased cerebral pressure. The head of the patient's bed should be elevated at least 30 degrees to promote cerebral venous drainage.

Stroke is the leading cause of seizures in the elderly. Seizures occur in 7% to 20% of patients after a stroke. They are most likely to occur in the first month. Seizures are more common as a complication of stroke when the stroke is the hemorrhagic type. Most seizures can be controlled by treatment with anticonvulsant therapy.

The recurrence rate for stroke is 7% to 10% per year and is highest in the first year after the first stroke (Gresham et al, 1995). Stroke recurrence was examined in a large population in the Framingham Study (Sacco et al, 1982). The researchers found that the cumulative recurrence rate of thrombotic brain infarction was 42% in men and 24% in women. It was noted that recurrences were primarily the same type as the initial stroke.

## Pneumonia

Pneumonia has been reported to occur in as many as 33% of stroke patients. Pneumonia can be caused by a number of factors. The stroke patient may suffer from atelectasis and poor mobilization of secretions as a result of remaining in a recumbent position for long periods. Impaired swallowing and the risk of aspiration caused by dysphagia or tube feeding can put the patient at risk for pneumonia. An impaired ability to cough and deep breathe resulting from muscle weakness also can contribute to respiratory infection.

Respiratory assessment of the stroke patient includes several observations. The nurse should observe the stroke patient's breathing patterns and make note of any changes in rate, rhythm, ability to handle secretions, and production of secretions. The stroke patient's ability to swallow should be assessed. The nurse also should assess for any signs of respiratory

distress such as cyanosis, restlessness, shortness of breath, nasal flaring, disorientation, or changes in mental status. Vital signs and temperature should be checked frequently in the acute stroke patient. The nurse should consult with the patient's physician when respiratory difficulties are suspected. Nursing interventions that can be used to prevent pneumonia in stroke include frequent position changes, encouraging coughing and deep breathing, early mobilization, and chest physical therapy. Carefully assessment for dysphagia and implementation of proper feeding techniques also can contribute to the prevention of pneumonia in the stroke patient.

## Circulatory Complications

Circulatory complications in stroke include **deep vein thrombosis (DVT)** and pulmonary embolism. Deep vein thrombosis is the formation of thrombi in any vein (Fowler, 1995). A pulmonary embolism (PE) occurs when a thrombus becomes dislodged and a clot travels into the lungs and occludes the pulmonary artery. Both are consequences of immobility, limb paralysis, and possibly comorbid conditions.

Thrombosis is likely to occur in patients with venous stasis, intimal injury, or hypercoagulability (Kinasewitz, 1993). Stasis is related to immobility, decreased leg musculature, varicose veins, and obesity. Intimal injury is related to vascular disease, which is also a risk factor for stroke and may be the cause of the stroke. Hypercoagulability might be the cause of a stroke and can also contribute to the risk of DVT and PE. The overall incidence of leg DVT in stroke patients is 47% (Clagett et al, 1992). Pulmonary embolism usually is a result of DVT. Pulmonary embolism has been reported to be responsible for up to 10% of deaths after a stroke (Silver et al, 1984). On average, the signs and symptoms of DVT appear 4 to 7 days after the onset of a stroke. These signs and symptoms include leg or calf pain, localized tenderness, or swelling and erythema of the affected leg. The symptoms of a pulmonary embolism can range from dyspnea to pleuritic chest pain (Box 31-4). Diagnosis of DVT and PE can be difficult because the symptoms can be so varied.

DVT and PE are preventable complications of stroke. Because the cause of pulmonary embolism in stroke usually is the result of DVT, the goal is to prevent DVT. The goal of DVT prevention is to empty blood from venous valve pockets and increase blood flow in the leg veins to restore deep venous circulation. Early mobilization of the stroke patient is critical. If the patient is bedridden because of medical or neurologic instability, active and passive range of motion exercises can be performed on a regular schedule. It is also important to enhance blood flow by assuring adequate hydration. Often the stroke patient may also

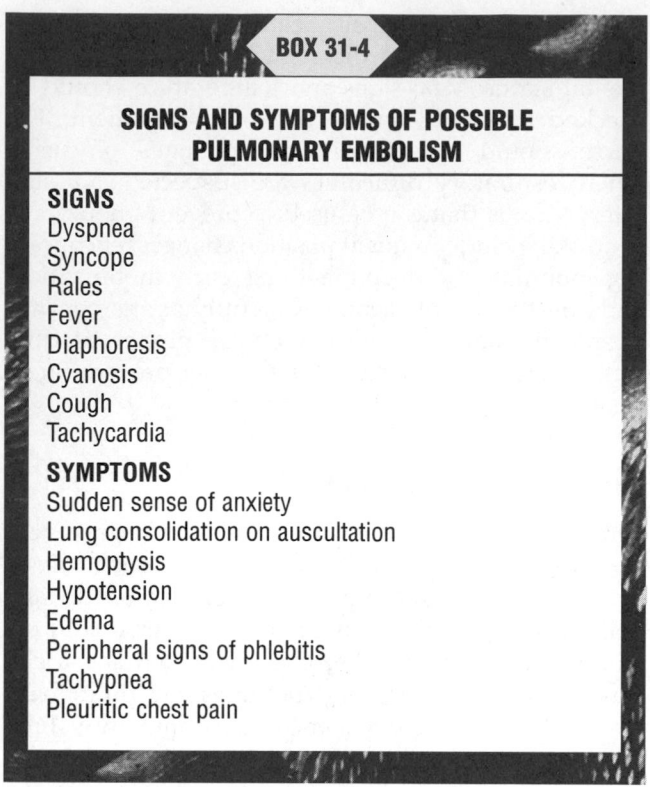

**BOX 31-4**

### SIGNS AND SYMPTOMS OF POSSIBLE PULMONARY EMBOLISM

**SIGNS**
Dyspnea
Syncope
Rales
Fever
Diaphoresis
Cyanosis
Cough
Tachycardia

**SYMPTOMS**
Sudden sense of anxiety
Lung consolidation on auscultation
Hemoptysis
Hypotension
Edema
Peripheral signs of phlebitis
Tachypnea
Pleuritic chest pain

require blood thinning medication such as low-dose heparin or low-molecular-weight heparin, which have proved useful in preventing DVT in stroke (Clagett et al, 1992). Pneumatic compression boots or elastic stockings might be prescribed as well, although the use of these methods has not been widely studied in stroke.

## Cardiac Complications

Cardiac dysfunction often is seen in conjunction with stroke. It sometimes is the cause of the stroke, as in atrial fibrillation, or is a coexisting disease. Cardiac complications can also be the result of a stroke. Cardiac arrhythmias are common in patients after a stroke. It has been demonstrated that arrhythmias are predominant in patients with hemispheric strokes (Mikolich, Jacobs, Fletcher, 1981; Myers et al, 1982). An increase in arrhythmias may be associated with stroke mortality (Broderick et al, 1992). A stroke patient's cardiac status should be monitored by telemetry in the acute phase to detect any life-threatening or sustained cardiac arrhythmias.

## Falls and Safety

Falls are the most common cause of injury in stroke patients in the hospital (Gresham et al, 1995). Stroke pa-

tients are at risk for falling because of poor balance and decreased mobility, which makes them dependent on walking devices or wheelchairs that require transfers. Impaired communication and possible confusion can interfere with the patient's ability to ask for help when he or she needs to get up for activities such as toileting. Changes in sensation and perception, such as visual field deficits, can contribute to difficulty in navigating the environment, which can lead to falls. Patients who have had a right hemisphere stroke are at particular risk of falling because of poor insight and judgment and impulsive behavior. The incontinent patient is at risk for slipping and falling because of urine on the floor. A stroke patient who falls is at risk for fractures, soft tissue injuries, and head injury.

The Agency for Health Care Policy and Research's Clinical Practice Guideline for Stroke (Gresham et al, 1995) suggests facility-wide fall prevention programs to reduce the risk of falls. A fall prevention program involves identifying patients at risk for falling. Some predictors of falls include a history of falling, restlessness, weakness, activity intolerance, impaired decision making, and impulsivity (Byers, Arrington, Finstuen, 1990; Rapport et al, 1993). To assess patients' risk of falling, several institutions devise a fall risk assessment tool or use already devised instruments such as the Downtown Index (Nyberg, Gustafson, 1996).

Once a patient has been identified as being at risk for falls, measures should be taken to reduce the risk. Frequent and timely assistance to the bathroom can help prevent falls. Removing clutter and potential slipping hazards, such as area rugs, and providing adequate lighting can help reduce environmental falling hazards. Technologic approaches such as bed and chair alarms, antitipping devices on wheelchairs, and wedge cushions can be of assistance in preventing falls (Gresham et al, 1995). Restraints should be used only as a last resort.

## Skin Integrity

Pressure sores occur in 14.5% of stroke patients, as estimated by the National Survey of Stroke (Gresham et al, 1995). Factors that put stroke patients at increased risk of pressure sores are immobility, incontinence of bowel or bladder, decreased sensation, decreased perception, decreased mental status, obesity, decreased nutrition, and muscle spasticity.

The goal is to initiate interventions that prevent pressure sores from forming. The patient's risk for pressure sores can be assessed by identifying some of the risk factors listed above. A risk assessment scale, such as the Braden scale (see Chapter 17), can be used in conjunction with nursing assessment to provide a reliable prediction of which patients are at risk for skin breakdown (Capobianco, McDonald, 1996; Vanden-Bosch et al, 1996). Inspection of the skin, with special attention given to bony prominences, should be integrated into the patient's daily care. Nursing interventions include assessment of nutritional status, repositioning of the relatively immobile patient, keeping the skin dry and free of urine or stool, and providing pressure-reducing equipment as needed. The patient and the family should be educated about skin care and should be taught techniques to prevent skin breakdown.

## Pain and Shoulder Injury

A stroke patient may experience pain for a number of reasons, either as a result of the stroke or because of premorbid conditions such as osteoporosis, arthritis, and peripheral vascular disease. Pain that might occur because of stroke complications includes muscle spasticity, muscle spasm, or soft tissue or joint injury in the paretic limb (Gresham et al, 1995), with the most common injuries being related to the shoulder. Some rare pain syndromes (e.g., reflex sympathetic dystrophy and thalamic pain syndrome) are associated with stroke, but these are beyond the scope of this chapter.

Initially an assessment can be made of the stroke patient's history of pain and the types of interventions the patient used to relieve the pain. Patient self-report and nursing assessment of signs and symptoms of discomfort are the main tools for assessment of pain.

The most common problem with pain in the stroke patient is shoulder pain caused by an injury to the shoulder. In the early phases of a stroke, the muscles that normally maintain the shoulder position in the joint capsule are flaccid. Thus normal gravity and pulling on the shoulder for repositioning can damage the shoulder. It is important that preventive measures be initiated to avoid any injury to the shoulder. Interventions include proper anatomic positioning of the shoulder while sitting or standing and use of pull sheets when positioning the patient in bed. Range of motion exercises should be performed on the affected joint, but the shoulder should not be ranged beyond 90 degrees of flexion and abduction (Gresham et al,

1995). If the patient reports pain in the shoulder, the interventions are the same (positioning, range of motion) but might include pain medication, antiinflammatory medication, application of heat, and ultrasound therapy. The nurse should work in conjunction with the physician and therapists in addressing pain in the stroke patient.

## Depression

Stroke survivors suffer from depression more often than other people with disabilities (Whitney et al, 1994). Depression after stroke is common and is seen in 11% to 68% of patients (Gresham et al, 1995). Roughly half of depressed stroke patients suffer from major depression and half from minor depression (Berk, Schall, 1991). The Agency for Health Care Policy and Research's Clinical Practice Guideline for Poststroke Rehabilitation lists etiologies of depression in stroke as follows: (1) a normal reaction to losses following stroke, (2) preexisting personality exacerbation, (3) a major depression, (4) a medical condition, (5) medications, such as sedatives or antihypertensives, or (6) organic brain damage (Gresham et al, 1995). A major depression is more common when the stroke is located in the left frontal lobe or left basal ganglia (Clothier, Grotta, 1991). The prevalence and severity of depressive disorders are highest 6 months to 2 years after the stroke (Robinson, Price, 1982).

A major complication of depression is diminished ability to participate in a rehabilitation program. This can lead to an overall decrease in level of functioning and may seriously affect discharge planning. Clothier and Grotta (1991) advise that depression should be seriously considered as a factor in the stroke patient who is not progressing in rehabilitation. A number of signs and symptoms that might indicate that a person is feeling depressed are described in the Agency for Health Care Policy and Research's Clinical Practice Guideline for Poststroke Rehabilitation (Gresham et al, 1995). A patient may appear consistently depressed and may have a decreased interest in his or her usual activities. Other indicators could be an agitated state or problems with sleep, loss of appetite, decreased energy, expression of feelings of worthlessness, poor concentration, or suicidal thoughts. If a patient displays these signs and symptoms, he or she should be evaluated by a qualified mental health professional. Depression in stroke may be treated with antidepressant medications, psychotherapy, or a combination of the two. Depressed patients can be additionally supported by encouragement and support from staff and family members. Overall, the goal is to identify and treat depression to increase the stroke patient's overall quality of life and his or her ability to participate in the recovery process.

> **NURSE ALERT**
>
> Never pull on a stroke patient's hemiplegic shoulder for positioning; use a pull sheet to assist with moving the patient in bed. A hemiplegic shoulder should always be kept in the anatomically correct position. These measures help prevent shoulder injuries.

# NURSING CARE PLAN

## CARE OF THE STROKE PATIENT

Mr. Roberts, a 64-year-old retired salesman, was admitted to the Emergency Department of an acute care hospital with hemiplegia, paralysis of the arm, trunk, and leg on the right side of his body. He was also unable to speak. He has a long history of hypertension and has been a diabetic for the past 16 years. He also has a long history of smoking and is significantly overweight. He was diagnosed as having a stroke and was transferred to the stroke unit.

During his first 24 hours on the stroke unit, Mr. Roberts was carefully assessed by the nursing staff. His vital signs were checked and a neurologic evaluation was completed every 2 hours. His cardiac status was monitored via telemetry. He was placed on bed rest and made NPO. He was given fluids intravenously. An MRI performed that day revealed that Mr. Roberts had not sustained a hemorrhagic stroke. He was diagnosed as having a thrombotic stroke, caused by the narrowing of his internal carotid artery.

The nurse's assessment indicated that Mr. Roberts had difficulty swallowing, therefore the head of his bed was raised 30 degrees to prevent aspiration. Occupational, physical, swallowing, and speech therapy consultations were requested. The social services department was notified of the patient's arrival.

On his second day in the hospital, Mr. Roberts was evaluated by all members of the interdisciplinary team, and the team met to plan his care. He was found to have severe paralysis of his right arm, with some improvement in the movement of his right leg. He was dependent in self-care activities. He was able to begin attempting some speech, although it was rather garbled. The swallowing therapist said that Mr. Roberts had some problems with swallowing because of weakness in the muscles of his face, as well as some delay in initiating swallowing. The nurse reported that Mr. Roberts was extremely fearful and that his wife and children were very anxious and worried. Mr. Roberts had been incontinent and had problems sitting up straight in bed. The social worker made plans to meet with the patient and family. The team identified the need to educate the Roberts family about stroke and the consequences of stroke, as well as describe the rehabilitation services available in the community.

Over the next few days Mr. Roberts made remarkable progress. He was able to sit on the edge of the bed, and with the assistance of the therapist and the nurse to stand and turn to sit in a chair. He was able to assist with his bath but not with dressing. He tired easily but was able to sit up in a wheelchair. He was started on a soft, solid diet, eaten under the nurse's supervision. He did well with this and did not appear to aspirate or choke. His speech became clearer, and his urinary incontinence resolved. He was screened and accepted by a local rehabilitation hospital.

The nurse discussed the outcome of stroke with Mr. Roberts and his family. They were given materials to read, and the nurse talked with them about ways to prevent another stroke. Mr. Roberts' medications were reviewed, and the nurse stressed the importance of his controlling his blood pressure, carefully monitoring his diabetes, losing weight, and quitting smoking.

After 6 days in the acute care hospital, Mr. Roberts was transferred to the rehabilitation hospital.

---

**NURSING DIAGNOSES**

Impaired physical mobility related to neurologic impairment
Self-care deficit related to impaired mobility
Impaired verbal communication related to neurologic impairment
Altered urinary elimination pattern related to neurologic impairment
Altered bowel elimination related to neurologic impairment
Risk for injury: falling related to impaired mobility
Risk for impaired skin integrity related to impaired mobility
Impaired swallowing related to neurologic impairment
Risk for activity intolerance related to impaired mobility
Body image disturbance related to neurologic deficits

## NURSING CARE PLAN
## CARE OF THE STROKE PATIENT—cont'd

### Days 1-2

| Assessment Data | Nursing Interventions | Patient and Family Teaching |
| --- | --- | --- |
| • *Neurologic:* Motor, sensory, and cognitive assessment; swallowing assessment<br>• *Cardiovascular* and *respiratory:* Vital sign monitoring every 2-4 hours; ECG monitoring; cardiac telemetry; monitoring of cardiac enzymes; respiratory rate and rhythm; breath sounds; ability to handle secretions<br>• Laboratory studies<br>• *Volume status:* I&O measurement; daily weight<br>• Consultations to be made within the first 24 hours include social services, physical therapy, and occupational therapy<br>• Additional consultations to be made within the first 24 hours based on neurologic findings include swallowing therapy, speech therapy, nutrition, and neuropsychology<br>• Monitoring for presence of deep vein thrombosis<br>• *Nutrition:* Swallowing and eating ability; weight and height; diet history and dietary requirements; baseline laboratory measures of nutritional status<br>• *Medical history:* Previous stroke, TIA, hypertension, diabetes, cardiac or pulmonary disease, history of smoking, excessive alcohol intake<br>• Medication history, medication compliance<br>• Functional status before admission, living arrangements before admission<br>• Assessment of family and social support<br>• *Beginning fall risk assessment:* History of falls before admission | • Notify physician of any changes in neurologic, cardiac, or pulmonary status or of any abnormal laboratory findings.<br>• Maintain optimum pulmonary function. Turn every 2-4 hours, encourage deep breathing and coughing to clear airway, provide chest physiotherapy and oxygen therapy as needed.<br>• Monitor blood pressure control within physician-designated parameters.<br>• Continue to monitor fluid and volume status.<br>• Monitor patient activity. The patient typically is confined to bed rest for the first 24 hours. Bed rest is maintained to rule out myocardial infarction and/or to provide adequate cerebral perfusion. The patient is turned and repositioned every 2 hours, with bony prominences and skin assessed with repositioning. Affected limbs should be positioned to protect joint mobility and prevent injury. The patient is carefully moved in bed to prevent injury to paretic limbs; a pull sheet is used to prevent pulling on hemiparetic limbs. Range of motion exercises are provided for involved limbs to promote movement and prevent formation of joint contractures. Splints are used as needed; splints are removed and skin is inspected frequently. Bed mobility is encouraged by having the patient assist with turning and moving in bed. Fall prevention strategies are initiated (e.g., bed alarms and toileting schedule).<br>• Institute measures to prevent deep vein thrombosis. | • Patient and family education about stroke begins on admission.<br>• Interdisciplinary team members collaborate and provide the family with initial information about stroke; the impact of stroke; and the rationale for initial medical, nursing, and therapeutic interventions.<br>• Evaluative procedures and the experience of acute care hospitalization are discussed.<br>• The family is provided with reading materials about stroke and invited to stroke education forums. |

*Continued*

## NURSING CARE PLAN

### CARE OF THE STROKE PATIENT—cont'd

| | **Days 1-2—cont'd** | |
| Assessment Data | Nursing Interventions | Patient and Family Teaching |
| --- | --- | --- |
| | • Monitor medications.<br>• Prepare patient and family for evaluative procedures (e.g., CT scan, MRI, Holter monitor, echocardiography). | |

| | **Days 3-4** | |
| Nursing Assessment | Nursing Interventions | Patient and Family Teaching |
| --- | --- | --- |
| • Assessment continues and depends on the severity and complications of the stroke.<br>• Neurologic assessment<br>• *Cardiovascular and respiratory assessment:* As the patient's activity level increases, endurance should be monitored through frequent checking of vital signs and assessment of the patient's appearance and complaints of fatigue.<br>• *Functional assessment:* Levels of functional ability (e.g., bed mobility, sitting balance, transfer ability, standing balance, and walking ability) should be evaluated. Orthostatic hypotension is evaluated before getting the patient out of bed. Self-care ability (i.e., bathing, grooming, feeding, dressing, and toileting) should be evaluated.<br>• Continued swallowing and nutritional assessment<br>• *Bladder and bowel assessment:* Indwelling catheters should be removed as soon as possible. For continued urinary incontinence, review additional factors such as history of incontinence, physical examination, urinalysis, functional ability, mental status, presence of urinary tract infection, and gynecologic or prostatic problems. Obtain a 24-hour incontinence record. Identify type | • The level of nursing intervention depends on the severity of the patient's stroke, the resultant functional and cognitive deficits, and the medical condition. Many of these interventions are initiated in the acute care setting and continued in the rehabilitation setting or home. Interdisciplinary collaboration is an integral aspect of planning interventions.<br>• Continue cardiac monitoring. Cardiac telemetry most likely will be continued if arrhythmias are present. Otherwise, telemetry generally is discontinued.<br>• Continue to monitor pertinent laboratory results.<br>• Continue respiratory monitoring.<br>• Continue to monitor the patient's activity. He should be out of bed and sitting in chair as soon as medically and neurologically possible. The patient's level of activity is determined by cardiac and respiratory status and level of endurance. Initiation of rehabilitation therapies (physical, occupational, speech, and swallowing) should begin as soon as possible. The patient should be encouraged to participate in as much self-care as possible.<br>• *Approaches to swallowing:* Identify needed changes in positioning: position of trunk and position of head. Identify the need for | • Patients and families need continued support and education. At this time, teaching should center on assessing the family's ability to be involved in the patient's care. Once the family's level of involvement has been determined, learning needs can be better established. During this time of great stress, explanations may require frequent repetition. Results of tests and procedures may be available and need to be shared with the patient and family. Further investigation of the patient's living situation and potential discharge plans should begin to be addressed. The social worker should be informed of the needs and involved in the planning. Discussion of the need for rehabilitation and the type of setting needed are initiated. |

# NURSING CARE PLAN

## CARE OF THE STROKE PATIENT—cont'd

| Nursing Assessment | Days 3-4—cont'd<br>Nursing Interventions | Patient and Family Teaching |
| --- | --- | --- |

of bowel dysfunction and evaluate cause: immobility and inactivity, inadequate fluid or nutritional intake, infection, cognitive deficit, impaired mobility.

- Continued fall risk assessment: If the patient's activity is increased, the patient's balance and stability while sitting and walking should be evaluated. Mental status evaluation and perceptual evaluation are other factors to consider.
- *Language assessment:* Speech therapist should be consulted if the patient shows any sign of having difficulty with the production or comprehension of language; reading, writing, or using gestures; or moving the lips, tongue, and mouth in a coordinated fashion to produce speech.
- *Perceptual assessment:* An occupational therapist should assist the nurse in identifying any perceptual deficits. Examples of some patient cues include lack of acknowledgment of one side of the environment; inability to recognize the function of an object by shape and/or touch; denial of one side of the body; denial of illness.

changes in food consistency, temperature, and bolus size. Identify environmental factors: need for decreased distractions and quiet and privacy during eating.

- *Approaches to urinary incontinence:* Involves early removal of indwelling urinary catheter and determination of postvoid residuals through catheterization. If residual is greater than 100 ml, determine need for intermittent catheterization. Place patient on scheduled program of toileting, with schedule based on 24-hour incontinence record. Ensure protection of skin through cleaning and use of skin barriers. When necessary, maintain containment of urine through condom drainage system for men.
- *Approaches to bowel care:* Establish a bowel program based on previous bowel pattern. Begin a high-fiber diet if possible. Encourage adequate fluid intake. Establish an elimination schedule. If necessary, use a stool softener and suppository regimen, but enforce judicious use of laxatives.
- *Approaches to language disturbance:* Collaborate with speech therapist in planning communication strategies. Keep communication with patient simple. Attempt to limit patient's frustrations with limitations in communication ability.
- *Approaches to perceptual deficits:* Collaborate with occupational therapist and all members of the interdisciplinary team in planning strategies of care.
- Identify methods to promote the patient's safety. Identify environmental factors that may enhance perceptual ability.

*Continued*

## NURSING CARE PLAN
### CARE OF THE STROKE PATIENT—cont'd

**Days 4-7 through Discharge**

**Nursing Assessment**

- The focus of nursing assessment is shifted to assessment of rehabilitation needs and discharge planning. Patient and family coping are continually addressed. Nursing assessment should continue to include all the previously discussed areas, with particular emphasis on neurologic and functional status, as well as continuous assessment of the patient's ability to swallow and nutritional status if a problem has been identified in these areas. Cardiac telemetry is discontinued if the patient has remained stable hemodynamically. Otherwise, it continues until any problems have been addressed. Monitoring of laboratory results continues throughout hospitalization, particularly if the patient is undergoing anticoagulation therapy or has an ongoing medical problem.

**Nursing Intervention**

- The patient's functional status and available family and community supports determine the need for continued rehabilitation services. Discharge planning is the major focus at this time. Members of the interdisciplinary team are actively involved in identifying the need for continued rehabilitation and the selection of the best type of facility or agency to provide those services.

## KEY CONCEPTS

➤ The two major categories of stroke are ischemic stroke, which involves a thrombotic or embolic mechanism, and hemorrhagic stroke, which involves bleeding into the brain tissue or subarachnoid space.

➤ Signs and symptoms of stroke include difficulty with speech, visual changes, dizziness, headache, confusion, and motor weakness.

➤ Acute stroke management focuses on maintaining cerebral circulation to prevent ischemia of cerebral tissue.

➤ Proper positioning, range of motion, and early mobilization of the stroke patient can reduce the risk of complications related to immobility.

➤ Nursing assessment of neglect includes noting whether the patient is ignoring one side of the body or not turning the head or eyes to one side of the room.

➤ Communication disorders most often occur in patients who have had a stroke in the left hemisphere.

➤ Newly acquired physical disabilities, the increased energy demands of rehabilitation, and increased metabolic requirements after a stroke all can make maintaining proper nutrition difficult.

➤ Impairments in mobility, sensation and perception, cognition, nutrition, hydration, and communication can contribute to altered elimination.

➤ Pain, incontinence, inability to move in bed, muscle spasms, and hospital disruptions can interfere with the stroke patient's ability to sleep.

➤ If families are coping poorly, it is difficult to expect compliance with education.

➤ Atelectasis, poor mobilization of secretions, impaired swallowing, and impaired ability to cough and deep breathe put the stroke patient at increased risk of pneumonia.

➤ The stroke patient is at risk for deep vein thrombosis and pulmonary embolism resulting from immobility and limb paralysis.

➤ Falls are the most common cause of injury in stroke. Patients are at risk for falls because of poor balance and diminished mobility.

➤ Depression is a major complication after stroke.

➤ A major complication arising from depression after stroke is a decreased ability to participate in rehabilitation.

# CRITICAL THINKING EXERCISES

1. What measures are taken to ensure that a stroke patient maintains adequate cerebral perfusion?
2. Communication deficits are a common complication of stroke. List some strategies for communicating with a stroke patient with altered communication.
3. Your 34-year-old patient is being discharged with a prescription for Coumadin for stroke prevention. What would be some points on which to educate her?
4. Mr. Milford is a 77-year-old man with a brainstem stroke. His major deficits include a decreased ability to swallow and dysarthric speech. He has been eating a soft diet but is taking in only small amounts. He recently had episodes of choking and coughing while eating, and there is concern that he will become malnourished and dehydrated. What might be a solution to this problem? Consider the following points: (1) How would you best assess Mr. Milford's nutritional status? (2) What interventions are needed to prevent pneumonia? (3) If a nasogastric tube is in place, what care is required? (4) What are some of the possible long-term issues if Mr. Milford's ability to eat does not improve?

## REFERENCES AND ADDITIONAL READINGS

Adams HP et al: Guidelines for the management of patients with acute ischemic stroke: a statement for healthcare professionals from a special writing group of the stroke council, AHA Medical/Scientific Statement Special Report, 1994, American Heart Association.

Agency for Health Care Policy and Research: Urinary incontinence in the adult, Pub No 92-0047, Rockville, Md, 1992, Public Health Service, US Department of Health and Human Services.

American Heart Association: *Recovering from a stroke*, Dallas, 1986, American Heart Association National Center.

Baggerly J: Sensory perceptual problems following stroke: the "invisible" deficits, *Nurs Clin North Am* 26(4):997-1005, 1991.

Berk SN, Schall RR: Psychosocial factors in stroke rehabilitation, *Phys Med Rehabil Clin North Am* 2(3):547-561, 1991.

Blissitt PA: Ticlopidine hydrochloride, *J Neurosci Nurs* 24(5):296-300, 1992.

Boss BJ: Managing communication disorders in stroke, *Nurs Clin North Am* 26(4):985-996, 1991.

Brocklehurst J et al: Incidence and correlates of incontinence in stroke patients, *J Am Geriatr Soc* 33(8):540-542, 1985.

Broderick JP et al: Relationship of cardiac disease to stroke occurrence, recurrence, and mortality, *Stroke* 23(9):1250-1256, 1992.

Bronstein K, Popovich J, Stewart-Amidei C: *Promoting stroke recovery: a research-based approach for nurses*, St Louis, 1991, Mosby.

Buelow JM, Jamieson DJ: Potential for altered nutritional status in the stroke patient, *Rehabil Nurs* 15(5):260-263, 1990.

Byers V, Arrington ME, Finstuen K: Predictive risk factors associated with stroke patient falls in acute care settings, *J Neurosci Nurs* 22(3):147-154, 1990.

Capobianco MC, McDonald DD: Factors affecting the predictive validity of the Braden scale, *Adv Wound Care* 9(6):32-36, 1996.

Clagett GP et al: Prevention of venous thromboembolism, *Chest* 4 (suppl):391S-407S, 1992.

Clothier J, Grotta J: Recognition and management of poststroke depression in the elderly, *Clin Geriatr Med* 7(3):493-506, 1991.

Culebras A: Neuroanatomic and neurologic correlates of sleep disturbances, *Neurology* 42(suppl 6):19-27, 1992.

Dyken ME et al: The relationship between stroke and obstructive sleep apnea, *Stroke* 27(3):401-407, 1996.

Emick-Herring B, Wood P: A team approach to neurologically based swallowing disorders, *Rehabil Nurs* 15(3):126-132, 1990.

Evans RL et al: Poststroke family function: an evaluation of the family's role in rehabilitation, *Rehabil Nurs* 17(3):127-132, 1992.

Fisher M: *Stroke therapy*, Newton, Mass, 1995, Butterworth-Heinman.

Fowler SB: Deep vein thrombosis and pulmonary emboli in neuroscience patients, *J Neurosci Nurs* 27(4):221-228, 1995.

Gillum RF: Strokes in blacks, *Stroke* 19:1-6, 1988.

Gresham GE et al: Poststroke rehabilitation, Clinical Practice Guideline No 16, Pub No 95-0662, Rockville, Md, 1995, Agency for Health Care Policy and Research, US Public Health Service, US Department of Health and Human Services.

Gross JC: Bladder dysfunction after stroke: it's not always inevitable, *Gerontol Nurs* 16(4):20-25, 1990.

Holas MA, DePippo KL, Reding MJ: Aspiration and relative risk of medical complications following stroke, *Arch Neurol* 51:1051-1053, 1994.

Horner J et al: Dysphagia following brainstem stroke: clinical correlates and outcome, *Arch Neurol* 48:1170-1172, 1991.

Keller C, Williams A: Cardiac dysrhythmias associated with central nervous system dysfunction, *J Neurosci Nurs* 25(6):349-355, 1993.

Kelly-Hayes M et al: Factors influencing survival and need for institutionalization following stroke: the Framingham study, *Arch Phys Med Rehabil* 69:415-418, 1988.

Kinasewitz GT: Thrombophlebitis and pulmonary embolism in the elderly patient, *Clin Chest Med* 14(3):523-536, 1993.

Korner E et al: Sleep alteration in ischemic stroke, *Eur Neurol* 25(suppl 2):104-110, 1986.

McDowell FH et al: Stroke: the first six hours, NSA Consensus Statement, 1993, National Stroke Association.

Metheny N: Minimizing respiratory complications of nasoenteric tube feedings: state of the science, *Heart Lung* 22(3):213-223, 1993.

Mikolich JR, Jacobs WC, Fletcher GF: Cardiac arrhythmias in patients with acute cerebrovascular accidents, *JAMA* 246(12):1314-1317, 1981.

Mohsenin V, Valor R: Sleep apnea in patients with hemispheric stroke, *Arch Phys Med Rehabil* 76(1):71-76, 1995.

Myers MG et al: Cardiac sequelae of acute stroke, *Stroke* 13(6):838-842, 1982.

Nyberg L, Gustafson Y: Using the Downtown index to predict those prone to falls in stroke rehabilitation, *Stroke* 27(10):1821-1824, 1996.

Nyswonger G, Helmchen R: Early enteral nutrition and length of stay in stroke patients, *J Neurosci Nurs* 19(2):106-109, 1992.

Rapport LJ et al: Predictors of falls among right hemisphere stroke patients in the rehabilitation setting, *Arch Phys Med Rehabil* 74(6):621-626, 1993.

Robinson RG, Price TR: Poststroke depressive disorders: a follow-up study of 103 patients, *Stroke* 13(5):635-640, 1982.

Robinson-Smith G, Mahoney C: Coping and marital equilibrium after stroke, *J Neurosci Nurs* 27(2):83-89, 1995.

Sacco RL et al: Survival and recurrence following stroke: the Framingham study, *Stroke* 13:290-295, 1982.

Shepard TJ, Fox SW: Assessment and management of hypertension in the acute ischemic stroke patient, *J Neurosci Nurs* 28(1):5-12, 1995.

Silver FL et al: Early mortality following stroke: a prospective review, *Stroke* 15(3):492-496, 1984.

Smithard DG et al: Complications and outcome after acute stroke: does dysphagia matter? *Stroke* 27(7):1200-1204, 1996.

VandenBosch T et al: Predictive validity of the Braden scale and nurse perception in identifying pressure ulcer risk, *Appl Nurs Res* 9(2):80-86, 1996.

Vanetzian E, Corrigan BA: A comparison of the educational wants of family caregivers of patients with stroke, *Rehabil Nurs* 20(3):149-154, 1995.

Victor M, Adams RD: *Principles of neurology,* ed 5, New York, 1993, McGraw-Hill.

Vingerhoots F et al: Atrial fibrillation after acute stroke, *Stroke* 24(1):26-30, 1992.

Watson PG: Stroke in the family: theoretical considerations, *Rehabil Nurs* 11(5):15-17, 1986.

Whitney F: Drug therapy for acute stroke, *J Neurosci Nurs* 26(2):11-117, 1994.

Whitney FW et al: Depression in stroke survivors: the relationship of laterality in right and left hemisphere strokes, *Rehabil Nurs Res* 3(4):130-140, 1994.

Wolf PA, et al: Probability of stroke: a risk profile from the Framingham study, *Stroke* 22(3):312-318, 1991.

# CHAPTER 32

# Head and Spinal Cord Injuries

## CHAPTER OBJECTIVES

1 Describe the principal mechanisms associated with head and spinal cord injury.
2 Discuss the physical findings noted with basal skull fracture.
3 Discuss the significant clinical differences between diffuse and focal brain injury.
4 List the three categories of subdural hematomas.
5 Describe the priorities of management in the Emergency Department following acute head injury.
6 Discuss the phenomenon of spinal shock.
7 Describe nursing interventions for patients with autonomic hyperreflexia.
8 Discuss common methods of conservative management following intervertebral disk herniation.

## KEY TERMS

| | |
|---|---|
| autonomic hyperreflexia | laminectomy |
| Battle's sign | nucleus pulposus |
| cerebral perfusion pressure | otorrhea |
| concussion | paraplegia |
| contrecoup injury | poikilothermy |
| contusion | postconcussive |
| coup injury | syndrome |
| diskectomy | quadriplegia |
| Glasgow Coma Scale | spinal shock |

Trauma, the leading cause of preventable death in persons between the ages of 1 and 44 years, causes a greater loss of productive years of life than heart disease and cancer combined. Central nervous system trauma, including injury to the brain and the spinal cord, contributes significantly to death in more than half of these trauma victims. Those that survive are often left with permanent disability, including paralysis, memory loss, personality changes, and speech disturbances. The incidence of central nervous system injuries is two to three times higher in males than in females, and over half are associated with alcohol and drug use. Victims are often young and therefore require care over many years after the injury. Public education in the prevention of accidents and the use of safety measures such as seat belts, air bags, and helmets is essential to lower the incidence of devastating injuries from trauma.

## HEAD INJURIES

The term *head injury* refers to any injury involving the scalp, the skull, or the brain. Nearly one half of all head injuries are caused by motor vehicle accidents. Other causes include violent acts such as assaults or gunshot wounds, falls, and sports-related injuries. The severity of the sequelae is largely related to the type of injury sustained and the age at the time of injury. Mortality rates are significantly higher with patients 60 years of age and older (Figure 32-1).

Health care providers aim to preserve the highest possible level of neurologic function in these individuals, as well as the best quality of life with the greatest degree of independence.

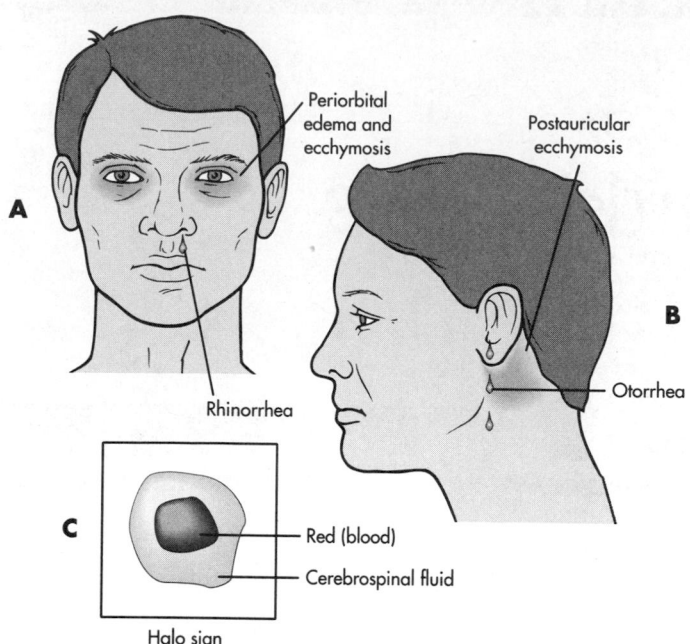

**Figure 32-1**  **A,** Raccoon eyes and rhinorrhea. **B,** Battle's sign (postauricular ecchymosis) with otorrhea. **C,** Halo or ring sign. (Redrawn from Barker E: Neuroscience nursing. In Lewis SM, Collier IC, Heitkemper MM: *Medical-surgical nursing: assessment and management of clinical problems,* ed 4, 1996, Mosby.)

## Mechanisms of Injury

Injuries to the cranium are classified as occurring by a variety of mechanisms. Direct blows to the head happen either when a moving object strikes a stationary head (acceleration injury) or when the head strikes a relatively immobile surface (deceleration injury). These injuries often result in deformation or distortion of the skull.

Rotation injury occurs with a lateral blow to the head, rotating the brain about the sagittal axis. These types of injuries cause brainstem contusion and white matter disruption.

Blunt blows to the head are usually nonpenetrating but can cause contusion to the underlying brain. Penetrating injuries such as gunshot wounds create open wounds that cause tissue laceration and destruction from expanding gases.

## Types of Head Injuries
### Scalp Injuries

Injuries to the scalp can be classified as abrasions, contusions, or lacerations. No specific treatment is required for abrasions or contusions with the exception of application of ice to reduce swelling.

Scalp lacerations require medical intervention. The bleeding that accompanies lacerations can be substan-tial, and all lacerations should be explored with a sterile gloved finger to rule out underlying skull fracture or the presence of a foreign body. Once bleeding is under control, either by direct pressure or by surgical intervention, the surrounding scalp is shaved. The wound is irrigated, debrided if appropriate, and sutured.

### Skull Fractures

The skull is the bony vault that encloses and protects the brain. Skull fractures are classified in several ways. Linear fractures of the skull resemble a single, non-displaced crack. They are the most common type of skull fracture and usually occur as the result of a low-velocity impact. Patients with linear fractures often develop swelling, tenderness, and ecchymosis over the fracture site. Treatment is symptomatic with the application of ice to the site and the use of analgesics to control headache.

A comminuted fracture refers to the fragmented disruption of the skull from multiple linear fractures. A displaced comminuted fracture or a depressed skull fracture involves inward depression of bone fragments. Depressed fractures may be associated with laceration of the dura and brain injury directly below the fracture. Dirt, hair and particles of the offending object may be found in the wound. Patients can exhibit bruising and laceration at the site of the fracture as well as neurologic changes, depending on the presence and degree of brain injury involved. Surgical elevation of a depressed fracture is necessary when the depression is greater than the thickness of the skull at the fracture site.

Basal skull fractures are linear, comminuted, or depressed fractures involving the base of the skull. Most often, however, the fractures are linear in nature and involve the frontal and temporal bones. These fractures carry greater consequences, particularly because they often result in tearing of the dura and subsequent leakage of cerebrospinal fluid (CSF). The nurse should carefully observe any patient with suspected basal skull fracture for serous or bloody drainage from the ear or the nose. Such an opening may allow infection to be introduced into the cranial cavity, thus causing meningitis.

Physical findings of basal skull fracture vary depending on the fracture site (see Figure 32-1). Anterior fossa fractures generally involve drainage of CSF through the nose (rhinorrhea) and periorbital ecchymosis (commonly called *raccoon's eyes*). With middle fossa fractures, drainage of CSF through the ear occurs, **(otorrhea).** Damage to cranial nerve VIII can cause tinnitus or deafness, and bleeding behind the ear drum can occur (hemotympanum). Ecchymosis behind the ear, or **Battle's sign,** is another hallmark of

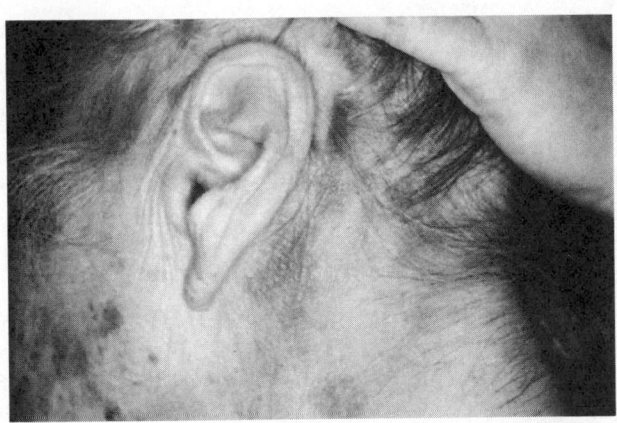

**Figure 32-2** Battle's sign. (From Bingham BJG, Hawke M, Kwok P: *Atlas of clinical otolaryngology*, St Louis, 1992, Mosby.)

middle fossa basal skull fracture (Figure 32-2). Patients with posterior fossa fractures can also exhibit Battle's sign as well as hearing loss and facial palsies as a result of cranial nerve damage.

Treatment of basal skull fractures involves a course of observation and bed rest. Prophylactic antibiotics may be used if CSF leakage is confirmed. Nasal procedures (such as insertion of nasogastric tubes or nasal suctioning) should be avoided in such patients. If frank drainage is observed, a sample of fluid should be checked for the presence of glucose, an indication of the presence of CSF.

## Brain Injuries

Injuries to the brain can be classified as diffuse or focal. Diffuse injuries include concussion and diffuse axonal injury. Focal injuries include contusion, hemorrhage, and hematoma formation.

**Diffuse injuries.** A **concussion** is considered a diffuse injury and is defined as a transient, temporary, neurogenic dysfunction caused by mechanical force to the brain (Hickey, 1992). Common signs and symptoms include a loss of consciousness that is often brief but may last for several hours, retrograde and antegrade amnesia, or the loss of the memory of events immediately before and after the injury. The degree of severity of a concussion is determined by the length of loss of consciousness and the persistence of memory deficits. Other symptoms include headache, drowsiness, confusion, dizziness, and irritability.

Concussion is diagnosed by history and neurologic examination. No focal lesions will be seen on a computed tomography (CT) or a magnetic resonance imaging scan. Treatment involves observation and patient education regarding the common after-effects of

minor head injury. Sometimes described as **postconcussive syndrome,** patients may experience headache, dizziness, irritability, fatigue, and memory and concentration problems. These symptoms can last from several weeks to a full year after the injury.

Diffuse axonal injury generally occurs as a result of the rapid acceleration and deceleration that occur in motor vehicle accidents. With this type of injury, damage occurs involving the axons of the cerebral white matter causing hemorrhagic lesions in the deeper structures of the brain. Following the event, patients are often in coma and are at high risk for succumbing to their injuries.

**Focal injuries.** A cerebral **contusion** is a bruising of the surface of the brain resulting in small areas of hemorrhage. The frontal and temporal poles are common sites of contusion, especially in association with acceleration-deceleration injuries. The area of injury that occurs directly below the point of impact is called a **coup injury.** This injury commonly occurs in the frontal area when, for example, the patient's head strikes the windshield in a motor vehicle accident. As the patient's heads is thrown back from the point of impact, injury occurs at the opposite point of impact, often the temporal lobe. This is called a **contrecoup injury.** The irregular structures that comprise the base of the skull in the anterior and middle fossae can lacerate the brain and are responsible for contusions in these areas.

The signs and symptoms of contusion are related to the anatomic structures involved. They may be relatively minor if the contusion is small, whereas larger contusions often produce significant deficits and problems with increased intracranial pressure (ICP). The treatment depends on the degree of injury. Severe injuries often require specialized head injury rehabilitation programs.

Traumatic intracranial hemorrhage is a common complication of head injury (Figure 32-3). Subarachnoid hemorrhage commonly occurs in association with severe head injury. The symptoms noted depend on the degree of hemorrhage and include headache, restlessness, changes in level of consciousness, nuchal rigidity, and temperature elevation. If the hemorrhage is severe and ICP is rising, hemiparesis and pupillary dilation may be seen. Treatment involves measures to control ICP and overall management of the patient with an injured head (Box 32-1).

An epidural hematoma refers to hemorrhage into the potential space between the inner table of the skull and the dura. Approximately 85% of epidural hematomas occur in association with skull fractures. The temporal bone is the most common site of fracture, causing laceration of the underlying middle meningeal artery and formation of the hematoma. As

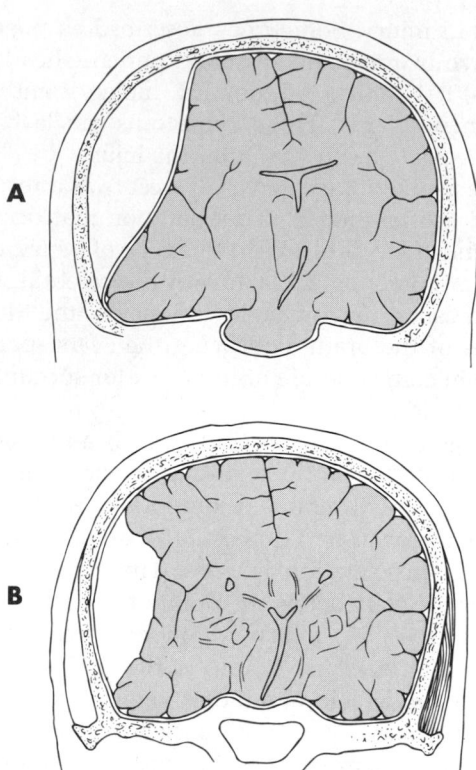

**Figure 32-3** **A,** Epidural hematoma in the temporal fossa, usually a result of laceration of the middle meningeal artery. **B,** Subdural hematoma, usually a result of laceration of the subdural veins. (Redrawn from Price S, Wilson L, editors: *Pathophysiology: clinical concepts of disease processes*, ed 4, St Louis, 1992, Mosby.)

bleeding occurs, the dura is separated from the inner table of the skull. The hematoma causes increasing pressure on the underlying brain and begins to exert mass effect locally. Left untreated, shift, herniation, and brainstem compression will result.

Signs and symptoms often include a brief loss of consciousness at the time of injury followed by a lucid period that can last for a number of hours or a day or two. A rapid deterioration in level of consciousness is then seen, with hemiparesis, ipsilateral pupil dilation, and possible progression to herniation. This decline is indicative of the ultimate failure of the protective mechanism of the brain, where the dura is no longer able to adhere to the skull.

Treatment of epidural hematomas is always surgical, and early diagnosis with the aid of CT scanning is imperative. The clot may be evacuated through a burr hole, or craniotomy may be done. The longer surgery is delayed, the poorer the prognosis. Because bleeding is often arterial, death can result if left untreated. Ongoing neurologic assessment of these patients is a key nursing intervention, particularly within the first 48 hours after the injury.

A subdural hematoma results from bleeding into the subdural space between the dural and the arachnoid layers. Bleeding is generally caused by rupture of the small vessels that bridge the subdural space. Subdural hematomas are divided into three categories based on the amount of time it takes for symptoms to appear following the injury. Acute subdural hematomas cause symptoms to occur immediately or within 72 hours following trauma. They are associated with major head trauma and often result in rapid neurologic deterioration. Patients may initially complain of headache and exhibit drowsiness and confusion that worsens. Ipsilateral pupil dilation and hemiparesis contralateral to the side of the hematoma also occur.

Subacute subdural hematomas occur as a result of less severe head injuries. Although the symptoms are the same, they are not exhibited for 48 to 72 hours after the injury occurs. Deterioration is slower with this population of patients, and treatment can often be initiated before the patient is severely compromised.

Chronic subdural hematomas cause patients to become gradually symptomatic over days, weeks, or months. The progression of symptoms is so slow, in fact, that the cause of the head injury is often forgotten. Symptoms include headache, drowsiness, confusion, personality changes, and bowel and bladder incontinence. Chronic alcoholics and elderly patients with cerebral atrophy commonly develop subdural hematomas that are chronic in nature.

Treatment of subdural hematomas depends on the size of the lesion. Small hematomas may be treated medically because they are often absorbed. Larger hematomas require surgical evacuation to prevent increased ICP and herniation. Acute subdural hematomas can generally be evacuated through burr holes. Subacute and chronic hematomas often require craniotomy for evacuation because the hematoma is sometimes thick and gelatinous.

Bleeding may also occur within the brain itself, resulting in intracranial hemorrhage or hematoma formation. They are often associated with serious brain injuries such as contusions, lacerations, and other types of hematomas. They most commonly occur in the frontal and temporal lobes. Signs and symptoms include headache, deterioration in level of consciousness, hemiplegia on the contralateral side, and dilation of the pupil on the side of the clot. Craniotomy is beneficial when there is a distinct clot that can be evacuated. Most of these patients are at risk for problems related to increased ICP.

## Early Management of Head Injuries

Initial prehospital management of the head-injured patient involves assessment and stabilization follow-

◁ **BOX 32-1** ▷                          **NURSING PROCESS**

## ACUTE HEAD INJURY

### ASSESSMENT

- Neurologic status (loss of consciousness, orientation, motor function, pupil size and reaction to light, EOMs, speech, thought processes)
- Vital signs
- Intracranial pressure (ICP), if indicated
- Cranial nerve function
- Respiratory status
- Oxygen saturation
- Fluid balance status
- Daily weight
- Swallowing ability, gag reflex, ability to cough
- Seizure activity
- Cerebrospinal fluid leak (nasal, ear, or head wound drainage)
- Pain/headache
- Attention span, memory, concentration, if applicable
- Nutrition status
- Individual/family coping and knowledge of status
- Laboratory studies: ABGs, electrolytes, BUN, CBC, serum osmolarity, albumin

### NURSING DIAGNOSES

- Altered cerebral tissue perfusion related to edema, increased ICP, hemorrhage, vascular spasm
- Risk for fluid volume deficit related to vomiting, diaphoresis, fever
- Fluid volume excess related to syndrome of inappropriate secretion of antidiuretic hormone
- Ineffective airway clearance related to decreased loss of consciousness
- Risk for injury (seizures, falls) related to intracranial bleed, electrolyte disturbance, motor impairment
- Altered nutrition: less than body requirements related to decreased level of consciousness, restriction of intake, impaired gag reflex, dysphagia
- Pain related to trauma
- Impaired physical mobility related to cerebral injury, activity restrictions
- Altered thought processes related to cerebral injury
- Ineffective individual/family coping related to change in health status and lengthy hospitalization
- Knowledge deficit related to new injury and long-term care

### NURSING INTERVENTIONS

- Record regular and frequent neurologic status to determine any change in condition.
- Report elevated ICP (>15 mm Hg), increased or decreased urine output (<30 ml/hr or <200 ml/hr).

- Defer nursing care as appropriate if elevated ICP.
- Elevate head of bed 30 degrees.
- Maintain head in midline position.
- Administer medications as prescribed (hyperosmotic agents, anticonvulsants, calcium-channel blockers, analgesics).
- Administer central nervous system depressants with caution.
- Protect from injury with seizure precautions, side rails up and bed in low position.
- Reorient as indicated.
- Explain all procedures and treatments.
- Restrain only if absolutely necessary.
- Restrict fluid and free water if indicated.
- Encourage deep breathing if capable.
- Administer oxygen as prescribed.
- Suction secretions prn only as necessary (hyperoxygenate and hyperventilate before event).
- Prepare for or provide care related to mechanical ventilation if indicated.
- Turn or reposition q 2 h.
- Administer tube feedings or total parenteral nutrition as prescribed.
- Avoid insertion of nasogastric tube until basal skull fracture ruled out.
- Minimize environmental stimuli.
- Avoid startling patient.
- Provide active/passive range of motion tid.
- Increase activity as tolerated when stable.
- Do not converse about patient at bedside.
- Encourage family to bring in pictures, favorite music, etc.
- Place familiar items within view.
- Encourage family involvement in care and provide support.
- Refer family to social service if indicated.

### EVALUATION OF EXPECTED OUTCOMES

- Absence of new neurologic deficit
- Overall improvement in neurologic status
- No evidence of fluid volume deficit/excess
- Urine specific gravity between 1.005 to 1.0025
- No evidence of respiratory distress
- Clear breath sounds
- Normal ABGs for patient
- No secondary injury or trauma
- Free from seizures
- Stable weight
- Family able to describe treatment/nursing care

ing the guidelines of advanced cardiac life support and advanced trauma life support. Neurologic assessment, including the **Glasgow Coma Scale** (see Chapter 30), will provide valuable information that may help direct the care of the individual even before he reaches the hospital. Once stabilized, the patient should ideally be transported to a trauma center equipped to provide the specialized care necessary in the management of a patient whose head is acutely injured.

On arrival in the emergency department, the priorities of management include maintenance of airway, breathing, and circulation. The patient's nose and mouth should be cleared of mucous, blood, and other secretions to prevent aspiration and ensure a patent airway. If the respiratory effort is inadequate or the patient is unconscious and cannot protect his or her airway, he or she should be intubated. To prevent further injury if a cervical spine fracture is suspected, hyperextension of the neck must be avoided during intubation. Once a patent airway is established, the patient should be mechanically ventilated with the aid of a respirator, if necessary.

Assessment of circulation involves blood pressure and electrocardiographic monitoring. If hypotension is present, hemorrhage (often in the abdomen) should be suspected.

A careful history and physical examination are carried out next. X-rays of the cervical spine, chest, and other suspected sites of fracture caused by trauma should be done. Laboratory testing including arterial blood gases, complete blood count, electrolytes, type and crossmatch, and toxicology screen should be obtained. A CT scan is done once the patient is hemodynamically stable. A detailed neurologic examination including pupillary responses, assessment of level of consciousness and assessment of best motor and best verbal responses should be done and repeated frequently because the level of consciousness is an important indicator of neurologic function.

Primary goals during this emergency phase of management include reducing and controlling cerebral edema and preventing compression of intracranial contents from depressed skull fractures, hemorrhage, or hematomas.

Intensive care unit management involves the continuation of these emergency care measures with a greater focus on the prevention of the major complications that occur as a result of this devastating type of injury. The management of intracranial hypertension and the assurance of adequate cerebral oxygenation are primary concerns initially.

Increased ICP following acute head injury is most often caused by cerebral edema. This edema, a normal response to injury, generally peaks at 72 hours posttrauma. Medical management of increased ICP in-

cludes a variety of measures. Normally, ICP is less than 10 mm Hg. With the head-injured patient, ICP readings greater than 15 mm Hg require treatment.

> **NURSE ALERT**
>
> Deterioration in a patient's level of consciousness accompanied by changes in pupillary response, motor weakness, headache, seizures, or vomiting may indicate that intracranial pressure is increasing.

Respiratory support and mechanical hyperventilation are important hallmarks in this management. The necessity of maintaining a clear and patent airway to ensure effective respirations cannot be overemphasized. Impaired respiratory function can result in decreased oxygen supply to the brain tissue and contribute to cerebral edema. The nurse should observe the patient closely for any changes in respiratory function, hyperventilation, hypoventilation, or irregular respiratory rate. Any signs of respiratory dysfunction should be reported immediately so that treatment can be initiated.

Mechanical hyperventilation is an effective adjunct in the management of increased ICP of the intubated patient. By maintaining the $pCO_2$ at a level of 28 to 35 mm Hg, cerebral vasoconstriction will reduce cerebral blood flow and ultimately reduce intracranial volume. This reduced volume also decreases ICP.

The use of osmotic diuretics such as mannitol helps draw water from the extracellular space of the cerebral tissue, resulting in a decrease in the overall volume of the brain. When using mannitol, serum electrolytes and osmolality must be carefully monitored. An indwelling catheter should be in place, and careful intake and output records must be kept. The response to mannitol is generally seen within 20 to 60 minutes following administration. Effects of the medication may be noted for 1 to 3 hours.

The control of temperature and blood pressure are also important aspects in the management of the patient whose head is acutely injured. Hyperthermia can occur as a result of injury to the hypothalamus. As cerebral metabolism increases when the patient is hyperthermic, it is important to monitor the temperature closely and treat fevers promptly with antipyretics.

Hypertension may add to the problem of cerebral edema, whereas hypotension can cause cerebral ischemia. More important than maintaining adequate blood pressure, however, is the maintenance of an adequate **cerebral perfusion pressure** (CPP). Defined as the blood pressure gradient across the brain, the CPP is calculated by subtracting the ICP from the mean arterial pressure and is an estimate of the adequacy of cerebral circulation.

$$CPP = MAP - ICP$$

Normal CPP in an adult is 70 to 100 mm Hg. In patients who have an injured head, the goal of treatment often involves maintaining CPP at a level greater than 60 mm Hg.

Limiting fluid intake to 1200 cc per 24-hour period also reduces brain swelling. Fluid and electrolyte balance should be monitored closely because sodium and water retention often occur as a result of increased secretion of antidiuretic hormone.

## Intracranial Pressure Monitoring

Continuous ICP monitoring following head injury is now common technology in intensive care units. ICP monitoring allows the caregivers to make more accurate treatment plans and witness the response to their interventions.

The most commonly used types of ICP monitoring devices include the following:
- The intraventricular catheter
- The fiberoptic transducer-tipped catheter
- The subarachnoid bolt or screw

The intraventricular catheter has the dual advantage of allowing continuous monitoring of ICP as well as a method for drainage of CSF as a means of reducing ICP. A catheter is inserted via a burr hole into the anterior horn of the nondominant lateral ventricle. The catheter is connected to a transducer, a monitor, and a recording device.

The fiberoptic transducer-tipped catheter can be placed within the ventricle as well as in the epidural space, the subdural space, or into the brain itself. It is the state-of-the-art technology with regard to ICP monitoring. It is easy to insert and is usually highly accurate.

The subarachnoid bolt and screw do not offer the ability to drain CSF and are often less accurate than the other two methods of monitoring. They are, however, easy to insert, and they are beneficial for short-term monitoring in a relatively stable patient.

Most patients with ICP monitors in place are cared for in intensive care unit settings. Nursing considerations important to these patients' care while undergoing ICP monitoring include monitoring the insertion site for drainage or loosening of the dressing (an occlusive dressing should always be in place over the insertion site), ensuring proper positioning of the patient and the equipment to optimize the accuracy of the readings, and reporting the readings to the physician.

## Other Considerations

The nutritional needs of the patient should be addressed early because the metabolic rate following head injury increases markedly. Patients may require long-term nutritional management via a gastrostomy or jejunostomy tube. Stress ulceration of the stomach and duodenum is also a concern in this population. These ulcers are thought to result from disturbances in the autonomic nervous system as a response to injury. Treatment and prevention are similar to that for any patient with an ulcer and include the use of $H_2$ blockers and antacids.

Prevention of constipation is an important consideration because increased intraabdominal pressure can cause a rise in ICP. The administration of stool softeners and a high-fiber diet or tube feeding will help prevent this problem.

Seizure activity is a concern in the early phase after head injury because it causes an increase in cerebral metabolism and an increase in ICP. In the months and years after the injury, seizures as a result of scar tissue may occur in some patients. Most patients receive prophylactic anticonvulsants such as Dilantin for a period following their injury. The current recommendation regarding the use of prophylactic anticonvulsants varies from 7 days to several months after the injury.

## Rehabilitation

The aftermath of brain injury depends on the severity of damage to the brain tissue. The majority of patients with minor injuries recover without any residual effects. However, some patients complain of headache, dizziness, and cognitive changes for several months following injury. These individuals need to be counseled regarding the impact of these symptoms on their personal and professional lives. Any persistent cognitive deficits should be further investigated by having the patient undergo neuropsychologic testing.

Moderate to severe head injury may result in more serious physical, cognitive, and personality changes and deficits. These individuals will require rehabilitation in an inpatient setting. Their families will need guidance and support during the search for an appropriate facility and program.

## SPINAL CORD INJURIES

Injuries to the spinal cord resulting in loss of motor and sensory function are by far one of the most devastating traumatic injuries that health care providers encounter. Recent studies indicate that traumatic spinal cord injuries occur most often between the ages of 16 and 30. Of all victims, 82% are male (Cochran, Kessler, Wittenborn, 1994). Motor vehicle accidents account for the majority of injuries, whereas falls and acts of violence are ranked second and third, respectively. Injuries resulting in complete transection of the spinal cord are more devastating and result in complete loss of motor and sensory function below the level of injury (Figure 32-4). An injury to the cervical or high-thoracic region may result in **quadriplegia,** whereas an injury in the thoracic or lumbar region results in **paraplegia.**

## Mechanisms of Injury

Injuries to the spinal cord can occur in a variety of ways. When external force is applied to the spinal column from the rear, the head and upper back are first bent sharply backward in hyperextension and then thrust forward. This action can result in an acceleration injury to the muscles and ligaments. This mechanism is often seen in a rear-end collision.

Deceleration injuries occur when the outside force is applied from the front, as in a head-on collision. The head is thrust forward, or hyperflexed, and strikes an object. The head then snaps backward in hyperextension.

Deformation injuries are injuries to the tissues or structures that enable the spinal cord to accommodate the normal movements of rotation, hyperextension, and hyperflexion. Axial loading or compression injuries occur when a vertical force is exerted on the spinal column such as when an object falls on one's

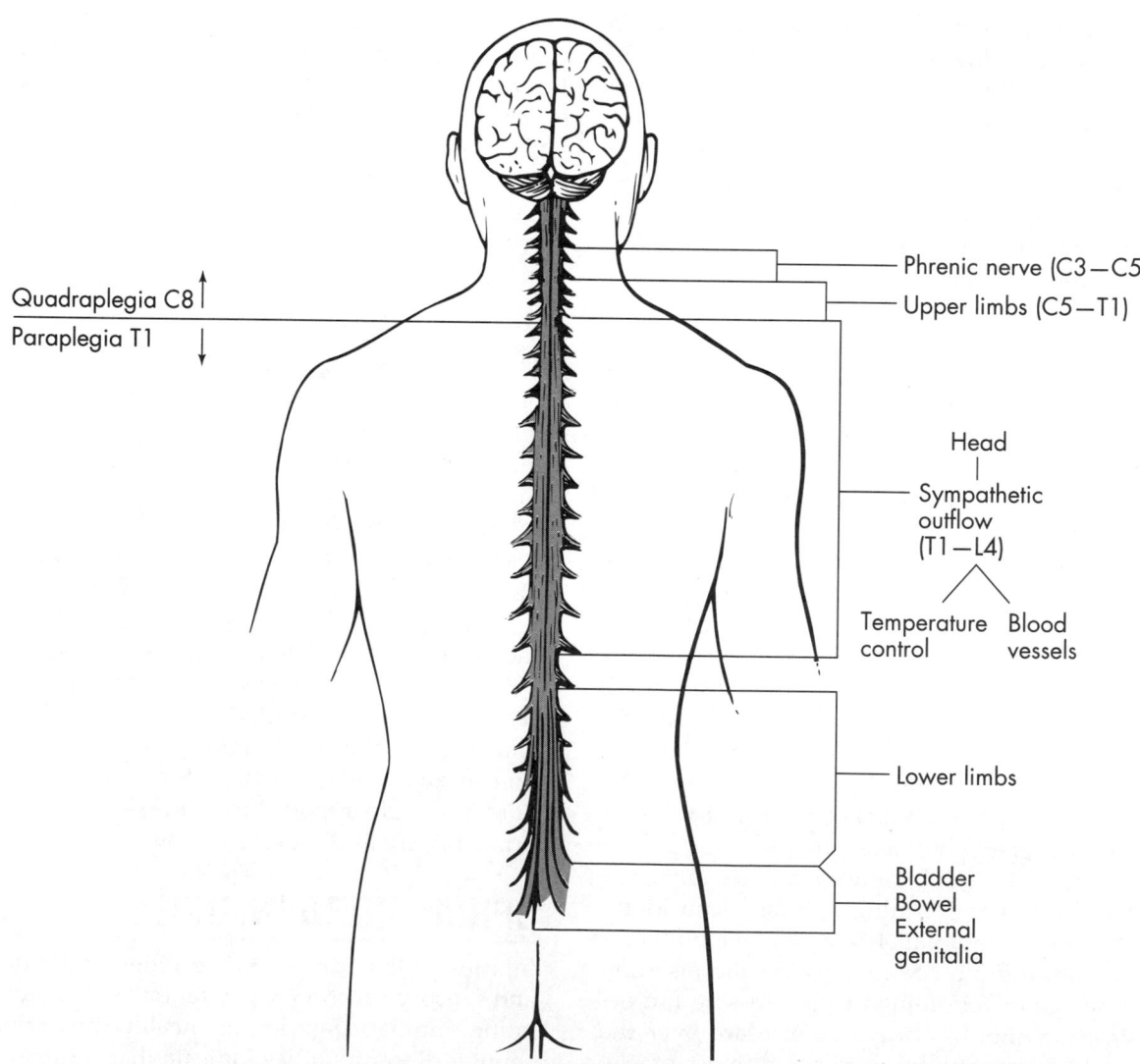

**Figure 32-4**  Symptoms, degree of paralysis, and potential for rehabilitation depend on the level of the lesion. (From Lewis SM, Collier IC, Hietkemper MM: *Medical-surgical nursing: assessment and management of clinical problems,* ed 4, St Louis, 1996, Mosby.)

head or when a person lands on his or her feet after falling. Penetrating wounds or missile injuries occur when bullets, shrapnel, or knives penetrate the spinal column, injuring tissue, bone, and the spinal cord.

> ### NURSE ALERT
> People with suspected spinal cord injuries should not be moved until trained emergency personnel can immobilize and stabilize the head, neck, and back with a cervical collar and back board.

> ### NURSE ALERT
> A decreasing heart rate of 40 to 50 beats/minute, decreasing blood pressure, and loss of reflexes below the level of the lesion can be life-threatening, early complications of spinal cord injury (neurogenic shock).

## Classification of Injuries

Injuries resulting from this type of trauma can be classified as soft tissue injuries, vertebral injuries, and spinal cord injuries.

### Soft Tissue Injuries

Soft tissue injuries are commonly seen in the cervical region in the form of whiplash. Whiplash occurs when the head is thrust forward in extreme hyperextension as in a rear-end collision. A stress and strain injury occurs involving the ligaments and muscles of the neck. Cervical spine x-rays are negative, and the diagnosis is based on history, signs, and symptoms. Patients complain of pain and stiffness in the neck and shoulders, limited range of motion, and muscle spasm. Headache is also commonly reported. Treatment is symptomatic with the use of a soft cervical collar, nonnarcotic analgesics and nonsteroidal antiinflammatory agents, muscle relaxants, local application of heat or cold, and rest.

### Vertebral Injuries

Vertebral injuries or fractures are further subdivided into three major categories: pure fractures, dislocations, and fracture-dislocations. Simple fractures involve a single break with the alignment remaining in-

tact. These injuries do not require surgery and are treated with immobilization in a hard collar when they occur in the cervical spine.

Comminuted fractures or burst fractures are caused by axial loading injuries, such as diving accidents. The vertebral body is shattered into many pieces, and fragments may be driven into the spinal cord. These injuries require surgical intervention for removal of bone fragments, spinal cord decompression, and stabilization with hardware.

Dislocations occur when one vertebra overrides another and unilateral or bilateral facet dislocation results. Damage to the supporting muscles, ligaments, and the spinal cord can, but does not always, result. Treatment consists of realignment with the use of traction and immobilization. Surgical stabilization is sometimes necessary.

Fracture-dislocations have the highest incidence of neurologic deficit. As the name implies, these injuries involve both a fracture and a dislocation that often causes ligamentous and spinal cord injury as well. Surgery is generally indicated to stabilize the spine and to decompress the spinal cord.

### Spinal Cord Injuries

Spinal cord injuries can result in complete loss of motor and sensory function or a partial loss of either function. Complete lesions occur as a result of transection of the spinal cord, whereas incomplete lesions result from partial cord transection, compression, or contusion of the cord. With incomplete lesions, some motor or sensory function is preserved below the level of injury. Often, these patients show some improvement in function over time, whereas patients with complete injuries often present with a fixed deficit.

Examples of incomplete spinal cord lesions include central cord syndrome and Brown-Sequard syndrome. Central cord syndrome is characterized by motor weakness that is more pronounced in the upper than the lower extremities. Sensory deficits and bowel and bladder dysfunction are also seen. This syndrome occurs as a result of injury or edema involving the central aspect of the spinal cord, where the fibers supplying the upper extremities are concentrated. Some functional improvement is usually noted with these patients over time. Rehabilitation efforts are focused on improving upper extremity function.

Brown-Sequard syndrome is seen in injuries that involve hemisection of the spinal cord (i.e., a gunshot or knife wound). These injuries result in a loss of motor function, position sense, and perception of light touch on the ipsilateral or same side as the lesion from the level of injury down. On the opposite or contralateral side, pain and temperature perception are lost.

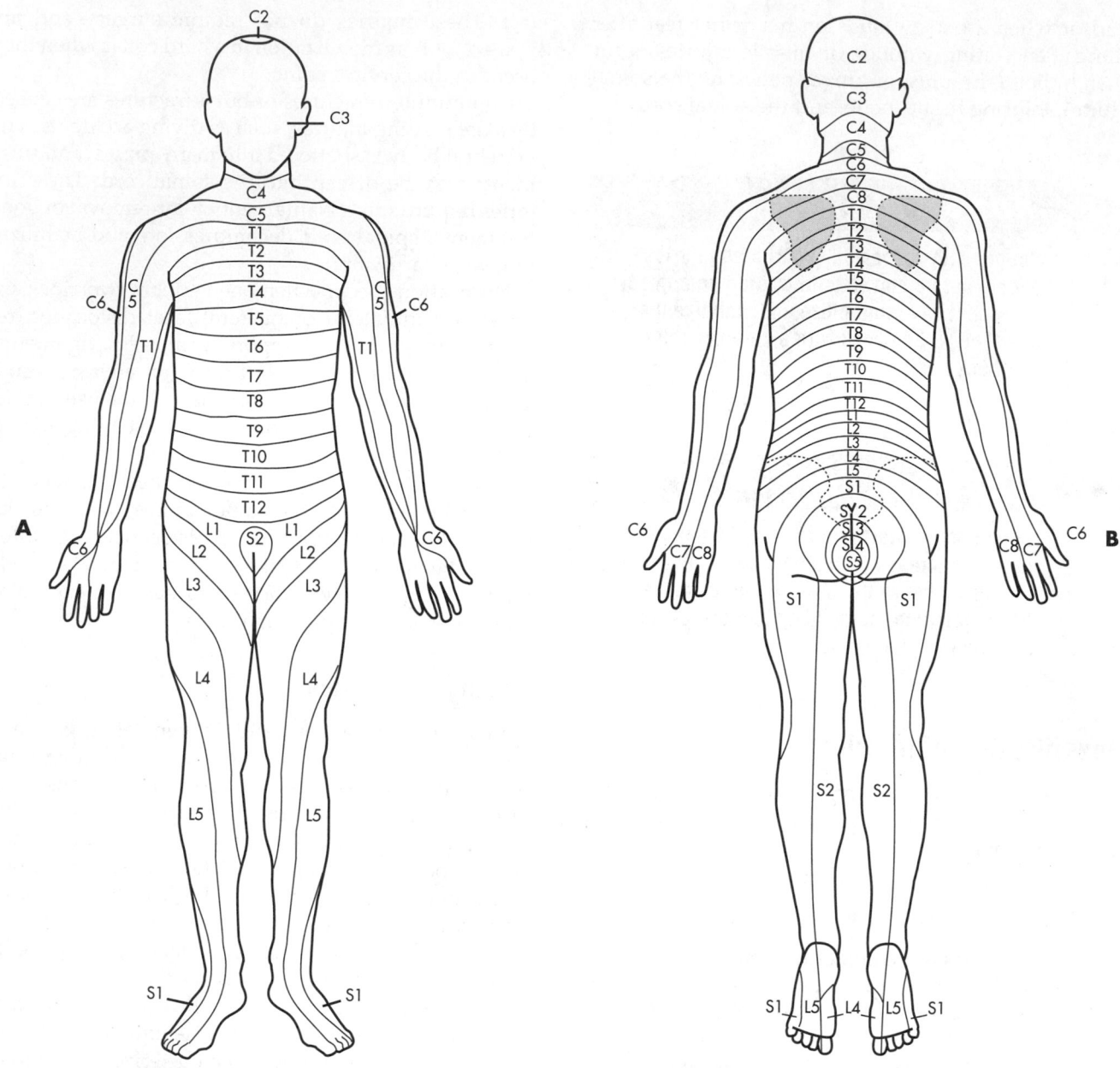

**Figure 32-5**    Sensory chart. **A,** Anterior aspect. **B,** Posterior aspect.

Although these individuals can often be functional, they too are in need of rehabilitation.

## Emergency Management

Initial management of the patient with a spinal cord injury is a collaborative effort involving emergency medical technicians, emergency room nurses, and physicians. Any person with a suspected spinal cord injury should be handled with extreme caution to prevent further damage to the cord. Until proven other-wise, every trauma patient should be treated as if he or she has a spinal cord injury. A spinal cord injury should also be highly suspected in any person who cannot move their arms or legs, who complains of tingling or lack of feeling in any extremity, or who complains of neck or back pain. The patient should not be moved until properly trained emergency personnel are available to immobilize and stabilize the head, neck, and back with a cervical collar and a back board. Minimizing the extent of spinal cord trauma is the primary goal during this phase of care.

Initial care of the patient in the emergency room with a spinal cord injury focuses on the principles of basic life support; maintenance of airway, breathing, and circulation. Once it is determined that respiratory function is adequate and vital signs are stable, a neurologic examination can be performed. The purpose of this initial examination is to determine the level of injury and to establish a baseline for further assessments. During the first 24 to 48 hours after the injury, deficits may ascend one or two levels as a result of vascular changes in the zone of injury. Therefore the precise level of motor and sensory involvement is important to document. Standard dermatome and myotome charts are useful aids for documentation (Figure 32-5). Deep tendon reflexes are also assessed.

The administration of high-dose intravenous methylprednisolone should also take place during this time. Therapy initiated within 8 hours of injury has been proven to reduce edema and subsequent cord damage, resulting in measurable improvement in both motor and sensory function.

## Diagnostic Studies

Plain x-rays of the spine with anteroposterior and lateral views provide information about possible areas of involvement. Myelography is still used in some centers; however, it has largely been replaced by CT scanning for complete assessment of spinal injury. Extreme caution should be taken with regard to moving the patient during these studies. Immobilization and proper handling are of paramount importance to avoid extending an already serious injury.

## Goals of Acute Management
### General Considerations

After the injury, a disturbance of the heat-regulating mechanism occurs, and the patient does not perspire below the level of injury. The loss of temperature regulation results in a phenomenon referred to as **poikilothermy**—the tendency of the body to take on the temperature of the surrounding environment. If the environment is hot, the patient's temperature rises; if the environment is cold, the patient's temperature falls. The patient should be instructed to avoid extremes in temperature to prevent the undesirable effects of hyperthermia or hypothermia. In addition, the skin must receive meticulous care. Powder should be avoided because it holds moisture and contributes to maceration of the skin. Wrinkles in sheets and clothing must be removed to ensure that pressure ulcers do not develop.

The patient with quadriplegia cannot use a traditional push-button bell signal to summon help. Special devices such as a bladder-type call bell should be ob-

tained to allow the patient the maximum amount of independence possible.

## Spinal Shock

Immediately after a spinal cord injury, a period of complete inactivity of the nervous system occurs below the level of injury. This period of **spinal shock** may last from 1 week to several months and is characterized by flaccid paralysis; loss of sensation, reflex activity, and autonomic function below the level of injury; and bowel and bladder dysfunction. Because of the loss of muscle tone, the patient is extremely susceptible to many of the complications of immobility, particularly pressure ulcers, thrombophlebitis, and renal calculi. Conscientious and expert nursing care during this acute period can help prevent many of these complications.

## Musculoskeletal System

Decompression, realignment, and stabilization are important early goals in the care of this population. These can be achieved with operative or conservative management. There are two schools of thought regarding which approach is best.

Physicians who advocate early surgery believe operation is necessary to restore alignment to as near an anatomically correct position as possible. Other benefits include complete decompression of neural tissue and stabilization of the spine by fusion. This in turn allows for earlier mobilization of the patient and shortens the time of acute care hospitalization and rehabilitation.

Those who favor conservative management with bed rest and immobilization say that unless an operation can be proven advantageous, it should not be done. They say that there is no need to remove fragments of bone or disk from the neural canal after cord trauma because it has never been demonstrated that they cause further injury.

---

### NURSE ALERT

Pounding headache, markedly elevated blood pressure, flushed face, "goose flesh," and a period of tachycardia followed by bradycardia may herald autonomic hyperreflexia. This is an emergency condition occurring in patients with cervical or high-thoracic injuries. The nurse should check immediately for bladder distention, obstruction of the Foley catheter, impaction, or other stressful conditions. Antihypertensive medications may be necessary.

BOX 32-2

**Guidelines for Care for Patient in Halo Brace**

| NURSING INTERVENTIONS | RATIONALE |
|---|---|
| 1 Explain routine care and procedure to patient. | Provides basis for patient cooperation and education regarding care while in halo |
| 2 Using proper body mechanics, position patient to perform care. Patient is flat on back to gain access to anterior aspect and side lying for posterior aspect. | Decreases risk of injury to patient. Patient is repositioned by grasping shoulders, lower extremities, and posterior portions of vest; patient is *never* lifted, turned, or pulled by strut bars |
| 3 Open one side of vest to visualize desired area. | Maintains vest stability |
| 4 Cleanse skin with soap and water. | |
| 5 Perform visual assessment, noting any reddened or open area. | Identifies any high risk or broken areas of skin |
| 6 Chest physiotherapy may be performed while patient is on side and vest is open. | Allows greater access to thorax, especially at lower lobes |
| 7 Auscultate breath sounds while vest is open. | Allows for identification of adventitious breath sounds over a greater area |
| 8 Rebuckle vest and reposition patient. | Maintains vest stability |
| 9 Open alternate side of vest and repeat hygiene and assessment measures. | |
| 10 Perform pin care every 8 hours. | To prevent crust formation and decrease risk of pin infection |
|   a Mix 1 oz each of hydrogen peroxide and sterile saline in sterile container. | Half-strength solution used for pin care; solution expires within 24 hours of mixing |
|   b Dip sterile cotton swab in solution and cleanse around pin. Repeat if necessary to remove old blood, crusts, or exudate. | Sterile technique used for pin care while patient is hospitalized; use clean swab for each pin site cleansed |
|   c Rinse with sterile cotton swab soaked in saline only. | Not necessary to apply povidone-iodine (Betadine) or antibacterial ointments at pin sites |
|   d Note pin integrity to insertion area. | Pin should be set tightly at insertion site; disengaged pin or tenting of skin beneath pin suggests patient is no longer in effective traction and should be reported immediately to the physician |
|   e Identify any signs and symptoms of localized infection. | Redness, swelling, pain, and exudate are symptoms to be reported to physician |

Modified from Beare PG, Myers JL: *Adult health nursing*, ed 3, St Louis, 1998, Mosby.

Restoration of alignment and stability of the cervical spine is accomplished with cervical tongs and the halo device. The halo (metal ring) is attached to the skull using four cranial pins. Once in place, the ring can be attached to traction or to a body jacket that allows for increased mobility (Figure 32-6 and Box 32-2). Some institutions also use the Rotorest kinetic treatment table (Figure 32-7) to care for patients who require a great degree of immobilization. These beds are particularly helpful when immobilizing patients with thoracic or lumbar injuries.

Both schools feel that surgery is indicated when it is impossible to restore acceptable alignment by closed methods or when a deficit progresses beyond two segments above the initial level of injury. In all cases, surgery is intended to correct an abnormality of the bony structure of the spinal column and thus prevent later deformity or instability.

Prolonged immobility has many negative effects on the bones, joints, and muscles. Keeping the body in functional alignment is essential to prevent contractures. The use of foot supports or high-top sneakers and hand splints can help maintain normal functional position of the joints. Passive range of motion to all joints and a regular turning schedule are imperative in the prevention of contractures and pressure ulcers. Involvement of rehabilitation services (physical and occupational therapy) is imperative during this period.

and vigorous pulmonary toilet must be part of the daily plan of care (Box 32-3). It is important to remember that during the acute phase, ascending edema can rapidly cause worsening of respiratory status. The patient who is not on ventilatory support needs particularly close monitoring during this early phase.

## Cardiovascular System

Because of the loss of input from higher centers in the brain, vasodilation of the blood vessels occurs below the level of injury. Blood pools in the lower extremities, causing problems with vasodilation, hypotension, vascular stasis, and edema. The use of thigh-high elastic stockings and abdominal binders can help control the pooling of blood in the abdomen and lower extremities. Elevation of the legs also helps control edema. The prophylactic use of heparin (if not contraindicated) is also helpful in the prevention of disseminated vascular thrombosis.

## Gastrointestinal System

Peristalsis is lost during the immediate postinjury phase, and paralytic ileus often develops. Abdominal distention can interfere with respiratory function; therefore decompression with a nasogastric tube is sometimes necessary. When the patient begins to eat, a high-protein, high-calorie diet is preferable. Fluid intake should be at least 3L per day to prevent urinary tract infections and renal calculi formation. $H_2$ blockers (Axid, Pepcid) and antacids are also used to prevent stress ulcers and upper gastrointestinal bleeding.

Because bowel function is affected, fecal incontinence and impaction should be guarded against. A bowel retraining program should be initiated soon after bowel sounds return. Stool softeners (Colace, Peri-Colace) should be used on a routine basis. Bisacodyl (Dulcolax) or glycerin suppositories should be administered every 1 to 2 days until bowel retraining is complete. Because the goal of the retraining program is to establish a predictable pattern of elimination for the patient, suppositories should be administered at the same time every day. Digital stimulation may be required, particularly during the early stages of the bowel program. Enemas should be avoided and should be used only when all other methods fail.

## Genitourinary System

In the patient with severe spinal cord injury, urinary retention often occurs. An indwelling catheter usually is inserted while the patient is in the emergency department. For the female quadriplegic patient, an indwelling catheter may be necessary if she is unable to

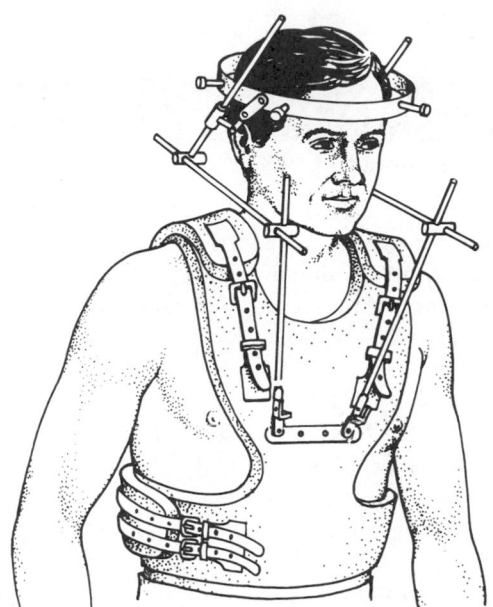

**Figure 32-6** Halo vest. (From Beare PB, Myers JL: *Adult health nursing,* ed 3, St Louis, 1998, Mosby.)

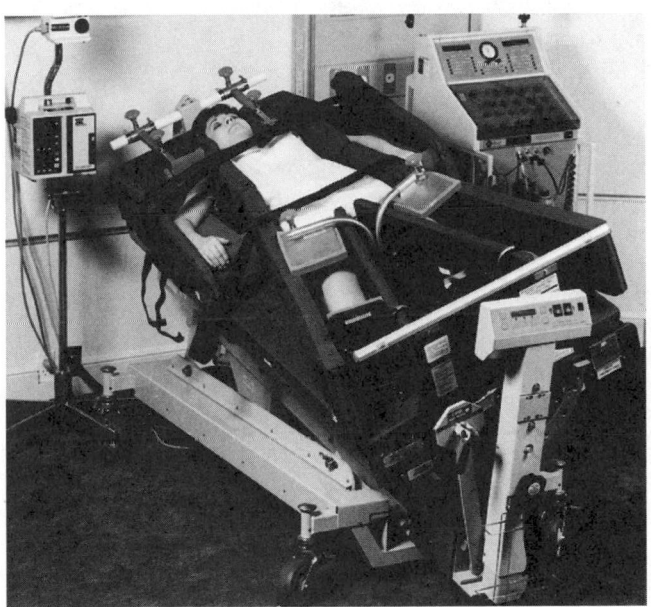

**Figure 32-7** Kinetic Therapy treatment table (Roto Rest Delta bed). (Courtesy Kinetic Concepts, Inc., San Antonio, Tex. In Lewis SM, Collier IC, Heitkemper MM, editors: *Medical-surgical nursing: assessment and management of clinical problems,* ed 4, St Louis, 1996, Mosby.)

## Respiratory System

Depending on the level of injury, the patient develops varying degrees of respiratory difficulty. Paralysis of the diaphragm occurs with injuries at the level of C4 and above. The patient with low-cervical or high-thoracic level lesions must also be monitored carefully,

| BOX 32-3 | **NURSING PROCESS** |

## SPINAL CORD INJURY

### ASSESSMENT
**Acute Phase**

- Respiratory status
- Ability to cough
- Oxygen saturation
- Vital signs
- Neurologic status (muscle movement of upper and lower extremities, sensation, proprioception, deep-tendon reflexes, sphincter contraction, and perianal sensation)
- Peripheral pulses, capillary refill
- Laboratory studies: ABGs, electrolytes, CBC

**Ongoing**

- Respiratory status
- Vital signs
- Neurologic status for change
- Ability to perform self-care activities
- Baseline range of motion
- Skin integrity
- For signs/symptoms of dysreflexia
- For complaints of excessive warmth or coolness below level of injury
- Coping skills
- Perception of illness on self and lifestyle
- Level of anxiety

### NURSING DIAGNOSES

- Inability to sustain spontaneous ventilation related to high-cervical injury
- Altered systemic tissue perfusion related to spinal shock
- Ineffective breathing pattern related to loss of abdominal and intercostal muscle function, immobility
- Impaired physical mobility related to paralysis, paresis
- Risk for impaired skin integrity related to immobility
- Ineffective thermoregulation related to loss of compensatory feedback to temperature change
- Altered urinary elimination related to injury effect on nerve innovation to bladder
- Constipation related to decreased mobility, decreased sensation, decreased control of defecation
- Risk for injury: dysreflexia related to loss of sympathetic nervous response below level of injury
- Anxiety related to sudden change in health status
- Body image disturbance related to paralysis, change in lifestyle
- Powerlessness related to dependence on others
- Knowledge deficit related to change in health status

### NURSING INTERVENTIONS
**Acute Phase**

- Administer oxygen as prescribed.
- Assist with intubation as indicated.
- Provide care related to mechanical ventilation as indicated.
- Suction prn.
- Maintain stability of neck with any movement.
- Administer IV fluids as prescribed.
- Avoid elevation of head of bed.
- Apply MAST suit as prescribed.
- Assist with application of spinal immobilizing device.
- Administer medications as prescribed (anticholinergics, sympathomimetics, corticosteroids).
- Provide information/reassurance as indicated.

**Ongoing**

- Logroll every 2 hours.
- Provide range of motion tid.
- Apply antiembolic stockings, remove for 30 to 60 minutes bid.
- Apply abdominal binder when out of bed if indicated.
- Provide support to prevent foot drop.
- Consult with physical and occupational therapists.
- Keep skin clean and dry.
- When up in wheelchair, shift weight every 30 minutes.
- Provide appropriate pressure reducing/relieving devices.
- Encourage deep breathing and coughing.
- Use assisted cough as indicated.
- Maintain room temperature at 70° F if indicated.
- Provide/remove blankets and clothing as indicated.
- Initiate bladder and bowel programs (intermittent catheterization, Crede or trigger techniques, rectal suppository).
- Encourage ventilation of feelings.
- Provide accurate information regarding status.
- Provide support as indicated.
- Include patient in decision making.
- Encourage independence.
- Encourage high-fiber and 2500-ml intake.
- Provide pin care if indicated.
- Prevent stimulation of sympathetic nervous system below level of injury (full bladder, pressure, trauma).

> **BOX 32-3**
>
> ### NURSING PROCESS
>
> ### SPINAL CORD INJURY—cont'd
>
> - Monitor BP for complaint of headache, flushing, diaphoresis, or blurred vision.
>
> **EVALUATION OF EXPECTED OUTCOMES**
>
> - Respiratory status stable
> - ABGs within normal limits for patient
> - Neurologic status stable
> - Vital signs within normal limits for patient
> - Palpable peripheral pulses
> - Maintenance of full range of motion
>
> - No evidence of foot drop
> - Skin intact
> - Urinary/bowel program established
> - Effective management of dysreflexia if it occurs
> - Discusses feelings and coping methods
> - Participates in self-care activities
> - Verbalizes beginning adjustment to injury and change in lifestyle
> - Verbalizes understanding of rehabilitation

manage self-catheterization. For the male quadriplegic and for the paraplegic patient, intermittent catheterization is the method of choice because it is less likely to result in chronic urinary tract infection.

Patients are catheterized intermittently to maintain urine volumes less than 500 ml for each void. Consistent volumes greater than this can result in overstretching the bladder and can increase the potential for the development of **autonomic hyperreflexia,** which is an emergency condition occurring in the patient with cervical or high-thoracic injury. It occurs as a result of an exaggerated and uncontrolled response of the sympathetic nervous system to external stimulation. Some of the common causes are bladder or bowel distention, enemas, digital rectal stimulation, bladder irrigation, infection, or skin ulcers. The condition is characterized by pounding headache, markedly elevated blood pressure (sometimes as high as 300 mm Hg systolic), flushed face, "goose flesh," and a period of tachycardia followed by bradycardia. Once the cause of the attack has been identified and corrected, the symptoms usually subside without further treatment. When the symptoms of hyperreflexia occur, the nurse should immediately check for bladder distention, obstruction of the Foley catheter, or other causes so the problem can be corrected. If the bladder is distended, the patient should be catheterized immediately. In cases of fecal impaction, a local anesthetic ointment should be inserted into the rectum before any attempt is made to remove the impaction. The preceding emergency nursing measures should be attempted immediately. The physician should be notified that the patient has had an episode of autonomic hyperreflexia or if these measures are ineffective. If the above interventions fail, rapid-acting antihypertensive medications such as metoprolol (Lopressor) are required. The patient and family should have a complete understanding of this problem and how to correct it before the patient is discharged.

## Rehabilitation

The process of rehabilitation begins immediately, and the primary objective of care is to assist the patient in achieving an optimum level of physical and mental function within the limits of the disability. The extent of functional return for patients with spinal cord injury depends on the type and extent of spinal cord damage. The higher the level of injury, the more muscles involved and the greater the degree of disability. With long-term physical and occupational therapy, the patient can learn to use remaining functional muscles and adaptive devices to achieve independence in daily activities. Ambulation with or without bracing may be attempted in select patients with lumbar and sacral injuries. The nurse plays an important role during this period in teaching the patient and family aspects of self-care so that many of the potential complications of chronic disability can be prevented.

Bladder and bowel reconditioning are considered major goals during rehabilitation. If the patient can regain continence of bladder and bowel function, self-confidence and potential for successful rehabilitation improves. Once spinal shock has passed, bladder and bowel reconditioning should be initiated. A rigid program of regulated fluid intake and attempts to void is begun. Many patients are able to empty their bladders through stimulation of the voiding reflex by tapping over the bladder area, stroking the inner thighs, or pulling pubic hairs. Catheterization for residual urine is done routinely to prevent distention and to determine the effectiveness of bladder emptying. The goal of bowel reconditioning is to achieve a regular schedule of emptying the bowel by methods previously cited. The time selected should be convenient for the patient after discharge. As soon as the patient can maintain an upright position, he or she should be assisted to the toilet to facilitate evacuation.

Sexual counseling has been an area commonly neglected in the past. Many patients with spinal cord injuries have concerns regarding their potential for normal sexual activity. The nurse should be aware that some patients may be embarrassed or reluctant to ask questions related to sexual functioning. If the nurse does not feel comfortable with or capable of answering questions, a referral to the appropriate resource person should be made.

Adjustments to disability are difficult, with extreme changes in body image being required. The grief process, including such emotions as anger, depression, denial, and withdrawal, can be anticipated. Often the patient does well when interacting with others who have similar problems.

## Intervertebral Disk Trauma

The intervertebral disks are fibrocartilaginous structures located between the vertebral bodies. Disks allow for limited flexibility of the spine and act as shock absorbers to protect the vertebrae from jars and jolts. Sometimes these disks rupture, and the soft, gelatinous substance in the center **(nucleus pulposus)** escapes (Figure 32-8). The disk material may compress the spinal cord or exert pressure on the nerve root, causing neurologic symptoms. The disks in the lumbar and cervical regions are most commonly affected.

Lower back pain is generally the initial symptom. The pain eventually radiates over the buttock and down the leg to the ankle or foot. The patient may ex-perience tingling or numbness in the foot and muscles spasms in the leg. Motor weakness may also occur.

Heavy lifting or twisting the back usually precipitates the onset of the pain. In cases of herniation of cervical disks, hyperextension of the neck (whiplash) may be the precipitating factor. Intervertebral disk rupture is now considered to be one of the major causes of severe, recurrent lower back pain and accounts for many lost days of work.

### Nursing Intervention

Conservative methods of treating ruptured intervertebral disks are tried initially unless symptoms of cord compression are present. A short period of bed rest followed by limitations in activity are necessary. Pain is often treated with nonsteroidal antiinflammatory drugs if the patient has no sensitivity or contraindication to the use of this class of drugs. In severe cases, stronger analgesics such as codeine or Percocet may be required.

Muscle relaxants such as cyclobenzaprine (Flexeril) and diazepam (Valium) often are helpful. Lying on the side with knees and hips flexed helps relieve the tension on the lumbar and sacral nerves. Another position of comfort for the patient with lower back pain is on the back with the head of the bed elevated and the knees elevated. This helps lengthen the muscles of the back and legs to prevent muscle spasms. A small pillow placed under the lumbar region of the back also helps relieve the tension. Physical therapy, applying moist heat or ice to the lumbar area, or light massage often is helpful in reducing symptoms. With cervical disk problems, a cervical collar usually is worn to keep the neck in a neutral or slightly flexed position. If con-

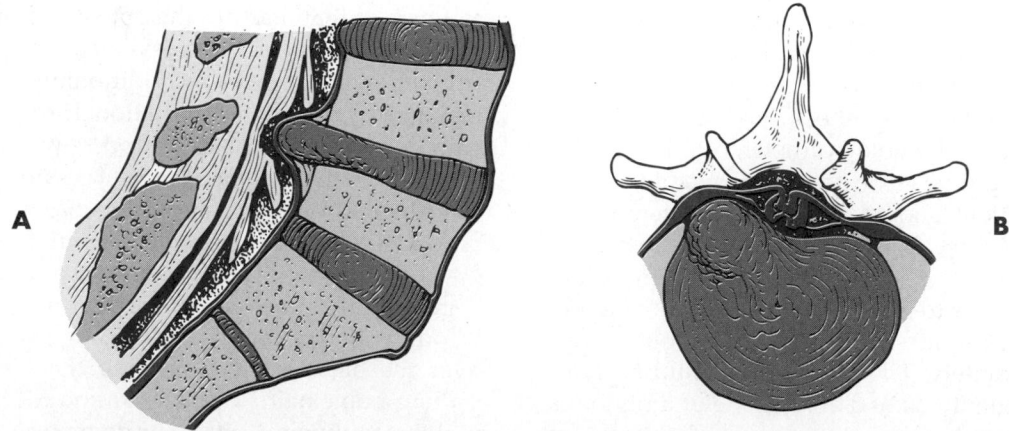

**Figure 32-8**  Ruptured intervertebral disk. Diagram shows herniation of the nucleus pulposus. **A,** Herniation presses on the structures of the spinal cord. **B,** Herniation may press on the exit of the spinal nerve and produce pain and other symptoms. (From Barker E: *Neuroscience nursing*, St Louis, 1994, Mosby.)

servative treatment is ineffective or neurologic symptoms increase, surgical intervention may be necessary.

The nurse can be helpful in teaching the patient correct body mechanics when bending, lifting, or turning in bed. The patient should be advised not to twist or strain the back during movement. General care of the patient is similar to that of any patient who is immobilized for a period of time (Box 32-4). Attention should be given to maintaining adequate fluid intake and elimination. Mild laxatives may be necessary.

## Surgical Intervention

**Laminectomy** and **diskectomy** are surgical procedures performed to remove bone, cartilage, or herniated intervertebral disk material. The posterior arch of the vertebra is removed so that the spinal cord or nerve root is exposed, and the disk material is removed. A spinal fusion also may be done during the procedure. Spinal fusion consists of the placement of a piece of bone (either from another area of the body, such as the hip, or from cadaveric bone graft) onto the vertebrae for grafting purposes. This provides a firm, bony union in a weakened area of the vertebral column. Metal wires or rods also may be attached to the vertebrae to provide additional support to the area. A laminectomy may involve the cervical, thoracic, or lumbar vertebrae. However, the thoracic vertebrae are less often involved. A partial laminectomy, or hemilaminectomy, can be performed to remove a herniated disk. In this case, a spinal fusion is unnecessary because the defect that results is negligible.

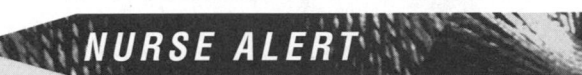

**NURSE ALERT**

Correct alignment is essential for the post-laminectomy patient.

---

| BOX 32-4 | NURSING PROCESS |
|---|---|

### POSTOPERATIVE CARE—LAMINECTOMY PATIENT

**ASSESSMENT**

- Neurovascular status to lower extremities
- Vital signs
- Respiratory status
- Bladder/bowel functioning
- Pain level
- Ability to perform self-care activities

**NURSING DIAGNOSES**

- Pain related to surgical procedure
- Impaired physical mobility related to surgical procedure
- Self-care deficit related to impaired mobility
- Risk for ineffective breathing pattern related to discomfort
- Sensory/perceptual alterations related to surgical procedure
- Risk for infection related to surgical intervention and immobility
- Risk for altered urinary elimination related to surgical procedure

**NURSING INTERVENTIONS**

- Check postoperative orders carefully.
- Place patient on firm mattress.
- Keep head of bed flat until ordered otherwise.
- Check patient's vital signs and monitor motor and sensory function in all extremities—report any muscle weakness and numbness or tingling to the surgeon.
- Observe dressing for signs of hemorrhage or cerebrospinal fluid leakage.
- If cervical laminectomy was performed, closely observe quality and rate of respirations.
- Maintain correct body alignment at all times.
- Turn patient in logroll fashion with a turning sheet every 2 hours; caution patient not to attempt to turn self.
- Check for urinary retention; catheterize patient as necessary.
- Assist patient to ambulate when ordered; encourage patient to walk erect and not to bend forward.
- Avoid having patient sit in chair for long periods— use only straight-back chair.

**EVALUATION OF EXPECTED OUTCOMES**

- Maximum pulmonary function maintained
- Aspiration prevented
- Infections prevented
- Participates in self-care as appropriate
- Demonstrates understanding of rationale for interventions
- Reports increased comfort following pain relief measures
- Maintains continence, voids voluntarily

# KEY CONCEPTS

➤ Head injuries can be classified by mechanism of occurrence. These include acceleration injuries, deceleration injuries, rotation injuries, blunt blows to the head, and penetrating injuries.

➤ Physical findings of basal skull fracture vary depending on the fracture site. With anterior fossa fractures, rhinorrhea and periorbital ecchymosis are exhibited. Middle fossa fractures cause otorrhea, ecchymosis behind the ear, and hemotympanum. Battle's sign, hearing loss, and facial palsies are associated with posterior fossa fractures.

➤ Subdural hematomas are divided into three categories based on the amount of time it takes for symptoms to appear following injury. These categories are acute, subacute, and chronic.

➤ The Glasgow Coma Scale is a tool available to nurses for accurate reporting of a patient's level of consciousness.

➤ Acute head injury often results in fracture of the skull, hemorrhage into cerebral tissue, and cerebral edema. Emergency management includes maintenance of the airway, breathing, and circulation.

➤ Cerebral edema results in increased intracranial pressure that must be controlled.

➤ Injuries to the spinal cord result in loss of motor and sensory function. Early intervention is aimed at reducing the effects of the injury, maintaining alignment of the spine, and providing stabilization to prevent further damage.

➤ Autonomic hyperreflexia is an emergency condition occurring in patients with cervical or high-thoracic injuries. Acute hypertension and tachycardia followed by bradycardia occur. Nurses should check immediately for stressful conditions such as bladder distention or catheter obstruction. Antihypertensive medications may be necessary.

➤ Rehabilitation of the patient with spinal cord injury begins immediately. Major goals are bladder and bowel reconditioning, sexual counseling, and psychologic support.

➤ Intervertebral disk trauma may compress the spinal cord or exert pressure on the nerve root, causing back and leg pain. A laminectomy may be performed to remove bone, cartilage, or herniated intervertebral disk material. Correct alignment is crucial during the postoperative period.

# CRITICAL THINKING EXERCISES

1. Discuss nursing considerations important in the care of the patient with an epidural hematoma. For how long is frequent neurologic assessment critical?
2. Why is mechanical hyperventilation an effective adjunct in the management of increased intracranial pressure. In what range should the $pCO_2$ be kept to achieve this benefit?
3. Discuss central cord syndrome. Identify areas of rehabilitation that would be necessary for a patient with this problem.
4. What are the important factors in the care of a patient with Halo traction? Why?
5. Based on the standard dermatome charts in Figure 32-5, where would a patient with an L5-S1 disk herniation note a sensory deficit?

## REFERENCES AND ADDITIONAL READINGS

Cochran JW, Kessel ES, Wittenborn R Jr: Neurologic disease: 5 scenarios to manage, *Patient Care* 28(10):32-36, 38, 41, 1994.

Eisenhart K: New perspectives in the management of adults with severe head injury, *Crit Care Nurs Q* 17(2):1-12, 1994.

Hall M, Brandys C, Yetman L: Multidisciplinary approaches to management of acute head injury, *J Neurosci Nurs* 24(4):199-204, 1992.

Hickey JV: *The clinical practice of neurological and neurosurgical nursing*, ed 3, Philadelphia, 1992, Lippincott.

Kerr ME, Brucia J: Hyperventilation in the head-injured patient: an effective treatment modality? *Heart Lung* 22(6):516-522, 1993.

Laskowski-Jones L: Acute SCI . . . spinal cord injuries, *Am J Nurs* 93(12):22-32, 1993.

Marshall SB et al: *Neuroscience critical care: pathophysiology and patient management*, Philadelphia, 1990, Saunders.

Martin KM: When the nurse says "he's just not right": patient cues used by expert nurses to identify mild head injury, *J Neurosci Nurs* 26(4):210-218, 1994.

Nayduch D, Lee A, Butler D: High-dose methylprednisolone after acute spinal cord injury, *Crit Care Nurs* 14(4):69-72, 77-78, 1994.

Richmond TS: Spinal cord injury, *Nurs Clin North Am* 25(1):57-69, 1990.

Richmond TS, Metcalf J, Daly M: Requirement for nursing care services and associated costs in acute spinal cord injury, *J Neurosci Nurs* 27(1):47-52, 1995.

Ross A, Pitts L, Kobayashi S: Prognosticators of outcome after major head injury in the elderly, *J Neurosci Nurs* 24(2):88-93, 1992.

Simmons B: What do you think? What are some strategies for managing the "difficult patient" on a spinal cord injury unit?, *Sci Nurs* 11(2):62-63, 1994.

Stamatos CA, Sorensen PA, Tefler KM: Meeting the challenge of the older trauma patient, *Am J Nurs* 96(5):40-48, 1996.

Walleck C, Mooney K: Managing craniocerebral trauma, *Am J Nurs* 95(3):52B, 52E, 1995.

Wirtz KM, La Favor KM, Ang R: Managing chronic spinal cord injury: issues in critical care, *Crit Care Nurse* 16(4): 24-35, 1996.

# CHAPTER 33

# Musculoskeletal Problems

## CHAPTER OBJECTIVES

1. Describe the structure and function of the musculoskeletal system.
2. Discuss the physiology of fracture healing, including the role of hematomas, granulation tissue, and callus formation.
3. Differentiate between osteomyelitis and tuberculosis of bone.
4. Compare and contrast the interventions for sprains, dislocations, and fractures.
5. Discuss the nursing assessment, care, and education needs of the patient in a Thomas splint with a Pearson attachment.
6. Identify the various types of fractures, as well as their medical interventions.
7. Discuss the assessment of and interventions needed for patients with newly applied casts.
8. Discuss the psychosocial and teaching needs of patients with casts.
9. Discuss the nursing measures for preparing a patient who has had an amputation and is being fitted with a prosthesis.
10. Describe the psychosocial and teaching needs of a patient who has had an amputation.
11. Differentiate between the assessment of muscular dystrophy and cerebral palsy.
12. Identify nursing measures, including psychosocial and teaching needs, that help prevent the complications associated with immobility.

## KEY TERMS

abduction
adduction
callus
compartment syndrome
countertraction
ecchymosis
external rotation

internal rotation
isometric
periosteum
prostheses
remodeling
synovial membrane
traction

## STRUCTURE AND FUNCTION OF THE MUSCULOSKELETAL SYSTEM

### Structure

The musculoskeletal system consists of bones, joints, and muscles. Within this system, muscles are attached to bones by fibrous cords called *tendons*. Bones are held together at the joints by bands of tough tissue called *ligaments*. Cartilage is a somewhat flexible tissue that connects bones and acts as a shock absorber. For example, cartilage is found between the vertebrae of the spinal column.

Bones are composed of living cells that are surrounded by an intercellular matrix infiltrated with calcium salts, which make bones hard and provide strength and rigidity. This calcified intercellular substance is permeated by a system of tiny canals that are filled with tissue fluid and through which bone cells are nourished and waste is removed.

Bones have various shapes. Long bones are found in the extremities, and short bones are found in the hands and feet. Flat bones protect vital structures, such as the brain and thoracic organs. Irregular bones include the vertebrae and other small bones throughout the body.

Long bones consist of the diaphysis, the long shaft of the bone, and the two epiphyses at either end. The medullary cavity is the space that is filled with bone marrow. In the adult, this cavity is filled with fatty, yellow marrow, and the ends of the long bones contain blood-forming red marrow. The medullary cavity is lined with the endosteum, which consists of cells that form new bone as needed. The **periosteum** is the fibrous membrane that covers the outside of the bone, except at the joints, and it contains blood vessels, lymphatic vessels, and nerves. The inner layer of the periosteum also contains bone-forming cells. Each end of a long bone is covered with articular cartilage, which cushions blows to the joint. The **synovial membrane** is the inner layer of the articular capsule. It secretes synovial fluid to lubricate the joint. Bursae (singular, bursa) are flattened sacs that are filled with synovial fluid. These sacs are located wherever it is necessary to reduce or eliminate the friction of a muscle or tendon against another muscle, tendon, or bone. The bursae also cushion certain muscles, as well as muscles that must move over bony prominences (Figure 33-1).

Bones in children are more flexible than those in adults. More calcium is deposited as bones grow, and they become rigid and inflexible. With advanced age, calcium may be lost from bones, which makes them porous and brittle.

To effectively put the patient's joints through a full range of motion, the nurse should have an understanding of joints. The range of motion for a joint is described as the degree or amount of motion that is possible for that joint (Figure 33-2). Some joints are freely movable, such as the hinge joints in the elbows and knees. The movements of these joints include flexion (bending at the joint) and extension (straightening the joint). Joint movement is also described by the terms **abduction,** which involves moving the extremity away from the midline of the body, and **adduction,** which involves moving the extremity toward the midline of the body. Shoulder and hip joints are ball-and-socket joints and have a rotating motion. The description of the rotating movement of a joint often includes information to indicate which way the joint is rotating, such as **external rotation** (away from the body's midline) and **internal rotation** (toward the body's midline). Other joints are slightly movable. For example, the joints between the vertebral bodies provide limited motion of the spine. Some joints are immovable and are found in places such as the cranium. Only those joints that are freely movable can be put through a full range of motion. Although movement of the body depends largely on muscle contraction, mobility is actually a cooperative function of bones, muscles, and joints.

## Function

The musculoskeletal system has other functions in addition to locomotion. The bony framework supports

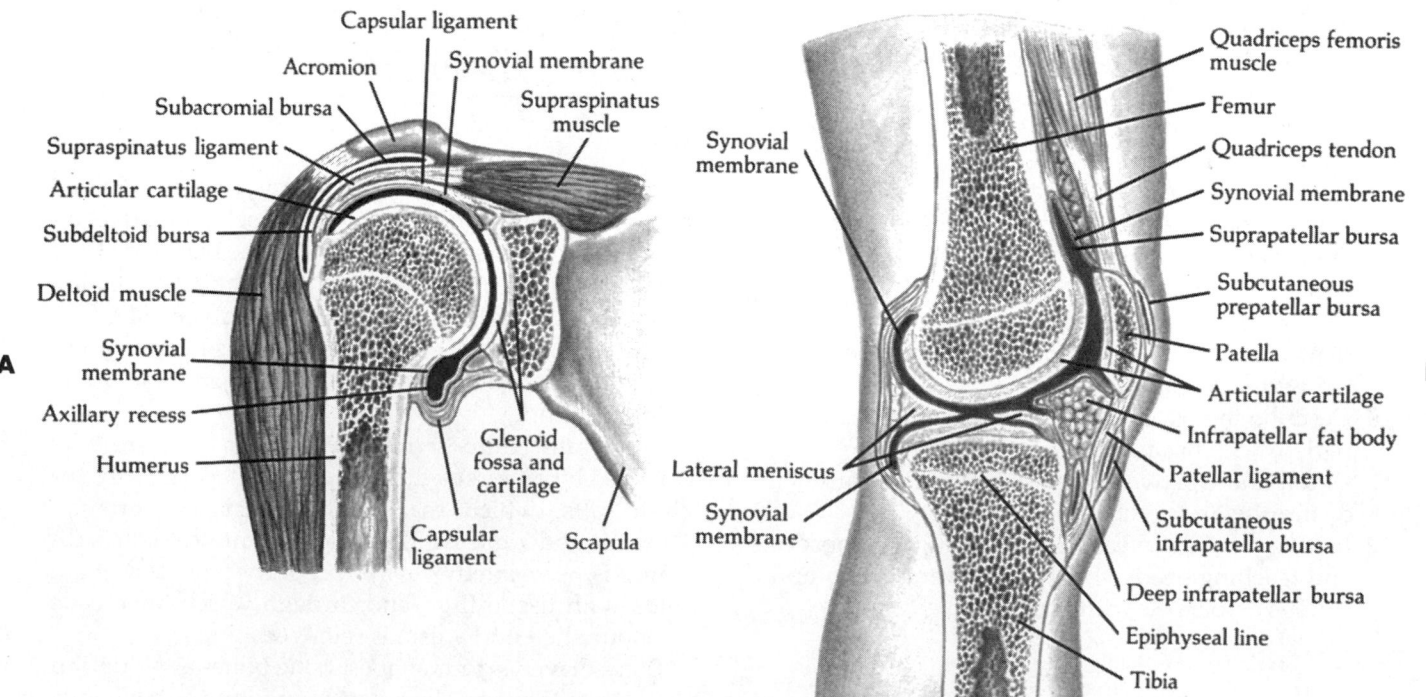

**Figure 33-1** **A,** Bursae of the shoulder joint. **B,** Bursae of the knee joint. (From Thompson JM et al: *Mosby's clinical nursing,* ed 4, St Louis, 1997, Mosby.)

SHOULDER

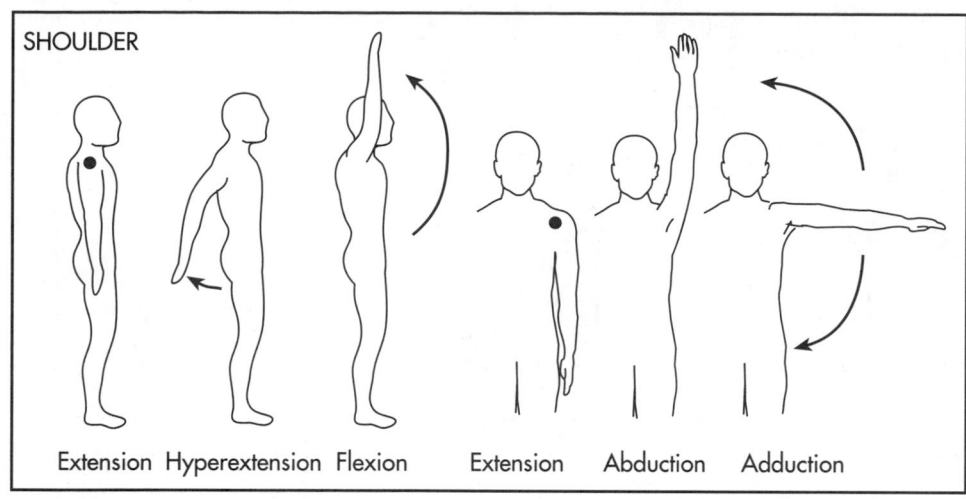

Extension  Hyperextension  Flexion     Extension    Abduction    Adduction

FOREARM

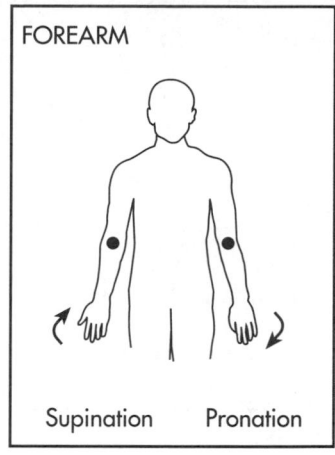

Supination  Pronation

FINGERS

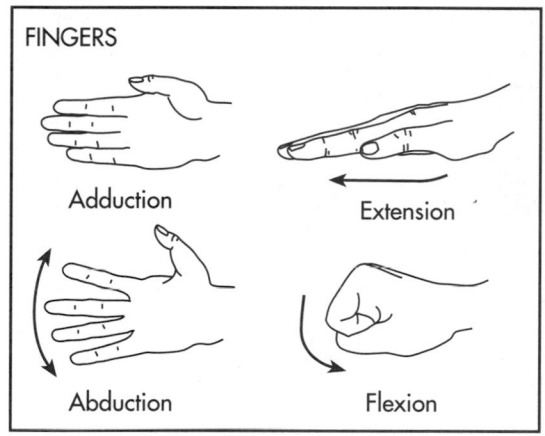

Adduction

Extension

Abduction

Flexion

THUMB

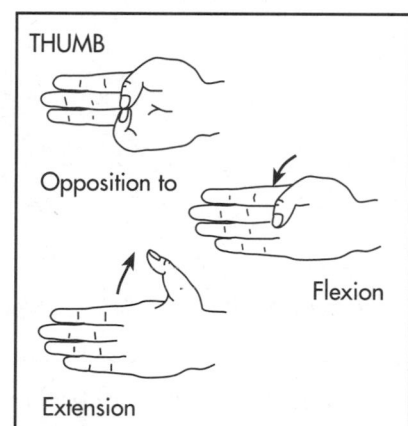

Opposition to

Flexion

Extension

ELBOW

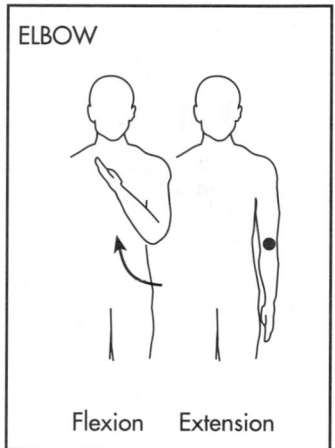

Flexion  Extension

ANKLE

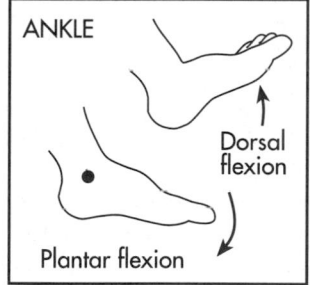

Dorsal flexion

Plantar flexion

HAND

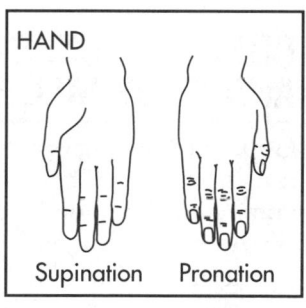

Supination  Pronation

WRIST

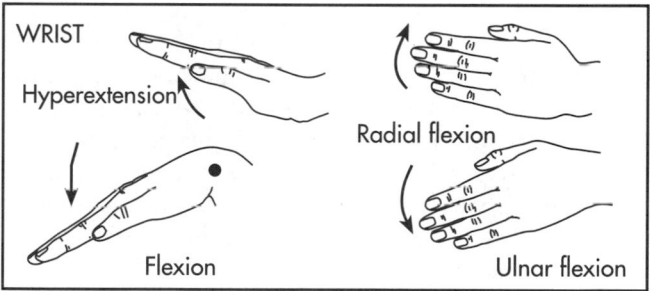

Hyperextension

Radial flexion

Flexion

Ulnar flexion

LEGS

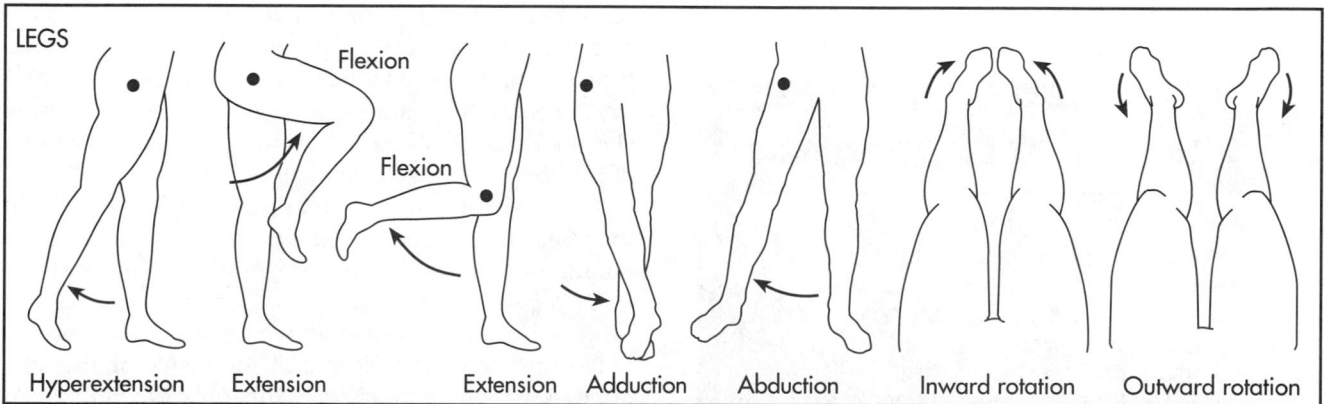

Hyperextension    Extension       Extension   Adduction    Abduction    Inward rotation   Outward rotation

**Figure 33-2**  Range of motion for joints in the body. (Redrawn from Beare PG, Myers JL: *Principles and practice of adult health nursing*, ed 2, St Louis, 1994, Mosby.)

*Continued*

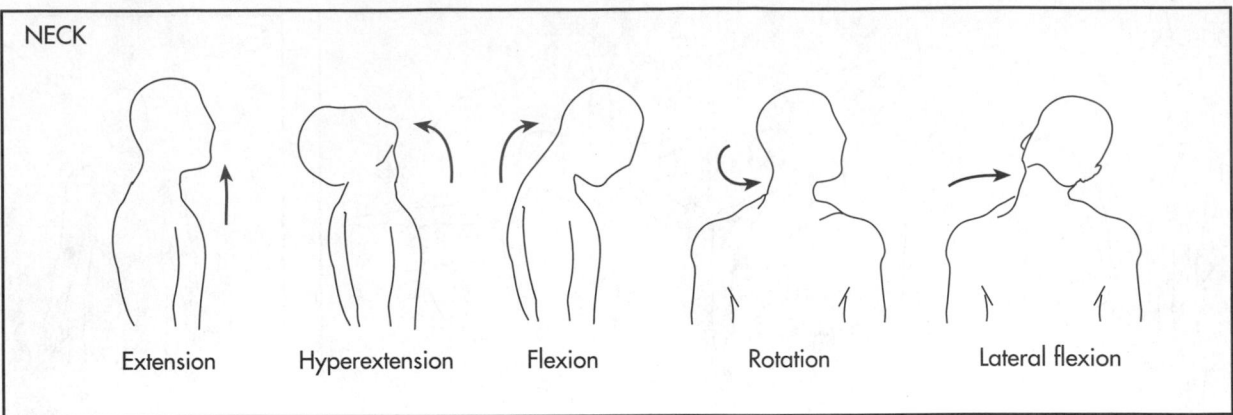

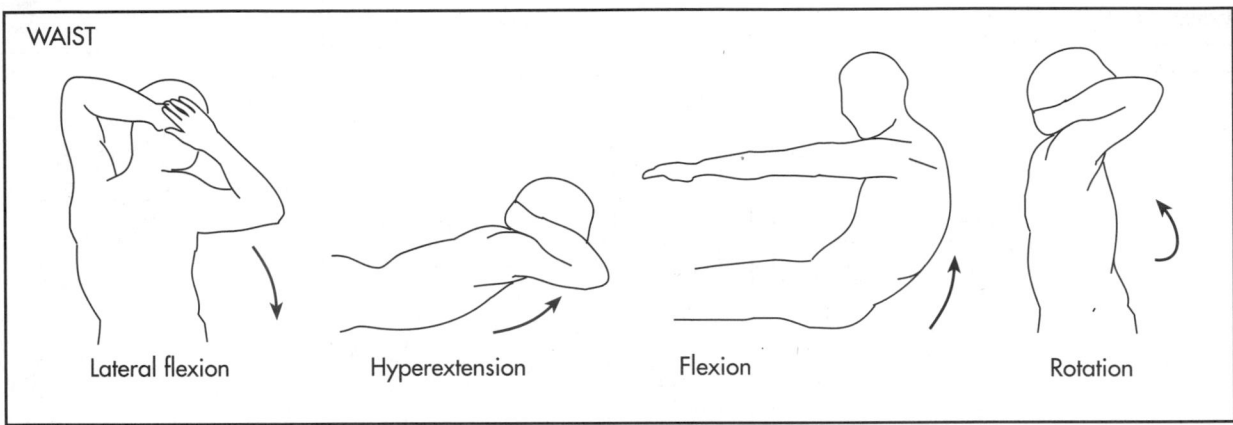

**Figure 33-2, cont'd** For legend see page 993.

the body in an upright position and protects vital organs. Blood cells are formed in the marrow of bones, and bones deposit calcium, which may be used to supply a deficiency in the body fluids. Injury and disease may affect any part of the system and may result in deformity or impairment of functions. Some disorders involve both nerves and muscles and are called *neuromuscular disorders*.

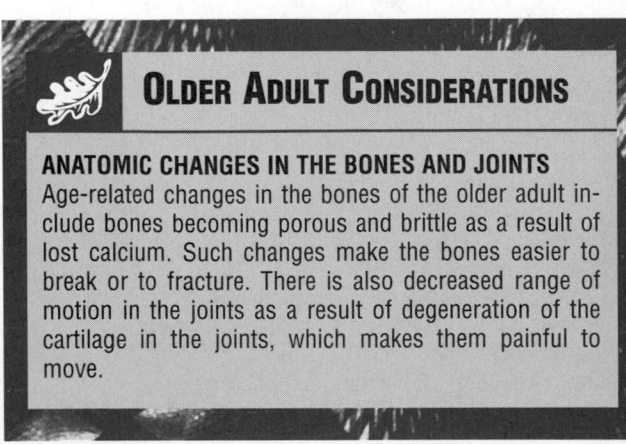

### OLDER ADULT CONSIDERATIONS

**ANATOMIC CHANGES IN THE BONES AND JOINTS**
Age-related changes in the bones of the older adult include bones becoming porous and brittle as a result of lost calcium. Such changes make the bones easier to break or to fracture. There is also decreased range of motion in the joints as a result of degeneration of the cartilage in the joints, which makes them painful to move.

# POSITION, EXERCISE, AND BODY MECHANICS

Proper positioning of a patient who is confined to bed rest is essential. Properly positioning a patient is a nursing intervention, and medical orders are not necessary except in those surgical procedures in which physicians' preferences vary. Orthopedic patients may be required to remain in plaster casts, traction, or other stabilization devices for prolonged periods. Nursing care must emphasize positioning to prevent contractures, deformities, or other complications of immobility. A contracture is a permanent shortening of muscles, tendons, and ligaments, and it reduces the range of motion in affected joints.

Active and passive exercise of the muscles of both the affected and unaffected extremities is essential for maintaining muscle tone, preventing complications, and preparing for ambulation. Active exercise is performed by the patient. Passive exercise does not involve muscle contraction, and the nurse or therapist often assists the patient with this type of exercise. An exercise program that is tailored to the individual is often initiated soon after immobilization. Active and passive movement of joints through their full ranges of motion should be incorporated into the daily activities of physical care and ambulation. Active range-of-motion exercises are performed by the patient, who moves the affected joint through its range of motion by using the muscles that surround that joint. Passive range-of-motion exercises require that the joint be moved through its range of motion by either the patient or someone else, but the muscles of the joint are not used. An example of passive range of motion is a patient using the left arm to move the right elbow through its range of motion. Patients may fear that doing the prescribed exercises or moving an extremity that is in a cast will cause further injury. The nurse should explain to these patients that the exercises stimulate bone growth and prevent muscle atrophy and thrombus formation.

Specific exercises that prevent thrombophlebitis and help maintain muscle tone include antithromboembolic exercises of the calf muscle, as well as quad-setting and gluteal-setting **isometric** exercises. Isometric exercises require the patient to consciously tighten the muscles, but no movement is involved. Antithromboembolic and isometric exercises are performed in the supine position. To encourage circulation and to prevent thrombus and embolus development in the calf muscle, patients fully extend their legs and push the backs of their knees down on the bed while dorsiflexing the feet. For quad-setting exercises, patients tighten their quadriceps muscles, with legs fully extended, and push the backs of their knees down on the bed. For gluteal-setting exercises, they tighten and pinch their buttocks together. With each of these exercises, patients may be advised to hold the position for a count of 10. They also may be advised to repeat these exercises 10 times every hour while awake.

Exercises that are designed to strengthen muscles in preparation for ambulation include prescribed weight-lifting and bridging exercises. To perform the bridging exercise, patients flex their unaffected leg at the knee. They push down on the bed with the sole of their foot while using the trapeze to lift their back and buttocks off the bed. They hold themselves in the lifted position with their backs straight for as long as possible. Patients also may be advised to do this 10 times each hour while awake.

Emphasis also has been placed on the importance of turning patients to prevent pulmonary complications. Too often a comfortable patient objects to being disturbed, and moving an obese or comatose patient or a patient who is in a body cast or in traction presents a special challenge for the nurse. However, research has confirmed that turning a patient as little as 12 degrees is sufficient to prevent pulmonary complications, stimulate circulation, and prevent decubitus ulcers. Therefore all immobilized patients should be turned at least every 2 hours.

The tilt table is a device that helps the patient adjust to an upright position before ambulation. Patients who have been confined to bed rest for long periods may develop hypotension when they sit or stand. Gradual elevation with a tilt table helps prevent this problem. The tilt table is used to prepare the patient for crutch walking and ambulation, as well as to reduce osteoporosis that develops from immobilization. The tilt table may also prevent urinary tract infections by decreasing the pooling of urine in the bladder, which results when the patient remains in a supine position. Because patients are discharged so quickly from acute care settings, tilt tables are more likely to be used in rehabilitation facilities.

After an injury to the musculoskeletal system, many patients need to be taught the proper methods of standing, sitting, walking, stooping, and lifting. Nurses who use their bodies skillfully are in a much better position to help teach their patients about body mechanics. The consideration of body mechanics conserves energy, prevents injuries to muscles, prevents fatigue, and promotes work efficiency.

> ### NURSE ALERT
>
> Nurses need to be very conscious about using good body mechanics because of the risk of injury to themselves while caring for their patients.

## NEUROVASCULAR INTEGRITY

Neurovascular impairment is a threat to patients with orthopedic conditions and must be relieved promptly. Impairment of circulation or nerve function can result in tissue necrosis or loss of the use of an extremity. Damage to nerves and blood vessels may result from trauma; surgery; or tight bandages, splints, and casts. Assessment and intervention for arterial vascular compromise are discussed later in this chapter in relation to the serious complications of compartment syndrome. Temporary impairment of the venous circulation in the extremities is more common and should be suspected when edema, coolness, pallor, cyanosis, pain, numbness, and tingling are observed in the fingers or toes. Edema is swelling that is caused by excess interstitial fluid. Pallor describes a whitish, grayish color of the skin. Cyanosis describes a bluish skin color. Cyanosis can be easily seen in the skin, nail beds, and mucous membranes. These symptoms may be accompanied by slow capillary refill in the nail beds, as well as by the absence of radial, pedal, or tibial pulses.

## Assessment

To perform an accurate neurovascular assessment the nurse should always compare color, movement, and sensation in the affected extremity with that of the unaffected extremity. Extremities should be positioned correctly, with the affected arm or leg elevated. An accurate description of sensations should be elicited from the patient. Using the same hand (rather than two hands) to access both extremities may provide a more accurate assessment. To determine true coolness in the affected extremity, the nurse must feel both feet because many people have cool feet under normal circumstances. The foot of the affected extremity may be warmer than the other extremity as a result of the normal inflammation that is associated with trauma and surgery.

Edema that is accompanied by warmth and normal color usually does not indicate harmful circulatory impairment, particularly if other signs are absent or if the edema occurs within 48 to 72 hours after trauma or surgery. This type of warmth and edema gradually subsides. However, edema that is accompanied by pallor, cyanosis, and coldness is a sign of circulatory impairment. If swelling is difficult to determine, a comparison of the wrinkles on the toes or fingers of both feet or hands may show stretching of the tissue on the digits in question, which indicates slight edema (Box 33-1).

The blanching sign is a test of the rate of capillary refill, which signals the adequacy of circulation. When the nail of each toe or finger is compressed and immediately released, the nail bed should rapidly change from white to pink. Slow or sluggish capillary refill indicates decreased circulation.

Each digit should be checked for sensation and motion because not all digits are innervated by the same nerve. Localized numbness and the inability to flex and extend the digits indicate nerve compression. Increased pain may accompany circulatory impairment. A clear description of the pain with regard to its precise location (e.g., along a nerve or over a bony prominence), intensity, and response to movement should be obtained from the patient before pain medication is given. Palpating the pedal, tibial, or radial pulse may be difficult or impossible when a cast or bandage renders these areas inaccessible. Sometimes the nurse may be able to reach under a bandage to locate the pulse. However, caution must be used if an incision or open wound is underneath the bandage, and sterile gloves are required to protect the nurse from accidental contamination. The presence and strength of the pulse in the affected extremity should be identified and compared to the pulse in the unaffected extremity.

Beginning immediately after surgery or the application of a cast, a neurovascular assessment should be performed every 30 minutes. Patients often describe a transient tingling and numbness in an extremity, which results from general immobility. Flexing the fingers and toes relieves this, and the patient should be

---

| BOX 33-1 | NURSING PROCESS |
|---|---|

### NEUROVASCULAR INTEGRITY

**ASSESSMENT**

- Alignment of body
- Peripheral tissue perfusion
- Wound/fracture site
- Pain/comfort level
- Peripheral nerve sensation

**NURSING DIAGNOSES**

- Risk for neurovascular dysfunction related to injury/treatment
- Impaired physical mobility related to injury/treatment
- Pain related to injury/treatment

**NURSING INTERVENTIONS**

- Position extremities in alignment; elevate affected extremity.

- Compare affected extremity with unaffected extremity; use the same hand for palpation.
- Test capillary refill.
- Check each digit for sensation and motion.
- Document the location and characteristics of pain.
- Palpate pedal, tibial, or radial pulses, and compare them to those of the unaffected extremity.
- Look for edema with pallor, cyanosis, and coldness.
- Elicit a description of sensations from the patient.

**EVALUATION OF EXPECTED OUTCOMES**

- Adequate neurovascular function
- Performs range of motion exercises and muscle-setting exercises
- Pain diminished or relieved by pain management protocol

encouraged to flex whenever these symptoms occur. Neurovascular assessments should be completely and accurately recorded. The previous assessment of the patient's circulation should be reviewed before each subsequent neurovascular assessment. This review provides a baseline for evaluating progress or deterioration of circulatory integrity.

The physician should be notified immediately when circulatory impairment is suspected. Repositioning, elevating, and applying ice packs to the extremity may alleviate the symptoms. The physician may loosen or remove a cast or bandage. Modification of a cast is discussed later in this chapter.

## PAIN

Specific types of musculoskeletal injuries or disorders produce specific types of pain. To effectively assess and alleviate the pain, the nurse must know the nature of the pain. The nurse must differentiate between pain as an expected outcome and pain as a diagnostic sign (see Chapter 11).

Patients with fractures often describe acute, deep, severe pain at the time of injury, which persists until the fracture is reduced and medication is given. When the fracture is reduced, the bone ends and fragments are realigned and stabilized in the proper position. Reduction and stabilization prevent further soft-tissue, nerve, and blood vessel damage by the ragged bone pieces, which is an expected outcome of traumatic fractures. The pain that accompanies a fractured hip can be severe because of muscle spasms and trauma to surrounding nerves. Once a fracture is reduced, the pain becomes more localized and gradually subsides as healing takes place.

A recurrence of severe pain after a fracture is reduced and stabilized indicates that something is wrong. A constant, aching pain may be the first sign that neurovascular integrity is being compromised. This pain may be increased with passive movement of the extremity and is accompanied by other signs of neurovascular impairment, such as numbness, paralysis, coolness, and paleness. These findings are diagnostic of a circulatory problem that must be corrected promptly.

Pain associated with spinal column disorders often accompanies a long-standing back problem. The pain ranges from being sudden and sharp to being constant or intermittently aching. The pain may extend down one or both extremities and often is influenced by voluntary movement or positioning of the patient. Ongoing precise assessment of the frequency, location, intensity, and influencing activity of the pain is necessary for determining progress in both the conservative and surgical treatment of spinal disorders.

Because pain associated with musculoskeletal disorders may be severe and persistent, the nurse can anticipate the patient's need for pain medications on a regular basis until the pain subsides. Pain medication should be given as soon as the pain has been assessed thoroughly. Have the patient use a pain scale to rate the level of pain (see Chapter 11). Additional measures to alleviate the pain by repositioning the affected body region should also be initiated.

## THE PATIENT WITH A CAST

Casts are applied to fractured extremities or to other parts of the body to maintain correct alignment of bones during healing. Casts can also be used to prevent or correct deformities and to immobilize the extremity. Casts are most commonly applied to fractures that are reduced by closed manipulation. Closed manipulation involves realignment of the bone ends by manipulation, manual traction, or both. Casts may also be applied following other surgical repairs, including realignments that involve surgical open reduction with internal fixation of the fracture (see the interventions for fractures later in this chapter). Usually the cast extends beyond the joints above and below the fracture site (Figure 33-3).

The application of a cast may be anticipated by the patient, but more often it accompanies an unexpected fracture. Once the cast is applied, the patient is faced with a frustrating limitation of movement and an interruption in fulfilling roles and responsibilities. The emotional adjustment may be difficult. The nurse should recognize the patient's and the family's need to ask questions and to be supported in their adjustment to a changed level of function.

### Care of the Cast

A newly applied plaster cast sets quickly but takes as long as 48 hours to dry completely. During this drying time, the cast must be handled with the palms of the hands rather than with the fingers to prevent indentations that could create pressure. Casts are positioned and elevated on pillows to reduce swelling and to prevent pressure from the firm mattress (Figures 33-4 to 33-6). The drying of the cast is accompanied by a considerable feeling of heat, which should be explained to the patient. To combat this heat and to help reduce swelling of the extremity, ice bags are placed beside the cast for 48 hours.

Once the cast has dried, it should be examined for rough edges that can be covered with adhesive petals. Petals are rectangular or oval pieces of adhesive with rounded corners and are approximately 1 inch × 3 inches. They are slipped under the edge of the cast,

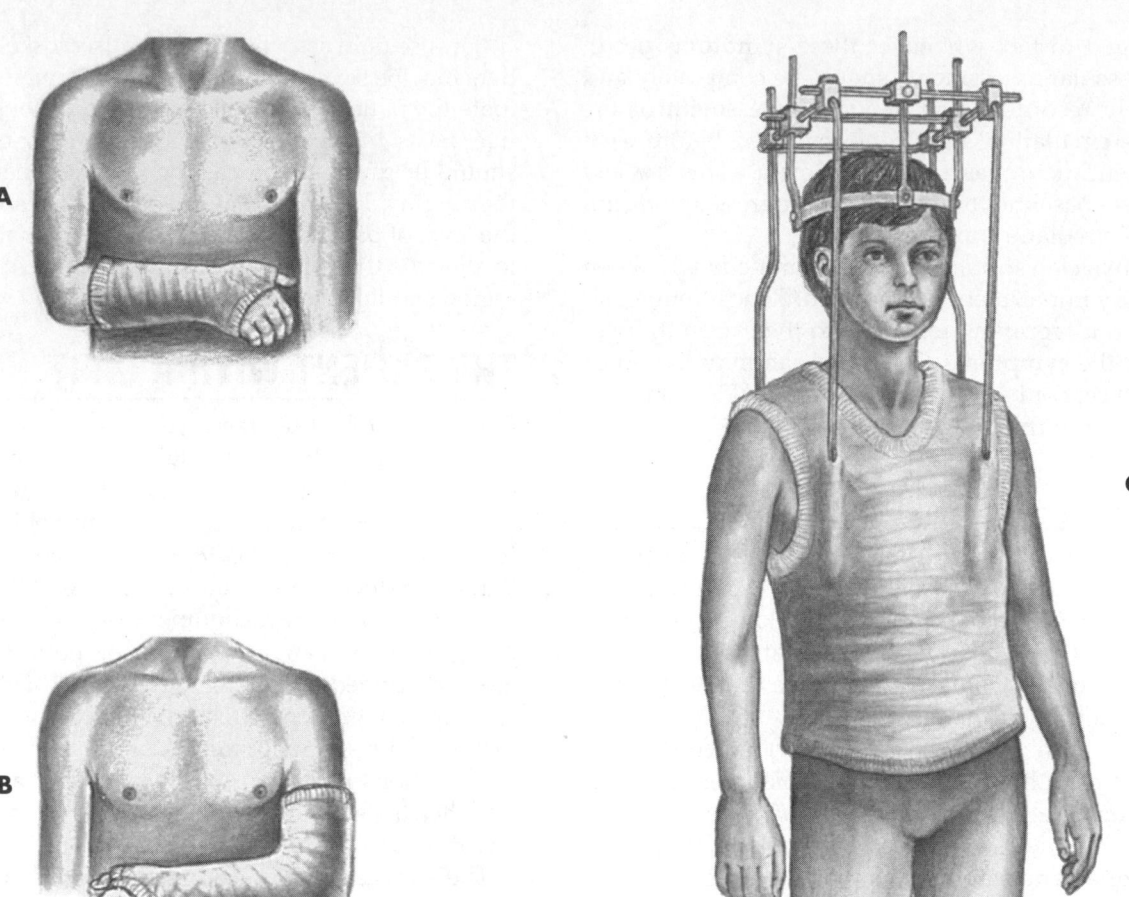

**Figure 33-3** Examples of casts for upper extremity injuries. **A,** Short arm cast. **B,** Long arm cast. **C,** Body jacket with halo apparatus attached; it may be used with a brace, not a cast. (From Thompson JM et al: *Mosby's manual of clinical nursing,* ed 2, St Louis, 1989, Mosby.)

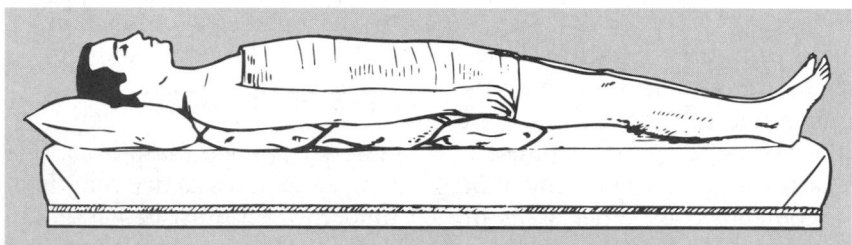

**Figure 33-4** Placement of pillows to receive patient in wet body cast.

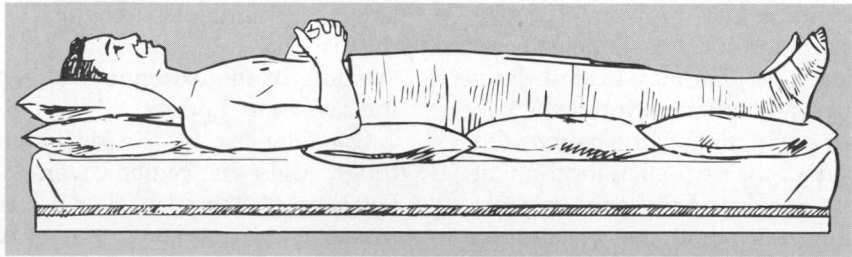

**Figure 33-5** Placement of pillows to receive patient in wet hip spica cast.

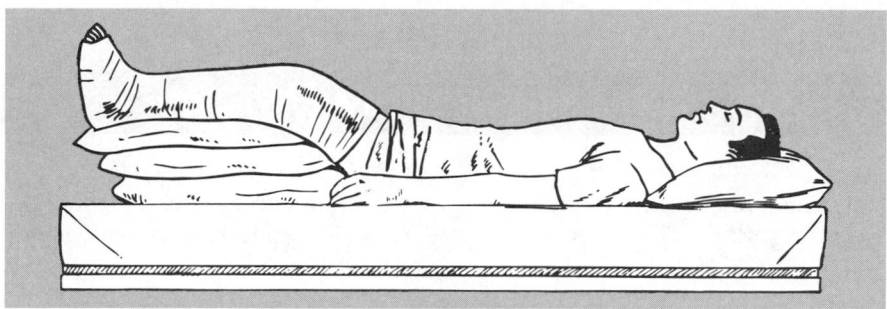

**Figure 33-6**    Placement of pillows to support extremity in long leg cast.

brought over the edge, and adhered to the top of the cast. Cotton wadding or a stockinette is applied under the cast during the application to provide smooth edges. Never trim cast edges without a physician's order.

A plaster cast must be kept clean and dry. Moisture may soften the plaster and cause the cast to crack. A cast around the genital area can be protected from urine and stool by tucking plastic or a disposable diaper inside the cast and taping it to the outside. If this procedure is done, the skin beneath the plastic must be checked regularly for evidence of irritation or maceration. Using powder under the cast should be avoided because moisture from the patient's body may cause the powder to clump, which results in pressure against the skin. Cleaning a plaster cast is difficult, but small stains on the outside of the cast can be removed by gently rubbing it with scouring powder on a slightly dampened cloth. Rubbing baby powder on a cast whitens it and gives it a pleasant smell. Spraying a cast with a plastic coating or painting it with white shoe polish is generally not recommended because such steps prevent the cast from "breathing." Bathing with a cast is possible if the cast is not submerged and if it is covered with a leak-proof plastic bag, such as a trash bag.

Fiberglass is a newer type of casting material that can be used instead of plaster. It may be referred to as a synthetic cast. A fiberglass cast is lighter and stronger than a traditional plaster cast. The fiberglass reaches full strength only minutes after it is applied. It is more expensive and is used for casts that do not require frequent changing, such as casts applied to nondisplaced fractures. A plaster cast may be used as a temporary cast if edema is present, removed after edema lessens, and then followed by application of a fiberglass cast.

Performing regular neurovascular assessments on all patients who have casts is a critical nursing function (Box 33-2). During the neurovascular assessment, the nurse should feel the entire cast for excessive local warmth and should sniff it for any foul odor. These signs, along with the patient's description of a localized burning sensation, signal the presence of tissue necrosis as a result of localized cast pressure. When a

cast is applied, bony prominences and areas with nerves close to the skin are usually well padded. However, these sites are particularly susceptible to cast pressure, local necrosis, or neurovascular impairment. In the arm, susceptible sites are the condyles and olecranon processes of the elbow and the radial and ulnar styloids. In the leg, susceptible sites are the popliteal space, the head of the fibula, the lateral aspect of the knee, the lateral and medial malleoli, the heel, and the small toe. To relieve circulatory impairment and localized pressure, the cast may be split lengthwise. To accomplish this procedure, an oscillating saw (cast cutter) is used by the physician, nurse, or trained assistant. The patient should be assured that the saw vibrates to cut the cast and is not a sharp blade that can cut into the skin.

A cast should also be observed for external bloody drainage, which may be expected with certain types of open reduction procedures. The area of drainage should be circled, dated, and timed on the cast with a permanent marker (not red ink); and its progression should be monitored, recorded, and reported. Because drainage may occur in the direction of gravity, careful examination of the underside of the cast is essential, even when the site of the incision is on the anterior surface of the extremity. The nurse should monitor the extremity carefully for other indicators of blood loss and tissue damage, because evidence of bleeding on the cast and development of odor from necrotic tissue may not occur until after considerable blood or tissue has been lost.

Skin care of the entire body and of areas that are close to the cast is important because casts can be heavy and patients may have difficulty moving in bed. Regular inspection of areas that usually rest on the bed is vital. Patients need assistance in regular turning and should be positioned in good body alignment with firm, supportive pillows. Itching under the cast as the wound heals is usually inevitable and is probably the patient's greatest annoyance. To alleviate itching, blow cool air from a hair dryer down the cast. The physician may order oral diphenhydramine (Benadryl). Patients should be

| BOX 33-2 | NURSING PROCESS |
|---|---|

## THE PATIENT WITH A CAST

### ASSESSMENT

- Neurovascular assessment of affected extremity
- Skin assessment
- Pain/comfort
- Elimination patterns
- Mobility
- Self-concept/role disturbance
- Home maintenance

### NURSING DIAGNOSES

- Pain related to bone displacement and muscle spasm
- Constipation related to inactivity and altered position for elimination
- Impaired home maintenance management related to restrictions on activity
- Risk for injury related to immobility
- Risk for neurovascular dysfunction related to cast
- Pain related to injury
- Diversional activity deficit related to alteration in recreation
- Knowledge deficit related to diet to promote bone healing and correct use of ambulatory assistive devices
- Impaired physical mobility related to cast
- Altered nutrition: risk for more than body requirements related to reduced activity
- Self-care deficit in feeding, bathing/hygiene, and dressing/grooming related to cast
- Actual or risk for impaired skin integrity related to trauma, cast irritation, or immobility
- Altered tissue perfusion related to edema and cast constriction
- Risk for impaired gas exchange related to imposed immobility or restricted respiratory movement secondary to body cast

### NURSING INTERVENTIONS
#### While Plaster Cast Dries

- Place patient on firm surface.
- Handle cast with palms of hands.
- Explain to patient that he or she will feel heat as the cast dries.
- Do not cover cast until it is completely dry.
- Do not speed drying with heat or lamps; the cast may dry on the outside but remain weak on the inside and crack.

- Elevate extremity on plastic-covered pillows, or support curves of body cast with small pillows.
- Avoid weight bearing on walking leg cast for 48 hours.

#### When Cast is Dry

- Attend to all complaints of pain, which may signal impending complications; do not medicate for pain until cause of pain is clearly identified.
- Observe for signs of pressure, such as pain, burning, and odor.
- Check circulation; observe for pain, numbness, tingling, edema, color, blanching and capillary refill, skin temperature, inability to move fingers or toes, and presence and rate of pulse; compare these signs to the other extremity.
- Use plastic sheeting to protect a cast in the perineal area from soiling.
- Cleanse cast with an almost-dry cloth and abrasive soap or cleanser; whiten and freshen it by rubbing in baby powder.
- Cover edge of cast with adhesive tape petals.
- Inspect skin under and at edge of cast for irritation.
- Instruct patient not to insert wire hangers, knitting needles, or other sharp instruments under cast to scratch skin.
- Assist patient with isometric exercises of affected extremities.
- In addition to isometric exercises, actively exercise unaffected joints.
- Allow patient to verbalize feelings about fracture, cast, and alterations in role performance and activity.

#### When Cast is Removed

- Explain to patient that the cast cutter vibrates and cannot cut or injure skin.
- Explain how affected extremity will appear when cast is removed.
- After cast is removed, support affected body part with pillows in same position as when the part was in the cast.
- Move extremity gently.
- Wash skin with soap and water, followed by a gentle massage with lanolin or baby oil.
- Assist patient in performing prescribed muscle-strengthening exercises.

◄ BOX 33-2 ►        **NURSING PROCESS**

**THE PATIENT WITH A CAST—cont'd**

- If lower extremity is involved, instruct patient to elevate foot when sitting to prevent edema; apply an elastic bandage or elastic stocking as ordered to provide support; reinforce physician's instructions about weight bearing, which is usually limited after removal of leg cast.

**EVALUATION OF EXPECTED OUTCOMES**
- Knows rationale for cast application
- Cast integrity maintained
- Neurovascular status intact
- Cares for cast and observes condition of skin and extremities
- Verbalizes feelings about altered self-concept
- Identifies appropriate accommodations for self-care and home maintenance

cautioned against using knitting needles, wire hangers, or foreign objects to scratch under the cast.

## Hip Spica and Body Casts

Hip spica and body casts are large, cumbersome casts (Figure 33-7). They are worn for long periods (5 months or longer) and require special techniques for turning and caring for the patient. These casts surround the entire trunk and may make the patient claustrophobic. The hip spica cast begins below the axilla and extends the entire length of one or both legs. It is applied to immobilize congenital hip dislocations or fractures of the hip and femur. The body cast extends from the upper chest to the groin or thigh. Confinement in these casts can be very frightening, and the patient must adjust to being confined within the cast. The patient may need to eat smaller or more frequent portions of food to be comfortable. A cast that is too tight can cause respiratory complications if the lungs cannot expand fully. The patient should be taught breathing exercises to prevent complications such as atelectasis while in the cast. The most serious complication of a tight body cast is the development of "cast syndrome," which occurs when the superior mesenteric artery presses on or obstructs part of the duodenum. Symptoms of nausea, vomiting, abdominal pain, or intestinal obstruction require removal of the cast to alleviate the condition. Body casts following spinal surgery have been replaced with synthetic rigid jackets (e.g., the thoracic, lumbar, spinal orthosis [TLSO]) that can be removed when the patient is supine (Figure 33-7).

## Cast Removal

When a cast is removed, the extremity should be moved carefully and supported at the joints. If the patient has been in a cast for a long time, some decalcification has

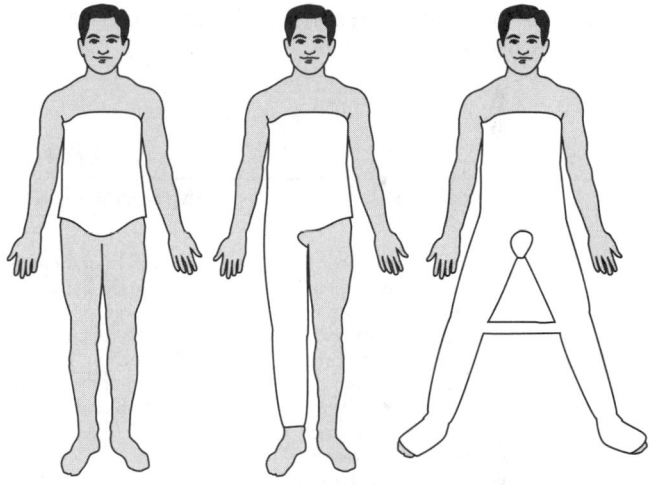

Body jacket cast    Single-hip spica    Double-hip spica

**Figure 33-7**    Common body casts. (Redrawn from Lewis SM, Collier IC, Heitkemper MM: *Medical-surgical nursing: assessment and management of clinical problems*, ed 4, St Louis, 1996, Mosby.)

occurred. The patient may experience some discomfort once the external support has been removed. The patient should be told that the appearance of the casted limb will differ from the unaffected limb. The skin should be cleansed gently to remove the dead skin. An emollient lotion should be applied to dry skin. Exercises to restore strength and mobility are begun. Weight bearing may be restricted until total bone healing has taken place.

## THE PATIENT WITH AN ORTHOPEDIC DEVICE

### Traction

**Traction** means "pulling." When traction is applied to a lower extremity because of a broken bone, the two ends of the bone are pulled into place (correct alignment). To relax or "stretch" the muscles of the affected extremity and allow the bone fragments to be brought into correct alignment, the force of the traction must be stronger than the force of the muscle contraction of the affected extremity. The physician decides on the type of traction, its placement, and the weight applied to achieve the desired results. When applied correctly, traction will be equal to countertraction. **Countertraction** pulls in the opposite direction and is applied either by the patient's own body weight or by other weights or devices. Traction may be applied to any of the extremities, the cervical area, or the pelvic region. The purpose of traction may be to relieve muscle spasm, which often occurs as a result of disease or injury. For patients with certain types of fractures, traction may be necessary to keep bones in place while healing of the bones and soft tissue occurs. Traction may also be used to reduce dislocations or to correct or relieve contractures.

> **NURSE ALERT**
>
> **Check that the weights are hanging freely and not resting on the bed or the floor. Make sure that the knots are secure. Be sure that the patient is positioned properly and not pulled to the end of the bed where the traction is attached.**

Traction may be applied as *skin traction*, in which some material with an adhesive surface is applied directly onto clean, dry skin, or as skeletal traction, in which traction is applied directly to the bone by surgically inserting a pin or wire into the bone (Figure 33-8). The Steinmann pin (Figure 33-9) and Kirschner wire are most commonly used. Weights are attached to the pin or wire while the patient is placed in suspension traction (see Figure 33-8).

### COMMON TYPES OF TRACTION

| Type | Indications | Nursing Implications | |
|---|---|---|---|
| **Skin** | | | |
| Buck's | Used for many conditions affecting hip, femur, knee, or back. It is generally used for temporary immobilization and stabilization of fractured hips or fractures of the femoral shaft. It can be unilateral or bilateral. | Assess for nerve and circulatory disturbances caused by circumferential bandages, especially over bony prominences, and for skin necrosis, an allergic reaction to the adhesive material, rotation of the extremity, and constant traction and countertraction forces. | 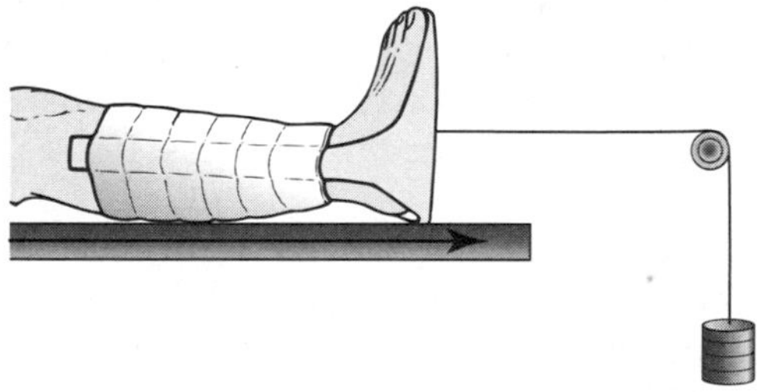 |
| Russell's | Used for fractures of femur and hip and certain knee problems. Known as balanced traction. | Same as above. Assess knee sling for smoothness and an overly tight edge. Because the arrangement of this traction may vary, be aware of initial setup and maintain it. | 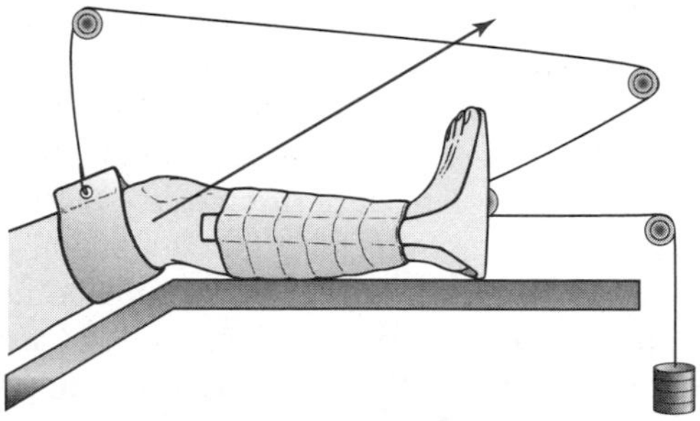 |
| Bryant's | Used for fractures of the femur, fractures in small children, and stabilization of hip joints in children under 2 yr or 30 lb (14 kg) in weight. | Be aware that with traction in place, buttocks should just clear the mattress. Check for undue pressure over the outer head and neck of fibula, dorsum of foot, Achilles tendon, scapulae, and shoulders. Check that bandages or boot has not slipped. Be aware that these are usually removed for skin care and assessment q 8 hr. | 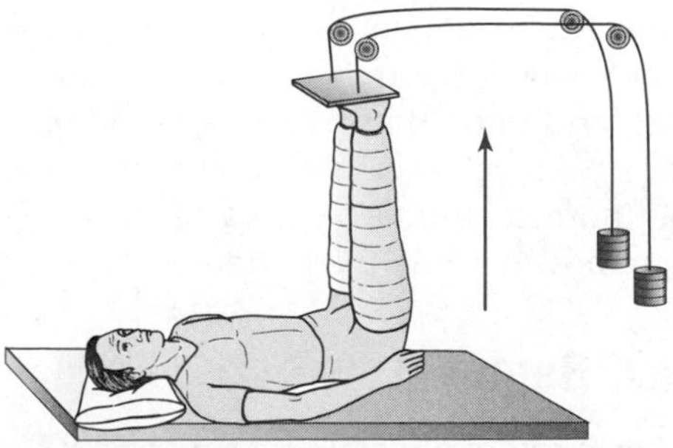 |

**Figure 33-8**   Common types of traction. (Modified from Lewis SM, Collier IC, Heitkemper MM: *Medical-surgical nursing: assessment and management of clinical problems*, ed 4, St Louis, 1996, Mosby.)

**COMMON TYPES OF TRACTION—cont'd**

| Type | Indications | Nursing Implications | |
|---|---|---|---|
| **Skin—cont'd** Pelvic | Used for sciatica, muscle spasms (low back), and minor fractures of the lower spine. | Check for security of the pelvic belt. Check frequently for skin irritation over iliac crests. Use measures to prevent skin breakdown. Check and adjust pelvic belt straps so that they are unrestricted and equal in length. Secure the straps with adhesive tape. Use a foot board to prevent footdrop. Maintain the correct angle of pull of the traction. Be aware that the physician orders the type of countertraction. | |
| **Circumferential** Head halter | Used for soft-tissue disorders and degenerative disk disease of the cervical spine. It is not commonly used for unstable fractures of the cervical spine. | Assess for alignment with trunk, areas of local pressure under the chin and occipital area, and pain or dysfunction in the temporomandibular joint. | |
| **Skeletal** Overhead arm (90 degrees and 90 degrees) | Commonly used for immobilization of fractures and dislocations of the upper arm and shoulder. | Be aware that the shoulder and elbow joint are maintained at 90-degree angles. | |
| Lateral arm | Commonly used in immobilization of fractures and dislocations of the upper arm and shoulder. | | |
| Balanced suspension traction | Used for injury or fracture of the femoral shaft of the femur, acetabulum, hip, lower leg, or any combination of these. | Be aware that this traction uses half-ring Thomas splint (1) and Pearson attachment (2) and that suspension of the extremity (A) and direct skeletal traction (B) are applied. Be aware that this type allows raising of the buttocks off the bed for bedpan use and in care without altering the line of traction. Use nursing assessments so that countertraction is maintained (e.g., position patient high in bed so that feet do not press on foot of bed, do not elevate the head of the bed >25 degrees if it causes continual movement toward foot of the bed). Encourage self-help in patient's performance of activities of daily living, movement in bed with help of trapeze, and flexion and extension of affected foot to prevent footdrop. Assess and care for skin of the groin (ischial) area, sacrum, and scapulae. Inspect the pin site and perform pin site care according to hospital policy. | |

**Figure 33-8, cont'd**    For legend see opposite page.

> ## NURSE ALERT
>
> Monitor the skeletal pin sites for signs of infection. Care of the pin site is ordered by the orthopedic surgeon or identified in protocols adopted by the hospital or clinic. Occasionally patients are placed in balanced suspension with a splint. This type of traction is generally used to maintain an extremity in a specific position after surgery and may or may not involve skin or skeletal traction. In all types of traction, ropes, pulleys, weights, and countertraction are used.

The pin or wire insertion site or sites must be inspected regularly, at least once daily. Care of the site is not always ordered by the physician. If it is, aseptic technique must be used while cleaning the area surrounding the site with sterile solution, usually normal saline, and drying it thoroughly. Evidence of redness, inflammation, or drainage from the pin site should be reported to the physician immediately.

## Pelvic Traction

Pelvic traction may be used to relieve pain from injury of the lower back, often in the lumbar region (see Figure 33-8). Sciatica, muscle spasms, and minor fractures of the lower spine may be treated with pelvic traction. The patient wears a canvas girdle or belt that fits snugly over the crests of the iliac and the pelvis. On either side are webbing straps that are joined to form one strap on each side at approximately mid-thigh. Ropes are attached to the straps and secured to a spreader bar. Another single rope is attached to the bar, threaded through a pulley at the end of the bed, and attached to the desired amount of weight. Pelvic traction can be adapted for home care. If traction does not have to be continuous, the girdle can be removed for hygiene care. The weight should be lifted before removing the pelvic girdle to avoid sudden and unequal pull on the pelvic area.

## Buck's Extension

Buck's extension is a type of skin traction that is applied to the lower extremities (Figures 33-8 and 33-10).

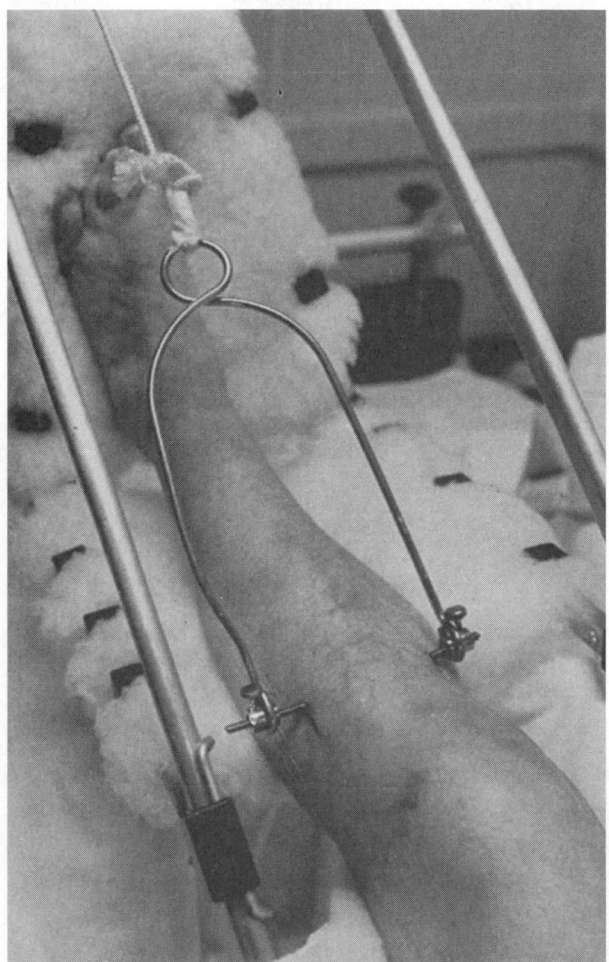

**Figure 33-9**  Tibial pin traction with Steinmann pin used in treatment of a distal femoral fracture. The bow attached to the pin provides a place of attachment for the rope that holds the traction weights. The pull exerted by the weight keeps the fracture fragments aligned. Pin sites must be inspected at least daily to detect signs of pin reaction or infection. (From Phipps WJ et al: *Medical-surgical nursing: concepts and clinical practice*, ed 5, St Louis, 1995, Mosby.)

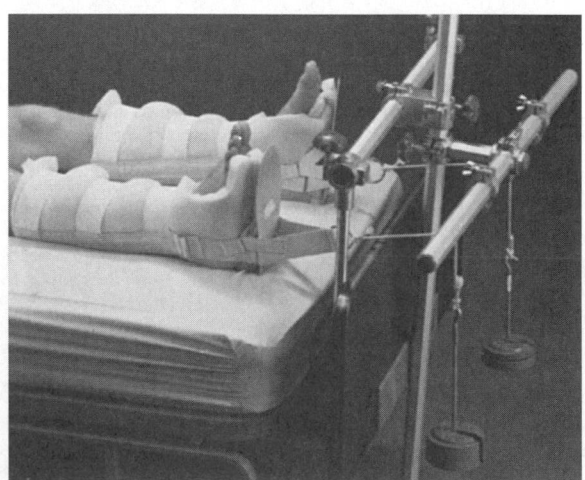

**Figure 33-10**  Buck's extension. Heel is supported off bed to prevent pressure on heel. Weight hangs free of bed and floor. Foot is well away from footboard of bed. The limb should lie parallel to the bed unless prevented as in this case by a slight knee flexion contracture. (From Thompson JM et al: *Mosby's clinical nursing*, ed 4, St Louis, 1998, Mosby.)

The traditional form requires the application of an adhesive material to the skin of the leg from a point 1 inch above the malleolus up to the knee. The adhesive material is attached to a footplate, which is attached to a rope. The rope is placed over a pulley at the foot of the bed, and the desired weight is attached at the end. More commonly seen today is Buck's boot. The patient's foot and lower leg are placed in a foam boot that is secured with Velcro straps. The foam boot grips the skin, a rope is attached to a footplate at the bottom of the boot, and a weight is attached to the rope, thus applying traction. When applied correctly, the edges of the boot come together or overlap completely. If the patient does not require continuous traction, the boot can be removed easily for bathing and ambulating. The weight must be lifted before removing the boot to avoid a sudden pull on the skin as the straps are released.

**Nursing intervention.** Regardless of the method used to apply Buck's extension, the nursing care of the patient is the same. Impaired circulation resulting from compression of the dorsalis pedis artery must be prevented. Decreased circulation to this area can result in ischemia (insufficient blood supply), which causes paralysis. The bony prominence of the foot and ankle must be observed for evidence of strap pressure, and cotton or felt should be used to protect the Achilles tendon, which is at the back of the ankle, from irritation.

The upper part of the calf should also be examined closely. The peroneal nerve lies close to the surface in this area, and compression against the bone can result in paralysis, plantar flexion (footdrop), and inversion of the foot. The foot should be observed daily for the tendency to turn inward toward the midline of the body. Any complaints of burning or pain should be reported immediately.

## Balanced Traction

Balanced traction (Russell's traction) consists of skin traction, often Buck's extension, as well as a sling under the knee that is attached to ropes and pulleys to provide suspension (Figure 33-11). The rope is brought overhead to a pulley and then down to a pulley at the foot of the bed. The same rope is brought back to a pulley on the footplate of Buck's extension and then back over the foot of the bed to a fourth pulley before dropping to the attached weight. This system of pulleys creates running traction plus a balanced traction or countertraction and may be used in fractures of the femur or hip. Countertraction is provided by elevating the foot of the bed.

With balanced traction, movement does not alter the position of the traction. The suspension apparatus takes up any slack in the traction caused by movement, and the line of the traction remains unchanged.

This suspension provides greater freedom of movement for the patient and greater ease for the nurse who is providing care. The affected limb may be suspended above the bed or may be resting on the bed with slight knee flexion, depending on how much weight is used for suspension, usually 5 to 7 pounds. Firm pillows can be placed crosswise under the calf, thus elevating the heel from the bed to prevent pressure and subsequent skin breakdown. The patient may be turned toward the limb in traction.

## Thomas Splint

A Thomas splint, either half ring or full ring, is often used in another type of suspension traction (Figure 33-12). This type of traction is used preoperatively to stabilize the fracture until surgery. When the half-ring splint is used, the half ring is positioned over the anterior aspect of the thigh. Proper weights and adequate countertraction prevent the half ring from causing pressure in the groin and on the anterior aspect of the thigh. The full ring of a Thomas splint is covered with smooth, moisture-resistant leather. Pressure from the ring on the adductor and ischial area must be avoided at all times. A Pearson attachment can be fastened to a Thomas splint to support the leg down from the knee. The Pearson attachment usually is horizontal to and just high enough to swing clear of the bed. The patient's knee should correspond with the point where the Pearson attachment is fastened to the splint. The limb is usually held in a neutral position or in slight internal rotation and abduction. The patient must be positioned straight in bed because traction is lost if the patient lies diagonally. The patient in suspension

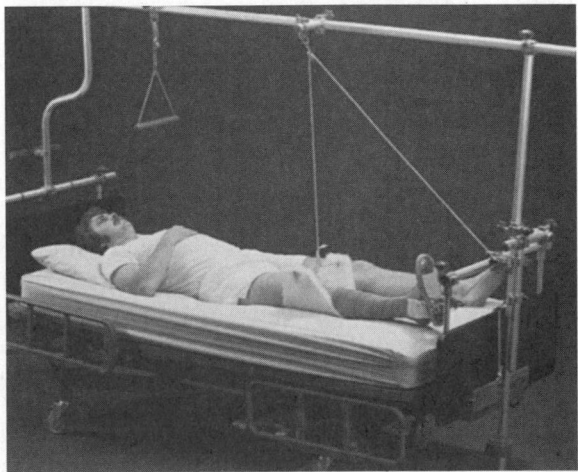

**Figure 33-11**    Balanced traction (Russell's traction). Hip is slightly flexed. Pillows may be used under lower leg to provide support and keep the heel free of the bed. (From Thompson JM et al: *Mosby's clinical nursing*, ed 4, St Louis, 1998, Mosby.)

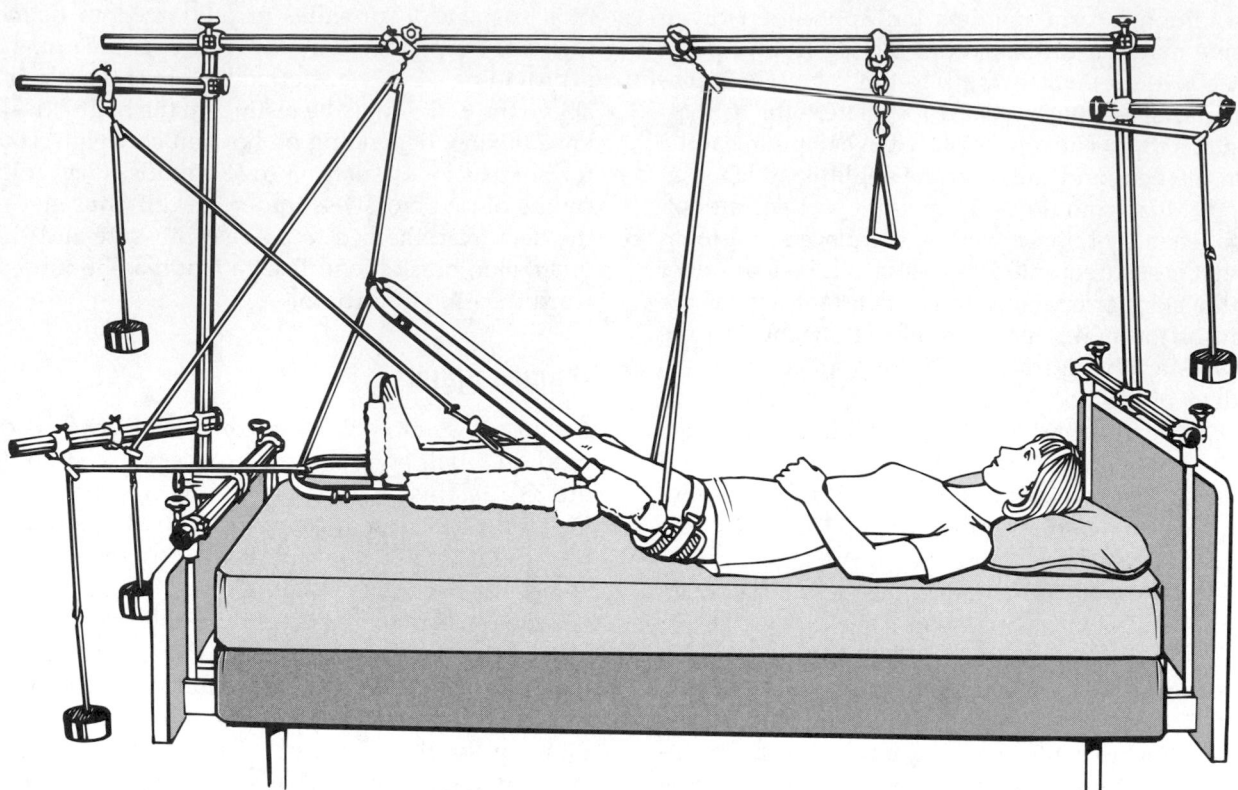

**Figure 33-12**    Balanced suspension with Thomas splint and Pearson attachment. This apparatus can be used alone or, as in this case, with skeletal traction. (From Phipps WJ et al: *Medical-surgical nursing: concepts and clinical practice*, ed 5, St Louis, 1995, Mosby.)

traction may turn toward the limb in traction. This traction is also described in Figure 33-8.

## Cervical Traction

Cervical traction may be used with injury to the cervical or upper thoracic vertebrae or spinal cord. Cervical fractures require skeletal traction. Tongs or pins, such as in the halo ring, are placed against the outer table of the skull and traction is applied. When tongs are used, the points of the tongs either rest against the skull or pierce it slightly (Figure 33-13). With the halo ring, the pins are placed approximately 0.05 mm into the skull (see Figure 33-3, *C*). Insertion of pins is generally performed with a local anesthetic. Severe sprains, strains, and mild trauma to the region of the cervical spine might be treated with a cervical halter, a circumferential form of skin traction (see Figure 33-8). A halter is never used with a cervical fracture.

When skeletal traction is required, the advantage of halo traction is that it can be attached to a rigid vest, which allows the patient to sit upright and to ambulate (see Figure 33-3, *C*). However, caution must be used when the patient is upright because peripheral vision is restricted and the patient's balance is affected by

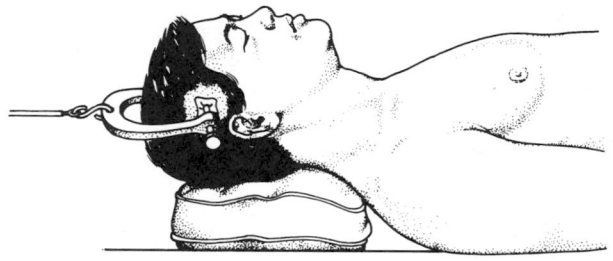

**Figure 33-13**    Gardner-Wells tongs. (From Beare PG, Myers JL: *Adult health nursing*, ed 3, St Louis, 1998, Mosby.)

the weight of the halo vest, which is approximately 7 pounds (Smeltzer, Bare, 1992; Maher et al, 1994).

Whenever skeletal traction is used, assessment of pin and wire insertion site is needed. Follow the physician's order for pin and wire site care. Pin care is not always ordered. If it is, aseptic technique must be used to prevent infection, which can be severe if bacteria enter the wound and infect the underlying bone. Pin care consists of cleaning the surrounding area with sterile solution (usually normal saline) and drying it thoroughly. Evidence of redness, inflammation, or drainage from the pin site should be reported to the physician.

## Nursing Intervention

The nurse is responsible for making sure that the traction is set up properly. Many hospitals have personnel who are trained and responsible for setting up the type of traction ordered by the physician. If such persons are not available, the nurse assumes responsibility for constructing the traction. The hospital's procedure manual and the manufacturer's manual can be used as a reference for traction construction. The nurse is responsible for monitoring the traction equipment for effectiveness (e.g., the weights are not resting on the floor) and safety (e.g., the knots are tight and taped).

In many instances the patient's position in bed may be limited. The nurse caring for patients in traction must be familiar with the amount of movement that the physician allows.

The skin around the edge of adhesive tape must be observed for irritation or abrasion. If the tape seems to be pulling or loosening, it must be reinforced or replaced. Neurovascular assessment of the extremities should be performed several times each day. The skin over the ankles and the heels must be watched for pressure areas and irritation.

The patient's position and body alignment in bed, as well as the avoidance of internal or external rotation of the extremities, are extremely important. The patient should be positioned in good alignment at all times. The traction, height of the backrest, and knee elevation should not be changed unless ordered by the physician. Although the patient usually is turned toward the affected side, specific turning instructions should be obtained from the physician before a regular turning schedule is begun. The skin beneath and around the traction splint or sling should be observed often for signs of pressure and irritation. In addition, the traction weights should hang free of the frame or bed and should never rest on the floor.

When giving care, several persons may be needed to lift the patient so that his or her back can be washed and massaged. The patient with an overhead trapeze should use the unaffected extremities to help lift himself or herself. The sacral area should be inspected for pressure points. The area should be massaged several times per day, which may be accomplished without lifting the patient by running a hand under his or her back. The bottom of the bed is changed from the unaffected side, or top to bottom, and small blankets, sheets, or split linen may be used to cover the patient when large ones interfere with the placement of ropes or mechanical devices.

If a bedpan is needed, a plastic-covered pillow should be placed lengthwise along the patient's back when he or she is lifted onto the pan. An overhead trapeze allows patients to assist in lifting by raising their hips.

Good oral care and a diet that is high in calcium, protein, iron, and vitamins are important. Foods high in roughage may help prevent constipation. Active and isometric exercises help prevent osteoporosis in the immobilized patient. Osteoporosis occurs when calcium leaves the bones of the immobilized patient. As it leaves the bones, it enters the serum and causes elevated levels of serum calcium. These high serum levels produce an alkaline urine, which can lead to the formation of urinary calculi. Fluids should be forced to help prevent this complication. The patient also should be encouraged to cough, deep breathe, and actively exercise the unaffected extremities. The affected extremity should not be exercised unless specifically ordered by the physician (Box 33-3).

Several new beds have been designed for the management of immobilized patients. The mattresses are filled with water, air, or air that is forced through silicone beads. These beds help the patient move, yet they minimize the potential for constant pressure against skin and bony prominences. *Kinetic beds* also are available and provide constant side-to-side movement of the patient while also maintaining proper alignment of fractures in the thorax, pelvis, spine, or extremities. Each type of bed has distinct advantages and certain

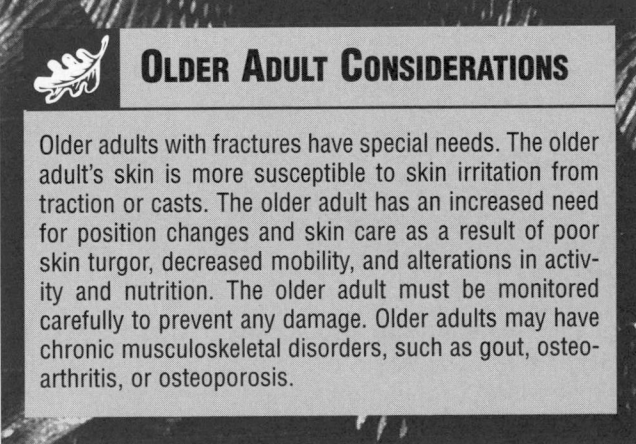

**OLDER ADULT CONSIDERATIONS**

Older adults with fractures have special needs. The older adult's skin is more susceptible to skin irritation from traction or casts. The older adult has an increased need for position changes and skin care as a result of poor skin turgor, decreased mobility, and alterations in activity and nutrition. The older adult must be monitored carefully to prevent any damage. Older adults may have chronic musculoskeletal disorders, such as gout, osteoarthritis, or osteoporosis.

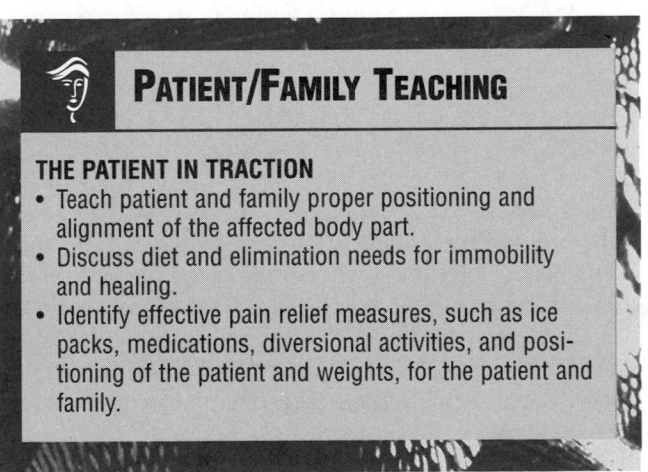

**PATIENT/FAMILY TEACHING**

**THE PATIENT IN TRACTION**
- Teach patient and family proper positioning and alignment of the affected body part.
- Discuss diet and elimination needs for immobility and healing.
- Identify effective pain relief measures, such as ice packs, medications, diversional activities, and positioning of the patient and weights, for the patient and family.

---

⟨ **BOX 33-3** ⟩        **NURSING PROCESS**

## THE PATIENT IN TRACTION

**ASSESSMENT**

- Neurovascular status
- Body alignment
- Traction apparatus
- Skin assessment
- Pain assessment
- Need for diversional activities
- Self-concept or role alteration
- Home maintenance
- Elimination needs
- Signs and symptoms of infection

**NURSING DIAGNOSES**

- Pain related to bone displacement, muscle spasm, and tissue trauma
- Constipation related to inactivity and altered position for elimination
- Diversional activity deficit related to restrictions imposed by traction
- Impaired home maintenance management related to hospitalization
- Risk for injury related to accidental disturbance of line of pull and weight of traction
- Knowledge deficit related to diet to promote healing and prevent urolithiasis and to exercises to promote circulation and bone healing
- Impaired physical mobility related to traction
- Altered nutrition: risk for more than body requirements related to decreased activity
- Self-care deficit: feeding, bathing/hygiene, dressing/grooming, and toileting related to traction
- Actual or risk for impaired skin integrity related to trauma, skin or skeletal traction, or immobility
- Altered tissue perfusion related to edema

**NURSING INTERVENTIONS**

- Keep patient in proper alignment.

- Never remove traction unless ordered by physician.
- Place patient on firm mattress.
- Ensure that ropes and pulleys are in straight alignment with fracture site.
- Check equipment often to ensure that ropes are not frayed, that the ropes are unobstructed and move freely in pulley grooves, that the knots are tied securely, and that the weights hang freely.
- Check pin or wire insertion site often when skeletal traction is used; be alert for odors, signs of local inflammation, or other evidence of osteomyelitis.
- Check skin at least every 2 hours for evidence of pressure or friction over bony prominences.
- Encourage active motion and exercise of unaffected joints.
- Check for circulatory impairment (e.g., numbness, cyanosis, edema, color, pain).
- Encourage self-help and independence within limitations of traction.
- Obtain specific orders on how patient can move; turning is not allowed with running traction; slight turning, usually to the affected side, is allowed with balanced suspension.

**EVALUATION OF EXPECTED OUTCOMES**

- Knows rationale for traction and observes condition of skin and extremities
- Traction alignment maintained
- Neurocirculatory status normal
- Elimination needs met
- Performs exercises properly as ordered
- No respiratory complications
- Verbalizes that comfort needs are met
- Verbalizes feelings about immobility, self-concept, and altered role performance
- Assists with as much self-care as possible

---

limitations. Because each type is expensive, the potential benefit to the patient should be evaluated carefully. Always check to determine whether the patient's medical insurance will cover the cost of the bed before ordering the bed for use. Whenever possible, the patient and family should participate in the final decision about the use of the bed. See Chapter 40 for a more complete description of specialty beds.

## Splints

Splints are used to support or immobilize an area of the body in a specific position. They are made of a variety of materials, such as plywood, lightweight aluminum, plastic, or casting materials. Plywood splints generally are used for first aid only. A tongue blade can be used to treat a fractured finger or an injury in which immobilization of the finger is desired. Aluminum splints are made for right or left extremities and support the foot or thumb. Many premolded splints are available for upper and lower extremities and are held in place by Velcro straps. Premolded splints are used for nondisplaced or incomplete fractures (e.g., a greenstick fracture) and sprains. Other splints may be held in place by elastic bandages or gauze and have the advantage of allowing the application of wet dressings to care for ulcers or other superficial injuries. These adjustable splints are also used when there is soft-tissue swelling at the fracture site. Plaster or fiberglass casts are occasionally bivalved (cut in two along both sides) and made into removable shells. This allows access to the affected area while also maintaining mobilization. When splints of any type are used, the nurse must observe the skin for pressure areas and must use care when handling the extremity involved. The patient and family must be taught how to care for the cast and how to prevent and monitor complications from the fracture and the cast.

## Other Orthopedic Devices

External fixation devices are used to reduce complex fractures that have bone fragments that need stabilization. These devices can be used on extremities and pelvic fractures (Figure 33-14). Preoperative and postoperative care is the same as for internal fixation of fractures, with frequent and accurate neurovascular assessments of the affected extremity. Before discharge, the patient and family need to be taught pin care, as well as the signs and symptoms of infection at the sites.

Plastic or rubber heels may be incorporated into a cast to allow the patient to walk on the extremity. Walking casts can be used with only certain types of fractures, and the orthopedic surgeon decides if such a cast can be used safely. An inflatable air cast may also be used as a walking cast. The patient must always be cautioned against outward rotation of the foot when walking.

Various types of collars or neck supports are designed to immobilize the head and to take the weight of the head off the spine. Collars and neck supports generally are used temporarily while healing occurs and may not be required at night. Corsets and back braces are used to immobilize the spine and to prevent the patient from engaging in activities that would further harm the spine. Braces may have steel supports in the back, and corsets usually lace in front. Patients are measured for the supports, which are made specifically for their needs. A cotton T-shirt is worn under the brace to prevent skin irritation and to absorb perspiration. The brace or corset should be put on patients while they are in a recumbent position before they arise in the morning.

## Interventions

The treatment of patients with orthopedic conditions is considered a surgical specialty because many patients require minor or major surgical procedures. Certain basic aspects of nursing care apply to most orthopedic patients, and many of these procedures have been referred to in this and other chapters.

All patients with fractures should have a firm mattress and an overhead trapeze. Cast care is the same for all patients regardless of the location of the cast. Extreme care must be taken to protect devices such as traction equipment, splints, or tongs so that the corrective procedure is not jeopardized. Skin care is a must for orthopedic patients. Because the immobilized patient may have problems with elimination, a diet high in roughage, as well as the use of mild laxatives or enemas, may be necessary. Adequate fluid intake must be ensured to promote bowel function and to prevent a urinary tract infection and the formation of urinary calculi (see Chapter 37). Isometric exercises slow the osteoporosis that accompanies immobility. Prescribed exercises should be carried out with the assistance of a physical therapist and members of the nursing staff. Maintaining muscle tone and function, as well as flexibility of unaffected joints, is important for preventing contractures and fostering rehabilitation. Open surgery may be performed on bones, tendons, or muscles, and the immediate postoperative care is essentially the same as that for any surgical patient. All wounds must be protected from contamination.

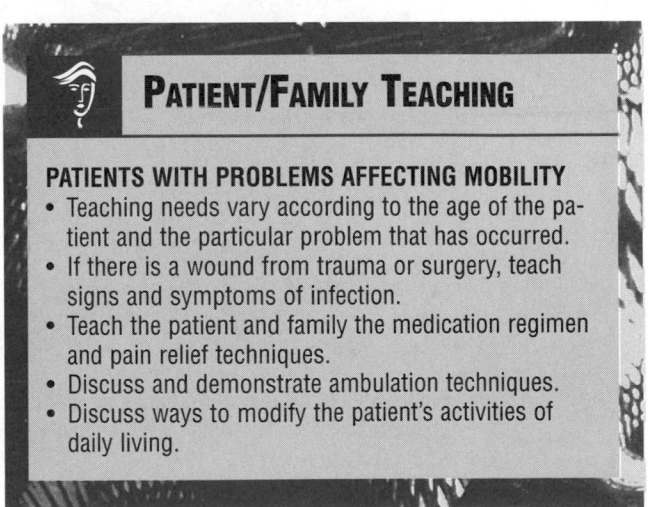

### PATIENT/FAMILY TEACHING

**PATIENTS WITH PROBLEMS AFFECTING MOBILITY**
- Teaching needs vary according to the age of the patient and the particular problem that has occurred.
- If there is a wound from trauma or surgery, teach signs and symptoms of infection.
- Teach the patient and family the medication regimen and pain relief techniques.
- Discuss and demonstrate ambulation techniques.
- Discuss ways to modify the patient's activities of daily living.

One of the most important interventions for patients with musculoskeletal conditions involves recognition and support of their psychosocial needs (Smeltzer, Bare, 1992). Individuals who suddenly are

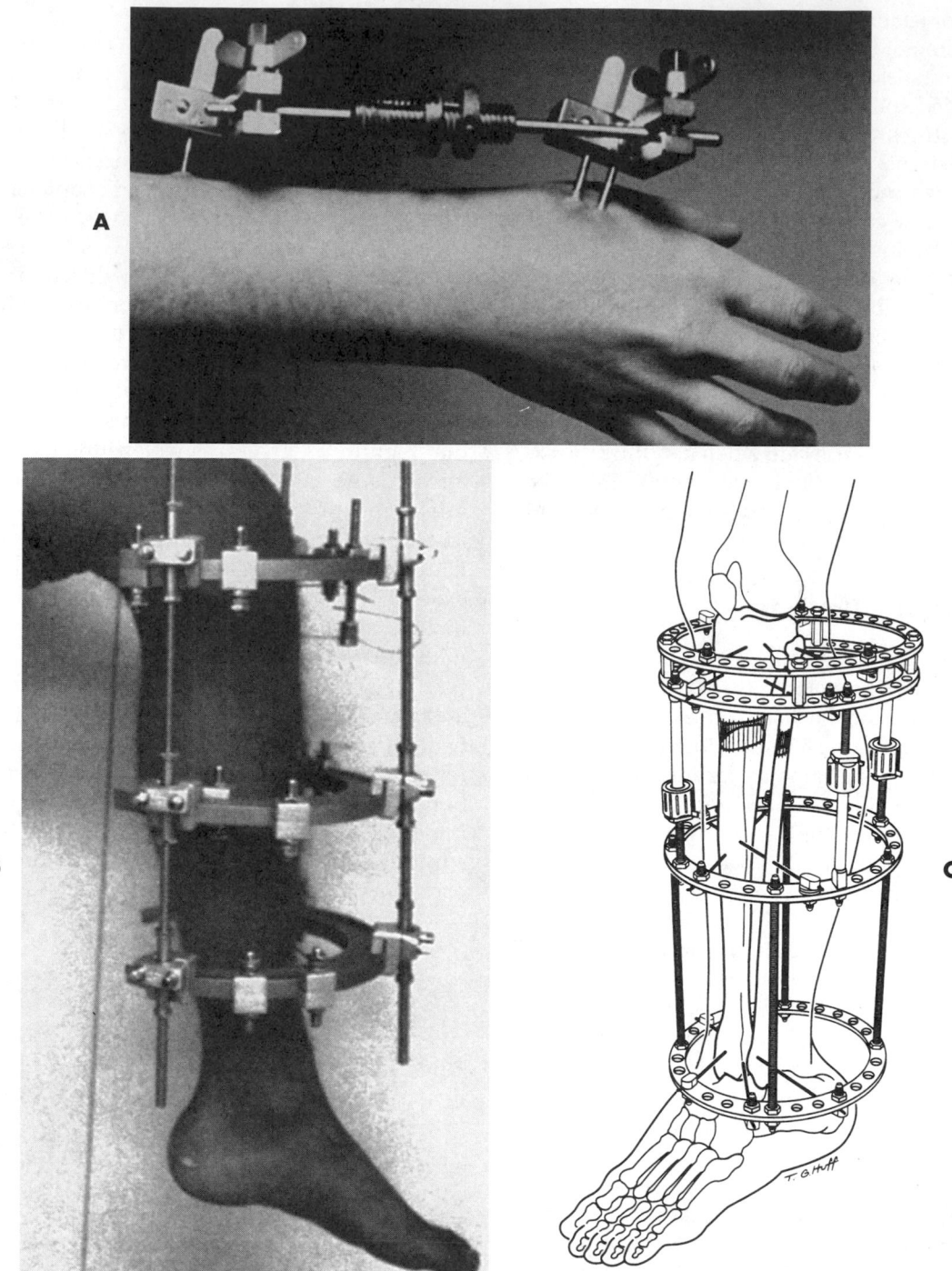

**Figure 33-14** External fixation devices. **A**, Hoffman. **B**, Monticelli-Spinelli Circular Fixator. **C**, Ilizarov apparatus with corticotomies for lengthening lower leg. (**A** from Thompson JM et al: *Mosby's manual of clinical nursing*, ed 2, 1989, Mosby; **B** and **C** from Thompson JM et al: *Mosby's clinical nursing*, ed 4, St Louis, 1998, Mosby.)

hospitalized as a result of injuries sustained during an accident, as well as those who are receiving medical care for chronic musculoskeletal disorders, are certain to have questions and concerns about how the injuries or illnesses will affect them and their families. In addi-

tion, patients who are elderly or who are hospitalized for long periods may show signs of confusion and disorientation. Consistent attention by the nurse to the patient's socialization and adaptation needs helps prevent or alleviate these concerns.

# OSTEOMYELITIS

*Osteo-* is a prefix that means "bone." Therefore osteomyelitis is inflammation of the bone. The most common cause of the disease is the introduction of pathogenic bacteria into the bone as a result of penetrating injuries, such as gunshot wounds, or as a result of compound fractures with protruding bones. Acute osteomyelitis may also result from infections elsewhere in the body when the pathogenic bacteria are carried to the bone by the bloodstream. Because many infections are now treated with chemotherapeutic drugs, fewer cases of osteomyelitis result from bloodstream infection.

Chronic osteomyelitis may recur throughout life. No uniform method of treating patients with osteomyelitis exists. For some patients, surgery may be performed to remove necrotic bone. Antibiotics generally are given, and immobilization may be helpful. Treatment depends on the age and condition of the patient (Maher et al, 1994).

Because the wounds caused by osteomyelitis are painful, the nurse should be gentle when moving the affected part. Wounds often have antibiotic beads implanted, and strict asepsis must be maintained. Contractures may occur unless care is taken to see that the patient is positioned properly. Because new foci of infection may develop, the patient should be observed for any sudden elevation of temperature, which should be reported at once. The diet should be high in calories, protein, and vitamins. Because osteomyelitis patients often are children, diversional activities should be planned.

# TRAUMATIC INJURIES

Among all age groups, traumatic injuries to the musculoskeletal system are responsible for a large number of hospital admissions. Many less severe injuries, including contusions, sprains, and strains, are cared for in outpatient clinics or in a physician's office.

## Contusions

Contusions are the most common and the simplest type of injury to the musculoskeletal system. *Contusion* is synonymous with *bruise* and is the result of an external injury to the soft tissues. Sharp blows to the eye, arm, or thigh are examples of injuries that can cause a simple contusion. The injury causes a rupture of small blood vessels and subsequent bleeding into tissues, which results in an **ecchymosis**, or the familiar discoloration that is often called a bruise or "black-and-blue spot." When the contusion is severe, a large amount of blood may collect in the tissue, resulting in a hematoma.

Treatment for contusions generally includes elevation of the part and the application of cold, which may be in the form of cold compresses or an ice cap. If there is no further bleeding after 24 hours, heat may be applied to relieve muscle soreness.

## Sprains

A sprain involves ligaments, tendons, and muscles and occurs as the result of twisting or wrenching a joint beyond its normal range of motion. When this occurs, ligaments are torn, and tendons may be pulled from the bone. Blood vessels are ruptured, which causes contusions with ecchymosis. Pressure on nerve endings results in pain. As the result of a disturbance of circulation and lymph drainage, muscle spasm occurs, and there is a tendency for edema to occur. Sprains of the ankle or wrist joint are common examples.

Immediately after the injury, weight bearing or other pressure on the joint should be avoided. Walking on a sprained ankle causes further bleeding into soft tissues. The involved extremity should be elevated to promote drainage away from the injury. Ice bags should be applied for the first 24 hours to constrict blood vessels and to ensure control of further bleeding. After 24 hours, mild heat may be applied to encourage circulation and healing and to relieve soreness in the area. Treatment should include an x-ray examination to rule out the possibility of a fracture. The joint is then immobilized by a splint and Ace bandage or a cast if the sprain is severe. Taping the foot occasionally provides enough immobilization for healing to occur. The support is removed in 2 to 3 weeks. If the ankle joint is involved, minimum weight bearing is permitted at first and is increased gradually as the discomfort subsides. If the ankle has been casted, active exercises should be performed after cast removal and before full weight bearing begins.

## Dislocations

A dislocation may be congenital, as in the case of a congenitally dislocated hip; it may be caused by a disease process in the joint; or it may be caused by trauma. A dislocation results in the temporary displacement of a bone from its normal position within a joint. It is accompanied by a stretching and tearing of ligaments and tendons, and a fracture may sometimes occur at the same time. A dislocation results in severe pain, deformity, and loss of function. The treatment of dislocations is usually done with the patient under sedation or general anesthesia. The displaced parts are manipulated manually into normal position. Sometimes a fluoroscope may be used to assist the surgeon. The affected joint is immobilized in splints, bandages, or a cast until the injured tissues have healed. When a fracture accompanies a dislocation, achieving an effective outcome may be more difficult than with dislocation alone.

Nursing care of the patient includes observing for signs of impaired circulation, such as pain, tingling, numbness, or loss of sensation. Cast care is reviewed earlier in this chapter.

## Fractures

A fracture is the same as a break and results from some force (blow, crushing, twisting) that places more stress on the bone than it can absorb. Decalcification and brittleness of bones (osteoporosis) occur in the aging process and make the bones increasingly unable to withstand external stresses. In elderly persons, this process may lead to fractures that occur with very little stress to bones and joints. Metastatic cancer and bone tumors also weaken bones and may result in fractures with little or no stress. These types of fractures are called *pathologic fractures*. Fractures may occur directly at the point at which stress is applied, or they may be some distance away from this point. Various types of fractures exist, and the method of treatment varies with the location and type. Some injury to the soft tissues and some bleeding occur whenever there is a fracture because the bones have their own blood supply.

Fractures are classified in four general categories. First, they are described as either open or closed, which means that the fracture either does or does not protrude through a break in the skin (Figure 33-15). Open fractures generally are more serious because they are accompanied by considerable soft-tissue damage, require surgical treatment to repair, and involve a break in the body's first line of defense against infection—the skin. An open fracture is compounded by injury to the skin and by the possibility of infection. Because closed fractures do not involve a break in the skin, bones may be realigned by external manipulation only.

Fractures are also described according to their appearance. Greenstick, complete, comminuted, impacted, transverse, oblique, and spiral fractures are examples of various types of fractures (Box 33-4 and Figure 33-16). Third, fractures are described according to their location on the bone, namely, proximal, midshaft, or distal (Figure 33-17). Fourth, fractures are described according to their displacement. Figure 33-18 shows that fragments may be displaced sideways, may override the opposite fractured surface, may angulate or create a bend in the bone, or may rotate away from the fracture site. Any displacement of bone fragments results in soft-tissue damage, and the patient is likely to experience severe pain, swelling, and muscle spasm in the early stages of healing.

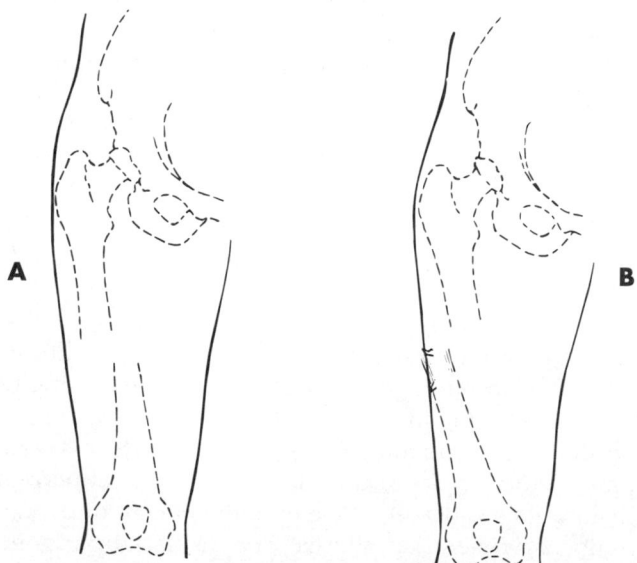

**Figure 33-15**  **A,** Closed fracture. **B,** Open fracture with bone protruding through skin.

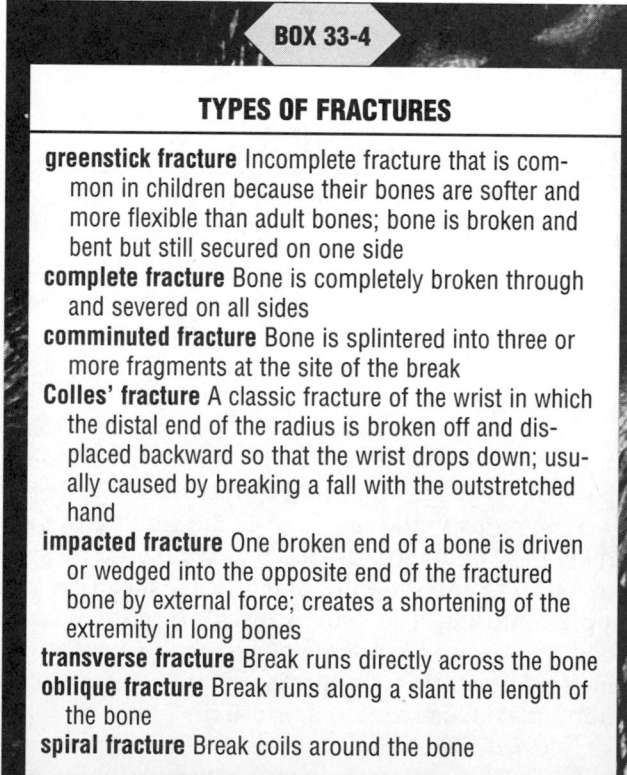

**BOX 33-4**

### TYPES OF FRACTURES

**greenstick fracture** Incomplete fracture that is common in children because their bones are softer and more flexible than adult bones; bone is broken and bent but still secured on one side

**complete fracture** Bone is completely broken through and severed on all sides

**comminuted fracture** Bone is splintered into three or more fragments at the site of the break

**Colles' fracture** A classic fracture of the wrist in which the distal end of the radius is broken off and displaced backward so that the wrist drops down; usually caused by breaking a fall with the outstretched hand

**impacted fracture** One broken end of a bone is driven or wedged into the opposite end of the fractured bone by external force; creates a shortening of the extremity in long bones

**transverse fracture** Break runs directly across the bone

**oblique fracture** Break runs along a slant the length of the bone

**spiral fracture** Break coils around the bone

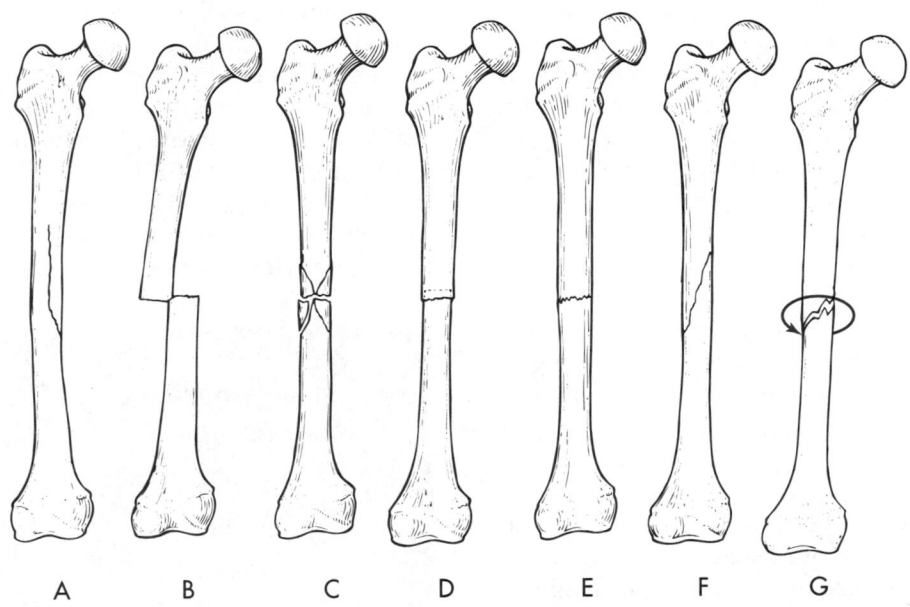

**Figure 33-16** Description of fracture by appearance. *A,* Greenstick. *B,* Complete. *C,* Comminuted. *D,* Impacted. *E,* Transverse. *F,* Oblique. *G,* Spiral.

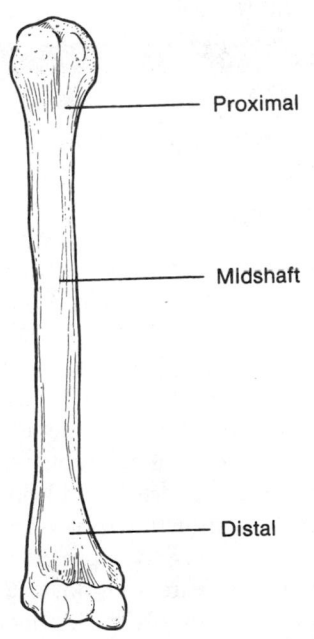

**Figure 33-17**   Location of fractures.

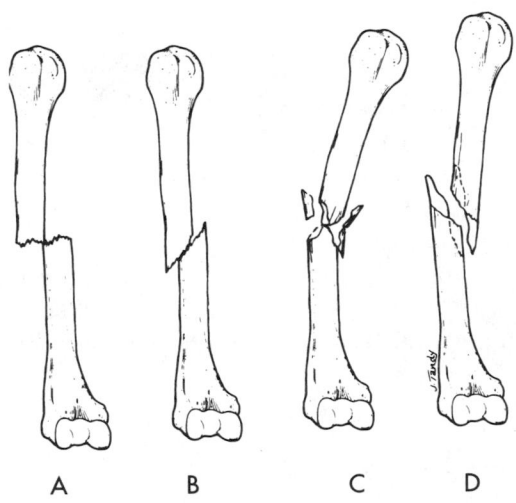

**Figure 33-18**   Displacement of fragments. *A,* Sideways. *B,* Override. *C,* Angulate. *D,* Rotate.

## Assessment

Signs and symptoms of a fracture vary with the type and location and may include pain and swelling (particularly at the time of injury), tenderness, muscle spasm, deformity, and loss of function. Sometimes symptoms may not be present at the time of injury. Often injury to other body parts occurs simultaneously, and the patient may be admitted unconscious and in severe shock. The treatment of any general systemic condition takes precedence over treatment of the fracture. Immobilization of the fracture as soon as possible prevents further injury.

An accurate diagnosis of the fracture is made by x-ray examination or by fluoroscopic examination. The physician will want to know exactly how the accident happened, because this information has a bearing on the type of fracture and the method of treatment.

## Intervention

To treat a fracture, the bone segments must be realigned. The realignment of a fracture is termed *reduction*. Fractures are reduced by closed or open methods. In closed reduction, the bones are externally manipulated into position and immobilized with external devices, such as casts, splints, or traction. In open reduction, the bones are exposed and aligned through a surgical incision and may be fixed in position with wires, nails, plates, screws, bolts, or any combination of these. The use of these devices is called *internal fixation*. As with closed reduction, external devices may be used for immobilization of the extremity.

### NURSE ALERT

After open reduction, check for drainage *under* the cast. Because of gravity, drainage from the wound flows around the extremity and soaks through the underside of the cast or dressing before appearing on the anterior surface of the extremity. Bleeding is to be expected because of the bone's vascularity.

## Fracture Healing

Whereas other parts of the body heal by the formation of scar tissue, bones heal by the formation of new bone. When a fracture occurs, the bone is broken, soft tissues are damaged, and the periosteum is torn. The bleeding that occurs results in the formation of a hematoma, which surrounds the area within 24 hours. The coagulation of this blood forms a loose fibrin mesh, which acts as a framework for the early stages of new bone growth.

An inflammatory reaction follows, which causes the fibrin mesh to be replaced by granulation tissue. Within 6 to 10 days the granulation tissue contains calcium, cartilage, and osteoblasts and is termed **callus**. Callus unites the bone so the cast can be removed, but the bone cannot withstand unprotected stress. The bone is immature and is gradually replaced by mature bone in the process of ossification. **Remodeling** of the bone is the process in which bone tissue consolidates and compacts the bone in relation to its function. This final step in fracture healing requires the stresses of muscle action and weight bearing. After remodeling, the bone is considered to be in union and may be used unprotected.

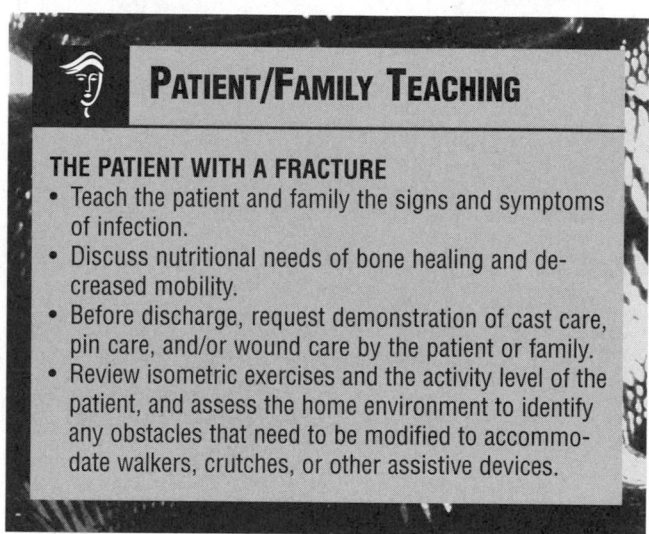

### PATIENT/FAMILY TEACHING

**THE PATIENT WITH A FRACTURE**
- Teach the patient and family the signs and symptoms of infection.
- Discuss nutritional needs of bone healing and decreased mobility.
- Before discharge, request demonstration of cast care, pin care, and/or wound care by the patient or family.
- Review isometric exercises and the activity level of the patient, and assess the home environment to identify any obstacles that need to be modified to accommodate walkers, crutches, or other assistive devices.

The time required for the healing of fractures varies and is influenced by the type of fracture, the bone involved, and the age and condition of the patient and his or her bones. For example, displaced fractures take longer to heal than those with no displacement of fragments. Bones of the arms heal in 3 months, but long bones of the leg take 6 months to heal. A solid callus may be present in the fracture of a child within 3 weeks but may take 6 to 8 weeks in a young adult, and that same fracture may not develop good callus formation for 3 to 4 months in an elderly person.

The complete union of fractured bones may be prevented or delayed by infection, poor circulation, inadequate nutrition, necrosis, and improper immobilization or fixation. When a fracture does not form a bony union within the usual amount of time, *delayed union* occurs, which requires extended immobilization. *Nonunion* results when healing fails to occur, which requires revision or bone grafting to stimulate callus formation. Faulty reduction or improper immobilization may cause *malunion* of a fracture and result in deformity and disability and require surgery for repair. *Aseptic* or *avascular necrosis* is literally a clean death of the bone that results from loss of blood supply to the fracture site.

## Fractures of the Hip

Because more people are living longer now, the incidence of hip fractures among older persons is increasing. Because of the brittleness of their bones, older people need only a slight fall to sustain a fracture of the hip or arm. Hip fractures occur spontaneously in older people, which means that the patient falls as a result of the fracture rather than suffering the fracture as a result of the fall. A spontaneous fracture usually occurs in the neck of the femur. Regardless of the cause, the patient with a fractured hip experiences pain in the fracture site, the affected extremity shortens, and the foot turns outward (external rotation). Healing of a bone as large as the hip takes a long time in elderly persons, which predisposes them to numerous complications. They are at risk for atelectasis and pneumonia, deep vein thrombosis, decubitus ulcers, urinary retention, constipation, and mental confusion or depression (Box 33-5).

Newer methods of treatment allow earlier and greater mobility than was previously possible after hip fracture. Because different types of fractures occur,

---

◁ **BOX 33-5** ▷      **NURSING PROCESS**

### HIP FRACTURE, TOTAL HIP REPLACEMENT, AND TOTAL KNEE REPLACEMENT*

**ASSESSMENT**

- Vital signs (often)
- Fluid volume status
- Dressing for evidence of bleeding
- Wound for healing and evidence of infection
- Drain output
- Tissue perfusion to affected extremity (often)
- Respiratory status
- Level of comfort
- Elimination patterns and bowel sounds
- Level of consciousness, orientation
- Leg position in bed, in chair, and during ambulation
- Laboratory studies (CBC, coagulation profile)
- Self-care ability
- Evidence of skin breakdown
- Signs and symptoms of thrombophlebitis
- Restlessness, confusion, sudden chest pain, dyspnea, tachycardia
- Signs of dislocation of hip
- Evidence of bleeding if taking anticoagulants

**NURSING DIAGNOSES**

- Pain related to bone and soft-tissue trauma and physical therapy
- Ineffective breathing pattern related to sedation, anesthesia, and immobility
- Impaired physical mobility related to pain and surgical procedure
- Risk for altered tissue perfusion to affected lower extremity related to surgical procedure, edema, immobility
- Risk for infection related to implanted prosthesis
- Risk for impaired skin integrity related to immobility, age, pain
- Self-care deficit related to pain and immobility
- Constipation related to analgesics and immobility

- Risk for injury: dislocation, deep vein thrombosis (DVT), pulmonary embolism related to improper positioning, surgical procedure, immobility
- Knowledge deficit related to new condition, mobility restrictions, memory impairment

**NURSING INTERVENTIONS**

- Prevent skin breakdown.
- Turn patient and encourage him or her to cough and deep breathe every 2 hours.
- Maintain affected extremity in alignment.
- Mobilize patient and weight bearing per physician's order and patient tolerance.
- Request occupational therapy consultation for help with activities of daily living.
- Perform range of motion exercises on all joints except affected leg.
- Provide trapeze.
- Request physical therapy consultation for transfer techniques and use of mobility aids.
- Administer intravenous fluids as ordered.
- Administer prophylactic anticoagulants as ordered.
- Apply antiembolism stockings as ordered.
- Encourage dorsiflexion and plantar flexion exercises.
- Provide high-protein, high-roughage diet.
- Provide diet and fluids as tolerated.
- Discuss use of patient-controlled analgesia for pain control with physician if not ordered and if appropriate.
- Administer analgesics as prescribed.
- Provide comfort measures (massage, relaxation, diversion).
- Administer medications before physical therapy.
- Encourage isometric exercises (quadriceps, gluteal sets per physical therapist's order).
- Maintain aseptic technique with dressing changes.

*See Chapter 34 for discussion of total hip and total knee replacement.

*Continued*

---

<BOX 33-5> **NURSING PROCESS**

## HIP FRACTURE, TOTAL HIP REPLACEMENT, AND TOTAL KNEE REPLACEMENT—cont'd

- Encourage participation in self-care activities.
- Encourage balance between rest and activities.
- Refer to social services for home physical therapy and nursing if indicated.

### Mobility for Total Hip Replacement

- Enforce mobility restrictions to prevent dislocation.
- Use abduction pillow at all times.
- Avoid extreme flexion of affected hip (>90 degrees), as well as adduction and external rotation.
- Teach patient to avoid bending at waist, crossing legs, and sleeping on operative side for 2 months.
- Use raised toilet seat and high, firm chair.
- Reinforce hip precautions often.

### Mobility for Hip Fracture

- When on unaffected side, support fractured extremity with pillows in alignment.
- Maintain pillow between legs.
- Prevent external rotation.
- Avoid adduction (especially with prosthesis).

### Mobility for Total Knee Replacement

- If prescribed, apply continuous passive motion machine.

- Maintain correct position and knee alignment at all times.
- Elevate leg on pillow when not in continuous passive motion machine; place pillow under calf to promote leg extension.
- Initiate weight bearing as prescribed.
- Instruct patient to sit with legs dependent to promote knee flexion.

### EVALUATION OF EXPECTED OUTCOMES

- Meets discharge criteria for postsurgical patient
- Affected extremity in alignment
- No evidence of dislocation
- No evidence of infection
- Pain controlled with oral analgesics
- Tolerates activity within limitations
- Demonstrates understanding of mobility limitations
- Demonstrates increased strength and function of affected extremity
- No evidence of thrombophlebitis
- Adequate tissue perfusion to affected extremity
- Verbalizes understanding of rehabilitation program

---

methods of treatment vary. The surgeon determines the method to be used on the basis of an x-ray examination. The care of patients in casts and traction is reviewed earlier in this chapter.

**Nailing.** *Nailing* means that a nail or rod made of stainless steel and a cobalt-chromium alloy (Vitallium) is inserted through the marrow cavity of one bone fragment and driven across the site of the fracture into the marrow cavity of another bone, thus holding the fractured bones in correct anatomic position. Not all fractures can be nailed, but when this procedure is possible, it allows many patients to be out of the hospital and walking on crutches in a few weeks. In some types of fractures a prosthetic device may be used. Prosthetic devices are usually inserted when the neck of the femur has been fractured and the blood supply that is necessary for healing has been disrupted. The head and neck of the femur are surgically removed and replaced with a ball and stem (bipolar, unipolar, or Batemann prosthesis), which fits into the shaft of the femur. This procedure enables the patient to bear weight directly on the leg in a short time. Nailing and

prosthetic devices offer the advantage of early ambulation and help to prevent complications commonly associated with immobility.

**Intervention.** The patient with internal fixation is given a general or epidural anesthetic for the procedure, after which vital signs are checked often until the patient is stabilized. After internal fixation, turning and moving the patient can begin. The patient's position should be changed from side to side every 2 hours. When the patient is turned on the unaffected side, the fractured extremity should be supported with pillows and should remain in the same line as the rest of the body. When the patient is in the supine position, the knee may be slightly flexed, and the extremity can be supported with a trochanter roll to prevent outward rotation. Pillows may be used to support the legs and keep the heels off the bed. Because physicians vary in what activities they permit, the nurse should understand exactly what the physician wishes to be done.

The elderly patient should be observed for fecal impaction, and mild laxatives or small enemas may be ordered. Intake and output records should be maintained. With the physician's permission, the patient may be taught muscle-setting exercises such as quadriceps setting, gluteal and abdominal muscle tightening, plantar flexion, and dorsiflexion of the feet. All joints except the affected leg should be exercised, and the patient may be encouraged to use the trapeze to move and exercise the arms. Exercise of the affected leg must be ordered by the surgeon. In most instances the patient is out of bed and in a chair on the day after surgery. Elderly patients may tire easily and should not be left sitting for long periods. Usually 1 hour two or three times each day is sufficient. Because the appetite may be poor, allowing the patient to be up at mealtimes may improve intake. Non-weight-bearing ambulation is allowed as soon as possible, and weight bearing is allowed when healing is complete.

When a prosthesis such as the bipolar, unipolar, or Batemann is inserted into the femur, the limb is kept in a neutral position, with slight abduction to prevent dislocation. The patient is lifted off the bed for back care or turned to the nonoperative side. The patient is placed on his or her unaffected side, and abduction is maintained by placing pillows between his or her legs. Muscle exercises are encouraged. Partial weight bearing may be allowed in a few days and full weight bearing in approximately 4 to 8 weeks. Specific exercises, activities, and weight-bearing restrictions must be ordered by the physician.

## Complications

Serious complications of fractures include pulmonary embolism, fat embolism (mostly occurs with long bone fractures), wound infection, tetanus, and **compartment syndrome.**

Because of prolonged immobility, patients with fractures of the lower extremities are particularly susceptible to pulmonary embolism, which may be secondary to thrombophlebitis or may occur spontaneously. Measures to prevent pulmonary embolism include prophylactic anticoagulation, early ambulation, exercises, and the use of elastic stockings. Sudden respiratory distress with acute substernal pain and signs of shock should alert the nurse to suspect pulmonary embolism. Treatment includes oxygen administration to support respiration, anticoagulant therapy, and general emergency measures.

Fat embolism develops most commonly in young adults who sustain multiple, crushing types of fractures, such as those occurring from motorcycle accidents or industrial injuries. Although rare, fat embolism is life threatening because the released fat droplets can effectively occlude capillaries of the pulmonary circulation and cause brain hypoxia and tissue death. Measures to prevent fat embolism include cau-

tious and minimum manipulation of bone fragments with immediate immobilization. Mental disturbances, respiratory distress, and signs of shock that occur within 72 hours after injury are signs of fat embolism. The classic appearance of petechiae on the upper chest and axillae, as well as the appearance of blood-tinged sputum, may accompany these early signs. Treatment includes the administration of high concentrations of oxygen, the control of shock, and all symptomatic measures to sustain life (Smeltzer, Bare, 1992; Black, Matassarin-Jacobs, 1993).

> ### NURSE ALERT
>
> The larger the bone involved, the higher the probability of fat embolism occurring. Watch for signs of respiratory distress when the femur is fractured.

Gas gangrene and tetanus occur rarely but must always be considered as possible complications when a compound fracture has been sustained through a small or puncture type of wound. Both gas gangrene and tetanus are caused by anaerobic bacteria, which produce rapid and life-threatening results. Gas gangrene is a rapid destruction of tissue and is signaled by an acute, fulminating infection with fever, wound pain, gas bubbles, and edema. If left untreated, the condition progresses to systemic toxemia and death. In tetanus, the bacteria affect the nerves, which causes muscle twitching, severe spasms, and inability to open the mouth (lockjaw). It progresses to severe seizures that can be stimulated by the slightest movement or noise. Treatment for both conditions includes wound debridement, hyperbaric oxygen, and antibiotic therapy. Anticonvulsive drugs are given for seizures. Amputation of the affected limb may be necessary.

Acute compartment syndrome (ACS) is a condition in which there is an increase in pressure within a muscle. The inelastic fascia that surrounds the muscle creates an enclosed space or compartment. Pressure within this space will rise from hemorrhage or edema associated with acute injury, such as a fracture or severe trauma, or with sustained external pressure on a limb from things such as constricting casts, dressings, and splints. Prolonged positioning in long surgical procedures can result in compartment syndrome, as can burns and snake and spider bites. Closed fractures of the tibia are a common cause of lower extremity compartment syndrome, and a supracondylar fracture of the humerus is often the cause in upper extremity compartment syndrome. The increase in pressure reduces circulation, resulting in muscle ischemia and tissue damage. A vicious cycle is set in motion in which histamine is released, capillaries dilate, additional swelling occurs, blood flow is decreased further, and more ischemia results. The condition can rapidly result in a permanent contracture deformity of the hand or foot, called *Volkmann's contracture* (Figure 33-19).

The signs and symptoms of ACS can be referred to as the five "Ps": pain, pallor, paresthesia, paresis, and pulselessness (Rockwood, Green, Bucholz, 1991). Pain is the first symptom to appear, and it is severe, deep, unrelenting, and unrelieved by analgesics. The pain is progressive and increases with passive stretching of the digits of the affected extremity, referred to as *stretch pain*. The patient may not be able to flex the fingers or toes. Pallor may be present, but there may be warmth or redness over the area. Paresthesia (numbness) and muscles weakness may be present, and the weakness may progress to paresis and even complete inability to move the affected extremity.

Pulselessness is a late and ominous sign (Stuart, Karaharju, 1994). Within 6 hours the condition can progress to irreversible muscle ischemia, with compression of the arteries, nerves, and tendons that enter the compartment. Paralysis and loss of sensation follow, and contracture and permanent disability of the extremity may be complete within 24 to 48 hours. The nurse's careful assessment of the neurovascular integrity of fractured extremities can interrupt the development of compartment syndrome.

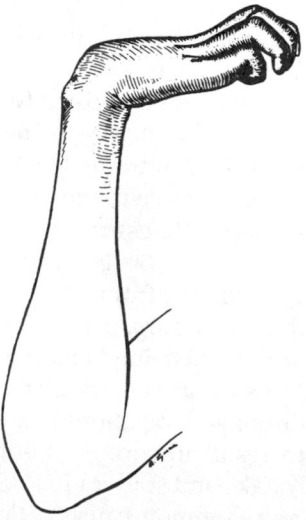

**Figure 33-19** Well-established Volkmann's contracture with claw-hand and flexion of wrist and fingers. (From Larson CB, Gould M: *Orthopedic nursing*, ed 9, St Louis, 1978, Mosby.)

Frequent assessment of the affected extremity is essential and should include observation of skin color and tension. Palpation detects changes in temperature, pulse rate, and capillary refilling time. Muscle strength of the extremity should be tested, and increased pain that is associated with muscle stretching should be reported. Tissue pressure measurements can be taken by a physician to determine the extent of tissue compression within the fascial compartment. Normally pressure is recorded at 0 mm Hg. Tissue ischemia begins when pressure rises to between 10 and 30 mm Hg less than the patient's diastolic blood pressure (Mourad, 1991; Gregory, 1994; Maher et al, 1994).

Continued elevated pressures in the presence of decreased sensory and motor function necessitate surgical intervention. A *fasciotomy* (surgical incision into the fascia) is performed to relieve pressure within the compartment and to allow return of normal blood flow to the area (Figure 33-20). After surgery, the patient is observed for signs and symptoms of infection in the open wound. The extremity is elevated above the level of the heart, and range-of-motion exercises are begun.

## General Nursing Interventions

The patient with a fracture needs a well-balanced diet, and opinions differ on the value of vitamin and mineral supplements in hastening bone repair. Fluids should be provided. Exercise of the unaffected joints, muscle-setting exercises, skin care, and elimination are important considerations in patient care. Although internal fixation has simplified nursing care for many patients with fractures and has shortened the period of hospitalization, many patients require several weeks of hospitalization. Some form of occupational therapy should be available for these patients. If activity is restricted, the complications that result from immobility must be anticipated and prevented.

## Whiplash Injuries

A whiplash injury to the musculoskeletal system is the result of a combination of severe flexion and extension of the neck. The injury may cause a compression fracture of the cervical vertebrae or result in tearing of muscles and ligaments. Although the injury can be severe enough to cause paralysis and loss of consciousness, most whiplash injuries do not produce immediate symptoms. Symptoms often do not appear until 4 or 5 days after the injury, at which time headache, spasm of neck muscles with loss of motion, and a drawing sensation in the back of the neck may be noted. Pain may be referred from one side of the head to the base of the skull, and vision may be disturbed. If

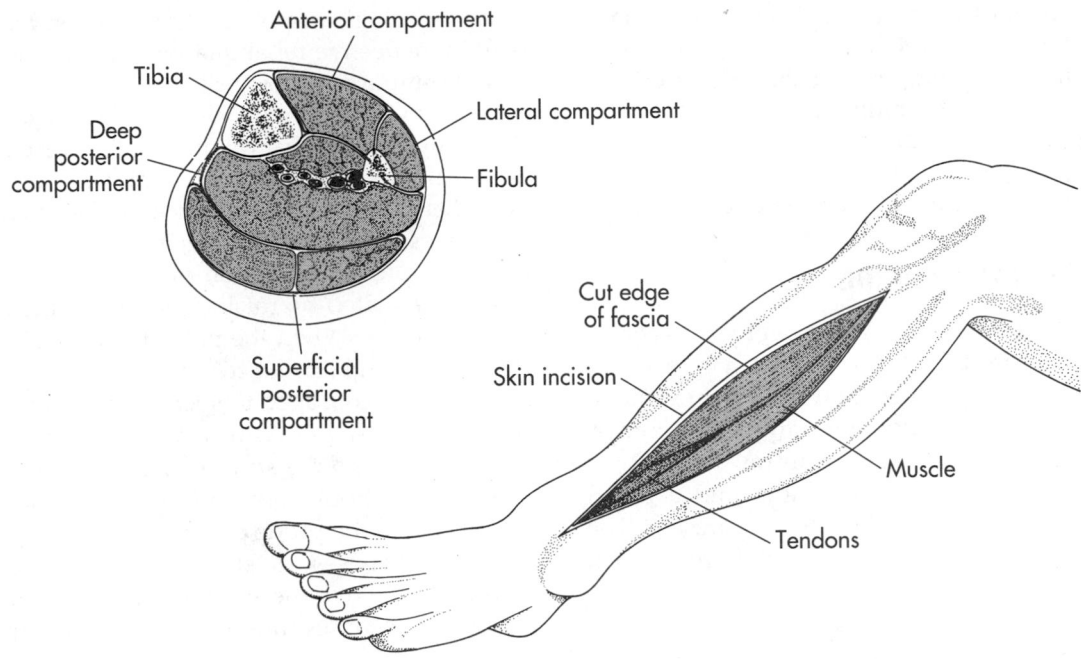

**Figure 33-20**    Compartment syndrome and fasciotomy to relieve pressure. Often more than one compartment is involved. (From Beare PG, Myers JL: *Principles and practice of adult health nursing,* ed 2, St Louis, 1994, Mosby.)

the injury has been severe enough to injure a nerve root, neurologic symptoms may occur.

Treatment should be obtained immediately after injury because without treatment, the condition may become chronic. Methods of treatment vary, and bed rest may be prescribed. Cervical traction with a head halter, as well as the application of heat and massage, may be used. The patient may be fitted with a neck support that is to be worn when out of bed. After approximately 4 weeks, physical therapy and exercise are begun to strengthen neck muscles.

## BONE TUMORS

Tumors of the bone may be primary or secondary and may be benign or malignant. Several types of benign tumors exist, and their cause is not always known. Benign tumors do not metastasize to other parts of the body and usually produce few symptoms, with the most common symptom being pain from pressure exerted on surrounding anatomic structures. Benign tumors are diagnosed by x-ray examination and biopsy, and most are removed surgically.

Several different types of malignant bone tumors exist. One type of primary malignant tumor, osteogenic sarcoma, occurs in younger persons and metastasizes to the lungs, from which the malignant cells are carried throughout the body by the bloodstream. The long bones are usually affected, and amputation generally is

required (Wyngaarden et al, 1992). Other types of malignant tumors affect the flat bones and often involve other types of tissues. Carcinoma of the prostate, lung, breast, thyroid, and kidney may metastasize to the bones, where destruction of the bone and spontaneous fractures result. In most cases of both benign and malignant bone tumors, pain and declining health are the primary symptoms. Anemia, temperature elevation, swelling, and platelet disturbance occur with some types of bone tumors. Treatment depends on the type of tumor, the extent of involvement, the location, and the presence of malignant lesions in other parts of the body.

## AMPUTATION

Amputation of an extremity or a portion of it may be necessary as a result of a malignant bone tumor, injury, diabetic gangrene, or any condition that threatens the patient's life unless the procedure is performed. Occasionally amputation is an emergency procedure that is performed when a severe accident has nearly severed the extremity, but generally it is an elective procedure, and the final decision rests with the patient. Deciding whether to exchange a leg for a life, particularly when life expectancy may not be too long, is not easy. Patients need as much emotional support and understanding as possible. Patients should know preoperatively about **prostheses,** and often a visit from a person who uses a prosthesis is helpful.

Advances in microsurgery techniques have made the reattachment of severed limbs possible. The equipment and skills for accomplishing this procedure are not available in many communities, and patients may need to be transferred to another hospital where these services are available. Upper extremities have a greater success of attachment than lower extremities.

## Preoperative Intervention

Before surgery, the patient's general physical condition is assessed carefully. If the patient has diabetes, his or her diabetic status is evaluated. Other examinations, such as electrocardiograms and chest x-rays, may be ordered by the physician. Intravenous fluids may be given to combat dehydration, and a blood transfusion may be ordered if anemia is present. The skin is prepared according to the hospital procedure.

## Postoperative Intervention

The months of stump wrapping and conditioning before being fitted with a prosthesis have now been eliminated. Patients are fitted with a rigid temporary prosthesis either immediately after surgery or when the stump is healed and the sutures have been removed. Every patient who has had an amputation should receive a temporary prosthesis as soon as possible after surgery. The patient benefits psychologically from a temporary prosthesis, and complications are prevented. After returning from surgery, the patient should be watched for signs of shock, and vital signs should be checked at frequent intervals until he or she is stabilized. The dressings should be observed for evidence of bright red blood. In cases of severe bleeding, the nurse should apply manual pressure to the site and contact the physician immediately. If oozing from the stump occurs, the nurse may reinforce the dressing but should never attempt to change it without a physician's order.

Because many amputations are performed on persons between 60 and 70 years of age, the patient must be observed carefully for shock, pulmonary complications, or cardiovascular collapse. Because elderly patients may have problems with urinary incontinence, the dressing may need to be protected to prevent contamination of the wound.

The postoperative care of the patient with an amputation is directed toward preparing the stump for a prosthesis, preventing contractures of the hip or nearest joint, maximizing wound healing, and facilitating adaptation to an altered life-style. Providing support to the patient is an important component of nursing care. The loss of a limb results in grieving and fear about how to function and interact with others. When the psychologic response to the loss is severe, it can result in ineffective rehabilitation (Novotony, 1991).

If a temporary prosthesis has not been applied, the stump is wrapped with elastic compression bandages to shrink and shape it (Figure 33-21). Once the original surgical dressing has been removed, a stump sock shrinker may be used in place of elastic compression bandages. Before healing occurs, every effort must be made to prevent infection of the wound. The stump may be elevated by raising the foot of the bed for the first 24 hours. When the patient is in the supine position, the stump should rest flat on the bed. The patient should be encouraged to spend some time each day in the prone position, with a pillow tucked under the lower trunk and the stump for support (Figure 33-22). The stump should not be flexed over the unaffected leg. When in the prone position, the patient may begin pushup exercises to strengthen arm and shoulder muscles. When in the supine position, the patient may begin leg exercises unless such exercises strain the suture line.

> **NURSE ALERT**
>
> Do not elevate the stump on pillows after the first 24 hours after surgery. This may cause flexion contractures.

If there is to be immediate postsurgical fitting of a prosthesis, a sterile stump sock is pulled over the stump when surgery is complete. Pressure areas are protected with felt pads. The stump is wrapped with elastic bandages to form a firm, snug dressing that prevents swelling and protects the stump from injury. The nurse must be alert for edema that may prevent weight bearing, and, if the dressing comes off or is damaged, the physician must be notified immediately and compression bandages applied until the physician arrives (Bending, 1993). Brief ambulation with limited weight bearing is possible within 24 hours. Gradually ambulation is increased, but weight bearing is limited until healing is complete (Black, Matassarin-Jacobs, 1993). Immediate postsurgical fitting of a prosthesis minimizes stump edema, reduces the risk of embolism, and prevents contractures that preclude subsequent use of a prosthesis. Pressure points must be inspected often for irritation that may progress to necrosis. The patient or family must be taught the signs and symptoms of infection at the incision site, as well as how to monitor the stump for pressure sores from the prosthesis.

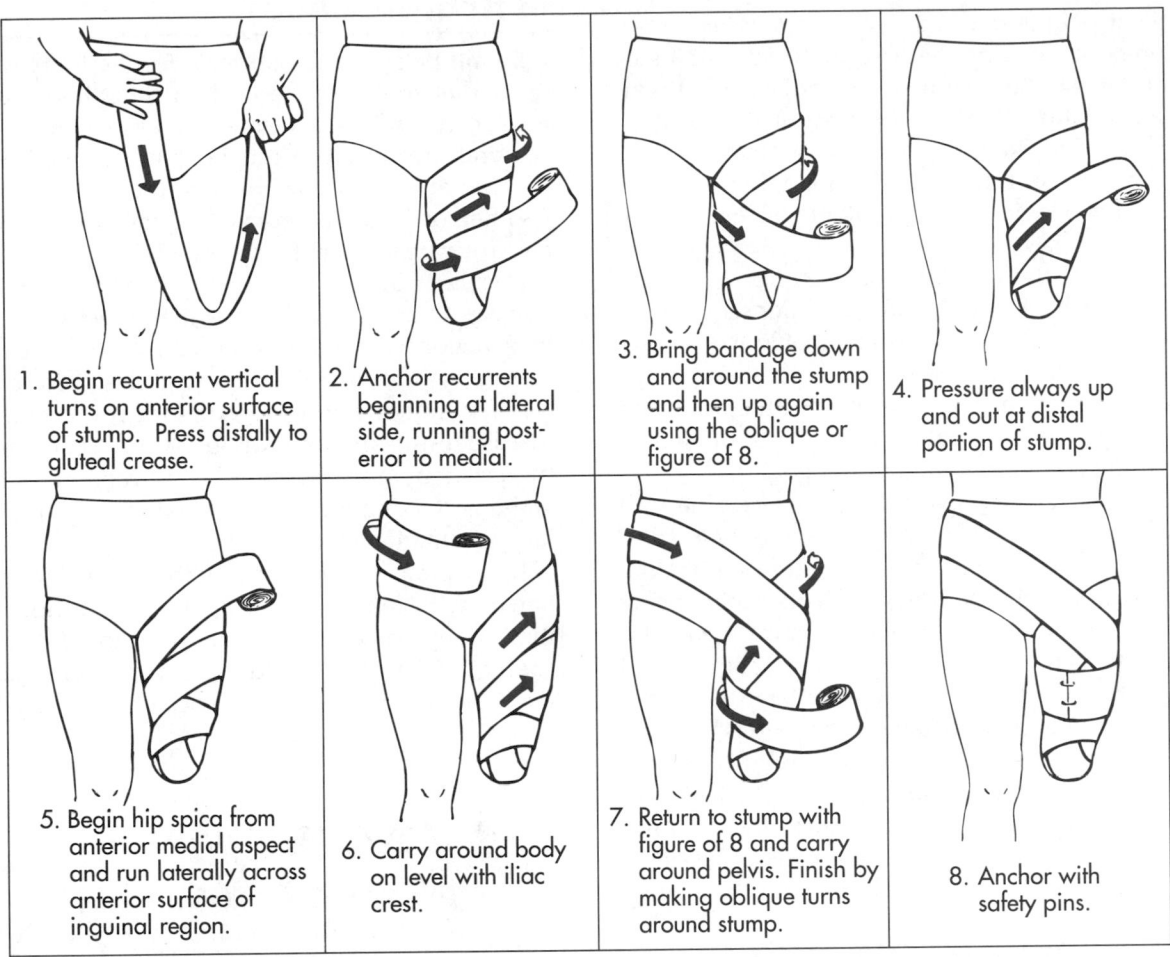

1. Begin recurrent vertical turns on anterior surface of stump. Press distally to gluteal crease.

2. Anchor recurrents beginning at lateral side, running posterior to medial.

3. Bring bandage down and around the stump and then up again using the oblique or figure of 8.

4. Pressure always up and out at distal portion of stump.

5. Begin hip spica from anterior medial aspect and run laterally across anterior surface of inguinal region.

6. Carry around body on level with iliac crest.

7. Return to stump with figure of 8 and carry around pelvis. Finish by making oblique turns around stump.

8. Anchor with safety pins.

**Figure 33-21**    Method of wrapping to help shape stump after above-the-knee amputation. (From Mourad LA: *Orthopedic disorders,* St Louis, 1991, Mosby.)

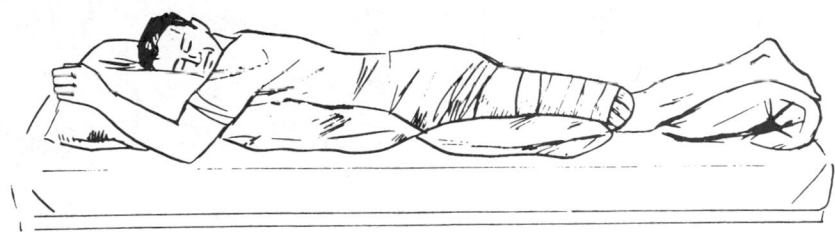

**Figure 33-22**    Patient in prone position following amputation. Note position of pillows.

If no complications occur and the wound has healed, the sutures are removed, and a temporary prosthesis that is made of plastic or plaster of Paris is provided 2 to 3 weeks after surgery. With the temporary prosthesis, the patient is allowed partial weight bearing. Unless complications develop, the patient may bear full weight on the prosthesis within 6 weeks, and a permanent prosthesis is supplied within 3 months. Patients may need to be taught balance and crutch walking before leaving the hospital. They often are re-ferred to the physical therapy department. The patient should be instructed to wash and dry the stump thoroughly once each day when healing is complete. If any abrasion occurs, the physician should be consulted immediately.

## Phantom Limb Sensation

Patients may have little pain from the surgical procedure or may complain of pain in the amputated limb.

This type of pain is referred to as *phantom limb sensation,* often occurs during the first few weeks after surgery, and is most intense during the initial 6 months after the amputation (Bowser, 1991; Rounseville, 1992; Davis, 1993). The exact mechanism of phantom limb sensation is not completely understood, but a combination of physiologic and psychologic factors may be involved.

Until recently, the measures used to treat phantom limb sensation have been ineffective. Consequently a number of individuals have been unable to be completely rehabilitated because of the extreme discomfort associated with the application of the prosthesis and their inability to participate in programs of muscle strengthening and ambulation training.

Encouraging results have been seen over the past few years with the use of transcutaneous electrical nerve stimulation (TENS) for the relief of phantom sensation (Katz, Melzack, 1991). Patients experiencing limb sensation after amputation are now being instructed to attach a TENS unit to the nonamputated limb at a site that is comparable to where the pain is felt in the amputated limb. Relief from pain is believed to be the result of the inability of the cerebral cortex to distinguish the origin of the impulse. The impulses generated by the TENS unit "override" the pain impulses, which breaks the cycle of pain and relieves the discomfort (Katz, Melzack, 1991).

## NEUROMUSCULAR CONDITIONS

A number of neurologic conditions affect the musculoskeletal system. Lower back pain may be caused by a ruptured intervertebral disk or by muscle strain that results from poor alignment of the vertebral column or excessive activity. Carpal tunnel syndrome and thoracic outlet syndrome both involve tingling and numbness of the upper extremities and impaired function (see Chapter 30).

## CEREBRAL PALSY

Cerebral palsy is a broad term for a variety of conditions that are characterized by impaired functional muscle control as a result of an abnormality in the cerebral areas that affect these functions. The cause may be any condition that produces cerebral anoxia and hemorrhage or trauma. The causal event may occur during the prenatal period, during or after delivery, or later in life. If the injury produces irreversible damage to any cerebral areas that affect neuromuscular function, cerebral palsy results. Many types of cerebral palsy exist, and the disease is classified on the basis of symptoms and the extent of involvement. The disease results in motor disability and is characterized by spasticity and involuntary movements related to walking, talking, or any activity that requires muscular coordination.

In addition to problems with motor function, the person with cerebral palsy may have multiple disabilities. Many have impairments of vision, hearing, and speech; convulsive disorders; and mental retardation. Psychologic, emotional, and social problems may also occur.

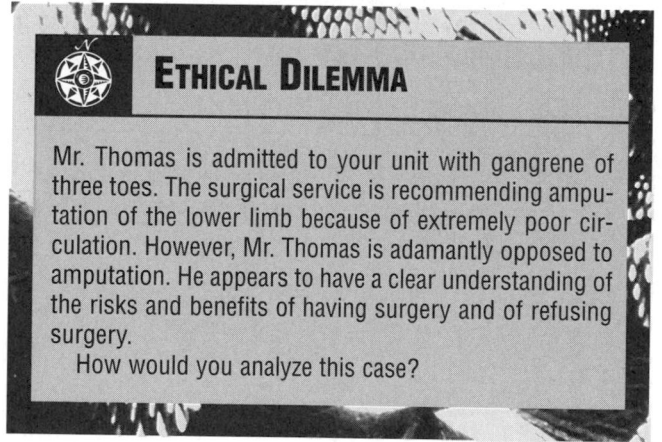

### ETHICAL DILEMMA

Mr. Thomas is admitted to your unit with gangrene of three toes. The surgical service is recommending amputation of the lower limb because of extremely poor circulation. However, Mr. Thomas is adamantly opposed to amputation. He appears to have a clear understanding of the risks and benefits of having surgery and of refusing surgery.

How would you analyze this case?

# NURSING CARE PLAN

## PATIENT WITH BELOW-THE-KNEE AMPUTATION

Mrs. Carter is an 88-year-old woman with a history of non-insulin-dependent diabetes mellitus (NIDDM, type II). She enters the hospital for a below-the-knee amputation of the left leg as a result of gangrene and poor circulation. She states that she has enjoyed good health until this "circulation" problem. Additional medical data reveal that she has a history of hypertension. She has never smoked or used alcohol. She had her left below-the-knee amputation 2 days ago.

| Medical History | Psychosocial Data | Assessment Data |
|---|---|---|
| Appendectomy at 17 years old | Currently resides in an extended care facility because of increasing difficulty in performing activities of daily living (ADL) and because of lack of available family resources | Patient alert and oriented × 3 |
| Total hysterectomy at 46 years old because of fibroid tumors | | Blood pressure stable at 130/70 |
| | | Afebrile |
| | | *Respiratory:* lungs clear, able to demonstrate effective cough, rate of 18-20 breaths/min, regular depth and rhythm |
| Fractured left femur at 55 years old after fall from bicycle; healed without sequelae | | *Abdominal:* soft, nontender, nondistended, bowel sounds heard in all four quadrants |
| Denies any respiratory or cardiac disease | Has been a widow for 9 years; no children | *Skin:* clear with the exception of a reddened area 2 × 3 cm on coccyx, with a 1-cm open area on left buttock |
| Diabetes discovered during routine physical at 62 years of age; takes chlorpropamide (Diabinese), 250 mg daily in the morning; follows American Diabetes Association (ADA) exchange diet with good control | Retired elementary school teacher; engaged in physical sports until 70 years of age | *Cardiovascular:* apical pulse 68-72 bpm; rate regular without thrills or murmurs; pulses on right leg palpable (femoral, popliteal, pedal); pulses on left leg thready and weak (femoral, popliteal) |
| | | *Wound assessment:* stump dressing dry, intact, and in good alignment; patient moving with only minor discomfort |
| | | ***Laboratory data*** |
| | | Hemoglobin (Hgb) 13.1, hematocrit (Hct) 40 |
| | | Electrolytes within normal limits (WNL) |
| | | Serum glucose 238 mg/100 ml |
| No known food or drug allergies; has received antibiotics and blood transfusions in the past without problems | | Urinalysis and other laboratory data within normal limits |
| | | Chest x-ray examination and electrocardiogram (ECG) within normal limits |

### NURSING DIAGNOSES

Self-care deficit related to surgical procedure
Impaired physical mobility related to pain and surgical procedure
Body image disturbance related to left below-the-knee amputation as evidenced by statements of depression and periods of crying

| NURSING INTERVENTIONS | EVALUATION OF EXPECTED OUTCOMES |
|---|---|
| Inform patient that feelings of depression are expected after loss of a body part. | Acknowledges a change in body image |
| Provide time to listen. | Takes an active role in planning aspects of daily care |
| Discuss fears. | Expresses her emotions associated with the change in body image |
| Encourage expression of feelings. | Expresses at least one positive feeling about herself daily |
| Explore resources among friends. | Participates in discussion with person who has had a similar change in body image |
| Arrange for patient to interact with others who have similar problems. | |

*Continued*

# NURSING CARE PLAN
## PATIENT WITH BELOW-THE-KNEE AMPUTATION—cont'd

**NURSING DIAGNOSIS**

Pain related to phantom sensations caused by nerve stimulation secondary to amputation as evidenced by complaint of soreness in left leg when moving and sensation of "feeling" blanket on missing foot

| NURSING INTERVENTIONS | EVALUATION OF EXPECTED OUTCOMES |
|---|---|
| Explain the sensation of phantom limb pain. | Verbalizes understanding of phantom sensations |
| Assess patient's physical pain. | Expresses relief from pain |
| Have patient describe the pain on a scale of 1 to 10. | |
| Provide comfort measures as indicated, including positioning, massage, ice packs, medications, diversional activities, and relaxation techniques. | |

**NURSING DIAGNOSES**

Impaired physical mobility related to left below-the-knee amputation as evidenced by need of assistance when moving and inability to assist with own ADL

Ineffective individual and family coping

| NURSING INTERVENTIONS | EVALUATION OF EXPECTED OUTCOMES |
|---|---|
| Maintain patient in proper body alignment; turn and position patient every 2 hours. | Properly demonstrates isometric and range of motion exercises |
| Increase mobility by having patient move into chair, commode, and geriatric chair; teach patient how to assist with these transfers. | Explains rationale for maintaining activity level and states at least five risk factors for activity intolerance |
| Teach patient to move self in bed; encourage use of unaffected leg. | Performs self-care activities with as little assistance as possible |
| Monitor deep breathing and coughing exercises. | Does not exhibit evidence of cardiovascular or respiratory complications during or after activities |
| Perform range of motion exercises every 2 to 4 hours; teach these exercises to patient. | |
| Encourage and praise independent behaviors. | |
| Encourage active movement using trapeze and other assistive devices. | |
| Assess patient's physiologic response to increased activity (monitor vital signs). | |

**NURSING DIAGNOSIS**

Impaired skin integrity related to decreased mobility and bed rest as evidenced by reddened and open skin

| NURSING INTERVENTIONS | EVALUATION OF EXPECTED OUTCOMES |
|---|---|
| Change patient's position at least every 2 hours. | No further breakdown in skin |
| Keep skin clean and dry | Reddened areas show signs of improved circulation |
| Avoid use of irritating soap; rinse skin well. | Mucous membranes remain intact |
| Use preventive skin care devices as needed, such as sheepskin pads and heel protectors. | Eats at least 80% of each meal |
| Protect bony prominences, and massage them gently every 2 hours to increase circulation. | Drinks at least 100 ml of extra fluids every 2 hours while awake |
| Keep linen clean, dry, and free of wrinkles or crumbs. | Remains clean and dry at all times |
| Monitor nutritional intake; encourage adequate hydration. | Position is changed at least every 2 hours |
| Leave reddened area exposed to air; turn patient from that area. | Weight remains within her established limits |
| Teach patient and family the importance of preventing pressure sores. | Lists preventive skin care measures |

# KEY CONCEPTS

➤ Proper patient positioning and active and passive exercises are essential for preventing permanent complications of prolonged immobility.

➤ Frequent assessment of neurovascular integrity of the injured limb will identify impairment of the neurovascular system and allow for early intervention to prevent damage.

➤ Edema with pallor, cyanosis, and coldness are signs of circulatory impairment.

➤ The blanching sign is a test of the rate of capillary refill, which is an indicator of adequacy of circulation in the extremity.

➤ A recurrence of severe pain after a fracture has been reduced and stabilized indicates that something is wrong.

➤ When traction is applied to an extremity because of a broken bone, the two bone ends are pulled into place.

➤ Skin traction uses the skin to maintain the pull of traction. Skeletal traction uses pins or wires, which are placed in the bone to hold the traction on the affected extremity.

➤ Aseptic technique is used when caring for the pin or wire sites of skeletal traction.

➤ Patients in traction should have skin care performed on pressure points at frequent intervals to prevent skin irritations and pressure sores.

➤ External fixation devices are used to reduce complex fractures that have bone fragments that need stabilization.

➤ Patients with fractures should eat a diet high in calcium, minerals, and fiber to promote healing of the fracture and normal elimination habits.

➤ A sprain involves ligaments, tendons, and muscles that have been torn or pulled from the bone as the result of twisting or wrenching a joint beyond its normal range of motion.

➤ A dislocation may be congenital or a result of disease or trauma. It is the temporary displacement of a bone from its normal position within a joint.

➤ Fractures are described as being open or closed. They are also described according to their appearance, location, and displacement.

➤ The time for healing of fractures varies and is influenced by the type of fracture, the bone involved, and the age and condition of the patient.

➤ Serious complications of fractures include pulmonary embolism, fat embolism, gas gangrene, tetanus, and compartment syndrome.

➤ Whiplash injury to the musculoskeletal system is the result of a combination of severe flexion and extension of the neck.

➤ Bone tumors may be primary or secondary and may be benign or malignant.

➤ An amputation of part or all of an extremity may be necessary because of a malignant bone tumor, injury, diabetic gangrene, or any condition that threatens the patient's life unless the procedure is performed.

➤ Cerebral palsy is a neuromuscular disorder that results in motor disability and is characterized by spasticity and involuntary movements related to walking, talking, or activities that require muscular coordination.

# CRITICAL THINKING EXERCISES

1. Prepare a list of instructions for a patient who is going home with a cast on his or her arm.

2. Your 35-year-old patient has a fractured femur and will be placed in skeletal traction. He asks you why that is necessary. Explain to him what traction does and why it is necessary to keep the weights hanging freely.

3. Describe three physiologic changes in the older adult that make bone healing more difficult.

## REFERENCES AND ADDITIONAL READINGS

Adams RD, Victor M: *Principles of neurology*, ed 5, New York, 1993, McGraw-Hill.

Altizer L: Total hip arthroplasty, *Orthop Nurs* 14(4):7-18, 1995.

Bending J: TENS relief of discomfort, *Physiotherapy* 79(11): 773-774, 1993.

Black JM, Matassarin-Jacobs E: *Luckman and Sorensen's medical-surgical nursing*, ed 4, Philadelphia, 1993, Saunders.

Bliven KA: An orthopedic emergency: compartment syndrome, *Nurs Spect* 10(8):14-16, 1997.

Bowser MS: Giving up the ghost: a review of phantom limb phenomena, *J Rehabil* 57(3):55-62, 1991.

Carpenito LJ: *Handbook of nursing diagnoses*, ed 5, Philadelphia, 1993, Lippincott.

Davis RW: Phantom sensation, phantom pain, and stump pain, *Arch Phys Med Rehabil* 74(1):79-91, 1993.

DeGeorge P, Dunwoody C: Transfer technique of lower extremity with an external fixator, *Orthop Nurs* 14(6):17-21, 1995.

Driscoll AH: When your patient wears an Ilizarov device, *Am J Nurs* 93(6):63-65, 1993.

Gregory B: *Orthopaedic surgery*, St Louis, 1994, Mosby.

Houston M: Care of the school-aged child in 90/90 traction, *Orthop Nurs* 15(2):57-63, 1996.

Katz J, Melzack R: Auricular transcutaneous electrical nerve stimulation (TENS) reduces phantom limb pain, *J Pain Symptom Manage* 6(2):73-83, 1991.

Lewis SM, Collier IC, Heitkemper MM: *Medical-surgical nursing: assessment and management of clinical problems*, ed 4, St Louis, 1996, Mosby.

Maher AB et al: *Orthopaedic nursing*, Philadelphia, 1994, Saunders.

Mikulaninec CE: An amputee critical path, *J Vasc Nurs* 10(2): 2-6, 1992.

Mourad LA: *Orthopedic disorders*, St Louis, 1991, Mosby.

Newman DM, Fawcett J: Caring for a young child in a body cast: impact on the care giver, *Orthop Nurs* 14(1):41-46, 1995.

Novotony MP: Psychosocial issues affecting rehabilitation, *Phys Med Rehabil Clin North Am* 2(2):373-393, 1991.

Olson R: Halo skeletal traction pin site care: toward developing a standard of care, *Rehabil Nurs* 21(5):243-246, 1996.

Piasechi P: Nursing care of the patient with metabolic bone disease, *Orthop Nurs* 15(4):25-33, 1996.

Rockwood C, Green D, Bucholz R: *Rockwood and Green's fractures in adults*, Philadelphia, 1991, Lippincott.

Ross D, editor: *National Association of Orthopedic Nurses scope and standards of orthopaedic nursing practice*, Pitman, 1996, AJ Janetti.

Ross D, editor: *Scope and standards of orthopaedic nursing practice*, Pitman, 1996, AJ Janetti.

Rounseville C: Phantom limb pain: The ghost that haunts the amputee, *Orthop Nurs* 11(2):67-71, 1992.

Salmond S et al, editors: *Care curriculum for orthopaedic nursing*, ed 3, Pitman, 1996, AJ Janetti.

Salmond S et al, editors: *National Association of Orthopedic Nurses core curriculum for orthopaedic nursing*, ed 3, Pitman, 1996, AJ Janetti.

Smeltzer SC, Bare BG: *Brunner and Suddarth's textbook of medical-surgical nursing*, ed 7, Philadelphia, 1992, Lippincott.

Smith M: Two legs to stand on . . . left above the knee amputation, *Am J Nurs* 93(12):42-44, 1993.

Stuart M, Karaharju J: Acute compartment syndrome: recognizing the progressive signs and symptoms, *Phys Sports Med* 22(3):908, 1994.

Styrcula L: Traction basics. I, *Orthop Nurs* 13(2):71-74, 1994.

Styrcula L: Traction basics. II. Traction equipment, *Orthop Nurs* 13(3):55-59, 1994.

Styrcula L: Traction basics. III. Types of traction, *Orthop Nurs* 13(4):34-44, 1994.

Styrcula L: Traction basics. IV. Traction for lower extremities, *Orthop Nurs* 13(5):59-69, 1994.

Tucker SM et al: *Patient care standards: collaborative practice planning*, ed 6, St Louis, 1996, Mosby.

Williams A, Denton S: Phantom limb pain: elusive, yet real, *Rehabil Nurs* 22(2):73-77, 1997.

Williams M et al: Family caregiving in cases of hip fracture, *Rehabil Nurs* 21(3):124-131, 1996.

Wyngaarden JB et al: *Cecil's textbook of medicine*, ed 19, Philadelphia, 1992, Saunders.

Yetzer E: Helping the patient through the experience of an amputation, *Orthop Nurs* 15(6):45-49, 1996.

# CHAPTER 34

# Arthritic and Rheumatic Problems

## CHAPTER OBJECTIVES

1  List common nursing diagnoses for arthritic disorders.
2  Describe the differences between rheumatoid arthritis and osteoarthritis.
3  Discuss medical treatment and nursing intervention related to rheumatoid arthritis and osteoarthritis.
4  Discuss the pathophysiology of gout, as well as the medical treatment, nursing process, and education for the patient with gout.
5  Define and describe the assessment of bursitis.
6  Describe reconstructive surgery of the hip, as well as the education for the patient recovering from total hip arthroplasty.
7  Describe the pharmacologic management and related nursing considerations associated with rheumatoid arthritis.
8  Describe the sequence leading to joint destruction with osteoarthritis.
9  Identify the nursing interventions required for the treatment of arthritis and related rheumatic disorders.

## KEY TERMS

| | |
|---|---|
| abduction | osteoarthritis |
| arthritis | osteotomy |
| arthrodesis | prosthesis |
| arthroplasty | rheumatoid arthritis |
| arthroscopy | sequential compression device |
| bursae | tophi |

## DISORDERS OF THE JOINTS

The American Rheumatism Association recognizes 13 groups of joint disease. Most of these disorders can be placed into two major categories: inflammatory and noninflammatory joint diseases. Inflammatory joint disease involves inflammation of the synovial membrane in the joint and is usually associated with systemic signs and symptoms. Noninflammatory disease is characterized by the absence of inflammation, and no systemic signs and symptoms are present.

## ARTHRITIS (INFLAMMATORY JOINT DISEASE)

Inflammatory joint disease is commonly called **arthritis**. There are various types of arthritis. Inflammatory joint disease is characterized by inflammatory damage or destruction in the synovial membrane or articular cartilage accompanied by systemic signs of inflammation such as fever, leukocytosis, malaise, anorexia, and hyperfibrinogenemia. Inflammatory joint disease can be infectious or noninfectious. Infectious inflammatory joint disease is caused by the invasion of pathogenic organisms through a wound or delivered by the bloodstream from sites of infection elsewhere in the body such as the bones, heart valves, or blood vessels. In noninfectious inflammatory joint disease, the inflammation is caused by either immune reactions or crystal deposits. Rheumatoid arthritis and ankylosing spondylitis are caused by immune reactions; gouty arthritis is caused by the deposit of crystals of monosodium urate in and around the joint.

## RHEUMATOID ARTHRITIS

**Rheumatoid arthritis** is the most serious form of arthritis. It is an autoimmune disease that causes chronic inflammation of connective tissue, primarily in the joints. The synovial membrane is affected first, and eventually inflammation may spread to the articular cartilage, fibrous joint capsule and surrounding ligaments and tendons, causing pain, joint deformity, and loss of function (Figure 34-1). The disease may occur at any age but most commonly affects persons between ages 20 and 50 years. It can also occur in children. It commonly affects the fingers, feet, wrists, elbows, ankles, and knees, but the shoulders, hips, and cervical spine may also be involved as well as the tissues of the lungs, heart, kidneys, and skin. It effects 1% to 2% of adults and develops in three women for every one man affected. In addition to joint involvement, there are systemic symptoms, including fever, malaise, rash, lymph node or spleen enlargement, and Raynaud phenomenon (transient lack of circulation to the fingertips and toes).

Research has failed to find a specific cause of rheumatoid arthritis. It is probably a combination of genetic, environmental, hormonal, and reproductive factors (Spector, 1990). It probably occurs because the individual responds abnormally to the presence of an antigen. Patients with rheumatoid arthritis often have a history of some type of recent infection.

## Pathophysiology

For reasons unknown, with long-term or intensive exposure to an antigen, the normal antibodies (immunoglobulins) of patients with rheumatoid arthritis become autoantibodies: antibodies that attack the tissues of the host. These transformed antibodies are called *rheumatoid factors*. These rheumatoid factors bind with their target self-antigens in the blood and synovial membrane, forming immune complexes (antigen-antibody complexes). Synovial inflammation (synovitis) occurs when immune complexes in the blood and synovial tissue trigger the inflammatory response, chiefly by activating the plasma protein complement. Complement activation stimulates kinin and prostaglandin release that increases the permeability of blood vessels in the synovial membranes and attracts leukocytes and lymphocytes to the synovial membrane. Several types of leukocytes are attracted from the blood to the synovial membrane. The phagocytes of inflammation (neutrophils and macrophages) ingest the immune complexes and release powerful enzymes that degrade synovial tissue and articular cartilage. The B lymphocytes are stimulated to produce more rheumatoid factor. The T lymphocytes produce enzymes that amplify and perpetuate the inflammatory response. The self-antigens are in constant supply and the immune system continues to act and form immune complexes, which triggers complement formation, and the inflammatory response is perpetuated.

The disease may develop insidiously, or it may have an acute onset. Remissions occur and symptoms subside, but subsequent attacks follow and a chronic state slowly develops. The inflammatory and immune responses have several damaging effects on the synovial membrane (Figure 34-2). The membrane swells as a result of leukocyte infiltration and it thickens as its cells proliferate and enlarge abnormally. The synovial inflammation progresses to involve its blood vessels, and small venues become occluded by the by-products of the inflammatory process: endothelial cells, fibrin, platelets, and inflammatory cells. Vascular flow to the synovial tissue is decreased. Reduced circulation and increased metabolic needs results in hypoxia and metabolic acidosis. Acidosis stimulates the release of hydrolytic enzymes from synovial cells into the surrounding tissue. This

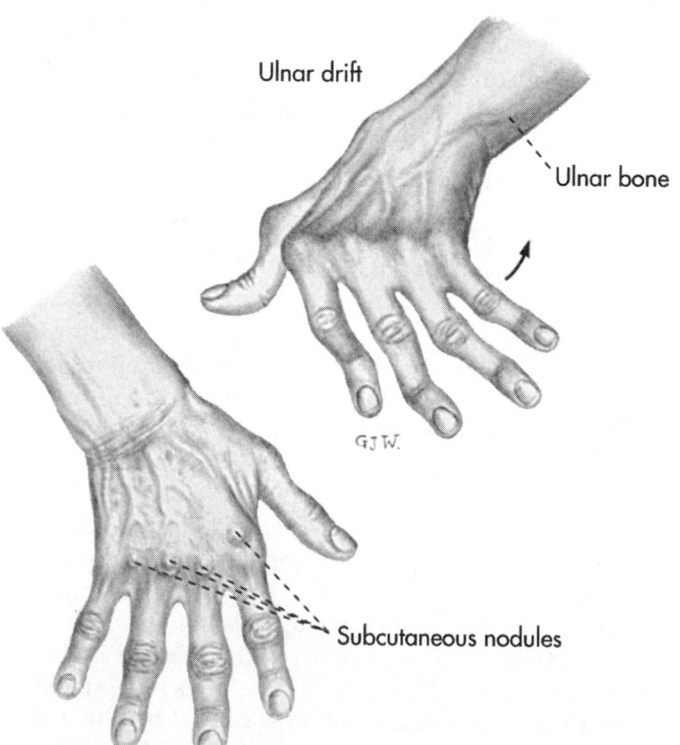

**Figure 34-1** Rheumatoid arthritis of the hand. Note swelling from chronic synovitis of metacarpophalangeal joints, marked ulnar drift, subcutaneous modules, and subluxation of metacarpophalangeal joints with extension of proximal interphalangeal joints and flexion of distal joints. Note also deformed position of thumb. Hand has wasted appearance. (From Mourad LA: *Orthopedic disorders: Mosby's clinical nursing series*, St Louis, 1991, Mosby.)

causes erosion of the articular cartilage and inflammation in the ligaments and tendons in the affected joints. As the disease progresses, granulation tissue called *pannus* fills the joint and the normal joint cartilage is destroyed. The joint cavities fill with scar tissue, which immobilizes the joints.

## Assessment

The early symptoms of rheumatoid arthritis are loss of weight; loss of appetite; muscle aches; malaise; fever; and swollen, painful joints. Complaints of joint stiffness, especially on rising in the morning, are common. During the early course of the disease, considerable muscle spasm occurs, and any effort to move the affected joints is painful. The diagnosis is established by a variety of findings. The rheumatoid factor (RF) titer is elevated, which indicates the presence of an abnormal serum protein concentration. The erythrocyte sedimentation rate is elevated, and x-ray films show progressive damage to the joints. Swan-neck deformities of the hands and fingers are seen in later stages (Figure 34-3).

## Intervention

The care of the patient with rheumatoid arthritis is directed toward maintaining function, relieving pain, and preventing deformities (Box 34-1). One of the most distressing factors in the treatment of rheumatoid arthritis is that some patients obtain unprofessional advice in hopes of relieving their symptoms. As a result, they may wear copper bracelets, drink potions of vinegar and honey, wear beans or potatoes around their necks, or sit in uranium mines. Patients hear about these "cures" through well-meaning friends and relatives who may be acquainted with someone whose symptoms seemingly disappeared with similar therapy. Because the disease is characterized by alternating periods of exacerbation and remission, a patient who adopts quackery as treatment may experience a normal remission and attribute the improvement to the "cure." As a result, the supposed cure is believed to be valuable despite medical advice to the contrary. Patients should seek medical attention early so that pain and joint deformity can be minimized.

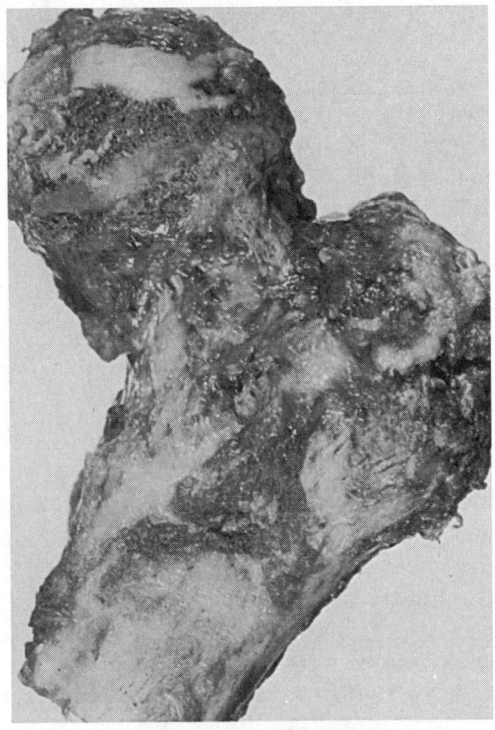

**Figure 34-2** Advanced rheumatoid arthritis involving femur. There is prominent proliferation of synovium and almost complete destruction of overlying articular cartilage. (From Rosai J: *Ackerman's surgical pathology* ed 8, St Louis, 1996, Mosby.)

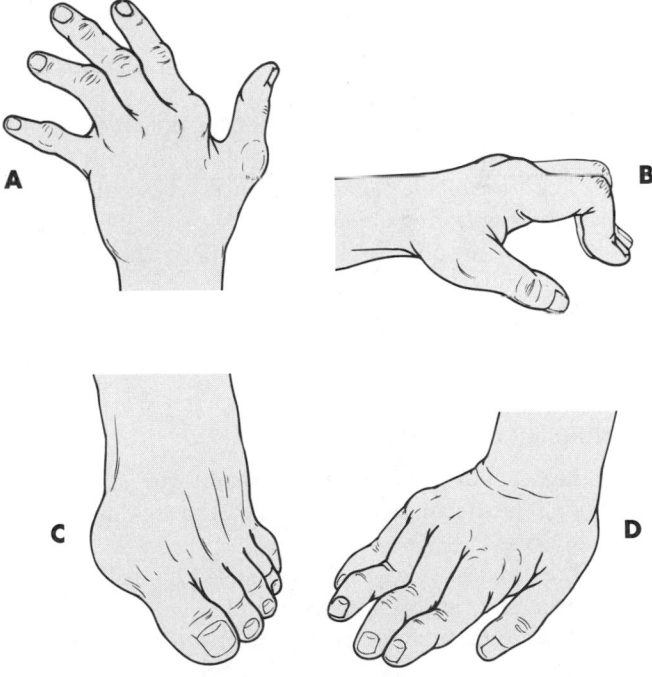

**Figure 34-3** Typical deformities of rheumatoid arthritis. **A,** Ulnar drift. **B,** Boutonniere deformity. **C,** Hallux valgus. **D,** Swan-neck deformity. (From Lewis SM, Collier IC, Heitkemper MM: *Medical-surgical nursing: assessment and management of clinical problems,* ed 4, St Louis, 1996, Mosby.)

Rest is important during acute attacks, and the nurse should give special attention to good body alignment. The mattress should be firm to provide adequate support. The extremities should be straight without pillows under the knees, and the knee gatch on the bed should not be raised. Sandbags or trochanter rolls should be used to prevent outward rotation of the extremities. The patient should be positioned so that the back is straight, and a small pillow should be placed under the head. Hip and knee flexion must be avoided. Some of the most severe joint deformities are caused by patients assuming a comfortably flexed position.

Aspirin or ibuprofen is generally considered to be the drug of choice to decrease both pain and inflammation. It may be given in fairly large doses and should be taken with food to avoid gastric upset. Other antiinflammatory drugs may be tried if the ibuprofen is ineffective. Gold compounds are selected for some patients, usually those who are not responding to other forms of treatment. These medications are slow acting, and the patient must be watched carefully for side effects while receiving the drug. Adrenocorticoids (e.g., cortisone, prednisone, and hydrocortisone) are given if more conservative treatment fails. These drugs may produce dramatic relief of symptoms but do not cure the disease. However, somewhat severe side effects can result, and, once the medication is discontinued, the patient may have a full return of original symptoms. Usually the patient is maintained on the lowest dose of corticosteroids that will produce an improvement in the condition. Hydrocortisone acetate injected into the joints results in immediate relief of pain and a temporary halt to the destructive process, which usually lasts for several weeks (Table 34-1). The use of heat is helpful in relieving pain and may include hot, moist packs; hot tub baths; electric blankets; paraffin baths; and whirlpool baths.

---

| BOX 34-1 | NURSING PROCESS |
|---|---|

## ARTHRITIC DISORDERS

### ASSESSMENT
- History of fatigue, malaise, weakness
- Joint comparison for size, shape, color, and symmetry
- Reports of joint pain and stiffness, especially in morning lasting at least an hour
- Muscle atrophy
- Peripheral pulses
- Muscle strength and function
- Joint mobility, crepitus, function, and sensation
- Level of pain using pain scale

### NURSING DIAGNOSES
- Self-care deficit caused by disease progression
- Pain (acute and chronic) related to inflammatory process
- Impaired physical mobility caused by disease process or surgical intervention
- Altered body image related to chronic disease activity
- Activity intolerance or fatigue related to disease process

### NURSING INTERVENTIONS
- Provide comfort measures to reduce or alleviate pain (acute and chronic)
- Maintain or increase mobility and muscle strength.
- Set up exercise program to maintain joint mobility.
- Assess need for assistive device for ambulation to maintain mobility.
- Promote patient participation in exercise program to maximize endurance.
- Modify home environment for ease of patient mobility.
- Encourage positive coping mechanism.
- Encourage range of motion exercises to prevent unnecessary mobility restrictions.

### EVALUATION OF EXPECTED OUTCOMES
- Pain decreased below current level on pain scale or relieved
- Mobility maintained, not decreased
- Muscle strength maintained or increased
- Balances activity and rest to limit pain or fatigue
- Home environment free of barriers to mobility
- Completes activities of daily living independently or with assistance
- Has increased range of motion of joints

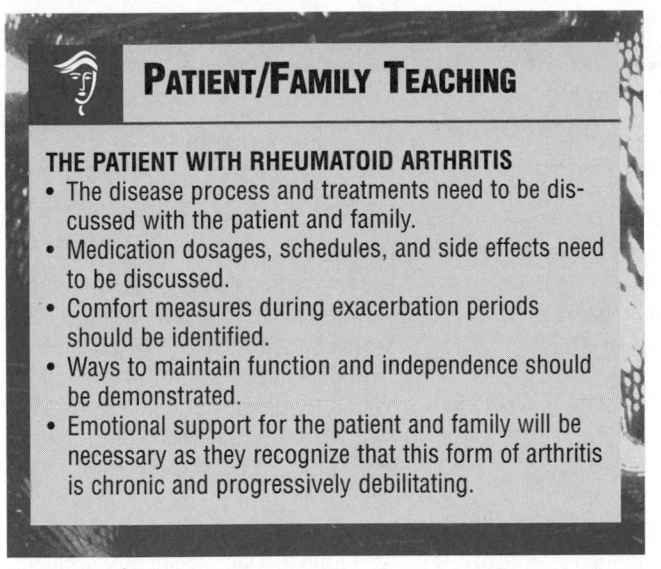

Once the acute stage is passed, a program of physical therapy must be established. A planned program of rest and activity is important. Active exercise should be a part of the therapeutic plan so that normal functioning of the joints is maintained. Exercises should be simple and may be taught by the nurse or physical therapist. No special diet is required for the patient with arthritis, but a well-balanced diet and adequate fluid intake should be encouraged. After recovery from acute attacks, the patient may return to work and should be encouraged to remain active. Many patients with rheumatoid arthritis remain independent and self-sufficient most of their lives.

# RHEUMATOID (ANKYLOSING) SPONDYLITIS

Rheumatoid (ankylosing) spondylitis is an inflammation of the vertebrae and sacroiliac joints and may affect part or all of the spine and lead to complete rigidity. The rheumatoid process may cause the thoracic spine to bow outward (kyphosis). Treatment of the condition is similar to that for rheumatoid arthritis except that the program of exercise is designed to prevent kyphosis. Exercises are planned to keep the spine straight and to maintain range of motion in the

---

**TABLE 34-1**

## Pharmacologic Management of Rheumatic Disorders

| DRUG | MECHANISM OF ACTION | SIDE EFFECTS | NURSING CONSIDERATIONS |
|---|---|---|---|
| **Salicylates** Aspirin, salsolate (Disalcid) Choline salicylate (Arthropan) Choline magnesium trisalicylate (Trilisate) Diflunisal (Dolobid) | Antiinflammatory Analgesic Antipyretic effect Act by inhibiting the synthesis of prostaglandins | GI irritation (ulcer, gastritis, hemorrhage), hypersensitivity, salicylism (nausea, tinnitus, dizziness, hyperpnea), prolonged bleeding time | When drug is taken for antiinflammatory effect, discontinue if pain decreases. Administer drug with food, milk, antacids as prescribed, or full glass of water or use enteric-coated aspirin. Report signs of bleeding (e.g., tarry stool, bruising, petechiae, melena). Need for frequent dosing decreases compliance. |
| **Nonsteroidal Antiinflammatory Drugs** Ibuprofen (Motrin, Advil, Rufen) Naproxen (Naprosyn, Anaprox) Piroxicam (Feldene) Indomethacin (Indocin) Sulindac (Clinoril) Tolmetin (Tolectin) Diclofenac (Voltaren) Meclofenamate (Meclomen) and many others | Antiinflammatory Analgesic Antipyretic effect Act by inhibiting the synthesis of prostaglandins | GI irritation (dyspepsia, nausea, and vomiting), GI bleeding, dizziness, rash, headache, tinnitus, prolonged bleeding time, elevated serum transaminases, drug-induced nephrotoxicity, exacerbation of asthma | Report signs of bleeding, edema, skin rashes, persistent headaches, or visual disturbances. |

From Lewis SM, Collier IC, Heitkemper MM: *Medical-surgical nursing: assessment and management of clinical problems,* ed 4, St Louis, 1996, Mosby.
*CBC,* Complete blood count; *GI,* gastrointestinal.

*Continued*

## TABLE 34-1

## Pharmacologic Management of Rheumatic Disorders—cont'd

| DRUG | MECHANISM OF ACTION | SIDE EFFECTS | NURSING CONSIDERATIONS |
|------|---------------------|--------------|------------------------|
| **Corticosteroids** **Intraarticular injections** Methylprednisolone acetate (Depo-Medrol) Triamcinolone hexacetonide (Aritsopan) | Antiinflammatory Analgesic Act by inhibiting the synthesis of prostaglandins | Local osteoporosis or neuropathic arthropathy from repeated injection | Use strict aseptic technique as joint fluid is removed and steroids are injected. Inform patient that joint may feel worse immediately after injection. Inform patient that improvement lasts weeks to months after injection and that weight bearing should be minimized for 2-6 wk after injection. |
| **Systemic** Hydrocortisone sodium succinate (Solu-Cortef) Methylprednisolone succinate (Solu-Medrol) Dexamethasone (Decadron) Prednisone Triamcinolone (Aristocort) | Antiinflammatory Analgesic | Cushing's syndrome, including fluid retention, GI irritation, osteoporosis, hypertension, diabetes mellitus, acne, menstrual irregularities, hirsutism, risk of infection, bruising | Use only when symptoms persist with less potent antiinflammatory drugs or in life-threatening situations. Administer for limited time only, tapering dose slowly. Be aware that exacerbation of symptoms occurs with abrupt withdrawal. Monitor blood pressure, weight, CBC, and potassium. Limit sodium intake. Report signs of infection. Instruct patient to report corticosteroid use to surgeon or dentist to avoid postoperative adrenal insufficiency. |
| **Immunosuppressive** Azathioprine (Imuran) | Acts as an immunosuppressant by inhibiting purine metabolism and decreasing DNA, RNA, and protein synthesis | GI irritation and ulceration, alopecia, oral lesions, dermatitis, blood dyscrasia, bone marrow depression, general increase in susceptibility to infection | Be aware of teratogenic potential that cautions against use for children or adults of childbearing age. Monitor CBC and urinalysis values. Be aware that drug should be used with great caution in patients with hepatic or renal impairment and should not be used in patients with a history of malignant tumors. |
| Cyclophosphamide (Cytoxan) | Acts as an immunosuppressant by cross-linking DNA and RNA strands and inhibiting the synthesis of protein | GI irritation and ulceration, alopecia, oral lesions, dermatitis, blood dyscrasia, bone marrow depression, oncogenicity, hemorrhagic cystitis, sterility | Be aware that therapy is limited to patients who are responsive to conventional therapy. Monitor CBC and urinalysis values. Be aware of teratogenic potential that cautions against use for children or adults of childbearing age. Inform patient that contraception should be used during therapy. Use usually limited to treatment of rheumatoid vasculitis. |
| Methotrexate | Acts as an immunosuppressant by inhibiting the metabolism of folic acid, thus inhibiting the synthesis of RNA and DNA | GI irritation, photosensitivity, oral lesions, hepatic toxicity, blood dyscrasia, infertility | Monitor CBC and liver enzyme values. Instruct patient to avoid alcoholic beverages and report signs of jaundice. Be aware of teratogenic potential that cautions against use for children or adults of childbearing age. Inform patient that contraception should be used during and 3 mo after treatment. |

**TABLE 34-1**

## Pharmacologic Management of Rheumatic Disorders—cont'd

| DRUG | MECHANISM OF ACTION | SIDE EFFECTS | NURSING CONSIDERATIONS |
|---|---|---|---|
| **Disease-Modifying Agents** | | | |
| *Chrysotherapy* | | | |
| Parenteral<br>   Gold sodium thiomalate<br>   (Myochrysine)<br>Oral<br>   Aurothioglucose (Solganal)<br>   Auranofin (Ridaura) | Unknown inflammatory suppressive effect, possibly caused by inhibition of macrophage function, complement activation, prostaglandin synthesis | Parenteral: dermatitis, pruritus, stomatitis, blood dyscrasia, nephrotoxicity, diarrhea<br>Oral: less toxic than parenteral; GI irritation, mucocutaneous, hematopoietic system, and kidney complications | Parenteral: test blood and urine regularly. Check urine for blood and protein before each dose and delay injection until negative. Mix drug well and give deep intramuscular injection in buttocks. Inform patient that symptomatic improvement is not expected for 3-6 mo and that therapy may be continued indefinitely.<br>Oral: institute new oral therapy with bulking agents. Do not taper oral dosage; be aware that laboratory testing is less frequent with oral drug. Instruct patient to not become pregnant while receiving chrysotherapy. Less toxic and less effective than parenteral gold. |
| *Antimalarials* | | | |
| Chloroquine (Aralen)<br>   Hydroxychloroquine<br>   (Plaquenil) | Unknown; has the ability to bind and alter DNA | Nausea, abdominal discomfort, rash, asymptomatic retinopathy, corneal opacity, headache, dizziness, blood dyscrasia | Inform patient that ophthalmologic examination including slit lamp studies is required every 3-6 mo. Instruct patient to take drug with meals, milk, or antacid as prescribed, to report all skin eruptions and visual disturbances, and to avoid excessive sun exposure. Be aware that drugs are contraindicated for patients with psoriasis. Monitor CBC and liver enzyme values periodically. Instruct patient to discuss condition with physician before pregnancy and breast-feeding. |
| *Other* | | | |
| Penicillamine (Cuprimine) | Unknown, disease-modifying effect | Blood dyscrasias, glomerulonephropathy, rashes, GI irritation, diarrhea | Give drug on empty stomach before meals (not with). Monitor CBC, urinalysis, and liver enzyme values. Report fever, sore throat, chills, bruising, or bleeding. Be aware that drug is contraindicated with gold therapy. Instruct patient to not become pregnant while taking drug. |

cervical spine. The patient should be positioned on a firm mattress and should only use a small pillow to keep the spine in alignment.

# OSTEOARTHRITIS (DEGENERATIVE JOINT DISEASE)

**Osteoarthritis** (OA) is a noninflammatory joint disease. Osteoarthritis is referred to as secondary when it occurs in relationship to known risk factors such as joint stress, congenital abnormalities, or joint instability caused by trauma. It is considered idiopathic osteoarthritis (formerly called *primary OA*) when it occurs in individuals who do not have a history of known risk factors. Osteoarthritis has been called degenerative joint disease in the past.

Idiopathic OA is the most common type of noninflammatory joint disease. OA exists in about 50% of all

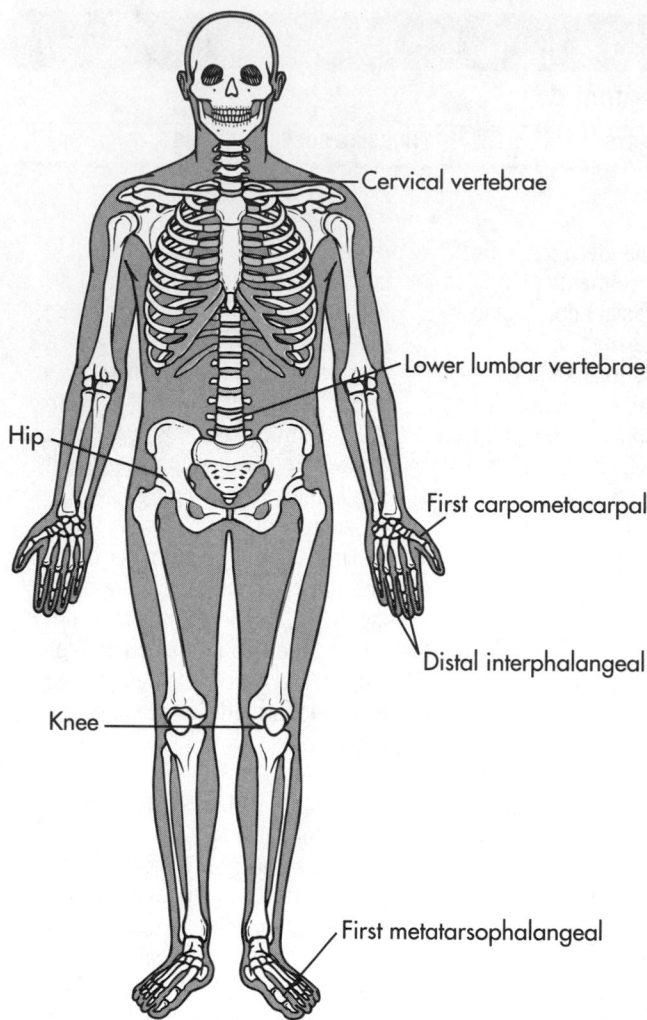

**Figure 34-4**  Joints most frequently involved in osteoarthritis. (From Lewis SM, Collier IC, Heitkemper MM: *Medical-surgical nursing: assessment and management of clinical problems*, ed 4, St Louis, 1996, Mosby.)

people by age 16 (Mankin, 1989) and in 70% of those over age 65 (Felson, 1990). The joints most often affected are those in the hand, wrist, neck (lower cervical spine), lower back (lumbar spine, sacroiliac), hips, knees, ankles, and feet (Figure 34-4). Aging is an important associated factor, and recently a genetic basis for the disorder has been described. With aging, the quality and quantity of proteoglycans in cartilage decrease. Proteoglycans are one of the essential components of the matrix of cartilage. A decrease in proteoglycans renders the cartilage more susceptible to breakdown. The genetic predisposition is linked to a defect in one or more of the genes encoding for the structural components of articular cartilage, thus causing premature cartilage degeneration (Jimenez, 1991). Secondary OA can be caused by any condition that

damages the cartilage, by chronic force or stress on joint surfaces or bones, and by injury that causes instability in the joint. Obesity may hasten the process.

## Pathophysiology

The loss of articular cartilage is the primary defect in both idiopathic and secondary osteoarthritis. Early in the disease the articular cartilage loses its glistening appearance and becomes yellow-gray or brownish-gray. With progression, surface areas of the articular cartilage flake off and deeper layers develop longitudinal fissures. The cartilage becomes thin and may be absent over some areas, leaving the underlying bone (subchondral bone) unprotected. The unprotected bone surface becomes sclerotic or dense and hard. Cysts sometimes develop within the subchondral bone and communicate with (extend into) the longitudinal fissures in the cartilage. Pressure builds in the cysts until the cystic contents are forced into the synovial cavity, breaking through the articular cartilage on the way. As the articular cartilage erodes, cartilage-coated osteophytes or "bone spurs" may grow outward from the underlying bone and change the contours of the bone. These spurlike bony projections enlarge until small pieces, called *joint mice*, break off into the synovial cavity. If osteophyte fragments irritate the synovial membrane, synovitis and joint effusion (an increase in synovial fluid) result. The joint capsule also becomes thickened and at times adheres to the deformed underlying bone, which may limit movement. Contour changes can lead to subluxation of the bone from the joint (McCance, Huether, 1994). Figure 34-5 depicts changes seen in osteoarthritis.

The process that triggers the loss of articular cartilage in osteoarthritis is still being studied. In cases where there is a genetic predisposition, articular cartilage is probably lost as a result of enzymes breaking down the cartilage matrix. The matrix consists of the proteoglycans, glycosaminoglycans, and collagen. The enzymes break down these macromolecules of the matrix into large, diffusible fragments. Then the fragments are taken up by the cells of the cartilage (chondrocytes) and are digested by the cell's own enzymes. A loss of proteoglycans results, which interferes with the pumping action that regulates movement of water and synovial fluid into and out of the cartilage. Without the regulatory action of the proteoglycan pump, cartilage imbibes too much fluid and becomes less able to withstand the stresses of weight bearing. Proteoglycan content also decreases with aging, causing the same increase in water content in joint cartilage that will affect its strength and ability to bear weight. Enzyme activity also causes a loss of collagen, which is

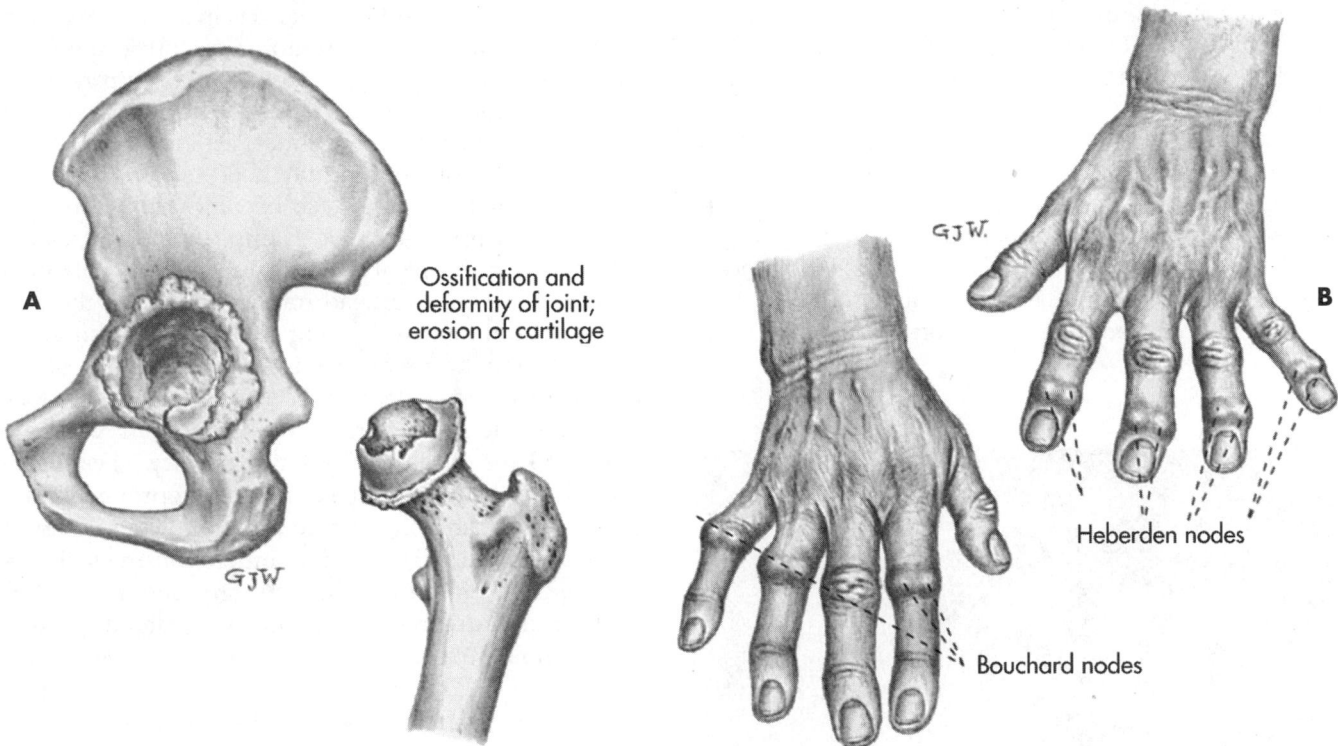

Ossification and deformity of joint; erosion of cartilage

Heberden nodes

Bouchard nodes

**Figure 34-5**    Osteoarthritis. **A,** Cartilage and degeneration of the hip joint from osteoarthritis. **B,** Heberden's nodes and Bouchard's nodes. (From Mourad LA: *Orthopedic disorders: Mosby's clinical nursing series*, St Louis, 1991, Mosby.)

essential for the tensile strength of the articular cartilage (McCance, Huether, 1994).

Treatment for osteoarthritis should include a reduction in weight (if obesity is present) and a regular program of exercise to maintain range of motion. Analgesics may be given three or four times daily to relieve pain. In patients with severe joint pain, hydrocortisone acetate may be injected into the synovial cavity and usually provides pain relief for several weeks. The patient should have a program of rest, and the joints should be protected from continuing wear and strain. The application of moist heat with baths, soaks, packs, or paraffin baths may provide temporary relief.

## SURGICAL INTERVENTION FOR ARTHRITIS

A variety of surgical procedures are available to prevent progressive deformities, to relieve pain, to improve function, and to correct deformities that result from rheumatoid arthritis or osteoarthritis. Tendon transplants can be done to prevent the progressive deformity caused by muscle spasm. An **osteotomy,** which is a cutting of bone to correct bone or joint de-

formities, may be performed to improve function or to relieve pain. Severe joint destruction may be treated with **arthrodesis,** which is a surgical fusion of the joint in a functional position. **Arthroplasty** involves surgery on a diseased joint, such as the elbow, hip, knee, or shoulder, to increase mobility. Sometimes an arthroplasty involves removing a portion of the joint and replacing it with a metal or synthetic **prosthesis.** **Arthroscopy** involves the introduction of an instrument or scope into a joint to examine it. Many surgical procedures can be performed through the arthroscope.

## TOTAL HIP REPLACEMENT

A hip arthroplasty is a common procedure that is performed when arthritis involves the head of the femur and the acetabulum. In this type of surgery the arthritic acetabulum is removed and is replaced by a Vitallium cup lined with plastic to receive the head of the femur, thus providing friction-free movement of the joint. A stainless steel or Vitallium ball on a stem replaces the head of the femur. The cup replacing the acetabulum is either cemented in place or placed in contact with the healthy bone surface and will become secure as the growth of new bone attaches the cup to the acetabulum. This is called a *bony ingrowth prosthesis*. The stem of the femur is either cemented in the femoral canal or the bony ingrowth prosthesis is used to secure it. When the bony ingrowth prosthesis is used, the patient is told that the acetabulum and femur stem may not be secure for 4 to 8 weeks and to limit weight bearing during this period.

The cement used in this procedure is a soft, surgical bone cement that hardens quickly and stabilizes the prosthesis to prevent future erosion of the surround-

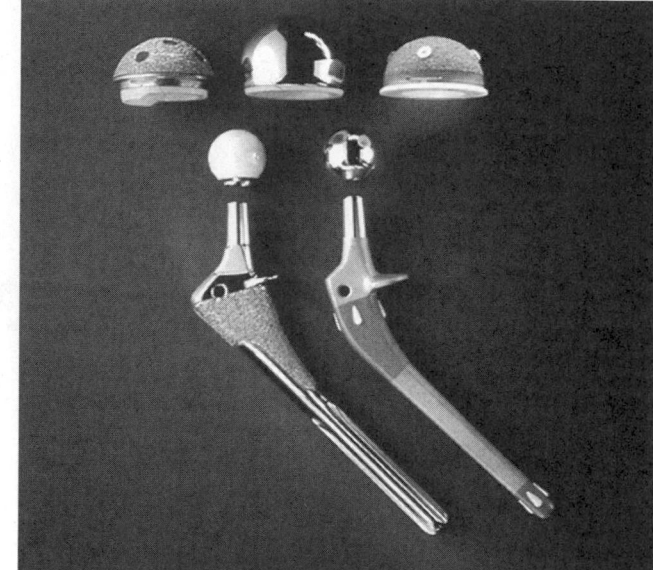

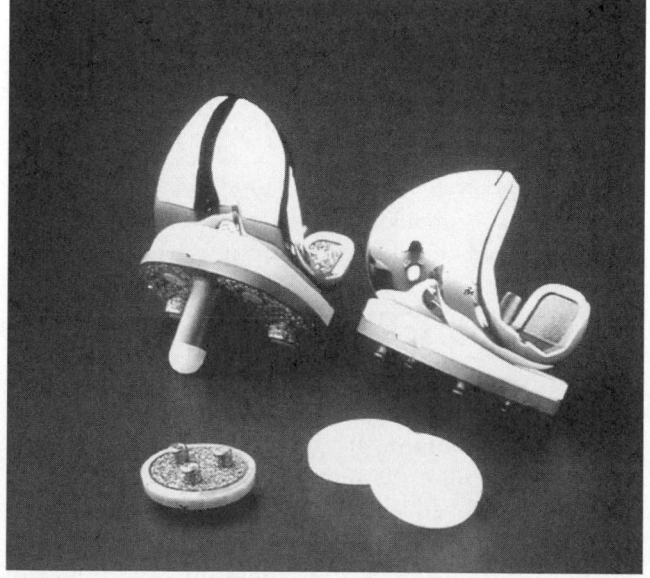

**Figure 34-6**    Total joint replacements. **A,** Hip. **B,** Knee. (Courtesy Zimmer, Inc, Warsaw, Ind. In Lewis SM, Collier IC, Heitkemper MM: *Medical-surgical nursing: assessment and management of clinical problems*, ed 4, St Louis, 1996, Mosby.)

ing bone. If the patient experiences an adverse reaction to the cement, which is a remote possibility, the prosthesis must be surgically removed. Total hip replacement is performed for damage that results from trauma or congenital deformities, as well as for arthritis. The joint replacement may need to be repeated in 15 to 20 years if the prosthesis becomes too worn to be effective. Figure 34-6 shows examples of joint prostheses used in arthroplasty. Before surgery, the patient is taught to use the overhead trapeze to elevate the buttocks. In addition to coughing and deep breathing, the patient is taught to perform isometric exercises of the quadriceps and gluteal muscles, to keep the toes pointed up, to flex the ankles often, and to flex and extend the knee of the unaffected extremity. These exercises are continued after surgery to improve circulation, prevent emboli, and reduce joint stiffness and muscle weakness. Thigh-high antiembolism stockings are applied before or during surgery and **sequential compression devices** (SCDs) may be ordered to assist with venous return, thus reducing the risk of thrombophlebitis. SCDs are plastic boots that are wrapped around the leg that alternately fill with air and then deflate. A wound drain is usually placed in the wound during surgery to provide closed wound suction. The patient is moved directly from the operating table to a bed to reduce the chance of dislocation during transfer at a later time.

## POSTOPERATIVE POSITIONING

After surgery, the affected extremity must be maintained in a position that will not cause dislocation of the operative hip. The ideal position is determined by the surgeon and is based on the approach used for the surgery. The operative hip is dislocated during surgery, and if the surgical position is repeated postoperatively, there is great danger of dislocating the hip prosthesis. The nurse must check the surgeon's orders postoperatively to determine the correct position. It is likely that the patient received instructions on positioning before surgery, and the nurse should evaluate the patient's understanding and reinforce instruction or provide teaching accordingly.

If the surgeon used the posterolateral approach, the patient would lie on the unaffected side during surgery with the operative hip internally rotated, adducted, and flexed. Postoperatively, the patient must be maintained in a position with the hip in external rotation, **abduction,** and extension—the opposite of the surgical position (Altizer, 1995). Some surgeons apply traction but more often they order the use of an abduction pillow between the legs to maintain abduction and extension. An abduction pillow is a large, hard, triangular pillow with Velcro straps on each side to wrap around each leg. The pillow is positioned and secured between the legs to maintain abduction while the patient is supine and is kept in place to maintain abduction while turning the patient to the unaffected side. Additional pillows may be needed to support the affected extremity in abduction while the patient is in a side-lying position.

If an anterior surgical approach is used, the patient is supine and the operative hip is externally rotated and extended during surgery. The safest postoperative position for the patient is to maintain the hip in a flexed position with limited external rotation (Altizer, 1995). To do this, pillows must be used to prop the extremity.

The patient should maintain the desired position when getting out of bed and may sit in a high chair as soon as the first postoperative day. Extreme flexion of the hip should be avoided regardless of the surgical approach used so sitting in a low chair or stooping must be avoided for several weeks to reduce the chance of dislocation. Exercises are performed while the patient is supine or standing (Maher et al, 1994). Because prosthetic devices and materials for hip replacement are continually being developed and improved, the therapy prescribed and the restrictions imposed will vary.

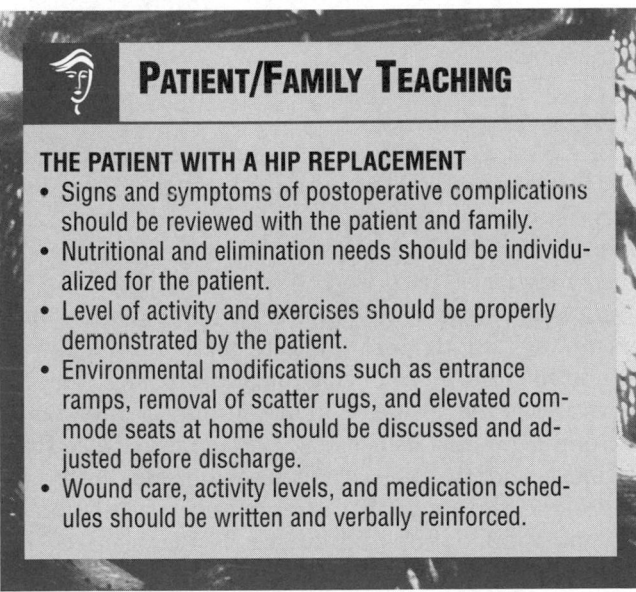

**PATIENT/FAMILY TEACHING**

**THE PATIENT WITH A HIP REPLACEMENT**
- Signs and symptoms of postoperative complications should be reviewed with the patient and family.
- Nutritional and elimination needs should be individualized for the patient.
- Level of activity and exercises should be properly demonstrated by the patient.
- Environmental modifications such as entrance ramps, removal of scatter rugs, and elevated commode seats at home should be discussed and adjusted before discharge.
- Wound care, activity levels, and medication schedules should be written and verbally reinforced.

## COMPLICATIONS

The patient must be observed for phlebitis, urinary retention, infection, and circulation and sensation in the affected leg, as well as any adverse reaction to the cement. Some elevation in temperature is expected, but a fever that persists longer than 3 or 4 days may indicate a problem. A plan of weight bearing and physical ther-

apy is ordered by the physician, and some patients get out of bed the day of surgery. Patients experience an immediate relief of joint pain after surgery and have relatively normal range of motion in the hip.

## TOTAL KNEE REPLACEMENT

Total knee replacements are done for arthritic conditions that involve the knee, and procedures have also been developed to replace shoulder, elbow, and finger joints (Gregory, 1994; Maher et al, 1994). Following knee replacement, continuous passive motion (CPM) may be ordered to exercise the joint. With CPM, the extremity is placed in a motorized splint that continually flexes and extends the knee to an angle predetermined by controls on the machine (Figure 34-7).

## GOUT (GOUTY ARTHRITIS)

Gout is a metabolic disease that results from an accumulation of uric acid in the blood. The disease may be primary and caused by a hereditary metabolic error, or it may be secondary to some other disease process and to certain drugs. The disease usually appears in middle life. It does not occur before puberty in the male or before menopause in the female. The disease almost exclusively attacks men (Wyngaarden et al, 1992). When the disease is primary, it takes approximately 20 years for sufficient urates to accumulate in the body before causing symptoms. However, when gout is the result of a negative response to drugs, its symptoms may develop rapidly over several days. Gouty arthritis can affect any joint in the body, but 20% of all first attacks occur in a joint of the great toe. First attacks may occur in other joints, but the great toe is involved

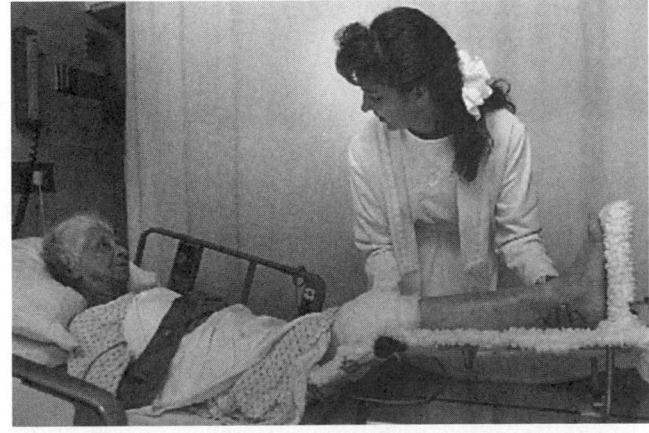

**Figure 34-7**  Continuous passive motion therapy device. (From Elkin MK, Perry AG, Potter PA: *Nursing interventions and clinical skills*, St Louis, 1996, Mosby.)

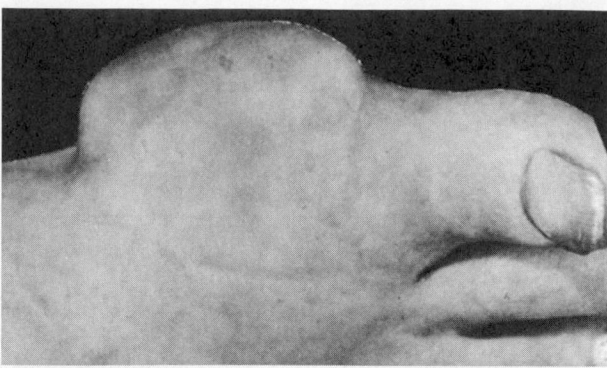

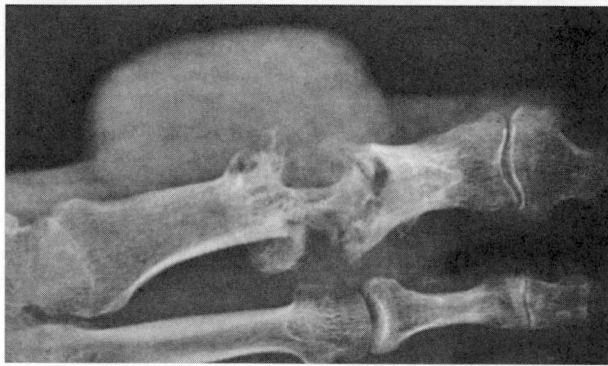

**Figure 34-8** Gout of long duration. Tophaceous mass at base of great toe, as well as destructive bone and joint changes shown in x-ray film, are associated with extensive urate deposits. (From Brashear H, Raney R: *Handbook of orthopaedic surgery*, ed 10, St Louis, 1986, Mosby.)

in 80% of all persons with the disease (Figure 34-8). Typically the onset occurs at night, with excruciating pain, swelling, and inflammation in the affected joint. The pain may be of short duration and return at intervals, or it may be severe and continuous for 5 to 10 days. The patient may never have more than one attack throughout his or her entire life, or attacks may continue at intervals of months and gradually occur closer together.

The diagnosis is made on the basis of finding the blood level of uric acid above normal (normal range is 2.5 to 8 mg/dl) (Smeltzer, Bare, 1992). Several drugs are used in the treatment of the disease. For acute attacks, colchicine is administered orally or may be given intravenously. When administered orally, 5 mg may be given hourly until 12 doses have been given. The drug is discontinued if gastrointestinal symptoms develop. Indomethacin (Indocin) is a potent anti-inflammatory drug that is useful for controlling gout in patients who suffer frequent attacks despite prophylactic dosages of colchicine. Because the high doses that are required tend to cause headache, dizziness, and epigastric pain, dosages should be reduced quickly and discontinued as soon as possible. In some

cases, daily doses prevent acute attacks (Wyngaarden et al, 1992).

One factor in the treatment of gout is the prevention of tophi and gouty arthritis. **Tophi** are deposits of uric acid that may form in various parts of the body, including the kidneys. Uric acid stones may develop here and destroy kidney tissue. Drugs may be given to prevent these disorders from occurring or to relieve them when they are present. Drugs in use include allopurinol (Zyloprim), probenecid (Benemid), and sulfinpyrazone (Anturane) (Wyngaarden et al, 1992). Allopurinol decreases the production of uric acid in the body and must be taken regularly to prevent acute attacks and tophi formation. Probenecid increases the excretion of uric acid by the kidney, thus reducing the amount in the body. It must be taken daily to be effective. Each patient is treated on an individual basis, and the period during which these drugs are to be administered depends on the stage of the disease and the practices of the individual physician. The patient may need to continue receiving drugs over several years. Although no special diet has been found to be effective, foods high in purine such as liver, kidneys, anchovies, sardines, and sweetbreads should be avoided. The diet should be well balanced, and water intake should be high. During an acute attack, the patient should be prescribed a regimen of bed rest, and painful joints should be protected from bedcovers by a bed cradle.

## BURSITIS

The **bursae** are small sacs that are located in the shoulder, elbow, knee, hip, and foot. They contain a small amount of fluid that lubricates areas in which movement may cause friction. The bursae may become inflamed and cause acute bursitis, or inflammation may extend over a long period and result in chronic bursitis and the formation of calcium salt deposits. Bursitis generally is the result of injury, strain, or prolonged use of the bursae, such as in active exercise. It also may occur secondary to infection elsewhere in the body. The subdeltoid region is the most common location of inflammation. Subdeltoid bursitis is characterized by severe pain that may radiate down the arm and into the fingers. Treatment consists of supporting the arm in a sling and administering an analgesic for pain. Hydrocortisone may be injected into the bursae. Several other methods of treatment may be used, including administering a local anesthetic before inserting needles and washing out the calcium deposits. Range-of-motion exercises should be started as soon as possible. In chronic bursitis, pain occurs during use of the affected part, and treatment includes analgesics and physical therapy. Surgical removal of hardened calcium deposits may be necessary.

# KEY CONCEPTS

➤ Arthritis involves inflammation of the joint, which results in pain and restrictive movement of the affective joint.

➤ Rheumatoid arthritis is considered an autoimmune disorder that affects the joints.

➤ Rheumatoid spondylitis is an inflammation of the vertebrae and sacroiliac joints.

➤ Osteoarthritis is the result of wear and tear that has been placed on the joints over the years.

➤ Aspirin or ibuprofen is generally the over-the-counter drug of choice for both pain and inflammation.

➤ Antiinflammatory medication must be taken with caution because they can result in gastric upset.

➤ Exacerbation of rheumatoid arthritis is common and treated with comfort measures.

➤ Osteoarthritis in some degree is seen in people by the time they reach 60 years of age.

➤ A regular exercise program is needed to maintain range of motion.

➤ A total hip replacement is a common procedure performed for arthritic changes of the head of the femur and acetabulum.

➤ Precautions to prevent prosthesis dislocation need to be followed for a minimum of 6 to 8 weeks after total hip replacement surgery.

➤ After total joint surgery the nurse works closely with the physical therapist, occupational therapist, physician, patient, and the patient's family to develop a plan of care.

➤ Gout is a metabolic disease that results from an accumulation of uric acid in the blood.

➤ The bursae are small sacs that are located in the shoulder, elbow, knee, hip, and foot.

➤ Bursae lubricate areas in which movement can cause friction.

➤ Range-of-motion exercises are essential to preserve joint function.

# CRITICAL THINKING EXERCISES

1. Prepare a list of instructions for a patient who is going home after a total hip arthroplasty.
2. Your 55-year-old patient has a diagnosis of gout. Explain the dietary restrictions he or she will need to follow.
3. Describe the difference between rheumatoid arthritis and osteoarthritis.

## REFERENCES AND ADDITIONAL READINGS

Alder SL et al: Collaboration: the solution to multidisciplinary care planning, *Orthop Nurs* 14(2):21-29, 1995.

Altizer L: Total hip arthroplasty, *Orthop Nurs* 14(4):7-18, 1995.

Felson DT: Osteoarthritis, *Rheum Dis Clin North Am* 16(3): 499-512, 1990.

Gray MA: NSAIDs revisited, *Orthop Nurs* 14(1):52-54, 1995.

Gregory B: *Orthopaedic surgery*, St Louis, 1994, Mosby.

Halverson PB: Extraarticular manifestations of rheumatoid arthritis, *Orthop Nurs* 14(4):47-50, 1995.

Jimenez SA: Molecular biological approaches to the study of heritable osteoarthritis, *J Rheumatol Suppl* 27(19):7-9, 1991.

Lewis SM, Collier IC, Heitkemper MM: *Medical-surgical nursing: assessment and management of clinical problems*, ed 4, St Louis, 1996, Mosby

Maher AB et al: *Orthopaedic nursing*, Philadelphia, 1994, Saunders.

Mankin HJ: Clinical features of osteoarthritis. In Kelley WN et al, editors: *Textbook of rheumatology*, ed 3, Philadelphia, 1989, Saunders.

McCance KL, Huether SE: *Pathophysiology: the biologic basis for disease in adults and children*, St Louis, 1994, Mosby.

Pastorino C: *Advanced clinics in orthopaedics: elder mobility*, Pitman, 1995, AJ Janetti.

Purdy KS et al: You are what you eat: healthy food choices, nutrition, and the child with juvenile rheumatoid arthritis, *Pediatr Nurs* 22(5):391-398, 1996.

Rankin JA: Pathophysiology of the rheumatoid joint, *Orthop Nurs* 14(4):39-46, 1995.

Ross D, editor: *Scope and standards of orthopaedic nursing practice*, Pitman, 1996, AJ Janetti.

Salmond S et al, editors: *Core curriculum for orthopaedic nursing*, ed 3, Pitman, 1996, AJ Janetti.

Smeltzer SC, Bare BG: Brunner and Suddarth's textbook of medical-surgical nursing, ed 7, Philadelphia, 1992. Lippincott.

Spector TD: Rheumatoid arthritis, *Rheum Dis Clin North Am* 16(3):513-538, 1990.

Spencer EH: The ROBODOC clinical trial: a robotic assistant for total hip arthroplasty, *Orthop Nurs* 15(1):9-14, 1996.

Wyngaarden JB et al: Cecil's textbook of medicine, ed 19, Philadelphia, 1992, Saunders.

Yandrich TJ: Preventing infection in total joint replacement surgery, *Orthop Nurs* 14(2):15-19, 1995.

## CHAPTER 35

# Digestive Tract Problems

## CHAPTER OBJECTIVES

1 Describe the pathway of food through the gastrointestinal tract.
2 Discuss the elements of a nursing assessment and physical examination of the gastrointestinal system.
3 Explain the following diagnostic tests, including purpose, procedure, and of the patient: esophagogastroduodenoscopy, colonoscopy, upper gastrointestinal series, lower gastrointestinal series, and gastrointestinal series.
4 Discuss the nursing care of the patient with the following gastrointestinal disorders: diverticulitis, inflammatory bowel disease, intestinal obstruction, and peptic ulcer.
5 Discuss the care of the ostomy patient, including skin care, application of appliances, psychologic aspects, and nutritional management.
6 Describe the nursing care of the patient with a gastric decompression and enteral feeding, including routine care measures, problem solving, and prevention of complications.
7 Discuss the purpose of total parenteral nutrition and the potential side effects of administering it too rapidly.
8 Discuss the management of the patients who have had a surgical procedure for peptic ulcers.
9 Develop a plan of care for the nursing management of a patient with ulcerative colitis and esophageal reflux disease.

## KEY TERMS

| | |
|---|---|
| anastomosis | hiatus hernia |
| colostomy | ileostomy |
| diverticulitis | paralytic ileus |
| dysphagia | peptic ulcer |
| enteric fistula | peristalsis |
| esophagogastroduodenoscopy | total parenteral |
| hernia | nutrition |

## STRUCTURE AND FUNCTION OF THE GASTROINTESTINAL SYSTEM

The gastrointestinal (GI) system, or alimentary tract, is also called the digestive system because its function is the digestion and absorption of food. The system begins in the mouth and terminates at the anus (Figure 35-1). The mouth is also called the *buccal* or *oral cavity.* Three sets of salivary glands secrete through ducts that open into the mouth. The teeth and tongue are considered accessory organs of digestion. The esophagus, which is approximately 10 inches long, leads from the mouth to the stomach. It descends through the thoracic cavity behind the trachea and the heart. A muscle, the *gastroesophageal sphincter,* controls the opening between the esophagus and the stomach. The muscle relaxes to permit the passage of food or fluids, after which it contracts to prevent backward flow.

The stomach is a pouchlike structure located in the right upper quadrant of the abdominal cavity under the liver and the diaphragm. It is divided into three parts: the *fundus,* the upper part nearest the esophagus; the middle section, or *body;* and the *antrum,* which is the lower part. Located between the stomach and

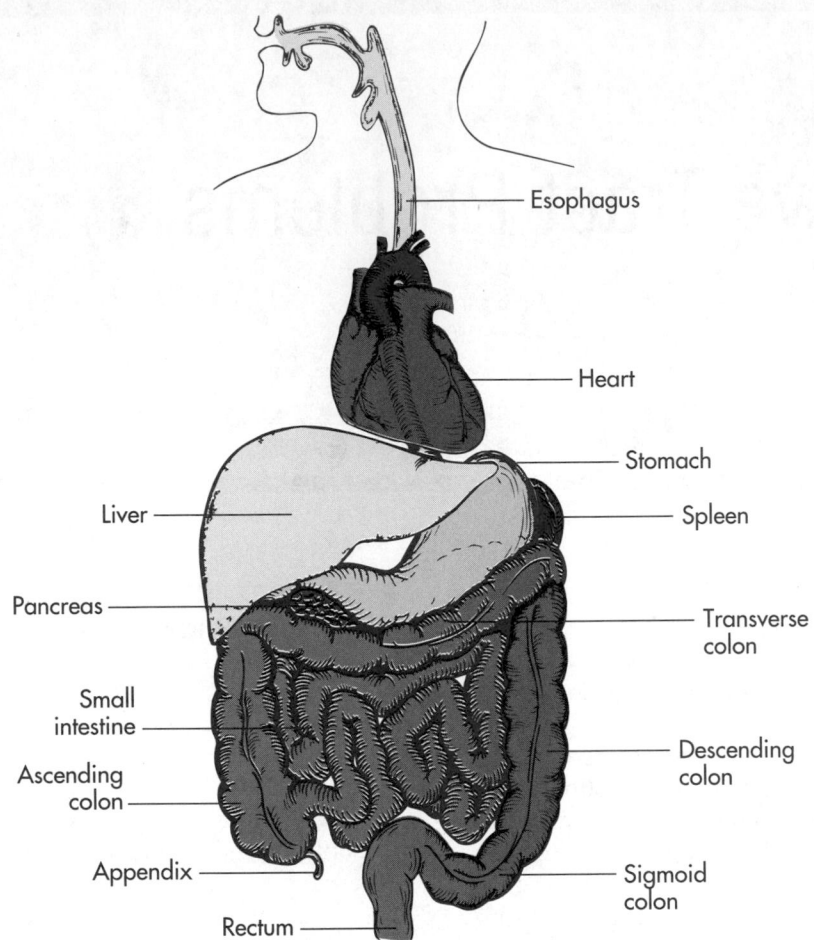

Esophagus

Heart

Liver

Stomach

Spleen

Pancreas

Transverse
colon

Small
intestine

Ascending
colon

Descending
colon

Appendix

Sigmoid
colon

Rectum

**Figure 35-1**    Anatomy of the gastrointestinal system. (From Potter PA, Perry AG: *Basic nursing*, ed 3, St Louis, 1995, Mosby.)

the small intestine is the *pyloric sphincter,* which relaxes to permit passage from the stomach into the small intestine and contracts to prevent the contents of the intestine from returning to the stomach.

The small intestine, which is approximately 20 feet long, is divided into three segments: the *duodenum,* the *jejunum,* and the *ileum.* Most of the digestion and absorption of food takes place in the small intestine.

The large intestine or colon extends from the ileocecal valve to the anus. It is divided into seven segments: the cecum, the *ascending colon,* the *transverse colon,* the *descending colon,* the *sigmoid colon,* the *rectum,* and the *anus.* The large intestine is responsible for the absorption of water and electrolytes and the transport and elimination of waste matter. The *ileocecal valve* is located at the junction between the last section of small intestine (the ileum) and the first section of the large intestine (the cecum). The valve regulates the forward passage of intestinal contents from the ileum into the cecum and prevents the reflux of contents backward into the small intestine. The *vermiform appendix,* a

small, wormlike appendage, is located at the lower end of the cecum. Two sets of sphincter muscles, the internal and external sphincters, are located within the anal canal and control defecation. The alimentary tract is lined with muscles that contract involuntarily to produce the wavelike contractions called **peristalsis.**

The liver, gallbladder, and pancreas are accessory organs of digestion. They assist the process of digestion by contributing specific secretions and enzymes essential for normal digestion and use. The liver, located in the right upper quadrant of the abdomen, under the diaphragm, is the largest of the organs. It has many digestive and metabolic functions. The gallbladder is shaped like a pear and lies under the liver. It stores and concentrates bile and releases it into the duodenum during the process of digestion. The pancreas is a slender organ, fishlike in shape, which is located at the back of the stomach with a portion extending into a C-shaped curve of the duodenum. Located within the pancreas are small masses of cells called *islets of Langerhans,* which secrete insulin.

Because much of the care of the patient depends on which specific parts of the gastrointestinal system are affected, the nurse is encouraged to review in greater detail the structure and function of the system.

## Digestion and Absorption

Digestion is the process by which food is prepared so that it may be absorbed and used by the body. Absorption is the process by which nutrients pass into the circulation so that they may be carried to the body tissues. Digestion is accomplished by two processes: mechanical digestion and chemical digestion.

During mechanical digestion, which begins in the mouth, food is cut and ground into small pieces (mastication). The passage of food from the mouth to the stomach is aided by lubricating mucus from the salivary glands and the mucus-secreting glands along the esophagus. Food entering the stomach from the esophagus passes through the gastroesophageal sphincter. The muscle relaxes to allow food to enter the stomach, then contracts to prevent its backward flow. Passage of the semi-liquid contents of the stomach (*chyme*) into the small intestine at the duodenum is controlled by the contraction and relaxation of the pyloric sphincter. Food is moved along the entire intestine by wavelike muscular contractions called *peristalsis.* Mechanical digestion is best described as a cutting, grinding, and churning process. As this action goes on, numerous enzymes are secreted that chemically act on the various food constituents.

Chemical digestion is the action of enzymes on proteins, carbohydrates, and fats, breaking them into simple compounds in preparation for absorption. Ptyalin is secreted in the mouth and acts on starches; however, this action is limited and largely stopped by the hydrochloric acid in the stomach. Several hormones are secreted into the blood and transported to the stomach and small intestine to assist with the process of digestion. The major hormones affecting digestion are secretin, gastrin, and cholecystokinin. The breakdown of proteins begins in the stomach. Hydrochloric acid is secreted in the stomach, and the acidity must remain at about pH 2 for enzyme action. There is little chemical digestion of fats in the stomach. The major part of chemical digestion occurs in the small intestine, where all of the food constituents are acted on by various enzymes. Pancreatic enzymes (amylase, lipase, trypsin, and chymotrypsin) secreted into the duodenum aid the digestion of carbohydrates, proteins, and fats. Bile produced in the liver and stored in the gallbladder is also released into the duodenum and is required to digest fats and fat-soluble vitamins. Other vitamins, minerals, and water that are present require no enzyme action.

When chemical action is complete, absorption begins. Carbohydrates and proteins enter the circulation through the portal system, whereas fats enter the lymph vessels and eventually reach the portal system near the thoracic duct. There are no digestive enzymes in the large intestine. After the residue from the small intestine passes through the ileocecal valve and enters the large intestine (colon), water and some electrolytes such as sodium and chloride are absorbed into the blood. Bacteria in the colon putrefy undigested foods, synthesize vitamin K and vitamins $B_1$, $B_2$, and $B_{12}$ and produce gas that assists in propelling the feces toward the anus. The urge to defecate is a reflex stimulated by distention of the rectum. Voluntary relaxation of the rectal sphincter assists defecation. It takes 24 to 40 hours for feces to pass through the large intestine. The liver plays an important role in the metabolism of carbohydrates, fats, and proteins. It assists in the regulation of blood glucose by converting carbohydrates to glycogen, storing glycogen, and then converting it to glucose as needed. When glycogen stores are low, the liver can also make glucose from proteins (amino acids) and fats. It synthesizes and catabolizes fatty acids and neutral fats to form ketone bodies and active acetate (sources of cell energy). Its role in protein metabolism includes synthesis of amino acids and supply of plasma proteins for tissue repair. It synthesizes the proteins, prothrombin, and fibrinogen necessary for blood coagulation. The liver stores vitamins, including vitamin K and the other fat-soluble vitamins, and is the primary site of vitamin $B_{12}$ storage.

There are many factors that affect the processes of digestion and absorption. Elderly persons who have lost their teeth and have no dentures or have poorly fitting ones will have problems with mastication. Thus the mechanical process of cutting and grinding will be compromised. The patient who must remain in a recumbent position may have difficulty in swallowing because food does not pass down the esophagus as easily as for a person in a sitting position. Emotions

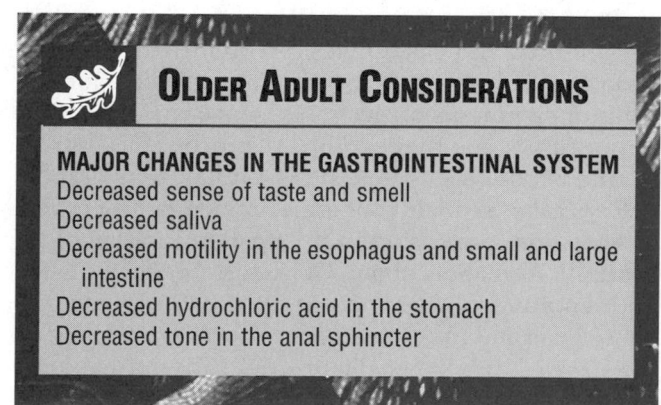

### OLDER ADULT CONSIDERATIONS

**MAJOR CHANGES IN THE GASTROINTESTINAL SYSTEM**
Decreased sense of taste and smell
Decreased saliva
Decreased motility in the esophagus and small and large intestine
Decreased hydrochloric acid in the stomach
Decreased tone in the anal sphincter

affect the secretion of enzymes or may cause severe and painful contractions of the sphincter muscles. Pathologic disease may affect any part of the system; some may be treated medically, whereas others may require surgery. The lack of specific nutrients or sufficient calories may result in malnutrition or starvation.

## ASSESSMENT OF THE GASTROINTESTINAL SYSTEM

### Health History and Physical Assessment

Many conditions can disrupt the normal functioning of the gastrointestinal system. Specific pathologic conditions, traumatic injury, metabolic abnormalities, immunologic alterations, as well as normal age-related changes can interrupt normal function. Medications and other treatment measures often have an effect on the gastrointestinal system as well. For example, some chemotherapy drugs and antibiotics are known to cause nausea, vomiting, and diarrhea. Similar symptoms may occur in several different diseases, and the nurse assists the physician by carefully eliciting, reporting, and recording the patient's complaints and the assessment findings.

The nurse performs a systematic assessment to ensure a thorough examination of the patient. The patient or the family should be questioned regarding the normal pattern for the patient and any significant changes noted in weight, diet and appetite, and bowel elimination. In addition, the nurse asks the patient about the use of laxatives or enemas to regulate bowel movements. The nurse should be conscious of the total patient and concerned with all systems.

The patient's mental state is observed for signs of depression, anxiety, apprehension, and restlessness. The nurse obtains specific information about the *onset*, *duration*, and *severity* of any GI symptoms or complaints. Key symptoms the nurse should ask the patient about include pain, distention, dyspepsia (indigestion), **dysphagia** (difficulty swallowing), nausea, vomiting, diarrhea, constipation, fecal incontinence, and bloody vomitus or stool. Because a serious imbalance of fluid and electrolytes can occur with many GI problems, it is essential for the nurse to assess for any signs or symptoms of electrolyte loss (see Chapter 27). Tissue turgor and the condition of mucous membranes should be assessed to determine the state of hydration.

Physical examination of the abdomen by inspection, auscultation, percussion, and palpation contributes essential information about GI status. When assessing and reporting information about the patient, the nurse should use and make reference to specific anatomic locations on the abdomen (Figure 35-2). The nurse records and reports all abnormal findings to the physician.

> ### NURSE ALERT
> When performing a physical examination of the abdomen, auscultation is done before percussion and palpation so as not to alter the characteristics of bowel sounds.

When assessing abdominal pain, the nurse asks the patient to describe the location and characteristics of the pain. Abdominal pain is usually described as throbbing, aching, stabbing, dull, intermittent, or constant. The nurse observes the abdomen for distention and notes whether the distention is localized to one or more areas of the abdomen or is generalized across the entire abdomen. If the patient complains of nausea, the nurse determines whether the nausea is constant or intermittent and whether the nausea is followed with vomiting. If the nausea is intermittent, does anything precipitate the nausea, like medications, hunger, or eating? If the patient is vomiting, the amount and characteristics of the vomitus are determined. Stools are observed for frequency, color, consistency, presence of mucus, bright red blood, coffee-grounds appearance (indicating old blood), odor, and macroscopic parasites (worms).

### Diagnostic Procedures

Several diagnostic tests and procedures are performed to evaluate GI and biliary function. Some are performed to aid the physician in establishing a diagnosis when symptoms of a disease are present. Tests may be done to rule out the existence of a specific disease, and some may be done as a preventive or screening measure to discover a disease before symptoms occur, when treatment may be most advantageous. There may be some variation in procedures among physicians and hospitals. The nurse must understand the physician's directions, orders, and laboratory or x-ray protocols. This will ensure safe and accurate testing. In addition, the nurse explains to the patient purpose of the procedure and any needed preparation for the procedure.

### Radiologic Examinations

**Abdominal x-ray examination.** The abdominal x-ray examination is noninvasive and is used to assess the size and position of organs, to determine the presence of any masses, and to determine the distribution of intestinal gas, fluids, or calcifications. No patient preparation is needed. Several different x-ray films may be taken to examine the abdomen from various direc-

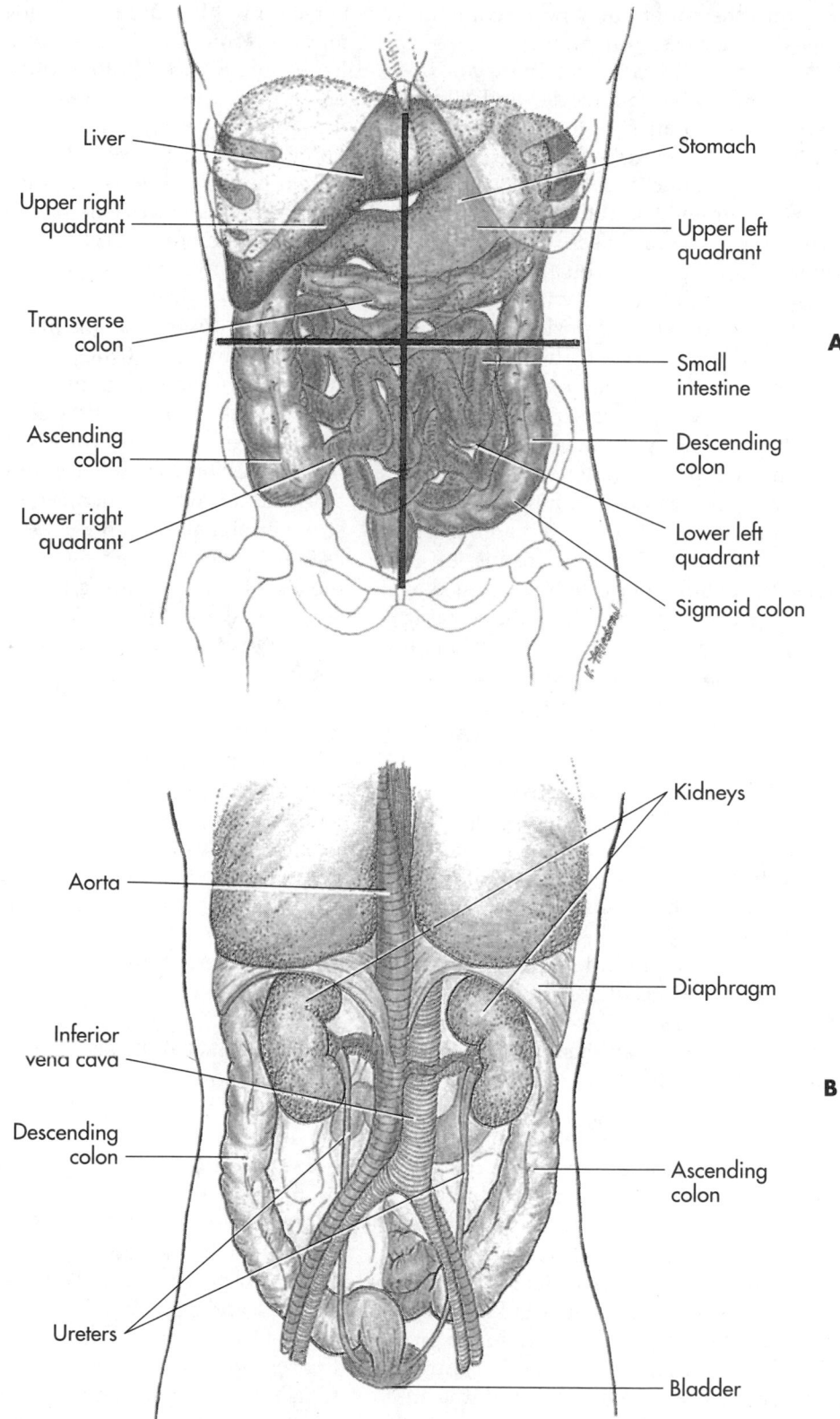

**Figure 35-2    A,** Anatomic areas of the abdomen described in *quadrants*—right and left upper quadrants; right and left lower quadrants. **B,** Posterior view. (From Potter PA, Perry AG: *Basic nursing,* ed 3, St Louis, 1995, Mosby.)

tions. Because of this, the patient may need to assume various positions during the examination.

**Ultrasonography.** Ultrasound examination may be ordered for examination of the gallbladder and biliary system, liver, spleen, and pancreas to determine the presence of abscesses or to evaluate the stage of rectal cancer. High-frequency sound waves are channeled into the region to be examined, and the echoes that result are converted to electric impulses, which are displayed as a pattern of spikes or dots on an oscilloscope screen. The pattern of the dots varies with tissue density and reflects the size, shape, and position of the organ being examined. There is no exposure to radiation. The ultrasound picture resembles an x-ray image, but closer examination will reveal the series of dots or spikes that create the image. When a good view is obtained, photographs are taken for later study.

The patient is instructed to take nothing by mouth before the examination. This reduces the amount of gas in the bowel, which could hinder transmission of ultrasound. When the gallbladder is to be examined as well, the patient is given a fat-free meal the evening before to promote accumulation of bile in the gallbladder. During the procedure the room may be darkened slightly to improve visualization on the oscilloscope. The test will take 15 to 30 minutes for each organ being examined. A water-soluble lubricant is applied to the face of the transducer, and then transverse scans are taken at frequent intervals and at angles appropriate for the organ being examined. After the procedure, the lubricant is washed from the abdomen and the patient may resume his or her usual diet. No other follow-up care is necessary.

The presence of barium within the GI tract will interfere with ultrasound, so the ultrasound should be performed before any barium studies or delayed for at least 48 hours after any barium studies.

**Computed tomography (abdominal).** Computed tomography (CT) involves the passage of multiple x-ray beams through specified portions of the abdomen while detectors record the strength of the x-ray beam as it is deflected off various tissues (tissue attenuation). This information is reconstructed by a computer as a three-dimensional image on an oscilloscope screen. Because attenuation varies with tissue density, CT can distinguish various tissues. The patient is kept NPO (nothing by mouth) for at least 8 hours before the procedure. CT may be done with or without contrast medium. When oral contrast medium is used it is administered approximately 2 to 4 hours before the procedure to accentuate different densities. Defects in the tissue are seen as density variations from normal tissue. Intravenous contrast may be given before the procedure as well. The patient is positioned supine on a radiographic table in the center of the scanner. Trans-

verse x-ray films are taken and recorded on magnetic tape. This information is fed into the computer, and selected images are photographed. The patient must be observed for an allergic reaction (iodine sensitivity) to the contrast medium. CT may be ordered for examination of the biliary tract, liver, and pancreas or to diagnose tumors or abscesses in the abdominal cavity. Barium interferes with visualization of tissues during CT scanning; therefore, CT scanning should be performed before barium studies or delayed for at least 4 days after barium studies.

**Magnetic resonance imaging (abdominal).** Magnetic resonance imaging (MRI) uses radiofrequency and a strong magnetic field to produce images of tissue. Different tissues produce different signals, and these variations are interpreted by the MRI computer to produce the images of various structures. Tissues with large amounts of water, such as blood vessels, produce stronger signals; whereas very dense structures, such as bone, produce weak signals. For this reason, MRI is most useful in evaluating soft tissue and blood vessels. Abdominal MRI is used to assist in evaluating abscesses, fistulas, and sources of GI bleeding. Patients are usually kept NPO for 6 to 8 hours before an abdominal MRI. Because of the strong magnetic field used in the MRI process, it is essential to determine whether the patient has any metallic devices or implants, such as earrings, rings, braces, pacemakers, or shrapnel. Some of these metal devices or implants may be contraindications to the use of MRI. The patient is instructed to remove any metal-containing devices. The nurse must report any metal-containing implants or devices that are not easily removed, such as braces or pacemakers, to the MRI department before beginning the procedure. No postexamination follow-up is required.

**Gastrointestinal series.** The gastrointestinal series (upper or lower) uses a radiopaque contrast material to provide an outline of the GI tract. These tests aid in the identification and diagnosis of abnormal conditions of the GI tract, tumors, ulcerative lesions, and problems with motility.

*Upper gastrointestinal series.* An upper GI series provides visualization of contrast material (usually barium) as it passes through the esophagus and into the stomach and small intestine, if needed. The actual passage of the contrast material can be visualized with a fluoroscope as it moves down the esophagus. X-ray films are taken over time as the stomach and small intestine fill with the contrast material. The contrast material may take up to several hours to pass through the small intestines. The patient is kept NPO for 6 to 8 hours before the examination. After the examination, the nurse monitors the color and consistency of stool to ensure that the barium contrast material is com-

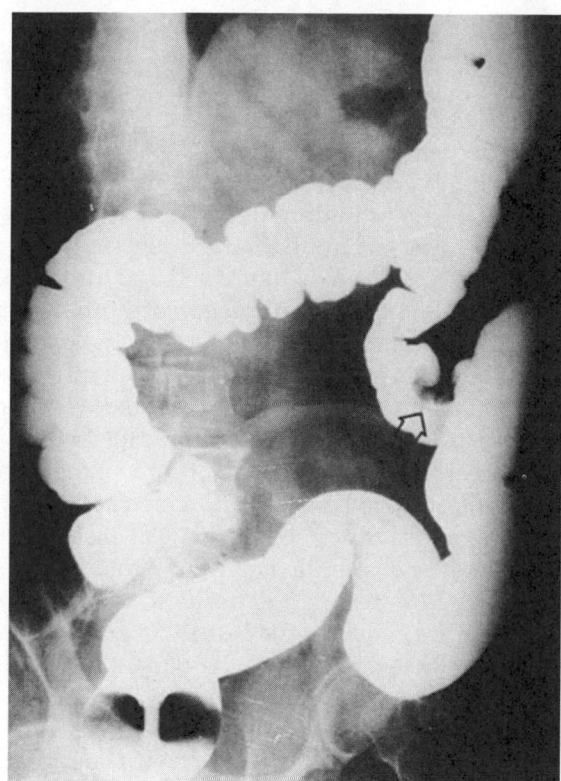

**Figure 35-3** Barium enema. (From Pagana KD, Pagana TJ: *Pocket guide to laboratory and diagnostic tests*, St Louis, 1986, Mosby.)

pletely passed. If the barium is not completely expelled within 2 to 3 days, a stimulant laxative (milk of magnesia, citrate of magnesia) is usually administered. If barium is not cleared from the GI tract, it can form a hard mass and lead to an impaction or an intestinal obstruction.

*Lower gastrointestinal series (barium enema).* When the physician needs to visualize the lower intestinal tract above the sigmoid, an enema containing barium is administered. The radiologist observes the filling of the colon with the fluoroscope, after which x-ray films are taken (Figure 35-3). If both upper and lower GI series are to be done, the patient should have the lower GI series first because it will take several days to completely eliminate the barium from the upper series.

A thorough bowel cleansing is necessary for a quality study of the lower GI tract. The patient is usually given a clear liquid diet for 24 hours before the lower GI series. Laxatives and enemas are administered to clear the colon of stool. After the examination, the nurse monitors for evacuation of the barium contrast and administers laxatives as needed as with the upper GI series.

In some clinical situations, it may be necessary to perform the study of the lower GI tract with a water-soluble contrast material (Gastrografin). For example, the use of barium contrast for a patient with suspected GI perforation is contraindicated because of the risk of peritoneal contamination. The procedure is the same as the barium enema but with a different contrast medium. Patient preparation is similar to that for barium studies, except that bowel cleansing will depend on the patient's diagnosis. Laxatives and enemas are usually avoided in the patient with a suspected bowel perforation. Gastrografin is iodinated, so the nurse determines whether the patient has any known allergies or sensitivity to iodine or other contrast materials. Postprocedure enemas or laxatives are not needed because the medium is not constipating and is easily eliminated.

## Endoscopy

The upper and lower gastrointestinal tract may be examined by means of endoscopy. The endoscope is an instrument containing a cluster of glass fibers that transmit light and return an image to a scope at the head of the instrument (fiberoptics). Pictures can be taken of suggestive lesions by attaching a camera to the head of the scope; a biopsy can be performed through the scope when desired. In addition to its use in diagnosing inflammatory, ulcerative, infectious, and neoplastic diseases of the gastrointestinal tract, it can be used for the removal of a foreign body. The **esophagogastroduodenoscopy** (EGD) allows direct visualization of the mucosal surface and luminal structures of the esophagus (esophagoscopy), the stomach (gastroscopy), or the duodenum (duodenoscopy). For a complete EGD or any portion of this examination, the patient is usually kept NPO for 6 to 12 hours before the procedure. An intravenous line is started or a heparin lock is inserted for intravenous administration of fluids, if needed, and medications. Before the patient is medicated, instruction should be provided on the purpose and procedure, and a procedural consent form must be signed. The patient is given a sedative such as diazepam (Valium) or midazolam (Versed) before the procedure. Atropine may be given to reduce secretions and to act as a vagolytic to protect the patient from profound bradycardia during the insertion and manipulation of the endoscope tube. Vital signs are taken before any medication is given and again before the patient is transferred to the examination room. Before insertion of the flexible tube of the endoscope, the vital signs are taken once more, and the blood pressure cuff is left in place to monitor the patient's blood pressure throughout the procedure.

The patient's throat is sprayed with an anesthetic, and a mouth guard is inserted to protect the teeth and keep the mouth immobile. The nurse maintains the patient on a cardiac monitor throughout the procedure because of the potential for cardiac arrhythmias. In addition, a finger or ear pulse oximeter is used to measure the transcutaneous oxygen levels to assess the patient for respiratory problems, especially during an upper endoscopy.

The patient is positioned on the left side with the head of the bed elevated. The tube is inserted through the mouth and into the esophagus with the head bent forward. The physician may instruct the patient to change the position of the head and chin as the tube is passed through the various parts of the gastrointestinal tract. Additional medication for relaxation is given intravenously if needed. Air is sometimes instilled to flatten tissue folds, and water or normal saline may be instilled to rinse materials from the lens or from a lesion. Suction may be applied to remove fluid and secretions. The patient will experience feelings of pressure as air is inserted. The tube is withdrawn when the physician has completed visualization or biopsy of the organ.

After the test is completed, the patient's vital signs are taken again to assess the condition of the patient at the end of the procedure. If the patient is an outpatient, further observation is performed in the recovery area. The hospitalized patient can be returned to his or her room. Until the patient is fully awake and stable, vital signs are taken frequently, and the patient is observed closely for respiratory problems. Food and fluid are withheld until the gag reflex returns. The gag reflex is assessed by touching the back of the throat with a tongue blade. With this stimulation, the patient will experience a gag if the reflex has returned. In the recovery period, the patient will experience a sore throat and some belching from the instillation of air. More severe pain in the throat, neck, stomach, back, or shoulder is not expected and could indicate perforation; the physician should be notified immediately and the patient's vital signs should be monitored frequently. An elevated temperature is another indication of possible perforation. Patients should be instructed to observe their vomitus or stool for blood and report it immediately to the physician.

Examination of the rectum alone (proctoscopy), the rectum and sigmoid colon (sigmoidoscopy), or the rectum and the entire colon to the ileocecal valve (colonoscopy) are endoscopic procedures performed on the lower GI tract.

**Colonoscopy.** The colonoscope is inserted via the rectum. The large intestine must be thoroughly cleansed to be clearly visible. The patient remains on a clear liquid diet for 24 hours before the examination. In addition, a thorough bowel cleansing with a laxative such as GoLYTELY or Colyte is given the evening before the examination. Two to three hours before the examination, tap water or saline enemas are administered un-

til clear returns occur. Soapsuds enemas are not given because they irritate the mucosa and stimulate mucous secretions that may hinder the examination. A sedative may be given intramuscularly or intravenously to help the patient relax. Vital signs, cardiac rhythm, and oxygen saturation are monitored as outlined for the patient undergoing EGD.

The patient is positioned on the left side, and the colonoscope is generously lubricated and inserted into the rectum. The patient will experience pressure and an urge to defecate. The nurse instructs the patient to breathe deeply and slowly through the mouth to relax the abdominal muscles. Air may be introduced to distend the intestinal wall. Flatus will escape around the instrument when air is instilled, and the patient is instructed not to try to control it. Suction can be used to remove blood or liquid feces. When the instrument is advanced to the descending sigmoid junction, the patient is assisted to the supine position, if necessary, to facilitate advancement of the instrument.

Following the examination, the patient's vital signs are monitored in a manner similar to that for the patient undergoing EGD, and the patient is observed for side effects of the sedatives and for perforation. Malaise, rectal bleeding, abdominal pain and distention, fever, and mucopurulent discharge are reported to the physician immediately. The patient will pass large amounts of flatus and may be embarrassed unless privacy is provided. A normal diet can be resumed after recovery from sedation. Some blood may be present in the stool if a polyp is removed. This procedure is contraindicated in patients who have diseases of the bowel that would predispose them to perforation, such as ischemic bowel disease, acute diverticulitis, peritonitis, and active colitis.

Proctoscopy and sigmoidoscopy are examinations that enable the physician to visualize the lower portion of the gastrointestinal tract. The proctoscope is used to examine the rectum alone, whereas the sigmoidoscope can be inserted further to visualize the lower 10 inches of the gastrointestinal tract. Preparation for both procedures includes the administration of an enema before the examination. Diet and fasting orders will vary with the physician; they should be checked and followed closely.

The procedure is performed with the patient in the knee-chest or lateral position. The patient usually assumes a kneeling position on a special proctoscopy table that "breaks" in the middle so that he or she can bend at the waist. The patient is secured to the table while it is rotated so that the head is lowered and the buttocks are elevated. This position eases the insertion of the instrument. The patient will feel pressure during insertion and advancement of the instrument and when air is instilled to distend the bowel lining. The position and procedure may be embarrassing to the patient. After the examination the patient is observed for signs of perforation as in the postoperative interventions for other endoscopic procedures.

## Miscellaneous Diagnostic Tests

**Gastric analysis and histamine test.** The test for gastric analysis is performed to examine the acidity of the stomach contents. Cells of the stomach secrete hydrochloric acid, which aids digestion. The specific value of acid measured in the stomach is useful in the diagnosis of diseases of the upper GI tract, such as peptic ulcers, carcinoma, and Zollinger-Ellison syndrome. The patient receives nothing by mouth after supper the evening before the test, and in the morning a tube is passed through the nose into the stomach. A large syringe is attached to the tube, and the contents of the stomach are aspirated. Usually several specimens are secured at intervals according to the physician's direction. Each specimen must be carefully labeled with the time it was taken, as well as its numerical order. A clamp is placed on the tube between specimens, and the tube is taped to the patient's face. The physician may order a subcutaneous injection of histamine or betazole (Histalog) to stimulate the flow of gastric secretions. This is known as the histamine test. The gastric secretions are then aspirated at 15-minute intervals for 1 hour or longer. Because some patients are sensitive to histamine and may have a reaction, a tray with a syringe containing a 1:1000 solution of epinephrine should be ready for emergency use.

The procedure is explained to the patient, and the patient is assured that, although the procedure may be uncomfortable, it is not painful. An emesis basin is given to the patient because gagging may produce vomiting during the procedure. The test may be performed in the physician's office or in an outpatient clinic. The procedure may be carried out by the nurse under the physician's direction, or it may be done by a laboratory technician.

**Stool (fecal) analysis.** Stools may be examined for bacteria, parasites, pus, fat, or blood. It should be noted that the process of digestion changes blood that might be coming from the stomach or the intestine so that it will not be observed in the stool on inspection. Chemical examination is then necessary to detect *occult* (hidden) *blood*. In some instances the patient may be given a meat-free diet for 3 days before the test because these substances may cause a false positive reaction, whereas in other situations any random stool may be sent to the laboratory. Stools may also be examined for other substances that may indicate disorders of the biliary tract, pancreas, or some problem of digestion of food.

Stool specimens may be examined for various types of parasitic infections. The specimen is obtained and kept in various ways, depending on the type of parasite sought. Most stool specimens must be taken to the laboratory as soon as they are obtained and must be kept warm.

**Manometry.** Manometry is a method that allows the physician to directly measure pressure within a tubular structure, like the GI tract. To assess GI muscle function, manometric pressure may be obtained in the esophagus, stomach, small intestine, rectum, and anus. A pressure-sensitive probe is inserted into the specific area of the GI tract to be measured, either from above (to measure esophageal, gastric, and small intestinal pressures) or from below (to measure anal and rectal pressure). Pressures may be obtained from a single area or from multiple, contiguous areas (mapping).

The patient having esophageal, gastric, or small intestinal manometry needs to be kept NPO for 8 to 12 hours before the procedure. Gastric and small intestinal measures may take up to 5 hours to complete. Anal and rectal manometry requires a preprocedure enema to evacuate stool.

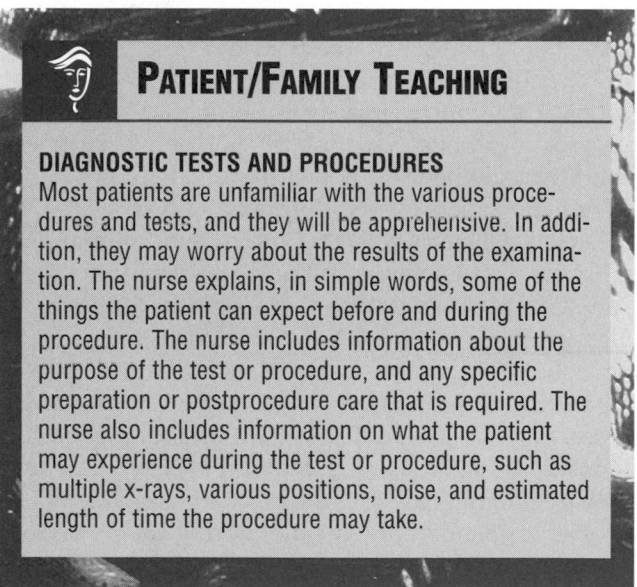

**PATIENT/FAMILY TEACHING**

**DIAGNOSTIC TESTS AND PROCEDURES**
Most patients are unfamiliar with the various procedures and tests, and they will be apprehensive. In addition, they may worry about the results of the examination. The nurse explains, in simple words, some of the things the patient can expect before and during the procedure. The nurse includes information about the purpose of the test or procedure, and any specific preparation or postprocedure care that is required. The nurse also includes information on what the patient may experience during the test or procedure, such as multiple x-rays, various positions, noise, and estimated length of time the procedure may take.

## Nursing Responsibilities for Diagnostic and Laboratory Tests

When the physician writes the order for examinations and tests, the forms must be properly completed and the laboratory or x-ray departments notified without delay. Several tests and procedures require special patient preparation before the procedure, such as diet modification, NPO status, or bowel cleansing. The nurse determines what specific preparation is necessary and initiates patient preparation procedures.

Specimens to be collected by the nurse are obtained promptly, labeled properly, and sent to the laboratory. The patient is prepared and transported to the x-ray department or laboratory at the scheduled time. If for any reason an appointment cannot be kept at the specified time, the department should be notified as early as possible. Medications ordered before and in preparation for tests and studies must be administered promptly and recorded. Any patient receiving intravenous dye is carefully assessed for allergies before the examination and for reactions after the procedure.

Many patients, especially the elderly, are at risk for fluid and electrolyte problems related to special preparations for these tests and procedures. Restricted dietary and fluid intake, as well as repeated bowel cleansing procedures, could result in severe dehydration and electrolyte depletion. The nurse must evaluate the patient for potential problems and discuss with the physician the need for intravenous fluid and electrolyte replacement in high-risk patients.

## Laboratory Studies

Laboratory studies of blood, urine, and stool provide information about gastrointestinal function. Serum electrolytes, hematocrit and hemoglobin, white blood cell count, and serum osmolarity and bicarbonate contribute valuable but nonspecific information about pathologic conditions. Some tests, however, provide more specific information about GI and nutritional status.

**Carcinoembryonic antigen.** Carcinoembryonic antigen (CEA) is a protein seen on the membrane of many tissues. CEA is also seen on some cancerous tissues of the GI system. However, elevated levels of CEA are not diagnostic of GI cancer because the level may be elevated with other cancers as well as noncancerous diseases. For this reason, CEA levels are not a good tool for identifying GI cancers. However, CEA levels are a valuable monitoring tool for evaluating a patient's response to treatment or for monitoring the patient for recurrence of disease.

**Nutritional status.** Dietary intake and GI function affect nutritional status. Selected laboratory tests are used to evaluate nutritional status. Blood levels of *albumin, prealbumin,* and *transferrin* depend on protein intake and the liver's ability to synthesize the specific proteins and are therefore markers of nutritional status. Decreased values reflect either inadequate protein intake or inability of the liver to synthesize proteins. Urine urea nitrogen (UUN) is also used to assess protein balance. The value is determined by subtracting the amount of protein excreted in the urine from the amount of dietary protein. Normal UUN is a positive

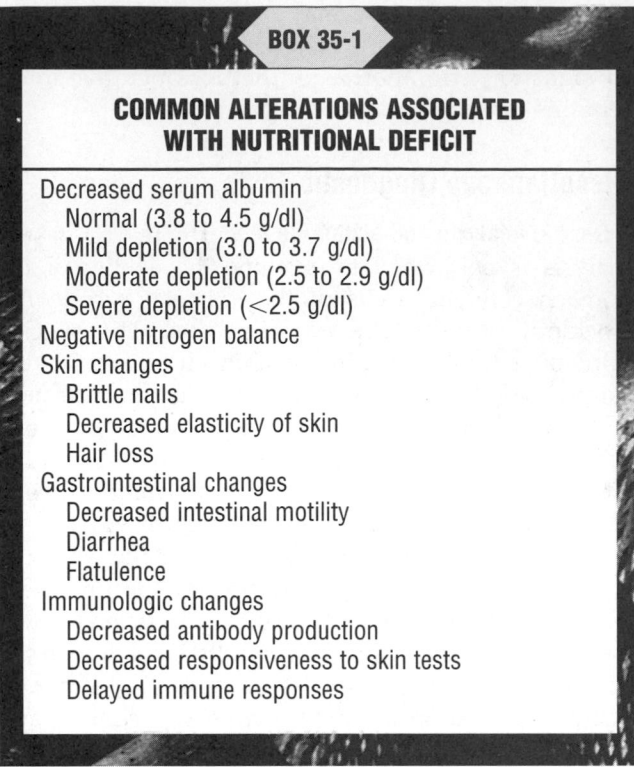

**BOX 35-1**

### COMMON ALTERATIONS ASSOCIATED WITH NUTRITIONAL DEFICIT

Decreased serum albumin
 Normal (3.8 to 4.5 g/dl)
 Mild depletion (3.0 to 3.7 g/dl)
 Moderate depletion (2.5 to 2.9 g/dl)
 Severe depletion (<2.5 g/dl)
Negative nitrogen balance
Skin changes
 Brittle nails
 Decreased elasticity of skin
 Hair loss
Gastrointestinal changes
 Decreased intestinal motility
 Diarrhea
 Flatulence
Immunologic changes
 Decreased antibody production
 Decreased responsiveness to skin tests
 Delayed immune responses

number, indicating that more protein was ingested than excreted (Box 35-1).

# THERAPEUTIC TECHNIQUES FOR THE GASTROINTESTINAL TRACT

## Gastric Lavage

Gastric lavage refers to the washing out of the stomach. Gastric lavage is used to remove large amounts of blood accumulated from upper GI bleeding, to remove ingested poisons, or to neutralize any ingested caustic agents. A large-bore tube is passed through the mouth into the stomach. Approximately 4000 ml of solution (which may be tap water, physiologic saline, 5% solution of sodium bicarbonate, or in case of poison, the specific antidote or activated charcoal) is used. Not more than 500 ml of solution is instilled into the stomach at one time. It is then siphoned back and the procedure is repeated. In the case of poison, the siphoned solution is usually saved for laboratory analysis. Emotional and physical support of the patient is very important during this procedure.

## Gastric Decompression

Gastric decompression is a process to remove air (gas) and fluids from the upper gastrointestinal tract. A nasogastric tube (Levin tube or Salem sump) is most

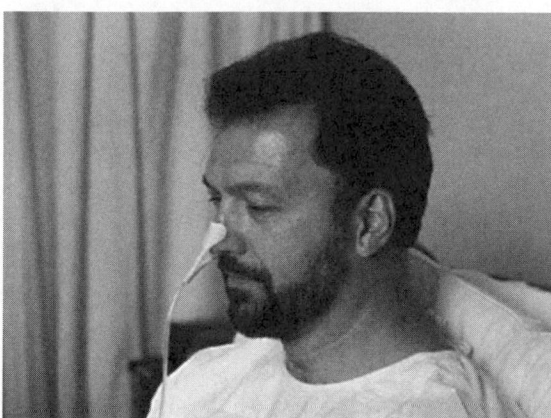

**Figure 35-4** The nasogastric tube is secured with tape to maintain correct placement and prevent damage to the nasal tissues.

commonly used for this purpose. The tube is generously lubricated with a water-soluble jelly and passed through a nostril, down the esophagus, and into the stomach. After the tube is inserted, placement in the stomach must be checked. There is no foolproof method of verifying correct tube placement other than a chest x-ray examination. Common bedside methods used to check for correct tube placement include aspiration of gastric contents, pH testing of contents, and air instillation. To check for tube placement by aspiration, the nurse should attach an irrigating syringe to the drainage port of the tube and attempt to aspirate stomach contents. The aspiration of stomach contents into the syringe suggests correct tube placement. The normal pH of stomach contents is low because of the presence of hydrochloric acid, so, if the result of pH testing of the contents aspirated from the tube is acid (a pH of between 2 and 4), correct placement of the tube in the stomach is assumed. If the nurse is unable to aspirate stomach contents, a small amount of air (10 to 30 ml) can be injected through the tube while auscultating the gastric bulb (upper middle abdomen) for the "rush" of air. After correct placement is confirmed, the tube is taped in place to secure its position. The tube should be taped in such a fashion as to prevent pressure injury to the nostril (Figure 35-4 and Box 35-2). The tube is then attached to either continuous or intermittent low suction (60 to 80 mm Hg).

Gastric decompression is commonly used to prevent or treat a postoperative ileus and to reduce pressure from accumulated fluid on anastomotic suture lines in the patient who has had upper GI surgery. Gastric decompression is also used for patients who have an intestinal obstruction with a large accumulation of secretions.

The length of time the tube is left in place depends on the patient's condition. It is dependent on the re-

---

**BOX 35-2**

**Guidelines of Care for the Patient with Gastrointestinal (Gastric) Decompression**

1  Maintain patency of decompression tube.
2  Irrigate tube as necessary with 30 ml normal saline. Check with physician before irrigating tube in patients with esophageal or gastric surgery.
3  Tape nasogastric tube to nose or cheek; *do not* tape long intestinal decompression tubes; ensure that no pressure is placed on nostril.
4  Administer nothing by mouth unless ordered; physician may permit sips of water, ice chips, or hard candy.
5  Cleanse nostril through which tube is passed at least once every 8 hours; lubricate with water-soluble jelly.
6  Administer mouth care every 2 hours; rinse mouth with water or alcohol-free mouthwash; lubricate lips and oral mucosa with water-soluble jelly or solution.
7  Pin nasogastric tube to gown to prevent displacement with turning; loop intestinal decompression tube on bed to prevent displacement.
8  Attach external end of the tube to low suction unless otherwise ordered.
9  Empty and measure drainage bottle every 8 hours and record.
10 Observe and record color, appearance, odor, pH, and presence of blood, bile, or mucus.
11 Notify physician if tube is not draining despite irrigation.
12 Assess for signs of fluid and electrolyte deficit; evaluate fluid balance (total fluid in minus total fluid out).

---

turn of peristalsis (bowel sounds) and the amount and characteristics of the drainage. As long as the patient has a gastric decompression tube in place, the nurse is responsible for maintaining tube patency, recording the amount and characteristics (color, odor, pH, and heme) of the drainage, and assessing for the presence of bowel sounds.

## Intestinal Decompression

Intestinal decompression may be necessary when an obstruction along the intestinal route is suspected or in the case of paralytic ileus. Several types of long tubes may be used for this purpose, including the Harris tube, Miller-Abbott tube, or Cantor tube. These are long, soft rubber tubes with a balloon at or near the end and openings through which secretions may be drained. The Miller-Abbott tube has two lumens; one opens into the balloon, into which mercury is placed, and the other is attached to suction. The tube is inserted through the nostril and is advanced along the intestine by peristaltic action or by the weight of the mercury. Secretions along the route are removed by low suction. The tube usually remains in the intestinal tract for several days and then is removed gradually (Figure 35-5).

All decompression tubes are generally attached to some type of suction apparatus, and it is important that the equipment used be in working order. The tubing for gastric suction is pinned or clipped to the patient's gown, allowing sufficient slack to permit the patient to turn without displacement of the tube. Care should be taken to prevent the tubing from becoming kinked or obstructed by the patient's lying on it. Patients usually complain of considerable discomfort from the nasogastric tube. The nostrils become dry and crusted from increased mucus secretions. The throat is irritated, and the mouth and lips are dry from mouth breathing. The patient often receives nothing

by mouth but should be allowed to rinse the mouth often with water or a mouthwash that does not contain alcohol. Water-soluble moisturizers, such as K-Y jelly or Mouth Moisturizer, are recommended for use on the lips and within the mouth to promote moisture. Lemon and glycerine swabs should be avoided. The acid in the lemon can cause tissue irritation as well as decalcification of the teeth; in addition, glycerine absorbs water, leading to drying and irritation of the mucous membranes. The nares around the tube are cleansed with cotton-tipped applicators and warm tap water or a water-soluble jelly. Some physicians may allow the patient to occasionally have chipped ice, sips of water, or hard fruit-flavored candy to relieve throat discomfort. The chewing of gum results in some swallowing of air; so it is generally discouraged.

Drainage tubes may become blocked with blood or mucus, which can obstruct the flow. The physician often orders irrigation of the tube with sterile physiologic saline solution every 2 hours or as necessary to keep it patent and draining. Not more than 30 ml of solution should be injected (gently) through the tube at one time. Careful aspiration of the solution may be necessary to ensure patency of the tube, but any vigorous effort to aspirate the tube should be avoided. Irrigating solution is *not to be aspirated from long intestinal decompression tubes.* If the suction apparatus is working properly and the tube is patent, the solution will return. Accurate records of irrigation solution used must be maintained, and the amount must be deducted from the total gastric drainage. The secretions in the drainage bottle are measured at least every 8 hours and recorded. The appearance, odor, and presence of blood, bile, or mucus are noted. If the nurse observes that the tube is failing to drain despite efforts to irrigate it, the physician is immediately notified.

When intestinal decompression tubes are used, they should *not* be taped to the nose because they are designed to move through the intestine by gravity and peristaltic action. Caution must be used in irrigating these tubes to ensure that the solution is injected into the opening that is attached to suction. The other opening leads into the balloon containing air or mercury and it is kept clamped shut. To avoid error, both outlets should be labeled. Measurement and observation of drainage are the same as for the gastric tube.

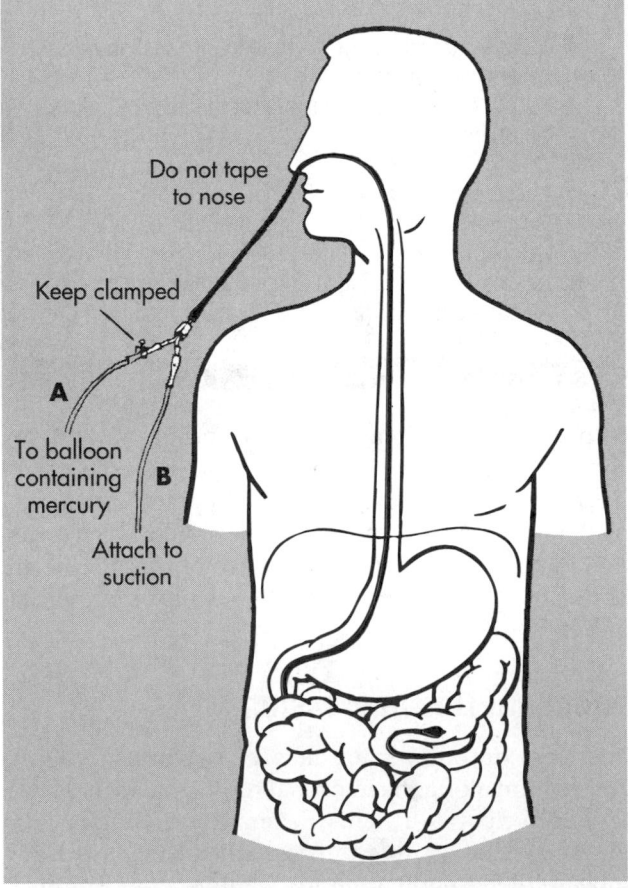

**Figure 35-5**   Intestinal decompression tube in place. Note that the tube is not taped to the nose. **A,** The arm of the Y tube leading to the balloon containing mercury or air must be kept clamped. **B,** The other arm of the Y tube is attached to rubber tubing leading to suction.

## Enteral Feeding

Enteral feeding is used to provide nourishment to patients who are unable to meet their nutritional needs with an oral diet. *Enteral* refers to any location within the GI tract, usually via the stomach, the duodenum, or the jejunum. Enteral feeding is the preferred alternative to normal eating for providing nutrition when the GI tract is able to tolerate and absorb an adequate amount of nutrients. *If the gut works, use it.* Enteral feeding may be administered as the sole source of nutrition or as a supplement to oral or intravenous nutrition. A tube for feeding may be inserted into the stomach or duodenum either through the nose (nasogastric, nasoduodenal) or directly into the stomach or duodenum (gastrostomy, duodenostomy). If the patient is to be fed into the jejunum, the tube is placed during surgery. Jejunostomy tube feeding is usually reserved for patients who have had extensive surgical resection of the upper GI tract, such as total gastrectomy or Whipple procedure. It allows the patient to receive nutrition via the GI tract while bypassing the surgical area.

A small-bore, flexible tube is preferred for nasoenteral feeding to minimize the discomfort and complications associated with the large-bore, hard tubes used for gastric drainage. The tube is introduced through the nose into the stomach in the same manner as a Levin tube or Salem sump. If the tube is to be placed into the duodenum, a slightly longer and weighted tube is used to help the tube move forward past the pylorus and into the duodenum. Placement of feeding tubes is confirmed by x-ray examination before administering feedings or medications. Tubes are flushed with 20 to 30 ml of water intermittently and after administering any medications to prevent clogging.

Enteral feeding may also be administered via a gastrostomy tube—a tube placed directly into the stomach with an exit site on the surface of the abdomen. *Percutaneous endoscopic gastrostomy* (PEG) is a method of placing a gastrostomy tube through the skin (percutaneous) with internal placement guided and visualized through an endoscope. PEG tubes are usually placed when long-term gastrostomy feeding is anticipated (Figure 35-6).

Displacement of the tube, perforation of the mucosa, and gastric reflux are potential complications of all types of enteral feeding tubes. Displacement of the tube, either inward or outward, is a complication that the nurse assesses. The nurse measures the length of the tube from the skin to the feeding adaptor and compares the length with previous measurements. If the tube migrates inward, it may obstruct the pyloric outlet, causing nausea and vomiting. Perforation of the gastric mucosa by the tube allows gastric contents to leak into the peritoneal cavity, causing peritonitis, with signs of temperature, abdominal pain, and rigidity. Reflux of gastric contents and enteral feeding material onto the skin causes chemical irritation to the skin. The nurse keeps the tube site clean and dry. The site is cleansed with mild soap and water, and initially a dry dressing is applied. After complete healing, a cover dressing is no longer necessary. If gastric contents leak onto the skin, the nurse applies a protective barrier ointment or wafer to protect the skin around the insertion site.

Liquid feedings or medications are introduced through the tube and may flow by gravity or be controlled by pump. Feedings may be administered continuously at a set rate or intermittently at a prescribed volume (bolus). Fewer complications are associated with continuous tube feeding. The patient is positioned with the head of the bed elevated at least

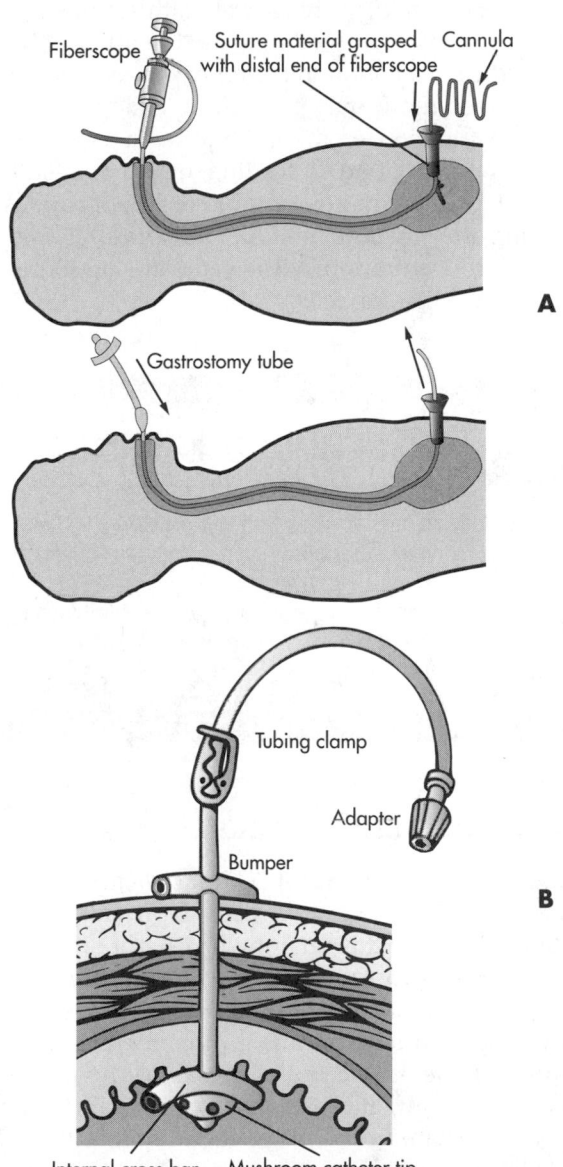

**Figure 35-6** Percutaneous endoscopic gastrostomy. **A,** Gastrostomy tube placement via percutaneous endoscopy. Using endoscopy, a gastrostomy tube is inserted through the esophagus into the stomach and then pulled through a stab wound made in the abdominal wall. **B,** A retention disk and bumper secure the tube. (Modified from Lewis SM, Collier IC, Heitkemper MM: *Medical-surgical nursing: assessment and management of clinical problems*, ed 4, St Louis, 1996, Mosby.)

30 degrees, if not contraindicated, or in the side-lying position to prevent aspiration. Signs of pain, gastric or abdominal distention, or vomiting are reported to the physician. Routine assessment of appropriate tube placement is completed by the nurse. For intermittent feedings, correct tube placement is checked by aspiration of intestinal contents or air instillation before each feeding. With continuous feedings, the nurse checks for correct tube placement at least once each shift. The nurse observes the patient for any changes in respiratory rate, breathing pattern, or breath sounds to assess for aspiration of the feedings into the lungs.

Diarrhea is a common complication associated with enteral feeding. It may occur from changes in the absorptive function of the GI tract as a result of prolonged periods of no GI feeding, or it may result from the high osmotic nature of tube feeding formulas. Decreasing the rate and volume and diluting the tube-feeding concentration with water are measures that may reduce the diarrhea.

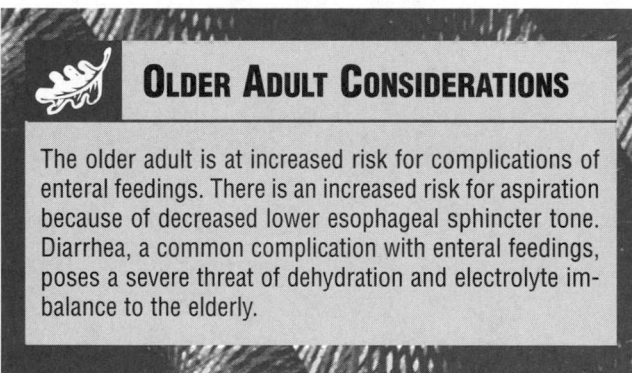

## OLDER ADULT CONSIDERATIONS

The older adult is at increased risk for complications of enteral feedings. There is an increased risk for aspiration because of decreased lower esophageal sphincter tone. Diarrhea, a common complication with enteral feedings, poses a severe threat of dehydration and electrolyte imbalance to the elderly.

## Total Parenteral Nutrition

**Total parenteral nutrition** (TPN), or *hyperalimentation,* is an intravenous technique used to provide for the nutritional needs of the patient who cannot or should not digest or absorb nutrients via the GI tract. The patient's nutritional deficits are carefully determined, and an appropriate formula is prepared for nutritional support. Patients selected for this procedure are generally poorly nourished as a result of surgery, trauma, or disease and are unable to adequately meet their own nutritional needs. Patients with gastrointestinal disorders often fall into this category because of an interruption of the normal digestion and absorption processes of the system.

TPN is administered as a concentrated solution of at least 10% dextrose in water, proteins, and electrolytes and trace elements. Emulsified fats may also be added to the formula. Because these solutions are so concentrated, a large vessel must be used so that the amount of plasma in the vessel can sufficiently dilute the solution to prevent complications. The infusion rate is kept constant for proper dilution to occur, as well as for the prevention of complications that could arise from sporadic infusion of such a concentrated solution so high in glucose. Nausea and headache are often early signs of too rapid administration. Later symptoms may include severe dehydration and seizures (Box 35-3).

### NURSE ALERT

Total parenteral nutrition should be administered using an intravenous pump to keep the rate of administration constant. The rate should not be sped up to catch up if the infusion falls behind schedule. Speeding up the rate may cause a dangerous increase in blood glucose.

# GASTROINTESTINAL MANIFESTATIONS OF ILLNESS

## Anorexia

Anorexia, or lack of appetite, is a nonspecific symptom that is associated with a variety of illnesses and diseases. Anorexia may appear in conjunction with other nonspecific GI symptoms such as nausea, diarrhea, or pain, or it may be an isolated presenting symptom. Multiple factors may cause anorexia. Emotional stress and psychologic disorders are often associated with lack of appetite. Anorexia may be a symptom of some specific GI problems, such as intestinal obstruction, and may also be associated with problems related to other illnesses and disease, such as chronic renal disease and heart disease. Prolonged anorexia can lead to severe nutritional deficits unless treatment is instituted.

## Nausea and Vomiting

*Nausea* is a subjective feeling of the need to vomit. Like anorexia, nausea may appear with other GI symptoms and may be caused by a variety of factors. Nausea may be a symptom associated with GI problems or may be associated with other systemic problems. The association of nausea with other symptoms, like vomiting, pain, anorexia, and abdominal distention, may be helpful in diagnosing the specific problem.

*Vomiting* is the forceful expulsion of gastric or duodenal contents through the mouth. Vomiting is a reflex that can be stimulated in a variety of ways. The vom-

| BOX 35-3 | NURSING PROCESS |
|---|---|

## TOTAL PARENTERAL NUTRITION

### ASSESSMENT

- Weight loss
- Fluid and/or electrolyte deficit
- Inadequate nutritional intake
- Abnormal laboratory values for albumin and prealbumin

### NURSING DIAGNOSIS

Altered nutrition: less than body requirements related to inability to ingest or digest food or to absorb nutrients

### NURSING INTERVENTIONS

- Monitor intake and output.
- Monitor vital signs.
- Measure blood glucose (fingerstick) every 6 hours.
- Maintain constant intravenous flow rate.
- Monitor insertion site and report any evidence of redness, swelling, oozing, or tenderness.
- Be familiar with additives to total parenteral nutrition (TPN) (especially insulin).
- Use sterile technique when caring for central line and TPN supplies.
- Maintain sterile occlusive TPN dressing.
- Change TPN solution and tubing at least every 24 hours.
- Change intravenous dressing per protocol.
- If infusion is interrupted, infuse 10% dextrose in water until TPN is restarted.
- When discontinuing TPN therapy, taper rate over 2 to 4 hours.
- Keep TPN solution refrigerated until needed.
- Never use TPN line for administering medications, drawing blood, or taking CVP readings.
- Use filter and infusion device per policy.
- Weigh patients at regular intervals.
- Monitor serum electrolytes and albumin and prealbumin levels.

### EVALUATION OF EXPECTED OUTCOMES

- Cessation of weight loss or weight gain
- Maintenance of fluid and electrolyte balance
- Normal blood glucose levels
- Absence of infection through the intravenous line or at venipuncture site

iting center lies in the cerebral medulla; stimulation of this center induces the vomiting reflex. Vomiting may be induced by direct stimulation of the cerebral vomiting center; by increased stimulation of the semicircular canals, as in motion sickness; or by stimulation of certain nerve fibers located in the pharynx, the stomach, the intestine, the kidneys, the heart, or the uterus. Vomiting is usually preceded by a wave of nausea. *Projectile vomiting* is spontaneous vomiting that is not preceded by nausea. Projectile vomiting is associated with cerebral tumors and cerebral aneurysms and with increased intracranial pressure.

## Assessment

The nurse assesses the patient for potential causes of nausea or vomiting, including stress, foods, medications, and disease. Associated symptoms such as pain, abdominal distention, constipation, or diarrhea must also be considered. The nurse measures the amount of vomitus and carefully inspects the contents for the presence or absence of undigested food particles, bile, and blood. The presence of blood in the vomitus is an indication that the patient is bleeding from some source in the upper GI tract. The blood may be bright red, which is usually indicative of recent or rapid bleeding, or it may appear as coffee grounds, with a dark red or black appearance, which is indicative of blood mixing with gastric secretions.

Any specific odor of the vomitus is also noted; fecal odor of the vomitus is associated with a longstanding intestinal obstruction. Prolonged vomiting predisposes the patient to dehydration, electrolyte and acid-base imbalances, weakness, and nutritional deficiency, so the nurse must monitor closely for these complications.

## Interventions

Nursing interventions for the patient with nausea and vomiting are aimed at preventing aspiration, maintaining fluid and electrolyte balance, and providing symptomatic relief. If the patient is able, the nurse places the patient in a sitting or in a side-lying position with the head slightly flexed forward to prevent aspiration during vomiting. Deep breathing and swallowing often can suppress the urge to vomit. Warm fluids such as weak tea or carbonated beverages may be given in sips if tolerated by the patient. Dry crackers or toast may be added if liquids are tolerated. Fried or spicy foods are to be avoided until all symptoms have resolved. If oral intake of bland fluids continues to produce vomiting, intake is withheld for a period and then reintroduced slowly. Intravenous fluid replacement may be necessary to maintain adequate fluid and electrolyte balance during prolonged vomiting. In some cases the patient is given nothing by mouth, and a nasogastric tube is placed to remove gastric contents to prevent further vomiting.

*Antiemetic agents* are used to relieve the symptoms of prolonged, severe nausea and vomiting (Box 35-4). Antiemetics may be administered orally, intramuscularly, intravenously, or rectally. The nurse monitors the patient for the effectiveness of the antiemetic agent. If the agent does not relieve the symptoms, the nurse notifies the physician. Additional nursing measures in caring for the patient with nausea and vomiting include keeping an emesis basin within easy reach and emptying the basin quickly after patient use. If clothing or linens are soiled by vomitus, clean replacements are provided immediately. Providing mouth care after vomiting and applying a cool cloth to the forehead or back of the neck may increase patient comfort.

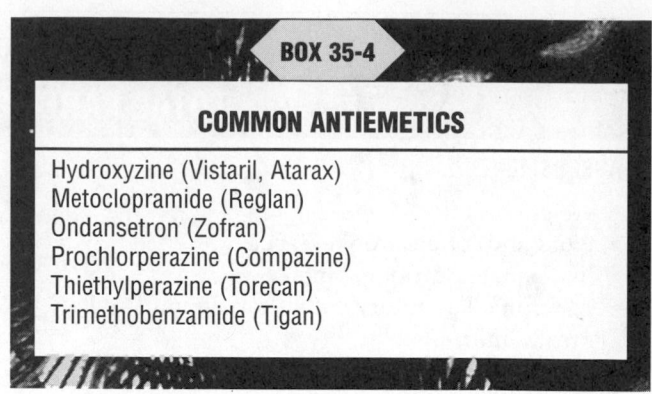

**BOX 35-4**

**COMMON ANTIEMETICS**

Hydroxyzine (Vistaril, Atarax)
Metoclopramide (Reglan)
Ondansetron (Zofran)
Prochlorperazine (Compazine)
Thiethylperazine (Torecan)
Trimethobenzamide (Tigan)

flammation of the mucosal (innermost) layer of the GI tract or from infections with toxin-producing organisms. Secretory diarrhea is usually high in volume (greater than 1 L/day) and high in sodium content.

*Osmotic diarrhea* is characterized by poor water reabsorption from the GI tract and occurs as a result of an increased amount of water being "pulled" into the GI lumen by hyperosmolar contents. This type of diarrhea may be caused by certain drugs, such as cathartics, sorbitol, lactulose, antacids, and some antibiotics, as well as certain surgical procedures or disease processes that increase the speed at which contents pass through the GI tract, reducing the time for water and electrolyte reabsorption. Osmotic diarrhea contains high levels of potassium.

*Mixed diarrhea* is associated with increased intestinal motility and a combination of secretory and osmotic factors. Increased motility decreases the time allowed for adequate water and electrolyte reabsorption by the intestine. It is believed that this increased motility stimulates factors that increase secretion and malabsorption of intestinal fluids.

The consequences of diarrhea depend on both the cause and the severity. Severe dehydration and electrolyte imbalance can result from prolonged loss of GI secretions through diarrhea. Major patient care considerations include fluid and electrolyte imbalance and perianal skin irritation.

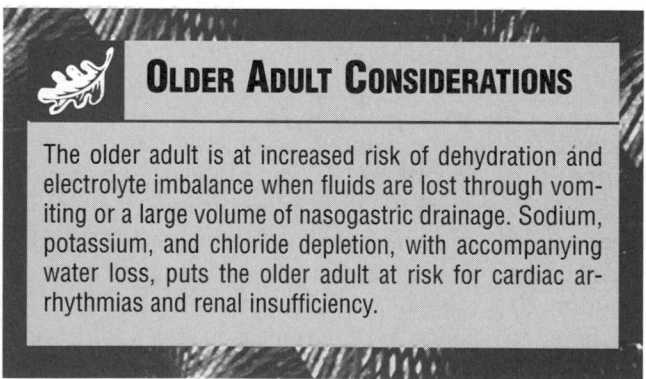

**OLDER ADULT CONSIDERATIONS**

The older adult is at increased risk of dehydration and electrolyte imbalance when fluids are lost through vomiting or a large volume of nasogastric drainage. Sodium, potassium, and chloride depletion, with accompanying water loss, puts the older adult at risk for cardiac arrhythmias and renal insufficiency.

## Diarrhea

*Diarrhea* is the passage of stool that is characterized by increased frequency and increased water content. The causes of diarrhea vary but are usually classified by how excessive water content gets into the GI tract: *secretory, osmotic,* or *mixed.* Water is either "pushed" into the lumen of the GI tract by secretion or it is "pulled" into the lumen by osmosis. Diarrhea is often a result of a combination of both secretory and osmotic factors. *Secretory diarrhea* is due to an abnormal increase in the production ("push") of intestinal secretions (water and electrolytes), which usually occurs as a result of in-

## Assessment

The nurse monitors the color, odor, volume, and consistency of diarrhea stool and inspects the stool for the presence of blood, mucus, or undigested food. In addition, the nurse assesses for any associative factors that relate to the occurrence of diarrhea. How often are the diarrhea stools occurring? How long has the diarrhea persisted? Are the episodes of diarrhea related to eating? What specific foods have been ingested? Has the patient recently traveled outside the country? What medications, especially new medications, is the

patient taking? Are any other symptoms associated with the diarrhea? Pain? Abdominal cramps? Nausea? Vomiting? Abdominal distention?

Stool samples may be obtained and sent for analysis to assist with determining the nature and cause of the diarrhea. Laboratory analysis of stool samples can determine the presence of bacterial toxins, ova and parasites, blood, fat, electrolytes and osmolarity, and white blood cells (WBCs). Upper and lower endoscopy or a barium enema may also be used to assist with the diagnosis.

General physical assessment parameters, including blood pressure, heart rate, and temperature, as well as assessment of hydration status and intake and output should be monitored. Serum WBC count may also be evaluated to assess for infectious causes; serum electrolytes are evaluated to assess the need for replacement therapy.

## Interventions

Care of the patient with diarrhea is directed at eliminating or controlling the cause, controlling symptoms, preventing complications, and providing for patient comfort. Specific foods or medications that are poorly absorbed or precipitate inflammation are discontinued if possible. Antibiotics are administered for infectious causes of diarrhea. Antiinflammatory agents are used in the treatment of diarrhea caused by inflammatory bowel disease. Antidiarrheal agents are used to control the frequency of diarrhea episodes by decreasing peristalsis; bulk-forming agents are used to reduce the water content of the diarrhea stool. Fluid and electrolyte maintenance or replacement therapy is administered as needed.

Careful cleansing and protection of the perianal skin area is essential to prevent skin breakdown caused by frequent soiling and the caustic nature of the diarrhea stool. Gentle washing with tap water, mineral oil, or special products available for perineal skin cleansing is used to remove stool from the skin surface. Topical application of skin sealants or moisture barriers can provide further protection. Agents with vitamin A, D, or E can also be applied to prevent or treat perianal skin breakdown. If severe diarrhea persists, the nurse may choose to apply a perianal pouch to provide for skin protection and to contain the stool. The use of rectal tubes to collect fecal drainage is discouraged because of the potential for injury to the rectal mucosa and anal sphincter. If possible the use of diapers in the adult patient should be avoided, because of the increased risk of skin irritation and demeaning and humiliating psychologic effect.

To provide patient comfort measures, the nurse ensures easy access to the bathroom or places a bedpan within easy reach. Room deodorizers are used to control odors. Soiled linen and clothing are changed immediately.

> **NURSE ALERT**
>
> Agents that control diarrhea by affecting peristalsis, such as codeine, diphenoxylate, or loperamide, should not be given to patients who have diarrhea from any type of infectious agent, ulcerative colitis, or pseudomembranous colitis because of the risks of toxic complications. In addition, always check with the physician before administering antidiarrheal agents to patients with acute abdominal pain, gastrointestinal bleeding, intestinal obstruction, or abdominal inflammation.

# FUNCTIONAL DISORDERS OF THE GASTROINTESTINAL TRACT

## Constipation

*Constipation* is best defined as the decrease in the frequency of bowel movements from what is normal for the patient. In addition, the patient will complain of difficulty passing stool; hard, dry stool; and a decrease in the amount of stool passed. Stool may be retained in the rectum but not passed. There is a wide variation in what is considered a normal stooling pattern, from as often as two or three times a day to once every two or three days. The existence and severity of constipation must be evaluated in terms of the patient's normal pattern.

Most commonly, constipation results from decreased dietary fiber (fruits, vegetables, whole grains, bran), inadequate fluid intake, and decreased physical activity and exercise. Dietary fiber adds bulk and volume to stool, which promotes good peristalsis and propulsion of intestinal contents toward the rectum. Adequate fluid intake prevents the stool from becoming excessively dry and hard as it passes through the GI tract. Physical activity and exercise promote GI motility.

There are several other factors that contribute to developing constipation, including medications, environmental changes, disease states, and psychologic factors. Some common medications known to contribute to constipation are iron supplements, anticholinergic agents, antidepressants and antipsychotic drugs, and antacids containing calcium and aluminum. Continued abuse of laxatives may cause the colon to become chronically dilated and atonic, leading to constipation.

Changes in day-to-day routines, including diet changes or changes in meal schedules, may lead to temporary changes in bowel habits and constipation. Constipation is also associated with several other disease states, usually because of the disease effect on intestinal motility. Hirshsprung's disease, spinal cord tumors or injuries, multiple sclerosis, and diabetes are some disease states that predispose the patient to constipation. Psychologic stress and depression may also cause constipation.

Ignoring the urge to defecate causes fecal matter to become dry as it sits in the rectum because the water content is absorbed. Dry, hard stool is more difficult to pass out of the rectum and can lead to constipation. Repeatedly ignoring the urge to defecate may lead to desensitizing the rectal muscles and mucosa to the presence of stool in the rectum, compounding the problem.

It must be kept in mind that constipation is a symptom of many organic diseases. During an acute illness constipation may occur because of reduced food intake and reduced intestinal motility. This type of constipation is usually relieved as soon as health returns. The patient in the hospital may repress the need to defecate because he or she does not want to use a bedpan. Privacy is essential for the patient. Constipation may occur during the latter part of pregnancy as a result of pressure on the lower bowel, or it may be a complication after delivery in the postpartum period. The patient may be able to relieve the disorder during the antepartum period by drinking more water and eating fresh fruit and vegetables and food containing roughage. Elderly people often suffer from constipation as a result of the slowing down of the digestive process, inadequate diet, and reduced fluid intake.

Complications associated with constipation include hemorrhoids, which develop secondary to venous engorgement caused by repeated straining at stool and venous compression caused by impacted stool, and obstipation, fecal impaction secondary to constipation.

## Assessment

A thorough history and physical examination is performed in order to determine the cause of constipation and to determine the appropriate intervention. The nurse determines the normal stooling pattern for the patient. In addition, the onset, duration, and severity of the constipation episode are elicited: When did the constipation start? Were there previous episodes? How long has this condition persisted? Assessing dietary habits, fluid intake, and activity level will assist in determining contributory factors. The nurse also gathers information about other diseases and health-related conditions the patient may have, such as a history of any colorectal disease, bowel obstruction, diabetes and neurologic and neuromuscular disorders. A list of current prescriptions and over-the-counter medications is also obtained.

The nurse examines the patient for the frequency and characteristics of bowel sounds and the presence of abdominal distention and fecal impaction, and tests a stool sample for occult blood. Abdominal x-rays, endoscopy, and anorectal manometry may be used to determine the cause of constipation.

## Interventions

Treatment must be based on the type of constipation and the patient's individual needs, and the presence of possible organic disease must be ruled out. In most cases medication, dietary, and behavioral interventions are successful in treating the patient with constipation. Laxatives should not be used regularly because chronic overuse may actually become a cause of constipation. Bulk-forming agents are useful in relieving symptoms of constipation (Box 35-5). Enemas act rapidly in relieving constipation and are useful in its immediate treatment but should also be avoided in long-term treatment of constipation.

Diet modifications are the easiest way to relieve constipation. Fresh fruits and vegetables, whole grains,

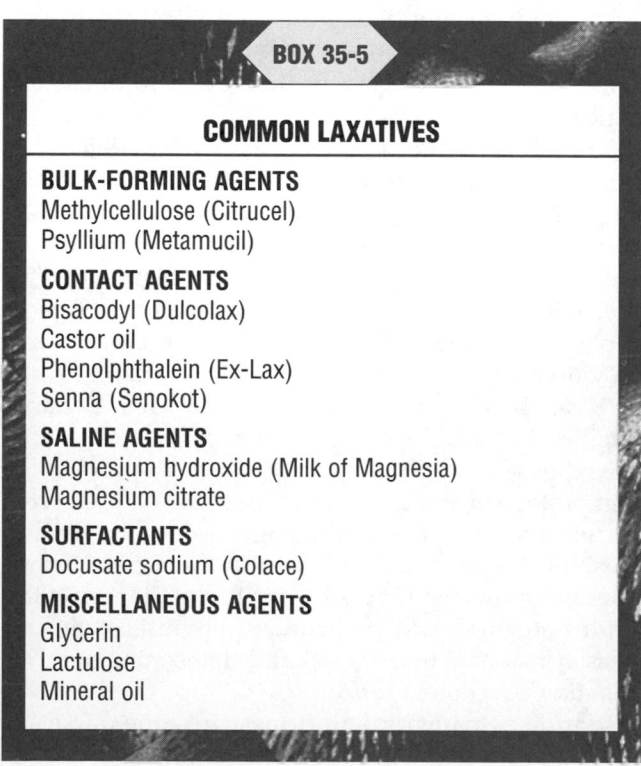

**BOX 35-5**

**COMMON LAXATIVES**

**BULK-FORMING AGENTS**
Methylcellulose (Citrucel)
Psyllium (Metamucil)

**CONTACT AGENTS**
Bisacodyl (Dulcolax)
Castor oil
Phenolphthalein (Ex-Lax)
Senna (Senokot)

**SALINE AGENTS**
Magnesium hydroxide (Milk of Magnesia)
Magnesium citrate

**SURFACTANTS**
Docusate sodium (Colace)

**MISCELLANEOUS AGENTS**
Glycerin
Lactulose
Mineral oil

and bran increase the fiber content of the diet and promote fecal evacuation. Adequate hydration is also important in preventing constipation; 6 to 8 glasses of water per day is appropriate for people with no fluid restrictions.

Patient education about the importance of diet, fluids, and exercise in preventing and treating constipation is a major role for the nurse. In the hospital setting, providing the patient with clean, accessible, and private toileting facilities will aid in the prevention of constipation. If the patient cannot get to a bathroom, the use of a bedside commode or adjusting the patient on a bedpan to a sitting position will help to normalize the process of defecation.

## Fecal Incontinence

Fecal incontinence is best defined as the *involuntary passage of stool.* Normal passage of stool involves adequate sensory and muscular activity in the rectum and anus. Sensory fibers are stimulated as stool enters the rectum. Intentional storage of stool in the rectum until it is convenient to defecate requires integrations of the internal and external anal sphincters. Fecal incontinence may occur as a result of fecal impaction, diarrhea, neurologic injury or disease, injury or surgery to the perirectal area, weakened pelvic floor muscles, or age-related loss of elasticity of the rectum. Fecal incontinence is preventable and curable in most patients. Even elderly, institutionalized patients with fecal incontinence can reduce or eliminate incontinent episodes with proper preventative or therapeutic interventions.

Treatment of fecal incontinence is aimed at treating the cause and preventing complications. Digital rectal examination is used to assess muscular tone in the anus and rectum and to evaluate the patient for fecal impaction. Endoscopy, barium contrast enema, and anal manometry are also used to examine the condition of the colon, rectum, and anus.

### Assessment

A thorough history and physical examination is performed in order to determine the cause of fecal incontinence and to direct appropriate intervention. The nurse determines the stooling pattern for the patient before the onset of incontinence and determines if there is any pattern to the incontinent episodes. When did the fecal incontinence begin? Were there previous episodes? When did this change in pattern first occur? Has the patient had injury or surgery in the rectal area? The nurse also evaluates the patient's mental status and determines the frequency and nature of the incontinent stool.

### Interventions

Nursing interventions for the patient with fecal incontinence are directed at bowel training programs and maintenance of perianal skin integrity. The purpose of bowel training programs is to establish bowel regularity in order to control fecal incontinence and prevent fecal impaction. Bowel training involves toileting at regular intervals, usually after breakfast. Bowel training programs are effective for patients whose fecal incontinence is associated with altered mental status, such as dementia, or those patients who ignore the urge to defecate and whose stool becomes impacted. Bowel regulating programs use cathartics, such as Dulcolax or glycerin suppositories, with or without a gentle enema, to aid in the evacuation of stool from the colon and rectum. Regulating programs are particularly effective in bowel management for patients with neurologic or neuromuscular disorders.

Maintaining perianal skin integrity for the patient with fecal incontinence is a major role of the nurse. Skin barriers applied to a clean, dry perirectal area protect the skin from injury. When the patient passes stool, prompt, gentle cleansing of the area decreases the risk of skin breakdown. The use of diapers for the adult patient with fecal incontinence should be avoided, because it is demeaning and humiliating, and because it does not provide for adequate skin protection. Perianal pouching may be used both to provide perianal skin protection and to provide for fecal containment.

Biofeedback and electrical stimulation are behavioral techniques that are used to train rectal and anal sphincter muscles to control the urge to defecate until proper facilities are available. Surgery is indicated only when all other measures fail to control the problem or when there is atony or altered anatomy in the anal and rectal areas causing incontinence.

## Indigestion

Indigestion may be the result of disease somewhere in the body, but, as a functional disorder, it does not have a pathologic basis. Some hypersensitive persons who are tense and anxious may become aware of normal sensations present in the stomach, usually related to the digestive process. These individuals may interpret such sensations as pain. They complain of pain in the upper abdomen, usually related to the eating of food. They may describe the pain in a variety of ways and often attribute their discomfort to specific foods. Often these individuals resort to the habitual use of sodium bicarbonate or some popularly advertised antacid, which may provide temporary relief. Treatment, however, is based on a thorough assessment, physical examination, and accurate laboratory studies to rule out physical disease.

## Cardiospasm and Pylorospasm

Sphincter muscles are located between the esophagus and the stomach (gastroesophageal sphincter) and between the stomach and its outlet into the duodenum (pyloric valve). Normally, these muscles contract to prevent the backward flow of food material and gastric secretions and relax to allow food to enter the stomach from the esophagus and to permit the passage of food from the stomach into the duodenum. Under certain conditions these muscles fail to relax at the proper time and may contract vigorously. These severe contractions are called *spasms*. They give rise to symptoms of inability to swallow, regurgitation of food, epigastric pain, and vomiting. Spasms of the pyloric sphincter may be associated with peptic ulcer, but emotional factors are believed to be the primary cause of *cardiospasm* and *pylorospasm*. Treatment may include regulation of the diet, administration of antispasmodic and sedative drugs, and psychologic support. If cardiospasm is severe, dilation of the constricted esophagus may be necessary.

## Anal Sphincter Spasm

Sphincter muscles surrounding the anus and rectum relax to permit defecation. When the individual has severe hemorrhoids or fissures (cracks) in the anus or mucous membrane of the rectum, spasms of the sphincter muscles may occur. Difficult and painful defecation may then result. The treatment is correction of the cause or dilation of the sphincter muscles.

## Hyperacidity

Hyperacidity, commonly called *heartburn,* may occur as the result of a pylorospasm that contributes to reverse peristalsis. The gastric juice in the stomach is forced up through the cardiac valve into the esophagus, which creates the characteristic burning sensation.

## Psychic Vomiting

Psychic vomiting occurs in persons with emotional and psychologic problems. It may occur after every meal or infrequently, particularly when the individual is faced with a tense situation and frequently occurs after breakfast. Often the amount of food vomited is small and is regurgitated rather than vomited; thus it does not interfere with normal nutrition. However, if large quantities of food are regurgitated at frequent intervals, the individual may become malnourished. Psychic vomiting is rare in children. If the child expects to face an unpleasant situation at school, it may provide a means of escape.

# SURGERY OF THE GASTROINTESTINAL TRACT

Surgical procedures of the GI tract and accessory organs usually involve an incision into the thoracic or abdominal cavity and sometimes into both. An incision into the thoracic cavity is called a *thoracotomy;* an incision into the abdomen cavity is called a *laparotomy.* The thoracic cavity may be entered for surgical procedures involving the esophagus and sometimes the stomach. The abdominal cavity is opened for most other surgical procedures involving the GI tract and accessory organs. Surgical procedures within the abdominal cavity include surgery on the stomach, the small intestine, the large intestine, and the accessory organs of digestion (liver, pancreas, gallbladder). In addition, the upper part of the uterus, fallopian tubes, and ovaries are within the abdominal cavity. Therefore the abdomen is opened for the surgical removal of any or all of the gynecologic pelvic organs. Abdominal surgery may also involve certain other structures within the abdominal cavity such as lymph nodes and blood vessels, or it may provide for drainage of blood or pus. An *exploratory* laparotomy is performed when it is not possible to make an accurate diagnosis before surgery.

## Preoperative Nursing Care

The preoperative nursing care of all patients who undergo surgery of the GI tract and accessory organs is essentially the same, with slight variations based on the specific surgical procedure. Most patients are admitted to the hospital on the day of surgery or may even have their procedures performed in an outpatient surgical center. Only patients who require more extensive preoperative assessments or procedures or are considered to be at high risk for complications are admitted to the hospital before the day of surgery. Therefore it is most common for patients to have their preoperative assessments, testing, and preparations completed outside the hospital setting. Coordination and communication of nursing assessments and interventions among nurses who work with the patient from preadmission through the surgical procedure are essential to ensure thorough patient preparation and continuity of care.

The nurse evaluates the patient's understanding of the surgery and identifies areas in which further clarification is needed. The patient's feelings and fears about the surgery are determined beforehand so that problems that may be encountered during the postoperative period are identified. During this time the nurse offers encouragement, relieves anxiety, and reassures the patient that efforts will be made to meet his or her individual needs.

Cleansing enemas are often completed before abdominal surgery, unless an inflammatory condition contraindicates this procedure. If the large bowel is to be entered during surgery, a laxative, such as GoLYTELY or Colyte, may be administered, and a series of cleansing enemas and oral antibiotics will be given to *sterilize* (a term commonly used for the process of reducing bacterial count in the lower gastrointestinal tract) the bowel and reduce the risk of postoperative peritonitis. The nurse ensures that the patient understands the rationale and steps for these preoperative procedures, especially if they will be completed before admission to the hospital. The nurse may wish to call the patient at home before the day of surgery to verify that the procedures are completed and to offer additional information and encouragement.

Required laboratory studies, chest x-ray examinations, ECGs, and any other diagnostic tests to be completed preoperatively are based on the patient's diagnosis and surgical procedure, age, and medical history. Laboratory studies commonly performed before major surgery on the GI tract are complete blood cell count; serum electrolyte, hematocrit, hemoglobin, and blood glucose levels; prothrombin and partial thromboplastin times; liver function tests; blood urea nitrogen and serum creatinine levels; and urinalysis. If the patient is at high risk for nutritional deficits (malnutrition, obesity, eating disorder, malabsorption), serum protein and prealbumin values are usually obtained.

The most important aspect of preoperative nursing care is patient teaching. The patient must know what to expect in preparation for surgery and the usual postoperative course and understand the method and importance of turning, coughing, and deep breathing; care of the wound and dressings; antiembolism exercises; pain control; and ambulation. The nurse evaluates the patient's understanding of the preoperative instructions by observing behavior. For example, a patient who has learned about coughing and deep breathing would be expected to demonstrate the technique and explain the importance of performing it regularly. All preoperative teaching and evaluation of patient learning is documented in the patient record.

## Postoperative Nursing Care

Postoperatively, the nurse observes the patient's vital signs (heart rate, respiratory rate, temperature, and blood pressure); observes for abdominal distention, nausea, and vomiting; and notes the passing of stool or flatus. Peristalsis is usually interrupted after abdominal surgery, producing a period of adynamic or paralytic ileus for 12 to 36 hours. Normal intestinal function usually resumes without treatment. Food and fluids are generally withheld until the patient has passed flatus. A nasogastric tube may be inserted to drain intestinal contents until peristalsis returns. Intravenous infusions are given to provide necessary fluids, electrolytes, and nutrients until oral feedings can be resumed. If a patient begins to vomit after surgery, oral intake is usually withheld, and any emesis or distention is reported to the physician.

Distention is detected by inspecting, percussing, and auscultating the abdomen. Accurate quantification of distention is difficult. Body position, elevation of the head of the bed, the presence of dressings, and caregiver variance may render measurement of distention unreliable. The characteristics of bowel sounds assist with diagnosing the cause of distention. For example, high-pitched bowel sounds are heard in the area proximal to an obstruction. To listen for bowel sounds, the diaphragm of the stethoscope is placed over all four quadrants, and sounds are listened to for 3 to 5 minutes. Normal bowel sounds are gurgling, swishing, or tinkling noises.

**Paralytic ileus,** or the inability of the intestinal tract to move its contents because of an absence of peristalsis, is a complication associated with abdominal surgery and inflammation or infection within the abdominal cavity. Bowel function is also affected by pH and electrolyte imbalance, anesthetics, narcotics and other drugs, the extent of the tissue trauma, and the concentration of albumin in the plasma. When normal intestinal function is slowed or stopped, gas, fluid, and waste products collect in the intestines. This results in a rapid increase of pressure within the intestine, distention, and pressure on surrounding areas such as the diaphragm. Gastric decompression is essential at this time to prevent atelectasis and life-threatening complications such as intestinal perforation.

Patients who have surgery of the GI tract are at high risk for fluid and electrolyte imbalance in the early postoperative period as a result of fluid losses from tubes and drains, bleeding, or leakage of fluid from the intravascular space to the interstitial space (third space fluid shift). The nurse maintains accurate records of fluid losses from all sources (e.g., urine, nasogastric and other drainage tubes, and dressings) as well as all fluids administered (e.g., intravenous lines, blood, and medications). The nurse also assesses other parameters of fluid status such as thirst, mucous membrane quality, skin turgor, serum osmolarity, and heart rate.

## COLOSTOMY AND ILEOSTOMY

Both **colostomy** and **ileostomy** provide an artificial opening for the elimination of fecal matter. A colostomy may be temporary or permanent. Until recently, an ileostomy was almost always permanent, but new surgical techniques may be used to create an *ileoanal reservoir* (a pouch that connects the ileum to the anus) that allows stool to be evacuated through the anus. Often a temporary ileostomy is the first stage of this reconstructive procedure.

The most common reasons patients require a fecal ostomy (either ileostomy or colostomy) are cancer, inflammatory bowel disease (Crohn's disease or ulcerative colitis), trauma, perforated diverticulum, **enteric fistula** (an abnormal connection between sections of the intestine, between the intestine and peritoneal cavity, or between the intestine and the skin), or intestinal obstruction. Part or all of the diseased or injured colon is removed, and a stoma is created for elimination of stool.

An ileostomy is created by bringing the distal end of the ileum out to the abdomen as a stoma. Colostomies can be constructed at any point in the large intestine but are most commonly constructed in the cecum (cecostomy), or the transverse, descending, or sigmoid sections of the colon. The location of the stoma usually depends on the part of the intestine that is being exteriorized. For example, an ileostomy or cecostomy stoma is usually located in the right lower quadrant of the abdomen; the descending and sigmoid colostomy stoma is usually located in the left lower quadrant; and the transverse colostomy stoma may be located in the right or left upper quadrant and occasionally in the midline position.

There are three types of stomas: an end stoma, a double-barreled stoma, and a loop stoma (Figure 35-7). An end stoma is created by cutting the bowel and bringing the proximal (functioning) end out to the skin as a single stoma. The distal end of the bowel may be removed or left in the abdomen. If the distal end of the bowel is left in the abdomen, it is sutured closed and left in place (Hartmann's pouch), or it may be sutured closed and affixed to the peritoneum near the end stoma. If the distal end of the bowel is surgically re-

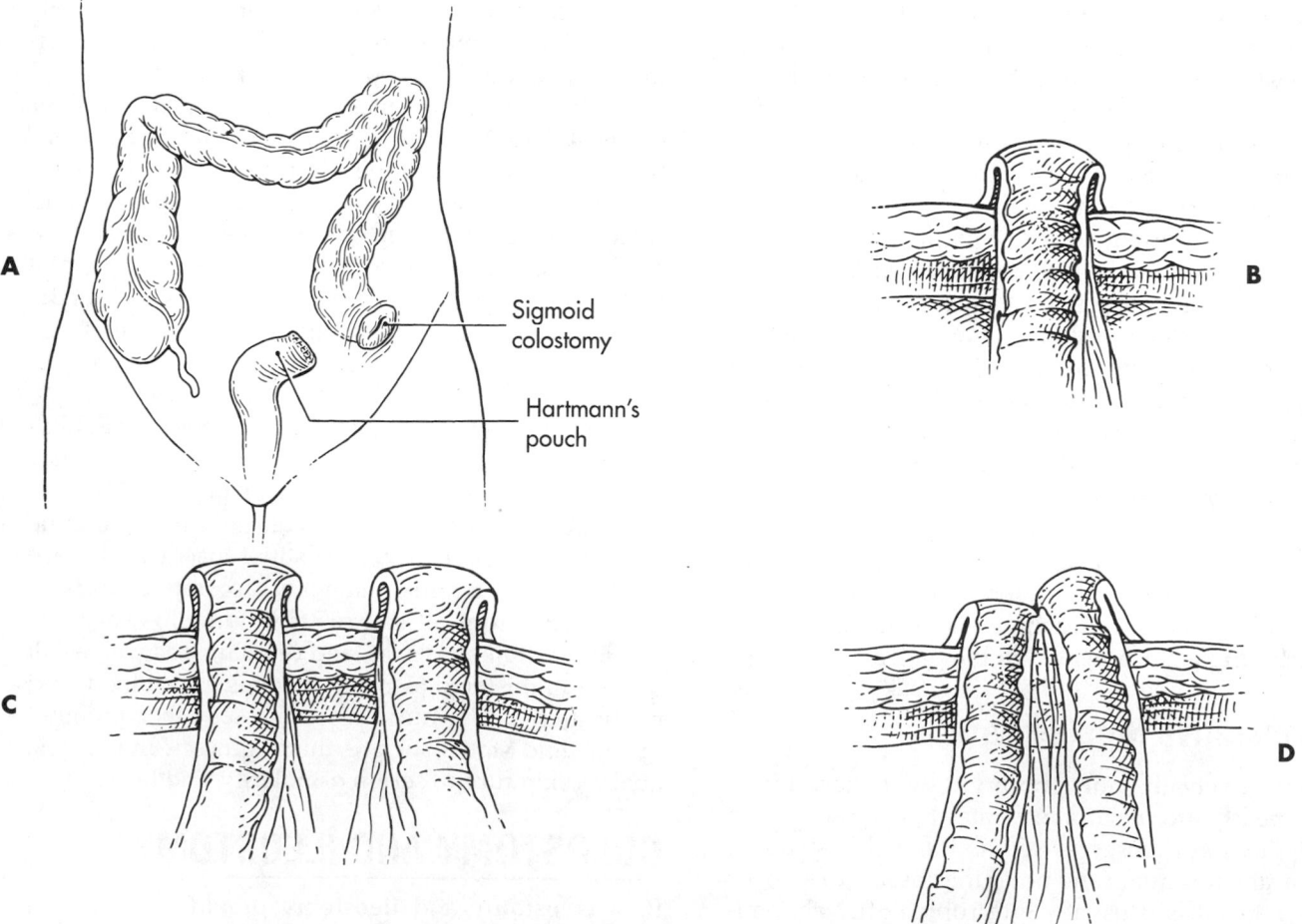

Sigmoid colostomy

Hartmann's pouch

**Figure 35-7**   Types of stomas. **A,** End stoma of sigmoid colostomy, anterior view. **B,** Cross-section view of end stoma. **C,** Cross section of double-barreled stoma. **D,** Cross section of loop stoma. (From Hampton BG, Bryant RA: *Osteotomies and continent diversion*, St Louis, 1992, Mosby.)

moved, the ostomy is likely to be permanent. However, some patients with ulcerative colitis may have the distal bowel removed and the rectal stump left in place for reconstructive surgery in the future (see the section on ileoanal reservoir). If the distal bowel is left in the abdomen, it is possible to reconnect the bowel and close the stoma (ostomy "takedown").

A double-barreled stoma is created when both the proximal and distal ends of the cut bowel are brought to the surface of the skin as two separate stomas. The proximal end is the functioning portion of the bowel; the distal end is called a *mucous fistula.*

With a loop stoma, a loop of bowel is brought up through the skin and an opening is made into the anterior wall of this bowel loop to provide for fecal drainage. The posterior wall of the loop stoma remains intact, so a single stoma has both a proximal and distal os. Usually a plastic rod or bridge is positioned beneath the loop of bowel to secure its position on the surface of the skin and to prevent it from retracting back into the abdomen. The ostomy pouch should be labeled "bridge underneath" so that the pouch is removed gently from the skin and the bridge is not accidentally displaced during pouch removal. The bridge is usually removed 7 to 10 days after surgery by the physician. A loop stoma is usually much larger than other stomas and is usually temporary.

The nursing care of the ostomy patient both preoperatively and postoperatively is generally the same as for all patients with GI surgery. Stoma assessment, GI function, and patient teaching are additional nursing considerations for the ostomy patient in the postoperative period. In the first few postoperative days, the nurse assesses the appearance of the stoma with each reading of vital signs. A normal, healthy stoma is red and moist. Changes in color of the stoma could indicate ischemia and potential necrosis. If the stoma appears blue or black, or if it is not visible (retracted), the nurse should notify the physician immediately. The stoma is pouched immediately after surgery or on the first postoperative day to protect the skin from drainage and to prevent contamination of the surgical wound. The mucous fistula, if present, is usually covered with an impregnated gauze, such as Xeroform, or a moist normal saline gauze. When applying an ostomy pouch, the skin is cleansed with plain water (Box 35-6). If petroleum jelly–gauze was applied in the operating room, it must be removed and the skin cleansed with water and defatted for the ostomy pouch to adhere. A drainable pouch instead of a closed-end pouch is used so that it can be emptied without being removed. The presence of flatus (expansion of the pouch with air) is assessed along with measuring and recording the amount, color, and consistency of the drainage.

Evacuation of stool from a descending or sigmoid colostomy may be regulated by using routine irrigation. After a period of daily irrigations, the patient may become regulated enough to wear a small, closed pouch or gauze dressing. Most patients prefer the security of the small pouch. Irrigations should not begin until approximately 6 weeks after surgery. Patients who have chemotherapy or radiation should not have irrigation. An enterostomal therapy (ET) nurse should evaluate the patient for the safety of routine irrigations (Box 35-7).

---

**BOX 35-6**

### Guidelines for Changing an Ostomy Pouch

1 Provide for patient privacy
2 Remove the old pouch by gently lifting the barrier and gently pushing skin away from barrier adhesive
3 Wash around the stoma using mild soap and water. Rinse and dry thoroughly
4 Measure stoma size to within ⅛ inch
5 Inspect stoma for color, moisture, and position at skin level. Inspect peristomal skin
6 Cut pouch or wafer to measured stoma size, or obtain pre-cut pouch or wafer to match measured stoma size
7 Remove protective backing from adhesive side of pouch or wafer
8 Place pouch or wafer around stoma on abdomen
9 Pat entire surface of barrier wafer to secure adhesion to abdomen

---

**BOX 35-7**

### Guidelines for Colostomy Irrigation

1 Provide for patient privacy
2 Remove ostomy pouch
3 Apply irrigation sleeve; direct drainage into toilet or close bottom of sleeve to collect irrigation returns
4 Use lukewarm solution for irrigation; use 500 to 1000 ml; fill and prime irrigation bag; attach cone tip adaptor
5 Lubricate cone tip adaptor; gently insert cone tip into stoma; hold cone tip in place to prevent back flow
6 Instill irrigating solution over 5 to 10 minutes; remove cone tip adaptor
7 Expect returns within 30 to 45 minutes
8 Remove irrigation sleeve; reapply ostomy pouch

Modified from Hampton BC, Bryant RA: *Ostomies and continent diversions,* St Louis, 1992, Mosby.

GI function normally returns within a few days after surgery. A small amount of serosanguinous drainage may flow from the stoma site immediately after surgery, but this drainage does not signal the return of GI function. Usually, the patient first begins to pass flatus, followed by the passage of stool. An ileostomy usually begins to function within 2 to 3 days after surgery. Stool draining from an ileostomy is initially watery and may amount to 1800 to 2000 ml each day. But after a period of time (a few days to a couple of weeks), it is expected that the drainage will decrease in volume to approximately 500 to 1000 ml each day and change in consistency to a loose, pastelike quality similar to that of toothpaste. The nurse closely monitors the ileostomy patient for signs of dehydration and electrolyte imbalance in the early postoperative period.

When a new colostomy begins to function is dependent on the location of the stoma within the colon; more proximal stomas regain function before the more distal stomas. Cecostomy function is likely to return within 2 to 3 days, as in an ileostomy, whereas it may take 5 to 7 days for a descending or sigmoid colostomy to begin to function. The amount and characteristics of stool from a colostomy depend on the location of the colostomy along the length of the large intestine. The large intestine normally absorbs approximately 900 to 1000 ml of the fluid that comes from the ileum. As stool passes along the length of the large intestine, more fluid is absorbed, and the stool volume decreases and becomes more formed. The cecum is adjacent to the ileum of the small intestine, so the amount and characteristics of the stool will be similar to those of ileostomy drainage. Stool from a transverse colostomy is usually "mushy" or partially formed because it has less water content than an ileostomy or cecostomy. Water content of stool from the descending or sigmoid colostomy is more similar to normal stool and may be partially or fully formed.

## Patient Education

Patient education begins as early in the preoperative period as possible and continues until the patient is secure and confident in the management of the stoma, diet, and lifestyle changes.

### Psychosocial

The nurse helps the patient to recognize and acknowledge the changes in body image that the new stoma presents. The patient may need to grieve the loss of "normal" body image and function and the loss of a body part. By talking with the patient and listening to the patient express fears and concerns about body and lifestyle changes, the nurse can help the patient to progress through periods of anger and denial and move toward acceptance. The patient should be asked about previous experiences with other people who have ostomies. Previous positive or negative experiences will often affect the way the patient views this change. The nurse also allows family members or significant others to discuss their reactions to the ostomy. Information about ostomy support groups should be provided to both the patient and the family (Box 35-8).

### Diet

Most ostomy patients require little or no modification in diet after surgery. The nurse emphasizes the importance of eating a balanced diet. The patient is instructed about which foods may cause problems with odor, gas, diarrhea, or obstruction. Each person reacts differently to foods; therefore new foods should be added gradually to the diet to identify any that stimulate bowel activity and gas formation. Fresh vegetables and fruits, nuts, whole grains, bran, and other high-fiber foods increase stool volume and gas; however, some people find that a steady high-fiber diet eventually decreases gas and fecal odor. Yogurt and buttermilk may reduce odor, probably because of the bacte-

---

**BOX 35-8**

## SUPPORT SERVICES FOR OSTOMY PATIENTS

**UNITED OSTOMY ASSOCIATION**
The United Ostomy Association helps ostomy patients return to normal life through mutual aid and moral support. It publishes *Ostomy Quarterly* and other educational materials. Contact the American Cancer Society for more information.

**OSTOMY VISITOR PROGRAM**
The Ostomy Visitor Program is a service of the American Cancer Society provided to ostomy patients. A trained volunteer who has an ostomy will visit the patient to provide support and assistance to the patient with an ostomy. Contact the American Cancer Society for more information.

**ENTEROSTOMAL THERAPY NURSES**
An enterostomal therapy nurse has specialized training in the care of patient with ostomies. This nurse provides assistance to patients and family members through preoperative and postoperative teaching and counseling, teaching about ostomy supplies, and skin and stoma problem management is included. Contact Wound, Ostomy, Continence Nurses Society (714) 476-0268 for more information.

ria normally present in these foods, as will green leafy vegetables like parsley and spinach that contain chlorophyll. Patients with ileostomies are at high risk for fluid and electrolyte imbalances because the fluid reabsorption function of the colon no longer exists. Symptoms of electrolyte imbalance include headache, fatigue, drowsiness, nausea, and anorexia. Some patients complain of muscle cramps, but they are more likely to complain of flaccid muscles, weakness, and fatigue resulting from a deficiency of potassium. These patients are encouraged to drink at least 6 to 8 glasses of water a day to prevent dehydration. Patients are instructed to notify the physician if there is a significant increase in drainage from the stoma.

## Sexual Dysfunction

Sexual dysfunction may result from various surgical procedures involving the creation of an ostomy. Male patients may be incapable of achieving an erection, and female patients may experience changes in vaginal lubrication and expansion when the surgical procedure involves the nerves and blood supply of the pelvis or resection of parts of the vagina. Surgical procedures that commonly affect sexual function include abdominal perineal resection and total proctocolectomy. The nurse discusses the changes in sexual function as a result of surgery with both the patient and the partner. More importantly, the nurse discusses with the patient alternative methods of achieving sexual pleasure with the partner. Ostomy support groups and sexual counseling may be particularly helpful for these patients.

## Care of the Stoma and Management of Fecal Drainage

The nurse instructs the patient on how to assess and care for the stoma and surrounding skin. The nurse emphasizes the appearance of a normal stoma and the surrounding skin and instructs the patient to call the nurse or physician if any changes occur. The pouch is emptied when it is one-third to one-half full to prevent it from pulling off from the weight of the drainage. Initially, the pouch is changed every 3 to 4 days or whenever it leaks. The size of the stoma normally decreases in the first 6 to 8 weeks after surgery, so the patient is instructed to change the size of the pouch opening as the stoma changes in size. After the stoma shrinks to its permanent size, the pouch can be changed every 5 to 7 days, or as needed. The patient may bathe or shower with the pouch on or off. Skin problems should be prevented, but, when they arise, the ET nurse should be consulted. Barrier wafers or topical medications are often helpful in treating ostomy skin

problems; sometimes specialized pouching equipment may be needed for stomas that are difficult to manage. There is no odor from a well-pouched stoma. If odor occurs, it is likely caused by leakage of drainage from around the pouching equipment. Patients should be informed that the only time they will have odor is when they open the pouch to remove flatus or to drain the contents.

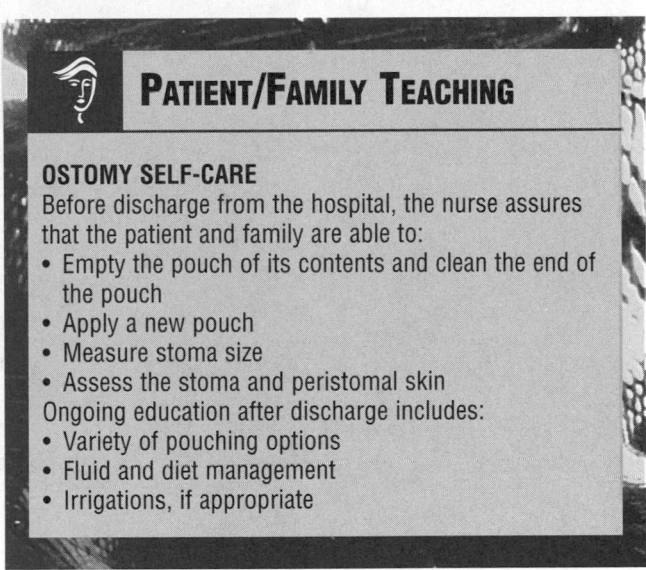

### PATIENT/FAMILY TEACHING

**OSTOMY SELF-CARE**
Before discharge from the hospital, the nurse assures that the patient and family are able to:
- Empty the pouch of its contents and clean the end of the pouch
- Apply a new pouch
- Measure stoma size
- Assess the stoma and peristomal skin

Ongoing education after discharge includes:
- Variety of pouching options
- Fluid and diet management
- Irrigations, if appropriate

## Enterostomal Therapy Nurse

The ET nurse is specialized in the care of patients with wounds, ostomies, and incontinence. The ET nurse is a resource for ostomy patients, their families, and other nurses involved in the care of the ostomy patient in both the hospital and the community setting. All ostomy patients should be referred to an ET nurse as early in their surgical course as possible. Before surgery, the ET nurse marks the site on the abdomen where the stoma should be placed. The ET nurse tries to select a site that avoids skin folds and scars that could interfere with good pouch adherence and makes it easier for the patient to perform stoma care and pouching.

The ET nurse plays a major role in preoperative and postoperative patient/family education and counseling. The ET nurse will provide information about the disease process necessitating the ostomy procedure and will discuss the surgical options, the effects of the surgical procedure, and postoperative care and management. The ET nurse also provides psychosocial support to patients and families throughout the preoperative and postoperative periods.

The ET nurse is an expert in ostomy supplies and ostomy management and is a resource for the selection

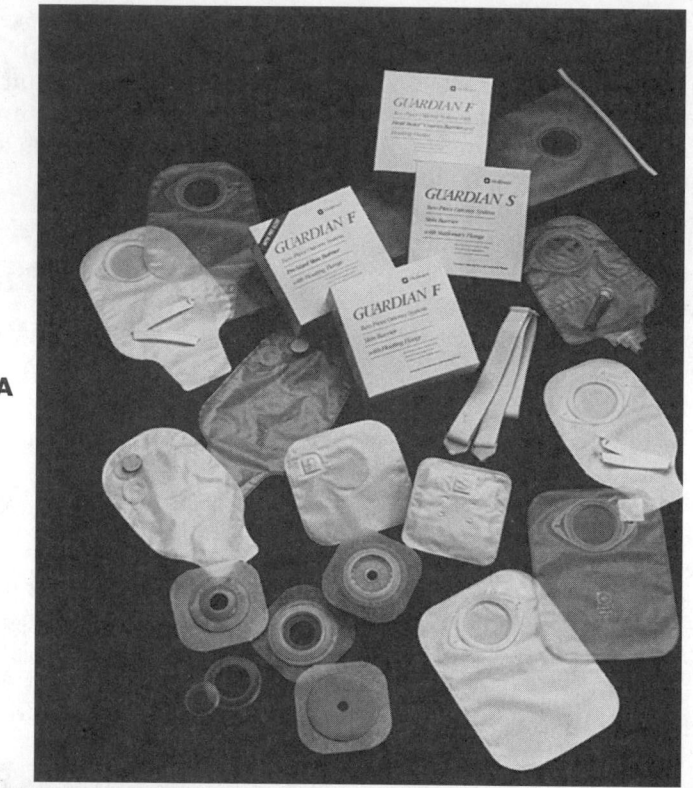

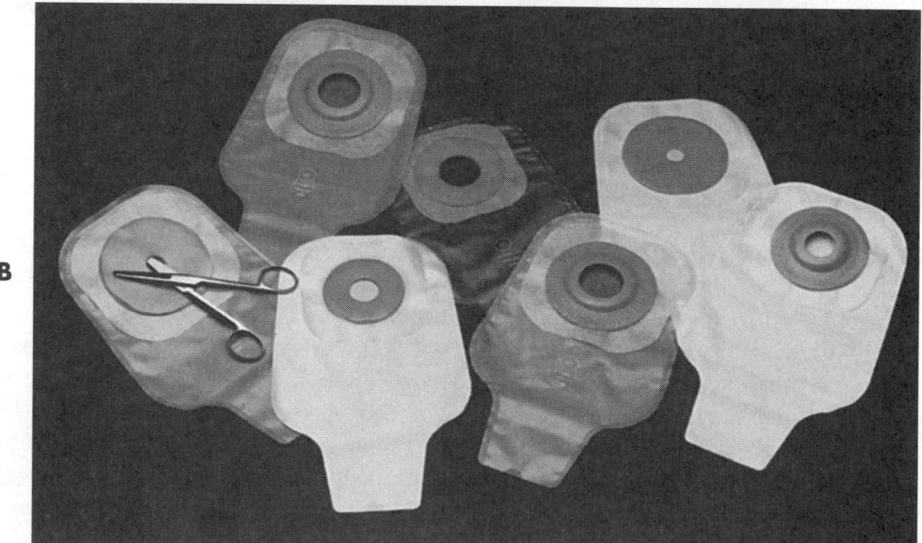

**Figure 35-8**   Ostomy equipment. **A,** The Guardian two-piece ostomy system by Hollister provides a complete selection of skin barrier styles (cut-to-fit, presized, convex, flat, floating flange, and stationary flange), pouch styles (drainable, closed, and urostomy), irrigator drains, and stoma caps. Drainable and closed pouches are available with transparent or opaque pouch film in small or full sizes. Guardian pouches securely attach to Guardian skin barriers and are used by people with colostomies, ileostomies, and urostomies. **B,** The FirstChoice one-piece drainable ostomy pouches by Hollister provide a complete selection of preattached skin barrier styles (cut-to-fit, presized, convex, and flat) with either transparent or opaque pouch film. FirstChoice drainable ostomy pouches are used by people with colostomies and ileostomies. (Courtesy Hollister, Inc., Libertyville, Ill.)

of pouching equipment and supplies that will maximize the patient's quality of life and facilitate self-care (Figure 35-8). If the patient develops problems with skin irritation or inadequate appliance adherence, the ET nurse can suggest appropriate additions or changes in stoma care to manage these difficulties.

# COMMON DISEASES AND DISORDERS OF THE GASTROINTESTINAL SYSTEM

## Eating Disorders

Eating disorders are abnormal eating behaviors that result in physical and psychologic illness or injury. Primary eating disorders are *anorexia nervosa* and *bulimia*. Eating disorders are essentially psychologic disorders that are associated with physical manifestations and physical complications. Psychologic disturbances associated with eating disorders are depression and obsessive-compulsive behavior.

### Anorexia Nervosa

Anorexia nervosa is characterized by an abnormal preoccupation with food and the fear of becoming fat. Patients with anorexia nervosa perceive themselves as overweight and react by severely restricting their food intake and inducing starvation to achieve a desired body image. Excessive exercising to achieve weight loss may also be evidence of anorexia nervosa. The major symptom of anorexia nervosa is marked cachexia; other symptoms include amenorrhea, sleep disturbances, intolerance of the cold, and skin changes. Patients may try to cover up their weight loss by wearing long sleeves, long pants, or long skirts despite the weather. The major complications are those related to prolonged starvation and severe fluid and electrolyte imbalances and can be associated with major damage to the heart and liver.

### Bulimia

Bulimia is also characterized by an abnormal preoccupation with food and eating. But unlike anorexia nervosa, bulimia is characterized not by starvation but by alternating episodes of eating abnormally large quantities of food and calories *(bingeing)* with induced intestinal *purging* by means of vomiting or laxatives or both. Patients with bulimia are not usually cachectic like those with anorexia nervosa. Generally symptoms and complications related to bulimia are associated with the metabolic alterations caused by bingeing and purging. Gum disease and dental caries are commonly seen and are caused by injury from acidic vomitus.

## Interventions

Treatment of patients with eating disorders includes nutritional management and psychologic intervention. Psychotherapy is instituted as a prime focus of the treatment plan. A consultation from a psychiatric nurse specialist is appropriate.

Nutritional management is guided by the findings of a thorough nutritional and metabolic assessment. Mild to moderate malnutrition may be managed outside the hospital, but severe malnutrition will require hospitalization. Oral nutrition is preferred, but if adequate nutrition cannot be provided by the oral route, enteral feeding must be initiated. Occasionally TPN is required as a primary or supplementary source for nutritional replacement. If the patient is not hospitalized, a home-care or visiting nurse referral is appropriate.

## Diseases and Disorders of the Oral Cavity
### Stomatitis and Candidiasis

Inflammation of the oral cavity results from several causes and may affect the entire mouth or only a small part of the mucous membrane. Among the causes of stomatitis are vitamin deficiency, infection by specific organisms such as fungi or bacteria, certain drugs including chemotherapy drugs, and some viral diseases. Symptoms may include a burning sensation; pain; formation of ulcers; the presence of membranes as in diphtheria; tender, bleeding gums; a disagreeable odor; and sometimes fever. Treatment depends on identifying and treating the cause. Vincent's stomatitis, commonly called *trench mouth*, often occurs in epidemics and is fairly common. The condition responds readily to penicillin and good oral hygiene.

Thrush (candidiasis) is caused by a fungal organism, *Candida albicans*. The disease appears as small, white patches on the mucous membrane of the mouth and tongue. The same organism is responsible for monilial vaginitis in the adult, and newborn infants may become infected as they pass through the birth canal. The infection may be spread in the nursery by the carelessness of nursing personnel. Handwashing, care of feeding equipment, and cleanliness of the mother's nipples are important to prevent the spread of bacteria. There are several methods of treatment, including 1 to 4 ml of nystatin (Mycostatin) dropped into the infant's mouth several times a day. Oral candidiasis is a side effect seen with adults who are receiving broad-spectrum antibiotics, particularly chlortetracycline or tetracycline, or immunosuppression therapy. Treatment for the adult is usually 5 ml of nystatin (Mycostatin) as an oral "swish and swallow" four times a day. The possibility of transmission of some inflammatory diseases of the mouth has been questioned. However, when bacterial disease is known to exist, nurses should use every precaution to protect themselves and all patients. Nursing care consists of cleansing the mouth and teeth of any foreign material, rinsing the mouth, and lubricating the lips. The mouth is inspected using a flashlight and tongue blade. The frequency of oral care depends on the patient's condition, and whatever procedure is used should meet the needs of the patient and should be consistent and effective. The nurse identifies patients who are in need of special mouth care and should encourage good oral hygiene in all patients.

## Cancers of the Oral Cavity

Tumors of the lips, tongue, and mouth may be benign or malignant; cancer of the tongue is the most common type of tumor of the mouth. Although the cause of mouth cancer is unknown, it is believed that irritation resulting from smoking, alcohol consumption, dental appliances, and rough, jagged teeth are predisposing factors. Malignant tumors of the mouth metastasize early to adjacent structures such as the lymph nodes in the neck and muscle tissue. Cancer of the mouth is often associated with leukoplakia, a condition characterized by the formation of white patches on the mucous membrane of the tongue or cheek. Cancer of the mouth is more common in men than in women and is responsible for 3% to 6% of deaths from cancer. With early diagnosis, the prognosis of the disease improves.

Malignant lesions may involve the lips, tongue, or mucous membrane lining the mouth, and surgery or radiation or both may be used in the treatment. Any surgery of the mouth interferes with the normal functions of respiration, speech, and eating and will involve certain nursing problems. The mouth cannot be rendered completely free of pathogenic organisms but should be kept as clean as possible to prevent infection.

*Preoperative care of the mouth* for patients with malignant tumors requires meticulous attention. The teeth should be brushed before and after meals, and dental floss should be used to remove any particles between the teeth. Dentures and bridges are cared for in the same manner. Warm mouthwashes or irrigations with an antiseptic solution may be ordered by the physician. If necrotic tissue is present, various preparations may be used to loosen the tissue and deodorize the mouth. A solution of 1 teaspoon of salt and 1 teaspoon of baking soda in 1 quart of warm water may be used for frequent mouthwashes. In addition, 1.5% hydrogen peroxide may be used as a mouthwash with moderate pressure irrigation. Depending on the site and the extent of the lesion, eating may be difficult. The diet should contain soft food and be free of acids and citrus foods, which may cause pain; frequent small feedings may be more desirable than three large meals a day. The emotional factors involved in this type of surgery require that the nurse have an understanding of the patient's feelings. The patient may fear permanent disability or disfigurement and should be given as much information before surgery as is necessary to help relieve his or her anxiety. If the malignancy involves the lymph nodes in the neck, a radical neck dissection may be done in an attempt to remove all affected tissue. After surgery, the patient's speech will be affected. To improve the patient's ability to communicate, a pad and pencil should be at the bedside. The patient may have a tracheotomy or a tracheostomy, and nursing care is the same as that outlined in Chapter 22. A nasogastric tube or gastrostomy tube will be in place and connected to suction. The physician will order the specific position in which the patient should be placed, including the elevation of the head of the bed and the position of the head and neck. Depending on the suture line and the extent of surgery, suction of secretions and mucus may be gently done, or a wick of gauze may be placed in the mouth and allowed to drain into an emesis basin. The physician may prescribe mouth irrigations, using a medicated solution with sterile equipment. Intravenous infusions will be given until other forms of fluid and nutritional therapy are instituted. If a radical neck dissection has been done, blood transfusions may be needed to maintain adequate hemoglobin and hematocrit levels, and a large pressure dressing may be applied to help prevent edema at the incision lines. Some patients may have a wound drain (Hemovac, Jackson-Pratt) placed to remove blood and serous drainage from the wound site. The method of feeding will depend on the site and the extent of the surgery. Enteral feeding is often required in the early postoperative period. When a portion of the tongue has been removed, a thread is often passed through the remaining portion of the tongue and fastened to the outside of the cheek with adhesive tape to keep it from obstructing the airway. The patient is watched carefully for hemorrhage and respiratory difficulty because edema may occur and obstruct the airway. A tracheostomy tray, suction and suction catheters, and oxygen should always be available for emergency use (Box 35-9).

Cancer of the mouth may be treated by external radiation or by implanting radium needles or radon seeds (see Chapter 12). When radium needles are used, they are attached to threads fastened to the outside of the cheek with adhesive tape, and the patient must be cautioned against pulling on the threads. The threads must be checked and counted several times a day and recorded on the patient's chart.

## NURSING PROCESS

## RADICAL NECK DISSECTION (POSTOPERATIVE)

### ASSESSMENT

- Vital signs
- Fluid volume status
- Airway and breathing pattern
- Breath sounds
- Clearance of secretions
- Level of comfort
- Laboratory values (WBC, hematocrit, hemoglobin, coagulation profile, electrolytes)
- Evidence of bleeding or swelling in head/neck region
- Wound drainage and surgical incision
- Nutrition

### NURSING DIAGNOSES

- Ineffective airway clearance related to artificial airway
- Risk of aspiration related to surgical procedure and artificial airway
- Risk of fluid volume deficit related to bleeding or hematoma
- Impaired swallowing related to surgical procedure
- Pain related to surgical procedure and required positioning
- Impaired verbal communication related to tracheostomy

- Body image disturbance related to disfigurement from surgical procedure

### NURSING INTERVENTIONS

- Suction airway as needed.
- Perform tracheostomy care.
- Maintain accurate intake and output from all sources.
- Position patient with head of bed elevated to promote venous drainage and to prevent aspiration.
- Administer analgesics to achieve satisfactory pain control.
- Provide for alternate means of communication (pencil and pad, chalk and chalkboard).
- Allow patient to verbalize fears and feelings.
- Assist patient with personal hygiene as needed.

### EVALUATION OF EXPECTED OUTCOMES

- Airway patent
- Absence of aspiration
- Clear lungs
- Vital signs stable and within normal limits
- Patient communicates effectively
- Patient verbalizes satisfaction with pain control
- Patient accepts change in body appearance

Oral hygiene is important, and a spray may be ordered and used while the needles are in place. Any equipment used must be carefully inspected for radium that may have become dislodged. The physician will give directions concerning food and fluids. The patient should be observed carefully for hemorrhage, edema, or choking.

## Diseases and Disorders of the Esophagus and Stomach
### Esophagitis

Esophagitis is an inflammation of the esophagus caused by various insults to the lining of the esophagus. The most common causes of esophagitis are chemical irritants (such as strong acids or alkali and lye), physical irritants (such as smoking), reflux of gastric acids back into the esophagus, and exposure to radiation therapy. Burning pain is the hallmark symptom and may also be associated with dysphagia.

Complications associated with esophagitis include esophageal ulceration and stricture. Endoscopy is used to confirm the diagnosis, evaluate the extent of tissue injury, and to rule out other causes of symptomatology. The treatment centers around relief of symptoms and removal of the cause.

### Gastritis

Gastritis is an inflammatory disorder affecting the mucosal surface of the stomach. The disease may be acute or chronic. Acute gastritis is usually caused by injury to the mucosal surface. This injury may be caused by irritating drugs or agents, such as aspirin, alcohol, or nonsteroidal antiinflammatory drugs (NSAIDs). Acute gastritis is also associated with uremia and liver disease. Clinical manifestations of acute gastritis include anorexia, vague abdominal distress, epigastric pain, and potential bleeding. Treatment consists of discontinuing the irritating drugs or substances and the use of antacids and acid-inhibiting drugs such as cimetidine, ranitidine, famotidine, and nizatidine. If bleeding is present, sucralfate may be used to promote healing. Healing should occur within a week.

Chronic gastritis is a progressive disease and often occurs in the elderly. Chronic gastritis causes the stomach mucosa to thin and atrophy. The most common type of chronic gastritis is called antral gastritis and exhibits the inflammatory changes associated with the bacterium *Helicobacter pylori*. Another type of chronic gastritis, called atrophic gastritis, is characterized by atrophy of the gastric mucosa and a decrease in acid secretion. The patient with chronic gastritis may report vague signs and symptoms, such as poor appetite, nausea, and epigastric pain. Bleeding may be the only symptom the patient reports. Treatment consists of avoiding irritating agents such as aspirin or alcohol; eating small, frequent meals; and adhering to a bland diet. Vitamin $B_{12}$ may be given if the patient has associated pernicious anemia.

## Hiatus Hernia

The **hiatus hernia** (*hiatus* meaning opening), or *diaphragmatic hernia,* is a common pathologic disorder of the upper gastrointestinal tract. It is the protrusion of part of the stomach through the diaphragm and into the esophagus caused by a weakness in the area where the esophagus passes through the diaphragm. Hiatus hernia occurs with conditions that cause increased intraabdominal pressure, such as obesity or pregnancy. It may also occur with aging because of the decrease in muscle strength. Diagnosis is made by esophagoscopy and barium and x-ray examination. Cytologic studies are usually made to eliminate a diagnosis of cancer.

**Pathophysiology.** Before entering the stomach, the esophagus passes through a small opening in the diaphragm. Under normal conditions the opening in the diaphragm encircles the esophagus securely. Thus the esophagus is held within the thoracic cavity, whereas the stomach remains in the abdominal cavity. For some reason, often congenital, the esophageal sphincter fails to remain tight, permitting the opening to become enlarged and relaxed. When this occurs, the upper portion of the stomach may protrude upward through the relaxed muscle into the thoracic cavity. Often this type of hernia may occur when the individual is in a prone position, and it will return to its normal position when the individual is in an upright position.

**Assessment.** When the patient is symptomatic, a hiatus hernia may cause considerable distress. The primary symptom is *heartburn* caused by the gastric contents of the stomach being regurgitated into the esophagus. There may be substernal or epigastric pain, most notably after eating, that may radiate, simulating

angina pectoris. Vomiting and abdominal distention may occur.

**Intervention.** Treatment includes dietary measures such as eating small meals and avoiding foods that increase the symptoms of heartburn. Antacids may be used if symptoms are not relieved. The patient is advised to stop smoking and to avoid wearing a girdle or tight-fitting belts or clothes. Sleeping with the head elevated on pillows at night may provide some relief of symptoms. Straining for bowel elimination, coughing, and bending are discouraged.

Hiatus hernias usually do not require surgical treatment. However, surgery may be necessary if the hernia is in danger of becoming strangulated. Strangulation occurs when the blood supply is markedly decreased or completely stopped.

## Gastroesophageal Reflux Disease

Gastroesophageal reflux disease (GERD) is a disorder that affects the lower esophageal sphincter (LES). The lower esophageal sphincter is a muscle that, through contraction and relaxation, plays a part in controlling the flow of food and fluids from the esophagus into the stomach. When the LES functions properly, it also prevents the backward, or upward, flow (reflux) of stomach contents into the esophagus. GERD occurs when the LES does not function properly, allowing the contents of the stomach to flow back up into the esophagus.

The presence of an hiatus hernia is associated with GERD. It is believed that the hiatus hernia weakens the LES, thus leading to reflux. In addition, diet and lifestyle play a role in the disease. Smoking is known to weaken the LES. It is believed that certain foods and fluids, such as fried and fatty foods, coffee, alcohol, chocolate, and peppermint, weaken the LES. Obesity and pregnancy are also associated with GERD.

The hallmark symptom of GERD is heartburn, a burning sensation usually in the mid-sternal area. This burning pain may worsen after eating. Lying down or bending over may initiate the pain. Since heartburn shares many characteristics of ischemic chest pain, it is essential to evaluate the pain and other associated symptoms to be sure the patient is not mistaking heartburn for angina.

Complications associated with GERD include esophagitis, esophageal ulceration and bleeding, esophageal strictures, and Barrett's esophagus, a condition that many consider a precursor to esophageal cancer.

**Treatment.** The goals of treatment are to reduce reflux and the associated pain and to prevent or minimize injury to the mucosal surface of the esophagus caused by the contents of the reflux. Lifestyle and dietary modifications are the foundations of treatment.

Eliminating foods that weaken the LES and minimizing food and liquids that can irritate the esophageal mucosa (citrus and tomato products and strong spices such as pepper) is recommended. Weight loss, if indicated, and smoking cessation are also recommended. Eating smaller portions at mealtime and avoiding eating close to bedtime may also help relieve symptoms.

Various diagnostic tests are used to diagnose and assess the severity of GERD. Upper GI series and endoscopy with biopsy are used to both diagnose GERD and to rule out other causes of symptoms. Esophageal manometry is a method used to evaluate the function and any abnormalities of the LES. Esophageal pH testing is a technique used to monitor esophageal pH over time to assist in identifying the frequency and severity of reflux episodes.

Antacids, histamine blockers, proton-pump inhibitors (omeprazole, lansoprazole) are used to control stomach acid. Other drugs, such as cisapride and bethanechol can decrease reflux.

Surgery is indicated only when dietary and life-style modifications and medication therapy have failed to control symptoms. Fundoplication is a surgical procedure to increase LES pressure.

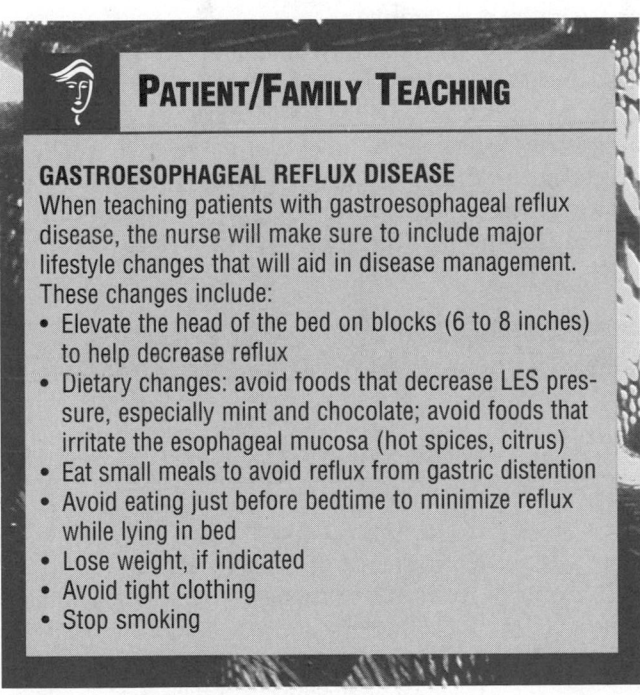

## PATIENT/FAMILY TEACHING

**GASTROESOPHAGEAL REFLUX DISEASE**
When teaching patients with gastroesophageal reflux disease, the nurse will make sure to include major lifestyle changes that will aid in disease management. These changes include:
- Elevate the head of the bed on blocks (6 to 8 inches) to help decrease reflux
- Dietary changes: avoid foods that decrease LES pressure, especially mint and chocolate; avoid foods that irritate the esophageal mucosa (hot spices, citrus)
- Eat small meals to avoid reflux from gastric distention
- Avoid eating just before bedtime to minimize reflux while lying in bed
- Lose weight, if indicated
- Avoid tight clothing
- Stop smoking

## Peptic Ulcer Disease

A **peptic ulcer** is an erosion of the mucosal and submucosal surface of the lining of the upper GI tract. Erosions may be confined to the mucosal or submucosal layers, or they may go as deep as the muscle layer and may penetrate the serosa into the abdominal cavity (perforated ulcer). Peptic ulcers most often occur in the upper duodenum just below the pylorus (duodenal ulcers) but also occur in the stomach (gastric ulcers) and in the lower esophagus—in other words, all the places that come in contact with gastric juices.

Approximately 20 million people, or 10% of the population, in the United States will develop at least one ulcer in their lifetime. Ulcers may develop at any age, but they are uncommon in children. Duodenal ulcers usually develop between 30 and 50 years of age and occur more frequently in men than women. Stomach ulcers develop more frequently in people over 60 years old and more frequently in women than men.

In the past it was believed that stress and diet were the cause of peptic ulcers, but research now indicates that the primary cause of peptic ulcers is the result of infection with the *Helicobacter pylori (H. pylori)* bacterium. Ulcers can also be caused by pancreatic tumors, which secrete excessive amounts of the hormone gastrin (Zollinger-Ellison syndrome). This leads to an imbalance between the amount of gastric acid secreted and the ability of the mucosal protective system. For reasons that are unknown, the incidence of both gastric and duodenal ulcers has declined over the last two decades.

While research indicates the primary role of *H. pylori* bacteria in the development of peptic ulcers, cigarette smoking, caffeine, alcohol, stress, NSAIDs, and physical stress are still believed to play some role in the development of peptic ulcers.

**Pathophysiology.** Peptic ulcers occur when the lining of the lower esophagus, stomach, and duodenum are injured by digestive juices, gastric acid, and pepsin. The lining is usually protected from its own juices by a barrier of mucus and epithelium. Erosion occurs when there is an increase in the concentration or activity of gastric acid or pepsin or when there is a decrease in the normal resistance of the protective barrier.

Gastric juices are released in three phases. The first is the cephalic, or psychic, phase, a reflex action in response to parasympathetic fibers in the vagus nerve. This reflex action takes place when food is seen, smelled, or even imagined. Second, in the gastric phase, juices are secreted in response to a hormone, gastrin, which is formed by cells in the antrum of the stomach. Gastrin is released when partly digested proteins are present. The third is the intestinal phase. When hydrochloric acid enters the duodenum, it stimulates the secretion of the hormone secretin. Secretin stimulates bicarbonate secretion by the pancreas, and these alkaline secretions enter the duodenum and neutralize the acid. Secretin also inhibits the production of gastric juices during the gastric phase.

The glands in the mucosa lining of the stomach secrete the substance that provides the protective barrier.

These mucous secretions are a mixture of muco-polysaccharides and mucoproteins. This mucus absorbs pepsin and protects the stomach by allowing hydrochloric acid to pass through to the surface of the gastric mucosa very slowly. This gastric mucosal barrier prevents the mucosa from being digested by its own secretions. The ability of the mucosa to resist digestive action is also influenced by blood supply, acid-base balance, the condition of the mucosal cells, and the ability of the epithelium to regenerate.

It was once thought that people with peptic ulcers simply secreted more acid than others. This has been found to be true for those with duodenal ulcers and gastric ulcers near the duodenum, but individuals with gastric ulcers seem to secrete subnormal amounts of acid.

In times of stress, the sympathetic nervous system takes over and prepares the body for "fight or flight" by inhibiting the blood flow to the digestive organs and decreasing the production of juices. In some individuals chronic stress seems to enhance the action of the parasympathetic system on the abdominal organs, thus stimulating gastric juice production and the entire digestive process. These individuals will develop a peptic ulcer in response to chronic stress.

**Stress ulceration.** Stress ulceration is a form of hemorrhagic erosion that may occur in patients experiencing severe injury or illness such as burns, head injury or intracranial disease, major surgery, or sepsis. Cushing's ulcer is a stress ulceration associated with injury to the central nervous system. This type of ulcer is usually a single, deep erosion found in the duodenum or in the stomach. Curling's ulcer, a stress ulcer associated with burn injuries, may appear in the esophagus, stomach, small intestine, or even the colon. The exact cause of stress ulceration is unknown, but it is thought to be caused by a decrease in blood supply, which in turn causes a decrease in energy metabolism within the gastric mucosa. The gastric mucosal barrier is disrupted, and its protective ability decreases. Gastric juices are then allowed to act on the mucosa, and multiple lesions (ulcers) develop very rapidly. Hypersecretion of acid is often implicated in the cause of stress ulceration, especially in patients with central nervous system and burn injuries. However, not all patients who have low gastric pH develop ulcerations. In addition, non-acidic pH values do not ensure prevention of these stress-induced ulcerations.

**Complications.** The major consequences of peptic ulcers are obstruction, bleeding, and perforation (Table 35-1).

**Assessment.** Patient symptoms may vary with the location and severity of the ulcer (see Table 35-1). If the ulcer erodes through a blood vessel, bleeding or severe hemorrhage may result. In the case of hemorrhage, the vomited blood has a bright red or coffee-grounds appearance. If slow bleeding occurs, the blood generally passes through the intestinal tract, and stools are dark and tarry in appearance.

Pain is a characteristic symptom of peptic ulcer disease and is described by the patient as dull, gnawing, burning, or boring and is located in the midline of the epigastric region. Pain most often occurs between meals and in the very early morning hours. This pain may awaken the patient from sleep. The pain is caused by the irritation of the ulcer by the gastric acid, ex-

---

## TABLE 35-1

## Comparison of Gastric and Duodenal Ulcers

|  | GASTRIC ULCER | DUODENAL ULCER |
|---|---|---|
| Location | In antrum of stomach | In first 1-2 cm of duodenum |
| Incidence | Usually between 40 and 70 years of age | Usually between 40 and 60 years of age |
|  | Common in elderly women | More common in men than women |
|  | Higher mortality rate than duodenal ulcers | Occurs more often than gastric ulcers |
| Risk factors | Stress, ulcerogenic drugs (ASA, NSAIDs), alcohol, smoking, gastritis | COPD, cirrhosis, pancreatitis, alcohol, smoking, chronic renal failure, stress |
| Pain characteristics | Occurs 1 to 2 hours after eating | Occurs 2 to 4 hours after eating |
|  | Described as heartburn or indigestion | Episodic (pain/eat/relief cycle) |
|  | May be relieved by food | Described as heartburn or back pain |
|  |  | Relieved by food or antacid |
| Effects | May cause weight loss | May cause weight gain |
|  | High recurrence; fewer remissions | Occurs seasonally (spring and fall) |
|  | May develop into gastric cancer | Remission and recurrence pattern |
|  | More likely to be associated with hemorrhage than duodenal ulcers | Seldom malignant |
|  |  | Likely to perforate |

posed sensory nerve endings at the edges and base of the ulcer, or increased motility and spasm of the muscle at the ulcer site. Although pain is the typical symptom, individuals may report variances in the character and duration of pain.

Nausea and vomiting may or may not be present. When present, they are often the result of pyloric obstruction, which may result from ulcerous inflammation or scarring. Many patients are anemic because of loss of blood but are usually well nourished because they eat to relieve the pain. Some patients, however, will experience loss of appetite and weight loss.

The diagnosis is established through a gastrointestinal series, endoscopic examinations, and examination of stool specimens for occult blood. The histamine test and cytologic examination of gastric washings may be done to rule out malignancy. If the patient with a suspected gastric ulcer fails to secrete hydrochloric acid after an injection of histamine, it is likely that he or she has a malignancy in the stomach. Confirming the presence or absence of *H. pylori* is essential in the diagnosing of peptic ulcer disease.

Blood, breath, and tissue testing are currently available to diagnose the presence of *H. pylori bacteria*. Enzyme-linked immunosorbent assay (ELISA) identifies and measures *H. pylori* antibodies in the blood. Carbon breath tests, which measure the amount of carbon exhaled via the lungs after the ingestion of urea, allow the physician to determine the presence of *H. pylori*. Tissue samples taken during endoscopy enable the physician to assess for presence of the bacteria's enzyme urease and to visualize the bacteria under a microscope.

**Interventions.** The goals of therapy are to relieve pain, heal the ulcer, prevent complications, and prevent recurrence (Box 35-10). Healing generally occurs in 4 to 8 weeks, with a reduction in pain during that time. The patient should be encouraged to complete the entire treatment plan even though the symptoms may disappear before the entire therapeutic plan is completed. Treatment includes rest, diet, medication (antacids, anticholinergics, histamine blockers), treatment for *H. pylori* bacteria, if present, and, in some cases, surgery.

---

| BOX 35-10 | NURSING PROCESS |
| --- | --- |

## PEPTIC ULCER DISEASE

### ASSESSMENT
- Vital signs
- Level of comfort (abdominal or epigastric pain, pain associated with meals, nausea)
- Stool and emesis for blood
- Abdomen for bowel sounds, contour, firmness
- Overall skin color
- Fluid volume status
- Laboratory studies (hemoglobin, hematocrit, coagulation profile)
- Stress management

### NURSING DIAGNOSES
- Pain related to action of gastric secretions on inflamed mucosa
- Knowledge deficit related to medications and diet prescribed to promote healing and over-the-counter drugs that must be avoided
- Sleep pattern disturbance related to pain at night
- Anxiety related to inability to manage stress
- Risk for fluid volume deficit related to sudden hemorrhage at ulcer site
- Risk for injury: peritonitis related to possible perforation

### NURSING INTERVENTIONS
- Offer and administer analgesics as needed.
- Administer medications as ordered (antacids, anticholinergics, histamine blockers).
- Provide oral hygiene as indicated.
- Provide quiet environment.
- Plan treatments to provide rest periods.
- Provide diversional activities as needed.
- Explain all procedures and anticipate needs.
- Maintain IV fluids as ordered.
- Reinforce dietary instructions and restrictions.
- If patient smokes, facilitate efforts to avoid smoking.

### EVALUATION OF EXPECTED OUTCOMES
- Absence of pain
- Absence of blood in stool
- Vital signs stable and within normal limits
- Patient is able to select and eat foods for well-balanced diet that complies with dietary modifications
- Patient understands medications
- Patient verbalizes fears and concerns

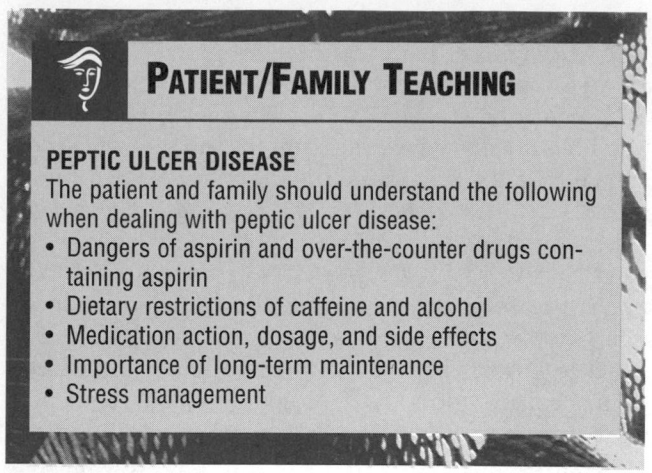

***Rest.*** The patient must have physical rest and relief of tension. Diversional activities such as reading, watching television, or making crafts are encouraged. Stress should be reduced for the patient whenever possible. Everything that is done, as well as the goals of treatment, must be carefully explained; being informed reduces the patient's anxiety. The patient must identify those factors that aggravate the condition, and a good listener is necessary for the patient to vent his or her feelings and examine his or her lifestyle. Referral to a physician, social worker, or other qualified counselors may be helpful for the patient.

***Diet.*** The traditional milk and cream (sippy) diet is no longer used, although patients will still ask about it. It has been found that although milk products do buffer gastric acid, the high protein and fat in milk stimulates further acid production. Some authorities recommend a diet that eliminates only those foods that stimulate secretion, highly seasoned foods, highly fibrous foods, and those that cause pain to the patient. An even more liberal approach eliminates only those foods that cause pain. When milk is prescribed, skim milk is used. In the early stages of healing, the patient will need to be more cautious and may be given small, frequent feedings. Foods that stimulate gastric acid secretion and motility, such as extremely hot or cold foods, coffee, alcohol, and seasonings, are avoided at first and then are used with moderation to test tolerance. Because gastric contractility is increased when the stomach is empty or overly full, small, frequent feedings are indicated.

***Drug therapy.*** Antacids are used to bring relief of symptoms, but there is no conclusive evidence that they promote healing. An antacid made of calcium carbonate (Dicarbosil, Tums) is not desirable because it produces rebound gastric secretion. The calcium carbonate also is absorbed into the bloodstream, producing hypercalcemia and possible renal damage with long-term treatment. A magnesium and alu-minum hydroxide mixture (Maalox) may cause loose stools, whereas magnesium trisilicate and aluminum hydroxide (Gelusil) and aluminum hydroxide gel (Amphojel) may be constipating. Some patients alternate these drugs to prevent problems in elimination. Camalox is a mixture of the two but also contains small amounts of calcium carbonate, which stimulates acid secretion. Antacids can affect the absorption of some drugs; therefore they should be given 1 to 2 hours before or after other drugs. In the event of constipation or diarrhea, the patient should consult his or her physician. Cathartics should be avoided because they increase peristaltic activity and thus are not therapeutic.

Anticholinergics, such as methantheline (Banthine) and propantheline (Pro-Banthine), may be prescribed with antacids because they block stimulation from the vagus nerve, which causes the secretion of hydrochloric acid. They also decrease gastric motor activity and permit antacids to remain in the stomach longer. Anticholinergics should be used with caution, however, because they can cause gastric obstruction.

The introduction of histamine 2 blocking ($H_2$ blockers) agents, such as cimetidine (Tagamet) in the late 1970s brought about dramatic results in treating ulcers. Cimetidine, ranitidine (Zantac), and famotidine (Pepcid) are classified as histamine blockers; they act by blocking the action of the histamine $H_2$ receptors, thereby inhibiting the secretion of hydrochloric acid. These drugs relieve the pain and promote healing of the ulcer. Their effectiveness in treating ulcers has greatly reduced the need for surgical intervention. Because antacids can decrease the absorption of cimetidine, they should not be given concurrently.

Other agents used in the treatment of peptic ulcer disease include sucralfate, omeprazole, and misoprostol. Sucralfate is a cytoprotective agent used to promote ulcer healing. The drug coats the surface of the ulcer and protects it from gastric secretions. Omeprazole (Prilosec) is an antisecretory agent that suppresses gastric acid production. Misoprostol (Cytotec) is a synthetic prostaglandin that serves to inhibit gastric acid secretion and provides mucosal protection (Table 35-2).

It is generally agreed that smoking, caffeine, and alcohol should be eliminated by the patient with an ulcer. Smoking reduces the bicarbonate content of pancreatic juice, which is the neutralizer of gastric acid in the duodenum. Both regular coffee and decaffeinated coffee stimulate acid output. Tea, cocoa, cola, and chocolate also contain caffeine and should be avoided. Alcohol reduces the ability of the mucosa to resist the effects of gastric secretions. It should be avoided while the ulcer is healing and taken only occasionally after the ulcer has healed. An ounce of liquid antacid taken half an hour before an alcohol drink limits the alcohol's effect on the mucosa.

| TABLE 35-2 |
| --- |

## Pharmacology of Drugs Used in Gastrointestinal Function

| DRUG (GENERIC AND TRADE NAME); ROUTE AND DOSAGE | ACTION/INDICATION | COMMON SIDE EFFECTS AND NURSING CONSIDERATIONS |
| --- | --- | --- |
| **Aluminum hydroxide** (Amphogel) **Route:** PO **Dosage:** 5-30 ml 3-6 times a day | Antacid. Used in the treatment of symptoms of hyperacidity, gastritis, esophagitis, GERD, peptic ulcer disease | Constipation; use cautiously with renal impairment and decreased bowel activity |
| **Aluminum hydroxide and magnesium hydroxide** (Maalox) **Route:** PO **Dosage:** 5-30 ml 3-6 times a day | Antacid. Used in the treatment of symptoms of hyperacidity, gastritis, esophagitis, GERD, peptic ulcer disease | Constipation and diarrhea; use cautiously with renal impairment and decreased bowel activity |
| **Aluminum hydroxide, magnesium hydroxide, and simethicone** (Mylanta) **Route:** PO **Dosage:** 5-30 ml 3-6 times a day | Antacid. Used in the treatment of symptoms of hyperacidity, gastritis, esophagitis, GERD, peptic ulcer disease | Constipation and diarrhea; use cautiously with renal impairment and decreased bowel activity |
| **Bethanechol** (Urecholine) **Route:** PO **Dosage:** 25 mg before meals and at bedtime | Cholinergic. Used in the treatment of GERD; increases lower esophageal sphincter pressure | Cramps and diarrhea; may increase gastric acid so not a good agent for patients with GERD and peptic ulcer disease |
| **Calcium carbonate** (Tums, Os-Cal) **Route:** PO **Dosage:** 0.5-2 g 4-6 times a day | Antacid. Used in the treatment of symptoms of hyperacidity, gastritis, esophagitis, GERD, peptic ulcer disease | Constipation and diarrhea; acid rebound; flatulence; contraindicated in hypercalcemia or hypercalciuria; use cautiously with decreased bowel activity |
| **Cimetidine** (Tagamet) **Route:** PO, IV **Dosage:** 300 mg 4 times a day; 400 mg 2 times a day; or 800 mg at bedtime; IV: 300 mg q 6-8 hr or 900 mg continuous infusion over 24 hr | Histamine 2 blocker. Used in the treatment of symptoms of peptic ulcer disease, gastritis, and hyperacidity and to promote healing of active peptic ulcers | Confusion; use with caution in patients with renal disease and in the elderly |
| **Cisapride** (Propulsid) **Route:** PO **Dosage:** 10-20 mg 4 times a day taken 15 min before meals and at bedtime | Used in the treatment of symptoms of GERD; increases lower esophageal sphincter pressure, lower esophageal peristalsis, and rate of gastric emptying | Diarrhea, abdominal pain, constipation |
| **Diphenoxylate, atropine** (Lomotil) **Route:** PO **Dosage:** 2.5-5 mg 3-4 times a day (not to exceed 20 mg/day) | Opioid. Used in the treatment of diarrhea | Dizziness, lightheadedness, constipation, nausea, dry mouth; use with caution in inflammatory bowel disease, in those addicted to opiates, and with atropine hypersensitivities |
| **Famotidine** (Pepcid) **Route:** PO, IV **Dosage:** 20 mg at bedtime; IV: 20 mg q 12 hr (higher doses may be used) | Histamine 2 blocker. Used in the treatment of symptoms of peptic ulcer disease, gastritis, and hyperacidity and to promote healing of active peptic ulcers | Diarrhea, constipation, headache, dizziness, confusion; use with caution in renal impairment |

*Continued*

### TABLE 35-2

## Pharmacology of Drugs Used in Gastrointestinal Function—cont'd

| DRUG (GENERIC AND TRADE NAME); ROUTE AND DOSAGE | ACTION/INDICATION | COMMON SIDE EFFECTS AND NURSING CONSIDERATIONS |
|---|---|---|
| **Loperamide** (Imodium)<br>**Route:** PO<br>**Dosage:** 4 mg initially, then 2 mg after each loose BM; 4-8 mg/day in divided doses (not to exceed 16 mg/day) | Opioid. Used in the treatment of diarrhea | Dizziness, lightheadedness, constipation, nausea, dry mouth; use with caution in inflammatory bowel disease, in those addicted to opiates |
| **Metoclopramide** (Reglan)<br>**Route:** PO<br>**Dosage:** 10-15 mg before each meal and at bedtime | Used in the treatment of GERD; increases rate of gastric emptying and increases lower esophageal sphincter pressure | Drowsiness, nervousness, extrapyramidal reactions, diarrhea, allergic rash |
| **Misoprostol** (Cytotec)<br>**Route:** PO<br>**Dosage:** 200 μg 4 times a day; 400 μg 2 times a day | Synthetic prostaglandin. Used in the prevention of gastric ulcers in patients taking NSAIDs and aspirin | Diarrhea, cramping abdominal pain, flatulence, headache; take with or after meals and at bedtime |
| **Nizatidine** (Axid)<br>**Route:** PO<br>**Dosage:** 150 mg 2 times a day or 300 mg at bedtime | Histamine 2 blocker. Used in the treatment of symptoms of peptic ulcer disease, gastritis, and hyperacidity and to promote healing of active peptic ulcers | Diarrhea, constipation, headache, dizziness, confusion; use with caution in liver renal impairment |
| **Omeprazole** (Prilosec)<br>**Route:** PO<br>**Dosage:** 20-40 mg/day | Proton pump inhibitor. Used for short term treatment of duodenal ulcers and GERD | No significant side effects noted in short-term therapy; risk of cancer when used over extended periods |
| **Ranitidine** (Zantac)<br>**Route:** PO, IV<br>**Dosage:** 150 mg 2 times a day or 300 mg at bedtime; IV: 50 mg q 6-8 hr | Histamine 2 blocker. Used in the treatment of symptoms of peptic ulcer disease, gastritis, and hyperacidity and to promote healing of active peptic ulcers | Headache, malaise; use with caution in liver renal impairment |
| **Sucralfate** (Carafate)<br>**Route:** PO<br>**Dosage:** 1 g 4 times a day for active ulcer; 2 times a day for maintenance | Used in the treatment and prevention of peptic ulcer disease; binds to ulcer site, forming protective coating | Constipation, metallic taste; take on empty stomach; antacid may decrease activity |

### TABLE 35-3

## Pharmacologic Agents Used in Peptic Ulcer Disease

| DRUG CATEGORY | ANTI-ULCER ACTIVITY | AGENT |
|---|---|---|
| Antacids | Neutralize gastric acid | Aluminum hydroxide, magnesium hydroxide, calcium carbonate, sodium bicarbonate |
| Antibiotics | Eliminate *Helicobacter pylori* bacteria | Amoxicillin, flagyl, tetracycline |
| Histamine blockers | Suppress secretion of gastric acid | Cimetidine (Tagamet), ranitidine (Zantac), famotidine (Pepcid), nizatidine (Axid) |
| Mucosal protectant | Creates protective barrier against the activity of acid and pepsin | Sulcrafate (Carafate) |
| Proton pump inhibitor | Inhibits production of enzyme that generates gastric acid | Omeprazole (Prilosec) |
| Synthetic prostaglandins | Suppress secretion of gastric acid, promotes secretion of bicarbonate, promotes submucosal blood flow | Misoprostol (Cytotec) |

Mucosal resistance is also reduced by many medications, including acetylsalicylic acid (aspirin), steroids, phenylbutazone, reserpine, indomethacin, and many over-the-counter drugs containing aspirin. Aspirin may also act as an anticoagulant and precipitate hemorrhage at the ulcer site. The patient must be alert to avoid medications that contain aspirin and should be taught to read labels thoroughly for ingredients (Table 35-3).

***Treating complications.*** The major complications occurring in peptic ulcer are hemorrhage, perforation, and obstruction. When a large hemorrhage occurs, measures are taken to control the bleeding and restore the volume of circulating fluid. The patient is transfused with red blood cells or plasma expanders, such as hetastarch (Hespan), and intravenous fluids are administered to maintain urinary output and electrolyte balance.

A nasogastric tube is inserted to remove acid and the protein load from the stomach, prevent nausea and vomiting, and monitor blood loss. While the tube is in place, the patient needs frequent mouth care and cleansing and lubrication of the nostril through which the tube is passed. The tube is checked often to see that it is patent and draining. All intake and output are recorded, with a description of the color and consistency of the gastric drainage. Nothing is given by mouth in order to promote physiologic rest and avoid further irritation to the stomach.

Fluids and electrolytes are given by intravenous infusion. Because gastric drainage removes fluids and electrolytes from the body, the nurse monitors the patient for signs of fluid and electrolyte imbalance. Dry skin, oliguria (urine output of less than 30 ml/hr), increased heart rate, and hypotension indicate a deficit in fluid volume (hypovolemia). Shallow respiration could indicate metabolic alkalosis, and muscle weakness may be a sign of potassium and sodium deficiencies.

Perforation occurs when an ulcer erodes through the wall of the stomach or the duodenum and the intestinal contents are released into the peritoneal cavity. The result is peritonitis. Emergency surgery is required to close the perforation. The gastric contents that have escaped into the peritoneal cavity are aspirated by suction during the operation. A solution containing antibiotics may be placed in the abdominal cavity before the abdomen is closed.

Surgical procedures include gastrectomy (gastric resection), vagotomy (resection of the vagus nerve to decrease secretion of gastric acids), and antrectomy (removal of a large amount of the acid-secreting mucosa of the stomach) or vagotomy and pyloroplasty (enlarging of the pyloric sphincter to allow reflux from the duodenum).

Another complication of peptic ulcer disease is obstruction of the pyloric sphincter (gastric outlet obstruction), which results from scarring and fibrosis caused by the healing or breakdown of an ulcer. The muscle becomes spastic, edematous, and stenosed, gradually obstructing the passage from the stomach to the pylorus. Surgery is usually required to relieve the condition, and vagotomy with pyloroplasty is the procedure most often used.

## Gastric Resection (Gastrectomy)

Peptic ulcers that do not respond well to medical management and chronic peptic ulcers may be treated surgically by performing a gastric resection or *gastrectomy*. A total or subtotal gastrectomy may be done, and several different types of surgical procedures may be used. Usually the ulcer and a large amount of acid-secreting mucosa of the stomach are removed (antrectomy), and the remaining portion of the stomach is anastomosed to the small intestine (gastroenterotomy). The remaining portion of the stomach may be joined to the duodenum (Billroth I) or jejunum (Billroth II) (Figure 35-9). A patient whose duodenum is abnormal or scarred as a result of a duodenal ulcer requires the remainder of the stomach to be joined to the jejunum, whereas a patient whose duodenum is normal may have the remainder of the stomach joined to the duodenum.

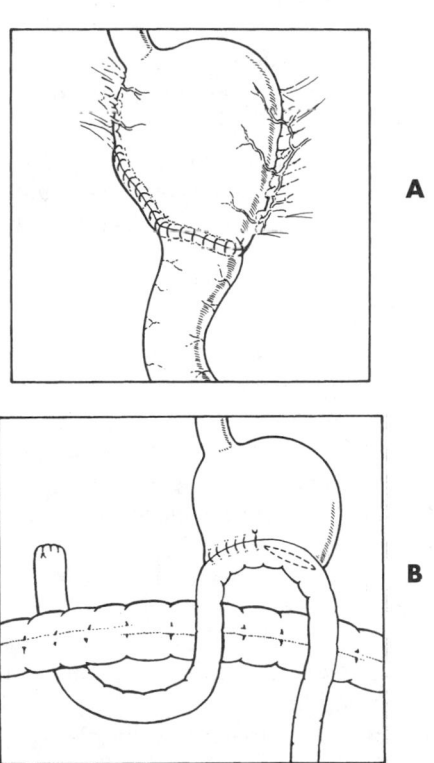

**Figure 35-9** **A,** Bilroth I operation: completed anastomosis. **B,** Bilroth II operation. (From Doughty DB, Jackson DB: *Gastrointestinal disorders*, St Louis, 1993, Mosby.)

A vagotomy may be done at the same time. This procedure includes resection of the vagus nerve to decrease secretion of hydrochloric acid and gastric motility. A vagotomy with a pyloroplasty or segmental resections is used because of the lower incidence of side effects and a low ulcer recurrence rate.

**Nursing interventions.** The patient who is preparing to have a gastrectomy has probably been ill for a long time and feels discouraged and worried, often fearing that the condition may be cancer. During this time an explanation of the various treatments and procedures and the reasons for them will help relieve tension and apprehension. During the preoperative period the patient is encouraged not to smoke and is given an explanation of what to expect after surgery.

After surgery, the patient has a nasogastric tube connected to suction and is given nothing by mouth for at least 24 to 48 hours. Drainage from the gastric tube is monitored carefully. Initially, the drainage may be bright red, but this changes to dark brown or dark red within 6 to 12 hours after surgery. Within 24 to 36 hours the drainage becomes greenish-yellow, indicating normal secretions containing bile. If large amounts of bright red blood continue, the physician should be notified. Dressings are observed for any evidence of bleeding, which should be reported promptly. The nurse monitors the nasogastric suction often to ensure that it is working properly. Distention of the stomach will strain the internal suture line and may cause the **anastomosis** to break open.

---

**BOX 35-11**

## NURSING PROCESS

## GASTRECTOMY

### ASSESSMENT

- Vital signs
- Level of comfort
- Abdomen for bowel sounds, contour, firmness, passage of flatus
- Surgical incision and/or dressing
- Surgical drains
- Fluid volume status
- Character and amount of nasogastric drainage
- Respiratory status
- Patterns of elimination
- Laboratory studies (electrolytes, hemoglobin, hematocrit, whole blood cell count, albumin, prealbumin)

### NURSING DIAGNOSES

- Altered nutrition: less than body requirements related to change in absorption of nutrients and passage of food and fluids
- Pain related to surgical incision, abdominal distention, presence of nasogastric tube
- Risk for fluid volume deficit related to excessive losses
- Risk for infection related to invasive procedure, nutritional deficit
- Risk for altered breathing pattern related to pain, high abdominal incision, sedation from analgesics, and immobility
- Anxiety related to surgery and lifestyle changes
- Knowledge deficit related to dietary and lifestyle modifications

### NURSING INTERVENTIONS

- Explain all treatments and procedures.
- Maintain suction of NG tube.
- Irrigate NG tube only if ordered.
- Do not reposition NG tube under any circumstances.
- Provide oral hygiene. Administer intravenous fluids as prescribed.
- Progress diet as tolerated, as ordered, advancing from clear liquids to bland diet with frequent, small feedings.
- Administer analgesics as needed.
- Provide comfort measures (massage, relaxation, diversion).
- Ambulate as soon as possible.
- Encourage coughing and deep breathing every 2 hours.
- Encourage to splint incision with turning or coughing.
- Provide aseptic wound care.
- Encourage expression of feelings and concerns.

### EVALUATION OF EXPECTED OUTCOMES

- Maintains stable weight
- Pattern of elimination is reestablished
- Diet is tolerated without nausea and vomiting
- No evidence of dehydration
- Wound healing without evidence of infection
- No respiratory distress
- Pain control is acceptable
- Patient verbalizes understanding of diet and lifestyle modifications

Vomiting usually indicates obstruction or kinking of the nasogastric tube; the surgeon is notified immediately. There may be an order to irrigate the tube with 30 ml of normal saline to keep the tube open. No irrigation should be performed unless it is specifically prescribed.

Intravenous fluids are given to maintain fluid balance in the body. All intake, including fluids, and all output, including gastric drainage, are measured and recorded. The mouth and the area of the nares near the tube require frequent care.

The nasogastric tube is removed when peristalsis returns and sutures begin to heal. The nurse determines the return of peristalsis by listening for bowel sounds with a stethoscope and by questioning the patient about passing flatus. Oral fluids are given, beginning with sips of water or other clear liquids. Oral intake is resumed gradually, usually beginning with small, frequent feedings, and increasing as tolerated by the patient. Any feeling of fullness, nausea, or vomiting is reported (Box 35-11).

When a total gastrectomy is performed, the entire stomach is removed and the small intestine (jejunum) is anastomosed to the esophagus. Patients having this procedure will require injections of vitamin B$_{12}$ for the rest of their lives. The stomach mucosa secretes the intrinsic factor that is essential for the absorption of this vitamin from the intestinal tract; without it, no vitamin B$_{12}$ will be absorbed. In addition, the patient will need to eat small, frequent meals.

A complication that occasionally occurs with some extensive gastric surgeries is the *dumping syndrome*, which is characterized by a sensation of nausea, weakness, and faintness after meals, commonly accompanied by profuse perspiration and palpitations and a sense of fullness in the epigastric area. It is believed that these symptoms may be caused by the rapid emptying of large amounts of food and fluid through the gastroenterostomy into the jejunum, rather than passing through the entire stomach and the duodenum before entering the jejunum. The intestinal contents are more hypertonic than they would be if they had passed through the entire stomach and the duodenum, and dilution is attempted by drawing fluid from the circulating blood volume into the intestine, consequently reducing the blood volume and producing a syncope-like syndrome. This may occur after many of the surgical procedures used to treat gastric ulcer, and approximately 20% of patients experience this reaction after gastric surgery. The dumping syndrome generally subsides within 6 months to 1 year and may be further avoided by eating frequent, small meals; avoiding chilled foods and fluids; lying down after meals; reducing carbohydrates in the diet; and taking fluids between meals rather than with meals. Sedatives and antispasmodics that delay gastric emptying may be prescribed.

**Patient and family teaching.** Before discharge from the hospital, the patient is given instructions concerning diet and the importance of eliminating irritants such as coffee, alcohol, tobacco, and aspirin. Foods that contain many spices may be prohibited. The patient needs to follow a regimen that is relatively free from tension. Specific teaching related to medications to be taken after discharge is be included. If the patient has had surgery as part of the treatment for ulcer disease, specific postoperative instructions pertinent to the particular surgery are given to the patient. Diet, activity, wound care, and symptoms that may occur are included in discharge teaching.

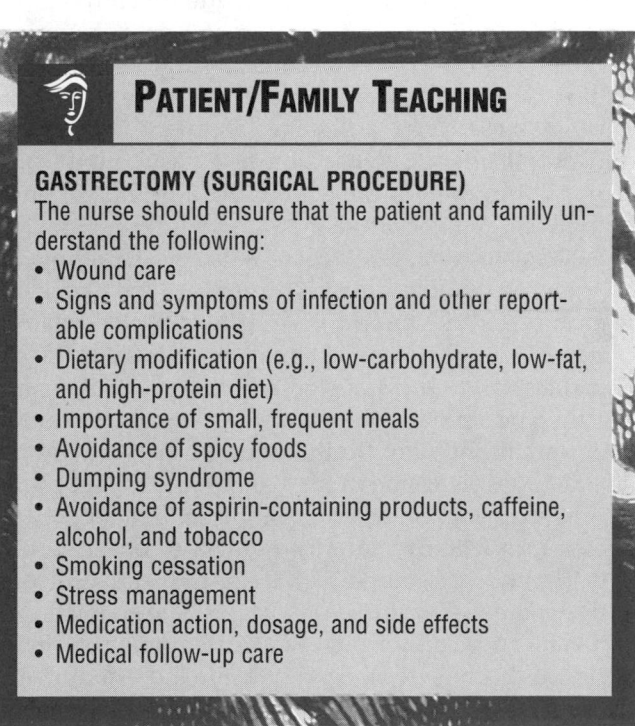

### PATIENT/FAMILY TEACHING

**GASTRECTOMY (SURGICAL PROCEDURE)**
The nurse should ensure that the patient and family understand the following:
- Wound care
- Signs and symptoms of infection and other reportable complications
- Dietary modification (e.g., low-carbohydrate, low-fat, and high-protein diet)
- Importance of small, frequent meals
- Avoidance of spicy foods
- Dumping syndrome
- Avoidance of aspirin-containing products, caffeine, alcohol, and tobacco
- Smoking cessation
- Stress management
- Medication action, dosage, and side effects
- Medical follow-up care

## Cancer of the Esophagus

Cancer of the esophagus occurs mostly in men and accounts for more than 6000 deaths each year in the

United States. Despite all therapy, the 5-year survival rate for esophageal cancer is poor—at only about 4%. In the majority of cases only palliation is possible.

Dysphagia (difficulty in swallowing) with the ingestion of solid foods is the prime symptom in 90% of cases; weight loss may also be reported. Because pain does not occur until the disease is well advanced, and swallowing difficulty may be intermittent early in the course of the disease, there is usually a delay in reporting symptoms to a health care provider. This is unfortunate because metastasis does not occur until after extensive local infiltration. Hence, the slightest dysphagia should be investigated promptly and thoroughly examined with *esophagoscopy*, esophagrams, and cytologic examinations of esophageal washings. The tumor metastasizes to the lymph nodes in the neck and chest and eventually to the liver and the bones. The patient becomes thinner and more malnourished as the disease progresses. Radiation may be used for palliation when metastasis has occurred. Early diagnosis and surgical removal of the lesion improve the prognosis. The surgery performed generally removes the tumor and surrounding lymph nodes. The esophagus is anastomosed to the stomach (esophagogastrostomy), or a portion of the intestine may be anastomosed between the remaining segment of the esophagus and the stomach after the tumor is removed (colonic interposition). In some cases, the patient is not a candidate for a major surgical procedure or if it is not possible to remove the tumor with surgery. In these cases, palliative treatment is provided and may include the insertion of a gastrostomy tube that will provide for the continuing administration of enteral feeding and fluids.

**Gastrostomy care.** The patient with a gastrostomy has an opening into the stomach through which a tube has been inserted for the purpose of feeding or drainage (Figure 35-10). The stomach may be sutured to the abdominal wall to prevent stomach contents from entering the abdominal cavity, and the catheter is secured into a small incision. Routine care of the gastrostomy site includes cleansing of the skin around the tube with a mild soap and water or an antibacterial agent. A dry dressing is usually placed around the tube insertion site. The tube is secured in place to prevent accidental dislodgement. The nurse follows specific hospital protocols for tube care. Should the gastrostomy tube inadvertently become dislodged or removed, the nurse is responsible for notifying the appropriate personnel.

Nursing management of the patient with a gastrostomy feeding tube includes caring for the skin, maintaining patency of the tube, providing good oral care, stabilizing the tube, and administering feedings as prescribed by the physician. Often there is a slight

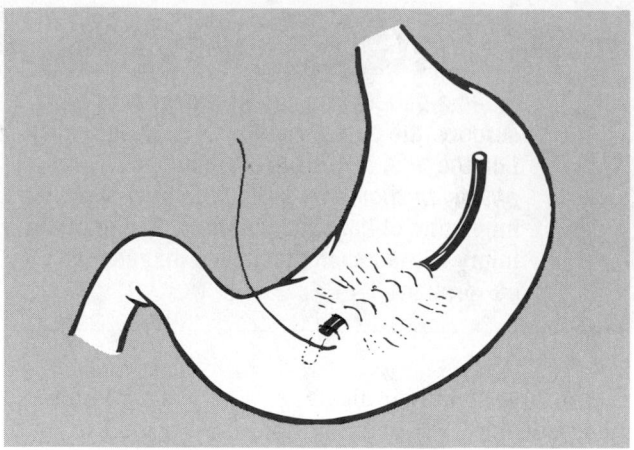

**Figure 35-10** Gastrostomy tube is inserted into the stomach and secured with sutures. The end of the tube or catheter is brought out through the opening in the abdomen so that feedings may be given.

seepage of secretions around the tube, which will cause excoriation of the skin. Careful washing with mild soap and water, thorough drying, and the application of a skin barrier will keep the skin in healthy condition. More aggressive treatment of the skin around the gastrostomy may be needed if routine care does not prevent breakdown. If the tube becomes blocked, it is gently irrigated with a bulb syringe and physiologic saline solution. Force should not be used to irrigate the tube. If patency is not restored, the physician should be notified.

Most institutions use commercially prepared feeding formulas. The specific formula, volume, rate, and concentration of the enteral feeding is prescribed by the physician. Formulas are administered at room temperature. Cold feedings may cause cramping and diarrhea. The patient is placed with the head of the bed elevated or in a side-lying position to prevent aspiration during feeding. The amount of feeding taken is recorded so that the physician may determine if the amount of food that the patient is receiving provides sufficient calories (refer to the section on enteral feeding).

> **NURSE ALERT**
>
> It is essential to keep the gastrostomy tube securely positioned to prevent the tube from moving around the site on the abdomen. Movement may cause the tract from the stomach to the abdomen to enlarge and can cause leakage of stomach contents into the abdomen.

The patient with a gastrostomy feeding tube has a difficult emotional adjustment to make. The realization that he or she will not be able to eat normally may be traumatic, and the patient will need a great deal of support and encouragement. As acceptance of this method of feeding occurs, the patient should be encouraged to participate in administering the feeding and caring for the skin. If this method of feeding will be long term or permanent, it is important to include a family member in the preparation of the diet and the skin care and feeding of the patient. After the patient leaves the hospital, the home health nurse will visit the patient to supervise, instruct, and provide continuing encouragement.

## Cancer of the Stomach

Cancerous lesions of the stomach cause obstruction, either into or out of the stomach, and bleeding, and can metastasize to adjacent or vital organs. The cause of cancer of the stomach is unknown, but environment, genetics, and the presence of the bacterium *H. pylori* are factors implicated in the disease. Diet is probably the most significant environmental factor associated with the development of cancer of the stomach. The incidence is high in parts of the world where there is heavy consumption of smoked fish and smoked meat, such as Japan, Iceland, Chile, and Hawaii. Diets rich in starch, pickled vegetables, salted meats and fish, as well as nitrates and nitrites, correlate with an increased risk for cancer of the stomach. *H. pylori* is a known cause of gastritis and atrophic changes associated with gastritis and has been implicated as a possible factor predisposing to gastric cancer. In addition, an increased incidence of cancer of the stomach is noted in patients with type A blood and a family history of gastric cancer.

**Assessment.** The early symptoms of cancer of the stomach are so poorly defined that most individuals delay medical treatment until the malignancy is well established. Symptoms related to metastasis prompt the patient to consult a health care provider. Symptoms include dysphagia, loss of appetite, a feeling of fullness after meals, epigastric distress, nausea, vomiting, weight loss, anemia, vomiting blood that has a coffee-grounds appearance, blood in the stools that appears dark and tarry, and pain. A palpable mass may be felt through the abdominal wall.

Early diagnosis is extremely important. Diagnostic tests include upper GI endoscopy and upper GI barium studies. Gastric analysis is performed, and cytologic examination using Papanicolaou's technique to determine the presence of cancer cells may be done following lavage. Emesis may be saved for examination, and stool specimens are examined for the presence of occult blood.

**Interventions.** The only surgical treatment is a subtotal or total gastrectomy. The malignant growth often causes severe malnutrition, and several days of preoperative nutritional support may be required before surgery. Chemotherapy and radiation therapy are part of the postoperative treatment plan.

Interventions for the patient after a total gastrectomy are slightly different from those after a subtotal gastrectomy because the chest cavity must be entered to remove the entire stomach. There will be little nasogastric drainage because secretions are normally formed in the stomach, which has been removed. Small, frequent feedings are given, beginning with tap water and slowly progressing to bland foods. Often a period of enteral tube feedings is required to provide or supplement oral nutrition. The patient should be given easily digested foods, eat slowly, and chew the food thoroughly. Because the intrinsic factor normally produced by the stomach is now missing, vitamin $B_{12}$ cannot be absorbed, and a regular injection of vitamin $B_{12}$ is necessary to prevent pernicious anemia. The patient may undergo chemotherapy. A combination of chemotherapeutic agents (5-fluorouracil, doxorubicin, and mitomycin C) has been found to be more effective than single-drug therapy. Radiation may be used with chemotherapy, but radiation alone has not proven effective against gastric cancer.

# Diseases and Disorders of the Small and Large Intestine
## Gastroenteritis

Inflammation of the intestine accompanying gastritis is called *gastroenteritis*. Enteritis occurs in conjunction with some infectious diseases, such as typhoid fever, dysentery, tuberculosis involving the intestines, and most cases of food infection. The severity of the condition depends on the virulence of the organism causing the condition. The primary symptoms are diarrhea and abdominal cramping. When the infection is from food, the symptoms occur within a few hours after the contaminated food has been eaten. Fever may or may not occur, but dehydration and weakness are usually present. Diarrhea is a common symptom of infection.

Treatment is based on identifying the cause by using stool examination or cultures from suspected food. Precautions should always be taken until the cause of the diarrhea has been established. Bed rest may be indicated, and only oral liquids are used. When vomiting is present, oral fluids may be withheld, and the appropriate electrolyte solutions replaced intravenously.

Antibiotic or sulfonamide drugs may be ordered by the physician in treating some types of enteritis.

## Irritable Bowel Syndrome

Irritable bowel syndrome (IBS) is characterized by cramping abdominal pain, flatulence, bloating, and constipation, diarrhea, or alternating bouts of each. This disorder does not involve the inflammatory process and should not be confused with inflammatory bowel disease.

The cause of IBS is not known. Although stress may worsen symptoms, it is not a cause of IBS. Research has found that the bowel of a patient with IBS tends to go into spasm after only mild stimulation. Certain foods, medications, or just the stimulation of simply eating or having gas in the GI tract may stimulate the reaction. Chocolate, milk products, alcohol, and caffeine are common agents that trigger the irritable response.

Some patients with IBS may pass mucus with their stool. However, bleeding, fever, weight loss, and continued pain are *not* symptoms of IBS. The patient with these symptoms requires further medical evaluation.

Dietary modifications may lessen symptoms or frequency of symptoms associated with IBS. Some patients have relief of symptoms with increasing dietary fiber, yogurt (if they have intolerance to milk and milk products), or eating smaller meals. Although medications to help treat diarrhea or constipation may help with symptom relief, there is no drug that is used to eliminate the condition.

## Inflammatory Bowel Disease

Inflammatory bowel disease (IBD) is an umbrella term that refers to a group of chronic disorders in the small and large intestine that cause inflammation or ulcerations of GI tissue. Most commonly, IBD refers to Crohn's disease and ulcerative colitis, but it may also include *colitis, enteritis, ileitis,* or *proctitis.* It is estimated that as many as 2 million people in the United States suffer from IBD. Recent research points to a complex interplay between genetic and environmental factors as the cause of IBD. These factors join to produce an exaggerated, inappropriate, or prolonged inflammatory response. Genetic markers for Crohn's disease and ulcerative colitis have been discovered. Environmental factors include infectious agents, food additives, and the use of birth control pills. The current hope in treating IBD is that, as the responsible genes are identified, medications can be developed to correct or neutralize the genes. Although the exact cause is unknown, it is known that IBD is not caused by emotional stress. Psychologic stress may cause exacerba-

tion of the symptoms of IBD or may alter the course of the disease, but it does not initiate the disease process (Box 35-12).

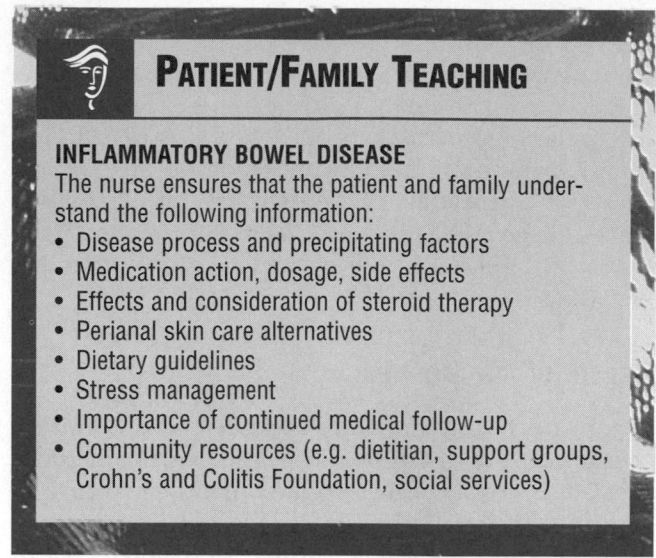

**PATIENT/FAMILY TEACHING**

**INFLAMMATORY BOWEL DISEASE**
The nurse ensures that the patient and family understand the following information:
- Disease process and precipitating factors
- Medication action, dosage, side effects
- Effects and consideration of steroid therapy
- Perianal skin care alternatives
- Dietary guidelines
- Stress management
- Importance of continued medical follow-up
- Community resources (e.g. dietitian, support groups, Crohn's and Colitis Foundation, social services)

**Ulcerative colitis.** Ulcerative colitis is one of the most serious diseases of the gastrointestinal tract. Although the disease has been reported since 1875, the specific cause is still unknown. There appears to be little evidence that the disease is caused by pathologic organisms. Possible causes include food allergies, immunologic reactions, infections, destructive enzymes, and autoimmune reactions. Like Crohn's disease, ulcerative colitis is a chronic disease characterized by episodes of exacerbation and remission. The disease usually attacks young adults and may be found in children and adolescents; it almost always occurs before 30 years of age.

Ulcerative colitis affects the mucosal surface of the colon and rectum. It begins in the rectum and spreads upward through the colon, eventually involving the entire colon. It is characterized by chronic, persistent inflammation, fibrosis, and narrowing of the bowel lumen. Because of the associated frequent diarrhea and poor absorption of nutrients, the disease can lead to chronic nutritional deficiency, anemia, and electrolyte imbalances. Cancer of the colon is a known complication of long-term chronic ulcerative colitis. The disease may be controlled medically but is cured only by surgical intervention and removal of the diseased colon.

**Assessment.** Ulcerative colitis is characterized by frequent loose, bloody, mucoid stool. Although pain is not the hallmark symptom associated with ulcerative colitis, patients often complain of a mild, cramping pain occurring in the left lower quadrant. This pain is often associated with the urge to defecate and is relieved with defecation. Symptoms begin rather insidi-

| BOX 35-12 | NURSING PROCESS |
| --- | --- |

## INFLAMMATORY BOWEL DISEASE

**ASSESSMENT**

- Vital signs
- Abdomen for pain, bowel sounds, contour, firmness
- Fluid volume status
- Weight
- Nutritional status
- Stool frequency and appearance
- Rectal bleeding
- Laboratory studies (electrolytes, $B_{12}$, folic acid, hemoglobin, hematocrit, WBC)
- Coping mechanisms
- Perianal skin integrity

**NURSING DIAGNOSES**

- Pain related to bowel inflammation, frequent diarrhea, perirectal excoriation
- Altered nutrition: less than body requirements related to malabsorption, diarrhea, anorexia
- Risk for fluid volume deficit related to excessive diarrhea, blood loss, or poor oral intake
- Risk for infection related to poor nutritional status and immunocompromised state
- Diarrhea related to inflammation of bowels
- Anxiety related to change in health status
- Ineffective individual coping related to stress, disease process, pain, lack of rest, or lack of support
- Knowledge deficit related to chronic disease, change in treatment, new information

**NURSING INTERVENTIONS**

- Administer medications as prescribed and evaluate effectiveness.

- Provide heating pad for abdomen if indicated.
- After defecation, cleanse anal area and apply skin sealant or barrier cream, if indicated.
- Keep room as free of odors as possible.
- Administer total parenteral nutrition or intravenous fluids as prescribed.
- Provide diet high in protein, calories, vitamins, and minerals.
- Provide small, frequent meals.
- Avoid food high in fat and fiber, spicy foods, milk products, and raw vegetables, fruits, nuts, or whole grains.
- Encourage optimal nutrition.
- Test stool for occult blood.
- Wash hands before providing nursing care.
- Provide or instruct on perianal hygiene.
- Promote skin and mouth care.
- Provide opportunity to discuss feelings, concerns, frustrations.
- Encourage diversional activities.

**EVALUATION OF EXPECTED OUTCOMES**

- Pain level is acceptable
- Weight is stable
- Diarrhea is controlled
- No evidence of dehydration
- No evidence of infection
- Patient and family understand disease and management
- Patient is able to verbalize anxiety and coping measures

ously, with increasing distress and frequency of stools until the individual may pass as many as 20 to 30 stools a day. The presence of ulcers on the lining of the intestine results in blood loss and anemia and possibly in severe hemorrhage. The patient becomes debilitated, pale, weak, and thin, and electrolytes are constantly being depleted because of the severe diarrhea. Because of the nutritional deficiency, symptoms of vitamin deficiency may occur. Diagnosis is made on the basis of the history and physical examination, including colonoscopy, biopsy, x-ray examination, and stool specimens.

The nurse assesses the patient for the occurrence and severity of abdominal pain and cramping, and the number and amount of diarrhea stools during periods

of exacerbation. Electrolyte balance and nutritional status are monitored. The nurse evaluates patient response to medical therapy. Like Crohn's disease, ulcerative colitis affects patient lifestyle and psychologic well-being. The nurse assesses the patient for adjustment to disease and adequacy of coping strategies.

**Interventions.** Treatment includes physical and psychologic rest; nutrition, fluid, and electrolyte management; control of inflammation; and prevention of infection.

***Pharmacologic therapy.*** Current pharmacologic therapy used in the treatment of ulcerative colitis is aimed at modifying the inflammatory response at the mucosal layer. In particular, drug therapy using aminosalicylates and corticosteroids is aimed at modifying the mediators of the inflammatory response. Sulfasalazine, mesalamine, and corticosteroids are the mainstays of therapy (Nassif et al, 1996).

Sulfasalazine is a combination of an antibiotic (sulfapyridine) and an antiinflammatory agent, 5-aminosalicylic acid (5-ASA). Sulfapyridine is absorbed in the colon and excreted in the urine; 5-ASA, however, is poorly absorbed, so it exerts primarily a topical effect in the colon and is excreted in the feces. The drug has been successfully used both in the treatment of acute disease and as maintenance therapy.

5-aminosalicylic acid, or 5-ASA, is an alternative to sulfasalazine in the treatment of active ulcerative colitis and as maintenance therapy. For oral therapy, 5-ASA is pharmacologically prepared for optimal delivery to the colon for activity in two forms, as enteric-coated/time-released preparations, or linked with another molecule as a pro-drug. Mesalamine is the generic name for the enteric-coated or time-released preparation; olsalazine, ipsalazide, and balsalazide are pro-drugs. Topical preparation of mesalamine (Rowasa) is available in enema and suppository form for use during acute episodes and as maintenance therapy (Procaccino, 1996).

Corticosteroids are the drug of choice during active disease, but there is no evidence supporting their use as maintenance therapy. They are available for administration in the oral, parenteral, and topical (as enema or suppository) forms. The method of administration is dictated by the severity of the disease and of the exacerbation. Prolonged use of steroids is limited both by its effectiveness and by adverse side effects. A usual course of steroid therapy in severe, acute exacerbations is a tapered dose lasting approximately 3 weeks.

Immunosuppressive agents are used by some physicians in the management of acute exacerbations, as well as in maintenance therapy. Azathioprine, 6-mercaptopurine, and cyclosporine have been studied and used in the management of selected patients with ulcerative colitis.

Antidiarrheal agents are used along with standard drug therapy in the management of acute and chronic diarrhea. However, antidiarrheals should be avoided if the patient is acutely ill or unstable due to the increased risk of developing toxic megacolon.

***Surgical intervention.*** Because of the association of ulcerative colitis with increased risk of colon cancer, at some point in the course of the disease the patient with ulcerative colitis is likely require a total colectomy. Current surgical options include total proctocolectomy with permanent-end ileostomy, Kock continent ileostomy, and ileoanal reservoir procedure. With the total proctocolectomy with permanent end ileostomy, the entire colon, rectum, and anal sphincter are removed and an end ileostomy is created. The stool drains into an external pouch through the abdominal stoma. The patient needs to wear an ostomy pouch at all times.

KOCK CONTINENT ILEOSTOMY. The Kock continent ileostomy and the ileoanal reservoir are two procedures developed to provide surgical alternatives that maintain fecal continence, thus eliminating constant stool drainage from an ileostomy. These procedures are being done on an increasing number of patients with ulcera-

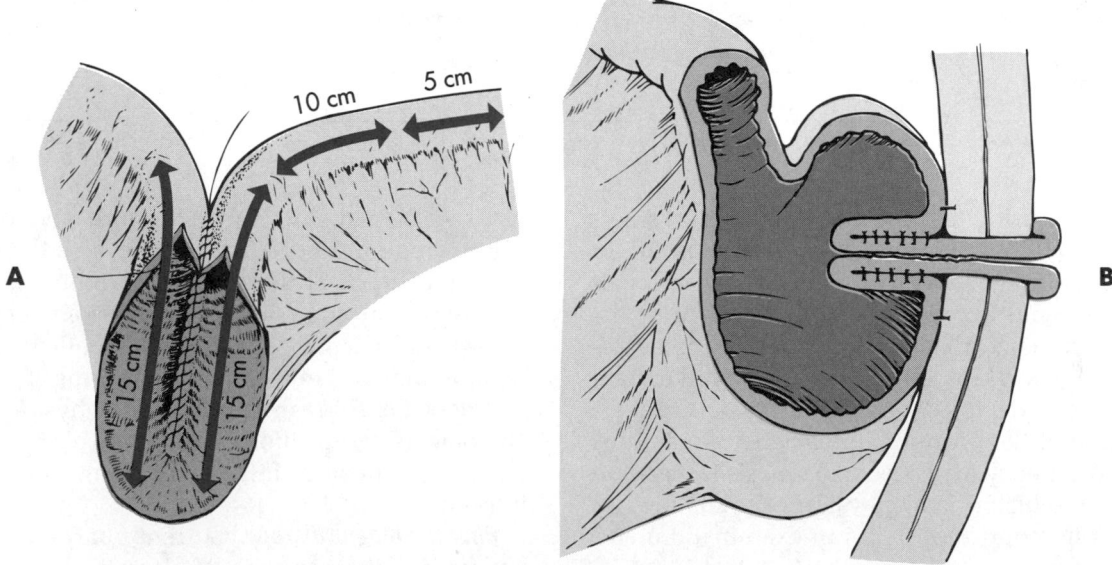

**Figure 35-11** Kock pouch for continent ileostomy. **A,** Pouch created from ileum. **B,** Nipple valve to control release of contents and provide for drainage by inserting tubing. (From Hampton BG, Bryant RA: *Ostomies and continent diversions,* St Louis, 1992, Mosby.)

tive colitis and familial adenomatous polyposis (FAP) who formerly required a permanent ileostomy.

With the Kock continent ileostomy, the entire colon, rectum, and anal sphincter are removed. The patient has a stoma but does not need to wear a stoma pouch because a reservoir to collect and hold the stool is surgically created using a section of the terminal ileum (Figure 35-11). The last few inches of ileum are used to create a *nipple valve,* which controls the release of stool from the stoma in much the same way as the anal sphincter controls the collection of stool in the normal bowel. A catheter is usually placed through the stoma into the pouch to allow for continuous drainage of stool from the ileum until the newly created pouch is fully healed (10 days to 3 to 4 weeks). During this time the catheter is irrigated to remove mucus from the pouch. Once the new pouch is healed and the catheter is removed, a tube is inserted into the pouch at gradually lengthening intervals to evacuate drainage from the pouch (every 2 hours, then every 3 hours, then every 4 hours). This process allows the pouch to gradually increase in capacity; eventually the pouch is able to hold 500 to 1000 ml and requires draining only two or three times a day. A small, absorbent dressing is taped over the stoma to protect it. Ultimately, the drainage procedure takes no more than 5 or 10 minutes (Box 35-13).

**ILEOANAL RESERVOIR.** With the ileoanal reservoir (IAR) procedure the entire colon and the inner lining of the rectum are removed. An internal reservoir, or pouch, is constructed from the ileum, similar to the Kock procedure. However, with the ileoanal procedure, the internal reservoir (pouch) is surgically attached to the anus. Stool collects in the reservoir and is expelled via the rectum in a normal toileting fashion.

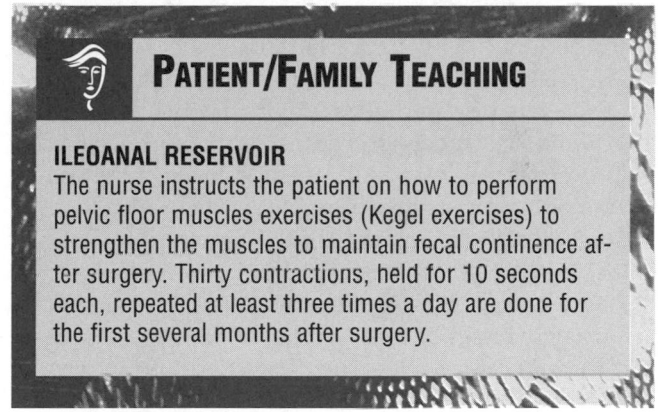

### NURSE ALERT

Nothing should be inserted into the rectum of a patient with a new ileoanal reservoir. Any object inserted into the rectum could damage the new reservoir.

### PATIENT/FAMILY TEACHING

**ILEOANAL RESERVOIR**
The nurse instructs the patient on how to perform pelvic floor muscles exercises (Kegel exercises) to strengthen the muscles to maintain fecal continence after surgery. Thirty contractions, held for 10 seconds each, repeated at least three times a day are done for the first several months after surgery.

---

### BOX 35-13

#### Guidelines of Care for Drainage of a Continent Ileostomy Pouch

1  Sit or stand at the toilet.
2  Lubricate the catheter (usually 28 F Silastic) generously with water-soluble jelly.
3  Slowly and gently insert catheter through the stoma and valve into the pouch to the premarked site on the catheter; if the catheter is difficult to pass, relax, take deep breaths, and gently advance the catheter during exhalation or instill a small amount of water or air into the catheter to relax the pouch valve.
4  Instill 20 to 25 ml lukewarm water into pouch to dilute thicker stool if needed.
5  Remove the catheter when drainage is complete; usually takes 5 to 10 minutes.
6  Clean the catheter thoroughly with mild soap and water, allow to dry; strong detergents may erode the catheter.
7  Store supplies in a plastic bag or kit for easy transport.

---

An IAR may be created in a single surgical procedure, but more commonly it is created in stages. When the procedure is performed in stages, the patient requires a temporary ileostomy to allow the reservoir to heal before making the final surgical connection. If the IAR is constructed in stages, the first stage involves removal of the entire colon, construction of the reservoir pouch from the ileum, connection of the reservoir pouch to the anus, and creation of a temporary ileostomy. Postoperative care is generally similar to that for patient with abdominal surgery and a new ileostomy. Because the ileostomy is created in a more proximal section of the ileum, output of effluent is 1500 to 2400 ml per day. The patient may have the urge to defecate and may pass mucus from the rectum. Fecal incontinence, usually mucoid in nature, may occur throughout the first few postoperative weeks. The physician may prescribe irrigations of the IAR in order to remove foul-smelling mucous secretions. When the IAR is completely healed, usually 8 to 10 weeks after the initial surgery, the temporary ileostomy is closed. Fecal output from the anus usually begins within 2 to 3 days. Fecal drainage is in fact ileostomy drainage via the rectum, so perianal skin irritation is a common complication of this procedure. Skin sealants and moisture barrier products must be used to prevent breakdown. Toilet paper and soap should not be used to cleanse the perianal area. Baby wipes provide a convenient, soothing method for cleansing. Soft tissues moistened with water can also be used to dab the perianal area clean. Initially the patient will have frequent bowel movements (10 to 12 a day), but the frequency should decrease over time. Patients often take a fiber supplement or an antidiarrheal such as Lomotil or Imodium to add bulk to the stool and to slow peristalsis to allow for more water to be absorbed before defecation.

Two other surgical alternatives, total colectomy with ileorectal anastomosis and total colectomy with ileoanal anastomosis, are available but have some major disadvantages. With the ileorectal anastomosis procedure, because the rectum is left intact, recurrence of the disease is possible and continued surveillance for rectal cancer is required. The major disadvantage of the ileoanal anastomosis procedure is the high frequency of stool evacuation resulting in subsequent perianal skin irritation or breakdown.

Pouchitis (inflammation of the pouch) can occur in patients with either a continent pouch ileostomy or an ileoanal reservoir. Symptoms associated with pouchitis are new onset of frequent bowel movements, pain, fecal urgency, and bleeding. The condition is usually treated with antibiotics.

### Nursing interventions

*Diet.* A diet high in protein, calories, and vitamins and minerals is encouraged. Foods that are high in fat, fiber, and residue are usually avoided. Because the appetite is poor, the patient needs encouragement to eat, and consideration should be given to the patient's food desires because he or she will often know which foods cause the most discomfort. Patients who are severely malnourished may require TPN.

*Psychosocial support.* The psychologic care of the patient with ulcerative colitis requires the empathic understanding of everyone concerned with his or her care. A thoughtfully prepared nursing care plan designed to provide for continuity of care is important in meeting the patient's needs for a feeling of security and a sense of well-being. Because the patient's behavior may be characterized by periods of depression and changes in mood, the nurse must be prepared to accept such changes and continue to provide personalized nursing care. The nurse should refer the patient to support groups for patients with IBD.

If medical management is unsuccessful, surgery is indicated to remove the diseased colon. Surgical alternatives for the patient with ulcerative colitis include colectomy with the creation of a permanent ileostomy, colectomy with the creation of a continent reservoir (Kock pouch), colectomy with the creation of an ileoanal reservoir, or colectomy with an ileoanal anastomosis. The decision to treat the patient medically or surgically is dependent on the severity of the disease, the patient's age, and the patient's preference.

*Patient and family teaching.* Because of the chronicity of IBD, patient teaching is integral to successful disease management. The patient is instructed on how to control diet and stress to reduce acute exacerbations of the disease. The nurse and dietitian work with the patient to make a list of do's and dont's for eating (e.g., do eat small frequent meals and eat food high in carbohydrates, proteins, and minerals; don't eat foods high in fat, fried foods, spicy foods, milk and milk products, raw vegetables, fruits, nuts, or whole grains). A complete and balanced dietary plan can be developed that incorporates the patient's food preferences.

The patient is taught the expected actions of medications in controlling the symptoms of the disease, as well as how to monitor response to the medical treatment. Instructing the patient in stress management techniques is a valuable adjunct to the medical and surgical management of IBD.

## Crohn's Disease

Crohn's disease is a chronic, progressive inflammatory disease that can affect any part of the GI tract from the mouth to the anus but most commonly involves the small and large intestines. The most common symptoms of Crohn's disease include abdominal pain and diarrhea. Although the mortality rate is low, the disease often results in a significant alteration in lifestyle and requires chronic medical therapy and sometimes surgery. All layers of the bowel wall are affected by this disease. The course of the disease is characterized by periods of acute disease and periods of remission.

Inflammatory lesions tend to appear in patches, with normal segments interspersed between diseased segments. It has been suggested that Crohn's disease is a disorder of the lymphoid tissue. This would explain the frequent involvement of the terminal ileum and anus, both of which have a rich lymph supply.

In addition to pain and diarrhea, fever, anorexia, weight loss, and malnutrition are commonly seen. Extension of the ulcerative lesions through all layers of the bowel predisposes the patient to abscess and fistula formation. Fistulae often involve other loops of the small intestine, the colon, the bladder, the vagina, or even the abdominal wall. Anal fissures, perianal abscesses, and partial bowel obstruction are other complications associated with Crohn's disease.

This disease occurs most often in young adults, and there is a higher incidence among Jews. The disease often results in disability and incapacity and requires long medical or surgical treatment. Crohn's disease is also associated with complications affecting other areas of the body—arthritis, kidney stones, gallstones, cutaneous manifestation of the disease (pyoderma gangrenosum), and inflammation of the eyes.

**Assessment.** The symptoms are mild and intermittent at first. Exacerbations often follow dietary indiscretions (e.g., milk, milk products, fatty foods), emotional upsets, or illness. Abdominal pain, cramping, tenderness, flatulence, nausea, fever, and diarrhea will occur in an acute attack. The more typical picture is the chronic type with diarrhea accompanied by mild pain. It may be aggravated by illness or emotional upsets but is usually less severe than diarrhea associated with ulcerative colitis. The stool is usually soft or semiliquid and may be quite foul smelling and fatty. Urgency to expel stools may awaken the patient at night. A large amount of flatus is also likely to be present. The passing of gross blood is rare and would indicate extensive ulceration.

Diagnosis of Crohn's disease is made by a series of x-ray examinations, including an upper GI series (barium swallow) and a barium enema. Colonoscopy with tissue sampling is used to confirm the diagnosis and to rule out other diseases such as ulcerative colitis or diverticulitis.

The nurse monitors the patient for the occurrence and severity of signs and symptoms of active disease, including abdominal pain, diarrhea, and fever. In addition the nurse works with the patient to try to identify factors that may have triggered an exacerbation.

The nurse assesses the patient for signs and symptoms of complications from Crohn's disease, including malnutrition, bowel obstruction, bowel perforation, and fistula formation.

**Interventions.** Treatment of Crohn's disease is neither specific nor curative but is supportive and palliative and is aimed at attaining remission of the disease. Goals of treatment are reducing inflammation and controlling symptoms. Medical treatment initially attempts to reduce active inflammation and is more likely to be successful early in the course of the disease before permanent structural changes have developed. Loperamide hydrochloride (Imodium) is used to treat abdominal cramping and diarrhea. As with ulcerative colitis, antiinflammatory (prednisone) and immunosuppressive (azathioprine) agents are used in the treatment plan. Although the exact mechanism of action in Crohn's disease is unknown, metronidazole (Flagyl) may also be used; it is suspected that the drug acts as an immunosuppressant. Following recent clinical trials, mesalamine (Pentasa) is used to reduce inflamma-

tion. Its antiprostaglandin activity is thought to be the effective action.

Nutritional support and dietary modifications are part of the treatment plan in Crohn's disease. A low-roughage, low-residue diet will reduce the diarrhea associated with the inflammatory process. Surgical intervention as a treatment for Crohn's disease is delayed until symptoms can no longer be controlled or significant complications have developed. Surgical treatment is aimed at correcting complications or removal of the affected portion of the intestinal tract or both. Strictures may require surgical treatment with stricturoplasty to increase the diameter of the bowel or resection to remove the stricture. An ostomy is performed only when the rectum and anus must be bypassed temporarily or removed (Doughty, 1994). Nursing interventions are centered around rest, relief of pain and diarrhea, monitoring response to drug therapy, patient education, and psychologic support.

## Appendicitis

One of the most common causes of an acute abdominal condition is appendicitis. The risk of fatal complications is increased when treatment is delayed. Factors that have helped reduce deaths from appendicitis during past years include early recognition of the disease, improvement in surgical techniques and anesthesia, the use of antibiotics, and intensive nursing care.

**Pathophysiology.** Appendicitis is an inflammation of the vermiform appendix, a projection of bowel tissue located at the apex of the cecum where the small and large intestine meet. The lumen of the proximal end of the appendix is shared with that of the cecum, whereas the distal end is closed. The walls of the appendix contain lymphoid cells, and, although the appendix has been generally considered to have no specific function, it is now believed to share with other lymphoid tissues of the body the function of preventing infection. The appendix fills and empties regularly in the same way as the cecum. However, the lumen is narrow and is easily obstructed. It is most commonly believed that appendicitis develops as a result of an obstruction of the lumen of the appendix and subsequent bacterial overgrowth. When the lumen becomes obstructed, the blood supply is disrupted, the appendix becomes distended and hypoxic, and inflammation occurs. Pathogenic bacteria present in the intestinal tract, often *Escherichia coli,* begin to multiply in the appendix, and infection develops with the formation of pus. If distention and infection are severe enough, the appendix may perforate, with spillage of intestinal contents and bacteria into the peritoneum. If this occurs, the infectious material may be walled off and the infection localized with an appendiceal abscess. If it is not localized, the infectious material spreads to the abdominal cavity and generalized peritonitis occurs. Perforation with subsequent peritonitis and abscess formation is the most serious consequence of acute appendicitis.

> ### NURSE ALERT
>
> **Patients who are suspected to have appendicitis should not be given cathartics or enemas. These agents could increase the pressure within the bowel lumen and cause a perforation.**

**Assessment.** Diagnosis of acute appendicitis is made based on the presence of a typical pattern of signs and symptoms. The symptoms most characteristic of acute appendicitis are pain, fever, elevated WBC, anorexia, and nausea and vomiting. Pain may be felt in the lower right quadrant of the abdomen, halfway between the umbilicus and the crest of the ileum *(McBurney's point)*, or experienced near the umbilicus. *Rebound tenderness* in the right lower quadrant may be present (Figure 35-12).

**Interventions.** Surgical removal of the appendix (appendectomy) is the definitive treatment for acute appendicitis. The procedure may be performed as an emergency operation. When appendicitis is suspected, surgery is usually done as soon as the diagnosis has been completed to prevent rupture and complications.

In a clean appendectomy (without rupture), recovery is usually rapid. The patient is discharged from the hospital quickly, often within 24 hours, and may re-

sume most normal activities within 5 to 7 days. If the appendix has ruptured before surgical intervention, intraoperative irrigations with balanced electrolyte and antibiotic solutions are used to cleanse the peritoneal cavity of intestinal spillage. Drains are often placed in the wound, and the wound is left open to heal by secondary intention to prevent abscess formation.

> ### NURSE ALERT
>
> **To test for the presence of rebound tenderness, the patient is placed in a supine position. The fingertips are extended at a 90-degree angle directly over the abdomen in an area away from the suspected area of tenderness. The fingers should be gently pressed deep into the abdomen and removed quickly. Quick removal of the fingers causes the abdominal organs to rebound to their normal position. If the patient has rebound tenderness, a sharp pain will be felt in the area of peritoneal irritation.**

The nurse closely monitors the patient for signs and symptoms of local and systemic infection following surgery for a ruptured appendix. Specific attention is given to monitoring temperature, heart rate, WBC count, pain, the appearance of the surgical wound, and the presence and characteristics of any wound drainage (Box 35-14).

Postoperative care is directed toward preventing wound infection and pulmonary complications. Ambu-

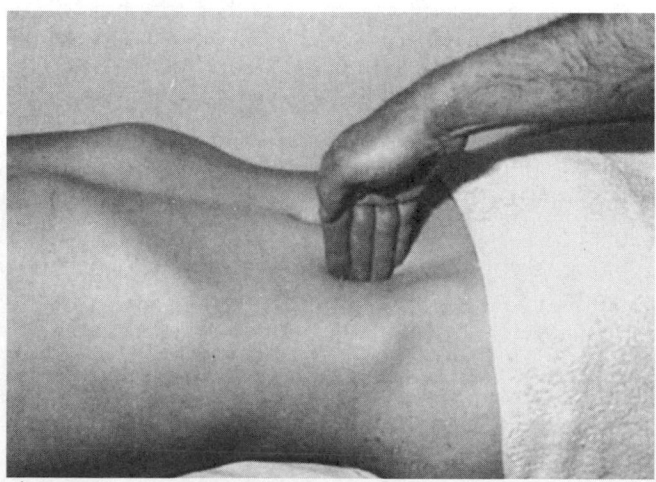
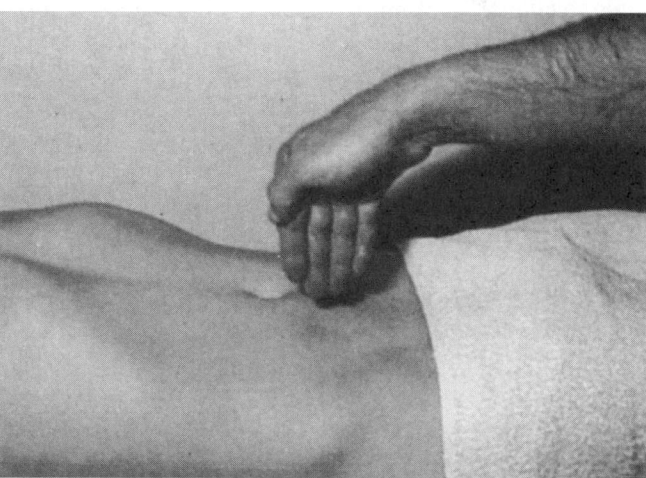

**Figure 35-12**  Testing for rebound tenderness. (From Seidel HM et al: *Mosby's guide to physical examination,* ed 3, St Louis, 1995, Mosby.)

lation usually begins the day of surgery. When drainage is necessary because of an abscess, dressings must be changed as necessary and disposed of carefully.

**Patient and family teaching.** Before being discharged from the hospital, the patient is taught how to assess the wound for signs and symptoms of infection, including redness, tenderness, and drainage, and to report these findings. Patients may require specific wound care instructions if the surgical wound is not closed before discharge. Any limitation on physical activity, especially lifting, is carefully explained.

## Peritonitis

Peritonitis is an inflammation of the peritoneum and the abdominal cavity and is a complication of a bacterial, fungal, or yeast infection. Infection may develop the leakage of GI contents into the peritoneum from a perforated or ruptured area. It may be caused by infection from the internal female organs. Although in-

frequent, it may occur from trauma to abdominal organs or may be carried by infection in the bloodstream. Peritonitis can also occur as a complication of peritoneal dialysis.

Every patient who has surgery of the GI tract is at risk for developing peritonitis. The inflammatory process may be localized, with abscess formation, or it may be generalized, with bacteria spreading throughout the entire abdominal cavity. Sometimes peritonitis occurs without any known cause.

**Assessment.** Generalized peritonitis is an extremely serious condition characterized mainly by severe abdominal pain. The patient usually lies on his or her back or side with the knees flexed to relax the abdominal muscles because any movement is painful. Nausea and vomiting occur. Constipation or diarrhea may occur early, but, as the condition progresses, peristalsis ceases and paralytic ileus develops. The abdomen becomes distended, tense, rigid, and very tender. The pulse is weak and rapid, and blood pressure falls. Leukocytosis

---

| BOX 35-14 | NURSING PROCESS |
| --- | --- |

### APPENDICITIS AND APPENDECTOMY

**ASSESSMENT**
**Preoperative**

- Abdominal pain
- Bowel sounds
- Contour, firmness, and rebound tenderness
- Vital signs
- Anorexia, nausea, or vomiting
- Whole blood cell count

**Postoperative**

- Vital signs
- Comfort level
- Fluid volume status
- Respiratory status
- Abdomen for bowel sounds, contour, firmness
- Surgical incision and drains, if present

**NURSING DIAGNOSES**

- Pain related to inflammation or surgery
- Risk for infection related to perforation of appendix
- Risk for fluid volume deficit related to preoperative vomiting, surgery, or third spacing
- Ineffective breathing pattern related to pain and analgesic effect
- Knowledge deficit related to new diagnosis, home care needs

**NURSING INTERVENTIONS**

- Administer analgesics as ordered.
- Provide comfort measures.
- Administer antibiotics if ordered.
- Provide aseptic wound care.
- Administer intravenous fluids as prescribed.
- Advance diet slowly; when oral intake is initiated, start with clear liquids.
- Maintain accurate input and output records.
- Encourage coughing, deep breathing, and ambulation.
- Instruct on splinting of incision with movement and cough.
- Help patient turn every 2 hours while in bed.
- Refer to visiting nurse for assistance with dressing changes if indicated.

**EVALUATION OF EXPECTED OUTCOMES**

- Evidence of wound healing without purulent drainage and erythema
- Temperature within normal limits
- No evidence of respiratory distress
- Lungs clear
- Tolerating diet without distress
- Tolerating diet without nausea
- Pain level acceptable
- Return to preoperative self-care level
- Bowel function returns

and marked dehydration occur. Without quick and appropriate intervention, early death may occur.

**Interventions.** Interventions for peritonitis include antibiotics to treat infection, fluid and electrolyte replacement, pain management, and relief of paralytic ileus. The patient is placed in a semi-Fowler's position for comfort. Pain medication, preferably morphine, is administered to relieve pain. The patient is maintained NPO. A nasogastric tube is inserted and connected to suction to keep the stomach empty and to help relieve the ileus. Intravenous fluids are administered to prevent dehydration and to maintain electrolyte balance. Antibiotic therapy is started. A broad-spectrum antibiotic is usually used until the exact infectious agent is identified through cultures. Further care or indications for surgery depend on the cause of the peritonitis and the patient's condition.

The nurse monitors all vital signs, including blood pressure, heart rate, and temperature, and examines the abdomen for distention, pain, and the presence of bowel sounds. In addition, the nurse carefully monitors and records all intake and output, including intravenous fluids, vomitus or NG drainage, and urine. The patient is observed for pain, and the type of pain and its location are described, recorded, and reported. The patient often realizes the seriousness of this condition, and the nurse should facilitate expression of fears by providing emotional support.

## Hernia

A **hernia** is the projection of a loop of an organ, tissue, or structure through a congenital or acquired defect. Most hernias have their origin in the abdomen.

One type of hernia is the *umbilical hernia,* which is often seen in infants as the result of a congenital weakness of the abdominal wall. A *femoral hernia,* more common in women, occurs at the point where the femoral artery passes into the femoral canal. An *inguinal hernia,* seen more commonly in men, occurs when part of the intestine projects through the inguinal canal. Hernias may also develop at the site of an incision *(incisional hernia);* they develop because of impaired wound healing. If the protruding structure can be returned by manipulation to its own cavity, it is called a reducible hernia. If it cannot, it is called an irreducible or *incarcerated* hernia. The size of the defect through which the organ passes largely determines whether the hernia can be reduced. When the blood supply to the structure within the hernia becomes occluded, the hernia is said to be *strangulated* and gangrene may result, requiring immediate surgery.

**Assessment.** There may be no symptoms associated with a hernia other than swelling or protrusion on the abdomen or groin when the patient coughs, stands, lifts heavy objects, or strains in any other way. The nurse looks for maneuvers that contribute to the protrusion, the degree (size) of the protrusion, and any pain noted with the hernia. Pain is an ominous sign with hernias and usually signals the need for surgical intervention.

**Interventions.** The treatment of choice for all hernias is surgery. However, because of risk factors surgery is sometimes inadvisable. If surgery is not performed, an abdominal binder, a girdle, or a mechanical appliance called a *truss* may provide some relief and prevent the hernia from enlarging.

The surgical procedure for repair of a hernia is called *herniorrhaphy.* To prevent recurrence of the hernia and facilitate closure of the defect, a *hernioplasty* may be performed, using fascia, filigree wire, mesh, or a variety of plastic materials to strengthen the muscle wall.

The preoperative care for the patient needing hernia repair is the same as that for any uncomplicated abdominal surgery. Postoperative care includes prevention of wound infection and avoidance of any strain on the wound for approximately 2 weeks. Early ambulation is encouraged to prevent abdominal distention. Food and fluids are usually permitted as soon as nausea ceases. Any evidence of abdominal distention or coughing after hernia repair is reported to the physician immediately. Hernia repair is generally performed in an ambulatory surgical center. The repair is completed in the morning, and the patient rests at home in the evening.

After repair of an inguinal hernia, tenderness and swelling of the scrotum may be reduced by applying ice packs. If scrotal edema does occur, the use of a suspensory belt may provide some relief. The urinary output is watched because retention sometimes occurs and catheterization may be necessary.

**Patient and family teaching.** The patient is instructed to avoid any strenuous activity, including lifting, to prevent recurrence of the hernia. The physician will advise the patient when normal activity can be resumed. Discharge instruction must also include a plan

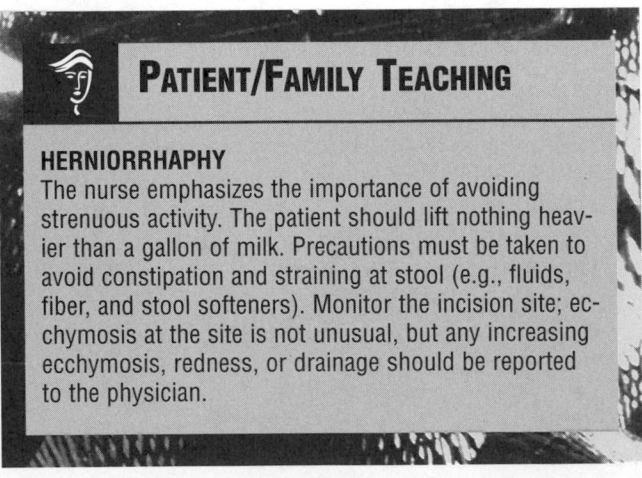

**PATIENT/FAMILY TEACHING**

**HERNIORRHAPHY**
The nurse emphasizes the importance of avoiding strenuous activity. The patient should lift nothing heavier than a gallon of milk. Precautions must be taken to avoid constipation and straining at stool (e.g., fluids, fiber, and stool softeners). Monitor the incision site; ecchymosis at the site is not unusual, but any increasing ecchymosis, redness, or drainage should be reported to the physician.

for avoiding constipation (straining). Increased fluids (6 to 8 glasses of water a day) and a balanced diet rich in bulk and fiber will help prevent constipation. Stool softeners or bulk-forming agents may be needed.

## Intestinal Obstruction

An obstruction of the small or large intestine may occur when any condition exists that prevents the free passage of bowel contents through the intestine. The obstruction may be partial or complete, but it is always considered serious. Some intestinal obstructions resolve or correct with only conservative medical treatment, whereas others require surgical intervention.

**Pathophysiology.** An intestinal obstruction has many causes, some of which include a strangulated hernia, volvulus (twisting of the bowel), cancer, postoperative adhesions, paralytic ileus, and stricture. The most common causes are postoperative adhesions and hernia. Obstruction may occur in the small or the large intestine. Obstruction in the large intestine is less dramatic than in the small intestine. Most obstructions occur in the small intestine and affect the normal homeostasis of the body. The continuous vomiting associated with small bowel obstruction causes loss of electrolytes and loss of hydrochloric acid from the stomach, leading to alkalosis. The loss of water and sodium from the body may cause acidosis and severe dehydration.

**Assessment.** The symptoms of obstruction vary according to location and extent of the obstruction. When the obstruction is high in the small intestine, symptoms appear earlier and are more acute than when the large intestine is obstructed. The early symptoms are abdominal pain, abdominal distention, vomiting, and constipation. The pain is often wavelike, and vomiting may be projectile. The gastric contents are first vomited, but, as peristalsis is reversed, bile and fecal matter from above the obstruction are vomited. When the obstruction is in the colon, vomiting may not occur. The patient may eliminate blood or mucus via the rectum, but no fecal matter or flatus passes if the obstruction is complete. Extreme thirst occurs; the tongue and mucous membranes of the mouth and lips become parched. Abdominal distention develops and is greater when the obstruction is in the colon. Signs of shock may appear, and, without treatment, the patient may die within a few hours.

**Interventions.** A nasogastric tube is inserted and attached to low suction to remove intestinal secretions and gas that have accumulated proximal to the obstruction. Some physicians may insert a long intestinal decompression tube, such as the Miller-Abbott, instead of the nasogastric tube. The patency of the tube is checked often and is maintained by irrigating the tube every 1 to 2 hours with 30 ml of normal saline.

The volume, characteristics, and consistency of the drainage are observed and recorded. Drainage is tested for the presence of blood (refer to the section on gastric decompression). A long intestinal decompression tube is intended to travel down the intestinal tract and should never be taped. The patient is given nothing by mouth. Intravenous fluids are administered to correct the dehydration and replace the electrolytes lost through vomiting or intestinal drainage. All vomitus or drainage is accurately described, and any fecal matter should be saved to be examined for occult blood.

Temperature, heart rate, blood pressure, and respiratory rate are taken at least every 4 hours; more frequent assessments are made if the patient exhibits signs of hypovolemic shock. The nurse may elevate the head of the bed 30 to 40 degrees to prevent respiratory difficulty that might occur as a result of abdominal distention, to help prevent aspiration, and to encourage passage of small intestine contents into the colon. Careful records of urinary output are maintained, and, if retention occurs, the patient should be catheterized. The patient is assisted with frequent cleansing of the mouth and changes in position. The environment is kept well ventilated and free of odors through prompt disposal of vomitus and the use of a deodorizer as necessary.

Surgery for intestinal obstruction depends partly on the cause of the obstruction, its location, and the condition of the patient. In some cases surgery may be relatively simple, whereas in other situations the cause may complicate the surgical procedure. In obstructions resulting from a strangulated hernia, cutting off the blood supply may have caused the bowel to become gangrenous, and resection of the affected bowel may be necessary. Before surgery, the patient may be given a small enema under low pressure. Intravenous fluids are administered to replace electrolytes lost through vomiting, and TPN may be initiated to provide nutritional elements. After surgery, if the bowel has been resected, oral feeding is withheld to give the anastomosis time to heal. A nasogastric tube attached to suction aids in keeping the stomach empty. Accurate intake and output records are maintained. Other postoperative care is the same as that for any abdominal surgery.

## Diverticular Disease
## (Diverticulosis and Diverticulitis)

A *diverticulum* is a pouch or sac arising from any tubular structure. Diverticula (plural of diverticulum) most frequently occur within the lumen of the large intestine, most commonly in the sigmoid area, but they may also occur in the esophagus, the stomach, and the small intestine. A *true diverticulum* involves all tissues layers of the GI tract, mucosa, submucosa, muscularis, and serosa. With a *false diverticulum* the mucosa and submucosa layers protrude or herniate through weak points in the muscular layer of the GI tract (Figure 35-13). Diverticula are rarely seen in persons younger than age 40, but it is estimated that one of every three persons over age 60 has some diverticula. There is increasing evidence that a low-fiber diet contributes to the development of diverticula. The disease was recognized in the United States just about the same time that processed foods were introduced and is common in industrialized nations where low-fiber diets are the norm. However, the disease is rare in countries where the general diet is rich in fiber. *Diverticulosis* refers to multiple *diverticula* scattered throughout the colon. **Diverticulitis** occurs when fecal matter penetrates the thin-walled diverticula, resulting in inflammation and abscess formation outside the bowel.

**Pathophysiology.** The exact cause of diverticular disease is unknown, but there appears to be a strong correlation with factors that contribute to increased colonic pressure and weakened points in the muscle wall of the colon. The role of diet in the development and progression of the disease is also a factor.

Diverticula develop when the muscles of the colon hypertrophy or become thickened. Both the circular and longitudinal muscles and the muscular fibers (teniae coli) are involved. Small sacs develop between these circular fibers. Increased pressure in the colon results in the protrusion of mucosa through the weakened muscle in the sacs, resulting in diverticula. Once diverticula develop, there is the possibility that the protrusion will continue and inflammation and perforation of the sac will occur, resulting in diverticulitis. This complication can be in the form of microperforations into the fat layer around the bowel or larger macroperforations opening into the peritoneal space. Microperforations result in the formation of abscesses and localized peritonitis. Macroperforations produce severe, generalized peritonitis. The body responds as it does to any inflammatory process, with pain, fever, and elevated WBC. Complications of diverticulitis include fistulas, abscesses, perforation, obstruction, bleeding, peritonitis, and septicemia.

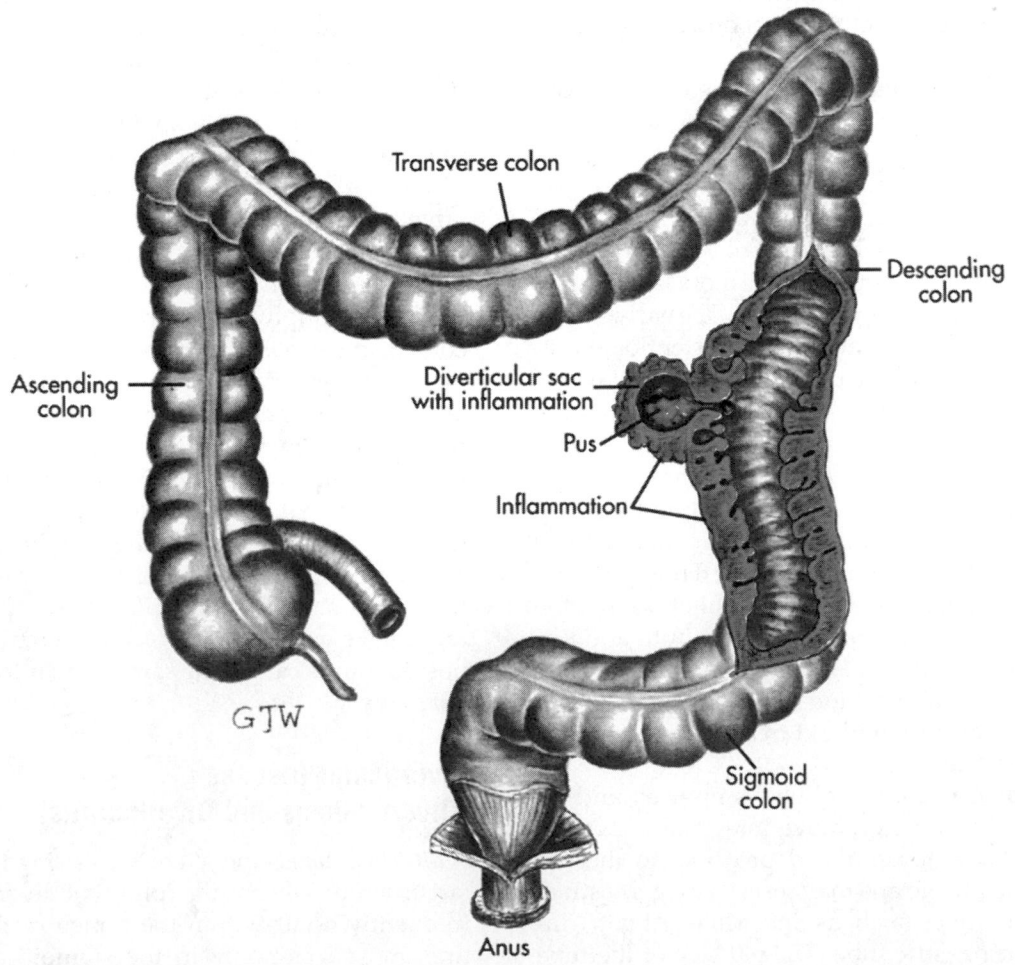

**Figure 35-13** Diverticula located in the descending colon. (From Doughty DB, Jackson DB: *Gastrointestinal disorders*, St Louis, 1993, Mosby.)

Those who theorize that diet plays a role in diverticular disease believe that a diet low in fiber causes muscle thickening that predisposes the individual to formation of diverticula. Reduced fiber in the diet results in less bulk in the stool. The lumen of the bowel is not forced to widen, and the pressure within that lumen is therefore increased (intracolonic pressure). The sigmoid is normally the narrowest segment of the large bowel and the most common site of diverticula. Fiber also affects stool transit time, the time it takes for stool to move through the bowel. Stool that moves faster will have less water absorbed and will thus be softer and easier to eliminate. Increased intracolonic pressure is believed to be the cause of the muscle hypertrophy that leads to the formation of diverticula.

**Assessment.** The patient with diverticulosis may not display any symptoms. Diarrhea, constipation, distention, or flatulence, along with mild to moderate complaints of cramping pain over the lower abdomen, are associated with diverticulosis. When diverticula perforate and diverticulitis develops, the patient will complain of mild to severe pain in the lower left quadrant of the abdomen and will have fever and an elevated WBC and sedimentation rate. If the condition goes untreated, septicemia and septic shock can develop. The septic patient will be hypotensive, have a rapid pulse rate and rapid respiratory rate, and may have a change in mental status. If obstruction occurs the patient will experience abdominal distention, nausea, and vomiting. Hemorrhage occurs in approximately 10% to 20% of patients; it may be mild and go unnoticed for some time or be severe and result in shock.

**Interventions.** Management of diverticulosis includes a high-fiber diet, including vegetables, fruits, and whole grains; fiber supplements (if needed); and a bulk-forming laxative. If mild to moderate inflammation develops, the treatment plan will change to a low-fiber diet and, likely, antibiotics. In more severe cares, the patient will require hospitalization, with intravenous fluid replacements and gastric decompression as necessary, and intravenous antibiotics. Microperforation resulting in localized abscess is treated with a combination of antibiotics effective against gram-negative, gram-positive, and anaerobic organisms. Fluids and electrolytes must be administered intravenously, and a nasogastric tube is inserted and attached to suction. Analgesics, usually morphine sulfate or meperidine, are given to manage pain. Surgical intervention is indicated for repeated bouts of diverticulitis, especially if the acute exacerbation results in a partial bowel obstruction. Macroperforations always require surgical intervention. A temporary or permanent colostomy or bowel resection with a reanastomosis may be performed, depending on the severity of the disease and the extent of complications.

Nursing intervention includes monitoring vital signs and fluid balance, providing relief of pain, and assessing the response to treatment. The patient is observed closely for signs of septicemia and shock. The schedule for antibiotic therapy is carefully followed. When surgery is necessary, nursing interventions follow the recommendations for the specific procedure performed (Box 35-15).

**Patient and family teaching.** Patients are taught the importance of dietary control of diverticular disease. Working with the patient, the nurse and the dietitian develop a dietary plan based on the stage of the disease. Diverticulosis is managed with a diet rich in fiber and whole grains. During episodes of acute inflammation, however, modifications in diet are needed. A low-fiber diet is used during these episodes to decrease irritation and minimize inflammation.

Patients are instructed on the importance of avoiding constipation through diet and fluid intake in order to avoid high intracolonic pressures that occur with straining at stool.

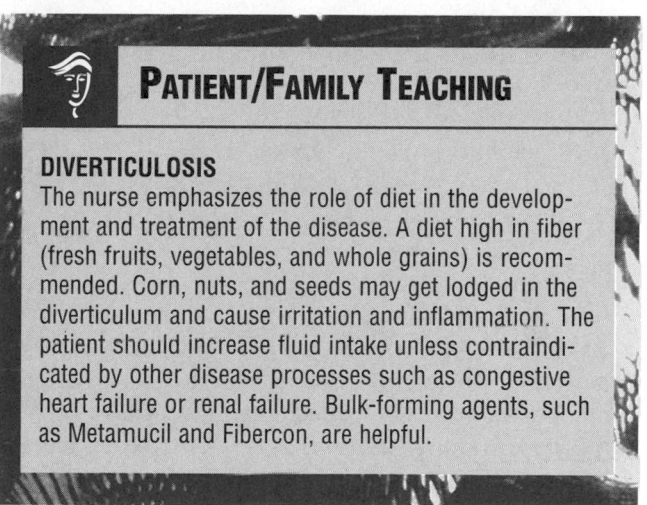

**PATIENT/FAMILY TEACHING**

**DIVERTICULOSIS**
The nurse emphasizes the role of diet in the development and treatment of the disease. A diet high in fiber (fresh fruits, vegetables, and whole grains) is recommended. Corn, nuts, and seeds may get lodged in the diverticulum and cause irritation and inflammation. The patient should increase fluid intake unless contraindicated by other disease processes such as congestive heart failure or renal failure. Bulk-forming agents, such as Metamucil and Fibercon, are helpful.

## Hemorrhoids

*Hemorrhoids* are dilated veins similar to varicose veins. They may occur outside the anal sphincter as external hemorrhoids or inside the sphincter as internal hemorrhoids. The small, bluish lumps characteristic of external hemorrhoids may disappear spontaneously, leaving a small skin tag. Occasionally the hemorrhoid will become thrombosed, and a blood clot will develop within the vein. In addition to hemorrhoids, anal fissures (cracks in the mucous membrane) and an anal fistula (a duct extending from one tissue surface to another) may be present. Hemorrhoids result from numerous factors, including prolonged constipation, heavy lifting, straining in an effort to defecate, and pregnancy or large pelvic tumors. Certain forms of liver disease and high blood pressure may also contribute to the disorder.

---

◄ **BOX 35-15** ► **NURSING PROCESS**

## DIVERTICULOSIS AND DIVERTICULITIS

**ASSESSMENT**

- Vital signs
- Abdomen for pain, bowel sounds, contour, firmness
- Dietary history
- Patterns of elimination
- Laboratory studies (whole blood cell count and sedimentation rate)

**NURSING DIAGNOSES**

- Pain related to bowel inflammation or micro-perforation
- Risk for infection related to bowel microperforation
- Risk for injury: peritonitis related to bowel perforation
- Constipation related to inadequate diet or fluid intake
- Anxiety related to life-style modification
- Knowledge deficit related to causative factors of disease and dietary modifications

**NURSING INTERVENTIONS**

- Provide comfort measures.
- Medicate as needed with analgesics.

- Promote relaxation and diversional activities.
- Administer intravenous fluid as ordered.
- Administer antibiotics as ordered.
- Provide dietary modification depending on acuity of illness (acute diverticulitis, nothing by mouth to clear liquids to low-fiber diet; diverticulitis, high-fiber diet).
- Refer to dietitian if indicated.
- Encourage liberal fluid intake if not contraindicated.
- Spend time providing emotional support.
- Encourage ventilation of feelings, fears, concerns.

**EVALUATION OF EXPECTED OUTCOMES**

- Absence of abdominal pain
- No evidence of infectious process
- Soft, formed bowel movements
- Patient identifies symptoms that indicate need for medical treatment
- Patient states necessary dietary modifications

---

**Assessment.** Symptoms may include an awareness of a mass in the rectum near the anus. Constipation is almost always present. Bleeding may occur and will appear as bright red blood that is not mixed with feces. The dilated veins may become thrombosed, causing severe pain. Although hemorrhoids rarely become malignant, bleeding and constipation are symptoms of cancer of the rectum. For this reason, all patients with these symptoms should have a thorough examination to rule out cancer, including a sigmoidoscopy and barium enema. Hemorrhoids do resolve without medical or surgical care. Individuals are often reluctant to talk about the problem and may delay seeking health care.

**Interventions.** When the patient comes in for an examination, the nurse should be aware that this has been a difficult decision and should assure the patient of absolute privacy and should protect the patient's self-respect. Medical treatment consists of warm compresses to stimulate circulation and healing and analgesic ointments such as dibucaine (Nupercaine). Sitz baths help to reduce pain and edema, and bulk stool softeners such as Metamucil or Fibercon, bran, and other natural food fibers are recommended to assist in

the passage of fecal material. Steroid suppositories may be given to relieve inflammation. External hemorrhoids are usually excised as an outpatient procedure. Internal hemorrhoids occasionally are treated with the injection of a solution that will cause sclerosing or hardening of the dilated vein. This causes the vein to shrink and adhere to underlying muscles as it heals with fibrous tissue.

Internal hemorrhoids may also be treated by ligating them with rubber bands. Tight bands are applied that cause constriction, necrosis, sloughing, and scarring. Fixation to underlying muscle is also accomplished with infrared photocoagulation, in which the tissue is destroyed by creating a small burn to cause inflammation. Scarring cryotherapy destroys the tissues by freezing. The Nd:YAG laser is also used for fixation and excision of hemorrhoids.

***Hemorrhoidectomy.*** Standard treatment involves surgical excision of the hemorrhoid (hemorrhoidectomy), leaving the wounds open or closed. A laxative may be given before surgery. After surgery the patient is often positioned on the stomach. If positioned on the back, buttock support is provided. Following surgery the pain may be acute, and narcotics may be given and analgesic ointments applied. Sitz baths are recommended to relieve pain and promote healing. If a spontaneous bowel elimination does not occur within 3 days, an oil retention enema may be given, followed by a cleansing enema. Dressings may or may not be used. Difficulty in voiding may occur. A soft diet is permitted on the evening of the surgery; a full diet is given on the first postoperative day. The patient is advised to include fiber and plenty of fluids and to exercise moderately to promote regular bowel function.

## Cancer of the Small Intestine

Malignant lesions develop less often in the small intestine than in other segments of the gastrointestinal tract. Symptoms, which include intestinal obstruction, bleeding, and upper abdominal pain, do not appear early in the course of the disease. Treatment is surgical removal of the tumor. The prognosis is poor because these tumors tend to metastasize early into the liver and local lymph nodes. A considerable portion of the bowel wall becomes involved before symptoms appear, making early diagnosis almost impossible.

## Colorectal Cancer

Cancers of the colon and rectum are the most prevalent internal cancers in the United States, occurring equally in men and women. Early detection and treatment lead to a good prognosis, but most patients are still diagnosed and operated on late in the course of the disease. Etiologic factors are not definite, but certain conditions appear to be more prone to malignant changes, including ulcerative colitis and diverticulosis. Evidence suggests that a low-fiber diet is related to the development of cancers of the colon and rectum. A diet rich in beef and saturated fats also appears to lead to an increased incidence of colorectal cancer. It is theorized that carcinogens are formed from degraded bile salts and that stool, which remains in the large bowel for a longer period as a result of too little fiber to stimulate its passage, may overexpose the bowel to these carcinogens. Another theory relates diverticulosis to low-fiber diets, proposing that the lack of fiber necessitates stronger muscle contractions to excrete hard stools, increasing pressure on the colon wall, which leads to outpouching, or diverticula. Thus the reduced weight of stool and the increased time it takes for stool to pass (transit time), which result from a low-fiber diet have been related to both diverticulosis and cancer of the colon. As stated earlier, the individual with diverticulosis is already considered more prone to malignant changes.

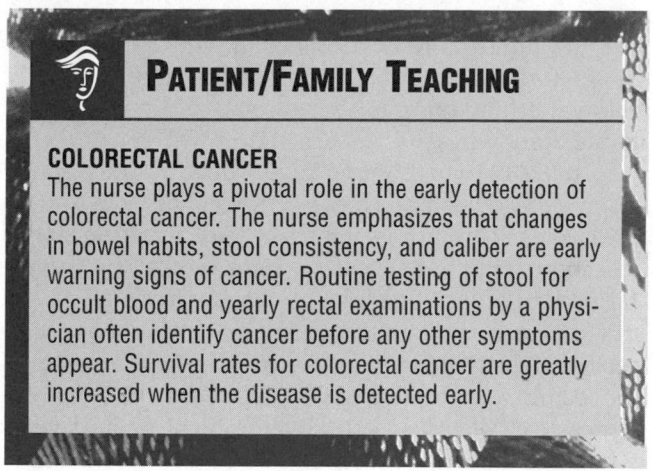

### PATIENT/FAMILY TEACHING

**COLORECTAL CANCER**
The nurse plays a pivotal role in the early detection of colorectal cancer. The nurse emphasizes that changes in bowel habits, stool consistency, and caliber are early warning signs of cancer. Routine testing of stool for occult blood and yearly rectal examinations by a physician often identify cancer before any other symptoms appear. Survival rates for colorectal cancer are greatly increased when the disease is detected early.

**Assessment.** Symptoms relate to the area of the colon and rectum involved in the disease. Rectal bleeding is still the most common symptom. Alternating constipation and diarrhea is common, along with excessive flatus, cramping pains in the lower abdomen, and abdominal distention. Obstruction is most likely to occur if the tumor is on the right side or in the transverse colon. The individual may complain of weakness, loss of appetite, and weight loss, and anemia may be present. Hemorrhoids and cancer often coexist. Rectal bleeding can never be assumed to be the result of hemorrhoids alone without an examination that rules out cancer.

The diagnosis is made on the basis of abdominal and rectal examinations, which include a barium enema and a GI series, colonoscopy, biopsy, and examination of stool for occult blood. Three fourths of all colon and rectum cancers can be detected with the aid of a colonoscopy, and it is important to include this examination in the routine physical examination for all adults over 50 years of age. Any change in normal bowel habits should be reported to the physician. The American Cancer Society (ACS) recommends early screening for colorectal cancer beginning at age 50 for both men and women. ACS recommends a yearly examination for fecal occult blood plus a sigmoidoscopy and digital rectal examination every 5 years. As alternatives to these screening measures, the ACS endorses either colonoscopy and digital rectal examination every 10 years, or a barium enema and digital rectal examination every 5 to 10 years. Individuals with a family history of colorectal cancer or polyps or a personal history of inflammatory bowel disease should begin cancer screening at an earlier age.

**Interventions.** Curative treatment is always surgical, but preoperative or postoperative radiation and chemotherapy may be part of the overall treatment plan. The specific type of surgery depends on the anatomic position and extent of the carcinoma. Whenever possible, the tumor is removed and an end-to-end anastomosis (bringing together the healthy sections of the colon after the tumor has been removed) is performed. If the tumor has obstructed the bowel, a temporary colostomy may be done to divert bowel contents, and resection is done after the obstruction has been decompressed. If the tumor is in the sigmoid or rectum, bowel resection with or without a colostomy may be performed. In order to remove all disease from the area, it may be necessary to perform an abdominoperineal resection (APR). This procedure involves the removal of the rectum and the diseased segment of bowel and constructing a colostomy on the abdominal wall. Patients who have inoperable disease may be treated with radiation therapy or chemotherapy. A colostomy may be performed to divert the bowel contents if an inoperable tumor is causing obstruction.

**Preoperative.** The psychologic preparation of the patient is extremely important. If the surgeon anticipates that a colostomy will be necessary, the patient should be prepared for it. The patient needs to understand that he or she may expect to lead a normal life (refer to *Colostomy and Ileostomy Nursing Care*).

**Postoperative.** Postoperative care includes the management of all tubes, such as a nasogastric tube, a urinary drainage catheter, or drains placed in the perineal wound. The character and appearance of all drainage is observed and recorded. Considerable bloody and serosanguinous drainage is expected to occur from the perineal wound for the first 24 hours after APR. Dressings are changed or reinforced often, and the patient is observed closely for signs and symptoms of hemorrhage or severe volume depletion. Antibiotics are usually administered after surgery to prevent or control infection for the first 24 to 48 hours. The patient receives nothing by mouth, but intravenous fluids are given to maintain hydration and replace electrolytes. If an abdominoperineal resection was done, the perineal wound may have been packed, and the packing is removed gradually by the physician within the first few days after surgery. When all packing has been removed, irrigation of the wound may be required once or twice a day. The physician prescribes the specific directions regarding how the wound is to be irrigated and what solution is to be used. Irrigation is a mechanical method of removing tissue and debris. Routine care is given for the colostomy.

Patients who have had an abdominal perineal resection usually have more difficulty with ambulation and sitting as a result of the perineal wound, and the nursing procedures of encouraging deep breathing and coughing, turning the patient, and giving leg exercises are of special importance. Postoperative pain control measures are essential to early ambulation and good pulmonary hygiene.

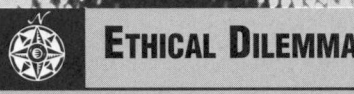

## ETHICAL DILEMMA

Mrs. Emory is an 82-year-old widow. She lives with her married daughter and the daughter's family. She was admitted to the hospital this afternoon. Mrs. Emory believes that she is going to have her gallbladder removed. However, she is actually scheduled to go to the operating room tomorrow for a permanent colostomy because she has cancer of the rectum. Her daughter has told you, the nurse, and the doctor not to tell Mrs. Emory that she will have colostomy surgery. "She doesn't want one. Let's just do it, then we'll tell her about it afterward." The doctor says, "The family knows her best, so we'll do what the daughter says."

How would you discuss this issue with the doctor? With the daughter? How would you do preoperative teaching with Mrs. Emory?

# KEY CONCEPTS

➤ A thorough bowel cleansing is necessary for study of the lower GI tract: clear liquid diet for 24 hours, laxatives, and enemas. Laxatives and liquids are necessary following barium studies to clear barium.

➤ Gastric decompression removes air and fluids from the upper gastrointestinal tract. The tube is secured to the nose to maintain position in the stomach.

➤ Intestinal decompression requires a tube that is not taped so it is free to descend into the lower gastrointestinal tract.

➤ Total parenteral nutrition is administered in a large vessel, and the rate of infusion must be kept constant because the solution is so high in glucose.

➤ When surgery involves the large bowel, antibiotics are given preoperatively to reduce the bacterial count and the risk of postoperative peritonitis. This is commonly referred to as "sterilizing" the bowel, even though the bowel is not actually sterile as a result.

➤ After gastrointestinal surgery, the patient must be observed for resumption of normal function: return of bowel sounds, passing flatus, absence of distention, and presence of nausea and vomiting.

➤ A normal, healthy stoma is red and moist and is visible above the surface of the skin. If it retracts below the skin or changes color, indicating ischemia and potential necrosis, the physician must be notified.

➤ A continent pouch ileostomy (Kock's pouch) does not require wearing a stoma pouch to collect stool because a reservoir has been created. It is drained continually until it heals, and eventually it will need to be emptied only two or three times a day by inserting a tube.

➤ Severe dehydration and electrolyte imbalance can result from prolonged loss of gastrointestinal secretions through diarrhea.

➤ The patient with anorexia nervosa or bulimia will require nutritional management and psychologic intervention.

➤ Crohn's disease involves sections of inflamed tissue anywhere in the gastrointestinal tract, causing pain and diarrhea. It is possibly a disorder of lymphoid tissue. The patient is predisposed to abscess and fistula formation and bowel obstruction.

➤ Ulcerative colitis involves the colon and rectum, and the inflammation results in fibrosis and narrowing of the bowel lumen. Cancer of the colon is a complication in the long term. The patient has frequent, loose, bloody, mucoid stools with some mild cramping pain in the left lower quadrant.

➤ Patients with inflammatory bowel disease need support in dealing with complications and in handling the difficulties associated with frequent, loose, foul-smelling stools.

➤ Signs and symptoms of appendicitis typically include fever, elevated whole blood cell count, anorexia, nausea and vomiting, and pain in the lower right quadrant of the abdomen, halfway between the umbilicus and the crest of the ileum (McBurney's point) or near the umbilicus. Rebound tenderness may be present in the right lower quadrant.

➤ Diverticula are pouches of mucosa and submucosa that protrude or herniate through the circular muscles of the intestinal wall. A low-fiber diet may contribute to the development of diverticula.

➤ Diverticulitis occurs when fecal matter penetrates the thin-walled diverticula, resulting in inflammation and abscess formation outside the bowel. The patient will have mild to severe abdominal pain in the left lower quadrant, fever, and elevated white blood cell count and sedimentation rate. Septicemia and septicemic shock can develop if the condition is untreated.

➤ Symptoms of bowel obstruction include abdominal pain, distention, vomiting, and constipation. Shock may develop. A nasogastric tube may be inserted to remove gas and secretions. Surgery may be necessary.

➤ Cancer of the tongue is the most common type of tumor of the mouth, believed to be predisposed by irritation resulting from smoking, consumption of alcohol, dental appliances, and rough, jagged teeth. Leukoplakia (white patches) may be seen on the mucous membrane of the tongue or cheek.

➤ Dysphagia (difficulty in swallowing) is the prime symptom of cancer of the esophagus.

➤ Nursing management of the patient with a gastrostomy tube includes caring for the skin, maintaining patency of the tube, good oral care, and administering the prescribed feeding. Force should not be used to irrigate the tube if it becomes blocked.

➤ The bacterium *Helicobacter pylori*, which is associated with chronic gastritis and peptic ulcer, is also a factor in the development of cancer of the stomach. Diet is probably the most significant environmental factor.

## KEY CONCEPTS—cont'd

➤ Evidence suggests that a low-fiber diet that is rich in beef and saturated fats leads to an increased incidence of colorectal cancer. Rectal bleeding is the most common symptom.

➤ Peptic ulcers are found in the stomach (gastric ulcers) and in the duodenum. Pain is a characteristic symptom, described as dull, burning, gnawing, or boring. It is located in the midline of the epigastric region. Gastric ulcer pain occurs 60 to 90 minutes after eating. Pain with duodenal ulcer occurs 2 to 4 hours after eating and is relieved by eating or antacids. There will be bright red bleeding or coffee-grounds emesis with hemorrhage and dark, tarry stools with slow bleeding.

➤ Pain with hernia signals the need for surgical intervention.

➤ Adequate hydration (6 to 8 glasses of fluids per day) and fresh fruits and vegetables, whole grains, and bran increase the fiber content of the diet, promote fecal evacuation, and prevent constipation.

## CRITICAL THINKING EXERCISES

1. What information is necessary to give the patient who is going to have a sigmoidoscopy?
2. What factors predispose the elderly to diverticular disease?
3. Abbey Johnson is a 24-year-old woman with ulcerative colitis. She is scheduled for ileoanal reservoir surgery next month. How can you help prepare her for her surgery and recovery?
4. James Clark, a 72-year-old man, is on the surgical nursing unit. He had surgery for cancer of the sigmoid colon 5 days ago and now has a permanent colostomy. Last evening he developed severe diarrhea with almost constant drainage of liquid stool from his colostomy. What can you do to assist Mr. Clark with this situation, considering (1) his dietary needs with a new colostomy and diarrhea, (2) fluid and electrolyte losses, and (3) management of ostomy drainage and stoma care?

## REFERENCES AND ADDITIONAL READINGS

Barnie DC, Currier J: What's that GI tube being used for? *RN* 58(8):45-49, 1995.

Brozenec SA: Ulcer therapy update, *RN* 59(9):48-50, 1996.

Chapman GM, Sinclair L, Langevin JM: *A patient handbook for the ileoanal reservoir procedure*, Princeton, NJ, Convatec, ER Squibb & Sons.

Cox J: Inflammatory bowel disease: implications for the medical-surgical nurse, *Medsurg Nurs* 4(6):427-434, 1995.

Cumbie B, Clement S: Actionstat: bowel obstruction, *Nursing* 26(1):33, 1996.

Doughty DB: What you need to know about inflammatory bowel disease, *Am J Nurs* 94(7):24-30, 1994.

Doughty DB, Jackson DB: *Gastrointestinal disorders*, St Louis, 1993, Mosby.

Giese LA, Terrell L: Sexual health issues in inflammatory bowel disease, *Gastroenterol Nurs* 19(1):12-17, 1996.

Hampton BG, Bryant RA: *Ostomies and continent diversions: nursing management*, St Louis, 1992, Mosby.

Lewis SM, Collier IC, Heitkemper MM: *Medical-surgical nursing: assessment and management of clinical problems*, ed 4, St Louis, 1996, Mosby.

Marchiondo K: When the Dx is diverticular disease, *RN* 57(2):42-46, 1994.

McCance KL, Huether SE: *Pathophysiology: the biologic basis for disease in adults and children*, ed 2, St Louis, 1994, Mosby.

Nassif A et al: Role of cytokines and platelet-activating factor in inflammatory bowel disease: implications for therapy, *Dis Colon Rectum* 39(2):217-223, 1996.

Pagana KD, Pagana TJ: *Mosby's diagnostic and laboratory test reference*, ed 3, St Louis, 1997, Mosby.)

Potter PA, Perry AG: *Basic nursing: theory and practice*, ed 3, St Louis, 1995, Mosby.

Procaccino F, Eysselein VE: Medical management of ulcerative colitis. In Snape WJ, editor: *Consultations in gastroenterology*, Philadelphia, 1996, Saunders.

Seidel HM et al: *Mosby's guide to physical examination*, ed 3, St Louis, 1995, Mosby.

Sleisenger MH, Fordtran JS: *Gastrointestinal disease: pathophysiology, diagnosis, management*, vols I and II, ed 5, Philadelphia, 1993, Saunders.

Weant CA: Easing the pain of esophageal surgery, *RN* 58(8):26-30, 1995.

Wilson R: Patient teaching for an ileoanal reservoir, *J ET Nurs* 20(5):199-203, 1993.

## CHAPTER 36

# Problems of the Liver, Gallbladder, and Pancreas

## CHAPTER OBJECTIVES

1  Describe the function of the liver, gallbladder, and pancreas in the digestive tract.
2  Explain the following diagnostic tests, including purpose, procedure, and preparation of the patient: liver function tests, cholangiography, and endoscopic retrograde cholangiopancreatography.
3  Discuss the care of the patient with the following disorders: hepatitis, hepatic coma, cirrhosis, cholecystitis, cholelithiasis, pancreatitis, and pancreatic cancer.
4  Discuss the care of the patient undergoing the following surgical interventions: laparoscopic cholecystectomy, open cholecystectomy, portosystemic shunts, and Whipple procedure.

## KEY TERMS

| | |
|---|---|
| biliary colic | esophageal varices |
| cholangiography | gastrectomy |
| cholecystectomy | hepatic coma |
| cholecystography | jaundice |
| cholelithiasis | pancreatitis |
| cirrhosis | |

## STRUCTURE AND FUNCTION OF THE LIVER, GALLBLADDER, AND PANCREAS

The liver, gallbladder, and pancreas (Figure 36-1) are the accessory organs of the digestive system. They assist the process of digestion by contributing specific secretions and enzymes essential for normal digestion, allowing the body to make better use of nutrients. An understanding of exactly how these important organs function will make the appreciation of the severity of consequences of dysfunction easier to understand and appreciate.

### Liver

The liver, located in the right upper quadrant of the abdomen, under the diaphragm is the largest of the accessory organs. The liver performs a wide range of functions each of which has a tremendous impact on the total function of the body. The liver plays an important role in the metabolism of carbohydrates, fats, and proteins. It assists in the regulation of blood glucose by converting carbohydrates to glycogen, storing glycogen, and then converting it to glucose as needed. When the glycogen stores are low, the liver removes the ammonia (deaminates) from amino acids to make glucose and glucagon or ketones for energy. The liver also breaks down fat to provide another source of energy to meet the body's demands. It synthesizes and catabolizes fatty acids and neutral fats to form ketone bodies and active acetate sources of cell energy. The liver converts excess carbohydrates and proteins into fat, which can be stored by adipose tissue for later use. Its role in protein metabolism includes synthesis of amino acids and supply of plasma proteins for tissue repair.

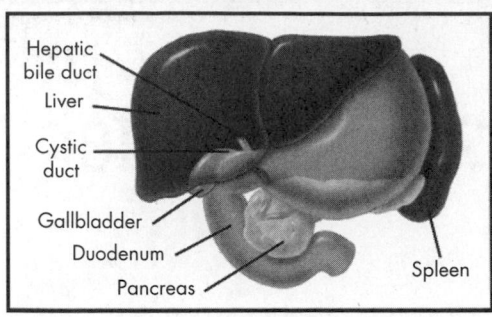

**Figure 36-1** Organs of gastrointestinal system. (From Thibodeau GA, Patton KT: *Anatomy and physiology.* ed 3, St Louis, 1996, Mosby.)

The liver is the organ responsible for the synthesis of cholesterol and lipids (Secor, 1996). Most of the cholesterol is converted into bile salts and is secreted into the bile. The other parts of the cholesterol and the lipids are used elsewhere in the body for other functions.

The liver also synthesizes the proteins, prothrombin, and fibrinogen necessary for blood coagulation. The liver stores vitamins, including vitamin K and the other fat-soluble vitamins, and is the primary site of vitamin $B_{12}$. It also plays a role in the detoxification of drug hormones and their products such as calcium, secreting them into the bile or into the urine.

## Gallbladder

The gallbladder is a small pear-shaped organ that lies under the liver. It serves as a concentrator of a storage compartment for bile, which it releases into the duodenum during digestion. Bile is required to dissolve fats and fat-soluble vitamins. Bile is a yellow-brown fluid produced in the liver that contains cholesterol, lipids, bile salts (natural detergents that break up fat), and bilirubin (the bile pigment that gives bile and stools their color). The liver produces as much as three cups of bile per day, and at any one time the gallbladder can store up to a cup of concentrated bile (National Digestive Diseases Information Clearinghouse [NDDIC], 1993). The bile is recirculated in the digestive tract by being reabsorbed in the intestine and returning to the liver in the bloodstream.

## Pancreas

The pancreas is a slender fish-shaped organ that is located posterior to the stomach with a portion extending into the C-shaped curve of the duodenum. The pancreas consists of three segments: the head, which lies within the curve of the duodenum; the body,

which is the portion that lies horizontally across the abdomen; and the tail, which is the portion that extends to the spleen.

The pancreas has both endocrine and exocrine functions. The endocrine function refers to the ability of the pancreatic islet cells or the islets of Langerhans to secrete insulin and glucagon directly into the blood. The exocrine function refers to the ability of the pancreas to produce pancreatic digestive juice, which helps in the digestion of proteins, carbohydrates, and fats. Approximately 1000 to 3000 cc/day is secreted into the duodenum through the pancreatic duct. It is a fluid that contains amylase, lipase, and other enzymes such as trypsin.

# DIAGNOSTIC PROCEDURES

There are several common tests that are used in the evaluation of the structure and function of the liver, gallbladder, and pancreas. The main purpose of these examinations is to aid the physician in establishing the problem that is causing the patient's symptoms.

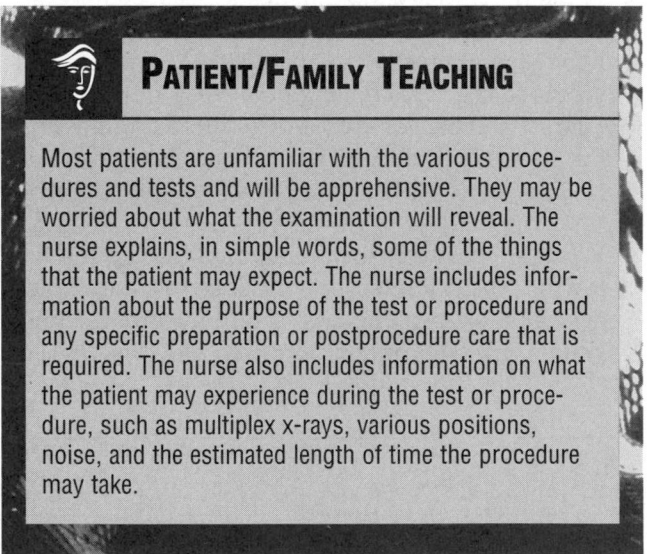

**PATIENT/FAMILY TEACHING**

Most patients are unfamiliar with the various procedures and tests and will be apprehensive. They may be worried about what the examination will reveal. The nurse explains, in simple words, some of the things that the patient may expect. The nurse includes information about the purpose of the test or procedure and any specific preparation or postprocedure care that is required. The nurse also includes information on what the patient may experience during the test or procedure, such as multiplex x-rays, various positions, noise, and the estimated length of time the procedure may take.

## Abdominal X-Ray Examination

Abdominal x-ray examination is a noninvasive evaluation that can be used to give some general, quick information about the abdomen. With abdominal x-ray examination, the physician can visualize some types of gallstones (10% to 15% of cases) and can assist in quick diagnosis when combined with the physical examination. An enlarged gallbladder can sometimes also be identified with this simple test (Way, 1996). Chest x-rays can be helpful in diagnosing pleural effusions, which are commonly seen in patients with pancreatitis. In general, pleural effusions are in the left side of the chest (Silen, 1987). There is no patient preparation needed for the standard x-ray.

## Ultrasonography

Ultrasound examination may be used to diagnose gallbladder disease, biliary system diseases, and diseases of the liver and the pancreas. Pulses of high frequency ultrasonic waves are passed into the body through its surface. The deflected waves are then recorded in a visual image, allowing for identification of the organs and abnormalities such as gallstones, tumors, cysts, and fluid collections.

The patient is instructed to fast for 8 to 12 hours before the examination to reduce the gas in the bowel, which hinders the transmission of the sound waves. In some cases the patient may be instructed by the radiologist to have a fat-free or a clear liquid meal the evening before the examination (Lewis, Collier, Heitkemper, 1996).

During the examination, the room is darkened and the patient lies on an examining table. The examination takes approximately 15 to 30 minutes. A water-soluble gel is applied to the abdomen, and an ultrasound transducer is gently rubbed over the abdomen to obtain the images. After the examination, the gel is wiped off and the patient may resume his usual diet. It is best if this test is scheduled before any abdominal studies that require the use of barium because it interferes with the ultrasound transmission. Ultrasound has no known side effects and does not contain radiation.

## Computed Tomography

Computed tomography (CT) scanning involves the passage of multiple x-ray beams through the upper abdomen while detectors record the strength of the x-ray beam as it is deflected off various tissues. A three-dimensional image of the organs is then constructed on an oscilloscope screen. CT scans are of greatest value in the detection of hepatic abscesses or tumors and can be used to confirm fluid collections detected on ultrasonic images. In some cases the use of contrast medium administered orally 4 hours before the procedure can assist in the diagnostic process by accentuating the difference between different tissues. Intravenous contrast medium may also be used.

CT scanning is performed with the patient positioned on a radiographic table in the center of the scanner. Transverse films are taken and fed into a computer from which selected images are taken. If intravenous contrast is given, the patient must be monitored for allergic reaction to the contrast medium. The presence of barium also interferes with a CT scan, so it is impor-

tant to delay CT scanning for approximately 4 days after barium studies are performed.

## Magnetic Resonance Imaging

Magnetic resonance imaging (MRI) is a process that involves the use of radiofrequency waves and a powerful magnetic field to produce images of tissue. Tissues with different content provide different signals, allowing for a clear anatomic picture of various structures. MRI of the abdomen can be useful for the detection of hepatic tumors, or metastases to the liver, and to evaluate abscesses.

Patients are generally instructed to intake nothing by mouth (NPO) for 6 hours before the procedure. Because of the powerful magnetic field, the patient is told to remove all metal jewelry before the examination and patients are carefully screened by the radiology technician concerning the presence of any metal in their body—such as pacemakers or braces. Patients should be instructed that the test will take approximately 30 minutes. They will lie on a radiographic table that will move, sliding their bodies into the MRI scanner. The space is tight and can be difficult for claustrophobic patients to bear. The patients are instructed to lie still throughout the examination. There is no follow-up necessary by the x-ray staff for the patients following MRI.

## Oral Cholecystography

Oral **cholecystography** allows for the visualization of the gallbladder and the extrahepatic biliary system. This examination can assist in the diagnosis of gallstones, inflammatory conditions of the gallbladder, and tumors of the gallbladder. The study helps determine the ability of the gallbladder to store bile and the patency of the biliary ducts. After a low-fat evening meal the patient is given an oral radiopaque drug (Telepaque, Bilopaque). The number of tablets is based on the weight of the patient. The tablets are taken one at a time at 5-minute intervals with sips of water. Following ingestion of the pills, the patient is NPO. If the patient vomits the tablets or shows any signs of intolerance to the dye such as itching, diarrhea, or flushing, the physician should be notfied. In some cases an enema is ordered in the morning of the examination to remove stool which may obstruct visualization of the gallbladder (Lewis, Collier, Heitkemper, 1996).

## Cholangiography

**Cholangiography** allows for the visualization of the biliary ducts. It may be used for patients who cannot tolerate oral agents. The contrast medium is injected into the blood, into a T-tube if present, or directly into the ductal system percutaneously.

The patient is NPO for 8 hours before the examination. The patient is informed that the procedure may involve being placed on a radiographic table that rotates into vertical and horizontal positions. In some cases the injection of the contrast dye causes nausea, vomiting, hypotension, flushing, and urticaria. Severe allergic reactions may cause anaphylactic shock. A careful history of hypersensitivity to iodine, seafood, or contrast medium is taken. The patient signs to give informed consent before the procedure. The patient is monitored during and after the procedure.

## Endoscopic Retrograde Cholangiopancreatography

Endoscopic retrograde cholangiopancreatography (ERCP) is a test that involves the oral insertion of a fiberoptic endoscope tube. The tube follows the digestive tract through the esophagus and stomach and into the duodenum. Finally the common bile duct and pancreatic ducts are visualized. Contrast medium can be injected through the tube into the ducts for direct visualization of the structures. In addition to its diagnostic ability, this technique can be used to retrieve gallstones lodged in the distal common bile duct, can dilate the ducts and sphincters, can allow for the biopsy of tumors, and can aid in the diagnosis of pancreatic pseudocyst (Lewis, Collier, Heitkemper, 1996).

The patient is NPO for 8 hours before the procedure. Informed consent is obtained. Sedation is administered to the patient before and during the procedure. In some cases antibiotics may be ordered before the examination. After the procedure the patient is monitored for signs of perforation of the intestine or infection. The most common complication of ERCP is pancreatitis, which will be discussed in depth later in the chapter. Before resuming the patient's diet, the presence of a gag reflex must be assessed.

## Radionuclide Scan

A radionuclide scan involves the intravenous injection of a radionuclide followed by images of the bile ducts and gallbladder with a radionuclide scanner. In patients with right upper quadrant pain and tenderness, this test provides an easy-to-perform method for diagnosing acute cholecystitis.

## LABORATORY STUDIES

Laboratory studies of the blood, urine, and feces can provide information about the function of the liver,

gallbladder, and pancreas and aid in the diagnosis of disease.

## Pancreatic Function
### Serum Amylase

A serum amylase blood test is the single most important measure for the diagnosis of acute pancreatitis. Serum amylase levels are generally two times the normal level in patients with pancreatitis Amylase levels are highest in the early stage of an attack of acute pancreatitis; they begin to return to normal after about 12 hours (Secor, 1996).

### Serum Lipase

Serum lipase measures the amount of lipase in the blood and enzyme secreted by the pancreas. Lipase remains elevated for a longer part of the duration of pancreatitis.

### Serum Glucose

Serum glucose is elevated in patients with pancreatitis because of altered function of the pancreatic islet cells.

### Fecal Analysis

Form, consistency, and color of the stool are noted. The specimen is examined for fat content, which may be high in the patient with diseases of the pancreas.

## Liver and Gallbladder Function
### Bilirubin Tests

Bilirubin tests may be performed on blood, urine, or feces. Bilirubin, a pigment resulting from the breakdown of hemoglobin, is excreted with bile into the small intestine, where it is converted to urobilinogen. Some of the urobilinogen is excreted, and some is returned to the liver, where it is converted to bilirubin. Normally, little bilirubin appears in the blood, but when obstruction of the bile ducts or liver cell damage occurs, the bilirubin is picked up in the blood, resulting in jaundice. In jaundice there is an increase of bilirubin in the blood. Bilirubin is normally excreted in feces and urine in the form of urobilinogen. Elevated levels of serum bilirubin are associated with hemolysis of red blood cells (indirect), liver damage, or biliary obstruction (direct and total) (Table 36-1).

### Liver Enzymes

**Alkaline phosphatase.** Alkaline phosphatase is synthesized primarily in the liver and bone. Elevated levels of

**TABLE 36-1**

## Laboratory Tests of GI, Hepatic, and Biliary Function

| TEST | NORMAL VALUE |
|---|---|
| Carcinoembryonic antigen | <5.0 ng/ml |
| Bilirubin | |
|    Indirect | 0.2-0.8 mg/dl |
|    Direct | 0.1-0.3 mg/dl |
|    Total | <1.0 mg/dl |
| Liver enzymes | |
|    Alkaline phosphatase | 30-85 ImU/ml or 42-128 U/L (SI units) |
|    Aspartate aminotransferase (formerly SGOT) | 8-20 U/L or 5-40 IU/L |
|    Alanine aminotransferase (formerly SGPT) | 5-35 IU/L or 8-20 U/L (SI units) |
|    $\gamma$-Glutamyl transpeptidase | 8-38 U/L men and women ↑ 45 years; 5-27 U/L women ↓ 45 years |
|    Lactate dehydrogenase | 45-90 U/L or 115-225 IU/L |
| Ammonia | 15-110 $\mu$g/dl or 47-67 $\mu$mol/L (SI units) |
| Serum proteins | |
|    Albumin | 3.5-5.0 g/dl |
|    Globulin | 2.0-3.5 g/dl |
|    Total | 6.4-8.3 g/dl |
| Clotting factors | |
|    Prothrombin time | 11.5-14 sec |
|    Partial prothrombin time | 25-40 sec |
| Nutritional factors | |
|    Albumin | 3.5-5.0 g/dl |
|    Prealbumin | 15-32 mg/dl |
|    Transferrin | 250-300 mg/dl |
|    Urine urea nitrogen | Positive balance |

alkaline phosphatase are seen in several processes such as bone fractures and bone metastases and are not specific to the gastrointestinal (GI) system, although elevated levels can reflect impaired excretory function of the liver. Test results are evaluated in light of the patient's history, symptoms, and physical assessment.

**Aspartate aminotransferase.** Aspartate aminotransferase (AST) is an enzyme found in cardiac, liver, skeletal muscle, kidney, and cerebral tissue. It functions in the synthesis of amino acids. When cell damage occurs, AST is released and serum levels rise.

**Alanine aminotransferase.** Alanine aminotransferase (ALT) is found in high concentrations in liver tissue. Lower concentrations are seen in cardiac tissue. Like AST, ALT is an enzyme that also functions in normal protein metabolism. Elevated levels of ALT are indicative of liver cell damage.

**Lactate dehydrogenase.** Lactate dehydrogenase is an enzyme found in almost all cells. It is found in the liver, heart, kidney, skeletal muscle, brain, and red blood cells. It is released when cells are damaged. It is nonspecific as to which tissue is damaged, but there are more specific isoenzymes that can be measured to locate which tissue it is that is damaged. The coordination of test results with the clinical picture is important.

## Ammonia

Ammonia is the end product of protein metabolism. Normally ammonia is absorbed into the blood from the intestine and transported to the liver via the portal vein. In the liver, ammonia is converted to urea for excretion by the kidneys. If liver cells are damaged and cannot convert ammonia to urea, or if portal blood is shunted away form the liver via collateral circulation, serum ammonia levels rise.

## Serum Proteins

Serum proteins (albumin, globulin, and transferrin) are synthesized in the liver. Therefore reduced levels of these proteins may be indicative of reduced liver function. Albumin, prealbumin, and transferrin depend on protein intake as well as the liver's ability to synthesize the specific proteins and are therefore markers of nutritional status. Decreased values can reflect liver damage or inadequate nutritional status, and correlation with the clinical presentation is important.

## Blood Clotting Factors

The liver plays a major role in coagulation by synthesizing coagulation factors. Additionally, bile salts in the GI tract arc required for the absorption of vitamin K, which is necessary for the liver to synthesize prothrombin. Abnormalities of the liver may alter the syntheses of coagulation factors. Prothrombin time (PT) and partial prothrombin time (PPT) are used to evaluate coagulation status, which may be altered in the presence of liver disease.

# DISEASES AND DISORDERS OF THE LIVER, GALLBLADDER, AND PANCREAS

## Jaundice

**Jaundice** is a yellowish discoloration of the skin, sclera, and mucosa that results from the inability of the liver to remove the bilirubin from the bloodstream. Jaundice can be a reflection of a problem within the liver or an obstruction in the ducts of the gallbladder and pancreas (the biliary duct system). The jaundiced patient has darkened urine as the kidney attempts to remove the excess pigment from the bloodstream. In some cases of jaundice, the stool is clay colored because no bile pigment is entering the intestines. Jaundice is a symptom, not a disease.

Jaundice can be caused by an increased breakdown of red blood cells, which might happen in patients who have blood transfusion reactions, sickle cell crisis, or hemolytic anemia. This is referred to as *hemolytic jaundice*. Jaundice that is caused by the liver's inability to excrete bilirubin is called *hepatocellular jaundice*. One might see this condition in those patients with hepatitis, liver cancer, or cirrhosis. Obstructive jaundice is caused by blocked bile flow at the level of the liver or biliary duct system (Lewis, Collier, Heitkemper, 1996). This type of jaundice can be caused by liver tumors, hepatitis, cirrhosis or gallstones, or cancer of the pancreas. Each of these conditions will be discussed in greater depth later in the chapter.

## Diseases and Disorders of the Liver
### Viral Hepatitis

Viral hepatitis is a disease that attacks the liver. A variety of similar viruses cause hepatitis. The mode or transmission and incubation periods differ among the various forms of the virus. The most common strains of hepatitis are types A, B, and C. Hepatitis D and hepatitis E are less common but can cause severe damage to the liver and cause liver failure (Lewis, Collier, Heitkemper, 1996) (Box 36-1). In the United States acute hepatitis is most often caused by hepatitis A virus (47% of cases). Hepatitis B is responsible for 34% and hepatitis C is responsible for 17% of acute hepatitis cases (Lemon, Thomas, 1997). Between 43,012 and 64,075 cases were reported annually between 1984 and 1993, but many cases of hepatitis are asymptomatic and therefore have remained undiagnosed. An estimated 16,000 people die each year from chronic liver disease associated with persistent hepatitis virus infection (Lemon, Thomas, 1997).

The source of the virus that causes type A hepatitis is primarily human feces. It is spread by oral intake of food, milk, or water contaminated by the virus. There is some evidence that the virus can also be transmitted by the parenteral introduction of the hepatitis virus through blood, blood products, or the equipment used for venipuncture or other procedures that require penetrating the skin. The virus is excreted in the feces long before clinical symptoms appear. The carrier is thought to be most infectious just before the onset of symptoms. An individual may have and carry the disease but may not be diagnosed because hepatitis can

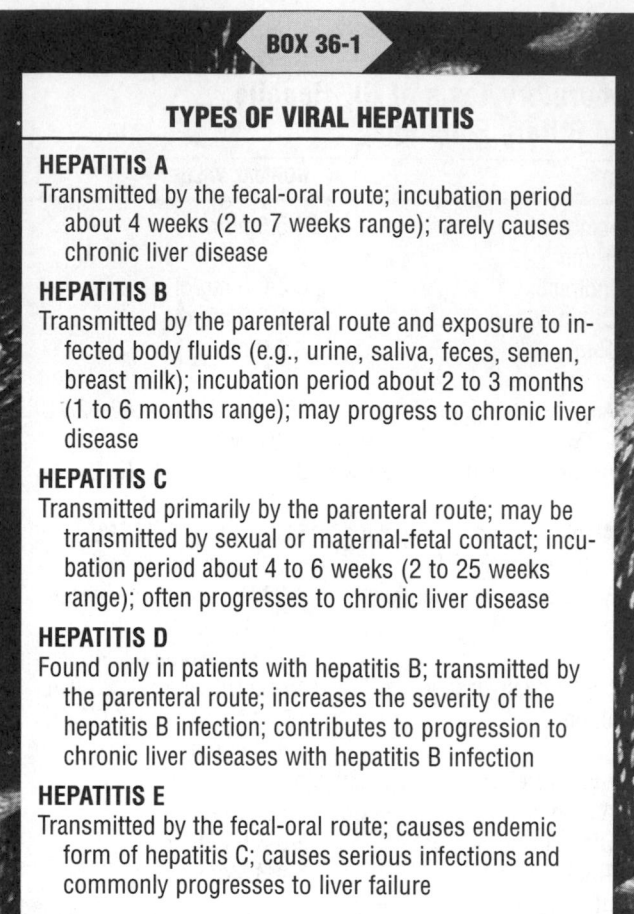

**BOX 36-1**

### TYPES OF VIRAL HEPATITIS

**HEPATITIS A**
Transmitted by the fecal-oral route; incubation period about 4 weeks (2 to 7 weeks range); rarely causes chronic liver disease

**HEPATITIS B**
Transmitted by the parenteral route and exposure to infected body fluids (e.g., urine, saliva, feces, semen, breast milk); incubation period about 2 to 3 months (1 to 6 months range); may progress to chronic liver disease

**HEPATITIS C**
Transmitted primarily by the parenteral route; may be transmitted by sexual or maternal-fetal contact; incubation period about 4 to 6 weeks (2 to 25 weeks range); often progresses to chronic liver disease

**HEPATITIS D**
Found only in patients with hepatitis B; transmitted by the parenteral route; increases the severity of the hepatitis B infection; contributes to progression to chronic liver diseases with hepatitis B infection

**HEPATITIS E**
Transmitted by the fecal-oral route; causes endemic form of hepatitis C; causes serious infections and commonly progresses to liver failure

occur in a mild form that is not severe enough to produce jaundice.

The source of the virus that causes hepatitis B is the blood of the person who has the infection or who is a carrier of the virus. The virus is present in semen, saliva, and blood and is transmitted by sexual contact or blood products usually through accidental needle sticks or the sharing of needles by intravenous drug users.

Hepatitis C is also transmitted in the blood and is the major cause of transfusion related to viral hepatitis. It is often seen in parenteral drug users, patients in chronic care institutions, health care workers, hemodialysis patients, and transplant recipients. Hepatitis C is the predominant type of hepatitis found in persons with chronic hepatitis (Lemon, Thomas, 1997).

Hepatitis D is also called *delta virus*. It can transform cases of hepatitis B into severe, chronic, active hepatitis and can also lead to fulminant hepatitis B.

Hepatitis E occurs primarily in developing countries. The diagnosis is made by exclusion because there are no blood tests as yet that are diagnostic of this particular form of hepatitis. Hepatitis E causes serious infections that commonly progress to hepatitis failure.

Vaccines are currently available for both hepatitis B and hepatitis A. Hepatitis B immunizations are generally scheduled so that a booster dose is administered at 1 to 2 months after the initial dose and then again 4 to 6 months later. In children the hepatitis B immunization begins in the hospital at birth, followed by injections at 4 months, and again at 18 months. Immunization for hepatitis B was initially only recommended for infants born to hepatitis B-positive mothers, homosexually active men, intravenous drug users, and health care workers exposed to blood. It is now required by Occupational Safety and Health Administration for all health care workers. The recognition of the difficulty in identifying high-risk persons has prompted recommendations for routine immunizations of all infants and "catch-up" immunizations of all children, adolescents, and high-risk adults in the United States. At present, 58% of all babies born in the United States are immunized by the age of 19 to 24 months.

Hepatitis A vaccinations are now also licensed in the United States. The vaccination is recommended for people at increased risk for hepatitis A infection, including travelers to regions where sanitation is poor and where hepatitis A is common; children living in communities where hepatitis A is common, homosexually active men, users of illicit drugs, and people working closely with nonhuman primates (Thomas, Lemon, 1997). Travelers should receive the immunization 1 month before they travel. At present, a one-time dose is all that is given. This relatively new vaccination is not yet licensed for children under 2 years old.

**Pathophysiology.** A diffuse inflammatory reaction occurs with the infection of hepatitis, and the liver cells begin to degenerate and die. As the liver cells degenerate, the normal functions of the liver are affected. Degeneration, regeneration, and inflammation may occur simultaneously and may distort the lobular pattern of the liver and create pressure within and around the portal vein areas. These changes may be associated with elevated AST and ALT levels, a prolonged PT and a slightly elevated serum alkaline phosphatase. In some cases, hepatic inflammation may cause interruption of bile flow.

In most instances of viral hepatitis, regeneration begins almost with the onset of the disease. The damaged cells and their contents eventually are removed by phagocytosis and enzymatic reaction, and the level returns to normal. The outcome of viral hepatitis is affected by such factors as the virulence of the virus, the preexisting condition of the liver, and the supportive care provided when symptoms appear.

**Assessment.** Symptoms may be mild or severe and include loss of appetite, fatigue, nausea and vomiting, chills, headache, and a temperature that may range form 38° C to 40° C (100° F to 104° F). Jaundice usually appears in 4 to 7 days but may be altogether absent in some patients. Temperature usually returns to normal when the jaundice appears, but anorexia and nausea persist. Children usually have a milder form of infectious hepatitis with no jaundice and with symptoms predominantly appearing as those of an intestinal or respiratory illness.

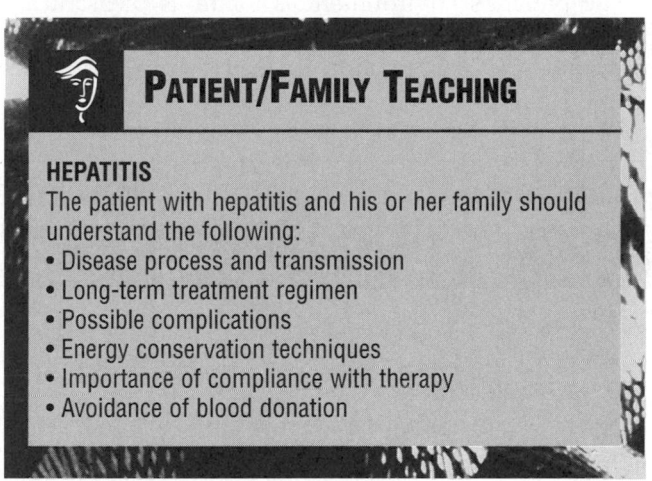

### PATIENT/FAMILY TEACHING

**HEPATITIS**
The patient with hepatitis and his or her family should understand the following:
- Disease process and transmission
- Long-term treatment regimen
- Possible complications
- Energy conservation techniques
- Importance of compliance with therapy
- Avoidance of blood donation

**Intervention.** There is no specific treatment for hepatitis. Therapy is planned to strengthen the patient's resistance to infection, and rest and nutrition are primary considerations. Antibiotics may be administered to prevent secondary infection, and antihistamines may be given to relieve the itching associated with jaundice. In some cases Interferon is used by patients to help boost the immune system and prevent infections. Fluid intake is encouraged during the acute stage, and, if a sufficient amount is not taken, intravenous infusions may be given.

Diet is of major importance and should provide all the necessary nutrients. Because the appetite is poor, the patient will need considerable encouragement to eat, and records of the intake and calorie count are maintained. Appetite tends to be best in the morning and throughout the day. If eating does not provide sufficient calories and nutrition, enteral feedings or parenteral nutrition is used to supplement or replace oral fluids. Many of these patients will be recovering in their homes with the support services of a home care agency. The visiting nurse is then responsible for accurately evaluating the nutritional status of the patient.

Prevention is the most important goal in controlling hepatitis. Patients, their families, and health care providers must be knowledgeable about how the virus is transmitted and take steps needed to prevent its spread. Handwashing is the mainstay for prevention of all disease transmission. Patients and family members must be instructed on proper handwashing techniques. Using standard universal precautions will control exposure to potentially contaminated blood and body fluids and excrement (Centers for Disease Control and Prevention, 1994). In the case of diapered infants and children or incontinent patients with hepatitis, contact precautions are implemented to prevent the spread of infection.

The patient's environment is made as pleasant as possible. Tepid baths, rubs, and oral care are important, and a soothing lotion is used to provide relief from skin pruritus associated with jaundice. The patient should be urged to keep fingernails short. Cotton gloves may also be indicated to protect the patient's skin from scratching. The patient may have concerns about the problems created by long illness and the resulting financial difficulties. The nurse makes appropriate referral to social services to explore financial options for the patient. The nurse may encourage the patient to engage in diversional activities to relieve the monotony of convalescence. With children the problems of a long convalescence may be greater and will require the help of everyone involved to keep them occupied and contented. Physical and emotional support is essential to recovery during this long convalescence (Box 36-2).

---

| BOX 36-2 | NURSING PROCESS |
| --- | --- |

## HEPATITIS

### ASSESSMENT

- Energy level
- Activity tolerance
- Vital signs before and after activity
- Weight
- Fluid volume status
- Skin
- Pruritus, anorexia, fatigue, jaundice
- Laboratory studies (liver enzymes, albumin)

### NURSING DIAGNOSES

- Activity intolerance related to viral infection, fatigue, weakness
- Altered nutrition: less than body requirements related to anorexia, fatigue, nausea, decreased metabolism of nutrients by liver
- Risk for fluid volume deficit related to vomiting, diarrhea, decreased intake
- Risk for infection related to malnutrition and inadequate secondary defenses
- Risk for impaired skin integrity related to accumulation of bile salts onto skin
- Risk for diversional activity deficit related to lack of energy, isolation, and lengthy course of disease
- Situational low self-esteem related to isolation, length of illness, jaundice
- Knowledge deficit related to new condition and unfamiliarity of disease

### NURSING INTERVENTIONS

- Prevent spread of disease by handwashing and proper handling of blood, body fluids, and feces.
- Use disposable dishes and utensils (hepatitis A).
- Provide quiet environment.
- Promote rest.
- Coordinate nursing activity in blocks of time.
- Increase activity as tolerated.
- Provide diversional activities when energy levels adequate.
- Determine food preferences.
- Provide diet high in calories and carbohydrates and limited in fat.
- Provide small, frequent meals.
- Monitor I&O.
- Weigh every day before breakfast.
- Encourage fluids.
- Provide comfort measures to skin (tepid bath, lotion).
- Avoid soap on skin.
- Encourage discussion of feelings.
- Discuss prolonged recovery.

### EVALUATION OF EXPECTED OUTCOMES

- Verbalizes understanding of disease process, transmission, and treatment
- Reports an increase in activity tolerance
- Able to perform self-care activities
- Stable weight
- No evidence of dehydration
- Skin intact
- Absence or decrease in pruritus
- Verbalizes self-acceptance

A more severe course will be seen in the patient with a fulminating viral hepatitis that involves a sudden and severe degeneration and atrophy of the liver that may lead to hepatic failure and death. Fulminating viral hepatitis causes acute massive necrosis, finally destroying enough of the liver to cause death. Fulminating hepatitis occurs in a small percentage of those patients with hepatitis.

Other complications of hepatitis are chronic viral hepatitis in which there is a delayed convalescent period. In chronic viral hepatitis the symptoms may persist for more than 6 months. Chronic viral hepatitis is the principal cause of chronic liver disease, cirrhosis, and liver cancer in the world and now ranks as the chief reason for liver transplantation in adults (Hoofnagle, di Bisceglie, 1997).

The only therapy known to have a beneficial effect in chronic hepatitis is interferon alpha. Interferon alpha is generally given as a subcutaneous injection in doses of 5 million or 10 million units three times per week. Interferon alpha can lower the concentration of the active hepatitis virus, decrease the degenerative changes in the liver, and help prevent complications such as renal failure or human immunodeficiency virus infection. The side effects of interferon are flulike symptoms. Low-grade fever, chills, headaches, and muscle aches, which begin approximately 6 to 8 hours after infection, may last for up to 12 hours. After several injections the side effects generally decrease. If the patient is working during the day, it is important to suggest to them that they might consider taking the medication in the evening to avoid the symptoms during their workday.

## Cirrhosis

**Cirrhosis** is a chronic liver disease in which diffuse destruction and regeneration of liver cells occur and in which there is an accumulation of fibrous connective tissue. This accumulated tissue distorts the normal lobular structure of the liver and obstructs the biliary and vascular channels in the liver. The basic cause is not clearly understood but appears to be repeated injury to the liver cells. Although the liver cells have a great potential for regeneration, repeated scarring decreases the ability of the cells to be replaced. Cirrhosis is more common in men who are middle aged or older, but it may occur in younger persons. The highest incidence occurs in the age range of 40 to 60 years, and men are affected twice as much as women (Lewis, Collier, Heitkemper, 1996). In the United States cirrhosis is the seventh leading cause of death by disease, with 25,000 people dying each year from this illness. There is also a great toll in terms of human suffering, loss of work, and hospital costs for people with cirrhosis (NDDIC, 1991).

Causes of cirrhosis include chronic hepatitis, as well as inherited diseases such as cystic fibrosis, hemochromocytosis, and Wilson's disease. A blockage in the bile duct can also cause cirrhosis. Other less common causes of the disease are severe reactions to prescribed drugs, environmental toxins, and repeated bouts of congestive heart failure. However, despite the initiating cause, the final result is essentially the same for each type. There are three primary classifications of types of cirrhosis: alcoholic (Laënnec's), biliary, and postnecrotic (named because of the initiating cause of the disease). The most common form of the disease in the United States is Laënnec's cirrhosis, which is caused by the effects of alcohol on the liver.

**Pathophysiology.** Cirrhosis is a disease that develops slowly and usually progresses gradually over a period of years. There is slow destruction of the functional cells of the liver (hepatocytes). As the cells degenerate, they become infiltrated with fat and the organ size increases (fatty cirrhosis). Eventually, irregular, disorganized regeneration, poor cellular nutrition, and hypoxia caused by inadequate blood flow and scar tissue result in decreased functioning of the liver (Lewis, Collier, Heitkemper, 1996). The damaged liver cannot metabolize protein normally; therefore protein intake may result in an elevation of blood cell ammonia.

Early symptoms of cirrhosis are anorexia, dyspepsia, nausea, flatulence, and bowel habit changes (diarrhea or constipation). A dull, heavy feeling in the right upper quadrant might also be present. As the disease progresses, jaundice; dilated blood vessels (spider angiomas) appearing on the face, trunk, and neck; and hematologic disturbances like anemia and thrombocytopenia; peripheral neuropathy; and some endocrine disturbances are common developments.

*Late complications.* Liver cell damage reduces the liver's ability to synthesize albumin. The progressive liver damage also obstructs the flow of blood through the liver. This obstruction of the circulation results in portal hypertension, or increased pressure in the veins that drain the GI tract. This increased pressure forces fluid and albumin into the peritoneal cavity, which is called *ascites*. Reduced synthesis of protein and the leaking of existing protein result in hypoalbuminemia (reduced protein or albumin level in the blood), which reduces oncotic pressure of the blood, leading to leakage of serum out of the blood vessels into the interstitial tissue. Protein must be present in adequate amounts to create colloidal osmotic pressure and to "pull" the fluid back into the blood vessels after it escapes from the capillaries. As fluid leaves the blood and the circulating volume decreases, the receptors in the brain signal the adrenal cortex to increase secretion of aldosterone to stimulate the kidneys to retain sodium and water. The normal liver inactivates the hormone aldosterone, but the damaged liver allows its effects to continue. Retention of fluid and sodium then results in increased pressure in the blood vessels and lymphatic channels, adding to the problem of portal hypertension. Ascites is, therefore, a result of portal hypertension, hypoalbuminemia, and hyperaldosteronism.

Because of the obstruction to blood flow through the liver, collateral vessels develop as a mechanism to divert the blood from the portal vein back to the inferior vena cava and the heart. These collateral vessels develop primarily in the esophagus **(esophageal varices),** the rectum (hemorrhoids), and on the surface of the abdomen (caput medusae). These vessels dilate and distend as a result of increased portal pressure and increased volume in the blood vessels. All of the collateral vessels, but primarily the esophageal varices, may rupture, causing severe hemorrhage.

Hepatorenal syndrome is a late complication of cirrhosis. It involves the development of functional renal failure with advanced azotemia, oliguria, and ascites. Although there is no structural problem with the kidneys, the low blood flow to the kidneys causes failure.

**Hepatic coma** or hepatic encephalopathy is a terminal complication of cirrhosis that involves degeneration of the brain as a result of rising levels of ammonia in the bloodstream. Symptoms include inappropriate behavior, confusion, and twitching that progress to stupor and coma.

**Assessment.** Early assessment may detect weight loss, gynecomastia, and a reported change in the patient's bowel habits. A blood test would reveal anemia caused by nutritional deficiency. Epistaxis, spider angiomas, purpura, and bleeding gums are also noted. The patient may be weak and feel depressed.

Later physical assessment would reveal ascites, hematologic disorders, and hemorrhage from esophageal varices or other distended veins. Mental status changes may also be detected. Ultimately, coma and death will result.

**Intervention.** Interventions used to manage the patient with cirrhosis vary with the symptoms and their severity, but there is no cure for the disease. Diet may be one intervention. Food is best served when the patient feels like eating. Small, frequent meals may be better tolerated by the patient.

Early in the disease process a high-protein diet is used to maintain body needs and to provide for tissue repair. The diet should include approximately 3000 calories per day. But a protein-limited diet will be needed if serum levels of ammonia become elevated. Salt (sodium) is restricted to reduce edema and ascites, and potassium supplements may be necessary to replace potassium lost as a result of diuretic therapy. Careful records of food intake and calorie counts are

maintained. Strict fluid intake and output records are maintained, and the patient is weighed daily.

Special attention to the skin is extremely important because poor nutritional status and tissue edema may contribute to the development of decubiti. Mouth care is given often and regularly. Use of an alcohol-free mouthwash before meals may make food a bit more appealing. The patient's environment should be quiet and conducive to rest, and precautions should be taken to prevent exposure to secondary infections.

Community nursing care stresses the importance of continuous health care. The patient and family are taught signs and symptoms of infection and about when to seek medical help. Instruction on proper diet, alcohol avoidance, and special attention of over-the-counter medication is reinforced (Box 36-3).

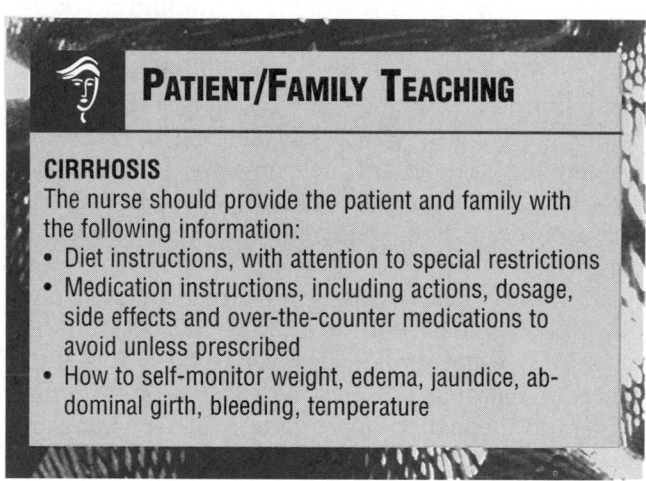

**PATIENT/FAMILY TEACHING**

**CIRRHOSIS**
The nurse should provide the patient and family with the following information:
- Diet instructions, with attention to special restrictions
- Medication instructions, including actions, dosage, side effects and over-the-counter medications to avoid unless prescribed
- How to self-monitor weight, edema, jaundice, abdominal girth, bleeding, temperature

Diuretic therapy is used in conjunction with a low-sodium diet, and fluid removal, ascites, and the peripheral edema associated with hepatic failure The sodium in the diet should be limited to 250 to 500 mg/day (Lewis, Collier, Heitkemper, 1996). Spironolactone (Aldactone) is a commonly used diuretic used in this population. The diuretic action reduces fluid and sodium. Spironolactone minimizes potassium loss associated with diuresis. Other potassium-sparing diuretics are amiloride (Midamor) and triamterene (Dyrenium). Furosemide (Lasix) is also frequently used in combination with other above potassium-sparing diuretics. Chlorothiazide (Diuril) or hydrochlorothiazide may also be used. Another method of relief of ascites is the removal of ascitic fluid by paracentesis. This involves a needle puncture of the abdomen and removal of fluid.

For the patient in a later stage of the disease and with encephalopathic changes, the goal of treatment is to reduce the amount of circulating ammonia in the blood. Neomycin may be given orally or rectally (as an

| BOX 36-3 | NURSING PROCESS |
| --- | --- |

## CIRRHOSIS

### ASSESSMENT

- Vital signs, including temperature, pulse, blood pressure, respirations
- Neurologic status, including state of arousal, mood alterations, confusion, neuromuscular activity
- Ascites
- Peripheral edema
- Fluid balance
- Laboratory values, including electrolytes, AST, ALT, bilirubin, ammonia, PT, PTT, platelets, hematocrit, WBC, BUN, and creatinine
- Active or occult bleeding
- Pain level on 0 to 10 scale
- Breath sounds and oxygenation
- Nutritional status
- Jaundice
- Compliance with therapeutic plan

### NURSING DIAGNOSES

- Risk for altered tissue perfusion related to ascites, fluid and electrolyte losses, or bleeding
- Fluid volume excess related to increased intraabdominal pressure and decreased osmotic gradient
- Pain related to ascites, liver inflammation
- Ineffective breathing pattern related to ascites, altered level of consciousness
- Risk for infection related to diminished immunologic response
- Altered thought process related to encephalopathy
- Risk for injury related to neurologic changes
- Altered nutrition: less than body requirements related to anorexia and fatigue
- Noncompliance with diet modification and alcohol restriction
- Risk for impaired skin integrity related to decreased activity, ascites, peripheral edema, and elevated bilirubin level

### NURSING INTERVENTIONS

- Check vital signs at least every 4 hours and more often if evidence of bleeding is noted.
- Observe mental status and neuromuscular activity; note and report any changes.
- Observe for edema by checking dependent areas for pitting (indentation) with pressure.
- Observe for ascites by measuring abdominal girth at least daily.
- Monitor laboratory values and note changes from baseline.

- Weigh daily.
- Check all gastrointestinal drainage for blood.
- Position patient in low or semi-Fowler's position to facilitate breathing.
- Administer oxygen, if ordered.
- Help patient to take deep breaths.
- Turn patient or help patient with turning every 2 hours while in bed.
- Maintain IV fluid therapy as ordered.
- Maintain accurate I&O records.
- Assist with paracentesis if performed by physician.
- Medicate patient for pain, as ordered.
- Assist with activities of daily living as needed to conserve energy.
- Provide adequate rest.
- Provide oral hygiene before meals.
- Give frequent, small feedings individualized to patient's preference and dietary restriction; provide nutritional supplements as needed.
- Cleanse skin with tepid water (avoid soap) and apply moisturizing lotions to relieve pruritus.
- Protect patient from harm.
- Orient to time, place, or person as indicated.
- Make referral for alcohol abuse treatment, if appropriate.

### EVALUATION OF EXPECTED OUTCOMES

- Maximum gas exchange maintained as evidenced by acceptable SaO$_2$ and clear breath sounds
- Adequate tissue perfusion and absence of elevated temperature
- Acceptable pain level
- Skin integrity maintained
- Adequate nutritional status maintained with stable weight and implementation of dietary modifications
- Demonstrates self-monitoring activities: weight, edema, jaundice, abdominal girth, bleeding, temperature
- Identifies signs and symptoms to be reported to physician immediately, including weight gain, increased abdominal girth, elevated temperature, bleeding or tarry stools, changes in memory or behavior
- Demonstrates knowledge and correct use of prescribed medications and reasons to avoid nonprescription medications
- Demonstrates knowledge of the dangers of alcohol use
- Alert and oriented

**Figure 36-2** LeVeen shunt showing placement of catheter. (Redrawn from Phipps WJ et al: *Medical-surgical nursing: concepts and clinical practice*, ed 5, St Louis, 1995, Mosby.)

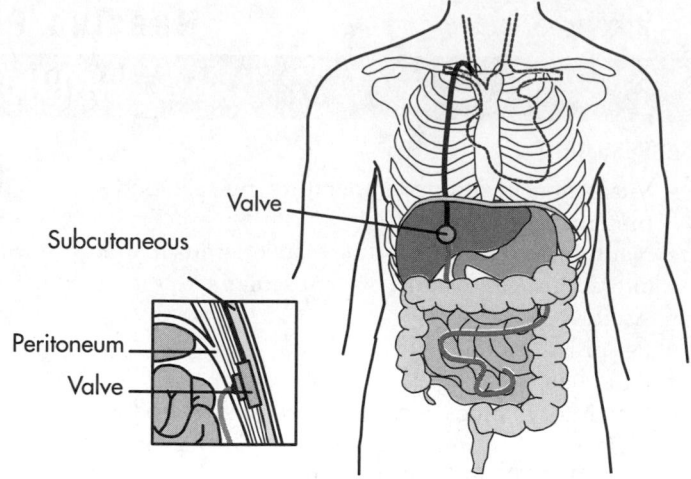

enema [infrequently]) to decrease the bacteria in the colon therefore reducing the production of ammonia. Lactulose (Cephulac) is used to trap ammonia in the gut and expel it from the colon with its laxative effect.

### Surgical interventions

**LEVEEN SHUNT.** When diet and medication fail to control the problem of ascites, a peritoneovenous shunt called a *LeVeen shunt* may be indicated. This surgical procedure involves the placement of a specially designed tube that contains a one-way valve. One end of the tube is placed in the peritoneum and the other into the jugular vein or superior vena cava (Figure 36-2). The tube is threaded through the subcutaneous tissue. The tube allows for ascitic fluid to pass into the perforations in the section of the tube in the peritoneum and flow through the tube upward, emptying into the vena cava where it is recirculated into the blood. The one-way valve is triggered by the patient's breathing and changing intraabdominal pressure. Inspiration causes the diaphragm to drop and causes an increase in the pressure in the peritoneum while simultaneously causing a decrease in the intravenous pressure in the superior vena cava. The pressure changes cause the one-way valve to open and the fluid to flow into the tube and upward to the superior vena cava.

Although this procedure controls ascites, there are risks involved. The tube may become occluded, ascitic fluid can leak from the incision site, and the blood can become too dilute from the circulating ascitic fluid. In addition, there is a risk of wound infection especially considering that those patients with ascites are generally debilitated and in a poor nutritional state.

**SENGSTAKEN-BLAKEMORE TUBES.** GI bleeding occurs in 40% to 60% of cirrhosis patients. Bleeding may occur secondary to erosive gastritis, peptic ulcer, or esophageal varices. When GI bleeding is apparent, the cause is determined immediately by endoscopy. Blood transfusions are given to replace blood loss. Severe hemorrhage may be treated by intravenous vasopressin

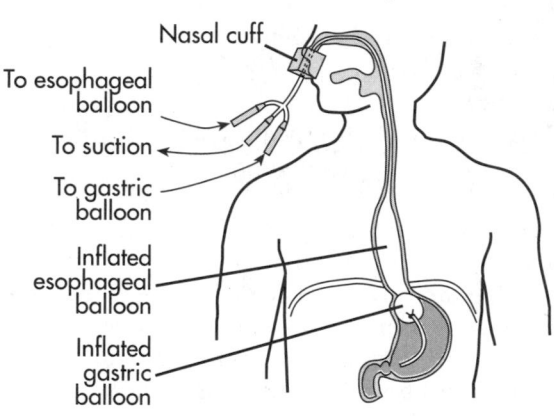

**Figure 36-3** Sengstaken-Blakemore tube. (Redrawn from Beare DB, Myers JL: *Adult health nursing*, ed 3, St Louis, 1998, Mosby.)

(Pitressin) or somatostatin. If medical treatment fails to stop the bleeding, an esophageal tamponade tube may be inserted. The tube (Figure 36-3) has two balloons that may be inflated to put pressure on the bleeding vessels in an attempt to stop the bleeding. In many cases these patients are treated in intensive care settings.

The tube is inserted in the mouth and through the esophagus into the stomach. When correct placement is ensured, the balloon in either the stomach alone or the stomach and esophagus is inflated to press against the bleeding varices and control the hemorrhage. The gastric drainage port is attached to low, intermittent suction to remove the blood and secretions from the stomach. If the gastric balloon alone or the gastric and esophageal balloons are inflated, the secretions above the balloon must be removed to prevent aspiration. A Salem sump may also be inserted through the nose or mouth and attached to low, intermittent suction to drain secretions. Tamponade therapy generally does not continue for more than 24 to 48 hours to prevent ischemia and necrosis to the mucosal surface of the stomach or esophagus.

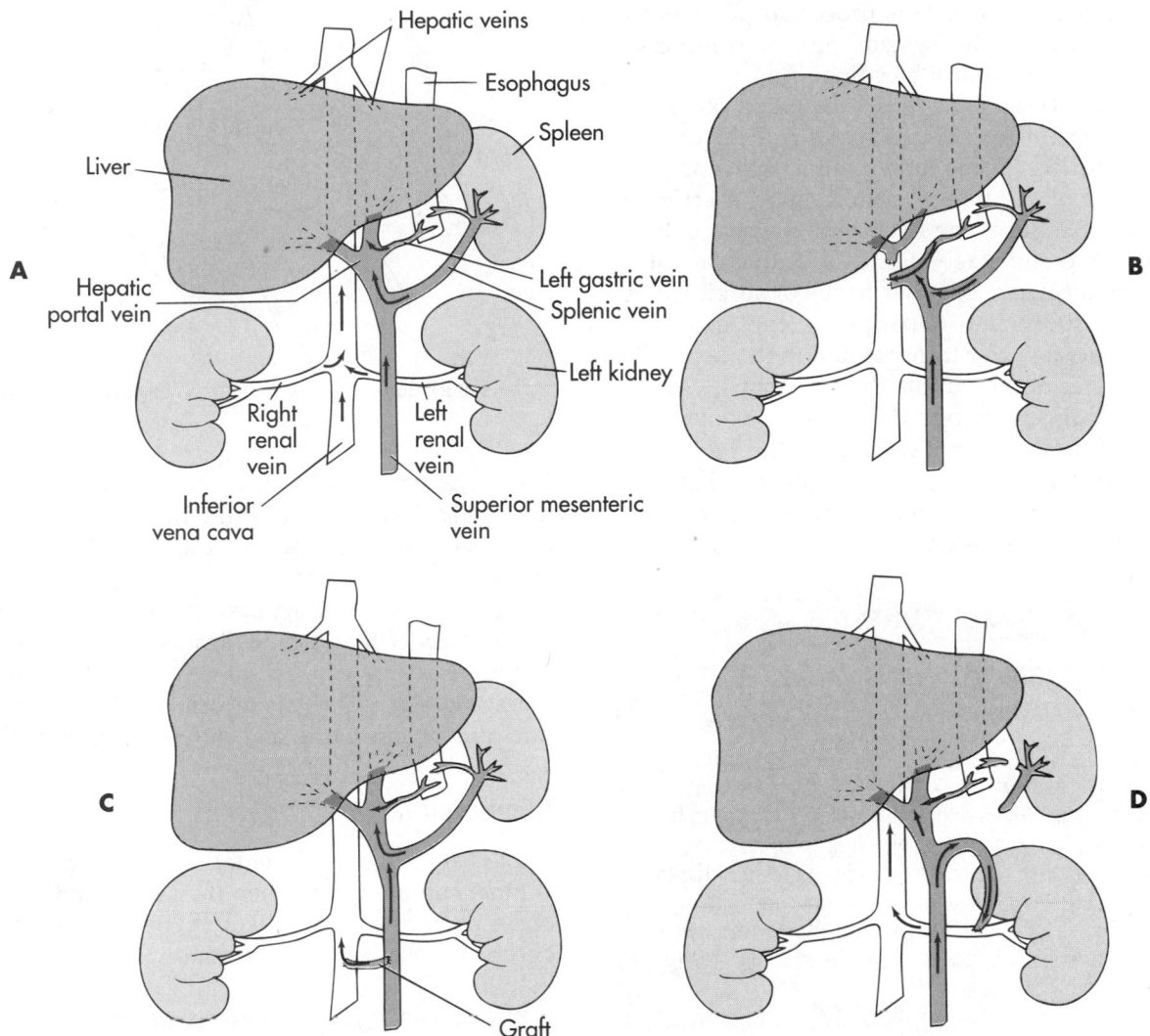

**Figure 36-4** Portosystemic shunts. **A,** Normal portal circulation. **B,** End-to-side portacaval shunt. Large amount of blood is diverted from its usual route to the liver and flows directly into the inferior vena cava. The portal vein and vena cava are anastomosed just outside the liver. Encephalopathy is a danger because ammonia and other toxins enter the systemic circulation directly instead of going to the liver for detoxification. **C,** Side-to side mesocaval shunt. In this more conservative procedure, a graft is added between the superior mesenteric vein and the inferior vena cava to reduce blood flow to the liver and to reduce pressure. **D,** Distal splenorenal shunt. In this selective shunt the splenic vein is connected to the renal vein to reduce the pressure in the varices without drastically decreasing liver perfusion via the portal vein. Often the spleen is removed with this procedure.

**PORTOSYSTEMIC SHUNTS.** Surgical and radiologic procedures may be performed to lower portal venous pressure or to treat ascites. The increased portal vein pressure, which occurs from the damage to the liver, may be reduced by shunting some of the portal blood directly into the inferior vena cava (Figure 36-4). In a portacaval shunt the portal vein is anastomosed directly to the inferior vena cava so that the liver is bypassed. In a splenorenal shunt the splenic vein is anastomosed to the left renal vein, and the spleen is removed. A more conservative procedure is the meso-

caval shunt in which the superior mesenteric vein and the inferior vena cava are connected with a small piece of graft material. This reduces blood flow to the liver and is a conservative palliative procedure.

An alternative procedure, used to reduce portal venous pressure, is the transjugular intrahepatic portosystemic shunt. This is a nonsurgical approach in which a tract is created between the systemic and portal venous system by placing a catheter into the right internal jugular vein and through the right atrium into the inferior vena cava. A stent is inserted between the hepatic and portal veins. This procedure reduces the pressure in the portal system and decompresses varices, which help control bleeding.

**LIVER TRANSPLANTATION.** Liver transplantation is considered the treatment for various forms of liver disease. Indications for liver transplantation include congenital abnormalities of the biliary system, inborn errors of metabolism that affect the liver, malignancy confined to the liver, and end-stage liver disease that cannot be cured by medical care or other forms of surgical care. Advanced cirrhosis and hepatitis are the most common indicators for liver transplantation in adults. The scarcity of liver donors limits those persons who can benefit from this therapy. The major postoperative treatment of these patients centers on the prevention of infection and rejection. Postoperatively these patients are cared for in intensive care units or in a highly specialized nursing care unit.

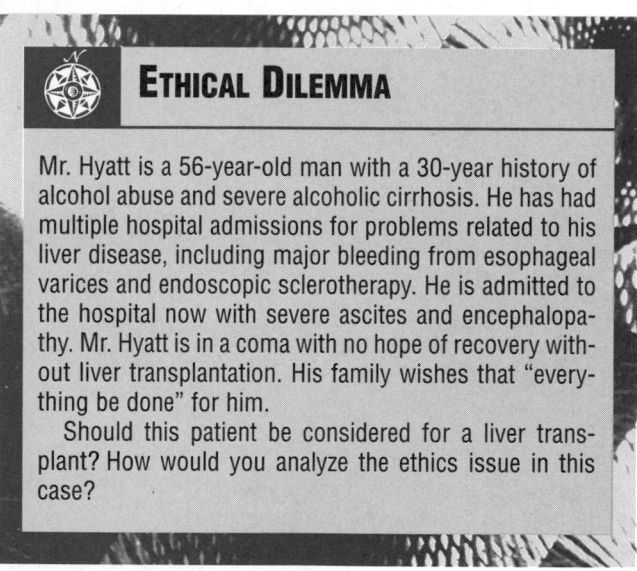

## ETHICAL DILEMMA

Mr. Hyatt is a 56-year-old man with a 30-year history of alcohol abuse and severe alcoholic cirrhosis. He has had multiple hospital admissions for problems related to his liver disease, including major bleeding from esophageal varices and endoscopic sclerotherapy. He is admitted to the hospital now with severe ascites and encephalopathy. Mr. Hyatt is in a coma with no hope of recovery without liver transplantation. His family wishes that "everything be done" for him.

Should this patient be considered for a liver transplant? How would you analyze the ethics issue in this case?

# Diseases and Disorders of the Biliary System

The biliary system consists of the gallbladder and the ducts leading from the liver to the duodenum. About 1 liter of bile per day is formed in the liver and secreted into the left or right hepatic ducts, which merge to become the common hepatic duct (Figure 36-5). Bile passes through the hepatic duct to the cystic duct that leads to the gallbladder where it is stored and concentrated. When needed for digestion, bile is released from the gallbladder and into the cystic duct, flows through the common bile duct, and empties into the duodenum. Bile salts are the metabolically active components of bile. In the intestine, they act on fat to make it more soluble and to break it up into tiny particles (emulsification) that can pass through the intestinal wall. Cholesterol and lecithin in bile keep bile salts in suspension.

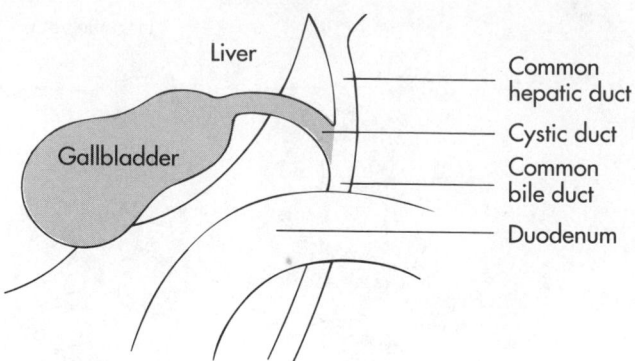

**Figure 36-5** Biliary system. Gallbladder and ducts.

Bile facilitates the absorption of fat-soluble vitamins, iron, and calcium and activates the release of pancreatic and intestinal enzymes (McCance, Huether, 1994; Way, 1996).

Disorders of the biliary system are responsible for approximately 800,000 hospitalizations per year. Diseases of the biliary system include cholecystitis (inflammation), **cholelithiasis** (stone formation), and the more rare tumors, infections, and congenital abnormalities.

## Cholecystitis

Cholecystitis is an inflammation of the gallbladder. It is more common in women than men, and sedentary, obese persons are more likely to be affected. The incidence increases with age, becoming highest in persons in their 50s and 60s.

**Pathophysiology.** Cholecystitis can be caused by an obstruction, a gallstone, or a tumor; however, it is associated with gallstones in almost every case (Way, 1996). In general, the term *cholecystitis* is applied to gallbladder disease whenever gallstones are present, regardless of the appearance of the gallbladder. A variety of organisms contribute to the inflammation of the gallbladder. Because the bile cannot leave the gallbladder during an inflammation or obstruction, more water is absorbed and the bile becomes more concentrated and irritates the wall of the gallbladder. A typical inflammatory response follows, and the gallbladder becomes enlarged and edematous. Chronic inflammation results in the thickening of the wall, which becomes fibrous, replacing normal muscle and mucosal tissue. This can further affect the ability of the gallbladder to empty and concentrate bile. As the tissues of the gallbladder become damaged, bacteria or other irritants can become trapped and contribute to antiinflammatory process. There is danger of rupture of the gallbladder and the spread of infection to the hepatic duct and the liver. When the disease is severe enough to interfere with the blood supply, the gallbladder may become gangrenous.

**Assessment.** Cholecystitis may be acute or chronic in nature. With an acute attack, there is sudden onset of nausea, vomiting, and severe right upper quadrant pain. The pain of **biliary colic** is usually steady, not intermittent like that of intestinal colic. It can begin and cease abruptly but may last for several minutes to several hours. Fatty food intolerance, indigestion, and heartburn are often associated with disease of the gallbladder. During an acute attack the patient may be febrile, usually up to 40° C. In some mild cases the patient may avoid medical attention until jaundice develops or until more severe pain from obstruction of the biliary tract occurs. Tests include abdominal x-ray, ultrasound, electrocardiogram, oral cholecystogram, and perhaps radionuclide scan and ERCP, depending on the presenting symptoms.

**Intervention.** Intravenous fluids are given on admission to the hospital, and the serum electrolytes are checked and corrected with the administration of parenteral supplementation. A nasogastric tube may be inserted and intravenous antibiotics ordered. There are two modes of treatment for the patient presenting with cholecystitis. One mode is to manage the patient with intravenous fluid and antibiotics with a plan to perform a cholecystectomy when recovery from the acute attack has occurred. The second mode is to perform a cholecystectomy immediately. The decision is made based on the general health of the patient, signs of complications of acute cholecystitis, and whether the diagnosis is firmly established (Way, 1996).

Pain management is a key medical and nursing issue in these patients. Meperidine is the traditional agent for managing these patients because it does not cause spasms of Oddi's sphincter. However, morphine sulfate provides far superior pain control. Nursing care includes monitoring intake and output, fluid and electrolyte status, vital signs, and efficacy of pain medication and management.

## Cholelithiasis

Cholelithiasis is the presence of stones in the gallbladder or bile ducts. Each year more than one million people in the United States learn that they have gallstones. They join the estimated 20 million Americans, roughly 10% of our population, that already have gallstones (USDHHS NDDIC, 1993). The profile of those most likely to get gallstones include women between the ages of 20 and 60 years (twice as likely as men), men and women older than 60, and pregnant women who have used birth control pills. Native Americans have the highest prevalence of gallstones in the United States. Mexican American persons of all ages are likely to develop gallstones, as are overweight men and women. Finally, crash dieters who lose a lot of weight quickly are at a higher risk for gallstones.

**Pathophysiology.** Gallstones are primarily comprised of cholesterol, bilirubin, and calcium. They may be large, measuring inches across, or small stones, referred to as gravel. The cause of gallstone formation is not fully understood, and there are numerous theories. Evidence suggests that gallstones form when bile excreted by the liver is abnormally high in cholesterol and lacks the proper concentration and proportion of salts. Individuals with an increased cholesterol level may be predisposed to the formation of gallstones.

When the balance of cholesterol, lecithin, and bile salts is disturbed, precipitation of bile salts may cause the formation of gallstones. Stasis of bile from delayed emptying may result in excess saturation of bile with cholesterol and may promote the precipitation of bile salts. Infection can create an area of irritation that may become a site for stone formation. Inflammation may cause gallstones, and stones may cause inflammation.

**Assessment.** Symptoms result from the inflammation of the gallbladder and the obstruction of the bile flow from the liver or the gallbladder. Pain occurs in the right rib cage in the upper right quadrant and may radiate to the back and shoulders. Decreased flow of bile results in fat intolerance, with symptoms of abdominal distention, flatulence, and nausea and vomiting. Symptoms may first appear after ingesting a meal high in fat. With severe disease, pain and tenderness are increased with elevation of temperature, increased white blood cell count, and increased pulse and respiratory rates. Pain is more severe when the bile passages are blocked. The obstruction of bile flow may cause jaundice. Diagnostic tests may include abdominal x-ray scan, CT scan, radionuclide scan, ultrasound, cholecystogram, and cholangiography.

**Intervention.** Some mild attacks of cholelithiasis may be treated medically. An avoidance of offending foods may be helpful. Anticholinergic drugs, which decrease secretions thereby decreasing biliary contractions, may be helpful in conjunction with analgesic agents. A nasogastric tube may be inserted in the patient with nausea and vomiting, and intravenous hydration is administered. The nurse keeps a careful record of the intake and output of the patient. Positioning of the patient with the head elevated at 45 to 60 degrees and the knees flexed or with the patient lying on his or her side in a knees-to-chest position helps management of pain.

Other medical treatments include the use of medication to dissolve the gallstones. This is helpful for the chronic treatment of cholesterol gallstones. Unfortunately this is a marginally effective therapy. Extracorporeal shock wave lithotripsy is the application of shock wave to the gallbladder to dissolve gallstones. This method is of limited value because the fragments of the stones remain in the gallbladder unless they can be dissolved by oral medication. This treatment has not been approved by the Food and Drug Administration.

Another type of intervention for cholelithiasis is retrieval of stones by endoscopic sphincterotomy (papillotomy). An endoscope is passed through the mouth to the duodenum, and, with a special instrument attached to the endoscope, Oddi's sphincter is widened. A basketlike instrument can then retrieve the gallstone from the duct, but more commonly, through the widened sphincter the stone passes into the duodenum and is expelled by the body in the stool (Lewis, Collier, Heitkemper, 1996).

## Cholecystectomy

**Surgical intervention.** Surgical removal of the gallbladder **(cholecystectomy)** is indicated when the patient had chronic or acute cholecystitis or cholelithiasis. Approximately 500,000 of these surgeries are done yearly in the United States (USDHHS, NDDIC, 1993). Careful evaluation and examination of the patient's general condition are made before the surgery.

In the open cholecystectomy method, an incision is made in the right upper quadrant and the gallbladder is excised. If the common bile duct is explored in the surgery, the surgeon places a T-tube in the common bile duct to allow adequate drainage during the healing of the duct (Figure 36-6). The T-tube also allows a route for postoperative T-tube cholangiogram, if desired.

Laparoscopic cholecystectomy is the preferred method of surgery and is done in approximately 80% to 85% of the cases (Lewis, Collier, Heitkemper, 1996). Laparoscopic cholecystectomy requires that four small incisions be made in the abdominal wall to allow the insertion of surgical instruments and a small video camera. The camera sends a magnified image from in-

side the patient's abdomen to a video monitor, giving the surgeon a close-up view of the organs. The surgeon watches the monitor and performs the operation using surgical instruments through the several other small incisions. The gallbladder is identified and carefully separated from the liver and the other structures. Finally the cystic duct is cut and the gallbladder is removed through one of the small incisions.

**Postoperative interventions.** Following laparoscopic cholecystectomy, the patient is discharged on the operative day or after a one-night stay in the hospital. Postoperative pain is minimal, and patients can usually return to work in 2 to 3 days. Patients who stay in the hospital overnight require monitoring of vital signs, administration of pain medication, and measurement of intake and output. The diet is advanced as tolerated, and the patient is able to ambulate with assistance once he or she feels awake enough to do so. There are generally small adhesive strips over the puncture sites that can be removed before discharge. The patient may shower.

Following open cholecystectomy, the patient will generally stay in the hospital for 3 days. Vital signs are monitored, and the surgical dressing is assessed for bleeding. Adequate intake and output are recorded. Intravenous fluid in administered as ordered. The patient is encouraged and assisted as necessary to turn in bed and to ambulate at least four times per day, beginning on the first postoperative day. Deep breathing exercises are extremely important, and an incentive spirometer is a helpful visual aid for the patients. Pain medication must be ordered in adequate amounts to allow the patient the ability to ambulate and take deep breaths. In some cases a nasogastric tube may be in place, and the patency of drainage is assessed by the nurse. Bowel function is assessed and, generally, a

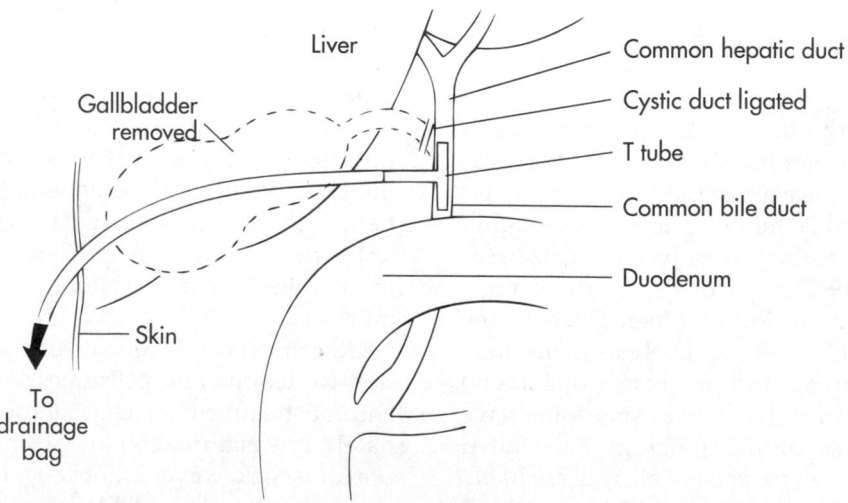

**Figure 36-6**   T-tube in common duct.

> ◁ **BOX 36-4** ▷   **NURSING PROCESS**
>
> ## CHOLECYSTECTOMY, CHOLECYSTOSTOMY, OR CHOLEDOCHOSTOMY POSTOPERATIVE CARE
>
> **ASSESSMENT**
>
> - Vital signs, including temperature, pulse, blood pressure, respirations
> - Pain level on 0 to 10 scale
> - Breath sounds and oxygenation
> - Abdominal distention
> - Surgical wound area and surgical dressing
> - Surgical tubes and drains, including nasogastric tube, T-tube, Penrose, or self-suction drain (Jackson Pratt)
> - Learning needs related to self-care and diet changes
>
> **NURSING DIAGNOSES**
>
> - Risk for altered tissue perfusion related to fluid and electrolyte losses or bleeding
> - Pain related to abdominal incision
> - Ineffective breathing pattern related to pain and splinting of abdominal incision
> - Risk for injury related to accidental obstruction of biliary drainage
> - Risk for impaired skin integrity related to wound drainage
> - Knowledge deficit related to diet modifications, activity restrictions, and signs of biliary obstruction after discharge
>
> **NURSING INTERVENTIONS**
>
> - Check vital signs every 15 minutes until stable, then at least every 4 hours.
> - Assist patient with taking deep breaths; help to splint incision with coughing.
> - Medicate patient for pain as ordered.
> - Assist patient with turning, or turn patient every 2 hours while in bed.
> - Assist patient with ambulation as early as permissible.
> - Maintain intravenous fluid therapy as ordered.
>
> - Maintain accurate I&O records.
> - Maintain patency of nasogastric tube, if in place.
> - Observe for nausea, vomiting, and abdominal distention.
> - Observe color of skin and sclera for jaundice, indicating obstruction of bile flow.
> - Note color and consistency of stool.
> - Observe surgical dressing for drainage; reinforce or change per hospital standards; avoid use of tape by using Montgomery straps if frequent dressing changes are needed.
>
> *If T-tube is in place:*
>
> - Maintain patency of T-tube and prevent tension of tube.
> - Place patient in low to semi-Fowler's position to promote drainage from T-tube.
> - Observe, describe, and record amount and characteristic of drainage at least every 8 hours.
> - Empty bag when half full.
> - Clamp tube in intervals prescribed by physician.
>
> **EVALUATION OF EXPECTED OUTCOMES**
>
> - Meets discharge criteria for postsurgical patient
> - Understands activity restrictions, such as driving and lifting limitations; signs and symptoms of wound infection; diet modifications (low fat)
> - Maximum gas exchange maintained as evidenced by no respiratory distress, acceptable $SaO_2$, and clear breath sounds
> - Adequate tissue perfusion and absence of elevated temperature
> - Acceptable pain level
> - Absence of bile duct injury
> - Skin integrity maintained
> - Evidence of wound healing
> - Adequate nutritional status maintained and implementation of dietary modifications
>
> Return to preoperative self-care level

clear liquid diet is ordered 24 to 48 hours after surgery and increased as tolerated (Box 36-4).

If a T-tube was inserted in the common bile duct, the nurse records the output of the drain at every shift, noting the color and consistency of the bile, and monitors the tube for patency. The bag must be positioned so that the tubing does not become kinked. The T-tube may be left in place for up to 10 days, and some pa-

tients are discharged home with the tube in place. Patients are taught how to empty the T-tube drainage bag and how to record the output. After open cholecystectomy the patient is instructed to avoid heavy lifting for 4 to 6 weeks.

Throughout the postoperative period the patient is monitored for complications. Jaundice will appear if the common duct is occluded by stones or there is a stricture of the duct. A decrease in the blood pressure and rise in the pulse may be a sign of bleeding. In some cases after cholecystectomy the patient will need to remain on a low-fat diet.

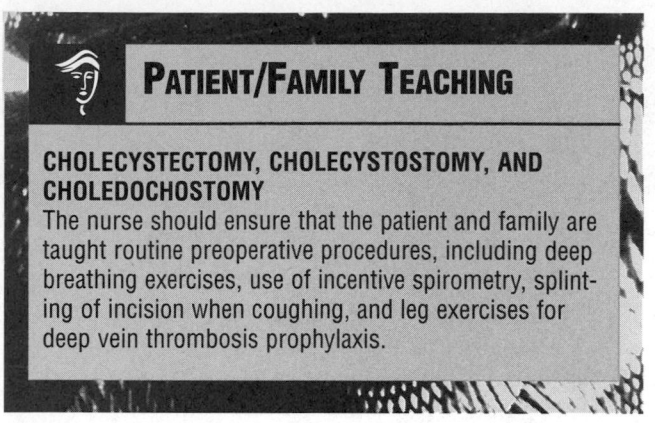

**PATIENT/FAMILY TEACHING**

**CHOLECYSTECTOMY, CHOLECYSTOSTOMY, AND CHOLEDOCHOSTOMY**
The nurse should ensure that the patient and family are taught routine preoperative procedures, including deep breathing exercises, use of incentive spirometry, splinting of incision when coughing, and leg exercises for deep vein thrombosis prophylaxis.

**Other interventions.** Less common interventions for cholelithiasis are cholecystostomy and choledochostomy. A cholecystostomy is an opening into the gallbladder for the retrieval of stones. An incision is made in the top of the gallbladder, and a large lumen tube is sutured to the gallbladder for drainage during the postoperative period. A choledochostomy is the opening and perforation of the common bile duct usually performed to remove stones. A T-tube is inserted for drainage (see Box 36-4).

## Cancer of the Gallbladder

Cancer of the gallbladder is an uncommon occurrence that occurs most frequently in elderly patients. It is twice more common in women than in men and is associated with gallstones in 70% of the cases. At the time of surgery, many of these cancers have spread, and the general areas of metastasis are common duct lymph nodes, the liver, and the lungs. About 85% of the patients are deceased within a year of diagnosis.

## Diseases of the Pancreas
### Pancreatitis

**Pancreatitis** is a common nonbacterial inflammation of the pancreas caused by activation of pancreatic enzymes that results in autodigestion of the pancreatic tissue. Most cases of pancreatitis are caused by gallstones (40%) and alcoholism (40%), but it may be caused by trauma, hypercalcemia, hyperlipidemia, or a genetic predisposition to the disease (Way, 1996). Many cases are idiopathic, and the exact cause and pathogenesis of this disorder are still unknown.

**Pathophysiology.** Biliary pancreatitis associated with gallstones gives rise to acute attacks that recur if left untreated. Chronic pancreatitis rarely results from biliary pancreatitis. In biliary type of pancreatitis, the cause is temporary blockage of the pancreatic duct by gallstones.

Alcoholic pancreatitis occurs in those people with a history of 6 or more years use of excess alcohol. It is more common in those individuals who consume wine and hard liquor, and less common in those who drink beer. In most cases of alcoholic pancreatitis, even with the first attack of pancreatitis, changes of chronic pancreatitis are evident on examination of the pancreas. In this type of pancreatitis, the cause is probably spasm of the pancreatic sphincter and a stimulation of pancreatic enzymes.

### Assessment

*Acute pancreatitis.* In acute pancreatitis there is a sudden upper abdominal pain that radiates to the back. The pain is unrelenting and usually associated with nausea and vomiting. Examination of the patient reveals decreased or absent bowel sounds and tenderness. Temperature may be slightly elevated. The white blood cell count may be slightly elevated as a sign of inflammation, and the hematocrit may be elevated as a sign of dehydration. The serum amylase level may be 2 to 2.5 times normal within the first 6 hours of the attack. Serum lipase levels may be elevated for several days. A simple abdominal x-ray will reveal abnormality in about ⅔ of the cases. The chest x-ray will demonstrate a left pleural effusion, which results from the inflammation of the pancreas. A CT scan of the abdomen will reveal the extent of the inflammation surrounding the pancreas, and the formation of abscesses or fluid collections (pseudocyst) can be identified.

Depending on the severity of the attack, there may be profound dehydration, tachycardia, and hypotension. The patient may collapse from shock. Acute pancreatitis may be complicated by multiple organ failure, principally adult respiratory distress syndrome, myocardial depression, and renal failure. These patients are frequently admitted immediately to the intensive care unit for management. The death rate associated with an attack of acute pancreatitis is about 10%, and nearly all deaths occur with the first attack.

If the patient with acute pancreatitis fails to recover within 1 week of treatment, a pseudocyst is suspected. Pancreatic pseudocysts are encapsulated collections of fluid with high enzyme concentration that arise from the pancreas. They develop in about 2% of the cases of pancreatitis. The principal treatment is to improve symptoms with pain medication. The cysts spontaneously resolve in about 40% of the cases. In some other cases, external drainage catheters are placed to drain the cysts, or internal drainage is established with an operation to connect a limb of the jejunum to the cyst wall to allow for drainage of fluid into the bowel.

**Chronic pancreatitis.** Chronic pancreatitis is characterized by chronic pain that waxes and wanes from day to day. It is pain in the upper abdomen radiating to the back. A pattern of chronic pain may lead to addiction to narcotics in some of these patients. X-ray examination reveals pancreatic calcification. ERCP is helpful in making the diagnosis of chronic pancreatitis. Steatorrhea and diabetes mellitus may result from the abnormal function of the pancreas. Attacks of acute pancreatitis often occur in cases of chronic pancreatitis. Except in advanced cases, alcoholics who can be persuaded not to drink can experience freedom from pain and from recurrent attacks of pancreatitis (Way, 1996).

**Intervention.** The treatment interventions of acute pancreatitis center on the reduction of pancreatic activity and the maintenance of fluid and electrolyte balance. A nasogastric tube is inserted to aspirate gastric secretions. Aggressive fluid replacement of third space fluid loss is essential. Electrolyte replacement therapy is administered based on the laboratory findings. Frequently, calcium and magnesium are needed. Oxygen is administered because hypoxemia is a frequent complication of pancreatitis. In some cases total parenteral nutrition is administered for the severely ill patient.

In biliary pancreatitis the person generally undergoes cholecystectomy soon after the acute attack resolves. However, in severe cases surgery is delayed for several months until the patient recovers from pancreatitis. In some severe cases of pancreatitis, surgical debridement of the dead tissue lowers the mortality rate. In this surgery all necrotic tissue is removed, and a T-tube is inserted in the bile duct if there is bile obstruction. Large drains may be left in the bed of the debrided areas, and these can be used for sterile lavage of the area.

In chronic pancreatitis the treatment centers on treating the steatorrhea and malabsorption. The patient is urged not to use alcohol. Dietary control and taking pancreatic extracts orally are indicated. The patient will require insulin administration and must be taught the skills of blood glucose monitoring and insulin administration.

In those patients with chronic pancreatitis, there may be surgical interventions aimed at controlling the pain. A pancreatoduodenectomy (Whipple's operation) is the operation of choice (Figure 36-7). Pain relief is achieved in 80% of the cases. When unsuccessful, a total pancreatectomy may be performed. In some patients a nerve block, called a *celiac plexus block,* may be used in an attempt to control the pain of chronic pancreatitis.

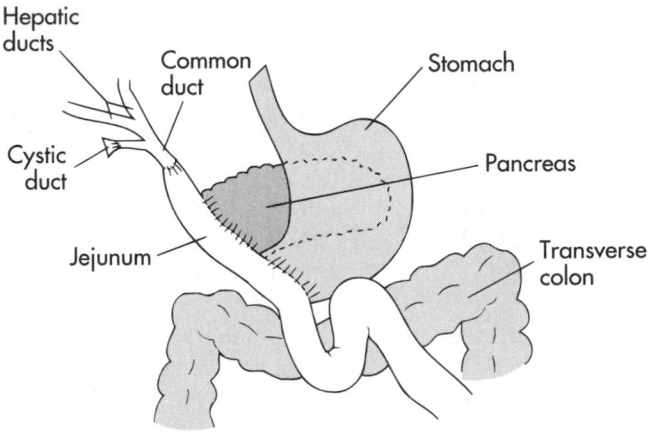

**Figure 36-7**    Whipple procedure includes resection of the distal portion of the stomach, the duodenum, and part of the pancreas. The gallbladder is removed and the biliary ducts are connected to the jejunum. The remaining stomach and pancreas are anastomosed to the jejunum.

## Pancreatic Cancer

Approximately 28,000 cases of pancreatic cancer are diagnosed in the United States each year. Pancreatic cancer is the third leading cause of tumors in men aged 35 to 54 (following lung and colon) (Way, 1996). Factors associated with pancreatic cancer are smoking, dietary consumption of meat (especially fried), and previous **gastrectomy.** It is more common among black men in the United States than white men.

**Pathophysiology.** Approximately 75% of the cases of pancreatic cancers are in the head of the pancreas, and the remainder are in the body of the pancreas. Of the cancers, 80% are ductal adenocarcinoma. It is characterized by early extension to the structures close to the pancreas and alters metastasis to the lymph nodes and liver. The mean survival after palliative therapy is 7 months. Following Whipple's operation the survival rate is approximately 18 months (Way, 1996). Of the patients who present with early stages of pancreatic cancer, 20% survive 5 years.

**Assessment.** The patient will present with weight loss, obstructive jaundice, and deep-seated abdominal pain. The pain may be described as boring into the back. Sudden onset of diabetes mellitus is present in about 25% of the cases. Serum levels of bilirubin and alkaline phosphatase may be elevated as a result of common bile duct obstruction or hepatic metastases. A CT scan will reveal a pancreatic mass in most of the cases. In cases where the CT scan is negative, an ERCP may be done to detect abnormalities in the pancreatic ducts.

**Intervention.** The surgical intervention for curable pancreatic cancer is the pancreatoduodenectomy

(Whipple's operation). This operation involves resection of the common bile duct, the gallbladder, the duodenum, and the pancreas to the midbody. This may also include a partial gastrectomy.

In cancers that are not resectable, the surgical intervention centers on providing relief of jaundice. Cholecystojejunostomy and choledochojejunostomy may be performed to allow bile to flow into the jejunum. Gastrojejunostomy will allow the patient to eat, bypassing the duodenum if the tumor is obstructing it. Biliary stents can also be placed as a palliative measure to treat jaundice. Radiation therapy and chemotherapy may also be used, but they have little curative value.

Nursing care of the patient with pancreatic cancer should provide symptomatic relief and supportive care to the patient and family. Medications to relieve pain should be provided as ordered. Psychologic support is essential. Nutritional support, including supplemental feedings, may be necessary.

Postoperative care of the patient undergoing Whipple's operation is similar to that of any postoperative abdominal surgery patient. The patient will be NPO, and a nasogastric tube will present. Intravenous fluid is administered, and strict input and output are recorded. A Foley catheter will be present for the first several postoperative days. The patient who has undergone a Whipple's operation may have a pancreatic drain or a biliary drain coming out of the abdominal wall. The output of these drains should be recorded every 8 hours. Pain medication should be administered as ordered. The patient is generally out of bed on the first postoperative day with progressive ambulation increased as tolerated. The total length of the hospital stay is generally 5 to 7 days. Many patients return home with indwelling biliary or pancreatic drains. Patient teaching concerning care of the drains and emptying the bags is done by the nurse. In many cases a referral to the visiting nurse in the community is made (Box 36-5).

---

### BOX 36-5

## RESOURCES FOR PATIENTS

***FACTS AND FALLACIES ABOUT DIGESTIVE DISEASES, 1991***
This fact sheet discusses commonly held beliefs about digestive diseases, including pancreatitis and gallbladder disease. Available from the National Digestive Diseases Information Clearinghouse, Box NDDIC, 2 Information Way, Bethesda, MD 20892-3570. (301) 654-3810.

American Liver Foundation
1425 Pompton Avenue
Cedar Grove, NJ 07009
(800) 223-0179 (973) 256-2550

United Network for Organ Sharing
1100 Boulders Parkway, Suite 500
P.O. Box 13770
Richmond, VA 23225-8770
(804) 330-8500

***YOUR GALLSTONES: DIAGNOSIS AND TREATMENT, 1991***
Digestive Disease National Coalition
507 Capitol Court, Suite 2
Washington, DC 20002
(202) 544-7497

Hepatitis B Coalition
1573 Selby Avenue, Suite 234
Saint Paul, MN 55104-6328
(612) 647-9009

Hepatitis Foundation International
30 Sunrise Terrace
Cedar Grove, NJ 07009-1423
(201) 239-1035

# KEY CONCEPTS

➤ The liver, gallbladder, and pancreas are the accessory organs of digestion. Together they assist the process of digestion by contributing specific secretions and enzymes for digestion, allowing the body to make better use of nutrients.

➤ The liver has multiple functions. It assists in the metabolism of carbohydrates, fats, and proteins. It helps regulate the blood glucose and break down fats to provide energy to meet the body's demands.

➤ The gallbladder is a storage compartment for bile, which is produced by the liver. Bile is released into the duodenum to assist with the digestion of fat.

➤ The pancreas is an organ with both endocrine and exocrine functions. The endocrine function refers to the ability of the pancreas to produce insulin. The exocrine function refers to the ability of the pancreas to produce digestive juices and amylase, which help in the digestion of carbohydrates and protein.

➤ The source of the virus hepatitis A is primarily human feces and is spread by oral intake of contaminated milk, food, or water. It may be transmitted through blood and blood products.

➤ The source of the virus that causes hepatitis B is the blood of the person who has the infection or who is the carrier of the infection. The virus is present in semen, saliva, and blood.

➤ The hepatitis C virus is also transmitted by blood and is the major cause of transfusion-related hepatitis.

➤ Hepatitis D is also called the *delta virus*. It primarily attacks those already infected with hepatitis B.

➤ Hepatitis E is a serious infection that primarily occurs in developing third-world countries.

➤ Cirrhosis is a chronic liver disease in which diffuse degeneration and regeneration of the liver cells occur when there is an accumulation of fibrous connective tissue that obstructs the normal biliary and vascular channels in the liver. The most common form is Laënnec's cirrhosis, which is caused by the effects of alcohol on liver disease.

➤ A LeVeen shunt may be performed to control ascites in the patient with cirrhosis when it cannot be controlled with diet and medication.

➤ Hepatic coma follows liver failure. The failing liver causes increasing levels of ammonia in the bloodstream, which results in hepatic encephalopathy.

➤ Cholecystitis is most often caused by a gallstone obstructing the bile duct. Accumulated bile becomes concentrated and irritates the walls of the gallbladder, causing edema and fibrous thickening of the walls and trapping bacteria and other irritants that are possibly interfering with the blood supply, thus resulting in gangrene. The infection can spread to the hepatic duct and the liver, and rupture can occur.

➤ Cholelithiasis is most commonly treated by cholecystectomy. Of cholecystectomies, 80% are now done with a laparoscopic approach.

➤ Pancreatitis is caused by the premature activation of pancreatic enzymes, which result in autodigestion of the pancreatic tissue and altered organ function.

➤ Whipple procedure (pancreaticoduodenectomy) is the surgery of choice for resectable pancreatic cancer.

# CRITICAL THINKING EXERCISES

1. What information would you give to the patient who is going to undergo an open cholecystectomy tomorrow morning?
2. What information would you give the patient who is going to have a laparoscopic cholecystectomy in the morning?
3. You are discharging a patient with hepatitis B. He will be taking interferon at home. What will your discharge instructions include?
4. Mr. Jones is a 49-year-old man admitted to your unit with acute onset of severe right upper quadrant pain that is boring into his back. He has a history of heavy consumption of vodka. Work out a scenario that includes the following: (1) What diagnostic tests will be done immediately, and how will you prepare him for those tests, (2) What are the immediate nursing considerations, (3) What do you expect of his intake and output? What do you expect of his electrolyte picture?

## REFERENCES AND ADDITIONAL READINGS

Adams L, Soulen MC: TIPS: a new alternative for the variceal bleeder, *Am J Crit Care* 2(3):196-201, 1993.

Bagg A: Whipple's procedure: nursing guidelines, *Crit Care Nurse* 8(5):34-45, 1988.

Centers for Disease Control and Prevention (CDC): Guidelines for preventing transmission of *Mycobacterium tuberculosis* in health care facilities, *Fed Reg* 59, October 28, 1994.

Folsch U et al: Early ERCP and papillotomy compared with conservative treatment for acute biliary pancreatitis: the German study group on acute biliary pancreatitis, *N Engl J Med* 336(4):237-241, 1997.

Hoofnagle J, di Bisceglie AM: The treatment of chronic viral hepatitis, *N Engl J Med* 336(5):347-356, 1997.

Jackson MM, Rymer TE: Viral hepatitis: anatomy of a diagnosis, *Am J Nurs* 94:43, 1994.

Lemon S, Thomas D: Vaccines to prevent viral hepatitis, *N Engl J Med* 336(3):196-203, 1997.

Lewis SM, Collier IC, Heitkemper MM: *Medical-surgical nursing: assessment & management of clinical problems*, ed 4, St Louis, 1996, Mosby.

McCance KL, Heuther SE: *Pathophysiology: the biologic basis for disease in adults and children*, ed 2, St Louis, 1994, Mosby.

McFadden DW, Reber HA: Indication for surgery in severe pancreatitis, *Int J Pancreatol* 15:83, 1994.

Secor VH: *Multisystem organ failure: pathophysiology & clinical implications*, ed 2, St Louis, 1996, Mosby.

Silen W: *Cope's early diagnosis of the acute abdomen*, ed 17, New York, 1987, Oxford University Press.

United States Department of Health and Human Services, National Digestive Diseases Information Clearinghouse: *Cirrhosis of the liver*, NIH Pub No 95-1134, Washington, DC, 1991, USDHHS.

United States Department of Health and Human Services, National Digestive Diseases Information Clearinghouse: *Pancreatitis*, NIH Pub No 95-1596, Washington, DC, 1992, USDHHS.

United States Department of Health and Human Services, National Digestive Diseases Information Clearinghouse: *Gallstones*, NIH Pub No 95-2897, Washington, DC, 1993, USDHHS.

United States Department of Health and Human Services, National Digestive Diseases Information Clearinghouse: *Digestive disease statistics*, NIH Pub No 95-3873, Washington, DC, 1995, USDHHS.

Way L: *Current surgical diagnosis and treatment*, ed 10, Norwalk, 1996, Appleton & Lange.

# CHAPTER 37

# Urinary Problems

## KEY TERMS

acute renal failure
anuria
blood urea nitrogen (BUN)
chronic renal failure
creatinine
cystitis
diuretic
glomerular capillaries
hematuria
hemodialysis
ileal conduit
lithiasis
micturition
nephron
nephrotoxic
peritoneal dialysis
pyuria
uremia
ureters
urinalysis

# STRUCTURE AND FUNCTION OF THE URINARY SYSTEM

## Structure
### Macroscopic Anatomy

The urinary system consists of two *kidneys,* two **ureters,** one urinary *bladder,* and one *urethra* (Figure 37-1). The kidneys are located in the posterior abdominal cavity, one on each side of the vertebral column, and are protected and surrounded by muscles, fascia, fat, and different abdominal organs. Additionally, the posterior upper portion of each kidney is protected by ribs. A thin, cellophane-like *capsule* covers

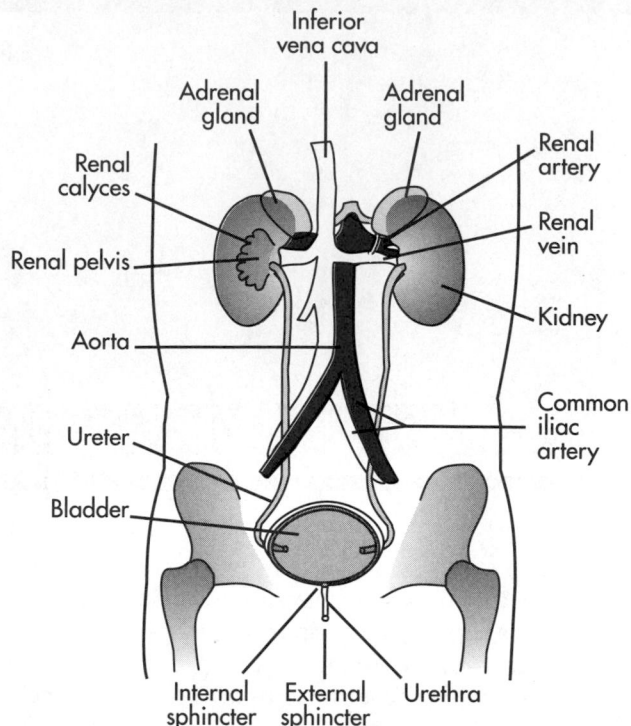

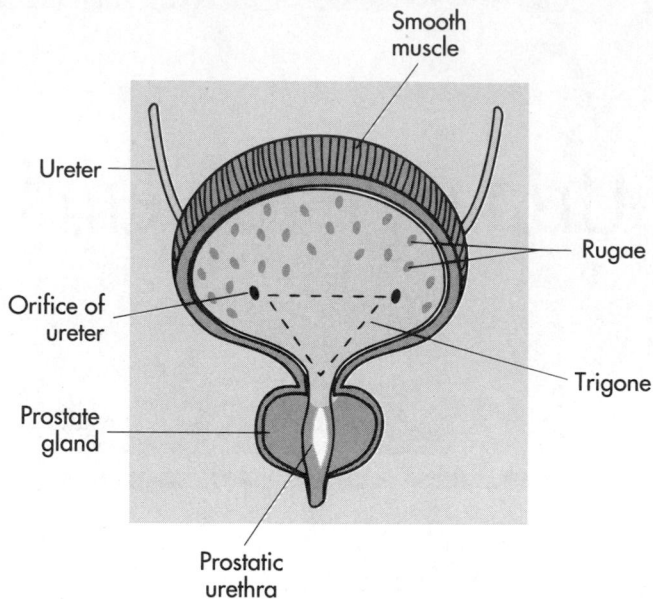

**Figure 37-1**   Organs of the urinary system and the vascular and surrounding structures. The kidneys are located between the twelfth thoracic vertebra and the third lumbar vertebra. The bladder is bisected to show placement of the ureter as it enters the bladder, and the right kidney is bisected to show the renal pelvis and calyces. Note that the renal vein is anterior to the renal artery, and an adrenal gland is located above each kidney.

**Figure 37-2**   Cross section of the male urinary bladder showing the trigone, a small, smooth area between the ureteral openings and the urethra.

each kidney and contains blood vessels, lymphatic vessels, and nerve fibers. Pain can be felt if the capsule is stretched or punctured (Richard, 1995a and 1995b).

The ureters are fibromuscular, mucosa-lined, narrow tubes approximately 25 to 30 cm (1 to 1⅕ inches) in length that originate in the kidneys and terminate in the bladder. The urinary bladder, a distensible muscular sac, holds approximately 300 to 800 ml (9 to 24 ounces) of urine and is located in the pelvis between the rectum and the pubic bone. The interior of the bladder consists of many folds, or *rugae,* when the bladder is empty. The rugae flatten when the bladder is full. The *trigone* is a small, triangular region between each ureteral opening (or orifice) and the urethra. The trigone is usually smooth, without rugae, and nondistensible, and it is located in the lower portion of the bladder (Figures 37-1 and 37-2).

The urethra is a mucosa-lined tube that connects the bladder to the urinary meatus. The urethra is shorter in the female, approximately 3 to 5 cm (1⅕ to 2 inches) in length, and longer in the male, approximately 20 cm (8 inches) in length. The internal urethral sphincter, a ring of muscle, is located at the beginning of the urethra and is controlled involuntarily. The external ure-

thral sphincter is located farther down the urethra and is controlled voluntarily.

Because the ureters, urinary bladder, and urethra are innervated with pain receptors, pain can be felt in any of these structures (Richard, 1995b). The kidneys produce urine that is transported unchanged via peristalsis through the ureters to the bladder, through the urethra, and out the urinary meatus.

## Microscopic Anatomy

The structural-functional unit of the kidney is the **nephron,** and there are more than a million in each kidney. Although nephrons are packed together closely, they are separated by interstitial tissue.

A nephron is composed of five parts: Bowman's capsule, a proximal convoluted tubule, the loop of Henle, a distal convoluted tubule, and a collecting duct (Figure 37-3). The nephron wall is one cell thick and is supported by a *basement membrane,* which is composed of collagen and glycoproteins (Richard, 1995b). The beginning of each nephron is shaped like a cup and is called *Bowman's capsule.* It surrounds a cluster of **glomerular capillaries,** which are also supported by a basement membrane (Figure 37-4).

Extending from each Bowman's capsule is the *proximal convoluted tubule.* It is proximal because it is the segment nearest the tubule's origin from Bowman's capsule; it is convoluted because it is twisted. The proximal tubule narrows and becomes the descending limb of the *loop of Henle;* it later becomes the ascending limb, widens, and becomes the *distal convoluted tubule.* The

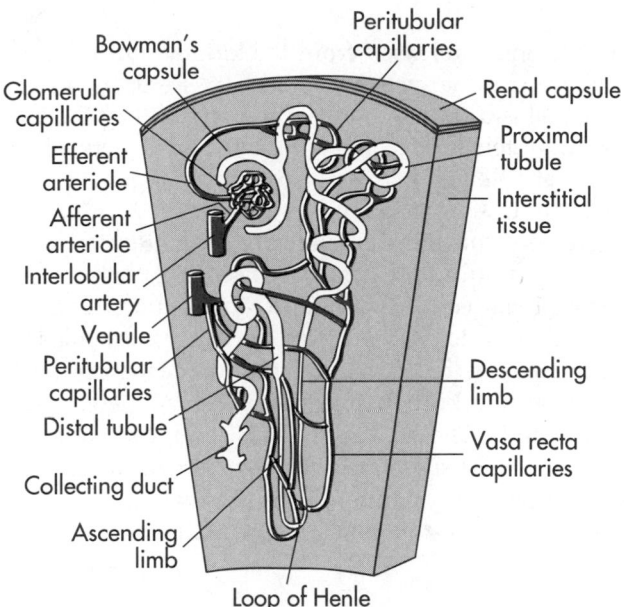

**Figure 37-3** A nephron and its vasculature. The nephron is composed of Bowman's capsule, a proximal tubule, the loop of Henle (descending and ascending limbs), a distal tubule, Many distal tubules empty into a collecting duct. Blood flows through the afferent arteriole and the glomerular capillaries into the efferent arteriole, which divides into peritubular capillaries (which surround the proximal and distal tubules) and the vasa recta capillaries (which surround the loop of Henle and the collecting duct). Both capillary systems drain into a venule.

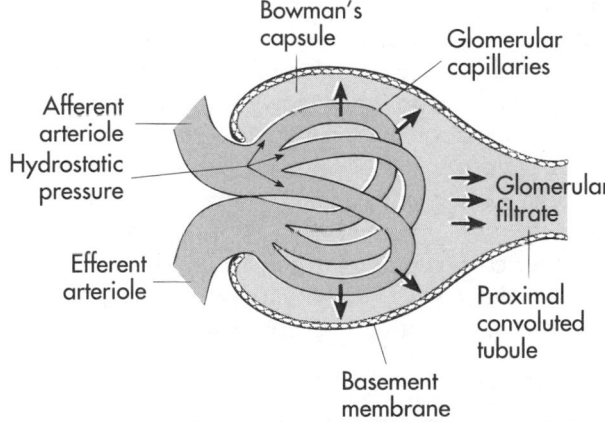

**Figure 37-4** Enlarged view of Bowman's capsule, glomerular capillaries, and the process of glomerular filtration. The afferent arteriole divides into the glomerular capillaries, which unite to form the efferent arteriole. The glomerular capillaries are surrounded by Bowman's capsule, which narrows into the proximal convoluted tubule. A continuous basement membrane supports the wall of Bowman's capsule, which is one cell thick, and the proximal convoluted tubule. Blood flows through the afferent arteriole into the glomerular capillaries, where filtration begins. The large arrows indicate the direction of filtration. Hydrostatic pressure is the main driving force for filtration. This pressure is a result of systemic blood pressure, which exerts a force against the walls of the glomerular capillaries *(small arrows)*. The solution filtered through the glomerular capillaries into Bowman's capsule is called the glomerular filtrate.

distal tubule terminates in the collecting duct. Many *collecting ducts* join and form the renal calyces and subsequently the kidney pelvis. The *kidney pelvis* is small, holding 3 to 5 ml of urine. It is the last intrarenal structure before the ureter begins (see Figure 37-1).

Blood flows to the kidney through the *renal artery*. This artery divides many times and eventually forms the *afferent arteriole* (see Figure 37-3). The afferent arteriole divides into glomerular capillaries, which unite to form the *efferent arteriole.* The efferent arteriole divides into two branches, the peritubular and the vasa recta capillaries. The *peritubular capillaries* surround the proximal and distal tubules, and the *vasa recta capillaries* surround the loop of Henle and collecting ducts. Both capillary systems drain into venules. The kidneys are very vascular and require a large blood supply for the high metabolic rate of the nephrons.

## Function

The kidneys are organs of *regulation.* They regulate many substances such as water, electrolytes, nitrogenous wastes, acids, and bases; they also regulate bodily processes, such as blood pressure, through the production of urine and hormones.

### Urine Formation

Urine formation is divided into two steps: glomerular filtration and tubular processes.

**Glomerular filtration.** As blood flows through the glomerular capillaries, water and many substances filter from the blood and pass through the capillary wall into Bowman's capsule (see Figure 37-4). The main driving force for filtration is *hydrostatic pressure* in the glomerular capillaries. This pressure is a result of systemic blood pressure, which exerts a force against the glomerular capillary walls. For glomerular filtration to occur, systemic blood pressure must be maintained. If systemic blood pressure falls significantly, glomerular filtration diminishes or even stops.

Another factor that influences glomerular filtration is the structural integrity of the glomerular capillaries and Bowman's capsule. Usually erythrocytes, leukocytes, platelets, and plasma proteins do not filter because they are too large to pass through the glomerular capillaries and Bowman's capsule. If these structures are diseased, blood cells and proteins may filter and may be found abnormally in urine. *Proteinuria,* or proteins in the urine, is one sign of glomerular capillary disease.

The solution that is filtered through the glomerular capillaries into Bowman's capsule is called the *glomerular filtrate.* It is composed mostly of water, electrolytes, creatinine, sugars, nitrogenous wastes, and bicarbonate. The *glomerular filtration rate* is the volume of glomerular filtrate and the rate at which it is filtered and is approximately 125 ml/minute. As glomerular filtrate leaves Bowman's capsule and enters the proximal tubule, the second step of urine formation, tubular processes, begins.

**Tubular processes.** Throughout the length of the nephron, the tubular processes of reabsorption and secretion selectively alter the reduce the glomerular filtrate to form urine. *Reabsorption* is the movement of substances from within the nephron to the surrounding capillaries (peritubular and/or vasa recta) and/or interstitial tissue, the cells between nephrons and blood vessels. *Secretion* is the movement of substances from within the capillaries and/or interstitium into the nephron. The following paragraphs briefly describe how tubular processes affect the glomerular filtrate as it flows through the nephron.

In the proximal tubule approximately 60% to 70% of the glomerular filtrate is reabsorbed; this includes water, most electrolytes, sugars, urea, and bicarbonate. Hydrogen ions and some drugs are secreted. In the descending loop of Henle, a small volume of water is reabsorbed and urea is secreted. In the ascending limb, chloride and sodium are reabsorbed and urea is secreted (Richard, 1995b).

In the distal tubule the transport of many substances is regulated by extrarenal hormones. Aldosterone causes sodium reabsorption and potassium secretion. Chloride follows sodium. Atrial naturetic hormone decreases sodium reabsorption (Gillenwater et al, 1996). Parathyroid hormone increases calcium reabsorption and decreases phosphate reabsorption. Calcitonin decreases phosphate and calcium reabsorption. Hydrogen ions and ammonia are secreted.

The collecting duct determines the final volume and composition of urine. *Antidiuretic hormone (ADH),* also called vasopressin, causes water reabsorption and forms a concentrated urine. Without ADH water is not reabsorbed, and a dilute urine is excreted. Urea is reabsorbed or secreted, or both, depending on its concentration in the tissues surrounding the collecting duct.

**Creatinine,** an end product of muscle metabolism, is a unique substance because it is freely filtered through the glomerular capillaries but minimally affected by tubular processes. Therefore the amount of creatinine filtered is found in the urine. Because creatinine is only excreted by the kidneys, it is very useful in diagnosing and evaluating renal disorders (Richard, 1995b).

The kidneys correct acid-base imbalances that blood buffers and lungs have started to correct. The kidneys regulate the bicarbonate level and neutralize and excrete acids. The urinary pH can vary from acidic to alkaline, depending on the body's needs.

## Renal Hormones

The hormones released from the kidney and their actions are summarized in Table 37-1. Renin is an enzyme that is produced, stored, and released by the kidney. Angiotensinogen is synthesized and secreted by the liver. Renin converts angiotensinogen to angiotensin I. As angiotensin I circulates through the lung, an enzyme there converts it to angiotensin II. Angiotensin II stimulates thirst, causes peripheral vasoconstriction, decreases renin secretion, and stimulates aldosterone release. Aldosterone causes the plasma sodium level to rise by stimulating the reabsorption of sodium in the kidney, intestine, salivary glands, and sweat glands. The above system is commonly referred to as the *renin-angiotensin-aldosterone system,* and its overall goal is to maintain sodium, water, and blood pressure balances (Richard, 1995b; Gillenwater et al, 1996).

## Urination

The process of releasing urine from the body is called urination, **micturition,** or voiding. When the bladder has 300 to 500 ml (9 to 15 ounces) of urine, the stretch receptors are stimulated and send a message to the spinal cord. The spinal cord sends a message to the cerebral cortex in the brain. The person is consciously aware that the bladder is filling and of the need to empty it soon. The cerebrum sends a message via the spinal cord to the bladder, which contracts and relaxes the internal urethral sphincter. When the person is ready to void, the external urethral sphincter is consciously relaxed and urine flows from the body. Usually once urination has begun, it continues until the bladder is empty. However, a person can stop urination midstream by consciously contracting the external sphincter.

Another component of urination is called the *spinal cord micturition reflex.* As described previously, with bladder filling the stretch receptors are stimulated and

---

**TABLE 37-1**

### Hormones Produced and/or Secreted by the Kidney

| HORMONE | ACTION |
| --- | --- |
| Erythropoietin | Stimulates formation of red blood cells in the bone marrow |
| Kinins | Vasodilation |
| Prostaglandins | Renal vasodilation; some cause constriction |
| Vitamin D | Increases calcium and phosphate absorption from the intestine, bone, and kidney |

send a message to the spinal cord. The spinal cord sends a message to the bladder, causing it to contract and the internal urethral sphincter to relax. Therefore bladder contraction and internal sphincter relaxation can be controlled by the spinal cord reflex or cerebral messages, or both. Examples of this reflex are seen in an infant who is not toilet trained or a comatose adult; both urinate whenever the bladder is full because they do not have cerebral control of the external urethral sphincter.

The terminal portion of the ureters are located within the bladder wall. As the bladder contracts, the ureters are squeezed shut, preventing backflow or reflux of urine up the ureters. The prevention of urine reflux is one the urinary tract's protective mechanisms for ensuring that contaminated urine does not reach the sterile kidneys (Gillenwater et al, 1996).

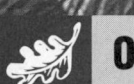

## OLDER ADULT CONSIDERATIONS

During the fourth decade, the kidneys begin to decrease in size and function and by the eighth decade have shrunk 30% and lost a proportionate amount of function. The change in kidney size is mostly a result of the loss of glomerular capillaries. A loss of these capillaries causes a decrease in glomerular filtration. In addition the kidney has a decreased ability to conserve water and salt. Actually the kidneys in the elderly meet their needs unless the elderly are stressed severely. Stressful situations include gastrointestinal fluid and electrolyte losses from vomiting and diarrhea, water loss associated with fever, water and electrolyte losses from diuretics, decreased fluid intake, and blood losses from surgery. During these stressful situations the kidney does not have the speed or capacity to respond as though it were in a younger body. Therefore it is important that the elderly be protected from rapid fluid and electrolyte shifts. The elderly are also more susceptible to renal damage from drugs, which means it is beneficial for older people to have their renal function evaluated while they are taking medication.

## NURSING ASSESSMENT—HISTORY AND PHYSICAL EXAMINATION

This section highlights aspects of the history and physical examination that are specific for the urinary system. A discussion of a complete history and physical can be found in the text *Health and Physical Assessment* by Barkauskas and colleagues (1996). Additional information on patient assessment for specific conditions is presented in the section Diseases and Disorders of the Urinary System. Important nursing responsibilities associated with caring for a patient undergoing an assessment are to explain all procedures and tests and to make sure that the patient understands, to his or her satisfaction, the results of all procedures and tests.

Because the kidneys and ureters are located deep within the abdominal cavity, they are difficult to examine physically. It is even more difficult to obtain information about their function from a physical examination. The urinary system, however, is assessed during an abdominal examination with the patient supine and the nurse on the right side of the patient. The nurse imagines the abdomen divided into four quadrants with the umbilicus as the center. The nurse inspects the entire abdominal region, diaphragm to symphis pubis, from a standing position and then at eye level for raised masses. Usually these abnormalities are not present. Enlarged kidneys may be visible in the upper quadrants, and an enlarged bladder may be visible in the lower quadrants across the midline. The nurse palpates and then percusses the abdomen. A distended bladder feels tense, smooth, round, and dull to percussion.

Pain associated with the urinary tract may be stimulated during a physical examination and can be felt from an area slightly below the ribs to the upper thighs. Typically, ureteral pain is felt in the groin or genital area, bladder pain is felt in the suprapubic to upper thigh area, and renal pain is felt at the *costovertebral angle* in the back. The costovertebral angle is slightly above the waist where the ribs join the vertebral column. If the person feels tenderness or pain in any of these areas, the nurse should be as gentle as possible when touching the areas.

Unfortunately, extensive damage and even complete loss of a kidney can occur without the person feeling any pain because most of the kidney has no pain receptors. The renal capsule, however, is innervated with pain receptors, and if it is punctured, distended, or inflamed, a dull to sharp pain is felt. The rest of the urinary tract has many pain receptors and responds according to the pathologic condition. For example, a sudden obstruction, such as a stone in the ureter, causes an abrupt onset of sharp pain (Richard, 1995a).

## DIAGNOSTIC TESTS AND NURSING RESPONSIBILITIES

### Collection of Urine Specimens
#### Methods

Urine can be collected by the clean-catch or voided-midstream method, bladder catheterization, or suprapubic aspiration of (bladder) urine. All procedures should be thoroughly explained to the patient whether the patient, the nurse, or someone else does the collection. The clean-catch or voided-midstream method is explained first. After washing the hands, the external genitalia are washed thoroughly with soap and water. With a female the labia are separated; with an uncircumcised male the foreskin is retracted before voiding. The patient voids approximately 100 ml (3 ounces) to wash out bacteria and leukocytes in the urethra, continues voiding, and then collects the urine in a sterile container. Only the outside of the container is touched, and it is covered as soon as the urine has been voided into it.

---

### NURSE ALERT

**Nurses are responsible for educating the patient about what will occur before, during, and after diagnostic tests.**

---

*Bladder catheterization* and *suprapubic aspiration* are invasive procedures that can cause urinary tract infections and are done when no alternative, noninvasive method is available. These procedures are discussed in the section Therapeutic Procedures and Nursing Implications. If the patient has a bladder catheter in place, a urine specimen can be collected using aseptic technique. Newly excreted urine is taken from the drainage system rather than old urine that has accumulated in the drainage bag. The exact method of urine collection can vary with the design of the drainage system; the manufacturer's instructions should be followed. Aseptic technique always is used. See the section Ileal Conduit (Ileobladder), p. 1160, for an explanation of the procedure for collecting urine from a urinary stoma.

### Timing

If the urine cannot be taken to the laboratory immediately after it is collected, it is refrigerated. Substances in the urine change at room temperature, making the results of the urinalysis inaccurate. For example, red blood cells hemolyze, bacteria grow and consume glucose, and the pH changes. The frequency of urine collection depends on the requirements of the test and is explained in the next section.

### Purposes

Although urine may be analyzed for many reasons, this section focuses on urinalysis as it relates to structures, functions, and diseases of the urinary system.

Additional information on urinalysis for specific conditions is presented in the section Diseases and Disorders of the Urinary System.

## Urinalysis

A *routine* or *baseline* **urinalysis** assesses urine color, clarity, odor, specific gravity and/or osmolality, pH, glucose, ketones, proteins and related substances, sediment (which includes cells, crystals, casts, and bacteria or other microorganisms), and possibly enzymes and electrolytes. The first urine of the day is the most concentrated from an overnite fast; therefore it is the best specimen to use for a routine/baseline urinalysis, especially to assess pH, osmolality, and sediment. The clean-catch method should be used to collect urine. Although usually a minimum of 15 ml (about ½ ounce) is required for routine urinalysis (the nurse should check with the laboratory doing the test because some can do the urinalysis with less), it is helpful to send more urine so that results can be double checked. If abnormalities are found, further testing can be done. Some patients with urinary tract disease may have less than 15 ml with any voiding; the nurse sends what there is.

A *24-hour urine collection* can measure the total quantity of a substance or substances excreted in a day. This is helpful for substances excreted in varying concentrations throughout the day, such as hormones, creatinine, protein, urea, and glucose. A 24-hour urine collection can be started at any time by using the following procedure:

1. Explain the entire procedure to the patient.
2. Prepare a collection container per laboratory instructions; for example, refrigerate, add preservatives or both.
3. Designate a time for collection to start. The patient voids at this time, and that urine is discarded.
4. Save all subsequent voidings. Using the clean-catch method, urine is voided into a receptacle and then poured into a collection container to prevent contamination with feces.
5. Collect the last urine specimen 24 hours from the starting time.
6. Send all urine in properly labeled containers to the laboratory immediately. If the collection is interrupted and some urine is omitted from the collection, the collection is stopped, the urine is discarded, and the procedure is restarted.

A *urine smear* or *culture* and *sensitivity* tests (or both) are done to assess the urine for microorganisms and accompanying cells and to identify medications or drugs to which the organisms are most sensitive. A few milliliters of urine collected by the clean-catch method and placed in a sterile container are required for these tests.

With a *serial urine collection* each voiding is saved in a separate container for a designated number of voidings, hours, or days or until some urinary characteristic is adequately assessed. For instance, after bladder surgery, hematuria (blood in the urine, which has a red tinge) can occur, and a serial urine collection is implemented. Each voiding is labeled with the patient's name and room number, as well as the date and time that the specimen was collected. Each voiding is saved and assessed for changes in **hematuria** (redness). The redness should diminish with each voiding, and the urine should become yellow. If the hematuria persists, specific treatment is implemented. With a serial urine collection, the clean-catch method is adequate, and specimens can be assessed in a patient's room or a utility room or sent to a laboratory, or any combination of these.

Urine is approximately 95% water and consists of excess water and excess substances that are end products of body metabolism. It is a valuable body fluid to assess because it reflects renal function as well as other bodily processes.

Freshly voided urine has a slight *odor* caused by the breakdown of urea to ammonia. If urine stands for a period of time or has a large bacteria population, it will have a strong ammonia smell. The ingestion and excretion of certain foods and medications, such as asparagus and vitamins, also causes urine to smell differently.

The pale yellow to amber *color* of urine is a result of the presence of urochrome pigments. Urine color can be changed by the presence of cells and by an increased urine concentration. The presence of red blood cells, hematuria, can cause urine color to range from yellow to bright red. White blood cells can make urine look whitish. Concentrated urine is usually dark yellow to orange.

Normally urine is clear and slightly acidic, although its pH range is 4.5 to 8. Urine becomes cloudy and alkaline upon standing because of the breakdown of urea to ammonia, which increases the pH. Cloudiness can result from the presence of cells, bacteria, crystals, casts, or fat substances.

The kidneys are significant in regulating overall body fluid balance. They excrete a concentrated urine when water needs to be conserved or a dilute urine when there is an excess of water. A measure of the kidneys' ability to concentrate or dilute urine is urine osmolality, which ranges from 300 to 1200 mOsm/kg water. A very dilute urine is 300 mOsm/kg water, whereas a very concentrated urine is 1200 mOsm/kg water. It is helpful to measure urine osmolality and blood osmolality (approximately 290 mOsm/kg water) simultaneously to determine if the kidneys are accurately regulating body fluid balance. Urine *specific gravity* varies with the amount of solids in the urine such as cells, casts, and microorganisms, but urine osmolality is not affected by these substances; this urine osmolality is a more accurate measure of the kidneys' ability to concentrate or dilute urine. The range for specific gravity is 1.005 to 1.030, with the higher number indicating a more concentrated urine. Usually urine osmolality and specific gravity vary somewhat throughout the day and from day to day. If they become fixed or remain the same for consecutive voidings and days, this could indicate renal disease (Richard, 1995a; King, 1997).

*Urea,* an end product of *protein* metabolism, is found in urine and varies with protein intake and fluid balance. A small amount of proteinuria is insignificant, but a quantity greater than 150 mg/24 hours should be investigated because this could indicate glomerular capillary disease. Proteinuria can produce a foamy urine.

The kidneys regulate *electrolyte* balance. They excrete a variable amount of electrolytes per day as well as throughout the day. Urinary electrolyte excretion is influenced by many factors and is accurately assessed with a 24-hour urine collection and analysis of blood electrolytes.

*Glycosuria* (glucose in the urine) is unusual except with hyperglycemia (elevated blood glucose), which can occur with diabetes mellitus or after excessive ingestion of sugar. Rarely does glycosuria indicate renal disease.

A few epithelial cells, erythrocytes, leukocytes, and bacteria are normally found in urine. An excess of any of these *cells* could indicate a pathologic condition anywhere along the urinary tract. The site of the pathologic condition can usually be identified with further assessment. For instance, erythrocytes that originate in the kidney are usually broken and found with red blood cell casts, whereas erythrocytes from the lower urinary tract are not as broken and not found with red blood cell casts. Eosinophils (not usually found in urine) indicate a hypersensitivity reaction such as rejection of a transplanted kidney.

*Crystals* and *stones* are not usually found in the urine, but either one can originate anyplace along the urinary tract. If found in the urine, their composition should be identified and the urinary tract assessed for more crystals and stones. They may not be the result of urinary tract disease but can cause it by obstructing the flow of urine.

*Casts* are formed within the nephron and are unique to renal disease. There are many types of casts, and each is associated with certain renal pathologic conditions. For example, white cell casts are composed of bits of leukocytes and are associated with renal inflammation, such as pyelonephritis (Price-Anderson, Wilson-McCarty, 1996).

## Creatinine Tests
### Plasma Creatinine

*Creatinine* is an end product of muscle metabolism and is excreted only by the kidney. Plasma creatinine averages approximately 0.7 to 1.3 mg/dl and is relatively constant throughout the day and from day to day. Creatinine levels are slightly higher in men than in women because of men's larger muscle mass. A rise in plasma creatinine indicates a decrease in renal function. A blood sample can be collected at any time to measure plasma creatinine.

### Creatinine Clearance

Like plasma creatinine measurement, *creatinine clearance* is a very specific test that assesses renal function, primarily the glomerular filtration rate. Creatinine is filtered through the glomerular capillaries and passes through the rest of the nephron unaffected. Therefore the rate at which creatinine is excreted in the urine is similar to the glomerular filtration rate. Normal creatinine clearance is approximately 110 to 125 ml/minute. To conduct the test, the nurse should collect a 24-hour urine specimen and one blood specimen at the midpoint (hour 12) of the urine collection. A decline in creatinine clearance indicates a decrease in renal function (Richard, 1995a).

## Blood Urea Nitrogen

Urea is an end product of protein metabolism. It is primarily excreted by the kidney and is measured in the blood as **blood urea nitrogen (BUN).** BUN averages approximately 10 to 20 mg/dl. It rises with a decrease in renal function or fluid volume and with an increase in catabolism and dietary protein intake. Because BUN is affected by multiple factors, it is correlated with changes in plasma creatinine to assess renal function. When renal function decreases, both plasma creatinine and BUN rise. A rapidly rising or very elevated BUN can affect the nervous system and the patient can experience loss of memory, disorientation, confusion, and convulsions. Nursing interventions focus on preventing injury by visiting and orienting the patient often, placing the call light within close reach, and possibly putting the side rails up on the bed.

## Kidneys, Ureters, and Bladder X-rays

An x-ray film is taken of the abdomen to visualize the kidneys, ureters, and bladder (KUB) and to serve as a screening test before most other procedures. A KUB visualizes the position, shape, size, and number of macroscopic or gross renal, ureteral, and bladder structures and surrounding bones. The only patient preparation required is an explanation of the procedure (Corbett, 1992).

## Pyelography
### Excretory Urography

Several methods that use a radiopaque dye are used to obtain x-ray films of the urinary system. In *excretory urography,* also called intravenous pyelography, dye is injected into a vein, circulates through the kidney, and is excreted in the urine. A series of x-ray films is taken at short intervals while the dye is being excreted. This test determines the size, shape, and location of urinary tract structures and evaluates renal excretory function. Patient preparation includes an explanation of the procedure and postexamination care; adequate fluid intake; a clear, empty gastrointestinal tract; an allergy history; and baseline information about renal function. The dye is **nephrotoxic** (poisonous to the kidney) and allergenic to some people (Shannon, Wilson, 1994). A hydrated state helps the dye pass through the kidney and prevents renal damage.

Because the intravenous dye usually contains iodine, the patient is questioned carefully concerning any allergies, especially to iodine or shellfish. A test dose is often given to determine the patient's sensitivity to the dye, but it is generally believed that such testing is not totally reliable. A negative reaction to a sensitivity test does not guarantee that the patient will not have a severe reaction to the injected dye. Therefore knowledgeable personnel are present during the test to observe for and treat an allergic response. Because fecal matter and gas in the intestinal tract interfere with the visualization of the kidneys and the ureters on the x-ray film, a laxative or enema may be indicated before the test.

When the test is completed, the patient needs to drink plenty of fluids to help eliminate any dye left in the body. The patient is also observed for signs and symptoms of an allergic response or decreasing renal function, or both (Richard, 1995b).

### Retrograde Urography

*Retrograde urography* is an invasive procedure that consists of passing a catheter or cystoscope into the bladder, passing small catheters into the ureters (*ureteral catheterization),* injecting a radiopaque dye, and taking x-ray films. More x-ray films can be taken as the catheters are removed and then 15 to 30 minutes after the initial x-ray examination to make sure all the dye is secreted. This test provides anatomic information about the urinary tract from the renal pelvis through the urinary meatus and is often done when an obstruction is suspected. If necessary, urine specimens may be obtained from each kidney before the dye is injected. Retrograde urography is often done in connection with cystoscopic examination.

**NURSE ALERT**

Dye used for excretory and retrograde urography is nephrotoxic. Have the patient drink 300 to 360 ml (10 to 12 ounces) of water every hour for 4 to 6 hours after the test to help excrete the dye and protect the kidneys from damage. Fluids can also be given intravenously.

After the test the patient must be observed for *urinary tract infection (UTI),* hematuria, allergic response to the dye, and changes in urine output. Urinary tract infection can result from retrograde movement of organisms with catheter insertion and dye injection. Hematuria can be associated with UTI or can result from injury to the urinary tract mucosa caused by the catheter or cystoscope. Ureteral edema can result from manipulation of the catheters and can obstruct urine flow. Signs and symptoms of this are decreased urine output and possibly pain.

Although excretory and retrograde urographic tests provide very useful information about urinary tract structures and function, they can be hazardous to the patient's urinary tract. The nurse can minimize the hazards by properly assessing and preparing the patient and implementing postexamination care that focuses on evaluating and preserving urinary tract function (Richard, 1995a; King, 1997).

## Bladder Studies
### Cystoscopic Examination

The cystoscopic examination directly visualizes the inside of the urinary bladder and may be done with retrograde urography. A cystoscope is a long, lighted, metal instrument that is passed through the urethra and into the bladder to observe the bladder and ureteral openings for abnormalities. The examination may be done while the patient is under a local or general anesthetic. Unless a general anesthetic is to be given, fluids are encouraged and the patient does not void before the examination. A sedative may be given shortly before the procedure to decrease anxiety. The nurse ensures that patients understand the procedure and their role in it, especially if only a local anesthetic is used.

After the procedure the urine may be blood tinged or sometimes colored blue or red from the dye used to evaluate kidney function (retrograde urography). The patient is taught that the discoloration is expected and that it will clear. The patient may also have some discomfort, such as burning on urination or pain in the back. Analgesics, warm sitz baths, and external heat to the back and abdomen may relieve the discomfort. Severe pain warrants further investigation. Patients having a cystoscopic examination are always observed for possible hemorrhage after the procedure (Gillenwater et al, 1996).

## Cystography

In cystography, a catheter is introduced into the bladder, urine is removed, a radiopaque substance is injected into the bladder, and x-ray films are taken. Stones, tumors, or any other pathologic condition is detected. Patient care is similar to that for the cystoscopic examination and retrograde urography (Richard, 1986).

## Urodynamic Studies

Various tests can be used to evaluate bladder, urethral, and sphincter functions and all phases of voiding; for example, a cystometrogram measures bladder pressure during bladder filling and voiding. Other urodynamic studies are urinary sphincter electromyography, urethral pressure studies, urinary flow rate determination, and urinary videofluoroscopy. The nurse can refer to Wozniak-Petrofsky (1997) for a thorough explanation of these tests and patient care.

## Radioisotope Studies
### Renography

In renography, a small amount of radioactive material is administered intravenously; it circulates through the kidney and is excreted in the urine. This test measures renal function. A graphic record (renogram) is made that traces the radioisotope through the kidney and assesses renal blood flow, glomerular filtration, and tubular secretion. Patient preparation includes an explanation of the test and an assessment of the patient's ability to sit or lie quietly for 30 to 60 minutes. No special postexamination patient care is required.

### Renoscan

The renoscan is a procedure that outlines the kidney by external scanning. After intravenous injection of a radioactive isotope, a scanning device, such as a scintillator, is passed over the patient's back directly above each kidney and counts the activity of the isotope. In the presence of tumors or nonfunctioning areas, the radioactive material is not detected by the scan. Patient care is the same as for renography.

## Ultrasonography

Ultrasound scanning is a noninvasive procedure that provides almost immediate information. High-frequency sound waves are reflected over the desired body areas, transmitted to an oscilloscope, and recorded. There is no discomfort associated with ultrasound. However, it is important to realize that the patient must be able to tolerate a prone position for approximately 30 minutes for a renal ultrasound.

## Computed Tomography

Computed tomography (CT) combines the basic principles of radiography with computer technology. Instead of broad x-ray beams passing through the patient to be captured on x-ray film, CT scanning uses a thin x-ray beam that is visualized on a computer screen. For a CT scan of the kidneys the patient is in a recumbent position. It is possible, however, to elevate the head with pillows if the patient has difficulty with a flat position. Thin x-ray beams are transmitted rapidly through the body and assembled and integrated by computers. This information is developed into a two-dimensional image that gives remarkable definition of body anatomy. A renal CT scan takes about 30 minutes. Images are obtained first without a contrast agent and again after intravenous injection of a contrast agent.

## Magnetic Resonance Imaging

Magnetic resonance imaging (MRI) is a noninvasive diagnostic study that provides better visual information about soft tissues than a CT scan does. However, the MRI does not differentiate benign from malignant tumors. The MRI scanner creates a strong magnetic field, then emits radio waves that cause the magnetic field to rotate or resonate. This activity is analyzed by a computer, and pictures or images are created. The threefold process of MRI is described accurately by its name, magnetic resonance imaging.

The patient must assume a recumbent position for the length of the test and must be able to tolerate being in a small space. Most closed MRI scanners are about 2.4 m (8 feet) long, and the body part to be scanned must be in the center of the circular space. For a renal MRI the entire body is inside the MRI scanner for approximately 40 to 90 minutes. A renal MRI can be done with or without contrast media (Figure 37-5).

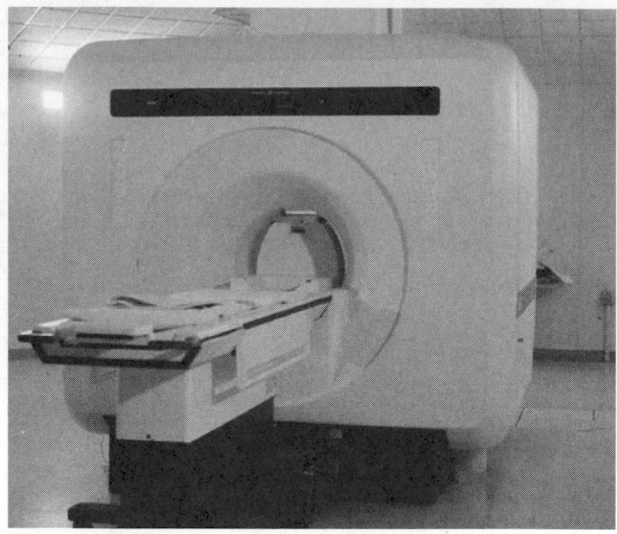

**Figure 37-5**   A closed magnetic resonance imaging (MRI) machine. In the foreground is a tablelike structure, called a trolley or bed; behind it is the magnet, a large, square structure with a hole in the middle. The patient lies on the trolley, which is slid into the bore of the magnet, and the MRI scan is taken. (From Lewis SM, Collier IC, Heitkemper MM: *Medical-surgical nursing: assessment and management of clinical problems*, ed 4, St Louis, 1996, Mosby.)

## Renal Biopsy

Tissue obtained from a renal biopsy is examined microscopically, which helps to determine the nature and extent of renal disease. Biopsy of renal tissue may be accomplished by the open or closed method. Both are invasive procedures that require sterile technique. An *open renal biopsy* requires an operation with general anesthesia. An incision is made, the kidney is exposed, the biopsy needle is inserted into the kidney, a piece of tissue is extracted, and the area is closed and sutured.

The procedure for a *closed renal biopsy* (also called a percutaneous renal biopsy) is as follows. A local anesthetic is given, and the patient is placed in a prone position with a pillow under the abdomen. A patient who has undergone a kidney transplant is positioned to maximize access to the transplanted kidney, which is usually in the groin area. The patient is instructed to hold his or her breath while the biopsy needle is inserted through the skin and into the kidney. Confirmation that the needle is in the kidney is provided when the needle moves when the patient breathes, because the kidneys are in contact with the diaphragm and move with ventilation. A small fragment of tissue is obtained, and the needle is withdrawn. After a specimen is obtained, pressure must be applied to the site, along with a pressure dressing.

With either method hemorrhage is the most common complication. The patient must be kept on bed rest for 24 hours in a supine position with a pressure dressing. The patient is assessed for pain and given analgesics as needed. Vital signs are evaluated often, as is the biopsy site and the dressing. The patient is encouraged to drink fluids to keep the urine diluted and prevent clot formation in the kidney, which could obstruct urine flow. Urine is evaluated for hematuria. The patient is also observed for signs and symptoms of urinary tract infection (Richard, 1995a). The patient may be fearful of the possible diagnosis, and waiting for the biopsy results may be stressful. Hence the nurse provides emotional support during this time.

## THERAPEUTIC PROCEDURES AND NURSING IMPLICATIONS

### Diuretics

**Diuretics** are substances or drugs that increase the urinary output. The excretion of large amounts of urine is called *polyuria,* and polyuria after the administration of a diuretic is called *diuresis.* Diuretics have different physiologic actions in the kidney and are classified according to their actions, whether the action occurs in the nephron, and if the diuretics are potassium sparing or potassium depleting. The more thoroughly renal physiology is understood, the easier it is to understand the action and side effects of diuretics and to take care of patients receiving them.

Table 37-2 lists several diuretics. Alcohol and caffeine suppress the release of antidiuretic hormone (ADH) from the pituitary gland. When ADH is not present in the collecting duct, a copious dilute urine is secreted. Spironolactone (Aldactone) inhibits aldosterone from causing sodium reabsorption and potassium secretion in the distal tubule. Because sodium attracts water, excess water is excreted with the sodium. Potassium is reabsorbed and is not excreted in excess in the urine. Ethacrynic acid (Edecrin) and furosemide (Lasix) inhibit the reabsorption of sodium, primarily in the ascending loop of Henle, and increase potassium excretion. An elevated concentration of electrolytes in the nephron attracts water, which increases the fluid volume and flow rate and decreases potassium reabsorption in the distal tubule (Shannon, Wilson, 1994; Hardman, Limbird, 1996).

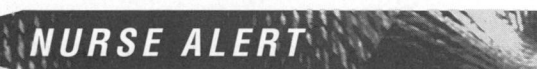

**NURSE ALERT**

**Diuretic therapy can result in water and electrolyte imbalances.**

Major side effects of diuretics are an exaggeration of their physiologic actions. For instance, all diuretics cause polyuria, and with prolonged polyuria there is water loss that can result in a fluid volume deficit. Dehydration, therefore, is an important side effect that nurses and patients need to watch for. Signs and symptoms of fluid volume deficit are weight loss, concentrated urine, hard stool, sunken eyeballs, dry mouth, poor skin turgor, dizziness, orthostatic hypotension, increased hematocrit, and increased plasma osmolality. If a fluid volume deficit becomes severe enough, blood flow to the kidney can be so reduced that renal failure results (Richard, 1995b; Holcomb, Simmons, 1997).

The most reliable method of assessing body fluid changes is weighing the patient. The patient is weighed daily and, if possible, fluid intake and output are recorded. The patient is weighed at the *same* time each day with the *same* amount of clothing and on the *same* scale. A good time to weigh is usually before breakfast, after the bladder has been emptied. The nurse balances the scale before each weighing and uses a metric scale, if possible, because it is easier to calculate fluid changes on a metric scale. Fluid intake and output changes are correlated with daily weight changes. For example, if the weight change from one day to the next is a loss of 1 kg, then the fluid change should also be a loss of 1 L (1 kg = 1 L = 2.2 lb).

Patients are taught how to weigh themselves and how to record fluid intake and output. Additionally patients are taught about the action, onset, and duration of diuretics so that they will not be alarmed at the increased voiding and will know when to expect it and how long it will last. Diuretics are administered at certain times so that the patient's sleep is not disturbed.

Most diuretics cause potassium depletion by interfering with its reabsorption. Some diuretics directly affect the potassium reabsorbing mechanisms. Other diuretics, especially those that act proximal to the distal tubule, increase the volume of fluid in the nephron. An expanded fluid volume increases the fluid flow rate, which sweeps potassium and other substances along so fast that they do not have time to be reabsorbed.

The nurse is alert to signs and symptoms of hypokalemia, such as undue fatigue, weakness, loss of appetite, loss of muscle tone, muscle cramping in the legs, arrhythmias, constipation, and abdominal distention. Blood levels of potassium often are evaluated. Dietary or drug potassium supplements, or both, are given as needed (Shannon, Wilson, 1994; Lancaster, 1995; Hardman, Limbird, 1996; Holcomb, Simmons, 1997).

**TABLE 37-2**

## Pharmacology of Drugs Used for Urinary Disorders

| DRUG (GENERIC AND TRADE NAME); ROUTE AND DOSAGE | ACTION/INDICATION | COMMON SIDE EFFECTS AND NURSING CONSIDERATIONS |
|---|---|---|
| **Acetazolamide** (Diamox)<br>**Route:** PO, IV, IM<br>**Dosage:** PO, glaucoma, 250-1000 mg/day in 1-4 divided doses or 500 mg/kg/day in 1-4 divided doses; IM, IV, 250-500 mg, may repeat in 2-4 hr | Inhibits carbonic anhydrase in the proximal tubule, resulting in increased excretion of sodium and water in the urine; used primarily as a diuretic to lower intraocular pressure in cerebral edema; also used as adjunct therapy in seizure disorders | Tiredness, weakness, metallic taste, anorexia, weight loss, and paresthesia; use with caution in diabetes mellitus and hepatic disease |
| **Belladonna and Extract of Opium** (B & O Supprettes)<br>**Route:** Rectal<br>**Dosage:** 1 q 3-4 hr/prn bladder spasms | Antagonizes the parasympathetic nervous system, resulting in bladder and urethral relaxation; used in the treatment and management of bladder spasm pain | Use with caution in addicted patients; store at room temperature |
| **Bethanechol** (Urecholine)<br>**Route:** PO, SC<br>**Dosage:** PO, 10-50 mg bid to qid; SC, 2.5 mg tid to qid | Enhances parasympathetic nervous system, resulting in bladder contractions; used for postpartum and postoperative urinary retention caused by neurogenic bladder | Heart block, abdominal discomfort, diarrhea, vomiting, salivation, urgency, flushing, and sweating; contraindicated in patients with obstruction of the GI or GU tract; use with caution in those with asthma, ulcers, epilepsy, or hyperthyroidism |
| **Bumetanide** (Bumex)<br>**Route:** PO, IV<br>**Dosage:** PO, 0.5-2 mg/day (up to 10 mg/day; larger doses may be required in renal insufficiency); IV, 0.5-1.0 mg, may give 1-2 more doses q 2-3 hr (not to exceed 10 mg/24 hr) | Inhibits sodium resorption in the loop of Henle, causing increased excretion of sodium and water in the urine; used as a diuretic in edema secondary to congestive heart failure or to hepatic or renal disease | Hypotension, hearing loss, metabolic alkalosis, hypovolemia, dehydration, hyponatremia, hypokalemia, hypochloremia, and hypomagnesemia; much more potent than Lasix; use with caution in patients with severe liver disease |
| **Cyclosporine** (Sandimmune)<br>**Route:** PO, IV<br>**Dosage:** PO, 15 mg/kg/day (first dose before transplant) for 1-2 weeks, taper by 5% weekly to maintenance dose of 5-10 mg/kg/day; IV, 5-6 mg/kg/day (⅓ PO dose) initially, change to PO as soon as possible | Suppresses helper T lymphocytes, resulting in decreased production of antibodies; used in the prevention and treatment of rejection in renal, cardiac, and hepatic transplantation (with glucocorticoids) | Tremor, hypertension, hirsutism, gingival hyperplasia, nausea, vomiting, diarrhea, nephrotoxicity, hepatotoxicity, infections, and hypersensitivity reactions; use with caution in patients with severe hepatic impairment, renal impairment, and any active infection; larger and more frequent doses may be required in children |
| **Epoetin Alfa** (Epogen)<br>**Route:** IV, SC<br>**Dosage:** SC, IV, 100 U/kg 3 times weekly initially, then adjust dosage by changes of 25 U/kg/dose to maintain target range of HCT; usual maintenance dose is 25 U/kg 3 times weekly | Stimulates the formation of red blood cells; used for the treatment of anemia associated with chronic renal failure; also used for the management of anemia secondary to zidovudine (AZT) therapy in HIV-infected patients | Hypertension; contraindicated in patients with uncontrolled hypertension; use with caution in those with history of seizures; rotate injection sites; bring solution to room temperature and inject slowly; works best with adequate iron stores |

**TABLE 37-2**

## Pharmacology of Drugs Used for Urinary Disorders—cont'd

| DRUG (GENERIC AND TRADE NAME); ROUTE AND DOSAGE | ACTION/INDICATION | COMMON SIDE EFFECTS AND NURSING CONSIDERATIONS |
| --- | --- | --- |
| **Furosemide** (Lasix)<br>**Route:** PO, IV<br>**Dosage:** PO, IV, 20-80 mg/day initially (up to 600 mg may be necessary; doses up to 1 g/day have been used in CHF and renal failure); when maintenance dose is determined, dose may be given every other day 2-3 times weekly | Inhibits sodium resorption in the loop of Henle, resulting in increased excretion of sodium and water in the urine; used in the management of edema secondary to congestive heart failure or to hepatic or renal disease; also used alone or in combination with antihypertensives in the treatment of hypertension | Metabolic acidosis, hypovolemia, dehydration, hyponatremia, hypokalemia, hypochloremia, and hypomagnesemia; use with caution in patients with severe liver disease, electrolyte depletion, diabetes mellitus, and anuria or increasing azotemia |
| **Hydrochlorothiazide** (Hydro-chlor, Hypodiuril, Thiuretic Esidrex)<br>**Route:** PO<br>**Dosage:** 25-100 mg/day in 1-2 doses (up to 200 mg/day); as a diuretic may be given every other day or 3-5 days/week | Reduces sodium resorption in the distal tubule, resulting in increased excretion of sodium and water in the urine; used alone or with other agents in the management of mild to moderate hypertension; also used alone or with other drugs in the treatment of edema associated with congestive heart failure, renal dysfunction, cirrhosis, and glucocorticoid and estrogen therapy | Hypokalemia and hyperuricemia; contraindicated in anuria; use with caution in patients with renal or severe hepatic impairment |
| **Mannitol** (Osmitrol)<br>**Route:** IV<br>**Dosage:** 50-100 g as a 5%-25% solution; may be preceded with a test dose of 0.2 g/kg over 3-5 min | Reduces water and electrolyte resorption in the proximal tubule, thereby increasing the volume of urine excreted; used as an adjunct in the treatment of acute oliguric renal failure; also used as an adjunct in the treatment of edema and in the reduction of intraocular and intracranial pressure | Transient volume expansion, hyponatremia, hypernatremia, hypokalemia, hyperkalemia, and dehydration; contraindicated in patients with anuria, dehydration, and active intracranial bleeding |
| **Neostigmine** (Prostigmin)<br>**Route:** SC, IM<br>**Dosage:** SC, IM, 250 mg-500 mg q 4-6 hr for 2-3 days for prevention and treatment of bladder atony and abdominal distention | Prolongs the effect of acetylcholine, resulting in increased gastrointestinal activity and bladder emptying; used in the prevention and treatment of postoperative bladder distention and urinary retention or ileus; also used to increase muscle strength in myasthenia gravis | Excess secretions, bronchospasm, bradycardia, abdominal cramps, nausea, vomiting, diarrhea, excess salivation, and sweating; contraindicated in patients with mechanical obstruction of the GI or GU tract; use with caution in those with asthma, ulcers, cardiac disease, epilepsy, or hyperthyroidism and in pregnant women |
| **Phenazopyridine** (Pyridium)<br>**Route:** PO<br>**Dosage:** 200 mg tid for 2 days | Has an analgesic effect on the urinary tract through an unknown mechanism; used to relieve urinary tract symptoms (pain, itching, burning, urgency, frequency) that may occur because of infection or after a urologic procedure | Bright orange urine; contraindicated in patients with glomerulonephritis, severe hepatitis, uremia, or renal insufficiency or failure |
| **Spironolactone** (Aldactone)<br>**Route:** PO<br>**Dosage:** 25-400 mg/day in 2-4 divided doses | Diminishes the effects of aldosterone in the distal tubule, resulting in increased excretion of sodium, potassium, and water; most commonly used to counteract potassium loss induced by other diuretics in the management of edema or hypertension | Nausea, vomiting, diarrhea, and hyperkalemia; contraindicated in patients with hyperkalemia, renal insufficiency, menstrual abnormalities, or breast enlargement; use with caution in those with hepatic dysfunction and in the elderly or debilitated |

## Provision for Urinary Drainage

There are several types of urinary drainage procedures. The most common method is to allow the urine to flow by gravity. It is recommended that a closed drainage system be used for all patients needing urinary drainage. Closed systems have the drainage tube sealed to the container, whereas open systems are not sealed and allow air and microorganisms to enter the system freely (Figure 37-6, *A*).

Collection sets in widespread use contain sterile drainage tubing that is permanently connected to plastic containers (Figure 37-6, *B*). Most containers are flexible bags with drains at the bottom of the bags to allow the urine to be emptied frequently. The end of the drain is protected by a cap, and the tube is fastened to the container when it is not being used. Most containers have valves at the top where the drainage tubing enters, to prevent bacteria from invading the drainage tubing and traveling upward toward the urethra and bladder. Filter air vents, located on the top of the containers, allow air to enter the system but prevent bacteria in the air from contaminating the urine.

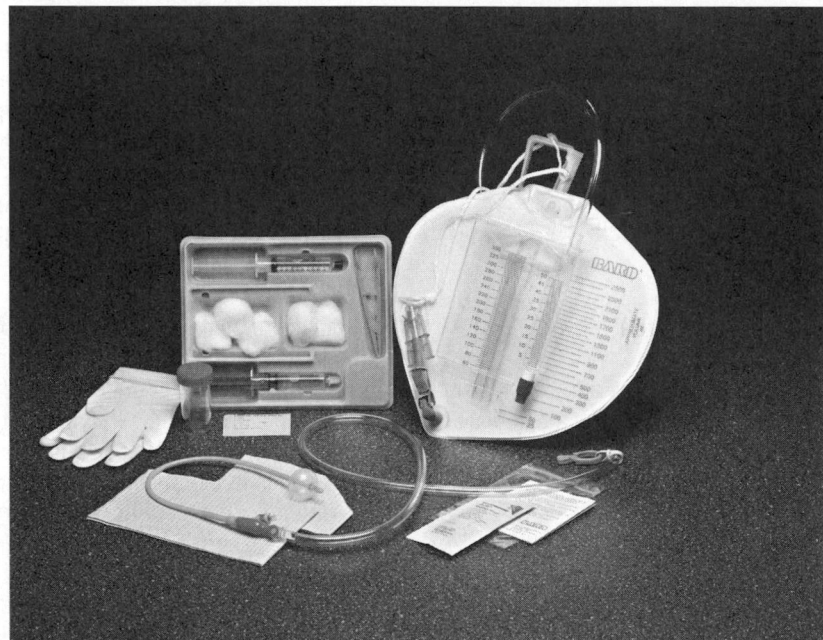

**A**

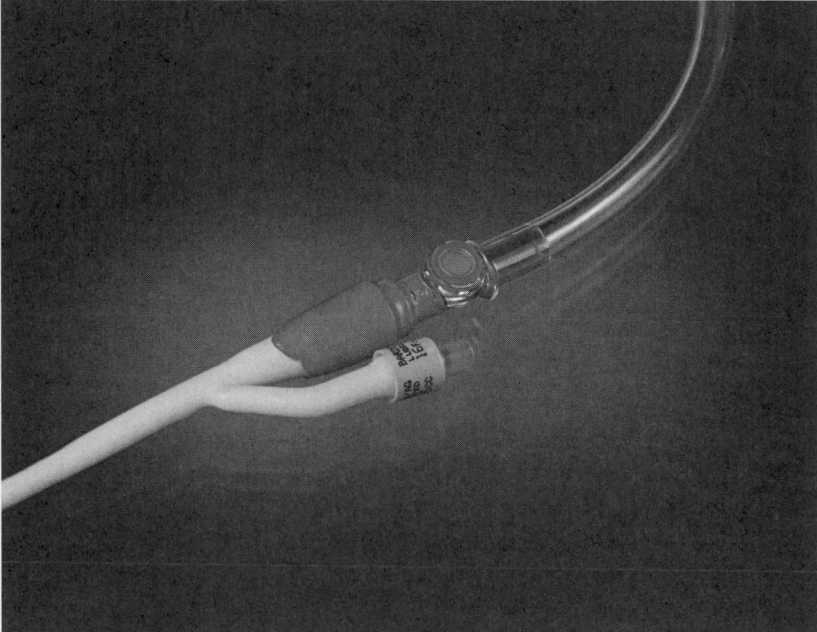

**B**

**Figure 37-6** Urine collection equipment. **A,** Equipment needed for bladder catheterization and urine drainage. A Foley catheter, showing the balloon inflated, is connected to drainage tubing that connects to a drainage bag with a 350-ml calibrated collection chamber. **B,** The catheter-drainage tubing junction is covered with an antitamper seal. The round area at the end of the drainage tubing is a port for obtaining urine. The short side arm of the catheter, labeled with the catheter size and balloon volume, is the lumen used to insert sterile water and inflate the balloon.

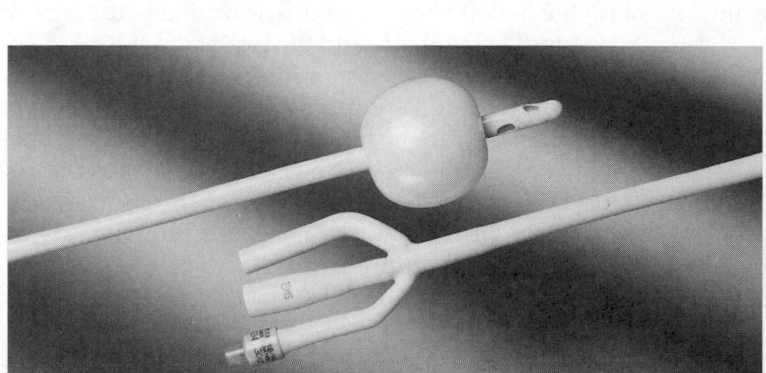

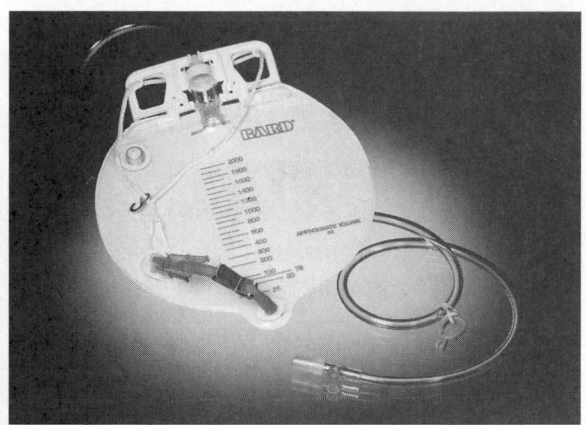

**Figure 37-6, cont'd** Urine collection equipment. **C,** Enlargement of the triple-lumen Foley catheter with balloon inflated. The lumens are used for urine drainage, irrigation solution, and balloon inflation. See Figure 37-8 for additional discussion of use of the triple-lumen catheter. **D,** A calibrated urinary drainage collection bag. **E,** Bard CritiCore system, an electronic monitoring device that measures core body temperature and urine output. (Courtesy Bard Medical Division, Covington, Georgia.)

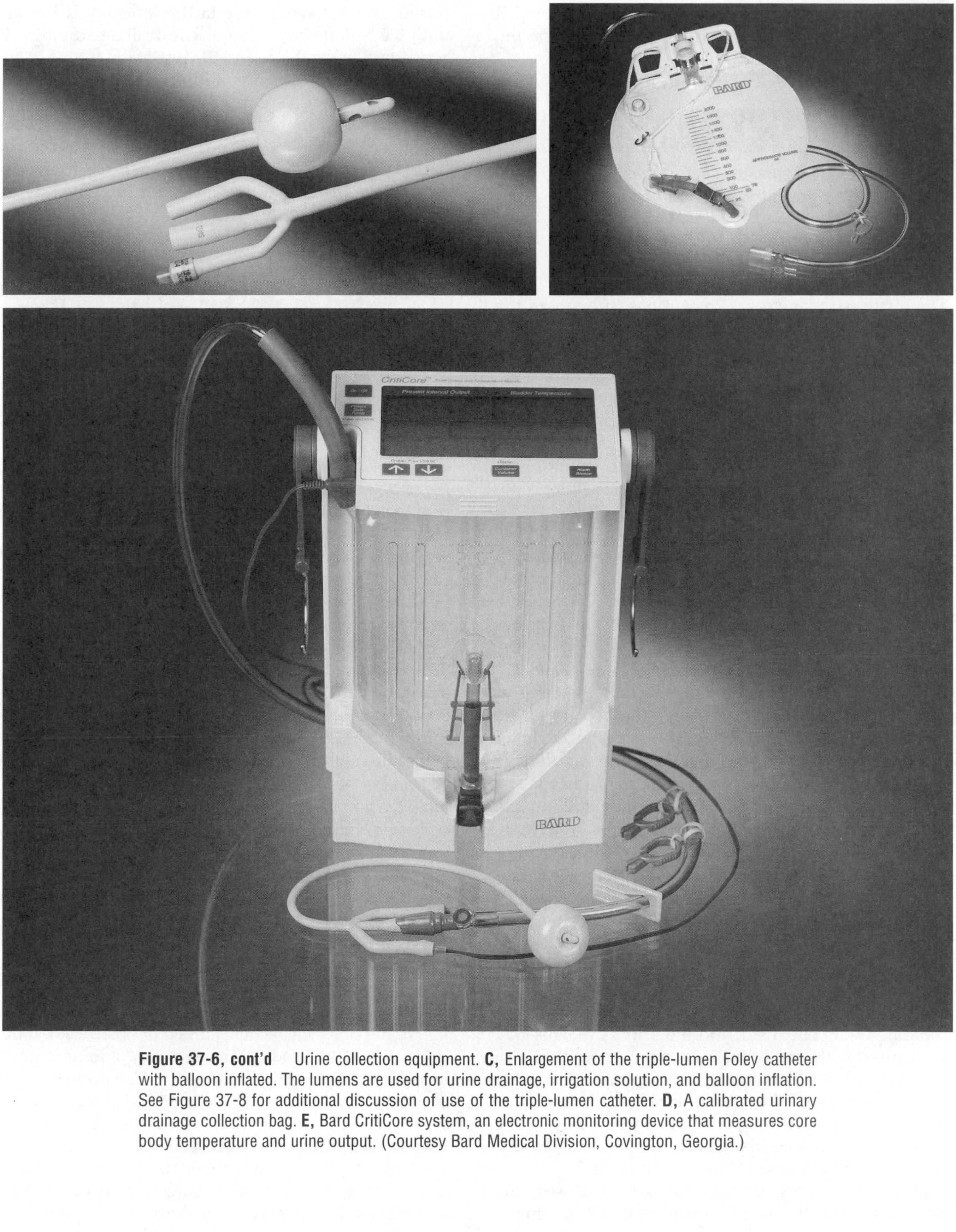

All collection containers have bed hangers, which keep the containers in an upright position and off the floor.

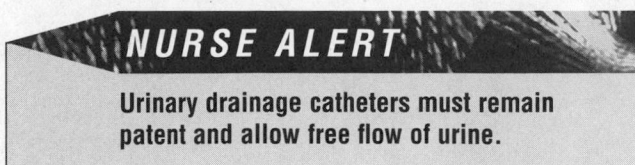

> **NURSE ALERT**
>
> **Urinary drainage catheters must remain patent and allow free flow of urine.**

### Inserting a Bladder Catheter

The nurse uses Universal Precautions throughout the procedure. The nurse explains the procedure to the patient, including the fact that catheterization usually does not hurt. Pain could be associated with a lower urinary tract obstruction and must be reported to a physician. Occasionally during catheter insertion men tighten their muscles and resistance is felt as the catheter is advanced. Men say this is uncomfortable and even painful. Deep, slow breathing helps people relax.

Although most bladder catheter insertion sets contain the equipment necessary, the nurse should read the list of what is in the set before beginning the procedure. A good light source is essential. The perineal area is washed with soap and water and dried. The patient is positioned as comfortably as possible, with the head of the bed as flat as possible. The legs and abdomen are draped with a sheet, and only the perineal area is exposed. The nurse brings the bed up to the center of gravity about waist level, so that good body mechanics are used during the procedure.

Sterile technique is used to insert the catheter. The nurse opens the insertion set and then follows the manufacturer's directions. The nurse puts on a mask, if necessary, dons gloves, and assesses all the equipment in the set (e.g., fills the balloon with the sterile solution to make sure it does not leak and then deflates the balloon) (Figure 37-6, C). The nurse positions all the cleaning items, lubricating jelly, catheter, and other equipment so that they can easily be reached with one hand. The nurse tells the patient what is being done throughout the procedure. With a female, the labia are separated with one hand, and the urinary meatus area is cleansed with single strokes that go from anterior to posterior. The goal is to have the urinary meatus as clean as possible. The area is cleansed three to five times. With a male, the penis should be held slightly upward and the foreskin retracted if present. The urinary meatus is cleansed three to five times.

Once the urinary meatus has been cleansed, the nurse lubricates the bladder catheter, inserts it into the meatus, and gently pushes it through the urethra until urine appears in the drainage tubing. The nurse

pushes the catheter a little farther and holds it there until the balloon has inflated. The drainage tubing can be secured to the thigh, and the rest of the tubing is positioned so that it is without kinks and lower than the bladder. The drainage bag is positioned so that it is lower than the tubing and off the floor. The nurse lowers the bed into its lowest position and makes the patient safe and comfortable. The nurse observes and records the urine characteristics and the patient's response to the procedure.

> **NURSE ALERT**
>
> **Bladder catheterization is done using only sterile technique and only when absolutely necessary.**

### Catheter Care

Most bladder catheters are made of rubber, whereas drainage tubing is clear plastic (see Figure 37-6, B). Determination of urine clarity or color is made by observing the urine in the tubing; the urine collected in the drainage bag does not give an accurate assessment. Specimens must be taken only from the port with a sterile syringe (see Figure 37-6, B).

Patients whose condition necessitates the presence of indwelling catheters over extended periods are very susceptible to infection. This is especially true of chronically ill patients. A point to remember to help prevent infection is that the catheter must provide free flow of urine and must be comfortable for the patient. It should be secured to the inner upper thigh in females to eliminate tension on the bladder, and laterally to the thigh or lower abdomen in males to avoid pressure on the urethra at the penoscrotal junction, which can cause the formation of a fistula. The drainage tubing may be placed over the thigh, downward between the legs, or under the patient's leg near the popliteal space. Excess tubing is coiled on the bed and not allowed to loop below the collection container. Many collection sets provide an apparatus so that the tubing can be attached to the sheets in a proper manner. Care must be taken that the tubing does not become kinked or obstructed. If the urine flow is blocked, stasis occurs, providing a good medium for the growth of bacteria. The entire system remains sterile and is not disconnected. The collection set and tubing are not lifted or elevated because urinary drainage may flow back into the bladder.

Using a catheter of the proper size is also important. If the catheter is too small, leakage may occur around it; if it is too large, it may be uncomfortable for the patient. Retention catheters are available in various sizes, with balloons of 5- and 30-cc capacity. For most patients a size 16 or 18 French catheter with a 5-cc balloon is satisfactory and will be both comfortable and adequate for free drainage.

Free urinary drainage is facilitated when the patient receives adequate amounts of fluid. Adequate fluid intake helps prevent accumulation of mucus, minerals, and exudate, which may adhere to the catheter and cause obstructions. Adequate fluids also eliminate the necessity for irrigation. Crusts and secretions around the vulva or penis and around the catheter should be removed and the general area cleansed as needed. There are differing opinions about cleansing methods, but washing the area gently with soap and water is now thought to be adequate. Trauma to the meatus is avoided.

When patients must have retention catheters indefinitely, the catheter and its tubing are changed every 7 to 10 days or more often if they become encrusted with organic deposits.

## Pyelostomy, Nephrostomy, Ureteral, and Cystostomy Catheters

Several surgical procedures performed on the urinary tract can result in the patient returning from the operating room with a catheter placed in the *kidney pelvis (pyelostomy)* or in the kidney (nephrostomy). The nephrostomy catheter or tube is brought out through an incision in the flank and sutured to the skin (Figure 37-7). *Ureteral catheters* are passed through the urethra and bladder and to the ureters and the kidney pelvis.

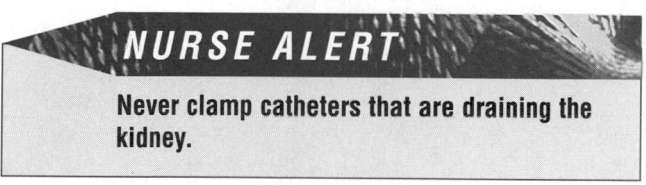

### NURSE ALERT

**Never clamp catheters that are draining the kidney.**

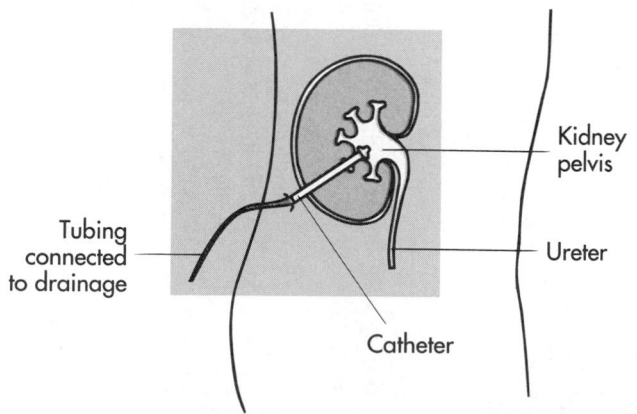

**Figure 37-7**   A nephrostomy catheter in the kidney pelvis. The catheter is brought out through a skin incision in the flank, sutured to the skin, and connected to tubing; the system uses gravity drainage.

These catheters are attached to free drainage. Any catheter placed in the kidney pelvis is never clamped, because obstructing the flow of urine causes increased pressure in the kidney pelvis, resulting in hydronephrosis and subsequent damage to the kidney. Care must be taken to prevent any displacement of these catheters because reinsertion may not be possible. The nurse observes the catheters often to be sure they are opening and draining, and any evidence of failure to drain must be reported to the physician immediately. All drainage is measured and recorded.

Sometimes a catheter is placed in the bladder through an abdominal incision (*cystostomy* or *suprapubic tube*) and is attached to drainage at the bedside. All equipment used for pyelostomy, nephrostomy, and ureteral and cystostomy drainage must be kept sterile (Table 37-3).

## Catheter Irrigation

A physician's order is needed for catheter irrigation. If the fluid intake is adequate and no blood clots occur, it should not be necessary to irrigate the urethral catheter unless the procedure is specifically ordered. Thirty milliliters of physiologic saline solution, 0.9% NaCl, is usually sufficient to determine the patency of the catheter. After irrigation, the solution returns by gravity. If the irrigating fluid flows in well but does not return, a clot is usually present at the end of the catheter. The nurse should remember that catheter irrigation is done to keep the catheter open and draining and not to irrigate the bladder.

If the patient has a bilateral pyelostomy and irrigations are ordered, separate equipment must be maintained for each catheter. The irrigating equipment and solution must be sterile; only 2 to 3 ml is used for the irrigation, depending on the physician's order. Remember the renal pelvis holds only 3 ml. The solution must be injected with extreme care and gentleness, and its return by gravity is observed. Failure of the solution to return must be reported, and additional solution is not injected.

If a urethral catheter needs frequent irrigation, it may be practical to set up closed intermittent irrigation using a Y connector (Figure 37-8). A bottle of sterile irrigating solution is elevated on a stand, and sterile tubing leads from the irrigating solution to the Y connector, which is attached to the catheter. The third arm of the Y connector is attached to the drainage tubing. By releasing a clamp on the tubing to the irrigating solution, the nurse allows the desired amount of solution to flow into the patient's bladder. A clamp on the drainage tubing prevents the solution from immediately draining into the collection set. When the desired solution has entered the bladder, that clamp is turned off, and the clamp on the drainage tubing is

**TABLE 37-3**

## Urinary Drainage System

| CATHETER AND ORIGIN | IRRIGATION | CLAMP | MEASURING OUTPUT | DRAINAGE TUBING | CARE OF SITE |
|---|---|---|---|---|---|
| Indwelling bladder catheter | Only if needed to assess or maintain patency; use sterile equipment with each irrigation; approximately 30 ml of sterile normal saline or an amount as ordered; gently instill saline and let it gravity drain. | To obtain specimen or as ordered, for example, with bladder retraining | Empty drainage bag every 8 hours or more often if filled to capacity. | Place over thigh and secure to avoid trauma to urethra; maintain closed system with drainage bag attached to bed. | Cleanse entire perineal area with soap and water as needed. |
| Cystostomy catheter (suprapubic tube) | If necessary to disconnect system; close three-way stopcock before disconnecting to maintain column of urine in catheter and to maintain siphon action. | On physician's order the suprapubic tube may be clamped 4 hours, then drained 30 minutes so bladder fills, and patient attempts to void through urethra while the tube is clamped | Empty drainage bag every 8 hours or more often if filled; measure and record voided urine on separate record if catheter is clamped and patient voids. | Secure to lower abdomen; attach catheter to closed drainage system. | Apply sterile, dry dressing to site; dressing may become saturated with leaking urine. |
| Ureteral catheters (through bladder and ureters to kidney pelvis) | Irrigate according to physician's order; irrigate with 2 or 3 ml of sterile solution. | Never | Measure and record separately for each kidney; observe output hourly. | Tape to thigh; maintain closed system and patency. | Care as for bladder catheter if it enters meatus; apply sterile, dry dressing if brought out on flank or abdomen. |
| Pyelostomy (kidney pelvis) | Only with physician's order; use 2 or 3 ml of sterile solution as ordered; irrigate gently with gravity return; separate sterile equipment for each catheter. | Never | Measure drainage from each kidney and record separately. | Secure to flank; maintain patency and closed system. | Apply sterile, dry dressing; change often to keep dry. |
| Nephrostomy (kidney) | Only with physician's order and sterile equipment | Never | Measure drainage and record separately. | Secure to flank; maintain patency and closed system. | Apply sterile, dry dressing; change often to keep dry. |

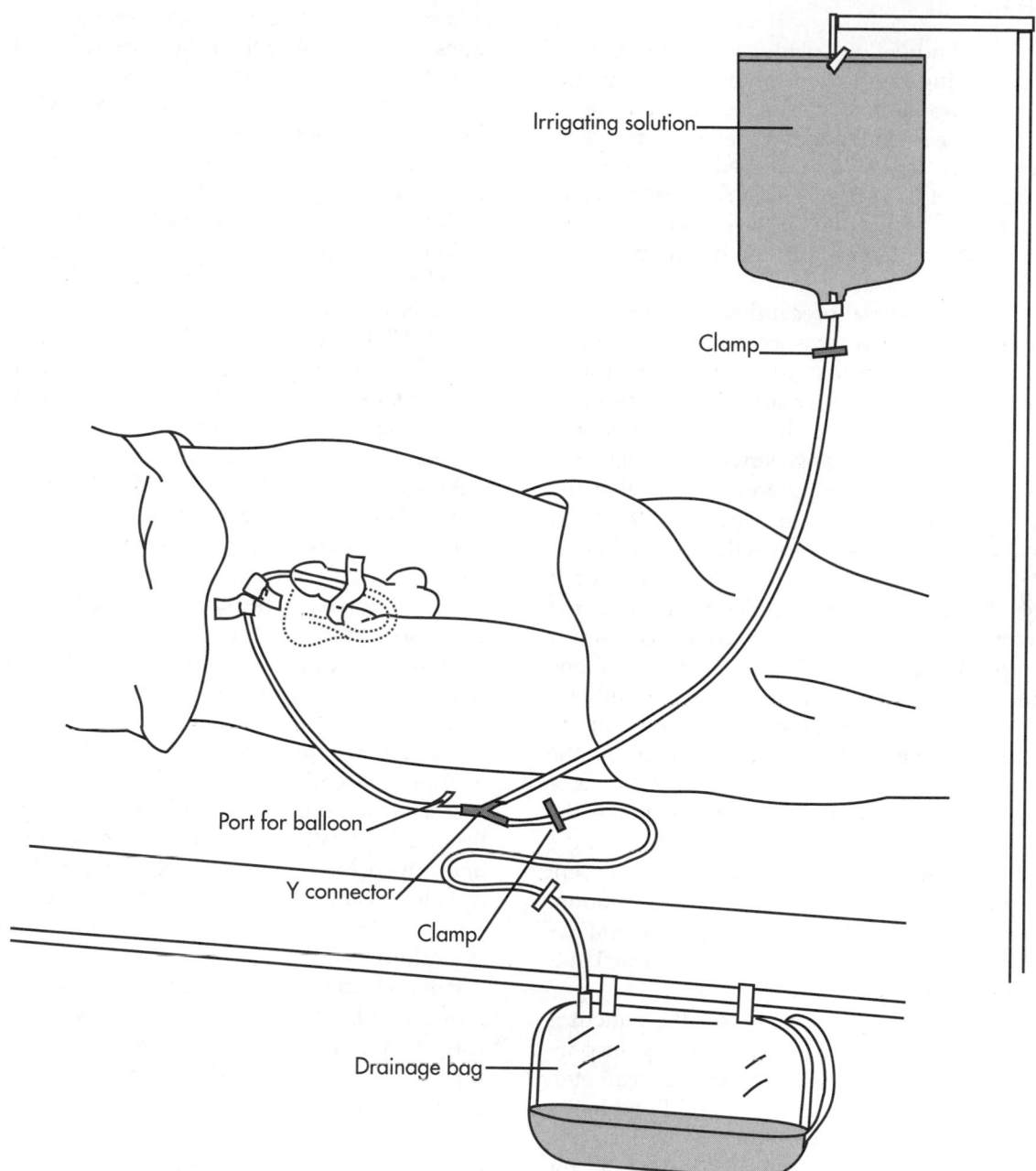

Irrigating solution

Clamp

Port for balloon

Y connector

Clamp

Drainage bag

**Figure 37-8** Retention catheter inserted for urinary drainage and a closed system with Y connector for intermittent irrigation. Continuous irrigation requires a triple lumen catheter. One lumen is used for instilling irrigating solution, another for draining urine and irrigation solution, and the third for instilling fluid to inflate the balloon.

released, allowing the solution to drain from the bladder under force of gravity. The drainage tubing is left unclamped until the next irrigation. The physician orders the kind of solution, the amount, and the interval for irrigation.

If continuous irrigation is necessary, the patient must have a triple lumen Foley catheter (or a cystostomy tube and a urethral catheter) in the bladder to provide for continuous flow into and out of the bladder (see Figure 37-6, C). The irrigation equipment is the same except that a drip-o-meter may be attached to the irrigating solution to regulate the rate of flow; the drainage tubing is left unclamped. In both intermittent and continuous closed bladder irrigation, it is important to keep an accurate record of the amount of irrigating solution used and to subtract this amount from the measurement of total drainage.

## Catheter Removal

Removal of the indwelling bladder catheter is preceded by explaining the procedure to the patient and collecting all equipment: gloves, absorbent pad (e.g., Chux, blue pad, or several paper towels), syringe, and bedside commode, urinal, and/or bedpan if the person is unable to get to a toilet. The syringe is the same size or larger than the balloon on the catheter. Usually the volume of the balloon is printed on the port that leads to the balloon.

The nurse uses universal precautions during the entire procedure. The nurse washes his or her hands, provides privacy, and places the commode, urinal, and/or bedpan within close reach. The nurse dons gloves and places the absorbent pad under the catheter and drainage tube and between the patient's legs. The nurse deflates the balloon by attaching the syringe to the balloon port and aspirating the fluid from the balloon. The nurse ensures that the balloon is entirely deflated by pulling strongly on the plunger of the syringe. A partially inflated balloon can injure the urinary tract as the catheter is removed. The nurse gently untapes the catheter from the skin, places one hand under the absorbent pad, and holds the catheter with the other hand. The patient is informed that the catheter is about to be removed. The nurse can ask the patient to take a long, deep breath through the nose and to slowly exhale through the mouth while the nurse gently pulls out the catheter. The purpose of the breathing exercise is to relax the patient. The absorbent pad is wrapped around the catheter, and the amount of urine in the collection bag is measured and recorded. The catheter is inspected, and the physician is notified if it is not intact.

After the catheter has been removed, the patient is instructed about and observed for urinary incontinence and retention. With prolonged bladder catheterization, the bladder is continually emptied and hence does not have an opportunity to function as a muscle, loses tone, and needs time to recover. Additionally, the urethral muscular sphincters, forced open by the presence of the catheter, lose tone and need time to recover. The loss of bladder and sphincter tone can result in a variety of situations. Flaccid bladder and sphincters result in incomplete bladder emptying and dribbling of urine. Sphincters that contract produce urinary retention. A contracted bladder with decreased capacity can result in frequent urination.

The nurse can encourage the patients to assist in keeping a record or diary of the amount and appearance of urine and the time voided. Patients are taught about the micturition process and that it is important to maintain their hydration status by drinking a glass of water every 1 to 2 hours. Patients are encouraged to void every 1 to 2 hours and to do Kegel exercises four times a day to strengthen the muscles used in urination. A Kegel exercise is done correctly when one can stop and start the flow of urine. These exercises, however, must be done when the patient is not urinating.

At the bedside a portable ultrasound machine can be used to scan the bladder for residual urine after voiding instead of catheterizing the bladder. The procedure is similar to other ultrasound procedures: a conductive gel is applied to the lower abdomen and a hand-held probe is moved gently over the area. Sound waves reflect off the bladder, and the volume of urine is recorded. Machines are accurate to approximately 1½ ounce (50 ml) of urine. Bladder ultrasonography is a quick, reliable, and noninvasive method that assesses for residual urine (Moore, Edwards 1997) (Figure 37-9).

Sometimes the patient is unable to void normally, and catheterization or replacement of the retention catheter, or both, may be necessary. The patient may void only small amounts because the bladder cannot empty completely. The bladder capacity is temporarily decreased, and the patient complains of abdominal discomfort shortly after removal of the catheter because he or she is unable to void and the bladder is full.

Bladder muscle retraining may be helpful before removing a retention catheter. The catheter is clamped and unclamped on a schedule for 12 to 48 hours. For instance, the catheter is clamped for 1 hour and then unclamped for 5 to 15 minutes for 4 to 6 hours. The catheter is clamped for two hours and then unclamped for 5 to 15 minutes for 6 to 8 hours, and so on (Mondoux, 1994).

If blood appears in the urine (hematuria) after removal of a bladder catheter, the physician is notified. It is often necessary to maintain fluid intake and output records for several days, especially if the patient has had urinary tract surgery.

## Patient and Family Teaching

Many patients are discharged from the hospital to their homes with indwelling catheters, draining wounds, and permanent appliances. A planned program must be available that teaches the patient self-care insofar as he or she is competent. This includes three steps: (1) observation, (2) participation, and (3) practice under supervision. The patient observes the nurse in the various procedures; at the same time the nurse explains, step by step, what is being done and the reason for it.

As the patient is able, he or she begins to assist the nurse or to participate in the procedures, gradually assuming more and more of the care. Finally the nurse

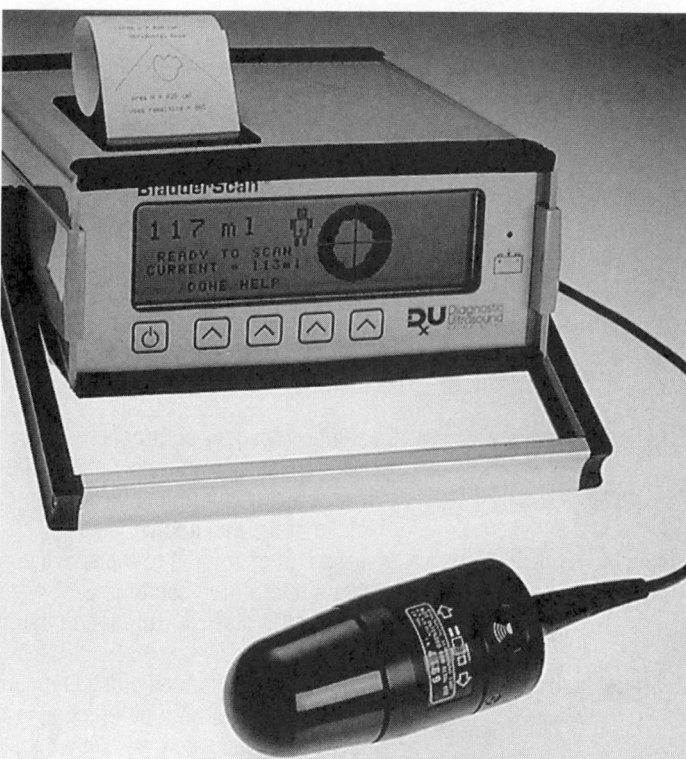

**Figure 37-9**    Bladder Scan procedure. **A,** Positions of the patient, health care provider, and Bladder Scan machine during the procedure. See the text for a description of the procedure. **B,** Enlarged view of the Bladder Scan machine and probe. (Courtesy Diagnostic Ultrasound Corp., Redmond, Washington.)

allows the patient to give all the care while observing to correct any mistakes and provide positive feedback.

When the patient leaves the hospital, he or she should feel secure about knowing what to do and how to do it. There may be catheters or dressings that the patient cannot reach, and a member of the family or another person should be instructed in the care. In addition, hospitals should provide written instructions with a list of the home equipment needed for the patient or the family. In planning care for patients with urologic conditions, it has been found that each patient has her or his own special needs.

There should be a referral system between the hospital and the home health agency, and when it can be arranged, the home health nurse should visit the patient in the hospital before discharge. Information is given to the home health nurse concerning the care needed and the instructions given the patient. The home health nurse supervises or assists with the necessary care after discharge. The continuity of care between the hospital and the home provides a feeling of security for the patient and facilitates the process of rehabilitation.

## URINARY INCONTINENCY

Urinary incontinency is the inability to retain urine, and it is a symptom and not a disease. Urinary incontinency can be temporary or permanent. There are many causes for incontinence, including side effects of drugs. Physiologic reasons could include injury or disease of some part of the urinary pathway such as the bladder, sphincters, spinal cord, and cerebral cortex. There could be psychologic or emotional reasons such as fear, stress, a feeling of loss of control of one's life, sorrow, and excitement. Table 37-4 summarizes the different types and causes of urinary incontinencies.

It is important to assess carefully for the cause of urinary incontinency and not just assume that it is some incurable physical problem. It may require multiple conversations with the person to determine the cause. Some people are uncomfortable and even ashamed to discuss their elimination problems because they think that urine is a socially unacceptable topic related to sex. The urinary tract is part of the male reproductive tract and very close to the female reproductive tract. Many people are uncomfortable discussing anything that remotely relates to sex. People believe myths, such

---

**TABLE 37-4**

## Classification of Urinary Incontinency

| TYPE | CAUSE | DESCRIPTION |
|---|---|---|
| Functional incontinency | Impaired mobility, musculoskeletal function, cognitive function, and physical and environmental barriers to toilet facilities | Urinary tract is intact and functional; unable to reach toilet facilities in time to void |
| Stress incontinency | Urinary sphincter dysfunction and/or weak pelvic floor muscles associated with obesity, multiple pregnancies, and prostatectomy surgery | Involuntary loss of urine with increased intraabdominal pressure such as coughing, sneezing, laughing, and straining with a bowel movement and with physical exertion such as lifting and jumping |
| Urge incontinency | Involuntary bladder contractions associated with neurologic disorders (stroke and Parkinson's disease), bladder irritation (infection and tumors), and large intake of alcohol and caffeine | Feels the urge to void, and shortly afterward has an involuntary loss of urine; incontinence can occur as often as every 2 hours |
| Reflex incontinency | Disease and/or trauma to the spinal cord above the sacral micturition center at S2-S4 associated with spinal cord disease (tumor and injury) and multiple sclerosis | Constant loss of urine without the sensation to void |
| Overflow incontinency | Bladder is overdistended and has not emptied completely because of an obstruction in the lower urinary tract associated with an enlarged prostate gland or constricted urethra | Continual and/or persistent loss of urine; also referred to as dribbling |

---

as the belief that with aging one automatically becomes incontinent of urine. People are humiliated and devastated by incontinency because they feel like an infant who cannot control urination. They feel that adults are supposed to void in appropriate places at appropriate times.

Urinary incontinency is a sensitive emotional and physical problem that must be approached with compassion and solved professionally. The nurse should sit down with these patients, provide privacy, express concern about their incontinency, and encourage them to vent their feelings. The nurse should demonstrate listening by repeating to them what they have said using their words. The nurse should ask the following questions: When did the incontinency start? What does the incontinency mean to you? Is it a problem for you? How has it altered your life? How do you think it can be changed? Do you want help with the incontinency? The nurse should encourage the person to keep a diary of when the incontinency occurs and the feelings associated with it. The information can help to identify the cause. Patients may need to undergo an examination and physical tests of the urinary tract to assess for a cause of incontinency.

Some general goals or outcomes of care for the person with urinary incontinency are to maintain self-esteem, self-worth, skin integrity, and fluid balance or hydration, as well as to increase their knowledge of

micturition and incontinency. When incontinency occurs, the nurse treats the person with respect. The skin is cleansed with soap and water and patted dry. Cornstarch and/or bag balm can be applied to reduce skin irritation. The nurse should change clothes and bed linens immediately and wash them or send them to the laundry. Urine containers are emptied immediately, and the room kept well ventilated. These interventions help keep the environment clean. The nurse can offer to take the patient to the toilet or can offer the bedpan or urinal to prevent incontinence. The nurse can encourage hourly fluids, except for 2 hours before sleep, which helps maintain fluid balance, keeps the urine dilute, and decreases fabric staining, odors, and skin irritation (Mondoux, 1994).

The nurse can set goals with the patient and create an individualized program based on what is most important to the patient. Many people socially isolate themselves, change their life-style drastically, decrease their fluid intake to dangerously low levels so that they will urinate less, and worry about incontinency all the time. Instead of worrying and imagining themselves being incontinent, patients can visualize and imagine their urinary tracts being healthy and being continent.

If hospitalized, patients may feel that they are a nuisance and are sometimes treated as such by the staff; they are put in diapers and further humiliated. The diapers cause skin breakdown, which is very painful to the patient and increases hospital stay and staff work. Some people are immediately catheterized and then are at risk for urinary tract infection, which is dangerous and costly and enhances urinary incontinency. Only as a last intervention should an absorbent pad be used with incontinency. The pad should be small, covering the perineal area only, and should be changed whenever wet or every 2 hours to preserve skin integrity.

### NURSE ALERT

Urinary incontinency, an inability to retain urine, is a symptom requiring investigation and not a disease.

## DISEASES AND DISORDERS OF THE URINARY SYSTEM

Pathogenic organisms may gain entrance to the urinary tract by the bloodstream or from infections elsewhere in the body. The result may be an inflammatory process or an infection that may spread from the urethra upward to other parts of the system. Obstructions may occur along the tract from stones, strictures, tumors, or a kinked ureter. Tumors, either benign or malignant, may result in serious injury to the bladder, urethra, or kidneys. Injuries elsewhere in the body may also affect the kidney. Some diseases of the kidney may be the result of allergic factors, and others may be the result of degenerative changes.

## Noninfectious Diseases

*Glomerulonephritis* is a term that encompasses several conditions affecting the glomerular capillaries of the kidney. Early classifications were based on the clinical picture of the disease. Since the advent of percutaneous renal biopsy and sophisticated techniques of electron microscopy, the newer classifications of the glomerulopathies are based on histologic and immunologic findings.

### Acute Poststreptococcal Glomerulonephritis

**Pathophysiology.** Acute poststreptococcal glomerulonephritis (APSGN) is usually preceded by a recent infection of the pharynx or the skin (impetigo) caused by beta-hemolytic streptococcus. Antibodies develop and combine with an unknown antigen, possibly a protein (M) of the streptococcus, and form an *immune complex*. These immune complexes become trapped in the glomerular basement membrane (GBM) and cause inflammation. The inflammatory response in the glomeruli results in the passage of red blood cells and protein into the urine.

It is not yet known why some people develop the immune complex and APSGN after a streptococcal infection and others do not. The disease is most common in children, appears suddenly, and usually clears up with no residual damage. It may progress to a chronic form of the disease, however, when the patient is an adult.

**Assessment.** Urine output is reduced (oliguria) and is rusty colored because of the presence of red blood cells. Edema results from increased capillary permeability and is seen in the face, eyelids, and hands in the morning and in the legs at night. A significant number of patients have circulatory congestion from fluid and sodium retention, resulting in dyspnea, cough, and pulmonary edema. Protein is found in urine, but blood levels of protein remain normal. The BUN and serum creatinine levels are elevated. Most patients have mild to moderate hypertension at the onset that diminishes as the body eliminates the excess fluid.

Some cases are more severe, resulting in **anuria** (absence of production of urine) and subsequent uremia. The prognosis is favorable if there is no preexisting renal disease or if proteinuria is not heavy or persistent. Patients may have some urinary abnormalities for several years after recovery. Follow-up studies are now revealing residual pathologic conditions, but evidence is not conclusive. Adults who develop the disease are more likely to develop chronic renal disease as a complication, resulting in end-stage renal failure (Price-Anderson, Wilson-McCarty, 1996).

**Intervention.** Treatment of acute glomerulonephritis is aimed at relieving the symptoms of hypertension, circulatory congestion, and edema. The patient probably will be allowed as much activity as can be tolerated. Bed rest is indicated in the acute stage until hematuria and proteinuria subside.

Fluids and sodium are restricted if there is circulatory congestion or hypertension. Diuretics can be used, but vigorous diuresis and dehydration should be avoided. Antihypertensives are used to reduce the elevated blood pressure. Treatment of hypertension prevents additional damage to the renal microvasculature. Protein intake must be restricted if nitrogenous protein waste levels in the blood rise (azotemia), but vigorous protein restriction is avoided.

Steroids and cytotoxic agents may help control the deposition of immune complexes (Lancaster, 1995). Antibiotics do not help the patient but may be given to the family to prevent them from having the antibody reaction to the antigen associated with the preceding infection.

An increase in urine output and a corresponding weight loss signal improvement. The urine begins to clear itself of albumin and red blood cells, the blood pressure decreases, and the patient feels better. This usually begins about 3 weeks after the onset of the edema. When the weight and blood pressure are stable, edema and hematuria are gone, and the BUN level is decreased, dietary and activity restrictions may be lifted (Box 37-1).

## Nephrotic Syndrome (Nephrosis)

**Pathophysiology.** The increased permeability of the glomeruli allows protein to leave the blood and enter the urine, producing proteinuria. The reduced serum protein level causes a decrease in plasma oncotic pressure. The inadequate plasma oncotic pressure reduces the natural force that draws fluid back into the capillary from the interstitial spaces. The excess fluid remaining in the interstitial space results in edema (see Chapter 27). An unknown factor stimulates hepatic lipoprotein synthesis, which results in hyperlipidemia. Cholesterol and low-density lipoproteins are the first to elevate, followed by triglyceride levels. Fatty casts are found in the urine.

**Assessment.** The term *nephrotic syndrome* is used to describe the patient with massive proteinuria, hyperlipidemia, hypoalbuminemia, and edema. The edema

---

> **BOX 37-1**

## NURSING PROCESS

### ACUTE POSTSTREPTOCOCCAL GLOMERULONEPHRITIS

**ASSESSMENT**

- Recent sore throat or skin infection
- Changes in urine volume and color
- Signs and symptoms of edema
- Elevated blood pressure, pulse, and respirations

**NURSING DIAGNOSES**

- Activity intolerance related to fatigue and weakness secondary to renal dysfunction
- Anxiety related to unknown prognosis
- Impaired physical mobility related to inactivity secondary to prolonged bed rest
- Fluid volume excess, edema related to decreased renal excretion
- Knowledge deficit: signs and symptoms of fluid and electrolyte imbalance and side effects of corticosteroids and cytotoxic agents
- Risk for infection related to increased susceptibility secondary to corticosteroid therapy, immobility, invasive procedures
- Risk for impaired skin integrity related to edema, bed rest
- Altered nutrition: less than body requirements, related to anorexia and restrictions of protein and sodium
- Altered urinary elimination related to decreased renal excretion of potassium.

**NURSING INTERVENTIONS**

- Maintain activity as tolerated.
- Measure and record intake and output—report reduced output.
- Measure urine output hourly if indwelling catheter is present.
- Observe urine for color and sediment and record.
- Test urine for protein (albumin).
- Restrict fluids as ordered, based on urinary output and body weight.
- Restrict protein intake as ordered, based on blood levels of nitrogenous wastes and urine output.
- Give high carbohydrate diet.
- Check temperature, pulse, and respirations every 4 hours; report elevated temperature, galloping or irregular pulse, dyspnea, and coughing.
- Check blood pressure every 4 hours—notify physician if systolic pressure is over 160 mm Hg or diastolic pressure is over 110 mm Hg.
- Weigh patient daily.
- Observe for edema and note location.
- Measure abdomen daily to evaluate ascites.
- Observe for signs of hyperkalemia; administer ion resin exchanges for hyperkalemia.
- Observe mental status at least once each shift and report changes, including confusion, headache, sleepiness, or tremors.
- Institute seizure precautions if mental changes are observed.
- Teach patient about disease process and treatment.

**EVALUATION OF EXPECTED OUTCOMES**

- Weight stable at level maintained before edema
- Blood pressure stable
- Urine negative for albumin and red blood cells
- Absence of edema
- Urine output appropriate for intake

accompanying the nephrotic syndrome causes a puffy face, distended eyelids, a bloated abdomen (ascites), and swelling in the lower extremities. The skin may have a waxy pallor because of the edema.

The syndrome has multiple causes and is characterized by increased glomerular permeability, which results in protein and fat found in the urine. Nephrotic syndrome is not a disease but is a group of symptoms found in many diseases affecting the glomeruli. It occurs with some infectious diseases, poisoning from chemical substances, toxemia of pregnancy, shock resulting from external burns, and coronary occlusion and may follow a transfusion with incompatible blood. It is seen in membranous, proliferative glomerulonephritis and poststreptococcal glomerulonephritis. It is also found in diabetic glomerulosclerosis, systemic lupus erythematosus, renal vein thrombosis, syphilis, and some neoplastic conditions (Lewis, Collier, Heitkemper, 1996; Price-Anderson, Wilson-McCarty, 1996).

**Intervention.** Treatment usually consists of administration of diuretics to decrease the edema. Dietary restraints depend on the severity of the symptoms, but the diet should include high-protein foods and restrictions on sodium. Corticosteroids and cyclophosphamide (Cytoxan) are used in severe cases. Intravenous albumin is not usually administered because it is rapidly lost from the permeable glomeruli, but it may be used if edema is severe and generalized (anasarca). The individual is encouraged to continue normal activity unless the edema is severe.

Prevention and control of infection are important because the patient is highly susceptible, and infection is one of the chief causes of death. Nursing care requires the monitoring of diuretic therapy; it includes weighing the patient daily as well as measuring the girth of the abdomen and extremities, intake and output, and the protein and sodium intake. The patient may be anorectic, and small, frequent feedings may be necessary to ensure an adequate protein intake. The disorder may be acute or chronic, and the primary causative disease must be cured or controlled to relieve the condition.

## Infectious Diseases

An infection can originate anywhere along the urinary tract and can spread from one area to any or all areas of the tract (Figure 37-10). Urinary tract infection (UTI) is a broad term that includes a variety of clinical diseases. Cystitis and pyelonephritis are discussed in the following sections.

The urinary tract has several defenses against infection. The major defense is micturition. Approximately 99% of all microbes are washed out with voiding, which is why it is so important for a person with a UTI to drink lots of fluids. Additionally, a large fluid intake can help to prevent a UTI. Other defenses are the acidity and high osmolality of urine, which retards bacterial growth; the bladder mucosa, which is somewhat resistant to bacterial attachment; prostate fluid, which

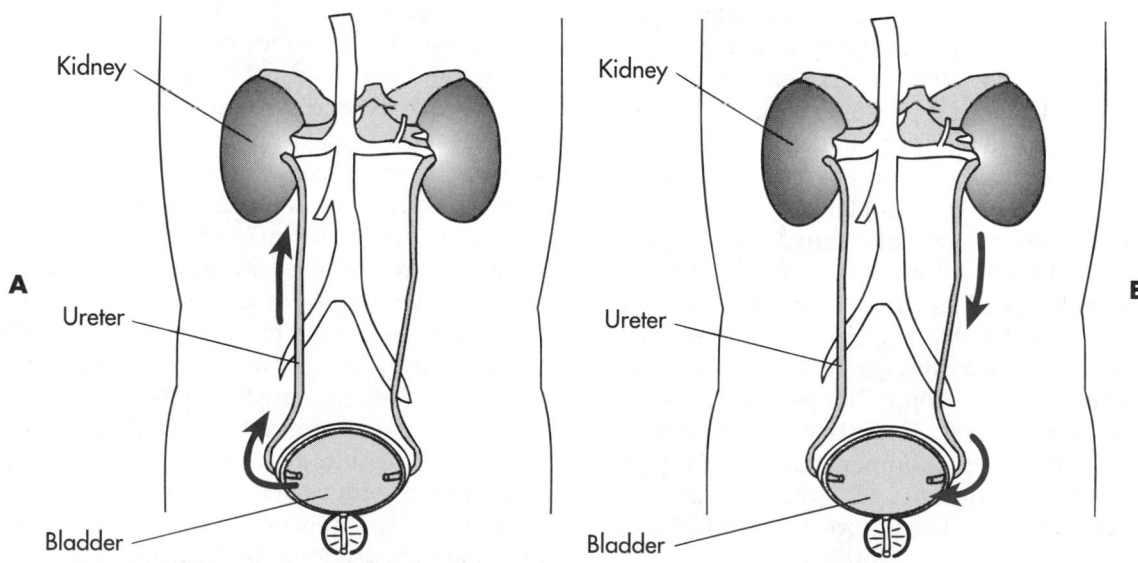

**Figure 37-10**    Urinary tract infection. **A,** Bacteria enter the bladder, ascend the ureter, and invade the kidney. **B,** Bacteria originate in the kidney and, with micturition, descend through the ureter and into the bladder. Arrows indicate the directions in which bacteria can move. (From Richard CJ: *Comprehensive nephrology nursing,* Boston, 1986, Little, Brown.)

contains an antibacterial substance; and the male urethra, which is longer than the female urethra.

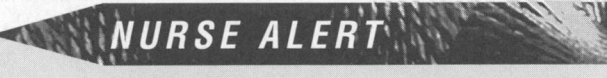

**NURSE ALERT**

**Urinary tract infections can best be prevented by drinking a lot of water and avoiding invasive urinary tract procedures.**

## Cystitis

**Pathophysiology.** **Cystitis** is an inflammation of the lining of the bladder. It may be acute or chronic and is more common in females than males. The female urethra is shorter and straighter than the male urethra and therefore can more easily contaminated. In addition, the prostatic secretions in the male have antibacterial properties. Cystitis may be caused by bacteria that enter through the urinary meatus, or it may occur through catheterization, during which organisms in the urethra are carried into the bladder. Cystitis in women may occur after sexual intercourse for unknown reasons. Infections may also be carried from the upper urinary tract, beginning with the kidney and involving the ureters and the bladder. In this instance the infectious organism gains entrance to the kidney by way of the bloodstream. Cystitis may result from nonbacterial factors such as injury to the lining of the bladder caused by instruments or a catheter.

**Assessment.** Symptoms are frequent urination, including nocturia, severe pain and burning in the urethra with urination, and a sensation of bearing down or pressure in the bladder and suprapubic area. Examination of the urine may show the presence of pus and may reveal blood. Specific pathogenic organisms are often not found (Lewis, Collier, Heitkemper, 1996).

**Intervention.** The first criterion of treatment is to establish the cause of the problem. Antispasmodic drugs, sulfonamide, or antibiotic drugs, and preparations to acidify the urine may be ordered. Nitrofurantoin (Macrodantin) inhibits bacterial enzymes, is effective against *Escherichia coli, Staphylococcus aureus,* and *Streptococcus faecalis* but can change urine to a brown color (Shannon, Wilson, 1994). The patient is encouraged to drink water freely. Hot sitz baths and the application of heat to the abdomen may relieve pain. Phenazopyridine (Pyridium), a urinary antiseptic, may be given to relieve discomfort, but it can change the urine to orange and stain clothing.

Nursing interventions include teaching the patient to prevent recurrence of cystitis. The patient is instructed to have regular follow-up examinations to rule out the presence of asymptomatic infections and

to take medications as prescribed with a full glass of water. The patient is advised to continue taking medication for the full time prescribed, even though symptoms may be relieved or disappear. Women who experience frequent urinary tract infections should be instructed to do the following:

1. Cleanse the perineal area from front to back after each voiding and bowel movement.
2. Increase fluid intake and void every 2 to 3 hours during the day to empty the bladder and reduce the growth of bacteria.
3. Void before and after sexual intercourse.
4. Wear absorbent cotton panties or those lined with cotton in the crotch.

## Pyelonephritis

Pyelonephritis is an acute pyogenic infection involving the parenchyma in one or both kidneys. Although *pyelitis* (infection of the kidney pelvis) may occur alone, it is considered rare.

**Pathophysiology.** Pyelonephritis is caused by bacteria: the *Proteus* group, *E. coli,* and *Pseudomonas;* less common causes are the *Streptococcus* and the *Staphylococcus* bacteria. The infection may be brought to the kidney by the bloodstream or the lymphatic system from infection elsewhere in the body. It may also spread upward from the bladder. Factors that contribute to the disorder include obstructions that restrict urinary flow and examinations, such as cystoscopy and catheterization. Pyelonephritis may occur in persons with some neurologic diseases or with conditions that require long periods of immobilization during which urinary calculi may develop.

**Assessment.** The kidney becomes edematous and inflamed, and the blood vessels are congested. The urine may be cloudy and contain pus, mucus, and blood. Small abscesses may form in the kidney. The diagnosis is made by microscopic examination of the urine and urine cultures; an intravenous urography may be done. The symptoms may occur abruptly with fever, chills, severe malaise, an elevated leukocyte count, aching, **pyuria,** and white blood cell cysts. There may or may not be pain in the back (Richard, 1995a).

**Intervention.** The treatment of the patient depends on locating and eliminating the cause. Sensitivity tests are done, and the appropriate antibiotic is administered. Bed rest is required during the acute period. Vital signs are recorded twice a day, and the patient is weighed daily. Fluid intake is encouraged, and all intake and output should be recorded. The patient is observed for any difficulty in voiding, such as pain and burning. Urine is observed for color. The patient is kept warm and protected from drafts or chilling and respiratory tract infections.

With proper intervention, the patient with pyelonephritis has a normal temperature, no abnormal urinalysis results, no back or flank pain, and no fatigue.

## Obstructions of the Urinary System

Obstructions of the urinary system can be caused by stones, tumors, kinking of a ureter, a congenital anomaly, or an enlarged prostate gland in a male (see Chapter 42) and be located anywhere from the kidney to the urinary meatus. Any prolonged obstruction will lead to serious anatomic and physiologic pathologic conditions.

With an obstruction, pressure develops in the urinary tract as urine backs up. The obstruction may be high enough to cause damage to the kidney, resulting in a decreased glomerular filtration rate; a decreased excretion of creatinine, urea, and other substances; and dilation of the kidney or ureter or both (Figure 37-11). Dilation of the kidney is called *hydronephrosis,* and dilation of the ureter is called *hydroureter.* Once hydronephrosis begins, it cannot be reversed. It can, however, be stopped by relieving the obstruction, which allows urine to flow freely. Hydroureter does not result in loss of function. Hydronephrosis, however, can result in renal failure as more and more kidney tissue is damaged (Figure 37-12) (Richard, 1995a).

## Renal Calculi

**Pathophysiology.** A stone is called a *calculus,* the formation of stones is called **lithiasis,** and the presence of stones in the kidney is called *nephrolithiasis.* When stones occur in any other part of the urinary system, the location determines the term used, as in ureteral calculi. The exact cause of the formation of renal calculi is unknown, but some factors that contribute to their formation are known. Paraplegic patients and patients who are required to remain on a regimen of bed rest for long periods are likely to develop calculi because of stasis of urine and the release of increased amounts of calcium from bone. Some common organisms that cause infection of the bladder and kidney cause the urine to become alkaline. Calcium phosphate, a compound readily excreted by the kidneys, cannot dissolve in the alkaline urine and forms crystals around a shred of tissue or other substance in the kidney, resulting in stone formation. Patients requiring continuous urinary drainage often develop kidney or bladder stones as a complication. Pathologic disorders such as senile osteoporosis, gout, infection, hyperparathyroidism, and disorders affecting the pH and concentration of the urine are believed to be contributing factors (Resnick, 1997).

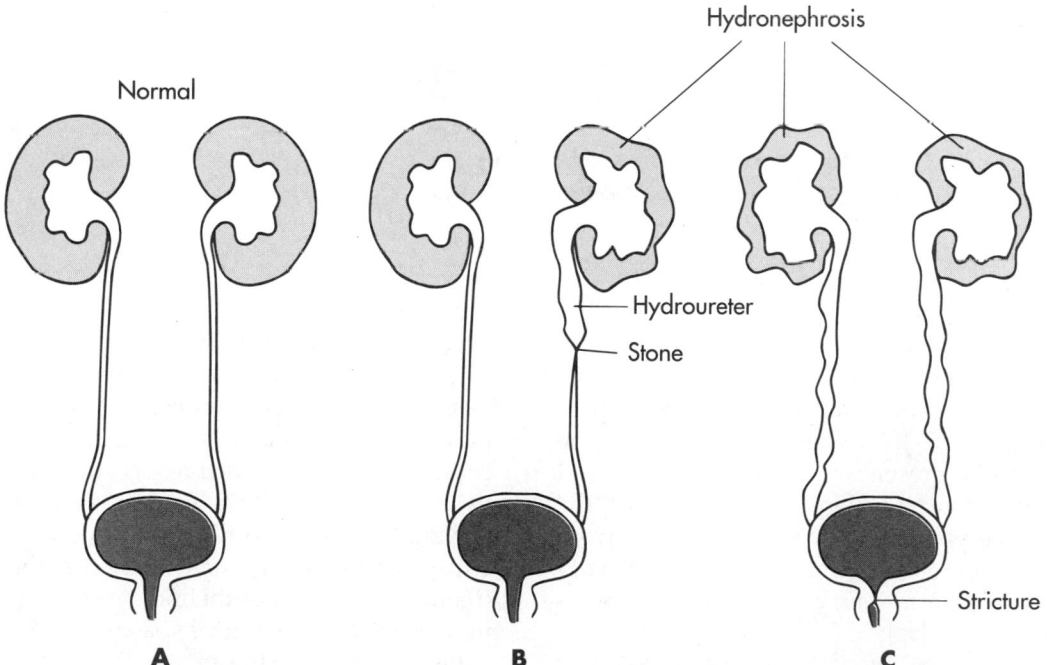

**Figure 37-11** Obstructions of the urinary tract. Dilation occurs above the point of obstruction. **A,** Normal urinary tract. **B,** Unilateral urinary tract obstruction from a stone in the left ureter, resulting in hydroureter and hydronephrosis. The right kidney and ureter are normal. **C,** Bilateral urinary tract obstruction from a urethral stricture caused by an enlarged prostate gland; this results in bilateral hydroureters and hydronephrosis. (From Phipps WJ et al: *Medical-surgical nursing: concepts and clinical practice,* ed 5, St Louis, 1995, Mosby.)

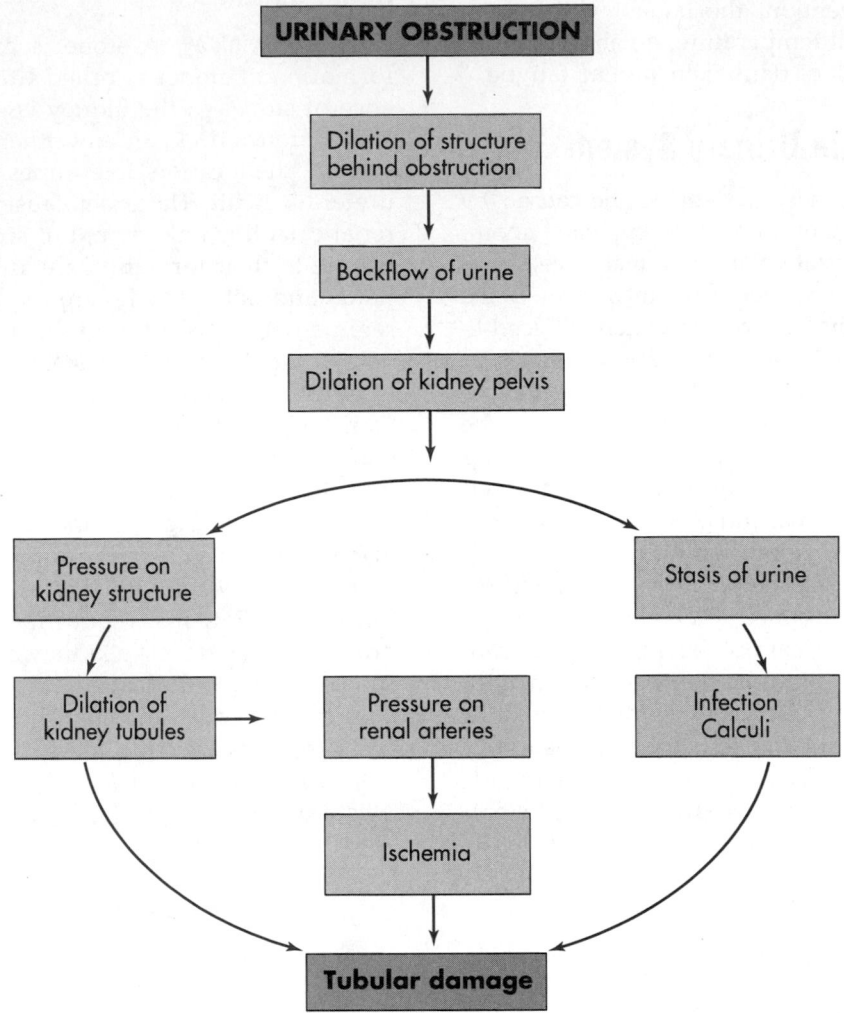

**Figure 37-12** Pathophysiology of uncorrected urinary obstruction. (From Phipps WJ et al: *Medical-surgical nursing: concepts and clinical practice,* ed 5, St Louis, 1995, Mosby.)

**Assessment.** Stones may be like tiny gravel, and the patient may be asymptomatic. Large stones with irregular branches may be present in the kidney pelvis; they are known as *staghorn calculi* and require surgical intervention (Figure 37-13). When stones occur in the kidney, pain may be present on the involved side and usually radiates from the flank to the crest of the ileum. Pus may be present in the urine, resulting from infection at the back of the stone. Hematuria, usually microscopic, results from injury to the mucous membrane from the rough, jagged edges of the stone.

*Ureteral colic* is caused by a stone passing down or becoming lodged in the ureter. The pain is excruciating and radiates down the ureter and may extend to the thigh and the urethra. Nausea, vomiting, and sweating occur, and the patient feels weak and may faint.

**Intervention.** All urine from patients with renal calculi is voided, poured through a straining device, and carefully inspected for stones. The patient is encouraged to drink at least 2½ quarts (3000 ml) of fluid in 24 hours because increasing urinary output facilitates passage of the stone. If infection is present, the appropriate antibiotic may be ordered. The patient is encouraged to remain active because stones are more likely to be passed if the patient is ambulatory.

Narcotics are required to relieve the pain, and an antispasmodic drug such as methantheline bromide (Banthine) or propantheline bromide (Pro-Banthine) may be ordered to relieve spasm (Box 37-2).

*Prevention* is also important. Patients confined to bed should be turned regularly every 2 hours. Long periods of immobilization result in a loss of calcium from the bones and an increase of calcium in the bloodstream. High levels of calcium in the blood contribute to the formation of kidney stones. Adequate hydration dilutes the urine so that stones are less likely to form

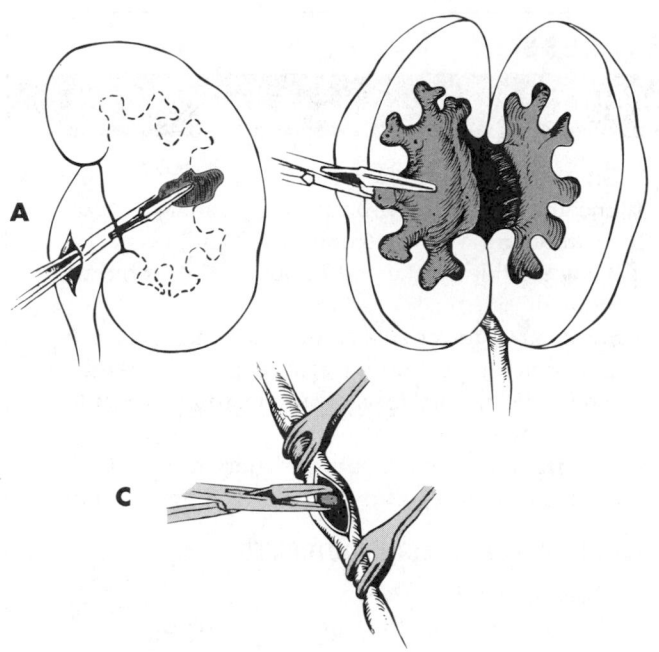

**Figure 37-13** Removal of renal calculi from the upper urinary tract. **A,** Pyelolithotomy. The stone is removed through the renal pelvis. **B,** Nephrolithotomy. A staghorn calculus is removed through a lateral bisection of the kidney. **C,** Ureterolithotomy. The stone is removed from the ureter. (From Phipps WJ et al: *Medical-surgical nursing: concepts and clinical practice*, ed 5, St Louis, 1995, Mosby.)

(Phipps et al, 1995). Isometric exercise and weight-bearing exercise reduce calcium loss from the bones. The use of the tilt table, the circle bed, rocking bed, and overhead trapeze provides exercise for the patient and helps in the prevention of stone formation.

Patients who require intervention for removal of large stones have several options. In place of conventional open surgical techniques, percutaneous stone removal and extracorporeal shock-wave lithotripsy are used successfully for stone removal or dissolution. Percutaneous stone removal is achieved through a nephroscope under fluoroscopy after the patient has received a local anesthetic. This method has the greatest success rate with renal pelvic and caliceal stones (Gillenwater, 1996). The nephrostomy tube is left in situ for several days.

Extracorporeal shock-wave lithotripsy is a noninvasive procedure that uses high-energy shock waves to pulverize renal stones into tiny fragments that are excreted in the urine (Lancaster, 1995). This procedure can be done with the patient in a tank of water or lying on a table similar to an x-ray table. Before the treatment begins, the procedure is explained and all questions are answered. Patients usually receive a sedative, maybe an epidural or general anesthetic, cardiac monitoring, and maybe oxygen, and have an IV

placed. Patients must lie still while the high-energy waves are directed toward the stone through electrodes. Patients experience different degrees of discomfort during the procedure, and appropriate analgesics are administered. X-ray examinations are performed throughout the procedure to evaluate the effectiveness of the treatment and assess for the position of the stone.

**Patient and family teaching.** The shock waves pulverize the stone into dust or small gravel. To facilitate passage of these particles through the urinary tract, the client is instructed to drink about 3 to 4 quarts (3 to 4 L) of water every day for at least a week. It is critical that patients understand the importance of drinking the fluid to pass the pulverized stone, because, without copious urine, the stone fragments can cause a urinary tract obstruction. Patients have discomfort, hematuria, and bruising at the electrode sites and are tired after treatment. Analgesics are prescribed for the pain. Although lithotripsy is done in outpatient settings, it can also be done in the hospital. Usually patients are advised to rest for several days before returning to work and daily routines.

## Tumors of the Urinary Tract
### Kidney

Tumors of the kidneys are generally malignant and usually result from metastasis from the lung. The malignancy is often spread to the lungs and bones by the bloodstream. The primary symptom is blood in the urine; other symptoms are weight loss and fatigue. The treatment is a nephrectomy, which may be only palliative because metastasis may have occurred.

### Bladder

Tumors of the bladder may be benign or malignant. A complete urologic examination, including cystoscopy and a biopsy, is done to diagnose the problem. Cancer of the bladder is more common in men over age 50. Smoking and exposure to dyes, chemicals, and ionizing radiation increase the risk of developing cancer of the bladder. The bladder is also a site of metastasis of cancer originating in the male prostate or female lower reproductive tract. The most common symptom is gross, painless hematuria. Urinary tract infection often develops as a complication of malignancy and produces symptoms of frequency, urgency, and dysuria. A distant metastasis may produce pelvic or back pain.

For malignancy, a partial or complete cystectomy may be performed. A complete cystectomy necessitates urinary diversion. Radiation therapy or chemotherapy may be initiated. Chemotherapy may be given systemically or locally by instilling a solution into the bladder.

---

<BOX 37-2>

## NURSING PROCESS
## RENAL CALCULI

**ASSESSMENT**

- Stone fragments when straining urine
- Decreased urine output
- Pain in the abdominal region, lower back, and/or upper thighs

**NURSING DIAGNOSES**

- Anxiety related to fear of disease process, invasive medical procedure
- Pain related to passage of calculi, invasive procedure
- Knowledge deficit related to limited understanding of disease process, prescribed treatment
- Altered urinary elimination related to obstructing calculi

**NURSING INTERVENTIONS**

- Teach patient about disease process and treatments.
- Encourage activity and ambulation.
- Encourage patient to verbalize fears and concerns.
- Explain all diagnostic tests, nursing measures, and physiology of ureteral colic and bladder spasm.

- Give analgesics as often as ordered to relieve pain.
- Encourage fluids to produce high urinary output of dilute urine—offer 6 ounces (200 ml) every 2 hours while awake and 12 ounces (100 ml) during night.
- Strain all urine and observe for sediment, crystals, and stones; report findings; save any solids and send to laboratory for analysis; instruct patient to do the same.
- Instruct patient and supervise dietary restrictions indicated by nature of stone as analyzed by laboratory.

**EVALUATION OF EXPECTED OUTCOMES**

- Absence of pain
- Urine output of 42 to 48 ounces (1400 to 1600 ml) every 8 hours
- Absence of calculi
- Can verbalize diet restrictions and be able to select appropriate foods for restricted diet

---

Immunotherapy is in the experimental stage but offers hope for the future. BCG (Bacille Calmette-Guérin) has been instilled into the bladder and allowed to remain a given time before withdrawal. This treatment offers the advantage of actual contact with the tumor.

## Traumatic Injuries

Injuries to the urinary system often occur in connection with injuries to other parts of the body. Injuries may be caused by gunshot wounds, penetrating wounds from sharp objects, and crushing injuries with fracture of the pelvis, which may cause rupture of the bladder or the urethra. Injuries resulting from external violence such as falls or blows may result in simple injury to the kidney or may completely shatter the kidney. All trauma victims should be observed for blood in the urine. The patient in shock has a reduced blood supply to the kidney, and urine output is be reduced. Initial interventions are aimed at stabilizing vital signs and maintaining circulation and oxygenation of tissues. Assessment of the extent of injury determines the method of treatment, which may be conservative or may require surgical intervention (Figure 37-14) (Richard, 1986).

## Renal Failure

Renal failure is a broad term for kidneys that are unable to meet the demands of the body. It is described as acute or chronic, according to the time required for the development of the condition and whether it is short-lived or prolonged.

### Acute Renal Failure

**Acute renal failure** may develop insidiously or suddenly, but the kidneys suddenly stop functioning. Acute renal failure proceeds through several well-defined stages.

**Pathophysiology.** The causes of acute renal failure are numerous, but decreased renal blood flow and nephrotoxins are the most common causes. Postoperative shock produces hypotension that prevents the kidney from filtering the blood adequately. This decreased flow and lack of oxygen to the kidney may cause acute renal failure. Other causes include burns, blood transfusion reactions, infections, antigen-antibody reactions (acute glomerulonephritis), and obstructions.

Changes that occur in the kidney include necrosis and a sloughing of the lining of the renal tubules. Areas of the nephron rupture, resulting in the formation

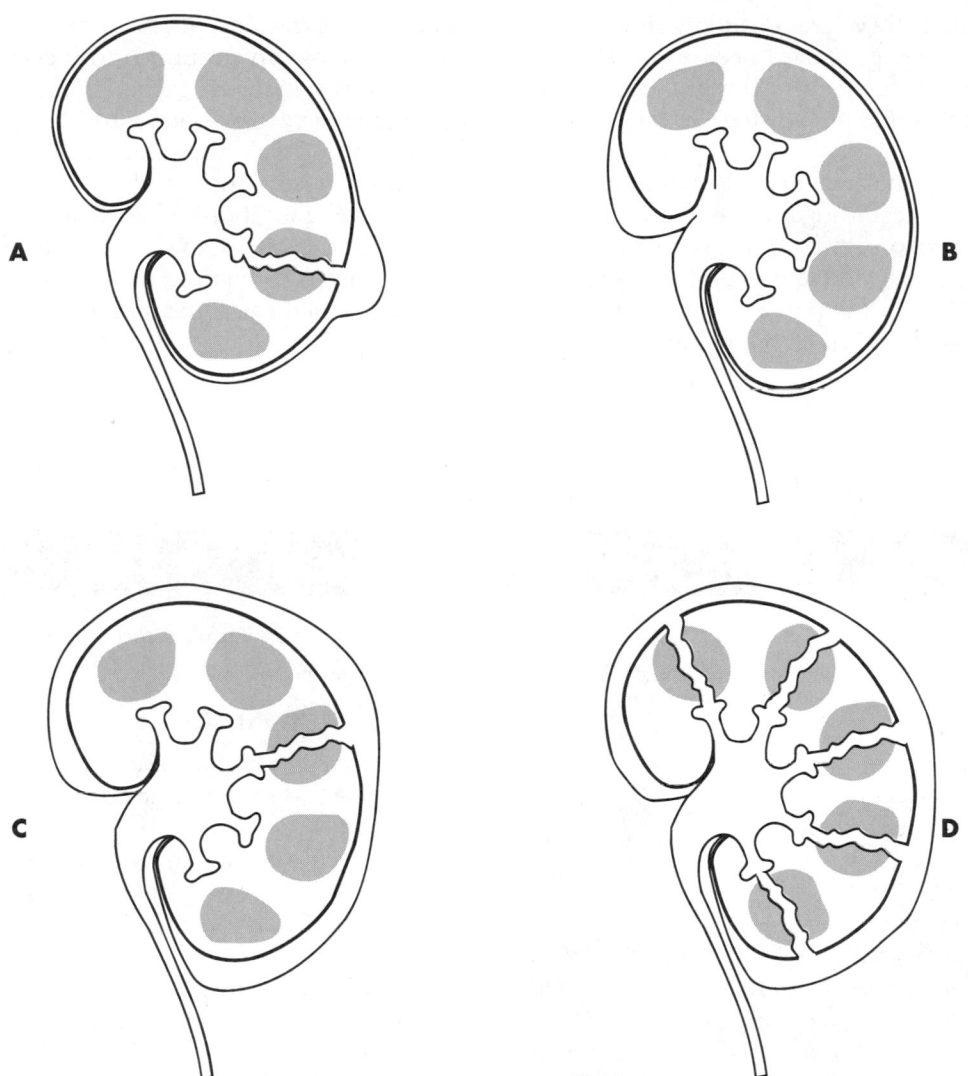

**Figure 37-14**    Four degrees of renal trauma. **A,** Urine extravasates through a split in the renal parenchyma but is confined under the renal capsule. **B,** Urine extravasates through a tear in the renal pelvis. **C,** Urine extravasates through a rent in the kidney and capsule and surrounds the kidney and the renal pelvis. **D,** The kidney is shattered, and urine is extravasating in all areas.

of scar tissue. Blood chemistries show an increase in the BUN, plasma creatinine, and potassium and a decrease in pH (acidosis) and bicarbonate. Generalized edema, pruritus, headache, disturbance of vision, hypertension, and vomiting occur, and there is an odor of urine on the breath. The patient appears acutely ill.

**Assessment.** The first stage is the *onset stage,* the time from the precipitating event to the onset of oliguria or anuria, usually a short period. Next is the *oliguric-anuric stage,* in which output is less than 12 ounces (400 ml) in 24 hours. This may last only for a day or two, or it may last as long as 2 weeks. Then the kidney starts to recover and enters the *diuretic stage,* when urinary output increases and the BUN level stops rising

and eventually falls to normal range. The *convalescent stage* begins when the BUN level is stable and ends when the patient returns to normal activity and urine output is normal. This may take several months, and some patients may develop chronic renal failure.

**Intervention.** Treatment begins with determining the cause and correcting it if possible. Management focuses on fluid balance, electrolyte balance, nutrition, preventing infection, and educating the patient. The patient is kept alive while the kidney heals itself. The mortality rate is approximately 50%, and the leading cause of death is infection (Richard, 1995a).

There is a tendency for nurses to become preoccupied with the patient's urine volume and blood chemistries and to forget that they are dealing with a very frightened human being. Nurses need to be alert for and respond to the patient's behavior and provide the support and understanding needed in this difficult time.

Because daily weights and fluid output guide fluid replacement, careful recording is done. The diet is high in carbohydrates to prevent the breakdown of fats, which produces ketosis, and low in protein and potassium to reduce BUN and hyperkalemia. Fluids are restricted. Protein is increased as the nephron units be-

gin functioning and BUN decreases. If the level of serum potassium continues to increase and becomes dangerously high, an exchange resin is administered to release the excess potassium. Medications are evaluated to determine potential buildup. Conservative treatment is continued, and dialysis is indicated when the clinical condition or biochemical state is deteriorating. Peritoneal dialysis may be used unless very rapid dialysis is required or repeated dialysis is anticipated; in such cases hemodialysis is used (Box 37-3) (Kelly, 1997).

---

**BOX 37-3**

## NURSING PROCESS

## ACUTE RENAL FAILURE

### ASSESSMENT

- Recent history of severe fluid depletion, exposure to nephrotoxins, and obstruction in the urinary tract
- Volume of urine
- Rise in plasma creatine and BUN
- Feelings of malaise

### NURSING DIAGNOSES

- Anxiety related to prognosis
- Decreased cardiac output related to arrhythmias, drug intolerance, stress on heart function
- Pain related to infection, muscle cramps
- Ineffective individual coping related to anger, anxiety, denial, dependent behavior, depression
- Altered family processes related to complex therapies, hospitalization, illness of family member
- Fear related to disease process, hospitalization, invasive medical procedure, powerlessness, real or imagined threat to well-being
- Fluid volume excess related to decreased output
- Grieving related to actual or perceived loss
- Knowledge deficit related to limited understanding of disease process or prescribed treatment
- Altered nutrition: less than body requirements related to dietary restrictions, loss of appetite, nausea and vomiting
- Powerlessness related to disease process, hospitalization
- Ineffective breathing pattern (impaired gas exchange) related to fluid overload
- Personal identity disturbance related to body image, personal identity, role performance, self-esteem
- Altered thought processes related to impaired perception of reality

- Altered urinary elimination related to decreased kidney function, decreased urine output

### NURSING INTERVENTIONS

- Teach patient about disease process and treatment.
- Measure and record urine output hourly; report if less than 30 ml/hr.
- Report any reduction in urine output.
- Restrict and regulate fluid intake as ordered and as permitted by output and weight gain.
- Weigh patient daily.
- Observe signs of fluid excess—dyspnea, tachycardia, pulmonary edema, distended neck veins, peripheral edema.
- Observe signs of elevated serum potassium (hyperkalemia) and administer ion exchange resins as ordered.
- Turn patient every 2 hours.
- Have patient cough and deep breathe every 2 hours.
- Provide emotional support, anticipating needs.
- Limit dietary protein as necessary during oliguric phase.
- Restrict sodium intake as ordered.
- Anticipate treatment with dialysis.

### EVALUATION OF EXPECTED OUTCOMES

- Blood chemistries to level before illness
- Urine output greater than 30 ml/hr
- Weight decreased to level maintained before illness
- Absence of edema and respiratory distress
- Lungs clear
- No signs or symptoms of infection
- Patient and family verbalize fears and concerns

# Chronic Renal Failure

Chronic changes in renal failure may be considered on a continuum that ranges from impairment to insufficiency to failure. *Renal impairment* is detected by changes in concentration and dilution of the urine. *Renal insufficiency* becomes apparent when the kidney cannot meet the demands of dietary or metabolic stress. *Renal failure* appears when the normal demands of the body cannot be met. As many as 80% of the nephrons may be lost before renal functional losses are detected. Hypertrophy and hyperplasia of the remaining nephrons permit an increase in their workload and in their ability to maintain function (Price-Anderson, Wilson-McCarty, 1996). **Uremia** is a term that has been used for years to describe terminal renal failure and literally means urine in the blood. Although it is less popular now, the term is still used.

**Pathophysiology.** As renal function diminishes, the kidney loses its ability to adapt to varying intakes of foods and fluids. Polyuria and an inability to concentrate the urine are early signs of chronic renal failure. Oliguria and anuria occur later. An output of less than 12 ounces (400 ml) of urine per day indicates failure.

The kidneys may be small and contracted or large and irregular in shape. The nature and extent of the underlying disease affect the rate of progression and the complicating factors. The most common causes are pyelonephritis, chronic glomerulonephritis, glomerulosclerosis, chronic urinary obstruction, severe hypertension, diabetes, gout, and polycystic kidney disease (Richard, 1995a; King, 1997).

**Assessment.** Patients with **chronic renal failure** have a characteristic dusky, yellow-tan, or gray color from retained urochrome pigments. The pallor of anemia is obvious. Pruritus and crawling or tickling sensations cause the patient to scratch the skin, producing excoriations that become infected. Abnormalities in clotting and capillary fragility permit large bruises and purpura to develop. The skin is dry and scaly because of a decrease in oil gland activity and in subcutaneous tissue. Uremic frost appears as white or yellowish crystals on the skin and is a late sign of chronic renal failure that is rarely seen if dialysis is implemented.

The patient develops a nonbacterial stomatitis caused by the action of the urea-splitting flora of the oral cavity on the increased urea in the tissues. This gives rise to a metallic taste in the patient's mouth. Anorexia, nausea, and vomiting are common. Metabolism of urea in the intestinal tract forms ammonia, which causes formation of ulcers that may then hemorrhage, causing melena. High levels of urea in the blood produce a general feeling of lethargy advancing to drowsiness, confusion, and eventual coma.

Elevation of the serum potassium level accompanies the loss of sodium and the elimination of hydrogen ions from the kidneys (the body's attempt to reduce acidosis). The high potassium level may cause arrhythmias. For some reason calcium is not absorbed in the gastrointestinal tract, and low levels of calcium may produce muscle irritability followed by tetany or convulsions if not corrected. Acidosis progresses, depleting bicarbonates and stimulating the respiratory center to increase respirations. Thus a deep sighing form of breathing is a symptom of renal insufficiency, whereas in the late stages of uremia, hyperventilation is amplified to rid the body of carbonic acid along with water in the form of carbon dioxide.

Anemia accompanies chronic renal failure because the kidney is unable to produce erythropoietin. This causes air hunger and a mild dyspnea. Belching and hiccups are also common.

Hypertension develops to compensate for the decreased oxygen-carrying capacity of the blood in anemia, and retinopathy may then occur.

**Intervention.** Ongoing teaching is the most important nursing intervention implemented for the patient with renal failure (Brundage, Swearingen, 1994). Chronic renal failure is treated by restriction of nutrients and fluids to levels that the kidneys are able to manage effectively, and by dialysis or renal transplantation. If dietary management is initiated early, the buildup of toxins can be prevented or minimized and the impaired functional abilities of the kidneys can be more effective for a longer time. Transplantation and dialysis are discussed later in this chapter.

Usually the diet is complex and is managed by a renal dietitian (Rodriguez, 1997). The diet contains enough protein to prevent tissue wasting but not so much as to contribute to the overload of its metabolic end products (urea). When even a minimum amount of protein cannot be handled by the kidneys, dialysis is required. The diet is high in calories from carbohydrates and fats, consisting of at least 2500 to 3000 calories daily. Without sufficient calories from carbohydrates and fats, the liver forms glycogen from amino acids (glyconeogenesis) and increases the metabolic end products of protein in the blood. Other dietary restrictions are related to the patient's degree of acidosis. Potassium is retained; therefore foods high in potassium could be restricted. Sodium is controlled at a level sufficient to replace sodium loss without causing fluid retention. Table salt is almost always eliminated, and commercially prepared low-salt foods are used. Boiling and processing fruits and vegetables removes potassium.

Fluid balance is of prime importance. The patient may have fluids equal to the amount excreted in the urine plus 9 to 15 ounces (300 to 500 ml) to compensate for insensible fluid loss (e.g., through the lungs, perspiration). Fluids in excess of the amount that can be eliminated are retained in the body, and the patient gains weight. Accurate records of all intake and output, as well as daily weights, are essential to the calculation of fluid replacement. Weighing the patient at the same time each day on the same scale with the same amount of clothes is important.

The patient often complains of thirst, but the thirst associated with renal failure cannot be relieved by ordinary means. Factors that the nurse must consider in relation to the patient's thirst include the total amount of fluid allowed, the condition of the patient's mouth, fluid output, diet, physical activity, and the patient's mental state. There are ways in which the nurse can space the fluid without giving more fluid than the amount permitted.

When fluids are restricted, the following methods of administering medications should be considered: (1) giving several medications at mealtime, (2) giving small pills and capsules rather than large ones that may require larger amounts of water to swallow, (3) using solid forms of medications rather than liquid forms, (4) using small glasses rather than large glasses (a small glass full of water has a better psychologic effect than a large glass with a small amount of water), and (5) realizing that a small amount of cold water is more satisfying than warm water.

Dietary and fluid restrictions may be eased once the patient begins dialysis, but some treatment plans continue rigid control on the premise that this prevents complications and improves the prognosis.

Thorough and frequent oral hygiene is necessary to relieve the effects of stomatitis and the metallic taste in the mouth. Vinegar (0.25% acetic acid) used as a mouthwash helps to neutralize ammonium. Hard candy, gum, and cold liquids help improve the taste in the mouth. The more critical the patient's condition, the more mouth care is required, and in some cases it may have to be given hourly. Whatever method is used must meet the needs of the patient. The mouth may be dry because of dyspnea or because of the effects of receiving oxygen. Humidification of the air provides moisture and relieves dryness.

Patients who are given a regimen of bed rest may develop decubiti or pulmonary complications and should be turned regularly and encouraged to breathe deeply. The use of an alternating air pressure pad may provide comfort for some patients. Skin care is extremely important in the care of patients with chronic renal failure. Mild soap such as Basis, a baking soda solution, or bath oil may be used to cleanse the skin. Lanolin or other ointments may be ordered to relieve itching. Nails should be kept short so that the patient does not scratch and traumatize the skin. Edematous areas should be supported with pillows and circulation stimulated

through active or passive exercises. Edematous extremities should be elevated above the level of the heart.

If the patient's vision is failing, care should be taken to prevent injury. Padded side rails should be used for patients who are confused or disoriented. The nurse ensures that an oral airway is kept at the bedside or nearby in case convulsions should occur.

The administration of Epoetin alfa, a form of recombinant human erythropoietin, has improved the signs and symptoms of anemia in many patients with chronic renal failure (Cutler, 1997).

Blood transfusions may be necessary, and only washed donor cells may be used, especially if the patient is awaiting transplantation. Antigens should not be introduced into the body unnecessarily because the formation of antigen-antibody complexes may limit the patient's ability to accept a donor kidney. Blood transfusions, with hyperkalemia, fluid retention, and hypertension, may result in congestive heart failure. In treating congestive heart failure, it must be remembered that drugs normally excreted by the kidney, such as digoxin, require reduced dosages and that diuretics that depend on glomerular filtration are not effective.

Patients with chronic renal failure should be encouraged to participate in self-care activities and to remain active if their condition permits (Brundage, Swearingen, 1994).

# DIALYSIS

## Hemodialysis

**Hemodialysis** is an extracorporeal mechanical method of removing waste products and establishing equilibrium of electrolytes and water when the kidneys are unable to perform their functions. Hemodialysis is accomplished by the use of the artificial kidney called a *dialyzer* and may be used in (1) chronic renal failure, (2) acute renal failure, and (3) drug poisoning. Hemodialysis does not cure the damage caused by renal disease but removes waste products from the body and prevents damage to other organs until further treatment can be instituted and healing of the kidney takes place.

The process of hemodialysis is as follows: blood leaves the body and flows through sterile tubing, a sterile *dialyzer* (also called an artificial kidney), more sterile tubing, and back to the body (Figure 37-15). The dialyzer is composed of two compartments that are separated by a semipermeable membrane, which is similar to cellophane. In one compartment is the patient's blood, and in the other compartment is the dialyzing solution that is chemically similar to blood. As the blood and the dialyzing solutions circulate on the two sides of the semipermeable membrane, waste products leave the bloodstream, cross the membrane,

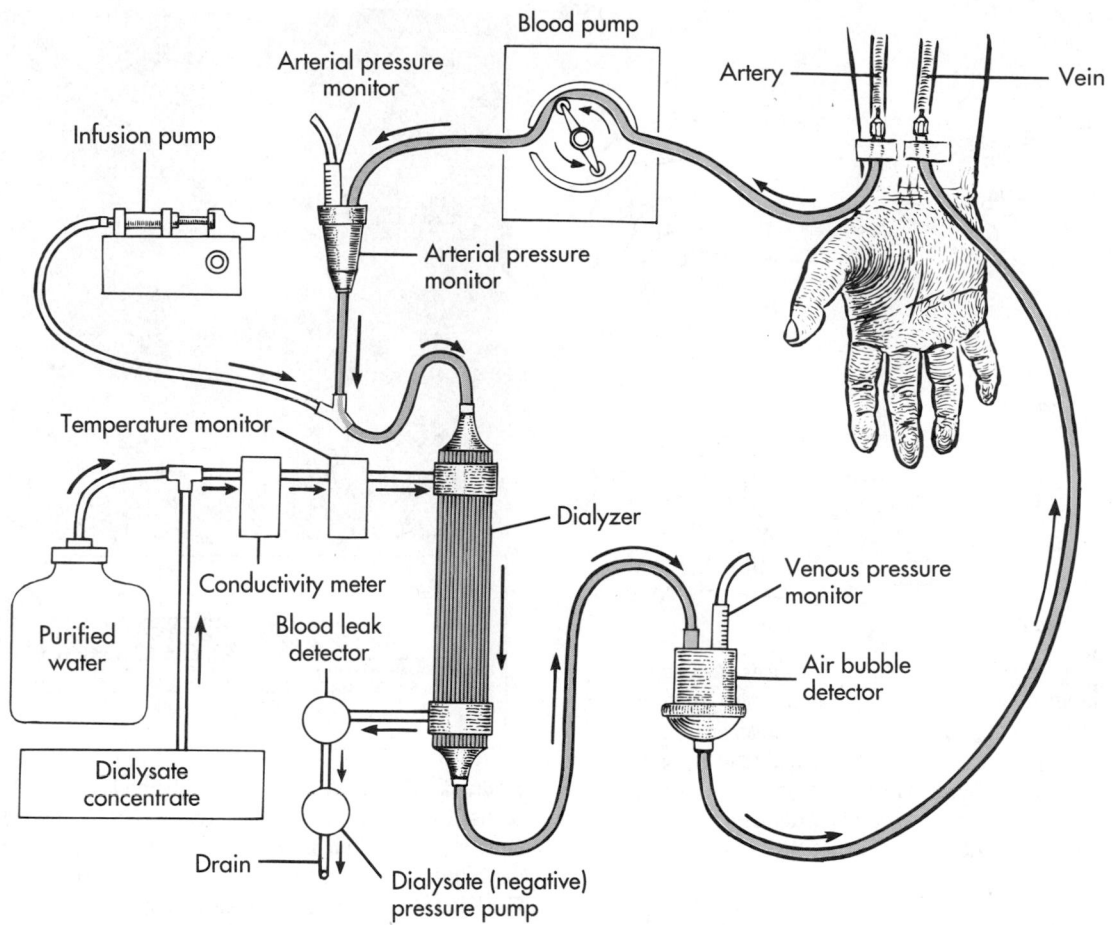

**Figure 37-15**    Components of a hemodialysis system. (From Thelan LA et al: *Critical care nursing: diagnosis and management,* ed 3, St Louis, 1998, Mosby.)

and enter the dialyzing solution, which is changed periodically. Therefore the dialysis process occurs across the semipermeable membrane inside the dialyzer. The dialyzer is attached to a hemodialysis machine that has different pumps and safety devices.

There are three basic circulatory accesses to remove and return the blood. The *external arteriovenous shunt* requires the insertion of cannulas in an artery and a vein, usually on the forearm (Figure 37-16). Cannulas are attached to the dialysis tubing during hemodialysis treatment, but otherwise they are attached to each other by a connector. This shunt is intended for short-term use.

An alternative to the arteriovenous shunt is the insertion of a specially designed, double lumen *catheter* through the subclavian or jugular vein. The catheter is designed so that blood is removed from a point proximal to the insertion site, routed through the dialyzer, and returned through a distal hole in the catheter (Figure 37-17). The subclavian or jugular site is easier to protect and maintain than the shunt site in the forearm. It can be used for a number of weeks. The site must be cleansed and redressed regularly, as for any

long-term infusion catheter. The other method used to conduct dialysis involves an *arteriovenous fistula,* in which a vein is surgically anastomosed to an artery. The vein then becomes distended, and the vessel wall thickens and can be palpated easily so that needles can be inserted for dialysis hook-up (see Figure 37-17).

Patients can be maintained on dialysis therapy and their lives prolonged pending the possibility of a kidney transplant. When long-term dialysis is necessary for end-stage renal disease, the patient may go to a dialysis center, usually two or three times weekly, and remain approximately 4 to 6 hours for the treatment. Some patients receive their treatment at night and go about their normal activities during the day. Smaller, portable units have been developed that allow the patient to be dialyzed anywhere. Many patients, with the help of an assistant, dialyze themselves at home.

Patients receiving dialysis therapy need a great deal of psychologic support and encouragement (Start, 1997). Most patients realize the seriousness of their condition. They may become depressed and question why they are being kept alive. The patient's family plays a most important role.

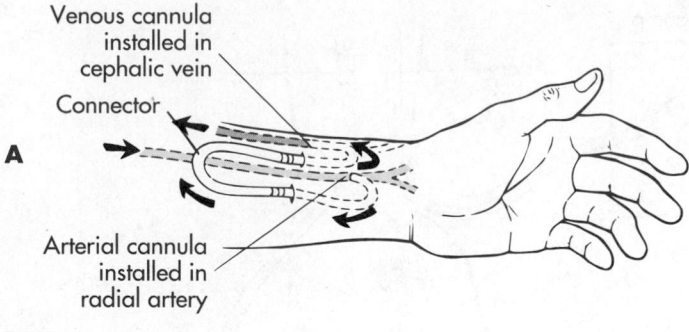

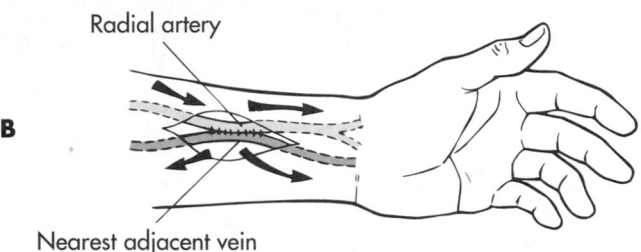

**Figure 37-16** Hemodialysis circulatory accesses. **A,** External arteriovenous shunt. A cannula is inserted into a vein, and another cannula is inserted into an artery. The two cannulas are joined by a connector. Arrows indicate the direction of blood flow. **B,** Arteriovenous fistula. An artery and a vein are surgically anastomosed. Blood flows through the artery into the vein and arterializes the vein. Arrows indicate the direction of blood flow.

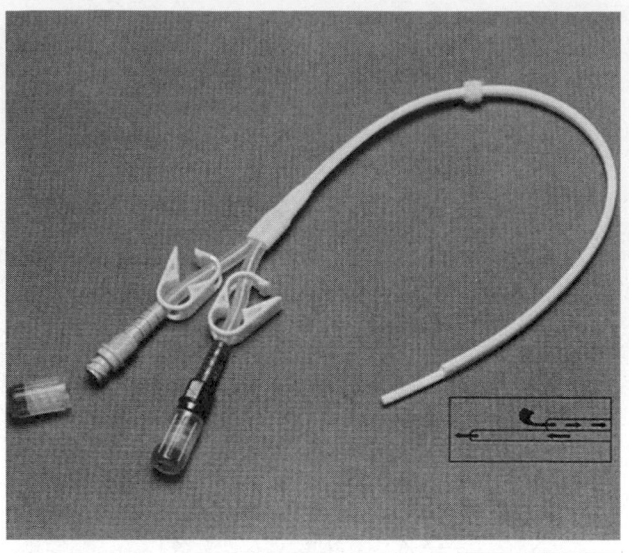

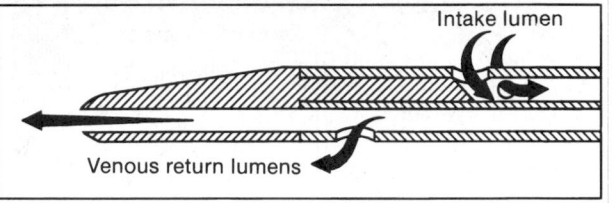

**Figure 37-17** **A,** A double-lumen hemodialysis catheter that can be used for subclavian and femoral insertion. **B,** (Enlargement of small inset in **A.**) The distance between the venous return lumen and the return intake lumen ensures minimal recirculation. (Courtesy The Kendall Company LP, Mansfield, Mass.)

Personnel who work with hemodialysis patients must be specially educated in anatomy, physiology, and pathology of the kidney and in pharmacology. Usually each dialysis center has its own education program, lasting 6 to 12 weeks (Richard, 1986; Lancaster, 1995; Start, 1997).

## Peritoneal Dialysis

**Peritoneal dialysis** was the original substitute for a nonfunctioning kidney. It can be performed in any hospital with minimum equipment, as well as when the patient is ambulatory. In all types of peritoneal dialysis, a fluid is instilled into the peritoneal space by gravity, allowed to remain there long enough to collect waste products and excess electrolytes that have been left in the blood by the nonfunctioning kidney, then drained from the space and discarded (Figure 37-18). While in the peritoneal space, the fluid, called *dialysate,* bathes the peritoneal membrane. The waste products and electrolytes pass through the capillaries in the membrane, by the processes of osmosis and diffusion, into the dialysate. The chemical composition of the dialysate is designed to promote removal of products from the blood in the same way it functions in hemodialysis.

The catheter is inserted into the peritoneal cavity using a technique that is similar to abdominal paracente-

sis. A trocar, a large needle with a large bore, is inserted through a tiny incision made in the skin of the abdomen. During insertion, a stylet is in place in the bore of the trocar; after insertion, the stylet is removed, and a catheter with tiny holes running the length of all sides is inserted through the trocar. The trocar is then withdrawn, and the catheter remains in the peritoneal cavity.

Next, 60 ounces (2000 ml) of dialyzing solution is allowed to run into the peritoneal cavity and remain for 30 to 60 minutes. The solution is warmed before it is instilled to improve its effectiveness and to prevent chilling of the patient. The fluid is then drained by gravity. When 3 to 6 ounces (100 to 200 ml) of solution remains in the cavity, another bottle of solution is connected, and the process is repeated. Sterile technique is observed when inserting the catheter and caring for the site. All connections to the tubing and the addition of bottles of solution must be done in a manner that prevents contamination of the inside of the tubing, the site, and the solution.

During the procedure the patient should be observed for signs of abdominal or respiratory distress, changes in vital signs, and bleeding. The amount of fluid in-

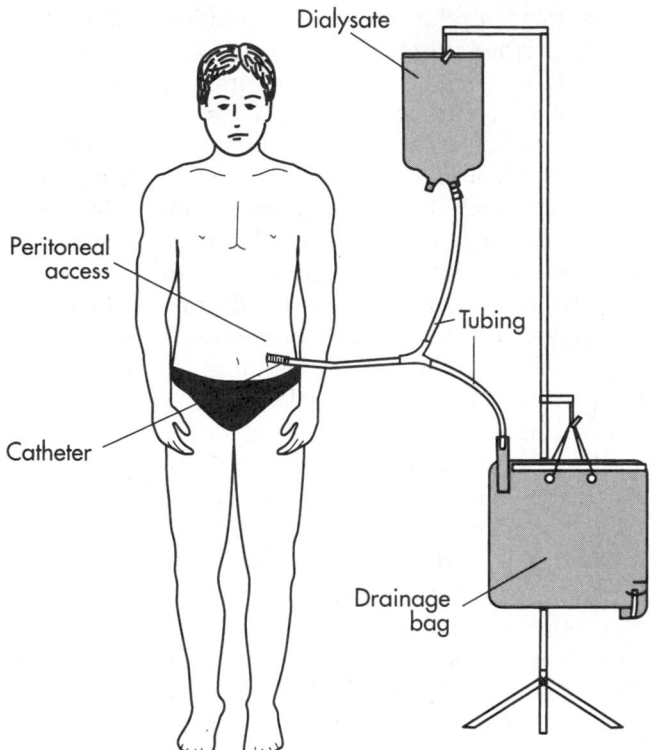

**Figure 37-18**    Peritoneal dialysis system.

stilled and drained should be carefully recorded. The patient should be weighed before and after the procedure. The catheter is removed when the process is completed. If the procedure is to be repeated in a day or two, the pathway to the peritoneal cavity may be kept open with a sterile plastic tube specially designed for this purpose. A sterile dressing is applied to the site; the incision is small and does not require repair with sutures.

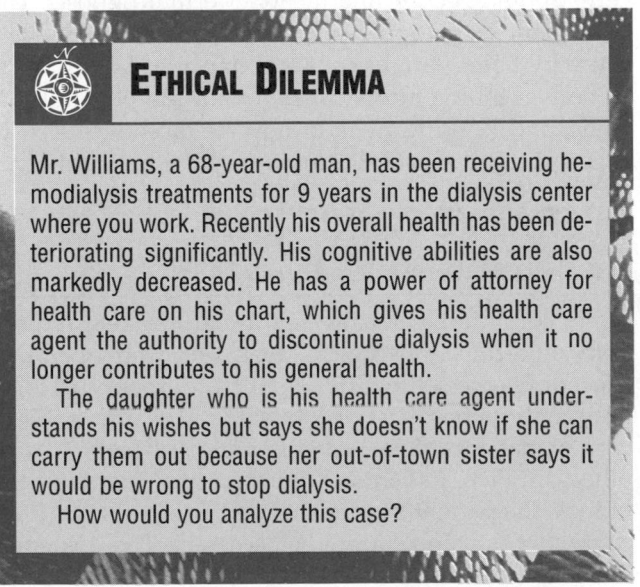

## ETHICAL DILEMMA

Mr. Williams, a 68-year-old man, has been receiving hemodialysis treatments for 9 years in the dialysis center where you work. Recently his overall health has been deteriorating significantly. His cognitive abilities are also markedly decreased. He has a power of attorney for health care on his chart, which gives his health care agent the authority to discontinue dialysis when it no longer contributes to his general health.

The daughter who is his health care agent understands his wishes but says she doesn't know if she can carry them out because her out-of-town sister says it would be wrong to stop dialysis.

How would you analyze this case?

Considering the time required for this procedure to remove the waste products, it is easy to see how hemodialysis came to be the preferred method for the patient with chronic renal failure. It is not practical to spend 24 hours every other day confined to bed or a hospital unit while receiving a peritoneal dialysis treatment. Although hemodialysis does restrict the patient, it is at least less time consuming (Gallagher, 1996).

## Continuous Ambulatory Peritoneal Dialysis

*Continuous ambulatory peritoneal dialysis* (CAPD) removes some of the restrictions from the patient with end-stage renal disease. It allows the patient to receive dialysis during the night while asleep at home or while ambulatory at home, work, or play. A catheter is inserted surgically and is left in place and covered by a sterile dressing. The catheter is placed in the peritoneal space through an incision, and the distal end is tunneled through a 7.5 to 10 cm (3 or 4 inch) section of subcutaneous tissue on the abdomen, then brought out to the surface of the abdomen. This tunnel creates a barrier to prevent infection of the peritoneal cavity if the catheter site should become infected. The patient is taught to meticulously care for the catheter and site, using a sterile technique. Before and after connecting the dialysate tubing, the connection is disinfected with a povidone-iodine (Betadine) soak for about 20 minutes.

For nighttime dialysis, the dialysate instillation is regulated by a machine that automatically starts the flow of solution, times the period it remains in the cavity, and then allows the fluid to drain by gravity. Safety mechanisms are built into the machine to prevent fluid from being instilled if the previous instillation has not drained adequately. Multiple bottles of dialysate are hooked up to the machine, and it automatically instills each bottle in sequence. Used dialysate is likewise collected in multiple bottles that are weighed by the machine to verify complete elimination before the next bottle is instilled. An alarm sounds to waken the patient if any problem is sensed by the machine.

For daytime dialysis with continuous ambulatory peritoneal dialysis, the patient attaches a small bag of dialysate to the catheter, instills it, then rolls it up and tucks it in an inconspicuous place while the dialysate is instilled. Later the dialysate is drained into the same bag and discarded. The procedure is repeated as necessary to maintain the waste products in the blood at a safe level, usually four times each day. Research and development of new products and techniques continue to make life more livable for the patient dependent on dialysis.

# RENAL TRANSPLANTATION

A renal transplantation is the procedure of placing a normal kidney from a donor into a person with non-functioning kidneys. The most successful transplants are those done with a sibling or family member with the same blood and tissue typing. By carefully matching the donor kidney with the recipient, kidneys from unrelated people and from cadavers are transplanted with fair success (Lancaster, 1995; Givliano, 1997).

The patient may undergo a bilateral nephrectomy in preparation for the transplant if the kidneys are severely infected or if the patient has severe diastolic hypertension. This patient will experience a sense of loss, even though the absent kidneys were not functioning. The kidneys may both be left in place for transplant surgery because the donor kidney is placed in the iliac fossa and receives its blood supply from the iliac arteries (Figure 37-19). Dialysis is necessary until the transplantation can be accomplished.

Postoperative care is centered around careful observation of hourly urine output and maintaining patency of the indwelling catheter along with the maintenance of intravenous fluid and electrolyte therapy. Massive diuresis or oliguria may be possible. Additional nursing measures are similar to those of any major surgical procedure. A central venous pressure line may be in place to monitor fluid needs. The patient is weighed daily to monitor fluid retention. The patient must be observed carefully for signs of *rejection* of the donor kidney, which include decreased urine output, increased blood pressure, fever, and swelling and tenderness at the site of the implanted kidney.

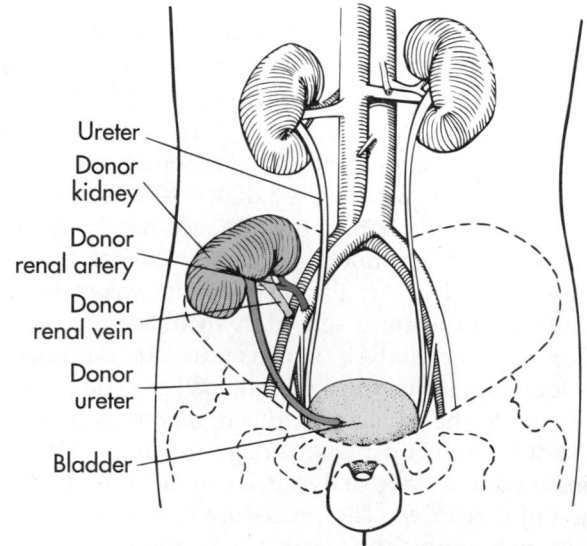

**Figure 37-19** Location of a transplanted kidney showing the anastomosis of the renal artery, the renal vein, and the ureter. (From Phipps WJ et al: *Medical-surgical nursing: concepts and clinical practice*, ed 5, St Louis, 1995, Mosby.)

The major problem in transplantation is that of rejection. Before surgery the patient's immunologic responses are suppressed, and immunosuppressive therapy is continued long after discharge. Cyclosporine (Sandimmune), a drug obtained from soil fungus, has revolutionized the success of organ transplantation, including kidney transplants (Hardman, 1996). Cyclosporine may be used as a single immunosuppressant agent or in conjunction with steroids. Cyclosporine may be administered intravenously or orally. Because cyclosporine is prepared in an oil base, patients may find it unpalatable. Administering it with food or diluting it in chocolate milk may help the patient ingest the drug. Therapeutic levels of cyclosporine are carefully monitored with a radioimmunoassay because, ironically, elevated levels of cyclosporine are nephrotoxic.

Other drugs that may be used are azathioprine (Imuran), prednisone, and methylprednisolone (Solu-Medrol). The visible side effects of steroid therapy, namely moon face and weight gain, may be the greatest problem for the patient during recovery. As immunosuppressive therapy is withdrawn, the physical appearance returns to normal.

The patient will also be given furosemide (Lasix) to control fluid retention, aluminum phosphate gel (Phosphaljel) to protect the stomach during steroid therapy, hydralazine (Apresoline) and methyldopa (Aldomet) for the control of blood pressure, and sulfisoxazole (Gantrisin) and nystatin (Mycostatin) to prevent infections.

Rejection of the transplanted kidney may occur soon after surgery, or it may be delayed for months or even years after transplantation. The possibility of rejection is a very important factor to the patient. The patient must be encouraged and facilitated in expressing concerns about rejection and the long-term prognosis. The patient must be prepared for discharge and convalescence by being taught the importance of taking medications, keeping appointments with the physician or clinic, and keeping track of how he or she feels. Psychologically, the patient must adopt the new kidney.

# OPERATIVE CONDITIONS OF THE URINARY SYSTEM

Many conditions affecting the urinary system require both medical and surgical treatment, and operative procedures are seldom done until a thorough urologic examination has been completed. The preoperative care of patients does not differ greatly from that of other surgical patients. When surgery involves the kidney, the patient's blood is typed and cross-matched in case transfusion should be necessary. The postoperative care differs from other kinds of surgery in that drains, tubes, or catheters are placed to remove urine (Meeker, Rothrock, 1995).

Many patients have draining wounds after surgery on the urinary system. Although patients may have understood this before surgery, when they are faced with the discomfort of wet dressings, the odor of urine, and the resulting skin irritation, they may become irritable and depressed and feel that adjustment is impossible. It may challenge the nurse to find ways to overcome these problems.

Because dressings need to be changed often, Montgomery straps or laced dressings could be used to avoid skin irritation from adhesive tape. Small dressings changed often keep the patient more comfortable than large, bulky ones that become saturated, heavy, and foul smelling. A ureterostomy cup may be applied and attached to free drainage, or the disposable plastic urostomy bags may be used for some patients. Wound drainage bags are available that may be effective in some drainage problems. Any device used is only an adjunct to good nursing care, which includes cleansing the skin and protecting wounds from infection.

## Cystectomy

A *cystectomy* is the surgical removal of the bladder and may be partial or complete. The surgery may be necessary because of malignant tumors involving the bladder and adjacent structures. When the bladder is removed, the ureters are transplanted by one of the methods discussed in the following section to provide for urinary drainage. The nursing care is the same as that for patients having abdominal surgery. The prostate gland may have been removed through a perineal wound, and such wounds must be observed for evidence of hemorrhage. The patient will have a nasogastric tube connected to suction siphonage and will be given nothing by mouth for several days. During this time the patient should receive special mouth care at frequent intervals.

If a partial resection of the bladder has been done, a catheter is inserted into the remaining bladder, and precautions must be taken to prevent any pulling on the catheter. The tubing should be pinned to the sheet and sufficient slack allowed to permit the patient to turn.

## Urinary Diversion: Ureteral Transplants

Several types of procedures are used to divert the flow of urine when required for treatment of bladder cancer, invasive cancer of the cervix, neurogenic bladder, and congenital anomalies. The *ureterosigmoidostomy* involves implanting the ureters into the large bowel, which is left intact so that both urine and feces are eliminated rectally. This technique is rarely used today because of the undesirable effects on the perianal skin resulting from chronically liquid stool. A variation of this procedure is the formation of an isolated rectal pouch into which the ureters are implanted while the remainder of the bowel is diverted to form a sigmoid colostomy.

A second procedure, *cutaneous ureterostomy*, involves direct implantation of the terminal ends of the ureters onto the skin (Figure 37-20). The ureters may be joined so that there is only one stoma, or each ureter may be brought to the skin separately, forming two stomas. A third procedure, the *ileal conduit*, is a common method of urinary diversion at present (Figure 37-21). In this procedure a section of the ileum is resected from the small bowel, and its blood supply is preserved. The remaining small bowel is then anastomosed so that normal bowel function is maintained. The resected segment of ileum is sutured closed at one end, forming a pouch, and the other end is sutured to the skin, forming a stoma. The ureters are transplanted into this segment of ileum, which forms a conduit that serves as a passageway for urine to flow from the body. It does not serve as a reservoir for urine.

A variation of the ileal conduit is the *continent urostomy* (or *Koch's pouch*), in which the pouch is formed from the ileum. In this instance the reservoir can hold up to 24 ounces (800 ml) of urine. A large segment of the

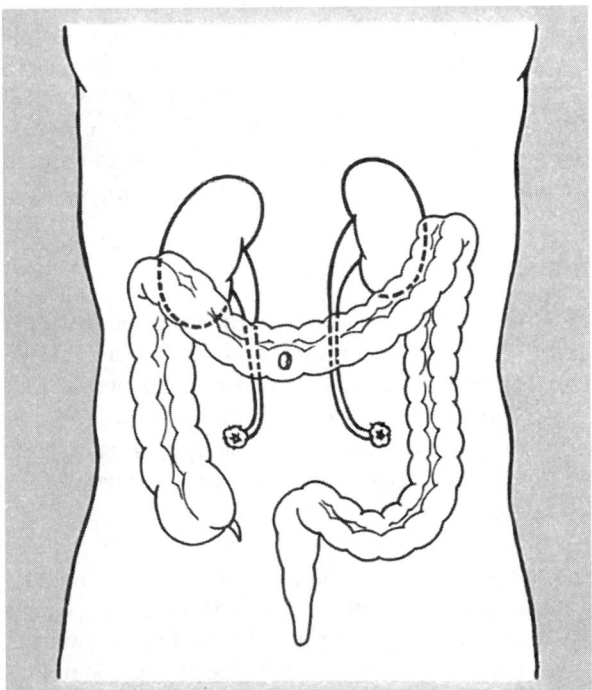

**Figure 37-20**   Cutaneous ureterostomy in which the ureters are brought through the skin onto the abdomen.

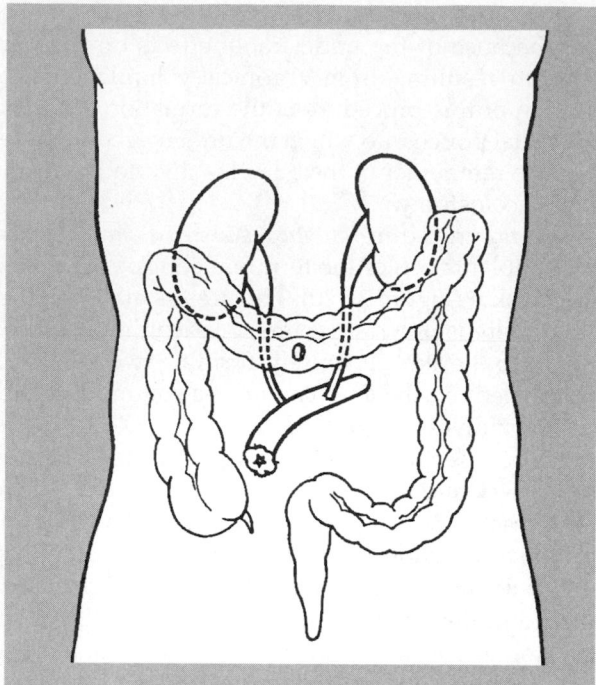

**Figure 37-21** Ileal conduit. A small section of the ileum is resected from the small intestine. One end of the resected portion is sutured closed, and the other end is brought to the skin surface. The ureters are transplanted into the resected ileum.

ileum is structured into an internal pouch with two nipple valves. The ureters are implanted into the reservoir, and a portion of the ileal reservoir is brought out transcutaneously and fashioned into a stoma. Patients are taught to catheterize this pouch approximately four times a day, and they do not need to wear an external urinary appliance. A small bandage over the stoma is sufficient (Lewis, Collier, Heitkemper, 1996).

## Cutaneous Ureterostomy

When the ureters have been transplanted to the abdominal wall a stent or soft catheter, is placed in each ureter for about 7 to 10 days. Stents provide a clear passageway for urine because the ureters are edematous from manipulation during surgery. It is important that the stents drain freely so that hydronephrosis does not develop.

If cutaneous ureterostomies heal properly, the patient can use ostomy bags instead of catheters for drainage. The bags can be applied to the skin with adhesive disks and may require changing only every 2 or 3 days. The technique for applying the bag is not difficult, but it does take practice. When the bag is first applied, the nurse must make sure that there is adequate drainage from the kidney. If the patient complains of

any back pain, the appliance should be removed at once and reapplied. Sometimes obstruction of drainage is caused by angulation of the ureter or by temporary ureteral edema.

If the ureter is angulated or if there is stomal stenosis, the kidney must be drained permanently with a catheter. If the patient must wear ureteral catheters, he or she is taught to irrigate these each day. Patients must return to the physician every 2 to 4 weeks to have the catheters changed, or they are taught to change their own catheters. The catheters are anchored to the skin with adhesive tape, or a catheter disk with a belt is used. The catheters are attached by tubing to a drainage receptacle. This procedure is not commonly used, since infections occur often, causing a series of complications.

## Ileal Conduit (Ileobladder)

The **ileal conduit** is a method of urinary diversion that results in few fluid and electrolyte problems and provides an added barrier to infection (the conduit). Preoperatively, the patient has little or no special preparation of the bowel because the ileum is considered sterile. Careful preoperative measurement and inspection of the abdomen for optimum placement of the stoma facilitates movement and application of an appliance for urinary drainage postoperatively.

The patient returns from surgery with stents in the ureters and a catheter in the ileal conduit covered with a temporary transparent appliance attached to the skin to collect urine. The appliance is attached to a drainage system to provide for continuous flow of urine. Urinary flow must be maintained; if it is allowed to distend the conduit, it will cause back pressure on the kidneys, damaging them, and/or it will rupture the suture lines. The nurse must watch closely for low abdominal pain and decreased urinary output. Urine output may be measured hourly in the early postoperative period.

Postoperative complications related to abdominal surgery are preventable. The abdomen is observed for any changes that might indicate inflammation. Paralytic ileus can occur as a result of manipulation of the bowel. A nasogastric tube is usually inserted to decompress the bowel until peristalsis returns. Oral intake is restricted or prohibited while the nasogastric tube is in place.

There is a possibility of urine leakage at the suture lines, which allows urine to enter the peritoneal cavity; the resultant inflammation causes pain, fever, nausea, and vomiting. The patient's abdomen will feel rigid and will be sensitive to the touch.

When the stoma has healed, a permanent (reusable) appliance is fitted to the patient. Disposable appliances are available (Figure 37-22) but expensive; therefore patients may choose a reusable appliance. Proper

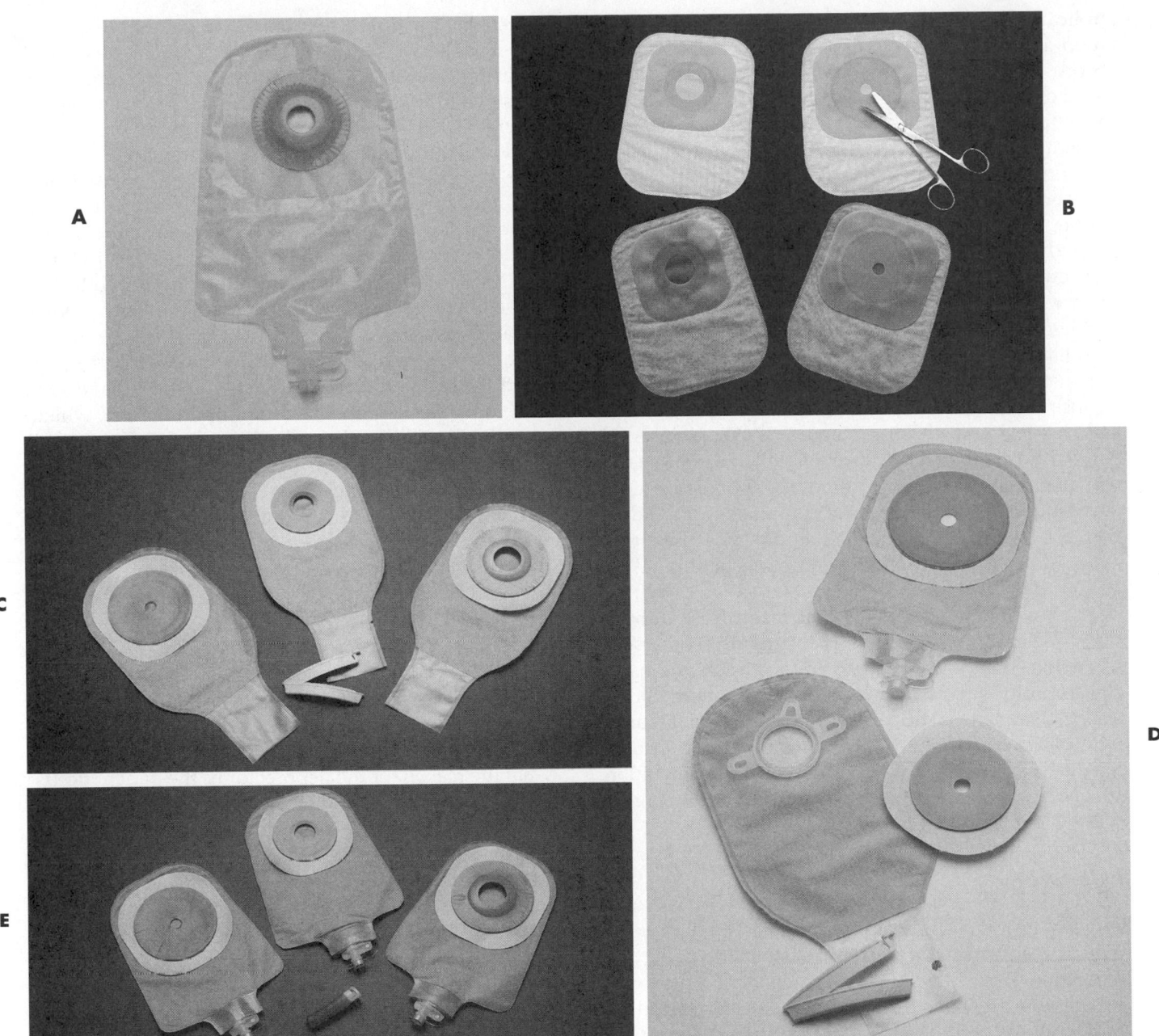

**Figure 37-22**     Urostomy pouches. **A,** First Choice Urostomy Pouch with a no-flowback valve and preattached skin barrier. **B,** First Choice Urostomy Closed Pouch with preattached skin barrier that can be cut to fit different size stomas. **C,** Premier series drainable pouches with a pouch clamp. Skin barriers from left to right are flat, cut to fit, and convex. **D,** Premier one-piece drainable urostomy *(top)* and two-piece drainable urostomy with built-in belt tabs and a pouch clamp. **E,** Premier series urostomy pouches with a no-flowback valve and drainage tube adapter. Skin barriers from left to right are flat, cut-to-fit, and convex. (Courtesy Hollister, Inc., Libertyville, Ill.)

application of the appliance prevents leaking and irritation of the skin. The stoma is covered with gauze to absorb urine while the area around the stoma is cleaned. It is essential to make sure the skin is dry before applying the appliance, or it will not adhere. Permanent appliances have a faceplate that is attached to the skin with cement or a double-faced adhesive. The collection pouch is attached to the faceplate. A permanent appliance can be worn for 3 to 7 days if applied properly. It is recommended that the patient purchase a second appliance so that one may be cleaned and aired while the other is worn (Box 37-4).

When a urine specimen is needed from a patient who has an ileal conduit, the stoma is catheterized using aseptic technique. After the stoma has been cleansed, a single lumen or double lumen catheter, a catheter inside a catheter (Figure 37-23), is inserted gently into the stoma, and urine is collected in a sterile container. The catheter is removed and disposed of and a pouch is reapplied. The container is labeled so that the laboratory personnel know that the urine came from an ileal conduit (Hampton, Bryand, 1992; Felton, 1993).

The psychologic problems that result from urinary diversion are similar to those occurring from diversion of the intestinal tract. The surgery is a traumatic experience, and the patient must adapt to an altered body image. The patient must be supported and reassured when learning to care for the urostomy and encouraged to continue everyday activities once recuperation from surgery has occurred. It is important to consult with an enterostomal nurse specialist.

## Cystotomy

A cystotomy is a surgical incision into the bladder. It may be performed for various reasons, including the correction of prostatic hypertrophy in connection with suprapubic prostatectomy. It may be performed to remove tumors or stones from the bladder.

The preoperative care of the patient is the same as that for other abdominal surgery. When the patient returns from surgery, a drainage tube will have been inserted into the bladder, which may be connected to a drainage bag. The dressings must be changed often to keep the patient dry and comfortable. The skin must be kept clean, and a protective ointment may be used to prevent irritation. Blood pressure and pulse must be checked often during the immediate postoperative period, and the patient must be turned from side to side to prevent pulmonary complications.

## Ureterotomy and Lithotomy

Surgery on the ureter is generally performed to remove a stone, to repair a severed ureter, or to do plastic repair of a stricture. If the stone is in the ureter, a *ureterolithotomy* is performed. Removal of the stone from the kidney is a *nephrolithotomy*, and removal of the stone from the kidney pelvis is a *pyelolithotomy* (see Figure 37-13). Patients having a stone removed from the lower third of the ureter have an abdominal incision, and care is similar to that for any patient with abdominal surgery. However, the incision will drain urine for several days after surgery because the ureter cannot be closed with watertight sutures or strictures will form. Stones removed from the upper two thirds of the ureter and the kidney necessitate a flank or kidney incision.

The postoperative care of the patient is directed toward the care of tubes and maintaining drainage. Occasionally a catheter is inserted into the ureter, which serves as a stent while healing occurs. It is important that the catheter be kept in place at all times. When there is urinary drainage onto the skin, there must be frequent change of dressings and cleansing of the skin to prevent irritation and maceration. All urinary drainage should be measured and recorded (Box 37-5) (Richard, 1995b; Lewis, Collier, Heitkemper, 1996).

## Nephrectomy and Nephrostomy

A *nephrectomy* is the surgical removal of the kidney. It may be done because of tumors or chronic infection or to provide a kidney for transplantation. No matter what the reason for the nephrectomy, the patient needs emotional support and an opportunity to express and discuss feelings about the loss of a body part.

A small drain may be placed in the wound for incisional drainage. When the patient has had a nephrectomy, there may be a minimal amount of drainage from the wound for the first 24 to 48 hours, which gradually diminishes.

Dressings are checked often for evidence of fresh bleeding because hemorrhage is always a possibility. Vital signs are watched, and any significant change in the pulse rate with restlessness should be reported to the physician. Gastrointestinal complications with nausea, vomiting, and abdominal distention may occur. Fluids by mouth may be restricted and a nasogastric tube inserted, which should be connected to suction drainage.

The most important postoperative concern is that good urinary drainage be established from the remaining kidney. The patient may have a retention catheter in place, which is connected to gravity drainage; if the patient does not void, catheterization may be ordered. All fluid intake and output must be carefully measured and recorded.

The patient will find it difficult to breathe deeply because of the location of the incision. In some cases the thoracic cavity may have been opened, and the patient

BOX 37-4     NURSING PROCESS

## URINARY DIVERSION—POSTOPERATIVE PHASE

### ASSESSMENT

- Signs and symptoms of urinary tract infection and systemic infection
- Decrease in urine volume and cloudiness
- Urinary tract pain
- Daily bowel movement

### NURSING DIAGNOSES

- Activity intolerance related to anxiety, pain, weakness, fatigue
- Anxiety related to fear, prognosis
- Constipation related to decreased activity, painful defecation
- Pain related to surgical procedure
- Ineffective individual coping related to anxiety, depression
- Fear related to disease process, hospitalization, powerlessness, real or imagined threat to well-being, surgical procedure
- Fluid volume deficit related to abnormal fluid loss, decreased fluid intake
- Impaired home maintenance management related to home environment obstacles, inadequate support system
- Knowledge deficit related to limited understanding of disease process, prescribed treatment
- Personal identity disturbance related to body image, role performance, self-esteem
- Sexual dysfunction related to altered bladder control, body image, depression, impotence, physiologic limitations
- Altered urinary elimination related to diversion

### NURSING INTERVENTIONS

- Administer standard immediate postoperative care, such as frequent vital signs.
- Measure and record intake and output.
- Report absence of urinary drainage immediately.
- Maintain intravenous fluid and electrolyte infusions.
- Provide mouth care every 4 hours while patient is awake.
- Maintain patency of nasogastric tube, and cleanse and lubricate nostril through which tube passes.
- Monitor return of peristalsis by observing for flatus, listening for bowel sounds once every 8 hours.
- Administer nothing by mouth until ordered, based on return of bowel function.
- Administer analgesics as ordered to relieve pain and facilitate movement.
- Turn patient every 2 hours and encourage coughing, deep breathing, and leg exercises.
- Ambulate as early as orders permit.
- Maintain patency of drainage tubes.

- Facilitate expression of feelings about altered body image.
- Assess integrity and color of the stoma every shift.
- Teach about disease process and treatment.

#### Cutaneous Ureterostomy

- Maintain patency of ureteral catheters.
- Put ureterostomy cups or urostomy bags in place after catheters have been removed.
- Dilate ureters with sterile catheters as ordered to ensure patency and prevent ureteral stricture.

#### Ileal Conduit

- Maintain drainage bag over stoma or catheter in stoma to collect urine; attach catheter to gravity drainage.
- Empty drainage bag every 2 hours; attach to gravity drainage bag at night.
- Control odor of urine and in appliance:
  Avoid odor-producing foods.
  Give cranberry juice.
  Add commercial deodorizers to bag.
  Wash permanent appliance with detergent and water and rinse in vinegar water; air dry overnight; patient uses two permanent appliances (alternating one each day) or uses disposable appliances.
- Change appliance and cleanse skin as follows:
  Remove appliance.
  Bend over to drain conduit before cleansing skin.
  Clean cement from skin with adhesive solvent.
  Wash skin with soap and water.
  Apply stomahesive skin barrier or powder for skin irritation.
  Apply cement or liquid adhesive or double-faced adhesive disks and appliance.
- Instruct patient and gradually involve the patient in care until self-care possible.

### EVALUATION OF EXPECTED OUTCOMES

- Adequate urinary drainage maintained
- Discomfort relieved
- No signs or symptoms of infection
- Actively participates in care
- Adequate nutritional and fluid states maintained
- Describes disease process, surgical intervention, and responsibility for care
- Relates less anxiety from fear of unknown, loss of control, or misinformation
- Shares feelings about control of elimination and bodily changes
- Patient and family verbalize fears and concerns
- Skin integrity maintained

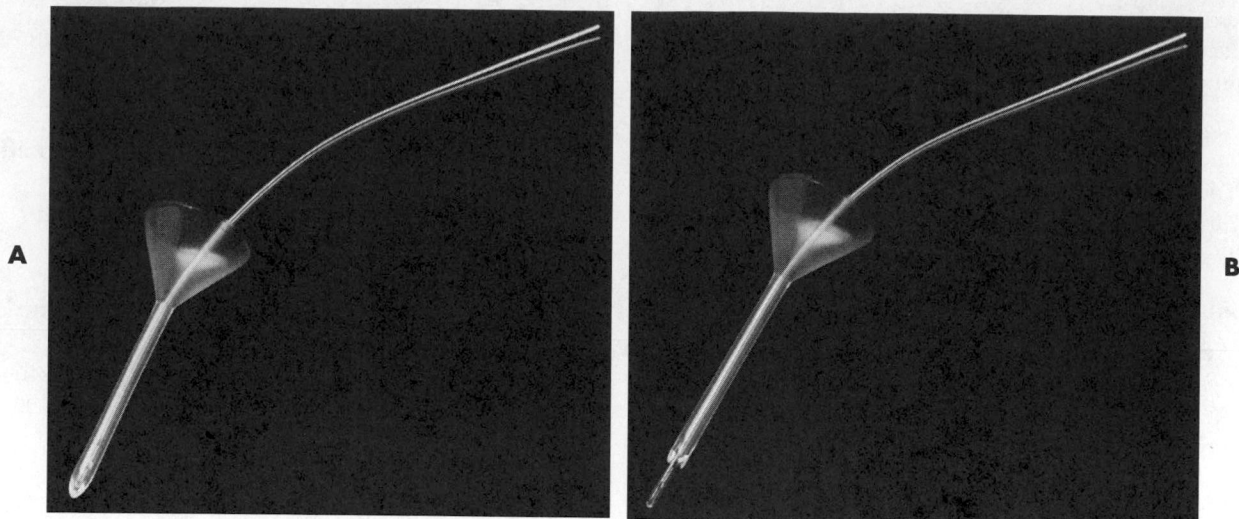

**Figure 37-23** Tele-Cath, a catheter within a catheter, is used to obtain urine from an ileal conduit/urostomy. **A,** The short outer sheath completely encloses a longer, narrow, inner catheter. **B,** The inner catheter has been advanced through the flexible tip of the outer sheath. The urinary stoma is cleansed, and the Tele-Cath is inserted as it appears in **A** into the stoma. The inner catheter is advanced, as depicted in **B,** until urine begins to flow. (See the text for further description.) (Courtesy Mentor Corp., Santa Barbara, Calif.)

will have a chest tube connected to underwater drainage. Medication for pain is given, the incision is splinted, and the patient is encouraged to breathe and cough deeply. The patient will be positioned according to the approach used for surgery. The patient is usually out of bed on the first postoperative day and ambulatory soon after. Most patients are able to tolerate a regular diet by the fourth postoperative day, with a fluid intake of approximately 2½ quarts (3000 ml).

When the patient leaves the hospital, he or she is advised to avoid heavy lifting and straining for 6 weeks, to maintain fluid intake, and to avoid alcohol. The patient should be advised to avoid respiratory tract infections and activities that might result in injury to the other kidney.

A *nephrostomy* is an incision into the kidney pelvis for the purpose of drainage. The postoperative care of the patient with a nephrostomy or pyelostomy is the same as that for nephrectomy except for the presence of catheters, which are attached to drainage (see Figure 37-8). The nurse watches carefully to be sure that the catheters do not become plugged with a blood clot. The physician's orders concerning turning the patient onto the affected side should be clearly understood. Drainage must be accurately measured and recorded, and dressings about the tubes or wound may need to be changed often. The skin may be kept clean by washing with mild soap and water and dried to prevent irritation. If tubes have been placed in both kidneys, both tubes should be placed on one side of the bed.

<BOX 37-5>

# NURSING PROCESS

## LITHOTOMY—POSTOPERATIVE PHASE
## (URETEROLITHOTOMY, PYELOLITHOTOMY, NEPHROLITHOTOMY)

### ASSESSMENT

- Decrease in urine volume
- Passing of stone fragments in the urine
- Healing of skin and operative site
- Signs and symptoms of urinary tract infection
- Pain
- Daily bowel movement

### NURSING DIAGNOSES

- Activity intolerance related to anxiety, pain, weakness, fatigue
- Constipation related to decreased activity, painful defecation
- Pain related to surgical procedure
- Ineffective individual coping related to anxiety, depression
- Fear related to disease process, hospitalization, powerlessness, real or imagined threat to well-being, surgical procedure
- Fluid volume deficit related to abnormal fluid loss, decreased fluid intake
- Knowledge deficit related to limited understanding of disease process, prescribed treatment

### NURSING INTERVENTIONS

- Weigh daily.
- Use standard immediate postoperative care.

- Anticipate drainage from wound; secure dressing with Montgomery straps.
- Change sterile dressing as often as necessary to keep dry; use caution to prevent displacement of penrose drain in wound.
- Maintain patency of bladder catheter.
- Measure and record intake and output.
- Observe color of urine.
- Relieve pain with analgesics as ordered.
- Splint incision during movement and coughing.
- Assist males to stand when voiding.
- Instruct on disease process and treatment.

### EVALUATION OF EXPECTED OUTCOMES

- Maintains adequate urinary drainage
- Discomfort relieved
- Actively participates in care
- Relates less anxiety from fear of unknown or misinformation
- Describes disease process, surgical intervention, and care
- Adequate nutritional fluid status maintained
- No signs or symptoms of infection

# NURSING CARE PLAN

## PATIENT WITH CHRONIC RENAL FAILURE

Ms. Barton is a 39-year-old female who comes into the outpatient dialysis unit for hemodialysis treatments three times per week because of chronic renal failure secondary to diabetic nephropathy. An internal arteriovenous fistula in her left arm is used as an access for dialysis. Physically, she has been tolerating the dialysis treatments well, with only mild dizziness at the end of each session.

The dialysis nurses have noted, however, that Ms. Barton gets irritated approximately 1 hour into the treatment. She calls to the nurses to check the machine, solutions, or her blood pressure, all of which are normal.

Ms. Barton has been on dialysis treatments on a regular basis for 6 months. She is on the transplant list, awaiting a matched donor.

| Medical History | Psychosocial Data | Assessment Data |
|---|---|---|
| Diagnosed as having juvenile diabetes (insulin dependent) at age 8 | Incomplete as to biologic family; adopted as an infant; is in the process of petitioning the courts to obtain birth records to identify genetic relatives in the hopes of locating a matched donor | Height 5' 4", weight 118 lbs |
| Good control until adolescence; multiple hospitalizations from age 12 to 19; periods of noncompliance, denial of the diabetes, and growth spurts | | Oriented × 3 (time, place, and person) |
| | | *Skin:* Dry and scaly; dusky color at times; usually pale but has been noted to be gray; signs of irritation from scratching evident on chest and arms; no signs of infection; small areas of broken skin on right chest wall; A-V fistula in left forearm (is right handed) |
| Appendectomy at age 16 | Currently a housewife; not employed outside of the home | |
| First pregnancy at age 21; baby a fetal demise at 39 weeks | Has completed 2 years of junior college; now attending a 4-year program, wants to obtain a degree as a counselor | *EENT:* Full extraocular movements (EOMs); wears glasses for nearsightedness; last ocular visit 3 months ago; teeth in good repair; visits dentist regularly |
| Second pregnancy at age 22; complicated by preeclampsia; C-sectioned at 36 weeks, viable male infant weighing 10 lbs | Divorced for 10 years; states she has a "friendly" relationship with her ex-husband due to the children | *Respiratory:* Regular rate and rhythm (18-20); all lung fields clear to percussion and auscultation |
| Third pregnancy at age 26; mild toxemia, repeat C-section at 36 weeks, viable female infant weighing 9 lbs 15 oz | Has 2 children: 17-year-old Dan Jr., a high school sophomore, and 13-year-old Lisa, who is in the 8th grade | *Breasts:* Firm; no nipple discharge; no masses or tenderness on palpation; practices breast self-examination monthly; had mammogram 6 months ago, negative findings |
| | Is living with her boyfriend David, who is supportive and caring | |
| Abdominal hysterectomy (uterus only) at age 29 | Current living situation for 6 years; both children spend every other weekend with their father and stepmother | *Abdominal:* Soft, nontender, nondistended; midline scar noted |
| Hospitalized at ages 30 and 37 for severe episodes of vomiting leading to ketoacidosis | Receives disability through Social Security, also on Medicaid (title 19) | *Cardiovascular:* Apical rate 68; best heard at apex; S1, S2 heard; all peripheral pulses felt |
| Major illness at age 38, characterized by intractable vomiting, diarrhea, ketoacidosis, and coma; diabetic nephropathy and retinopathy identified at that admission; being followed closely by specialists for both conditions | Ex-husband is a lawyer, contributes child support payments on a regular basis | *Musculoskeletal:* Full range of motion; joints not inflamed or painful; steady gait |
| | Owns own home—multilevel split style, but master bedroom on first floor | ***Laboratory data*** |
| | Quality relationships with adoptive parents, siblings and ex-in-laws | Blood sugar (fasting) 128; does own blood sugar daily |
| | *Religion:* Lutheran, active in church, sings in the choir | Hgb 9.4, Hct 27, WBC 8500, Platelets 300,000 |
| | | Electrolytes within normal limits now; before dialysis, potassium was high |

## Nursing Care Plan

## PATIENT WITH CHRONIC RENAL FAILURE—cont'd

| Medical History | Psychosocial Data | Assessment Data |
|---|---|---|
| Immunizations up-to-date; last tetanus booster 3 years ago<br>No known food or drug allergies<br>Has never smoked | *Hobbies:* Likes to read, garden, knit, and draw; is an avid hockey fan, has season tickets to local professional team<br>Does not feel well enough to drive after dialysis treatments, so David brings her to the dialysis center during his lunch hour at noon and returns to pick her up at 6 PM (treatment time is from 1 to 6 PM, Monday, Wednesday, and Friday) | Screened on a weekly basis<br>BUN 38; had been as high as 76<br>Creatinine clearance varies depending on when tested in relation to dialysis; felt to have some residual nephron function<br>*Medications*<br>NPH insulin 46 units daily<br>Regular insulin 8 to 10 units on a sliding scale<br>Colace 100 mg PO prn<br>Centrum vitamin tab 1 PO daily |

### NURSING DIAGNOSIS

Diversional activity deficit related to long hours of treatment and relative immobility during treatment, as evidenced by statements of boredom and frequent turning of the channel selector of the television set

| NURSING INTERVENTIONS | EVALUATION OF EXPECTED OUTCOMES |
|---|---|
| Encourage patient to discuss drawing and sketching in detail.<br>Ask her what parts of these activities are most meaningful.<br>Initiate a discussion of past artwork and have her describe specific details that give her pleasure.<br>Focus on what patient *can* do with one hand and her other senses while sitting for 5 hours, rather than on what she *cannot* do.<br>Encourage patient to use her analysis of the meaningful aspects of gardening to find something related to these activities.<br>If necessary, prompt patient with ideas related to her analysis, such as listening to tapes on gardening, drawing plans for use of oils or colored pencils, writing stories about painting, or planning hockey moves.<br>Let patient know that the environment can be adapted for her use (such as moving a larger table nearby, allowing her time to set up before hooking up the dialysis machine).<br>Have patient identify what she needs for her chosen daily activities and plan together how to obtain the materials.<br>Observe for periods of frustration and assist.<br>Let patient know that changes in her plans are possible (e.g., adding new activities). | Feels free to discuss the prolonged immobility and her negative feelings toward it<br>Identifies the personal meaning of her usual diversional hobbies and incorporates these into her treatment times<br>Identifies those diversional activities that appeal to her while immobilized<br>Selects certain activities to engage her time and mind while immobilized<br>Plans a range of diversional activities and feels comfortable in asking for assistance in setting them up<br>Chooses a desired activity that she can engage in<br>Satisfactorily engages in her chosen diversional activity during periods of immobility |

## NURSING CARE PLAN

### PATIENT WITH CHRONIC RENAL FAILURE—cont'd

**NURSING DIAGNOSIS**

Fluid volume excess related to compromised regulatory mechanisms, as evidenced by changes in neurologic, cardiovascular, respiratory, and renal status

| NURSING INTERVENTIONS | EVALUATION OF EXPECTED OUTCOMES |
|---|---|
| Assess for and report signs and symptoms of fluid volume excess: significant weight gain (greater than 0.5 kg/day), elevated BP and pulse (BP may not be elevated if fluid has shifted out of vascular space), development of an S3 or S4 gallop rhythm, change in mental status, crackles and diminished or absent breath sounds, dyspnea, orthopnea, peripheral edema, distended neck veins, or elevated central venous pressure. | At home, or in the dialysis center, does not experience symptoms of fluid volume excess |
| If respiratory difficulty, help patient into a semi-Fowler's position to facilitate breathing. | Can cite the importance of self-monitoring and self-regulating all necessary parameters (e.g., weight, fluid intake and output) |
| Administer oxygen as needed. | Identifies what symptoms to report to her physician and the dialysis center |
| Remind patient of the necessity of restricting fluids to 15 ounces (500 ml) plus amount of urine output daily. | States the importance of immediately reporting any changes to either her physician or the dialysis center |
| Discuss the importance of weighing herself daily and comparing and contrasting findings. | Does not experience fluid volume excess as evidenced by stable weight, stable BP and pulse, absence of gallop rhythm, usual mental status, normal breath sounds, absence of dyspnea, peripheral edema, distended neck veins, and central venous pressure within the normal range |
| Remind her to phone the dialysis center if her weight gain is over 1.8 kg (4 lb) per day. | |
| Reinforce teachings regarding measuring specific gravity testings. | |
| Discuss a sodium- and potassium-restricted diet. | |
| List foods that are to be avoided. Refer her to a dietitian to incorporate food restrictions into the ADA diet exchanges. | Avoids any complications of excess fluid volume |
| Teach patient to test all stools for occult blood. Have her give a return demonstration. | Has normal skin turgor |
| Provide a diet high in calories from carbohydrates and fats. | Electrolytes within the normal range |
| Reinforce with patient the importance of monitoring I&O. Remind patient of the need for frequent oral hygiene. | States her ability to breathe comfortably |
| Discuss the use of hard sugarless candy, gum, and cold liquids to help improve the taste in her mouth. | Takes the responsibility of teaching her children and significant other these untoward changes |
| | Keeps her fluid intake at 15 ounces (500 ml) plus the amount of urine output daily |
| | Baseline weight of 53.1 to 54 kg (118 to 120 lb) maintained |
| | Urine specific gravity remains within 1.005 to 1.020 |

## NURSING CARE PLAN

## PATIENT WITH CHRONIC RENAL FAILURE—cont'd

**NURSING DIAGNOSIS**

Powerlessness related to chronic illness, as evidenced by statements of ambivalent feelings about dependence on others

| NURSING INTERVENTIONS | EVALUATION OF EXPECTED OUTCOMES |
|---|---|
| Encourage patient to express her feelings. | Describes strategies for decreasing anxiety |
| Set aside time for meaningful discussions regarding daily happenings. | Demonstrates increased control by participation in decision making related to health care |
| Accept her feelings of powerlessness as normal. | |
| Plan to be present (if possible) during situations where feelings of powerlessness are likely to be greatest, and offer therapeutic use of self. | Actively participates in planning and carrying out some aspects of care and treatment; communicates a renewed sense of power and control over the current situation |
| Identify and develop patient's coping strategies, strengths (sense of humor), and resources (extended family) for support. | |
| Discuss situations that provoke feelings of anger, anxiety, and powerlessness to search for areas that she can control. | Acknowledges her fears, feelings, and concerns about the current situation |
| Encourage participation in self-care; provide positive reinforcement for her attempts; make her feel like a member of the health team by asking her opinion. | Participates in self-care activities such as personal hygiene |
| Provide opportunities for her to make decisions relating to care, treatment, positioning, and ambulation. | Decreases her level of anxiety by citing stressors and identifying ways to change responses (control for her) |
| Encourage family and significant other to support her without taking control. | Expresses feelings of regained control |
| Explain rules, policies, procedures, and schedules to decrease areas of potential conflict. | Accepts and adapts to lifestyle changes |
| Modify the environment when possible to promote a sense of control. | Projects and daydreams about the time when her kidney transplant will alter her illness and treatment needs |

**NURSING DIAGNOSIS**

Altered sexuality patterns related to illness and medical treatment as evidenced by statements of concern about sexuality

| NURSING INTERVENTIONS | EVALUATION OF EXPECTED OUTCOMES |
|---|---|
| Initiate a trusting therapeutic relationship with patient. | Describes crying episodes, the treatment plan, and all the effects on her sexual desire |
| Provide time for privacy. | |
| Encourage her to express her feelings openly in a nonthreatening, nonjudgmental atmosphere. | Identifies at least three activities to enhance pleasure and communication with significant other |
| Discuss with patient and significant other expressions of affection to enhance their relationship, as well as past supportive roles, especially in times of crisis. | Indicates a willingness to follow through with a referral if the sexuality problem remains unresolved |
| Offer a referral to counselors or support persons or groups (e.g., I Can Cope). | Voices her feelings about potential or actual changes in sexual activity and desire |
| | Identifies ways to enhance pleasure and improve interpersonal communication with significant other |
| | Regains a sexual desire after recovery from depression |

## KEY CONCEPTS

➤ The nephron is the structural-functional unit of the kidney.

➤ The nephron forms urine by filtering the blood and altering the filtrate to return necessary substances to the blood and excreting unnecessary substances in the urine.

➤ The kidney produces four hormones: erythropoietin, which stimulates the formation of erythocytes; vitamin D, which increases calcium and phosphate absorption from the intestine, bone, and kidney; kinin, which causes vasodilation; and prostaglandin, which causes vasodilation and vasoconstriction.

➤ Micturition is the process of releasing urine from the body and is controlled by voluntary and involuntary influences.

➤ Urinalysis provides important information about kidney function.

➤ A sterile urine specimen is collected by catheterization and clean-catch, and routine specimens are collected during voiding.

➤ Diagnostic tests such as x-ray, pyelography, ultrasonography, computed tomography, and magnetic resonance imaging provide information more about structure than function.

➤ Renal biopsy is an invasive test that obtains kidney tissue for microscopic examination and that provides information about renal structure and function.

➤ An important nursing responsibility associated with all diagnostic tests is to educate the patient about pretest procedures, what occurs during the test, and posttest care.

➤ Major side effects of diuretic therapy are fluid loss and electrolyte imbalances.

➤ Bladder catheterization is done using only sterile technique and when absolutely necessary because of the risk of urinary tract infection.

➤ Urinary incontinency is the inability to retain urine, is a symptom and not a disease, and needs to be investigated for the cause.

➤ Acute poststreptococcal glomerulonephritis is a disease that affects the glomerular capillaries and usually follows a recent sore throat.

➤ A urinary tract infection can best be prevented by drinking large quantities of water and by avoiding invasive procedures into the urinary tract.

➤ Cystitis is an infection of the bladder, and pyelonephritis is an infection in the kidney.

➤ Obstructions of the urinary tract can be caused by stones, tumors, kinking of a ureter, a congenital anomaly, or an enlarged prostate gland and can be located anywhere in the urinary tract.

➤ Acute renal failure is the sudden loss of renal function, and the focus of patient care is to keep the patient alive until the kidney heals, especially by preventing infection.

➤ Chronic renal failure is when renal function is lost over a period of time, and the focus of patient care is implementing treatments that substitute for the lost kidneys.

➤ Dialysis is a treatment that cleans the blood of waste products and excess water. Peritoneal dialysis is done within the body, and hemodialysis is done outside the body.

➤ Renal transplantation is the procedure of placing a normal kidney from a donor into a person with nonfunctioning kidneys.

➤ After surgery on the urinary tract, it is highly possible that drains, tubes, and/or catheters will be placed to drain urine. A major nursing responsibility associated with these devices is that they remain patent and allow the free flow of urine.

➤ People relate to their urinary tract in a variety of ways because of its association with the reproductive system and because it produces urine, a socially unacceptable topic to some people.

➤ It is important that nurses assess each patient's psychologic and emotional responses to a urinary tract problem.

## CRITICAL THINKING EXERCISES

1. What is the difference between voluntary control and the spinal cord reflex of urination?
2. Why is urinary incontinency a symptom and not a disease?
3. How does the urinary tract change with the normal aging process?
4. Why is it important for people who have had excretory urography or lithotripsy to drink a lot of water?

## REFERENCES AND ADDITIONAL READINGS

Barkauskas VH et al: *Health and physical assessment,* St Louis, 1994, Mosby.

Brundage DJ, Swearingen PA: Chronic renal failure: evaluation and teaching tool, *ANNA J* 21(5):265-270, 1994.

Corbett JV: *Laboratory tests and diagnostic procedures with nursing diagnosis,* ed 3, Norwalk, Conn, 1992, Appleton & Lange.

Cutler M: Administration of epoetin alfa, *ANNA J* 24(4):459-466, 1997.

Dossey BM et al: *Holistic nursing: a handbook for practice,* ed 2, Gaithersburg, Md, 1995, Aspen.

Driver DS: Renal assessment: back to basics, *ANNA J* 23(4):361-367, 1996.

Droller M: Immunotherapy and genitourinary neoplasia, part III, *Infect Control Urol Care* 16(4):12, 1992.

Felton R et al: Urostomy specimen of urine: technique of collection, *Br J Urol* 72(2):255-256, 1993.

Gallagher J: Peritoneal dialysis, *Nurs 96* 26(5):58-61, 1996.

Gillenwater JY et al: *Adult and pediatric urology,* ed 3, St Louis, 1996, Mosby.

Givliano KK: Organ transplants: tackling the tough ethical questions, *Nurs 97* 27(5):34-40, 1997.

Goshorn J: Clinical snapshot: kidney stones, *Am J Nurs* 96(9):40-41, 1996.

Hampton BG, Bryand RA: *Ostomies and continent diversions,* St Louis, 1992, Mosby.

Hardman JG, Limbird LE: *Goodman and Gilman's the pharmacological basis of therapeutics,* ed 9, New York, 1996, McGraw-Hill.

Holcomb SS, Simmons S: Understanding the ins and outs of diuretic therapy, *Nurs 97* 27(2):34-41, 1997.

Kelly M: Chronic renal failure, *Am J Nurs* 96(1):36-37, 1996.

Kelly M: Acute renal failure, *Am J Nurs* 97(3):32-33, 1997.

King B: Preserving renal function, *RN* 19(8):34-41, 1997.

Lancaster LE, editor: *Core curriculum for nephrology nursing,* ed 3, Pitman, NJ, 1995, American Nephrology Nurses Association.

Lewis SM, Collier IC, Heitkemper MM: *Medical-surgical nursing: assessment and management of clinical problems,* ed 4, St Louis, 1996, Mosby.

Meeker MH, Rothrock JC: *Alexander's care of the patient in surgery,* ed 10, St Louis, 1995, Mosby.

Mondoux LC: Patients won't ask, *RN* 15(2):35-40, 1994.

Moore DA, Edwards K: Using a portable bladder scan to reduce the incidence of nosocomial urinary tract infections, *MedSurg Nurs* 6(1):39-43, 1997.

Phipps WJ et al: *Medical-surgical nursing: concepts and clinical practice,* ed 5, St Louis, 1995, Mosby.

Porush JG, Faubert PF: *Renal disease in the aged,* Boston, 1991, Little, Brown.

Price-Anderson S, Wilson-McCarty L: *Pathophysiology: clinical concepts of disease processes,* ed 5, St Louis, 1996, Mosby.

Richard CJ: *Comprehensive nephrology nursing,* Boston, 1986, Little, Brown.

Richard CJ: Assessment of renal structure and function and causes of renal failure. In Lancaster LE, editor: *Core curriculum for nephrology nursing,* ed 3, Pitman, NJ, 1995a, American Nephrology Nurses Association.

Richard CJ: Renal function. In Copstead LE, editor: *Pathophysiology,* Philadelphia 1995b, Saunders.

Rodriquez D, Lewis SL: Nutritional management of patients with acute renal failure, *ANNA J* 24(2):232-243, 1997.

Shannon MT, Wilson BA: *Govoni and Hayes drugs and nursing implications,* ed 8, Norwalk, Conn, 1994, Appleton & Lange.

Start J: Dialysis choices, *Nurs 97* 27(2):41-48, 1997.

Wozniak-Petrofsky J: Urodynamic tests: client preparation, assessment, and follow-up, *Nurse Pract* 22(3):70-91, 1997.

# CHAPTER 38

# Vision

## CHAPTER OBJECTIVES

1 Correlate each anatomic part of the eye and its associated structures with its function in achieving sight.
2 Identify the purpose and procedure for common diagnostic tests involving the eye.
3 Describe the normal versus the abnormal refraction of the eye.
4 Explain the importance of screening for amblyopia in children.
5 Explain why and how to detect and remove contact lenses from an injured or unconscious patient.
6 Discuss the methods of interacting with visually impaired people.
7 Describe the method of punctal occlusion in the administration of ophthalmic medications.
8 Differentiate the signs and symptoms of conjunctivitis and acute glaucoma.
9 Discuss the relationship between injury to the cornea and corneal ulcers.
10 Describe the medical and surgical treatment for glaucoma.
11 Identify the symptoms of cataracts and describe the nursing considerations that follow cataract surgery.
12 Identify the signs and symptoms of retinal detachment.
13 List the conditions that are considered true ocular emergencies.
14 Describe potential hazards in the environment that may result in eye injuries, and list ways to prevent them.
15 Identify normal eye changes in the aging process.

## KEY TERMS

amblyopia
astigmatism
cataract
conjunctivitis
emmetropia
epiphora
glaucoma
hyperopia
keratoplasty
myopia

ophthalmologist
opticians
optometrist
phacoemulsification
photophobia
pseudophakic
refraction
tonometry
trabeculoplasty
vitrectomy

## STRUCTURE AND FUNCTION OF THE EYE

The eye is a highly specialized sense organ, a large portion of which lies protected within a bony cavity, with only the anterior portion exposed (Figure 38-1). The eye has three coats. The external, or fibrous, coat comprises the white, opaque *sclera*, covering four fifths of the eye, and the *cornea*, a transparent, avascular, curved layer covering the anterior one fifth of the eye. The cornea bends light rays entering the eye and focuses the resulting images on the retina. The sclera, the protective outer layer of the eye, has an opening at the back of the globe through which the optic nerve and blood vessels pass. The anterior surface of the sclera and the posterior surface of the eyelids are covered by the *conjunctiva*, a transparent mucous membrane that aids in tear-film dispersion.

The middle, or vascular, coat is also known as the *uveal tract* and consists of the choroid, iris, and ciliary body. The *choroid* lies between the sclera and retina

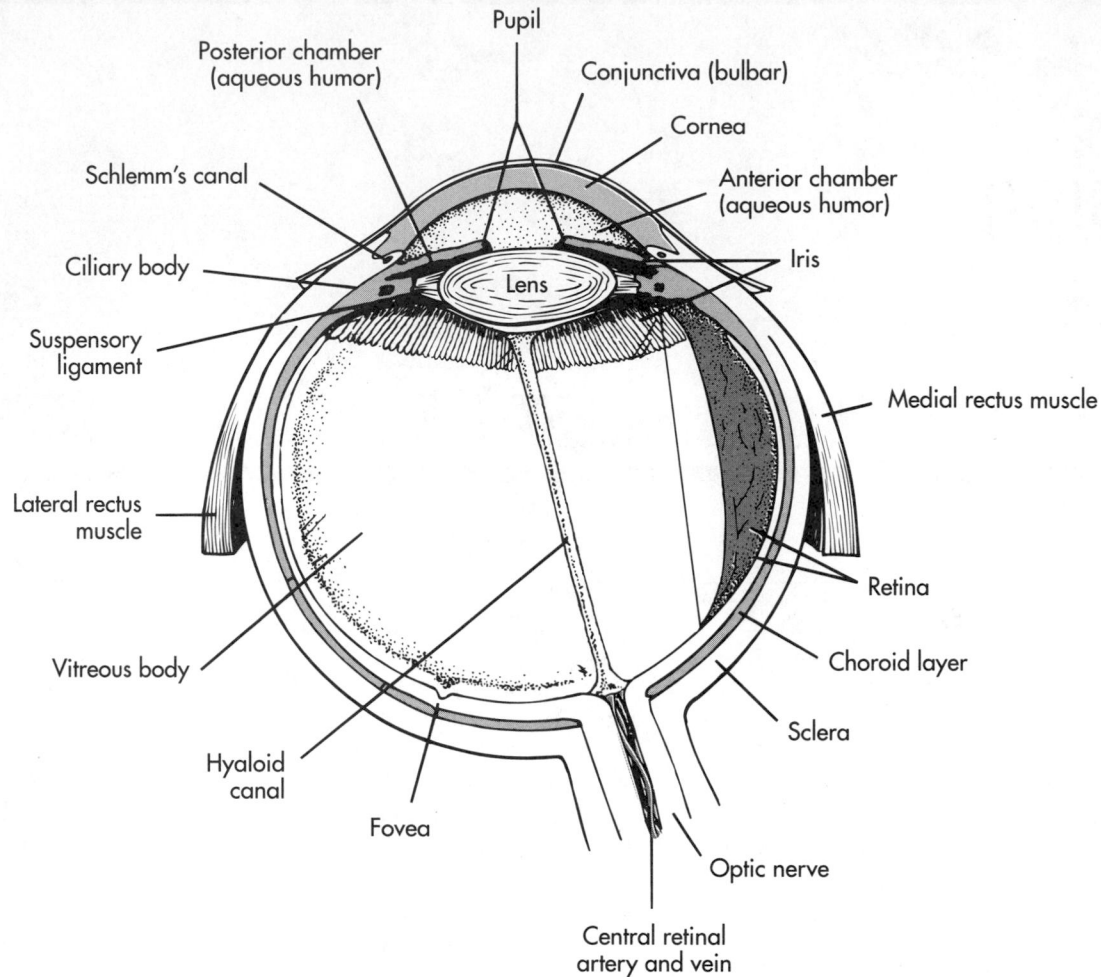

**Figure 38-1** Cross section of the eye. (From Phipps WJ et al: *Medical-surgical nursing: concepts and clinical practice*, ed 5, St Louis, 1995, Mosby.)

and is firmly attached on its inner surface to the retina. The blood supply of the choroid nourishes the retina, and the choroid's dark pigmentation prevents internal reflection of light. The *iris* is the colored part of the eye that can be seen through the cornea. It is composed of muscle fibers that regulate the amount of light entering the eye by changing the size of the *pupil,* the circular opening in its center. Behind the iris lies the crystalline *lens,* a biconvex, transparent structure enclosed within a transparent capsular membrane. The shape of the lens is controlled by the ciliary muscle contained in the external aspect of the *ciliary body.* This ability to change shape of the lens allows light rays to focus near or distant images precisely onto the retina. The internal surfaces of the ciliary body secrete *aqueous humor,* the watery fluid that fills the anterior and posterior chambers of the eye—the spaces in front of and behind the iris. The fluid passes from the posterior chamber through the pupil to the anterior chamber and then flows through spaces at the angle formed by the iris

and cornea through the *trabecular meshwork* and into a complex circular venous channel called *Schlemm's canal.* The ciliary body connects the choroid with the periphery of the iris.

The third and inner coat is the *retina,* a delicate membrane lined with pigmented epithelium. The retina contains a complicated network of nerve cells called *rods and cones* that transmit visual messages through the optic nerve to the brain. The rods are responsible for peripheral and night vision, whereas the cones are for central and color vision. The posterior portion of the retina is called the *optic fundus.* Near its center lies a circular, depressed, white to pink area where the optic nerve enters the eyeball; this is the *optic disc.* It contains no photoreceptor cells; thus it is insensitive to light and is known as the blind spot. Just lateral to the optic disc is a small, oval, yellowish area called the *macula lutea,* or macula. At the center of the macula is a depression known as the *fovea centralis,* the area of most acute vision. Blood is supplied to the

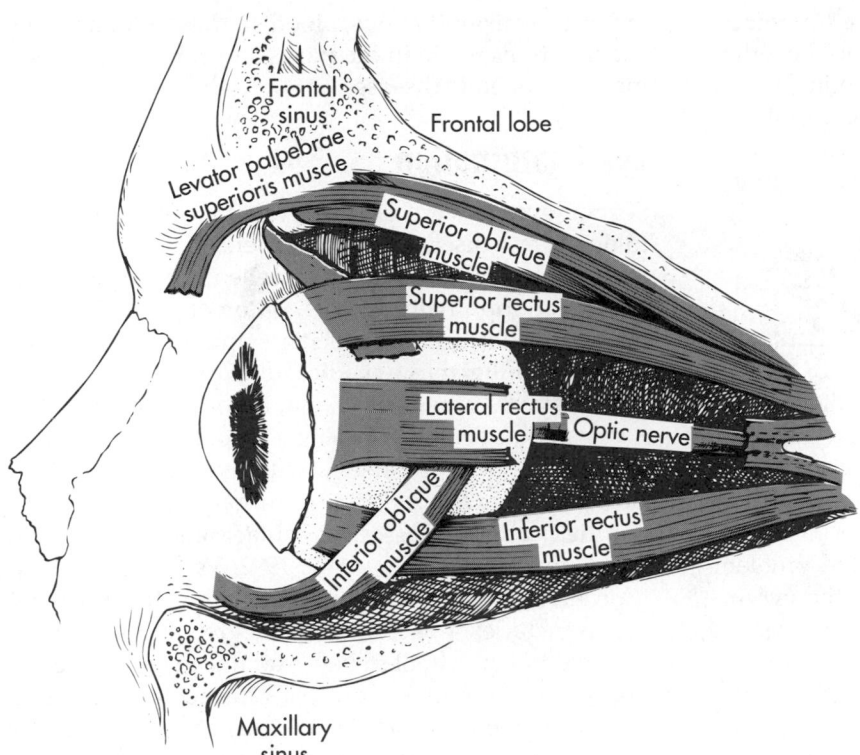

**Figure 38-2**  Extraocular muscles of the eye. Both oblique muscles insert behind the equator of the globe. The inferior oblique muscle passes inferior to the body of the inferior rectus muscle but beneath the lateral rectus muscle. (From Newell FW: *Ophthalmology: principles and concepts*, ed 8, St Louis, 1996, Mosby.)

retina by its central artery, which enters the eyeball alongside the optic nerve. Venous drainage flows through a corresponding system of retinal veins into the central retinal vein, which also exits along the path of the optic nerve. The space between the lens and the retina is the *vitreous chamber*, which comprises four fifths of the volume of the eye. It contains a colorless, transparent gel called the *vitreous gel,* or *vitreous humor.*

Vitreous gel maintains the shape of the eye and provides structural support for the retina. If the vitreous is lost and not replaced, as in a penetrating eye injury, the globe collapses.

The eye rests on a cushion of fat within its bony orbit. Six voluntary *(extrinsic)* muscles attached to the outside of the sclera control the movements of the eyes. The action of these extraocular muscles is coordinated to allow binocular vision, the concerted use of both eyes working together. Branches of several cranial nerves control these muscles. Involuntary *(intrinsic)* muscles within the eye control the shape of the lens and the size of the pupil (Figure 38-2).

The accessory organs of the eye include the eyebrows, eyelids and their muscles, eyelashes, bulbar and palpebral conjunctivae, lacrimal glands and tear ducts, and sebaceous glands. The eyebrows and eyelids protect the eyeball and help spread the tear film over the eye. Muscles within the lid help close the lid. The lacrimal glands secrete tears, which flow across the eye into the lacrimal sac. The fluid passes openings

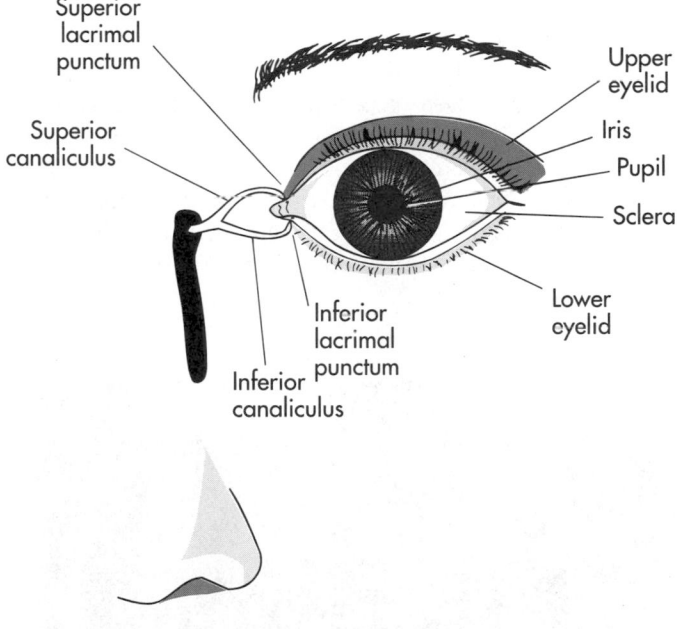

**Figure 38-3**  External landmarks.

in the nasal aspect of the upper and lower lids, called *puncta*. From this point, tears flow through the nasolacrimal duct into the back of the nose (Figure 38-3).

Vision is the result of light rays passing through the eye and focusing on the retina. The cornea is responsible for two thirds of this bending, or **refraction,** of light. The lens is responsible for the other third. When an image is produced on the retina, visual receptors are stimulated and cause a nerve impulse to be transmitted via the optic nerve to the visual center in the brain, the occipital lobes (Vaughan, Asbury, Riordan-Eva, 1995).

# NURSING ASSESSMENT OF THE PATIENT WITH EYE PROBLEMS

The assessment for conditions and diseases of the eye begins with a thorough nursing history that includes general medical health, family history, and allergies. Previous surgery, current medications, visual aids, glasses, contact lenses, and visual symptoms should be noted. The chief complaint (e.g., change in vision, floaters, discharge) and the duration of the problem are documented. Clinical observations of the eye include (1) general condition of the lids and lashes; (2) eye movement; (3) color of the sclera; (4) tear function; (5) pupil size, color, and shape; (6) position of the eye within the orbit; (7) systemic complaints of nausea and vomiting; and (8) level of cognizance (Hunt, 1992).

## Physical Examination

A complete physical examination is important in the treatment of many diseases of the eye (Figure 38-4). Often systemic diseases can be diagnosed by their ocular manifestations. When the underlying cause is diabetes, hypertension, rheumatoid arthritis, thyroid dysfunction, or leukemia, treatment of the underlying condition must accompany any treatment of the eye. The ophthalmologist may consult an internist or may

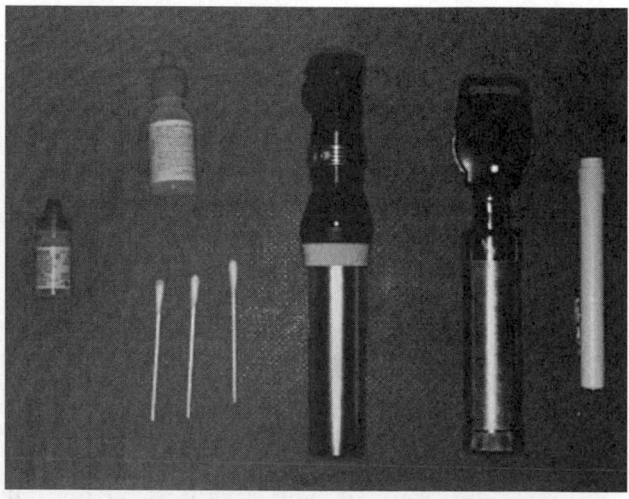

**Figure 38-4**   Examination instruments and supplies.

order x-ray examinations, blood studies, or neurologic examinations to aid in diagnosis and subsequent treatment of systemic disease.

## Eye Examination

Several eye tests are used to evaluate visual acuity or to detect eye diseases and disorders. A variety of professionals provide these comprehensive services. Included are ophthalmologists, optometrists, opticians, nurses, orthoptists, technicians, and photographers. **Ophthalmologists** are medical doctors who have completed 4 years of residency and, in some instances, 1 to 3 years of additional training in a subspecialty. They diagnose and treat patients with eye disease and vision problems by performing surgery or by prescribing medications, glasses, or contact lenses (American Academy of Ophthalmology, 1992; Vaughan, Asbury, Riordan-Eva, 1995). **Optometrists'** educational preparation includes a baccalaureate degree and 4 years in an optometry school. They examine eyes, prescribe glasses and contact lenses, check intraocular pressure, and prescribe exercises for various eye-muscle problems. They provide low-vision examinations, visual devices, and adaptive training for patients with limited vision (American Academy of Ophthalmology, 1992; Vaughan, Asbury, Riordan-Eva, 1995). **Opticians** are technicians who make and fit eyeglasses, contact lenses, and vision aids as prescribed. Some states require formal licensing to practice as an optician.

The eye examination begins with an evaluation of the general health and appearance of the external structures of the eye. Obvious defects of the orbit, eyelids, eyelashes, and lacrimal system should be noted (Hunt, 1992). Visual assessment follows the general examination.

### Visual Acuity

Visual acuity is the measurement of the smallest object a person can identify at a given distance from the eye. The most common method for determining acuity of distance vision is testing with *Snellen's eye chart*, a method used in schools, industry, physicians' offices, and screenings (Figure 38-5). The chart consists of rows of letters arranged in various sizes that a person views from a measured distance to the chart—usually 20 feet. By use of a mirror projection system, the actual distance can be less. If individuals are able to read the letters marked 20 at a distance of 20 feet, they have 20/20 ("normal") vision. However, if only rows marked at 30, 40, or 200 are read correctly, the person is said to have 20/30, 20/40, or 20/200 vision. If lenses are used to correct the vision to 20/20, the person has no vision loss. If visual acuity can be corrected to no better than 20/50, the person has a vision deficit. It is not unusual for each eye to have a slightly different acuity. If a person normally wears glasses or contact lenses, the test is performed both with and without the corrective lenses.

In younger children, illiterate adults, or those with language problems, a chart with the letter E can be used. With this E chart, the person points in the direction faced by the open side of the E, which may be rotated to be open at the top, bottom, right, or left. Various other object charts have been designed for use with children. Near-distance visual acuity is tested with *Jaeger's eye chart* (Vaughan, Asbury, Riordan-Eva, 1995). The procedure is similar to that of Snellen's chart but uses smaller graduated letter sizes on a hand-held card. The distance is measured at 14 inches (Figure 38-6).

## Refractometry

The phorometer *(Phoroptor)* is a machine that houses various combinations of prescriptive lenses in an apparatus. The patient looks through the Phoroptor so that the amount of refraction (bending of light) needed to focus images on the retina to achieve normal (20/20) vision can be determined (Figure 38-7). The patient's response to changes in lens power is used subjectively to determine the best achievable vision.

## Retinoscopy

The instrument for objectively measuring the visual acuity of the eye is a retinoscope. A streak of light is passed across the eye, and the reflex of the pupil is noted. Because it is an objective measurement, it is most useful for small children and for adults with

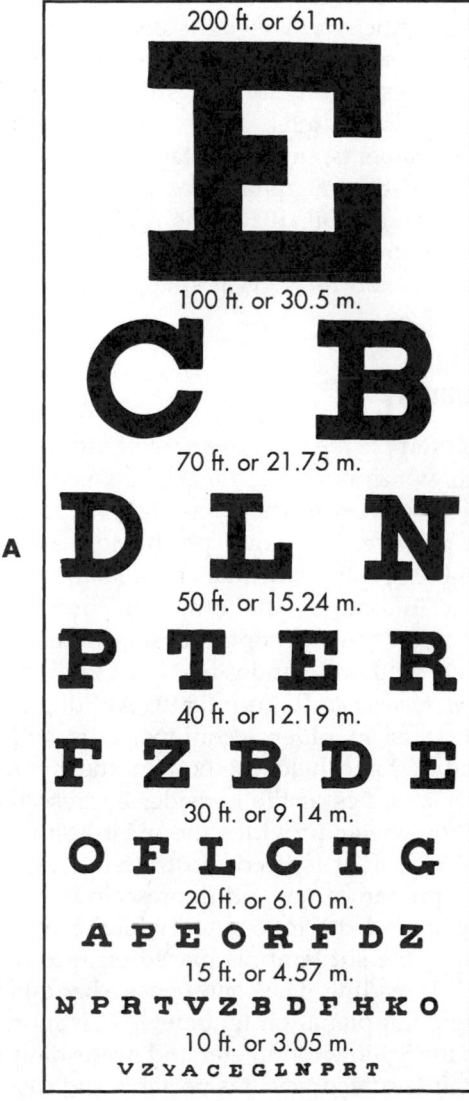

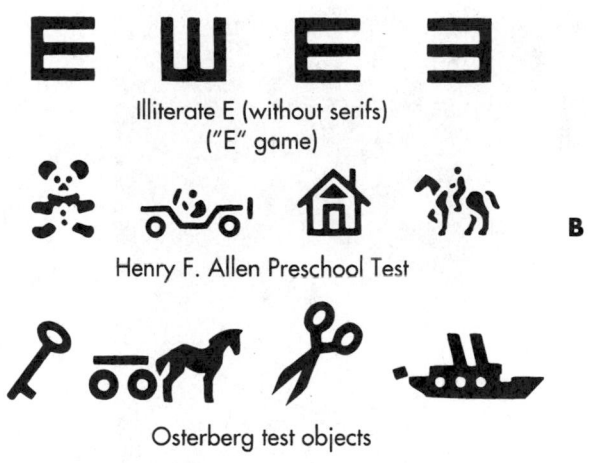

**Figure 38-5    A,** Snellen's chart used in testing vision. **B,** Symbols used in testing distance vision in children and illiterate adults. (Modified from Newell FW: *Ophthalmology: principles and concepts,* ed 8, St Louis, 1996, Mosby.)

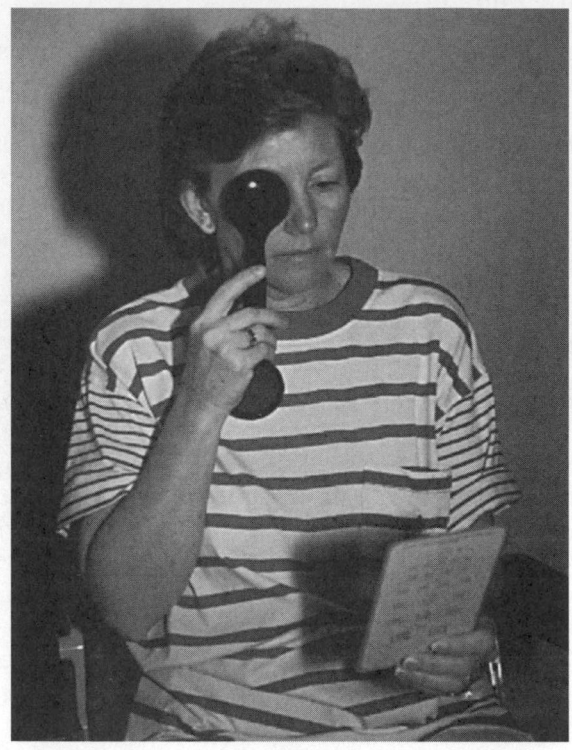

**Figure 38-6**  Assessing near vision with Jaeger's chart.

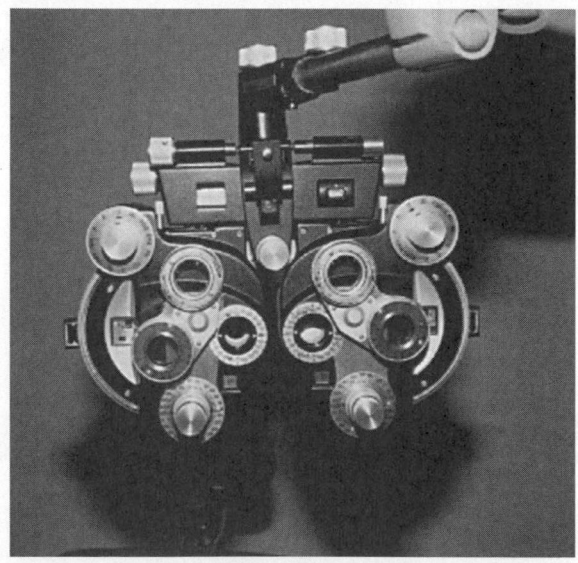

**Figure 38-7**  Phorometer (Phoroptor) stores lenses used in determining the refraction error of the eye.

disease conditions of the eye (Vaughan, Asbury, Riordan-Eva, 1995).

## Slit-Lamp Examination

The slit lamp is a lighted binocular microscope (Figure 38-8). The light beam can be projected onto the eye

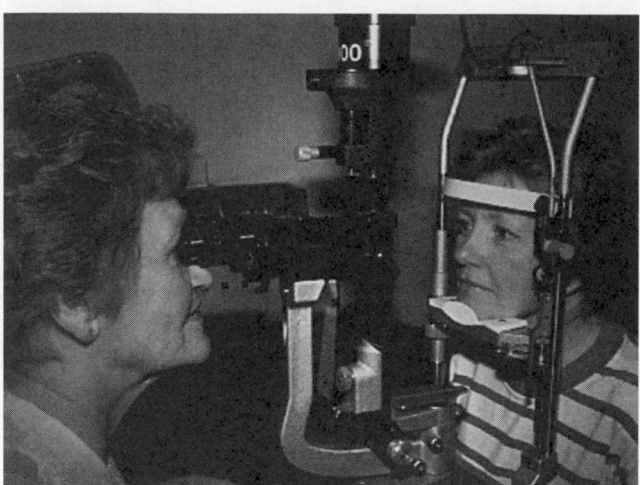

**Figure 38-8**  Examination of the eye with slit lamp.

in various widths and intensities. It is used to assess all the structures within the eye, as well as the lids, lashes, and conjunctiva. The light beam provides a three-dimensional view of the eye and helps determine abnormalities in any of the structures, including the aqueous fluid, lens, and vitreous. With additional lenses, cameras, or laser attachments, other examinations and treatments are possible. Dilating drops are used when pupil dilation is needed in the examination. Fluorescein stain is used to diagnose corneal abrasions and ulcers (Vaughan, Asbury, Riordan-Eva, 1995).

## Tonometry

**Tonometry** is the measurement of intraocular pressure (IOP), which normally ranges between 12 and 21 mm Hg (Berson, 1993). This pressure is the result of the balance between aqueous production and absorption from the eye. In glaucoma an imbalance results from a defect in one or the other of these mechanisms. Tonometry can be a contact or noncontact method. The contact method includes the *Schiötz tonometer* or *applanation tonometer* (Figure 38-9). Although the Schiötz method is an older technique, it is still used as a portable, hand-held method in the operating room and sometimes at the bedside. Because the applanation tonometer provides the most accurate measurement of IOP, it is used most often. Anesthetic drops (0.5% proparacaine) and fluorescein dye are placed in the eye, and the tonometer, which can be an attachment to the slit lamp, is placed on the cornea for the numeric reading. The Tono-pen is a hand-held, battery-powered applanation tonometer. It is more expensive than the Schiötz tonometer and needs daily calibration to maintain accuracy. It is portable and easy to use and

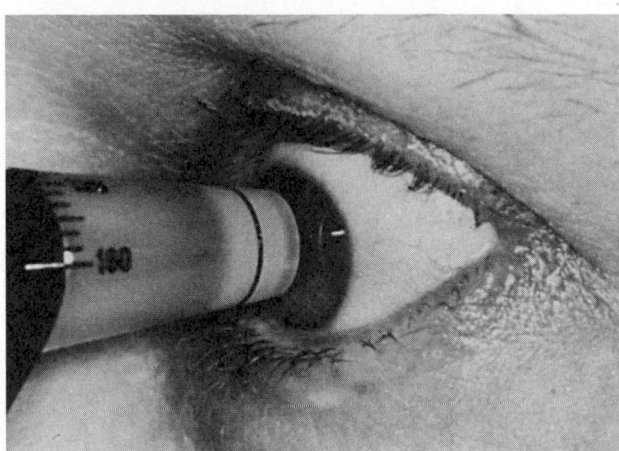

**Figure 38-9** Applanation tonometer provides a more precise measurement of intraocular pressure. (From Havener WH et al: *Nursing care in eye, ear, nose, and throat disorders,* ed 3, St Louis, 1974, Mosby.)

has a disposable cover for the tip. The *noncontact tonometer,* or "air-puff" method, is less precise but does not require anesthetic drops. Pressure from air on the cornea is calibrated by the machine. It can be used by a variety of trained ophthalmic personnel (Vaughan, Asbury, Riordan-Eva, 1995).

## Fundus Photography

Special cameras are used to provide documentation of the retina and fundus of the eye. This is particularly important in observing the progression of optic nerve damage associated with glaucoma.

## Perimetry

Perimetry is used to assess central and peripheral visual fields. It is used to measure the progression of glaucoma, to help determine the location of a brain lesion, or to establish loss of vision as a result of a cerebro vascular accident. Three methods are used: *tangent screen, Goldmann perimetry,* and *computerized automated perimetry.* The tangent screen is the fastest and simplest method for determining the loss of central field vision (central 30 degrees). An examiner uses a test object brought in from the periphery, and the patient signals when the object is seen. The Goldmann perimeter, a more accurate test, evaluates all the peripheral vision (Figure 38-10). The patient faces a hollow, white, spherical bowl. Lights of variable size and intensity are presented by the examiner, and the patient indicates when they are seen. The computerized automated perimeter uses the same method as Goldmann perimetry but with a computer program, which elimi-

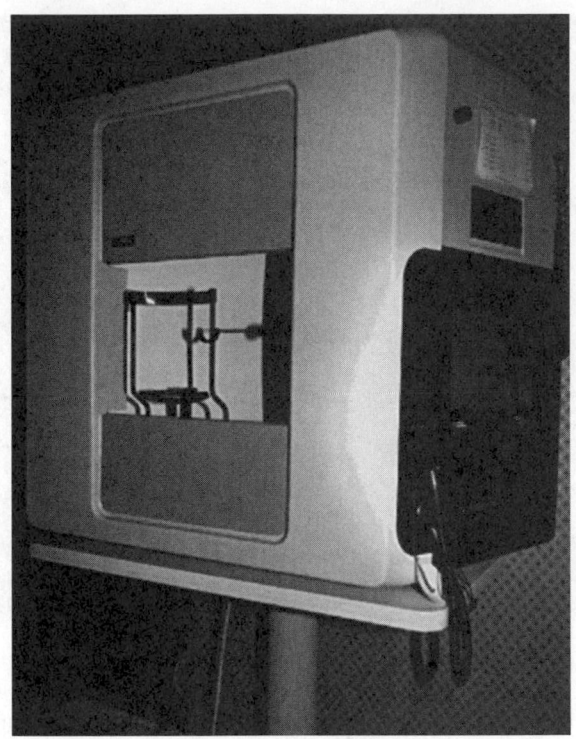

**Figure 38-10** Perimeter used to evaluate the visual fields of patients with glaucoma and tumors.

nates examiner bias. This sophisticated equipment is the most sensitive of all the perimetry methods and has the advantage of comparing recent results with previous testing of the patient (Vaughan, Asbury, Riordan-Eva, 1995).

## Ophthalmoscopy

The ophthalmoscope is used to visually examine the vascular and nerve tissue in the fundus of the eye, including the retina, retinal vessels, optic disc, and macula (Figure 38-11). With the hand-held or *direct ophthalmoscope,* no dilating drops may be necessary if room lighting can be reduced enough for pupillary dilation. Mydriatic drops may be instilled if pupil dilation is necessary for appropriate visualization. The direct ophthalmoscope provides a highly magnified view (×15) of the entire fundus. It also is used to check the red reflex of the eye, and if a slit lamp is unavailable it can be used to view the conjunctiva, cornea, and iris. The *indirect ophthalmoscope* provides a less magnified, wider view of the fundus. The examiner uses a hand-held lens and head-mounted ophthalmoscope. Because the examiner uses both eyes for the test, a three-dimensional view can be accomplished, which is helpful in diagnosing elevations or tumors in the back of the eye. The indirect ophthalmoscope is used to

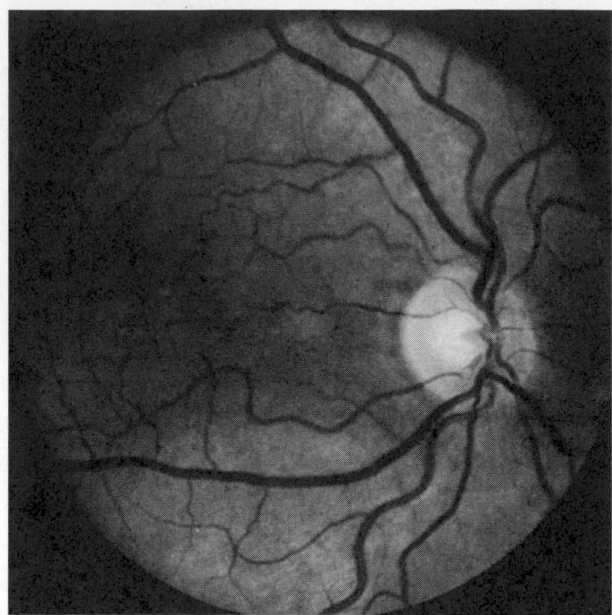

**Figure 38-11** Normal fundus photograph. Optic nerve and retinal blood vessels as seen with ophthalmoscope. (From Saunders WH et al: *Nursing care in eye, ear, nose, and throat disorders,* ed 4, St Louis, 1979, Mosby.)

diagnose retinal detachments, vitreous hemorrhages, and other diseases of the retina or vitreous. It is also used intraoperatively for retina or vitreous surgery. The intensity of the light source is not well tolerated by the patient.

## Keratoscopy

To determine the surface condition of the cornea, a keratoscope is used. Concentric circles, or "rings," are projected onto the cornea. If the distance between the circles is uniform, the cornea is considered normal. Distortion of the rings indicates corneal abnormalities. Keratoscopy is used for penetrating keratoplasties and refractive surgeries as well as corneal examination.

## Pachymetry

The central thickness of the cornea is measured by pachymetry. Patients with corneal edema are monitored to evaluate changes in corneal thickness.

## Keratometry

The keratometer measures the curve of the cornea in two 90-degree meridians to determine the spheric shape of the cornea. An uneven corneal curvature is called **astigmatism.** Contact lens fitting and intra-

ocular lens power calculations require keratometer measurements.

## Specular Microscopy

Corneal endothelial cell counts are determined by specular microscopy. Corneal decompensation can occur when there is a low cell count. Patients with corneal decompensation are at a higher risk for corneal edema or inflammation after intraocular surgery (Cataract Management Guideline Panel, 1993).

## Glare Testing

Glare testing determines the disturbance in vision that light can cause when striking opacities in the ocular media. Patients with complaints of glare in daylight or while gazing at oncoming traffic may have normal vision in a darkened room. Glare symptoms are found in patients with cataracts and corneal abnormalities (Cataract Management Guideline Panel, 1993; Vaughan, Asbury, Riordan-Eva, 1995).

## Contrast Sensitivity Testing

Contrast sensitivity testing determines the ability of the patient to detect subtle shading differences between lines and their background. The ability to determine contrast differences can be affected before visual acuity changes can be determined by Snellen's chart. Cataracts, retinal lesions, and optic nerve disease can be the causes. The U.S. government's Cataract Management Guideline Panel (1993) has suggested that research be done in older adults to determine the usefulness of this technique for diagnosing functional impairment in a cataract patient.

## Fluorescein Angiography

The technique for visually examining retinal circulation is fluorescein angiography. Fluorescein dye is injected through a vein in the arm. Fundus photographs are then taken in rapid sequence to document the flow of blood through the vessels of the retina. These black-and-white photographs are essential for diagnosis and treatment of retinal conditions, especially diabetic retinopathy. Patient preparation for the test includes an assessment for allergies to the dye. Fluids or a light meal is allowed. The pupils are dilated with mydriatic drops. Normally, blood vessels of the retina fill with dye in 12 to 15 seconds after injection. However, delayed photographs may be taken 20 minutes after the initial dye injection to diagnose leakage from the vessels. A small percentage of patients may be nauseated and vomit. For 24 hours the urine will be yellow-

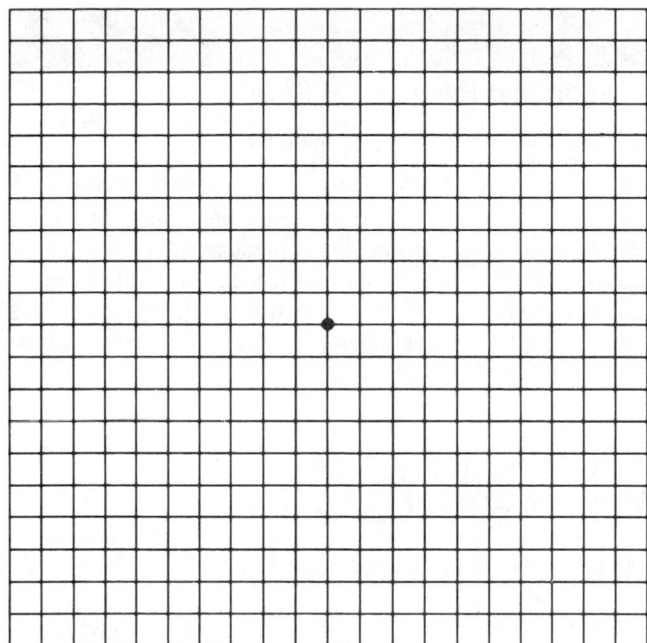

**Figure 38-12**  The Amsler grid. (From Phipps WJ et al: *Medical-surgical nursing: concepts and clinical practice*, ed 5, St Louis, 1995, Mosby.)

orange. An increase in oral fluids will hasten excretion of the dye. Dark glasses will lessen sensitivity to light caused by pupil dilation (Smith, Folk, Losch, 1992).

## Ocular Ultrasonography

Ocular ultrasonography involves transmitting high-frequency sound waves through the eye and the measurement of their reflection from ocular structures. A-scan is used to measure the axial length (cornea-to-retina measurement) of the eye—a measurement needed for calculating the intraocular lens power for cataract surgery. It is also used to determine tumor growth. B-scan provides a view of ocular structures when opacities in the cornea, lens, or vitreous make a view of the fundus difficult. Lesions within the eye and retinal detachments can be diagnosed with this technique.

## Amsler Grid Test

The Amsler grid is composed of horizontal and vertical lines that form 5-mm squares. It is used to detect scotomas, or blind spots, in the central 20 degrees of visual field and to evaluate the presence, stability, or progression of macular degeneration (Figure 38-12). Covering one eye and wearing any corrective lenses usually worn, the patient is instructed to stare at a dot centrally located on the grid. The patient should be

able to see the dot, and the lines on the grid should appear straight. All four sides of the grid should be visible. The patient is asked to describe and outline any area where the grid is distorted or absent. A pathologic condition of the macula is suggested if the patient describes a gray area or an area where lines are missing or distorted (*metamorphopsia*). This test is for initial screening only and must be followed by ophthalmoscopy, visual field testing, and fluorescein angiography to further evaluate the presence of disease.

## Schirmer's Tearing Test

The function of the major lacrimal glands responsible for tearing can be tested by inserting a strip of filter paper into the lower conjunctival sac. The amount of moisture absorbed by the paper is timed, measured, and compared to the normal level. The accessory lacrimal glands of Krause and Wolfring, responsible for maintenance of adequate corneal moisture, can be tested by instilling a topical anesthetic before inserting the paper. The anesthetic inhibits the reflex tearing by the major lacrimal glands that is caused by the filter paper so that only the basic tear film produced by the accessory glands is measured.

## Exophthalmometry

Exophthalmometry uses an instrument called an exophthalmometer to measure the forward protrusion of the eye and to evaluate an increase or decrease in the condition known as exophthalmos, the abnormal forward protrusion of the eye. This condition is seen in thyroid diseases and other conditions that displace the eye in the orbit.

## Tensilon Test

To evaluate ptosis (drooping) of the eyelids that is caused by myasthenia gravis, an edrophonium (Tensilon) test is done. A positive response (eliminating the lid droop) after injection of the edrophonium confirms the diagnosis of myasthenia gravis.

## Cardinal Fields of Gaze

To evaluate the extraocular muscles of the eye for possible abnormalities, the patient is asked to look in each of six directions known as the cardinal fields, or positions, of gaze (Figure 38-13; Table 38-1).

## Cover/Uncover Test

The cover/uncover test for evaluating strabismus requires a cooperative patient able to fixate on an object.

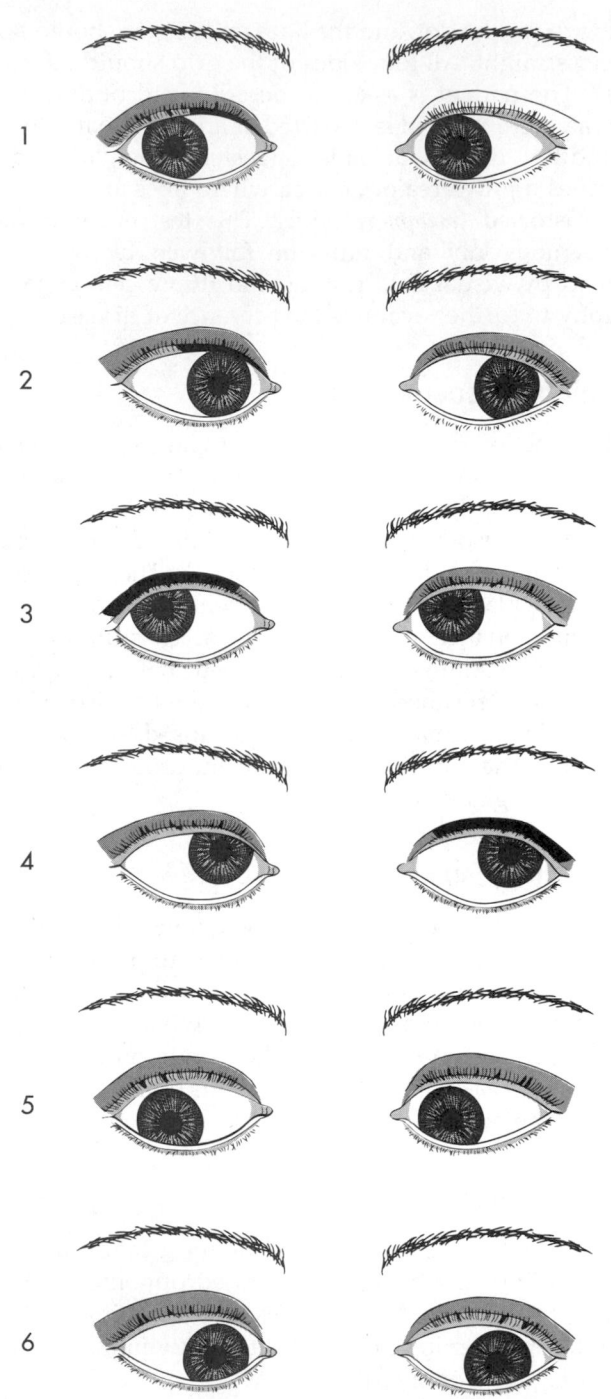

**Figure 38-13** Six cardinal positions of gaze and eye positions contracting to produce that eye rotation.

TABLE 38-1

**Six Cardinal Positions of Gaze**

| DIRECTION OF GAZE | MUSCLES INVOLVES |
| --- | --- |
| Right | Right lateral rectus, left medial rectus |
| Left | Left lateral rectus, right medial rectus |
| Up and right | Right superior rectus, left inferior oblique |
| Up and left | Left superior rectus, right inferior oblique |
| Down and right | Right inferior rectus, left superior oblique |
| Down and left | Left inferior rectus, right superior oblique |

# THE PATIENT WITH VISION PROBLEMS

## Refractive Errors of the Eye

Light rays enter the eye through the cornea, which is responsible for two thirds of the refractive or light-bending power of the eye. Light passes through the anterior chamber; the pupil; the lens, which is responsible for the remaining one third of the eye's refractive power; and the vitreous cavity. The light rays must focus directly on the retina for normal vision, also known as 20/20 or **emmetropia** (Figure 38-14). If this does not happen, the defect is known as a *refractive error*. The patient may complain of eyestrain, headache, and blurring of distance or near vision. To correct a refractive error, a person should have a thorough eye examination and be fitted with appropriate lenses. This examination, called a *refraction*, can be done by an ophthalmologist or optometrist.

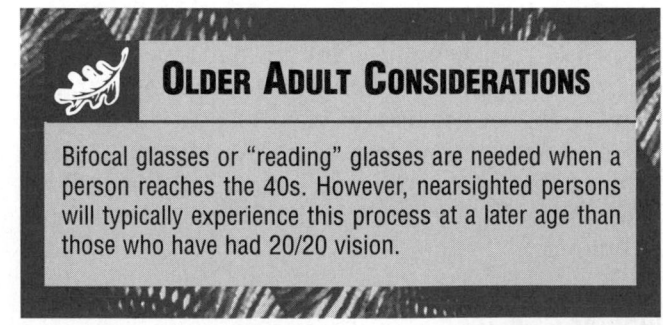

### OLDER ADULT CONSIDERATIONS

Bifocal glasses or "reading" glasses are needed when a person reaches the 40s. However, nearsighted persons will typically experience this process at a later age than those who have had 20/20 vision.

## Myopia (Nearsightedness)

Persons with **myopia** usually have a longer eyeball than normal. Incoming light from distant objects focuses in front of the retina. Near vision is fine, but distance vision is poor. A concave lens corrects the focus. Myopia may continue to progress in young persons,

When the "fixing" eye is covered, the fellow eye is checked for movement, either inward or outward. A deviation is present if the uncovered eye moves. Each eye is checked individually.

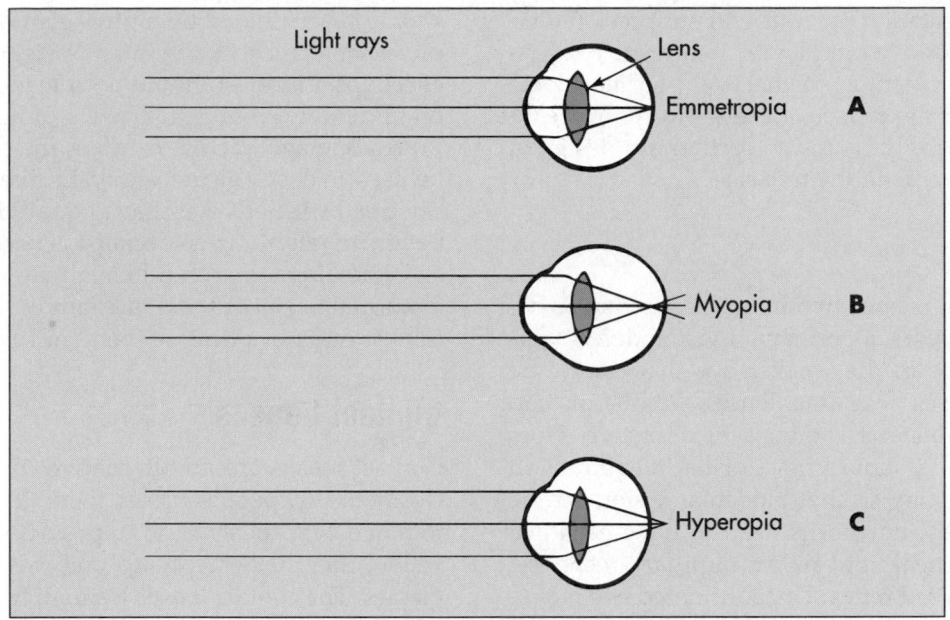

**Figure 38-14**    Refractive conditions of eye. **A,** Light rays entering eye are brought to focus directly on retina, resulting in normal vision (emmetropia). **B,** Light rays focus in front of retina, resulting in near-sightedness (myopia). **C,** Light rays focus at back of retina, resulting in farsightedness (hyperopia).

and frequent increases in lens strength may be required until the condition stabilizes. Techniques to correct this condition surgically are radial keratotomy and laser keratectomy (see p. 1197).

## Hyperopia (Farsightedness)

**Hyperopia** is less common than myopia. The eyeball is often shorter than normal, which causes the light rays to focus on a spot behind the retina. Distance vision is clear, but near objects are blurred. A convex lens corrects the focus. Examination with Snellen's chart may not show this condition, so Jaeger's chart should be used for testing a near-vision defect.

## Presbyopia

The ability to focus on near objects (accommodation) diminishes with age. This inability, called presbyopia, is caused by a loss of elasticity of the lens and ciliary body muscles. Consequently, most people older than 40 years require magnifying glasses or bifocals for reading and close-up work. Bifocal glass styles are designed to individualize patient needs. The flat-top design is used for close-up work. For tasks that require not only close work but also a wide field of vision, Franklin bifocals, which extend the magnifying portion of the lens all the way across the bottom of the lens, are better suited. Progressive lenses provide a gradual lens-power change from top to bottom, with no visible line. They give a distance, mid-range, and close vision range. However, they may be harder to adjust to for some people and are more costly.

## Astigmatism

Astigmatism is an irregularity or defect on the corneal surface or lens of the eyeball that blurs vision. Slight defects occur in most people, but they are not significant enough to cause any vision problem. However, when the irregularity is pronounced, light rays do not bend equally, and the patient experiences eyestrain and blurred vision. These patients tend to see better if glasses are worn at all times.

## Strabismus

Strabismus is a misalignment of one or both eyes. Children are primarily affected, but adults may also have the condition. The deviation or turning can be inward (esotropia), outward (exotropia), upward (hypertropia), downward (hypotropia), or in a rotary direction. If the deviation is present under binocular viewing conditions (using both eyes at once), it is called a *tropia*. If the deviation is present only after binocular vision is interrupted by covering one eye, it is called a *phoria*. Strabismus affects 2% to 3% of the population. It should be noted that to avoid the double vision caused by the deviation, a child will suppress the vision of the weaker eye (lazy eye). Treatment for strabismus includes patching of the eye, pharmacologic drugs, and motility exercises or glasses to stimulate vision. Surgical procedures for correction are designed to strengthen or weaken the muscles.

### Amblyopia

If a child does not receive treatment for strabismus before the age of 7 years, a permanent vision defect (**amblyopia**) develops in the weaker eye that cannot be treated with glasses or contact lenses. Amblyopia can be caused by strabismus, cataracts, or refractive errors in children. A child should have visual rehabilitation started without delay so that binocular vision can be preserved. Initially, newborns need to have each eye evaluated for corneal light reflex, pupillary response, and presence of a red reflex. Uncoordinated eye movements may be present until an infant is 3 to 4 months of age (Berson, 1993). However, persistent deviations

should be evaluated by a physician. The primary care physician can check the infant's vision during routine checkups. The eyes should be able to follow and fixate on an object. From 2 to 4 years of age, or during the prereading age, picture cards or the single E chart can be used to check visual acuity. Each eye is checked individually. If both eyes have equal vision of 20/40 or better, no referral to a specialist is necessary. However, an ophthalmologist should evaluate vision if there are abnormalities or if there is a family history of strabismus or other eye disease (Berson, 1993).

## Contact Lenses

Contact lenses are an alternative to wearing glasses. Cosmetically, people prefer them. They are designed to move with the eye and to provide better peripheral vision, depth perception, and visual acuity than glasses. The contact lens is a small, thin, polished plastic, silicone, or cellulose disc whose outer surface is shaped or ground to correct the vision abnormality. It

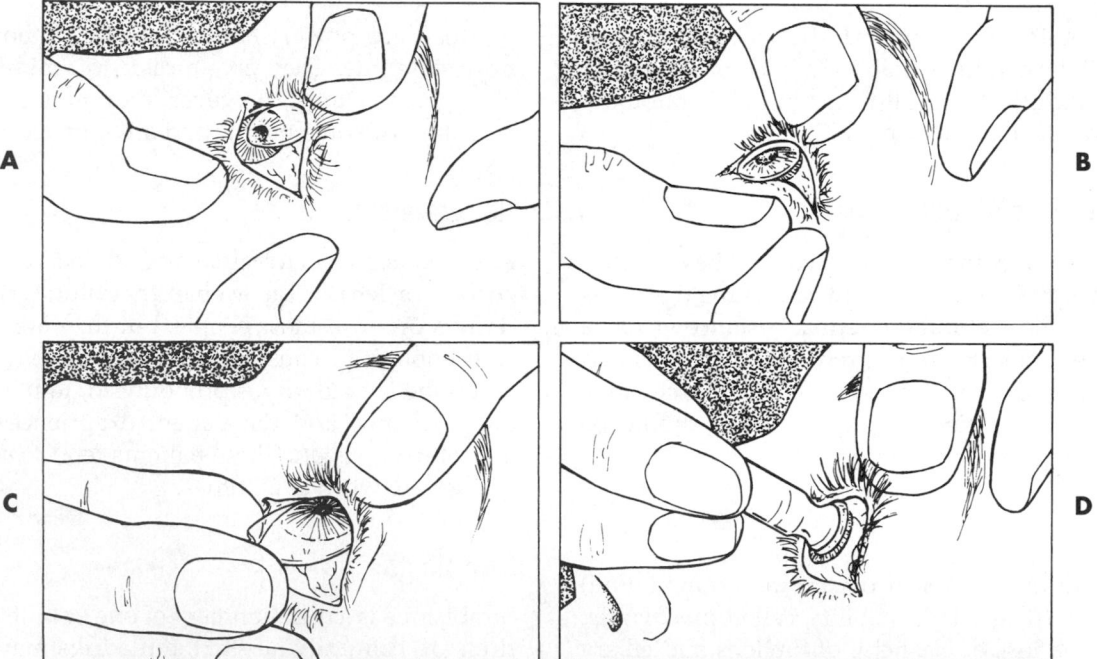

**Figure 38-15** **A,** To remove hard lens, place thumb or finger directly on margin of lid at base of eyelashes and raise lid. Use same procedure with other hand to lower bottom lid. Recenter lens before removing. **B,** Slowly bring lids together, trapping contact lens between lid margins. Eyelid will break tearlayer adhesion of contact lens, which will be ejected as lid forces it outward. **C,** Soft lens will move as lids are manipulated. If it does not seem slippery, it must be moistened with saline solution before attempting to remove it to avoid peeling epithelial tissues from corneal surface. To remove soft lens, raise upper lid with one hand and pinch lens with fingers of other hand. It will be removed easily if it is moist and may be removed even if it is off center in eye. **D,** Kits that contain contact lens suction cup are available in many emergency rooms. Suction cup is effective for removing hard and scleral lenses but cannot be used with soft lenses.

rests on the tear film over the corneal surface and is held in place by capillary traction and the upper lid. A variety of contact lens styles are available today. The original hard lenses are worn by relatively few users today. Soft and gas-permeable lenses are most common. Hard lenses, designed to be removed daily, are easy to care for and are less expensive, but they do not allow oxygen to reach the cornea. Soft and gas-permeable lenses do allow oxygen to reach the cornea. Soft lenses offer little correction for astigmatism and require greater care than gas-permeable and hard lenses. Wearing time for soft lenses is longer, and the cost is higher.

Contact lenses have been associated with corneal abrasions and infections. Among the risk factors for these injuries are prolonged wearing time, improper fit of the lens, scratched or torn lenses, hyposecretion of tears, improper hygiene, and decreased oxygen to the corneal surface. "Bandage," or therapeutic, soft lenses are used to treat lid disorders, corneal epithelial defects, corneal erosions or ulcers, wound leaks, and small corneal perforations. A contact lens may be prescribed to correct the vision of a patient who has had cataract surgery on one eye but did not receive an intraocular lens implant (Vaughan, Asbury, Riordan-Eva, 1995).

Patients should not wear contact lenses when taking eye medications. Certain medications, such as fluorescein, can stain the lenses. Also medications may be absorbed into soft lenses, causing overdose problems.

Contact lenses should be removed in an injured or comatose patient to prevent damage (abrasions) to the corneal epithelium (Figure 38-15; Box 38-1). If the eyes are not fully closed, the contact lenses may begin to adhere to the corneal surface. This happens because the tear film is not spread over the eye with normal lid blinking. Prolonged lens wear with decreased oxygen to the cornea can lead to keratitis and scarring.

## Vision Loss

Blindness is legally defined by the U.S. Internal Revenue Service as a visual acuity that is not correctable to at least 20/200 in the better eye or a visual field no greater than 20 degrees at its widest diameter. The area of vision lost can be the central field, the peripheral field, or a portion of the peripheral field in one or both eyes. Generally, vision loss can be thought of as a decrease in vision significant enough to prevent a person from performing activities of daily living without dependence on others or on visual aids. Vision loss may be congenital or acquired, and it may occur suddenly or gradually over time. Macular degeneration, glaucoma, diabetic retinopathy, cataract, and optic atrophy are major causes of blindness in the United States. Worldwide, blindness is attributed to cataract, trachoma, glaucoma, onchocerciasis (river blindness), xerophthalmia (nutritional blindness caused by vitamin A deficiency), and trauma (Grimes, Scardino, Martone, 1992; Vader, 1997).

## Color Blindness

The inability to distinguish colors may be congenital or acquired, and it may be partial or complete. Red-blue–sensitive and green-sensitive pigments in the retina are responsible for normal color vision. Defects in one or more of these pigments are responsible for color blindness. Congenital defects are gender linked and occur mostly in males. Retinal or optic nerve disease can also cause color vision abnormalities. The most common type of color blindness is red-green blindness, in which persons see these colors as yellow or blue. One or both eyes can be involved. Awareness of this defect is important to drivers, who must use some feature other than color to distinguish the difference in traffic lights. Some states require color vision testing when applying for a driver's license. Color vision testing can be accomplished with the Ishihara test (polychromatic plates). A person with normal color vision can identify all patterns or symbols on the test field, whereas a patient with a deficiency cannot. This problem affects approximately 8% of males and less than 1% of females. True color blindness, called

### BOX 38-1

**SUGGESTED EMERGENCY CARE FOR PATIENTS WEARING CONTACT LENSES**

**DETERMINE IF PATIENT IS WEARING CONTACT LENSES:**
Ask
Check I.D. card
Check Medic Alert medallion
Look for contact lenses

**IF YOU SUSPECT THE LENSES ARE STILL ON THE EYE:**
Apply adhesive tape strip to patient's forehead or adjacent area and label "Contact Lenses"
Consult emergency aid file when time permits

**IF THE LENSES ARE FOUND:**
Place in a case or bottle and label with patient's name (Mark "right" or "left," if known)
Record on emergency tag

Provided as a public service by the American Optometric Association. Reprinted with permission of the American Optometric Association, St Louis.

achromatopsia (the inability to see any colors), is rare (Vaughan, Asbury, Riordan-Eva, 1995).

# NURSING INTERVENTIONS FOR EYE DISORDERS

Several specific procedures are necessary for the patient with eye problems. The nurse should be familiar with these procedures and understand the basis for using each one on a selected patient. Hand washing and clean equipment are essential. In some instances, sterile supplies and equipment may be required.

Normal pupillary response is the response of the pupil to light (hence the acronym *PERRLA: p*upils *e*qual, *r*ound, *r*eactive to *l*ight, and *a*ccommodation). The pupil of one eye should constrict simultaneously when the opposite pupil is exposed to light, even when the unexposed eye is blind. To check the pupils, the nurse dims the lights and uses a pen light. The

nurse stands in front of the patient and has the patient look straight ahead at an object. The nurse directs the flashlight beam onto one pupil from the side and then repeats for the other eye. Head trauma, eye medications, and other drugs—therapeutic or recreational—can affect pupil size and response (Hunt, 1992).

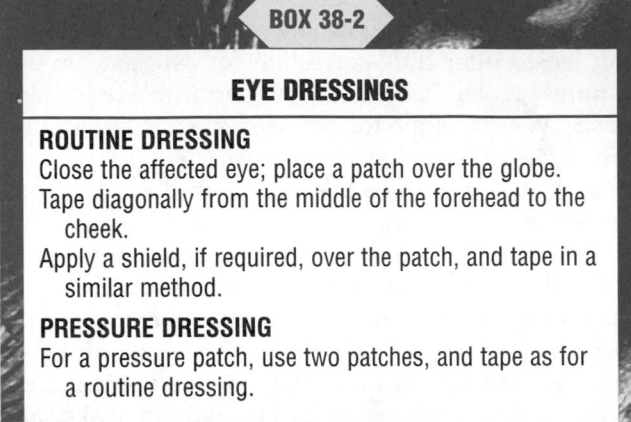

**BOX 38-2**

### EYE DRESSINGS

**ROUTINE DRESSING**

Close the affected eye; place a patch over the globe.
Tape diagonally from the middle of the forehead to the cheek.
Apply a shield, if required, over the patch, and tape in a similar method.

**PRESSURE DRESSING**

For a pressure patch, use two patches, and tape as for a routine dressing.

**BOX 38-3**

### INSTILLATION OF EYE DROPS

1 Wash your hands before and after doing any procedure on the eye.
2 With one hand, put a finger on the patient's cheek just below the eye on the bony socket. Gently pull down until a small pocket is formed between the eyeball and lower lid.
3 Have the patient tilt his or her head back and look up. Put a drop into the pocket that you have formed (conjunctival sac).
4 Have the patient gently close both eyes for 1 minute to let the drop absorb.
5 If another drop is to be instilled, wait 3 to 5 minutes before the next one is put in.
6 The same procedure is followed for putting in ointments. A strip of ointment approximately ½ inch long is squeezed into the conjunctival sac from the inner to outer side of the eye. If drops and ointment are given at the same time, the ointment goes in last.
7 Avoid touching any part of the eye with the medication container.
8 To prevent systemic absorption of drugs, the puncta (small openings to the nasolacrimal ducts located on the medial aspect of the upper and lower lids) should be occluded. After instilling the drop, press the index finger over the inner canthus until you can feel the bone beneath the skin. Release after 30 seconds.
9 Store medications properly.
NOTE: Some medications need to be refrigerated or stored away from light.

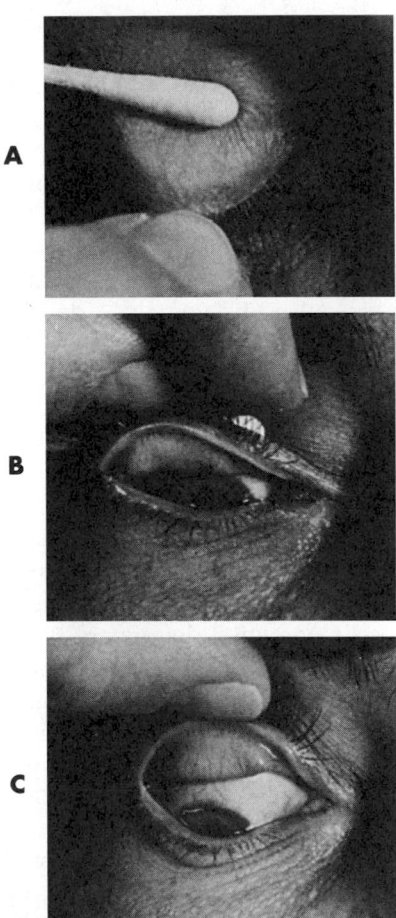

**Figure 38-16** Eversion of upper eyelid. Patient is instructed to look downward, and lashes of upper eyelid are grasped between thumb and index finger. **A,** Cotton-tipped applicator is placed at level of tarsal fold. **B,** Eyelid is folded back on applicator while patient continues to look downward. **C,** Applicator is removed. (From Newell FW: *Ophthalmology: principles and concepts,* ed 8, St Louis, 1996, Mosby.)

Other procedures include routine or compression eye dressings, medication application, lid hygiene and irrigation, everting the lids, and warm and cold compresses (Figure 38-16; Boxes 38-2 to 38-6).

## Overview of Ophthalmic Medications

Medications for ophthalmic diagnosis and treatment are used in many forms (Table 38-2). Topically, they are applied as drops or ointment. Ointments tend to cloud the vision, so they are better used at night or when the eye is closed. They do provide better lubrication than drops. Drops should be instilled before an ointment if both are ordered. Some drops may produce local irritation, causing redness, blurred vision, stinging, foreign body sensation, or tearing. Discolored solutions should be discarded. Special storage, such as refrigeration or storing away from light, is required for some

eye medications. Combinations of antibiotics with antiinflammatory medications are prescribed for external diseases such as blepharitis and bacterial corneal ulcers. Separate bottles or tubes of medication should be used for each eye if both are infected, and each bottle should be labeled properly (McCoy, 1992).

Parenteral or oral medications are used for systemic effect in various conditions. Injections are given subconjunctivally or intraocularly into the anterior chamber or the vitreous cavity. Doses for these injections are calculated and given with great care. An incorrect dosage can be toxic, and corneal decompensation or retinal tissue destruction is possible.

As with all treatments, meticulous hand washing before and after applying medications is a must. Universal precautions should be followed with all patients, according to U.S. Occupational Safety and Health Administration (OSHA) guidelines. The following drugs that are used for treatment of systemic disease can be toxic to the eye and cause irreversible damage:

1. Corticosteroids cause cataract formation. Children are more susceptible than adults.
2. Isotretinoin (Accutane), a vitamin A analog used for treating acne, can cause increased intracranial pressure and damage the optic nerve. A vision check needs to be done within 6 weeks of initial therapy.
3. Hydroxychloroquine (Plaquenil), an arthritis and lupus drug, is toxic to the rods and cones in the retina. A baseline examination should be followed by checks every 3 to 6 months while medication is being taken.
4. A tuberculosis drug, ethambutol (isoniazid), can cause optic neuropathy.

*Text continued on page 1193.*

---

### BOX 38-4

#### LID HYGIENE FOR POSTOPERATIVE CARE

1 Wash hands before and after the cleansing.
2 Assemble the solution (normal saline or tap water) and cotton balls, gauze, or a clean washcloth.
3 Position the patient sitting comfortably, possibly near the sink if tap water is used.
4 Wipe the eye with a moistened cotton ball or gauze from the nasal to the temporal side of the eye. Avoid getting solution into the unaffected eye.
5 Each time the procedure is done, use fresh, clean supplies.

---

### BOX 38-5

#### EYE IRRIGATION/CLEANSING

1 Wash hands before and after the procedure. Use gloves.
2 Assemble necessary equipment, including cotton balls, normal saline or other solution, and kidney basin or towel to absorb the solution.
3 Position the patient comfortably with the head turned to the affected side.
4 Direct the irrigating solution over the eye from the nasal to the temporal side of the eye. Avoid getting solution into the unaffected eye.
5 Use a separate set of supplies for each eye if both eyes are involved.
6 Do not instill the solution forcefully. The eyelid can be gently held open for a thorough cleansing.

---

### BOX 38-6

#### EVERTING THE LIDS

This procedure is done to inspect the eye for a foreign body or to irrigate the lid margins.
1 Assemble equipment, including cotton-tipped applicators, irrigation solution, fluorescein strips, and a light source (a slit lamp if available).
2 Gently pull down the lower lid on the orbital rim to expose the conjunctival sac of the lower lid.
3 For the upper lid, use a cotton-tipped applicator. Grasp the lashes with the finger and thumb, and gently fold the lid back over the applicator.
4 Once the lid is folded, remove the applicator so the lid can rest against the conjunctiva for inspection.
5 To close the eyelid, the patient need only blink or close eyelids slowly and reopen again (see Figure 38-16).

**TABLE 38-2**

## Pharmacology of Drugs Used for Vision

| DRUG (GENERIC AND TRADE NAME); ROUTE AND DOSAGE | ACTION/INDICATION | COMMON SIDE EFFECTS AND NURSING CONSIDERATIONS |
|---|---|---|
| **ANTIBIOTICS** | | |
| **Bacitracin Ointment (Ak-tracin)**<br>Route: Ocular<br>Dosage: ½-inch strip of 500 units/g ointment 2-4 times daily | Antibacterial used for minor gram-positive infections | Do not use with silver nitrate; can delay wound healing |
| **Ciprofloxacin (Ciloxan)**<br>Route: Ocular<br>Dosage: 1-2 drops q 15-30 min until infection is controlled, then 1-2 drops 4-6 times daily | Quinolone antibacterial used for corneal ulcers and bacterial conjunctivitis | Watch for local irritation; not to be used for *Pseudomonas* |
| **Erythromycin (Ilotycin)**<br>Route: Ocular<br>Dosage: 0.5% ointment to conjunctiva 1 or more times daily | Used for treatment of superficial ocular infections and for prophylaxis in ophthalmia neonatorum; useful when penicillin-based ophthalmic drug cannot be used because of hypersensitivity | Staph resistance may develop |
| **Gentamicin (Garamycin, Genoptic)**<br>Route: Ocular<br>Dosage: 1-2 drops of solution q 2-4 hr, or ointment 2-3 times daily | Bacteriocidal used for *Pseudomonas,* gram-negative infections, and other localized infections | Incompatible with erythromycin, chloramphenicol, and not effective against streptococci; use with caution in renal patients |
| **Norfloxacin (Chibroxin)**<br>Route: Ocular<br>Dosage: 1-2 drops q 2 hr for 2 days; then q 4 hr for 5 days | Quinolone antibacterial used for corneal or bacterial conjunctivitis | **Hypersensitivity** possible; overgrowth of nonsusceptible organisms possible; do not use with soft contact lenses; DO NOT inject |
| **Ofloxacin (Ocuflox)**<br>Route: Ocular<br>Dosage: 1-2 drops q 2 hr for 2 days; then q 4 hr for 5 days | Quinolone antibacterial used for corneal or bacterial conjunctivitis | **Hypersensitivity** possible; overgrowth of nonsusceptible organisms possible; do not use with soft contact lenses; DO NOT inject |
| **Polymyxin B Sulfate (Aerosporin)**<br>Route: Ocular<br>Dosage: 1-3 drops q 1 hr; dosage interval may be increased as response occurs | Bacteriocidal used for *Pseudomonas* and gram-negative infections | Not effective for gram-positive infections; may be toxic to renal patients |
| **Tetracycline (Achromycin)**<br>Route: Ocular<br>Dosage: Thin strip of ointment q 2-4 hr, or 1 drop of suspension q 6-12 hr (may be used more often); single dose for ophthalmia neonatorum | Bacteriostatic used against gram-positive and gram-negative infections and for prophylaxis in ophthalmia neonatorum | Use with caution in hepatic or renal failure |
| **Tobramycin (Tobrex)**<br>Route: Ocular<br>Dosage: 1 cm of ointment 2-3 times daily (q 3-4 hr for severe infections), or 1-2 drops of solution q 4 hr (q 30-60 min for severe infections) | Bacteriocidal used for *Pseudomonas, Staphylococcus,* and gram-negative infections | Prolonged use may result in overgrowth of nonsusceptible organisms |

*IOP,* Intraocular pressure; *BP,* blood pressure; *MAO,* monoamine oxidase.

**TABLE 38-2**

## Pharmacology of Drugs Used for Vision—cont'd

| DRUG (GENERIC AND TRADE NAME); ROUTE AND DOSAGE | ACTION/INDICATION | COMMON SIDE EFFECTS AND NURSING CONSIDERATIONS |
|---|---|---|
| **ANTIFUNGALS** | | |
| **Amphotericin B** (Fungizone) **Route:** Ocular **Dosage:** 3% ointment 1-2 drops daily or as ordered | Used against *Candida,* histoplasmosis, and blastomycosis | Use with caution in renal or electrolyte abnormalities; watch closely for adverse reactions; give test dose before maintenance dose |
| **Flucytosine** Ancobon **Route:** Oral, ocular **Dosage:** Oral, 50-100 mg/kg body weight in 4 equal doses; ocular, 1% solution | Used for *Candida, Cryptococcus* | May cause nausea or vomiting (space tablets at intervals); lower dosages with renal or liver impairment; excreted by kidneys |
| **Natamycin** (Natacyn) **Route:** Ocular **Dosage:** 1-2 drops q 4-6 hr | Used for treatment of fungal keratitis, blepharitis, or fungal conjunctivitis | |
| **ANTIVIRALS** | | |
| **Idoxuridine** (Herplex, Stoxil) **Route:** Ocular **Dosage:** 0.5% ointment; 0.1% solution, 1 drop q 1 hr when awake and q 2 hr at night | Used for herpes simplex keratitis | Refrigerate solution and keep from light; should not be mixed with other eye solutions; watch for signs of hypersensitivity |
| **Trifluridine** (Viroptic Ophthalmic Solution, 1%) **Route:** Ocular **Dosage:** 1-2 drops q 2-3 hr initially, then q 4 hr when awake | Used against primary keratoconjunctivitis and recurrent epithelial keratitis caused by herpes simplex virus, types I and II | Stinging on instillation; use with caution in pregnancy |
| **Vidarabine** (Vira-A Ophthalmic) **Route:** Ocular **Dosage:** ½-inch strip of ointment into lower conjunctival sac 5 times daily at 3-hr intervals | Used against herpes simplex keratitis and herpes zoster keratitis | Use cautiously with steroids; not for long-term use |
| **GLAUCOMA** | | |
| **Acetazolamide** (AKZol, Diamox) **Route:** PO, IV **Dosage:** PO 250-500 mg 1-2 times daily; IV 250-500 mg daily | Carbonic anhydrase inhibitor used in treatment of narrow-angle glaucoma | Nausea, vomiting, diarrhea, anorexia, headache, skin rash, confusion, and paresthesia; do not give to sulfa-sensitive patients; contraindicated in kidney or liver dysfunction |
| **Apraclonidine** (Iopidine) **Route:** Ocular **Dosage:** 1 drop of 1% solution, total of 1-2 drops/day; or 1 drop before and after laser therapy | Alpha-adrenergic agonist; decreases IOP (thought to decrease aqueous formation) | Use with caution in hypertensive, renal, or severe cardiovascular disease; protect from light; store at room temperature; contraindicated if using MAO inhibitors |
| **Betaxolol** (Betoptic) **Route:** Ocular **Dosage:** Instill 1 drop of 0.5% solution or 1-2 drops of 0.25% suspension bid | Beta-blocker, decreases aqueous formation | Local irritation and insomnia; contraindicated in pulmonary, renal, or cardiac disease, including congestive heart failure |

*Continued*

TABLE 38-2

## Pharmacology of Drugs Used for Vision—cont'd

| DRUG (GENERIC AND TRADE NAME); ROUTE AND DOSAGE | ACTION/INDICATION | COMMON SIDE EFFECTS AND NURSING CONSIDERATIONS |
|---|---|---|
| **GLAUCOMA—cont'd**<br>**Carteolol** (Occupress)<br>**Route:** Ocular<br>**Dosage:** 1 drop of 1% solution 2 times daily | Beta-blocker, decreases aqueous formation | Contraindicated in pulmonary, renal, or cardiac disease; can mask symptoms of hypoglycemia |
| **Dichloryhenamide** (Daranide)<br>**Route:** Oral<br>**Dosage:** 100-200 mg initially; then 100 mg q 12 hr until desired response; maintenance dose 25-50 mg/day | Carbonic anhydrase inhibitor; decreases intraocular pressure, given in conjunction with topical ocular hypotensive agents | Contraindicated in hepatic insufficiency, renal failure, chronic obstructive pulmonary disease; monitor potassium levels; may cause gastrointestinal disturbances |
| **Dorzolamide** (Truscopt)<br>**Route:** Ocular<br>**Dosage:** 1 drop of 2% solution 3 times daily | Carbonic anhydrase inhibitor; decreases aqueous humor secretion | Contraindicated with allergy to sulfa; additive effects with other carbonic anhydrase inhibitors; use with caution in renal patients; remove soft contact lenses before administering; some local irritation |
| **Glycerin** (Osmoglyn)<br>**Route:** PO, ocular<br>**Dosage:** PO, 1-1.5 g/kg as a single dose, may be followed by 500 mg/kg q 6 hr; ocular, 1-2 drops q 3-4 hr | Osmotic agent (oral) used for management of edema of the superficial layers of the cornea and reduction of IOP | Use with caution in diabetic patients; onset is 10 min and duration 45 min; serve over ice with lemon |
| **Levobunolol** (Betagan)<br>**Route:** Ocular<br>**Dosage:** 1-2 drops daily or bid | Beta-adrenergic blocking agent used for short-term reduction of IOP caused by glaucoma | Decreases heart rate; may cause headaches, nausea, dizziness, and depression; contraindicated in asthma, emphysema, diabetes, and bradycardia |
| **Mannitol** (Osmitrol)<br>**Route:** IV<br>**Dosage:** 5%-10% solution continuously up to 200 g IV, while maintaining urine output of 100-500 ml/hr and a positive fluid balance | Osmotic agent used for angle-closure glaucoma and preoperative or postoperative control of IOP | Nausea, vomiting, urine retention; contraindicated in pulmonary edema, congestive heart failure, and renal disease |
| **Metipranolol** (Opti pranolol)<br>**Route:** Ocular<br>**Dosage:** 1 drop of 0.3% solution daily | Beta-blocker; decreases IOP; does not affect pupil size | Local irritation, burning, redness, tearing; has additive effect when used with systemic beta-blockers |
| **Timolol Maleate** (Timoptic)<br>**Route:** Ocular<br>**Dosage:** Initially 1 drop of 0.25% solution bid; reduce maintenance dose to 1 drop daily | Beta-adrenergic blocking agent used for chronic open-angle glaucoma, secondary glaucoma, aphakic glaucoma, and optic hypertension | Nausea, vomiting, urine retention; not for use in pulmonary edema, congestive heart failure, or renal disease; does not affect pupil size or visual acuity; can cause apnea in infants |

**TABLE 38-2**

## Pharmacology of Drugs Used for Vision—cont'd

| DRUG (GENERIC AND TRADE NAME); ROUTE AND DOSAGE | ACTION/INDICATION | COMMON SIDE EFFECTS AND NURSING CONSIDERATIONS |
|---|---|---|
| **NONSTEROIDAL ANTIINFLAMMATORY** | | |
| **Diclofenac** (Voltaren) <br> **Route:** Ocular <br> **Dosage:** 1 drop of 0.1% solution 4 times/ day × 2 wk, beginning 24 hr after procedure | For management of inflammation after cataract extraction | May enhance digoxin, methotrexate, cyclosporin, and lithium |
| **Flurbiprofen** (Ocufen) <br> **Route:** Ocular <br> **Dosage:** Instill 1 drop into eye undergoing surgery approximately q ½ hr, beginning 2 hr before surgery; give total of 4 drops | Given preoperatively to inhibit miosis during intraocular surgery | May increase incidence of bleeding postoperatively; do not use with anticoagulants such as warfarin (Coumadin) |
| **Ketorolac Tromethamine** (Acular) <br> **Route:** Ocular <br> **Dosage:** 1 drop of 0.5% solution 4 times daily | Antiinflammatory, antipyretic analgesic; used for ocular itching; conjunctivitis | Contraindicated in patients with soft contact lenses; potentiates cross sensitivity to aspirin; can increase bleeding times—do not use preoperatively |
| **Suprofen** (Profenal) <br> **Route:** Ocular <br> **Dosage:** 1-2 drops of 1% solution 5 times on day before surgery, 3 times on the day of surgery | Inhibits intraoperative pupil constriction | Local burning; cross sensitivity to aspirin; increases bleeding time <br> Contraindicated for epithelial herpes simplex keratitis |
| **MIOTICS** | | |
| **Carbachol Intraocular** (Miostat) <br> **Route:** Ocular <br> **Dosage:** Physician instills 0.5 ml into the anterior chamber before or after securing sutures | Used to produce pupillary miosis during ocular surgery and for open-angle glaucoma | Prolonged constriction contraindicated in acute iritis and corneal abrasion |
| **Echothiophate Iodide** (Phospholine Iodide) <br> **Route:** Ocular <br> **Dosage:** Instill 1 drop of 0.03%-0.125% solution into conjunctival sac daily | Used in treatment of primary open-angle glaucoma and conditions obstructing aqueous flow | Discontinue several weeks preoperatively; causes respiratory depression with succinylcholine |
| **MYDRIATICS AND CYCLOPLEGICS** | | |
| **Atropine** (Atropisol, Isopto Atropine) <br> **Route:** Ocular <br> **Dosage:** 1 drop 2-4 times/day | Anticholinergic agent used for treatment of uveitis, amblyopia, iritis, posterior-segment surgery, and some anterior-segment surgery | Systemic reactions (tachycardia, increased blood pressure); side effects may last up to 2 wk; antidote is physostigmine |
| **Cyclopentolate Hydrochloride** (Cyclogyl, AK-Pentolate) <br> **Route:** Ocular <br> **Dosage:** 1-2 drops, up to 3 doses | Used for diagnostic procedures requiring mydriasis and cycloplegia | Photophobia and local irritation; onset 15-30 min, with up to 24-hr duration; use with caution if patient hypertensive |

*Continued*

**TABLE 38-2**

## Pharmacology of Drugs Used for Vision—cont'd

| DRUG (GENERIC AND TRADE NAME); ROUTE AND DOSAGE | ACTION/INDICATION | COMMON SIDE EFFECTS AND NURSING CONSIDERATIONS |
|---|---|---|
| **MYDRIATICS AND CYCLOPLEGICS—cont'd** | | |
| **Epinephrine** Route: Ocular Dosage: 1:1000 to 1:40,000; used in irrigation solution for intraocular injection | Adrenergic agent dilates pupil intraoperatively | Use with caution in cardiac, diabetic, and hypertensive patients |
| **Phenylephrine** (AK-Dilate, Mydfrin, Neo-Synephrine 2.5% or 10% drops) Route: Ocular Dosage: 1-3 drops, up to 3 doses, for refraction; 1 drop qid for uveitis | Adrenergic agent used for diagnostic tests, preoperatively, and for uveitis | Onset 5-10 min, with duration 3-5 hr; can cause systemic hypertension; monitor BP and pulse; use with caution with MAO inhibitors |
| **Scopolamine** (Isopto-Hyoscine 3% drops) Route: Ocular Dosage: 1-2 drops tid | Used for diagnosis, to induce refraction, and for iridocyclitis | Onset in 40 min, with duration 3-5 days |
| **Tropicamide** (Mydriacyl, Tropicacyl 1% drops) Route: Ocular Dosage: Instill 1 drop of 1% solution; may repeat in 5 min; additional drop in 20-30 min if necessary | Used for diagnosis, to induce refraction, and for fundus photography | Onset in 20-30 min, with duration 4-6 hr; local irritation and blurred vision |
| **STEROIDAL ANTIINFLAMMATORY** **Dexamethasone** (Decadron, Hexadrol, Maxidex) Route: Ocular, IV Dosage: Ocular, 1-2 drops 4-6 times daily, or hourly as prescribed; IV, 2-mg doses up to 12 mg daily | Used for ocular inflammation in intraocular surgery | Contraindicated for viral or fungal infections; can increase IOP or cause cataracts |
| **Fluorometholone** (Flarex) Route: Ocular Dosage: 1-2 drops 4 times daily | Cortisone preparation, suspension | DO NOT inject; contraindicated in herpes and other viral diseases and fungal infections; shake well |
| **Hydrocortisone** (Cortisol) Route: Ocular Dosage: 1-2 drops 4-6 times daily, or hourly as prescribed | Antiinflammatory and immunosuppressant used for treatment of sympathetic ophthalmia, chemical burns, corneal graft rejection, intraocular lens surgery, and conjunctivitis | Retards corneal regeneration; contraindicated for fungal and viral conditions and glaucoma; increased susceptibility to fungal and viral infections with long-term use; to discontinue drug, it must be tapered slowly |
| **Medrysone** (HMS) Route: Ocular Dosage: 1-2 drops of 1% solution | Antiinflammatory, antiallergic for treating allergic conjunctivitis, episcleritis, epinephrine sensitivity | DO NOT inject; prolonged use may cause cataract formation and increase intraocular pressure; contraindicated for fungal or viral conditions |

**TABLE 38-2**

## Pharmacology of Drugs Used for Vision—cont'd

| DRUG (GENERIC AND TRADE NAME); ROUTE AND DOSAGE | ACTION/INDICATION | COMMON SIDE EFFECTS AND NURSING CONSIDERATIONS |
|---|---|---|
| **STEROIDAL ANTIINFLAMMATORY—cont'd** | | |
| **Prednisone** (Deltasone, Meticorten) **Route:** Ocular **Dosage:** 1-2 drops 4 to 6 times daily and then taper properly to discontinue; may be ordered every hour | Same as for hydrocortisone | Same as for hydrocortisone |
| **Prednisolone** (Pred-Mild, Inflamase, AK-Pred, Econopred) **Route:** Ocular **Dosage:** Same as for prednisone | Same as for hydrocortisone | Same as for hydrocortisone |

The nurse should monitor the vision closely in any patient taking any of these medications.

## Conjunctivitis

**Conjunctivitis** is an inflammation of the conjunctiva of the eye. Symptoms include a burning or scratching sensation, foreign-body sensation, tearing, swelling, drainage, and increased blood in the vessels (hyperemia). It may result from an allergy or a viral or bacterial infection. *Allergic conjunctivitis* usually subsides when the allergen is removed, but the itching and redness can be treated with vasoconstrictive drops and cold compresses. Severe cases may require systemic antihistamines or steroids. *Viral conjunctivitis* is caused by herpes simplex, herpes zoster, adenovirus, and other viruses. After the causative organism is identified, topical antiviral drugs are used. It should be noted that although steroids can be used in allergic conjunctivitis, they are contraindicated in viral conjunctivitis.

The most common type of conjunctivitis is often referred to as *pink eye*. In temperate climates, it is often caused by the pneumococcus organism. In tropical climates, the Koch-Weeks bacillus is the most common cause. It is often encountered as an epidemic among school children and is spread through droplet infection. There is redness, burning, and mucopurulent discharge. The infection starts in one eye and rapidly spreads to the other (Vaughan, Asbury, Riordan-Eva, 1995). The eyelids are usually stuck together in the morning; warm, moist compresses may be applied to separate the lids. Eye irrigations using physiologic saline may be ordered, and once the specific organism is identified, the disease is treated with a sulfonamide or other antibiotic drug (see Box 38-5). Steroid therapy

is contraindicated before the infection is identified. Drops are used during the day, and an ointment is used at night. Lid hygiene should be performed before medication is applied (see Box 38-4). Persons with the infection should use their own towels and washcloths and avoid public pools. Children should not attend school until the infection has cleared (approximately 1 week). Meticulous hand washing is necessary to prevent the spread of infection. *Bacterial conjunctivitis* is caused by staphylococcus, streptococcus, diplococcus, *Escherichia coli*, and other bacteria. Universal precautions, including use of gloves for patient care during irrigations, lid hygiene, and medication application, are required.

*Ophthalmia neonatorum* refers to any purulent conjunctivitis of the newborn acquired from an infected birth canal. State laws require that erythromycin 0.5% or tetracycline 1% ophthalmic ointment or drops be instilled in the eyes of all newborn infants to prevent the disease. Prophylactic drugs are given no later than 1 hour after birth. Although ophthalmia neonatorum can occur as a result of maternal gonorrhea, it is now most commonly caused by chlamydia. Silver nitrate does not prevent chlamydial infections. If mothers have a known disease, infants may require systemic therapy as well as prophylaxis.

Untreated chlamydia causes *trachoma*, identified by the World Health Organization as the leading cause of blindness in the world (Vaughan, Asbury, Riordan-Eva, 1995). Initially, this infection leads to scarring of the conjunctiva and interferes with tear film. This leads to corneal infections, scarring, and eventual blindness. Treatment is with sulfonamides, tetracycline, or erythromycin administered orally for 3 to 5 weeks. All members of the family must be treated if they are infected. Proper hygiene practices and improved sanitation can eliminate trachoma. Evaluation of a "red eye" as a result of conjunctivitis should not be confused with angle-closure glaucoma (Table 38-3).

## Corneal Disorders

The cornea, or clear window at the front of the eye, has five layers. One or more of these layers can be involved in a disease process or injury that will necessitate replacing the defective cornea with a human donor cornea. Because the cornea has no blood supply or lymphatics, tissue typing is normally not required. *Corneal abrasions* and *ulcers* destroy the normal barrier of corneal epithelium and expose the other layers to infection from a variety of organisms. Included are yeasts, viruses, fungi, protozoa, and gram-positive or gram-negative organisms. *Pseudomonas,* a gram-negative organism, is one of the most common contaminants in used bottles of eye drops and used tubes of mascara. Invasion by the herpes simplex virus is easily identified, with the aid of fluorescein stain, by its characteristic appearance resembling a linear branch with feathered edges (Ostler, 1993; Vaughan, Asbury, Riordan-Eva, 1995).

Symptoms of abrasions and ulcers include pain, **photophobia** (light sensitivity), and **epiphora** (tearing). Symptomatic diagnosis is confirmed by slit-lamp examination with fluorescein staining. Correctly identifying the source of the infection is most important. A variety of medications are available for use, and the choice of drug depends on the causative organism. Initial treatment for an abrasion includes antibiotic drops or ointment, cool packs, and dark glasses to decrease the photophobia. With a larger abrasion or severe pain, a pressure dressing is applied for comfort and to limit eye movement. This patch also prevents the lid from opening and closing and rubbing over the abraded area. Pain medication may be prescribed. Serious abrasions and ulcers are treated more aggressively with topical and periocular antiinfective agents. Occasionally, systemic drugs are given. Most superficial ulcers heal without complications when the ulcers are treated. Deep ulcers may perforate and tend to scar.

Strict adherence to the regimen of drop administration for corneal ulcers is vital to preserve the cornea and prevent scarring. Initially, "fortified" eye drops (individualized to the patient's ulcer) are prepared by the pharmacist or the physician and are given every 5 minutes for 30 minutes and then every hour around the clock until the cornea improves. Nighttime drops may be given every 2 hours. After 72 to 96 hours, a commercial drop is substituted. Patient compliance with this regimen is difficult because the frequency of drops conflicts with normal activities and sleep. Usually hospitalization is required to achieve this type of therapy. Patients need to understand how important the schedule is in preserving vision.

Other treatments for persistent defects that fail to heal are *bandage contact lenses* or adhesives (Vaughan, Asbury, Riordan-Eva, 1995). Lateral tarsorrhaphy or suturing the eyelids closed can be a temporary or permanent procedure used to treat corneal complications as a result of trauma, coma, dry-eye syndrome, neurologic lid diseases, or strokes.

## TABLE 38-3

### Evaluating a Red Eye

| | ACUTE GLAUCOMA | BACTERIAL CONJUNCTIVITIS | VIRAL CONJUNCTIVITIS | ALLERGIC CONJUNCTIVITIS |
|---|---|---|---|---|
| Corneal opacity | Yes | No | 0 to + | 0 |
| Hyperemia (increased blood in vessels) | ++ | +++ | ++ | + |
| Pupil | Mid-dilated; nonreactive | Normal | Normal | Normal |
| Anterior chamber depth | Shallow | Normal | Normal | Normal |
| Intraocular pressure | High | Normal | Normal | Normal |
| Discharge | None | ++ to +++ | ++ | + |
| Preauricular nodes | None | None | + | None |
| Signs and symptoms | No exudates; itching, blurred vision, pain, photophobia, colored halos, nausea and vomiting affect one eye | Large amount of discharge—mucopurulent, yellowish exudate—affects one or both eyes | Moderate exudate—watery or yellow tinged—affects one or both eyes | Small amount of exudate—white, stringy—affects one or both eyes |

# Dystrophies and Degenerative Corneal Diseases

Other abnormalities of the cornea can be congenital or acquired. In all conditions, an opacity is found in one or more layers. This clouding interferes with vision. *Keratoconus,* or coning of the cornea, is a degenerative disease of unknown cause. The onset is in the teenage years. *Xerophthalmia,* a condition caused by vitamin A deficiency, is found primarily in Africa and Latin America. Symptoms can progress from night blindness to actual decompensation of the cornea. *Corneal dystrophies* are bilateral hereditary conditions of the cornea that appear later in life, after the second decade. They may progress slowly or be stationary for long periods and not require treatment. However, corneal decompensation accompanied by a decrease in visual acuity may require a full-thickness graft (penetrating keratoplasty [PKP]) (Ostler, 1993). *Pseudophakic bullous keratopathy,* or edema of the cornea as a result of an intraocular lens implant, accounts for approximately 40,000 PKP procedures per year in the United States. Acquired conditions that require surgery include trauma and lacerations that leave a scar across the visual axis (pupil) of the cornea (Figure 38-17).

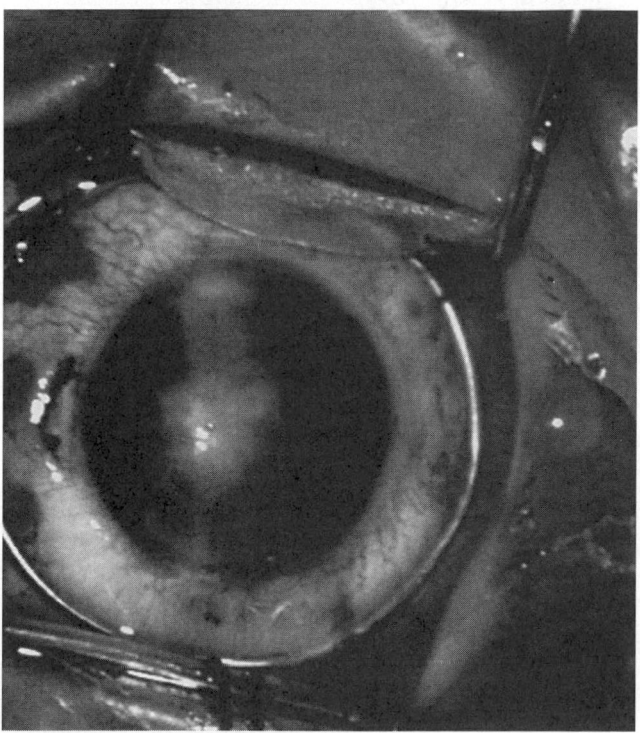

**Figure 38-17**    Preoperative view of corneal scar across the visual axis. (Photo courtesy Dr JB Rubenstein, Chicago.)

# Corneal Transplantation

Corneal transplantation **(keratoplasty)** is the surgical technique of replacing the patient's cornea with a human donor cornea (Box 38-7). A full-thickness graft is called a *penetrating keratoplasty (PKP).* A partial-thickness graft (lamellar keratoplasty) is seldom used today. Donor tissue is stored in a preservative medium that extends tissue viability to 10 days after the death of the donor (Box 38-8) (Ostler, 1993). This extension of viable storage has significantly decreased the number of patients on waiting lists. Scheduling for surgery procedures can be done on an urgent basis rather than on an emergent one. The patient can follow a normal routine without staying by a phone for news about the availability of tissue. Depending on the individual city or state, donor tissue may be in a limited supply.

A network of eye banks is set up by cities, states, and regions across the United States. This efficient and cost-effective linking of patient and tissue information ensures that the cornea is where it is needed when it is needed.

Preoperative evaluation of the patient includes a complete eye examination with keratometry readings, pachymetry, specular microscopy, and assessment of tear function if indicated. Routinely, surgery is performed with the patient under local anesthesia, with sedation and monitoring. Occasionally, general anesthesia may be indicated for reasons similar to those requiring general anesthesia for cataract extraction surgery. During the operative procedure the diseased central portion of the patient's cornea is removed and replaced with the donor tissue. The graft is sewn in place with a 10-0 or 11-0 suture in a running (continuous) or interrupted (individually tied) suture technique (Figure 38-18). When the procedure is completed, antibiotic and steroid injections are given subconjunctivally to prevent infection and inflammation. A patch and shield are routinely placed over the eye, and regular eyeglasses may be worn during the day to protect the eye.

Depending on the reason for the procedure, the patient is usually an outpatient or 23-hour observation patient. Uncomplicated cases are usually done on an outpatient basis similar to that for cataract surgery. Patients need to have a thorough understanding of postoperative medication orders and drop administration. They also need to know that compliance with this regimen and daily vision checks are equally important. Signs of rejection are redness, sudden loss of vision, or pain (RSVP), and any one of these must be reported to the ophthalmologist immediately. Follow-up visits are weekly for 2 to 3 weeks, every other week for 2 months, and then monthly until 6 months after surgery. Because the cornea is avascular, it heals slowly and sutures remain in place for up to 1 year. For this reason, seat belts

BOX 38-7

# NURSING PROCESS

## INTRAOCULAR SURGERY (CATARACT EXTRACTION, PENETRATING KERATOPLASTY, TRABECULECTOMY, VITRECTOMY

### ASSESSMENT

- Vital signs per routine
- Eye dressing
- Level of comfort
- Ability to care for self
- For signs of disorientation

### NURSING DIAGNOSES

- Anxiety related to fear of loss of sight or to symptoms of disease and prospective treatment
- Pain related to surgical inflammation or increased intraocular pressure (IOP)
- Self-care deficit related to decreased visual acuity or physical limitations
- Noncompliance to surgical protocol related to memory impairment, anxiety, or instructions not heard or seen well
- Knowledge deficit related to condition, treatment, medication administration, or activity restriction
- Risk for infection related to invasive surgery
- Sensory/perceptual alterations: visual related to disease and to surgical dressing postoperatively (especially important if both eyes are involved or if patient is monocular)
- Diversional activity deficit related to decreased vision

### NURSING INTERVENTIONS
#### Preoperative

- Review previous teaching done by the physician and staff, including written postoperative instructions for outpatients.
- Orient the patient to the surroundings, admission routine, and surgical environment.
- Facilitate the patient's expression of fear about the possibility of decreased vision.
- Ensure that the patient has followed restrictions to take nothing by mouth.
- Inform patient that a patch and shield will be worn immediately after surgery and that glasses may be substituted during waking hours.
- Review administration of drops or ointment as ordered.
- Inquire who will take the patient home.

#### Postoperative

- Orient the patient to the surroundings.
- Position the patient for comfort in bed or a recliner: supine with the head of the bed elevated 30 degrees or more.
- Ensure that the patient complies with activity restrictions on the basis of procedure or the physician's order.
- Allow the patient to watch television but prohibit reading.
- Provide a light diet the first day.
- Announce your presence when entering the room.
- Approach from the unoperated side.
- Place a call bell or signal within easy reach of the patient.
- Raise side rails as needed to protect the patient from injury.
- Administer medications as prescribed.
- Keep the eye patch or shield in place as ordered.
- Help the patient with meals, ambulation, and personal hygiene as needed.
- Report severe pain to the physician immediately.
- Question whether the home environment will be manageable and whether help will be needed.

### EVALUATION OF EXPECTED OUTCOMES

- Meets discharge criteria for the postsurgical patient (see Box 20-10)
- Expresses fears and concerns
- Vision improved or maintained (not applicable for enucleation patients)
- Able to ambulate with help
- Uses other senses to avoid bumping eye when patched
- Verbalizes understanding of instructions
- Demonstrates ability to administer own medications
- Able to return to normal activity or has assistance until normal activity resumes
- Knowledgeable about modifications at home to enhance safety

## CORNEAL DONOR CRITERIA

- Age between 1 and 75 years
- Negative medical history for the following:
  Acquired immunodeficiency syndrome (AIDS) or risk for human immunodeficiency virus (HIV) infection
  Active hepatitis
  Sepsis
  Lymphoma or active leukemia (other cancer types are okay)
- Ventilator support not required before tissue retrieval
- Routine testing of donors for the following:
  AIDS
  Hepatitis B and C
  Serology
- Donation within 6 to 12 hours after cardiopulmonary death (dependent on circumstances); keep lightweight eye packs over upper orbit
- Verbal consent by next of kin, followed by signed consent

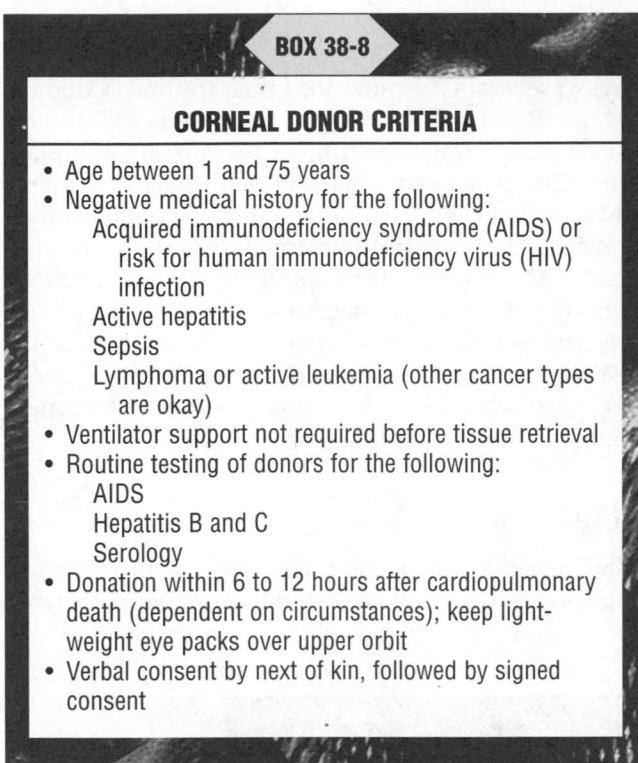

**Figure 38-18**    Sutures placed in corneal transplant. (Photo courtesy Dr RJ Epstein, Chicago.)

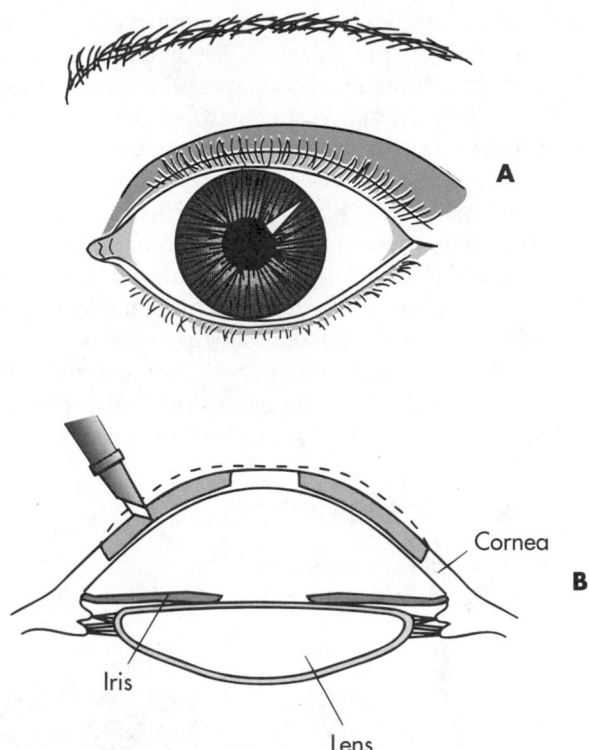

**Figure 38-19**    Radial keratotomy for myopia. Nearly full-thickness incisions of the cornea are made with a calibrated diamond blade in a radial fashion with sparing of the central cornea. **A,** Frontal view. **B,** Axial view.

are recommended every time the patient is in a car, and contact sports should be avoided (see Box 38-7).

Other surgical procedures on the cornea are designed to correct refractive errors of the eye. They include astigmatic keratectomy and radial keratotomy and laser keratectomy. *Radial keratotomy (RK)* consists of 4 to 16 pie-shaped cuts into the cornea, from a clear optical zone in the center to the outer portion of the cornea but not as far as the corneoscleral junction (limbus) (Figure 38-19). The amount of correction desired determines the number and depth of incisions. This reshaping or flattening of the cornea is done with a calibrated diamond knife.

Lasers are also used for treatment of "mildly" myopic eyes and central superficial corneal opacities. Combined automated lamellar keratoplasty (ALK) and laser keratectomy are other new techniques used for refractive surgery. (Controversies surround these procedures, whose goal is to have the patient be less dependent on eyeglasses.) After the procedure the patient may experience pain or discomfort, photophobia, or foreign-body sensation. Complications include corneal perforation, fluctuation in vision, persistent glare, regression of the correction, hyperopia, astigmatism, infection, and the need to continue wearing glasses or contact lenses. Long-term follow-up will determine risk and benefit factors more clearly. Most insurance companies consider refractive surgery a cosmetic procedure, so the expenses incurred are the patient's responsibility. This practice of nonreimbursement for expenses is changing with time.

## Uveitis

The uveal tract includes the ciliary body, iris, and choroid. Anterior uveitis refers to inflammation of the iris and ciliary body. Posterior uveitis refers to inflammation of the choroid. Uveitis usually affects one eye, and it is more common in younger people. Symptoms depend on the structure involved. They include photophobia, blurred vision, irregular pupil, and deposits on the posterior corneal surface. Uveitis is found in patients with toxoplasmosis, tuberculosis, sarcoidosis, and syphilis. Treatment is with appropriate antiinfective drugs, steroids, and dilating drops. Atropine or cyclopentolate prevents the formation of synechiae (adhesions). Children are sensitive to atropine, and toxicity may occur unless precautions are taken. Medications should be kept out of reach, and parents who will be giving atropine should be instructed on the toxic effects of an overdose and on the use of punctal occlusion to prevent systemic absorption of topical eye medications.

## Sympathetic Ophthalmia

*Sympathetic ophthalmia* is a rare bilateral condition occurring after a penetrating injury to the eye. The exact cause of the uveitis is not known, but it is thought to be an autoimmune response to the injury. It can occur 10 days to several years after the initial trauma (Vaughan, Asbury, Riordan-Eva, 1995). In rare instances it has occurred after intraocular surgery for cataract and glaucoma. The patient complains of photophobia, redness, and blurred vision. Local and systemic steroids and atropine can be given as initial treatment. However, enucleation is recommended for severely injured, sightless eyes to prevent inflammation in the "sympathizing" eye. The patient needs a thorough explanation of the treatment and risks involved. Complete bilateral blindness can develop over time without treatment (Vaughan, Asbury, Riordan-Eva, 1995).

## Glaucoma

**Glaucoma** is a disease that is characterized by a gradual, painless loss of peripheral vision that results in a tunnel-

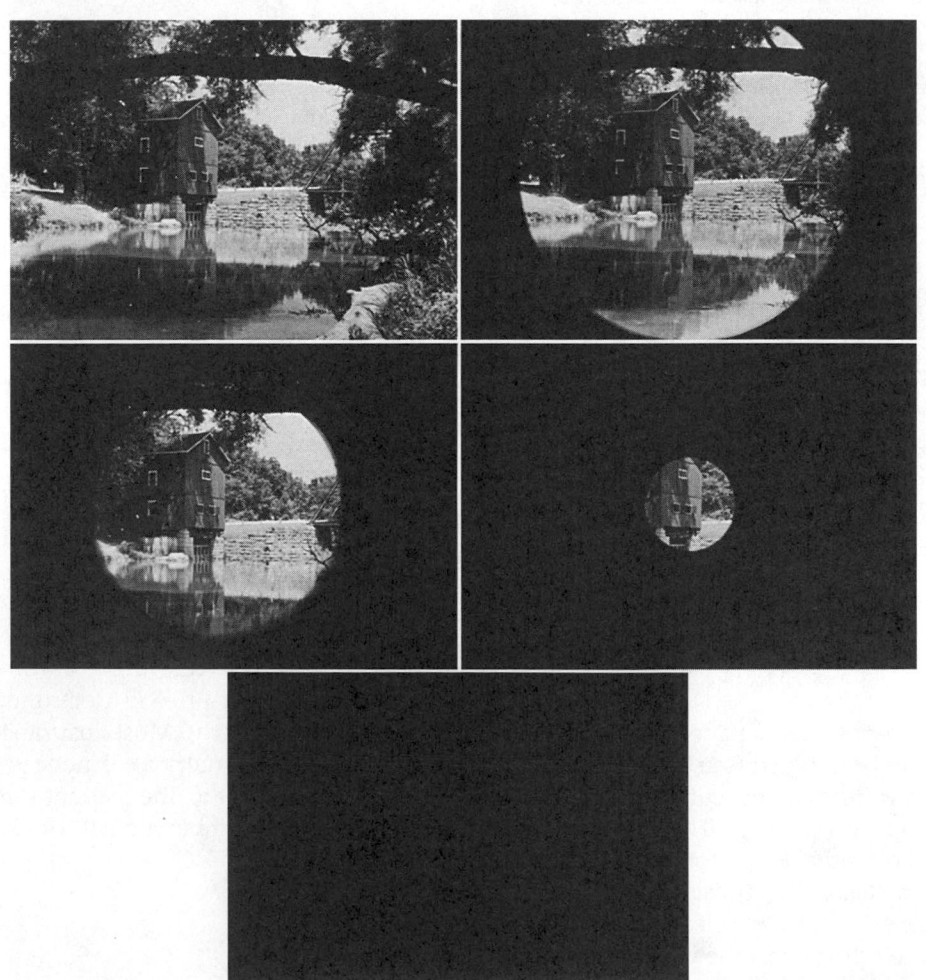

**Figure 38-20** Gradual loss of sight from glaucoma so insidiously destroys vision that the person is unaware of impending blindness until extensive and irreversible damage is present. Note loss of peripheral vision. (From Havener WH et al: *Nursing care in eye, ear, nose, and throat disorders,* ed 3, St Louis, 1974, Mosby.)

vision effect (Figure 38-20). It affects 0.4% to 0.7% of persons older than 40 years in the United States and 2% to 3% of those older than 70 years (Vaughan, Asbury, Riordan-Eva, 1995). Vision loss is caused by an increase in IOP, which damages the optic nerve. This damage is referred to as cupping of the disc. In a normal fundus examination, the ratio of cup size to optic disc diameter is less than 1:3. The optic disc has a depression (cup) that relates to the size of the optic nerve sheath fibers. In glaucoma the optic disc increases in depth and diameter. The blood vessels are also displaced.

Because peripheral vision is lost slowly, the patient is not aware of any changes until much vision is lost. This is why glaucoma is commonly referred to as the sneak thief of sight. Testing for glaucoma is done with a tonometer (see Figure 38-9), which measures IOP. Persons 40 years and older should have their IOP measured every 2 or 3 years during their regular eye examination. More frequent testing is recommended when there is a family history of glaucoma. The local chapter of Prevent Blindness America (PBA; formerly the National Society for the Prevention of Blindness) regularly provides information about the disease and about free testing in the community.

### ETHNIC/CULTURAL CONSIDERATIONS

Ten percent of African Americans older than 65 years have glaucoma. Three percent of Caucasian Americans 65 years and older have this disease.

## Types

The two main types of glaucoma are angle-closure (narrow-angle) glaucoma and open-angle (chronic open-angle) glaucoma (Figure 38-21). In angle-closure glaucoma, the iris pushes up against the cornea and blocks the flow of aqueous, which is an ocular emergency.

In chronic open-angle glaucoma, the blockage is located near the trabecular meshwork and Schlemm's canal. Symptoms are apparent only after vision is lost and may include frequent mild headaches, halos around lights, intermittent blurred vision, difficulty with night vision or adaptation to dark rooms and movie theaters, loss of peripheral vision, and frequent changes in vision. Diagnosis of the disease is made by assessing intraocular pressure (normal range is 12 to 20 mm Hg), optic disc abnormalities, and visual field loss. Treatment is designed to decrease the IOP medically by decreasing the pupil size (miotic drops) or by decreasing aqueous production (carbonic anhydrase inhibitors) or both (Table 38-2). When maximum medical therapy fails, laser treatments or operative procedures are needed to preserve the remaining vision.

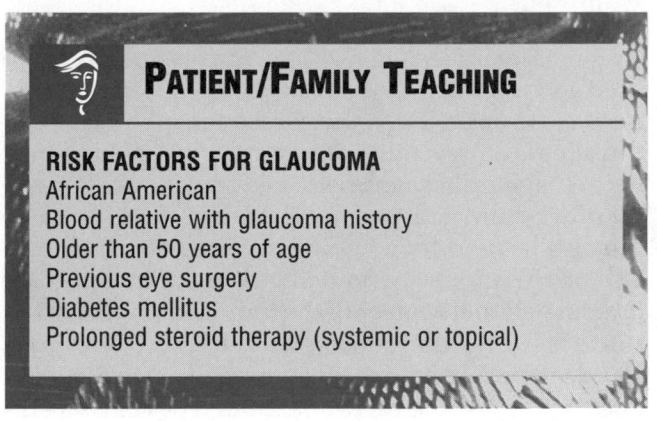

### PATIENT/FAMILY TEACHING

**RISK FACTORS FOR GLAUCOMA**
African American
Blood relative with glaucoma history
Older than 50 years of age
Previous eye surgery
Diabetes mellitus
Prolonged steroid therapy (systemic or topical)

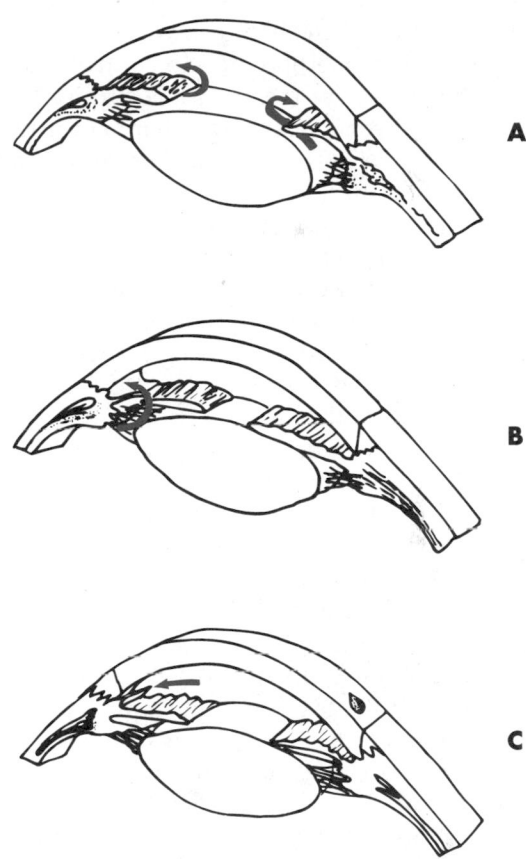

**Figure 38-21   A,** In the normal eye, aqueous produced by ciliary body flows through trabecular meshwork into Schlemm's canal to return to general circulation. **B,** In acute congestive (narrow-angle) glaucoma, angle of anterior chamber is too narrow and aqueous cannot enter canal. Treatment includes use of miotics to constrict pupil and widen angle, as well as laser trabeculoplasty and peripheral iridectomy to provide supplementary channel. **C,** In chronic (wide-angle) glaucoma, the problem is overproduction or decreased absorption of aqueous by the trabecular structures. When maximum medical therapy is no longer effective or tolerated or if there is a compliance problem, laser trabeculoplasty or filtration surgery may be indicated to improve aqueous outflow. (Modified from Kornzweig AL: *Hosp Pract* 12(7); Reichel W, editor: *The geriatric patient*, New York, 1978, HP Publishing.)

## Treatment

Argon laser iridectomy is a noninvasive procedure used to treat angle-closure glaucoma. For this procedure to be done easily, the cornea must be clear. It is considered a preventive procedure when used to treat narrow-angle glaucoma before an actual attack. Surgical iridectomies are rarely done today. The argon laser can also be used for a noninvasive procedure called a laser **trabeculoplasty.** Initially, an area covering approximately 180 degrees of the trabecular meshwork is treated. If pressure remains elevated, the remaining 180 degrees can be treated in a similar fashion. Frequently, the IOP increases after both types of laser surgery. The pressure is checked before the patient is released, approximately 1 to 2 hours after the procedure (Nowell, 1990).

Surgical *trabeculectomy* or filtration surgery may be required if other methods fail to control IOP. A portion of the trabecular meshwork is surgically incised to create an alternate drainage channel for the aqueous (Spires, 1991). This fistula then allows aqueous to be absorbed underneath the conjunctiva. Nursing interventions are those stated for intraocular surgery in Box 38-3, with an additional consideration: strict aseptic administration of eye drops is essential. The intraocular contents are now separated from external contamination by one layer, the conjunctiva, and bacteria have easier access to the inner eye. Complications of the procedure include a flat anterior chamber, soft eye, failure to filter, hyphema, endophthalmitis, cataract formation, and corneal decompensation. Failure to filter (drain) after the surgery has been attributable to scar tissue forming and blocking the site. Two antimetabolite drugs, mitomycin and 5-fluorouracil (5-FU), have been used to decrease the scarring, but dosage levels and administration techniques have not yet been established. Glaucoma implants to shunt aqueous from the anterior chamber to a disc sewn to the sclera are in the developing stages and are being used on some patients.

As a last resort for uncontrolled glaucoma, *cyclocryopexy* or cryosurgery is done. A freezing probe is used to destroy a portion of the ciliary body that produces the aqueous. Because of the tissue destruction, patients undergoing this procedure experience much pain. Treatment includes pain medication, steroids, and atropine.

Compliance with prescribed regimens is important to glaucoma patients, but it is difficult for many reasons: (1) daily drops do not improve existing vision; a patient who also has a cataract may experience decreased vision because of pupil constriction; (2) systemic medications have bothersome or toxic side effects; (3) drops may be difficult to administer because of physical limitations such as arthritis; and (4) treatment is a lifelong concern (Box 38-9).

## Cataract

A **cataract** is an opacity in the lens of the eye that may cause a loss of visual acuity and loss of the ability to function autonomously (Figure 38-22). The Agency for Health Care Policy and Research (AHCPR) describes functional impairment as a result of a cataract in the adult as the decreased ability to (1) perform everyday activities such as driving, using the phone, and taking medicine; (2) engage in hobbies and leisure activities such as reading and viewing television; and (3) work at one's occupation (Cataract Management Guideline Panel, 1993).

Because the lens focuses light rays on the retina, a clouding of this structure causes a painless loss of vision that can progress over time. Cataracts associated with the aging process are called *senile cataracts.* Other causes are congenital defects, intraocular infections, and trauma—surgical, blunt, or radiation. Factors that may influence formation of cataracts are diabetes, drugs, ultraviolet (UV) radiation, and nutritional deficiencies. Most cataracts are not visible to the naked eye until they become very dense, but an ophthalmoscopic examination or slit-lamp examination can detect the opacities at earlier stages (Ruehl, Schremp, 1992).

Symptoms of cataract formation include difficulty in reading, driving at night, and seeing well in bright light; increased sensitivity to glare; decreasing color vision; and double vision.

Diagnosis of cataract begins with a thorough patient history, including medical, surgical, and family history, as well as medications taken. The nurse should document allergies and when visual changes were first noted. The eye examination includes visual acuity tests for distance vision and near vision. Contrast sensitivity and glare disability may be assessed. However, the AHCPR panel believes that more research is necessary to corroborate the need for these tests (Cataract Management Guideline Panel, 1993). The direct ophthalmoscope and slit lamp are used to examine the lens and other structures in the eye so that the general health of the eye can be evaluated. If an intraocular lens implant is to be used to replace the natural lens, A-scan and keratometry are performed to determine the correct lens implant strength.

The cure for a cataract is surgical removal. Cataract extraction is not considered an emergency for the most part, and nonsurgical treatments can be tried. These may include stronger eyeglasses, magnification devices, and better illumination. The best judge for surgery is the patient, as well as quality-of-life issues as they relate to his or her visual and functional needs.

# NURSING PROCESS

## GLAUCOMA

**ASSESSMENT**

- Visual loss
- Loss of peripheral vision
- Level of comfort
- Ability to care for self

**NURSING DIAGNOSES**

- Sensory/perceptual alterations: visual related to disease process
- Anxiety related to possible loss of vision
- Self-care deficit related to decreased visual acuity
- Pain related to sudden increased intraocular pressure (IOP)
- Diversional activity deficit related to decreased vision
- Risk for injury (trauma) related to decreased vision
- Knowledge deficit related to new condition, treatment, and medications

**NURSING INTERVENTIONS**

- Listen actively to patient concerns.
- Help patient manage visual limitations.

- Assist with personal hygiene as indicated.
- Reduce clutter in the immediate environment.
- Administer medications as ordered.
- Provide analgesics as needed for acute glaucoma.
- Prepare patient for surgical intervention as indicated.
- Recommend that family members be examined regularly.

**EVALUATION OF EXPECTED OUTCOMES**

- Maintains current vision without further loss
- Expresses concerns and anxiety
- Verbalizes understanding of condition and treatment
- Demonstrates correct instillation of eye medications
- Able to care for self with assistance if necessary
- Exhibits safety measures in home environment
- Maintains acceptable level of comfort

## Cataract Surgery

Cataract surgery is usually performed on an outpatient basis except when there is a preexisting medical condition. Conditions requiring inpatient care include (1) surgery on the only eye, (2) mental disturbances, (3) physical disability preventing immediate postoperative care, and (4) a medical condition needing observation by a nurse or skilled professional. Most cataract surgery is performed with the patient under local anesthesia. However, general anesthesia is indicated in cases of extreme anxiety, a known allergy to local anesthetics, skeletal or other disorders preventing lying still, a language barrier, or inability to cooperate for other reasons (Cataract Management Guideline Panel, 1993).

There are two surgical types of cataract extraction: intracapsular and extracapsular. In intracapsular cataract extraction, the lens and surrounding capsular layer are removed intact. Approximately 98% of all cataract surgery is done by extracapsular extraction, and this procedure can be performed by either of two techniques: planned extracapsular cataract extraction or **phacoemulsification** (Ruehl, Schremp, 1992). In planned extracapsular extraction, the anterior portion of the capsule surrounding the lens is removed before

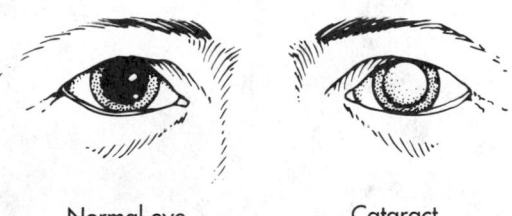

Normal eye          Cataract

**Figure 38-22**   Cataract, visible in left eye as white opacity of lens, is seen through pupil. (From Phipps WJ et al: *Medical-surgical nursing: concepts and clinical practice*, ed 5, St Louis, 1995, Mosby.)

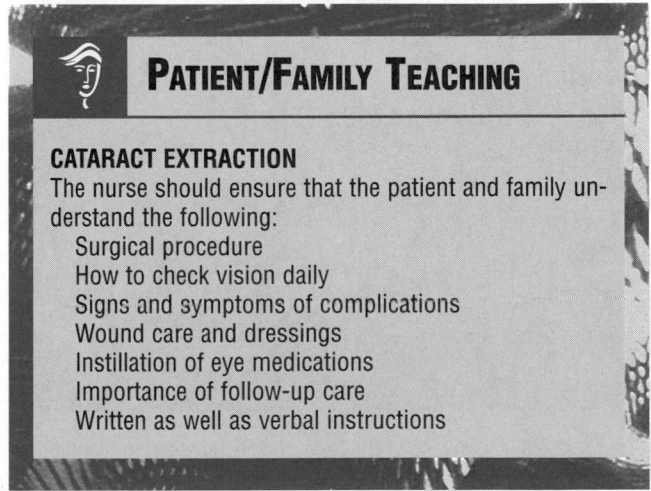

**PATIENT/FAMILY TEACHING**

**CATARACT EXTRACTION**
The nurse should ensure that the patient and family understand the following:
- Surgical procedure
- How to check vision daily
- Signs and symptoms of complications
- Wound care and dressings
- Instillation of eye medications
- Importance of follow-up care
- Written as well as verbal instructions

the lens nucleus is extracted. The cortex of the lens is then removed, leaving behind the posterior portion of the capsule. In phacoemulsification, the surgical incision is smaller because the lens nucleus is fragmented ultrasonically and irrigated and aspirated from the eye. The cortex is removed in a manner similar to extracapsular technique. The lens implant is placed in the posterior remnant of the capsule with either technique (Figures 38-23 and 38-24).

The normal eye is described as being phakic because it has a lens. When the lens is removed, the eye becomes *aphakic* (absence of lens) and cannot accommodate or refract light properly. Therefore a replacement lens is needed. Glasses or a contact lens can be used after cataract surgery, but the usual lens choice is the intraocular lens implant (IOL). With the IOL the eye is considered **pseudophakic** (having an artificial lens). Lens implants are manufactured from polymethylmethacrylate (PMMA), silicone, hydrogel, or acrylic material. They are designed in various sizes and shapes with structures to hold them in a stable posi-

tion within the eye (Ruehl, Schremp, 1992). The artificial lens is not able to accommodate (change focus) so glasses may still be needed by the patient to achieve the best near or distance vision. Most lens implants are placed in the posterior capsule today. However, anterior chamber lenses, those placed in front of the iris, are used in certain cases where support of the capsule is absent (Ruehl, Schremp, 1992).

Complications of cataract surgery include vitreous loss, inflammation, increased IOP, macular edema, retinal detachment, hyphema, endophthalmitis, and expulsive hemorrhage. After cataract surgery a patch and shield may be placed over the operative eye. Written instructions from the physician should be reviewed with the patient. Because depth perception is compromised, mobility guidance is needed.

Discharge instructions vary and may include leaving the dressing in place with a protective shield and avoiding strenuous activity. Reading should be avoided, but viewing television and eating moderately are allowed. The physician should be notified if the patient experiences any severe pain. Heavy lifting or straining, contact sports, and swimming are examples of activities to avoid. Lid hygiene should be done daily. Common sense instructions are to wash hands before and after drop/ointment instillation, avoid falling or bumping the eye, and wear sunglasses for glare or photophobia. The ophthalmologist examines the patient on the first postoperative day and at 1 week, 3 weeks, and 6 weeks after surgery unless there are complications. Total visual rehabilitation takes 6 to 12 weeks.

## Vitreous Pathologic Conditions

Normal vitreous can be observed by means of a slit-lamp examination. This transparent, colorless gel can become clouded with cell debris or membranes from acquired systemic diseases such as diabetes and hypertension. "Floaters" or "flashing lights" are often symptoms that a patient describes to the physician. This light flash is caused by cells floating across the pupillary space and casting a shadow on the retina. This can occur normally with age as the vitreous gel liquefies or as blood cells or pigments float into the gel. However, persistent floaters or showers of neon-type lights need to be evaluated for possible treatment (Vaughan, Asbury, Riordan-Eva, 1995). An immediate decrease in vision could be a symptom of vitreous hemorrhage, especially in patients with diabetic retinopathy. Inflammation or infection also can cause the vitreous to cloud.

*Endophthalmitis*, an extensive intraocular infection, may occur after penetrating injuries to the globe or as a postoperative complication of intraocular surgery. To properly diagnose and treat endophthalmitis, a vitreous tap is done to identify the cause of the infection.

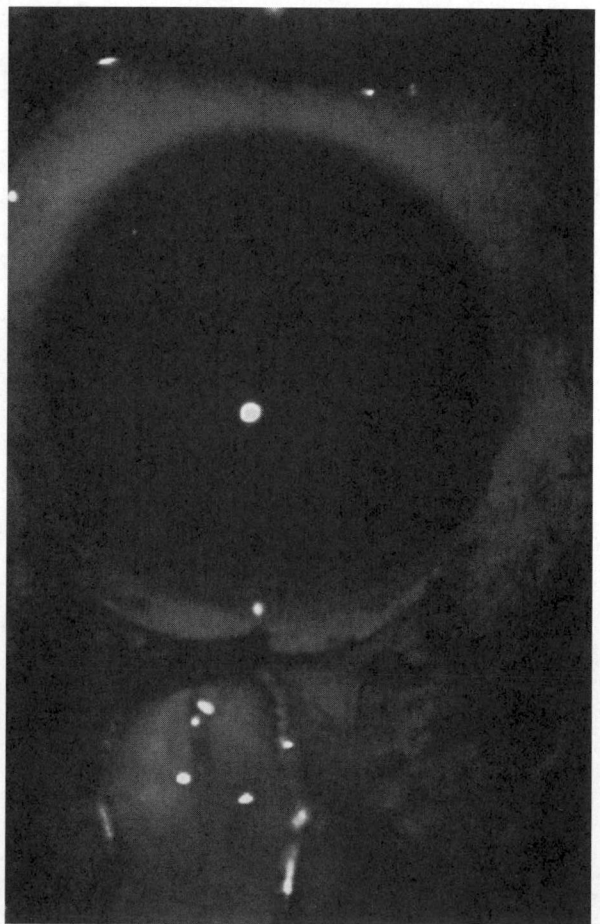

**Figure 38-23** Delivery of the lens nucleus as seen in planned extracapsular surgery. (Photo courtesy Dr JB Rubenstein, Chicago.)

Current treatment for endophthalmitis includes antibiotic therapy (systemic, intraocular, intravitreal, and topical), with or without **vitrectomy** (removal of diseased vitreous). Symptoms include pain and decreased vision, although pain is not always present. Signs are corneal haze, periorbital bruising, haze or cells in the anterior chamber, hypopyon (pus or cells in the anterior chamber), and decreased red reflex.

## Vitrectomy

Conditions for which vitrectomy may be necessary include endophthalmitis, vitreous hemorrhage, retinal membranes, cytomegalovirus (CMV) retinitis, and traction retinal detachment. It is also done in conjunction with scleral buckling for retinal detachment repair. In cases with dense vitreous opacities, B-scan ultrasonography can be used to locate membranes and intraocular foreign bodies, as well as normal vitreous and retinal structures.

Pars plana vitrectomy is a microscopic technique in which three incisions are made in the globe. One provides infusion to maintain the pressure within the eye, and the other two are for an illumination probe and the vitreous cutting instrumentation (Figure 38-25). Laser or cautery may also be used through one of these

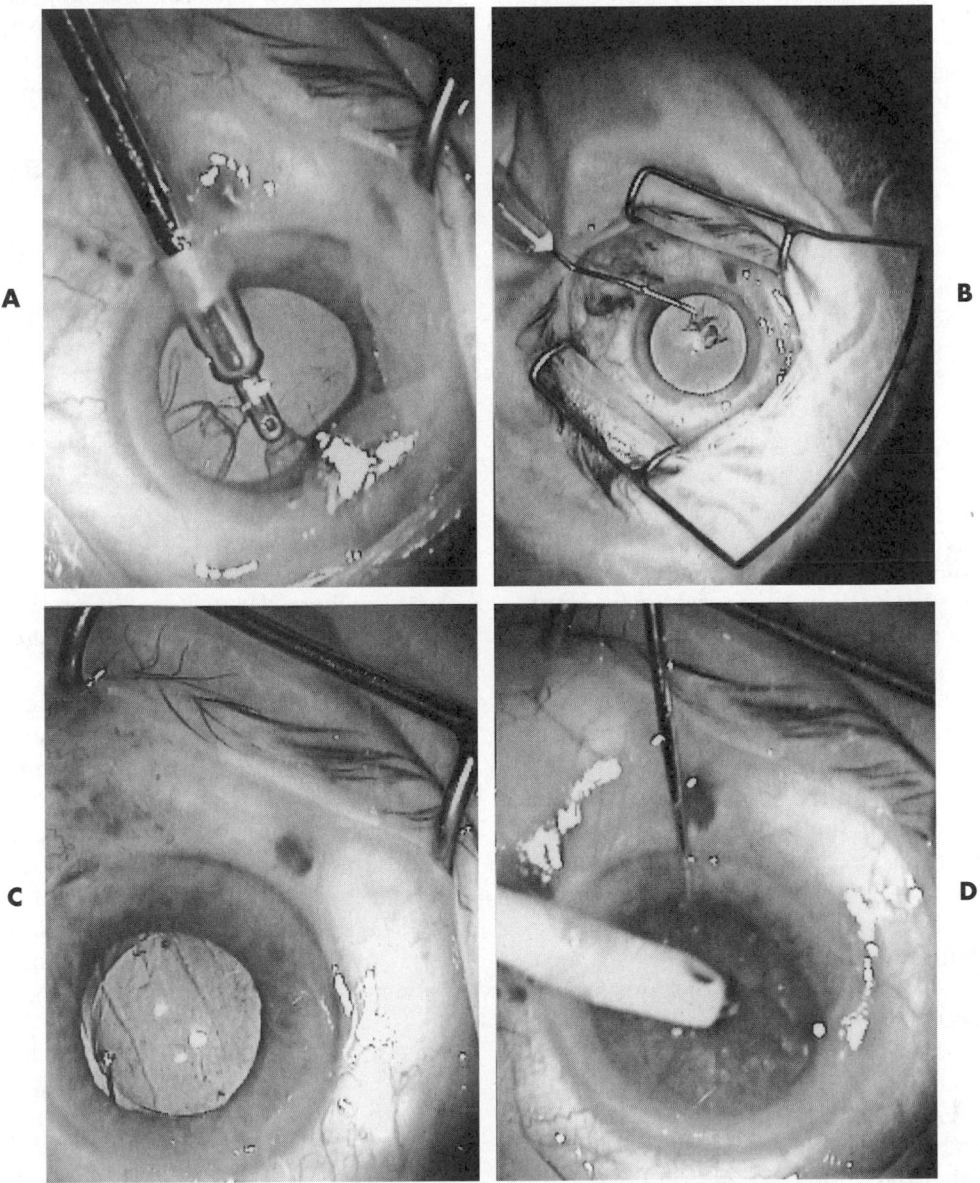

**Figure 38-24**   Phacoemulsification procedure with lens implantation. **A,** Incision into capsule of lens. **B,** Ultrasonic (phacoemulsification) removal of lens nucleus. **C,** Aspiration of lens cortex. **D,** Intraocular lens implant in position. (Photos courtesy Dr JB Rubenstein, Chicago.)

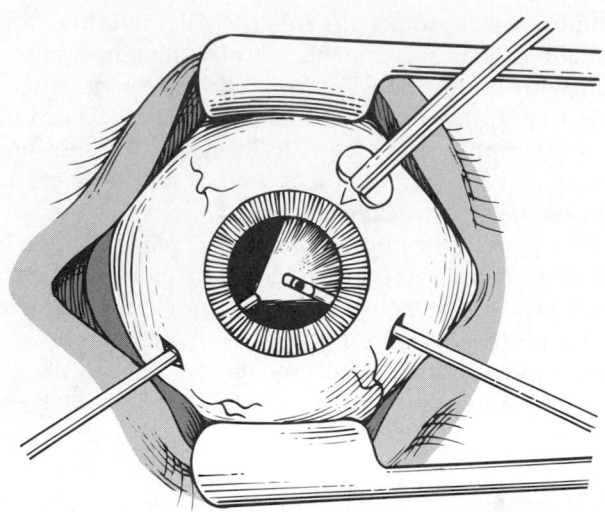

**Figure 38-25** The vitrectomy instrument and fiberoptic illuminator are positioned in the anterior vitreous cavity and visualized through the pupil.

incisions. Contact lenses are used on the cornea during the surgery to provide a better view of the inside of the eye. Air, surgical gases, or silicone oil can be instilled through the infusion port to provide pressure to the retina. Unlike air, some of these gases expand after a few days. Therefore IOP is carefully monitored during this time. Slowly the gases are resorbed and replaced by intraocular fluids. Changes in air pressure may influence the gas bubble, so flying in airplanes is to be avoided.

Vitrectomy patients may require a 23-hour observation period or hospitalization postoperatively. However, many patients go home the same day. Compromised health status because of systemic disease problems may necessitate preoperative as well as postoperative care, especially for patients with diabetes or hypertension. The ophthalmologist, internist, and anesthesiologist coordinate the plan of care to minimize the surgical risks. Patient education for activity, postoperative positioning, comfort (expectations relating to pain or nausea), and eye medication orders should be provided before surgery. It is important to support the patient emotionally and to allow him or her to express fears concerning visual prognosis.

Vitrectomy is an intraocular procedure (see Box 38-7). The eye is dilated preoperatively and kept dilated postoperatively. Other drops following surgery include an antibiotic/antiinflammatory medication. Patients with an air or gas bubble in the eye may need to position the head so that the bubble presses on the area of the retina that needs to be compressed. This may require prone position with the head down or turned to the side. While the patient is awake, the bedside table

can be used to help maintain this face-down position. A foam head donut provides additional comfort. Marking the eye shield with an arrow indicating the desired bubble position is also helpful. Ice packs can reduce some of the swelling. Additional considerations for vitreous surgery include medication for nausea and for pain caused by edema and increased pressure on the eye.

Strenuous activity is limited for 2 weeks. Driving a car is not allowed, but riding as a passenger is. A patch may be needed for comfort because of epiphora or photophobia. Dark glasses can be worn during the day to protect the eye, but the shield is preferable at night. Aching or cramplike pains may be common and can be relieved with a nonaspirin medication. Severe pain or change in vision needs to be reported to the physician. Lid hygiene can be followed (see Box 38-4). The visual acuity outcome depends on several factors. If the macula is involved, central vision is compromised.

## Retinal Pathologic Conditions

The entire retina can be visualized with the direct or indirect ophthalmoscope. Abnormalities of the vessels or retinal tissues can be seen, and systemic diseases often reveal themselves by producing characteristic changes in the retina. Treatment of the eye involves treatment of the underlying causes as well. The most common findings are complications related to diabetes mellitus and hypertension. Sickle cell disease, histoplasmosis, leukemia, lupus erythematosus, human immunodeficiency virus (HIV), and metastatic disease can be diagnosed by fundus examination. Abnormalities of the arteries and veins in the retina indicate disease elsewhere. The test for diagnosing retinal circulation abnormalities is called *intravenous fluorescein angiography* (Boyd-Monk, 1990).

*Diabetic retinopathy* is a progressive disease affecting the blood vessels in the retina. Initially, the blood vessels become more narrow and at times occlude. The narrowed vessels can develop aneurysms that can leak or rupture. New abnormal vessels grow to supply needed oxygen to the tissue, but these vessels also leak fluid. This continuing process results in decreased vision as a result of scar tissue formation. The amount of visual loss depends on the location of the disease (central versus peripheral vision) (Smith, 1992).

 **ETHNIC/CULTURAL CONSIDERATIONS**

African Americans and Hispanic Americans develop diabetes and hypertension more frequently than Caucasian Americans. Therefore they are at higher risk for diabetic retinopathy.

Patients who have had diabetes for 15 years or longer are more likely to develop diabetic retinopathy. Research reported by the American Diabetic Association indicates that diabetic persons are 25 times as likely to experience vision loss and blindness as the general population. Diabetic retinopathy is classified as *background diabetic retinopathy (BDR)* and *proliferative diabetic retinopathy (PDR)*. Microaneurysms, hard exudates, hemorrhages, and cotton-wool spots are signs of background diabetic retinopathy. The vision loss is a result of macular edema from the leaking vessels. In PDR, new blood vessels grow (neovascularization) to supply oxygen to the tissues. These new vessels grow over the macula and retinal surface. Fibrovascular tissue develops because of the continued leakage of blood from these vessels. These newly formed fibrous membranes are attached to the retina and to the posterior vitreous. The pulling of this scarlike tissue may cause a vitreous hemorrhage or a traction retinal detachment, which are the causes for vision loss in PDR.

Treatment for BDR is laser therapy on the specific leaking vessels to reduce the macular edema. This can be done with topical anesthesia only, and more than one treatment may be necessary. Panretinal photocoagulation (PRP), a therapeutic procedure involving scattered laser spots to the peripheral retina, is used for PDR. Local and topical anesthetics are necessary for this procedure (Smith, 1992; McEvoy, 1994), which helps stabilize vision if the neovascularization regresses. Vitrectomy surgery is recommended for longstanding vitreous hemorrhage, traction retinal detachment, or fibrous membranes pulling on the retina or vitreous. Persons with diabetes who experience vision loss as a result of diabetic retinopathy need a planned educational program to help manage their diabetes. With decreased vision, it is more difficult to monitor blood sugar and identify and administer their insulin. Methods for shopping, preparing meals, and instilling eye drops properly need to be individualized. Patient compliance and improved patient outcomes can be increased by appropriate nursing interventions. Patient understanding and knowledge, personal indepen-

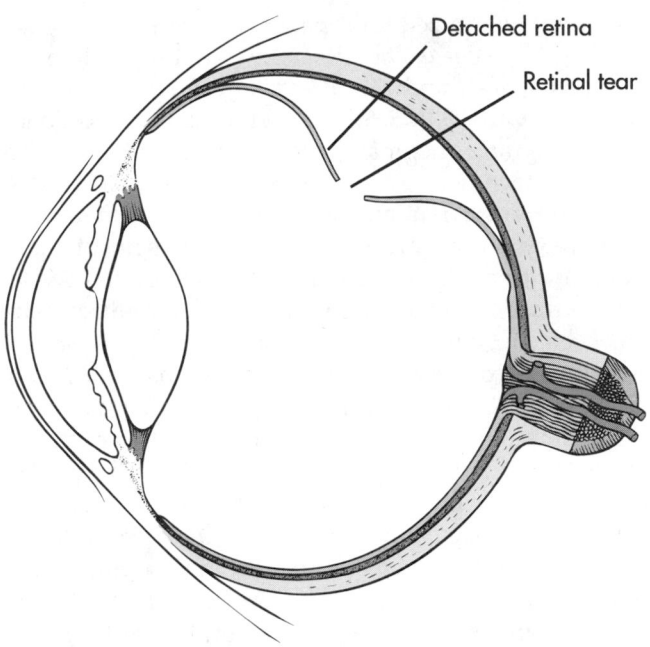

**Figure 38-26**   Retinal detachment. (From Phipps WJ et al: *Medical-surgical nursing: concepts and clinical practice*, ed 5, St Louis, 1995, Mosby.)

dence, and patient/family use of community resources are areas in which nurses and diabetes educators can collaborate to ensure the best overall health of the individual. A thorough eye examination by an ophthalmologist is recommended for people with type I or type II diabetes. This baseline evaluation can be used to monitor changes that may occur later. Routine yearly examinations are recommended unless vision changes noticeably (Smith, 1992).

## Retinal Detachment

A retinal detachment is a separation of the sensory retina from the pigmented layer with a subsequent subretinal fluid accumulation between the layers (Figure 38-26). Unless the retina is reattached, total blindness will develop. Predisposing factors include lattice degeneration, advanced myopia, cataract surgery, glaucoma, trauma, retinal detachment in the fellow eye, and a family history of retinal detachment.

Symptoms include a "shower" or "flashes" of light, floaters, or visual field defects. Vision is sometimes described as seeing through a veil or cobweb. The vision loss experienced depends on the location of the detachment. Peripheral vision is affected first, and then the central vision if the macula becomes involved. There can be one or more breaks or holes in the retina, and all breaks need to be found and repaired. Three

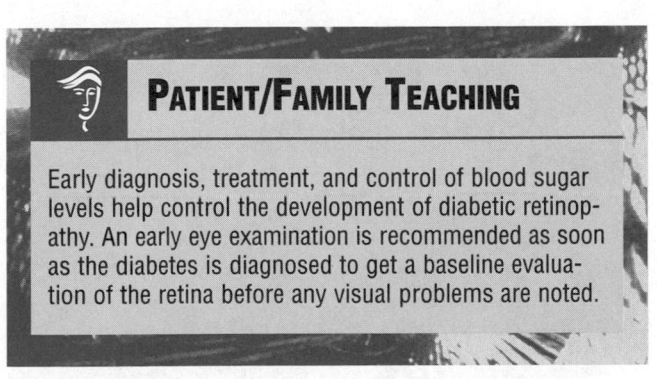

**PATIENT/FAMILY TEACHING**

Early diagnosis, treatment, and control of blood sugar levels help control the development of diabetic retinopathy. An early eye examination is recommended as soon as the diabetes is diagnosed to get a baseline evaluation of the retina before any visual problems are noted.

methods can be used for repair: (1) *scleral buckling* (Figure 38-27), (2) *pneumatic retinopexy* (injecting air into the vitreous space), and (3) *vitrectomy* (Vaughan, Asbury, Riordan-Eva, 1995). Scleral buckling is the traditional technique for a rhegmatogenous (break or hole in the retina) detachment. It is indicated for multiple breaks, lattice degeneration, and vitreous traction. Pneumatic retinopexy is not a procedure that requires hospitalization, but it has drawbacks in that it cannot be used to relieve traction of the vitreous or to repair multiple retinal breaks. However, with either technique—scleral buckling or pneumatic retinopexy—transconjunctival cryotherapy or laser is applied to the break or hole. Patient compliance is required for postoperative positioning of the air. Follow-up is required at 1, 2, and 4 weeks. Complications include recurrent detachment, increased IOP, more breaks, and endophthalmitis. Vitrectomy is used for complicated detachments, giant retinal tears, detachment as a result of macular holes, and vitreous traction with membranes. Other conditions that may require vitrectomy are recurrent detachments after scleral buckling and opacities in the vitreous.

Scleral buckling procedures can be done with local or general anesthesia. The physician locates the breaks in the retina by using the indirect ophthalmoscope, and cryotherapy is applied to the breaks and other areas of weakness. Various silicone implants are used to reattach the retina. These can be encircling bands to "belt buckle" the globe or radial components sewn to the sclera. Subretinal fluid that has collected may then

be drained through a small incision under the "buckle." Complications include redetachment, increased IOP, central retinal artery occlusion, deep sutures, choroidal detachment, infection, extrusion of the implant, and eye muscle disturbance. Prognosis for visual outcome is decreased if the macula is involved. When a patient has a retinal detachment and the macula is still attached, surgery is urgent if central vision is to be preserved. Follow-up examinations are scheduled for 1 week, 3 weeks, and 6 weeks postoperatively (Box 38-10).

## Macular Degeneration

Age-related macular degeneration (ARMD) is a disease associated with central vision loss that affects people 50 years and older. The two types of ARMD are dry (atrophic) and exudative (neovascular). Atrophic macular degeneration accounts for 70% to 90% of the cases (Vaughan, Asbury, Riordan-Eva, 1995). It is caused by a weakening and deterioration of the retinal cells and is seen as visible changes in the retina. Visual changes are variable and may be minimal. These changes may progress or stabilize. No treatment is available. Because the exudative stage can develop later, patients are advised to have their vision monitored with an Amsler grid (Boyd-Monk, 1990). Exudative macular degeneration accounts for 10% of the cases of ARMD but is responsible for 90% of all legal blindness as a result of ARMD. In exudative ARMD, abnormal blood vessels in the retina leak fluid, which results in scar tissue formation. This is followed by a proliferation of more abnormal new vessels (neovascularization). Early symptoms include difficulty with reading, blurred vision, and distortion of straight objects and straight lines. Eventually the entire central vision may be affected in one or both eyes. Peripheral vision, however, is not affected (Vader, 1997). Laser treatment of subretinal neovascularization in selected patients where the fovea is not involved has been done (Olk, 1992). Because this laser treatment itself destroys part of the retinal tissue, some central vision will be af-

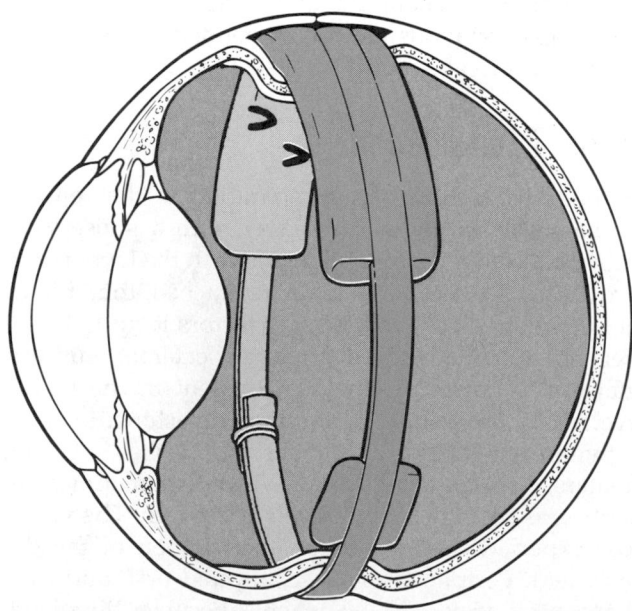

**Figure 38-27** Scleral buckle. (From Phipps WJ et al: *Medical-surgical nursing: concepts and clinical practice*, ed 5, St Louis, 1995, Mosby.)

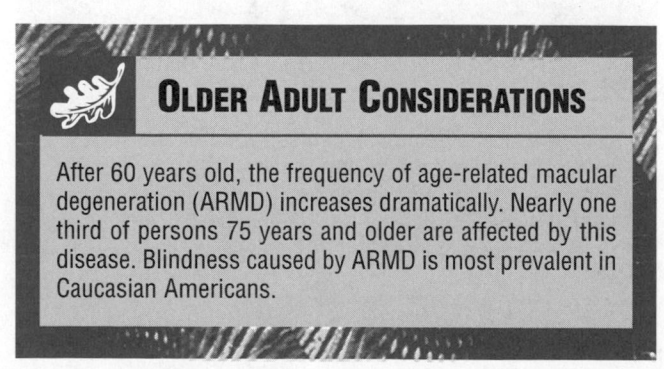

### OLDER ADULT CONSIDERATIONS

After 60 years old, the frequency of age-related macular degeneration (ARMD) increases dramatically. Nearly one third of persons 75 years and older are affected by this disease. Blindness caused by ARMD is most prevalent in Caucasian Americans.

fected. Even after successful therapy, recurrent neo-vascularization may develop within 2 years. Eventually many patients with exudative ARMD become legally blind and will need to alter their patterns and habits of daily living. Assessment of the patient's understanding and desire for help is essential for individualized care.

Low-vision referral and evaluation can help the patient use the remaining peripheral vision to the maximum. Recognizing that grieving over vision loss is a natural process, the nurse should encourage the patient to participate in support groups that include other members of the family, who also need help in coping with the loss (Woods, 1992). Low-vision care is available and needs to be a part of ophthalmic health care (Boxes 38-11 and 38-12). Centers designed for rehabilitation teach the patient how to maintain independence and function in activities of daily living. Special services are individualized to each patient. Optical and nonoptical aids are available. Mobility training, educational assessment, job rehabilitation, and counseling help the patient and the family to adjust to the vision loss. National, state, and local agencies provide special services. Catalogs and literature are available from the U.S. Department of Health and Human Services. Among the other agencies that provide resources are the American Foundation for the Blind, American Printing House for the Blind, Guide Dogs for the Blind, and Prevent Blindness America.

## Retinopathy of Prematurity

Retinopathy of prematurity (ROP), previously called retrolental fibroplasia (RLF), is a bilateral retinal disease that has been increasing. This is attributed to the increased survival rate of low-birth-weight (<1000 g) infants and the possibility that premature birth may trigger the onset of ROP (American Academy of Ophthalmology, 1994-95). Other factors may include high oxygen concentration and increased partial pressure of carbon dioxide ($PCO_2$) (Spires, 1991). Retinal vessels begin to develop at 16 weeks of gestation and are complete

---

### BOX 38-10 — NURSING PROCESS

## EXTRAOCULAR SURGERY (EYE MUSCLES, EYELIDS, ORBIT, LACRIMAL-DUCT PROBING, SCLERAL BUCKLING, ENUCLEATION)

**ASSESSMENT**

- Vital signs per routine
- Eye dressing
- Level of comfort
- Ability to care for self for signs of disorientation

**NURSING DIAGNOSES**

- Anxiety related to decreased vision, cosmesis, or surgical outcome
- Impaired physical mobility related to vision or postoperative positioning
- Risk for injury related to visual deficit and to decreased depth perception
- Knowledge deficit related to surgical repair and to activity restrictions
- Sensory/perceptual alterations: visual related to patching and ointment in the eye
- Risk for infection related to surgical procedure
- Pain related to light sensitivity and to the surgical procedure

**NURSING INTERVENTIONS**

- Listen actively to the patient's concerns.
- Provide information and reassurance.
- Position the patient according to physician's order.
- Ambulate patient with assistance.
- Speak slowly and clearly, and repeat if necessary.
- Protect the eye with a patch, if needed, to reduce lid edema, to contain drainage, or to shield the eye from light.
- Administer medications as ordered.
- Provide ice packs to reduce edema.
- Provide comfort measures.
- Dim the room lights if dilating drops are used.
- Provide light meals the first day.

**EVALUATION OF EXPECTED OUTCOMES**

- Meets discharge criteria for the postsurgical patient (see Box 20-10)
- Expresses fears and concerns
- Vision improved or maintained (not applicable for enucleation patients)
- Able to ambulate with help
- Uses other senses to avoid bumping eye when patched
- Verbalizes understanding of instructions
- Demonstrates ability to administer own medications
- Able to return to normal activity or has assistance until normal activity resumes
- Knowledgeable about modifications at home to enhance safety

---

### GUIDELINES FOR INTERACTING WITH VISUALLY IMPAIRED PERSONS

- When approaching, announce yourself each time and call the person by name. State the time of day if appropriate.
- Explain procedures before you begin. Do not touch the person before you speak.
- Let the person know when you are leaving so that the embarrassment of speaking when no one is present can be avoided.
- Remember that hearing is not impaired. Speak in a normal tone.
- When walking, the person grasps your arm and walks a half step behind you.
- Note obstacles on either side when walking.
- Before seating the person, place his or her hand on the back or arm of a chair. Stay nearby while the person sits down.
- At mealtime explain the menu. Arrange the food at clock hours. Explain the hot foods, and place them where they will not be spilled.
- In the hospital, orient the patient thoroughly to the environment. Note placement of furniture, phone, and call light.
- Place a sign on the door or over the bed indicating the person's visual status so that all personnel can approach correctly.

---

### HOME HELPS FOR VISUALLY IMPAIRED PERSONS

- Encourage family and friends to keep furniture and objects in the same place.
- Place food, cooking utensils, and supplies in specific locations in the refrigerator and cupboards.
- Place clothing in specific locations in the closets and drawers, or label with identifying or distinguishing marks.
- Arrange money in wallet compartments according to denomination, or fold different denominations in different ways.
- Investigate low-vision aids that may be of help, including magnifiers, large-print books and magazines, colored lenses, high-contrast paint, voice-activated phones, calculators, tapes, clocks, and watches. Also investigate special radio receivers that provide programming on a full range of subject matter, such as employment, news, business, and sports.

---

at 40 weeks. In a premature infant, an attempt to complete this vascularization process results in development of abnormal vessels. These vessels may then bleed and form scars, which may result in retinal detachment.

Careful screening for ROP in all premature infants should begin in the neonatal intensive care unit at 4 to 6 weeks after birth. Follow-up examinations are done every 2 weeks thereafter until the retina is fully vascularized. Most early stages of ROP resolve spontaneously. Cryotherapy is used to help regress the proliferation of abnormal vessels that cause retinal detachment, and some of the newer treatments for ROP show some promise. A study is being done to evaluate the effectiveness of indirect laser photocoagulation as a treatment alternative to cryotherapy. Repair of total retinal detachment through a vitrectomy approach is becoming more successful, and studies show that early cryotherapy reduces the rate of retinal detachment. Parent education while the infant is hospitalized is most important. ROP can lead to blindness, and there is a high risk for myopia, amblyopia, strabismus, glaucoma, and cosmetic defects. Parents need to know early in the premature infant's life that appropriate follow-up by an ophthalmologist gives the infant the best chance for visual rehabilitation.

## Ocular Malignancies

Although it is rare and affects relatively few people, *choroidal melanoma* is the most common adult primary intraocular tumor. It is found mostly in patients between 53 and 60 years, but it has been documented in teens and older adults (Servodidio, Abramson, 1992). Symptoms include blurring of vision, defects in the visual field, "floaters," pain, or "flashing" of light. Decrease in visual acuity and defects in the visual field are the most common presenting signs. The size of the tumor is determined by A-scan ultrasonography and fundus examination. After the diagnosis has been made, a metastatic workup that includes a liver scan is done to determine whether the disease has spread into the orbit or through the sclera into the blood. Treatment options include enucleation, radiation, or radioactive plaque therapy. Follow-up is required every 6 to 12 months for life (Servodidio, 1991). Teaching aids to demonstrate the location of the tumor inside the eye can also be used to explain the plaque placement if that is the treatment used. Ocular prostheses should be available to show patients if they so desire. Written postoperative instructions that can be individualized need to be used in conjunction with the verbal teaching plan.

## Retinoblastoma

The most common childhood intraocular tumor is retinoblastoma (1 per 17,000 live births). Most cases appear by the age of 3 years, and the tumor can affect one or both eyes. A parent who has the disease has a 50% chance of having an affected child. The most obvious sign is the characteristic "cat's eye reflex," a bright reflection from the pupil. Other signs are strabismus, tearing, inflammation, pain, and poor vision. A metastatic workup should follow a positive diagnosis. Treatment includes enucleation, external beam radiation, or irradiation plaque therapy. Vision prognosis in the fellow eye is excellent. Discharge planning involves teaching the parent how to care for the enucleation site by maintaining lid hygiene and instilling ointment or drops. Follow-up appointments are essential for evaluating a recurrence. Support groups and counseling help the parents to deal with guilt feelings associated with the disease, and genetic counseling can be suggested (Servodidio, 1993). Changes in the visual fields of successfully treated retinoblastoma patients can challenge the child's ability to keep up in school. With limited peripheral vision, reading can be a problem. Maximizing available vision helps the child cope with daily activities, school, and sports in ways that maintain safety.

## Eye Conditions Associated with Human Immunodeficiency Virus

Infectious or noninfectious ocular conditions develop in 75% of persons with HIV (Plona, Schremp, 1992). Kaposi's sarcoma, which produces lesions on the eyelids and conjunctiva, is not infectious. Non-Hodgkin's lymphoma and HIV retinopathy also are considered noninfectious. Keratitis, particularly that caused by herpes simplex or herpes zoster, is one of the opportunistic infections that develop because AIDS patients are immunosuppressed.

*Cytomegalovirus (CMV) retinitis* is a sight-threatening infectious disease involving the retina. It usually begins in one eye but progresses to the other. Characteristic granular spots are evident in the retina. These spots enlarge, denoting retinal necrosis and vision loss. Current treatments for CMV retinitis are ganciclovir and trisodium phosphonoformate through a central venous line to provide a therapeutic dose to the retina. Both drugs are available for oral as well as parental administration and are monitored for bone marrow toxicity. A method for dispensing ganciclovir directly into the vitreous cavity has been developed. This requires a surgical procedure (a limited vitrectomy) and implantation of a disc with time-released medication into the eye (Figure 38-28). This allows the patient to remain on oral medication for other AIDS-related problems. It also helps the patient with quality of life issues relating to life-style and independence with a venous access line in place. These include difficulties with the

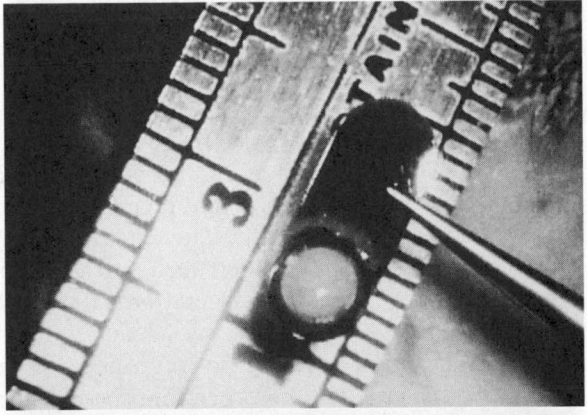

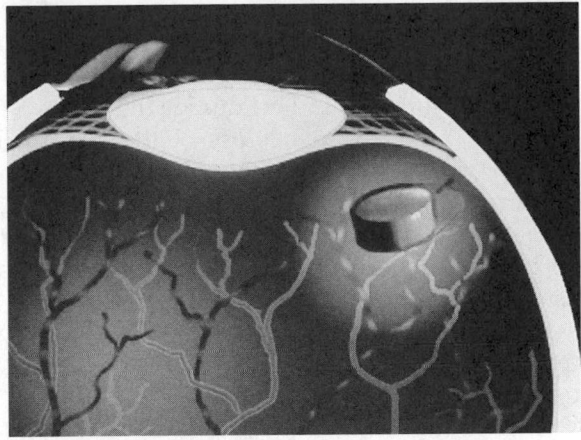

**Figure 38-28     A,** Ganciclovir (Vitrasert) implant. **B,** Ganciclovir (Vitrasert) implant within the eye for treatment of cytomegalovirus (CMV) retinitis. (**A** courtesy Dr Jack A Cohen, Chicago; **B** courtesy Chiron Vision Corp.)

catheter remaining patent, the risk of infection, limited mobility, and adherence to a strict time schedule. This drug implant therapy lasts 6 to 8 months and is more cost effective than providing therapeutic ocular levels by other means. Replacing the implant does require another surgery. (This implant technology has opened the door for developing similar treatment for other ocular conditions.) When medical therapy fails, a total vitrectomy procedure with silicone oil injection may be needed to treat retinal detachment caused by this virus (Martin et al, 1994; Spector, 1996). (See also Chapter 16 on HIV infections and AIDS.)

Treatment for Kaposi's sarcoma may be indicated for cosmesis or to allow better closing of the eyelids. Other treatment includes radiation or injection of chemotherapeutic drugs into the lesion.

Knowledge of ocular manifestations of AIDS and the treatment protocols will help in the total care of the AIDS patient. Nurses also should encourage patients to maintain their independence for as long as possible by using the resources available for educating low-vision persons and their families (Plona, Schremp, 1992).

## Enucleation

Indications for surgical removal of the eyeball (enucleation) include severe trauma; malignant tumors; a painful, blind eye; and cosmesis. The surgery may involve the entire eye and related structures or only the contents of the eyeball (evisceration). Before the surgery takes place, the patient's knowledge of the diagnosis and treatment needs to be confirmed. Discussion of the permanence of the procedure should be accompanied by an explanation of the postoperative appearance, orbital implant, prosthesis, and the fitting procedure. A sympathetic, understanding approach is essential. The nurse should encourage questions. Self-concept will be changed by loss of the eye, so the grieving process is normal in these individuals. However, in cases in which the eye has caused severe pain, the patient may look forward to the relief provided by this surgery. Immediate postoperative care includes a pressure dressing for 24 hours. The patient should be assessed for pain or hemorrhage, and if anticoagulants are part of the patient's preoperative routine, they are

withheld during the immediate postoperative period. Excessive coughing and sneezing should be avoided. Ice packs may be applied to reduce swelling and pain.

When the eye socket has healed (2 to 6 weeks), the patient is fitted with a prosthesis (Figure 38-29). The prosthetic eye shell is made to fit over the ball implant that was surgically placed under the conjunctiva and Tenon's layer of the orbit. The prosthetic eye is made of plastic and is fitted and crafted by an oculist to match the iris, sclera, and veins of the other eye. Plastic is preferred to glass because it is more durable and lasts longer. Care, cleaning, insertion, and removal instructions need to be given to the patient. If the prosthesis needs to be stored, it should be stored in saline. For routine cleaning of surface deposits, use a mild soap or toothpaste and fingers. Avoid a brush or cloth that may damage the surface. Heavier deposits on the surface can cause lid irritation. They can be removed by soaking in a denture cleaner for 20 minutes, followed by rinsing thoroughly in water. This can be done every 6 to 8 weeks as needed (American Society of Ophthalmic Registered Nurses, 1996).

Occasionally, people with artificial eyes will complain of a dry eye, which can be treated with artificial tears or lubricant. The following points should be reinforced with the patient:

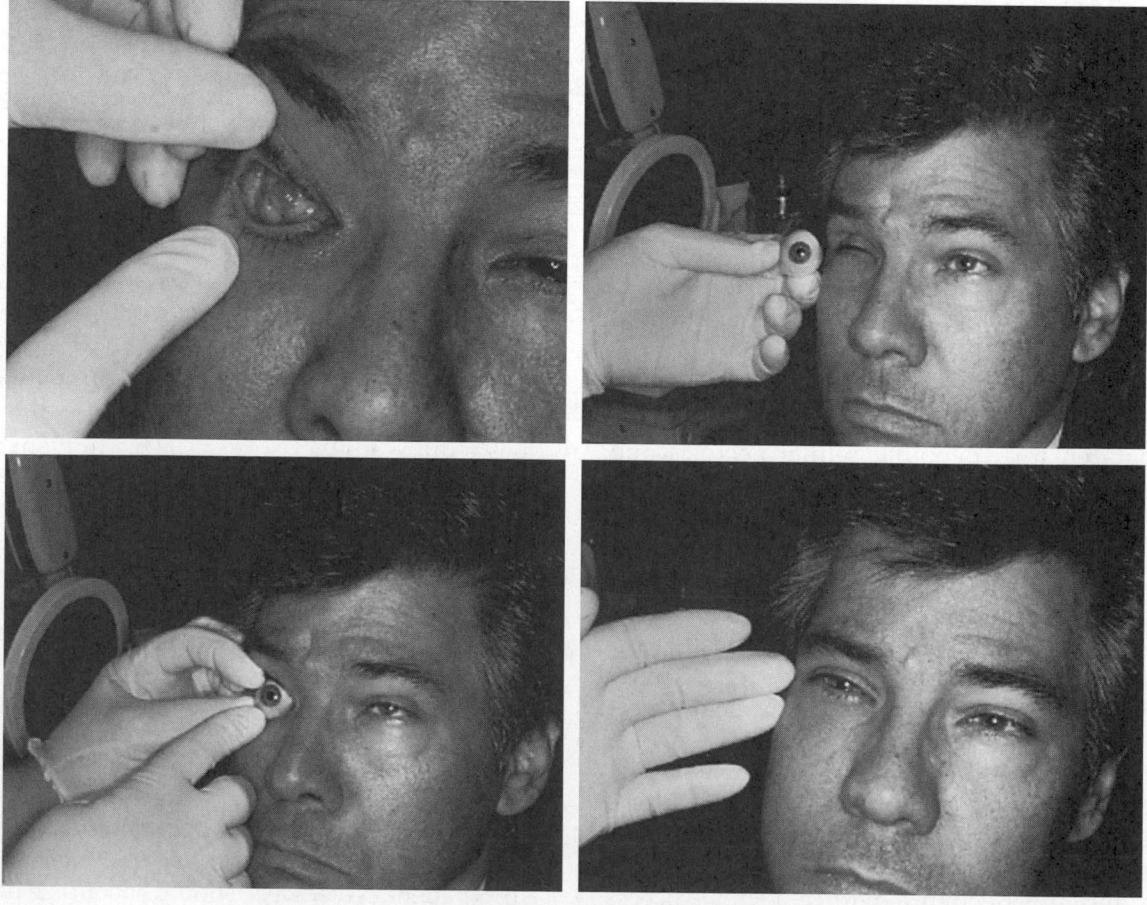

**Figure 38-29**   Artificial eye placement.

1. When wiping the eye, wipe toward the nose with the eyes closed; this procedure prevents the prosthesis from dislodging.
2. Alcohol, ether, chloroform, and other abrasive agents can damage the prosthetic eye.
3. When participating in water sports, the eyes should be protected with goggles, or the prosthesis should be removed.
4. The remaining seeing eye should be protected with safety devices, such as safety glasses, even if no eyeglass correction is needed.
5. At yearly visits to the oculist, the cells and protein build-up on the artificial eye can be cleaned.

Vision loss is more than just loss of sight. Body image, loss of a familiar life-style, occupational considerations, and financial concerns need to be addressed. Learning to live with the loss requires adjusting and adapting.

## Lid Disorders and Defects

*Marginal blepharitis* is a chronic inflammatory process involving the margin of both eyelids and may be caused by bacteria, allergy, or degenerative diseases. The most common type of blepharitis is seborrheic. The patient often has a history of a similar scalp condition commonly known as dandruff, and the skin and scalp are often excessively oily. The first symptoms of the eyelids may be itching and burning. The lids are red and inflamed, with fine crustlike scales at the base of the eyelashes. Ulceration of the lids may develop. Treatment consists of application of warm, moist compresses and lid scrubs to remove the crusts. Medications, such as sulfacetamide ointment, may be prescribed for bedtime application in patients susceptible to the disease. Cleanliness of the hair, skin, and scalp is important in controlling the disease. Severe lid infections (cellulitis) require systemic antibiotics to prevent spread of the infection into the orbit and then to the brain.

*Blepharospasm* is the involuntary spasm of the eyelid. It usually occurs bilaterally and is most common in elderly persons. Although the cause is not known, it can be made worse by fatigue or emotional stress. Rest and biofeedback are recommended initially. Treatment for persistent cases includes a botulinum A toxin injection to paralyze the lid muscle. Severe cases may need surgical intervention.

A *sty* (external hordeolum) is an infection of Moll's gland as a gland of Zeis in the eyelid. An internal hordeolum is an infection of a meibomian gland. Sties are characterized by a small, inflamed swelling at the edge of the eyelid. As the swelling increases, the sty may rupture spontaneously and drain, after which healing occurs. *Staphylococcus* is often the causative organism, and systemic antibiotic therapy may be necessary. The condition can become chronic, and some cases require incision and drainage.

*Chalazion* is a sterile, granulomatous inflammation of a meibomian gland. It is found in the upper and lower eyelids and begins with an inflammation and tenderness. It does not have the acute signs of inflammation seen in a sty. The most common symptom is a painless swelling that develops over several weeks. In the early stages, warm, moist compresses may help reduce the inflammation. Antibiotics or steroids also may be injected into the lesion. Chalazions may need to be removed surgically, and any recurrences need to have biopsies performed to rule out malignancy.

*Anatomic lid defects* have the potential to interfere with vision. Turning in of the lid (*entropion*) can be the result of aging, scar formation, or a congenital defect. Surgery is needed to prevent corneal irritation and damage caused by the lashes rubbing over the corneal surface. Turning out or sagging of the lid (*ectropion*) is also common in older people and is corrected by shortening the lower lid. Patients with this defect experience symptoms of exposure keratitis, tearing, and irritation. *Ptosis*, or drooping of the upper eyelid, can be congenital or acquired. The lid droop associated with myasthenia gravis can be diagnosed with the edrophonium (Tensilon) test. Surgery can correct either congenital or acquired ptosis. Postoperative care includes ice compresses to decrease swelling and antibiotic ointment to prevent infection and to keep the cornea moist.

## Lacrimal System Disorders

Dry-eye syndrome (*keratoconjunctivitis sicca*) is the result of abnormalities of the tear film, eyelid surface, or corneal surface. Patients complain of a foreign-body sensation, itching, unusual mucous secretion, and burning. This condition is often associated with rheumatoid arthritis and autoimmune diseases. Schirmer's test is done to assess tear production. Punctal occlusion, temporary or permanent, may be done to keep tears in the conjunctival sac. *Punctal obstruction* can be a congenital defect or the result of scarring as a result of infections, topical medications, or systemic chemotherapy. Blockage of the tear ducts causes a slight discharge and irritation of the eye. Patency needs to be established for normal tear flow. Dacryocystitis is an infection of the lacrimal sac. It can be the result of chronic infection, trauma, or a stone in the duct. Symptoms are purulent discharge and tearing (epiphora). Acute cases are treated with systemic antibiotics. Chronic cases may require surgery in which an opening is made between the lacrimal sac and the nose (Vaughan, Asbury, Riordan-Eva, 1995).

## EYE EMERGENCIES AND TRAUMA

It is important to know which eye emergencies and trauma need immediate or urgent treatment and which ones can be referred. Treatment for chemical burns and sudden painless loss of vision should be assessed within minutes to preserve sight. Chemical burns should be irrigated immediately with copious amounts of water or noncaustic liquids such as milk for 15 to 20 minutes. The patient can then be transferred to a physician's office or emergency room. Here the injury and visual acuity are assessed and testing for the type of chemical is done with litmus paper. More irrigating solution will be used. To prevent injury to the other eye, the head should be turned toward the affected eye (Figure 38-30 and Box 38-13). Other treatment includes cycloplegic medication, steroids, and antibiotics. To prevent *sudden vision loss* as a result of an occlusion of the central retinal artery, attempts to vasodilate the patient's retinal circulation should be made. Vasodilation can be accomplished by rebreathing into a paper bag, increasing the carbon dioxide level to help dilate the vessels. Also, intermittent pressure on the globe for several seconds with sudden releasing of the fingers may alter the IOP enough to dislodge the embolus. The chance of restoring sight is negligible after 30 minutes. For other eye emergencies treated in the office or emergency room, the first step is to assess the visual acuity of the injured eye. Although the patient may not want to cooperate,

it is essential for medical and legal reasons. The actual ability to see may allay the anxiety related to the injury. Both eyes should be tested and the visual acuity before the accident documented.

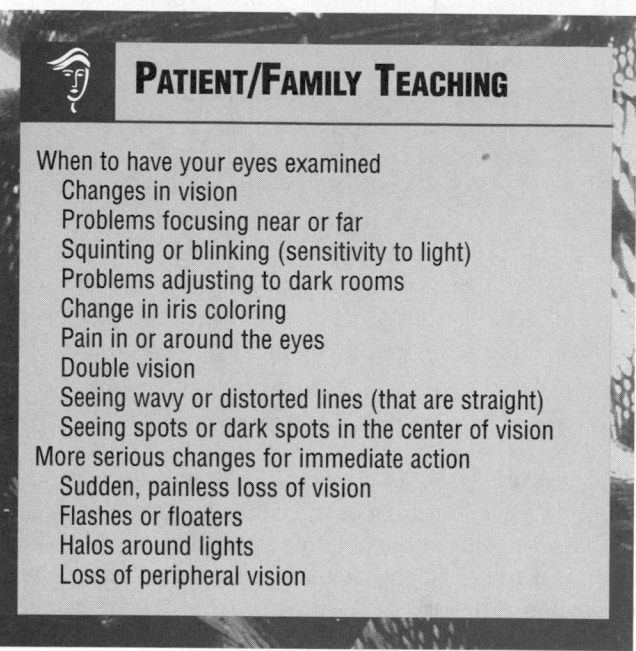

**PATIENT/FAMILY TEACHING**

When to have your eyes examined
    Changes in vision
    Problems focusing near or far
    Squinting or blinking (sensitivity to light)
    Problems adjusting to dark rooms
    Change in iris coloring
    Pain in or around the eyes
    Double vision
    Seeing wavy or distorted lines (that are straight)
    Seeing spots or dark spots in the center of vision
More serious changes for immediate action
    Sudden, painless loss of vision
    Flashes or floaters
    Halos around lights
    Loss of peripheral vision

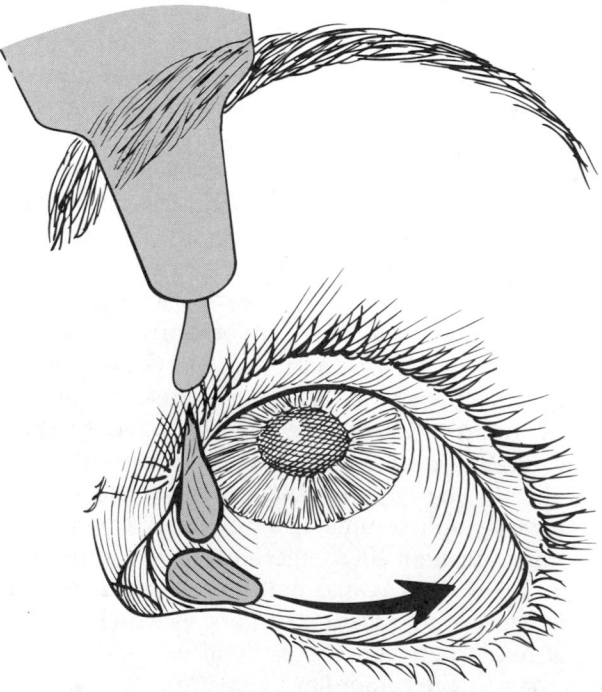

**Figure 38-30** Irrigating the eye. Fluid is directed along conjunctiva and over eyeball from inner to outer canthus. (From Long BC, Phipps WJ, Cassmeyer VL: *Medical-surgical nursing: a nursing process approach,* ed 3, St Louis, 1993, Mosby.)

**BOX 38-13**

**EYE IRRIGATION FOR CHEMICAL INJURIES (TRAUMA)**

1 Assemble equipment necessary, including 1000 ml IV irrigating solution (normal saline, lactated Ringer's, or balanced salt), IV tubing, lid retractors, cotton applicators, and topical anesthesia per physician or ER standing protocol.
   NOTE: Water is the most available fluid and should be used initially if other solutions are not readily available.
2 Position patient in a reclining position with head turned toward affected side.
3 Place a towel or kidney basin near the lateral canthus.
4 Hold the eye open if necessary. NOTE: Often the patient cannot hold the eye open because of severe pain.
5 Direct the flow of irrigating solution from nasal to temporal side of eye (inner to outer canthus).
6 If both eyes are affected, irrigate them alternately. Have a second liter of fluid available. Use 1000 ml of solution for each eye.
7 Have patient evaluated by an ophthalmologist.

Sudden vision loss as a result of *angle-closure glaucoma* or *temporal arteritis* needs to be treated within hours. In addition to decreased vision, the patient with angle-closure glaucoma will have pain, headache, and vomiting as a result of increased IOP.

> **NURSE ALERT**
>
> Eye injuries caused by the rapid deployment of automobile air bags and their contents include chemical and blunt trauma to the eye. Reported injuries are corneal burns or abrasions, orbital fractures, intraocular hemorrhages, dislocated lens, cataract formation, and retinal detachment.

*Lacerations* and *rupture of the globe* need to be evaluated by the ophthalmologist. No one should attempt to remove a protruding foreign object from the globe or apply pressure to the globe. A protective shield made from a cup or box can be used to protect the eye from further injury during transport to a medical facility. The fellow eye should be patched to decrease movement of both eyes with this type of injury. The patient needs to be instructed not to eat or drink anything until he or she is seen by the physician. Immediate surgery may be necessary to repair the eye. The incidence of infection is high, and extensive trauma may require enucleation.

*Blunt trauma* to the eye is evaluated by x-ray or other radiographic tests to rule out orbital fractures. The shock wave created by the trauma may have caused internal damage to the eye. This trauma includes hyphema, vitreous hemorrhage, and retinal detachment (Vaughan, Asbury, Riordan-Eva, 1995).

*Corneal abrasions* and *foreign bodies* cause significant discomfort to the patient in the form of pain, photophobia, *epiphora,* and conjunctival redness. Fluorescein dye is used to evaluate abrasions. Because this dye stains contact lenses, they should be removed before the dye is used. Foreign bodies often can be removed with a small needle or instrument after the cornea is anesthetized. The eyelids are everted and inspected when foreign objects are present (see Box 38-6). Treatment includes antibiotic drops, a pressure patch, and often a cycloplegic agent. The unconscious patient is at greater risk for corneal damage when the eyelids do not close properly. Within hours the patient can develop necrosis and permanent scarring. Closing the lids and applying lubricants decrease this danger.

*Lid lacerations* need to be treated in the same way as lacerations elsewhere. The lids are vascular and bleed freely. Foreign material in the wound needs to be debrided before repair is done. If the lid injury is on the nasal side, injury of the tear duct system should be evaluated. Other structures that may be injured are the lacrimal gland and levator muscle of the lid. Realignment of tissues in lid margin lacerations prevents a "notched" appearance of the lid. Postoperative treatment includes antibiotic ointment, patching, and ice to decrease swelling. If indicated, a tetanus injection may be given.

*Swollen lids* can be an indication of *orbital cellulitis,* or inflammation of the fatty tissue of the orbit. The patient may have a history of blunt trauma, dental infection, or sinusitis. Hospitalization and intravenous therapy with a broad-spectrum antibiotic are required to prevent the infection from traveling through the orbit into the brain, where it can cause meningitis or a brain abscess.

## EYE SAFETY

Eye safety needs to be everyone's concern. Nurses can provide vital information for prevention of eye injuries. Figures reported by Prevent Blindness America (PBA) indicate that 2 to 3 million people every year have an eye injury. It is estimated that 90% of these are preventable and that 45% occur around the home (Berlew, 1991). Prevention is the most effective way to save sight, and identifying potential hazards in the environment is the first requirement. Infants and children—more boys than girls—sustain more injuries than adults, and toys are a frequent cause of their injuries. Sharp, pointed toys or those with projectiles are the most dangerous to the child and other playmates. BB guns and pellet rifles cause irreparable damage (Hunt, 1993b). Sports-related injuries can be reduced by use of protective goggles or sunglasses. Children engaged in contact sports should wear helmets and face protection. If sight in one eye has been lost, eyeglasses with high impact–resistant prescription or nonprescription safety lenses are recommended at all times to protect the remaining eye.

Chemicals in the home are dangerous for infants, children and adults. Dangerous substances should be kept out of the reach of infants and children. Protective glasses should be worn when using chemicals, painting, or plastering. Contact lenses can trap chemicals under them, and mixing cleaning products can produce toxic gases. Steam from cooking can burn the cornea as well as the face. Bags of microwave popcorn have been reported to cause injury. Aerosols contain chemicals that are harmful to the eyes. Power tools, weed whackers, and lawn mowers can project rocks and other debris into the eyes. Ultraviolet (UV) light from the sun, sun lamps, or arc welding can cause symptoms similar to corneal abrasions. UV exposure also has been associated with cataract formation (Hunt, 1993; Vaughan, Asbury, Riordan-Eva, 1995).

In the workplace and schools, safety eyewear should be worn if there is a possibility of flying debris, chemical injury, or radiation exposure. Health care personnel need to shield their eyes from biohazards when giving patient care. Contact lenses should be avoided in areas of intense heat, flying debris, chemical fumes, and molten metal. Special eyewash stations need to be accessible to everyone in hazardous environments. To avoid injury from sparks or battery acid explosions, protective goggles should be worn when repairing cars. Fireworks should be avoided. Over 15,000 eye injuries per year are caused by fireworks, and 60% of these injuries affect children. PBA figures indicate that 40% of the injuries result in permanent damage to the eye (Berlew, 1991). Seventy-five percent of all fireworks injuries are caused by bottle rockets (Hunt, 1993b).

## NORMAL AGING AND THE EYE

Because Americans are living longer, health care providers can expect to see more of the normal vision changes associated with advanced age, as well as pathologic changes. Loss of vision in elderly persons can be caused by cataracts, glaucoma, macular degeneration, or diabetic retinopathy, but poor vision should not be equated with the aging process (Hunt, 1993a). A normal decrease in visual acuity is attributed to diminished elasticity of the lens and the muscles in the ciliary body, both of which affect accommodation. This change occurs at varying rates and times for different people, but it usually becomes noticeable in people who are in their 40s and tends to increase in those who are 50 to 59 years of age before it stabilizes (Vaughan, Asbury, Riordan-Eva, 1995). Other causes for decreased vision are a reduction in the function of the rods and cones, cataract formation, or a miotic pupil. To help improve vision, bifocal glasses, magnifiers, large print books, and easily brightened lighting sources (three-way) can be used. Visual-field loss can be caused by a miotic pupil, lid relaxation, or a decrease in the amount of orbital fat. People who notice this problem should exercise greater caution while driving and crossing streets. Turning the head instead of just moving the eyes will help, as will using the senses of touch and hearing to compensate for the reduced peripheral vision.

Yellowing of the lens and cornea and a decrease in cone function make colors seem less bright and affect depth perception. To offset this deficit, warmer colors can be used. Reds and yellows are seen better. The first and last stair can be painted a lighter color for better

visibility, and all stairways should have handrails. Night-vision impairment, dark-adaptation time, and glare problems increase with age because a slowing retinal metabolism and miotic pupil provide less light to the retina. Flat paint on surfaces decreases glare. Sunglasses should be used during the day, and looking directly into car headlights at night should be avoided. Sources of indirect lighting in the home should be positioned appropriately (Woods, 1992).

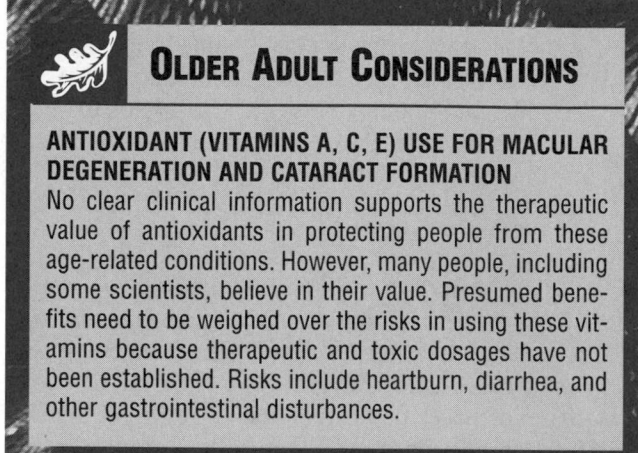

**OLDER ADULT CONSIDERATIONS**

**ANTIOXIDANT (VITAMINS A, C, E) USE FOR MACULAR DEGENERATION AND CATARACT FORMATION**
No clear clinical information supports the therapeutic value of antioxidants in protecting people from these age-related conditions. However, many people, including some scientists, believe in their value. Presumed benefits need to be weighed over the risks in using these vitamins because therapeutic and toxic dosages have not been established. Risks include heartburn, diarrhea, and other gastrointestinal disturbances.

Vitreous "floaters" or "spots" occur more often in myopic people. As the vitreous liquefies with age, the frequency can increase. A retinal evaluation is advised if the amount and frequency increase noticeably. Tear quality and quantity decrease, and this causes problems associated with dry eyes (Gilchrist, Hunt, 1993). Artificial tears and lubricants to ease this problem are available commercially. The skin of the eyelid thins and loses elasticity, which may cause the eyelid to droop. No treatment is indicated unless symptoms interfere with vision or the person desires cosmetic surgery.

The American Academy of Ophthalmology recommends that adults 65 years and older have an eye examination every 2 years or sooner with certain risk factors. Reasonably good vision can be expected as people age, and nurses can educate older people to seek early diagnosis and treatment so that their quality of life as it relates to vision can be preserved.

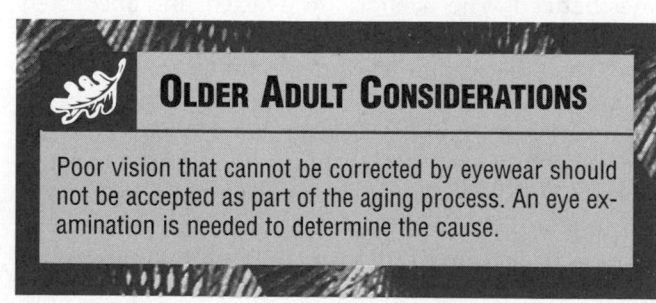

**OLDER ADULT CONSIDERATIONS**

Poor vision that cannot be corrected by eyewear should not be accepted as part of the aging process. An eye examination is needed to determine the cause.

# NURSING CARE PLAN

## PATIENT WITH PROLIFERATIVE DIABETIC RETINOPATHY SURGERY SCHEDULED: VITRECTOMY, MEMBRANECTOMY

The patient is a 54-year-old, insulin-dependent man who has had laser therapy on both eyes for his diabetic retinopathy. His right eye has progressed to blindness because of complications after cataract surgery. Now he has experienced a vitreous hemorrhage in his left eye. His vision has returned to counting fingers (CF) at 2 feet.

The patient is a slightly overweight, middle-aged man who has been on disability and supplemental social security insurance (SSSI) benefits because of his visual problems. He lives with his wife, who works during the day but is able to help with his insulin preparation. He is able to feed and dress himself and maintain his hygiene. He needs assistance in meal preparation, climbing stairs to the bedroom, shopping, and keeping doctors' appointments and social activities.

His ophthalmic examination revealed that he has a clearing vitreous hemorrhage with membrane formation in his left eye. His overall health status has been declining because of his 23-year history of diabetes. He has no known allergies to medications but is allergic to chocolate and bee stings.

| Medical History | Psychosocial Data | Assessment Data |
|---|---|---|
| Poor historian for early childhood problems | Mother (78 years old) lives nearby | Height 5' 9"; weight 175 lbs |
| Hernia repair at 42 years old | Wife (51 years old) works as cashier in local bank | Oriented × 4 |
| Wears glasses for near-sightedness | Two children: 23-year-old, single son, lives alone; 28-year-old, married daughter, with 2 children, lives 150 miles away | Moderate depression |
| Cataract surgery at 49 years old, with complications: blind right eye | No siblings alive; brother died in Vietnam | Good historian for recent history |
| Mild numbness in both lower legs | Lives in suburban area, "good" neighbors | *Skin:* intact, bluish coloring of feet and ankles |
| Never smoked | One year of technical school after 2 years in the army | *Respiratory:* regular rate and rhythm (18 breaths/min); clear to auscultation and percussion |
| Moderate use of alcohol, likes beer | Worked as school maintenance man 22 years | *Cardiovascular:* rate and rhythm regular (76 bpm); no bruits; blood pressure 176/94 |
| Diabetic for 23 years; diet modification and oral agents failed | Goes to church regularly, used to help with repairs | *Abdominal:* no distention; bowel sounds equal in all four quadrants |
| Takes 20 units NPH insulin daily | Avid fisherman; likes sports on TV | *Musculoskeletal:* full range of motion for all joints; gait unsteady at times; fine tremors of fingers when extended |
| ADA diet (1500 calories) not followed closely | Has been on disability and SSSI for 3 years | *Laboratory data* |
| | Likes to travel to see grandchildren | Electrocardiogram (ECG): occasional premature ventricular contractions (PVCs), unchanged for 3 years |
| | Depression for 15 months | Chest x-ray normal |
| | | Hemoglobin (Hgb) 11.6 g/dl; hematocrit (Hct) 37 ml/dl; white blood cell count (WBC) 8500/mm$^3$; platelets 325,000/mm$^3$ |
| | | Blood urea nitrogen (BUN) 30 mg/100 ml; potassium 3.3 mEq/L |
| | | Blood sugar 165 |
| | | *Urinalysis:* trace acetone |
| | | *Medications* |
| | | NPH insulin, 20 units subcuticular qd |
| | | Hydrochlorothiazide, 100 mg PO qd |
| | | Diazepam (Valium), 5 mg PO bid |

## NURSING CARE PLAN

### PATIENT WITH PROLIFERATIVE DIABETIC RETINOPATHY SURGERY SCHEDULED: VITRECTOMY, MEMBRANECTOMY—cont'd

**NURSING DIAGNOSIS**

Anxiety related to potential permanent vision impairment and being in unfamiliar surroundings with vision impairment

| NURSING INTERVENTIONS | EVALUATION OF OUTCOMES |
|---|---|
| Orient to surroundings: include bed controls, call light, phone, and TV. | Patient demonstrates level of comfort in surroundings and level of trust in nurses and other caregivers |
| Keep call light near at all times. | Able to express concerns about current visual status and prognosis for the future |
| Knock on door and speak when entering room. | Cooperates with eye treatment regimen |
| Announce when you are leaving. | |
| Tell him when to expect meal delivery, and ask when he would like afternoon and evening snacks. | |
| Offer to dial the phone as he wishes. | |
| Reorient to room as necessary. | |
| Reassure him appropriately. | |
| Speak with wife and family members. | |
| Give tranquilizers as needed. | |

**NURSING DIAGNOSIS**

Risk of injury and/or infection related to bilateral eye patches, unsteady gait, and delayed healing associated with diabetes

| NURSING INTERVENTIONS | EVALUATION OF OUTCOMES |
|---|---|
| Keep bed at lowest level to floor. | Patient's eye remains free of pain, excessive drainage, or signs of infection |
| Instruct patient on need for side rails. | Vital signs and laboratory values remain within patient's baseline data |
| Immediately postoperatively take vital signs every 15 minutes until stable and then every shift. | Discusses need of safety measures, such as side rails and assistance to bathroom |
| Position head of bed and patient's head and face per physician's orders. | Remains in desired head position postoperatively |
| Leave eye dressing in place. | Cooperates in self-care activities within limitations imposed by his patched eyes and "blind" status |
| Encourage deep breathing and movement of extremities. | Notifies staff if he feels reaction to insulin (decreased blood sugar) |
| Monitor for signs of pain or nausea, and medicate appropriately. | |
| Have appropriate eye drops at bedside to begin on postoperative day 1. | |
| Monitor glucose level (finger stick) before meals and at bedtime. | |
| Advance diet as tolerated. | |
| Administer sleep medication as needed. | |

## NURSING CARE PLAN

### PATIENT WITH PROLIFERATIVE DIABETIC RETINOPATHY SURGERY SCHEDULED: VITRECTOMY, MEMBRANECTOMY—cont'd

**NURSING DIAGNOSIS**

Risk for self-care deficit related to restricted activity level and visual impairment

| NURSING INTERVENTIONS | EVALUATION OF OUTCOMES |
|---|---|
| Assist with activities of daily living (ADL) as needed. | Patient identifies areas of self-care as well as areas for assistance |
| Help patient and wife identify self-care deficits and ways to accommodate them. | Patient and wife have quality discussions on effects of illness and life-style changes that may be necessary |
| Identify alternative caregivers (e.g., neighbors, friends from church). | Patient expresses desire to learn new ways to accomplish ADL |
| Refer to community agencies for support and resources as needed. | |

## KEY CONCEPTS

➤ The eye is a highly specialized sense organ that functions much like a camera, focusing light images that fall on the retina into electrical impulses that travel through the optic nerve to the brain, where the image is developed.

➤ The ophthalmoscope enhances visual examination of the fundus of the retina, including blood vessels, optic disc, and macula. The slit lamp provides a three-dimensional view of all internal structures of the eye. It is also used to view the lids, lashes, and conjunctiva.

➤ Ocular manifestations of systemic disease can be found during a fundus examination. The blood vessels and retinal pathologic conditions reveal the state of vessels elsewhere in the body.

➤ Visual acuity is measured for distance vision and near vision by various charts that are placed at a measured distance from the viewer. The viewer reads the graduated lines of letters or symbols on the charts, and his or her vision is stated in terms of its relation to normal, or 20/20.

➤ When light rays enter the eye and focus at a point in front of the retina, it is called myopia, or nearsightedness. If the light is focused at a point behind the retina, it is hyperopia, or farsightedness. Corrective lenses are prescribed to refract, or bend, the light rays to focus on the retina to achieve normal vision.

➤ Extraocular muscle imbalance in children may cause amblyopia, or "lazy eye." This condition may not always appear as "crossed eyes," so early vision screening is important. If amblyopia is not treated by the age of 8 years, useful binocular vision will never develop.

➤ Contact lenses that are not removed from an unconscious victim can adhere to the corneal surface if the eyes are not fully closed. This may cause severe damage to the corneal surface.

➤ Vision loss can be central, peripheral, or a combination of the two and may affect one eye or both. Adult vision loss in the United States is attributed to cataracts, diabetic retinopathy, glaucoma, and macular degeneration.

➤ Resources for persons with functional vision loss, or low vision, are available in all states. Schools and special clinics provide training for home and work settings. Patients who experience vision loss normally go through the grieving process.

➤ Punctal occlusion, pressing the finger over the inner canthus to obstruct the inner puncta, is used to prevent systemic absorption of topical eye medications.

➤ Angle-closure glaucoma can be mistaken for conjunctivitis. Both conditions exhibit increased blood in the superficial vessels, but the patient with acute glaucoma will have a shallow anterior chamber, high IOP, a mid-dilated nonreactive pupil, and no discharge.

➤ Injury to the corneal epithelium or corneal ulcers destroy the barrier that normally protects the

KEY CONCEPTS—cont'd

other layers from infection. These infections can cause severe scarring that leads to decreased vision or possible blindness.

➤ Medical therapy for glaucoma includes drugs that decrease aqueous production or increase aqueous outflow. When maximum medical therapy fails or is no longer tolerated, surgical procedures are indicated for open-angle glaucoma. These include laser iridectomy and trabeculoplasty, glaucoma filtering procedures, and glaucoma shunt insertion.

➤ Ophthalmic surgical procedures can be divided into intraocular and extraocular procedures. Intraocular procedures include cataract extraction, corneal transplantation, glaucoma filtering procedures, and vitrectomy. Extraocular procedures include surgery on the eye muscles, eyelids, lacrimal system, and orbit.

➤ A painless loss of vision progressing over time can be a sign of cataract formation. Symptoms include difficulty with reading or driving, with seeing well in bright sunlight, or with discriminating colors. The only cure for a cataract is surgical removal of the diseased lens, which is replaced with an artificial lens implant.

➤ Symptoms of a retinal detachment include seeing a "shower" or "flash" of light. Vision can be described as seeing through a curtain or veil. Complete loss of central vision occurs only when the macula is involved.

➤ Ocular malignancies are rare. The most common adult primary intraocular tumor is a choroidal melanoma. Retinoblastoma is the most common type in children.

➤ Most people with HIV develop infectious or noninfectious ocular conditions. Opportunistic infections affect the cornea because immunosuppression allows invasion by numerous organisms.

➤ Cytomegalovirus retinitis can be treated with an intraocular ganciclovir implant. This dispensing method increases drug level to the retina and decreases systemic toxicity problems.

➤ True ocular emergencies should be treated within minutes to preserve sight. Emergencies include chemical burns and sudden, painless loss of sight. The first step in assessing an injury is determining visual acuity of the eyes.

➤ Preventing eye injuries is the most important step in saving sight. Nearly half of all eye injuries occur around the home. Toys are a common cause of children's injuries, and chemicals or flying debris injure adults as well as children.

➤ Visual changes commonly associated with aging include diminished ability to focus on near objects, decreased peripheral vision and color vision, an increase in the frequency of "floaters" or "spots" in the vitreous, and dryness as a result of decreased tear formation.

➤ Eye examinations every 1 to 2 years help diagnose and treat potential problems that may affect sight.

## CRITICAL THINKING EXERCISES

1. Your patient needs to have a fluorescein angiogram. Explain the procedure and its purpose to your patient.
2. Develop a list of postoperative instructions for your patient who is being discharged after cataract removal and lens implantation.
3. Explain the action of the types of drugs used to treat open-angle glaucoma.
4. Identify accommodations that must be made by the older adult to adjust to changes in vision associated with normal aging.

## REFERENCES AND ADDITIONAL READINGS

Allen M, Buse E: Stigmatism and blindness, *J Ophthal Nurs Technol* 10(4):147-152, 1991.

American Academy of Ophthalmology: *At first sight—drugs that are toxic to the eye.* San Francisco, 1989, The Academy.

American Academy of Ophthalmology: *Introducing ophthalmology,* San Francisco, 1992, The Academy.

American Academy of Ophthalmology: Basic clinical and science course, Section 6, *Pediatric ophthalmology and strabismus;* Section 12, *Retina and vitreous,* 1994-95.

American Society of Ophthalmic Registered Nurses: *Standards of ophthalmic clinical nursing practice,* San Francisco, 1992, The Society.

American Society of Ophthalmic Registered Nurses: *Ophthalmic procedures: a nursing prospective,* vols I and II, San Francisco, 1994, 1996, *The Society.*

American Society of Ophthalmic Registered Nurses: *Core curriculum for ophthalmic nursing,* Dubuque, Iowa, 1997, Kendall/Hunt.

Arky R, medical consultant: *Physicians' desk reference,* ed 48, Montvale, NJ, 1994, Medical Economics Data Production Co.

Bartley GB, Liesegang TJ: *Essentials of ophthalmology,* Philadelphia, 1992, Lippincott.

Berlew JA: Preventing eye injuries—the nurse's role, *Insight* 16(6):24-28, 1991.

Berson FG, editor: *Basic ophthalmology for medical students and primary care residents,* ed 6, San Francisco, 1993, American Academy of Ophthalmology.

Boyd-Monk H: Assessing acquired ocular diseases, *Nurs Clin North Am* 25(4):811-822, 1990.

Bulachek GM, McCloskey JC: *Nursing intervention: essential nursing treatments,* Philadelphia, 1992, Saunders.

Bumpus S, Merchant M: Planning for high-risk ophthalmic ambulatory patients, *Insight* 18(2):16-19, 1993.

Burden N: *Ambulatory surgical nursing,* Philadelphia, 1993, Saunders.

Cataract Management Guideline Panel: *Cataract in adults: management of functional impairment. Clinical practice guideline 4,* Rockville, Md, 1993, Agency for Health Care Policy and Research, publication no. 93-0542, US Department of Health and Human Services.

Clinical guidelines: cataract surgery and its alternatives, *Am J Nurs* 93(1):59-61, 1993.

Doane JF, Koppes A, Slade SG: A comprehensive approach to Lasik, *J Ophthalmic Nurs Technol* 15(4):144-147, 1996.

Eichenbaum JW: Vitamins for cataracts and macular degeneration, *J Ophthalmic Nurs Technol* 15(15):65-67, 1996.

Fairchild SS: *Perioperative nursing principles and practice,* Boston, 1993, Jones & Bartlett.

Gallagher CM: The young adult with recent vision loss: a pilot case study, *Insight* 16(6):8-14, 1991.

Gilchrist V, Hunt L: Assessment and education of the diabetic with vision loss, *Insight* 18(3):9 12, 1993.

Glynn-Millay C, Mackay J: Home care for the postoperative cataract patient, *Insight* 20(4):21-25, 1995.

Goldblum K: Knowledge deficit in the ophthalmic surgical patients, *Nurs Clin North Am* 27(3):715-725, 1992.

Grimes MR, Scardino MA, Martone JF: Worldwide blindness, *Nurs Clin North Am* 27(3):807-816, 1992.

Hunt L: Caution: systemic adverse reactions from eye drops medications, *Insight* 16(4):5, 1991.

Hunt L: Ophthalmic nursing assessment, *Insight* 18(3):9-11, 1992.

Hunt L: Aging and the visual system, *Insight* 18(3):6-7, 18, 1993a.

Hunt L: Ocular emergencies, *Insight* 18(2):24-25, 1993b.

Langseth F: The use of 5-fluorouracil in glaucoma filtration surgery, *Insight* 18(2):11-13, 1993.

Lewis SM, Collier IC, Heitkemper MM: *Medical-surgical nursing: assessment and management of clinical problems,* ed 4, St Louis, 1996, Mosby.

Martin DF et al: Treatment of cytomegalovirus retinitis with an intraocular sustained-release ganciclovir implant, *Arch Ophthalmol* 112:1531-1539, 1994.

McCoy K: Ophthalmic drug use in the OR, *Insight* 17(4):10-21, 1992.

McEvoy GK: American hospital formulary service, *EyeENT* 52:1766-1867, 1994.

Nowell P: Lasers in ophthalmology, *Nurs Clin North Am* 25(3):635-643, 1990.

Olk RJ: New approaches to vitreoretinal surgery, Boston, 1992, Little, Brown.

Ostler HB: *Disease of the external eye and adnexa,* Baltimore, 1993, Williams & Wilkins.

Plona RP, Schremp PS: Nursing care of patient with ocular manifestations of human immunodeficiency virus infection, *Nurs Clin North Am* 27(3):793-805, 1992.

Reeves W: Surgical experiences of the ophthalmic patient, *Insight* 18(1):16-22, 1993.

Richard JM: *A manual for the beginning ophthalmology resident: eye emergencies,* ed 3, San Francisco, 1978, American Academy of Ophthalmology.

Ruehl CA, Schremp PS: Nursing care of the cataract patient: today's outpatient approach, *Nurs Clin North Am* 27(3):727-743, 1992.

Sandler RL: Glaucoma, *Am J Nurs* 95(3):34-35, 1995.

Servodidio CA: Teaching aids for patients diagnosed with choroidal melanoma, *Insight* 16(6):21-23, 1991.

Servodidio CA: Nursing implications of visual fields in successfully treated retinoblastoma patients, *Insight* 18(1):11-16, 1993.

Servodidio CA, Abramson DH: Choroidal melanoma, *Nurs Clin North Am* 27(3):777-791, 1992.

Smith SC: Diabetic retinopathy, *Nurs Clin North Am* 27(3):745-759, 1992.

Smith SC, Folk JC, Losch ME: Effects of collaborated education on patient satisfaction and knowledge, *Insight* 17(1):20-24, 1992.

Spector SA: Spectrum and treatment of cytomegalovirus disease in persons with AIDS, *J Int Assoc Physicians AIDS Care* 2(5):9-21, 1996.

Spires R: Retinopathy of prematurity, *J Ophthalmic Nurs Technol* 10(4):166-170, 1991.

Spires R: Glaucoma filtration surgery and the shell tamponade technique, *J Ophthalmic Nurs Technol* 13(1):17-20, 1994.

Stein HA, Scott BJ, Stein RM: *A primer in ophthalmology,* St Louis, 1992, Mosby.

Vader L: Vision and vision loss, *Insight* 22(1):13-19, 1997.

Vaughan DG, Asbury T, Riordan-Eva P: *General ophthalmology,* ed 14, Norwalk, Conn, 1995 Appleton & Lange.

Weisbacker CA, Naidoff M, Tippermann R: *Physicians' desk reference for ophthalmology,* ed 25, Montrale, NJ, 1997, Medical Economics Data.

Wong EK, Wang S, Leopold IH: How ophthalmic drugs can fool you, *RN* 43(3):37-44, 1980.

Woods S: Macular degeneration, *Nurs Clin North Am* 27(3):761-775, 1992.

# Hearing

## CHAPTER OBJECTIVES

1 Associate the anatomic parts of the ear to the functions of hearing and balance.

2 Identify the purpose and procedure for common diagnostic tests involving the ear.

3 List common complaints associated with ear problems.

4 Differentiate between conductive and sensorineural hearing loss.

5 Describe behavioral signs and symptoms of hearing loss in the adult.

6 Discuss methods to facilitate communication with the hearing-impaired person.

7 Describe methods that may be used to remove a foreign body from the external ear canal.

8 Discuss nursing interventions for the patient with otitis media.

9 Discuss both the preoperative and postoperative nursing care of the patient having ear surgery.

10 Define otosclerosis and describe the surgical procedure (stapedectomy) used to correct the condition.

11 Discuss both preoperative and postoperative care of the patient having a mastoidectomy.

12 Identify activity restrictions for the patient following tympanoplasty.

13 Differentiate between labyrinthitis and Ménière's disease, including signs/symptoms and nursing interventions.

## KEY TERMS

| | |
|---|---|
| auditory canal | nystagmus |
| auricle | otitis media |
| cochlea | otosclerosis |
| deafness | otoscopy |
| endolymph | perilymph |
| equilibrium | presbycusis |
| eustachian tube | saccule |
| incus | semicircular canals |
| labyrinthitis | stapedectomy |
| malleus | stapes |
| mastoiditis | tympanic membrane |
| Ménière's disease | tympanoplasty |
| myringotomy | vestibule |

The ears are a highly specialized, complex set of sense organs responsible for the functions of both hearing and balance. The ear consists of three structural parts: external, middle, and inner (Figure 39-1). Each structure has a distinct function that contributes to the processes of hearing and balance.

## STRUCTURE AND FUNCTION OF THE EAR

### External Ear

The external portion of the ear is composed of the visible **auricle** (pinna) and a passageway called the external **auditory canal** or external auditory meatus. The auricle is made up of cartilage and connective tissue covered with epithelium. It acts as a collecting trumpet for sound waves, directing them toward the external auditory canal (external acoustic meatus). The external auditory canal is lined with epithelium and

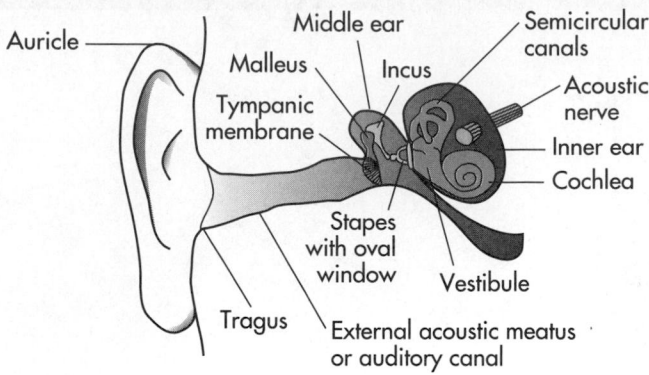

**Figure 39-1** Diagram of the ear.

ceruminous (wax-producing) glands and hair follicles. The purpose of the cerumen and hair follicles is to protect both the tympanic membrane and the middle ear. The hair follicles protect the external auditory canal from foreign debris. The ceruminous glands provide lubrication for both the tympanic membrane and the middle ear. During the aging process the hair follicles become coarse, causing a buildup of cerumen (wax). Impacted cerumen is a potential source of hearing loss, particularly for the older adult. The external ear is supplied by the fifth (trigeminal) and tenth (vagus) cranial nerves and the cervical nerves. The function of the auricle and external auditory canal is to collect and transmit sound waves to the tympanic membrane.

The **tympanic membrane** (eardrum) covers the end of the external auditory canal, separating the external ear from the middle ear. The external surface of the tympanic membrane is covered with the same ceruminous glands and hair follicles as the external auditory canal. The internal surface of the membrane is covered with a thin, hairless mucous membrane. Normally this membrane appears "pearly" gray and shiny. The tympanic membrane protects the middle ear and vibrates with incoming sound waves to facilitate hearing. It receives its innervation for this vibratory function from a small auricular branch of the vagus nerve, as well as from a portion of the glossopharyngeal and facial nerve fibers.

## Middle Ear

The middle ear, or tympanic cavity, is a small air-filled cavity located in the petrous portion of the temporal bone (toward the face). It is separated from the external ear by the tympanic membrane. The middle ear contains the ossicles, the oval and round windows, and the eustachian tube. The ossicles (auditory ossicles) are three small bones that traverse the middle ear. Each has been named to describe its shape: the **malleus** (ham-

mer), **incus** (anvil), and **stapes** (stirrup). The malleus is attached to the inner surface of the tympanic membrane, the incus is attached to the malleus, and the stapes is attached to the incus. These bones, or ossicles, are linked together in a chain, although not rigidly, which allows them to receive sound vibrations from the tympanic membrane and transmit them to the inner ear. The oval and round windows are membrane-covered openings leading from the middle ear to the inner ear. The oval window (fenestra ovalis) is attached to the stapes. The round window (fenestra rotunda) is located below the oval window. These windows provide an exit for sound vibrations from the inner ear, while protecting the middle ear from the inner ear.

The **eustachian tube** connects the middle ear with the nasopharynx. Its function is to equalize the pressure in the middle ear with the atmospheric pressure. The slitlike ending of the eustachian tube is normally closed. During swallowing or yawning, the tube can be opened, allowing air to enter or leave the tympanic cavity in order to balance the pressure on both sides of the tympanic membrane. This allows free movement of the tympanic membrane and prevents it from rupturing. A normally functioning eustachian tube keeps the middle ear free of contaminants from the nasopharynx.

## Inner Ear

The inner ear (labyrinth) consists of a system of interrelated cavities. Included in this system is the bony (osseous) labyrinth, membranous labyrinth, **vestibule,** cochlea, and semicircular canals. The membranous labyrinth lies within a portion of the bony labyrinth. Within the membranous labyrinth are housed the semicircular canals, utricle, and saccule. The **semicircular canals** contain fluid and hair cells. They are connected to the sensory nerve fibers of the vestibular portion of the eighth (vestibulocochlear) cranial nerve. The semicircular canals help to maintain a sense of balance or equilibrium. The utricle and **saccule** (two small sacs) separate the semicircular canals from the cochlea. These sacs are suspended within the vestibule. They serve as vestibular receptors that respond to the changing positions of the head. The **cochlea** is a snail-shaped tube containing the organ of Corti, the receptor end organ of hearing.

Important to the protection and maintenance of the inner ear are two fluids—perilymph and endolymph. **Perilymph** is contained within the space between the bony and the membranous labyrinths. It is also found in a portion of the cochlea. **Endolymph** is found within the utricle, saccule, and a portion of the cochlea. These fluids protect both the cochlea and the semicircular canals by cushioning them against abrupt movements of the head.

## Process of Hearing

The auditory center for hearing is located in the temporal lobe of the cerebrum. Stimulation of this center results in hearing. Sound waves enter the ear through the auditory canal, causing the tympanic membrane to vibrate. These vibrations are transmitted from the tympanic membrane through the ossicles of the middle ear. One of those ossicles, the stapes, moves against the oval window, causing the vibrations to be transmitted through the fluids in the cochlea to the round window. At the round window these vibrations dissipate. The passing of these vibratory waves from the oval to the round window stimulates the hair cells of the organ of Corti to move, sending a stimulus to the membrane of Corti. These impulses are received by the cochlear branch of the auditory nerve, where they are transmitted to the brain and perceived as sound.

## Maintenance of Balance

The vestibular system (saccule, utricle, and semicircular canals) is responsible for the maintenance of **equilibrium** and balance. The semicircular canals contain both endolymph fluid and hair cells. When an individual moves, this endolymph fluid also moves, causing the hair cells to bend. As the hair cells within the semicircular canals bend, they release impulses that stimulate the vestibular branch of the eighth cranial nerve. This allows the brain to reorient the individual and maintain balance. If an individual is stationary, the pressure of gravity on these hair cells maintains balance. Separating the semicircular canals from the cochlea are the utricle and saccule. They also function as vestibular receptors that respond to changes in head position.

# NURSING ASSESSMENT OF HEARING LOSS

A nursing assessment should include a thorough patient history of both current and past medical conditions, identification of the patient's chief complaints, a visual examination, and an observation of the patient for signs of hearing loss.

## Patient History

A patient history should include questions regarding past or current hearing or ear-related problems. For example, symptoms such as vertigo (the sensation of moving in space), ear pain, discharge, or recent ear trauma may be important in identifying a structural or hearing problem. The history should include questions regarding hearing acuity and any occupation or hobbies that may involve exposure to excessive noise.

A thorough medication history is crucial because some drugs are toxic to the cochlea and vestibule and may cause permanent damage. Other drugs can cause dizziness, which could be confused with an ear disorder. The existence of current medical conditions and their medical treatments not directly associated with the ear also should be identified. Conditions such as allergies or upper respiratory infections may cause hearing or equilibrium problems. Information about the patient's ability to hear also can be obtained during this interview by noting positioning of the patient's head and the appropriateness of response.

## Visual Examination

The external structure of the ear should be inspected for any signs of injury, redness, swelling, or drainage. The normal external canal is free from lesions and is dry, clean, and not reddened. The presence of any of these symptoms could indicate a possible infectious process, trauma, or the presence of a foreign object and should be reported to the physician for further evaluation. Visual examination also includes **otoscopy.** Otoscopy is the direct visualization of the external auditory canal and the tympanic membrane through an instrument called an otoscope (Figure 39-2). Otoscopy may reveal signs of common conditions such as a perforated tympanic membrane or acute **otitis media.** Otoscopy is performed before any other auditory or vestibular testing is done.

# DIAGNOSTIC TESTING

Various testing methods are used to assess for disorders of the ear. These testing methods are categorized according to their purpose. Auditory testing methods are used to determine hearing acuity. Vestibular testing methods are used to assess for dysfunction of the vestibular system, which affects equilibrium, resulting in dizziness, loss of balance, or **nystagmus** (involuntary rhythmic movement of the eyeball).

## Auditory Tests
### Voice Tests

Voice tests to determine hearing acuity may be done by whispering or speaking in a lower tone of voice. The individual being tested is placed at a distance of 20 feet and turned sideways. The ear to be tested is directed toward the examiner; the other ear is covered. The individual is asked to repeat each whispered or spoken word. Voice testing is insensitive to disorders of central auditory processing. This testing method is of value only as a simple screening tool to identify individuals who require a more thorough examination.

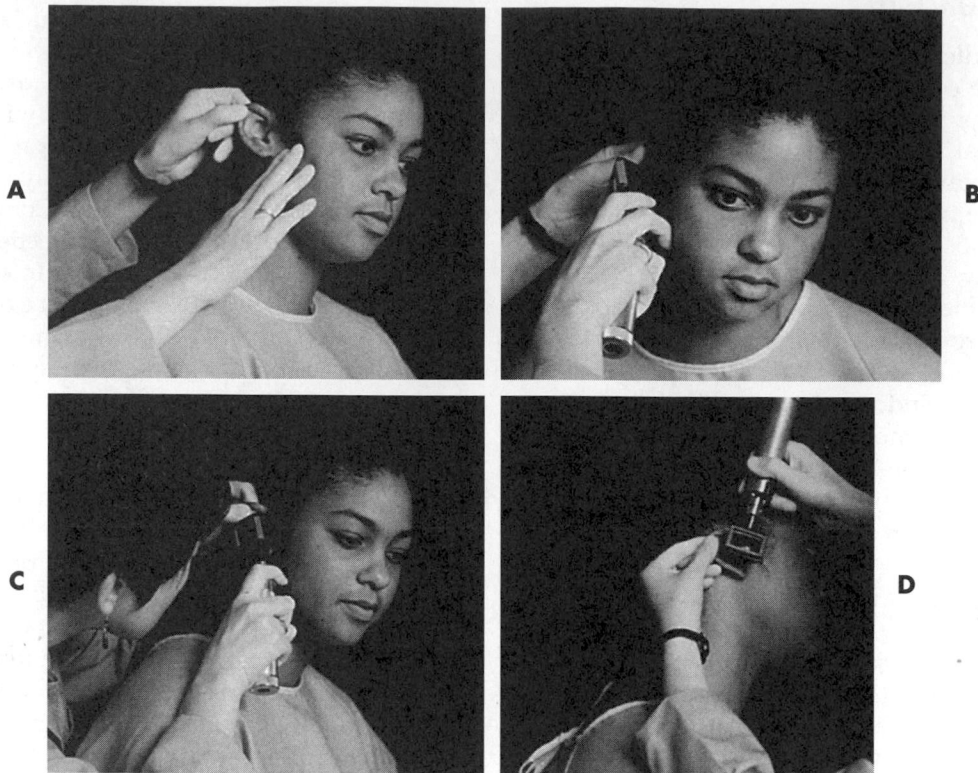

**Figure 39-2**    Examination of the ear with the otoscope. **A,** Inspection of the meatus. **B,** Patient's head is tipped toward the opposite shoulder. **C** and **D,** Two ways of holding the otoscope. (From Barkauskas VH et al: *Health and physical assessment,* St Louis, 1994, Mosby.)

Patients found to have evidence of hearing loss by screening should be referred to a specialist.

## Audiometry

A more accurate examination is done with an audiometer, an instrument that produces tones of varying pitch and intensity. The patient wears earphones that are attached to the audiometer. The individual listens to various tones and is asked to indicate when each sound is heard. Audiometry testing provides information concerning both quantitative and qualitative measurements of hearing. It provides the audiologist and the otologist (physician who specializes in diseases of the ear) with information that can help determine the type of treatment needed.

## Tuning Forks

Hearing acuity may also be tested through the use of a tuning fork (Figure 39-3). The tuning fork is made to vibrate and is then placed at various locations near the ear. There are several tuning fork tests used to differentiate between conductive and sensorineural hearing

loss. One method is called the Weber test. The Weber test is used to determine hearing loss in one or both ears. It is performed by placing the vibrating tuning fork in the middle of the individual's head at the midline of the forehead (Figure 39-4). The individual is asked whether the sound is heard equally in both ears or is louder in one ear than the other. The test results are considered normal if the individual hears equally well on both sides. The results are considered to be abnormal if the sound is heard in one ear only. If the individual's hearing loss is of a *conductive* nature, the sound will be louder in the diseased ear. If the hearing loss is of a *sensorineural* nature, the sound will be louder in the normal ear. Another method of tuning fork testing is the Rinne test. In the Rinne test the base of the vibrating tuning fork is shifted between two positions (Figure 39-5). First it is placed on the mastoid process of the temporal bone. While it is still vibrating, the tuning fork is then placed in front of the ear. As the position of the tuning fork is changed, the patient is asked to identify which tone is louder. The patient is also asked to identify when one of the tones is no longer heard. Under normal circumstances the sound will be heard longer in front of the ear. This is consid-

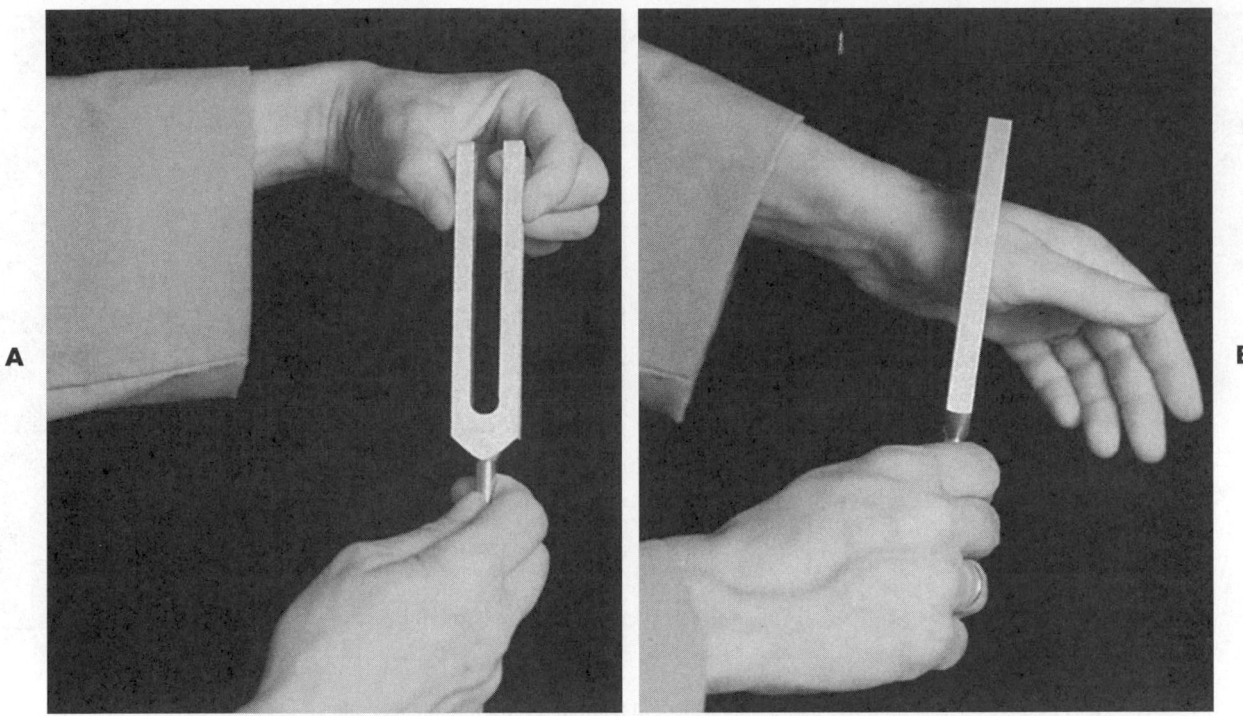

**Figure 39-3**    Activating tuning fork. **A,** Stroking the fork. **B,** Tapping the fork on the knuckle. (From Barkauskas VH et al: *Health and physical assessment,* St Louis, 1994, Mosby.)

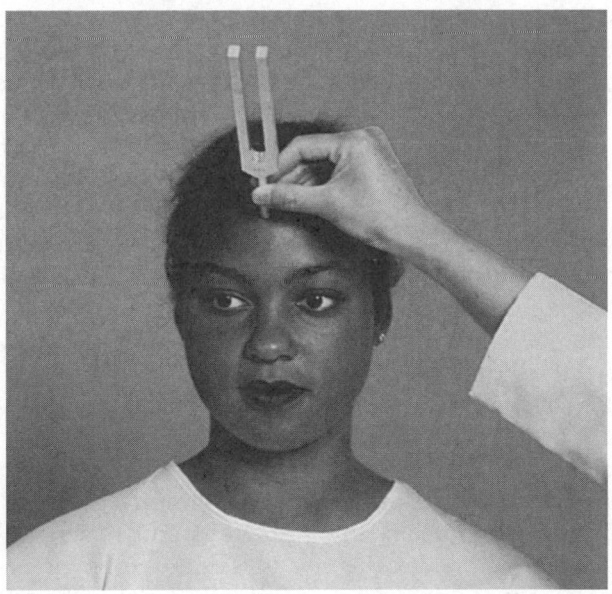

**Figure 39-4**    Weber test. (From Barkauskas VH et al: *Health and physical assessment,* St Louis, 1994, Mosby.)

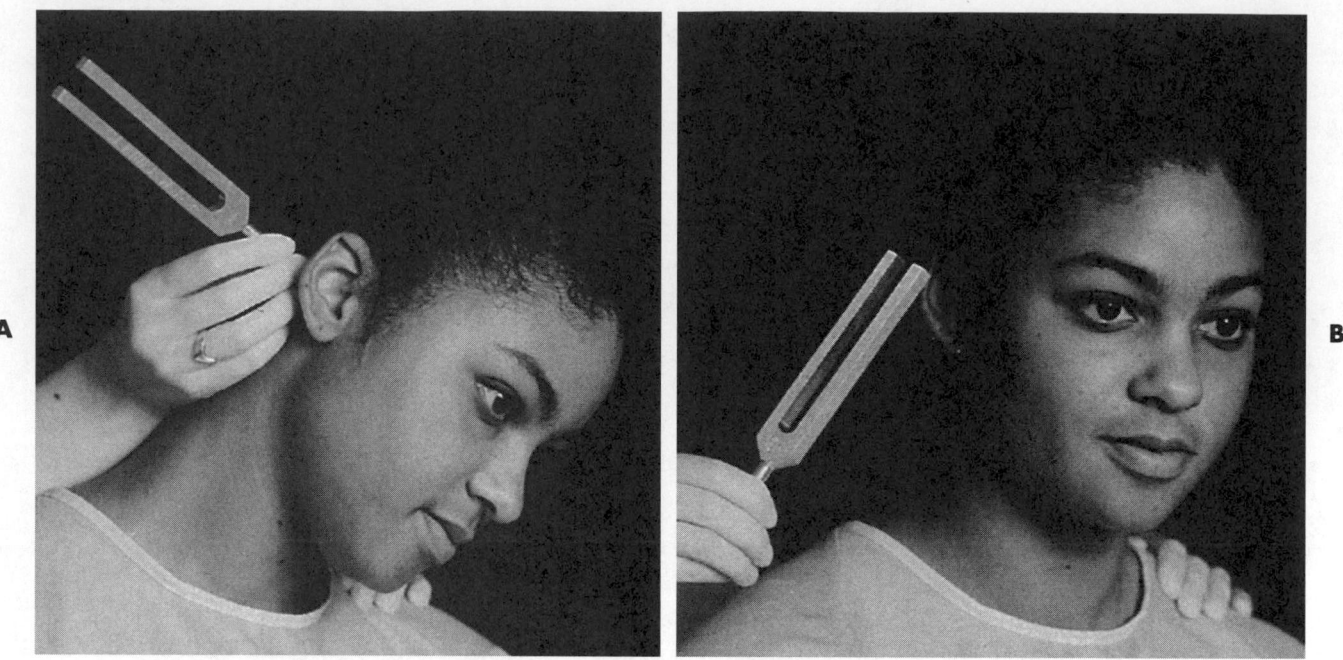

**Figure 39-5**    Rinne test. **A,** Tuning fork placed on mastoid process to check bone conduction. **B,** Air conduction. (From Barkauskas VH et al: *Health and physical assessment*, St Louis, 1994, Mosby.)

ered to be a normal or positive Rinne tuning fork test result. If the individual is unable to hear the sound through the air in front of the ear, the test is considered to be abnormal or negative. A negative Rinne test result indicates a conductive hearing loss on the side being tested.

## Vestibular Tests

Dysfunction in the vestibule or the cerebellum may result in dizziness, loss of equilibrium, or nystagmus. Individuals can be tested for vestibular and/or cerebellar dysfunction by using either the falling test or the past-pointing test. In the *falling test* the individual is instructed to stand with feet together, stand on one foot, stand heel to toe, and then walk forward and backward heel to toe. Each of these exercises is first performed with eyes open and then with eyes closed. Marked swaying or falling indicates dysfunction. In the *past-pointing test* the examiner holds an index finger out at shoulder level. The patient is instructed to reach out and touch the examiner's index finger. The patient is then asked to raise and lower both of his or her arms, attempting to return to the examiner's index finger (point of reference). The patient should be able to return to that point of reference. This would be considered a "normal" test result. Patients with vestibular dysfunction lack a "normal" sense of position. They are unable to return to the point of reference. Instead

they deviate to the right or the left of the examiner's index finger.

Recently, posturography and rotational chair testing have been used to determine vestibular dysfunction. Each test requires the patient to be placed in a series of alternating positions. Through these testing methods it is possible to isolate one semicircular canal from the other in order to determine the site of a lesion causing the vestibular disturbance. Although useful, these tests are time-consuming and may not be tolerated by the patient with a vestibular disability.

## Electronystagmography

Electronystagmography is a procedure used to evaluate both spontaneous and induced eye movements referred to as nystagmus. The purpose of electronystagmography is to distinguish between normal nystagmus and nystagmus caused by vestibular lesion. Nystagmus following a head turn is normal for a short period. Prolonged nystagmus is abnormal. The procedure uses a variety of stimuli, including position changes and hot and cold to elicit nystagmus. The eye movements in response to each stimulus are recorded and evaluated. Electronystagmography is also helpful in diagnosing unilateral hearing loss of unknown origin and identifying the cause of dizziness, vertigo (the sensation of moving in space), or tinnitus (ringing in the ears).

# HEARING LOSS

*Hearing loss,* or hearing impairment, is a generic term that means "a decrease in one's auditory acuity" (McLeod, Bently, 1996). Hearing loss can be partial or total. It can also occur in low, medium, or high frequencies or in combinations of frequencies. Hearing loss can occur in one or both ears, depending on the cause. It may be congenital, or it may occur later in life as a result of disease or injury.

Hearing is measured in decibels (dB). A decibel is a ratio that compares the relationship between two sound intensities. According to the American Medical Association, a hearing loss of 40 dB below normal (which is equal to a 22.5% hearing impairment) usually impairs a person's ability to function normally in a social situation and requires intervention, such as a hearing aid or other device that amplifies the sound. True **deafness** is defined as 85 to 90 dB below normal.

Presbycusis is a progressive bilateral hearing loss commonly occurring with age. Approximately one fourth of adults age 65 to 74 years and one half of adults 85 years and older report some degree of hearing loss. Hearing loss, particularly when it develops later in life, can compromise the ability to perform many daily activities. It may also lead to withdrawal and depression (Box 39-1).

In addition to the large population of older adults experiencing hearing loss, approximately 1 of every 500 adults in the United States is hearing impaired. Individuals who are hearing impaired may be profoundly deaf and use only American sign language as their primary language, or they may have a wide range of hearing abilities and may use other methods for communication, including lip reading and, in some cases, normal speech. There are many myths and misconceptions about deafness. Often the assumption is made that all individuals who are deaf cannot talk, cannot attend school, and are not as intelligent as hearing people. Although there have been many advances made in the treatment of deafness, there is still much to be done to educate and dispel these myths.

## Types

Hearing loss may be conductive, affecting only the external or middle ear, or it may be sensorineural (nerve deafness), in which the inner ear is involved. Conductive deafness may be caused by an obstruction of the auditory canal that prevents sound waves from reaching the inner ear. The problem may be an accumulation of cerumen in the auditory canal, or it may be caused by otosclerosis in the middle ear, which prevents transmission of sound vibrations from reaching the inner ear (Figure 39-6). For persons affected by otosclerosis, surgery may restore hearing. In some cases

## BEHAVIORAL SIGNS/SYMPTOMS OF HEARING LOSS

**fatigue** Straining to hear conversations is tiresome and often leads to irritability.

**speech deterioration** "Flat voice," incorrect pronunciation, or omitting words may occur because sounds are produced incorrectly.

**indifference** Lack of hearing can cause disinterest and depression.

**social withdrawal** Inattentiveness and withdrawal occur when the person is unable to hear correctly.

**insecurity** Improper hearing may cause the person to say or respond in the wrong manner, leading to feelings of embarrassment and insecurity.

**indecision/procrastination** Hearing problems lead to loss of self-confidence, which in turn makes decision making more difficult.

**suspiciousness** When only parts of conversations are heard, hearing-impaired people suspect that they are being talked about.

**false pride** Pretending to hear normally to avoid embarrassment often causes others to believe that the person has normal hearing.

**loneliness and unhappiness** Enforced silence can lead to many frightening experiences, giving the person a sense of not belonging.

**dominating conversations** By dominating conversations, the hearing-impaired person has control of the group, which eliminates embarrassment.

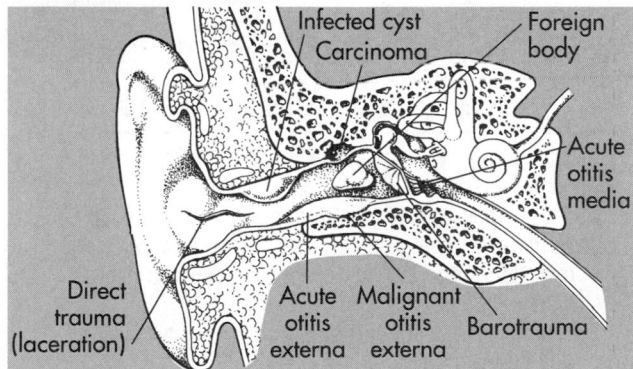

**Figure 39-6**   Disorders that contribute to conductive hearing loss. (From Beare PG, Myers JL: *Adult health nursing,* ed 3, St Louis, 1998, Mosby.)

there may be a congenital absence of the auditory canal or the tympanic membrane. In conductive deafness only the intensity of sound is affected. Disorders that lead to conductive hearing loss can often be corrected with no damage to hearing or only minimal hearing loss.

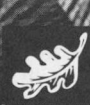

## OLDER ADULT CONSIDERATIONS

**Presbycusis**, impairment of hearing as a result of degenerative changes, is a common cause of sensorineural hearing loss associated with aging. In this case hearing loss is bilateral. Progression of the disease is gradual. Often the older adult will state that hearing is normal but that he or she cannot understand the words. The affected person can hear the spoken word, but it is muffled and often sounds as if the speaker is mumbling. This hearing loss is caused by degeneration or atrophy of several areas of the ear structure, especially the cochlea (Box 39-1).

In sensorineural deafness the auditory canal and the middle ear receive the vibrations normally, but the vibrations go no further. This is because of degeneration of the nerve fibers of the auditory nerve or the hearing center in the brain. Damage may result from tumors, head injuries, or other causes (e.g., congenital syphilis) that affect the eighth cranial nerve. Nerve deafness may occur in infants born to mothers who had rubella during the first trimester of pregnancy. A type of nerve deafness that usually involves high-frequency sounds may occur as part of the aging process (Box 39-2).

### BOX 39-2

#### CHANGES ASSOCIATED WITH AGING

Pinna becomes elongated because of loss of subcutaneous tissue and decreased tissue elasticity.

Hair becomes coarse and longer, especially in men.

Cerumen-producing glands decrease in number; cerumen becomes drier and impacted, causing hearing loss.

Tympanic membrane loses its elasticity and appears dull and retracted.

Ossicles decrease movement as a result of calcification.

Cochlea experiences degenerative changes.

Vestibular function becomes disturbed, causing vertigo and sensations of being unsteady.

Hearing acuity diminishes with increased age. Loss of hearing acuity includes loss of ability to hear high-frequency sounds, decreased speech reception (particularly the *f*, *s*, and *sh* sounds), and increased auditory reaction time.

## Management

Persons with sensorineural deafness experience distortion of sounds along with poor speech discrimination. Often they will speak loudly in an attempt to compensate. When sensorineural deafness is congenital or acquired during infancy or early childhood, speech is generally affected. Such children usually need training in lip reading and education in American sign language. Sensorineural or nerve deafness is permanent and irreversible, but research offers hope for finding a treatment in the future. An electronic cochlea has been devised that is implanted in the inner ear and conducts impulses to the higher centers in the brain. The development of this artificial cochlea has helped and will continue to do so as the implantation technique becomes more refined. However, for the present, most individuals with nerve deafness must be helped to live without the ability to hear.

A common method of improving conductive hearing loss is the use of a hearing aid. The hearing aid is a tiny electronic device designed to amplify sound. Those persons with conduction deafness (in which the problem is intensity of sound) generally benefit from the use of a hearing aid. The hearing aid, however, is of little value to the individual with sensorineural deafness.

The hearing aid consists of three parts: a microphone that picks up sound and converts it into electric signals, an amplifier that intensifies the signal, and a receiver that converts the signal back into an intensified sound. The amplifier can be worn in one or both ears. In the individual with bilateral hearing loss, use of bilateral amplifiers stimulates a stereo effect, which aids in speech discrimination. There are various types of hearing aids, including those that may be used about the head. Hearing aids can be built into glasses,

## PATIENT/FAMILY TEACHING

**CARE OF A HEARING AID**

1. The hearing aid should be kept dry and away from heat at all times.
2. It is unnecessary to wear the hearing aid at night.
3. When not in use, remove the hearing aid battery or open the battery door.
4. Store the hearing aid in a covered container, labeled with the patient's name.
5. To prevent the buildup of cerumen, the hearing aid should be cleaned daily. When cleaning, wipe the earmold (BTE) or body of the aid (ITE) using a moistened soft cloth or tissue.
6. Caution should be taken when removing a meal tray, changing the patient's bedding, or changing the battery to avoid loss of the battery or the hearing aid itself.

worn behind the ear, or worn in the auditory canal. (Figure 39-7) Other types may be worn on the torso.

The successful use of a hearing aid depends on the individual's feelings about the disability and the use of the device. Hearing aids amplify all sound, including background noise, which can cause confusion and actually make it more difficult to hear conversation. Not all persons will be able to adjust to this as well as the other aspects of the device. Older adults especially may find it more difficult.

Deafness, whether progressive or sudden in onset, produces anxiety and fear. The possibility of becoming cut off from familiar surroundings, losing friends, losing a job, and becoming isolated often leads to withdrawal. Many individuals deny the disability and refuse assistance. Early detection and appropriate intervention, including the use of a hearing aid, can promote increased independence and preserve the ability of the individual to interact with the environment. A hearing aid can play an important part in improving residual hearing, thus lessening the emotional impact of hearing loss, but only if it is used.

Proper care of a hearing aid can eliminate problems and increase an individual's confidence in using the device. Individuals should be taught to use the hearing aid only at times and places in which it improves hearing, not at those times when there is a great deal of background noise. Whistling noises can indicate a loose or improperly worn mold. Poor amplification can result from dead batteries, wax buildup, or incorrect volume control. Pain while wearing the mold may indicate an improper fit or may be a sign of an infection in the ear itself or the surrounding area (Box 39-3).

In addition to the hearing aid, there are other devices that are often helpful for individuals with hearing loss. Telephone amplifiers and flashing lights are available. A telephone amplifier increases the volume of the sound being carried by the telephone. Flashing lights alert the individual visually rather than through an auditory method. A small portable audio amplifier is another alternative. This device consists of a headset and an amplification device. The person with the hearing loss wears the headset. Anyone wishing to communicate with this individual speaks into the amplifier. The sound is then heard more loudly. Cochlear implantation has become successful for some individuals with sensorineural hearing loss. The artificial cochlea is a small computer device capable of converting sound waves into electronic impulses, which in turn stimulate the nerve fibers. Although still somewhat experimental, the cochlear implant has improved hearing by 50% in some cases (Figure 39-8). Lip reading and sign language are two additional tools that can enhance communication.

Communication for the individual with a hearing loss can become a hardship. There are several helpful tips that can facilitate communication and assist the individual with the hearing loss:

- Always face the individual so that the lips are visible. This is important if the person is relying on lip reading to aid communication.

---

**BOX 39-3**

### Guidelines for Troubleshooting Hearing Aid Problems

1 Check the placement (seating) of the hearing aid 2 times each day (best after meals since chewing may dislodge the aid).
2 Check the volume level occasionally if the wearer inserts the aid or tends to manipulate the settings.
3 If the aid squeals:
   a Check the seating (may be loose fitting).
   b Check the volume (should never need to be on full volume).
   c Check for cerumen in the ear mold, or do an otoscopic evaluation to check the ear canal.
   d Check the wearer's position in bed (if the aid is too close to the pillow or other solid object, this can cause feedback).
4 If the hearing aid is not working, the problem may be:
   a A "dead" battery. Many aids mark the battery door with a plus (+) to match the battery for proper insertion. Replace the old battery with a new one (most last 2 weeks ± if worn 8 hr/day).
   b The ear canal portion of the aid may be plugged with cerumen. Return the device to the dealer for removal of the wax.
   c Mechanical failure. Return the device to the dealer for repair.
5 If you suspect decreased hearing, consult an audiologist. Hearing can change with illness, some medications, and over time.

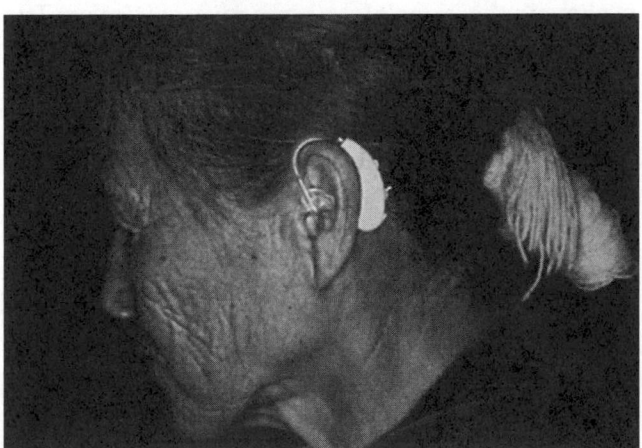

**Figure 39-7**   One type of hearing aid that is worn behind the ear.

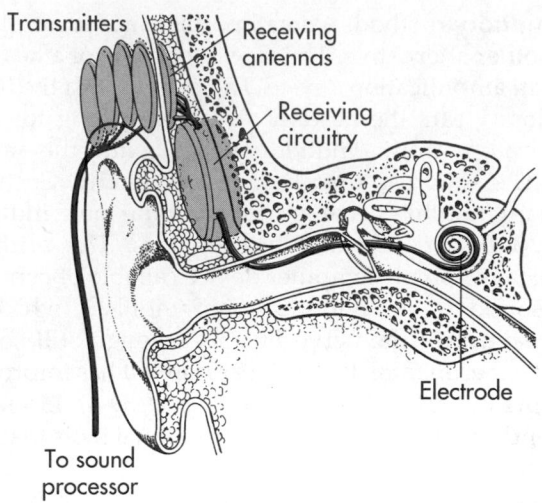

**Figure 39-8** Cochlear implant. (From Beare PG, Myers JL: *Adult health nursing,* ed 3, St Louis, 1998, Mosby.)

- Do not raise the voice to any great extent, but do speak more slowly and distinctly than usual.
- Avoid using high tones because they are more difficult to hear for the deaf person.
- If the individual does not understand what has been said, rephrase the statement using different words to say the same thing.
- Point to the object being talked about whenever possible.
- Be aware that some letters and sounds are more difficult to distinguish than others.
- If the individual cannot hear at all and cannot read lips, write out the message.

It is important to communicate in some way with the hearing-impaired person to prevent isolation. Sign language is a useful tool. The use of a sign language interpreter may make communication easier. Interpreters are now being used in a variety of educational, social, and medical settings. The nurse who works often with the hearing impaired should learn how to sign.

# DISORDERS OF THE EXTERNAL EAR

Certain disorders of the external ear may affect hearing while causing pain and discomfort (Box 39-4). Common disorders include infection, obstruction, injury, and perforation of the eardrum.

## Infections
### Boils

Boils are one common type of infection. If large enough, they may obstruct the auditory canal and cause some degree of temporary hearing impairment.

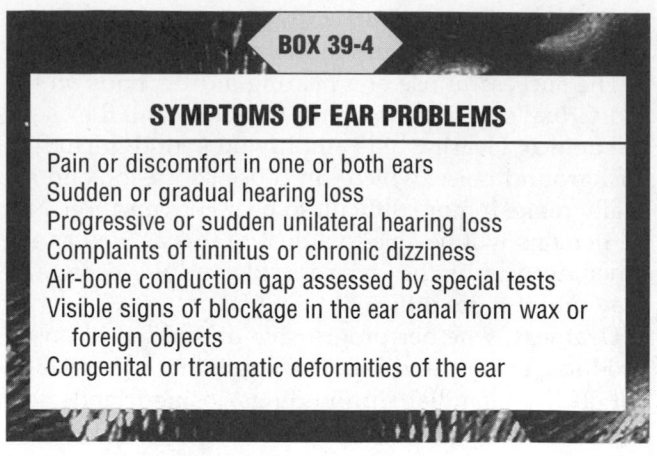

**BOX 39-4**

### SYMPTOMS OF EAR PROBLEMS

Pain or discomfort in one or both ears
Sudden or gradual hearing loss
Progressive or sudden unilateral hearing loss
Complaints of tinnitus or chronic dizziness
Air-bone conduction gap assessed by special tests
Visible signs of blockage in the ear canal from wax or foreign objects
Congenital or traumatic deformities of the ear

**BOX 39-5**

### EAR INSTILLATIONS

1  Turn the patient's head to the side, with the affected ear upright.
2  In adult patients, the auricle should be pulled upward and backward.
3  In children, the auricle should be pulled downward.
4  Instill the prescribed number of drops (usually 3 or 4) into the ear opening without touching the meatus.
5  Pump the tragus once or twice to remove the air locks and drive the solution forward.
6  To improve contact with the inner ear, have the patient lie on the side, with the affected ear upright, for 5 to 10 minutes before the medication is instilled.

The infectious agent that causes the boil is usually a staphylococcal bacteria. The bacteria gains entrance to the subcutaneous tissue through a scratch or injury that occurs while removing ear wax or a foreign body from the external ear canal. As the infection develops, swelling in the lining of the auditory canal occurs. This swelling in some cases actually leads to closure of the canal. Boils can be extremely painful. The severe pain occurs as a result of the swelling because there is no room to accommodate the tissue expansion in the bony canal. Relief may be obtained by the application of nonsterile warm compresses or an electric heating pad. Treatment may include instillation of drops containing antibiotics or cortisone (Box 39-5, Table 39-1). If the infection extends to the regional lymph nodes, oral or intravenous administration of antibiotics may be required. Drugs such as acetaminophen or acetaminophen with codeine may be needed for pain relief for those patients with a severe infection. Boils have a tendency to recur unless properly treated. Patients should

**TABLE 39-1**

## Pharmacology of Drugs Used in Hearing

| DRUG (GENERIC AND TRADE NAME); ROUTE AND DOSAGE | ACTION/INDICATION | COMMON SIDE EFFECTS AND NURSING CONSIDERATIONS |
|---|---|---|
| **Amoxicillin** (Amoxicillin)<br>**Route:** PO<br>**Dosage:** 250-300 mg q 8 hr | Used in treatment of otitis media | May cause rash and diarrhea; use with caution in severe renal disease; contraindicated in patients with hypersensitivity to penicillins |
| **Bacitracin**<br>**Route:** Topical—solution and ointment<br>**Dosage:** 1-3 drops or thin layer of ointment 2-3 times daily for 7-10 days | Bacteriostatic/bactericidal agent used against gram-positive and gram-negative bacteria found in cutaneous infections | Apply enough ointment to cover lesion completely; store at room temperature in a dry place; hypersensitivity reaction is rare with local application |
| **Carbamide Peroxide** (Auro Ear Drops, Debrox Drops, Murine Ear Drops)<br>**Route:** Topical<br>**Dosage:** Instill several drops in ear canal at bedtime, and plug with cottonball to hold solution in place; remove ear plug in AM; perform twice daily if wax is thick | Commercial ceruminolytics used to soften ear wax for removal | Common products such as baby oil, mineral oil, and vegetable oil are less expensive and can also be used for this purpose |
| **Clotrimazole** (Lotrimin)<br>**Route:** Topical<br>**Dosage:** Apply cream, solution, or lotion twice daily for 1-4 wk | Topical antifungal used for a variety of cutaneous infections | Local burning, itching, stinging, or redness or local hypersensitivity reactions |
| **Dimenhydrinate** (Dramamine)<br>**Route:** PO, IM, IV, rectal<br>**Dosage:** PO, rectal: 50-100 mg q 4-6 hr (not to exceed 400 mg/day); IM, IV: 50 mg q 4 hr | Used in treatment and prevention of nausea, vomiting, dizziness, and vertigo accompanying motion sickness | May cause drowsiness and anorexia; use with caution in patients with seizure disorder, glaucoma, or benign prostatic hypertrophy |
| **Fluocinonide** (Lidex, Flurosyn)<br>**Route:** Topical<br>**Dosage:** Ointment, cream, solution, gel (topical) 0.05%; thin layer 2-4 times daily | Topical corticosteroid used to decrease swelling and inflammation, relieve itching | Burning, dryness, itching; apply only to affected areas; do not use on weeping or infected wound; store at room temperature; can cause hypersensitivity reaction; may cause skin sloughing; if fever develops, discontinue |
| **Hydrochlorothiazide** (Dyazide)<br>**Route:** PO<br>**Dosage:** Adults 25-100 mg/day | Diuretic used in treatment of Ménière's disease to decrease fluid retention | Administer early in day to avoid nocturia; give with food if nausea occurs; may cause muscle weakness, cramps, nausea; instruct patient to eat foods that are high in potassium |
| **Hydrogen Peroxide**<br>**Route:** Topical<br>**Dosage:** 1.5% and 3.0% solutions—use as needed; fill ear canal, wait until bubbling stops, and then drain | Destroys bacteria by chemical action | Can be diluted with water or saline solution (1:1); monitor for irritation, rash, skin breaks, or dryness |
| **Isopropyl Alcohol**<br>**Route:** Topical<br>**Dosage:** 70%-85% solutions—use as needed | Used in management of dermatitis and eczema to dry ear canal | Toxic reactions rare |

*Continued*

**TABLE 39-1**

## Pharmacology of Drugs Used in Hearing—cont'd

| DRUG (GENERIC AND TRADE NAME); ROUTE AND DOSAGE | ACTION/INDICATION | COMMON SIDE EFFECTS AND NURSING CONSIDERATIONS |
|---|---|---|
| **Meclizine** (Antivert)<br>**Route:** PO<br>**Dosage:** 25-100 mg q day or 1 hr before exposure | Used in management and prevention of motion sickness; used to treat labyrinthitis or Ménière's disease | Use with caution in older adults and patients with glaucoma or benign prostatic hypertrophy; may cause drowsiness, headache, dry mouth, or blurred vision |
| **Neomycin Sulfate**<br>**Route:** Topical<br>**Dosage:** Instill 1-3 drops 3-4 times daily for 7-10 days | Antibiotic used to break down protein synthesis, causing death of bacteria | Warm to body temperature before administration; doses should be evenly spaced to maintain blood levels |
| **Prochlorperazine** (Compazine)<br>**Route:** PO, IV, IM, rectal<br>**Dosage:** PO: 5-10 mg 3-4 times daily; IM: 5-10 mg q 4 hr (not to exceed 40 mg/day); IV: 2.5-10 mg (not to exceed 5 mg/min); may be repeated in 30 min; single dose not to exceed 10 mg (not to exceed 40 mg/day); rectal: 25 mg bid | Antiemetic used in management of nausea and vomiting related to motion sickness | Extrapyramidal reactions (involuntary movement, changes in muscle tone, abnormal posture), dry eyes, blurred vision, constipation, dry mouth, and photosensitivity; contraindicated in patients with glaucoma and severe cardiac or liver disease |
| **Promethazine** (Phenergan)<br>**Route:** PO, IV, IM, rectal<br>**Dosage:** For motion sickness: 25 mg 30-60 min before departure; may repeat in 8-12 hr | Treatment and prevention of nausea, vomiting, and motion sickness | Excess sedation, confusion, and disorientation; contraindicated in patients with coma, benign prostatic hypertrophy, or glaucoma; use with caution in patients with sleep apnea or epilepsy and in older adults |
| **Scopolamine** (Transderm-Scōp)<br>**Route:** Transdermal<br>**Dosage:** Transdermal patch 1.5 mg delivers 0.5 mg over 72 hr and should be applied 4-5 hr before travel | Prevention of motion sickness | Drowsiness, blurred vision, tachycardia, dry mouth, and urinary hesitancy; contraindicated in patients with glaucoma or tachycardia; use with caution in older adults and in patients with chronic renal, hepatic, respiratory, or cardiac disease |

therefore be instructed to complete taking all antibiotics as prescribed.

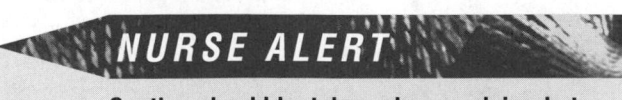

**NURSE ALERT**

**Caution should be taken when applying hot compresses or a heating pad to avoid injury to the ear.**

## External Otitis

External otitis is another common infection of the external ear. It can be the result of an infective, inflammatory, or allergic agent that comes in contact with the tissue of the external ear. External otitis is often called "swimmer's ear." Swimming tends to remove cerumen from the ear. Cerumen's primary function is to protect the external ear from bacteria. As the cerumen is removed, bacteria are introduced, causing an infection. Symptoms of external otitis include redness, swelling, and pain of the auditory canal. Treatment consists of a topical antibiotic and steroid, usually in the form of drops. Oral or intravenous antibiotics are administered in severe cases, especially if a cellulitis is present. Acetaminophen can be given, and heat may be applied locally to relieve pain.

Other types of infections include those caused by fungi, but such infections are rather uncommon. Various forms of dermatitis may occur, particularly in persons with diabetes. Other generalized infections such as erysipelas or eczema may involve the external ear.

## Obstructions

Children often put foreign bodies into their ears, obstructing the auditory canal. Parents and nurses should not attempt to remove foreign bodies because of the danger of pushing them farther into the canal. When the foreign body consists of vegetable matter such as corn, peas, or beans, irrigation should not be done because the fluid will cause the object to enlarge.

Another common cause of obstruction is the accumulation of cerumen, which may plug the auditory canal. Sometimes the cerumen pushes against the eardrum and hardens, causing pain and irritation. Not only is cerumen impaction potentially painful, but it physically obstructs sound transmission and can interfere with the ability to hear. Cerumen can be removed through the use of irrigation, ceruminolytic agents, or currettage. Cerumen removal involves potential hazards. Impaction should first be verified by otoscopic examination. The patient should be asked several questions regarding any history of ear disease or tympanic membrane perforation. Irrigation would be contraindicated under these circumstances.

Most cerumen can be removed by simple irrigation. Always use body temperature water (98° to 99° F). Any variation in water temperature, hotter or colder, can stimulate the semicircular canals, resulting in nausea, vomiting, and vertigo. If a syringe is being used, the tip of the syringe should be placed at the auditory meatus and aimed toward the side of the ear canal for best results. Dental irrigation devices can be used at low settings to achieve the same result. Irrigation should be performed under the direction of a physician.

A ceruminolytic agent such as Debrox may also be used. Debrox is a nonprescription solution containing glycerin and carbamide peroxide. It both softens and loosens cerumen, allowing for easy removal. Mineral oil, baby oil, or vegetable oil is less expensive and also can be used. The ceruminolytic agent is instilled in the affected ear with a dropper and is allowed to remain there. In most cases the cerumen will dissolve and be removed.

If the impaction persists, removal done by a physician with a curette may be required. The curette—a small, blunt spoon—is advanced beyond the point of cerumen impaction. Using extreme caution to prevent nicking of the tympanic membrane, the physician pulls the cerumen out of the auditory canal.

Insects such as moths can also cause an obstruction, resulting in discomfort and temporary hearing loss. An insect in the auditory canal can generally be killed by instilling a few drops of warm oil into the ear and then irrigating the canal with warm water. If the insect is alive, the physician may gently spray lidocaine in the ear to cause the insect to exit.

## Injury

Injury to the external ear may result from a contusion, abrasion, or laceration, or it may be congenital in nature. Occasionally there is loss of the pinna without interference with hearing. However, the congenital absence of the pinna may include absence of the canal and eardrum, resulting in total deafness in the ear.

## Perforation

Perforation of the eardrum may occur as a result of a fracture of the skull or a severe blow to the ear. It may also result from a loud noise or from otitis media (infection in the middle ear), in which there is a spontaneous rupture of the eardrum. At the time of the rupture, the individual may experience a sharp pain accompanied by some degree of hearing loss. Generally diagnosis of a perforation is made on the basis of the individual's symptoms as well as an otoscopic examination of the tympanic membrane. Most injuries to the eardrum heal without requiring medical intervention. However, if the perforation is a result of an infection, antibiotic treatment is initiated. Acetaminophen or other analgesics may be given for pain.

# DISORDERS OF THE MIDDLE EAR

The middle ear is connected with the posterior part of the nose by the eustachian tube. Equalization of air pressure on both sides of the eardrum is maintained by air entering the middle ear through this tube. Infection from the nose and throat may reach the middle ear through the eustachian tube. Sometimes the tube may become inflamed or plugged with mucus, resulting in diminished hearing. The middle ear contains the organs for transmitting sound to the inner ear, and, if they become diseased, deafness may result.

## Otitis Media

Otitis media is an inflammation of the middle ear. It is caused by either fluid or bacteria that enter the middle ear through the eustachian tube. Children are more susceptible to otitis media than adults are because during the early years of life the eustachian tube is more horizontal in position than in later years. This situation favors the transmission of fluid or bacteria from the respiratory passageways into the middle ear. Otitis media is most common in infants. Not only is the eustachian tube of infants horizontal, but it is also shorter, wider, and straighter. In addition, the infant lies flat most of the time, which allows fluid or bacteria to move easily from the respiratory tract to the middle ear. Both children and adults should be taught to keep the mouth open during nose-blowing to reduce the possibility of forcing fluid or bacteria from the respiratory tract into the middle ear.

There are several common forms of otitis media: acute, chronic, and serous. Each type affects the structures of the middle ear, varying in cause and incidence. Acute otitis is sudden in onset, affecting one or both ears. Bacteria is the most common cause of acute otitis. Untreated or repeated attacks of acute otitis media may lead to chronic otitis media. Chronic otitis media is characterized by a purulent, foul-smelling discharge. Serous otitis media is caused by an accumulation of sterile fluid in the middle ear. This fluid can be thin or mucoid and is located behind the tympanic membrane.

## Assessment

In all three types of otitis media, a foreign agent—fluid and/or bacteria—is introduced into the middle ear, causing inflammation of the mucous membranes. This inflammation leads to swelling and irritation of the ossicles. In addition, the tympanic membrane becomes red and swollen.

Signs and symptoms of otitis media vary depending on the causative agent. Acute otitis is bacterial in origin. It is characterized by ear pain, fever, malaise, headache, and reduced hearing. Untreated or repeated episodes of acute otitis media may lead to chronic otitis. Chronic otitis media is also bacterial in origin. Similar to acute otitis, chronic otitis media is characterized by fever, malaise, and some level of hearing loss. Ear pain may or may not be present. Chronic otitis media is usually painless. The presence of pain indicates fluid under pressure in addition to the causative bacteria. Serous otitis media, or middle ear effusion, results from the collection of sterile fluid in the middle ear. Complaints associated with serous otitis include a feeling of fullness in the ear, pressure, and decreased hearing. The individual with serous otitis media does not experience pain, fever, or ear discharge.

## Intervention

The aim of treatment of otitis media is to rid the middle ear of inflammation and/or infection and to prevent perforation of the tympanic membrane. In those cases in which bacteria are the causative agent, treatment consists of a 10-day course of oral antibiotics. In addition, acetaminophen is prescribed for fever and pain. Antihistamines are prescribed for treatment of serous otitis media to remove the excess fluid. However, antihistamines have not been proven effective in the treatment of both acute and chronic otitis media unless allergy is an accompanying factor.

---

| BOX 39-6 | NURSING PROCESS |
| --- | --- |

### OTITIS MEDIA

**ASSESSMENT**

- Comfort level
- Vital signs
- Outer ear for drainage and skin integrity
- Patterns of sleep
- Hearing
- Dizziness

**NURSING DIAGNOSES**

- Pain related to pressure and inflammation in the ear
- Risk for injury related to vertigo and diminished hearing
- Sensory/perceptual alterations related to disruption in conduction of sound
- Sleep pattern disturbance related to ear discomfort
- Risk for impaired skin integrity related to ear drainage

**NURSING INTERVENTIONS**

- Provide comfort measures.
- Encourage diversional activities.
- Provide soothing music at night.
- Administer analgesics, antibiotics, and antihistamines as ordered.
- Apply localized heat if indicated.
- Cleanse outer ear at frequent intervals to keep free of irritating drainage, if indicated.
- If ear is draining, place cotton loosely in external ear outside the canal and change often.
- Offer reassurance that hearing loss is usually temporary.
- Speak in a slow, soft voice (loud voices can cause distortion of sound).
- Maintain an environment that promotes sleep.

**EVALUATION OF EXPECTED OUTCOMES**

- Ear pain reduced or eliminated
- Outer ear clean and dry
- Hearing maintained
- Reports restful sleep
- No dizziness

There is much controversy surrounding the management of otitis media in children, especially chronic otitis media. Treatment options include medical management with antibiotics and surgical insertion of tympanostomy tubes. In some children with recurrent or persistent otitis media, prophylactic treatment with antibiotics is also indicated (Box 39-6).

Untreated or inadequately treated otitis media can result in the formation of a cholesteatoma or an abcess. A cholesteatoma is a cyst that forms after perforation of the tympanic membrane. It is made up of both epithelial cells and cholesterol. Unless surgically removed, a cholesteatoma can cause damage to the structures of the middle ear.

If the infection is severe and an abcess forms, the condition is called purulent otitis media (Figure 39-9). Purulent otitis media is treated with antibiotics and analgesics for pain. Because the mucous membrane lining the middle ear is continuous with parts of the mastoid process, the added danger of extension of the infection is always present.

If the pain from otitis media continues despite antibiotic therapy and the tympanic membrane continues to bulge because of excess fluid, a myringotomy is usually performed. A **myringotomy** is a surgical incision made into the tympanic membrane to release the increased pressure and exudate in the ear. It can be done with the patient under a local anesthetic using an ionesthetizer. The ionesthetizer anesthetizes the eardrum through ion transfer with the use of a local anesthetic solution and an electrode in the ear canal. The procedure is usually performed in a physician's office or an outpatient setting.

A myringotomy results in drainage of the middle ear and almost immediate pain relief. Drainage from the ear is generally bloody at first but becomes purulent. Small tissues should be used to remove the drainage, or cotton should be placed loosely at the external opening of the auditory canal so as not to obstruct the flow of drainage. The area around the external ear should be kept clean because the drainage will cause irritation if allowed to remain on the skin. The patient should be observed for pain or fever after the surgical procedure, which may indicate the need for an additional incision or may be a sign of extension of the infection.

> ### NURSE ALERT
>
> **Gloves should be worn and universal precautions observed when handling ear drainage.**

## Mastoiditis

The mucous membrane lining of the middle ear is continuous with parts of the mastoid process embedded in the temporal lobe. If an infection in the middle ear, such as chronic or acute otitis media, is untreated or inadequately treated, it can continue to the mastoid process and cause **mastoiditis,** an inflammation of those cells in the mastoid process. If severe enough, the infection may continue to extend to the brain, causing the formation of a brain abscess or the development of meningitis. In the days before antibiotic therapy, mastoiditis was a leading cause of death in children and of hearing loss in adults. Because of aggressive antibiotic therapy of otitis media, it is now rare for the infection to progress to mastoiditis.

Symptoms of mastoiditis include an elevated temperature, pain, general malaise, anorexia, and

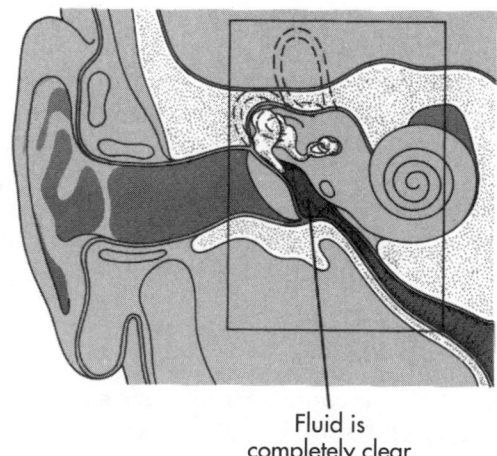
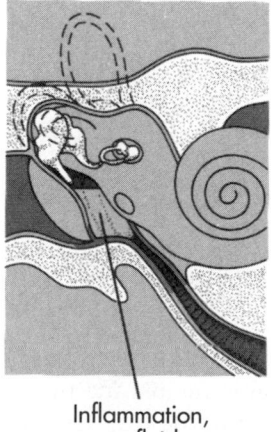
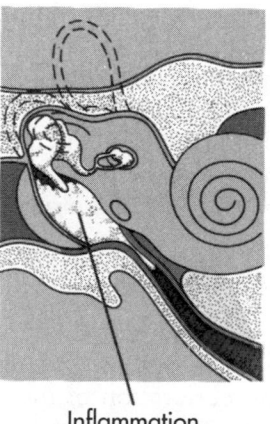

Fluid is completely clear

Inflammation, no fluid

Inflammation, with bacterial infection

**Figure 39-9** Anatomy of otitis media: clear fluid accumulation, inflammation but no fluid, and inflammation with bacterial infection. (From Beare PG, Myers JL: *Adult health nursing*, ed 3, St Louis, 1998, Mosby.)

tenderness over the mastoid area. The tenderness is due to tissue swelling, which tends to push the ear forward. A myringotomy and large doses of oral antibiotics will usually cure mastoiditis. A mastoidectomy, or surgical removal of the infected tissue, is necessary if there is evidence of bone destruction and the infection does not improve with antibiotic therapy.

## Mastoidectomy

### Preoperative Intervention

The preoperative care of the patient undergoing a mastoidectomy is the same as that for the other surgical patients. In addition, particular attention should be focused on hair removal because of the location of the surgery. A careful explanation should be given to all patients concerning removal of hair, and only the necessary amount of hair should be removed. An area of approximately $1\frac{1}{2}$ to 2 inches around the ear is shaved.

### Postoperative Intervention

When the patient returns from surgery, the ear is covered with a large pressure dressing that is secured with bandages around the head. The patient is placed in a semi-Fowler's position. As soon as nausea subsides, oral fluids and a diet as tolerated may be given. Fluids will be administered by the intravenous route if nausea persists. Medication is given to relieve pain as necessary. Antibiotics are administered prophylactically to prevent postoperative infection. Temperature, pulse, and respiration rates are measured every 4 hours and recorded.

Some drainage may occur, causing the dressing to become saturated. However, evidence of hemorrhage, which would appear as bright-red blood on the dressing, is not normal and should be reported to the surgeon immediately. If necessary, the nurse may reinforce the dressing, but in most cases the dressing is changed only by the surgeon. In addition, stiffness of the neck may occur. Stiffness alone can result from the positioning during surgery. The patient should be instructed that this effect is normal and should subside in several days. However, stiffness accompanied by headache, visual disturbances, or facial paralysis is not normal and should be reported to the surgeon immediately.

## Tympanoplasty

**Tympanoplasty** is the name given to a group of surgical procedures designed to restore hearing after loss caused by perforation of the tympanic membrane or necrosis of one of the ossicles of the middle ear, usually following chronic otitis media. The simplest form is a myringoplasty, in which the perforation in the eardrum is closed and reinforced with a tissue graft.

Other types of tympanoplasty are more extensive and involve the bones of the middle ear.

Diseased tissue is removed, and the ossicles are examined to determine the method that will restore the ability to conduct sound. Partial or total ossicular prosthesis may be used. If the tympanic membrane is perforated, it may be repaired with a fascia graft. The incision may be made within the ear canal (endaural) or behind the ear (postauricular). A mastoidectomy may be performed at the same time to remove diseased tissue and the source of infection.

### Preoperative Intervention

There is little preoperative care needed if the patient will be having a simple tympanoplasty such as a myringotomy. The procedure is done with the patient under local anesthesia in an outpatient setting. The preoperative care for a patient undergoing a more extensive tympanoplasty is the same as that for other surgical patients. In either case the patient should be given an explanation of the surgery and should know what to expect postoperatively.

### Postoperative Intervention

Immediately after the surgery, the patient will have an inner dressing located in the ear canal and an outer dressing covering the external portion of the ear. Some drainage can be expected. The inner dressing should be changed only by the surgeon. The outer dressing can be changed or reinforced as needed by the nurse. The patient should lie on the unaffected side with the affected ear upward for 12 hours after surgery. After 12 hours have elapsed, the patient may ambulate. Caution should be taken during ambulation because the patient is likely to experience vertigo. Antiemetics are often prescribed to decrease this vertigo and associated nausea. Antibiotics are given for 5 to 7 days postoperatively to reduce the risk of postoperative infection. The patient must keep the ear dry and avoid sneezing and blowing the nose. If it is necessary to blow the nose or if a sneeze occurs, the nurse should instruct the patient to maintain an open mouth to avoid a buildup of pressure in the ear. The patient may not swim or travel by air until healing is complete; however, once the healing is complete, the patient will have few restrictions.

## Otosclerosis

The middle ear contains three ossicles, whose function is to transmit sound to the inner ear. Normally the stapes vibrates against the oval window, through which sound reaches the inner ear. In otosclerosis a new growth of bone forms, causing the footplate of the stapes to become fixed in the oval window, preventing it from transmitting sound.

**Otosclerosis** is the most common cause of conductive deafness. The cause of otosclerosis is unknown, but it is believed that there is a hereditary predisposition to the disorder. Diagnosis is made through evaluation of symptoms and an examination of the family history. The loss of hearing may first be detected during the adolescent years and may be discovered through audiometer testing. Usually, the loss affects both ears, although one ear may be more severely involved than the other. The hearing impairment continues to increase slowly until the person reaches 40 years of age or older, by which time the loss may be great. There is currently no medical treatment that cures the disorder or impedes its progress. A surgical procedure called a **stapedectomy** restores hearing in approximately 90% of patients.

## Stapedectomy

The stapedectomy is considered the treatment of choice for otosclerosis. In this procedure the stapes is removed and replaced by a small piece of wire or a plastic piston. This is attached to a graft of fat, vein, or Gelfoam fashioned to cover the oval window. Occasionally the footplate of the stapes is left in place and the prosthesis is placed through it. Sound travels from the incus to the wire or plastic piece, which vibrates the tissues of the oval window. Liquids of the inner ear then pick up the vibrations, and nerve impulses are initiated.

### Preoperative Intervention

Preoperative preparation of the patient is the same as that for other ear surgery. The procedure is performed with the patient under local anesthesia, and a sedative is administered before and during surgery. The patient should be advised to wash the hair before entering the hospital to avoid the danger of getting water into the ear after surgery. The patient should be given an explanation of the surgery as well as what to expect postoperatively.

### Postoperative Intervention

For the first 24 hours postoperatively, the patient is kept flat in bed and once again instructed not to blow the nose. All head movements should be kept to a minimum. After the initial 24-hour period, the patient may be allowed up but should not get up alone. The patient should be helped to get out of bed and walk slowly, keeping the head and torso in line and the head level.

There will be packing in the auditory canal and a dressing covering the ear. Slight drainage may appear on the dressing but any bright-red blood should be reported to the surgeon immediately. The patient should be instructed to keep the dressing dry and to avoid getting water in the ear (thus hair washing and swimming are not allowed) and is taught to maintain a sterile technique while changing the dressing. Situations that involve air pressure changes, such as traveling on airplanes, should be avoided until healing has occurred.

The patient is hospitalized for the first 24 hours after surgery. During this time the patient should be carefully observed for signs that might indicate complications, such as meningitis or facial paralysis. Facial nerve paralysis may occur immediately postoperatively because of injection of anesthetic near the nerve. Function should return in about 4 hours. Dryness of the mouth or decreased taste sensation may occur from injury to the chorda tympani nerve during surgery. These symptoms will eventually pass but may last for several months. Vertigo may occur from trauma, loss of perilymph, or labyrinthitis. In addition, the patient may experience some hearing loss. Hearing will return gradually over several weeks. Postoperative nursing care should include education regarding each of these changes.

A sensation of sloshing in the ear may indicate a collection of serous fluid in the middle ear. Otitis media can also occur as a complication of the surgery. Because eating may be painful, administration of an analgesic before meals will increase comfort. A liquid diet is given postoperatively, with a gradual increase to soft foods as tolerated. If nausea and vomiting occur, antiemetics may be ordered.

## DISORDERS OF THE INNER EAR

### Labyrinthitis

The labyrinth is a system of cavities within the inner ear that communicate with one another. **Labyrinthitis** is an inflammation of these structures and usually results from an extension of infection from the middle ear. The characteristic symptom is severe dizziness (vertigo), causing a disturbance of equilibrium. In patients with severe cases of labyrinthitis, nausea and vomiting may occur. There is generally some hearing impairment as well. Labyrinthitis is usually treated with antibiotics. In addition, the individual is instructed to remain in bed as much as possible and to avoid getting out of bed without assistance because of the danger of falling. If nausea and vomiting are severe, intravenous fluids and antiemetic drugs to control vomiting may be administered.

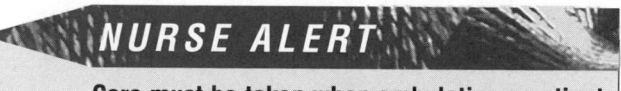

**NURSE ALERT**

Care must be taken when ambulating a patient who is experiencing vertigo.

# Ménière's Disease
## Assessment

**Ménière's disease** is a chronic progressive disorder of the inner ear characterized by intermittent vertigo, tinnitus, sensorineural hearing loss and the sensation of pressure in the ear. Symptoms are usually unilateral, but one third of those affected eventually have bilateral involvement. The symptoms result from an accumulation of endolymph in the membranous labyrinth, which causes an increased pressure in the inner ear. The cause of the increased endolymph is unknown. However, any factor that increases endolymphatic secretion, such as viral or bacterial infections, allergic reactions, or endocrine disorders, could potentially be the cause of Ménière's disease. Vascular changes in the circulation of the labyrinth due to vasospasm, sodium retention, and/or stress and anxiety have also been suggested as possible causes of the disease.

Symptoms of Ménière's disease tend to recur at varying intervals. Some individuals have weekly episodes, and others have symptoms monthly or less frequently. The episodic symptoms usually have a sudden onset. Common complaints include impaired hearing accompanied by roaring or hissing noises and a feeling of fullness in the ear. These symptoms, along with nausea, vomiting, and vertigo, may continue for several hours, generally resolving on their own. Hearing usually returns to normal once the symptoms subside. However, with recurrent symptoms permanent hearing loss may occur over time.

## Intervention

Ménière's disease is managed conservatively through a combination of drug and diet therapy. Drug therapy is aimed at controlling the vertigo and vomiting and restoring normal balance. Acute episodes are treated with bed rest, sedation, antiemetics, and/or drugs for motion sickness. Management between attacks may include administration of additional drugs to control the vertigo and nausea, diuretics and antihistamines to decrease the amount of fluid, and vasodilators to improve circulation in the ear. Many individuals with Ménière's disease experience less severe symptoms or longer periods of remission in response to a low-sodium diet and limited caffeine intake.

Surgical treatment aimed at controlling the vertigo may be performed. Surgical treatment includes several options: labyrinthectomy, endolymphatic sac decompression, or selective vestibular nerve section. Labyrinthectomy involves removal of the stapes and aspiration of the endolymph. During endolymphatic sac decompression, fluid is diverted from the inner ear to the subarachnoid space through a surgical shunt. Selective vestibular nerve section is performed during a craniotomy. The surgeon separates the cochlear and vestibular portions of the eighth cranial nerve, rendering the vestibular portion nonfunctional.

All these surgical procedures are controversial because they either further diminish or destroy hearing in the affected ear or cause facial nerve injury. For these reasons surgery is performed only when Ménière's disease is unilateral and incapacitating and shows no signs of remission with medical treatment.

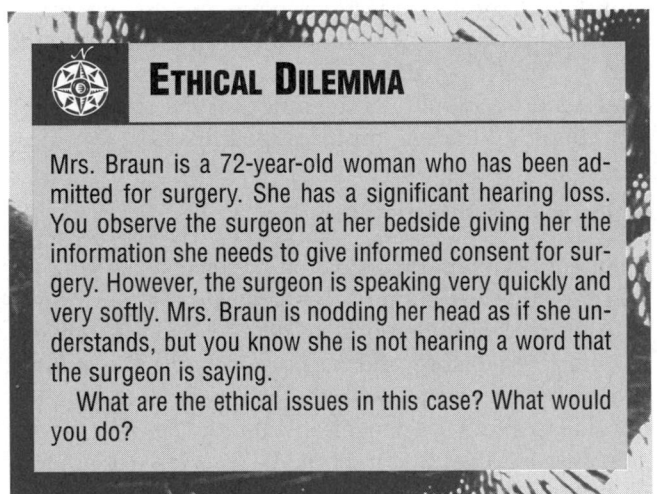

## ⊕ ETHICAL DILEMMA

Mrs. Braun is a 72-year-old woman who has been admitted for surgery. She has a significant hearing loss. You observe the surgeon at her bedside giving her the information she needs to give informed consent for surgery. However, the surgeon is speaking very quickly and very softly. Mrs. Braun is nodding her head as if she understands, but you know she is not hearing a word that the surgeon is saying.

What are the ethical issues in this case? What would you do?

## NURSING CARE PLAN

## PATIENT WITH TYMPANOPLASTY

Mrs. R.T., age 72, has a history of chronic otitis media, resulting in a conduction hearing loss in the left ear. She is scheduled for tympanoplasty. The necrotic ossicles of the inner ear will be reconnected by inserting a prosthesis to correct her conductive hearing loss. She has had preadmission bloodwork, ECG, and chest x-ray examination and arrives at the hospital the morning of surgery.

### Medical History

Has history of mild hypertension; takes Zestril, 5 mg daily

Has taken Premarin and Provera daily for estrogen replacement therapy since age 49.

Takes antioxidants and minerals daily: vitamin C, 500 mg; vitamin E, 400 IU; beta-carotene, 25,000 U; calcium, 1000 mg; magnesium, 500 mg; zinc, 25 mg

Has Crohn's disease: experienced first symptoms at age 16

Had total colectomy with ileorectal anastomoses at age 21 (at that time Crohn's disease was commonly misdiagnosed as ulcerative colitis and total colectomy was recommended treatment for ulcerative colitis)

Has had rectal surgery for strictures and perianal abscesses and fistulas; one perianal fistula could not be repaired without affecting sphincter control and fistula drains regularly

Daily sitz baths and use of baby wipes for perineal cleansing after elimination controls irritation

Must limit dietary intake of skins and seeds to prevent obstruction

Has had four pregnancies and has delivered four full-term infants, all living today

Had mastoidectomy at age 2 following acute ear infection (prior to development of antibiotics); had no noticeable hearing loss as a result of this childhood illness and surgery

Has been troubled with chronic sinusitis and frequent sinus infections for past 18 years and left eustachian tube becomes occluded frequently

Changes in pressure while flying require precautions to prevent tube from becoming blocked, which causes pain and hearing deficit

### Psychosocial Data

Married; lives in townhouse with husband of 49 years

Has four grown and married children, three of whom live within 20- to 60-minute radius

Active couple who walk or use exercise equipment at least 3 times/week

Mrs. T. retired teacher; receives pension

Mr. T. retired self-employed; receives income from investments and Social Security

Health care expenses covered by Medicare and supplemental insurance purchased annually

### Assessment Data

Oriented ×3 (time, place, and person)

Vital signs: T—98.2; P—72, regular; R—20, regular

Weight on admission: 114 lb

Height: 5′ 2″

*Skin:* Clear, well hydrated

*Respiratory:* Lungs clear to auscultation

*Cardiovascular:* Apical pulse—72, regular

*Abdomen:* Bowel sounds present, hyperactive; midline scar, previous bowel resections

Hearing deficit in left ear: patient reports about 50% deficit

Wears one contact lens (left eye) for presbyopia (monovision); needs no correction for distance in right eye

*Continued*

# NURSING CARE PLAN

## PATIENT WITH TYMPANOPLASTY—cont'd

### NURSING DIAGNOSES

Anxiety related to threat to health status resulting from chronic middle ear disorders and changes in auditory acuity preoperatively

Sensory/perceptual alterations (auditory) related to altered status of sense organs resulting from preoperative disease and postoperative edema and surgical packing in the ear

| NURSING INTERVENTIONS | EVALUATION OF EXPECTED OUTCOMES |
| --- | --- |
| Assess for level of anxiety, feelings about hearing loss and expectations of surgery. | Optimal auditory acuity maintained preoperatively and acuity improved postoperatively as evidenced by comprehension of communications, correct responses to communications, verbalization of decreased anxiety, and ability to hear |
| Identify methods to communicate effectively. | |
| Assess for ability to perform daily activities and perception of effect of hearing deficit on quality of life. | |
| Assess dressing for drainage, and maintain in place to protect ear postoperatively from trauma or contamination. | |
| Monitor, describe, and record characteristics of ear drainage, including results of cultures to determine infectious agent. | |
| Assist with audiometric hearing tests to measure hearing loss. | |
| Provide quiet, supportive environment; answer questions honestly and clearly; clarify information as needed to reduce anxiety and fear of unknown. | |
| Offer paper and pencils, cards, magic slate to provide alternative methods of communication if hearing deficit is severe. | |
| Face patient when talking, speaking into unaffected ear—slowly and slightly louder than normal—using simple, short sentences to enhance hearing and facilitate communication. | |
| Inform patient that dressing will be in place to protect the operative ear and that diminished hearing will last several weeks postoperatively because of the presence of edema and blood accumulation in the ear. | |

## NURSING CARE PLAN

## PATIENT WITH TYMPANOPLASTY—cont'd

### NURSING DIAGNOSES

Risk for infection related to disturbance in primary defenses resulting from ear surgical incision and frequent middle ear infections

Risk for injury related to (1) dislodgment of prostheses, (2) leakage of perilymph around the prostheses, causing vertigo and potential falls, (3) increased pressure on middle ear, (4) edema causing facial nerve paralysis

Pain related to surgical incision and localized pressure edema

### NURSING INTERVENTIONS

Assess for pain severity and duration in ear, edema, drainage, and auditory changes preoperatively.

Assess for pain severity and relief achieved by use of analgesics.

Assess for feeling of pressure, vertigo, tinnitus, changes in hearing, and foul-smelling purulent drainage from ear postoperatively.

Monitor, describe, and record temperature every 4 hours.

Monitor white blood cell count.

Administer antibiotics, antiinflammatory agents, analgesics, and antipyretics as ordered.

Provide bed rest for 12 hours with restricted movements (with patient lying on unoperated ear postoperatively).

Ambulate with assistance after 12-hour postoperative period. Vertigo is likely, so use caution.

Instruct/supervise patient on slow position changes, moving head and upper body at same time, not looking down when walking, and avoiding quick movements to reduce vertigo and risk of falls.

Observe ear dressing for serosanguineous drainage. Do not change inner dressing located in the ear canal. Outer dressing covering the entire ear can be changed and reinforced by the nurse. Dressing may be behind the ear if postauricular approach was used by surgeon.

Inform patient that noises such as cracking or popping or some pain in the ear or side of the face is to be expected immediately postoperatively.

Instruct patient to cough or sneeze with mouth open and to blow nose one side at a time to prevent increased pressure within the ears.

Use sterile technique for dressing changes and administration of ear medications or irrigations ordered to prevent transmission of pathogens.

To prevent falls, advise patient to hold onto rails or furniture or to sit down immediately if vertigo is present.

### EVALUATION OF EXPECTED OUTCOMES

Absence of infectious process and injury as evidenced by operative ear free from edema, pain, pressure, and purulent drainage and absence of tinnitus or trauma resulting from falls caused by vertigo.

*Continued*

# NURSING CARE PLAN

## PATIENT WITH TYMPANOPLASTY—cont'd

**NURSING DIAGNOSIS**

Knowledge deficit related to care after discharge: ear care, medications, activity restrictions, prevention of complications, identification of signs and symptoms that must be reported to the physician, and schedule for physician follow-up

| NURSING INTERVENTIONS | EVALUATION OF EXPECTED OUTCOMES |
| --- | --- |
| *Teach patient and family:* | Able to perform ear care procedures: administer ear medications and change ear dressings using sterile technique. Can perform return demonstration and state desired frequency, amount, and length of time to ingest or apply medications. |
| Purpose and side effects of medications | |
| Technique of instilling ear medications (allow return demonstration) | |
| How to change of cottonball daily, noting drainage or bleeding | |
| Characteristics of drainage that must be reported to physician | |
| To cover ear to protect from noise and prevent introduction of infectious agents | |
| To keep dressing dry and in place for 2 weeks; insert 2 cotton balls and coat outer ball with petroleum jelly to repel water to prevent contamination of wound | Able to identify signs and symptoms that must be reported to physician. |
| To avoid swimming, diving, and flying for at least 1 week to prevent infection and pressure changes | Able to list activities not allowed and specify time that they will be restricted. |
| To avoid physical activity for 1 week and strenuous exercise for 3 to 4 weeks to prevent trauma to ear | |
| To blow nose gently, one side at a time; to sneeze or cough with mouth open; and to avoid straining at defecation for 1 to 2 weeks to prevent increased pressure in ear | |
| To report decreased hearing, pain, or drainage from ear to allow early intervention in the event of complications | |
| To avoid exposure to upper respiratory disease to reduce risk of contamination via eustachian tube | |
| To keep appointments with physician as scheduled | |

# KEY CONCEPTS

➤ Hearing loss can occur as a result of an inflammatory process, an obstruction in the external or middle ear, or damage to the inner ear or auditory nerve.

➤ Loss of hearing has an impact on both the patient and the family.

➤ Hearing loss often contributes to feelings of anxiety, loneliness, and isolation. Nursing interventions should be aimed at supporting the patient and assisting him or her to explore the various avenues of communication.

➤ Older adults are more susceptible to hearing loss as a result of degenerative changes in many of their ear structures.

➤ The scope and type of testing performed on a patient with an ear disorder depend upon the symptoms presented.

➤ Successful use of a hearing aid depends on the patient's type of hearing loss, desire, and level of understanding of how to properly use the hearing aid.

➤ Conditions such as an upper respiratory tract infection or allergies can contribute to problems with hearing or equilibrium.

➤ The pain associated with many of the disorders of the external ear is caused by swelling in the lining of the auditory canal. There is no room to accommodate this tissue expansion in the bony canal.

➤ The location, characteristics, intensity, and duration of ear pain are important nursing assessments.

➤ Nursing care of the patient with otitis media is aimed at reducing pain and inflammation, keeping the outer ear clean and dry, and maintaining hearing.

➤ Postoperative care of the patient with ear surgery involves providing a safe environment, pain management, dressing care, positioning, providing hydration and nutrition, psychologic support, and monitoring for infection.

➤ A patient recovering from ear surgery should be instructed to avoid sneezing and nose blowing or told to maintain an open mouth when sneezing or blowing the nose to avoid middle ear pressure.

➤ An inner ear disorder is recognized by characteristic symptoms, including vertigo, tinnitus, nystagmus, and hearing loss.

➤ Potential for injury and sensory/perceptual alterations are two important considerations when caring for a patient with an inner ear disorder.

# CRITICAL THINKING EXERCISES

1. Mrs. Smith, age 82, has noticed a progressive loss of hearing. She tells you that she has come to see her physician because of her son's insistence. She thinks that her loss of hearing is just a part of old age and that nothing can be done to correct it. What changes in ear structure and function are associated with aging that might be causing Mrs. Smith's hearing loss? What tests and examinations would need to be done to determine the cause of her hearing loss?

2. Immediately after a myringotomy Mrs. Kazen tells you that she is unable to hear clearly. She raises questions about whether the surgery was a success. How would you respond?

3. Why is effective preoperative communication and teaching especially important for the patient who is undergoing ear surgery?

## REFERENCES AND ADDITIONAL READINGS

Alho O et al: Risk factors for chronic otitis media with effusion in infancy: each acute otitis media episode induces a high but transient risk, *Archin Otolaryngol Head Neck Surg* 121(8):839-843, 1995.

Barkauskas VH et al: *Health and physical assessment,* St Louis, 1994, Mosby.

Belkengren R, Sapala S: Pediatric management problems, *Pediatr Nurs* 21(3):304-305, 1995.

Brown AS: Early intervention for sensory impairment, *Semin Hearing* 16(2):115-208, 1995.

Chen HL: Hearing in the elderly, relation of hearing loss, loneliness, and self-esteem, *J Gerontol Nurs* 20(6):22-28, 1994.

Chmiel R, Jerger J: Hearing aid use, central auditory disorder, and hearing handicap in elderly persons, *J Am Acad Audiol* 7(3):190-202, 1996.

Erber NP: Communicating with elders: effects of amplification, *J Gerontol Nurs* 20(10):6-10, 1994.

Hanson MJ: Acute otitis media in children, *Nurse Prac* 21(5):72-74, 1996.

Katsarkas A: Hearing loss and vestibular dysfunction in Ménière's disease, *Acta Otolaryngol (Stockh)* 116(2):185-188, 1996.

Lewis SM, Collier IC, Heitkemper MM: *Medical-surgical nursing: assessment and management of clinical problems,* ed 4, St Louis, 1996, Mosby.

Lindblade DD, McDonald M: Removing communication barriers for the hearing-impaired elderly, *Medsurg Nurs* 4(5):379-385, 1995.

Margolis RH et al: Tympanic electrocochleography for diagnosis of Ménière's disease, *Arch Otolaryngol Head Neck Surg* 121(1):44-55, 1995.

McAllen PA: Hospital extra: managing Ménière's disease, *Am J Nurs* 96 (6 Nurse Pract Extra), 1996.

McLeod RP, Bently PC: Understanding deafness as a culture with a unique language and not a disability, *Adv Pract Nurs Q* 2(2):50-58, 1996.

Meador JA: Clinical outlook. Cerumen impaction in the elderly, *J Gerontol Nurs* 21(12):43-45, 1995.

Moores DF: Cochlear implants and hearing aids, *Am Ann Deaf* 140(3):245-246, 1995.

New guidelines question drug therapy for otitis media, *RN* 58(1):66, 1995.

Pollock KJ: Ménière's disease: a review of the problem, *ORL Head Neck Nurs* 13(2):10-13, 1995.

Practice guidelines. Chronic otitis media/chronic mastoiditis/cholesteatoma, *ORL Head Neck Nurs* 13(2):22-23, 1995.

Schuring LT et al: ORL–Head and Neck Nursing practice guidelines: stapedectomy, *ORL Head Neck Nurs* 12(4):22-23, 1994.

Seidel HM et al: *Mosby's guide to physical examination,* ed 3, St Louis, 1995, Mosby.

Sherman I, Drake-Lee A: Wound management in ear, nose and throat surgery, *J Wound Care* 4(4):186-188, 1995.

# CHAPTER 40

# Skin Integrity

## CHAPTER OBJECTIVES

1 Identify the functions of the skin.
2 Describe the correct methods for applying open and closed wet dressings and for administering a soak or therapeutic bath.
3 Identify measures to prevent and treat pressure ulcers.
4 Differentiate between the signs and symptoms of folliculitis, furuncles, and carbuncles, and identify the usual causative organism of each.
5 Describe the lesions and transmission of impetigo.
6 Differentiate signs, symptoms, and intervention for the various forms of ringworm (tinea).
7 Differentiate the causes of chafing, prickly heat, plant poisoning, exfoliative dermatitis, and drug dermatitis.
8 Describe lesions and interventions for psoriasis and eczema.
9 Discuss the facts essential to teaching the patient to control systemic lupus erythematosus.
10 Differentiate between herpes simplex types 1 and 2 and herpes zoster.
11 Describe nursing measures to provide relief for the patient with pruritus.
12 Differentiate between the appearance of malignant and benign skin lesions.
13 Describe methods for the prevention and treatment of pediculosis.

## KEY TERMS

| | |
|---|---|
| atopic | nodule |
| atrophy | papule |
| bleb | periungual |
| bulla | pressure ulcer |
| comedones | pustule |
| crust | sebaceous |
| debridement | seborrhea |
| dermis | sebum |
| emergent | shear |
| epidermis | shearing force |
| exfoliate | telangiectasia |
| fissure | tinea |
| gumma | urticaria |
| lichenification | vesicle |
| macule | wheal |

## STRUCTURE AND FUNCTION OF THE SKIN

The skin is the largest organ of the body and is often referred to as the integumentary system. It is considered an organ because of its physiologic structure and its many functions (Table 40-1). The functions of the skin are sensory reception, protection, excretion, thermoregulation, communication, vitamin synthesis, maintenance of homeostasis, processing of antigenic substances, and cosmetic adornment. Each function correlates to specific structures and properties in the epidermis and dermis (Hill, 1994).

The skin is usually thought of as having two distinct layers: the epidermis and the dermis (Figure 40-1); however, a third layer of tissue, the subcutaneous, may

TABLE 40-1

## Functions of the Skin

| FUNCTION | EPIDERMIS | DERMIS | SUBCUTANEOUS |
|---|---|---|---|
| Protection from dehydration | Keratin renders skin impervious to water, preventing undue water loss | Sebaceous glands render skin impervious to water, preventing undue water loss | |
| Protection from mechanical injury | Mechanical strength protects underlying structures; layer is thicker where subject to more friction (palms, soles of feet) | Mechanical strength from collagen fibers, elastic fibers, ground substance | Mechanical shock absorber |
| Protection from infection | Dry external surface inhibits growth of microorganisms | Lymphatic and vascular tissues capable of inflammatory and immune response; first line of defense against microorganisms | |
| Protection from ultraviolet light | Melanin absorbs UV light and protects subepidermal layers | | |
| Temperature regulation | Sweat glands secrete sweat, taking energy from the skin to reduce skin temperature by evaporating sweat, thus reducing core body temperature | Dilation or constriction of blood vessels will promote or inhibit heat conduction, convection, radiation, and evaporation | |
| Vitamin synthesis | When exposed to sunlight, synthesizes vitamin D from dehydrocholesterol in malpighian cells; supplements vitamin D taken with food | | |
| Sensory organ | Transmits sensations through neuroreceptor system | Relays sensations to brain | Contains large pressure receptors |
| Communication | Blushing and facial expressions communicate wide range of emotions | | |
| Preservation of self-image | Epidermal diseases such as psoriasis can alter body image and self-esteem | Dermal diseases such as scleroderma can alter body image and self-esteem | |

be included because of its function in helping to protect other body tissues. The **epidermis** is the outermost layer, and it actually has four layers or regions, sometimes called *strata* (stratum basale, stratum spinosum, stratum granulosum, stratum corneum). The three outermost regions consist of dead cells that are constantly being pushed to the surface and shed while new cells are being developed in the innermost region. The principal substance of the outside layer of the epidermis is keratin. Keratin is a protein that provides a waterproof covering that prevents the skin from drying. It has a slightly acidic action, which is the source of the skin's acidity and serves as a barrier to invading pathogens. Hair and nails are a specialized form of keratin that has become dry and firm. The epidermis also contains the pigment melanin, which provides the coloring of the skin and helps prevent skin cancer by shielding the skin from excessive exposure to sunlight. There is an increased synthesis of melanin on exposure to ultraviolet light, and this is the process involved in

suntanning. Dark-skinned people have larger melanin pigment granules than light-skinned people. There are no blood vessels in the epidermis, so it receives its nourishment and fluids through seepage of lymph from blood vessels below.

The **dermis,** or true skin, is closely attached to the epidermis and consists of two layers. The uppermost (superficial) layer contains small elevations that project upward into the epidermis. The reticular or deeper layer contains numerous capillary blood vessels and nerve fibers. This is why bleeding and pain occur when a person pricks a finger. Some of the nerve fibers have receptors for hot and cold, others for touch and pressure, and some are concerned with vasodilation and vasoconstriction. The dermis also contains the sudoriferous (sweat) and **sebaceous** (oil) glands. All the structures are held together by fibrous and elastic connective tissue. The elasticity of this tissue decreases with the aging process, which causes the skin to take on a wrinkled appearance.

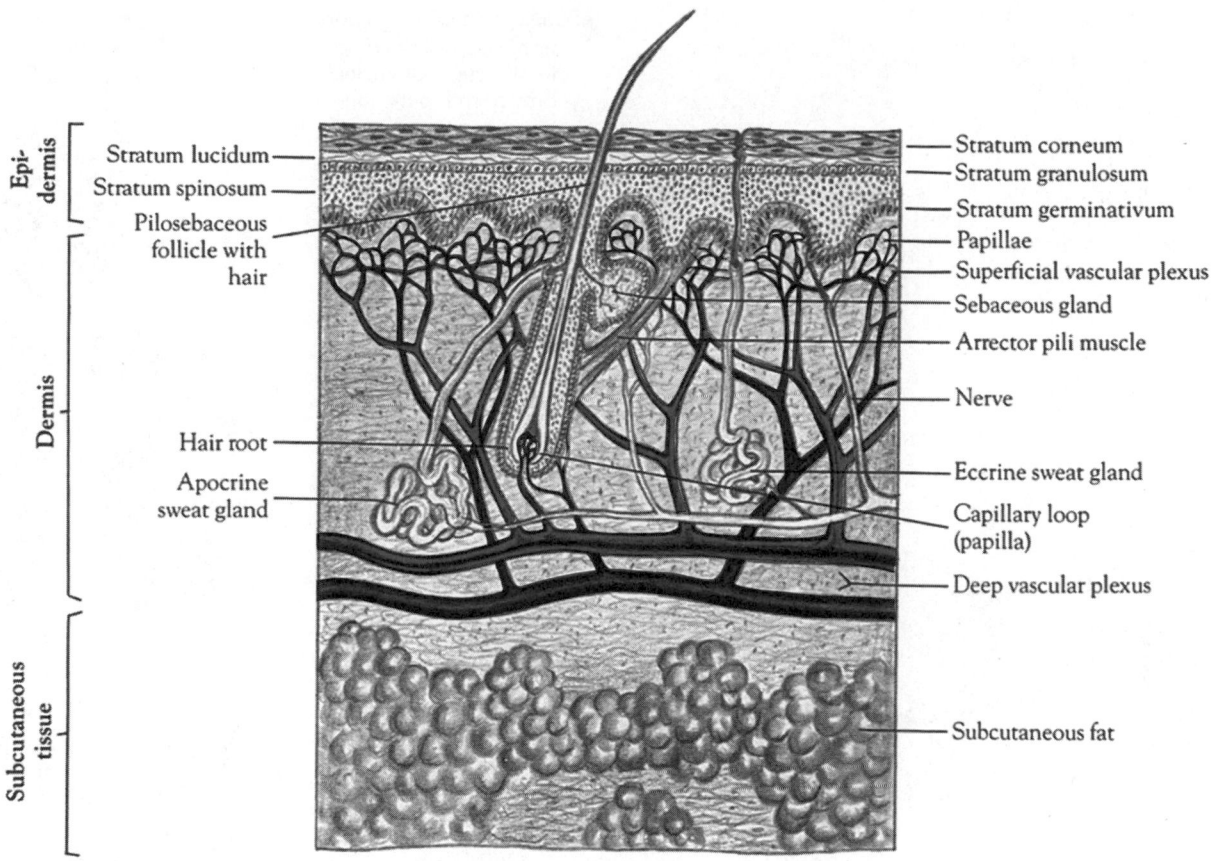

**Figure 40-1**    Structures of the skin. (From Thompson JM et al: *Mosby's clinical nursing,* ed 4, 1997, St Louis, Mosby.)

Beneath the dermis is a layer of subcutaneous tissue, also called superficial fascia. The subcutaneous tissue, closely adherent to the dermis, provides support and, through small arteries and lymphatics, maintains a blood supply to the dermis. Subcutaneous tissue contains large amounts of fat and some sweat glands. The thickness of the skin and the amount of subcutaneous tissue vary on different parts of the body.

The nails, hair, and sebaceous and sudoriferous glands and their ducts are appendages of the skin. The sebaceous glands secrete an oily substance called **sebum,** which keeps the hair from becoming brittle. Sebum also functions to waterproof the hair and skin, promote the absorption of fat-soluble substances into the dermis, and synthesize vitamin D. It may have some antibacterial function (Hill, 1994). The acid coating (pH 4.0 to 6.8) on the surface of the skin is provided by sebum. The vernix caseosa on the newborn infant is an accumulation of sebum from the sebaceous glands. The sebaceous gland may open into a hair follicle or may open directly onto the skin.

The sweat glands originate as blind coiled tubes with ducts that ultimately open on the surface of the skin as pores. These glands are distributed over the entire body but are more numerous on the forehead, palms of the hands, and soles of the feet. The sweat glands are important because they function in regulating body heat through evaporation of water from the skin surface.

The hair and nails are subordinate to the skin. The appearance of the nails changes during illness, and they may become brittle and easily broken, whereas in old age they may be rough and thickened.

Because of the numerous nerve endings in the skin, its function as a sense organ is of primary importance. Through the sense of touch, the nurse is able to feel the patient's pulse or the temperature of the skin. Any disruption of this function can have negative effects. The classic example is the patient with diabetes who develops a foot ulcer because the pain from the incorrectly fitted shoe is not perceived.

The unbroken skin is the first line of defense against pathogenic organisms. The skin protects deeper tissue from injury and loss of body fluids. The excretory function of the skin is limited, but one of its most important functions is to help regulate body temperature. This regulation is accomplished in two ways: (1) evaporation of sweat from the body and (2) dissipation of excess heat into the air when blood vessels dilate, bringing more blood, and thus increased heat, to the skin surface.

Lesion

Macule—flat; nonpalpable; circumscribed; less than 1 cm in diameter; brown, red, purple, white, or tan
Examples: Freckles, flat moles; rubella; rubeola; drug eruptions
Note: Classified as patch if greater than 1 cm in diameter

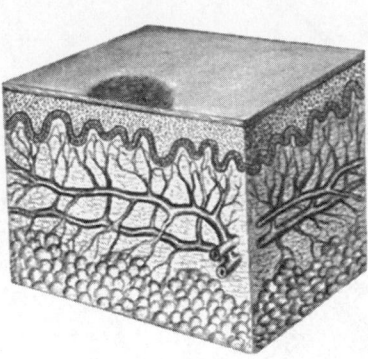

Papule—elevated; palpable; firm; circumscribed; less than 1 cm in diameter; brown, red, pink, tan, or bluish red
Examples: Warts; drug-related eruptions; pigmented nevi; eczema

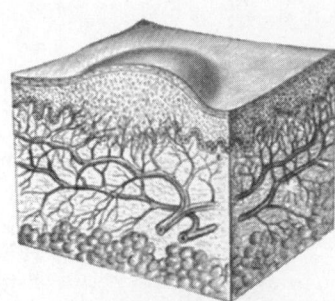

Plaque—elevated; flat topped; firm; rough; superficial papule greater than 1 cm in diameter; may be coalesced papules
Examples: Psoriasis; seborrheic and actinic keratoses; eczema

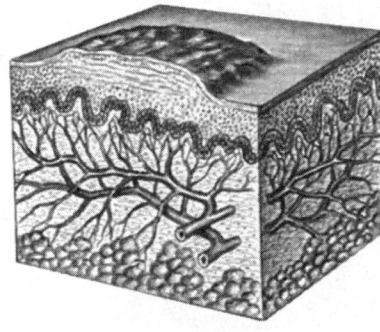

Wheal—elevated; irregular-shaped area of cutaneous edema; solid, transient, changing; variable diameter; pale pink
Examples: Urticaria; insect bites

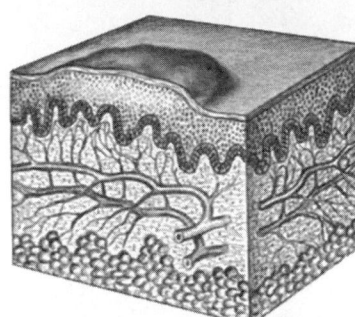

Nodule—elevated; firm; circumscribed; palpable; deeper in dermis than papule; 1 to 2 cm in diameter
Examples: Erythema nodosum; lipomas

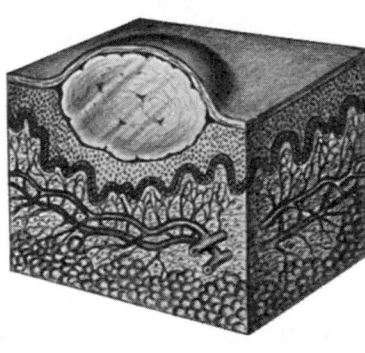

Vesicle—elevated; circumscribed; superficial; filled with serous fluid; less than 1 cm in diameter
Examples: Blister; varicella
Note: Classified as bulla if greater than 1 cm

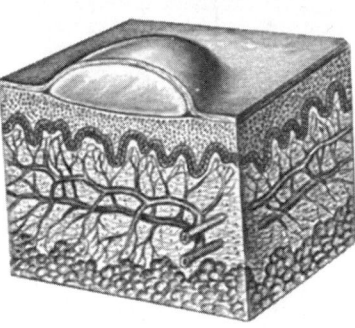

Pustule—elevated; superficial; similar to vesicle but filled with purulent fluid
Examples: Impetigo; acne; variola; herpes zoster

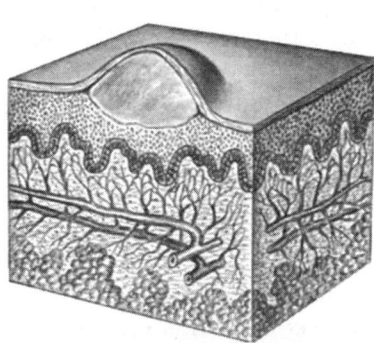

Scale—heaped-up keratinized cells; flaky exfoliation; irregular; thick or thin; dry or oily; varied size; silver, white, or tan
Examples: Psoriasis; exfoliative dermatitis

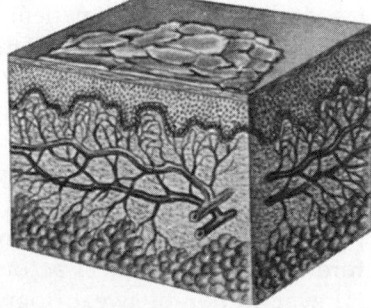

Crust—dried serum, blood, or purulent exudate; slightly elevated; size varies; brown, red, black, tan, or straw
Examples: Scab on abrasion; eczema; impetigo

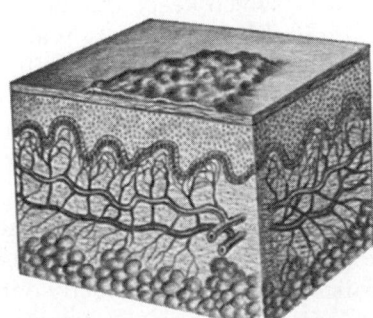

**Figure 40-2**   Common skin lesions. (From Thompson JM et al: *Mosby's clinical nursing*, ed 4, St Louis, 1997, Mosby.)

# NURSING ASSESSMENT OF THE SKIN

In health or disease the normal skin tells many things about an individual, and in many situations it may provide valuable diagnostic clues to disease. Nursing personnel should routinely observe the color of the skin, its texture, presence of rashes or lesions, and characteristics of the hair and nails. Cyanosis, pallor, profuse sweating, and skin rashes are some of the conditions observed that may help to identify disease. In a state of optimum health most persons take their skin for granted and pay too little attention to it, but when disease affects the skin, they become greatly disturbed. Skin that is well cared for and free from disease is a psychologic, social, and economic asset. It contributes to a feeling of well-being, to social acceptance, and to educational and employment opportunities.

# ASSESSMENT AND DESCRIPTION OF SKIN LESIONS

Certain types of skin lesions are peculiar to specific disorders and help the dermatologist identify the disease (Figure 40-2). Some diseases are characterized by an orderly sequence of skin lesions. For example, with chickenpox, red macules surmounted by vesicles first appear (lesion is described as a "dew drop on a rose petal"), then umbilication, and finally crusting. Several different types of lesions may be present in an individual at the same time (Boxes 40-1 and 40-2).

---

**BOX 40-1**

## TYPES OF SKIN LESIONS

**bleb** An irregular elevation of the epidermis filled with serous or seropurulent fluid; may be large in size and is seen in certain forms of severe dermatitis

**bulla** A vesicle greater than 1 cm in diameter

**crust** A dry exudate, commonly called a *scab*, as seen in impetigo, smallpox, chickenpox, and eczema

**excoriation** An abraded or denuded area of skin

**fissure** A groove, crack, or slit in the skin

**gumma** A tumorlike lesion similar in appearance to an abscess; characteristic of late syphilis

**macule** A discolored spot on the skin that may be of various colors and shapes; is neither raised nor depressed

**nodule** A raised, solid lesion that is deeper in the skin than a papule

**papule** A small, solid elevation varying from the size of a pinhead to a pea; may be seen in eczema, measles, smallpox, and syphilis

**pustule** A small elevation filled with pus; characteristic of impetigo and acne vulgaris

**scale** A small, thin flake of dry epidermis as seen in eczema and psoriasis

**scar** The mark left on the skin after repair of deep tissue loss

**ulcer** An open lesion on the skin with loss of deep tissue (epidermis and part of dermis), classic example is decubitus ulcer; stasis ulcers

**vesicle** A blisterlike elevation on the skin containing serous fluid; occurs in herpes simplex, chickenpox, and impetigo

**wheal** Elevation of varying size and irregular shape; if extensive, may run together; characteristic of various allergic reactions (i.e., hives/urticaria.)

---

**BOX 40-2**

## ASSESSMENT OF SKIN IN DARK-SKINNED INDIVIDUALS

1 Inspection and palpation are equally important in assessing the dark-skinned patient. Skin color changes are best observed in the sclera, conjunctiva, oral mucosa, tongue, lips, nail beds, palms, and soles. Normal variations in pigmentation should be considered when assessing for skin color changes. The oral mucosa may have areas of darker pigmentation in the gums, the cheeks, and borders of the tongue. The lips may have a normal dark blue color. The presence of edema may cause dark skin to appear lighter in color. Changes in skin texture assessed by palpation may be the only indication of the presence of skin rashes.

2 In dark-skinned patients, pallor results in the loss of normal red tones in the skin. The brown-skinned person may have yellow-tinged skin when pallor is present. In the black-skinned patient, pallor produces an "ashen gray" color.

3 Jaundice is best observed in the sclera closest to the center of the eye. The dark-skinned patient may have normal yellow pigmentation present in the sclera. Inspection of the hard palate for a yellow color can confirm the presence of jaundice.

4 Cyanosis may be difficult to detect in the dark-skinned patient. Inspection in areas of lightest pigmentation will often indicate the presence of cyanosis, such as the nail beds, conjunctivae, palms, and soles.

5 Petechiae are best observed in the conjunctiva and oral mucosa. They may also be seen in areas of lighter pigmentation over the abdomen, gluteal folds, or inner aspect of the forearm.

6 Erythema is determined by palpating for increased skin temperature that is usually associated with conditions that produce this skin color change.

From Beare PG, Myers JL: *Adult health nursing*, ed 3, St Louis, 1998, Mosby.

# NURSING RESPONSIBILITIES FOR DIAGNOSTIC TESTS AND PROCEDURES

Most skin disorders can be diagnosed from a carefully taken history, the patient's complaints, and observation of the lesion. A personal history should include allergies and their specific manifestations, sleep habits, occupation, medications, recent travel, contact with others, and level of anxiety. It is also important to find out when and where the lesion first appeared and the direction of its spread, whether it is constant or comes and goes, whether it is wet or dry, and whether pruritus (itching) is present. Four important observations must be made: identification, distribution, shape, and arrangement of the lesion. Careful observation and recording of this information can be of great value to the physician in making the correct diagnosis.

Sometimes the dermatologist may wish to make a bacteriologic study, in which case scraping or swabbing the lesion is necessary. Various types of fungi can be identified by this method. At other times a biopsy may be done for pathologic examination. The nurse's primary responsibility for any diagnostic procedure is to inform the patient of the procedure and answer any questions the patient may have. Skin biopsy is an invasive, though minor, procedure and requires a signed consent. After explaining the procedure to the patient, the nurse should remain with the patient during the procedure to help relieve any anxiety that the patient may have. Postprocedure instructions, which vary according to physician preference, should be carefully explained, and the patient should be told that the nurse is available by phone for assistance if any concerns or questions arise.

# NURSING RESPONSIBILITIES FOR THERAPEUTIC PROCEDURES

Nursing care of the patient with skin disorders may involve several nursing procedures, including therapeutic baths, wet dressings, soaks, and the application of various topical medications.

## Therapeutic Baths

Therapeutic baths are used for several purposes, including disinfecting and deodorizing, relieving pruritus, achieving a soothing effect, and softening and lubricating the skin. Soap, oils, medications, or a variety of substances such as oatmeal, cornstarch, baking soda, or a combination of these may be used (Table 40-2). One cup of either cornstarch or baking soda may be added to a tub of tepid water to provide a soothing bath for patients suffering from pruritus. For an oatmeal bath, prepare the oatmeal by placing 2 cups of oatmeal and 1 quart of boiling water in a double boiler and cook for approximately 45 minutes. The oatmeal mixture is then put in a gauze bag, and the bag is swished in a tub of water. The cooled oatmeal may be expressed and applied directly to the patient's body, to be washed off before the patient exits the tub. Commercial oatmeal preparations, such as Aveeno, are available and ready to add to the bath water. To prevent the commercial mixtures from lumping, they should be dissolved under running water and then dispersed throughout the bath water.

The temperature of the water for therapeutic baths should be 35° C to 37.8° C (95° F to 100° F), and the tub

## OLDER ADULT CONSIDERATIONS

**INTEGUMENTARY ASSESSMENT**
**General Approach**
- Allow more time than for a younger adult.
- Articulate clearly; the geriatric patient may be hearing impaired.
- Impaired sight, comprehension, or mobility may result in less than optimum cooperation.
- Provide clear, concise directions.

**History Collection**
- Be alert for answers that do not appear appropriate; the patient may not have understood the question correctly because of impaired hearing or comprehension.
- Some questions may need to be repeated in a different manner.

**Physical Assessment**
- The physical examination itself is not different, but the approach needs to be altered such that the appropriate information is assessed without undue discomfort or embarrassment for the patient.
- Maintain an environment with minimal noise, distractions, and interruption.
- Decreased elasticity (turgor) is found even in patients with adequate hydration and causes wrinkles.
- Dry skin is common secondary to decreased sweat and sebaceous gland production.
- Hyperpigmented macules may often be observed and are sometimes referred to as "age" or "liver" spots.
- Progressive thinning of all body hair occurs.
- Thinning of the epidermis and dermis leads to capillary fragility and therefore easy bruising.
- Onychomycosis, a fungal condition of the nails, is a common finding.

From Beare PG, Myers JL: *Adult health nursing*, ed 3, St Louis, 1998, Mosby.

**TABLE 40-2**

## Balneotherapy

| TYPE OF BATH | AGENTS | DISEASE | PURPOSE |
|---|---|---|---|
| Antibacterial | Potassium permanganate (1:32,000; 1:64,000)<br>Acetic acid<br>Hexachlorophene<br>Povidone-iodine | Infected eczema<br>Dirty ulcerations<br>Furunculosis | Lower skin bacterial load |
| Colloidal | Starch and baking soda (1 cup each/tub)<br>Aveeno Colloidal Oatmeal (1 cup each/tub)<br>Aveeno Oilated Colloidal Oatmeal | Any red, irritated, oozing condition (e.g., atopic eczema) | Relieve itching<br>Soothe |
| Emollient* | Bath oils: Alpha Keri, Lubath<br>Mineral oil | Any dry skin condition | Cleanse and hydrate the skin |
| Tar* | Bath oils with tar: Balnetar, Zetar, Polytar<br>Coal tar concentrate (liquor carbonis detergens) | Scaly dermatoses (e.g., psoriasis) | Loosen scale<br>Relieve itching<br>Potentiate UVA/UVB light therapy |

From Hill MJ: *Skin disorders: Mosby's clinical nursing series,* St Louis, 1994, Mosby.
*For emollient and tar baths, 3 to 6 capfuls of therapeutic agent are added per standard size bathtub.

should be three-fourths full or sufficiently full to cover the involved area. The bath may be given for 10 to 20 minutes several times a day. Warm water should be added to maintain a constant temperature, but the temperature should not exceed 37.8° C (100° F). Very hot water is not good for the skin because of the drying and vasodilation effects, and it is particularly inadvisable for persons with skin diseases.

Because some preparations may cause the tub to be slippery, extreme care should be taken to prevent the patient from slipping in the tub. When the patient is removed from the tub, the skin should be patted dry to avoid irritation or damage, and medication, if ordered, or a bland emollient, should be applied to the moist skin. Measures should be taken to prevent chilling the patient.

## Wet Dressings

Wet dressings are used for many types of skin diseases. They may be open or closed and warm or cold depending on the therapeutic effect desired (Table 40-3). Evaporation of the solution in an open dressing initiates vasoconstriction, which provides a cooling effect and relieves the pruritus that accompanies some disease. The moisture will soften crusts and stimulate drainage. Some solutions, such as Dakin's solution, will retard the growth of bacteria on the skin and help prevent infection. Open wet dressings should not be covered with impermeable materials. Because of rapid evaporation, frequent changing or wetting is

necessary. Pieces of soft old muslin, fluffs, or abdominal gauze are preferred to cotton, which has a tendency to pack down. Dressings must be clean but not necessarily sterile unless indicated by the overall condition of the patient (e.g., immunocompromised) or the presence of an open wound.

Wet dressings under occlusion (closed wet dressings) are used to help hydrate the epidermis to allow more effective absorption of topical medications. The dressings may be used on an isolated area or as total body treatment (mummy wrap) for patients with extensive or generalized involvement. If the area being treated is limited, the nurse should wet the dressing in the prescribed medicated solution and apply it directly to the area. The surrounding skin should be protected from moisture and from the medicated solution by applying petroleum jelly or other suitable protective substances. Wet dressings should be thoroughly saturated but should not drip. Dry towels are wrapped around the closed wet dressing.

A warm, moist dressing is wrapped in thin plastic material and secured. A constant-temperature heating pad may be used to keep the dressing warm, but in that case the dressing should not be wrapped in plastic because of the danger of burning the patient. The nurse should rewet the dressing as needed with an Asepto syringe. However, if drainage is present, it is preferable to remove the entire dressing and reapply a new one. Solutions often used for wet dressings include physiologic saline, magnesium sulfate solution, 0.5% aluminum acetate (Burow's) solution,

| TABLE 40-3 | | |
|---|---|---|
| **Solutions for Soaks and Wet Dressings** | | |
| **SOLUTION** | **PURPOSE** | **DILUTION** |
| Tap water | To cool and relieve pruritus<br>To loosen eschar and crusts | Tap water at approximately body temperature |
| Aluminum acetate (Domeborro, Aluwets, Burow's solution) | Same as tap water<br>To promote drying<br>To provide a mild antiseptic effect | Mix 1 tablet with 1 qt (1 L) water (1:40)<br>Mix 1 tablet with 1 pt (500 ml) water (1:20) |
| Potassium permanganate ($KMnO_4$) | Same as tap water<br>To provide astringent effect<br>To provide antimicrobial effect (especially effective against *Pseudomonas aeruginosa*) | Prepared by pharmacist at dilutions of 0.25% to 0.5% |
| Normal saline | Same as tap water<br>To provide isotonic solution to skin for cooling and antipruritic effect | 0.9% saline solution |
| Silver nitrate ($AgNO_3$) | Astringent and antibacterial | Prepared by pharmacist at 1:1000 to 1:10,000 |

From Hill MJ: *Skin disorders: Mosby's clinical nursing series*, St Louis, 1994, Mosby.

dilute sodium hypochlorite (Dakin's) solution, and 1:4000 potassium permanganate solution. Boric acid should not be used for widespread, raw areas because of its toxic effects, but it is safe and soothing for small, irritated areas. This limited use of boric acid is a major disadvantage. Even continuous wet dressings should be removed periodically to allow the skin to dry and to observe the status of the affected area. Cold dressings should be removed every 6 hours for at least 30 minutes. The bed and pillow should be protected when wet dressings are used. Because of the risk of maceration and the decreased frequency of wound observation, continuous wet dressings should be used cautiously and on a limited basis.

When topical medicines such as medicated creams need to be applied, the nurse should wet the dressing material with warm tap water and apply it over the medicine (Tables 40-4 to 40-7). Dry towels (for limited areas) or bath blankets (for mummy wraps) are placed on top of the dressing, which not only keeps the moisture in but also provides warmth for the patient as the dressings begin to cool. These dressings usually are left in place for 20 to 30 minutes, and a lubricating agent is applied over the affected areas to provide occlusion until the next wet dressing is applied. A mummy wrap is the dressing of choice when treating patients with generalized skin disorders that are erythematous, eczematous, or exfoliating (e.g., psoriasis, eczema, mycosis fungoides).

## Soaks

Soaks may be ordered to loosen necrotic tissue, promote suppuration, or hydrate the skin to increase the absorption of topical medications. When an extremity is involved, a basin or tub large enough to submerge the part should be secured. The solution, temperature, and frequency and duration of the treatment are prescribed by the physician. Patients with burns may be placed in physiologic saline soaks for the purpose of debridement. Whirlpool treatments can serve the same purposes as soaks.

## Paste Boots

Boots are often used for patients with certain types of dermatitis and ulcers on the lower extremities. Several commercial preparations containing water, gelatin, glycerin, and zinc oxide are available. One preparation known as Unna's boot (Dome-paste bandage) is impregnated with the materials, which simplifies its application. The extremity is elevated approximately 30 minutes before applying the boot. An ointment may be applied to the skin lesions and covered with a thin gauze dressing. The paste bandage is then applied from the ankle to the knee, with greater pressure on the ankle and reduced pressure near the knee. This increases venous return and is particularly beneficial in patients with venous stasis ulcers. Two layers of stockinette or an elastic bandage is applied as an outer dressing. The boot is changed every 5 to 8 days.

*Text continued on p. 1256.*

**TABLE 40-4**

## Topical Medications

| CLASS/CONTENT | PURPOSES | DISADVANTAGES | INERT EXAMPLES |
|---|---|---|---|
| **Cream**<br>Oil-in-water emulsion; water content 60% or more | Ease of application<br>Ease of removal<br>Lubrication<br>Delivers medication | Removed by perspiration<br>Low penetration of medication | Dermatology formula<br>Nutraderm |
| **Ointment**<br>Water-in-oil emulsion; water content 40% or less | Marked lubrication<br>Maintains a layer of medication on skin<br>Delivers medication with enhanced penetration | Greasy sensation<br>May stain clothing<br>May inflame hair follicles | Aquaphor<br>Eucerin<br>Nivea<br>Petrolatum<br>Lanolin |
| **Gel**<br>Semisolid mixture; between cream and ointment in content; often contains alcohol | Ease of application<br>Greaseless layer of medication | May cause burning on eroded skin | |
| **Powder**<br>Finely ground solid particles | Absorbs moisture, thereby promoting drying<br>Decreases skin friction<br>Delivers medication best in intertriginous areas | Wears off easily | Talcum<br>Bentonite<br>Cornstarch<br>Zinc oxide |
| **Lotion**<br>Powder suspended in liquid (water, alcohol, oil) | Cooling effect on evaporation<br>May absorb moisture, promoting dryness<br>Delivers medication as uniform residual film<br>Useful in hairy areas | Wears off easily<br>Can overdry skin | Ken<br>Lubriderm<br>WIBI<br>Cetaphil |
| **Solution**<br>Powder dissolved in liquid medium | Similar to lotion<br>Useful in hairy areas | Similar to lotion | Vehicle-N<br>C-solve |
| **Aerosol Spray**<br>Lotion delivered by airborne propellant | Similar to lotion but even more drying<br>Useful in hairy areas | Similar to lotion | |
| **Paste**<br>Powder mixed in ointment; 50% or more powder content | Leaves a protective coating while delivering medication | Low rate of penetration<br>Messy to use | Zinc oxide paste (Lassar's) |

From Hill MJ: *Skin disorders: Mosby's clinical nursing series,* St Louis, 1994, Mosby.

**TABLE 40-5**

## Pharmacology of Drugs Used for Skin Integrity

| DRUG (GENERIC AND TRADE NAME); ROUTE AND DOSAGE | ACTION/INDICATION | COMMON SIDE EFFECTS AND NURSING CONSIDERATIONS |
|---|---|---|
| **Acyclovir** (Zovirax ointment)<br>**Route:** Topical<br>**Dosage:** 5% ointment apply to lesions q 3 hr while awake, 6 times daily for 1 wk | Antiviral, interferes with DNA replication; used for simple mucocutaneous herpes simplex and herpes zoster; also used in immunocompromised patients with initial genital herpes | Rash, urticaria, stinging, burning, pruritus, and vulvitis |
| **Aluminum acetate** (Burow's Solution)<br>**Route:** Topical<br>**Dosage:** 1:20 or 1:40 solution as wet dressing q 15-30 min for 4-8 hr, or soak for 15-30 min 3 times daily | Used as an astringent for soothing effects of cooling and vasoconstriction; also used for relief from painful inflammation of skin | For external use only; avoid using near eyes |
| **Griseofulvin**<br>**Route:** PO<br>**Dosage:** Microsize tablets, 250-500 mg q 12 hr or 500 mg once daily; ultramicrosize tablets, 330-375 mg/day in 1 or 2 divided doses | Antifungal antibiotic used for various tinea infections, including ringworm | Headache; contraindicated in severe liver disease; possible cross-sensitivity with penicillin; should not be used for superficial infections that may respond to antifungals |
| **Hydrocortisone** (Hytone and many others)<br>**Route:** Topical<br>**Dosage:** Apply several times a day as ordered | Corticosteroid used as antipruritic and antiinflammatory for psoriasis, eczema, contact dermatitis, and pruritus | Contraindicated in hypersensitivity to corticosteroids; do not use on weeping, denuded, or highly infected areas; avoid sunlight on treated areas |
| **Isotretinoin** (Accutane)<br>**Route:** PO<br>**Dosage:** 0.5-1.0 mg/kg/day (up to 2 mg/kg/day) in 2 divided doses for 15-20 wk | Keratolytic agent used for management of cystic acne resistant to more conventional therapy, including topical therapy and systemic antibiotics | Epistaxis, conjunctivitis, cheilitis, dry mouth, nausea, vomiting, pruritus, decreased hemoglobin, decreased hematocrit, hypertriglyceridemia, hypercholesterolemia, decreased high-density lipoproteins, bone pain, and arthralgia; use with caution in diabetes, alcoholism, obesity, and inflammatory bowel disease |
| **Ketoconazole** (Nizoral)<br>**Route:** Topical, PO<br>**Dosage:** Topical 2% cream, apply 1 or 2 times daily; PO, 200-400 mg/day as single dose | Antifungal used to treat a variety of fungal infections, including dermatologic infections such as tinea corporis; also used for seborrheic dermatitis | Nausea and vomiting; use with caution in severe liver disease and alcoholism |
| **Lindane, gamma benzene hexachloride**<br>**Route:** Topical<br>**Dosage:** Apply 1% cream to all infested areas. May repeat in 1 wk | Miticide used in the treatment of scabies, head lice, body lice, and crab lice | Contraindicated in history of seizures |

## TABLE 40-5

## Pharmacology of Drugs Used for Skin Integrity—cont'd

| DRUG (GENERIC AND TRADE NAME); ROUTE AND DOSAGE | ACTION/INDICATION | COMMON SIDE EFFECTS AND NURSING CONSIDERATIONS |
|---|---|---|
| **Mafenide acetate** (Sulfamylon) **Route:** Topical **Dosage:** Apply topically $\frac{1}{16}$ inch to an affected area 1-2 times daily, and reapply as needed | Sulfonamide, interferes with bacterial wall synthesis; used as an adjunctive treatment in 2nd- and 3rd-degree burns | Bone marrow suppression, fatal hemolytic anemia, and eosinophilia; contraindicated in inhalation injury; use with caution in impaired pulmonary and renal function and in fluid loss and decreased urine output |
| **Minoxidil** (Rogaine) **Route:** Topical, PO **Dosage:** Topical, Rub into scalp daily; PO, 5 mg/day not to exceed 100 mg daily; usual range 10-40 mg/day in single dose | Antihypertensive with side effect of stimulating hair growth; used to treat alopecia; also used for severe hypertension not responsive to other therapy | Severe rebound hypertension, drowsiness, dizziness, and sedation; contraindicated in acute myocardial infarction and used with caution in renal disease and congestive heart failure; do not discontinue drug abruptly |
| **Mupirocin** (Bactroban) **Route:** Topical **Dosage:** Apply 2% ointment to affected area tid | Nonpenicillin antibiotic used dermatologically to inhibit bacterial protein synthesis; used against impetigo and other infections | Burning, stinging, and itching |
| **Silver nitrate** **Route:** Topical **Dosage:** Apply as ordered to area affected | Used as antiinfective and astringent and for cauterization of lesions, warts, and burns (low concentration) | Skin discoloration; use a wet dressing for burns; store in cool area; avoid contact with clothing to prevent discoloration |
| **Tretinoin, viramin A acid, retinoic acid** (Retin-A) **Route:** Topical **Dosage:** Apply once daily at bedtime | Keratolytic agent used in management of acne vulgaris | Photosensitivity; use cautiously around the mouth, eyes, angles of the nose, or other mucous membranes |

## TABLE 40-6

## Choosing Topical Vehicles

| DESCRIPTION OF SKIN CONDITION | EXAMPLE | TOPICAL VEHICLE OF CHOICE |
|---|---|---|
| Red, hot | Exfoliative erythroderma | Dermatologic wet dressing |
| Red, irritated, sore, oozing | Contact dermatitis | Lotions or sprays |
| Acute, red, wet skin; not painful to touch | Atopic eczema | Creams, gels |
| Chronic, scaly skin with redness | Seborrheic dermatitis | Creams, gels |
| Thick, hyperkeratotic skin | Psoriasis | Ointments |

From Hill MJ: *Skin disorders: Mosby's clinical nursing series,* St Louis, 1994, Mosby.

## Potency of Topical Corticosteroids

| POTENCY | GENERIC NAME | TRADE NAME |
|---|---|---|
| Very high | Fluocinonide | Lidex, Topsyn |
| | Halcinonide | Halog, Halciderm |
| High | Betamethasone benzoate | Benisone |
| | Betamethasone dipropionate | Diprosone |
| | Betamethasone valerate | Valisone |
| | Diflorasone diacetate | Maxiflor, Florone |
| Medium | Fluocinolone acetonide 0.025% | Synalar, Synemol |
| | Triamcinolone 0.1% | Aristocort |
| | Triamcinolone acetonide 0.1% | Kenalog |
| | Flurandrenolide | Cordran |
| Low | Desonide | Tridesilon |
| | Hydrocortisone valerate | Westcort |
| Very low | Hydrocortisone | Hytone, Nutracort, Cortril, Synacort |

From Hill MJ: *Skin disorders: Mosby's clinical nursing series*, St Louis, 1994, Mosby.

## Emotional Support

Patients with skin disorders may have a long road to travel before recovery is complete. Serious skin problems often become chronic, and the patient must learn to live with this disability. When lesions are on the face and exposed parts of the body, the fear of disfigurement is always present. The patient is concerned about what others think and that they may fear that the disease is contagious. Real or imagined feelings of being shunned may cause the patient to become isolated and withdrawn. In children and adolescents the impact on personality may be serious. Although few patients with skin disorders may be admitted to the hospital, they are everywhere. Probably few persons escape the experience of some type of skin disorder during their lifetime.

The nurse can be a source of encouragement to patients, whether they are in or out of the hospital. First, nurses should know that skin disease is rarely fatal and that few skin diseases are contagious. Next, nurses should analyze their own feelings toward the patient. If they find the patient repulsive, they will be unable to give support when it is needed. The nurse must care for the patient with warmth and understanding and convey a feeling of acceptance. Gentleness in removing and applying dressings, keeping wet dressings wet, and carrying out treatments on time will help make the patient feel secure. The nurse should avoid a "hurry-up" attitude and should spend enough time with the patient to reassure him or her of interest and acceptance and encourage expression of his or her feelings about the disease.

# PRESSURE ULCERS

**Pressure ulcers** are defined as local areas of necrosis as a result of vascular insufficiency in an area under pressure (Makelbust, Siegreen, 1996). These ulcers may appear anywhere on the body, but the greatest incidence is over bony prominences (Figure 40-3). Pressure over these areas cuts off the blood supply to the tissue, deprives the cells of nutrition, and prevents elimination of waste from the cells. Anything that hinders the normal cellular functioning will eventually lead to cellular death (necrosis). This results in a pressure ulcer (decubitus ulcer, pressure necrosis). Tissue destruction can occur rapidly. When the skin is broken, there is a rapid destruction of the underlying tissues. The ulcer may become secondarily infected, or the underlying bone may become infected (osteomyelitis). Either of these events complicates the healing process. Pressure ulcers are a cause of considerable morbidity, discomfort, and cost, and they require time-consuming, well-directed nursing interventions.

Sustained pressure is the major cause of pressure necrosis. Both the amount and duration of pressure are important factors. Skin may be able to experience high pressure for a short time without breaking down, whereas low to moderate pressure for an extended period will often result in skin breakdown. For example, the surgical patient may develop a pressure ulcer after a prolonged period on the operating table.

The prevalence and incidence of pressure ulcers vary among populations. In 1989 the National Pressure Ulcer Advisory Panel sponsored a pressure ulcer consensus development conference. It was reported that pressure ulcer prevalence in United States hospitals settings ranged from 3.5% to 29% on any given day. In 1990 the prevalence rate was reported as 9.2%, then in 1994 the rate was reported as 11.1%. It has been estimated that from 2.7% to 29.5% of patients in acute care facilities develop new ulcers during their hospital stay (Makelbust, Siegreen, 1996).

## Risk Factors

The most common risk factors for development of a pressure ulcer are existing disease states such as diabetes mellitus, cardiovascular disease, anemias, neuropathies, renal disease, immune deficiencies, and pulmonary disease; immobility; nutritional deficiencies; moisture; friction; shear; and incontinence (Makelbust, Siegreen, 1996).

1.3 cm                                    3 cm

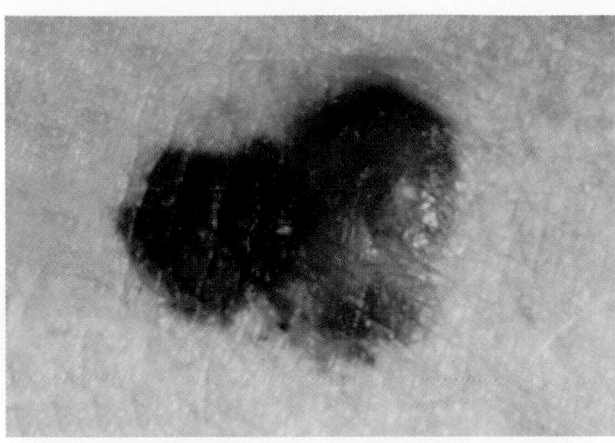
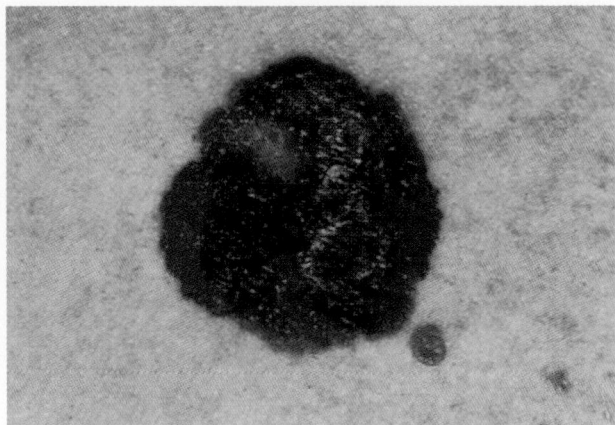

**Plate 1**  Superficial spreading melanomas. (From Habif TP: *Clinical dermatology,* ed 2, St Louis, 1990, Mosby.)

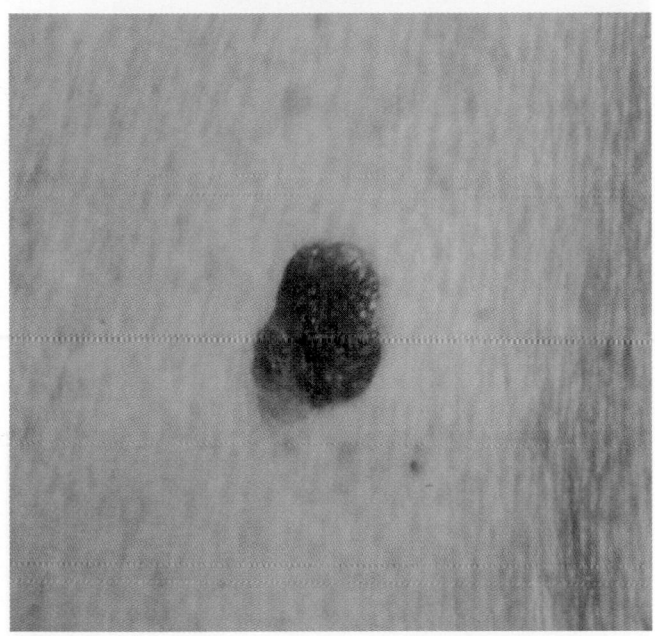

**Plate 2**  Seborrheic keratosis. (From Barkauskas VH et al: *Health and physical assessment,* ed 2, St Louis, 1998, Mosby.)

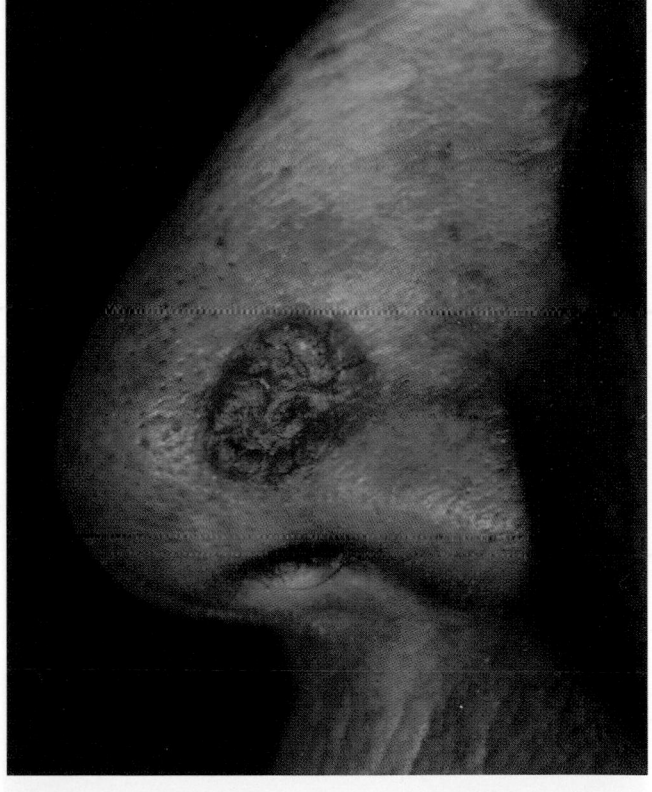

**Plate 3**  Squamous cell carcinoma. (From Habif TP: *Clinical dermatology,* ed 3, St Louis, 1996, Mosby.)

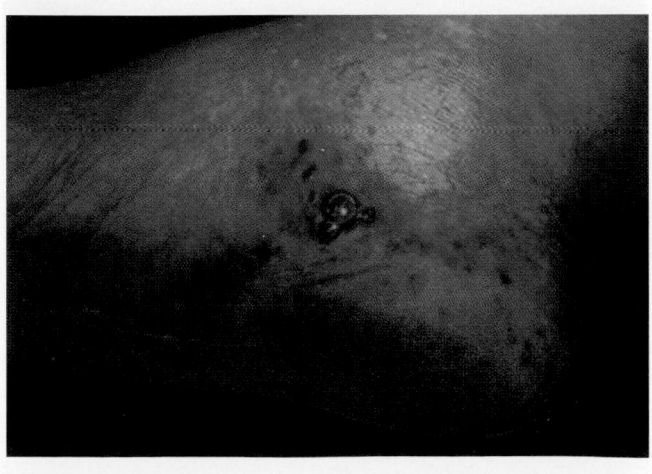

**Plate 4**  Kaposi's sarcoma. (From Habif TP: *Clinical dermatology,* ed 3, St Louis, 1996, Mosby.)

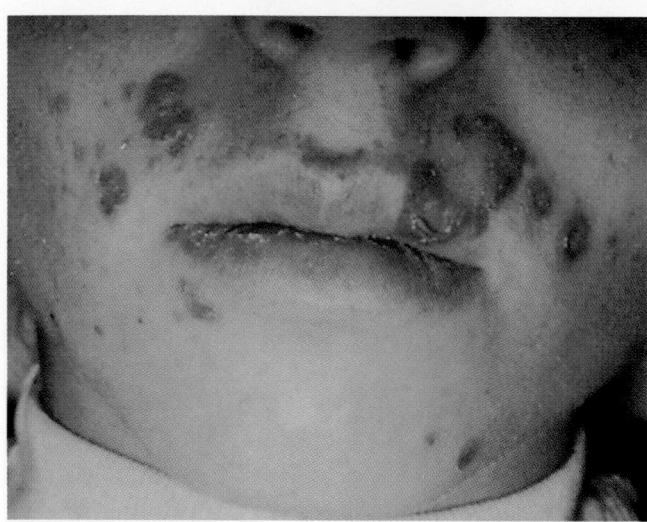

**Plate 5** Impetigo (bullous). (Courtesy American Academy of Dermatology and Institute for Dermatologic Communication and Education, Schaumburg, Ill.)

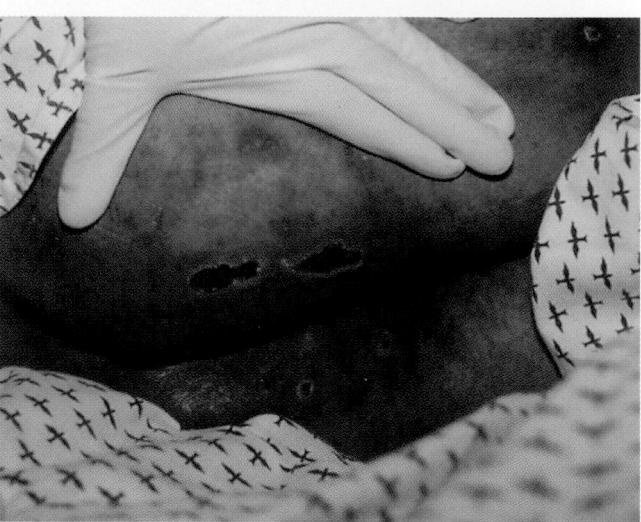

**Plate 6** Pressure ulcers. (From Potter PA, Perry AG: *Fundamentals of nursing: concepts, process and practice,* ed 4, St Louis, 1997, Mosby.)

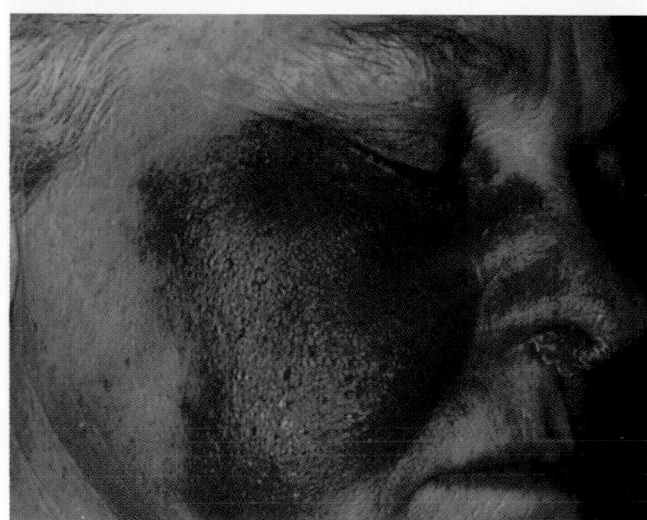

**Plate 7** Streptococcal cellulitis: acute phase with intense erythema (erysipelas). (From Habif TP: *Clinical dermatology,* ed 3, St Louis, 1996, Mosby.)

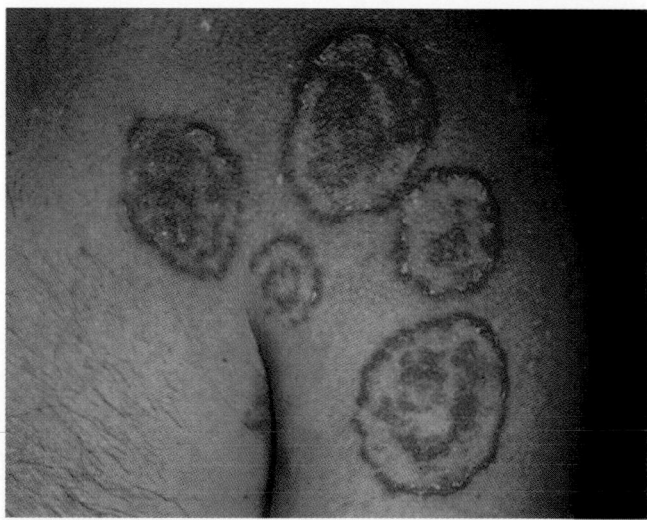

**Plate 8** Tinea corporis. (From Habif TP: *Clinical dermatology,* ed 3, St Louis, 1996, Mosby.)

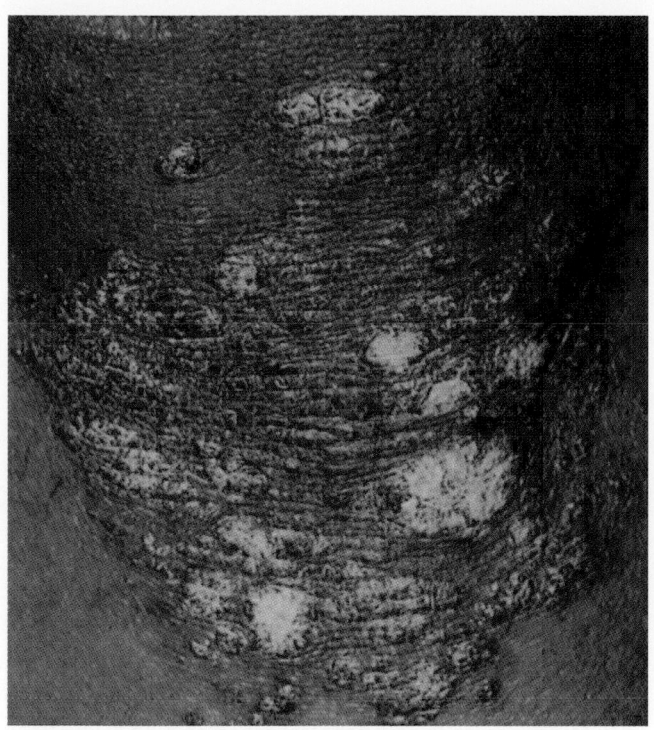

**Plate 9** Psoriasis. Note characteristic silvery scaling. (From Habif TP: *Clinical dermatology,* ed 3, St Louis, 1996, Mosby.)

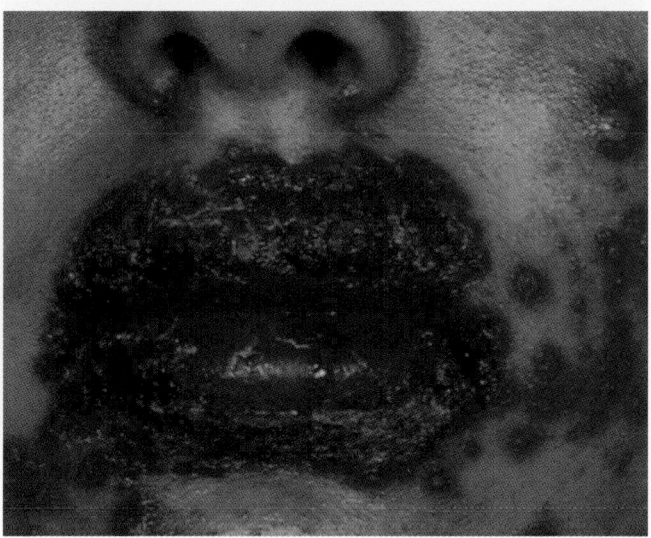

**Plate 10** Oral herpes simplex. (From Habif TP: *Clinical dermatology,* ed 3, St Louis, 1996, Mosby.)

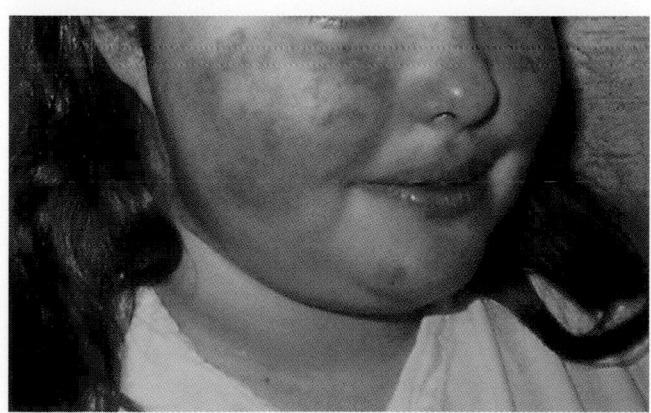

**Plate 11** Butterfly rash of systemic lupus erythematosus. Note butterfly-shaped rash over malar surfaces and bridge of nose. Either a blush with swelling or scaly, red, maculopapular lesions may be present. (Courtesy Walter Tunnessen, MD, The American Board of Pediatrics, Chapel Hill, NC.)

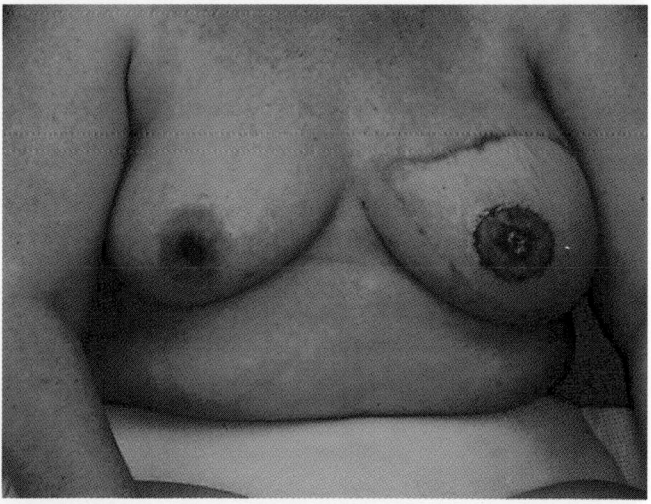

**Plate 12** Reconstructed breast, nipple, and areola. (Courtesy Michael A Epstein, MD, Elk Grove Village, Ill.)

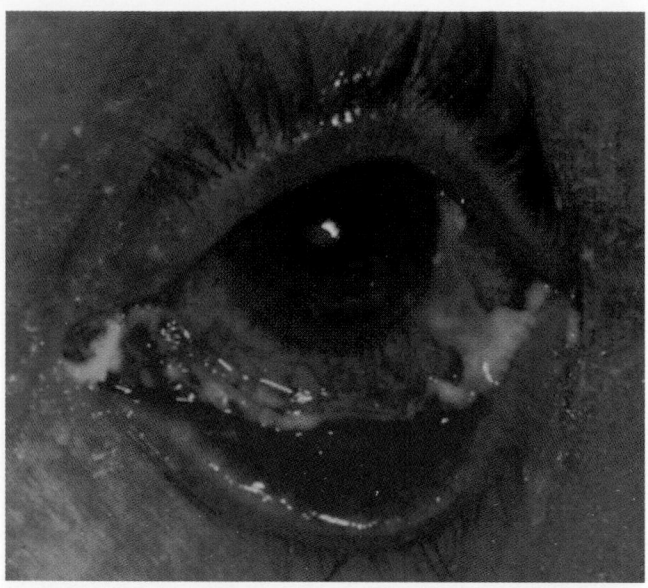

**Plate 13** Acute purulent conjunctivitis. (From Newell FW: *Ophthalmology: principles and concepts,* ed 8, St Louis, 1996, Mosby.)

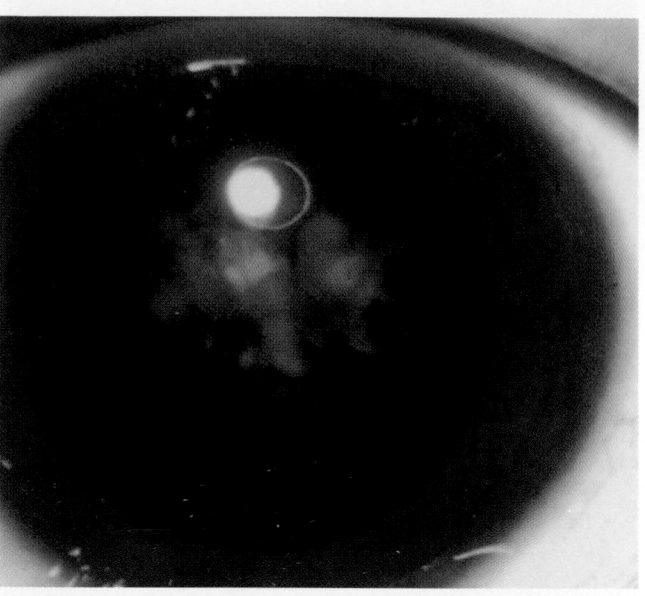

**Plate 14** Snowflake cataract of diabetes. (From Donaldson DD: Atlas of diseases of the anterior segment of the eye. In Seidel HM et al: *Mosby's guide to physical examination,* ed 4, St Louis, 1999, Mosby.)

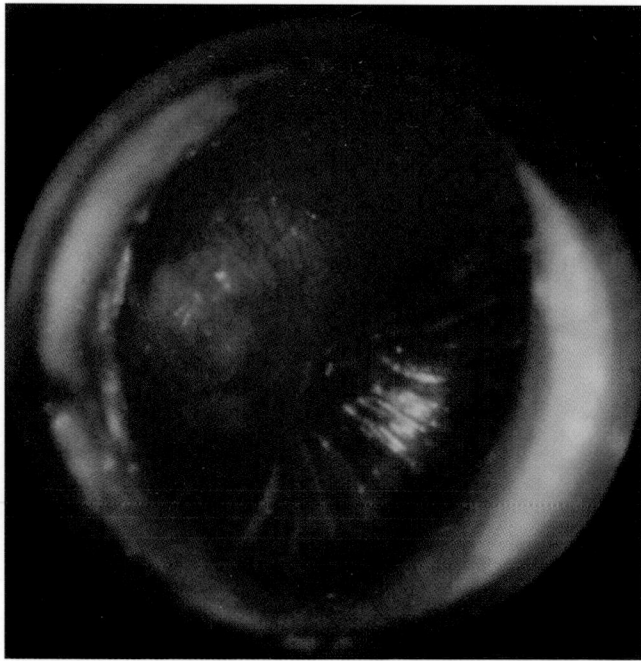

**Plate 15** Acute otitis media: red, nonmobile tympanic membrane with loss of bony landmarks and light reflex. (Courtesy Dr. Richard A Buckingham, Clinical Professor, Otolaryngology, Abraham Lincoln School of Medicine, University of Illinois, Chicago, Ill. In Barkauskas VH et al: *Health and physical assessment,* ed 2, St Louis, 1998, Mosby.)

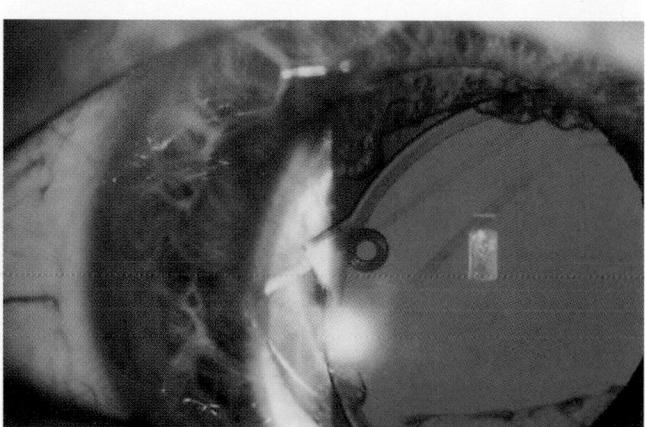

**Plate 16** Intraocular lens implant following cataract extraction. (Courtesy Dr. RJ Epstein, Chicago, Ill.)

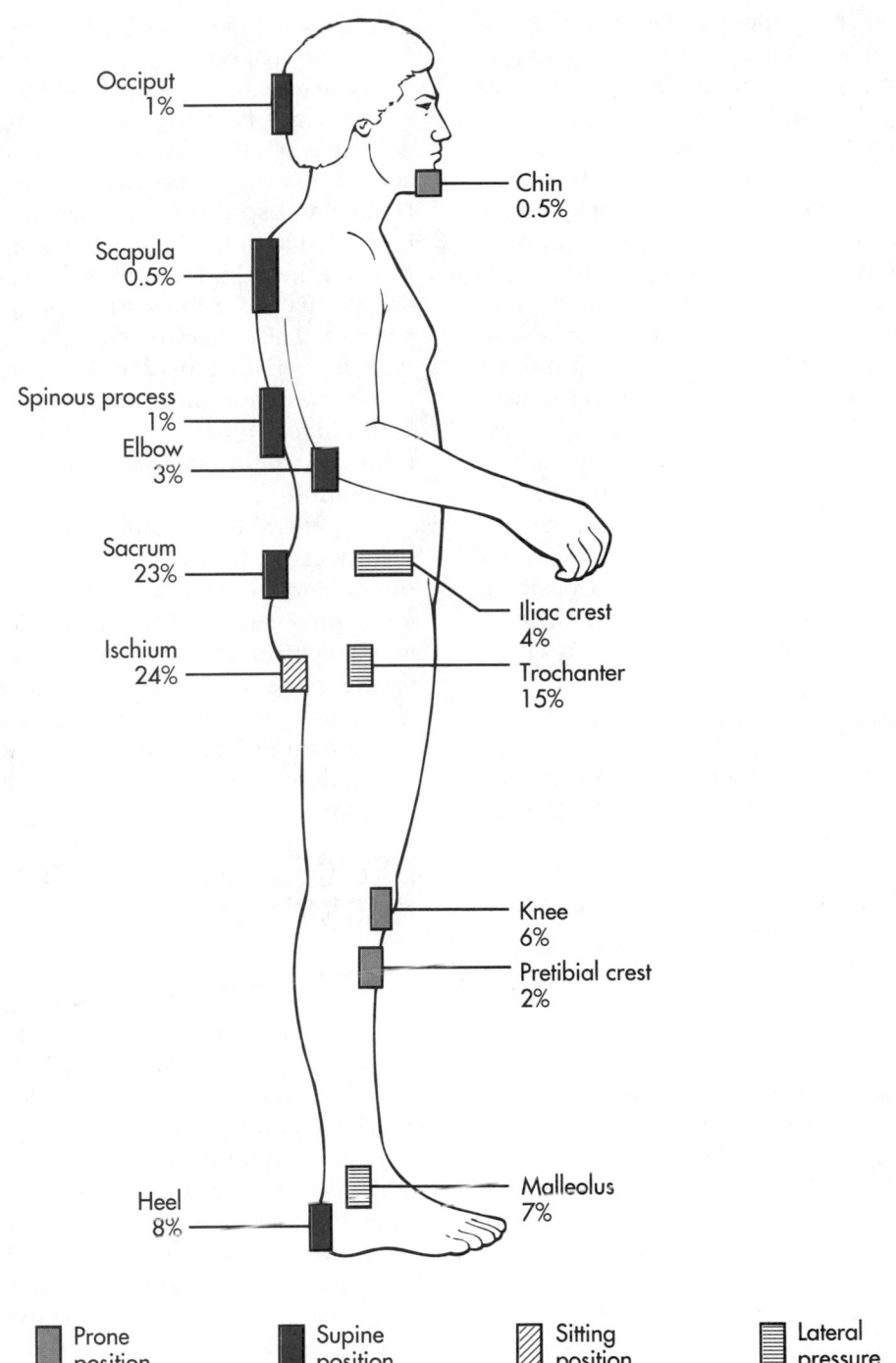

Occiput 1%
Chin 0.5%
Scapula 0.5%
Spinous process 1%
Elbow 3%
Sacrum 23%
Iliac crest 4%
Ischium 24%
Trochanter 15%
Knee 6%
Pretibial crest 2%
Malleolus 7%
Heel 8%

Prone position

Supine position

Sitting position

Lateral pressure

**Figure 40-3**   Common sites for pressure ulcers and frequency of ulceration per site. (Data from Agris J, Spira M: *Clin Symp* 31(5):2, 1979. In Bryant RA: *Acute and chronic wounds,* St Louis, 1992, Mosby.)

Preventing the conditions that aggravate pressure ulcers—moisture, friction, and shear—becomes solely the nurse's responsibility in the acute care setting and the caregiver's responsibility in the home. Sustained moisture (incontinence, diaphoresis) overhydrates the skin and results in maceration (softening of the skin as a result of moisture). The protective function of the skin is therefore impaired, which puts the patient at risk for further breakdown and infection. In addition, urinary or fecal incontinence increases the risk of breakdown by chemical irritation.

Friction occurs when a patient is pulled over a surface. This action can strip the epidermis and leave an open erosion. Using lifting devices to move patients rather than pulling them across the sheets greatly decreases this risk factor. The fragile skin of elderly patients is particularly susceptible to friction tears that may lead to infection and further tissue breakdown. Shear is another factor related to development of pressure ulcers. **Shear** occurs when two or more tissue layers slide in opposite, parallel directions and cause subcutaneous blood vessels to become kinked or stretched. This obstructs blood flow to and from the area supplied by those vessels and results in necrosis. Every patient in a hospital bed experiences shear when the head of the bed is elevated 30 degrees or more. As the head of the bed is raised, the patient slides toward the foot of the bed. Those tissues attached to bony structures move with the patient, but the outer skin layers tend to stay in a fixed position, which exerts **shearing force.** The resulting diminished blood flow to the sacral area causes tissue necrosis.

## Prevention of Pressure Ulcers

The total national cost of pressure ulcer treatment has been estimated to exceed $1.335 billion. Cost estimates to heal one pressure ulcer range from $14,000-$40,000 and can lengthen a patient's stay by a factor of 3.5 to 5. Daily ulcer treatment cost was 2.5 times the cost of prevention (Makelbust, Siegreen, 1996). Despite guidelines for preventive measures, pressure ulcers continue to occur. Prevention depends on early recognition of the patient at risk and prompt institution of the appropriate measures necessary to prevent breakdown. Nursing procedures include (1) identifying the patient at risk by use of a risk-assessment scale (e.g., Braden, Gosnell, or Norton); (2) maintaining a dry, unwrinkled bed; (3) using the appropriate pressure-reduction or pressure-relief surface; (4) repositioning the patient at least every 2 hours while in bed and encouraging weight shifts every hour for patients in wheelchairs; (5) constant attention to the overall health status of the patient; and (6) continued observation and reassessment of the skin. A reddened (erythematous) area is the first sign of pressure. In the light-skinned patient a red color change is seen; in the dark-skinned patient the erythematous area may be detected by an increase in skin temperature or by a darkening or lightening of that patient's normal skin color. All patients should be assessed for edema at the suspected pressure site. Edematous skin will feel slick and tight when touched with the back of the finger. Erythema should disappear within a short time after pressure is relieved if no skin damage has been done. If edema occurs and redness remains for 30 minutes after pressure is relieved, pressure ulcer development should be suspected.

Erythematous areas over pressure points should not be massaged because this may cause damage to vasculature. Massaging skin around existing ulcers should be avoided because it may cause unnecessary trauma and spread infection. The use of soap should be limited because the alkali in soap will produce dryness, cracking, and chapping. The old method of using doughnuts and rubber rings is no longer acceptable practice. These devices create rings of pressure that further restrict circulation. Preventing pressure ulcers in long-term and older adult patients requires consistent, diligent nursing care. Ulcers may occur quickly from only slight pressure; this is especially true in the older adult.

The general health and nutritional status of the patient does contribute to the development of pressure ulcers. Protein, vitamin C, and vitamin B are essential for normal cell growth and healing. Inadequate vitamin C contributes to capillary fragility, which makes tissues more susceptible to trauma and interrupted blood flow. Poor nutrition leads to an increased risk of breakdown or impaired healing. Adequate hydration is also necessary to maintain skin turgor and prevent infection.

## DEVICES THAT AUGMENT NURSING CARE

Increased concern for the development of pressure ulcers has resulted in development of products for both the prevention and care of pressure ulcers. To avoid confusion, the products should be looked at generically (e.g., high air loss, low air loss, overlays, beds), which may simplify choices.

Equipment for pressure reduction/relief varies considerably in both effectiveness and cost. Pressure-relieving devices work by redistributing pressure at bony prominences over the larger surface of the entire body. The desired goal is to obtain the largest possible support surface with the lowest possible contact pressure (Makelbust, Siegreen, 1991).

## Mattress Overlays

The first level of intervention is classified as mattress overlays. These may be convoluted-foam or air products and are either static or dynamic. Overlays provide *pressure reduction* as opposed to *pressure relief*. Convoluted-foam, water-filled, gel, and air-filled overlays are classified as static products. Static products decrease pressure by spreading the weight over a larger area (Bryant, 1992). Convoluted-foam overlays must be at least 4 to 6 inches thick to provide pressure reduction

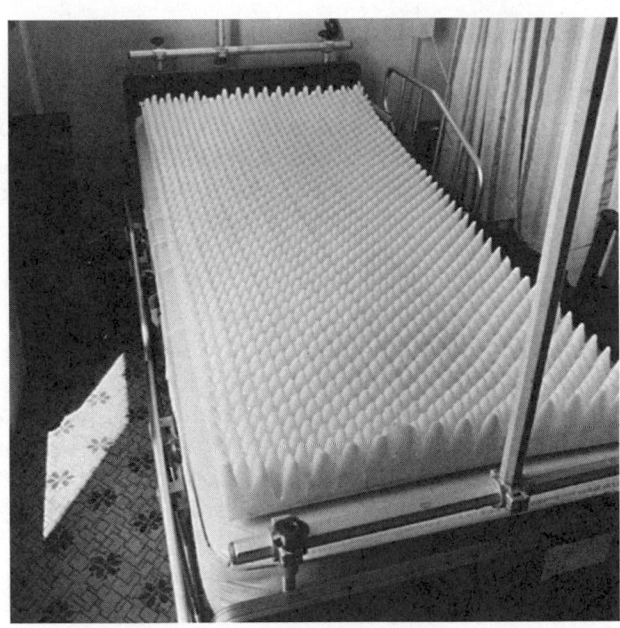

**Figure 40-4** Convoluted foam mattress. (From Perry GA, Potter PA: *Clinical nursing skills and techniques,* ed 3, St Louis, 1994, Mosby.)

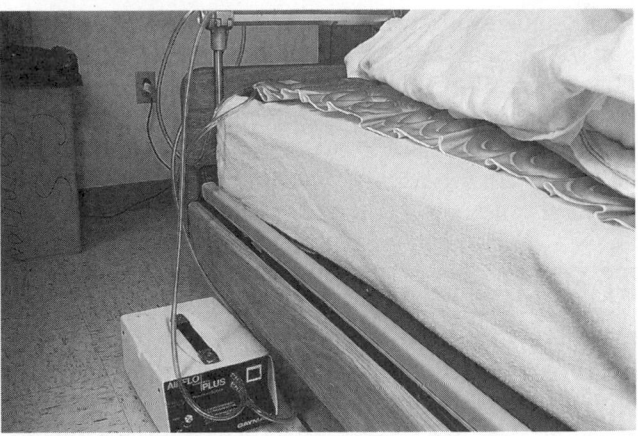

**Figure 40-5** Inflated air mattress. (From Perry AG, Potter PA: *Clinical nursing skills and techniques,* ed 4, St Louis, 1998, Mosby.)

(Figure 40-4). Anything less than 4 inches provides comfort but no significant pressure reduction. Water-filled overlays distribute body weight over the entire support system. Gel flotation pads provide flotation with pressure reduction.

Dynamic products (e.g., alternating air-filled overlays) prevent constant pressure against the skin and enhance blood flow by creating high-pressure and low-pressure areas (Bryant, 1992). These products are indicated for the patient with limited mobility who is at risk for further skin breakdown or who has a stage I, II, or III pressure ulcer. If the patient has documented stage I or stage II pressure ulcers along with excessive moisture (e.g., incontinence, perspiration), an air mattress overlay is indicated (Figure 40-5). Nursing care that includes a turning schedule must be implemented along with the use of any support surface. Patients who have a stage III or IV pressure ulcer or who have multiple stage II pressure ulcers that involve more than one surface can benefit from a low-air-loss mattress.

## Specialty Beds

Specialty beds have the technology to allow the bed surface to conform to the body contours, which reduces tissue-interface pressure below capillary closing pressure, thus providing pressure relief. Specialty beds also relieve shear and friction. Specialty beds may be classified as high air-loss, low air-loss, or kinetic.

High-air-loss beds have bactericidal properties because of their temperature, alkalinity (pH 10), and entrapment of the microorganisms by the beads in the bed. High-air-loss beds are recommended for patients with burns or multiple stage III or IV pressure ulcers. They may also be used to rewarm the patient with hypothermia. High-air-loss beds are not recommended for patients with pulmonary disease or unstable spines or for patients who are ambulatory. Low-air-loss beds help reduce moisture and manage pain. They are indicated for patients who need pressure relief and are contraindicated for patients with unstable spines. Patients with stage III or stage IV pressure ulcers, multiple stage II pressure ulcers involving more than one surface, multiple risk factors, end-stage cancer, pulmonary complications, or sepsis, as well as those who need pain management, should be placed on an oscillating low-air-loss bed (kinetic bed). This particular bed provides programmable turning of patients to promote drainage of lung secretions, enhances venous return from lower extremities, and facilitates urine flow. Oscillating support beds provide continuous turning of the patient from side to side to prevent and treat the complications of immobility. This bed may be used with spinal cord injury (Bryant, 1992).

A special function bed has a pressure-relieving surface that provides continuous pulsating air suspension. It has the same indications as the low-air-loss bed, with the addition of pulsation. It is indicated for the patient who needs pain management. Use of this bed is contraindicated for patients in cervical or skeletal traction.

Air-fluidized therapy provides pressure relief on a high-air-loss surface. This specialty bed is indicated for the patient who requires minimal movement to avoid skin damage by shearing forces (posterior grafts, or flaps). Turning schedules are highly recommended. This bed is also contraindicated for patients with unstable spines. The nurse must be aware of fluid intake of patients on air-fluidized therapy because the circulating air will promote evaporation of body fluid. Fluid intake should be sufficient to prevent dehydration.

# TREATMENT OF PRESSURE ULCERS

Many of the wound care products available for treating pressure ulcers must be used in conjunction with the appropriate pressure-reducing or pressure-relieving product. Factors affecting treatment, including the condition of the wound and the general health status of the patient, are continuously changing variables, and treatment choices must be made on the basis of an accurate and ongoing assessment of the wound and patient. Among the products available for treating pressure ulcers are agents for cleansing and debridement, topical medications (antimicrobials, antiseptics, antibiotics), exudate absorbers (beads, pastes), and multiple categories of dressings.

## Wound Cleansing

The goals of wound cleansing are (1) removal of bacteria and surface contaminants such as slough, foreign bodies, and purulent exudate, and (2) protection of the healing wound (Bryant, 1992). The body's own healing mechanism is very efficient, so any intervention should be aimed at enhancing that mechanism. Effective wound healing can be inhibited by indiscriminate use of some agents. Therefore the choice of cleansing method must be based on the type of wound and the stage of healing.

Hypochlorite solutions, such as Dakin's solution, or chlorpactin, will dissolve necrotic tissue and control odors, but they are toxic to fibroblasts in normal dilutions. Povidone-iodine preparations have broad-spectrum effectiveness when used on intact skin or small wounds, but they are toxic to fibroblasts in normal dilutions, have questionable effectiveness in infected wounds, and may cause iodine toxicity when used in large wounds over a prolonged time. Acetic acid is effective against *Pseudomonas aeruginosa* in superficial wounds but is toxic to fibroblasts in standard dilutions and changes the color of exudate, which gives a false assurance of elimination of infection. Lastly, hydrogen peroxide will provide mechanical cleansing and some debridement through effervescent action, but it can cause ulceration of newly formed tissue, is toxic to fibroblasts, and can cause air embolism when used to pack sinus tracts. Moreover, if used for forceful irrigation, hydrogen peroxide can cause subcutaneous em-

physema, which mimics gas gangrene (Bryant, 1992). There are several prepared wound cleansers available on the market. Most contain a wetting agent and a blend of moisturizers that help soften eschar (scab) and augment debridement. Each product should be used according to the recommendations of the manufacturer. Normal saline is appropriate and safe for all wounds.

## Debridement

To enhance the healing process, **debridement,** the removal of devitalized tissue, must be performed particularly in contaminated ulcers. Devitalized, or necrotic, tissue slows the wound-healing process. Debridement can be classified as chemical (topical agents/enzymes), mechanical (surgical, wet-to-dry, hydrotherapy), or autolytic (occlusive dressings).

Chemical debridement is accomplished through the use of enzyme preparations that dissolve necrotic tissue. The enzymes require a moist environment for activation. Enzymatic preparations are made to act on specific necrotic tissue. For example, fibrinolysin-deoxyribonuclease dissolves fibrin clots and hydrolyzes proteinaceous exudate. Sutilains is a proteolytic enzyme, and collagenase digests collagen and denatured protein (Eaglstein et al, 1990). Chemical debridement also may be accomplished by using gauze soaked with Dakin's solution to dissolve necrotic tissue.

Mechanical debridement is accomplished by the use of a scalpel and scissors, irrigation (whirlpool, syringe), or wet to dry dressings. Surgical debridement is aggressive, fast, and selective. Necrotic tissue is removed down to, or just above, viable tissue. Viable tissue is recognized when there is bleeding present. This type of debridement provides a wound bed that stimulates granulation. Carbon dioxide lasers have been used to accomplish this type of debridement. Another form of mechanical debridement is irrigation. Irrigation may be accomplished by putting the patient in a whirlpool tub, by having the patient stand in a shower, or by manual irrigation. Irrigation must be done gently so as not to disturb fragile, healing tissue. Once the wound has begun to granulate, irrigation should be discontinued. Lastly, wet-to-dry dressings are used for mechanical debridement. Although one of the purposes of wet to dry dressing is to debride the dead tissue, the nurse must be careful not to damage healthy new tissue growth while removing the old dressing. If the dressing adheres to healthy tissue, a syringe filled with sterile normal saline solution can be used to direct the solution at the adhered area so that it can be loosened and removed without damaging the tissue. Wet to dry dressings can be painful.

Autolytic debridement is accomplished with the use of an appropriate occlusive dressing. The dressing uses enzymes normally present in the wound fluid to liquefy the necrotic debris. Dressings that accomplish this goal are occlusive or semiocclusive (hydrocolloidal wafers, paste, or beads).

The choice of the debridement method to be used should be based on the condition of the wound, the amount of exudate present, and the condition of the patient. A patient with a large (stage III or IV) necrotic pressure ulcer who is at very high risk for secondary infection may benefit greatly from aggressive surgical (mechanical) debridement to augment the wound healing process.

## Topical Medications

Antimicrobials, antiseptics, and antibiotics can be in the form of a cream, ointment, solution, or spray. Topical agents should be chosen for their antibacterial effectiveness and for their ability to enhance healing. An occlusive ointment may cause maceration or encourage the growth of resistant organisms. Some topical agents interfere with neutrophils, fibroblasts, and endothelial cells in the healing process (see Tables 40-4 and 40-5).

## Exudate Absorbers

Exudate absorbers (absorption dressings) include, but are not limited to, dextranomer beads, hydrophilic powders, pastes, granules, calcium alginates, and other hypertonic dressings. Absorption dressings remove necrotic fluid, obliterate dead space (sinus tracts, undermining), and maintain a moist wound environment. Dead space impairs the wound-healing process and predisposes the patient to abscess formation. All of these dressings expand when they come in contact with the wound fluid, so it is not necessary to pack them tightly into the wound bed. Packing too tightly may impair circulation and damage healthy tissue. Absorptive dressings are suitable for stage III and stage IV pressure ulcers.

## Dressing Materials

Dressing materials are numerous and varied and should be chosen for their individual actions on the basis of the wound assessment. For simplification they are classified as transparent film dressings, hydrocolloids, foam dressings, hydrogels, and protective barriers. Transparent film dressings are semipermeable adhesive dressings that allow exchange of oxygen and moisture vapor but do not allow passage of fluids or bacteria. They enhance epithelial migration and are indicated for use in superficial (stage I or stage II) dermal ulcers, skin grafts, donor sites, and minor abrasions.

Hydrocolloids are adhesive dressings that absorb small to moderate amounts of exudate while interacting with the wound to form a liquid gelatinous substance that maintains a moist healing environment. They may be used on superficial pressure ulcers and skin tears that produce minimum amounts of exudate. Hydrocolloids may be either occlusive and impermeable to gases or semipermeable. The occlusive hydrocolloids are not suitable for infected wounds, deep wounds with tunnel tracts, or undermining. Semipermeable hydrocolloids are mechanically protective and properly humidify the wound. Hydrocolloids are excellent for autolytic debridement and may be used in stage I, stage II, and some stage III ulcers.

Hydrogels are water-polymer gels that act to provide a moist wound healing environment while absorbing excess exudate. Hydrogels also clean and debride the wound. This type of dressing is appropriate for all stages of wound healing but is most often indicated in stages II and III. Hydrogels may be used in necrotic wounds. They also have the added feature of relieving pain through their cooling properties. They are especially good for burns.

Foam dressings are nonadherent hydrophilic or hydrophobic polyurethane that provide thermal insulation and a moist wound environment. This type of dressing is atraumatic and is indicated for use in stage III and granulating stage IV wounds with a moderate amount of exudate. If the wound has depth or dead space, the foam dressing should be used with packing.

Protective barriers (skin sealants) provide a protective coating, usually in alcohol solution, that is applied to intact skin. This coating forms a second skin and is useful to prep skin before an adhesive is applied. Skin sealants may be applied on stage I wounds because the skin is intact.

## Nursing Care
### Assessment

A thorough assessment of the patient must be undertaken before any interventions are begun. An individualized plan is then formulated in accordance with the specific needs and condition of the patient. The plan of care must be consistent with goals for patient management, and the goals must be realistic. Several objective factors must be considered when assessing the patient at risk. These factors include general state of the skin, general state of health, mental status, degree of mobility and activity, level of sensory perception, nutritional status, and aggravating factors such as moisture, friction, and shear. Contributing factors must also be taken into consideration when interventions are being developed. These factors include predisposing disease states (diabetes mellitus, cardiovascular disease,

## RISK ASSESSMENT SCALES

### PRESSURE ULCERS

**Norton Scale**
- Consists of five parameters: physical condition, mental state, activity, mobility, and incontinence
- Each parameter is rated on a scale of 1 to 4, with one- or two-word descriptions for each parameter
- Scores may range from 5 to 20, with the lower scores indicating increased risk (12 or below)

**Gosnell Scale**
- Consists of five parameters: mental status, continence, mobility, activity, and nutrition
- Each parameter is rated on a scale of 1 to 4 except for mental status, which is rated from 1 to 5, and nutrition, which is rated from 1 to 3, with two- or three-sentence descriptive statements
- Additional variables measured include body temperature, blood pressure, skin tone and sensation, medication, and medical diagnoses (no weight given to these parameters)
- Scores may range from 5 to 20, with the lower scores indicating increased risk (16 or below)

**Braden Scale**
- Consists of six subscales that reflect (conceptually) degrees of sensory perception, skin moisture, physical activity, nutritional intake, friction and shear, and ability to change and control body position
- Each parameter is rated on a scale of 1 to 4 except for friction and shear subscale, which is rated from 1 to 3; each parameter is accompanied by a brief description of criteria for assigning the rating
- Scores may range from 4 to 23, with the lower scores indicating increased risk (16 or below, or in older population a score of 17 or 18 may be more predictive)

Modified from Bryant RA: *Acute and chronic wounds: nursing management*, St Louis, 1992, Mosby.

anemias, neuropathies, renal disease, pulmonary disease), age, weight, medications, allergies, serial laboratory values (albumin, total protein, hemoglobin, hematocrit, total lymphocyte count), and dietary restrictions. There are several risk-assessment tools in the literature to assist the nurse in this assessment. Some of the tools are the Norton scale, the Gosnell scale, and the Braden scale (Box 40-3).

## Prevention

If a patient is found to be at risk and has no skin breakdown, interventions should be aimed at prevention. Interventions should include placing the patient on a pressure-reducing/relieving surface, inspecting the skin regularly—at least every 8 hours—for redness or evidence of breakdown, instituting measures to reduce shearing forces and friction (keeping head of bed flat or below a 30-degree angle), using a draw sheet to turn the patient, applying cornstarch or powder to surfaces coming in contact with the skin, avoiding direct contact with plastic or vinyl surfaces such as chux or vinyl chairs, and encouraging and assisting ambulation. If the patient is incontinent or diaphoretic, measures must be implemented to prevent tissue breakdown caused by moisture. Breathable absorptive pads, fecal incontinence collectors, and external urinary catheters may be used to help manage incontinence. A regular skin cleansing regimen should be instituted and should include use of a skin protectant. Adult absorbent garments are available but should be used judiciously, and the patient should be assessed at least every 2 hours for changing the garment. Poor nutrition and hydration must be addressed if present. Intake and output records should be initiated, fluid intake should be encouraged if not contraindicated, and a dietary consult should be requested for nutritional assessment.

## Intervention

When a pressure ulcer is already present, the previously mentioned interventions and an individualized plan for treatment of the ulcer must be instituted (Box 40-4). Before any plan of care can be initiated, the ulcer must be staged (Figure 40-6). In addition to staging, a classification system is utilized for making decisions regarding wound care. It is the red-yellow-black system of wound classification (Cuzzell, 1988). It allows the nurse or physician to look at a wound and quickly assess the interventions needed (debridement, cleansing, dressing type). Red wounds may be acute or chronic. Acute red wounds may be caused by traumatic or surgical injury with frank bleeding or evidence of recent hemostasis. Chronic red wounds have clean pink, bright red, or dark red granulation tissue, which is seen after necrotic tissue is removed. The goal with a red wound is protection, which is accomplished with an atraumatic dressing (hydrogel, hydrocolloid) or appropriate topical medication. Cleansing of a red wound is not necessary in most cases.

Yellow wounds have soft necrotic tissue, "slough," or thick, tenacious exudate ranging in color from creamy ivory to yellow green. The goal with a yellow wound is debridement, cleansing, and protection. Debridement by using mechanical or autolytic methods is appropriate.

The black wound is a wound covered by thick necrotic tissue (eschar). The primary goal with this

STAGE                                                    APPEARANCE

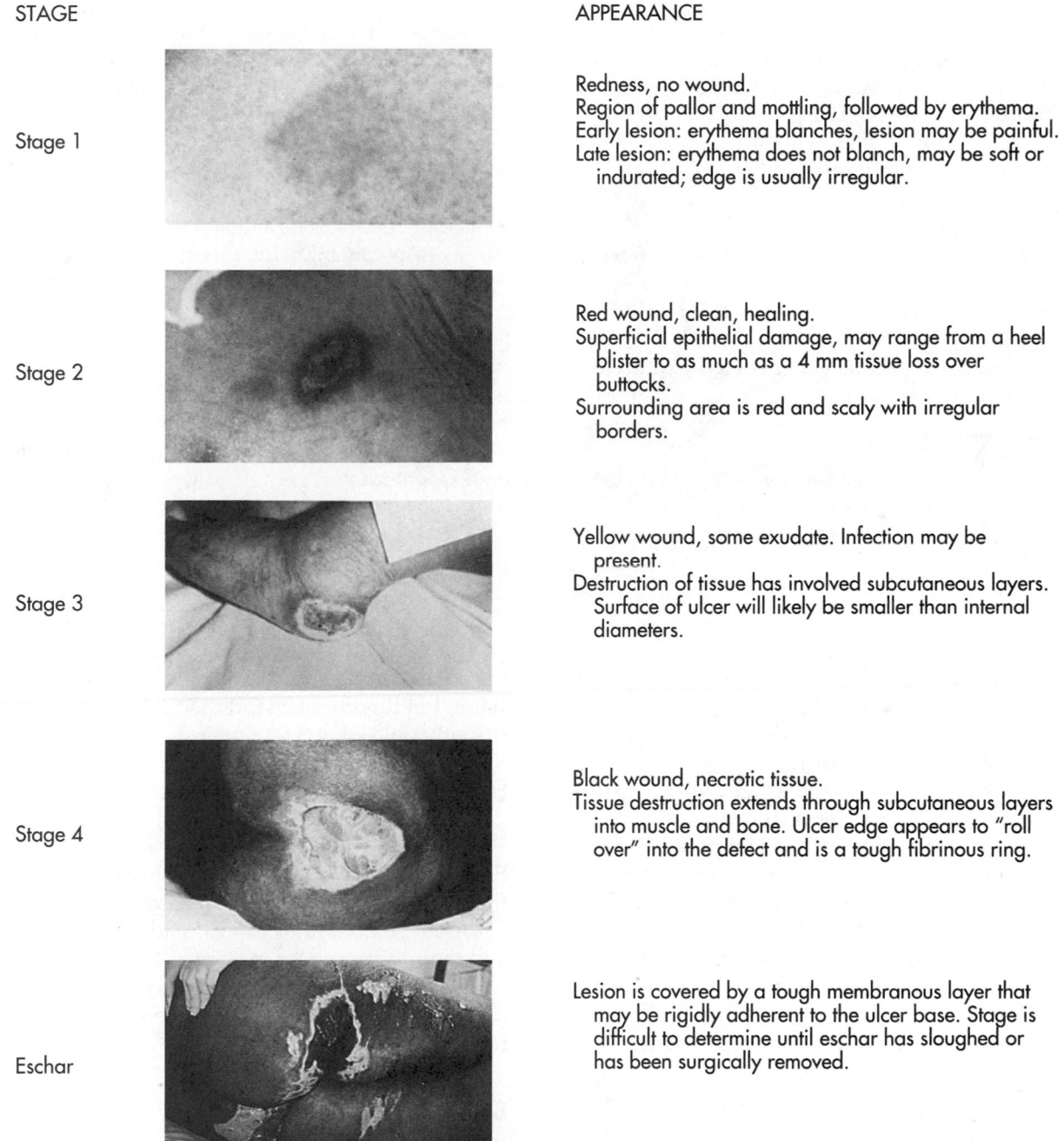

**Stage 1**

Redness, no wound.
Region of pallor and mottling, followed by erythema.
Early lesion: erythema blanches, lesion may be painful.
Late lesion: erythema does not blanch, may be soft or
    indurated; edge is usually irregular.

**Stage 2**

Red wound, clean, healing.
Superficial epithelial damage, may range from a heel
    blister to as much as a 4 mm tissue loss over
    buttocks.
Surrounding area is red and scaly with irregular
    borders.

**Stage 3**

Yellow wound, some exudate. Infection may be
    present.
Destruction of tissue has involved subcutaneous layers.
    Surface of ulcer will likely be smaller than internal
    diameters.

**Stage 4**

Black wound, necrotic tissue.
Tissue destruction extends through subcutaneous layers
    into muscle and bone. Ulcer edge appears to "roll
    over" into the defect and is a tough fibrinous ring.

**Eschar**

Lesion is covered by a tough membranous layer that
    may be rigidly adherent to the ulcer base. Stage is
    difficult to determine until eschar has sloughed or
    has been surgically removed.

NOTE: Stages describe layers of tissue visually involved. It is important to remember that even at the early stages (1 and 2) what is seen is only a small part of the damaged, swollen tissue underneath.

**Figure 40-6** Pressure ulcer stages. (From Perry AG, Potter PA: *Clinical nursing skills and techniques,* ed 3, St Louis, 1994, Mosby.)

◀ BOX 40-4 ▶     **NURSING PROCESS**

## PRESSURE ULCERS

**ASSESSMENT**

- Risk factors (age, mobility, continence, nutrition)
- Pressure ulcer for size, depth, drainage, presence of infection, evidence of healing
- Bony prominences after each turn
- Vital signs (temperature)

**NURSING DIAGNOSES**

- Impaired skin integrity related to shearing force as evidenced by ulcerated area over point of pressure
- Risk for injury and infection related to loss of skin barrier
- Impaired home maintenance management related to long-term treatment

**NURSING INTERVENTIONS**

- Relieve pressure on the pressure ulcer at all times.
- Turn the patient at least every 2 hours.
- Apply support surface appropriate to patient's needs.

- Keep skin free of excessive moisture, urine, and feces.
- Use a draw sheet to lift and turn the patient.
- Maintain the head of the bed below a 30-degree angle.
- Provide dressings, cleansing, and medication as ordered.
- Assist patient and family in setting realistic goals for healing, mobility, and overall recovery.
- Refer the patient for in-home nursing care when indicated.

**EVALUATION OF EXPECTED OUTCOMES**

- Ulcer decreased in size
- Ulcer free of infection
- Pink, healthy granulation tissue apparent, continues to increase
- Verbalizes understanding of home care

---

wound is debridement, which may be accomplished mechanically, chemically, or through autolysis. After the eschar is removed, the condition of the wound bed can be accurately assessed for further interventions.

Wounds should be assessed continuously so that treatment procedures can be changed as the wound progresses. For example, a yellow wound will become a red wound when exudate is no longer present and the wound exhibits a red, granulating base. The treatment should then be adjusted to that of a red wound. A wound may possess the characteristics of two different classifications. For example, a wound may have some granulation tissue evident, but slough is also evident. In this case the wound is considered a yellow wound and is treated accordingly. Interventions are always based on the worst scenario, with red being the optimum and black being the worst scenario. The rationale is that the goal of wound care is to have a red wound and that if any part of the wound is not at that stage, interventions must be aimed at advancing the entire wound to the red wound stage.

## DISEASES AND DISORDERS OF THE SKIN

Although most diseases and disorders of the skin are treated by the dermatologist as medical or dermatologic conditions, some require surgical treatment. Both the medical and surgical aspects of the disease are considered in this chapter, and discussion is based on basic pathophysiology.

## Disorders of Pigmentation
### Lentigo (Freckles)

Freckles are collections of skin pigment that result from quantitative changes in melanin. They may occur in certain persons after exposure to the sun in summer and tend to disappear in winter. Persons with severe cases may have the freckles removed by dermal abrasion, but assurance cannot be given that they will not return.

### Chloasma (Melasma)

Patches of pigmentation that may be yellowish brown, brown, or black occur on various parts of the body. They are more common in women and are often seen during pregnancy, at the time of menopause, or with the use of oral contraceptives.

No treatment is necessary unless the lesions occur on the face and the person is sensitive about them for cosmetic reasons. They may be removed with various bleaching preparations, but the procedure is not recommended. Laser therapy is now being used to treat these areas. Several treatments are usually necessary.

# DISORDERS OF THE GLANDS

## Seborrhea (Oily Skin)

Seborrhea is an excessive secretion of oil from the sebaceous glands. It is accentuated on the face, neck, and scalp, where the oil glands are most abundant. It is often associated with other conditions such as acne vulgaris, seborrheic dermatitis, eczema, and seborrheic warts. Although the condition is normal for some persons, particularly women, it not only detracts from personal appearance but also predisposes one to other, more serious skin conditions.

Treatment consists of washing often and thoroughly with soap and water and avoiding the use of greasy creams. Preparations containing salicylic acid or sulfur or both may be rubbed into the affected areas several times a day.

## Sebaceous Cyst (Wen)

A sebaceous cyst, commonly called a *wen,* is often seen on the scalp and may become large. It is the result of obstruction of the sebaceous duct in the presence of continued secretions from the gland. These lesions contain an accumulation of sebum, which develops an offensive odor. The treatment is surgical incision, with measures to prevent infection.

## Hyperhidrosis (Excessive Sweating)

Excessive sweating occurs in conjunction with several conditions, including diseases such as tuberculosis and hyperthyroidism, conditions involving severe pain such as that in renal colic, and certain acute heart attacks. It may also occur in some shock states and toxic conditions or after the administration of antipyretic drugs. Under normal conditions excessive sweating usually occurs when a person is exposed to extremes of heat or severe physical exercise. Excessive sweating may predispose the individual to skin disease or irritation.

Treatment is directed toward removing the cause, and nursing care should concern keeping the bed and clothing dry, sponging and drying the skin, and protecting the patient from exposure.

Axillary hyperhidrosis may be controlled by topical application of most of the commercial antiperspirant agents on the market. These preparations act by closing the pores and may occasionally cause a mild irritation. Excessive hyperhidrosis of the feet can be relieved by washing several times daily, drying thoroughly, and dusting with a medicated foot powder.

## Anhidrosis (Absence of Sweating)

Anhidrosis is a normal result of the aging process accompanied by decreased activity of the sebaceous glands, which causes dryness of the skin. It can also be a very serious condition seen in younger individuals in whom the temperature-regulating mechanism (sweating) is disturbed. If temperature regulation is severely affected, the chance of heat prostration increases. This disorder is characteristic of diabetes mellitus, nephritis, hypothyroidism, and several skin diseases and may follow the administration of drugs such as atropine.

There is no specific treatment for the condition except for the use of superfatted soaps and the application of creams or oils. Treatment of the causative factor may provide relief.

## Pruritus (Itching)

Pruritus is a symptom that accompanies many disorders, including a variety of skin diseases, systemic diseases, allergic reactions, and anhidrosis in the elderly person. The response of the individual is to scratch, and it is generally useless to tell the person not to scratch because the reply will probably be, "I can't help it." In fact, scratching is almost an automatic, unconscious act.

Whenever possible, treatment is based on removing or treating the cause. In treating small children, splinting of the arms or the use of mitts may be necessary to prevent scratching. Cold wet dressings, emollient baths, and emollient lotion containing phenol or menthol may be used, or the physician may prescribe a lotion containing a steroid drug. Some patients may benefit from antihistaminic drugs.

The nurse should do everything possible to provide comfort for the patient and to relieve the emotional tension often associated with pruritic conditions. Maintaining a cool, even room temperature and providing a quiet environment and some diversional activity will help to relieve itching.

# TUMORS OF THE SKIN

Tumors of the skin are among the most common of all tumors and generally affect exposed parts of the body such as the face and backs of the hands. Persons whose occupations expose them to wind, sun, and frost are often affected. Most patients with skin tumors are in the older age group. Skin tumors may be benign or malignant, and most malignant tumors can be easily diagnosed and cured. Benign tumors include the keloid, angioma, nevus, wart, and keratoses.

## Keloid

The keloid is an overgrowth of fibrous tissue occurring at a scar site. The shape may be irregular and small, or it may increase to the size of the hand. The tumor may develop after inflammation or ulceration from burns or traumatic injuries. It is not known why the condition occurs. It is more common in dark-skinned persons.

There is no uniform opinion concerning treatment. The lesion may be erythematous, irritated, and painful. Pain may be relieved by injection of a glucocorticoid (Aristocort, Kenacort) diluted 1:5 with lidocaine (Xylocaine). Surgical removal followed by x-ray therapy will be effective in approximately half the cases.

## Nevus (Mole)

The mole is a nonvascular tumor, many of which are pigmented and may be present at birth. There are many different types of nevi, almost all of which are harmless. However, the raised black mole, although benign, may become malignant if it is located where it is subjected to constant irritation. It is generally advisable for these moles to be excised as a precautionary measure.

## Angioma

Angioma is a benign skin tumor that consists of dilated blood vessels. There are several types of angiomas—one is congenital, called a birthmark by many people. The skin may have an area of purplish color known as port-wine stain. The stain is not elevated and may be large. Port-wine stains are commonly found on the face and may cover an entire side of the face. Treatment is usually for cosmetic purposes only and may consist of electrolysis, x-ray therapy, or laser removal.

The spider angioma is an acquired condition and consists of a network of venous capillaries that radiate outward in a spiderlike fashion. It may be related to liver disease and usually fades and disappears as the primary condition improves.

## Keratoses

Keratoses are generally considered precancerous lesions, of which there are many types. Some occur in older persons as senile keratoses and are most likely to become malignant. Surgical removal is generally indicated. Some forms of keratoses, such as solar or actinic, appear in persons who have been exposed to the sun and whose skin has been damaged by it. Others are found as seborrheic dermatoses in persons past middle age. These are less likely to become malignant but should be kept under observation.

## Malignant Tumors

Skin cancer can be prevented, and if diagnosed early, can be cured. The thousands of skin cancer deaths each year can be partially attributed to public ignorance about prevention and to laxity among professionals in assessing skin lesions. Skin cancer may be caused by frequent contact with carcinogenic chemicals such as those found in coal tar, pitch, and pesticides; overexposure or chronic exposure to the sun's ultraviolet rays; repeated scar-producing injuries, especially burns; and radiation treatment. Fair-skinned people are more susceptible to cancer from sun exposure because they have less melanin, which keeps the sun's ultraviolet rays from penetrating the skin. The ultraviolet rays are believed to set off a genetic reaction that results in skin cancer. There are three types of skin cancer: basal cell, squamous cell, and malignant melanoma. The first two types are the most common and are easily cured if detected and treated early. Malignant melanoma is rarer but is the most dangerous to the patient.

### Assessment

Assessment begins with a determination of the patient's risk for developing skin cancer. An investigation of life-style, occupation, geographic location, and hobbies will reveal factors that predispose the patient to skin cancer. Careful assessment of the skin of the entire body is important, including hidden areas between the toes and fingers and in the folds of the skin.

*Basal cell carcinoma* is seen most often in fair-skinned people who have had overexposure to the sun. It is usually found on the nose, eyelids, cheeks, rim of the ear, or trunk. There are two forms: nodular and superficial. The nodular form is elevated and firm to palpation and has an ulcerated center, raised margins, and a waxy or pearly border. The superficial type is flat and has a crusted or red center and a raised or pearly border.

*Squamous cell carcinoma* usually develops on areas exposed to radiation, mainly the head (especially on the lips) and hands. It can be an elevated, nodular mass or a large, fungus-like mass. It spreads more rapidly than basal cell carcinoma.

*Malignant melanoma* may appear without warning, beginning in or near a mole or other dark spot in the skin. The important warning signs are the ABCDs of melanoma. *A*symmetry: one side does not match the other; *B*order irregularity: the edges are notched, ragged, or blurred; *C*olor: the pigmentation is not uniform; shades of tan, brown, or black appear; dashes of red, white, or blue may be seen in the lesions; and *D*iameter: generally greater than 6 mm (about the size of a pencil eraser). The patient should see a physician if any of the following conditions are observed in a mole: the ABCDs, scaling, oozing, bleeding, spreading of pigmentation, or a change in sensation.

There is an inherited tendency to develop malignant melanoma, and melanoma-prone families can be identified by the presence of numerous large and unusual nevi on the skin. Now known as *dysplastic nevus syndrome (DNS),* this condition often leads to the development of malignant melanoma and is characterized by many large and unusual moles. The moles often number more than 100 and are usually larger than 5 mm. Their pigmentation is unusual, combining brown, black, red, and pink in a single mole. They are found on the back and chest and may even be found in the scalp and on the breast. Patients with DNS or multiple nevi should be seen regularly by a physician to detect changes warning of malignancy. The patient also must be instructed to regularly and systematically observe the moles so that early detection of change is possible. Any change in size or color of a mole, flaking, ulceration, bleeding, or sudden elevation of a previously flat mole should be reported immediately to the physician. Patients with fewer or no moles must likewise be alert for changes in warts, moles, scars, and birthmarks. Any unusual finding should be documented completely, including location, size, color, surface characteristics, and appearance of surrounding area. Documentation also should include the patient's observations of the lesion, including time of appearance, recent changes, irritation from clothing, and past treatment.

## Intervention

Skin cancer is treated with a number of methods, including excision by standard or laser surgery, radiation, cryosurgery, and electrodesiccation and curettage. More resistant and larger lesions are treated more effectively with a method called Mohs' surgery, named after Frederich Mohs, who developed the technique more than 30 years ago. The technique originally involved the application of a chemical fixative to the visible part of the skin cancer to eliminate blood flow during excision. Modern laboratory procedures and improved surgical techniques have eliminated the need for chemical fixation, and the technique is now performed on fresh tissue. The tissue is examined microscopically (by frozen section) as it is removed and the surgeon continues to remove tissue until microscopic malignancy is excised. The wound can be reconstructed immediately, which was not possible when the chemical fixative was used. It is relatively painless and can be performed on an outpatient basis under local anesthesia. The procedure is now known as *microscopically controlled excision,* or *Mohs' surgery fresh-tissue technique.*

After surgery, instruction in wound care is necessary. If the wound is left open to heal by secondary intention, it will be dressed postoperatively with an appropriate dressing (e.g., hydrocolloid, hydrogel, polyurethane foam, gauze). A topical antibiotic may be applied to the wound before dressing if desired. If the wound is dressed with a hydrocolloid, hydrogel, or a foam, the dressing needs to be changed only every 3 days unless signs of infection or heavy exudate are apparent. If a gauze dressing is used, it should be changed at least once daily. Because the wound is a clean surgical wound, cleansing is not necessary. If cleansing is desired or mandated by protocol, saline is the cleanser of choice. Hydrogen peroxide used to be the cleanser of choice for many years, but because of its cytotoxicity it should be used judiciously, if at all. If a gauze dressing is used, an antibiotic ointment is needed to help maintain a moist wound environment, help provide atraumatic removal of the gauze, and to provide some protection from bacteria. Some antibacterial ointments may cause sensitivity reactions, so the nurse should inform the patient to be aware of any redness, itching, or edema. As is true with any procedure, good handwashing is essential.

The most important intervention in skin cancer is prevention. (Box 40-5). Patients should be instructed on the use and importance of sunscreens. The minimum skin protection factor (SPF) that an individual should use is 15. Wearing broad-brimmed hats and limiting sun exposure should be advised. Individuals who are light skinned and have blue eyes and red or blonde hair are at higher risk for development of skin cancer. Dark-skinned individuals may have a false sense of protection because of their skin color. It

---

**BOX 40-5**

### Guidelines for Protecting the Skin Against Excessive Exposure to the Sun

- Avoid intense sunlight between 10 AM and 3 PM, when ultraviolet rays are the strongest.
- Plan such outdoor activities as walking, gardening, and other hobbies for early morning or late afternoon.
- Wear protective clothing such as hats and long-sleeved shirts.
- Use a sunscreen with a sun protection factor of 15 or higher. The sunscreen should be applied 15 to 30 minutes before going out into the sunlight and every 2 to 3 hours during exposure (it may need to be applied more often because of heat, humidity, and sweating). Sunscreen should be applied liberally to the head and neck, with special attention to the nose, rims of the ears, cheeks, and forehead.

From Hill MJ: *Skin disorders: Mosby's clinical nursing series,* St Louis, 1994, Mosby.

---

**BOX 40-6**

### ABCD RULE FOR EARLY DETECTION OF MELANOMA

A = Asymmetry

Most true moles tend to be symmetric.

Melanomas tend to be asymmetric (one half does not match the other).

B = Border

Most true moles have a clear-cut border.

Melanomas tend to have a notched, scalloped, or indistinct border.

C = Color

True moles may be dark or light, but they usually are uniform in color. Early melanomas have an uneven or variegated color (may range from various hues of tan and brown to black, with red and white intermingled).

D = Diameter

Once they have the A, B, and C characteristics, most melanomas are larger than 6 mm in diameter. Moles tend to be smaller. A sudden or progressive increase in the size of a mole should be reported.

From Hill MJ: *Skin disorders: Mosby's clinical nursing series*, St Louis, 1994, Mosby.

---

**BOX 40-7**

### SKIN CANCER SCREENING AND DETECTION

Perform monthly self-examination of skin or with other person.

With good lighting, use two mirrors to visualize the abdomen, perineal area, and back.

Use blow hair dryer and mirror to visualize scalp.

Observe each body part carefully, especially hidden areas such as between toes and folds of skin.

Use of body chart facilitates documentation of changes and suspected lesions to report.

Persons with two or more family members with a history of malignant melanoma should be examined by a dermatologist every 6 months.

Recognize and report symptoms or changes in skin characteristics promptly to physician, such as:

A, Asymmetry of shape

B, Border irregularity

C, Color variegation (black, brown, white, blue, red)

D, Diameter larger than 5 mm

From Otto SE: *Oncology nursing*, ed 3, St Louis, 1997, Mosby.

---

should be emphasized that even though their pigmentation offers some protection, they should still use a sunscreen and limit sun exposure. The use of tanning beds is discouraged.

Early detection of a skin cancer is also very important (Boxes 40-6 and 40-7). Patients should be informed of the five signs that should alert them to seek medical intervention. The five signs of skin cancer are (1) a persistent, nonhealing, open sore that bleeds, oozes, or crusts and remains open for 3 weeks or longer; (2) a reddish patch or irritated area, usually on the chest, shoulders, or limbs, that may or may not itch or hurt; (3) a smooth growth with an elevated, rolled border and indented center; (4) a shiny bump or nodule that is pearly or translucent and colored pink, red, white, tan, black, or brown; and (5) a scarlike area that is white, yellow, or waxy and often has poorly defined borders (Hill, 1994).

# DISORDERS OF THE APPENDAGES

## Alopecia (Loss of Hair)

Loss of hair may result from several causes, including the normal thinning of hair that is part of the aging process. Hair is sometimes lost after long and debilitating disease or high fever. A characteristic alopecia occurs in early syphilis and is marked by loss of hair in round patches; it may progress until the scalp presents a moth-eaten appearance. Alopecia areata results in patches of baldness that may appear suddenly and tend to spread from the edges. After several round patches of baldness occur, regrowth of hair begins but may not be permanent. Finally, however, the hair is replaced, and spontaneous recovery takes place after several months.

## Hypertrichosis and Hypotrichosis

Hypertrichosis is an excessive growth of hair in a masculine distribution. It may be congenital, acquired (hormonal dysfunction, porphyria, drugs), or result from a hereditary tendency. In congenital hypertrichosis, hair may cover moles or the skin over a spina bifida. Acquired hypertrichosis that is a result of endocrine disturbance is commonly seen as a growth of hair on the upper lip and on the chin of women. It also may be the result of a hereditary predisposition that is similar in character but not in effect to that which controls male pattern baldness. The most satisfactory method of removing superfluous hair is by electrolysis.

Hypotrichosis is an absence of hair or a deficiency of hair. The condition may be the result of heredity (alopecia universalis), skin disease, drugs, or endocrine factors. When the cause is endocrine disturbance, correction should be made if possible.

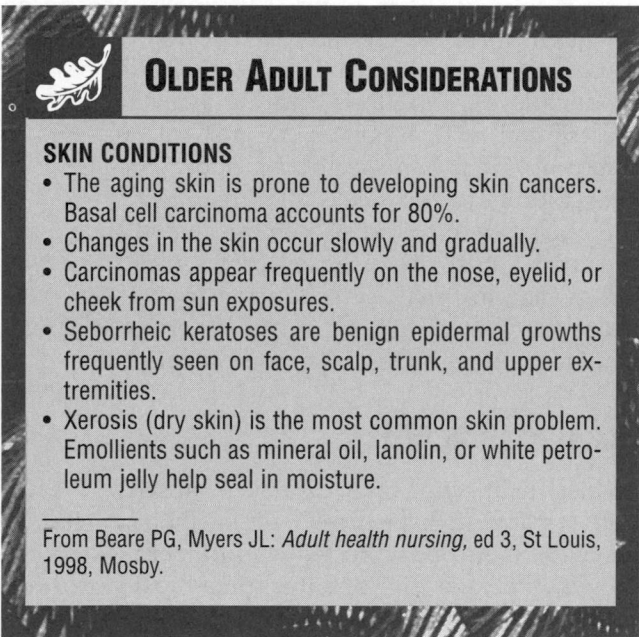

## OLDER ADULT CONSIDERATIONS

### SKIN CONDITIONS
- The aging skin is prone to developing skin cancers. Basal cell carcinoma accounts for 80%.
- Changes in the skin occur slowly and gradually.
- Carcinomas appear frequently on the nose, eyelid, or cheek from sun exposures.
- Seborrheic keratoses are benign epidermal growths frequently seen on face, scalp, trunk, and upper extremities.
- Xerosis (dry skin) is the most common skin problem. Emollients such as mineral oil, lanolin, or white petroleum jelly help seal in moisture.

From Beare PG, Myers JL: *Adult health nursing,* ed 3, St Louis, 1998, Mosby.

### TABLE 40-8

## Common Skin Manifestations of Ectoparasites

| ECTOPARASITE | SKIN MANIFESTATION |
| --- | --- |
| Scabies mite | Irregular, linear, gray-brown or pearly burrows less than 1 mm wide, often with a spot at the end; more prominent in the web spaces of the hands, on the flexor surfaces of the wrists, in the axillary folds, and on the buttocks; vesicles and papules may be present; in children, nodular lesions may be present on the upper back, chest, and genitals and in the axillary folds; disseminated papular eruption or crusted exfoliative areas with fissures may be seen in immunocompromised individuals |
| Lice | Small, erythematous papules and wheals, often with nits attached to hair shaft; cervical adenopathy may indicate severe involvement on the head and often is accompanied by purulent dermatitis, with matting of the hair; louse generally is visible on close observation |

From Hill MJ: *Skin disorders, Mosby's clinical nursing series,* 1994, St Louis, Mosby.

## Hair Transplants

The problem of baldness is more common in men than in women. As an alternative to wearing hairpieces, it is now possible to elect to have a hair transplant for cosmetic purposes. Most balding males retain healthy hair on the back and sides of the head. These hair follicles can be relocated by a transplant procedure in which dozens of small plugs of hair are removed and relocated to the areas where hair is thin or absent. Patterns of grafts are removed from the balding area and replaced by the healthy growing hair grafts from the donor area. Treatment is usually performed in two or three sessions, and each session lasts 1 or 2 hours. Sessions are spaced at least 2 weeks apart to allow adequate healing and to establish circulation through the transplant area. New hair should begin to appear about 12 weeks after the transplant.

## Nail Disorders

Disorders of the nails may be associated with diseases elsewhere in the body, nutritional status, congenital defects, drugs, or infection. The nails may be soft or brittle. Changes in the shape and contour may occur, and nails may grow into the soft tissues at the sides (ingrown nail). *Paronychia* is an infection in the fold of skin at the margin of the nail. The infection begins on the side of the nail, often from a hangnail or injury, and finally encircles the whole nail. The infection loosens the nail from the matrix and may cause pain. Surgical removal of the affected part of the nail is often necessary. Wet dressings using 1:2000 to 1:10,000 potassium permanganate and the application of neomycin ointment may relieve the condition. Fungal infections of the nails respond poorly to ordinary methods of treatment and may take months to cure.

# INFESTATIONS

## Pediculi (Lice)

Three types of pediculi infest human beings: *Pediculus humanus capitis, P. humanus corporis,* and *P. pubis.* Table 40-8 lists the common skin manifestations.

*P. humanus capitis* is the head louse, which lives on the scalp and attaches its eggs (nits) to the hair. The nits are attached to the hair by an adhesive substance that makes them difficult to remove. The louse bites the scalp to seek nutrition by sucking blood, which causes severe itching and scratching. Severe infestations may result in secondary infections that are associated with enlargement of lymph glands in the neck (Box 40-8). Immediate treatment is required. For many years, the treatment of choice was Kwell shampoo, which contained the active ingredient lindane. Kwell is no longer sold, but generic products containing lindane are available by prescription. Lindane is known to be cerebroneurotoxic, and other preparations such as 1% permethrin (Nix) or pyrethrin (RID) are considered less toxic and have proven as effective as lindane while causing fewer adverse reactions. Nix and RID are available without prescription (University of California at Berkeley, 1995).

*P. humanus corporis* is a body louse that may be found in the seams of underclothing. Scratch marks may appear on the skin in the area of the involved clothing seams. For both head lice and body lice, all personal items such as clothing and bedding must be washed in hot water. With body lice, the extra precaution of ironing the seams of clothing should be recommended. Hats, scarves, hair ornaments, combs, and brushes also must be cleared of lice and their eggs. Although lice can live only approximately 10 days after

separation from the host, the eggs may hatch in up to 30 days if kept near body temperature. Body lice are treated with 1% permethrin, pyrethrin, or lindane. Any one of the three pediculicides is applied to the affected skin/scalp after bathing and shampooing, with particular care to avoid the eyes. Lindane is applied to the total body and left on for 2 hours. The treatment may be repeated if necessary. If pyrethrin or permethrin is used, it is left on for 10 minutes, then rinsed thoroughly. This application is repeated daily for 3 consecutive days. As mentioned earlier, RID and Nix produce less toxic effects and are available without prescription. A fine-toothed comb should be used to comb nits from hair (scalp and pubic). Itching may persist for up to two weeks after treatment.

*P. pubis* is found primarily in the genital area; however, it may infect the axilla, eyebrows, beard, and eyelashes. The lice may be contracted from toilet seats, bedclothes, clothing, and sexual intercourse. Treatment is the same as for *P. humanis corporis*.

## Scabies (Itch Mite)

Scabies, an infectious skin disease, is caused by the itch mite, a parasite that burrows under the skin (see Table 40-8). A warm, protected environment fosters the growth of the parasite, and it is spread easily by direct contact with another person who is infested. Even handholding or simply shaking hands can transmit scabies from one individual to another. Contact with infected clothing or linens can spread scabies, but the mite does not jump from one person to the other and does not survive very long in clothing or linens. Outbreaks of scabies were common until World War II and then began a decline, only to make a vigorous comeback in recent years. It is not uncommon to find scabies on patients in nursing homes and hospitals.

Scabies may occur as epidemics or endemics. An individual can develop immunity to the disease, but the mechanism of this immunity is not clearly understood.

### Assessment

The nurse can prevent the spread of the disease to other patients and also avoid contracting the disease by being alert to the symptoms. A person is more likely to contract scabies from someone whose disease is not diagnosed than from one who has been identified and treated. The disease is recognized by the presence of intense itching and multiform lesions (lesions of many shapes). Papules and vesicles are common, and characteristic S-shaped burrows are often, but not always, present. Secondary bacterial infection and scratching may result in pustules and edema (see

---

**BOX 40-8**

## COMPLICATIONS OF ECTOPARASITE INFESTATION

- Because of the intense pruritus and scratching associated with scabies, secondary bacterial infections may occur. In immunocompromised individuals, the mite multiplies, unchecked by the cell-mediated response that normally kills a percentage of the mites. As the mites multiply, hyperkeratotic plaques form and fissuring develops. Normal skin flora may be introduced into the blood, resulting in bacteremia, sepsis, and occasionally death.

- Lice infestation may be the source of keratoconjunctivitis, photophobia, and secondary pyoderma, caused by *Pediculus humanus capitis*. Other complications include eczematization, pyodermas, nodular granulomas, urticaria, acarophobia, and delusions of parasitosis. *P. humanus corporis* serves as a vector for epidemic typhus fever *(Rickettsia prowazekii)*, relapsing fever *(Borrelia recurrentis)*, and trench fever *(Rickettsia quintana)* (Hill, 1994).

From Hill MJ: *Skin disorders: Mosby's clinical nursing series*, St Louis, 1994, Mosby.

Box 40-8). Delay in treatment may lead to an eczematous condition.

The characteristic location of the lesion varies with age. Children have involvement of the palms, soles, head, and neck. Adults rarely have lesions in these areas but do have them on the flexor surfaces of the wrist and elbows, on the waist, buttocks, genitalia in males, and on the breasts in females. Burrows can be found between fingers and around the umbilicus. The characteristic itching intensifies at night. A definite diagnosis may require examination of scrapings taken from lesions on the skin to isolate the mite.

Treatment requires use of an insecticide by the patient and all close contacts. Insecticides may include 5% permethrin cream (Elimite), 1% lindane, or crotamiton (Eurax). The permethrin cream is massaged into the skin from the head to the soles, left on for 8 to 14 hours, and washed off thoroughly. Lindane is applied the same way as permethrin cream, but because of evidence of neurotoxicity with infants and small children, the application time for them is shortened to 2 hours. In addition, if the lindane is applied to the hands of these very young patients, precautions should be taken to keep them from putting their hands in their mouths. Lindane should not be used in pregnant or lactating women. Treatment may be repeated in 7 days if indicated. Crotamiton (Eurax) is applied for 2 to 5 consecutive nights. The patient can bathe 24 hours after the last application. Crotamiton is contraindicated in pregnant or lactating women. Patients should be advised that itching may persist for up to 2 weeks and that they should not use this medication repeatedly to help control the itching because this increases the risk of absorption. Medication may be prescribed specifically to help control the itching (Hill, 1994).

# INFECTIONS

## Bacterial Infections

*Folliculitis* is inflammation of a hair follicle secondary to staphylococcal infection. It commonly occurs on the scalp, the extremities, or the bearded areas of the face. Chronic folliculitis of the beard is called *sycosis barbae.* If hair follicles are permanently damaged, hair will not grow from them.

A *furuncle* (boil) is an acute infection of a hair follicle or sebaceous gland. It usually is caused by a staphylococcus bacterium that produces an abscess of the skin in subcutaneous tissue. The lesion appears with central necrosis and accumulation of pus. Initial lesions are small, indurated, and painful. As the lesions progress, they become elevated, tender, shiny, and

bright red, and the patient complains of throbbing pain. Furuncles may resolve spontaneously, but incision and drainage gives almost immediate relief from pain and does hasten healing. Patients may also have fever, malaise, and regional lymphadenopathy. Lesions are most commonly seen on the back of the neck, face, buttocks, thighs, perineum, and breasts, or in the axillae. There may be single or multiple lesions. A carbuncle is similar to a boil, except that the infection infiltrates into the surrounding tissue and results in several boils. Carbuncles are also caused by a staphylococcus bacterium.

A *felon* is an infection of the end of a finger. It may result from a puncture wound such as a pinprick, or it may occur without a known cause. A streptococcus bacterium is a common cause of felons. Clinically, an abscess usually is seen on the distal phalanx of a finger.

Cellulitis is an acute streptococcal or staphylococcal infection of the skin and subcutaneous tissue. The skin becomes erythematous, edematous, hot, and tender to the touch. Lymphatic streaks may develop proximal to the infection (Hill, 1994).

Impetigo is skin infection that is categorized as impetigo contagiosa, caused by group A beta-hemolytic streptococci, or as bullous impetigo, caused by group II *Staphylococcus aureus.* Impetigo contagiosa is found most often in children and may be endemic (Hill, 1994). The initial clinical lesion of impetigo is a vesicular or pustular lesion with a "honey-colored crust" that is considered a definitive sign of impetigo. Lesions of impetigo may be seen on the lower extremities, face, or hands (Figure 40-7). The bacteria are easily spread through direct or indirect contact. It is common for an

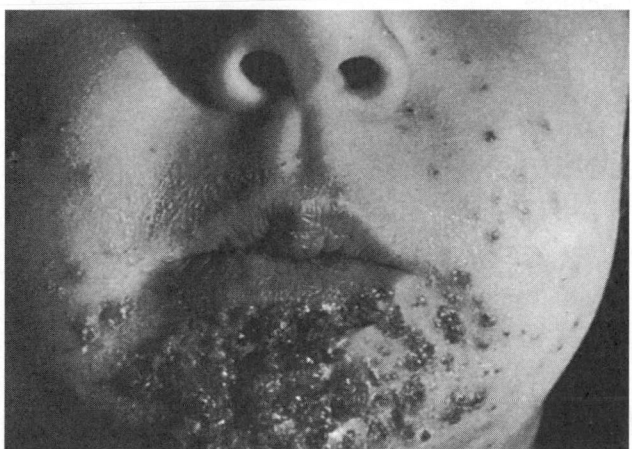

**Figure 40-7**    Impetigo contagiosa. (From Stewart WD et al: *Dermatology: diagnosis and treatment of cutaneous disorders*, ed 4, St Louis, 1978, Mosby.)

insect bite to become infected by the staphylococcus or streptococcus organism. Poor health and nutrition, a warm, humid environment, and preexisting pruritic skin eruptions may also predispose a patient to impetigo (Yotter, 1990). Definitive identification of the causative organism may be done by bacterial culture.

## Assessment

Nursing assessment of patients suspected of having a bacterial skin infection includes assessing current health status and performing a physical examination to identify lymphadenopathy and existing skin lesions. Patients with impetigo, cellulitis, furuncles, or carbuncles may appear healthy but complain of fever, chills, headache, and malaise. Lymphadenopathy may be present with any of these infections.

The lesion of *folliculitis* consists of a pustule surrounded by an area of erythema and appears as a raised dome around the follicle. The pustule weeps, forming a crust, and the hair seems to be growing from the center of the crust. Pain will occur if the infection spreads to the dermis surrounding the follicle.

A *furuncle* begins as a small, red, edematous, painful area on the skin of the face, neck, axilla, forearm, buttocks, groin, or legs. It may appear as only a tiny pimple and abate spontaneously, or it may continue to increase in size and exhibit pus formation within a few days. *Carbuncles* are most commonly found on the back of the neck and upper back. As the infection gradually comes to the surface from the deeper tissue, there will be several openings discharging pus. The site of a *felon* on a finger is red and edematous, and there is severe, throbbing pain. Both carbuncles and furuncles occur most often in poorly nourished and debilitated individuals and may be a sign of uncontrolled diabetes mellitus.

*Cellulitis* appears as an erythematous, edematous, hot, and tender area of skin with or without lymphangitic streaks. It may or may not be associated with another skin lesion. *Impetigo* begins as a vesicopustule on the skin that ruptures and leaves a red, oozing erosion. The erosion becomes covered by a characteristic yellow (honey-colored) crust. The infection may spread from an existing lesion to other parts of the body, so several lesions may be present at the same time.

## Interventions

Early treatment of these localized infections prevents complications and systemic spread. General management of these infections includes cleansing of the involved area with an antibacterial soap. The surrounding skin also should be cleansed carefully to prevent spread of the infection.

Warm, moist compresses are used to promote suppuration in folliculitis, furuncles, carbuncles, and felons. If the furuncles or carbuncles do not rupture spontaneously, surgical incision and drainage is necessary. Most patients with folliculitis, furuncles, carbuncles, and felons are cared for in the physician's office.

General management of cellulitis includes immobilization and elevation of the affected limb, hospitalization if necessary, cool compresses for discomfort, or warm compresses to increase circulation. General measures for the management of impetigo include removal of crusts with soap and water, application of cool compresses, and nutritional interventions as indicated. Patients should be instructed to avoid sharing of clothing, towels, or washcloths.

All skin infections require either topical or systemic antibiotics, depending on the severity. The nurse must educate the patient about any medication, proper use, and possible side effects.

Universal precautions—use of gloves, handwashing, and proper disposal of all contaminated dressings—should be followed at all times when dealing with skin infections. Patients should be instructed to use the same precautions at home to prevent cross contamination while lesions are still draining. Patients should also be instructed not to share clothing and linen while infection is still evident (Box 40-9).

## Fungal Infections

Fungal infections **(tinea)** are superficial infections of the skin and are classified by body region (tinea corporis, tinea capitis, tinea cruris, tinea barbae, tenia pedis). Fungi can infect and survive in the dead keratin of the stratum corneum (horny layer) of the epidermis. They also affect the hair and nails. Fungal infection rarely invades deep tissues or involves other organs except in the immunocompromised patient.

Fungal infections must be diagnosed by laboratory examination (KOH wet mount, wood's lamp, or culture). A potassium hydroxide (KOH) wet mount is done by taking a scraping of the suspected lesion, placing it on a microscope slide, adding a drop of KOH, applying a cover slip, heating it slightly, and examining it under the microscope. Hyphae of fungi may be detected under magnification with this technique. A wood's lamp, when shined on suspected lesions, causes the fungus to fluorescence a blue-green. Fungal culture is done by taking scrapings from the suspected lesion and putting them into the appropriate medium. If fungal growth is seen within 1 week, the patient can be told that the culture is positive.

Even though fungal infections are superficial, there are some complications that may occur. These include

> ◁ **BOX 40-9** ▷      **NURSING PROCESS**
>
> ## BACTERIAL INFECTION
>
> **ASSESSMENT**
>
> - Current health status
> - Skin lesions for characteristics, distribution, and severity
> - Level of discomfort
> - Temperature
> - Lymphadenopathy
>
> **NURSING DIAGNOSES**
>
> - Impaired skin integrity related to inflammatory process
> - Risk for impaired skin integrity related to exudate
> - Risk for infection related to inadequate primary or secondary defenses
> - Body image disturbance related to reaction of others to lesions
> - Pain related to infectious process
>
> **NURSING INTERVENTIONS**
>
> - Provide local treatment of lesions as ordered.
> - Use good handwashing technique and instruct the patient in the procedure.
> - Use antibacterial soap and instruct the patient to use it.
> - Administer analgesic medication as ordered and evaluate its effect.
>
> **EVALUATION OF EXPECTED OUTCOMES**
>
> - Skin integrity improved
> - No infection is evident
> - Pain is relieved

secondary infections, id reactions, pruritus, and infections that are atypical, generalized, or invasive (usually in immunocompromised patients). An id reaction is a cutaneous response elicited in other areas of the body distant from the primary infection (Hill, 1994).

## Tinea Capitis

Tinea capitis, better known as ringworm of the scalp, occurs primarily in preadolescent children. The lesion is easily recognized and appears as a scaly bald spot with hairs breaking off at the surface (Figure 40-8, *A*). Occasionally the patient will develop an inflammatory reaction to the fungus and will develop boggy areas with pus called *kerion.* Treatment of ringworm is usually successful with oral griseofulvin. If kerion are present, they should be treated topically with compresses and hydrogen peroxide at the same time that the oral steroids are given. Patients receiving cortisone should not be given griseofulvin at the same time. When the infection is severe, there may be patches of baldness on the scalp. This loss of hair is usually temporary, and the hair will return when the infection subsides. This infection is contagious, so all members of the family should be examined. The patient's personal toilet articles, such as combs and brushes, should not be used by other members of the family. The individual with tinea capitis is usually treated in the physi-

cian's office or in a clinic; however, the patient may have been admitted to the hospital for another condition. If tinea capitis is discovered in a hospital patient, it should be called to the physician's attention, and the nurse should take protective precautions.

## Tinea Corporis

Tinea corporis is a form of ringworm that occurs on the nonhairy areas of the body, face, neck, and extremities. The characteristic lesion is a papulosquamous annular lesion with raised borders, scaly borders, and central clearing (Figure 40-8, *B*). The lesion increases in size gradually, expanding peripherally. Tinea corporis is more common in hot and humid climates, more common in rural areas, and occurs in both adults and children (Hill, 1994). Treatment with a topical fungicide is satisfactory if only a few lesions are present. For more extensive cases, griseofulvin is used.

## Tinea Barbae

Tinea barbae, or barber's itch, occurs in the beard and is characterized by a soft nodular type of lesion with accompanying edema of the face. The nodules may break down and become suppurative. The hairs of the beard become loose and slip out, leaving bald areas. Several preparations have been used in the treatment

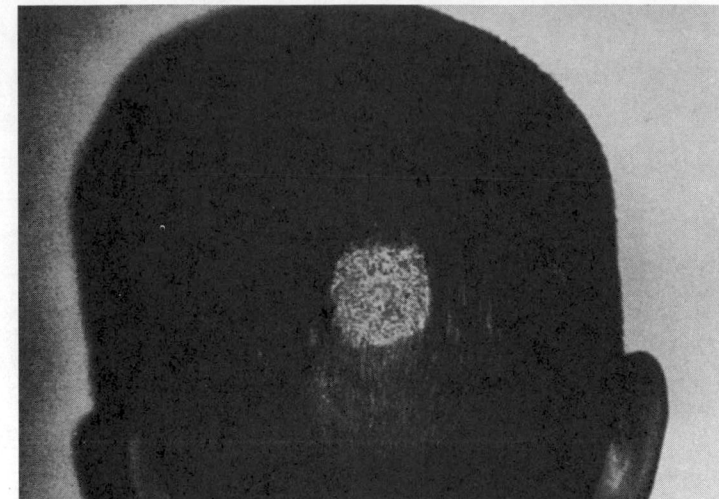

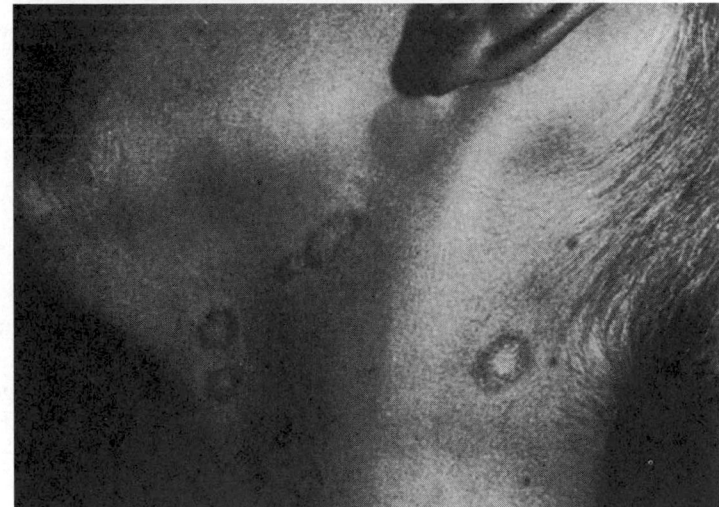

**Figure 40-8** **A,** Tinea capitis. **B,** Tinea corporis. (From Stewart WD et al: *Dermatology: diagnosis and treatment of cutaneous disorders,* ed 4, St Louis, 1978, Mosby.)

of the condition, including ammoniated mercury ointment, griseofulvin, and copper undecylenate.

## Tinea Cruris

Tinea cruris is commonly called jock itch and is found in the groin or inner thigh. It is more common in hot weather and is aggravated by friction caused by tight-fitting clothing. The lesion usually affects both sides of the groin equally and may extend to cover the entire groin area, giving a butterfly appearance. The lesions are either hypopigmented or erythematous, and they are well-demarcated, with scaling and central clearing. Pruritus is the main complaint. Maceration of the skin in the skin folds occurs, and secondary bacterial or candidal infection is common. Treatment involves keeping the area cool and dry, wearing loose, absorbent clothing, and applying an antifungal preparation as prescribed.

## Tinea Pedis

Tinea pedis, or athlete's foot, is a common disorder affecting the feet, although it may be spread to other parts of the body, particularly the hands (tinea manuum). It is rare in children and is not transmitted by simple exposure. It is generally believed that the infection is contracted in showers, around swimming pools, and in similar moist places, but absolute proof of this method of transmission is lacking. Clinical lesions vary and include maceration, scaling, fissuring of interdigital space, erythema of the plantar surfaces, and brittle, discolored nails. Pruritus is a common complaint.

General management of tineas includes keeping intertriginous areas clean and dry and using a medicated powder. With tinea pedis, white cotton socks should be worn. Application of the prescribed topical medication or adherence to the prescribed systemic medication schedule must be emphasized (Table 40-9 and Box 40-10).

**TABLE 40-9**

## Summary of Tinea

| TYPE | DISTRIBUTION | OCCURRENCE | CLINICAL FEATURES |
|---|---|---|---|
| Tinea corporis | Nonhairy parts of body, face, neck, extremities | More common in hot and humid climates; more common in rural than in urban settings; occurs in both adults and children | Pruritus; papulosquamous annular lesions with raised borders; lesions expand peripherally with central clearing |
| Tinea cruris | Groin, inner thigh, scrotum or labia not involved | More common in adult men; tends to recur; flare-ups common in summer; aggravated by tight clothes, perspiration, and physical activity | Pruritus; hypopigmented, well-demarcated lesions; dryness and scaling; pustules present at margins; central clearing sometimes present; secondary bacterial or candidal infection and maceration common |
| Tinea capitis | Scalp | More common in children; contagious | Lesions vary; small, gray scaly patches with short broken hairs; mild, erythematous papules; raised, boggy, inflamed nodules dotted with perifollicular abscesses; thick, yellow, suppurative lesions; lesions may be small and coalesced or may cover entire scalp; hairless patches |
| Tinea pedis | Feet; begins in third and fourth interdigital spaces and spreads to involve plantar surface; may involve nails | Rare in children; not transmitted by simple exposure | Lesions vary; maceration, scaling, fissuring of interdigital space; vesicular scaling, erythema of plantar surface; chronic, noninflamed, diffuse scaling; nails brittle, discolored; pruritus |
| Tinea unguium | Toenails and (less commonly) fingernails | | Nails thickened, lusterless, and discolored; subungual debris; nail plate crumbling or absent |

From Hill MJ: *Skin disorders: Mosby's clinical nursing series,* St Louis, 1994, Mosby.

**BOX 40-10** | **NURSING PROCESS**

## FUNGAL INFECTION

**ASSESSMENT**
- Skin lesions for characteristics, distribution, and severity
- Level of discomfort
- Signs of secondary infection

**NURSING DIAGNOSES**
- Impaired skin integrity related to presence of lesions
- Risk for infection related to loss of skin's protective barrier
- Pain related to skin lesions

**NURSING INTERVENTIONS**
- Cleanse lesions as indicated.
- Discourage scratching.
- Keep skin surfaces dry.
- Administer antihistamines or analgesics as indicated.
- Apply topical medications as ordered.
- Administer systemic medications as ordered.

**EVALUATION OF EXPECTED OUTCOMES**
- Skin integrity improved
- No infection is evident
- Pruritus/pain has been relieved

# VIRAL INFECTIONS

Viral infections that are contained in or manifested in the skin have distinct symptoms that allow clinical diagnosis without further testing. Rubella, rubeola, human papillomaviruses (warts), herpesviruses (simplex, zoster, and varicella), and human immunodeficiency virus (HIV) are all commonly seen on the skin (Hill, 1994).

## Rubella

*Rubella* (German measles, 3 day measles) is a viral infection that appears as erythematous macular/maculopapular lesions that last up to 3 days. Low-grade fever, coryza (rhinitis), malaise, headache, and conjunctivitis may precede the development of a rash by 1 to 5 days. These prodromal symptoms may not appear at all, especially in children. Mode of transmission is airborne, and the virus invades through nasopharyngeal secretions. The incubation period for rubella is 14 to 21 days from infection to presentation of rash. Lymphadenopathy may accompany the presentation of the rash. The rash characteristically begins on the face and spreads from the head toward the hands and feet. Petechial lesions may be seen on the soft palate and uvula. Pharyngitis (inflammation of the pharynx) may also be present (Hill, 1994).

## Rubeola

An acute, highly contagious viral disease that is spread by respiratory exposure is *rubeola* (red measles). The prodromes include fever, conjunctivitis, coryza, bronchitis, and Koplik's spots (small, red spots with bluish-white centers) on the buccal mucosa. A red, macular/maculopapular rash appears on the face 3 to 7 days after infection with the virus. The rash will generalize and last from 4 to 7 days. Desquamation is a common occurrence after the rash has resolved (Hill, 1994).

## Papillomavirus (Warts)

Human papillomaviruses cause benign skin growths called *warts*. Warts can be seen in all age groups. They commonly develop at sites of trauma, on the hands, in the **periungual** region (around the nail), and on the plantar surfaces, and they usually resolve spontaneously. Individuals with immunosuppression (HIV, drugs), atopic dermatitis, and lymphomas have more severe cases of warts when infected (Hill, 1994). Warts may appear on the genitalia in adults and are transmitted through sexual contact. If genital warts are seen in children, sexual abuse may be the cause.

## Herpesviruses

*Herpesviruses (Herpesvirus hominus)* cause opportunistic infections. Opportunistic infections are a consequence of defective functioning of one or more components of the immune system (Beare, Myers, 1994). Herpesvirus hominus is subdivided into *herpes simplex virus type 1* and *herpes simplex virus type 2*.

### Herpes Simplex

*Herpes simplex 1 (HSV-1)* is the most common form of herpes simplex and is found in gingivostomatitis (cold sore, fever blister) (Figure 40-9). *Herpes simplex 2 (HSV-2)* causes genital herpes and is found in lesions of the penis and cervix and in disseminated herpes in the newborn (see Chapter 14).

Each of the two forms of herpes has a primary and a secondary presentation. Primary infections are usually subclinical, but they can become severe and may be life threatening. Secondary presentations, or recurrences, are generally milder and of shorter duration. Subclinical primary infections appear as small vesicles that evolve into ulcerations, then crusts, with healing taking from a few days to 3 weeks. Pain and lymphadenopathy may be associated. Recurrences may have prodromes of tingling or pain in the area of involvement. Recurrent lesions reappear in the same site as the primary lesions (Hill, 1994).

HSV-1 is characterized by the appearance of a group of small vesicles on an erythematous base. It was originally thought that HSV-1 could be found only on the skin and mucous membranes of the lip or nose (see Figure 40-9). This has since been proven incorrect. HSV-1 has been cultured from lesions on the genitalia. The disease often occurs when other acute infections are present but may occur in the absence of any other condition. It was once thought that chancre sores (aphthous ulcers) on the mucous membrane of the mouth were also caused by this same virus, but it has now been demonstrated that they are not herpetic lesions. Herpes simplex is usually of short duration, but it is a recurring condition. The virus has the ability to persist in a latent state in certain tissues and to cause repeated infection despite the presence of circulating neutralizing antibodies. The appearance of the lesion, often called a cold sore, is often associated with certain stimuli such as sunlight, menstruation, fatigue, and emotional stress, all of which are thought to trigger viral replication and result in disease.

HSV-2 is found in approximately 20% of the adult population and is more prevalent in lower socioeconomic groups and in sexually active persons. The virus produces genital herpes and results in ulcerative or necrotizing lesions of the uterine cervix or the vul-

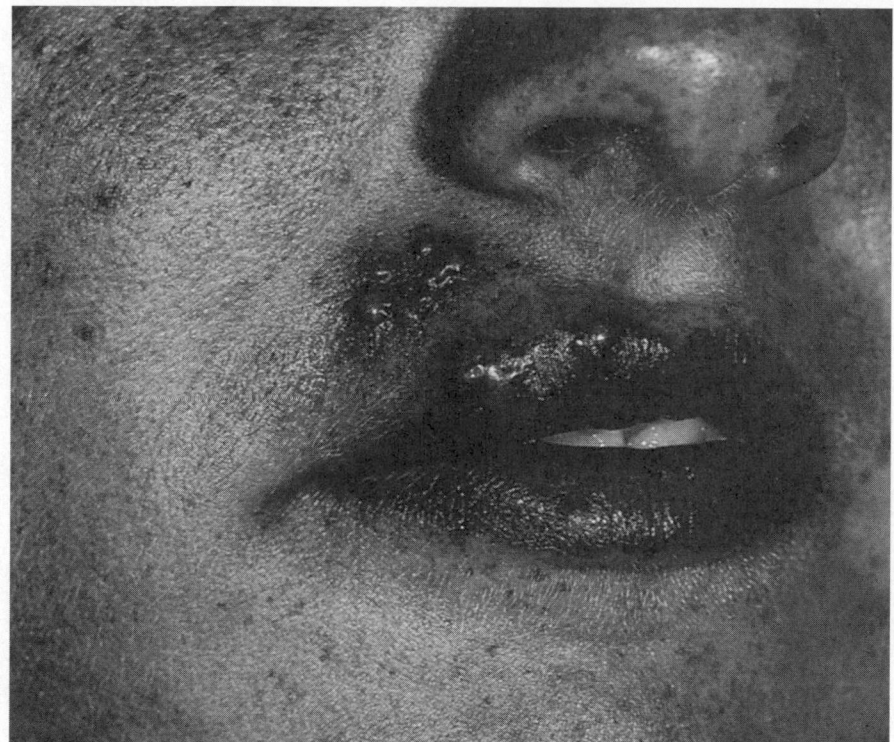

**Figure 40-9** Herpes simplex type I. (From Habif TP: *Clinical dermatology*, ed 3, St Louis, 1996, Mosby.)

var area in women. In men it produces ulcerations on the penis. The ulcerations are painful and tend to recur. It must be remembered that women may have asymptomatic lesions of the cervix that continually shed the virus. It is extremely important to evaluate pregnant women to determine whether vaginal delivery is safe.

## Herpes zoster

*Herpes zoster* and *varicella (chickenpox)* are caused by the herpesvirus varicella. Varicella is an acute, highly contagious viral infection. A maculopapulovesicular exanthem that has centripetal distribution is the presentation of varicella (chickenpox). The characteristic lesion is called "dew drop on a rose petal" because of its appearance—a singular vesicle on an erythematous base. Lesions develop in crops, so at any one time there may be primary and secondary (crusted or resolving) lesions present. Varicella is self-limiting, and healing is complete within 2 weeks. In immunocompromised patients, however, varicella is a life-threatening disease. Pruritus is the most disturbing symptom associated with varicella. Treatment is directed at alleviation of symptoms and includes soothing baths

(Aveeno, cornstarch), antihistamines, and topical drying agents (calamine, shake lotions).

*Herpes zoster,* also known as shingles, often classified as a neurologic disorder because the lesion is located in one or more of the spinal ganglia, with involvement of the skin area supplied by the nerve fibers. The virus can lie dormant in exposed individuals, including those who have developed chickenpox after exposure. Herpes zoster occurs when the dormant virus is activated. Individuals who have not had varicella may develop it (varicella) after exposure to the vesicular lesions of persons with herpes zoster. Herpes zoster can be a serious condition in any adult and may even lead to death from exhaustion in the older adult and the debilitated. It often occurs in persons with Hodgkin's disease or other cancers because of reduced cell-mediated immunity.

The skin lesions usually follow the dermatomes, which are the segments of the skin surface that are divided according to the nerves that innervate them (Figure 40-10). Because the lesions follow these nerve pathways, they rarely cross the midline of the body and may appear on only one side.

Herpes zoster can be precipitated by trauma, x-rays, or ultraviolet light, or it may be associated with a

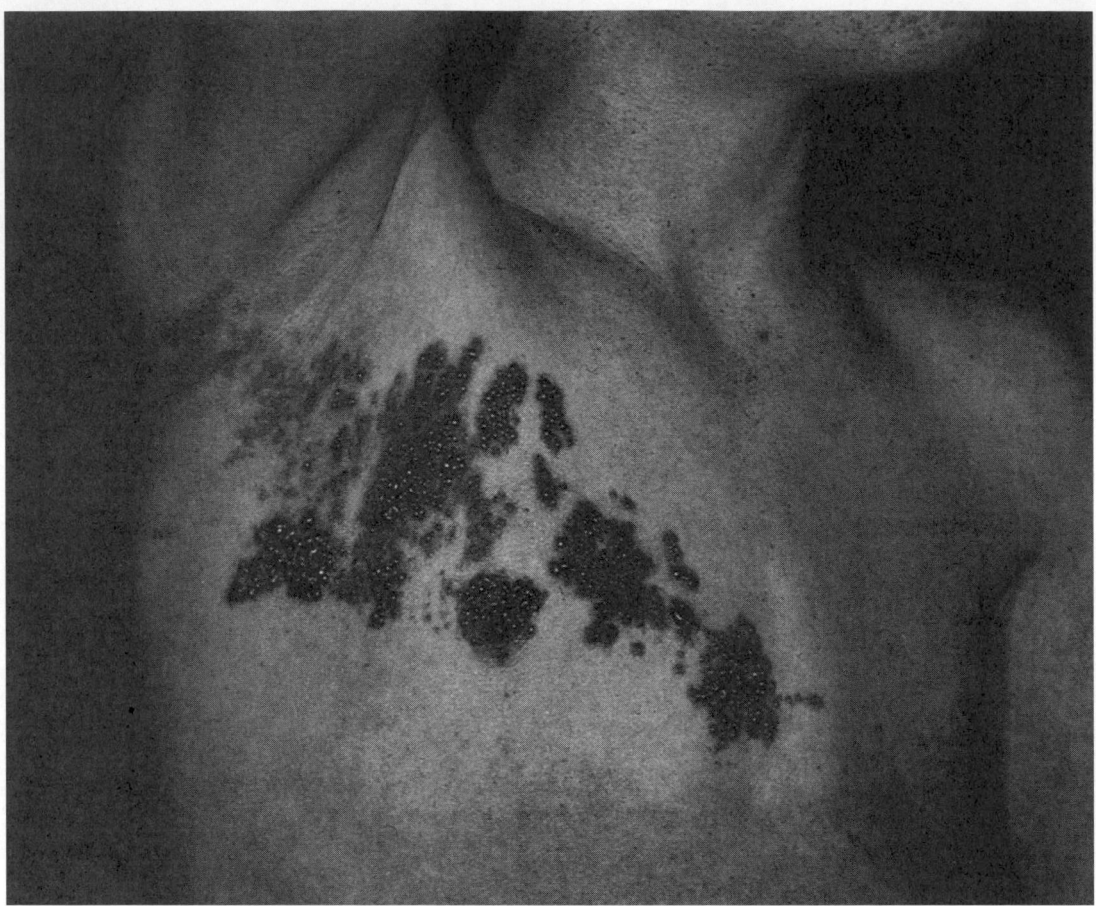

**Figure 40-10**    Herpes zoster. (From Habif TP: *Clinical dermatology*, St Louis, 1985, Mosby.)

malignancy. The patient may experience pain or burning, hyperesthesia (extreme sensitivity to pain or touch), or headache and malaise (uncommon) 1 to 10 days before lesions develop. The patient may also experience a slight fever and loss of appetite before the lesions appear. When the lesions are 1 or 2 days old, an inflamed, edematous area appears where papules are turning into vesicles and are arranged in groups following the sensory nerves from the posterior to the anterior. The most common location of the lesions is the thoracic region, but they may occur on the thighs, lower abdomen, or forehead. Approximately one third of the patients have involvement of cranial nerve V (trigeminal nerve), with lesions on the face, eyes, and scalp. If the lesions do occur along the branch of cranial nerve V, the patient should be observed for facial paralysis and eye or ear disturbances. A neurologic pain occurs in paroxysms and is worse with movement and at night. The pain may persist long after the skin manifestation has subsided; it is then called *postherpetic neuralgia.*

> ### NURSE ALERT
>
> **Zoster that crosses the midline, or disseminates, is a sign that the patient may be immunocompromised or may have an internal malignancy.**

**Intervention.** Herpes zoster is self-limiting, and acyclovir and vidarabine are used in severe cases and in immunocompromised patients. Analgesics are given for pain, and narcotics may be required for severe pain. The injection of a local anesthetic agent into the nerve has been attempted to control pain by blocking its transmission. If begun early enough, this method also seems to provide protection against the development of postherpetic neuralgia. Systemic corticosteroids are used to decrease inflammation and may

<BOX 40-11> **NURSING PROCESS**

## VIRAL INFECTIONS

**ASSESSMENT**

- Characteristics, distribution, and severity of lesions/rash
- Signs of secondary infection
- Lymphadenopathy
- Temperature
- Nutritional needs

**NURSING DIAGNOSES**

- Impaired skin integrity related to presence of lesions
- Risk for infection related to impaired skin integrity
- Pain related to skin lesions
- Hyperthermia related to disease process
- Altered nutrition: less than body requirements related to presence of oral lesions

**NURSING INTERVENTIONS**

- Cleanse the lesions.
- Apply topical medications as ordered.
- Discourage scratching.
- Administer analgesics as needed.
- Administer systemic medications as ordered.

**EVALUATION OF EXPECTED OUTCOMES**

- Skin integrity is improved or has been maintained
- No evidence of infection
- Pain has been relieved
- Nutritional status is adequate

reduce postherpetic neuralgia. Systemic steroids have no effect on the healing of the skin lesions. Topical shake lotions (calamine, zinc oxide mixture) will help to dry the lesions. If secondary infection is present, antibiotics are given.

Patients with herpes zoster may be hospitalized, and emotional depression often accompanies the disease. The nurse may find the patient irritable and uncooperative. Patience and understanding are needed in caring for these patients.

General management of patients with viral infections are supportive and are directed toward alleviating symptoms (Box 40-11). For pruritus, tepid baths with cornstarch, Aveeno, or baking soda is helpful. Bed rest during febrile periods is suggested. Lesions of herpesvirus should be kept clean and dry, and the patient and family should be educated about the transmission of viral diseases. Persons who have never had chickenpox (varicella) or the vaccine should not be exposed to or involved in the care of persons with herpes zoster because it would put them at risk for contracting varicella. Immunity is determined by varicella titer.

Patients with human immunodeficiency virus (HIV) have increased susceptibility to both superficial and disseminated infections (Box 40-12). Superficial infections include scabies, a variety of papillomavirus infections, herpes simplex, and herpes zoster. Chronic pruritic eruptions, bacterial infections, and fungal infections are common. Malignant lesions develop at a much higher rate in these patients (Hill, 1994).

# DISEASES OF EPIDERMAL ORIGIN

Diseases of epidermal origin have distinctive characteristics, including erythema and scale. Included in this category are dermatitis (eczema), exfoliative dermatitis (erythroderma), and psoriasis.

## Dermatitis (Eczema)

The terms dermatitis and *eczema* are used interchangeably, although they do have slightly different meanings. Dermatitis is an inflammatory condition of the skin resulting from a wide variety of causes such as allergy, stress, and unknown factors. In most cases it is characterized by erythema, pruritus, edema, and weeping/crusting on the skin surface in the acute stage and scaling, fissuring, and **lichenification** (thickening, bark-like) in the chronic stage. Eczema is a reactive process rather than a disease. Allergic contact dermatitis is caused by allergy to poison ivy, sumac, oak, or a proven allergen such as nickel. Irritant dermatitis is another cause of eczema. Irritant dermatitis is a result of direct contact with cosmetics, chemicals, dyes, or detergents. Other examples of eczema include nummular eczema (coin-shaped, oozing, crusting patches), seborrheic dermatitis (yellowish-pink scaling of the scalp, face, and trunk), and atopic dermatitis (characteristic distribution of eczema in individuals with a family history of allergic disease) (Hill, 1994).

Eczema/dermatitis exhibits three distinct stages: acute, subacute, and chronic. All three stages may be

## COMPLICATIONS OF VIRAL INFECTIONS

**RUBELLA**
Arthritis/arthralgia
Thrombocytopenic purpura
Myocarditis/pericarditis (rare)
Congenital rubella syndrome (frequent)
Deafness
Growth retardation
Cataracts
Retinitis
Meningoencephalitis
Microcephaly
Mental retardation
Myocarditis
Structural defects of the heart
Death

**RUBEOLA**
Photophobia
Clear rhinorrhea
Pharyngitis
Gastrointestinal symptoms (diarrhea)

**WARTS**
Contagious

**HERPES SIMPLEX**
Nutritional problems (gingivostomatitis)
Contagious
Recurrent
Aseptic meningitis (seen in some primary infections of genital herpes)
Possibly fatal in immunocompromised patients

**VARICELLA**
Primary varicella pneumonia
Superimposed bacterial infection
Bacterial sepsis/focal abscesses (rare)
Reye's syndrome

**HERPES ZOSTER**
Scarring
Varicella pneumonitis
Postherpetic neuralgia
Motor weakness (with involvement of cranial nerves)
Bell's palsy
Conjunctivitis
Iritis
Corneal ulcers
Blindness

**ACQUIRED IMMUNODEFICIENCY SYNDROME**
Opportunistic infections
Neoplasia
Central nervous system disease

From Hill MJ: *Skin disorders: Mosby's clinical nursing series*, St Louis, 1994, Mosby.

present at any one time. Acute dermatitis (acute eczema) appears as extensive exudative erosions or as pruritic erythematous papules and vesicles. Subacute dermatitis (subacute eczema) appears as erythematous, excoriated (traumatized by scratching), or scaling papules or plaques (flat or raised patches). Chronic dermatitis (chronic eczema) is characterized by lichenified (thickened, bark-like) skin caused by continuous rubbing or scratching, excoriated papules, nodules, and postinflammatory hyperpigmentation and/or hypopigmentation.

## Atopic Dermatitis

*Atopic dermatitis* (also known as endogenous eczema) is a chronic eczema marked by remissions and exacerbations. **Atopic** refers to the group of allergic diseases involved with this form of eczema, such as asthma, allergic rhinitis (hay fever), and atopic dermatitis. The exact etiology of atopic dermatitis is unknown, although it is known that it occurs in individuals with a family history of allergic diseases (Hill, 1994). Atopic dermatitis represents a hyperreaction to any one of a number of common environmental factors. Variations of atopic eczema include adult dermatitis (a continuation of the childhood disease), pompholyx (occurrence of irritant vesicles on the hands and feet), and discoid or nummular eczema (characterized by papules and raised lesions on the limbs) (GlaxoWellcome, 1995).

Clinical manifestations of atopic dermatitis include dry, lackluster skin; excoriations; erythema; and lichenification. It may appear as early as 2 to 6 months of age and may continue into adulthood. In infants the rash characteristically appears on the face and scalp, and it may develop on the extensor surfaces of the extremities. In older children and adults the rash tends to have a predilection for the large folds of the extremities. Pruritus is the major symptom of the disease. In most cases the pruritus precedes the development of the rash, leading to the statement that atopic dermatitis is "an itch that rashes." Lichenification, excoriation, and secondary infections are the major complications associated with atopic dermatitis.

## Exfoliative Dermatitis

Another form of dermatitis is *exfoliative dermatitis (erythroderma)*. This form of dermatitis involves large areas of skin. It appears as generalized erythema, edema, and desquamation (sloughing of the stratum corneum). Severe exfoliative dermatitis may affect the mucous membranes of the upper respiratory tract and the conjunctivae. Hair loss is not uncommon during the disease process, but hair regrows after the condition is brought under control. Exfoliative dermatitis is seen only in association with other skin diseases such as severe psoriasis, with systemic disease such as malignancy, or as secondary to drug hypersensitivity. With severe erythroderma, the patient experiences fever, chills, malaise, fatigue, skin tightness, and severe pruritus. Because of the generalized vasodilation and shunting of blood to the skin surface, patients must be observed for high cardiac output failure. Water and protein losses caused by the desquamation will lead to dehydration and negative nitrogen balance (Hill, 1994). Exfoliating dermatitis is treated with topical corticosteroids, antihistamines, and bland emollients. Systemic steroids are indicated only in extremely severe cases.

## Contact Dermatitis

*Contact dermatitis* (also known as exogenous eczema) manifests as primary irritant dermatitis or allergic contact dermatitis. It is usually found on the face, neck, backs of the hands, forearms, male genitalia, and lower legs. The borders of the reaction are commonly well defined, which aids in determining the cause. The lesions may be red, oozing, or scaly. A careful history is essential in determining the cause of contact dermatitis. Removal and avoidance of the offending agent must precede or accompany treatment with antihistamines, bland emollients, cool compresses, and topical steroids. If cutaneous reaction is severe, systemic corticosteroids may be added to the treatment regimen.

## Dermatitis Venenata

*Dermatitis venenata (plant poisoning)* occurs as the result of contact with certain plants and is referred to as ivy poisoning, sumac poisoning, or poisoning by other specific types of plants. Individual susceptibility is an important factor in this type of dermatitis. Although many different plants and shrubs may cause the condition, some of the more common ones are poison ivy, poison sumac, poison oak, and poison elder. Symptoms vary from a mild redness to severe systemic reactions and gangrene. The primary lesions are found on the parts of the body contacted by the irritant, usually the hands, arms, face, and legs. The skin may become erythematous, which may be followed by formation of papules, vesicles, and pustules in a characteristic linear distribution. Facial edema can be seen in patients exposed to airborne allergens (e.g., when the plant is burned). The tissue may be edematous, and severe itching and burning may occur.

When the individual is aware of contact with a poisonous plant, the exposed parts of the body should be washed immediately with soap and water. However, soap and water should not be used once lesions are present. Cool, open wet dressings of 1:20 solution of aluminum acetate (Burrow's solution) or physiologic saline solution may be applied 3 times a day for 30 minutes to cool and relieve pruritus. Topical steroid creams and antihistamines may be needed. If lesions and edema are present on the face, systemic steroids may be necessary.

## Dermatitis Medicamentosa

*Dermatitis medicamentosa (drug dermatitis)* is the term applied to skin eruptions caused by drugs, regardless of the method of administration. Almost any drug may cause a reaction in certain individuals, and, with the development of many new drugs and their increased use, the incidence of such reactions can be expected to increase. Drug reactions range from mild erythema to severe, life-threatening conditions. Every type of skin lesion reviewed in this chapter may be seen in various reactions to drugs. Therefore any rash must have drugs considered as a possible cause. A thorough history that includes questions regarding prescribed and over-the-counter drugs must be obtained by any patient showing a rash. The nurse must educate the patient and family about the possible side effects of any drugs that have been prescribed and the importance of reporting any reactions immediately. Dermatitis caused by drugs will usually subside after withdrawal of the medication, but resolution may take up to 2 weeks. Treatment is directed at relief of symptoms.

## Psoriasis

*Psoriasis* is a chronic, genetically determined disease of epidermal proliferation. The disease usually begins between the ages of 10 and 35 but may be seen at any age. The exact cause is unknown, but the disease is not contagious. There is no cure, and patients with this disease have episodes of remission and exacerbation. Psoriasis tends to improve during the summer months when the lesions are exposed to ultraviolet rays of the sun. Emotional stress, systemic infections, obesity, excessive alcohol ingestion, injury to the skin, and pregnancy exacerbate the disorder.

### Assessment

Clinically, psoriasis is most commonly seen as well-demarcated erythematous patches or plaques with silver scale, but it may exhibit generalized erythroderma (exfoliative dermatitis) or generalized pustules (Figure 40-11). Removal of scale may result in pinpoint bleeding known as Auspitz sign. Pruritus, if present, is generally severe. There are four basic types of psoriasis: plaque, guttate (drop-like lesions), psoriatic erythroderma, and pustular. Plaque type is the most commonly seen. Guttate psoriasis often occurs after an infection, usually streptococcal, and is commonly seen in school-aged children, so it is often initially misdiagnosed as one of the childhood diseases. Psoriatic erythroderma and pustular psoriasis are the most severe presentations of the disease and may involve the entire body surface. These forms of psoriasis are often resistant to treatment and may last for long periods. Lesions appear symmetrically on the body. Elbows, knees, scalp, genitalia, and the gluteal cleft are the areas most often affected. Lesions may be initiated in areas that have undergone trauma, which is called Koebner's phenomenon. Common complications of psoriasis include psoriatic arthritis and nail dystrophy.

## Intervention

Psoriasis can be treated topically with steroids, tar preparations, anthralin, salicylic acid preparations, ultraviolet light, bland emollients, and oral cipotriene (synthetic vitamin D). It is not uncommon for a combination of topical therapies to be used. The use of ultraviolet light B (UVB) and tar in combination is known as Goeckerman treatment. Psoralen and ultraviolet light A (PUVA) are also used. Psoralen is a photosensitizing agent that makes the patient sensitive to the ultraviolet-A spectrum of light. Psoralen is given 2 hours before the patient is exposed to UVA. Nausea, sunburn, headache, and photosensitivity may be side effects of the treatment. Patients must be instructed to wear sunglasses that shield against UVA, to wear sunscreens, and, ideally, to avoid sun exposure on the days of treatment.

In severe cases systemic medications may be used: antimetabolites such as methotrexate or hydroxyurea, retinoids (vitamin A derivatives) such as etretinate or Accutane, and in some cases antibiotics for secondary infection. Because of the liver toxicity seen when antimetabolites are given, patients receiving drugs in this category must have a pretherapy liver biopsy and must be monitored during therapy for liver and renal function, white blood cell count, hemoglobin, and hematocrit. Etretinate (synthetic vitamin A or aromatic retinoid) is indicated only for adults and is used with extreme caution in women of childbearing age. Retinoids and vitamin A are not the same compounds, and people should be cautioned not to take large doses of vitamin A in the hope of duplicating the effects of these synthetic drugs.

Systemic steroids are contraindicated as treatment for psoriasis because they produce a "rebound effect," which is a worsening of the psoriasis after withdrawal of the steroids.

Most patients with diseases of epidermal origin may be treated as outpatients, but occasionally the severity or extent of involvement warrants confinement for supervised care (Box 40-13). Most often the patients requiring hospitalization are those with erythroderma or pustular psoriasis. The most important part of therapy is the education of the patient regarding the disease process, its symptoms and appearance, and the fact

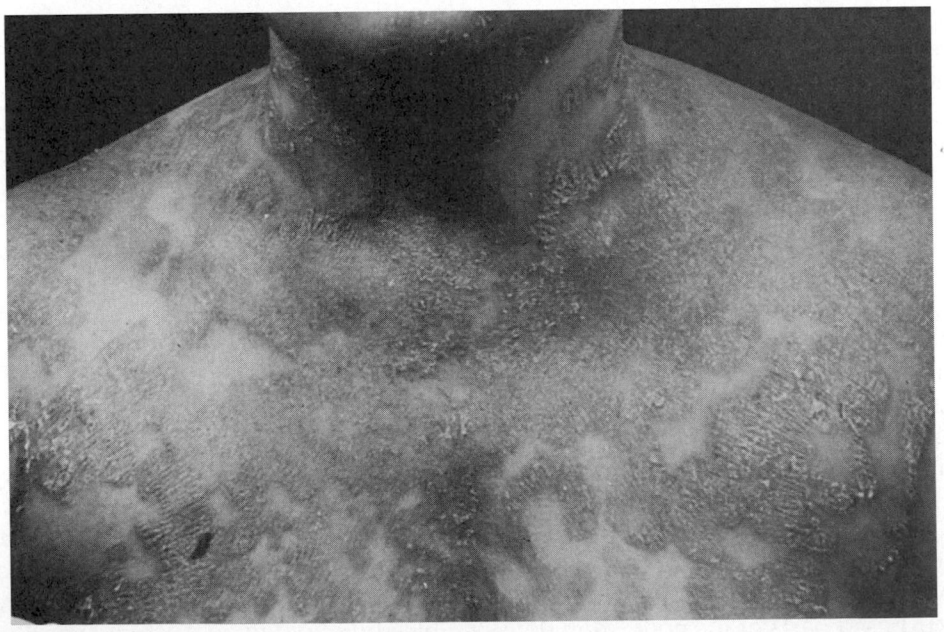

**Figure 40-11** Generalized psoriasis. (From Rosai J: *Ackerman's surgical pathology*, ed 8, St Louis, 1996, Mosby.)

that it is chronic. Patients must feel accepted by the caregiver, and treatment must be individualized.

General management of diseases of epidermal origin include the application of bland emollients to soothe and relieve skin irritability and to provide a temporary barrier, as well as wet wraps or occlusion to help hydrate the skin and to increase absorption of topical medications. In diseases where an allergen or irritant is the cause or suspected cause, the offending agent should be removed or avoided (Box 40-14).

## Acne

Acne is an inflammatory disorder of the pilosebaceous unit of the skin. It appears as eruptions of papules or pustules and is caused when oil delivered to the skin's surface meets with resistance (Hill, 1994). It mainly affects the face, chest, back, and shoulders. Adolescents are most widely affected by the disease, and severe cases may require medical intervention. The disease usually declines in the early twenties, but it can continue into the forties and fifties. It is not uncommon for the first case of acne to occur in the patient's forties, fifties, or even sixties (Laudano, Leach, Armstrong, 1990). Both men and women may be affected, with the higher incidence occurring in males.

### Assessment

The acne begins with the appearance of **comedones** (blackheads) that plug the ducts of the sebaceous glands and are the result of increased secretion of sebum from the glands. The inflammatory process within the duct soon leads to the formation of papules and pustules on the skin.

The papules, pustules, and comedones that characterize acne are found on the face and back. In addition to assessing the location and severity of the lesions, the nurse must assess the patient's reaction to the disorder and understanding of the causes. The psychologic effects are often more serious than the disease. Acne vulgaris occurs at a time when adolescents are concerned with personal appearance, and the unsightly skin condition may seriously interfere with personality development. It is also important to evaluate the patient's understanding of the treatment prescribed.

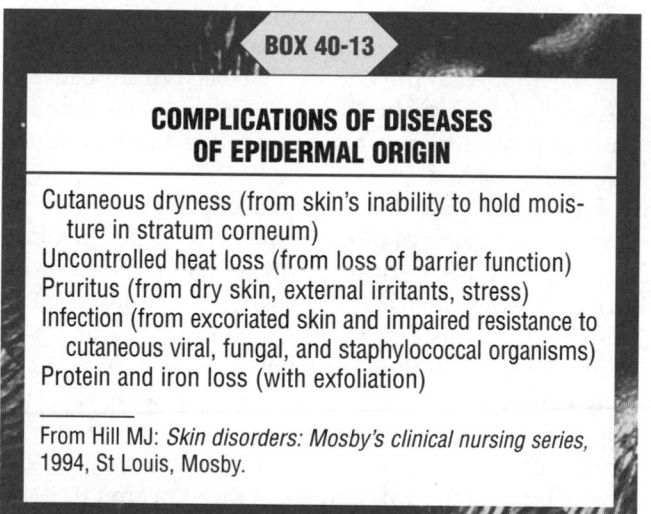

**BOX 40-13**

### COMPLICATIONS OF DISEASES OF EPIDERMAL ORIGIN

Cutaneous dryness (from skin's inability to hold moisture in stratum corneum)
Uncontrolled heat loss (from loss of barrier function)
Pruritus (from dry skin, external irritants, stress)
Infection (from excoriated skin and impaired resistance to cutaneous viral, fungal, and staphylococcal organisms)
Protein and iron loss (with exfoliation)

From Hill MJ: *Skin disorders: Mosby's clinical nursing series*, 1994, St Louis, Mosby.

---

**BOX 40-14** | **NURSING PROCESS**

## DISEASE OF EPIDERMAL ORIGIN

**ASSESSMENT**

- Lesions for characteristics, distribution, and severity
- Signs of secondary infection
- Temperature

**NURSING DIAGNOSES**

- Impaired skin integrity related to pathologic process and mechanical factors
- Risk for impaired skin integrity related to pruritus
- Risk for infection related to skin excoriation and impaired barrier function

**NURSING INTERVENTIONS**

- Apply cool compresses for wet skin or emollients for dry skin.
- Apply topical medications as ordered.
- Keep room at comfortable temperature to address poor tolerance to temperature changes.
- Administer antihistamines as ordered.

**EVALUATION OF EXPECTED OUTCOMES**

- Skin is well hydrated, and inflammation has been reduced
- Pruritus has been alleviated
- Ability to regulate temperature is restored
- No evidence of infection

## Intervention

Treatment for acne is nonspecific and is directed toward reducing inflammation and infection, reducing blackhead formation, and developing a program of good personal hygiene. The skin should be kept scrupulously clean by washing with soap and water several times a day. A preparation containing hexachlorophene will help to reduce the staphylococcus population on the skin. Keratinous agents that cause drying, such as salicylic acid and resorcinol, may be used to produce a peeling of the skin and the removal of keratinous plugs to prevent the development of comedones and cysts. Cleansing agents are used to remove excess sebum from the skin and thus prevent the development of comedones. Tetracycline, minocycline, or erythromycin may be prescribed by the physician to prevent infection and thus reduce the probability of scarring. Existing comedones can be removed with an extractor by the physician, and pustules can be opened with a blade every week or two. Small doses of estrogens administered to girls just before the menstrual period help relieve the oily condition of the skin and retard the formation of sebum. The patient should be advised against squeezing the lesions, which may worsen the condition and lead to scarring. Emphasis should be placed on developing a program of adequate diet, sleep, and wholesome physical activity. The restriction of certain foods in the diet, such as chocolate or fried foods, does not seem to have any effect on the prevention or treatment of acne. Iodized salt will make acne worse in sensitive people.

The most severe cases of acne, cystic acne, can be treated with isotretinoin (Accutane), a vitamin A derivative called a *retinoid*. This oral medication has potentially serious side effects and must be used with caution. A female who becomes pregnant while taking the drug is at high risk for having an infant with birth defects. Other possible side effects include dry skin, hair loss, eye irritation, nosebleeds, and muscle and joint pain. Increased blood levels of cholesterol and triglycerides occur in 25% of patients and increase the risk of heart disease. The cost is approximately $150 per month for the medication alone. After a few months of treatment the condition can be cured.

## Treatment of Scarring

When scarring is severe, the physician may recommend removal of the scars by chemical face peeling or dermabrasion. Chemical face peeling is also performed in the treatment of fine wrinkles, and both procedures are used to remove abnormal pigmentation, freckles, or scars caused by trauma or other skin diseases as well as by acne. Chemical face peeling involves the application of a phenol-base chemical to the entire face, followed by a mask of waterproof adhesive. The medication causes a burning sensation, and the patient will require medication to control apprehension and relieve pain. After 6 or 8 hours the face becomes edematous. The patient is not allowed to move about for 48 hours, except to go to the bathroom. The dressings are removed after 48 hours, and the appearance of the skin will be similar to that of a second-degree burn. During the next 24 hours a bacteriostatic medication, thymol iodide powder, is applied with a cotton applicator to the entire surface three or four times. After this series of treatments, a lubricating ointment such as A and D ointment is applied to facilitate the separation of the crust that forms on the skin. After an additional 24 hours the face may be washed with plain water. Facial redness will persist for several weeks, and the patient will not feel comfortable being seen by others for as long as 3 or 4 weeks. Cosmetics may be applied at the end of 3 weeks, but exposure to the sun is not permitted for 3 to 6 months because the natural protective mechanism against the sun, melanin, is diminished.

An alternative to chemical face peeling is dermabrasion, or surgical planing. This procedure involves scraping, sand papering, and brushing the skin to remove the epidermis and some superficial dermis. The remaining dermis produces new cells and forms a new epithelial layer in the dermabraded areas. The procedure can be performed by hand with coarse, abrasive paper or mechanically by using a rapidly rotating wire brush. The patient must be fully informed about the procedure and the appearance of the skin after its completion. After the procedure, pressure dressings may or may not be used, depending on the physician's preference. If dressings are used, they are removed after 48 hours, and the skin has the appearance of a recent sunburn. A crust begins to form, and petroleum jelly or cocoa butter may be used to relieve tightness. The crust separates in about 14 days, and the skin appears red. The patient must avoid direct sunlight for 3 to 4 months and use a sunscreen to protect the skin from exposure to the sun. It should be emphasized to the patient that even with repeat treatment deep scarring may not be completely eliminated, only improved. All patients who are candidates for dermabrasion should be questioned as to their expectations of the outcome of treatment. Some patients set their expectations too high, and these expectations need to be addressed before the procedure is undertaken.

## Rosacea

Rosacea (acne rosacea, or adult acne) is a fairly common inflammatory condition that affects the blood vessels in the central part of the face. It may resemble and be associated with acne, appearing as a rosy red pustular eruption without comedones (Hill, 1994). Rosacea primarily affects women over 30 years of age. When it is seen in men, it is more severe. Clinically it appears as erythema and dilated vessels (telangiectasia) with a predilection for the center of the face. Patients have a pronounced tendency to flushing or blushing that is generally pronounced with the intake of alcohol, hot drinks, or spicy food, as well as with exposure to external irritants and extremes of hot or cold. Rhinophyma (pronounced enlargement of the nose) may be seen in men in the later stages of rosacea. Rhinophyma is an overgrowth of sebaceous tissue and can be surgically corrected. Other complications that accompany rosacea include ocular disorders, including blepharitis, conjunctivitis, keratitis, and iritis.

Rosacea may be treated with topical acne medications and systemic antibiotics. A primary component of treatment is the avoidance of aggravating factors.

# CUTANEOUS DISORDERS

## Lupus Erythematosus

Lupus erythematosus is not strictly a disease of the skin and could be appropriately placed in a number of chapters in this text. It is a chronic inflammatory disease involving the connective tissues of the body. Because these tissues are found in almost all regions and areas of the body, almost any part or organ may be affected. The disease may be confined to the skin, as in discoid lupus erythematosus (DLE), or may become generalized, as seen in systemic lupus erythematosus (SLE).

**Discoid lupus erythematosus.** Discoid lupus erythematosus (DLE) is a skin ailment characterized by disklike lesions with raised, reddish edges and sunken centers. They are most likely to appear on the arm, neck, face, and scalp and may leave scars when they subside. DLE is rarely fatal, but it is irritating and painful. Few patients with the discoid form go on to develop the systemic form.

**Systemic lupus erythematosus.** The cause of systemic lupus erythematosus (SLE) is unknown, but theories include autoimmunity, predisposition, and drugs. The autoimmune theory proposes that SLE is an abnormal reaction of the body against its own tissues. The predisposition theory identifies such factors as physical or mental stress, streptococcal or viral infection, exposure to sunlight or ultraviolet light, vaccines, and x-ray treatments as predisposing certain persons to this disease. Because it has been observed in successive generations of some families, genetics may also be a predisposing factor. The drugs suspected of triggering

SLE include sulfa forms, penicillin and other antibiotics, certain birth control pills, and individual drugs such as hydralazine and procainamide. Women are 10 times as likely to have SLE as men, and most of these women are of childbearing age. These patients are more susceptible to having miscarriages, premature births, and stillbirths. The fetus who reaches full term is not usually affected by the mother's disease. The disease is also more common in blacks than whites, and it is rare in Asia. The incidence has been estimated at somewhere between two and five people per 100,000 persons.

SLE can affect the skin, kidneys, central nervous system, heart, lungs, blood vessels, serous membranes, joints, and muscles, either singly or in combination. The inflammation occurs in connective tissue common to all organs, so involvement usually becomes more widespread with time. Because it can affect so many organs, it is difficult to describe a classic group of symptoms and to distinguish it from other diseases. The Diagnostic and Therapeutic Criteria Committee of the American Rheumatism Association has issued a list of 14 preliminary criteria. The presence of four or more of the 14 criteria either serially or simultaneously during any interval of observation constitutes a diagnosis of SLE (Box 40-15).

Pregnant women who demonstrate signs of preeclampsia should be tested for SLE because this may be one of the early signs of the disease. Approximately 75% of all patients with SLE live 5 years or longer after diagnosis, and this disease is most likely to prove fatal in the patient with kidney or neurologic involvement. Early diagnosis and treatment improve the prognosis, and developments in hemodialysis and renal transplant techniques are improving the outcome for those who experience renal failure. The life expectancy following diagnosis has almost doubled in the last 15 years.

**Assessment.** Symptoms vary from patient to patient because the same organs may not be involved. The patient who has not been instructed well enough to understand this may become confused and lose confidence in the physician when discussing treatment with other SLE patients. The earliest symptoms often include fatigue, chills, occasional fever, and stiff aching joints on arising, usually followed several months later by a rash on the face and scalp and loss of hair in patches (alopecia). Approximately 70% of patients develop skin eruptions, and approximately 40% develop a characteristic butterfly rash over the bridge of the nose and the cheek. The rash and hair loss become worse on exposure to the sun. The rash sometimes spreads to the arms, trunk, or legs, causing a flushed, sunburned look or a scarred, patchy, coinlike look. Chest, stomach, and muscle pain may occur, or fluid may accumulate in the feet, ankles, or chest.

## SYSTEMIC LUPUS ERYTHEMATOSUS

Systemic lupus erythematosus (LE) is indicated by the presence of four or more of the following symptoms:

1 Facial erythema (butterfly rash)—diffuse flat or raised rash over the bridge of the nose; may be present on only one side of the face

2 Discoid LE—patches of redness or thickened red, raised, coin-shaped patches covered with scales and involving plugged follicles; may be present anywhere on the body, including the face

3 Raynaud's phenomenon—intermittent attacks in which the hands or some of the fingers of each hand become cold, pale, painful, and then deeply cyanotic; symptoms are relieved by warming the hands

4 Alopecia—rapid loss of large amounts of scalp hair

5 Photosensitivity—an unusual skin reaction from exposure to sunlight

6 Ulcers in the mouth or nose

7 Arthritis without deformity but involving pain on motion, tenderness, swelling in the joints of the feet, ankles, knees, hips, shoulders, elbows, wrists, hands

8 LE cells—an unusual cell can be identified in the blood of patients with systemic LE; if one of these cells is seen in two or more specimens, or two in one specimen, the test is considered positive

9 Chronic false-positive serologic test for syphilis

10 Profuse proteinuria—over 3.5 g of protein excreted in the urine per day

11 Cellular casts—examination of the urine reveals casts that may be red blood cells, hemoglobin, granular, tubular, or mixed in type. When casts are found in the urine, they indicate a pathologic condition in the kidney. They are named to reflect their composition and shape; for example, red blood cell casts are composed of red blood cells, indicating a leakage of red blood cells into the urine. Many contain albumin because albumin often pours out into the urine in diseases involving the kidney. Because systemic LE sometimes causes a type of glomerulonephritis, the presence of casts in the urine can be considered one of the criteria for diagnosis

12 Pleuritis or pericarditis or both—patient experiences pleuritic pain, a pleural rub is heard by the physician, or x-ray examination reveals thickening and fluid in the lungs; pericarditis is detected by electrocardiogram or can be heard by the physician as a rub

13 Psychosis or convulsions or both—uremia and drugs must be ruled out as a cause

14 One or more of the following—hemolytic anemia, leukopenia (white blood count less than 4000/mm³ on two or more occasions), thrombocytopenia (platelet count less than 100,000/mm³)

Pericarditis is the most frequent cardiac involvement. Women may experience irregular menstrual periods and may have difficulty in conceiving a child during an exacerbation of the disease. Pregnancy is less safe when there are kidney or neurologic abnormalities, so the pregnant patient with SLE must be watched closely. The blood pressure may become highly elevated. Protein, casts, and red blood cells in the urine indicate renal involvement. The site of the renal involvement usually is the glomeruli, which become inflamed as a result of the deposit of immune complexes in the glomerular basement membrane. Convulsions, cranial nerve involvement, and psychoses may occur with central nervous system involvement. Symptoms tend to come and go, and most can be relieved and even reversed with proper treatment.

Because of the widespread effect of the disease, a number of laboratory tests are performed to aid in diagnosis. In addition to routine blood work, chest x-ray examinations, electrocardiograms, and urinalysis, the urine is examined for creatinine clearance to evaluate kidney function. More specific tests include blood tests for the LE cells, as well as the ANA (antinuclear antibody) and the anti-DNA test, which are positive.

**Intervention.** Treatment is aimed at reducing the inflammatory process. High doses of aspirin are prescribed, often in combination with magnesium-aluminum hydroxide (Ascriptin) to reduce stomach distress. Indomethacin (Indocin) is also an antiinflammatory and should be taken at bedtime with a snack to prevent stomach distress and provide maximum relief from early morning joint stiffness and pain. Corticosteroids such as prednisone are used for more severe symptoms. The topical steroid flurandrenolide 0.05% is prescribed in ointment form (Cordran ointment) for the facial lesions and as a lotion (Cordran lotion) for the scalp. The patient must use a sunscreen when outdoors. Hydroxychloroquine (Plaquenil), an antimalarial drug whose action in the treatment of SLE is unknown, is prescribed only for severe skin lesions and may cause macular degeneration, which results in permanent blindness. Frequent eye examinations must be made to detect the early signs of this side effect. Immunosuppressive therapy is being used experimentally with patients who do not respond to conservative treatment. Patients must consult their physicians before receiving any immunizations or before taking birth control pills and over-the-counter drugs such as vitamins. The patient who is receiving steroids should be instructed to wear a Medic Alert bracelet. Hot baths or showers are used to relieve joint pain and stiffness, and an exercise program is prescribed to maintain mobility, strength, and endurance.

In addition to providing measures to relieve pain and supervising prescribed exercises, nursing care is concerned with patient education. The patient must understand the disease, its symptoms, and the treatment prescribed in order to control the disease. Return of symptoms or the onset of new symptoms must be reported immediately. The response to drug therapy must be carefully observed and reported to the physician. The patient must make alterations in life-style to obtain more rest and avoid exposure to the sun. It may be necessary for the patient to wear clothing that completely covers the body and head, to use a sunscreen on those small areas of exposed skin, and to avoid the sun at midday, when it is strongest. Fluorescent lighting is another source of ultraviolet light that may need to be avoided. The patient's self-concept may be affected by the disease as well as by the restrictions imposed with treatment. It is important to make the patient feel comfortable and free to express concerns and ask questions. The patient's family must also understand the disease and its treatment to be able to provide the support necessary for the patient to live with the disease. It is important to inform the patient of community groups available for supplying information and support. The Lupus Foundation of America and the Arthritis Foundation are two national sources. There may be a local "lupus club," and, if so, the patient should be advised of its availability but not pressured to join. With early diagnosis and control of the disease, aided by discoveries resulting from research into its causes and treatment, the patient will be able to make the most of the years ahead.

## Erythema Intertrigo (Chafing)

Chafing occurs when two skin surfaces rub together. It results in redness and may cause maceration of the skin. Common sites are the areas between the thighs, in the axillae, and under the breasts. In infants, chafing may occur in the folds of the skin, particularly around the neck. Obese persons are more likely to be affected. Treatment includes cleansing with mild soap and water, patting the area dry, and powdering with cornstarch. Good personal hygiene and avoidance of strong or irritating soaps are important practices. In extreme cases the application of hydrocortisone cream (Hytone) may be required. Before applying a hydrocortisone cream, the area should have a KOH prep done to rule out fungal infection.

## Miliaria (Prickly Heat)

Miliaria is a condition in which the flow of sweat from the eccrine sweat glands, which are found on all skin surfaces, is hindered. The cause of miliaria includes both environmental and physiologic factors. Persons exposed to extremes of temperature and humidity for long periods, those overprotected by clothing, those with high body temperature, and obese persons are most likely to suffer from attacks of prickly heat. Infants swathed in excessive clothing and blankets are especially susceptible. The condition occurs more commonly during hot weather.

**Assessment.** Tiny red papules appear on the skin, usually on the trunk but sometimes covering the entire body. The lesions are accompanied by burning, prickling, and itching. An infant with prickly heat will be restless and fretful.

**Intervention.** Treatment consists of cooling or soothing baths and thorough drying by patting. Emollient baths such as the starch bath may provide relief for persons with severe cases. The application of calamine lotion is generally effective, and cornstarch or other nonirritating powders may be used. The condition is usually of short duration and can be prevented by avoiding extremes of heat and humidity and by wearing absorbent and porous clothing.

# HYPERSENSITIVITY REACTIONS

## Urticaria

**Urticaria** is the presence of hives or wheals (Figure 40-12). The condition may be associated with a number of systemic diseases, such as hepatitis, Hodgkin's disease, lupus erythematosus, leukemia, rheumatic fever, dental and sinus infections, and infestations. It may be seen as a cholinergic response to heat, cold, or ultraviolet light, or as a reaction to certain foods. Genetic predisposition and psychogenic factors have also been seen as causative agents. Often the cause is not readily apparent, which is disturbing to patient and health care workers alike. Urticaria may be acute, lasting less than 12 hours, or chronic, lasting

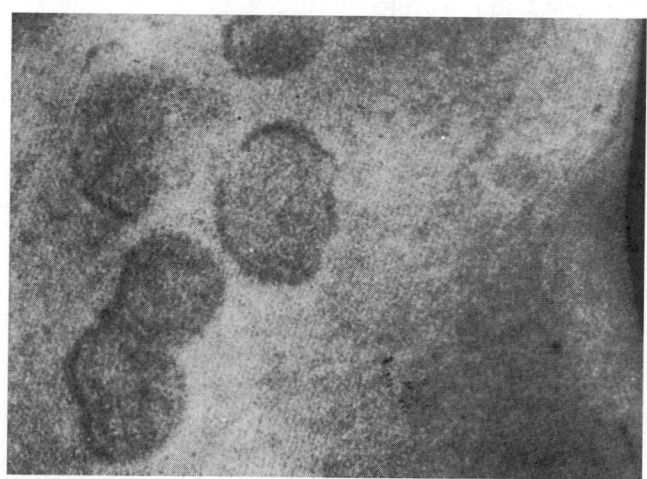

**Figure 40-12**    Urticaria. (From Stewart WD et al: *Dermatology: diagnosis and treatment of cutaneous disorders,* ed 4, St Louis, 1978, Mosby.)

more than 6 weeks. Select cases of urticaria may be accompanied by respiratory distress, hoarseness, abdominal pain, vomiting, diarrhea, arthralgia, headaches, or central nervous system dysfunction. Angioedema (swelling of the face) is the most severe complication seen with urticaria. This is a medical emergency, and the patient should seek treatment immediately. When urticaria appears suddenly, it should be determined whether the patient is taking any new drugs. If so, they should be stopped immediately and the physician notified.

## Erythema Multiforme

Erythema multiforme is a reactive skin disorder in which the individual lesions have a characteristic target (iris or bullseye) configuration (Figure 40-13). The lesions can be caused by drugs or by viruses such as herpes simplex and vaccinia. They also can be caused by systemic infections such as pneumonia, meningitis, or measles, and in some cases the cause cannot be identified. The lesions may last long enough to cause erosion of the lips, eyelids, and genitalia. Large areas of skin may eventually slough, and the disease can be fatal. Stevens-Johnson syndrome, the most serious form of erythema multiforme, has a mortality rate of 15% to 20%.

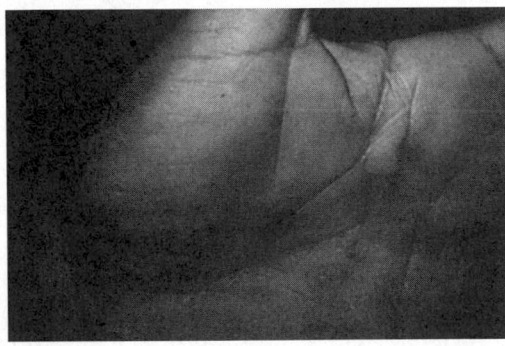

**Figure 40-13**   Erythema multiforme. (Courtesy Stephen B Tucker, MD, Department of Dermatology, University of Texas Health Science Center at Houston.)

### Assessment

The lesions are called iris or bullseye lesions because they are depressed in the center and have a raised, reddened border. They are found on the skin and the mucous membranes. Fever, chest pain, and joint pain may precede the eruption.

### Intervention

The underlying cause must be discovered and eliminated, if possible. If the patient is taking any drugs, all except those essential to life should be discontinued. Large doses of steroids are given, and the lesions will disappear within 2 weeks if a drug is responsible. Baths, soaks, and dressings are used to reduce the discomfort of the lesions. Adequate fluids and nutrition promote healing. Special mouth care is needed if lesions appear there.

# KEY CONCEPTS

➤ The skin is a protective organ consisting of the epidermis, dermis, and subcutaneous tissue layers.

➤ The unbroken skin is the first line of defense against pathogenic organisms. It protects deeper tissue from injury and loss of body fluids and regulates body temperature.

➤ Skin lesions must be assessed by size, shape, color, distribution, and sequence or arrangement.

➤ Diagnosis of skin disorders requires a careful history that should include allergies, sleep habits, occupation, medications, recent travel or contact with others, level of anxiety, time or appearance of lesions, and direction of their spread.

➤ A therapeutic oatmeal bath can be prepared by placing 2 cups of oatmeal and 1 quart of boiling water in a double boiler to cook for 45 minutes, then placing the mixture in a gauze bag and swishing it in a tub of water at 100° F.

➤ Open wet dressings initiate vasoconstriction to cool the skin and relieve pruritus (itching).

➤ Closed wet dressings hydrate the epidermis and increase absorption of topical medications.

➤ Warm moist dressings can be wrapped in plastic to stay warm, but plastic should not be used if a heating pad is applied to keep temperature constant.

➤ Individuals with skin disorders may experience real or imagined feelings of being shunned, which may prompt withdrawal and lead to isolation.

➤ Sustained pressure over bony prominences cuts off blood supply to the tissue, which causes local areas of necrosis called pressure ulcers.

➤ Moisture, friction, and shear contribute to pressure ulcers and can be prevented.

➤ Specialty beds can be used to prevent and reduce pressure and should be selected with specific patient needs in mind.

## KEY CONCEPTS—cont'd

➤ Wounds of pressure ulcers are treated by cleansing, debridement, and use of topical medications, exudate absorbers, and dressings. Patients who are at risk for formation of pressure ulcers can be identified by use of one of the three risk-assessment scales: Norton, Gosnell, or Braden. Specific measures can be instituted to reduce the risk of pressure ulcer formation.

➤ Decisions for wound care can also be made after classifying the wound as red, yellow, or black.

➤ Disorders of pigmentation include lentigo (freckles) and chloasma (patches of pigmentation).

➤ Disorders of the glands include seborrhea (oily skin), sebaceous cyst (wen), hyperhidrosis (excessive sweating), and anhidrosis (absence of sweating).

➤ Pruritus (itching) accompanies many skin disorders. Treatment involves removing the cause and reducing irritating factors.

➤ Skin tumors include keloids (overgrowth of fibrous tissue at scar sites), nevi (moles), and angiomas (benign tumors of dilated blood vessels). Keratoses are precancerous lesions.

➤ Basal cell carcinoma is seen most often in fair-skinned people who have had overexposure to the sun.

➤ Squamous cell carcinoma usually develops on areas exposed to radiation.

➤ Malignant melanoma is recognized by the ABCDs of melanoma: **A**symmetry, **B**order irregularity, **C**olor, **D**iameter greater than 6 mm.

➤ Pediculi (lice) are found on the head, on the body, and in the pubic area. Treatment is Nix, RID, or lindane lotion/shampoo.

➤ Scabies is an infectious skin disease caused by the itch mite, a parasite that burrows under the skin. It is recognized by intense itching and multiform lesions, papules, and vesicles, and a characteristic S-shaped burrow is sometimes present. Location of the lesion varies with age. It is treated with Elimite, Eurax, or 1% lindane.

➤ Skin infections require topical or systemic antibiotics, and the patient must receive instruction on use and side effects. Universal precautions should be employed when dealing with skin infections.

➤ Tinea capitis (ringworm of the scalp), tinea corporis (ringworm on the body, face, neck, and extremities), tinea barbae (barber's itch), tinea cruris (jock itch), and tinea pedis (athlete's foot) are caused by fungi.

➤ Viral infections can be confined to the skin, or they may be systemic and produce skin lesions, as in rubella and rubeola. The human papillomavirus causes warts. Those found in the genital area are transmitted through sexual contact.

➤ Herpes simplex 1 causes cold sores, and herpes simplex 2 causes genital herpes.

➤ Herpes zoster and varicella (chickenpox) are caused by the herpes virus varicella. The characteristic lesion is described as a "dew drop on a rose petal" because it is a single vesicle on an erythematous base.

➤ The lesions of herpes zoster (shingles) are located in one or more of the spinal ganglia, and the skin area supplied by the affected nerve fibers becomes involved. Herpes zoster can occur when a dormant virus becomes activated or when there is contact with lesions of persons with herpes zoster. The lesions follow the dermatomes (nerve pathways).

➤ Dermatitis is an inflammatory condition of the skin; eczema is a reactive process. The terms are often used interchangeably. Psoriasis is a chronic, genetically determined disease of epidermal proliferation. It improves with exposure to ultraviolet rays of the sun and is exacerbated by emotional stress, infection, and alcohol. It appears as well-demarcated erythematous patches or plaques with silver scale, generalized exfoliative dermatitis, or pustules.

➤ Acne is an inflammatory disorder of the pilosebaceous unit of the skin. It appears as eruptions of papules or pustules that are formed when oil delivered to the skin's surface meets with resistance. The nurse must assess the patient's reaction to the disorder and his or her understanding of the treatment prescribed. Severe cases are treated with a retinoid of vitamin A.

➤ Rosacea affects the blood vessels in the central part of the face. Rhinophyma (pronounced enlargement of the nose) may be seen in men in later stages of rosacea.

➤ Lupus erythematosus is a chronic inflammatory disease involving the connective tissues of the body. Discoid lupus erythematosus (DLE) is confined to the skin. Systemic lupus erythematosus (SLE) is generalized and affects many organs.

➤ Hypersensitivity reactions appear as urticaria identified by hives or wheals, or as erythema multiforme, characterized by iris or bull's-eye lesions. The underlying cause must be eliminated.

# CRITICAL THINKING EXERCISES

1. Explain the fact that patients with skin disorders are more likely to experience emotional problems than those with other types of disorders.
2. Develop a list of instructions to give a patient with pigmented moles.
3. Develop a list of instructions for the patient with impetigo. Include methods of treatment and methods of preventing spread of the disease to others.

## REFERENCES AND ADDITIONAL READINGS

Agency for Health Care Policy and Research: *Urinary incontinence in adults,* Rockville, Md, March 1992, Public Health Service, Pub No 92-0038, US Department of Health and Human Services.

Agency for Health Care Policy and Research: *Pressure ulcers in adults: prediction and prevention,* Rockville, Md, May 1992, Public Health Service, Pub No 92-0047, US Department of Health and Human Services.

Beare PG, Myers JL: *Adult health nursing,* ed 3, St Louis, 1998, Mosby.

Bryant RA: *Acute and chronic wounds: nursing management,* St Louis, 1992, Mosby.

Carroll P: Bed selection: help patients rest easy, *RN* 58(5):44-51, 1995.

Cuzzell J: Wound care forum: the new RYB color code, *Am J Nurs* 88(10):1342-1346, 1988.

Eaglstein WH et al: *New directions in wound healing,* Princeton, 1990, ER Squibb and Sons.

Erwin-Toth P, Hocevar BJ: Wound care: selecting the right dressing, *Am J Nurs* 95(2):46-51, 1995.

Hill MJ: The skin: anatomy and physiology, *Dermatol Nurs* 2(1):13-17, 1990.

Hill MJ: *Skin disorders: Mosby's clinical nursing series,* St Louis, 1994, Mosby.

Krasner D, editor: *Chronic wound care: a clinical source book for healthcare professionals,* King of Prussia, Pa, 1990, Health Management Publications.

Krasner D: Wound care: how to use the red-yellow-black system, *Am J Nurs* 95(5):44-47, 1995.

Krasner D: Managing pain from pressure ulcers, *Am J Nurs* 95(6):22-24, 1995.

Laudano JB, Leach EE, Armstrong RB: Acne: therapeutic perspectives with an emphasis on the role of isotretinon, *Dermatol Nurs* 2(6):328-336, 1990.

Makelbust J, Siegreen M: *Pressure ulcers: guidelines for prevention and nursing management,* Springhouse, Penn, 1996, Springhouse.

O'Hanlon-Nichols T: Commonly asked questions about wound healing, a quick review of the physiology of healing and the essentials of good wound care, *Am J Nurs* 95(4):22-24, 1995.

Phipps WJ et al: *Medical-surgical nursing: concepts and clinical practice,* ed 5, St Louis, 1995, Mosby.

University of California at Berkeley: *Wellness Letter* 11(8):6, 1995.

Whittington K: Debunking wound care myths, *RN* 58(8):32-33, 1995.

Willey T: High-tech beds and mattress overlays: a decision guide, *Am J Nurs* 89(9):1105-1252, 1989.

Yotter M: Contact dermatitis: nursing intervention, *Dermatol Nurs* 2(5):267-269, 1990.

# CHAPTER 41

# Burns

## CHAPTER OBJECTIVES

1 Identify the causes of the various types of burn injuries.
2 Discuss the historical aspects of the creation of burn units in the United States.
3 Describe the burn classification system.
4 Evaluate the location, size, depth, and severity of the burn wound.
5 Describe the prevention of airway obstruction and the treatment of burn shock.
6 Describe the three phases of burn care: emergent, acute, and rehabilitative.
7 Describe the following methods of treatment for burns: open (exposure), closed (occlusive) dressings, and antimicrobial topical agents.
8 Describe the role of the nurse in caring for a patient with skin or artificial grafts.
9 Identify the information to be included in discharge teaching for the burn patient and family.

## KEY TERMS

| | |
|---|---|
| autograft | escharotomy |
| carbonaceous sputum | fluid resuscitation |
| circumferential | full-thickness skin graft |
| closed method | heterograft |
| contracture | homograft |
| debridement | hydrotherapy |
| dermis | inhalation injuries |
| emergent | split-thickness skin graft |
| epidermis | total body surface area |
| eschar | (TBSA) |

Burns are the result of tissue injury to the skin resulting from excessive exposure to thermal, chemical, electrical, or radioactive agents. Eighty-five percent 85% of all burns occur in the home—in the kitchen, bathroom, and bedroom. Burns are the third leading cause of accidental death in the United States, especially for individuals between the ages of 15 and 45. There are approximately 2 million burn cases each year in the United States, and approximately 7% to 8% of these patients require hospitalization. Approximately one fourth of those hospitalized have major burns or significant associated injuries that require treatment in a specialized burn unit or burn center.

## HISTORY OF BURN CENTERS

The knowledge that has been gained about the treatment of burn wounds was acquired after World War II and the dropping of the atomic bomb. The U.S. Army Medical Division was sent to Japan to care for the victims after this disastrous event. It was here that doctors and scientists studied fluid shift changes, cosmetic surgery, and radiation therapy. When the division returned, it advised the government that this group of acutely ill patients had special needs. It was decided at this time that the U.S. government would give 138 contracts to emergency centers around the nation to establish specific units where all burn victims would be treated. The first of these units or centers was the Brooke Army Medical Center in San Antonio, Texas. The second center was established at the Shriners Hospital for Children in Boston, Massachusetts. In 1958 the University of Michigan, in Ann Arbor, became the site of the National Institute of Burn Medicine, where the American Burn Association is now housed. All research is kept on file at this institution and is available to anyone who wishes to study the treatment of burns.

# TYPES OF BURNS

Burns are usually acquired in two ways: (1) by involvement in an uncontrollable fire or explosion, and (2) through contact of some part of the body with a hot object or liquid, acid, or flaming substances. Thermal burns, the most common type, are usually caused by flammable liquids and clothing, space heaters, explosions from reignited gas pilot lights, and scalding from hot coffee or overheated tap water spilled directly on the victim.

Electrical burns occur when the electrical sparks or an electrical current passes directly through the body. This can occur with downed power lines, unprotected wall sockets, lightening, or defective wiring. Radiation burns are caused by exposure to the sun or treatment for cancer. Chemical burns result from contact with mixtures of acid, alkali, and phosphorus found in paint removers, disinfectants, and drain cleaners.

# CLASSIFICATION BY SEVERITY

The American Burn Association classifies a burn as minor, moderate, or major, depending on the basis of the criteria described in Table 41-1.

# CLASSIFICATION BY BURN DEPTH

Burns are classified as partial-thickness or full-thickness, depending on which layers of the skin have been damaged (Table 41-2 and Figure 41-1). Partial-thickness burns destroy and damage tissue in the **dermis.** A superficial or shallow partial-thickness burn will be red, warm, and painful. An example of this is a mild sunburn reaction. The **epidermis** is damaged, but this keratinized layer is rapidly replaced by underlying cells. Because the nerves are intact, there is pain

with this type of burn. This was previously classified as a *first-degree burn.*

A deep partial-thickness burn involves the dermis and the epidermis and is characterized by redness and blisters that usually increase immediately in size. There are enough epithelial cells remaining around the hair follicles and sweat glands to produce new skin, provided that the cells are not destroyed during treatment. The length of time to heal without complications is from 10 days to 2 weeks. This type of burn can be identified easily if the patient's skin blanches after slight fingertip pressure is applied. This type of burn was previously classified as a *second-degree burn.*

Full-thickness burns destroy all the layers of the skin, extending into the subcutaneous tissue, and may involve muscles, tendons, and bone. If the patient's hair can be pulled out easily, the burn is considered to be a full-thickness type. Full-thickness burns appear leathery and may be white, brown, tan, red, or black. Small thin-walled vesicles may be present. There is no sensation of pain at first because sensory nerve fibers in the dermis have been destroyed. Sensation and pain do return as the tissues recover. Because burns are usually a mixture of full-thickness and partial-thickness injuries, some pain is present. Full-thickness burns must be grafted to heal because there are no skin cells remaining and regeneration is therefore impossible. These burns were previously classified as *third-degree* and *fourth-degree burns.*

# DETERMINATION OF BURN EXTENT

Various methods are used to estimate the amount of body surface area affected by a burn injury. Regardless of the estimate method used, the extent of the injured area is expressed as a percentage of the **total body sur-**

---

| TABLE 41-1 |
|---|

## American Burn Association Adult Burn Classification

| MAGNITUDE OF BURN INJURY | PARTIAL THICKNESS* (SECOND-DEGREE) | FULL THICKNESS* (THIRD-DEGREE) | OTHER FACTORS |
|---|---|---|---|
| Minor | <15% | <2% | Does not involve special care areas (eyes, ears, face, hands, feet, perineum); excludes electrical injury, inhalation injury, complicated injury (fractures), all poor-risk patients (extremes of age, concomitant disease) |
| Moderate, uncomplicated | 15-25% | <10% | Excludes electrical injury, inhalation injury, complicated injury, all poor-risk patients; does not involve special care areas |
| Major | >25% | >10% | Includes all burns involving hands, face, eyes, ears, feet, or perineum; includes inhalation injury, electrical injury, complicated burn injury, and all poor-risk patients |

From Lewis SM, Collier IC, Heitkemper MM: *Medical-surgical nursing: assessment and management of clinical problems,* ed 4, St Louis, 1996, Mosby.
*Figures indicate percentage of total body surface area involved.

**face area (TBSA).** This measurement is used to determine fluid and nutritional needs of the burn patient. The "Rule of Nines" and the Lund-Browder classification (Figure 41-2), are methods commonly used to *estimate* the extent of the burn wound. Different burn centers around the country have their own pictorial representations for estimating the extent of burns. For all methods the person making the estimate colors a chart by using red for areas of full-thickness (third-degree) burns and blue for deep partial-thickness

## TABLE 41-2

### Causes and Factors Determining Depth of Burn Injury

| DEPTH | CAUSE | APPEARANCE | COLOR | SENSATION |
|---|---|---|---|---|
| Superficial partial-thickness (first-degree) | Flash flame, ultraviolet light (sunburn) | Swollen and red<br>Dry, no blisters<br>Minimal or no edema<br>Blanches with fingertip pressure and refills when pressure is removed | Increased redness | Painful |
| Deep partial-thickness (second-degree) | Contact with hot liquids or solids<br>Flash flame to clothing<br>Direct flame<br>Chemicals<br>Ultraviolet light | Large moist blisters that will increase in size<br>Skin blanches with fingertip pressure and refills when pressure is removed | Mottled with dull, white, tan, pink, or cherry-red areas | Very painful<br>Sensitive to pressure |
| Full-thickness (third-degree) | Contact with hot liquids or solids<br>Flame<br>Chemicals<br>Electrical contact | Hard and dry with leathery eschar<br>Charred vessels visible under eschar<br>Blisters rare, but thin-walled blisters that do not increase in size may be present<br>No blanching with pressure | White, charred dark tan<br>Black<br>Red | Little or no pain<br>Hair easily pulls out<br>Insensitive to touch |

Modified from Phipps WJ et al: *Medical-surgical nursing: concepts and clinical practice,* ed 5, St Louis, 1995, Mosby.

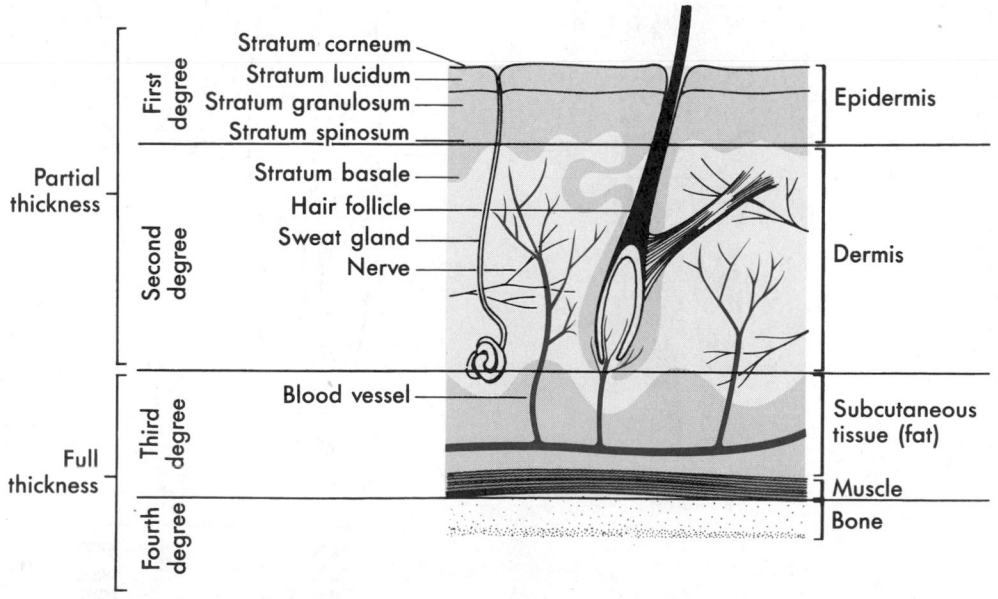

**Figure 41-1**    Layers of skin involved in burn injury. (From Beare PG, Myers JL: *Adult health nursing,* ed 3, St Louis, 1998, Mosby.)

## The Rule of Nines

| | |
|---|---|
| Head and neck | 9% |
| Right arm | 9 |
| Left arm | 9 |
| Posterior trunk | 18 |
| Anterior trunk | 18 |
| Right leg | 18 |
| Left leg | 18 |
| Perineum | 1 |
| | **100%** |

## Lund and Browder Chart

| Area | AGE-YEARS 0–1 | 1–4 | 5–9 | 10–15 | ADULT | % 2° | % 2° | % TOTAL |
|---|---|---|---|---|---|---|---|---|
| Head | 19 | 17 | 13 | 10 | 7 | | | |
| Neck | 2 | 2 | 2 | 2 | 2 | | | |
| Ant. Trunk | 13 | 17 | 13 | 13 | 13 | | | |
| Post. Trunk | 13 | 13 | 13 | 13 | 13 | | | |
| R. Buttock | 2½ | 2½ | 2½ | 2½ | 2½ | | | |
| L. Buttock | 2½ | 2½ | 2½ | 2½ | 2½ | | | |
| Genitalia | 1 | 1 | 1 | 1 | 1 | | | |
| R.U. Arm | 4 | 4 | 4 | 4 | 4 | | | |
| L.U. Arm | 4 | 4 | 4 | 4 | 4 | | | |
| R.L. Arm | 3 | 3 | 3 | 3 | 3 | | | |
| L.L. Arm | 3 | 3 | 3 | 3 | 3 | | | |
| R. Hand | 2½ | 2½ | 2½ | 2½ | 2½ | | | |
| L. Hand | 2½ | 2½ | 2½ | 2½ | 2½ | | | |
| R. Thigh | 5½ | 6½ | 8½ | 8½ | 9½ | | | |
| L. Thigh | 5½ | 6½ | 8½ | 8½ | 9½ | | | |
| R. Leg | 5 | 5 | 5½ | 6 | 7 | | | |
| L. Leg | 5 | 5 | 5½ | 6 | 7 | | | |
| R. Foot | 3½ | 3½ | 3½ | 3½ | 3½ | | | |
| L. Foot | 3½ | 3½ | 3½ | 3½ | 3½ | | | |
| | | | | | **TOTAL** | | | |

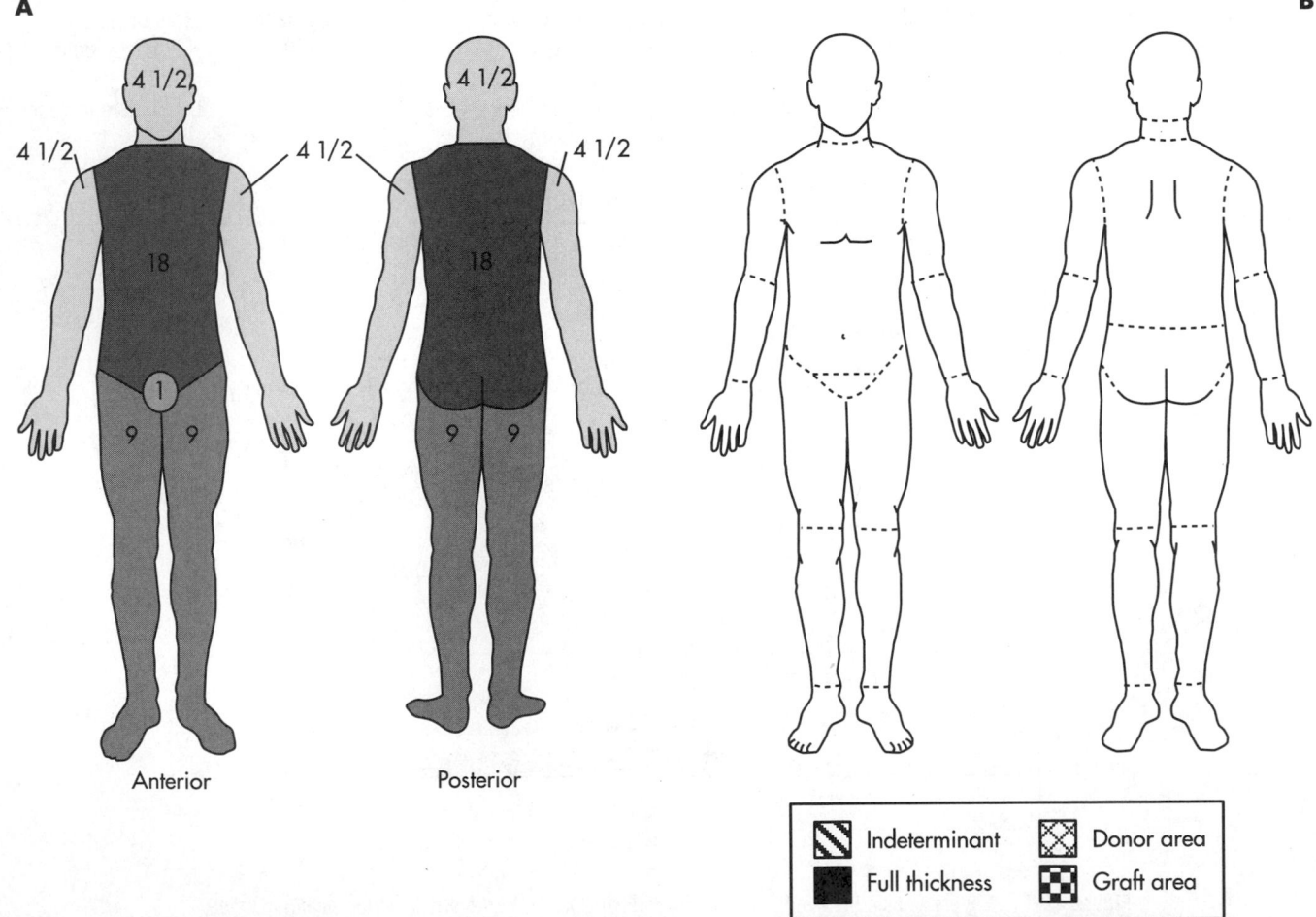

**A** 4 1/2 4 1/2 4 1/2 4 1/2 18 1 9 9 4 1/2 4 1/2 4 1/2 4 1/2 18 9 9

Anterior    Posterior

**B**

Indeterminant    Donor area
Full thickness    Graft area

**Figure 41-2** Estimating burn size. **A,** Rule of nines. **B,** Lund-Browder classification. (Modified from Lund C, Browder N: *Surg Gynecol Obstet* 1944.)

(second-degree) burns. With the Rule of Nines one adds the percentages listed for each burned area. For example, burns on the right arm and anterior trunk would total 27% TBSA.

A child who is age 12 or older is considered to be an adult and can be measured by the Rule of Nines to estimate the burned area. However, when a younger child is burned, these measures must be adjusted. The percentage of TBSA represented by an infant's head is twice the percentage represented by the head of an adult, whereas the percentage of a 10-year-old child's head is about one and one half times that of an adult. The trunk is considered approximately two thirds that of an adult. The Lund-Browder classification is considered more accurate for all patients because it divides the body into more sections and makes adjustments for age-related changes in body size. To use the Lund-Browder classification, the nurse should note the red- and blue-colored areas, find the column that reflects the patient's age, and then add the percentages for each area of the body burned. A 2-year-old child with burns on the right upper arm, the right hand, and the anterior trunk would have burns on 26.5% of the body, whereas the percentage for an adult with burns in the same areas would be estimated at 22.5% TBSA.

## PHASES OF BURN CARE

The care of the burned patient is classified into three phases: the **emergent** period, the acute period, and the rehabilitative period. The emergent period begins with the burn injury and includes the first stage and initial care as determined by the severity of the injury. This period ends when the patient is stable and begins to diurese and no longer requires fluid therapy.

The acute period is directed toward continuous care of the wounds to promote grafting, prevent infection, and promote healing. Rehabilitation involves all that is required to help that patient return to his or her previous or optimal level of functioning. Many aspects of rehabilitation, however, must be initiated from the time of admission and during the emergent care of the patient. The following sections on burn care deal with the patient's total needs throughout these periods.

### Emergent Phase

The first priority is to prevent further injury by extinguishing any flames still present or by removing the victim from the source of the burn, such as the electrical current in the event of an electrical burn. The patient must never be touched with metal or the rescuer's hands after an electrical burn. The current may still be active. Something nonmetallic such as a rope or wooden broomstick handle should be used to move the victim away from the electrical current.

Flames should be smothered by wrapping the patient in a blanket, rug, or coat and rolling the victim on the ground. The rule of thumb is to *"Stop, Drop, and Roll"* the patient until the flames are out.

In the case of a chemical burn, all contaminated clothing should be removed if it is *not* adhered to the skin. The skin is rinsed generously with cool water to remove the chemical. Any rings, watches, belts, ties, or other items that restrict circulation around any part of the body should also be removed because the patient will become edematous later from fluid shifts.

The size of any burn can be decreased by the application of cool water, which reduces the temperature of the skin, lessens tissue destruction, and may prevent a full-thickness burn from occurring. The application of ice or ice water to the wound is now contraindicated because of the potential harm from hypothermia and frostbite. *No* attempt should be made to apply ointments (petroleum jelly, cold cream, butter, or lard) because ointments allow the heat from the burn to be contained and intensified, causing deeper tissue destruction.

No medications should be given because the patient will probably go into *burn shock.* Burn shock is the combination of hypovolemic, cardiogenic, and neurogenic shock seen only in a patient who is burned. The victim should be wrapped in a clean sheet or blanket and taken immediately to the hospital or a burn center for emergency treatment.

Once the cause of the burn has been identified and initial treatment has begun, the next priority is to maintain or provide a patent airway. Any bleeding that is present should be stopped. Burn shock may also be present and should be treated. The burn victim is usually conscious and in pain. The rescuer should reassure the victim and provide information about what is happening.

On the way to the burn center, a brief history of the victim should be taken. The following information should be obtained from the patient or a family member and given to the burn team:

1. The patient's previous state of health and mental status
2. Any allergies to drugs or foods
3. Last tetanus immunization
4. Current height and weight
5. Detailed account of the accident identifying whether the victim was in an open or confined space at the time of contact with the flame, the duration of exposure to the burning agent, and the first aid treatment performed
6. The patient's age
7. Any other injuries that occurred
8. Any preexisting conditions, such as diabetes, hypertension, renal disease, cardiac disease, or metabolic disease

A further detailed head-to-toe assessment is performed after burn shock has been treated.

## Assessment and Intervention

During the emergent period, burn shock is a major problem for the victim. The shock can be treated with fluid therapy, which is discussed later in this chapter. Suctioning may be necessary to remove aspirated secretions in maintaining a patent airway. Humidified oxygen at 100% should be administered.

Smoke inhalation by the victim may also result in damage to the respiratory tract and may produce laryngeal edema. This type of damage is more likely when the victim inhales toxic chemical by-products from the combustion of synthetic materials or from prolonged exposure to smoke during the rescue operation. Early postburn pulmonary damage can be assessed by the following observations:

1. Look for burns around the neck and mouth. They will look like *soot* at the mouth-nose and red on the neck.
2. Look for singed nasal hairs.
3. Inspect the mouth for burns of the oral and pharyngeal mucous membranes (they will look white in color).
4. Observe for continual coughing, **carbonaceous** (sooty) **sputum,** or voice changes such as hoarseness.

The patient with **inhalation injuries** is at great risk for developing bronchial pneumonia because the alveoli can be charred and destroyed. Therefore an immediate bronchoscopy is performed at the bedside by the burn physician.

## Fluid Shift to Tissues (Edema)

Damage to the capillary system occurs in the burn area at the same time as damage to the body cells. Both injuries cause water and electrolytes to shift from the plasma to the interstitial fluid. This fluid accumulation causes edema, and in partial-thickness burns it is evidenced by blisters. In full-thickness burns the same process occurs, but the destroyed layers of the skin, or **eschar,** may trap the fluids beneath them. If the wounds are **circumferential,** covering all sides of an extremity, a tourniquet effect is created. Circumferential wounds on the torso can affect respiration by restricting diaphragmatic movements. Those involved in the neck may obstruct the airway. Pulses distal to the wound, respirations, and airway patency must be checked hourly. If edema causes complications in any of these areas, an **escharotomy**—cutting through the burned skin layers—is performed to relieve the constriction.

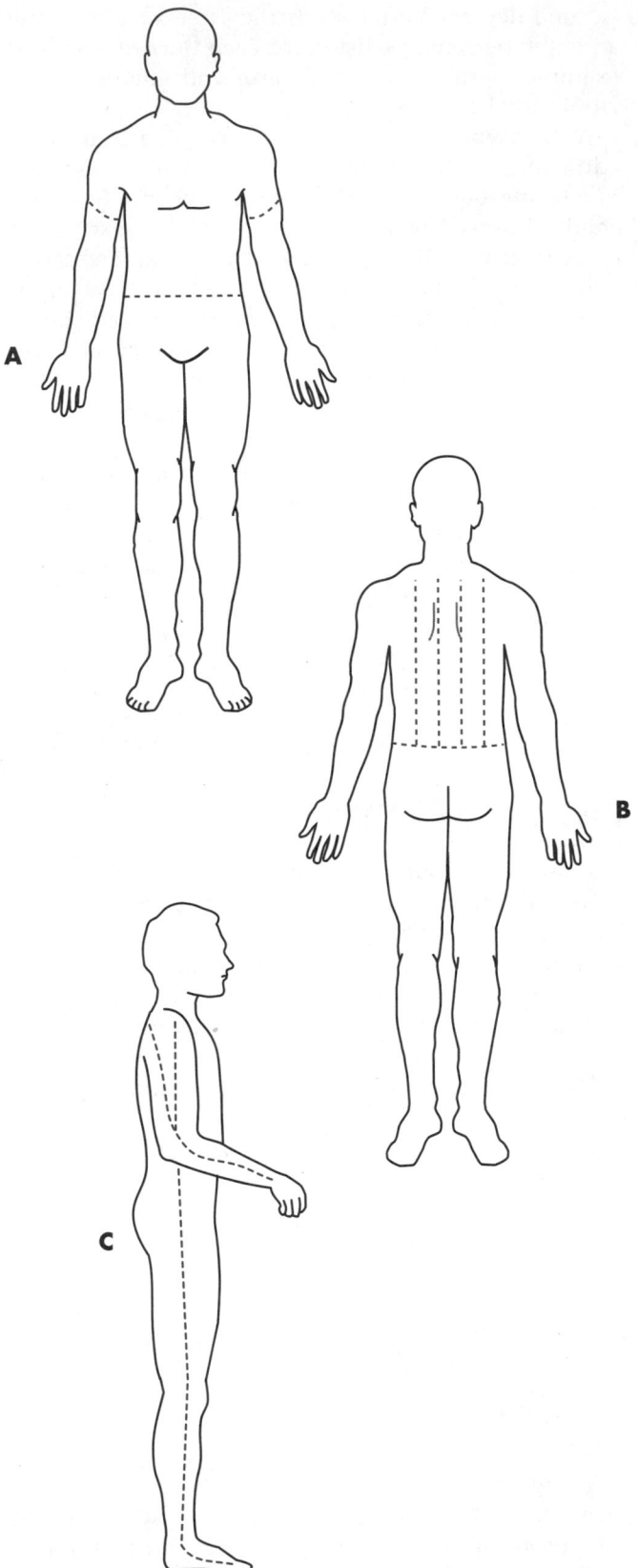

**Figure 41-3**  Escharotomy sites to prevent tourniquette effect of circumferential burn wounds. **A,** Circumferential. **B,** Tangential. **C,** Full-body.

The escharotomy, or incision of the hard layers of the burn wound, can be performed circumferentially (around the arm or waist), **tangentially** (down the chest wall or on each breast), or full body (down both sides of the body) (Figure 41-3).

## Burn Shock

It can be expected that an adult with 15% of the body burned or a child with 10% burned will be suffering from some degree of shock. The accumulation of edema fluids in the burned area and the loss of fluids from injured tissues result in a decrease in the amount of circulating blood plasma. When the volume of the bloodstream falls, blood pressure drops, circulation decreases to the vital organs, and less oxygen is available to all body tissues. This process leads to shock. If treatment is not instituted, acute renal failure and damage to the kidneys and other organs will occur. Metabolic acidosis may result. This shift of fluids, electrolytes, and albumin from the capillaries to the burned tissues occurs in the first 24 to 48 hours following the injury.

The nurse caring for a newly burned patient must be constantly alert for symptoms of burn shock. Restlessness is a common sign of hypoxia and may indicate onset of shock. The pulse increases before the blood pressure falls, and respirations also increase. Urine flow is scant or absent. To prevent burn shock, **fluid resuscitation** is usually the first emergency treatment given to the severely burned patient. Many combinations of fluids may be used, depending on the physician's preference (Table 41-3). Ringer's solution plus albumin may be given to combat protein loss. Fluids may be administered rapidly until urine flow is established, then regulated to maintain a urine output of 30 to 50 ml per hour. An indwelling catheter is inserted, and it is the nurse's responsibility to measure the output, urinary pH, and specific gravity each hour.

The specific gravity and hematocrit value may be elevated because of the shift of fluid from the circulating blood in the vascular spaces to the burn tissue. Almost every burn patient is extremely thirsty but must not be allowed to drink water because this tends to add to the massive fluid shifts. The patient is given nothing by mouth; intravenous fluids are administered instead. Fluid resuscitation criteria are reviewed to determine whether the patient is adequately hydrated (Box 41-1). If hydrated, the patient should not complain of thirst.

## Fluid Return to Bloodstream

With time, the capillary walls return to normal and the fluids accumulated in the tissues reenter the bloodstream. The electrolytes return with the fluid. This process is detected by a marked increase in urinary output or diuresis. If the kidneys are damaged or diseased, the patient is at great risk for kidney failure. This shift of fluid and electrolytes back into the

**BOX 41-1**

### CRITERIA FOR FLUID RESUSCITATION

Patient mentally alert and clear
Urine volume 30-50 ml/hr for an adult; 1 mg/kg body wt/hr for a child
Rectal body temperature = 99.6° F to 100° F
Central venous pressure normal (5-15 cm)
Slightly high pulse: <120 bpm for an adult; <160 bpm for a child
Slightly high but normal blood pressure
Absence of nausea, paralytic ileus, and thirst

Created by D. Starsiak, Loyola University, Chicago, 1994.

**TABLE 41-3**

### Formulas for Estimating Fluid Replacement of an Adult Burn Patient

| | FIRST 24 HOURS | SECOND 24 HOURS | |
| FORMULA | CRYSTALLOIDS | COLLOIDS | GLUCOSE IN WATER |
|---|---|---|---|
| Brooke (modified) | Lactated Ringer's solution: 2.0 ml/kg/% burn; ½ given during first 8 hr; ½ given during next 16 hr | 0.3-0.5 ml/kg/% burn | Amount to replace estimated evaporative losses |
| Parkland (Baxter) | Lactated Ringer's solution: 4 ml/kg/% burn; ½ given first 8 hr; ½ given each next 8 hr | 20%-60% of calculated plasma volume | Amount to replace estimated evaporative losses |

From Lewis SM, Collier IC, Heitkemper MM: *Medical-surgical nursing: assessment and management of clinical problems,* ed 4, St Louis, 1996, Mosby.

vascular system also puts an extra volume load on the heart and lungs. Patients with a prior history of heart or lung problems should be monitored very closely for signs of congestive heart failure or pulmonary edema. Because electrolytes are also returning to the bloodstream, it would be dangerous to administer additional electrolytes to the patient in the intravenous fluids. The fluids, however, are still needed, so dextrose and water are administered.

## Diuresis

The onset of diuresis signals the end of the emergent period of care. The nurse, continuously observing the patient, notes this change in status and reports to the physician so the treatment plan can be modified. Formulas such as Parkland's and Brooke's have been developed to help determine the volume of fluid replacement. The formulas serve as guidelines and must be adjusted according to the patient's response. Precise monitoring by the nurse should be performed as necessary to determine the patient's response. Determining the fluid needs of the burn patient requires accurate checking of intake, output, and vital signs every hour and frequent monitoring of weight and hematocrit levels.

## Support of Gastrointestinal Function

In patients with major burns, a nasogastric tube is inserted to prevent gastric dilation because peristalsis slows or stops altogether as a normal body response to stress.

## Wound Care

Initial treatment of the wound involves cleansing with a dilute solution of povidone-iodine (Betadine), pHisoHex (one part povidone-iodine or pHisoHex to three or four parts water), or chlorhexidine gluconate (Hibiclens) solution. The wound should then be rinsed thoroughly and covered with moist saline dressings until the physician can thoroughly estimate the percentage of TBSA that is burned. If the wounds cover a great deal of the body, the saline should be warm and the patient should be kept covered with a sheet to prevent excessive heat loss. After all the wounds are cleansed, the saline dressings may be covered with dry dressings or may be replaced with dry sterile dressings. If the wound is a result of a chemical injury, it is washed with copious amounts of warm water before it is cleansed and covered with a dry dressing (Calistro, 1993).

Strict asepsis is essential to avoid wound contamination and subsequent infection. Morphine sulfate may be given to reduce pain and apprehension. Medications are not given intramuscularly because tissue absorption is poor in the burn patient as a result of the reduced blood supply to the tissues. Reduced dosages given intravenously have been found effective. Antibiotics and tetanus toxoid prophylaxis are usually given because the burn wound is considered contaminated.

## Transfer From Emergency Department

The initial treatment of the patient takes place in the hospital emergency department. If a burn treatment center is available, the patient with major burns is transferred there as soon as the initial needs are met. The patient's clothing should be placed in a bag and sent with the patient to the burn center, where the staff may need to examine its composition. If admitted to the general hospital, the patient is placed in an intensive care unit or a regular medical or surgical unit. The patient should be placed in *reverse isolation* in a private room in a clean area of the hospital (Box 41-2).

## Expected Outcomes

The following should be observed in the burn patient after proper interventions during this emergent period:
- The burning process has stopped.
- A patent airway is maintained.
- Initial fluid resuscitation has been started using Ringer's lactate solution.
- Urinary output is greater than 30 ml/hour.
- Arterial blood gases are within normal limits.
- Peripheral pulses are palpable.
- Blood pressure is above 100/70 mm Hg.
- Apical pulse is slightly tachycardic.
- Bowel sounds are present, with passing of flatus.
- Lungs sounds are clear, and respirations are within normal limits.
- Temperature is afebrile at 99° F to 100° F.
- The patient expresses feelings of safety and comfort.

## The Acute Phase

The acute phase of burn injury begins with the return of fluid from the cells (intracellular fluid) and between the cells (interstitial fluid) to the intravascular space. Increased intravascular volume results in increased urine output, diuresis. The acute phase is concluded when the wounds are healed or covered with grafts. This process may take weeks to months.

> **NURSE ALERT**
>
> **Any patient under age 2 or over age 72 has less chance of surviving a burn injury than does a younger or middle-aged person.**

| BOX 41-2 | NURSING PROCESS |
|---|---|

## BURN INJURIES

### ASSESSMENT

- Burn area for drainage, evidence of healing, evidence of infection
- Vital signs
- Fluid volume status
- Weight
- Urine specific gravity
- Respiratory status, including lung sounds
- Overall skin color
- Pain level on a scale of 0 to 10 (often)
- Gastrointestinal function, bowel sounds, appetite
- Level of orientation, anxiety, restlessness
- Coping abilities and support systems
- Laboratory studies: electrolytes, complete blood count, albumin, arterial blood gases

### NURSING DIAGNOSES

- Impaired skin integrity related to thermal injury
- Risk for infection related to burn wound and inadequate nutrition for healing
- Fluid volume deficit/excess related to fluid shifts, loss of skin integrity
- Risk for impaired gas exchange related to inhalation injury, immobility
- Pain related to tissue injury, wound care
- Altered nutrition: less than body requirements related to increased metabolic needs, impaired gastrointestinal function, loss of body fluid
- Fear related to pain, hospitalization, and unknown outcome of burn injury
- Body image disturbance related to burn injury, potential long-term dependency, and therapy

### NURSING INTERVENTIONS

- Provide appropriate wound care (hydrotherapy, topical medications, dressings) as ordered.
- Maintain aseptic technique with wound care.
- Prevent trauma to the burn area.
- Elevate extremities, if affected.
- Obtain and monitor wound cultures if ordered.
- Administer antibiotics if ordered.
- Administer IV fluids as prescribed.
- Encourage patient to drink prescribed fluid amounts.
- Position patient for optimal breathing.
- Administer oxygen as ordered.
- Reduce oxygen need by using pain- and anxiety-reduction techniques.
- Pace activities according to patient's tolerance.

- Encourage use of incentive spirometer.
- Administer analgesics as ordered.
- Premedicate before dressing change.
- Use a variety of comfort measures such as positioning and massage.
- Teach relaxation, distraction, and guided imagery techniques.
- Consult with the physician, occupational therapist, and others to assist in pain management.
- Encourage high-protein, high-calorie diet, if permitted.
- Arrange consultation with dietitian.
- Encourage family to bring in preferred foods, if allowed.
- Modify environment to provide pleasant mealtime experience.
- Encourage patient and family to verbalize feelings, fears, and grief.
- Identify patient supports and coping strategies and use in planning care.
- Explain hospital resources such as counseling, social service, and pastoral care, and initiate referrals as requested.
- Provide care that maintains privacy and personal dignity.

### EVALUATION OF EXPECTED OUTCOMES

- No evidence of fluid deficit.
   Vital signs within normal limits for individual
   Balanced input and output
   Serum electrolytes, hematocrit within normal limits
   Mucous membranes moist, denies thirst, supple tissue turgor
- No evidence of fluid excess:
   No evidence of edema
   Weight constant
   Lung sounds clear
   Specific gravity within normal limits
   Vital signs within normal limits for individual
- Afebrile
- WBC within normal limits
- Burn area healing with no evidence of infection
- Verbalizes signs and symptoms of infection and risk factors
- Daily intake of 3000 to 5000 calories
- Serum albumin, nitrogen levels within normal limits

*Continued*

<table>
<tr><td colspan="2">

BOX 41-2

**NURSING PROCESS**

**BURN INJURIES—cont'd**

- Describes prescribed diet and indicates willingness to follow it
- Lungs clear, no congestion or hoarseness
- Skin pink, no cyanosis
- Demonstrates ability to deep breathe and use supportive oxygen equipment if indicated
- Able to rest, sleep 6 to 8 hours at night, and participate in care and decision making
- States pain as 0 to 5 on scale of 10 and reports relief after analgesic

- Demonstrates ability to use noninvasive techniques for pain relief
- Identifies strategies to reduce fear
- Able to verbalize fears and concerns
- Acknowledges actual change in appearance and function
- Maintains relationship with significant others
- States willingness to use identified resources after discharge

</td></tr>
</table>

## Objectives of Treatment

Each patient must be considered individually. The cause, depth, and extent of the burn; the patient's age; preexisting diseases or conditions; and the patient's emotional reaction to the injury determine the methods of treatment selected by the burn team. Although different methods are employed, the basic objectives are always the same:

1. Prevent and treat burn shock.
2. Relieve pain.
3. Prevent infection.
4. Heal open wounds.
5. Restore normal functioning and appearance.
6. Preserve emotional equilibrium.
7. Return to the social and work environment.

## Medical Management

Initially the burn wounds are cleansed and debrided in the burn ICU or the tub room. Hair is clipped or shaved to reduce the risk of infection. If a burn wound is to heal without surgical intervention, various treatment plans are needed to keep the area free of dead tissue and bacteria. Wound healing is slow, taking anywhere from 2 weeks to 18 months, with the dangers of infection, scarring, and **contracture** formation ever present. This form of burn treatment generally includes the use of hydrotherapy, topical antimicrobials, and leaving the burns open to the air or covered with dressings **(closed method).**

**Hydrotherapy.** **Hydrotherapy,** or tubbing the burn victim, is used to cleanse and debride the wound. It is used in combination with other treatment methods. Once a day, for no more than 30 minutes, the patient is immersed in a solution of normal saline, plain water, or a balanced electrolyte solution. Nonirritating cleansing agents also may be used. The patient rou-

> **OLDER ADULT CONSIDERATIONS**
>
> 1. Be aware that the older adult is less likely to withstand the rapid changes in fluid volume associated with burns because of preexisting cardiopulmonary diseases.
> 2. Older adults experience a decrease in pain sensation and sensitivity to touch; therefore an increased pain threshold may negatively affect the older adult's response time to the pain of the burn injury, thus increasing the depth of the burn.
> 3. Morbidity and mortality are increased in the older adult because of:
>    a. Preexisting malnutrition
>    b. Impaired sensory system
>    c. Decreased coordination and reaction time
>    d. Side effects of medications
>    e. Peripheral neuropathy
>    f. Thinning and drying of skin caused by the loss of elasticity to the tissues
>
> Modified from Trofino RB: *Nursing care of the burn-injured patient,* Philadelphia, 1991, FA Davis.

tinely receives pain medication before the procedure because debridement is painful. Dressings are removed before the patient is placed in a tub unless they adhere to the wound. Immersion in the solution facilitates removal of dressings that have adhered and loosens sloughed tissue, eschar, exudate, and topical medications. The tub also provides an excellent place for the patient to exercise the extremities. A whirlpool provides the ideal form of hydrotherapy.

The tub must be cleaned thoroughly with bleach between uses, and the use of plastic liners for the tub can save time and prevent cross-contamination. The patient is placed on a narrow frame called a plinth, for which plastic covers are available. Long plastic gloves are worn by the person working with the patient in the tank, and plastic aprons, masks, and caps must be worn if the patient's wounds are exposed. The patient must be observed for chilling. Patients with newly grafted areas are not usually given full-body baths until the graft is healed, which takes 3 to 7 days. If there is a fine-mesh inner gauze over a fairly fresh grafted area, it should be left in place while the patient is in the tub. The gauze over a donor area also is not disturbed unless it loosens; then it is trimmed off.

### Topical antimicrobials

***Mafenide acetate (Sulfamylon acetate).*** Organisms most often involved in infection of burn patients include *Staphylococcus aureus,* hemolytic streptococci, and *Pseudomonas aeruginosa.* Mafenide has been found to be a safe, effective adjunct in preventing infection, and some believe that it is more effective than silver nitrate.

***Silver nitrate.*** The use of silver nitrate for treating burns is based on its bacteriostatic and infection-preventing properties. After thorough cleansing of the wounds, the burns are wrapped with dressings saturated with a solution of distilled water containing 0.5% silver nitrate. The dressings must be thoroughly soaked and thick enough to hold large amounts of solution. The entire dressing is then covered with two layers of prebleached stockinette. The dressings must be rewet every 2 to 4 hours so that the solution is in direct contact with the skin at all times. The silver nitrate solution hardens the eschar, which then serves as a pseudo-skin covering to protect the underlying tissues.

***Povidone-iodine ointment.*** Povidone-iodine 10% ointment and solution (Betadine) are now being used in the care of burn wounds because of their broad spectrum of microbicidal action. The ointment can be used alone or in conjunction with the solution and may be used with or without dressings. This solution is used if a patient is allergic to sulfa drugs.

***Silver sulfadiazine 1%.*** Silver sulfadiazine 1% (Silvadene) was approved for general use in the United States in 1974. It is a water-soluble cream that can be applied directly to the burn area by a sterile-gloved hand. It can also be used to impregnate Kerlix rolls or thick back pads so it can be applied directly to the burned area without touching the patient with a gloved hand. Patients have reported that this method is preferred because less pressure is placed on the burn wound. The wounds may be left exposed, and the cream may be reapplied, as necessary, when it is rubbed off. A layer of cream 2 to 4 mm thick should be applied so that the wound is not visible through the cream. A single-layer gauze dressing can be impregnated with the cream and applied to the wound and secured with stretch gauze or tube dressings. If the wounds are draining heavily or are infected, the dressings may be changed as often as three times a day. Silver sulfadiazine cream can be bactericidal for up to 48 hours. It does annihilate *Pseudomonas* and *Candida* organisms. The area covered by the cream must be cleansed thoroughly to prevent buildup (Table 41-4).

**Surgical management.** Surgical care of burn wounds may involve only periodic **debridement** (removal of dead tissue) of an area that is being treated by the medical methods described here. If the burn wound is severe and no dermis remains to allow tissue regeneration, skin grafting is necessary. This approach involves removal of dead tissue and possibly the underlying fatty tissue and the application of a skin graft or an artificial covering. Closing a burn wound quickly decreases the potential for infection and scarring. It also results in decreased pain and fluid loss. The only permanent graft is an **autograft,** which is skin that is removed from a donor site on the burn victim. Any other form of wound cover is temporary and eventually will be rejected by the burn victim's immune system. Because the burn victim is initially medically unstable and unable to withstand autografting procedures, temporary grafts play a major role in early therapy. There are four major types:

1. *Autograft* is skin taken from the victim.
2. **Homograft** (allograft) is skin from another person. This skin may be from a living relative or, more commonly, from a cadaver or skin grown in a culture. These grafts may remain in place 3 to 5 weeks before rejection occurs.
3. **Heterograft** (xenograft) is skin from another animal species. Pig skin is the most common, and the major disadvantage is early breakdown and potential for infection.
4. Synthetic grafts involve the use of synthetic skin substitutes such as collagen dressings (Biobrane). They have a long storage life and can provide wound cover for 2 months or longer until autograft is possible.

In addition to classification by material, grafts are also categorized by depth (Figure 41-4). A **full-thickness skin graft** includes the epidermis and all the dermis and is the type used for reconstruction. When a full-thickness graft is taken, the donor site will also need grafting. A **split-thickness skin graft** leaves some dermis at the donor site, which allows that site to heal. The split-thickness graft may be applied to the burn wound as a sheet graft (without being altered) for the best cosmetic result. It may also be altered after removal from the donor site by a mechanical device

**TABLE 41-4**

## Pharmacology of Drugs Used as Topical Antimicrobials

| DRUG (GENERIC AND TRADE NAME); ROUTE AND DOSAGE | ACTION/INDICATION | COMMON SIDE EFFECTS AND NURSING CONSIDERATIONS |
|---|---|---|
| **Mafenide Acetate** (Sulfamylon)<br>**Route:** Topical<br>**Dosage:** Apply topically $\frac{1}{16}$ inch to affected area 1-2 times daily; reapply as needed | Sulfonamide, interferes with bacterial wall synthesis; used as adjunctive treatment in second- and third-degree burns | Bone marrow suppression, fatal hemolytic anemia, and eosinophilia; contraindicated in inhalation injury; use with caution in impaired pulmonary and renal function and in fluid loss and decreased urine output |
| **Povidone-Iodine 10%** (Betadine)<br>**Route:** Topical<br>**Dosage:** Apply as ordered to area affected | Used as antiinfective against gram-positive and gram-negative organisms and fungal organisms (especially *Candida*) | Use cautiously in patients with sensitivity since solution and ointment both sting. Avoid contact with clothing to prevent appearance of bleeding. Use sparingly when resoaking bandages |
| **Silver Nitrate 0.5%**<br>**Route:** Topical<br>**Dosage:** Apply as ordered to area affected | Used as antiinfective and astringent and for cauterization of lesions, warts, and burns (low concentration) | Brown skin discoloration; use as wet dressing for burns; store in cool area; avoid contact with clothing to prevent discoloration |
| **Silver Sulfadiazine 1%** (Silvadene)<br>**Route:** Topical<br>**Dosage:** Apply 1% cream 1 or 2 times daily in layer 1.5 mm thick | Topical antiinfective used in prevention and treatment of infection in second- and third-degree burns | Use cautiously with sensitivity to sulfonamides and with renal and hepatic disease; may need to premedicate with analgesic before application |

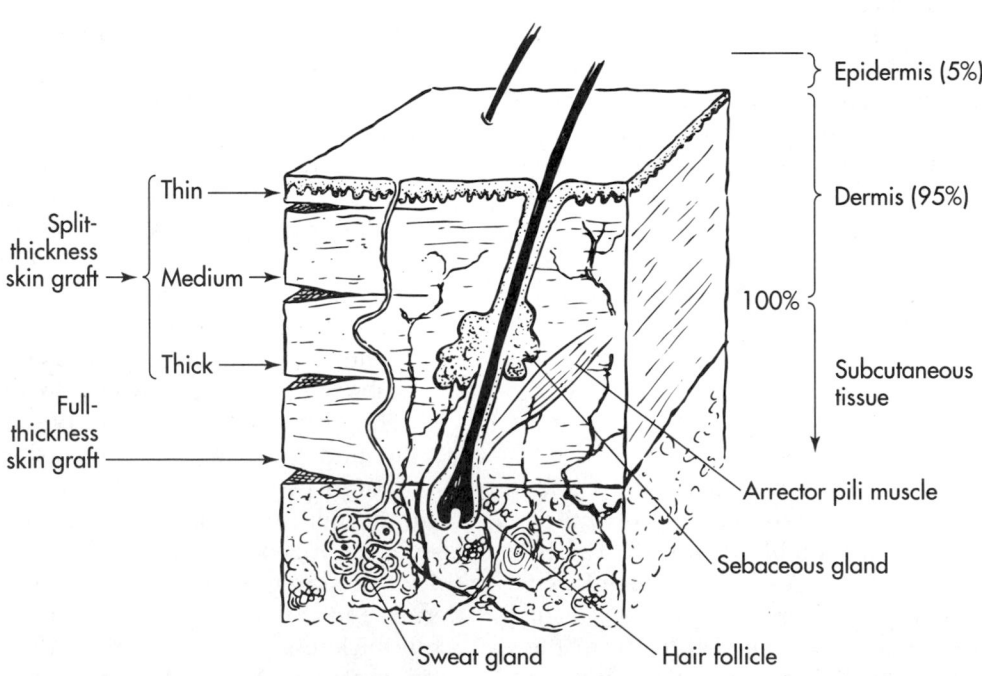

**Figure 41-4** Layers of skin involved in various types of skin grafts. Thickness of epidermis and dermis shown here is typical of that found on lateral thigh of adult.

that creates a mesh pattern of small slits (Figure 41-5). This mesh graft can be expanded to cover a larger surface area and allows drainage from the wound side.

The patient receives a general anesthetic for the grafting procedure, and on return from the operating room he or she will have two surgical sites that require care: the donor site and the grafted area. There are various types of dressings used for the grafted area, including fine-mesh gauze held in place by cotton pads and bandages. Some physicians prefer that the area be left open to the air. Most physicians staple the graft in place first, then apply a pressure dressing to ensure that the graft remains in close contact with the burn site. Care must be taken by the nursing staff during the first 48 hours not to move the patient in any manner that would disrupt this surface contact. If dressings are used, the nurse never removes them unless told to do so by the physician. In other cases dressings are removed daily to inspect for evidence of infection. Because many methods are used, the nurse will need to become familiar with the particular procedure desired by the surgeon.

The care of the donor site also varies. It may be covered with gauze and pressure bandages or it may have a layer of fine-mesh gauze and be left open to the air. This gauze remains in place until it starts to peel off by itself. Analgesics may be needed for pain, and the ambulatory patient often finds that there is more discomfort from the donor site than from the grafted area. When the donor site is the thigh, walking may be difficult. Repeated grafts can be taken from the same donor site if it has healed.

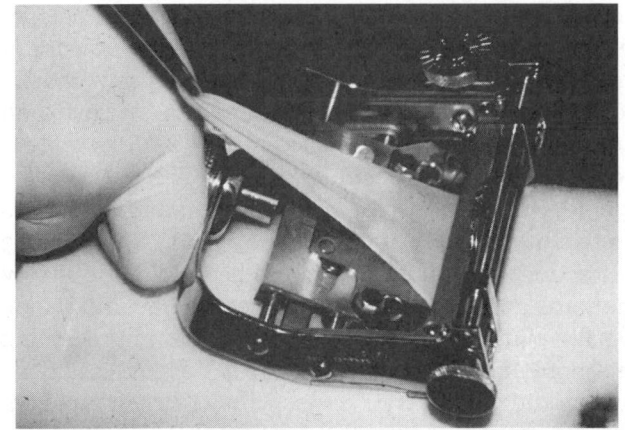

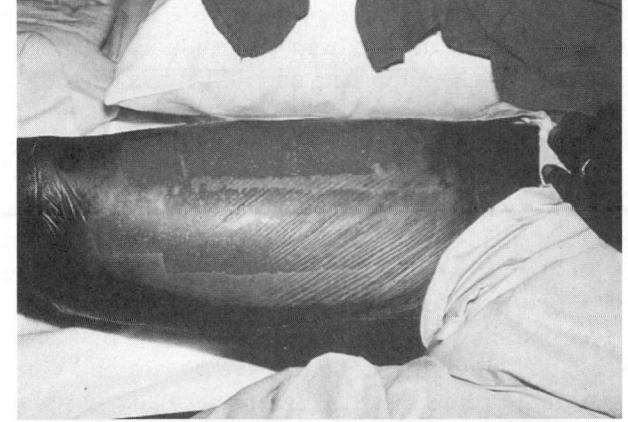

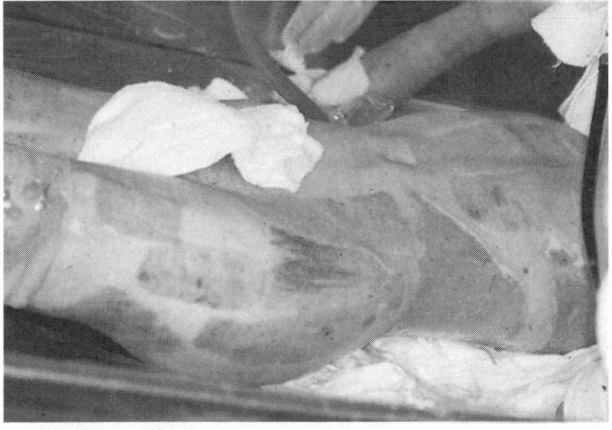

**Figure 41-5**   **A,** Surgeon harvests skin from a patient's thigh using a dermatome. **B,** Appearance of donor site after harvesting split-thickness skin graft. Donor site is covered with transparent occlusive dressing. **C,** Healed donor site. (From Lewis SM, Collier IC, Heitkemper MM: *Medical-surgical nursing: assessment and management of clinical problems,* ed 4, St Louis, 1996, Mosby.)

> **NURSE ALERT**
>
> If you remove or pull off the fine-mesh gauze over a donor site, you will leave a scar that is as severe as the original burned tissue. The area will not reepithelize. Trim the edges off carefully with scissors when they begin to dry and curl up.

 **ETHNIC/CULTURAL CONSIDERATIONS**

Cadaver homografts supplied through an organ donor skin bank *can* be used on any recipient in the emergent phase, regardless of skin color, since it will slough off in 5 to 7 days and is *not* permanent. Grafting with synthetic materials, such as Biobrane or Integra, may be done without having any type of cosmetic effect on the patient.

The use of a Jobst pressure stocking or garment is necessary after the final grafting has taken place. This is measured specifically for the patient's body or body parts by the company. It is an elastic material that increases circulation of the blood to the grafted site, provides compression for the graft site itself, and prevents contractures. The patient must be instructed before discharge on the care of this garment. Each person receives two garments; one is to wear 23 hours a day while the other one is washed. The garment can be removed only once a day for the patient to inspect his or her skin bathe and change into the other garment. These garments are worn by the patient for 1 to 2 years.

---

### NURSE ALERT

When caring for the eyelids of a patient, remember that they are *not* debrided because of the thinness of the tissues. Clean the eyelids with normal saline soaks, and assess daily for eyelid contractures. Lubricating eyedrops or ointments may be used to prevent corneal abrasions.

---

### Nursing management

*Monitoring weight and intake and output.* Careful measurement in recording fluid intake and urinary output is important for determining proper fluid replacement and preventing complications. The nurse should obtain and record a preburn weight for the patient because it will assist the burn team in determining the patient's fluid needs.

*Positioning.* Proper positioning of the patient is important in preventing contractures, decubitus ulcers, foot drop, and pulmonary complications. Care of the patient may be facilitated by using a specialty bed that alternates pressure on body surfaces. Flotation therapy also has been used successfully for severely burned patients. Flotation prevents pressure areas and allows blood flow to all areas of the body. This enhances nourishment of the cells, promotes healing, and helps to prevent pressure ulcers. The sensation of floating is soothing and relaxing and lessens pain and tension, and the patient is able to move about more freely. The physical therapist may assist with both passive and active range-of-motion exercises, and the patient should be encouraged to assist with his or her own exercises. The patient should not be placed in Fowler's position, and the knee gatch of the bed should not be elevated because both will contribute to contractures. When the patient is in the supine position, hyperextension of the head will help to prevent contractures when the neck is burned. Pillows should *not* be used under the patient's head because a neck contracture could result. Splinting and exercise programs may be instituted to prevent deformities. A major objective of care is to encourage patients to participate actively in their own care when their individual condition has stabilized. If

the patient's condition allows it, early ambulation is encouraged.

*Prevention of infection.* Some hospitals maintain rooms in which dressings are changed under aseptic conditions, or sometimes patients are taken to the operating room for dressing changes, and light anesthetics are administered. Medical centers and large hospitals are developing self-contained surgical suites in the burn units. Regardless of the method of treatment used, all personnel caring for the patient should observe the practice of thorough hand washing before providing any care. A gown, mask, and sterile gloves must be worn for all dressing changes and for all care if the burns are exposed (as in the exposure method). The patient also should wear a mask for protection against organisms present in his or her own respiratory tract. If visitors are allowed in the room, they should be required to follow the same gown-mask-gloves procedure. Antibiotics are usually administered to the patient to aid in preventing infection. Treatment depends partly on the conditions surrounding the injury. Persons with respiratory tract infections should not be allowed near the patient. When there are burns about the perineal area, care must be taken to prevent infection from fecal contamination. This may be especially important, and difficult, in children.

*Relief of pain.* When burns are severe, the patient will need medication for pain. When severe edema is present, medication to relieve pain should be given intravenously. Morphine may be given intermittently or as a continuous infusion. Medication should be given 15 to 30 minutes before any treatment or procedure that will be painful to the patient.

*Diet.* Nothing is given by mouth for the first 24 to 48 hours. Many burn patients have nausea and vomiting, and a nasogastric tube is usually inserted to prevent abdominal distention and paralytic ileus. After 24 hours, if there is no vomiting, the tube is clamped or removed and oral fluids started. When the physician orders a clear-liquid diet, the nurse offers 30 to 60 ml of fluid an hour and increases the amount as tolerated. If the patient can tolerate it, a high-calorie, high-protein diet is started in 7 to 10 days. Caloric requirements may exceed 5000 kcal daily. Until the patient is able to consume a diet that can provide the required calories, a supplemental nasogastric tube feeding (i.e., Vivonex) is given to deliver a high concentration of calories and proteins. Even the patient consuming a full general diet may lack the appetite to eat the amount and variety of foods needed to deliver the total calorie requirement. Small, frequent feedings should be given. The use of between-meal, high-protein drinks is helpful in meeting caloric requirements.

*Supportive care.* After admission of the patient, the bed linens may be changed by using 4 to 8 individuals to assist. Medication for pain should be administered 30 to 45 minutes before beginning the procedure. The patient needs special mouth care, with sponges dipped in water or diluted mouthwash. If the lips are not burned, cold cream or petroleum jelly should be applied. A retention catheter is usually inserted to measure hourly output, and care should be taken to prevent urinary tract infection by maintaining a sterile closed system of drainage.

If the feet have not been burned, ambulation is generally ordered as soon as possible for the patient. Ambulation helps to improve appetite and elimination. Soaks or tub baths may be ordered to remove dressings and to prevent damage to the tissues or to remove eschar before skin grafting. The tub should be thoroughly scrubbed with soap and water and disinfected with bleach, and the temperature of the water should be 37.8° C (100° F).

**Emotional care.** The burn patient has many emotional problems, especially fear of death and disfigurement. If the burn is the result of carelessness, there are bound to be feelings of guilt. Most patients realize that long weeks of recovery lie ahead, and the worry over loss of income and expenses may cause endless anxiety. The patient's family may have emotional problems and guilt feelings. Both the patient and the family need opportunities to talk about their problems, and these opportunities may be provided by the nurse, the hospital social worker, or a spiritual counselor. Plans to assist a family financially may relieve worry. Diversional activities should be provided for the patient to help fill unused time, and they may be helpful in preventing contractures by promoting muscle movement.

**Expected outcomes.** The following results should be seen in the burn patient during the acute period of hospitalization after proper intervention:

- Infection-free granulation tissue forms on burn sites.
- Graft sites and donor sites are free of infection.
- No pressure sores are formed.
- Patient consumes full diet without nausea or distention.
- Temperature, pulse, and respirations are normal.
- Patient has full range of motion in the burn area.
- Self-esteem is intact.
- Patient expresses concerns regarding changes in body image.

## The Rehabilitation Period

The patient with major burns usually leaves the hospital with the prospect of a long period of rehabilitation. In addition to further pain, grafting, and reconstruction in the years ahead, the burn victim must deal with the social and emotional trauma of a profoundly altered body image and the changes in social relationships that may result. Many burn victims are young children and are particularly affected by the social stigma of being "different" from their peers. Long-term physical, so-

cial, and psychologic therapy and the financial burdens that these services impose require careful coordination and planning by the burn unit staff before discharge.

At the time of discharge a number of factors must be considered to smooth the transition. These are not solely nursing responsibilities, but the nurse may need to coordinate home care activities. Discharge planning should include consideration of the following areas (Box 41-3):

- *Emotional-adjustment.* The patient and family may experience problems during the rehabilitative period. If the hospital social worker does not intervene, the nurse should arrange for psychologic follow-up.
- *Dressing procedures.* Instructions and supplies should be provided if the family is to continue changing dressings at home. What seems simple in the hospital setting may be problematic in the patient's kitchen or bathroom, so home care follow-up and supervision should be provided.
- *Exercise, splinting, and activities of daily living.* The nurse should observe the patient doing these activities before discharge. The physical therapist and/or occupational therapist may make follow-up visits to help with these programs.
- *Medications.* All medications, dosage, effects, and possible contraindications should be fully explained to the patient and family, and their level of understanding should be evaluated.
- *Return visits and phone numbers for problems.* The patient should be given written instructions for scheduling follow-up care. Arrangements for transportation should be made before discharge. Phone numbers of burn unit personnel should be given to the patient for use in case of questions or problems.
- *Home care or community agency follow-up.* If the hospital does not have a follow-up procedure, arrangements should be made with a community home care agency to provide these services.

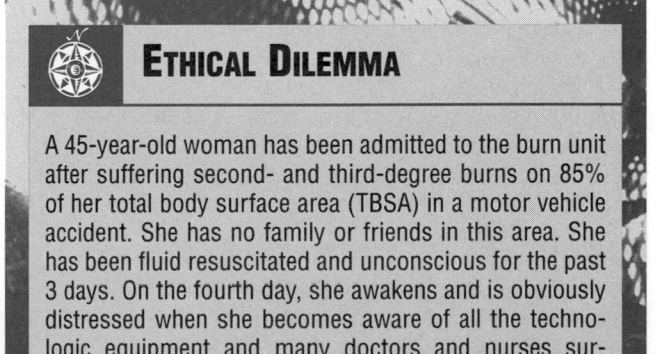

### ETHICAL DILEMMA

A 45-year-old woman has been admitted to the burn unit after suffering second- and third-degree burns on 85% of her total body surface area (TBSA) in a motor vehicle accident. She has no family or friends in this area. She has been fluid resuscitated and unconscious for the past 3 days. On the fourth day, she awakens and is obviously distressed when she becomes aware of all the technologic equipment and many doctors and nurses surrounding her bed. She frantically shakes her head to her primary nurse signifying, "Stop! No more!"

How would you analyze and resolve this dilemma?

BOX 41-3

## DISCHARGE INSTRUCTIONS FOR BURN PATIENT

We on the burn team are happy to see that you are able to go home. To ensure you the speediest possible recovery, it is important that you are able to care for yourself and recognize problems that may interfere with your complete recovery.

If any of the following occur, please call the hospital and ask for the Burn Clinic. The nurse will be able to assist you.

1 Healed area breaking open. Cover with clean dressing.
2 Formation of blisters.
3 Signs of infection:
   a Fever, temperature over 37.2° C (99° F).
   b Redness, pain, swelling, hardness, or warmth in or around wound or any other part of body.
   c Increased or foul-smelling drainage from wound.
4 Problems with your Ace bandages or Jobst garment such as improper fit, formation of blisters, or opening of healed area underneath.

Your first clinic appointment will be on _____. If a family member can come with you, they can register for you, and you may go to the Burn Clinic waiting room.

### BATHING

Bathing or showering daily in your usual manner cleans the wounds, especially the ones that are still open.

1 Check the water and be sure to adjust the temperature to a warm and comfortable level. Your skin is more sensitive to extra heat or cold and can be easily injured.
2 Wash gently with a clean, soft washcloth, using a mild detergent soap such as Dreft or Ivory Snow, approximately 2 tsp. Be careful not to rub too hard so as not to disturb the grafted areas. Avoid harsh or deodorant soaps.
3 Rinse skin thoroughly after washing.
4 Dry thoroughly.
5 Apply specific dressing as instructed.

### CARE FOR BURN WOUND

These are your guidelines for the care of your burn wound. During this time, look at the involved areas and note if there are any changes that need to be reported.

1 Wash hands.
2 Remove dressing and dispose in paper bag or wrap in newspaper.
3 Wash hands.
4 Wash open area with gauze using solution of Dreft (or Ivory Snow) and water. Add 1 tbsp Dreft to a basin of water; 2 tbsp Dreft, if you use the bathtub. Use a clean towel and washcloth with each dressing change.
5 Rinse skin well.
6 Wash hands.
7 Apply dressings as described below.
8 Wear gloves. Wash basin or bathtub with a disinfectant such as Lysol.
9 Wash hands.

### CARE OF CLOTHING

When you are discharged, you may find that healed burn areas are sensitive to harsh detergents, fabric softeners, and clothing dyes. If you are sensitive, we suggest the following:

1 Launder new clothing before use by machine or hand with Dreft or Ivory Snow.
2 Rinse clothes twice.
3 Do not use fabric softeners.
4 If you have open burns or a healed area that opens, wash all clothes separately from other family members.
5 Scarlet red ointment will permanently stain clothing.
6 If dyes used in clothing cause irritation, wear white articles.

### ACE BANDAGES

You have been taught to put on your own Ace bandages while in the hospital, but if you have a problem with this, please notify the Burn Clinic. It is also important that you know how to care for them and understand problems that occur.

1 If they are too loose, they will be ineffective and must be rewrapped.
2 If they are too tight, they will cause discomfort, numbness, tingling, and puffiness and must be rewrapped.
3 They must be worn for a long period of time, probably 6-12 months to be effective, so please do not stop wearing them until your doctor tells you.
4 To care for your Ace bandages:
   a Hand wash with Dreft or Ivory Snow in cold water.
   b Towel dry.
   c Lay flat or place over rod or clothesline.
   d Do *not* use clothespins.

### JOBST GARMENT

You have been taught to put on your Jobst garment while in the hospital, but if you have a problem with this, please notify the Burn Clinic. It is also important that you know how to care for it and understand problems that can occur.

1 If it is too loose, it will be ineffective and you will require a new garment.
2 If it is too tight, it will cause discomfort, numbness, and tingling. Do not wear it if this occurs, but notify the Burn Clinic as soon as possible.
3 To care for your Jobst garment:
   a Hand wash with Dreft or Ivory Snow in cold water.
   b Towel dry.
   c Lay flat or place over rod or clothesline.
   d Do *not* use clothespins.

Courtesy Burn Service, MetroHealth Medical Center, Cleveland. From Phipps WJ et al: *Medical-surgical nursing: concepts and clinical practice,* ed 5, St Louis, 1995, Mosby.

# KEY CONCEPTS

➤ Burns are classified by type or source as thermal, electrical, radiation, or chemical.

➤ Burns are classified by severity as minor, moderate, or major, depending on thickness (depth of the burn injury) and extent (amount of body surface involved).

➤ Extent of burn injury is estimated by either the Rule of Nines or the Lund and Browder Chart. The latter is more accurate because it accounts for differences in age.

➤ The care of the burned patient is divided into three phases: the emergent period, the acute period, and the rehabilitative period.

➤ The priorities in the emergent phase of burn care are to prevent further injury and maintain or provide a patent airway, stop bleeding, and treat burn shock.

➤ The goals of treatment during the acute phase of burn care are to relieve pain, prevent infection, heal open wounds, restore normal functioning and appearance, preserve emotional equilibrium, and return to the social and work environment.

➤ A severe burn wound that has no dermis remaining to allow tissue regeneration will require skin grafting. An autograft from the patient's own skin is the only graft that will not be rejected. Other grafts are used on a temporary basis until the patient's condition allows autografting.

➤ A full-thickness graft removes epidermis and dermis and is used for reconstruction. A split-thickness graft leaves some dermis and allows that site to heal. A specially made elastic stocking or Jobst garment may be worn for 2 years to compress the graft site, increase circulation, and prevent contractures.

➤ The rehabilitation period can be lengthy and may include further pain, cosmetic grafting, and reconstruction. The burn victim must deal with the social and emotional trauma of a profoundly altered body image and with the changes in social relationships that may result. Long-term physical, social, and psychologic therapy are required and must be coordinated before the patient is discharged.

# CRITICAL THINKING EXERCISES

1. Describe the interventions that the nurse may use in the management of pain in the burn patient.
2. Develop a list of the signs and symptoms that the patient experiences in the emergent phase of burn injury and relate them to the pathophysiologic changes in that phase.
3. Explain the reasons for the use of hydrotherapy for the burn patient.
4. Describe the additional dangers that exist with circumferential burns.

## REFERENCES AND ADDITIONAL READINGS

Baker RAU: Degree of burn, location of burn, and length of hospital stay as predictors of psychosocial status and physical functioning, *J Burn Care Rehab* 17(4):327-333, 1996.

Bayley EW: Wound healing in the patient with burns, *Nurs Clin North Am* 25(1):205-222, 1990.

Beare PG, Myers JL: *Adult health nursing,* ed 3, St Louis, 1998, Mosby.

Bryant RA: *Acute and chronic wounds: nursing management,* St Louis, 1992, Mosby.

Burgess MC: Initial management of a patient with extensive burn injury, *Crit Care Nurs Clin North Am* 3(2):165-179, 1991.

Calistro AM: Burn care basics and beyond, *RN* 56(3):26-32, 1993.

Dyer C: Burn wound management: an update, *Plastic Surg Nurs* 8(1):6-12, 1988.

Greenhalgh DG: The healing of burn wounds, *Derm Nurs* 8(1):13-23, 1996.

Hill MJ: The skin: anatomy and physiology, *Dermatol Nurs* 2(1):13-17, 1990.

Kinzie V, Lace C: What to do for the severely burned, *RN* 43:47-51, 1989.

Marvin JA: Burn nursing history: the history of burn care, *J Burn Care Rehab* 14(2pt2):252-256, 1993.

Phipps WJ et al: *Medical-surgical nursing: concepts and clinical practice,* ed 5, St Louis, 1995, Mosby.

Taddiono TE et al: A survey of wound monitoring and topical antimicrobial therapy practices in the treatment of burn injury, *J Burn Care Rehab* 11(5):423-427, 1990.

Trofino RB: *Nursing care of the burn-injured patient,* Philadelphia, 1991, FA Davis.

Walther PH: Burn wound management, *AACN Clin Issues Crit Care Nurs* 4(2):378-387, 1993.

Weber JM, Thompkins DM: Improving survival: infection control and burns, *AACN Clin Issues Crit Care Nurs* 4(2):414-423, 1993.

# CHAPTER 42

# Men's Reproductive Health

## STRUCTURE AND FUNCTION OF THE REPRODUCTIVE SYSTEM

The major function of the reproductive system is to create new life. The reproductive system includes the external **genitalia** and the internal organs associated with reproduction. Sexual and reproductive development are influenced by the endocrine system, and the nervous system is involved in human sexual response.

The male reproductive organs include the penis, **testes,** vas deferens, **seminal vesicles,** and accessory glands. The penis and the **scrotum** are the external genital organs of the male. The internal structures or organs include the testes **(gonads)** and seminiferous tubules, **epididymis,** ductus deferens (vas deferens), seminal vesicles and ejaculatory ducts, urethra, **prostate gland,** and bulbourethral glands **(Cowper's glands).** The penis is comprised mostly of erectile tissue that is divided into three sections: two corpora cavernosa and one corpus spongiosum. The penis is the primary organ of sexual pleasure in the male. It also contains the urethra (Figure 42-1). The urethra is a long channel that runs from the floor of the bladder through the corpus spongiosum to the external opening called the *urinary meatus.* The meatus is normally found at the end of the penis in the center of the **glans penis,** which is a bulging structure covered by a loose, retractable skin called the **prepuce,** or foreskin. The upper section of the urethra passes through the center of the prostate gland. The prostate secretes an alkaline

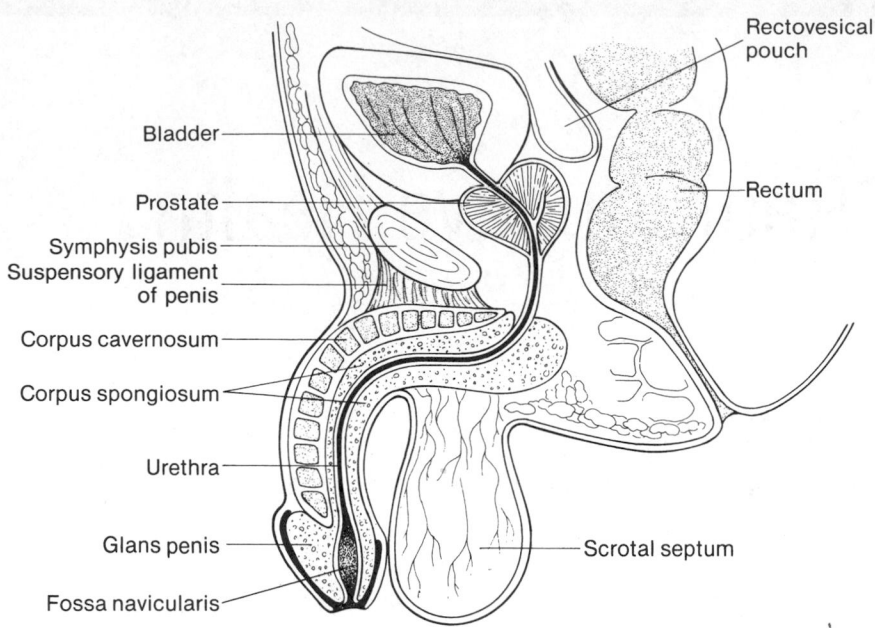

**Figure 42-1**  Male reproductive organs.

fluid that is transported by ejaculatory ducts that pass through it.

The testes are enclosed in and supported by the scrotum. Their location outside of the body allows them to maintain the sperm at a temperature lower than the rest of the body, which is essential for fertility. The testes produce **sperm** and **testosterone.** As sperm are produced, they collect in the epididymis, located along the upper side of the testes. The sperm are transported through the vas deferens to the ejaculatory ducts, where they are mixed with fluids from the seminal vesicles and the prostate gland to form **semen.**

Penile erection is controlled by the central, autonomic, and somatic nervous systems working together. The erection is caused by engorgement of the erectile tissue with blood. During coitus the seminal fluid and sperm are ejaculated into the upper urethra near the prostate and travel through the penis and into the vagina.

The breasts of the male do not contain the milk-producing glands or the subcutaneous and fatty tissue found in the female breast but do contain a small amount of glandular tissue. This glandular tissue is located under the nipple area.

# NURSING ASSESSMENT OF MEN WITH REPRODUCTIVE SYSTEM PROBLEMS

The history is a particularly important part of the assessment of the reproductive system. The nurse must be aware that the patient and his partner may be reluctant to discuss sexual habits with a nurse. This is particularly true of older couples and people who live in conservative parts of the country. Some religions and cultures may have taboos against discussing sexual matters. The nurse needs to be sensitive to the patient's needs in this area of the history taking.

Many factors affect men's reproductive health. A careful history should include patient's exposure to environmental or occupational chemicals, a medication review, and a medical history for conditions that may affect reproductive health. A history of vascular, neurologic, respiratory, and endocrine disorders may have an affect on the patient either by the direct disease process or by the treatment modalities used to control the disease.

If the patient's reading and writing levels are adequate, he is often provided with a form so that he may write out his own history. In other cases the nurse must be able to get the history verbally from the patient. In all cases the nurse's questions must be tactful and clear so that a complete sexual history can be obtained (Box 42-1).

Male patients must be assessed for signs and symptoms of prostate enlargement. Signs include (1) difficulty in voiding, (2) reduced urine stream pressure, (3) difficulty in starting or stopping the urine stream, (4) a feeling of bladder fullness after voiding, or (5) dribbling of urine. The nurse should also determine whether there has been any change in the size of the testes and whether there is any pain during voiding.

When assessing sexual functioning, the nurse should know that chronic illnesses such as hypertension, arthritis, and diabetes, as well as medication therapy

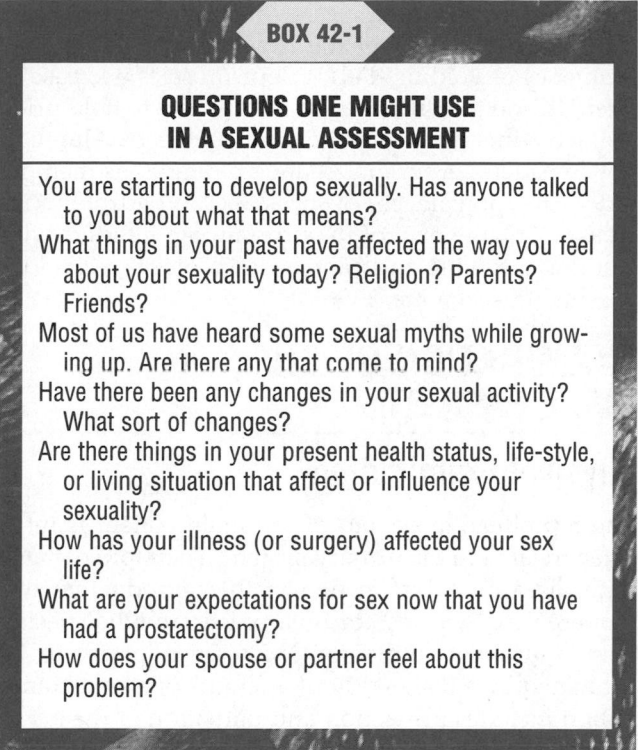

## QUESTIONS ONE MIGHT USE IN A SEXUAL ASSESSMENT

You are starting to develop sexually. Has anyone talked to you about what that means?

What things in your past have affected the way you feel about your sexuality today? Religion? Parents? Friends?

Most of us have heard some sexual myths while growing up. Are there any that come to mind?

Have there been any changes in your sexual activity? What sort of changes?

Are there things in your present health status, life-style, or living situation that affect or influence your sexuality?

How has your illness (or surgery) affected your sex life?

What are your expectations for sex now that you have had a prostatectomy?

How does your spouse or partner feel about this problem?

can decrease sexual desire and sexual ability. Many individuals who take antihypertensives such as propranolol (Inderal) and methyldopa (Aldomet) may find that they have a diminished libido. Men may have difficulty establishing an erection. The nurse should inform these individuals that their illness or medication may affect sexual desire and performance and that they should notify the physician if problems occur. Many times a solution to the problem can be found, such as lowering the dose or changing the medication.

The nurse should ask about the presence of any unusual discharge from the penis and any itching or lesions on the genitalia. Changes in the breast also should be documented. The breasts of the male may enlarge in response to hormonal changes during puberty or certain diseases. Medications such as digoxin also may cause breast enlargement. This abnormal enlargement is referred to as *gynecomastia.* Pain during intercourse (dyspareunia) or sexual dysfunction also should be investigated.

Topics such as reproductive health and sexual function or dysfunction are not easily approached without establishment of a good rapport between the nurse and the patient. The nurse may use the patient's self-history to facilitate discussion and gather pertinent information. The self-history may be one that the patient has already filled out, or it may be a self-history form that the nurse helps the patient fill out. In either case the indication of sexual problems in a self-history allows the patient to take the initiative and gives the

nurse the opportunity to verbalize and assess these areas. Patients differ greatly in the degree of openness with which they will discuss symptoms related to reproductive and sexual function. This method gives the patient the opportunity to set the pace.

# PHASES OF REPRODUCTIVE FUNCTION THROUGHOUT THE LIFE CYCLE

## Puberty

**Puberty** is the period during which the body prepares for reproductive ability. In males, puberty begins at about age 12, and secondary sex characteristics begin to make their appearance then. The size of the external reproductive organs increases, axillary and pubic hair grow, and the voice deepens.

With the increase in size of the sexual organs in the male at puberty, continuous production of sperm begins in the testes in response to the follicle-stimulating hormone (FSH) secreted by the anterior pituitary. When the reproductive system begins to function, the male experiences nocturnal seminal emissions (NSEs), or wet dreams, usually around age 14. NSEs are a physiologic benchmark of puberty in males, and they are characterized by a release, or ejaculation, of semen during sleep. The muscles of the body become larger and give the male a more mature appearance.

All children need preparation for puberty through sex education. From the moment of birth, infants begin to respond to and reflect the attitudes of others who care for them. Parents are usually the most influential caretakers during the developing years, so they have a great impact on their children's attitudes toward sexuality. Young children are curious and need direct, truthful answers to their questions. Although sex education in schools still arouses controversy, it is generally being accepted and incorporated into elementary and junior high school curricula. Often it is the school nurse or health teacher who is requested to teach basic sex education.

## Sexual Role Behavior

At each stage of physical and emotional growth there are learned skills that are related to behavior patterns associated with the particular sexual role. Any condition or situation that interferes with the mastery of these skills may affect the development of sexual role behavior, but the process continues and evolves throughout the lifetime of an individual.

Sexual role or gender role is the public expression of behavior that implies masculinity or femininity. *Gender identity* is defined as the private or personal experience of one's maleness or femaleness. It is usually, but not always, congruent with the individual's gender or biologic sex. The development of gender identity and sexual role behavior is a complex process influenced by biologic, psychologic, and social factors.

Gender identity begins with the biologic event of conception, when the X or Y chromosome from the male parent combines with an X chromosome from the female parent. An XY pair of chromosomes influences the undifferentiated gonad of the embryo to become a male at a gestational age of approximately 6 weeks, whereas an XX pair of chromosomes differentiates the gonad as a female at approximately 12 weeks' gestation. If the fetus develops testes, two hormonal secretions of the testes initiate the masculinization of the external genitalia. The first hormone, müllerian-duct inhibiting factor, suppresses development of the uterus, fallopian tubes, and upper vagina. The second hormone, testosterone, promotes the growth of the wolffian ducts, from which develop the internal male reproductive structures and external genitalia. The appearance of the external genitalia is the next factor in the development of sexual role behavior. The parents tailor child-rearing practices in accordance with their perception of a daughter or son. The child eventually becomes aware of his or her body, including genitalia. The child's body and the responses of others to it influence juvenile gender identity.

At puberty the production of hormones affects sexual desire and further development of the genitals. These changes at puberty, combined with social influences, determine adult gender identity. Gender identity and sexual identity are sometimes the same, but sexual identity is also used to indicate sexual orientation (e.g., heterosexual, homosexual, and bisexual).

## Climacteric

Climacteric occurs in males but is usually less pronounced than in women, and many men will exhibit no symptoms. Climacteric in males refers to the midlife changes that take place in the body both physiologically and psychologically. It is the normal pattern of reproductive aging or changes in men, which is different from that in women. It begins at about age 45 and continues until the man is 80 to 90 years of age. Some men may associate their approaching retirement with a loss of sexual power. Although sperm production may diminish, it does not stop completely. Some men do experience flushing and chills and may exhibit psychologic symptoms.

## Age-Related Changes

With age, bladder capacity decreases, involuntary bladder contractions or spasms increase in frequency, and urine production increases at night. These changes can increase feelings of the urgency to void and the frequency of voiding. Pelvic floor muscles decrease in strength and tonicity, affecting the ability to hold urine in the bladder and to control the sphincters. Although not considered a normal change of aging, as men get older the prevalence of prostatic hypertrophy increases. Enlargement of the prostate can interfere with bladder emptying and can cause involuntary bladder spasms (Lueckenotte, 1996).

# EXAMINATION OF THE MALE PATIENT

## Physical Examination

The reproductive system of the male patient is intricately related to the urinary system. Therefore patients with disease or dysfunction of the reproductive system are usually cared for by a physician who specializes in urology (urologist). Most men prefer to be examined by a male without a female present. Examination includes inspection and palpation of the external genitalia for abnormalities of structure, for signs of infection such as discharge and swelling, and for skin lesions. The penis is inspected for the presence and position of the urinary meatus. In the uncircumcised male the prepuce, or foreskin, must be retracted and the glans examined. If the foreskin does not retract easily, the patient may have **phimosis** (a tight prepuce that cannot be retracted).

The scrotum should be examined for size, symmetry, and the presence and size of both testes. The testes are also examined for masses, swelling, and movability. Examination often finds that the left testis is lower than the right, and this is normal. The scrotum contracts and becomes smaller when cold, so it is easier to examine the testes when the scrotum is relaxed. For this reason, men are advised to examine the testes monthly while in a warm tub or shower. Routine self-examination is of great value in early detection of testicular cancer and is recommended as a monthly procedure for all men age 15 and older.

The prostate gland is examined through the rectum by digital rectal examination. A gloved and lubricated finger is inserted into the rectum to palpate the prostate and determine its size, shape, and consistency.

Breasts of the male are examined for enlargement, lesions, discharge, and masses. The incidence of breast cancer in males is less than 1%, but men should be instructed to observe and report any discharge, masses, or changes in size, shape, and color of the breast and nipple area.

If sterility is suspected, several examinations may be performed. Among the first are an examination of semen to determine the presence and characteristics of spermatozoa and a physical examination to locate obstructions along the tubal route. A voided urine specimen may be collected after digital massage of the prostate gland for examination for cancer cells or tubercle bacilli. A biopsy of the prostate gland or the testes may also be done.

# TYPES OF DIAGNOSTIC PROCEDURES

## Laboratory Tests

The laboratory tests include urinalysis, a complete blood cell count, and usually a serologic test for syphilis. Blood levels of prostatic specific antigen (PSA), serum acid phosphatase, and alkaline phosphatase are reviewed. Elevated levels of PSA may indicate the presence of prostate cancer. The PSA levels do increase with age, thus more definitive diagnosis is needed. Two new tests of PSA have been added to help distinguish between normal and abnormal elevations. PSA density relates the prostate level to the prostate size, and the PSA velocity compares the rate of PSA levels over time (Black, Matassarin-Jacobs, 1997). The PSA tests are being used more and more as the accepted screening test for prostate cancer. The serum acid phosphatase and alkaline phosphatase tests are not as widely used any more.

Smears and cultures from urethral drainage are examined for both infectious and noninfectious organisms. Prostatic smears also may be obtained through massage of the prostate gland by a gloved finger placed in the rectum, after which a urine specimen is collected for laboratory examination.

Semen analysis is a relatively simple and inexpensive procedure for evaluating fertility in the male. It is also used to detect semen in a rape victim, to identify the blood type of an alleged rapist, or to prove sterility in a paternity suit. After a vasectomy, semen is analyzed to determine whether the surgical procedure was effective.

Semen may be collected after masturbation, after coitus, or by interrupting coitus. If the man prefers to collect the sample at home, the specimen must be protected from direct sunlight and extremes in temperature to avoid killing the sperm. When evaluating fertility, the physician may recommend refraining from intercourse from 2 to 5 days before collecting the specimen. The specimen must be brought in for examination within 3 hours after collection. The male is instructed either to masturbate and ejaculate into a clean container; to interrupt coitus just before ejaculating, withdraw the penis, and deposit the ejaculate in a container; or to collect the ejaculate during coitus by using a condom that has been washed with soapy water and dried to remove any spermicide. The entire specimen must be collected. The specimen is analyzed for volume of seminal fluid and for microscopically determined sperm count, sperm motility, and shape (morphology) of the sperm. When collecting semen from a female after rape or for evaluation of fertility, the physician uses a vaginal speculum and aspirates the specimen by using a small syringe without a cannula or needle.

## Diagnostic Studies

The nurse should be familiar with the following procedures and patient preparation for each so adequate patient teaching can occur.

Transrectal ultrasound of the prostate is performed to assess the size of the prostate gland. Scrotal ultrasound is used to assess for testicular abnormalities. Ultrasound can be used to distinguish between an abscess, a solid tumor, or cystic mass.

Computed tomography (CT) scanning is used to stage prostate and testicular cancer. CT scanning can be done with or without contrast medium. If contrast medium is used, the patient should be asked about allergies to such things as dyes and seafood. Magnetic resonance imaging (MRI) can be used to obtain a three-dimensional image of the prostate, seminal vesicles, and testicles.

A prostate biopsy removes a small amount of prostate tissue for cytologic examination. The biopsy sample can be obtained transurethrally, transrectally, or perineally. A cystoscope will be used if the biopsy is obtained transurethrally. Urodynamic assessments are used to find the cause of urinary frequency and decreased urinary stream in men. (See Chapter 38 for more information on urodynamic testing.)

# CONDITIONS AFFECTING THE MALE GENITALIA

## Congenital Malformation
### Epispadias and Hypospadias

Epispadias is a condition in which the male's urethra is open somewhere along the upper surface (dorsal) of the penis, whereas in hypospadias the urethra is open at some point along the undersurface (ventral) of the penis (Figure 42-2). Most cases of hypospadias are minor and require no corrective surgery. Severe urethral defects require extensive urethroplasty and plastic surgery.

### Cryptorchidism (Undescended Testicles)

During embryonic life the testes are in the abdomen, and during the last 2 months before birth they descend into the scrotum. In some instances they remain in the

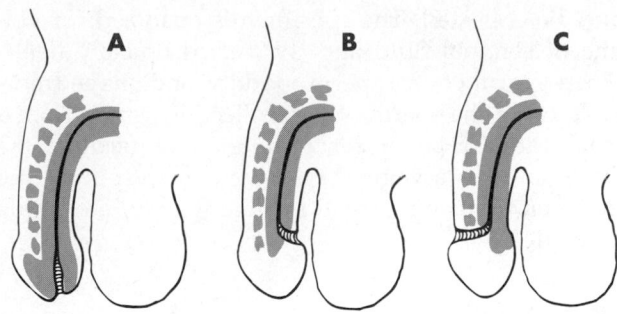

**Figure 42-2    A,** Normal urethral opening in the male. **B,** Hypospadias and, **C,** epispadias. (From Price SA, Wilson LM: *Pathophysiology: clinical concepts of disease processes,* ed 4, St Louis, 1992, Mosby.)

abdomen or the inguinal canal. One or both testicles may be involved. They sometimes descend during the first few weeks of life. By 1 year of age the incidence of undescended testes is less than 25%. If the testes fail to descend, treatment with certain hormones is usually initiated. If results are not secured, surgery may be done, but it is not always successful. Although the condition is fairly common in newborn infants, only a small number of adults are seen with an undescended testicle, which indicates that the condition is generally self-correcting.

### Ectopic Testes

*Ectopic testes* means that undescended testes are outside the normal path for descent. Because their location may subject them to greater risk of injury, intervention to place them into the scrotum is done early. Hormone treatment has no effect on ectopic testes.

## CONDITIONS AFFECTING THE TESTES AND ADJACENT STRUCTURES

### Epididymitis

The epididymis is a coiled tube approximately 20 feet long that lies on top of the testes in the scrotum and collects the spermatozoa. Any of several bacteria may cause an infection, including the streptococcus, staphylococcus, and colon bacilli. Infection of the epididymis **(epididymitis)** may occur after prostatitis or an infection of the urinary tract, and it often occurs as a complication of gonorrhea. The patient may be ill with fever, chills, headache, nausea, and vomiting. Painful swelling of the scrotum occurs, and it may be unilateral (involving one testes) or bilateral (involving

both testes). Treatment is to place the patient on a regimen of bed rest and support the scrotum. Heat or cold may be applied, and the appropriate antibiotic is given. If abscesses form, incision and drainage may be required.

### Orchitis

Orchitis, an infection of the testicles, may result from injury or from any one of several infectious diseases such as influenza, pneumonia, or gonorrhea. It may also occur as a complication of mumps. Symptoms include fever, nausea, and painful swelling of the testicles. The treatment is the same as that for epididymitis.

### Hydrocele and Varicocele

A **hydrocele** is a collection of fluid between the testes and their outermost covering, the tunica vaginalis testis. The condition is often associated with some other disease or injury. Several methods of treatment are used, including aspiration of the fluid; injection of a sclerosing solution, which causes the walls of the sac containing the fluid to adhere; and surgical removal of the sac, which is often the treatment method most likely to ensure cure. The scrotum should be supported with bandages, an athletic scrotal support, or a commercial suspensory.

A **varicocele** is a form of varicosity that involves the veins of the spermatic cord. It is usually a painless and harmless condition, but if it causes pain, the scrotum should be supported. If support fails to relieve the discomfort, ligation of the veins may be done.

### Tumors

Tumors of the male reproductive tract are usually malignant. They commonly occur in the testes, the prostate, and on the penis. Penile tumors account for a small percentage of cancer in men. They are usually the result of poor hygiene practices and are rarely seen in men who were circumcised as infants. Treatment involves removal of the cancerous tumor, and partial or total removal of the penis may be necessary.

Testicular tumors are the most common malignancy in men between the ages of 15 and 35 years of age. The incidence of testicular cancer is higher in men with cryptorchidism (undescended testes). It is less common in African-American and Asian men (Black, Matassarin-Jacobs, 1997). However, the disease does occur in the general population of men in most age groups, thus all men should be aware of the symptoms (Box 42-2). Regular testicular self-examination (TSE) is currently recommended as an effective method for detecting cancer in its early stages (Figure 42-3). All

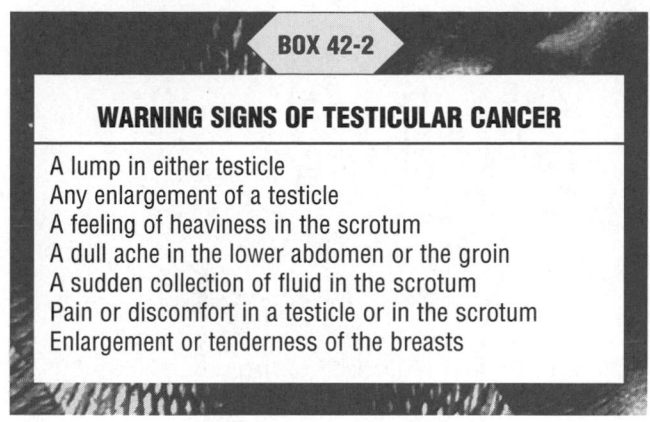

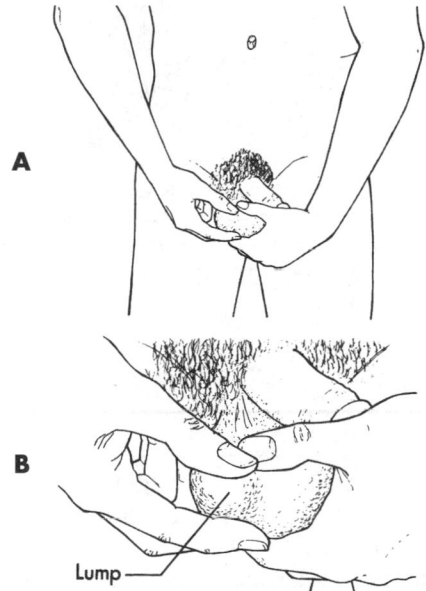

**Figure 42-3**    Testicular self-examination (TSE). **A,** Hold testis with both hands; palpate gently between thumb and forefingers. **B,** Abnormal lumps or irregularities should be reported to physician. Monthly TSE is recommended for all men age 15 and older and is most effective when performed during a warm bath or shower. (Modified from Phipps WJ et al: *Medical-surgical nursing,* ed 5, St Louis, 1995, Mosby.)

males age 15 and older should perform TSE once a month during a warm bath or shower.

Treatment for testicular carcinoma includes surgical removal of the testes (radical orchiectomy) and radiation therapy. After surgery, a prosthetic testis is placed in the scrotum. Chemotherapy is used in metastatic disease. A primary role for the nurse in caring for these patients would include providing emotional support. These men may express fear and anxiety about their sexual functioning, their ability to have children, and the outcome of cancer treatment. They may also experi-

ence alterations in role performance and may grieve over the cancer diagnosis and the upcoming treatments.

Postoperative care includes assessing the dressing over the scrotal wound, maintaining patency of the catheter if present, providing scrotal support, and maintaining the patient in a comfortable position. Men who have been treated for cancer in one testicle have approximately a 1% chance of developing cancer in the other testicle. They should be checked yearly by their doctors and should be encouraged to do TSE monthly.

## Phimosis

Phimosis is a condition in which the orifice of the prepuce is too small to allow retraction over the glans penis. The condition may be congenital but can result from local inflammation or disease. The condition is rarely severe enough to obstruct the flow of urine, but it may contribute to local infection because it does not permit adequate cleansing of the glans penis. The male may experience dyspareunia (painful intercourse) because of phimosis, urinary tract infection, or insufficient lubrication. A surgical procedure **(circumcision)** may be performed in which part of the foreskin is removed, leaving the glans penis uncovered. This reduces infections, allows for repair and healing of damaged tissue, and allows for additional lubrication during intercourse.

To prevent phimosis resulting from inflammation, circumcision is often performed on newborn infants before they leave the hospital. The procedure is also performed in a ritualistic ceremony, known as a *bris* in the Jewish religion. Uncircumcised boys and men should be taught how to retract the foreskin for cleansing of the glans penis as part of their daily hygiene.

## Torsion of the Spermatic Cord

A kinking and twisting of one of the spermatic cords also twists the enclosed artery and interrupts the blood flow to the testicle being supplied (Figure 42-4). This sequence of events can lead to ischemia of the testes and severe pain, and the pain may be aggravated by scrotal elevation. The patient with torsion of a spermatic cord is prepared for surgery, and the testicle is surgically fixed to the scrotal wall. If gangrene is present, the testicle is removed. The opposite testis (testicle) is usually anchored to its adjacent wall at the same time to prevent torsion of the spermatic cord on that side.

## Sterilization

When a man wishes to voluntarily become sterile (i.e., no longer father children), he can have a vasectomy

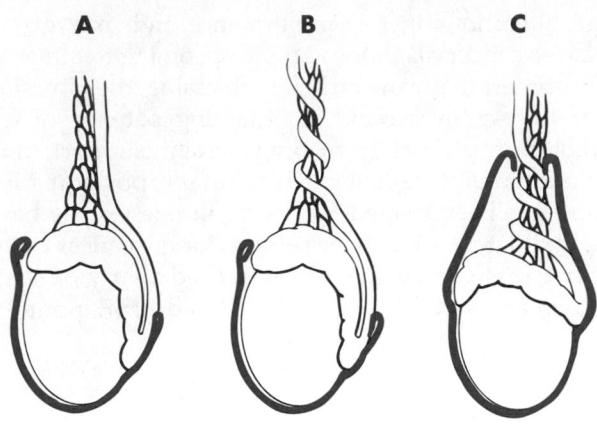

**Figure 42-4** Testicular torsion. **A,** Normal tunica vaginalis insertion. **B,** Extravaginal torsion. **C,** Intravaginal torsion with abnormally high vaginal insertion. (From Price SA, Wilson LM: *Pathophysiology: clinical concepts of disease processes,* ed 4, St Louis, 1992, Mosby.)

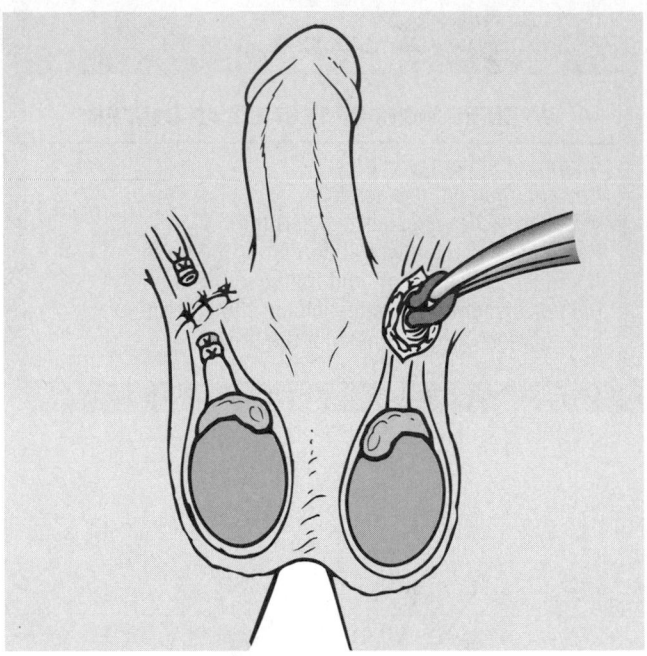

**Figure 42-5** Vasectomy procedure. The vas deferens is ligated or resected for the purpose of sterilization. (From Lewis SM, Collier IC, Heitkemper MM: *Medical-surgical nursing: assessment and management of clinical problems,* ed 4, St Louis, 1996, Mosby.)

performed. This surgery is the surgical ligation or resection of the vas deferens and is considered a permanent form of sterilization (Figure 42-5). In some cases a reversal of the vasectomy, a vasovasostomy, has been performed, but the return of fertility does not always occur.

After the vasectomy the patient should not notice any difference in the appearance or amount of ejaculate because its primary component is seminal fluid. An alternative form of contraception will have to be used for at least 10 ejaculations or 6 weeks. After this time the semen will be examined to be sure all of the sperm distal to the surgical site have been ejaculated. The testes continue to produce sperm cells, but they are absorbed by the body.

Sterilization by vasectomy does not affect any of the physiologic functioning of erection or ejaculation. There may be some psychologic adjustment because some men equate vasectomy with castration. This will affect their self-esteem and self-image. The nurse needs to be aware of this and discuss the procedure thoroughly with the patient before the surgery (Lewis, Collier, Heitkemper, 1996).

## Penile Ulceration

Ulceration on the penis may result from many sexually transmitted conditions, including syphilis, herpes virus, chancroid, and tuberculosis (see Chapter 14). Penile ulceration may also occur from poor hygiene habits of uncircumcised males. Examination should be made as soon as possible so that proper diagnosis and treatment may be started immediately.

# CONDITIONS AFFECTING THE PROSTATE GLAND

The prostate is a firm, partially glandular, partially muscular body that surrounds the urethra at the bladder neck. It has five lobes. Conditions affecting the prostate include prostatitis, cancer, and benign prostatic hypertrophy (BPH).

## Prostatitis

**Prostatitis** is a bacterial or viral infection of the prostate gland. It can occur in an acute or in a chronic form. Symptoms of acute prostatitis include fever, chills, lower back pain, perineal discomfort, dysuria, and urinary urgency and frequency. After the diagnosis is confirmed by culture of the urine and prostatic secretions, the patient is treated with antibiotics, rest, increased fluid intake, and analgesics.

Chronic prostatitis may affect as many as 80% of all men between the ages of 30 and 50. It may go undiagnosed for years until the patient seeks medical treatment at the onset of symptoms such as pain in the perineum, lower back pain, or persistent urinary tract infections. Treatment includes antibiotic therapy and periodic digital massages of the prostate to increase the flow of infected prostatic secretions. Sexual intercourse also helps increase prostatic secretions. The chronic inflammation may cause an increase in prostate size, which may result in obstruction of urinary flow requiring surgical correction.

Another form of prostatitis does not involve bacterial infection. It is a chronic prostatitis that is also called *prostatosis*. It may be caused by excessive consumption of alcohol or caffeine and may also be a psychologic problem in a man with sexual dysfunction. There is congestion in the prostate gland that is found on physical examination to be nontender and of normal consistency. The patient experiences mild urinary frequency and urgency, lower back pain, and discomfort in the rectum, urethra, and perineal area. The patient also may experience a moderate loss of libido. The symptoms are usually self-limiting, and treatment involves removing the cause of the problem.

## Cancer of the Prostate Gland

The prostate gland is the second most common site of cancer among men 55 to 74 years of age in the United States. It is the third leading cause of death from cancer in men of that age group. Prostate cancer is the most common type of cancer found in African-American men. It is catching up with lung cancer as the leading cause of cancer-related deaths in men of African descent. Prostate cancer tends to occur at an earlier age in African-American men, and by the time it is diagnosed, almost 50% of the patients in this group already have advanced disease. As a result of this delayed diagnosis, the survival rate among African-American prostate cancer patients is lower than in the overall group of men with prostate cancer (American Cancer Society, 1994).

Early detection, surgery, radiation therapy, hormone therapy, and chemotherapy drugs have improved the prognosis for prostate cancer during the last 15 years. Ninety-two percent of those with localized disease and 78% of those with metastatic disease survive 5 years or more (American Cancer Society, 1994).

Early detection of prostate cancer by routine rectal examination of prostate nodules can lead to early treatment. For this reason, all men over age 40 should have annual routine rectal examinations done by their physicians. The American Cancer Society recommends that men age 50 and older have an annual PSA blood test in addition to the rectal examination. If the PSA blood level is elevated, it is considered an indicator of possible prostate cancer.

Detection of firm nodules on the posterior lobe of the prostate indicates malignancy. The lesion may be the size of a marble before it can be palpated. Newer diagnostic techniques that use ultrasound can detect lesions as small as 2 mm. Early symptoms are rarely present, but the patient may complain of dysuria and frequent urination. Later the patient will experience a sciatic type of pain, urinary retention, and hematuria. The disease is usually far advanced by the time these symptoms appear (Gray, 1992). Laboratory findings in the advanced stages include an elevated serum acid phosphatase. Acid phosphatase is an enzyme that is normally present in large concentrations in the prostate gland. If metastatic carcinoma of the prostate gland ruptures the capsule surrounding the gland, the enzyme is released into the bloodstream. An elevated alkaline phosphatase indicates bony metastases.

If the diagnosis is made while the malignancy is still a small nodule within the gland and no metastasis has occurred, a radical resection of the prostate gland is usually curative (Gray, 1992). Radiation therapy involving implantation of seeds is an alternative to surgery for localized prostate cancer. However, when cancer of the prostate gland is extensive, treatment may be only palliative. The goal of treatment at this stage is to slow the growth rate of malignant cells and to provide relief from pain. Several procedures may be used, including cryosurgery (freezing prostatic tissues) and radiation therapy. Surgical removal of the testes (orchiectomy) eliminates the male sex hormones (testosterone) that contribute to growth of prostate cancer cells (Newman, 1996).

Hormone therapy is used to slow the growth of the prostate cancer. Estrogen therapy has been used in the past to control growth and to relieve symptoms of prostate cancer. This treatment is declining in use

## OLDER ADULT CONSIDERATIONS

Certain problems of the urinary tract and reproductive system are commonly found in the elderly male population. Many of the urinary problems are directly related to an enlarged prostate. Overflow incontinence, urinary tract infection, and urinary retention are three of the most common ones. Impotence can be related to medications that the elderly male may be taking for health problems such as cardiac ailments or hypertension. A careful voiding history and medication record is important when assessing urinary and reproductive problems in the elderly male. Fluid intake and output estimates are important to obtain because the patient who is dribbling urine may have limited his fluid intake in an attempt to control the problem on his own. This self-imposed fluid limitation may cause dehydration in the elderly.

because of the side effects. New therapies using leuprolide and goserelin that block androgen production at the pituitary level are being used more frequently. The medication is given monthly by subcutaneous injection (Newman, 1996).

## Benign Prostatic Hypertrophy

**Benign prostatic hypertrophy** is a common and treatable disease found in more than half of all men over the age of 50. It is simple nonmalignant enlargement of the prostate gland. As the gland enlarges, it presses the urethra and causes urinary symptoms to develop. The urinary stream begins to slow, and urination becomes frequent and painful, eventually progressing to complete urinary retention. The major complications of BPH are urinary retention and incontinence. Urinary retention can lead to urinary tract infections, kidney inflammation, septicemia, and acute renal failure (Morley, 1996). Most men have some symptoms by age 55, and many will eventually require surgery (transurethral resection of the prostate [TURP]) to remove blockage of the urethra.

Treatment options for BPH vary from doing nothing to performing surgical removal of the prostate gland. Symptoms can be relieved with medication (see Table 42-1). Procedures that are nonsurgical that are used to control the prostate gland growth include the use of laser to remove excess tissue transurethrally, stents and coils placed to hold the urethral passage open, heat to remove excess tissue, and balloon dilation to compress the excess tissue (Lewis, Collier, Heitkemper, 1996).

## Prostatectomy

The prostate gland may be removed by several methods, and the physician determines which method is best suited for the particular patient and his diagnosis. Nursing care is determined by the type of surgery (Box 42-3 and Figure 42-6).

Each situation will present certain special problems of nursing care. Additional problems may occur because most patients are men who are well past age 50 and who may have other diseases from degenerative changes.

### Preoperative Intervention

The patient is usually admitted to the hospital before surgery. Because of the urinary frequency, the patient should be shown the location of the bathroom and given a urinal on admission to the clinical unit.

Numerous laboratory tests are completed either before admission or upon admission to the hospital. Among the first are urinalysis and urine culture. These

---

**BOX 42-3**

### FOUR METHODS OF PROSTATECTOMY

1. Suprapubic prostatectomy is accomplished by an incision through the abdomen; the bladder is opened, and the prostate gland is removed with the finger from above.
2. Transurethral prostatectomy is done by approaching the prostate gland through the penis and bladder using a resectoscope, a surgical instrument with an electric cutting wire for resection and cautery, to cut the lobes away from the capsule.
3. Perineal prostatectomy requires an incision through the perineum between the scrotum and the rectum.
4. Retropubic prostatectomy is the method in which an incision is made into the abdomen above the bladder, but the bladder is not opened. The prostate gland is removed by making an incision into the capsule that encases the gland.

---

tests often indicate infection since one third of the patients with prostatic hypertrophy have infected urine because of urinary retention. Blood urea nitrogen and serum creatinine tests are done to determine renal function. Hemoglobin and coagulation time texts are done to evaluate the ability to withstand blood loss and to control bleeding. Acid phosphatase and alkaline phosphatase are done to determine metastases if malignancy is suspected. An intravenous pyelogram is done to rule out renal mass or other abnormalities. An electrocardiogram, as well as a cystoscopic examination with biopsy, may also precede a prostatectomy. Because the prostate gland is extremely vascular, blood loss during surgery may be extensive. Blood typing and cross matching are usually ordered in case transfusion therapy is necessary. The nurse should be sure that the physician's orders for the various examinations are understood and that the request forms are properly completed and routed to the appropriate departments.

Catheter drainage may or may not be ordered before surgery, but accurate records of urinary output must be maintained and should include the interval and the amount of urine voided. Many patients, if properly instructed, can help with maintaining the record. This allows them to participate actively in their care, which improves their feelings of helplessness. An enema will be given the night before the surgery to reduce the risk of straining during defecation, which could cause bleeding after surgery. Antiembolism stockings will be applied the morning of surgery. Nursing diagnoses and interventions commonly seen in patients after prostatectomy appear in Box 42-4.

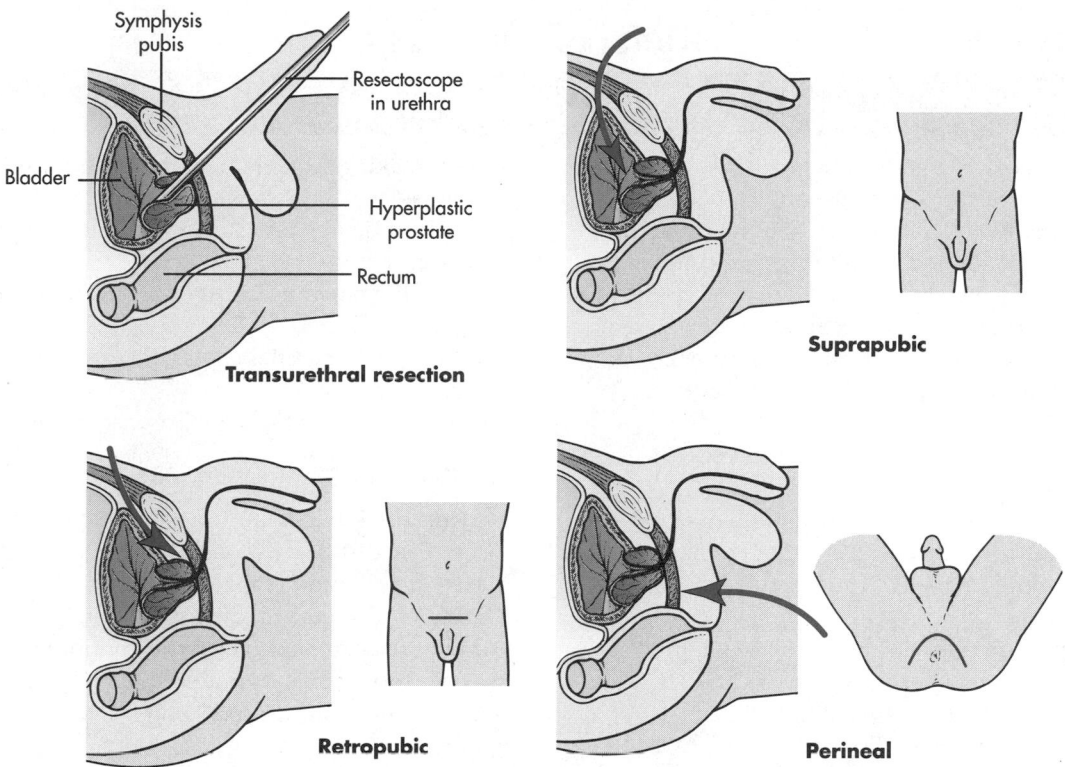

**Figure 42-6** Four types of prostatectomy. (From Lewis SM, Collier IC, Heitkemper MM: *Medical-surgical nursing: assessment and management of clinical problems,* ed 4, St Louis, 1996, Mosby.)

---

**BOX 42-4**

# NURSING PROCESS

## PROSTATECTOMY

**ASSESSMENT**

- Vital signs as indicated
- Incision and surgical dressing, if present
- Surgical drains and tubes
- Level of comfort
- Breath sounds and oxygenation
- Extremities for adequate tissue perfusion
- Fluid volume status
- Patency of urinary catheter
- Bleeding/clots from urinary catheter, hourly
- Mental status for confusion or disorientation
- Understanding of possible impact of surgery on sexual functioning
- Laboratory studies: hemoglobin, hematocrit, and electrolytes (especially sodium)

**NURSING DIAGNOSES**

- Anxiety related to uncertain outcome of surgery
- Pain related to bladder spasms or surgical incision
- Risk for altered peripheral tissue perfusion related to hemorrhage or deep vein thrombosis

- Risk for injury related to straining during defecation
- Risk for infection related to indwelling urinary catheter
- Risk for altered urinary function related to urinary retention from edema of urethra after catheter removal
- Risk for fluid volume excess related to excessive absorption of irrigating solution
- Risk for body image disturbance related to surgery involving reproductive organs
- Sexual dysfunction: impotence related to actual or perceived effects of prostatectomy on sexual functioning
- Sexual dysfunction: retrograde ejaculation and altered fertility related to surgical procedure

**NURSING INTERVENTIONS**

- Maintain NPO until a diet is ordered.
- Maintain IV fluids as ordered.
- Measure and record intake and output.

---

◁ **BOX 42-4** ▷　　　　　　　　**NURSING PROCESS**

## PROSTATECTOMY—cont'd

- Maintain patency of indwelling catheter.
- Instruct patient not to void around catheter.
- Maintain gentle traction for 24 hours if ordered.
- Administer continuous or intermittent catheter irrigation as ordered.
- After the catheter is removed, instruct the patient to perform perineal exercises: press buttocks together, hold as long as possible, relax and repeat 10 to 20 times per hour.
- Encourage the patient to void whenever he feels the urge.
- Inform the patient to expect dribbling of urine.
- Observe for urinary retention or incontinence.
- Maintain fluid intake of 2000 ml/day if not contraindicated.
- If dressings are present, change as needed to keep dry.
- Ambulate as ordered; avoid sitting.
- Administer antispasmodics and analgesics as ordered.
- Provide a low-residue diet during the healing period following perineal prostatectomy; provide a regular diet 24 to 48 hours postoperatively after other procedures as ordered.
- Administer a stool softener and mild laxatives as ordered.

- Avoid taking rectal temperatures and use of enemas.
- Apply antiembolism stockings while the patient is in bed.
- Allow the patient time to express his feelings and fears.
- Discuss the potential effects of surgery on sexual functioning.
- Refer the patient for sexual counseling as indicated.

### EVALUATION OF EXPECTED OUTCOMES

- Meets discharge criteria for the postsurgical patient (see Box 20-10)
- Hematocrit and hemoglobin stable
- Urinary drainage reddish-pink to light pink 24 hours postoperatively with continuous irrigation; cherry red and clear with intermittent irrigation; urine clear in 7 to 10 days
- Free of bladder spasms
- Absence of pain and pallor in lower extremities
- Absence of symptoms of fluid and electrolyte imbalance
- Maintains self-esteem as evidenced by attention to personal hygiene and appearance
- Verbalizes fears, concerns, and feelings

## Postoperative Intervention: TURP

A TURP has three major advantages: the patient is ambulatory soon after the surgery, recovery is generally rapid, and a shorter hospitalization is required. Postoperatively the patient will have a Foley catheter connected to continuous closed-bladder irrigation (CCBI, or CBI) to reduce clot formation (Figure 42-7). Gentle traction may be applied to the catheter by taping it against the thigh. This action pulls the catheter balloon down against the bladder and helps control bleeding (Figure 42-8). The irrigation system should be assessed every hour to be sure that patency is maintained and obstruction is prevented. Closed drainage with intermittent irrigation by 20 to 30 ml normal saline is sometimes used, but clots are more likely to form and obstruct the catheter or cause painful bladder spasms. The patient should be advised not to try to void around the blocked catheter because doing so will contribute to bladder spasm. The patient must be observed closely for hemorrhage, which is always a pos-

sible complication. Careful monitoring of the catheter drainage will alert the nurse if hemorrhage occurs.

When CCBI is used to clean the bladder, the drainage is expected to be reddish-pink to light pink within 24 hours after surgery. Without continuous irrigation the urine will be cherry red but clear. A deeper color indicates hemorrhage. Bright red drainage with numerous clots and viscous consistency accompanied by a falling blood pressure indicates arterial bleeding. This usually requires that the patient return to the operating room for further cautery of blood vessels to control hemorrhaging.

Venous bleeding is more common, causing the urinary drainage to be darker and less viscous than arterial bleeding. It can usually be controlled by applying traction to the catheter so that the ballooned end inside the bladder applies pressure to the prostatic fossa (see Figure 42-7). This technique should be done by the physician but may be done by an experienced nurse who has been trained in the procedure. Traction is rarely maintained longer than 24 hours, and this limitation avoids trauma to the external urinary sphincter.

If continuous irrigation is not ordered or maintained, a blocked catheter may result, causing bladder distention and spasms. If drainage stops, the catheter is usually irrigated with a sterile catheter tip (Toomey)

syringe and sterile normal saline. If gentle suction dislodges clots or tissue remnants, irrigation should be repeated after the initial sterile saline instillation has drained. Irrigation should be repeated at least every 4 hours until the drainage is entirely free of clots. If the catheter will not clear, the urologist may need to remove it and insert another.

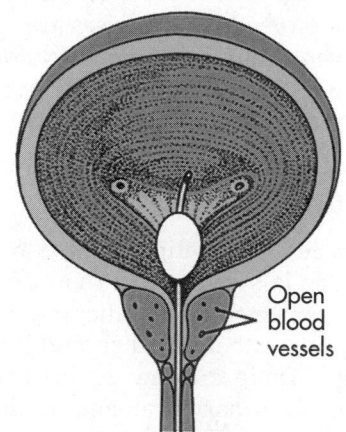

**Figure 42-7**  Continuous irrigation of the bladder requires a three-way Foley catheter that allows simultaneous infusion and drainage of irrigating solution (normal saline) through the bladder. The solution, infused rapidly into the bladder and drained into a bedside drainage bag, is assessed for evidence of excessive bleeding. The drainage bag should be emptied every 1 to 2 hours. (From Beare PG, Myers JL: *Adult health nursing,* ed 3, St Louis, 1998, Mosby.)

### NURSE ALERT

After prostatectomy, monitor for and report any signs of hemorrhage. Observe urinary drainage and report bright red bleeding in larger-than-expected quantities. Monitor blood pressure, pulse, and respirations, and report any abnormalities. Maintain catheter drainage. Do not perform any rectal treatments such as enemas or rectal temperatures (except B&O suppositories as ordered). Teach patient not to strain during bowel movements and to limit ambulation and chair sitting to 15 minutes three times a day.

As the urinary drainage clears, continuous irrigation is discontinued and straight drainage is maintained. The drainage may become deeper pink because there is no irrigation solution to dilute the color. With increased fluid intake, the color lightens and eventually returns to normal in 7 to 10 days.

Stool softeners and mild laxatives are ordered to prevent constipation. Straining must be avoided for 6 weeks after discharge to prevent pressure of the rectum against the prostatic fossa, which delays healing.

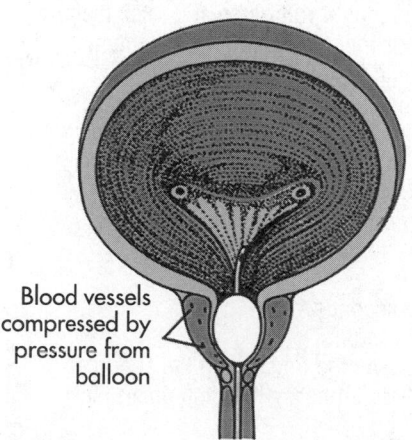

**Figure 42-8**  Gentle traction is maintained against the prostatic vascular bed to prevent excessive bleeding following transurethral resection. (From Beare PG, Myers JL: *Adult health nursing,* ed 3, St Louis, 1998, Mosby.)

Most complications are likely to occur in the first 24 hours postoperatively. Blood pressure should be taken every 2 hours. Temperature should be taken every 4 hours; a temperature above 38.3° C (101° F) by mouth indicates infection. A pulse rate below 60 beats per minute should be reported because bradycardia can result if spinal anesthesia was used for a prolonged time. An elevation in pulse accompanied by a drop in blood pressure indicates hemorrhage and shock.

The patient is ambulated on the first postoperative day. He should avoid sitting because it increases intraabdominal pressure and promotes bleeding. Ambulation should be increased to frequent short walks, and the patient should wear antiembolism stockings while in bed. He should be helped to turn and deep breathe at frequent intervals. When the catheter is removed, the patient will normally void small amounts (approximately 15 to 30 ml), and the amount of each voiding will remain small until the bladder is stretched to normal capacity.

## Patient and Family Teaching

Because the bladder capacity is small, the patient should void whenever he has the urge for at least 2 months. This will prevent pressure of a full bladder on the surgical site before it is fully healed. The patient may experience dysuria, which may be helped by warm tub baths. Some patients have difficulty voiding, and others are incontinent after the catheter is removed. Incontinence usually is caused by bladder

irritation and weakened sphincter muscles. Perineal exercises performed by tightening and releasing the gluteal muscles should improve control. Voiding problems usually disappear with time.

After discharge the patient should void whenever he has the urge, avoid straining during defecation, and avoid constipation by taking prescribed stool softeners and laxatives or by eating adequate fiber and fluids. Spicy foods should be avoided. The patient should be encouraged not to limit fluid intake to avoid urination. Fluid intake should be six to eight 8-oz glasses of fluids per day. Sexual activity can be resumed in 6 to 8 weeks. Erectile function should not be permanently affected but may be temporarily altered.

## Suprapubic Prostatectomy

When a suprapubic prostatectomy has been done, the surgeon may place some agent such as gauze packing or a hemostatic bag in the depressed area where the gland was located to prevent hemorrhage. In addition, there will be some provision for urinary drainage through the abdominal incision. Drains or tubes such as a cystostomy tube may be used. Not all urologists use this method. If only small drains are used, a ureterostomy bag may be used to collect urine and to keep the patient dry.

In other cases, large abdominal dressings may be used. The abdominal dressings may need to be changed often to keep the patient dry, and enclosing them in some type of impervious material may help. With any procedure used, the patient must be watched closely for hemorrhage.

The patient also will need medication for pain because bladder spasms may be severe and painful. Belladonna and Opium (B&O) rectal suppositories are often prescribed to prevent bladder spasms. The nurse should help and encourage the patient to turn often, and deep breathing exercises are especially important to prevent pulmonary complications. Ambulation for these patients is delayed. The catheter must be kept open and draining.

## Retropubic Prostatectomy

The patient recovering from a retropubic prostatectomy has less discomfort than do patients who have had prostatectomies by other methods. The patient has a retention catheter and should be observed for hemorrhage. There are few or no bladder spasms, and there is no urinary drainage on the abdominal dressing. If urinary drainage is noted on the abdominal dressing or if purulent drainage, fever, or increased pain with ambulation occurs, the physician should be notified. These symptoms may indicate deep wound infection or pelvic abscess.

---

### 👤 PATIENT/FAMILY TEACHING

**PERINEAL MUSCLE EXERCISES**
The patient should be taught to tighten and relax the perineal or pelvic floor muscles to strengthen them. The instructions should include the following:
1. Do 45 perineal muscle exercises every day.
2. Do the exercises in 3 sets: 15 at a time, 3 times a day.
   - Do 15 lying down in the morning.
   - Do 15 standing up in the afternoon.
   - Do 15 sitting in the evening.
3. For each exercise:
   - Squeeze for 10 seconds.
   - Relax for 10 seconds.
4. Remember to relax all the muscles in the abdomen and continue to breathe normally when doing these exercises.

From Lueckenotte AG: *Gerontologic nursing*, St Louis, 1996, Mosby.

## Perineal Prostatectomy

Perineal prostatectomy involves removal of part or all of the prostate gland through a perineal incision. It may be performed because of BPH or for cancer of the prostate gland. When the surgery is for cancer, radical prostatectomy may be performed, removing the entire prostate gland including the capsule, seminal vesicles, and the adjacent tissue. The remaining urethra is anastomosed to the bladder neck. Because the internal and external sphincters of the bladder lie close to the prostate, the patient is likely to experience some degree of urinary incontinence. He will also be impotent and sterile. Both the patient and his sexual partner must be made aware of the consequences of radical prostate surgery.

A modified radical approach may also be performed for cancer of the prostate gland. In this procedure the nerves controlling erection are saved. Erectile function may be disturbed for 6 to 12 months, but most patients will eventually regain erection capabilities. This greatly improves the patient's outlook on the effects of the procedure. It is recommended only for well-localized prostatic lesions.

The preoperative preparation of the patient for perineal prostatectomy is essentially the same regardless of whether the underlying disease is benign or malignant. The bowel is prepared by giving a laxative and enemas. An antibiotic or sulfonamide drug is often given preoperatively, and only clear liquids are allowed on the day before surgery.

When the patient returns from surgery, he will have a retention catheter, which should be connected to sterile closed drainage. Extreme care should be taken to ensure that the catheter does not become blocked or displaced. There is less possibility of hemorrhage and bladder spasms in the perineal approach to the prostate gland. Urinary drainage that may appear on the perineal dressings will gradually decrease over a period of a few hours. In a perineal prostatectomy, temporary fecal incontinence may occur. The patient should be taught perineal exercises, and beginning them early will strengthen the rectal and urethral sphincter muscles. Patients who have had simple perineal prostatectomy for BPH have no problem with urinary control.

For some patients the catheter is removed in approximately 1 week, whereas for others it may not be removed for several weeks. The patient should be instructed to perform perineal exercises and to void whenever he feels the urge. All patients should receive at least 3000 ml of fluid daily. After the first 24 to 48 hours most patients, except for those recovering from a perineal prostatectomy, are allowed to eat solid food. During the immediate postoperative period the patient receives nothing by mouth. Liquids or a low-residue diet may be given later and should continue until there has been time for healing.

## Cryosurgical Ablation for Prostate Cancer

A new surgical procedure known as *cryosurgical ablation* has been performed since 1993 as an investigational procedure in cases of prostate cancer. It involves freezing the entire prostate gland and the portions of the seminal vesicles closest to the prostate. The prostate is turned into an iceball, whereas the prostatic urethra is maintained above core body temperature by irrigation with water heated to 44° C (110° F). The areas to be treated are located by the physician with transrectal ultrasound. Cryosurgical ablation is used as an alternative to radiation therapy for patients with localized tumors and for those whose medical condition contraindicates radical prostatectomy. If it is proven successful, this procedure could be used instead of the radical prostatectomy, which would leave the patient with fewer complications.

Cryosurgical ablation of the prostate is believed to cause the death of prostate cells by dehydration. Freezing the cells causes hypovolemia, and the reduced fluid in the cells results in concentrations of electrolytes in the cells high enough to reach toxic levels. As the freezing continues, the cell membranes rupture. Thermal shock causes cell protein to change in structure. Blood flow to the area ceases, and the result is vascular necrosis.

After cryosurgery, the bladder needs to be retrained. Urine drains through a suprapubic tube, which is inserted during surgery. On the first postoperative day the tube is clamped and the patient attempts to void when he feels the need. After voiding, the patient unclamps and drains the tube and measures any urine remaining in the bladder. Any urine obtained after voiding is called *postvoiding residual (PVR)* urine. Eventually, the amount of PVR will be minimal. The patient must be taught to care for the suprapubic

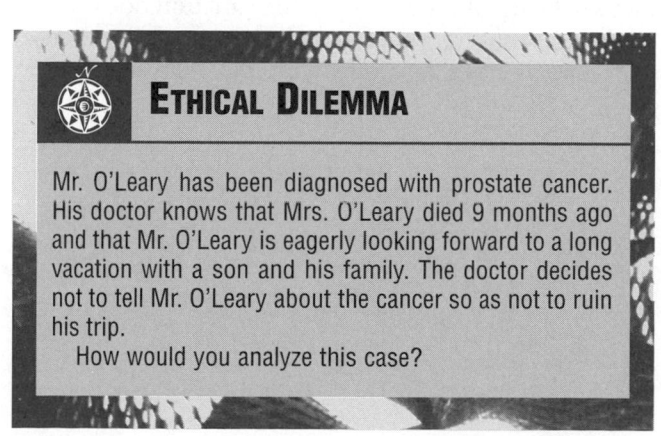

### ETHICAL DILEMMA

Mr. O'Leary has been diagnosed with prostate cancer. His doctor knows that Mrs. O'Leary died 9 months ago and that Mr. O'Leary is eagerly looking forward to a long vacation with a son and his family. The doctor decides not to tell Mr. O'Leary about the cancer so as not to ruin his trip.

How would you analyze this case?

catheter and site, to empty and measure PVR, to drink plenty of fluids, and to take stool softeners to avoid straining at stool. The patient can expect to be discharged on the second postoperative day, and he goes home with the suprapubic tube in place (Brenner, Krenzer, 1995).

## CONDITIONS AFFECTING ERECTILE FUNCTION

Any condition affecting erectile function causes the male to experience a period of impotence. Erectile dysfunction is the failure to achieve penile erection in a manner sufficient for successful intercourse. This condition has many causes, and the incidence tends to increase with age. It is estimated that 10 to 20 million men in the United States have erectile dysfunction (Skolnick, 1997). Hormonal disorders that disturb the hypothalamic-pituitary-gonadal circuit often cause erectile dysfunction. (Vascular disorders have a major effect on penile erection because it is a vascular event.) Both arterial and venous disorders can be responsible for erectile dysfunction. Neurologic disorders of erectile function are caused by conditions that affect the brain, spinal cord, or peripheral nervous system. Other causes include advanced syphilis, amyotrophic lateral sclerosis, and diabetes. Surgical procedures can compromise peripheral neural tissue or vascular erectile tissue in the penis. Radical prostatectomy is an example of a surgical procedure that may cause impotence. Trauma to the lower urinary tract and pelvis also can cause erectile dysfunction (Skolnick, 1997).

## METHODS FOR TREATING ERECTILE DYSFUNCTION

Treatment of erectile dysfunction is based on the cause of the impotence and is planned after a complete history and physical examination are done. The nurse should remember that sexual dysfunction might be a result of physiologic, psychologic, and sociocultural factors. Restoration of the erectile function does not remove underlying psychologic causes of impotence, nor does it have any effect on the man's ability to achieve orgasm or ejaculation. The female nurse must realize that the male patient may be embarrassed and hesitant to speak to or be examined by a female nurse.

Erectile dysfunction caused by hormonal abnormalities can be treated by medications. Exogenous **androgens** can be given orally or parenterally to correct this disorder. If infertility is also involved, a combination of drugs is used to treat both (Table 42-1 and Figure 42-9).

When erectile dysfunction is caused by vascular disorders, surgery can sometimes be done to correct or increase the blood supply to the penis. Vascular studies are done to identify the source of the vascular problems. Surgical correction of vascular erection problems has not been successful over the long term for these patients and other methods of treatment are generally used (Lewis, Collier, Heitkemper, 1996).

Some patients respond well to vasodilation medications. The patient is taught to inject a vasodilator, usually papaverine, into the corporal bodies of the penis. Side effects of injected vasodilators include sustained painful erection (priapism) and fibrous plaque development at the injection sites.

Other methods of treating erectile dysfunction make use of mechanical devices. One type is the vacuum pump device that uses suction to pull blood into the cavernous bodies (see Figure 42-9). To keep the blood in the penis and maintain the erection, a restrictive device is then placed at the base of the penis. Prosthetic devices can be surgically implanted in the corporal bodies on either side of the penis (see Figure 42-9). They are easy to use, but some devices are difficult to conceal in clothing. The main complications with these devices are infection and erosion of the device through the skin. Postoperative care includes assessing the penile or scrotal incision for infection and noting the amount and type of drainage during dressing changes. Penile and scrotal swelling usually lasts 3 to 5 days.

The patient who has had a penile implant should be advised that healing will proceed faster if he avoids strenuous exercise and sexual contact for at least 3 weeks. The patient should operate the device under direct supervision of his doctor to be sure that he is able to do it properly, and he should be instructed to promptly report any dysfunction in the device or any signs of infection.

**TABLE 42-1**

## Pharmacology of Drugs in Men's Reproductive Health

| DRUG (GENERIC AND TRADE NAME); ROUTE AND DOSAGE | ACTION/INDICATION | COMMON SIDE EFFECTS AND NURSING CONSIDERATIONS |
|---|---|---|
| **Diethylstilbestrol (DES)** **Route:** PO, IV **Dosage:** PO, 1-3 mg/day; IV, 500 mg-1 g/day initially until response is obtained (5 or more days), then 250-500 mg 1-2 times/wk | Hormone and antineoplastic agent used palliatively in advanced, inoperable metastatic prostate and breast carcinoma | Headache, edema, hypertension, intolerance to contact lenses, nausea, weight changes, breakthrough bleeding in females, dysmenorrhea, amenorrhea, testicular atrophy, impotence, acne, oily skin, gynecomastia, and breast tenderness; contraindicated in thromboembolic disease and undiagnosed vaginal bleeding; use with caution in renal, cardiac, and hepatic disease; may increase risk of endometrial carcinoma |
| **Finasteride (Proscar)** **Route:** PO **Dosage:** 5 mg once daily | Used in treatment of benign prostatic hyperplasia | Use with caution in hepatic impairment or obstructive uropathy; can cause impotence or decreased libido |
| **Papaverine (Cerespan, Pavabid)** **Route:** PO, IM, IV **Dosage:** PO, 100-300 mg 3-5 times daily; IM, IV, 30 mg initially, then 30-120 mg q 3 hr if necessary | Adjunct treatment with alpha-adrenergic blockers in the management of male impotence due to organic causes | Contraindicated if history of heart block; use with caution in glaucoma and in sickle cell, liver, and coagulation-defect diseases |
| **Prazosin (Minipress)** **Route:** PO **Dosage:** 1 mg 2-3 times daily initially (give first dose at bedtime); increase gradually to maintenance dose of 6-15 mg/day in 2-3 divided doses (not to exceed 20-40 mg/day) | Treatment for mild to moderate hypertension; also used in the management of urinary outflow obstruction in patients with BPH | Dizziness, drowsiness, headache, weakness, first-dose orthostatic hypotension, palpitations, and nausea; use with caution in renal impairment, angina, and with diuretics |
| **Terazosin (Hytrin)** **Route:** PO **Dosage:** 1 mg at bedtime, may be increased gradually to 5-10 mg/day | Antihypertensive used in the treatment of mild to moderate hypertension and in the management of outflow obstruction in patients with prostatic hypertrophy | Dizziness, weakness, headache, nasal congestion, and nausea |
| **Testosterone** **Route:** IM **Dosage:** 25-50 mg 2-3 times/wk | Used for treatment of hypogonadism in androgen-deficient males; also used for erectile dysfunction and as palliative treatment of androgen-responsive breast cancer | Edema, clitoral enlargement, change in libido, decreased breast size, acne, priapism, facial hair, oligospermia, impotence, and gynecomastia; contraindicated in males with breast or prostate cancer, hypercalcemia, or severe liver, renal, or cardiac disease |

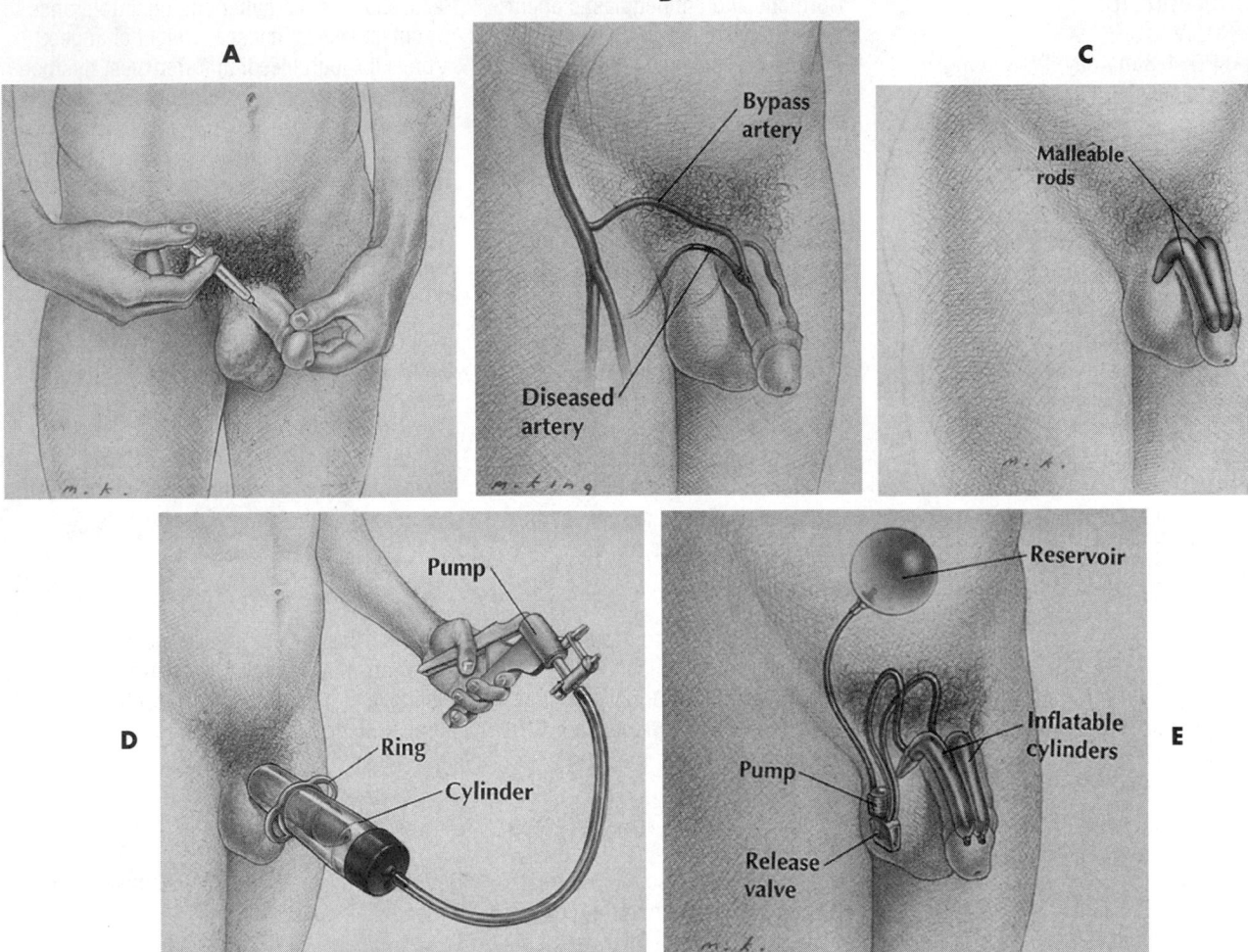

**Figure 42-9    A,** Self-injection therapy involves injecting a medication directly into the penis. This increases blood flow and causes an erection. **B,** A bypass operation can restore blood flow and sometimes cure erectile dysfunction. Unfortunately, it is rarely appropriate and long-term success has been disappointing. **C,** A semirigid implant is always erect but can be bent close to the body for concealment. **D,** With the vacuum device in place, blood can be drawn into the penis by means of a hand pump. This creates an erection. For intercourse, the ring is slipped to the base of the penis and the cylinder is removed. **E,** Inflatable implants consist of cylinders in the penis, a small pump in the scrotum, and a reservoir in the lower abdomen. When activated, the pump fills the cylinders with fluid from the reservoir. A small release valve permits the fluid to drain back into the reservoir after intercourse. (Courtesy of Mayo Clinic Health Letter with permission from Mayo Foundation for Medical Education and Research, Rochester, MN. In Lewis SM, Collier IC, Heitkemper MM: *Medical-surgical nursing: assessment and management of clinical problems,* ed 4, St Louis, 1996, Mosby.)

# NURSING CARE PLAN

## PATIENT HAVING SURGERY FOR IMPLANTATION OF PENILE PROSTHESIS

Mr. Bartlett is a 58-year-old male with a history of insulin-dependent diabetes for the last 20 years. He is entering the hospital for implantation of a penile prosthesis after a history of impotence for the last 2 years. His wife of 32 years accompanies him to the hospital. Additional medical data reveal that he has a history of hypertension controlled by medication. He does not drink alcohol and stopped smoking 15 years ago.

| Medical History | Psychosocial Data | Assessment Data |
|---|---|---|
| Transurethral resection of prostate for benign prostatic hypertrophy 1 year ago; no complications postoperatively | Lives locally with wife, in a two-story house with a small yard | Patient is alert and oriented × 3 |
| | | Afebrile |
| | | *Respiratory:* Lungs clear, able to demonstrate effective cough, rate 18-20, regular depth and rhythm |
| Follows ADA diet with good control | Has 4 adult children; two live locally; the other two are no more than 4 hours away | *Abdominal:* Soft, nontender, nondistended, bowel sounds present in all four quadrants. |
| Takes 15 units of regular insulin with 25 units of NPH insulin q AM | | Skin clear with no lesions present |
| | | *Cardiovascular:* Apical pulse 72-80, rate regular, pedal pulses palpable bilaterally |
| Takes methyldopa (Aldomet) 25 mg/day for his blood pressure | High school graduate and is retired from a local textile factory; wife works part-time at the library | **Laboratory data** |
| | | Hgb 14, Hct 42, electrolytes within normal limits, serum glucose 156 |
| No known allergies to food or drugs | Plays golf, fishes, and takes walks for recreation | Urinalysis and other laboratory data within normal limits |
| | | Chest x-ray and ECG within normal limits |

---

### NURSING DIAGNOSIS

Pain related to penile incision, postoperative edema, and indwelling urinary catheter

| NURSING INTERVENTIONS | EVALUATION OF EXPECTED OUTCOMES |
|---|---|
| Assess the patient's pain. | Describes pain on scale of 1 to 10 |
| Have patient describe pain on a scale of 1 to 10. | Verbalizes need for comfort measures |
| Provide comfort measures as needed: repositioning, ice packs, and analgesics. | Able to provide self-care measures such as positioning |
| Anticipate need for analgesics, administer as per orders. | Verbalizes decrease of pain after comfort measures |
| Use bed cradle to keep bed linens off the operative site. | |
| Tape catheter to abdomen to keep penis perpendicular to body. | |

---

### NURSING DIAGNOSIS

Risk for infection related to surgical incision and indwelling urinary catheter

| NURSING INTERVENTIONS | EVALUATION OF EXPECTED OUTCOMES |
|---|---|
| Assess dressing for drainage and odor. | No infection at surgical site |
| Change dressing as needed, using sterile technique. | No urinary tract infection |
| Monitor vital signs for elevations/changes. | Able to demonstrate incision care and dressing change before discharge |
| Provide catheter care at least bid. | |
| Monitor urinary drainage for changes in color and clarity. | Able to verbalize signs and symptoms of infections at surgical site before discharge |
| Encourage fluid intake of at least 2000 ml/day. | |
| Administer antibiotics as per orders. | Able to verbalize signs and symptoms of urinary tract infection before discharge |

*Continued*

## NURSING CARE PLAN

### PATIENT HAVING SURGERY FOR IMPLANTATION OF PENILE PROSTHESIS—cont'd

**NURSING DIAGNOSIS**

Body image disturbance related to need for penile prosthesis and need for exposure of genitalia to health care professionals

| NURSING INTERVENTIONS | EVALUATION OF EXPECTED OUTCOMES |
|---|---|
| Assess patient's verbalization about the prosthesis, the level of participation in his own care, and embarrassment. | Patient and wife discuss feelings about prosthesis and altered body image |
| Assess whether patient's expectations of surgery have been met or unmet. | Discusses and participates in self-care |
| When inspecting the surgical site, maintain a professional demeanor to decrease embarrassment. | Verbalizes both negative and positive feelings about implant |
| Allow patient time for expressions of feelings. | |

**NURSING DIAGNOSIS**

Altered sexuality patterns related to preoperative impotence, placement of prosthesis, expectations of self and partner after surgery

| NURSING INTERVENTIONS | EVALUATION OF EXPECTED OUTCOMES |
|---|---|
| Assess patient's and his wife's behavior when discussing expectations after surgery. | Patient and wife openly discuss expectations of surgery on their sexual relationship |
| Assess patient's and wife's knowledge and expectations for their sexual relationship after surgery. | Patient and wife verbalize concerns and feelings about surgery |
| Allow time for patient and wife to verbalize concerns and feelings about surgery. | Patient and wife have clear understanding of differences among erection, ejaculation, fertility, and orgasm |

# KEY CONCEPTS

➤ The major function of the reproductive system is the creation of new life.

➤ The reproductive organs of the male include the penis, testes, vas deferens, seminal vesicles, and accessory glands.

➤ Penile erection is controlled by the central, autonomic, and somatic nervous systems working together.

➤ The patient history is particularly important when assessing problems with the reproductive systems. A patient's culture and religious background may make it difficult for him to talk to the nurse about his problems.

➤ Chronic illnesses and their medications can affect sexual functioning.

➤ Puberty is the period of growth and development when secondary sex characteristics begin to appear.

➤ Nocturnal seminal emissions are a physiologic sign of puberty in males.

➤ Sexual role or gender role is the public expression of behavior that implies masculinity or femininity.

➤ Gender identity is the private or personal experience of one's maleness or femaleness. It is not always congruent with the individual's gender role.

➤ Climacteric in males refers to the midlife physical and psychologic changes that take place in males.

➤ Physical examination of the male patient includes inspection and palpation of the external genitalia for abnormalities of structure and signs of infection such as discharge, swelling, and skin lesions.

➤ Congenital malformations of the male involve the bladder, the urethra, and the penis.

➤ Tumors of the male reproductive tract are usually malignant.

➤ Testicular tumors are the second most common malignancy in men between the ages of 25 and 35.

➤ Regular testicular self-examination is recommended as an effective method for detecting cancer in its early stages.

➤ A primary role for the nurse when dealing with patients with testicular cancer is to provide emotional support.

➤ A vasectomy is a form of voluntary sterilization.

➤ Conditions affecting the prostate gland include prostatitis, cancer, and benign prostatic hypertrophy.

➤ Many urinary problems of the elderly are signs of prostate enlargement.

➤ Cancer of the prostate gland is the second most common site for cancer among men between the ages of 55 and 74.

➤ Prostate cancer is the most common type of cancer found in African-American men.

➤ Benign prostatic hypertrophy is simple, nonmalignant enlargement of the prostate gland.

➤ Erectile dysfunction is the failure to achieve penile erection in a manner sufficient for successful intercourse.

➤ Erectile dysfunction can be caused by hormonal, vascular, or neurologic disorders or by surgical procedures, trauma, and psychologic problems.

➤ Correction of the erectile dysfunction does not have an effect on the ability to achieve orgasm or ejaculation, nor does it remove underlying psychologic problems.

# CRITICAL THINKING EXERCISES

1. Develop a teaching plan for a patient undergoing a transurethral prostatectomy.
2. What instructions would you give to your patient to help him decrease his chances of developing a urinary tract infection following prostate surgery?
3. Discuss the possible complications of continuous bladder irrigation. What are the signs and symptoms you would monitor?
4. Discuss at least three reasons why a patient might have difficulty talking with the nurse about his expectations of sexual performance after penile implantation.

## REFERENCES AND ADDITIONAL READINGS

Acute Pain Management Guideline Panel: *Acute pain management: operative or medical procedures and trauma: clinical practice guideline,* Rockville, Md, February 1992, Agency for Health Care Policy and Research, Public Health Service, Pub No 92-0032, US Department of Health and Human Services.

American Cancer Society: *Cancer facts and figures,* New York, 1994, The Society.

Black JM, Matassarin-Jacobs E: *Medical-surgical nursing,* ed 5, Philadelphia, 1997, Saunders.

Brenner ZR, Krenzer ME: Update on cryosurgical ablation for prostate cancer, *Am J Nurse* 95(4):44-49, 1995.

Gray ML: *Genitourinary disorders,* St Louis, 1992, Mosby.

Greifzu S, Tiedemann D: Prostate cancer: the pros and cons of treatment, *RN* 58(6):22-27, 1995.

Greiner KA, Weigal JW: Erectile dysfunction, *Am Fam Physician* 54(5):1678, 1996.

Lewis SM, Collier IC, Heitkemper MM: *Medical-surgical nursing,* ed 4, St Louis, 1996, Mosby.

Lueckenotte AG: *Gerontologic nursing,* St Louis, 1996, Mosby.

Morley JE: Update on men's health, *Generations* 20(4):13, 1996.

Newman J: Epidemiology, diagnosis and treatment of prostate cancer, *Radiol Technol* 68(1):39, 1996.

Otto SE: *Oncology nursing,* ed 3, St Louis, 1996, Mosby.

Price SA, Wilson LM: *Pathophysiology,* ed 5, St Louis, 1996, Mosby.

Skolnick A: Guidelines for treating erectile dysfunction, *JAMA* 277(1):7, 1997.

Thibodeau GA: *Textbook of anatomy and physiology,* ed 2, St Louis, 1995, Mosby.

Walbrecker J: Start talking about testicular cancer, *RN* 58(1):34, 1995.

Yeo G: Ethnogeriatrics: cross-cultural care of older adults, *Generations* 20(4):72, 1996.

## CHAPTER 43

# Women's Reproductive Health

## CHAPTER OBJECTIVES

1 Explain the physiology of menstruation and menopause.
2 Identify the physiologic changes of puberty and discuss the teaching role of the nurse in the care of the teenage girl.
3 Contrast the efficacy, risks, and benefits of the various contraceptive options.
4 Identify patients at high risk for osteoporosis, and discuss the risks and benefits of hormonal replacement.
5 Discuss the use of open-ended questions in assessing sexuality.
6 Give an example of a physical change in the genitalia of the older woman.
7 Contrast the treatment of vaginitis caused by the *Trichomonas* organism with that caused by *Candida albicans*.
8 Identify the primary goal of nursing care after colporrhaphy.
9 Define endometriosis.
10 Discuss the risk factors for cervical cancer and the recommended screening interval for Papanicolaou smears.
11 Discuss the relationship between pelvic inflammatory disease and ectopic pregnancy.
12 Discuss medical indications for vulvectomy. Discuss the effect of vulvectomy on female sexuality.
13 Describe the goals of care for the patient after hysterectomy.
14 Compare possible treatments for breast cancer, and discuss methods of breast reconstruction after a mastectomy.
15 Discuss the need for abortion counseling and the use of active listening to support the patient's decision-making process.

## KEY TERMS

| | |
|---|---|
| amenorrhea | mastectomy |
| colporrhaphy | mastitis |
| colposcopy | menarche |
| culdoscopy | menopause |
| dilation and curettage | menorrhagia |
| dysmenorrhea | ovulation |
| endometriosis | Papanicolaou (Pap) smear |
| hysterectomy | pelvic exenteration |
| laparoscopy | puberty |
| mammography | vaginitis |

## STRUCTURE AND FUNCTION OF THE REPRODUCTIVE SYSTEM

The reproductive system includes the external genitalia of the female, as well as the internal organs associated with reproduction. The female breasts also play a role in sexuality and breastfeeding. Sexual and reproductive development are influenced by the endocrine system, and the nervous system is involved in human sexual response.

### Female Reproductive System

The region encompassing the female external genitalia is usually referred to as the *vulva* (Figure 43-1). The vulva includes the mons pubis, a pad of fatty tissue that protects the pubis. During puberty the mons becomes covered by hair, and its sebaceous glands become more active. The labia majora are two elongated folds of skin extending from the mons to the perineum (Figure 43-1). At puberty, hair begins to grow along the outside surfaces of the labia, while the inside surfaces start to

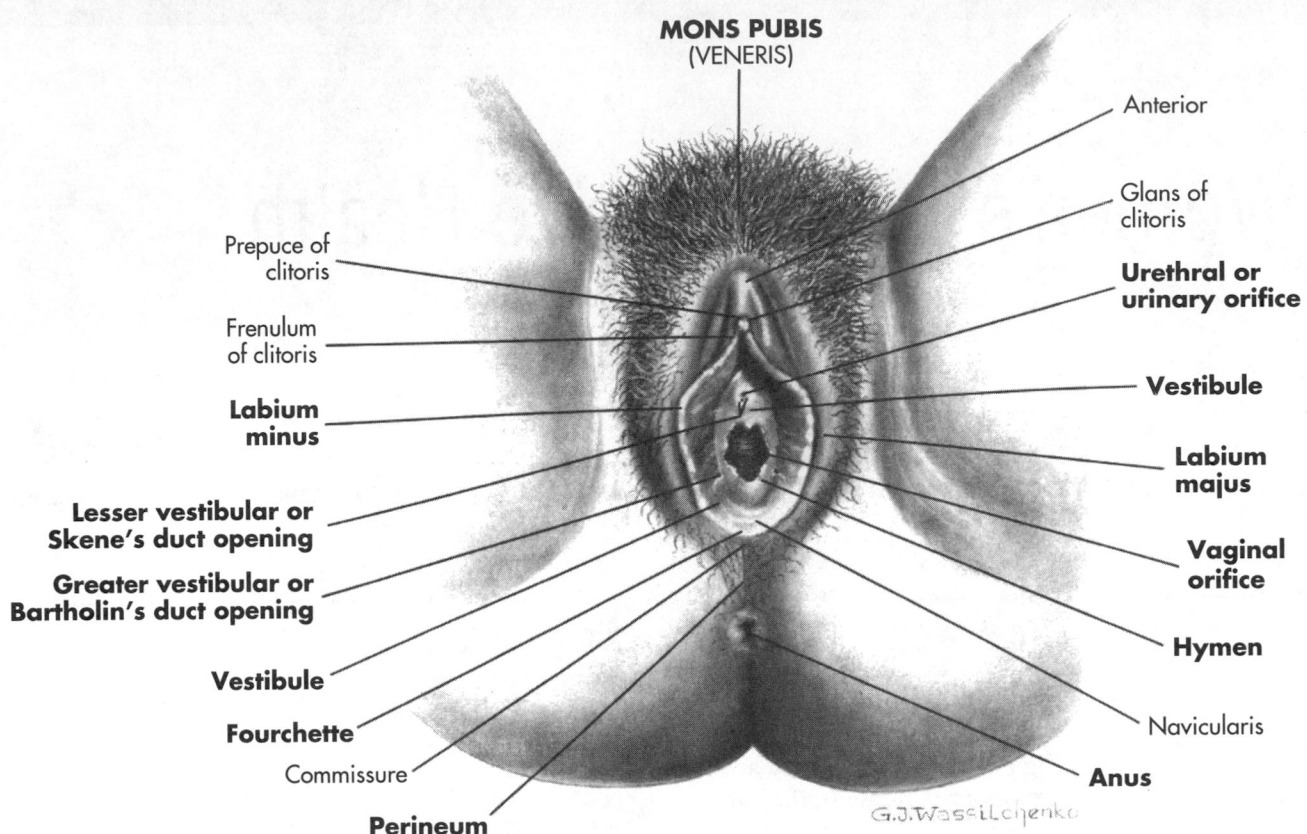

**Figure 43-1** External female genitalia. (From Bobak IM, Jensen MD: *Maternity and gynecologic care,* ed 5, St Louis, 1993, Mosby.)

secrete lubricants from their sebaceous glands. Lying within the labia majora are two thinner, hairless folds of skin known as the labia minora. The labia minora are richly supplied with sebaceous glands, nerves, and blood vessels. During sexual excitement they become engorged with blood and lubricated by secretions. The upper folds of the labia minora meet to form the clitoral hood or prepuce, which shields the clitoris beneath. The clitoris consists of spongy erectile tissue that becomes swollen with blood during sexual arousal. The clitoris is exquisitely sensitive because of a rich network of nerves, but only a small part of the clitoris is visible, since the deeper shaft lies beneath the skin. The labia minora protect an area called the vestibule, within which lie the urinary meatus (urinary opening) and below it the introitus (vaginal opening). The hymen is a fragile band of tissue that encircles or covers the introitus. Even in virgin girls the hymen allows the passage of menstrual blood and will usually accommodate a tampon without tearing. However, the hymen can be torn accidentally during exercise, trauma, and digital examination as well as during intercourse, and thus it is an unreliable indicator of virginity. The *perineum* is a muscular area that lies between the anus and the vaginal outlet. The area of the perineum where the labia minora join posteriorly is called the *fourchette.* The vagina is an elastic, muscular canal that extends from the introitus to the cervix. The space

surrounding the cervix is called the vaginal fornix. During the childbearing years the epithelium that lines the vagina is arranged in transverse folds called *rugae.* These folds allow the mucosal layer to stretch during coitus and childbirth. The vagina is lubricated by secretions from two sets of glands, *Bartholin's glands* and *Skene's glands,* located near the introitus. During sexual stimulation the vagina becomes engorged with blood, and this pushes some fluid to the surface of the epithelium, providing additional lubrication. Before puberty the vaginal pH is nearly neutral (7.0), but after puberty and until menopause it is more acidic (4.5). This acidity helps to protect women from infection during their most sexually vulnerable years. After menopause the vaginal pH becomes more alkaline and the epithelium thinner and less protective. The vagina acts as an outlet for menstrual flow, serves as the birth canal during childbirth, and functions as an organ of sexual pleasure. Although the vaginal walls are only sparsely supplied with nerves, the introitus is sensitive and can be highly excitable.

The *uterus* is a pear-shaped, hollow, muscular organ composed of three layers: the inner, *endometrial* layer, which is shed during menstruation; the muscular middle layer, or *myometrium,* which contracts during childbirth; and the outer layer, or *perimetrium.* The bulging, upper part of the uterus is called the *fundus* (Figure 43-2). The lowest portion of the uterus extends

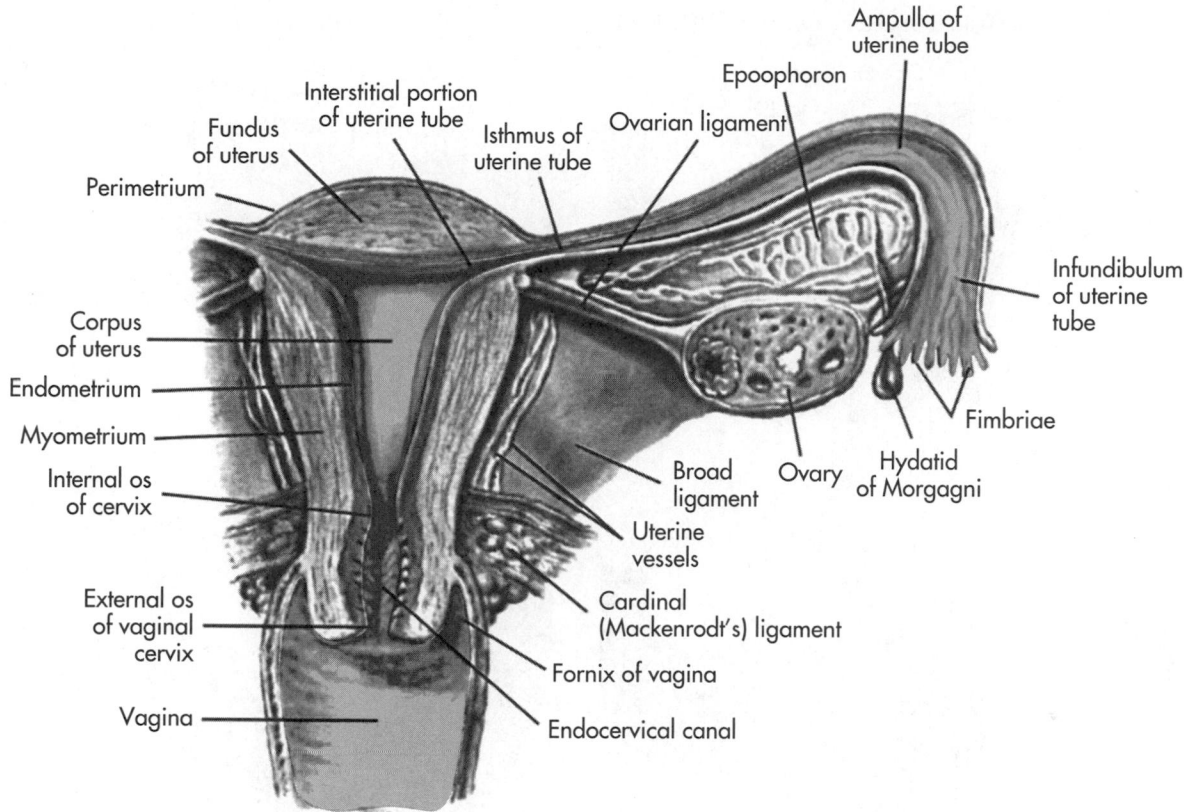

**Figure 43-2**     Cross sections of uterus, fallopian tube, and ovary. (From Bobak IM, Jensen MD: *Maternity and gynecologic care,* ed 5, St Louis, 1993, Mosby.)

downward into the vagina and forms the cervix. The cervix has a narrow canal with openings at the entrance and exit, called the *internal os* and *external os.* This passageway is called the *endocervical canal.* Usually the endocervical canal is less than an inch in circumference, but during childbirth the canal widens to 10 cm to permit passage of the fetal head. The endocervical canal is lined with columnar epithelial cells. These cells are taller and softer than the squamous epithelial cells that line the vagina and outer cervix. The junction of these cells, called the *transformation zone,* is usually within the endocervical canal and thus is not visible during the pelvic examination. The squamocolumnar junction (transformation zone) is the area where most cervical cancer begins. In young girls or in women taking birth control pills the transformation zone may extend from the endocervical canal and may be visible during the pelvic examination as a red, plush, circular area on the cervix. This is considered a normal finding. The endocervical canal also contains a thick plug of cervical mucus that acts as a barrier to infection. The uterus is not a fixed organ but lies suspended in the pelvic cavity by the round, broad, and uterosacral ligaments. Typically the uterus is anteverted (tilted forward) (Figure 43-3), but it may also be found midline or retroverted (tilted backward). The two fallopian tubes are at-

tached to and open into the upper part or fundus of the uterus. The distal end of the tubes flares out and is known as the *infundibulum.* It has a fimbriated or fringed end and opens into the abdominal cavity; the ovaries are near the distal end of each tube. At ovulation the fringed ends of the fallopian tubes move, producing a current that helps draw the ovum into the tubes. Fertilization usually occurs in the distal third of the fallopian tubes. Cilia and muscular contractions of the tubes keep the fertilized ovum moving toward the uterus for implantation. If fertilization does not occur, the ovum disintegrates and is shed during menstruation.

The white, almond-shaped ovaries are attached to the uterus by a ligament. In a woman of reproductive years each ovary is approximately 1 to 1½ inches long, 1 inch wide, and 1 inch thick. After menopause the ovary becomes smaller and is not typically palpable during the pelvic examination. Each ovary consists of a cortex and a medulla; the ovarian follicles form within the cortex. During the menstrual cycle one follicle matures more quickly than the others and releases an ovum that is transported down the fallopian tube toward the uterus. The follicle then becomes a structure known as the *corpus luteum,* the function of which is to secrete hormones that maintain pregnancy should the ovum be fertilized. If the ovum is not fertilized, the

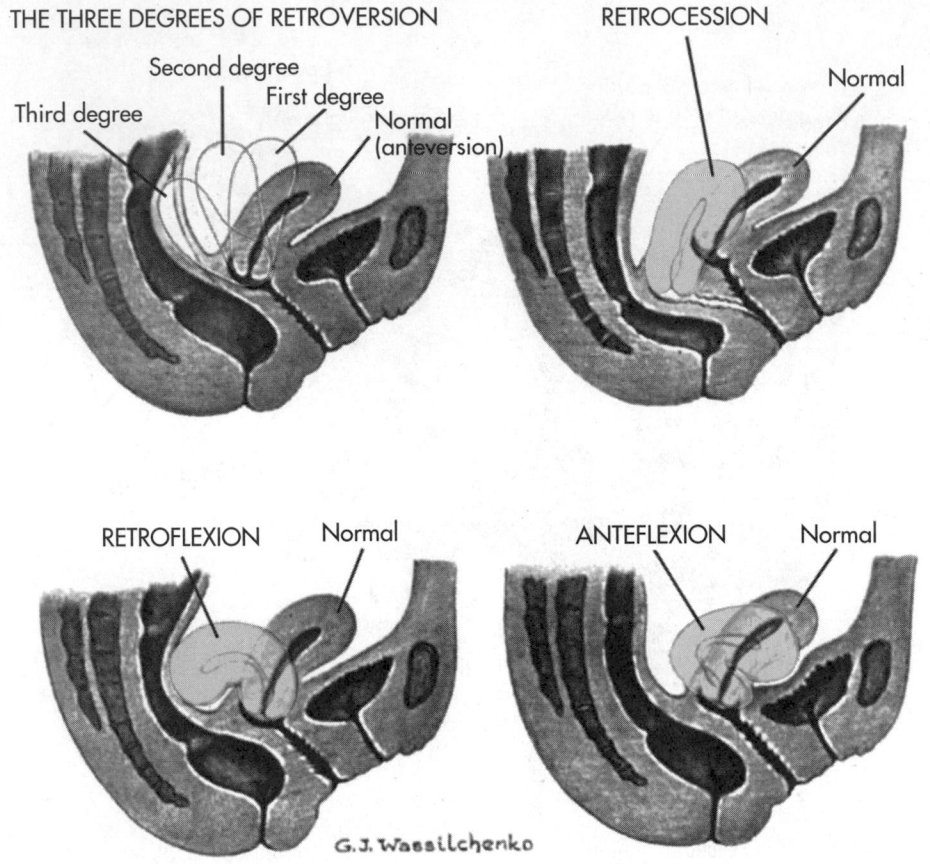

THE THREE DEGREES OF RETROVERSION

Third degree
Second degree
First degree
Normal (anteversion)

RETROCESSION

Normal

RETROFLEXION    Normal

ANTEFLEXION    Normal

G.J. Wassilchenko

**Figure 43-3**    Uterine positions. (From Bobak IM, Jensen MD: *Maternity and gynecologic care,* ed 5, St Louis, 1993, Mosby.)

corpus luteum disintegrates after a few days and menstruation occurs shortly afterward.

The female breast is composed of milk-producing glands called *acini;* the lactiferous ducts, which collect and deliver milk during lactation; and the nipple. The nipple is surrounded by a darkened area called the *areola.* The pigment of the areola deepens during pregnancy and with the use of oral contraceptives. The nipple is composed of erectile tissue and responds to tactile stimulation and cold temperatures by becoming erect. Nipples are usually everted but are occasionally inverted (pushed inward). Nipple inversion usually has no effect on breastfeeding because the nipple becomes everted by the infant's sucking. *Montgomery's glands,* small elevations on the areola surrounding the nipple, secrete a lubricating and protective substance during lactation. The form of the breast is provided by subcutaneous and fatty tissue supported by the pectoralis major and pectoralis minor muscles. A girl's breasts may develop unevenly during puberty, although the breasts usually become approximately equal in size. In some normal women a noticeable disparity in breast size persists. As women age, the breasts tend to stretch and become less firm. The female breast has a rich lymphatic system that drains from the breast to various nodes in the axilla.

## Menstrual Cycle

Menstruation is a cyclic process in females, occurring at fairly regular intervals between puberty and menopause and spanning a period of approximately 30 to 35 years (Figure 43-4). The onset of menstruation, or **menarche,** is a normal physiologic process and does not indicate a state of illness or disability. The average age of menarche in the United States is 12 years, with the normal range of onset between 10 and 16 years.

A wide variation exists in the cycle and duration of the menstrual flow. A cycle of every 28 days is normal for some women, but for others it may be shorter or longer. Menstrual cycles ranging between 21 and 35 days are normal for most women. The usual blood loss is 1 to 6 ounces. **Ovulation** is the discharge of an ovum from a follicle in the ovaries. It occurs approximately 2 weeks before the onset of menstruation, regardless of the duration of the menstrual cycle. Ovulation begins some time after menarche, and a girl may not ovulate for up to 2 years after her first period. Ovulation ceases at some time during menopause. The first day of bleeding is considered the first day of the menstrual cycle (see Figure 43-4). As levels of estrogen and progesterone decline from the preceding cycle, the

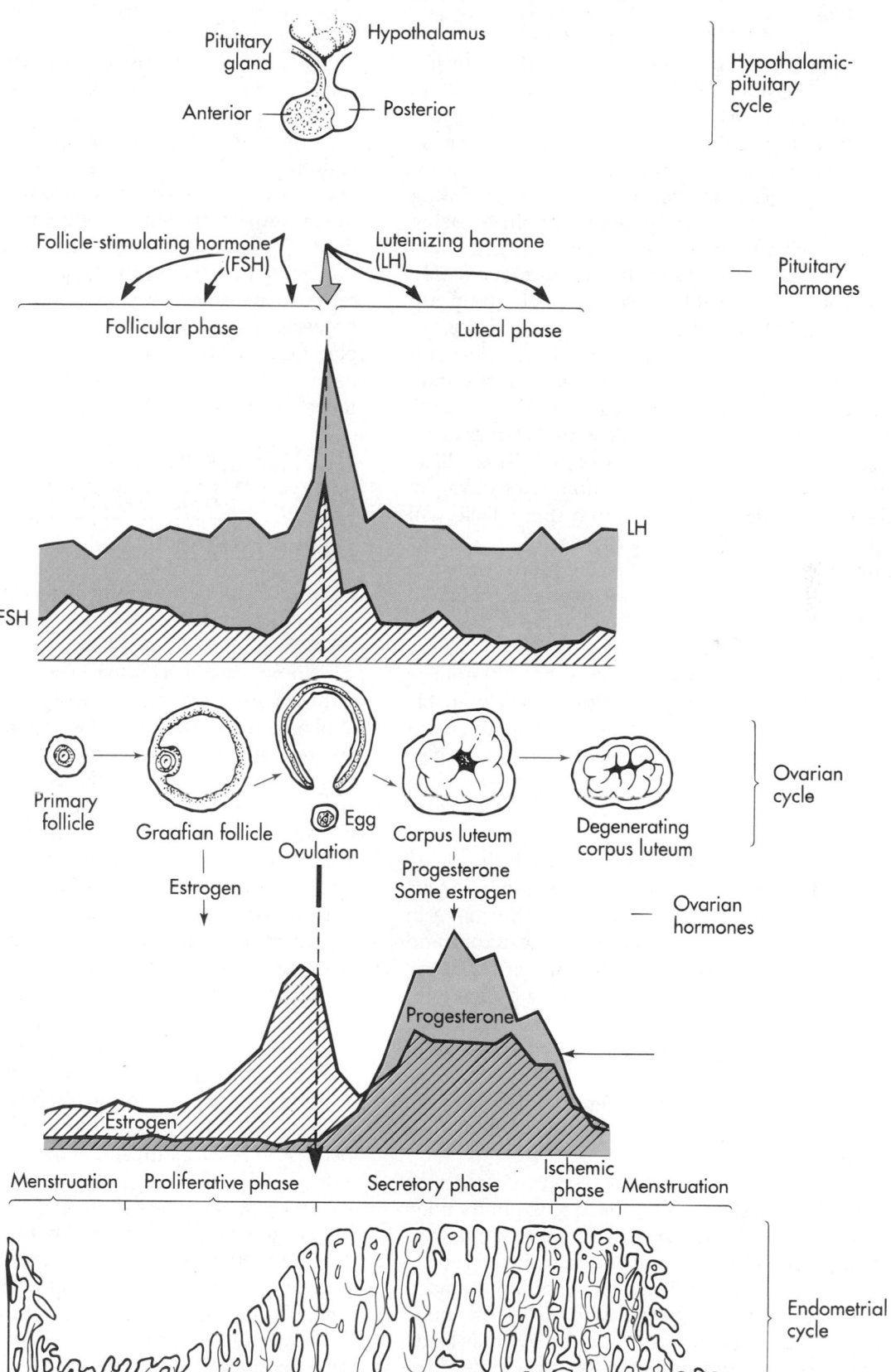

**Figure 43-4** Menstrual cycle: hypothalamic-pituitary, ovarian, and endometrial. (From Bobak IM, Jensen MD: *Maternity and gynecologic care,* ed 5, St Louis, 1993, Mosby.)

lining of the uterus (endometrium) is shed during menstruation. Usually this is accomplished in 2 to 7 days. Simultaneously several follicles begin to develop in the ovary during these first few days of the cycle. As the hypothalamus of the brain senses the low estrogen and progesterone levels from the preceding cycle, it responds by secreting gonadotropin-releasing hormone, which acts on the anterior pituitary gland and causes it to release follicle-stimulating hormone (FSH). This hormone helps the follicles to mature. In the group of developing follicles, one will become dominant because of its greater receptivity to FSH. All the developing follicles produce estrogen, which acts on the anterior pituitary gland to decrease FSH. As the level of FSH declines, only the dominant follicle with its larger number of FSH receptors can continue to thrive. This follicle continues to produce increasing amounts of estrogen, and the other follicles atrophy. From this follicle will come the mature ovum (egg) for the cycle.

Meanwhile the endometrium of the uterus becomes thicker in response to increased estrogen production in the ovary. Increasing estrogen also changes the character of the cervical mucus to a copious, stretchy, clear secretion that aids sperm transport. When the mucus may be stretched into a strand several inches long, it is known as *spinnbarkheit mucus*. This period in the menstrual cycle is known as the *follicular phase* with reference to the follicular development occurring in the ovary and as the *proliferative phase* with reference to events occurring in the uterus.

As the ovum and follicle near maturity, the rising levels of estrogen trigger the release of luteinizing hormone (LH) by the pituitary gland. This hormone in turn stimulates the ovary to produce progesterone and androgen a few days before ovulation begins. When the increasing level of estrogen produced by the follicle reaches a critical threshold, it causes a surge in LH production. This surge assists the final maturation of the egg and allows the follicle to rupture so that the ovum may enter the fimbriated end of the fallopian tube. This phase of the menstrual cycle is known as ovulation.

After the ovum is released, the ruptured follicle is transformed into the *corpus luteum,* a small body filled with yellow fluid. If the ovum is fertilized by a spermatozoon in the fallopian tube, it descends the tube to implant in the thick, vessel-rich lining of the uterus. If fertilization does not occur, the ovum leaves the body through the vagina. Whether or not the ovum is fertilized, the endometrium prepares for a possible pregnancy. After the follicle ruptures and becomes the corpus luteum, it produces the hormone progesterone, which makes the endometrium more vascular and glandular, enabling it to secrete glucose to an embryo. The production of FSH is now inhibited. This period is known as the *luteal phase* in reference to ovarian events and as the *secretory phase* in reference to endometrial changes. If the ovum is fertilized, the developing embryo produces the hormone human chorionic gonadotropin (HCG), which sustains the corpus luteum and allows it to continue producing estrogen and progesterone until the placenta can assume these functions. The corpus luteum must remain functional for the first 7 to 9 weeks of the pregnancy until the placenta can assume production of sufficient estrogen and progesterone. If the ovum is not fertilized, the prepared endometrium degenerates and menstrual flow begins approximately 2 weeks after ovulation. After menstruation the cycle begins again.

# DISTURBANCES OF MENSTRUAL FUNCTION

## Dysmenorrhea

Painful menstruation **(dysmenorrhea)** is the most common complaint associated with the menstrual process; at least half of all women experience some degree of physical discomfort. The discomfort may occur with or without the presence of a pathologic condition. When pain and discomfort are severe enough to incapacitate the individual, a medical examination should be performed to rule out disease. Sometimes pain may result from fibroid tumors of the uterus, ovarian cysts, chronic inflammation of the fallopian tubes, pelvic inflammatory disease, displacement of the uterus, endometriosis, or narrowing of the cervical canal.

Hypercontractility of the uterus resulting from higher than normal levels of prostaglandins may be the cause of dysmenorrhea. Prostaglandins stimulate smooth muscle contraction, and the uterus is composed of smooth muscle.

The discomfort of cramps, backache, and leg pain can often be relieved by rest, a heating pad or hot-water bottle applied to the abdomen, and medication (Table 43-1). Heat is an especially effective treatment because it reduces muscle tone and increases circulation, thereby increasing the oxygen supply to the muscle and relieving the ischemia.

Recent studies have shown that drugs inhibiting the production of prostaglandin (antiprostaglandins) reduce or eliminate pain or other undesirable symptoms that sometimes accompany menstruation. Several over-the-counter preparations are available for the treatment of dysmenorrhea. Aspirin, a drug commonly recommended to relieve dysmenorrhea, has been identified as having antiprostaglandin activity, which explains its effectiveness. Other drugs known to have antiprostaglandin action include ibuprofen (Motrin) and naproxen (Anaprox). They are

**TABLE 43-1**

## Nonsteroidal Antiinflammatory Agents for Dysmenorrhea

| ANTIINFLAMMATORY AGENT | DOSAGE |
| --- | --- |
| ibuprofen (Motrin and others) | 400 mg every 4 hours |
| ketoprofen (Orudis) | 25-50 mg every 6-8 hours |
| mefenamic acid (Ponstel) | 500 mg initially, followed by 250 mg every 6-8 hours |
| naproxen (Naprosyn) | 500 mg initially, followed by 250 mg every 6-8 hours |
| naproxen sodium (Anaprox) | 550 mg initially, followed by 275 mg every 6-8 hours |

thought to be more effective than aspirin in reducing the production of prostaglandins. These drugs were previously used primarily for their antiinflammatory action in diseases such as arthritis. In addition to reducing uterine cramping, antiprostaglandin drugs are thought to reduce the gastrointestinal symptoms of indigestion, nausea, vomiting, and diarrhea that accompany menstruation in some women. Prostaglandin activity is also thought to increase contractility in the gastrointestinal tract, which also causes these symptoms.

Antiprostaglandins should be taken with the onset of menstruation and only for the second, third, or fourth days of the menstrual cycle in which the individual normally experiences discomfort. These drugs should be taken only to control symptoms. If the dose is limited, the chance of side effects is reduced.

Little research has been conducted in the area of dysmenorrhea although it occurs to some degree in many women and regularly incapacitates many others.

## Amenorrhea

**Amenorrhea** is the absence of menstruation, which is normal before puberty, after menopause, and during pregnancy and lactation. Amenorrhea may occur with some diseases, such as tuberculosis, nephritis, anorexia nervosa, and certain endocrine disturbances. It may also result from change of climate, emotional factors, or strenuous exercise. Nurses must be aware that nongynecologic surgery may cause amenorrhea for a period of time. A woman of the appropriate age who has never menstruated is said to have primary amenorrhea, whereas suppression of menstruation once it has become established is called secondary amenorrhea. The treatment is based on the underlying cause and must be determined on an individual basis.

## Menorrhagia

**Menorrhagia** refers to menstrual flow that is excessive in amount or duration. The condition can be associated with some pelvic pathologic conditions such as uterine fibroids or an endocrine disturbance. It may also be associated with sexually transmitted diseases, spontaneous abortion, use of an intrauterine device (IUD), or anovulatory cycles. Medical examination is always indicated, and, if bleeding is severe, the individual may need endometrial biopsy or dilation and curettage (D&C) of the endometrium.

## Metrorrhagia

Metrorrhagia is bleeding that occurs between regular menstrual periods and usually indicates the presence of some abnormal pathologic condition. It may be associated with a malignant condition of the reproductive system or may result from benign lesions of the cervix or the uterus. It may also be caused by trauma, ectopic pregnancy, cervicitis, oral contraceptive use, vaginal infections, or IUD use. Postcoital spotting is often associated with benign or malignant lesions of the cervix and infections. A medical examination is indicated.

## Oligomenorrhea

Oligomenorrhea is infrequent menses (i.e., menses occurring less often than every 40 days). Oligomenorrhea may occur normally with anovulatory cycles, as in the young girl just beginning menstruation. It can also occur at times of stress or change, such as leaving home for college and during the perimenopausal period. Marathon runners, athletes, and women with anorexia nervosa may experience oligomenorrhea because of changes in muscle and fat distribution. A woman whose menses are more than 90 days apart may need to have menstruation regulated to prevent buildup of the endometrial lining, which can predispose her to endometrial cancer. Oral contraceptive pills and medroxyprogesterone (Provera) are sometimes used to regulate menses.

## Toxic Shock Syndrome

Although not related to menstrual function, *toxic shock syndrome* (TSS) may affect healthy young women during their menstrual periods. This illness was first reported to the Centers for Disease Control and Prevention in 1980. TSS also occurs in nonmenstruating women and in men, but it is especially associated with the use of high-absorbency tampons by women who have *Staphylococcus aureus* colonized in the vagina. Nonetheless, approximately 45% of TSS cases are not related to menstruation. Each year TSS occurs in an estimated 1 to 17 per 100,000 menstruating women (Colbry, 1992). TSS is characterized by the sudden onset of fever of 39° C (102° F) or higher, an erythematous macular rash (usually on the palms and soles) that desquamates in 7 to 24 days, systolic blood pressure below 90 mm Hg (in an adult), and involvement in three or more other organ systems. The systems most commonly involved are the gastrointestinal, muscular, mucous membrane, renal, hematologic, hepatic, central nervous, and cardiopulmonary. Nausea, vomiting, and diarrhea are common.

> ## NURSE ALERT
>
> The danger signs of toxic shock syndrome are a sudden onset of fever (39° C [102° F] or higher); hypotension (systolic pressure below 90 mm Hg); and a diffuse, erythematous, macular rash.

Danger signs of TSS may include a sore throat, headache, decreased urine output, and confusion. Laboratory studies reveal elevated levels of blood urea nitrogen, serum creatinine, creatine phosphokinase, serum glutamic-oxaloacetic transaminase, bilirubin, and leukocytes in the blood (leukocytosis).

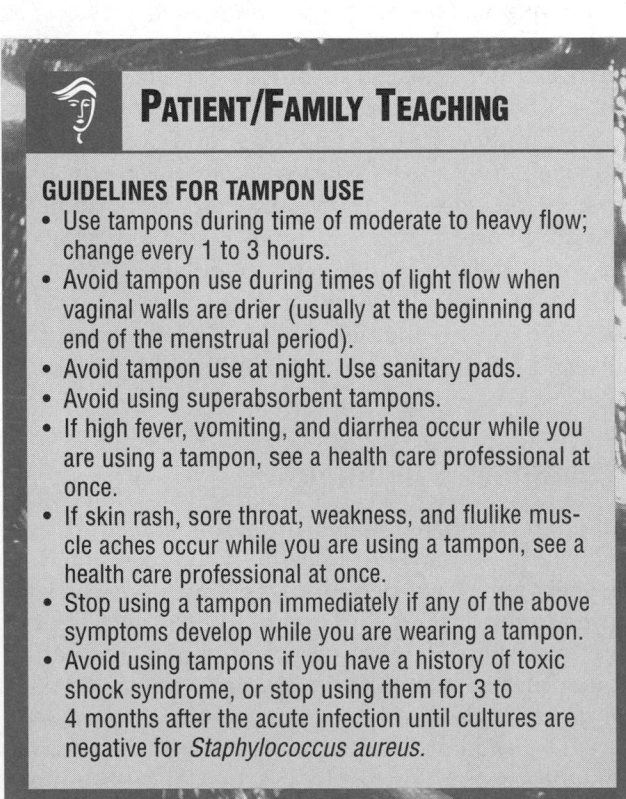

## PATIENT/FAMILY TEACHING

**GUIDELINES FOR TAMPON USE**
- Use tampons during time of moderate to heavy flow; change every 1 to 3 hours.
- Avoid tampon use during times of light flow when vaginal walls are drier (usually at the beginning and end of the menstrual period).
- Avoid tampon use at night. Use sanitary pads.
- Avoid using superabsorbent tampons.
- If high fever, vomiting, and diarrhea occur while you are using a tampon, see a health care professional at once.
- If skin rash, sore throat, weakness, and flulike muscle aches occur while you are using a tampon, see a health care professional at once.
- Stop using a tampon immediately if any of the above symptoms develop while you are wearing a tampon.
- Avoid using tampons if you have a history of toxic shock syndrome, or stop using them for 3 to 4 months after the acute infection until cultures are negative for *Staphylococcus aureus.*

Treatment involves antibiotic therapy with beta-lactam antistaphylococcal antibiotics such as nafcillin, oxacillin, or cephalosporin and fluid and electrolyte replacement. Careful monitoring of fluid intake, urinary output, and vital signs is necessary. Early detection and treatment improve the prognosis. Women who recover from TSS should be instructed to avoid tampon use altogether or until eradication of *S. aureus* in the vaginal flora can be documented. Previously unaffected women can reduce their risk of TSS by wearing tampons during only part of the day or night and during only part of their menstrual cycle. All women should be warned about the danger of high-absorbency tampons.

## Premenstrual Syndrome

*Premenstrual syndrome* (PMS), also called premenstrual tension, has been the subject of many research studies. However, the cause of PMS remains unknown and no universally accepted treatment has been developed. PMS is a set of physical and emotional symptoms that begin approximately 7 to 10 days before the beginning of the menstrual period. Symptoms commonly associated with PMS include irritability, depression, insomnia, fatigue, weight gain, edema, mastalgia, abdominal distention, headache, and backache. These symptoms usually disappear with the onset of the menstrual period. PMS symptoms may occur as a woman gets older and may worsen with time.

Because PMS is highly individualized, a nurse should help a woman to identify her symptoms. The nurse should advise her to keep a log of her symptoms and note their severity on her calendar over several months. The nurse might inquire whether certain events in the patient's life trigger symptoms and counsel her accordingly. The patient can be encouraged to anticipate days that may be especially difficult and plan low-stress activities at these times. Women may also find that open communication with their families on this subject increases their understanding.

Since the exact cause of PMS is unknown, a variety of methods are used to treat the condition. Nutritional supplements such as calcium, vitamins, and evening primrose oil have been suggested for relief of PMS. The nurse could suggest that the woman eat a diet low in sodium and high in complex carbohydrates 7 to 10 days before the beginning of the menstrual cycle and avoid use of caffeine and alcohol. Improved nutrition and exercise have been suggested as a means to control symptoms. Joining a self-help group may be useful to women who have low self-esteem from lack of understanding of PMS. Medication may be prescribed for the relief of the more severe symptoms. A diuretic such as chlorothiazide (Diuril) may relieve the edema resulting from water and sodium retention. Other medications that have been tried are progesterone, oral contraceptives, bromocriptine, and aldosterone.

# PHASES OF REPRODUCTIVE FUNCTION THROUGHOUT THE LIFE CYCLE

## Puberty

**Puberty** is the period during which the body prepares for reproductive ability. In females it begins at about age 10. Secondary sex characteristics begin to appear. The size of the external reproductive organs increases, axillary and pubic hair grows, and the breasts become larger. In the female the first menstrual period is termed *menarche.* There is some variation in age at onset of puberty and menarche. The first menstrual period usually occurs between the ages of 12 and 13, but it may occur anytime from age 10 to 15 years. Menarche usually occurs after the peak of the growth spurt. The average girl continues to grow about 2 to 3 inches in height after menarche. The first menstrual cycles are usually anovulatory, and they are likely to be irregular for the first 1 to 2 years after onset of menstruation. Menstrual cramps are uncommon during these first cycles. If menses has not begun by age 15 or 16 years, a gynecologist should be consulted to rule out endocrine imbalance, an imperforate hymen, or congenital anomalies. The hymen normally has an opening that allows menstrual flow to occur, but, if it is imperforate, there is no opening and the flow is held back.

The sequence of physical changes in girls during puberty varies by individual. Typically the first sign of puberty is the appearance of the breast bud (Figure 43-5). The development of pubic hair usually follows, with axillary hair appearing approximately 2 years after pubic hair (Figure 43-6). There are increases in height and weight, as well as changes in body contour and genital development. Puberty is considered precocious if menarche begins before age 10 or secondary development occurs before age 8. Precocious puberty may be a result of early physiologic maturation, but it could also result from an ovarian or adrenal tumor. Reassurance can be offered once pathologic causes of precocious puberty have been explored.

## Menstruation and Hygiene

The nurse may be involved in counseling and teaching girls about menstruation. This process must begin with an assessment of the individual's knowledge and feelings about menstruation. The nurse can then clar-

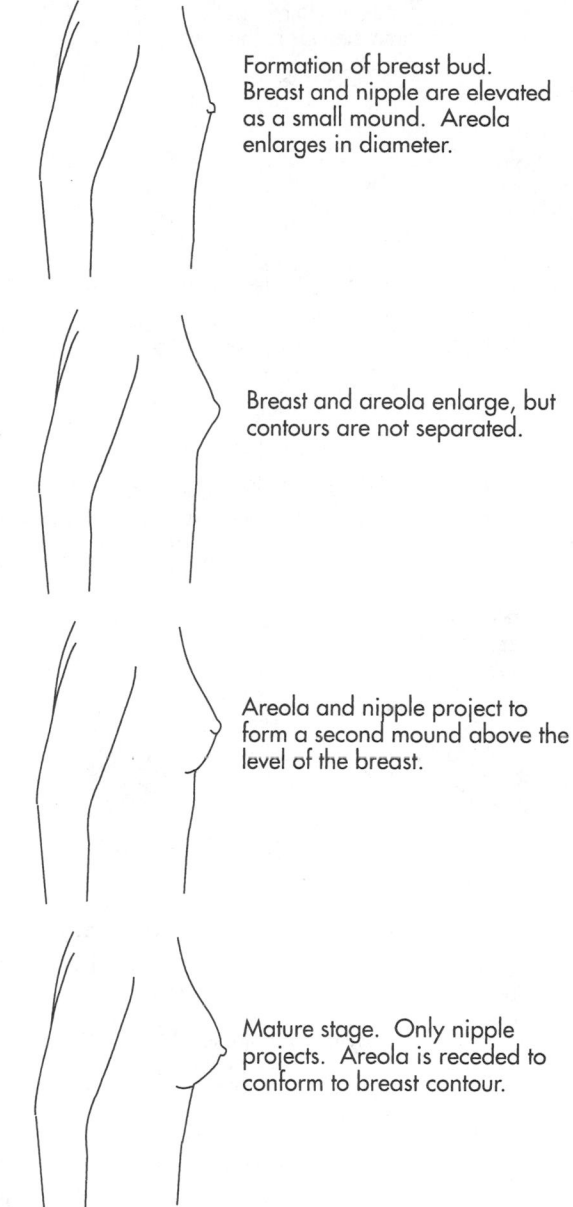

Formation of breast bud. Breast and nipple are elevated as a small mound. Areola enlarges in diameter.

Breast and areola enlarge, but contours are not separated.

Areola and nipple project to form a second mound above the level of the breast.

Mature stage. Only nipple projects. Areola is receded to conform to breast contour.

**Figure 43-5**    Development of breasts in girls.

ify any misconceptions and provide additional knowledge appropriate to the girl's age and developmental level. In addition to basic information regarding the process of menstruation, instruction should include hygiene measures and methods of sanitary protection. Either tampons or sanitary pads can be safely used by females of any age (see the Patient/Family Teaching box on p. 1338). However, the possibility of toxic shock syndrome (TSS) has resulted in some specific guidelines regarding tampon use (see discussion on toxic shock syndrome earlier in this chapter). A young girl may need to lubricate the tampon before she can insert

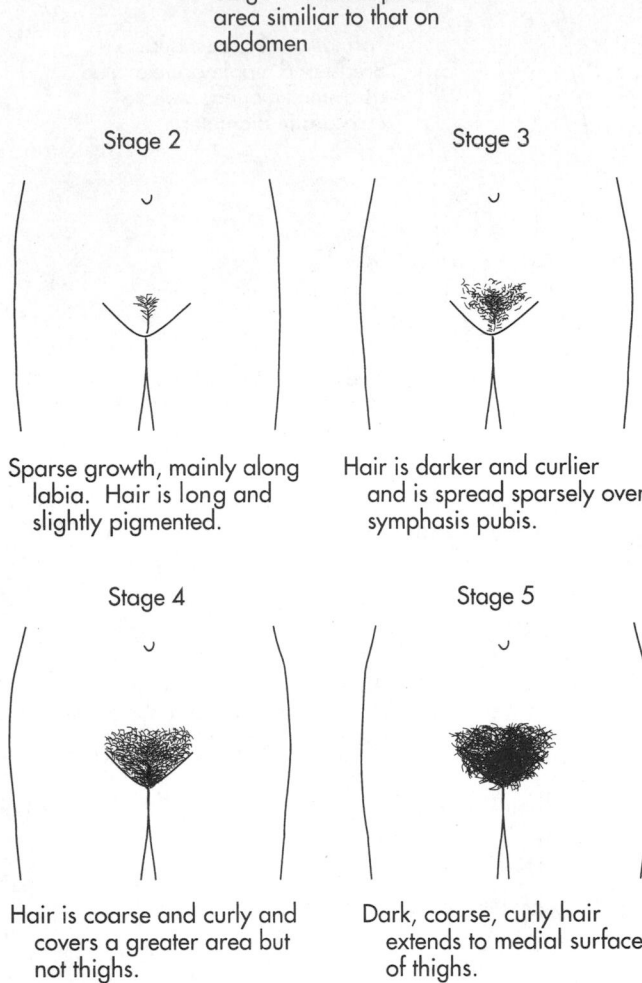

Stage 1: Hair in pubic
area similiar to that on
abdomen

Stage 2

Sparse growth, mainly along
labia. Hair is long and
slightly pigmented.

Stage 3

Hair is darker and curlier
and is spread sparsely over
symphasis pubis.

Stage 4

Hair is coarse and curly and
covers a greater area but
not thighs.

Stage 5

Dark, coarse, curly hair
extends to medial surfaces
of thighs.

**Figure 43-6**   Development of pubic hair in girls.

secreted by the skin of the vulva. Old menstrual blood and seminal fluid remaining after coitus sometimes produce odor. A simple and effective douching solution can be prepared using 30 ml of white vinegar in a quart of warm water. The solution is placed in a douche bag and instilled into the vagina under gentle pressure. Commercial preparations are *not* more effective and may contain perfumes that irritate the vaginal mucosa. Significant odor or discharge may indicate a retained tampon, a foreign body, or infection and should be further assessed. Soap and water cleansing of the perineal area is all that is normally necessary for feminine hygiene.

All females should be encouraged to lead a normal life during menstruation. Exercise, with a few exceptions, is considered helpful in relieving minor discomfort. Although many taboos previously existed concerning swimming or bathing, no harm has been shown to result from these activities. A daily warm bath or shower is important because the sweat glands are often more active at this time. Coitus may be objectionable to women during their periods, and they may choose to avoid it for aesthetic reasons. Women may also be at higher risk for sexually transmitted infections during menses because the cervical os is dilated slightly to allow the passage of blood.

Recent research has linked the discomfort associated with menstruation to the activity of prostaglandins, and treatment with antiprostaglandin drugs has been successful (see the discussion on dysmenorrhea earlier in this chapter).

## Psychosocial Development in Adolescence

Adolescence is a period of rapid physical growth, body change, and psychosocial development (see the Patient/Family Teaching box on p. 1341). Teenagers feel a need to assert their independence from family and experiment with new behaviors. Peer relationships assume greater importance, and adolescents are preoccupied with issues of body image, peer groups, and self-esteem. Adolescents also tend to believe that they are invulnerable to harm. This belief allows them to take greater physical and emotional risks. Girls, for instance, may engage in unprotected sex and become pregnant. They may avoid using birth control because doing so would indicate that they were planning to engage in sexual activity. They may also become pregnant to fill a sense of personal emptiness, resolve a dependency conflict with a parent, find an excuse to leave home, or achieve self-individuation (Trad, 1994). Sexual risk taking and exploration are common among adolescents, and teenage pregnancy is a significant problem in the United States. Adolescent girls are also

it comfortably. Even if not completely saturated, sanitary pads and tampons should be changed about every 4 hours to prevent leakage and odor. However, if tampons are changed too frequently, removing the dry tampon can irritate vaginal walls and increase the risk of TSS. The nurse should encourage hand washing before and after changing a tampon or pad to prevent infection.

The nurse has numerous opportunities to instruct patients in personal hygiene measures. Cultural differences influence the habits and opinions of an individual; some cultures place great importance on cleanliness, others do not. The practice of douching was once considered by some to be essential to feminine hygiene. Routine douching is now discouraged because it is known to irritate the vaginal mucosa and upset the normal protective flora of the vagina that resist infection. Genital odor rarely comes from the vagina but instead stems from the interaction of bacteria with oils

more susceptible to sexually transmitted disease because of the cellular structure of vaginal and cervical tissue in adolescence. Nurses may play an important role in assessing emerging sexuality and risk-taking behaviors. They can offer appropriate preventive measures such as birth control and condoms and provide education about physical and emotional changes.

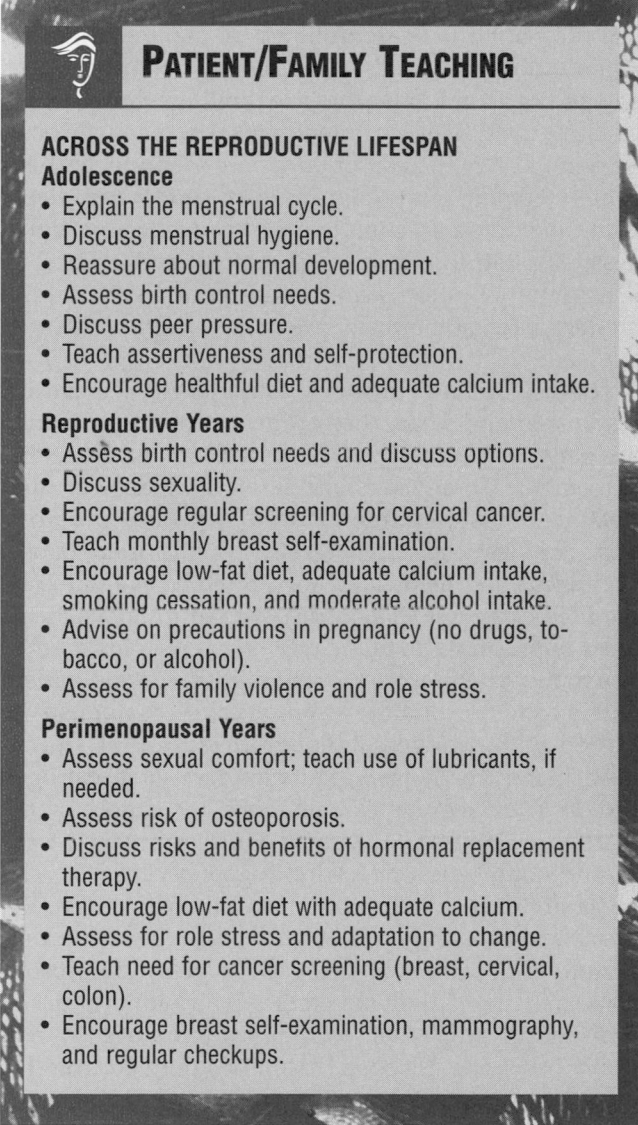

**PATIENT/FAMILY TEACHING**

**ACROSS THE REPRODUCTIVE LIFESPAN**
**Adolescence**
- Explain the menstrual cycle.
- Discuss menstrual hygiene.
- Reassure about normal development.
- Assess birth control needs.
- Discuss peer pressure.
- Teach assertiveness and self-protection.
- Encourage healthful diet and adequate calcium intake.

**Reproductive Years**
- Assess birth control needs and discuss options.
- Discuss sexuality.
- Encourage regular screening for cervical cancer.
- Teach monthly breast self-examination.
- Encourage low-fat diet, adequate calcium intake, smoking cessation, and moderate alcohol intake.
- Advise on precautions in pregnancy (no drugs, tobacco, or alcohol).
- Assess for family violence and role stress.

**Perimenopausal Years**
- Assess sexual comfort; teach use of lubricants, if needed.
- Assess risk of osteoporosis.
- Discuss risks and benefits of hormonal replacement therapy.
- Encourage low-fat diet with adequate calcium.
- Assess for role stress and adaptation to change.
- Teach need for cancer screening (breast, cervical, colon).
- Encourage breast self-examination, mammography, and regular checkups.

## Gender Development

In each stage of physical and emotional growth there are tasks related to the development of behaviors associated with the particular sexual role. Any condition or situation that interferes with the completion of these tasks may affect the development of sexual role behavior, but the process continues and evolves throughout the lifetime of an individual.

Sexual role or gender role is the public expression of behavior that implies masculinity or femininity. Gender identity is defined as the private or personal experience of a person's maleness or femaleness. It is usually, but not always, congruent with the individual's gender or biologic sex. The development of gender identity and sexual role behavior is a complex process influenced by biologic, psychologic, and social factors.

Gender identity begins with the biologic event of conception, when the X or Y chromosome of the male combines with the X chromosome of the female. An XY pair influences the undifferentiated gonad of the embryo to become a testis at a gestational age of about 6 weeks; an XX pair differentiates the gonad as an ovary at about 12 weeks.

The appearance of the external genitalia is the next factor in the development of sexual role behavior. The parents tailor child-rearing practices in accordance with their perception of their child's gender. The child eventually becomes aware of his or her body, including the genitalia. The child's body and the responses of others to it influence juvenile gender identity.

At puberty the production of hormones affects sexual desire and further development of the genitals. These changes at puberty, combined with social influences, determine adult gender identity.

## Reproductive Years

Patterns of childbearing are different for women of different cultural and economic circumstances. Some women bear children in their early teens, and others postpone motherhood until their late 30s or early 40s. Still others decide not to have children at all, and some women who want to have children eventually prove to be infertile. "Women of reproductive years" is thus a wide category, ranging from early teens to menopause. During this period women are concerned with establishing and maintaining intimate relationships and most women also have concerns about contraception. Decisions about birth control are needed to space childbearing or prevent it. Homosexual women do not share these concerns about birth control but may have different issues centering on becoming pregnant by the use of donor semen.

For a majority of women in their reproductive years, contraception is a significant concern. The well-informed nurse can provide much of the education and counseling that women need to make contraceptive decisions. A complete discussion of obstetrics is outside the scope of this book, and the nurse is advised to consult a comprehensive obstetric text (see the abortion and ectopic pregnancy discussions later in this chapter).

# Menopause

**Menopause** is defined as the cessation of menses associated with reduced ovarian function. It is diagnosed when a year has passed since the last menstrual period. The perimenopausal period is a transition during which reproductive function gradually diminishes and is eventually lost. Menopause is often referred to as "the change of life"; however, many women have no appreciable change in the normal pattern of living. Menopause is a normal physiologic process and simply means that the period of female reproductivity has come to an end.

In the majority of women menopause occurs between 45 and 55 years of age, but it may occur earlier or later. Artificial menopause may be induced by the surgical removal of the ovaries or by deep internal radiation and radium placed in the vaginal canal. Although some women stop menstruating abruptly, the usual pattern is a gradual tapering off. The flow may gradually decrease, with some irregularity of periods. When the production of the ovarian hormone (estrogen) falls below the level necessary to stimulate the endometrium, menstruation ceases. The uterus, vagina, and ovaries decrease in size.

Several changes in the epithelial cells occur in the postmenopausal woman that affect the vagina and urinary tract. Vaginal dryness, urinary frequency, and dysuria may result. Urinary tract infections may also occur more often in the menopausal woman because of thinning of the epithelial layer. At menopause the vaginal epithelium becomes pale and fragile and more susceptible to infection or trauma. The gradual loss of rugae and elasticity of the vagina and the decrease in lubrication may lead to complaints of dyspareunia. Because of atrophied tissue of the external genitalia, women may have vulvar pruritus. These changes are caused by the loss of estrogen and resolve with estrogen replacement. Loss of tone in the supporting ligaments may promote uterine prolapse or bulging of the uterus through the vaginal wall (rectocele, cystocele). Atrophic changes in breast glandular tissue result in altered shape and diminished size of the breasts.

Lack of estrogen contributes to the development of osteoporosis and a rise in heart disease risk. Cardiovascular disease is the leading cause of death among women over the age of 50 in the United States (Moore, Noonan, 1996). Metaanalysis of several studies suggests that estrogen replacement reduces the risk of cardiovascular disease by 35% to 50% in menopausal women (Thomas, 1996). Estrogen replacement also markedly reduces the risk of osteoporosis. Alternatively, osteoporosis may be treated by increased calcium intake, vitamin D supplements, and weight-bearing exercises, which prevent some loss of bone density after menopause. Most postmenopausal women are calcium deficient. The recommended intake of calcium for postmenopausal women not on hormone replacement therapy (HRT) is 1500 mg daily, which is equivalent to five 8-ounce glasses of skim milk. For a woman receiving HRT, 1000 to 1200 mg of calcium daily should be adequate.

With the cessation of menses many women do not experience symptoms severe enough to require medical care, but others are troubled by many symptoms. Hot flashes, which are warm feelings about the face and neck accompanied by sweating, are experienced by 50% to 87% of postmenopausal women (Moore, Noonan, 1996). These often occur at night and for some women may significantly interrupt sleep. Some women also complain of headaches, nervousness, palpitation, dizziness, insomnia, and irritability. When the symptoms are severe enough to require medical care, some form of estrogen therapy is often advised.

The use of supplementary estrogens to prevent osteoporosis and heart disease in menopausal women has generated a great deal of discussion and some disagreement. There is no single correct answer, and treatment must be individualized. Risk of osteoporosis and coronary disease, together with menopausal symptoms and medical history, must be evaluated by the medical provider and the woman to arrive at the most appropriate plan. *Estrogen therapy* is most effective in relieving hot flashes and night sweats. A patient with a history of uterine or breast cancer is not usually treated with estrogen, although this point of view is now being challenged. Patients receiving estrogen should have regular examinations for cancer of the uterus and breast. A woman with an intact uterus should not take unopposed estrogen, because this significantly increases the risk of endometrial cancer. For most women estrogen is usually prescribed with progesterone to eliminate this risk. If prescribed, estrogens may be administered orally, vaginally, or by transdermal patch. One form in common use is a naturally occurring estrogen (Premarin) derived from the urine of pregnant mares. When Premarin is administered in combination with Provera, a progesterone preparation, the excess risk of uterine cancer is eliminated. However, a woman may continue to have menses while receiving this combined therapy, and some women find this an unappealing side effect. Mild sedatives, tranquilizers, or mood-elevating drugs may be prescribed to alleviate psychologic symptoms. Emphasis should be placed on the normalcy of menopause, and women should be encouraged to pursue interests, hobbies, activities, and careers.

# NURSING ASSESSMENT OF THE PATIENT WITH PROBLEMS OF THE REPRODUCTIVE SYSTEM

The nursing assessment of female patients should include information on the onset of menses and menopause, a record of all pregnancies and their outcomes, the type of birth control (if used), and the date of the last Papanicolaou (Pap) smear. If the woman is still menstruating, the date of the first day of her last menstrual period should be recorded, as well as the length in days and the frequency and character of flow of each period or any bleeding between periods. The nurse should also note any of the symptoms related to PMS the woman is experiencing. These symptoms include weight gain, abdominal bloating, pelvic fullness, and a variety of emotional responses. (PMS is discussed in more detail earlier in this chapter.) The type and character of any pain or discomfort accompanying menstruation should be reported. In the menopausal female, symptoms of hot flashes, headache, nervousness, palpitation, dizziness, insomnia, and irritability should be identified, if present. Urinary symptoms such as stress, incontinence, urgency, or frequency are indicative of gynecologic problems.

Nursing is concerned with total patient care. Illness or disease can adversely affect a person's interest in sex or ability to function sexually. If a patient's condition or treatment raises sexual concerns or limits sexual ability, the nurse should provide an opportunity to discuss the situation with the patient. An attitude of nonjudgmental concern and caring on the part of the nurse creates an atmosphere conducive to discussion. Privacy when discussing sexual concerns is also important so that the patient knows confidentiality will be maintained. When privacy is provided and there are no distractions, the patient is better able to focus on sexual questions.

Nursing assessment of the patient with problems of the reproductive system is used to help the patient talk about sexual concerns and to help the nurse plan care, give information, or make referrals on the basis of the patient's problems. The assessment is best accomplished late in the interview when a nurse-patient relationship has been established. The assessment does not need to be long and detailed. Its primary focus is to help the patient identify sexual concerns (Box 43-1).

When assessing sexual functioning in the female, the nurse should know that chronic illnesses such as hypertension, arthritis, and diabetes, as well as medications, can decrease sexual desire and sexual response. Many individuals who take antihypertensives such as propranolol (Inderal) and methyldopa (Aldomet) may find that they have a diminished libido.

---

**BOX 43-1**

## QUESTIONS USED IN A SEXUAL ASSESSMENT

**TEENAGER**

You are starting to develop sexually. Has anyone talked to you about what that means?

Some girls your age have questions about the ways their bodies are developing. Do you have any?

What is the sexual climate at your school like? Are lots of kids sexually active?

Do you feel pressured by your friends to be sexually intimate?

Do you need a birth control method now?

Do you have any questions about birth control methods that I might answer?

**ADULT WOMAN**

Are you satisfied with your sexual life?

Do you think your partner is satisfied with your sexual life?

Do you experience pain or discomfort during intercourse?

Have you felt forced or pressured by your partner to have sex?

Have you ever or are you now being sexually abused?

**OLDER WOMAN**

In addition to the questions for the adult woman above:

What are your expectations for sex now that you are past menopause? Are things different than you expected?

Are there any illnesses that affect your sexuality?

Has your partner had any illnesses or surgeries that have affected your sex life?

---

This effect of medication on libido has been better studied among men than women, but problems of sexual function affect both partners. A woman may have suffered sexual abuse or rape at some time in her life and have subsequent difficulty enjoying sexual intimacy. Women may experience depression, anxiety, and sexual dysfunction for months to years after a sexually traumatic event. Referral for group or individual therapy or to a rape crisis center may be helpful.

Women may be troubled by sexual dysfunction but find it difficult to approach the topic with a health care provider. Nurses can introduce the subject by simply inquiring whether a patient is satisfied with her sexual life. Keeping questions open ended and allowing the patient to take the lead in the discussion promotes privacy and a sense of concern for the individual. The nurse should remember that words, tone of voice, and the phrasing of questions are important when assessing sexual function. The nurse should not reveal personal sexual value systems when asking questions or making comments. Clarification or additional information should be sought when an answer is unclear or incomplete. Words that the patient understands should be used. In some cases this means using slang or "street words." Both the patient and the nurse should be comfortable with word choices so that each understands what the other is saying. Patients differ greatly in the degree of openness with which they will discuss symptoms related to reproductive and sexual function. Learning to talk about sexual concerns and feelings is often difficult for both the nurse and the patient. For the nurse it is a skill that develops with careful practice.

Women often have problems they wish to discuss. The most common problem presented to the nurse is discomfort during intercourse. Pain occurring predominantly at the beginning of coitus may be caused by lack of lubrication, and the nurse can suggest that the couple engage in a longer period of foreplay until the woman is aroused or that she use a water-based lubricant such as K-Y Jelly to lubricate the introitus. A physical examination should rule out other causes such as herpes simplex, fissures, or other genital lesions. Pain during the thrusting phase of intercourse may be caused by the penis striking against the cervix or uterus. Some women have relatively short vaginal vaults or a position of the uterus that causes this type of discomfort. Changing position so that the woman has more control over the angle of coitus can help this problem. Of course, infections, pelvic inflammatory disease (PID), and uterine fibroids should be excluded. Other problems that women may report are anorgasmia (inability to have an orgasm) and decreased libido. Assessment of these problems can be complicated, and both physical and psychologic causes, including issues within the relationship, should be considered.

# NURSING RESPONSIBILITIES FOR DIAGNOSTIC PROCEDURES

## Physical Examination

Examination of the patient begins with a complete history, which includes the menstrual history, history of any pregnancies or past illnesses, and history of the present illness. The physical examination of the patient includes palpation of the breasts for evidence of cysts or tumors and examination of the pelvis. Nurses are employed in many ambulatory care offices, and it is important for them to be familiar with the procedure for pelvic examination and their responsibilities in assisting the health care provider.

## Breast Examination

The clinician palpates the breasts during the breast examination. In recent years emphasis has been placed on teaching women to palpate their own breasts monthly. Early cancer of the breast is curable, and if every woman would take time to examine her breasts carefully at regular intervals, many benign and malignant tumors would be discovered early. Nurses should become familiar with the procedure of breast self-examination so that they may teach patients, friends, or members of their families (Figure 43-7).

## Pelvic Examination

The nurse must understand that the pelvic examination may not be easy for the patient and may have been long delayed. The nurse should try to relieve the patient's anxiety, fears, and embarrassment by maintaining a caring attitude and explaining the procedure to her.

In preparation for the examination the patient should be instructed to void and evacuate the bowel, if necessary. Clothing below the waist should be removed to allow visualization of the genitalia and palpation of the abdomen. If the breast examination will be performed at the same time, all clothing should be removed and the patient should be dressed in an examination gown.

## Positioning the Patient

The patient is usually placed in the lithotomy position with both legs elevated in stirrups and the lower third of the table pushed back and out of the way. The patient is then asked to slide her buttocks down so that they extend just over the edge of the table. If an examination table is not available or the patient cannot be moved to one, the examination can be performed in bed with the buttocks elevated on a firm surface such as a wrapped bedpan. The patient should be carefully draped, and unnecessary exposure should be avoided. A sheet or bath blanket positioned diagonally should cover the chest, abdomen, and both legs; the lowest corner can be lifted to visualize the genitalia.

### Examination Procedure

The procedure begins with a visual inspection of the external genitalia. A speculum examination is performed to visualize the cervix and obtain the Pap smear. A sample of cells is obtained and placed on a slide or immersed in alcohol to fix the cells to the slide. Other cultures or a wet prep may also be obtained at this time, depending on the patient's symptoms and risk factors. Then a bimanual examination of the uterus

**How to do BSE**

*1. Lie down and put a pillow under your right shoulder. Place your right arm behind your head.*
*2. Use the finger pads of the three middle fingers on your left hand to feel for lumps or thickening. Your finger pads are the top third of each finger.*

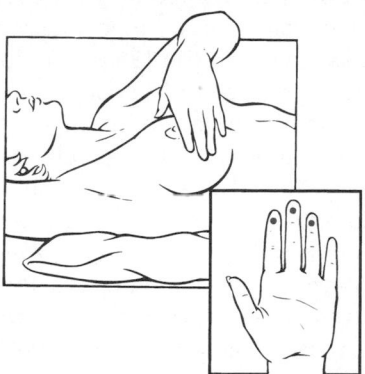

*3. Press hard enough to know how your breast feels. If you're not sure how hard to press, ask your health care provider. Or try to copy the way your health care provider uses the finger pads during a breast exam. Learn what your breast feels like most of the time. A firm ridge in the lower curve of each breast is normal.*

*4. Move around the breast in a set way. You can choose either the circle (A), the up and down line (B), or the wedge (C). Do it the same way every time. It will help you to make sure that you've gone over the entire breast area and to remember how your breast feels each month.*

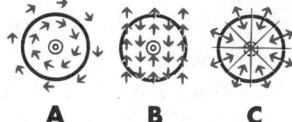

**A          B          C**

*5. Now examine your left breast using right hand finger pads.*
*You might want to check your breasts while standing in front of a mirror right after you do your BSE each month. You might also want to do an extra BSE while you're in the shower. Your soapy hands will glide over the wet skin making it easy to check how your breasts feel.*

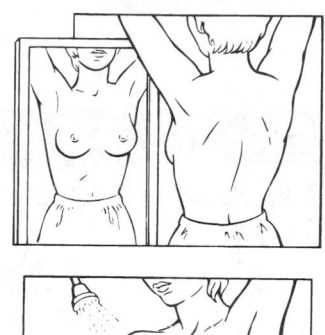

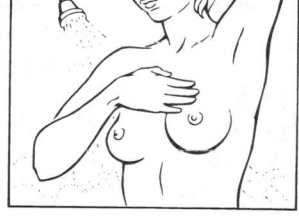

**Figure 43-7**    Breast self-examination. (Courtesy of American Cancer Society.)

is performed. The clinician inserts two fingers of a gloved hand into the vagina up to the cervix while using the other hand to place gentle pressure on the lower abdomen over the uterus. Pressure on the abdomen applies pressure to the fundus. The position of the uterus and the condition of the ovaries are checked at this time. Cervical motion tenderness might indicate a pelvic infection. Finally a bimanual rectovaginal examination is performed by inserting the second finger into the vagina and the third finger into the rectum. The other hand is placed on the abdomen to palpate rectal and pelvic abnormalities. A clean glove should be used because infections from the vagina, such as gonorrhea, can be inadvertently transmitted to the rectum by the clinician. The nurse stays during the procedure to offer support to the patient, assist the examiner, focus the light, and provide instruments or equipment as

needed. When the examination is complete, the patient should be cleansed of any lubricating jelly or offered tissues. The patient can then be assisted to sit on the table and should be encouraged to stay sitting until she is sure she is not dizzy. The clinician may speak to the patient at this time or may return after the patient has dressed to discuss further treatment.

Handling and cleaning of examination equipment, cultures, wet preps, or Pap smears should be performed with caution and while wearing latex gloves because many pelvic diseases are infectious. Clinicians do not always follow clean technique and subsequently contaminate objects in the room with their gloved hands. The light, fixative spray, and tube of lubricating jelly are most likely to be contaminated. The nurse should discuss with the clinician how to prevent this from occurring so that objects do not need to be discarded because of contamination. Care should be taken with a reusable tube of lubricating jelly that the clinician's gloved hand does not touch the dispensing end of the tube.

# BIRTH CONTROL (CONTRACEPTION)

Birth control, or contraception, is the voluntary prevention of pregnancy. The selected method of birth control depends on individual preferences, religious beliefs, and cultural considerations. A complete history, physical examination, and laboratory tests may precede the prescription of some forms of contraception. Methods of birth control include hormonal methods such as oral contraceptives, Norplant, and Depo-Provera; IUDs; diaphragms; cervical caps; condoms; foams; suppositories; jellies; and natural family planning (Table 43-2).

## Combined Oral Contraceptives

Combined oral contraceptive pills (OCPs) were approved by the U.S. Food and Drug Administration (FDA) in 1960. Since then they have been extensively studied and found to be safe and effective. Although brands differ, all combined oral OCPs contain some form of estrogen and progestin. Since the early research on the pill in the 1960s, the dose has been lowered considerably, and most women choosing this method today are started on a low-dose birth control pill. Although the serious side effects are theoretically possible at low doses, the likelihood of their occurrence is extremely low. Nonetheless, according to a 1980 Gallup poll, approximately 75% of women who are 35 years or younger consider the use of oral contraceptives to be very risky (Kaunitz, 1992). Most women named cancer as their chief concern. In fact, oral contraceptives have been shown to markedly *de-*

---

### TABLE 43-2

### Pharmacology of Drugs Used for Women's Reproductive Health

| DRUG (GENERIC AND TRADE NAME); ROUTE AND DOSAGE | ACTION/INDICATION | COMMON SIDE EFFECTS AND NURSING CONSIDERATIONS |
|---|---|---|
| **Clomiphene** (Clomid)<br>**Route:** PO<br>**Dosage:** PO 50-100 mg q × 5 days or 50-100 mg q beginning on day 5 of the cycle; may be repeated until conception occurs or 3 cycles of therapy have been completed | Ovulation stimulant used in female infertility | Headache; depression; nausea; vomiting; constipation; rash; and dermatitis; contraindicated in hepatic disease or undiagnosed vaginal bleeding; use with caution in hypertension, depression, convulsions, or diabetes |
| **Danazol** (Danocrine)<br>**Route:** PO<br>**Dosage:** Endometriosis, initial dose 500 mg bid, then decrease to 400 mg bid × 3-9 mo; fibrocystic breast disease, 100-400 mg q in 2 divided doses × 2-6 mo | Androgen used in the treatment of endometriosis, prevention of hereditary angiodema, and fibrocystic breast disease | Cholestatic jaundice; contraindicated in severe renal, cardiac, or hepatic disease; use with caution in seizures or migraine headaches; may increase effects of anticoagulants |
| **Estradiol, Estradiol Cypionate, Estradiol Valerate**<br>**Route:** PO, IM, topical<br>**Dosage:** Menopause, ovarian failure, PO 1-2 mg q × 3 wk on, 1 wk off or 5 days on, 2 days off; or IM 0.2-1.0 mg q wk; breast cancer, PO 10 mg tid × 3 mo or longer; atrophic vaginitis, vaginal cream 2-4 g qd × 1-2 wk, then 1 g 1-3 times a week; kraurosis vulvae, IM, 1-1.5 mg 1-2 wk | Nonsteroidal synthetic estrogen used for menopause, breast cancer, prostatic cancer, atrophic vaginitis, kraurosis vulvae, hypogonadism, castration, primary ovarian failure, and prevention of osteoporosis | Gynecomastia, testicular atrophy, impotence, thromboembolism, stroke; pulmonary embolism, myocardial infarction, and cholestatic jaundice; contraindicated in breast cancer, thromboembolic disorders, and reproductive cancer; use with caution in hypertension, asthma, blood dyscrasias, gallbladder disease, congestive heart failure, diabetes, bone disease, depression, migraine headaches, convulsant disorders, hepatic and renal disease, and family history of cancer of the breast or reproductive tract |

| TABLE 43-2 | | |
| --- | --- | --- |

## Pharmacology of Drugs Used for Women's Reproductive Health—cont'd

| DRUG (GENERIC AND TRADE NAME); ROUTE AND DOSAGE | ACTION/INDICATION | COMMON SIDE EFFECTS AND NURSING CONSIDERATIONS |
| --- | --- | --- |
| **Leuprolide** (Lupron) **Route:** SC **Dosage:** 1 mg/day | Antineoplastic gonadotropin-releasing hormone used in the management of endometriosis | Edema, hot flashes, impotence, decreased libido, amenorrhea, vaginal dryness, gynecomastia; contraindicated in thromboembolic disorders, pregnancy, and undiagnosed vaginal bleeding; use with caution in edema, hepatic, cerebrovascular accident, myocardial infarction, seizures, hypertension, or diabetes; monitor liver function tests |
| **Levonorgestrel Implant** (Norplant System) **Route:** Subdermal caps implanted in the upper arm **Dosage:** Implanted during first 7 days after onset of menses; may remain × 5 yr | Synthetic progestin contraceptive used in the prevention of pregnancy over a 5-yr period | Possibly a change in appetite or weight gain; no common side effects; contraindicated in thrombophlebitis, undiagnosed genital bleeding, liver tumors, breast carcinoma, and liver disease; use with caution in depression, psychosis, lactation, fluid retention, and contact lens wearers |
| **Medroxyprogesterone Acetate** (Depo-Provera) **Route:** PO, IM **Dosage:** Secondary amenorrhea, PO 5-10 mg q × 5-10 days; endometrial/renal cancer, IM 400-1000 mg/wk; uterine bleeding, PO 5-10 mg q × 5-10 days starting on 16th day of menstrual cycle | Progesterone derivative used for uterine bleeding, secondary amenorrhea, endometrial and renal cancer, and as a contraceptive | Depression, nausea, gynecomastia, testicular atrophy, impotence, spontaneous abortion, thromboembolism, stroke, pulmonary embolism, myocardial infarction, or cholestatic jaundice; contraindicated in breast cancer, thromboembolic disorders, reproductive cancer, or genital bleeding; use with caution in lactation, hypertension, asthma, blood dyscrasias, gallbladder disease, congestive heart failure, diabetes, bone disease, depression, migraine headache, convulsive disorders, hepatic or renal disease, and family history of cancer of the breast or reproductive tract |
| **Norethindrone** **Route:** PO **Dosage:** 5-20 mg q days 5-25 of menstrual cycle; endometriosis, 10 mg q × 2 wk, then increased by 5 mg q × 2 wk, up to 30 mg/day | Progesterone derivative used to control abnormal uterine bleeding, amenorrhea, and endometriosis | Nausea, thromboembolism, stroke, pulmonary embolism, myocardial infarction, cholestatic jaundice, and spontaneous abortion; contraindicated in breast cancer, thromboembolic disorders, reproductive cancer, and genital bleeding; use with caution in lactation, hypertension, asthma, blood dyscrasias, gallbladder disease, congestive heart failure, diabetes, bone disease, depression, migraine headache, convulsive disorders, hepatic or renal disease, and family history of breast or reproductive tract cancer |
| **Norgestrel** **Route:** PO **Dosage:** 1 tablet q day | Progesterone derivative used as a contraceptive | Nausea, gynecomastia, testicular atrophy, impotence, thromboembolism, stroke, pulmonary embolism, myocardial infarction, cholestatic jaundice, and spontaneous abortion; contraindications and precautions same as above |

*Continued*

**TABLE 43-2**

## Pharmacology of Drugs Used for Women's Reproductive Health—cont'd

| DRUG (GENERIC AND TRADE NAME); ROUTE AND DOSAGE | ACTION/INDICATION | COMMON SIDE EFFECTS AND NURSING CONSIDERATIONS |
|---|---|---|
| **Tamoxifen Citrate** (Nolvadex)<br>**Route:** PO<br>**Dosage:** 10-20 mg bid | Antineoplastic, antiestrogen hormone used in advanced breast carcinoma that has not responded to other therapy in estrogen-receptor-positive patients (usually postmenopausal) | Nausea, vomiting, rash, hot flashes, headache, and lightheadedness; use with caution in leukopenia, thrombocytopenia, lactation, and cataracts; withhold drug if WBC is <3500 or platelet count is <100,000 |
| **COMMON DRUGS FOR VAGINITIS**<br>**Clotrimazole** (Lotrimin)<br>**Route:** Topical, intravaginal<br>**Dosage:** Topical, rub into affected area bid × 1-8 wk; intravaginal 1 applicator × 1-2 wk hs | Local antifungal, antiinfective used for infections of the vagina and vulva | Infrequent burning, itching, stinging, redness, and local hypersensitivity reactions |
| **Metronidazole** (Flagyl)<br>**Route:** PO, IV, topical<br>**Dosage:** Anaerobic infections, PO, 7.5 mg/kg q 6 hr (not to exceed 4 g/day), IV, initial dose 15 mg/kg, then 7.5 mg/kg q 6 hr (not to exceed 4 g/day); trichomoniasis, PO, 250 mg q 8 hr for 7 days (single 2 g dose or 1 g bid for 1 day may be used); bacterial vaginosis, topical, 5 g bid for 5 days | Antiinfective used for treatment of anaerobic infections, including such gynecologic infections as trichomoniasis, and bacterial vaginosis | Headache, dizziness, nausea, vomiting, abdominal pain, anorexia, and diarrhea; contraindicated in first trimester of pregnancy; use with caution in blood dyscrasias, history of seizures or neurologic problems, and severe hepatic impairment; PO administrations should be administered with food |
| **Nystatin** (Mycostatin)<br>**Route:** Intravaginal, topical<br>**Dosage:** Intravaginal, one tablet (100,000 units nystatin) daily for 2 wk; topical, cream and ointment applied liberally to affected areas bid or as indicated until healing complete | Antifungal used in the treatment of vaginal *Candida* infections | Nystatin is well tolerated by all age groups; insert vaginal tablets high into the vagina with applicator |
| **Terconazole** (Terazol 3, Terazol 7)<br>**Route:** Intravaginal, topical<br>**Dosage:** Intravaginal, 1 suppository (80 mg) administered at bedtime × 3 consecutive days; topical, 0.4% or 0.8% vaginal cream is administered with applicator intravaginally at bedtime × 3 consecutive days | Antifungal, antiinfective used for vaginal and vulvovaginal candidiasis | Headache; patients with recurrent vulvovaginal infections may indicate a chronic illness requiring other interventions |

crease a woman's risk of developing ovarian and endometrial cancer. Oral contraceptives used for 1 year reduce a woman's risk of ovarian cancer by 40%, and OCPs used for 10 years reduce the risk of ovarian cancer by 80%. Furthermore, this protection appears to last for more than a decade after discontinuation of use (Kaunitz, 1992). Endometrial cancer risk is reduced by 50% after 12 months of OCP use, and this protective effect persists for more than 15 years after use is discontinued. No clear evidence of increased risk of breast cancer with use of the birth control pill has been presented. Thus the nurse can perform an important role in dispelling myths about the risks of cancer with use of the birth control pill.

> ## NURSE ALERT
>
> **Contraindications to oral contraceptive pills include cerebrovascular accident, myocardial infarction, deep vein thrombosis, uncontrolled hypertension, liver disease, and pregnancy.**

**Mechanism of action and effectiveness.** The combined birth control pill prevents pregnancy primarily by suppressing ovulation. In addition, progestin in the pill thickens cervical mucus, making it less possible for sperm to ascend the endocervical canal. The birth control pill is 97% to 99.9% effective. No differences in effectiveness among brands have been described. A higher potency pill is sometimes recommended for women who are taking medications for seizure disorder because these medications decrease the effectiveness of the pill (Table 43-3).

**Risks, benefits, and side effects.** Cardiovascular complications such as stroke, heart attack, blood clots, and hypertension are extremely rare, as are hepatic adenomas. The risk of cardiovascular complications increases in women over age 35 who smoke. Smokers over the age of 35 should be encouraged to consider other birth control methods.

Side effects are usually minimal but may occur in certain women, especially in the first few months of OCP use. These include nausea, headache, dizziness, spotting, weight gain, breast tenderness, and cholasma (increased pigmentation of the face). Taking the OCP at bedtime or with food should minimize nausea. Taking pills at the same time each day may help to prevent breakthrough bleeding. Occasionally a change in the OCP is needed to find the right match for the individual woman. Since many brands are available, this can be easily accomplished.

The nurse should take side effects seriously because patients may discontinue OCP use if they experience troublesome side effects. The noncontraceptive benefits in terms of cancer protection have been described previously. In addition, birth control pills protect the patient from uterine fibroids, benign breast masses, PID, and ovarian cysts. The pill also decreases menstrual blood loss and lessens menstrual cramps. OCPs may help to protect fertility by preventing PID and ectopic pregnancy. No delay in return to fertility is to be expected when a woman discontinues OCP use.

**Patient use.** Birth control pills are prescribed in 21- or 28-day cycles. In the 28-day pack the pills for the last week are inactive and may contain small amounts of iron. These inactive pills allow the woman to stay in the habit of taking a daily pill. A woman may be instructed to start her first pack on the first day of menses or on the first Sunday after the onset of menses. If she is prescribed a 21-day pack, she takes pills for 3 weeks and waits 1 week to begin the next pack. She can expect her period in the week she is not taking pills. If she is prescribed a 28-day pack, she begins a new pack immediately after finishing all the pills in the previous pack. She can also expect her menses in the week before starting a new pack of OCPs. Women should be

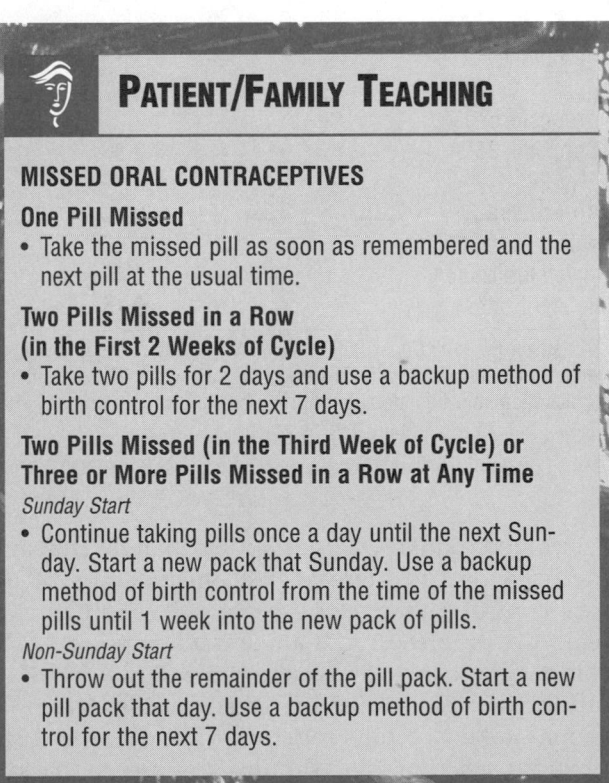

> ## 👤 PATIENT/FAMILY TEACHING
>
> ### MISSED ORAL CONTRACEPTIVES
>
> **One Pill Missed**
> - Take the missed pill as soon as remembered and the next pill at the usual time.
>
> **Two Pills Missed in a Row
> (in the First 2 Weeks of Cycle)**
> - Take two pills for 2 days and use a backup method of birth control for the next 7 days.
>
> **Two Pills Missed (in the Third Week of Cycle) or Three or More Pills Missed in a Row at Any Time**
> *Sunday Start*
> - Continue taking pills once a day until the next Sunday. Start a new pack that Sunday. Use a backup method of birth control from the time of the missed pills until 1 week into the new pack of pills.
> *Non-Sunday Start*
> - Throw out the remainder of the pill pack. Start a new pill pack that day. Use a backup method of birth control for the next 7 days.

**TABLE 43-3**

## Percentage of Women Experiencing a Contraceptive Failure During the First Year of Typical Use and the First Year of Perfect Use and the Percentage Continuing Use at the End of the First Year, United States

| METHOD | PERCENTAGE OF WOMEN EXPERIENCING AN ACCIDENTAL PREGNANCY WITHIN THE FIRST YEAR OF USE | | PERCENTAGE OF WOMEN CONTINUING USE AT 1 YEAR |
|---|---|---|---|
| | TYPICAL USE | PERFECT USE | |
| Chance | 85 | 85 | |
| Spermicides | 21 | 6 | 43 |
| Periodic abstinence | 20 | | 67 |
| Calendar | | 9 | |
| Ovulation method | | 3 | |
| Symptothermal | | 2 | |
| Postovulation | | 1 | |
| Withdrawal | 19 | 4 | |
| Cap | | | |
| Parous women | 36 | 26 | 45 |
| Nulliparous women | 18 | 9 | 58 |
| Sponge | | | |
| Parous women | 36 | 20 | 45 |
| Nulliparous women | 18 | 9 | 58 |
| Diaphragm | 18 | 6 | 58 |
| Condom | | | |
| Female (Reality) | 21 | 5 | 56 |
| Male | 12 | 3 | 63 |
| Pill | 3 | | 72 |
| Progestin only | | 0.5 | |
| Combined | | 0.1 | |
| IUD | | | |
| Progesterone T | 2.0 | 1.5 | 81 |
| Copper T 380A | 0.8 | 0.6 | 78 |
| LNg 20 | 0.1 | 0.1 | 81 |
| Depo-Provera | 0.3 | 0.3 | 70 |
| Norplant (6 capsules) | 0.09 | 0.09 | 85 |
| Female sterilization | 0.4 | 0.4 | 100 |
| Male sterilization | 0.15 | 0.10 | 100 |

From Hatcher RA et al: *Contraceptive technology*, ed 16 revised, New York, 1994, Irvington.
**Emergency contraceptive pills:** Treatment initiated within 72 hours after unprotected intercourse reduces the risk of pregnancy by at least 75%.
**Lactational amenorrhea method:** LAM is a highly effective, *temporary* method of contraception.

encouraged to take OCPs at approximately the same time each day to increase the effectiveness of the birth control pill and decrease the likelihood of breakthrough bleeding. If a woman misses a pill, she should take it as soon as she remembers or take it with the next scheduled pill. If she misses two pills, she may take two pills together for 2 days until she is caught up, but she should also use a backup method of birth control (such as condoms and foam) for 1 week (see the Patient/Family Teaching box on

p. 1349). Because some antibiotics decrease the effectiveness of birth control pills, a woman should be advised to use a backup method of contraception when antibiotics are prescribed. Birth control pills become effective for contraception after 1 week. Therefore a backup method of contraception should be used during the first week of use if the woman begins on the Sunday after her menses. If she begins on the first day of menses, a backup method of contraception is not considered necessary.

## Progestin-Only Pills (Mini Pills)

Progestin-only pills are not as effective as combined OCPs and tend to cause irregular menstruation. However, they can be used by lactating women without disruption of milk production, and they may be an appropriate alternative for women who should not take combined contraceptive pills. Thus women at risk for the estrogen-related side effects of the combined pill may be advised to use a progestin-only pill. In the older woman (ages 35 to 50) whose fertility is diminished, the lessened efficacy may not be as great an issue as for the younger woman. The effects of mini pills are immediately reversible. They have no effect on long-term fertility.

**Mechanism of action and effectiveness.** Progestin-only pills thicken cervical mucus, so that sperm have greater difficulty penetrating the endocervical canal and ascending into the uterus. The progestin-only pill does not inhibit ovulation as reliably as combined OCPs. It does, however, promote a thin, atrophic endometrium that is inhospitable to the fertilized ovum. In the first year of typical use the proportion of women becoming pregnant while taking the progestin-only pill ranges from 1.19% to 13.29% (Hatcher et al, 1994). Taking pills even a few hours late markedly reduces efficacy, as does use of anticonvulsants. Because lactation tends to inhibit ovulation, the progestin-only pill is almost 100% effective for lactating women.

**Risks, benefits, and side effects.** Because mini pills do not contain estrogen, they do not cause the estrogen-related complications that may occur with the combined pill. They are more likely to cause menstrual disturbance, which may include frequent bleeding or amenorrhea. Mini pills possibly decrease bone density, adding to a woman's risk of osteoporosis later in life, although this has not been thoroughly studied. Mini pills may cause lighter bleeding patterns or amenorrhea, which lessens a woman's risk for anemia. They may also lessen the cramping associated with endometriosis. Thickening of cervical mucus helps protect a woman from PID. Mini pills are also thought to protect women from endometrial and ovarian cancer, as do combined OCPs.

**Patient use.** Women who have contraindications to estrogen (Box 43-2) or who have severe headaches or hypertension while taking estrogen may consider use of progestin-only pills or other progestin-only methods (see Norplant and Depo-Provera discussions later in this chapter). For lactating women the progestin-only pill is an excellent choice. The nurse should counsel women to take progestin-only pills at exactly the same time each day to promote their effectiveness. If a woman tends to be forgetful about taking pills, the progestin-only pill may not be an effective method of contraception for her.

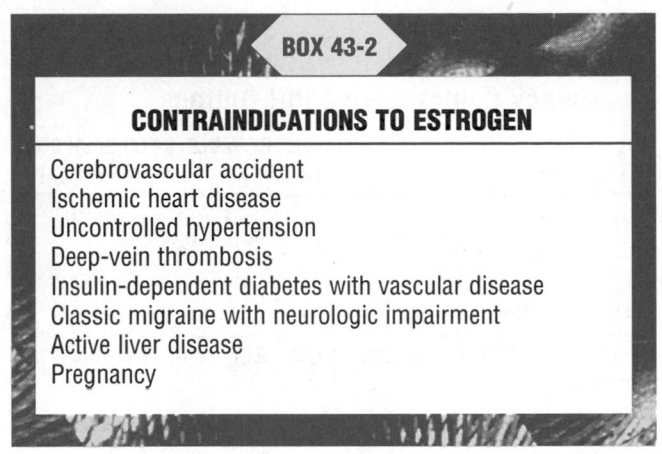

**BOX 43-2**

### CONTRAINDICATIONS TO ESTROGEN

Cerebrovascular accident
Ischemic heart disease
Uncontrolled hypertension
Deep-vein thrombosis
Insulin-dependent diabetes with vascular disease
Classic migraine with neurologic impairment
Active liver disease
Pregnancy

## Emergency Contraception: Postcoital Pill

Emergency contraception is safe and effective. It has been available for two decades but remains an underused form of birth control. Some clinicians are disinclined to offer it because the FDA has not approved birth control pills for this use and because they believe women will come to rely on it for contraception. These assumptions should be challenged. "As long as condoms break, inclination and opportunity unexpectedly converge, men rape women, diaphragms and cervical caps are dislodged, people are so ambivalent about sex that they need to be swept away, IUDs are expelled, and pills are lost or forgotten, we will need emergency postcoital contraception" (Hatcher et al, 1994). The contraceptive method most often used in an emergency involves commonly available but specifically formulated birth control pills given in two doses 12 hours apart (Table 43-4). Other birth control pills have not been used for this purpose. Postcoital insertion of an IUD can also be used as an emergency contraceptive, and high-dose progestin-only pills are available outside the United States for emergency contraception. Treatment should be initiated as early as possible (12 to 14 hours) after unprotected intercourse is ideal, but treatment may be given up to 72 hours after intercourse.

**Mechanism of action and effectiveness.** Hormonal methods interrupt ovarian hormone production and interfere with the preparation of the endometrium for implantation. These methods may also have an effect on transportation of the egg in the fallopian tube and thus inhibit fertilization (Hatcher et al, 1994). Effectiveness for an individual may be difficult to estimate because the risk of pregnancy varies depending on the timing of intercourse with relation to the menstrual cycle. At midcycle the risk of pregnancy is the highest. One act of intercourse at ovulation has been estimated to carry a 15% to 26% risk of pregnancy (Hatcher et al,

**TABLE 43-4**

## Emergency Contraceptive Pill Options

| BRAND NAME | NUMBER OF TABLETS FOR EACH DOSE (TWO DOSES, 12 HOURS APART) |
|---|---|
| Ovral | 4 |
| Lo/Ovral, Nordette, or Levlen; Triphasil or Tri-Levlen (yellow pills only) | 4 |

From Hatcher RA et al: *Contraceptive technology*, ed 16, New York, 1994, Irvington.

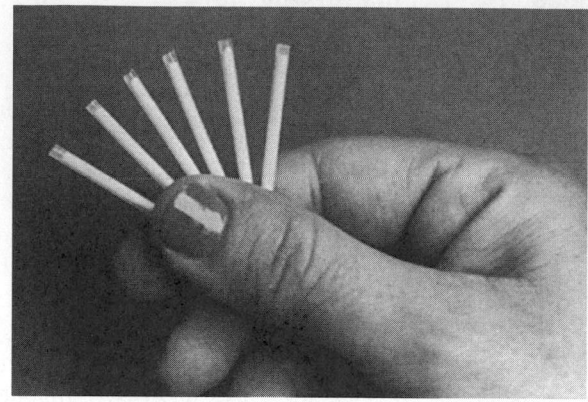

**Figure 43-8** Norplant System implants. (Courtesy of Wyeth-Ayerst Laboratories, Philadelphia.)

1994). Use of emergency contraception pill treatment reduces the risk of pregnancy by approximately 75% (Hatcher et al, 1994).

**Risks, benefits, and side effects.** Women who cannot take birth control pills should also not use hormonal emergency contraception. The most common side effects of this method are nausea and vomiting. Dizziness, headache, and abdominal pain occur less often. Menses usually occurs within 1 week of a woman's regular, expected period.

**Patient use.** The largest barrier to use of the postcoital pill is making women aware of its availability. The nurse should counsel all patients about the availability of emergency contraception. In particular, women using barrier methods should be informed that this method is available if they experience a failure of the barrier method. Women should be advised to return for a pregnancy test if menses does not begin within 3 weeks of treatment. Women should also be told that they may experience nausea and vomiting. Some clinicians advise that an extra dose be taken if the patient vomits within 1 hour of a dose. To use this method comfortably, women need careful instruction and preparation about what to expect.

## Norplant

The Norplant system is a long-acting, reversible method of birth control. Research and development for Norplant began in 1966, and the first clinical trials took place in Chile in 1974. Norplant was approved for use by the FDA in 1989 and first marketed in 1990 by Wyeth-Ayerst Laboratories.

The Norplant system provides effective and continuous contraception for up to 5 years. Six thin, flexible capsules made of Silastic tubing are filled with levonorgestrel (Figure 43-8). These capsules are inserted in a fan-shaped pattern just under the skin on the inside of a woman's upper arm. Small amounts of levonorgestrel continuously diffuse through the capsule walls to maintain an effective blood level of the hormone. Although the capsules may be palpable, they are usually invisible under the skin. Norplant may be a good choice of contraception for women who cannot remember to take birth control pills and who want a contraceptive method that does not depend on special action at the time of intercourse.

**Mechanism of action and effectiveness.** Norplant maintains a constant low level of hormone in the body. It prevents pregnancy by inhibiting ovulation, thickening cervical mucus, and decreasing the receptivity of the endometrium toward implantation. With an annual failure rate of 0.09% in the first year of use, Norplant is one of the most effective contraception methods available (Hatcher et al, 1994). The chance of accidental pregnancy rises only slightly with subsequent years of use. Women taking antiseizure medication should be advised to consider alternative contraception because most antiseizure medications induce hepatic enzymes that break down levonorgestrel, the hormone contained in Norplant.

**Risks, benefits, and side effects.** The most commonly reported side effect is a change in the menstrual bleeding pattern. Some women have prolonged bleeding, others have erratic spotting, and still others amenorrhea. The type of bleeding pattern a woman will experience with Norplant cannot be predicted. Usually the monthly blood loss does not exceed that of normal menses. Some women using Norplant also complain of headaches. More rarely women have complained of nervousness, nausea, dizziness, acne, weight change, mastalgia, hirsutism, and hair loss. The average weight gain with Norplant over 5 years is under 5 pounds, which is a typical pattern for women irrespective of contraceptive choice. There is a small risk of infection at the insertion site. A patient may also have a 1/4-inch scar at the site of insertion; no sutures are required.

**Noncontraceptive benefits.** The noncontraceptive benefits of Norplant use are similar to those of the progestin-only pill.

**Patient use.** Norplant is inserted under local anesthetic during minor, in-office surgery. Usually insertion can be accomplished within 15 minutes, although removal may be more difficult and time consuming. An incision of about ¼ inch is made in the skin, and the capsules are inserted by use of a trocar. A Steri-Strip is applied to close the incision, and a dry sterile dressing with a gauze bandage is placed over the incision. Patients should be advised to leave the dressing in place to protect the arm for 3 to 5 days. A woman may notice substantial bruising after the dressing is removed. She should be advised to return if she finds pus or bleeding at the insertion site.

Before having the Norplant inserted, the patient should have been advised of the likelihood of a change in menstrual periods and the possibility of other side effects (see the previously discussed risks, benefits, and side effects). Women with Norplant insertions should be told to call back in the event of frequent bleeding because a cycle of low-dose oral contraceptive pills or conjugated estrogens can be prescribed temporarily to control bleeding. Norplant becomes effective for contraception within 24 hours. Normally it is inserted during menses to ensure that the woman is not already pregnant at the time of insertion. If it is inserted at another time, a pregnancy test is performed before insertion and an alternative method of contraception should be used for the remainder of that cycle.

## Depo-Provera

Depo-Provera (DMPA) is a long-acting, injectable contraceptive that acts to prevent pregnancy for 3 months per injection. DMPA was used by 8 to 9 million women worldwide before it was approved in the United States (Hatcher et al, 1994). It is available as a 150-mg dose of medroxyprogesterone acetate suspension suitable for injection into the deltoid or gluteus maximus muscles. In the United States it is typically provided in single-dose vials of 150 mg of DMPA in 1 ml of fluid.

**Mechanism of action and effectiveness.** DMPA is given by intramuscular injection every 12 weeks. It inhibits ovulation by suppressing FSH and LH levels. Like other progestin-only contraceptives, it promotes a thick cervical mucus that functions as a barrier to sperm and an atrophic endometrium that resists implantation of a fertilized ovum. DMPA has a first-year failure rate of 0.3%. Its efficacy continues beyond the 12-week dosage regimen, and women may be given a subsequent injection up to 14 weeks after the prior dose.

**Risks, benefits, and side effects.** Because DMPA does not contain estrogen, it may be suitable for women who have contraindications to oral contraceptive pills. Its side effect profile is similar to those of Norplant and the progestin-only pill. The most prominent side effect is menstrual cycle disturbance. During the first year of use women may be more likely to experience frequent bleeding or spotting. However, the longer a woman continues to take DMPA, the more likely she is to experience amenorrhea. Weight gain is more likely than with other progestin-only contraceptives. An increase of 2 to 5 pounds is possible in the first year of use. DMPA provides a higher dose of hormone than Norplant and so is less likely to be adversely affected by antiseizure medication. In addition, it may improve seizure control. Some concern exists about the effect of DMPA on bone density over time. More research is needed to clarify this effect. The noncontraceptive benefits of DMPA use are similar to those of the progestin-only pill.

**Patient use.** Injections should be scheduled every 3 months. If the first injection is given within 5 days of the onset of menses, no backup method of contraception is necessary because DMPA becomes effective within 24 hours. If it is given at another point in the cycle, backup contraception must be used for 2 weeks. Although DMPA is reversible, patients should be advised that a 6-month delay in return to fertility is possible. Injection should be given intramuscularly in the deltoid or gluteus maximus muscles. The nurse should *not* massage the area of injection because this may decrease the effectiveness of DMPA (Hatcher et al, 1994).

Women using this method should be prepared to expect menstrual changes. Patients can be told that troublesome spotting or breakthrough bleeding can usually be managed by a cycle or more of combined OCPs. Patients should also be told that amenorrhea is likely to increase the longer they remain on DMPA but that this is not harmful.

## Intrauterine Device

The intrauterine device (IUD) was developed in the 1930s, but its use first became widespread in the 1960s. Only two kinds of IUDs are available in the United States. Lawsuits by women who became infertile because of PID caused other IUDs to be withdrawn from the market. In particular, an IUD known as the Dalkon Shield was associated with a greater chance of infection and infertility. Despite its current low popularity in the United States, the IUD remains popular worldwide and is an important option for selected women.

The CuT 380A (ParaGard) intrauterine copper contraceptive is approved for 10 years of use. It is manufactured in a polyethylene T-shape with barium sulfate added to create x-ray visibility. Thin copper wire is wound around the vertical arm of the T, and a single filament string is looped through the bottom of the T. In contrast, the progesterone T (Progestasert system), which releases small amounts of progesterone, is approved for only 1 year of use. Because it must be replaced annually, it offers no advantage over the copper T but is an option for women allergic to copper.

A new IUD called the levonorgestrel IUD is available in Europe and is likely to be approved for use in the United States soon. It releases 20 mg of levonorgestrel into the uterus daily and is designed for 5 years of use.

**Mechanism of action and effectiveness.** The manner in which the IUD works is unclear, although it appears to immobilize sperm, speed transport of the egg through the fallopian tube, and effect changes in the endometrium that make implantation unlikely. Its efficacy depends on many factors, including age and parity of the user and clinical experience in inserting the IUD. The first-year failure rates for typical IUD users are 0.8% for the ParaGard and 2% for the Progestasert system (Hatcher et al, 1994). The new levonorgestrel IUD has a better efficacy rate and may also reduce the incidence of PID and lessen menstrual bleeding.

**Risks, benefits, and side effects.** Women with IUDs are at increased risk for PID. Because the risk is slightly higher just after the time of insertion, the long-acting copper T rather than the Progestasert system, which needs annual replacement, is preferable. Women who are not in mutually monogamous relationships have a higher risk of PID and subsequent infertility. Whether the IUD puts a woman at greater risk for contracting HIV is unknown. A small risk of uterine perforation at the time of insertion is directly related to clinician experience. Approximately 2% to 10% of first-time IUD users spontaneously expel their IUDs (Hatcher et al, 1994). If expulsion is undetected, pregnancy can result. Pregnancy with the IUD in place results in spontaneous abortion half the time, but if the IUD is removed in early pregnancy, this rate of abortion can be halved. The IUD should not be left in place during pregnancy because severe pelvic infections with a high mortality rate can result. Most IUD users notice that menses are heavier, and between 10% to 15% of women choose to have their IUDs removed because of heavy bleeding or cramping during their periods (Hatcher et al, 1994).

**Patient use.** The IUD is usually inserted during the menses after a bimanual examination to rule out pregnancy and determine the position of the uterus. An analgesic before the procedure is helpful, and sometimes a local anesthetic is used. Because the material of the IUD has shape memory, it can be inserted by means of a narrow, plastic inserter high up into the fundus of the uterus where it resumes its original shape when released. The IUD usually is easily re-moved by steady traction on the string extending through the cervical canal. The nurse should counsel women to check for the IUD strings often during the first few months after insertion. Thereafter a woman should check the IUD string after each menses or with any unusual cramping. Patients should be advised to return for care if the IUD string feels longer or the plastic tip of the IUD is felt. Women should be advised that pelvic pain and fever could indicate a serious infection and that they should seek treatment immediately. Likewise they should seek attention if they learn that they have been exposed to a sexually transmitted disease. The IUD appears to be best tolerated by women who have borne children and who are in mutually monogamous relationships.

## Surgical Contraception

In the past 20 years improved surgical techniques and the use of a local anesthetic with light sedation have contributed to the safety of female sterilization. Approximately 1 million women now choose this method of contraception annually in the United States (Hatcher et al, 1994). The couple should consider both vasectomy (see Chapter 42) and female sterilization. Vasectomy is a safer, simpler procedure that can be performed during an office visit. Sterilization for both men and women should be considered permanent because current techniques to reverse the procedures are not dependable.

**Mechanism of action and effectiveness.** Sterilization involves tying or blocking the fallopian tubes to prevent sperm from reaching and fertilizing the ovum (Figure 43-9). Efficacy is quite high but varies slightly depending on the surgical procedure used and the skill of the surgeon. The failure rate for all techniques

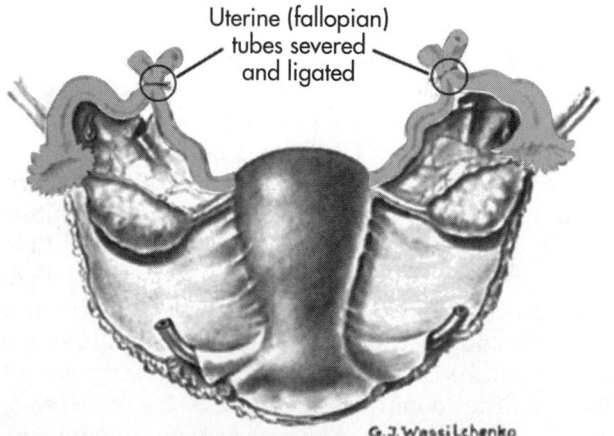

**Figure 43-9** Tubal sterilization (tubal ligation). (From Bobak IM, Jensen MD: *Maternity and gynecologic care*, ed 5, St Louis, 1993, Mosby.)

is 0.49% of women becoming pregnant in the first year of use (Hatcher et al, 1994). Different surgical techniques and incision sites may be used in the postpartum period.

**Risks, benefits, and side effects.** Sterilization for women is a safe procedure. Fatality rates in the United States are approximately 3 deaths per 100,000 women, which compares favorably with maternal mortality rates of 7.9 deaths per 100,000 women (Hatcher et al, 1994). Local anesthesia with light sedation can be used for both minilaparotomy and laparoscopic procedures. Local anesthesia has fewer complications than general anesthesia. Possible complications to surgery include infection, uterine perforation, and injury to the bladder or intestine. However, complications to surgery occur in less than 1% of sterilizations (Hatcher et al, 1994). New evidence suggests that tubal sterilization reduces a woman's risk of contracting ovarian cancer by 70% (Edwards, 1994). Even when researchers adjusted for influences that reduce a woman's risk of ovarian cancer, such as parity, use of the birth control pill, and age, the results were upheld. A biologic explanation for this effect has not been proposed, nor has a comparison of the effects by different tubal ligation techniques.

**Patient use.** Women should consider sterilization a permanent contraceptive method because procedures to reverse it are difficult and often unsuccessful. Patients should discuss how their plans might change if they were to divorce or lose their present children to death or illness.

Patients should not eat for 8 to 12 hours before the surgery and should be instructed to bathe or shower just before arrival for surgery. Because 1-day surgery will be performed, a patient arriving for surgery should have someone with her to drive her home. In addition, she should arrange for an adult to be with her at home for at least 24 hours after surgery in case complications develop. Women with small children will need assistance caring for their children on the day of surgery and a day or two immediately following. Women should be advised that the pain after surgery is usually managed with oral analgesics. After surgery, women should be advised to rest for at least 24 hours and to resume normal activities gradually over the next week. They should be counseled to avoid heavy lifting and sexual intercourse for 1 week after surgery. Typically the sutures dissolve, and women are allowed to bathe 2 days after surgery. Warm baths may relieve the gaseous distention that can occur with laparoscopy. A follow-up visit is usually scheduled for 1 week after surgery. Patients should be counseled to report signs of infection such as fever, syncope, or increasing abdominal pain. Abnormal bleeding or pus or other fluid from the incision site should also be reported. Women should be advised to seek medical attention immediately if they believe they have become pregnant because a high rate of ectopic pregnancies is associated with failure of the procedure.

## Barrier Methods of Contraception

Barrier methods of contraception include the diaphragm, cervical cap, female condom, male condom, spermicides, foam, and vaginal contraceptive film (VCF). Except for the cervical cap and diaphragm, which must be fitted by a clinician, all these methods are available without prescription. This may enhance their use by teenagers or women without access to medical care. Without exception, these methods are use dependent; that is, a woman or man must choose to use them at the time of intercourse. Use dependence often affects compliance.

**Mechanism of action and effectiveness.** Most barrier methods rely on a mechanical barrier together with a spermicide to prevent migration of sperm through the endocervical canal. Some methods, such as condoms, depend principally on a mechanical barrier, whereas others, such as foam and VCF, rely on a spermicide for their effectiveness. Efficacy rates vary depending on use. Typical failure rates for barrier methods range more widely from the perfect-use failure rate than with contraceptives such as Norplant, Depo-Provera, or the IUD (see Table 43-2). The diaphragm may offer greater efficacy for parous women than the cervical cap.

**Risks, benefits, and side effects.** Aside from a generally higher risk of pregnancy, barrier methods are quite safe, with few if any side effects. Some couples may be allergic or irritated by the latex in condoms or the nonoxynol-9 in spermicidal products, but these problems are uncommon. TSS is a rare possibility with use of vaginal barrier methods. The syndrome is caused by the toxins released by a strain of *Staphylococcus* bacteria and is more often associated with tampon use during menses (see TSS discussion earlier in this chapter). Two or three cases of TSS per 100,000 women annually may be attributed to using vaginal barrier methods (Hatcher et al, 1994).

Of the contraceptive methods available, the male and female condoms afford the greatest protection from sexually transmitted disease. All women at risk should be encouraged to use condoms, regardless of other contraceptive methods employed, to protect themselves from infection. Although spermicides have a bactericidal action, which offers some protection against sexually transmitted infections such as gonorrhea and syphilis, they do not offer the protection afforded by barrier methods such as condoms. Nor is there general agreement on whether spermicides decrease the transmission of HIV because of their spermicidal activity or possibly increase it because of the

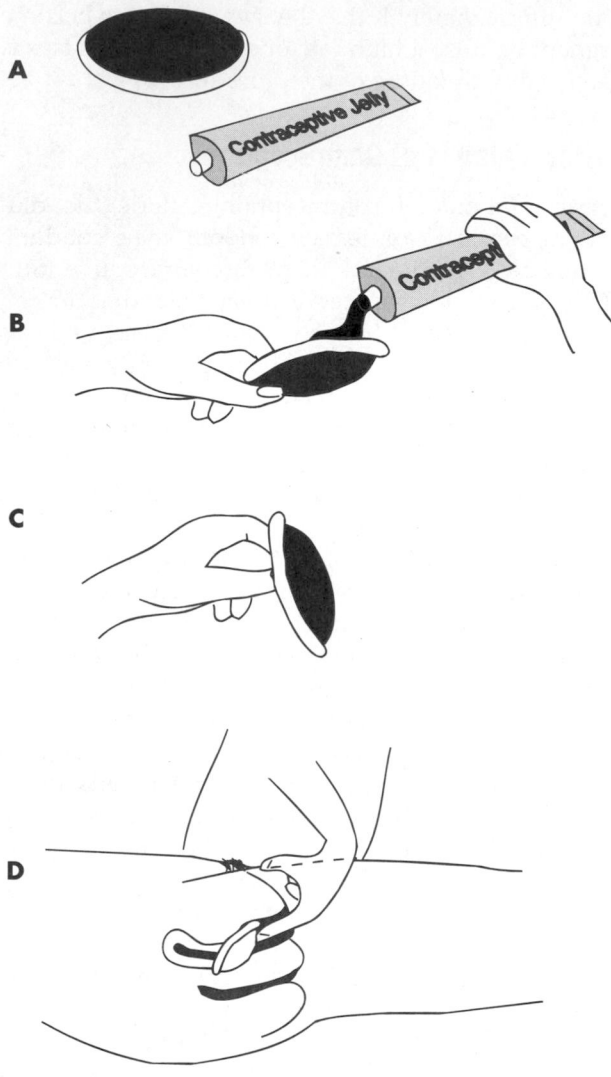

**Figure 43-10** Diaphragm insertion technique.

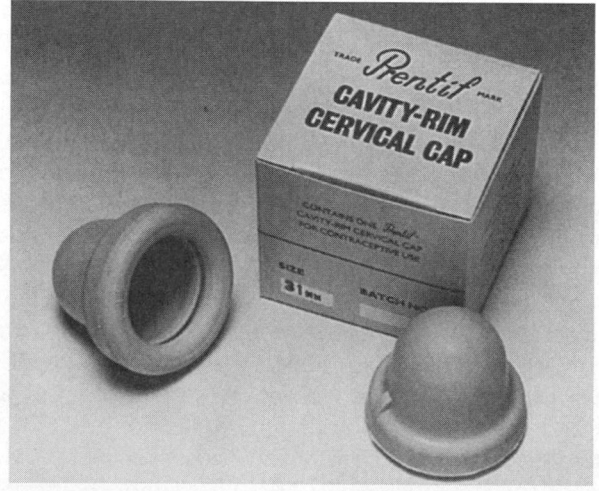

**Figure 43-11** Cervical cap. (Courtesy of Cervical Cap Ltd, Los Gatos, Calif.)

irritant effect of spermicides on vaginal and cervical mucosa that would facilitate entry of HIV.

### Patient use

***Diaphragm.*** The diaphragm has been in use for more than 60 years in the United States. The diaphragm is a dome-shaped rubber cup with a compressible rim that must be sized to the individual woman. The woman should be instructed in its use and allowed to practice inserting it before the office visit is concluded. Before insertion the woman should apply about a tablespoon of contraceptive jelly or cream into the cup of the diaphragm and spread it around the rim and interior surface of the dome. Then she should fold the diaphragm in half and push it gently into the vagina. The anterior rim should be tucked up behind the public bone and the posterior rim behind the cervix, thus covering the cervix (Figure 43-10). This can be checked by having the patient palpate for the cervix, which will feel somewhat firm and rubbery behind the dome. The diaphragm should be left in place for 6 to 8 hours after intercourse. If intercourse is desired again before the diaphragm should be removed, a second application of contraceptive cream should be inserted with an applicator and the diaphragm left in place for an additional 6 to 8 hours. The woman should check the diaphragm for tears or holes before each use and clean it with mild soap and warm water after use. When fitted correctly, the diaphragm should be completely comfortable for the woman. Her partner is usually unable to feel the device during coitus. The nurse should follow recommended cleaning and disinfecting practices for all fitting rings (diaphragms) used to size women during the fitting procedure.

***Cervical cap.*** The Prentif cervical cap is the only cap approved for use in the United States (Figure 43-11). It is devised to fit snugly over the cervix. Before insertion the dome is filled with approximately 1 tablespoon of contraceptive jelly or cream. A cervical cap can be more difficult to fit than a diaphragm. Insertion and removal may be slightly more difficult for the woman as well. Some women are unable to be fitted for a cap because of their cervical anatomy. The cervical cap may be left in place up to 48 hours, and repeated applications of spermicides with subsequent acts of intercourse are not necessary. It must be left in place for at least 6 hours after the last act of intercourse. Care of the cervical cap is similar to that of the diaphragm, and the same precautions should be followed by the nurse for disinfecting caps used for fitting and sizing.

***Female condom.*** The Reality female condom is a thin polyurethane sheath with a flexible ring at either end. The open ring is intended to lie outside the vagina, and a ring at the end of the pouch serves to anchor the device deep inside the vagina (Figure 43-12). The female condom is less likely to tear than the male condom, but, like the male condom, it may become dislodged during intercourse.

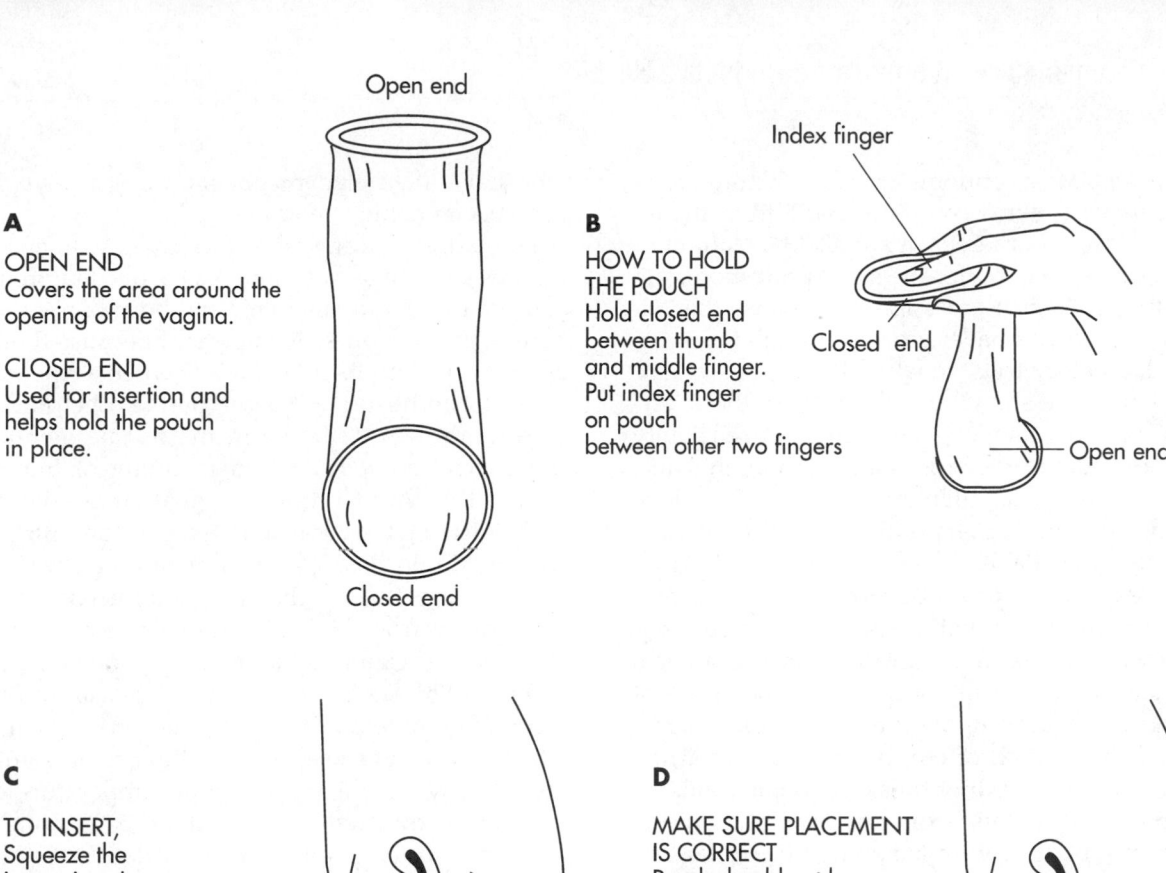

**A**

**OPEN END**
Covers the area around the opening of the vagina.

**CLOSED END**
Used for insertion and helps hold the pouch in place.

Open end

Closed end

**B**

Index finger

**HOW TO HOLD THE POUCH**
Hold closed end between thumb and middle finger. Put index finger on pouch between other two fingers

Closed end

Open end

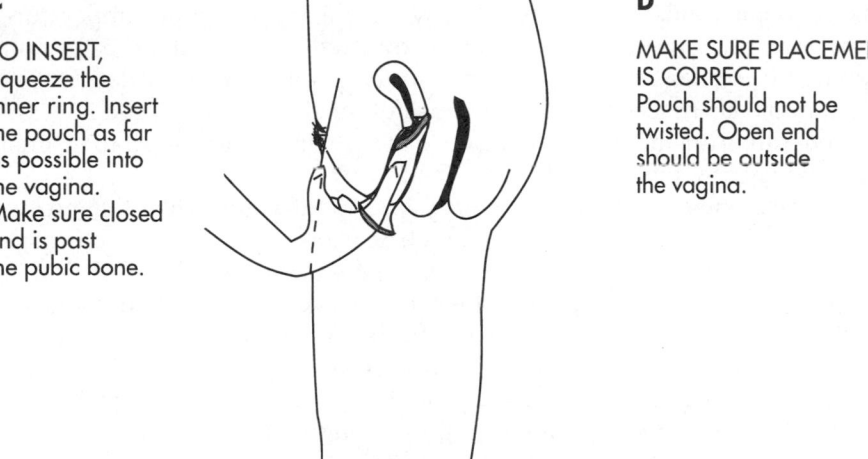

**C**

**TO INSERT,**
Squeeze the inner ring. Insert the pouch as far as possible into the vagina. Make sure closed end is past the pubic bone.

**D**

**MAKE SURE PLACEMENT IS CORRECT**
Pouch should not be twisted. Open end should be outside the vagina.

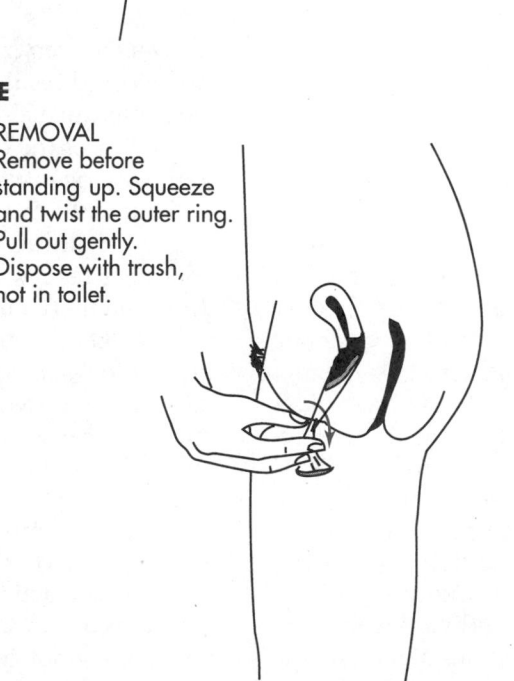

**E**

**REMOVAL**
Remove before standing up. Squeeze and twist the outer ring. Pull out gently. Dispose with trash, not in toilet.

**Figure 43-12**    Female condom.

***Male condom.*** Most condoms are manufactured from latex, but natural "skin" condoms made from the intestinal membranes of lambs are available. Natural or "skin" condoms do not offer the same protection from sexually transmitted diseases (STDs) because they allow passage of some smaller viruses through the membrane. In laboratory tests hepatitis B, herpes simplex, and HIV have been shown to pass through the "skin" condoms. For men and women with latex sensitivity the female condom, which is made of polyurethane, may be suggested as an alternative. Two new kinds of condom made of polyurethane and natural rubber are expected to be available in the near future. Alternatively, a latex condom could be worn under or over a natural skin condom so that the partner with sensitivity to latex is shielded from direct contact. Condoms should be unrolled carefully over the erect penis before any contact between penis and vagina occurs. It is recommended that ½ inch of empty space be left at the end of the condom to reduce breakage. Some condoms are designed with a "reservoir tip" for this purpose. The condom should be unrolled so that the rolled rim is on the outside of the condom. If a condom is unrolled incorrectly, using a new condom is better than attempting to reverse the first one because potentially infectious body fluids could otherwise be transmitted.

## Natural Family Planning

Natural family planning includes the basal body temperature, rhythm, and cervical mucus methods. Since the couple must abstain from intercourse during carefully calculated times, these methods require planning and dedication to be effective.

## Infertility

Infertility is usually defined as the inability of a couple to conceive after 1 year of sexual relations without contraceptive measures. Approximately 40% of infertility problems are a result of male factors, and approximately 40% are a result of female factors. Combined male and female factors account for 10% of problems, and 10% are unexplained. Aging has only a moderate effect on female fertility, and this effect is demonstrated only for women in their late 30s and older (Hatcher et al, 1994). The probability of conception remains roughly the same for an individual couple as long as health and sexual behavior remain constant. Because fecundity peaks in a given population at the age most women choose to bear children, statistics on fecundity do not give an accurate indication of the possibilities for pregnancy in an individual woman. Also, statistics for pregnancy in couples older than the norm are affected by including in this group women who have attempted pregnancy for many years and have been unable to conceive.

The causes of diminished fertility in women are numerous and range from simple lack of coital frequency and poor timing to anatomic and hormonal problems. Timing of intercourse is important because there may be only a few hours in each cycle when a ripe ovum is ready for fertilization. Sperm, on the other hand, survive more than 72 hours in the female genital tract (Hatcher et al, 1994). Optimal timing of intercourse around the expected time of ovulation can be assisted by monitoring the basal body temperature (BBT) of the woman. To do this, a woman must take her temperature at approximately the same time each morning before arising from bed. She should use a special BBT thermometer calibrated in tenths of a degree from 97° to 99° F. With such a thermometer she can record fine distinctions in temperature on a menstrual cycle chart, which can then be used as an aid to predict ovulation. For most women a slight dip in temperature occurs just before ovulation, followed by a sustained and sharp rise in temperature after ovulation. BBT monitoring is useful for timing intercourse and for coordinating tests that a woman may need to evaluate infertility further.

PID may lead to infertility when the infection is severe enough to cause scarring and blockage of the uterus or fallopian tubes. The risk of PID is increased by untreated STDs, postpartum and postabortion infections, and use of an IUD. Infections of human papillomavirus (HPV) may cause chronic cervicitus, cervical dysplasia, or cervical cancer, and treatment of any of these conditions may damage the mucus-producing cells of the cervix, affecting sperm transport or causing cervical incompetence. Cervical incompetence could result in pregnancy loss or preterm delivery. Infertility also results from surgery (necessitated by cancer of the cervix, endometrium, or ovaries) that removes the organs of reproduction.

Structural causes of infertility can be found in women with an absent or bicornuate uterus. Endometriosis results in implantation of endometrial tissue from the uterus in ectopic locations, which then swell and bleed at menses. This may lead to adhesions and tubal blockage significant enough to prevent conception in some women. Abdominal or pelvic surgery may also cause adhesions and contribute to infertility. Fibroid tumors may cause difficulties in implantation and subsequent pregnancies.

Endocrine imbalances in the thyroid, pituitary, and ovaries can contribute to infertility. Thus hypothyroidism, prolactinoma, polycystic ovarian disease, and premature ovarian failure all affect fertility. Some women do not ovulate with each cycle (anovulatory cycles), which decreases their chances of becoming pregnant. Both women and men can develop antibodies that immobilize sperm and cause them to clump rather than ascend the uterus. Other causes of infertility are malnutrition, extreme weight gain or loss, excessive exercise, exposure to toxic agents or radiation, and use of certain drugs.

Infertility of whatever cause can be an emotionally devastating diagnosis for a couple. A woman may feel acutely the potential loss of her role as a mother. The diagnosis may even affect her sense of femininity and sexual identity. It can cause feelings of grief, shame, and anger. Certainly the evaluation and treatment of infertility invade the private domain of a couple's sexual life. A detailed sexual history must be taken, and the couple is advised to time intercourse to coincide with ovulation, which may decrease their sense of pleasure and spontaneity. The inability to conceive in cycle after cycle adds to the couple's growing sense of futility and failure, which may affect their desire for coitus. Clinical tests that the couple may find invasive or embarrassing cause further stress.

Infertility can rightly be called a life crisis. Women may resent other women who have children and feel isolated from others who, they believe, cannot understand their feelings. Family members and friends may ask intrusive questions or make insensitive comments that cause further anguish. Sometimes women feel their lives are on hold while they are trying so hard to become pregnant. They may not feel that they can make long-range plans or commitments. One partner may blame the other for being the "cause" of infertility, or one partner may care more about resolving the problem, increasing the stress in the relationship. It is important for the nurse to explore the emotions of both partners and to help them understand their responses to this crisis. Self-help groups can also be of great benefit. When infertility is untreatable, couples may need assistance with adoption or reconceptualizing their lives without children.

The assessment of infertility should proceed from basic concerns such as frequency and timing of intercourse to a physiologic assessment of both partners. Thus both partners should have focused physical examinations that look for contributing causes of infertility at the same time the woman begins to keep BBT records. Assessment of the male is done first because it is noninvasive. Semen is usually analyzed twice for live sperm count as well as for morphology and motility. If the semen is normal and the couple have still not conceived after 2 to 3 months of BBT monitoring, a postcoital test is performed to assess adequacy of the semen when exposed to vaginal secretions. The couple is instructed to have intercourse the evening before or the morning of the examination. The examination is scheduled for 1 to 2 days before ovulation according to

BBT records. A specimen is obtained from the cervix and examined microscopically for particular characteristics conducive to sperm transport. Motility and the number of sperm are also assessed. If a cause is not found, subsequent visits may assess the woman's hormonal status, adequacy of the endometrium, and patency of the fallopian tubes. Blood tests, endometrial biopsy, and hysterosalpingogram are commonly used in this further assessment. Counseling and encouragement should occur on each visit, and the workup should proceed in a logical fashion from least invasive to more invasive examinations.

Female infertility is treated with a range of approaches, according to the cause. Cervical mucus disorder can be treated by placing sperm directly into the uterus. Hormonal imbalances are alleviated by treating the underlying cause. Ovulation can also be induced by drugs, if necessary. Uterine and tubal abnormalities or obstructions may be treated by surgical intervention. In other cases procedures such as gamete intrafallopian transfer or in vitro fertilization can offer success when more conventional methods fail.

# TYPES OF DIAGNOSTIC PROCEDURES

## Laboratory Tests

The laboratory tests conducted along with a pelvic examination include urinalysis; the **Papanicolaou (Pap) smear** for cancer; and smears and cultures from the vagina, cervix, and urethra, which may be examined for both infectious and noninfectious organisms. A complete blood count and a serologic test for syphilis also are usually performed.

Pap smears are used to detect early cases of cervical cancer. For women of average risk, routine smears are recommended once yearly for 3 years and then, after three negative tests, once every 2 or 3 years. The patient's or her family's history may reveal high risk and indicate more frequent testing. Patients with more than three lifetime sexual partners, who had first intercourse before age 20, who smoke, or who have a history of HPV infection are at higher risk for cervical cancer and should be screened yearly. Many providers recommend that their patients have a Pap smear and vaginal examination every year. A woman should begin routine testing at age 20 or before if sexually active. After an abnormal test, annual Pap smears are recommended thereafter. The woman must understand the purpose of the test and the interpretation of results. Douching 24 hours before the test is contraindicated because cellular discharges to be examined may be washed away and negate the test. Sexual intercourse should also be avoided, and the Pap smear should not be performed at the menses. The patient should void, be placed in the dorsal lithotomy position, and then be draped. The nurse may be asked to assemble the proper equipment for the clinician, including a glass slide, vaginal speculum, wooden swab or spatula, a fixing solution of alcohol or formalin, and a cytology laboratory requisition. Several Pap smear classification systems are in use, but currently the Bethesda system is the predominant one. Sometimes minor infections affect the Pap smear. Atypical Pap smears usually are repeated at 3, 6, and 12 months after the first atypical result. If the Pap smear is more seriously abnormal, colposcopy can be performed. Minor abnormalities often resolve without treatment.

## Colposcopy

**Colposcopy** involves the examination of the cervix and vagina with an instrument called a colposcope, which contains a magnifying lens and light. The test is used after an abnormal Pap smear or to further examine suggestive lesions seen during a vaginal examination. A biopsy may be performed, and photographs may be taken of suggestive lesions with the colposcope and its attachments. Patients whose mothers received diethylstilbestrol during pregnancy are monitored regularly with the colposcope. The patient is positioned in a lithotomy position, and the colposcope is used to inspect the vagina. If a biopsy has been performed, the patient must be instructed to abstain from sexual intercourse and to avoid inserting anything into the vagina except a tampon until healing of the biopsy site is confirmed.

## Cervical Biopsy

A cervical biopsy is the surgical excision of tissue from the cervix for histologic examination. Samples are taken from three or more sites around the cervix. The sites are determined by direct visualization with colposcopy or by iodine staining (Schiller's test). Cervical biopsy is indicated for women with suggestive cervical lesions and should be performed when the cervix is least vascular, usually 1 week after menses. If findings indicate advanced dysplasia or carcinoma in situ, a cone biopsy may be performed with the patient under general anesthesia to obtain a larger tissue specimen and allow a more accurate evaluation of the extent of dysplasia. Before biopsy a consent form must be signed and the patient should void. The patient is instructed to avoid strenuous exercise for 8 to 24 hours after the biopsy. She should be allowed to rest briefly before going home. A tampon may be inserted by the physician after biopsy to help stop bleeding. The patient should be instructed to leave it in place for the time ordered by the physician, usually 8 to 24 hours. Some bleeding is expected, but bleeding heavier than menstrual flow should be reported to the physician. Douching and intercourse should be avoided for about 2 to 6 weeks, as instructed. A foul-smelling, grayish green vaginal discharge will appear in a few days and remain for as long as 3 weeks. This discharge is caused by the healing of the cervical tissue, and the patient should be told to expect it.

## Culdoscopy

A culdoscope is a long, metal, lighted instrument that can be inserted into the vagina and through Douglas' cul-de-sac, a pouch that lies between the uterus and the rectum. **Culdoscopy** is usually performed in the operating room with the patient in the knee-chest position. An incision is made in the posterior fornix of the vagina, and the culdoscope is introduced through this incision to provide visualization of the pelvic organs. Preparation is routine for minor vaginal surgery, and postoperative care includes checking vital signs and observing for hemorrhage and infection. The incision usually heals rapidly, and douching and sexual activity are to be avoided for about 1 week or until permitted by the physician. Air embolism is a rare complication of this procedure.

## Laparoscopy

A laparoscope is a small, fiberoptic instrument that is inserted through a small incision in the anterior abdominal wall. **Laparoscopy** is used to detect abnormalities and to perform minor surgical procedures, such as lysis of adhesions, ovarian biopsy, tubal sterilization, removal of foreign bodies, and treatment of sites of endometriosis. Because laparoscopy is performed under anesthetic, the patient must fast for at least 8 hours before surgery. There is a danger of hemorrhage after the test and the possibility of peritonitis after the spilling of intestinal contents if a visceral organ is accidentally punctured. The patient will experience pain at the puncture site following the test. There also will be pain in the shoulder resulting from the air that was introduced into the peritoneal cavity to allow better visualization of the organs.

After the test, vital signs should be monitored according to routine postoperative instructions, urinary output should be checked, and the patient should be ambulated. A normal diet may be resumed gradually, and activity will be restricted for 4 to 7 days as ordered by the physician. The pain in the abdomen and shoulder should disappear within 24 to 36 hours and will be relieved by aspirin or acetaminophen as ordered.

# Hysterosalpingography

Hysterosalpingography is an x-ray examination used to visualize the uterine cavity, the fallopian tubes, and the area around the tubes. To detect tubal and uterine abnormalities, fistulas, and adhesions, a radiopaque substance is injected into the uterus and up into the fallopian tubes as fluoroscopic x-ray films are taken. The structure and patency of the tubes may be examined. The presence of foreign bodies can also be detected; however, pelvic ultrasound is more commonly used for this purpose. After the test the patient may experience cramps and a vagal reaction resulting in a slow pulse rate, nausea, and dizziness. These symptoms should subside quickly. The patient must be watched for signs of infection, such as fever, pain, increased pulse rate, malaise, and muscle ache.

# Pelvic Ultrasonography

In pelvic ultrasonography, high-frequency sound waves are passed into the area to be examined and are reflected to a transducer. The transducer converts the sound energy into electric energy and forms images on an oscilloscope screen, which is similar to x-ray film. Pelvic ultrasonography is used to detect foreign bodies; to distinguish between cysts and tumors; to measure organ size; to detect multiple pregnancies or fetal abnormalities; to evaluate the size, gestational age, growth rate, position, and viability of the fetus; and to determine the location of the placenta and the fetus during amniocentesis. The patient must have a full bladder during the examination to improve the image produced by the sound waves and to provide a landmark for defining pelvic organs. The patient is asked to drink approximately 6 to 8 glasses of water before the test and is instructed not to void. Immediately after the test the patient should be allowed to empty her bladder. Alternatively a transvaginal ultrasound can be used, which is performed with the bladder empty. A narrow probe is inserted into the vagina, and the sound waves are emitted directly into the pelvis. There is some question about the effects of ultrasound. Although no evidence of harm to the fetus or the mother has been found during the 20 years it has been in use, a hypothetical risk exists that cannot be ignored. The patient must be fully informed regarding the benefits and potential risks of ultrasonography.

# Mammography

**Mammography** is a radiographic (x-ray) technique used to detect breast cysts or tumors, especially those not palpable on physical examination. The test uses relatively low radiation levels but is contraindicated during pregnancy. The patient stands and is asked to place one of her breasts on a table above an x-ray cassette. A compressor is placed on the breast, and the patient is instructed to hold her breath while a picture is taken from above. The machine is rotated, the patient is repositioned, and a lateral view is taken. The procedure is repeated on the other breast. Abnormal tissues are evident on the developed films. The current recommendations of the American Cancer Society (1997) are as follows: Women 40 years of age and older should have an annual mammogram. A woman who has a family history of breast cancer in a first-degree relative or who has other risk factors should have annual mammograms starting at an earlier age.

# Needle Localization Biopsy

Needle localization biopsy uses the skills of both a radiologist and a surgeon. The radiologist places a needle in a solid breast mass with the use of x-rays to aid in placement. The needle is left in place, and the patient is transported to 1-day surgery, where a surgeon performs an open biopsy. This technique is useful for small, nonpalpable breast masses discovered by mammography.

# Pregnancy Tests

The most common tests for pregnancy are based on finding human chorionic gonadotropin (HCG) in serum or urine. The urine tests are widely available in kit form and are fairly accurate, simple, and inexpensive. The manufacturers of these kits claim that HCG can be detected in urine 42 days after the last menstrual period. Improper collection of the specimen, proteinuria, hormone-producing tumors, and other factors can produce false-positive or false-negative readings.

# Dilation and Curettage

**Dilation and curettage** (D&C) is a procedure in which the cervical os is dilated and the inside of the uterus is scraped with a curette. There are three basic reasons for this procedure: to secure tissue from the lining of the uterus (endometrium) for examination, to control uterine bleeding, and to clear the uterine cavity of any residue left after an incomplete abortion. D&C is a surgical procedure requiring an anesthetic. Preoperative preparation of the patient is the same as that for most other surgical patients. Postoperative care includes observation of the patient for excessive vaginal bleeding and urinary retention. The surgery is usually scheduled on an outpatient basis, and the patient is discharged the same day that surgery is performed.

# DISEASES AND DISORDERS OF THE REPRODUCTIVE SYSTEM

## Conditions Affecting the Female External Genitalia and Vagina

### Vulvitis

Vulvitis may be either an acute or a chronic inflammatory condition of the vulva. There are many causes, including an irritating vaginal discharge, infectious diseases, untreated diabetes, contraceptive pills, and trauma caused by scratching. There usually is severe itching and burning with redness and, in some patients, ulceration. Treatment consists of identifying and treating or removing the cause. Clothing that rubs or irritates the condition should be eliminated. Patients should be questioned about overzealous hygiene because excessive washing may be a cause of vulvitis.

### Vaginitis

**Vaginitis** is one of the most common disorders affecting the female. This condition affects females of any age group, from infants to the elderly.

**Pathophysiology.** Vaginitis is an inflammation of the vagina. Many factors are associated with its occurrence. *Trichomonas vaginalis* is a flagellated protozoan and is a common cause of vaginitis. It is considered to be sexually transmitted in most cases. Vaginitis may also be caused by *Candida albicans*, a yeastlike fungus. This form is commonly found in women with diabetes and during antibiotic or steroid therapy. Atrophic vaginitis occurs after menopause and is caused by low levels of estrogen, resulting in a thinning of the vaginal lining. Bacterial vaginosis is caused by a proliferation of one or more bacterial anaerobes in the vaginal flora. Vaginitis may be caused by faulty hygiene, tight clothing, illness, or emotional stress.

**Assessment.** The patient with vaginitis complains of burning and itching of the vulva and vaginal discharge and may report that she has pain on urination or with intercourse. Examination of the vaginal walls often shows a profuse foamy (bubbly) exudate if the cause of the vaginitis is *T. vaginalis*. If *C. albicans* is the causative agent, a thick, cheeselike discharge is more typical. Bacterial vaginosis produces a milklike discharge with a foul or fishy odor.

**Intervention.** Most patients with vaginitis caused by *Trichomonas* organisms are treated with metronidazole (Flagyl) in a 2-g single dose (see Table 43-2). Both partners should be treated at the same time to avoid reinfection. Douches using 1 tablespoon of vinegar to 1 pint of warm water may be ordered to remove excessive discharge and provide local comfort. Many treatment preparations for vaginitis caused by *C. albicans* can be purchased over the counter. The vaginal cream is inserted at bedtime with a specially designed applicator. Terazol vaginal cream may be prescribed for 7 days or Terazol double-strength suppositories for 3 days. Bacterial vaginosis is treated with a 2-g single dose of metronidazole (Flagyl) or with 500 mg given twice a day for 7 days. Patients should be advised to avoid drinking alcohol while taking this medication. Use of Flagyl should be avoided during pregnancy. Atrophic vaginitis in women past menopause is treated with estrogen vaginal creams. Pain during intercourse can be relieved with the use of vaginal lubricants. In all cases of vaginitis, patients should be instructed to maintain adequate cleanliness, especially after elimination; to ingest or apply medications as ordered; and to restrict sexual activity to allow the vagina to heal.

### Bartholinitis

Bartholinitis is inflammation of Bartholin's glands, which are located on either side of the vaginal opening. The condition may result from any of several pathogenic bacteria and can be seen in untreated gonorrhea. The ducts from the glands may become occluded by the inflammatory condition, resulting in abscess formation. The abscess may rupture spontaneously, or an incision and drainage may be necessary. Treatment includes administration of the appropriate antibiotic and hot sitz baths. The patient is usually treated in the physician's office or in an outpatient clinic. In some women Bartholin's cysts are not painful and may remain untreated. If they become markedly enlarged, minor surgery can be performed to remove the them.

### Vesicovaginal and Rectovaginal Fistula

A vesicovaginal fistula is an abnormal opening from the bladder to the vagina. Rectovaginal fistula is an abnormal opening between the rectum and the vagina. A fistula can occur congenitally, be caused by injury during childbirth or vaginal surgery, or result from tissue damage produced by Crohn's disease or invasive carcinoma. Surgical repair is indicated if the fistula does not heal. Healing is promoted by an increase in dietary vitamin C and protein, cleansing of the area with douches and enemas, rest, and oral antibiotics. A temporary colostomy may be necessary to keep the site clean. Soiling from leakage of urine or stool into the vagina is disturbing for the patient. Sitz baths, deodorizing douches, perineal pads, and protective pants are necessary preoperatively. For those with an irreparable fistula, hygiene and comfort are ongoing concerns. Daily sitz baths and use of "baby wipes" to cleanse the perineum after elimination reduce irritation. If the fistula is repaired surgically, a Foley catheter may be inserted postoperatively to prevent strain on the suture line caused by a full bladder.

## Relaxation of the Pelvic Musculature: Rectocele, Cystocele, and Uterine Prolapse

**Pathophysiology.** The uterus is normally supported by pelvic muscles. These muscles can atrophy with age or weaken with childbearing, allowing the uterus to descend, impinge on other structures of the bladder or rectum, and protrude through the vaginal wall. A rectocele is the bulging of the rectum against the vaginal wall; a cystocele is the bulging of the bladder against the vaginal wall; and uterine prolapse is the collapse of the uterus into the vagina. In severe cases of uterine prolapse the cervix may protrude through the external vaginal opening.

**Assessment.** These conditions cause a feeling of downward pressure, especially when the patient stands or walks. Stress incontinence and urinary frequency and urgency accompany cystocele. Rectal pressure, constipation, heaviness, and hemorrhoids are associated with rectocele. Uterine prolapse produces more severe urinary symptoms such as incontinence and retention. Constipation, backache, and vaginal discharge result from the increased pressure exerted by the prolapsed uterus. Some degree of prolapse occurs in many women, but treatment is not usually initiated unless symptoms are problematic.

**Intervention.** Uterine prolapse can be treated by insertion of a pessary to support the uterus, by transvaginal surgical correction, or by removal of the uterus (hysterectomy). Surgery is the preferred treatment, but a pessary is used if the woman plans further pregnancies or is unable to withstand surgery. A pessary is a small appliance placed in the vagina to reposition the uterus. A sterile lubricant is applied for insertion, and the pessary is removed and cleaned about every 2 months by the physician to prevent infection. The pessary may cause vaginal irritation or erosion. Therefore frequent and regular examinations by the physician are important. The patient must immediately report any unusual vaginal discharge or changes in voiding.

Pelvic floor exercises (Kegel exercises) are prescribed for women who experience prolapse after childbirth. The women alternately contracts and relaxes both the gluteal and perineal floor muscles to strengthen muscle tone. Hysterectomy may be necessary in severe cases of uterine prolapse. (See the section on care of the patient with vaginal or abdominal hysterectomy later in this chapter.)

Surgical repair of a cystocele involves shortening the muscles that support the bladder through a procedure called anterior **colporrhaphy;** repair of a rectocele is called posterior colporrhaphy (Box 43-3). Performing both repairs at the same time is referred to as an anteroposterocolporrhaphy or anteroposterior repair.

*Preoperative intervention: colporrhaphy.* Preoperative care for colporrhaphy is especially important in ensuring as clean an operative area as possible. Patients may be admitted to the hospital before surgery and given a cathartic, followed by enemas to be sure the bowel is completely empty. A liquid diet for 24 hours before surgery helps to keep the bowel empty. The surgeon may order a cleansing vaginal douche on the evening before and the morning of surgery. The entire vaginal area is shaved, including the pubis and rectal area.

*Postoperative intervention: colporrhaphy.* The postoperative care of the patient having colporrhaphy includes checking vital signs and observing often for hemorrhage. A retention catheter is usually inserted into the urinary bladder to keep it empty and to prevent pressure on sutures. It is important to keep the fecal residue as soft as possible. Some physicians order a liquid diet for several days or prescribe stool softeners to be given every night. An oil retention enema may be ordered, but cleansing enemas should not be given. A small, soft rubber tube should be used for the oil retention enema, and the patient must be instructed not to strain when defecating. External sutures may or may not be present, depending on whether perineal repair has been done. The nurse should understand the physician's orders concerning perineal care because some physicians want the area kept completely dry. The heat lamp may be used two or three times a day for 20 to 30 minutes. If a solution rather than plain water is to be used in giving perineal care, the physician will order it. All equipment and supplies must be sterile to prevent infection.

The patient is usually kept in a low Fowler's position to prevent pressure or strain on the sutures. When ambulation is allowed, the patient should be taught to roll out of bed. After discharge from the hospital the patient should be advised against standing for long periods or lifting heavy objects for several weeks. Coitus must be avoided until healing is complete, which takes approximately 6 weeks.

## Malignant Lesions of the Vulva

Malignant lesions of the vulva are relatively rare and occur most often in women after menopause. Although these lesions are easily visible, many women wait years before seeking medical attention. Cancer of the vulva is also diagnosed in women between 20 to 40 years ◆ of age. There may be a correlation between

> **BOX 43-3**   NURSING PROCESS
>
> ## COLPORRHAPHY (REPAIR OF RELAXED PERINEAL MUSCLES)
>
> **ASSESSMENT**
>
> - Vital signs (often)
> - Dressing/vaginal drainage (often)
> - Intake and output
> - Elimination patterns
> - Lung and bowel sounds
> - Level of comfort
> - Self-esteem and self-concept
>
> **NURSING DIAGNOSES**
>
> - Pain related to inflammation at surgical site
> - Risk for injury (strain on sutures at site of surgical repair) related to full bladder, straining during defecation
> - Risk for infection related to contamination by fecal material and obstruction of vaginal drainage
> - Urinary retention related to inflammation of bladder, bladder neck, and urethra
> - Altered sexuality patterns related to postoperative restrictions on sexual intercourse for 6 weeks
> - Knowledge deficit related to restrictions on physical activity
> - Alteration in self-concept related to hospitalization
> - Altered role performance related to surgery and restricted activity level
> - Risk for impaired skin integrity related to decreased activity level
> - Risk for respiratory infection related to anesthesia and decreased activity level
>
> **NURSING INTERVENTIONS**
>
> - Monitor routine vital signs until stable.
> - Maintain patency of indwelling urinary catheter.
> - Have patient void every 4 hours after catheter is removed to prevent strain on sutures from full bladder.
> - Give and instruct patient on low-residue diet to promote soft stool.
> - Avoid use of cleansing enemas.
> - Apply ice pack to perineum first 24 hours postoperatively; heat lamp to perineum 20 minutes tid beginning second postoperative day if prescribed.
> - Administer perineal care with sterile solution qid and after each voiding or defecation.
> - Apply anesthetic and antiseptic sprays to perineum as prescribed.
> - Maintain low Fowler's position.
> - Encourage deep breathing exercises every 2 hours; however, discourage coughing.
> - Encourage expression of feelings and concerns.
> - Inform patient that loss of vaginal sensation is usually temporary.
>
> **EVALUATION OF EXPECTED OUTCOMES**
>
> - Meets discharge criteria for the postsurgical patient (see Box 20-10)
> - Has soft, formed stool
> - Voids in adequate amounts without difficulty
> - Verbalizes ways to decrease the risk of reherniation of the bladder
> - Selects foods from a menu that complies with restrictions of a low-residue diet and promotes bowel function
> - Correctly performs perineal care
> - Identifies restrictions on activity and coitus during recovery

onset of this disease and a history of infection with herpes simplex virus and papilloma viruses. These cancers grow slowly and metastasize late. Chronic vulvar dystrophies such as leukoplakia are considered premalignant. Malignant lesions can be of the in situ variety, involving only the tissues at the site of origin, or the invasive type. If lesions are invasive, extensive local spread occurs, particularly into the lymphatic channels.

**Assessment.** The most common complaint of patients with early vulvar cancer is pruritus (itching). The precancerous lesions of leukoplakia may be present and are seen as thickened white patches on the mucous membranes of the vulva. The patient often gives a history of having used various salves, ointments, and lotions for symptoms of mild soreness before finally seeking medical care. Cardiovascular and degenerative diseases are often present because of the typical older age of these patients. Later symptoms include edema of the vulva and pelvic lymphadenopathy.

**Intervention.** Radiation therapy may be used if the disease has progressed beyond the operable stage. If the malignancy can be surgically removed, a vulvectomy is indicated.

Vulvectomy is the removal of the external female genitals. It may be a partial procedure for biopsy purposes, a simple procedure for removal of a benign or an in situ-type lesion, or a radical procedure for invasive malignant lesions. A simple vulvectomy is the removal of the vulva along with a margin of skin adjacent to the vulva. A radical vulvectomy includes the excision of skin from the symphysis pubis to the anus and may include removal of the inguinal lymph nodes in the groin on both sides. The excised areas are covered with a skin flap.

Preoperative care includes the same care as reviewed in Chapter 20. Wide areas of skin preparation should include the inguinal regions, vulva, and pubic and perineal areas. The emotional preparation of the patient is important, and the nurse should listen to any apprehension or fears that the patient expresses. Fear of disfigurement and loss of a body part is common. Both before and after surgery the patient may show signs of a grief reaction, such as depression, anger, denial, or withdrawal.

When the patient returns from surgery, a Foley catheter will be in the urinary bladder to prevent constriction of the urethra. Dressing changes may be needed for several days because of serous drainage from the wounds. A T binder may be used to hold dressings in place. The patient is placed in a low Fowler's position to prevent strain on the sutures. She should be turned every 2 hours, and when on her side a pillow should be placed lengthwise between her legs to support the upper leg and prevent strain. The wound is cleansed according to the physician's orders. Solutions often used for cleansing include hydrogen peroxide and warm physiologic saline solution. The surgeon may prefer that wounds be exposed and that a heat lamp be used because it stimulates circulation and promotes healing. Some physicians order sitz baths, whereas others believe that such baths increase the danger of wound infection. The patient is usually given a low-residue diet. Analgesics are required for several days, and recovery is generally slow. The patient may be ambulatory by the third day, but the nurse should remember that ambulation must be gradual for the older person. Leg edema is common after surgery and may become chronic. Elastic stockings, elevation of the legs, and avoidance of long periods of sitting or standing improve venous return. An important nursing function is the prevention of wound infection. Care should be taken to provide privacy when caring for the wound and to avoid any unnecessary exposure of the patient.

The patient's acceptance of and adjustment to her change in appearance may be difficult, and she may need support in helping her partner accept the change. The patient may experience difficulty in coitus because of loss of tissue in the supporting structures of the labia and vagina and possible constriction of the vaginal orifice. Constriction may require dilation or surgical revision.

**Expected outcomes.** With proper intervention the patient with a vulvectomy does the following:

- Preserves her self-esteem as indicated by attention to personal hygiene and appearance
- Verbalizes concerns about the change in appearance of her vulvar region and shares concerns with her husband or significant other
- Has approximation and healing of the wound with no signs of infection
- Voids regularly in amounts greater than 150 ml
- States plans for restricting activity postoperatively that will strain the operative area
- States plans for restriction of sexual activity until permitted by the physician
- Verbalizes understanding that constriction of the vaginal orifice may occur postoperatively and may require reconstructive surgery
- States plans for a follow-up visit to the physician

## Vaginal Cancer

Cancer of the vagina, particularly in young women, is rare. The incidence is higher in women who were prenatally exposed to diethylstilbestrol.

Early detection allows complete removal of the malignant area in the vagina. The vagina can then be reconstructed using a split-thickness graft from the buttocks applied to a Silastic mold, which is sutured to the labia. The mold is removed a few days postoperatively, after the graft shows evidence of taking. A lighter, more comfortable mold can be created with a condom filled with tampons that is inserted until healing is complete.

## DES Syndrome

Diethylstilbestrol (DES) is a synthetic form of estrogen that was prescribed for approximately 5 to 6 million women in the United States between 1941 and 1971. It was commonly used to treat women who were pregnant and who had one prior miscarriage, diabetes, toxemia, or slight bleeding during pregnancy. A prescription audit showed that DES was still being prescribed during pregnancy as late as 1974, despite the FDA's announcement in 1971 that the drug was contraindicated in pregnancy. This FDA restriction followed the discovery that adenocarcinoma of the vagina developed in several young women, each of whom was the daughter of a woman who had ingested DES during pregnancy. Studies were conducted on other young women who had been exposed to DES in utero, and characteristic benign genital tract abnormalities were found in the majority. Follow-up studies continue to determine the risk of malignancy in these women. Daughters of women who took DES are encouraged to have a yearly gynecologic examination and frequent colposcopy to screen for cervical and vaginal cancer.

# CONDITIONS AFFECTING THE CERVIX AND UTERUS

## Cervicitis

Cervicitis may be the result of an acute inflammatory condition of the vagina, or it may be a chronic condition resulting from lacerations occurring at the time of delivery, erosion, cysts, or a specific infection such as gonorrhea. The cause of erosion is not always known. Cervicitis may occur in any woman. Often it produces no symptoms and is detected only during a routine pelvic examination. Most physicians believe that untreated chronic cervicitis predisposes women to cancer of the cervix. Treatment includes examination and studies to exclude cervical cancer. Cervical erosions may be cauterized or treated with cryotherapy (freezing). If the condition does not respond to conservative treatment, the patient may be admitted to the hospital and placed under general anesthesia to have the cone-shaped portion of the cervix removed (conization).

## Endometriosis

**Endometriosis** is the growth of endometrial tissue in abnormal sites, usually in the peritoneal cavity. The ovaries and the peritoneum are the most common sites. The uterus is an organ that sheds cells periodically. These are endometrial cells, and occasionally they become seeded throughout the pelvis and other organs. The exact cause is unknown. Although these endometrial cells are not in the uterus, they are stimulated by the ovarian hormones and bleed into the nearby tissue, resulting in an inflammatory process. Adhesions, strictures, cysts, and infertility can result.

The patient is usually asymptomatic until she is between 25 and 40 years of age. Symptoms that gradually begin to occur are pain during menstruation that becomes progressively worse, fatigue, pressure in the pelvic organs, and general discomfort. Treatment with drugs that suppress ovulation for a time delays the stimulation of the cells and increases the chance of fertility when administration of the drug is stopped. When endometriosis is severe, removal of the uterus, fallopian tubes, and ovaries may be necessary.

## Tumors
### Fibroid

A fibroid, or myomatous tumor, is a benign growth of muscle tissue of the uterus. It occurs in 20% to 30% of women and develops slowly between the ages of 25 and 40. Menorrhagia, abnormally long or heavy bleeding with menstrual periods, is the characteristic symptom. If the fibroid tumor becomes large enough to cause pressure on other structures, backache, constipation, and urinary symptoms may occur. Treatment is surgical removal. If the fibroid tumor is small, a myomectomy is performed to remove just the tumor. If the tumor is large or produces excessive bleeding, a hysterectomy is performed, preserving the ovaries if possible.

## Cervical and Uterine Cancer

Cervical cancer is the second most common form of malignancy affecting the female reproductive organs. Postcoital spotting is the predominant symptom, but this is common with any kind of cervical lesion or inflammation and is not restricted to cervical carcinoma. Unfortunately, cancer of the cervix may not cause symptoms during the early stages and the condition may be far advanced before signs appear. Although cervical cancer may occur in young adults, the incidence increases with age and is greatest between 30 and 50 years of age. The incidence of cervical carcinoma is increased in young women whose mothers took DES during pregnancy as treatment to prevent spontaneous abortion. The Pap smear test is widely used and has had a primary effect in the decreasing the mortality associated with cervical cancer. Carcinoma in situ (CIS) is a preinvasive, asymptomatic carcinoma that can be diagnosed only by microscopic examination. Once it is diagnosed, it can be treated early without radical surgery. CIS of the cervix is essentially 100% curable. All women who are over 18 years of age or sexually active should have a pelvic examination and Pap smear every 3 years after three negative examinations 1 year apart. High-risk women should be examined more often, and many gynecologists prefer to see their patients yearly. Risk factors for cervical cancer include first sex partner at an early age, multiple sex partners, smoking, history of HPV infection, and history of irradiation of the pelvis. Uterine cancer occurs somewhat later in life, usually affecting postmenopausal women. The most common symptom is vaginal bleeding. There is no relationship between the amount of bleeding and the existence of cancer. Sometimes only slight spotting occurs.

Treatment of cervical and uterine cancer varies with the extent of the cancer and age of the patient. For cervical CIS a conization or laser surgery may be performed, which removes a portion of the cervix. Other patients may have a hysterectomy. Radical surgery and radiation therapy are used for more advanced cancer (see Chapter 12).

# CONDITIONS AFFECTING THE OVARIES AND FALLOPIAN TUBES

## Cysts and Tumors

Many different types of ovarian tumors and cysts are benign. However, others may be malignant. Ovarian cysts may cause no symptoms or may result in a disturbance of menstruation, a feeling of heaviness, and slight bleeding. If a pedicle (a stemlike structure) is present, the cyst may become twisted on the pedicle, cutting off the blood supply. If this occurs, immediate surgery is required.

Cancer of the ovary represents 4% of all cancer seen in women and ranks second in number among reproductive cancer diagnoses in women (American Cancer Society, 1997). The risk of ovarian cancer increases with age, with the highest rates occurring in women age 65 to 84. It has been called the silent disease because early warning signs that prompt medical attention rarely occur. As a result, ovarian cancer causes more deaths than cancer of the uterus. Vague lower abdominal discomfort and mild digestive complaints are early symptoms for some women. Later symptoms include pelvic pain, anemia, and ascites. The ovary may be the primary site of the cancer, or the cancer may occur as a result of metastasis from the gastrointestinal tract, breast, pancreas, or kidneys. Treatment for cancer of the ovary depends on the severity of the malignancy. Surgical removal of the tumor is the preferred treatment. This may include radical excision of the uterus, ovaries, tubes, and omentum. Chemotherapy follows surgery.

## Pelvic Inflammatory Disease

Pelvic inflammatory disease (PID), also termed pelvic infection, is an inflammatory condition of the pelvic cavity that may involve the fallopian tubes (salpingitis), ovaries (oophoritis), pelvic peritoneum, or pelvic vascular system. The disease can be acute or chronic and can be caused by gram-negative bacteria, *Staphylococcus*, *Streptococcus*, or sexually transmitted organisms such as gonorrhea or chlamydia. It can be confined to one structure or be widespread in the pelvic cavity (see Chapter 12). Pathogens invade the pelvic organs during sexual intercourse, childbirth, the postpartum period, or abortion, or they may spill into the cavity after rupture of an infected organ such as the appendix. PID is more common in women using IUDs.

**Pathophysiology.** Pathogenic organisms are usually introduced from the outside and enter the cervix from the vagina, move up through the uterus to the fallopian tubes, exit from the tubes, and enter the pelvic cavity. They may also enter the pelvis through throm-

bosed uterine veins or through the lymphatics of the uterus. When the pathogens lodge in the fallopian tubes, the inflammatory process results in purulent material and subsequent adhesions, strictures, and obstruction. Infertility results when the tubes become occluded. Partial tubal obstruction predisposes the woman to ectopic pregnancy. Whereas the sperm may be small enough to pass through the stricture or obstructed area, the fertilized ovum is too large to make the return trip to the uterus and remains in the tube, where it begins to develop. Adhesions may produce symptoms severe enough to require removal of the uterus, fallopian tubes, and ovaries.

**Assessment.** Acute PID is characterized by severe abdominal pain, pelvic pain, malaise, nausea, vomiting, and fever with leukocytosis. A foul-smelling, purulent vaginal discharge may be present. The symptoms may be so mild that the woman ignores them. They may subside before the patient seeks medical care, and the disease then goes untreated. Lack of treatment or inadequately treated acute PID results in the chronic form. The patient then complains of a chronic dull pain in the lower abdomen, backache, constipation, malaise, low-grade fever, and menstrual disturbances. Acute symptoms can also appear during periods of exacerbation. The patient's complaints are often vague and nonspecific. Examination reveals pain and tenderness in the lower abdomen, which increases with a vaginal examination. Masses are felt if the fallopian tubes or ovaries are enlarged or if an abscess is present. Abscess formation is common in Douglas' cul-de-sac. If adhesions are present, the pelvic organs will be less movable. Smears and cultures are taken from the vagina, cervix, or Douglas' cul-de-sac to identify the causative organism and determine the most effective antibiotic. Laparoscopy may be performed to diagnose the disease. In this way the physician is able to visualize the reproductive organs and surrounding tissues.

**Intervention.** Hospitalization may be required so that the patient can receive intensive antibiotic therapy. Activity is restricted to bed rest, and the patient is placed in a mid-Fowler's position to prevent upward flow of drainage and the formation of abscesses high in the abdomen. Intravenous fluids may be necessary if the patient's condition requires restricted intake. The antibiotics are given intravenously at first to ensure that blood levels of the drug are adequate to be effective against the causative organism. Heat to the abdomen or hot sitz baths may be ordered to improve circulation and provide comfort. Analgesics are necessary for pain. Blood pressure, temperature, pulse, and respirations should be taken every 4 hours until the fever subsides. The patient should be observed for any increase or decrease in pain and any change in amount, color, odor, or consistency of vaginal drainage. Surgical removal of involved organs may be necessary.

**Expected outcomes.** After proper intervention the patient with PID:

- Is afebrile
- Has absence or reduction of pain and vaginal drainage
- Identifies the point of entry and route of travel of organisms causing PID
- Identifies signs and symptoms of recurrence
- Lists all medications to be taken after discharge, including time and frequency of each dose
- Demonstrates compliance with restrictions on activity, medication regimen, and recommendations for follow-up care

# SURGICAL INTERVENTION FOR CONDITIONS AFFECTING THE CERVIX, UTERUS, OVARIES, AND FALLOPIAN TUBES

## Hysterectomy

**Hysterectomy** is the surgical removal of the uterus. A hysterectomy may be performed through an incision into the abdominal cavity (abdominal hysterectomy), or the uterus may be removed through the vagina (vaginal hysterectomy). In premenopausal women the ovaries are usually not removed unless some abnormal condition exists. Depending on the existing condition, the physician may remove one or both ovaries or one or both fallopian tubes. Removal of both ovaries is called *bilateral oophorectomy,* and removal of both fallopian tubes is called *bilateral salpingectomy.* When the entire uterus, tubes, and ovaries are removed, the operation is called *panhysterosalpingo-oophorectomy,* or *panhysterectomy.* It may also be referred to as a *total abdominal hysterectomy with bilateral salpingo-oophorectomy* (TAH BSO). Removal of the body of the uterus, leaving the cervix in place, is termed a *subtotal hysterectomy.* In a total hysterectomy the entire uterus is removed but the tubes and ovaries are left in place. The patient should understand that a hysterectomy does not necessarily mean that any organs will be removed other than the uterus. However, if there is evidence of disease affecting other organs, those organs are removed at the same time as the uterus.

Surgery involving the female reproductive tract is upsetting to most women. Often the patient perceives the procedure as a threat to her femininity. If the patient is of childbearing age, she may be disappointed because she can no longer have children. Patients often worry about the process of healing and the resumption of sexual activity. If cancer is suspected or found, she may have a fear of death. The more thoroughly the patient is prepared for the surgery, the more satisfactorily she will recover, both physically and emotionally (Box 43-4).

## Abdominal Hysterectomy

**Preoperative intervention.** Preoperative care for the abdominal hysterectomy patient is the same as that for patients having other types of abdominal surgery. The surgical preparation of the skin includes the abdomen, pubis, and perineum. The physician may order an antiseptic vaginal douche, and a Foley catheter may be inserted to keep the bladder from filling during surgery and causing strain postoperatively.

**Postoperative intervention.** Postoperative nursing care is concerned with the prevention of urinary retention, intestinal distention, and venous thrombosis. If a retention catheter was inserted, it should be kept patent and attached to closed drainage. If it is not, the patient must be checked often for bladder distention. The incidence of urinary retention is greater after a hysterectomy than after other types of surgery because some trauma to the bladder unavoidably occurs. Urinary retention leads to discomfort from distention and increases the danger of urinary tract infection. Before administering drugs for pain, the nurse should be sure that the discomfort is not from an overdistended bladder. Most patients are given intravenous fluids for 1 or 2 days, and the additional fluid may contribute to bladder distention. Every method should be used to assist the patient to void before catheterization. Efforts should be instituted early, not delayed until the patient is miserable because of an overdistended bladder. If the patient does not have an indwelling catheter and is unable to void, catheterization every 8 hours may be necessary. Intestinal distention is common after a hysterectomy. A nasogastric tube may be inserted. Early ambulation helps to return the bowel to normal function. As soon as bowel sounds have returned and flatus is being expelled, the patient is allowed liquids by mouth with a gradual return to solid food.

Patients undergoing pelvic surgery are more susceptible to venous stasis and phlebitis because of trauma to blood vessels. Patients who have varicose veins in the extremities must be carefully observed. The nurse should *not* raise the knee gatch, place pillows under the knees, or place the patient in a high Fowler's position. Active exercise should be started as soon as the patient is fully conscious because early ambulation helps prevent venous stasis. Some surgeons order pneumatic compression devices or antiembolism stockings for the lower extremities to prevent stasis and to support venous flow.

| BOX 43-4 | NURSING PROCESS |
|---|---|

## HYSTERECTOMY

### ASSESSMENT

- Vital signs (often)
- Dressing/vaginal drainage (often)
- Intake and output
- Elimination patterns
- Lung and bowel sounds
- Level of comfort
- Signs and symptoms of menopause

### NURSING DIAGNOSES

- Pain related to surgical incision and abdominal distention
- Altered sexuality patterns related to restrictions on sexual intercourse
- Ineffective individual coping related to loss of reproductive function
- Dysfunctional grieving related to loss of reproductive organ
- Knowledge deficit related to onset of menopause and postoperative limitations
- Risk for infection related to interruption in integrity of skin or vaginal mucosa
- Disturbance in self-concept (body image, self-esteem, or role performance) related to loss of reproductive organ and function
- Urinary retention related to pelvic edema and discomfort
- Altered peripheral tissue perfusion related to venous congestion in pelvis

### NURSING INTERVENTIONS

- Administer routine nursing care immediately after anesthesia.
- Check abdominal or perineal dressing for hemorrhage; change as needed according to hospital policy.
- Maintain intravenous infusion, as ordered.

- Administer nothing by mouth until peristalsis returns.
- Maintain patency of indwelling catheter or check for bladder distention every 8 hours; perform straight catheterization, as necessary.
- Catheterize for residual urine after voiding, if ordered.
- Apply heat to abdomen for gas pains, if ordered.
- Encourage deep breathing and coughing every 2 hours.
- Apply plastic or pneumatic stockings, if ordered.
- Avoid sharp flexion of knees or thighs.
- Do not place pillows under the knees.
- Have the patient dangle legs the evening of surgery.
- Encourage leg exercises until the patient is ambulating.
- Provide emotional support.
- Encourage ventilation of fears and concerns related to loss of reproductive capacity.

### EVALUATION OF EXPECTED OUTCOMES

- Meets discharge criteria for the postsurgical patient (see Box 20-10)
- Voids regularly, with amounts greater than 150 ml and residual amounts less than 60 ml
- Tolerates regular diet without nausea or distention
- Has no signs and symptoms of complications
- Demonstrates self-esteem evidenced by attention to personal hygiene and appearance
- Expresses fears and concerns regarding loss of reproductive capacity and sexual identity
- Identifies restrictions on activity and coitus during recovery
- Verbalizes an understanding of surgical menopause

Medication will be ordered for relief of pain. Slight vaginal drainage may occur for a day or two, but any unusual bleeding should be reported to the physician. The nurse should routinely check vital signs and observe the abdominal dressing for evidence of bleeding. Most patients without complications are released from the hospital in approximately 3 to 4 days (Box 43-4).

## Vaginal Hysterectomy

**Preoperative intervention.** Skin preparation involves shaving the pubis and perineum. Some physicians or-

der prophylactic antibiotics and some an antiseptic vaginal douche. A primary source of postoperative infection is the vaginal vault. A Foley catheter is inserted to drain the bladder during surgery, and an enema is given.

**Postoperative intervention.** If a repair has been done along with the hysterectomy, the Foley catheter remains in place for 4 or 5 days to prevent pressure on the sutures. Otherwise it is removed postoperatively, and the patient must be observed for bladder distention and assisted to void. Other postoperative nursing care is essentially the same as that for repair of relaxed muscles.

## Discharge Teaching: Hysterectomy

Before the patient is discharged, she should know what changes to expect. She will no longer menstruate, and she should not have coitus until after the first checkup in 4 to 6 weeks. She may have worries concerning her ability to continue to share sexual pleasure. When a hysterectomy is performed, the vaginal floor is reconstructed with ligaments, and most women should have the same capacity for sexual stimulation after surgery as before. Pain experienced during intercourse (dyspareunia) should be reported to the physician. Normal physical activity and light work may be done when the woman returns home. However, lifting heavy objects and more difficult activity must be avoided for a few weeks.

## Pelvic Exenteration

Complete or total **pelvic exenteration** consists of removal of the rectum, distal sigmoid colon, urinary bladder and distal ureters, internal iliac vessels and their lateral branches, all pelvic reproductive organs, lymph nodes, peritoneum, levator muscles, and perineum. Urinary and fecal diversions are done. *Pelvic evisceration* and *pelvic sweep* are terms used interchangeably with pelvic exenteration.

The procedure is sometimes modified. An anterior pelvic exenteration removes the bladder and distal portion of the ureters while the proximal portions are implanted in an ileal conduit. The normal bowel structure is preserved. In posterior pelvic exenteration the colon and rectum are also removed. Pelvic exenteration is indicated for carcinomas that are locally destructive and capable of growing to great size but that do not tend to metastasize and for tumors that are radioresistant or incurable by less radical surgery. The tumor must be confined to the pelvis without metastatic spread to distant sites and must be operable within the pelvis. The patient should be of an age and general physical and mental condition that make rehabilitation a reasonable goal. Exenteration is an alternative to lethal disease, but the patient and spouse or supportive partner must have a strong desire to live in order to cope with altered methods of elimination and sexual intercourse. Their psychologic and sociologic status must be carefully evaluated preoperatively.

Preoperative care must focus on the patient's psychologic needs, as well as physical preparation of the bowel with a low-residue diet, laxatives, a saline enema, and antibiotic therapy. A sulfonamide drug regimen for bowel cleansing may be used, but controversy exists regarding the use of antibiotics for bowel cleansing. Antiembolism stockings are applied, and a nasogastric tube may be inserted the morning of surgery.

Before surgery the woman douches daily with an antiseptic solution. Vitamin K therapy to promote blood coagulability may begin 2 to 3 days before surgery. The patient must be prepared to remain in bed for up to 1 week postoperatively as healing begins.

After surgery the vital signs and blood pressure are taken every hour for approximately 48 hours. Then they are assessed every 4 hours for 7 days or as long as necessary. Rectal temperature measurement is contraindicated. Intravenous therapy is maintained up to 4000 ml daily. All intake and output are measured. The operative site, the dressings, and all drainage tubes are also assessed hourly for the first 48 hours. Dressings should be reinforced and changed as ordered. Specific nursing care is indicated by the extent of the procedure, the status of the wounds or ostomies that were created, and the patient's response to the surgery.

### Self-Worth

Exenterative surgery has a drastic effect on body image. Loss of the reproductive organs and the ability to have sexual intercourse may be a major handicap to the patient's rehabilitation. Society's emphasis on physical attractiveness makes it even more difficult for the patient to maintain a positive self-concept and strong sexual role identity after the loss of the ability to function in a reproductive capacity. Sexual readjustment may be a problem of great magnitude for the patient and her sexual partner. Vaginal reconstruction is possible, but it is usually done as a follow-up procedure. Segments of colon or ileum or skin grafts over a stent can be used. It is important for the nurse to facilitate the patient's expression of fears and concerns and to communicate the patient's needs to other members of the healthcare team and community resources. Ostomy clubs can be of help to patients in their efforts to regain social mobility and maintain a realistic yet hopeful outlook on life.

# CONDITIONS AFFECTING THE BREAST

## Acute Mastitis

**Mastitis** is an inflammation of the mammary gland (breast) that often occurs during lactation but may occur anytime. It is usually the result of the entrance of bacteria through a crack or fissure in the nipple. The infection may block one or more of the milk ducts, causing the milk to stagnate in the lobule. The infection may spread throughout the breast tissue and cause abscess formation. The infection usually causes an elevation of temperature, with pain and tenderness of the breast. The treatment consists of administration of antibiotic drugs, application of heat or cold, and support of the breast. Incision and drainage of an abscess may be necessary. Because the invading organism in mastitis is often *Staphylococcus,* isolation and care as outlined in Chapter 15 should be followed.

## Physiologic Nodularity (Fibrocystic Breast Disease)

Physiologic nodularity is a common occurrence in premenopausal women. It is characterized by the formation of a nodular type of benign cyst in the breast. The exact cause is unknown. Many women go through life unaware of the condition or neglect diagnosis and treatment. The condition is benign and does not produce an inflammatory condition. Although it generally involves both breasts, it may be accentuated in one breast. The cysts may occur singly or may be numerous and vary in size and tenderness over the menstrual cycle. Pain may be present and may become worse during the menstrual period. Treatment is usually conservative after cancer has been ruled out. However, the patient should examine her own breasts monthly and remain under medical supervision. In most instances there is no increased risk of breast cancer.

## Tumors

Tumors of the breast can be benign or malignant. Benign tumors are not tender and are freely movable. An exact diagnosis can be made only by careful microscopic examination of the cells. Benign tumors should be surgically removed.

## Breast Cancer

Breast cancer is the most common cancer in women, but it is now second to lung cancer in the number of deaths from cancer in women. An estimated 1 of every 9 women in the United States will have cancer of the breast in her lifetime. One of every 100 cases is seen in males (American Cancer Society, 1997). Women who do not bear children or who bear children after the age of 35 have a slightly increased risk of breast cancer. The incidence of breast cancer appears to be lower among women who breast-feed their infants for at least 3 months. However, some authorities question this factor. A small proportion of breast cancers appear to run in families. The most significant risk factor is age; risk increases with each decade. The cause of breast cancer is poorly understood despite extensive research (Box 43-5).

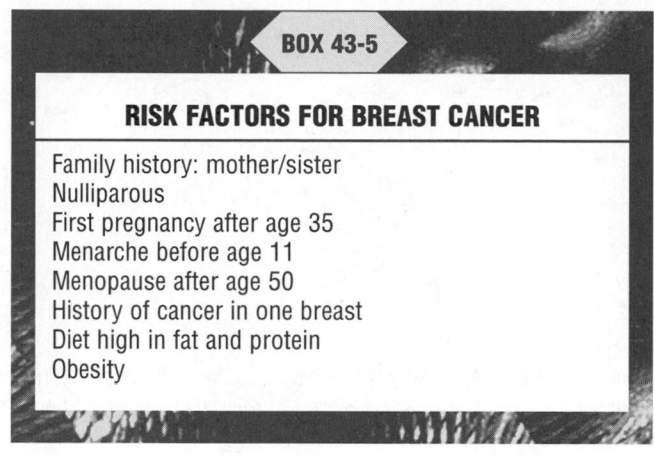

**BOX 43-5**

### RISK FACTORS FOR BREAST CANCER

Family history: mother/sister
Nulliparous
First pregnancy after age 35
Menarche before age 11
Menopause after age 50
History of cancer in one breast
Diet high in fat and protein
Obesity

Time is an important factor in the diagnosis and treatment of breast cancer. If the disease discovered in the early stages, the probability of cure is high. When it is localized in the breast, 97% of patients survive 5 years or longer (American Cancer Society, 1997). The 5-year survival rate is 76% when axillary nodes are involved and 20% when distant metastases are involved (American Cancer Society, 1997).

## Assessment

The American Cancer Society has outlined a program for breast self-examination and has sought to encourage women to examine their breasts monthly to detect abnormalities (Figure 43-7). Women are advised to begin monthly self-examination of their breasts at age 20. Annual examinations by a clinician are recommended for women over age 40. Women between the ages of 20 and 40 should be examined at least every 3 years. The American Cancer Society (1997) recommends annual mammograms after the age of 40. However, mammography screening is not 100% effective: 10% to 14% of breast cancers found by physical examination are missed by mammography (Baird, 1992). Nurses should therefore continue to teach and encourage breast self-examination.

The development of breast cancer is insidious, and pain is usually absent in the early stages. The only sign that may be present is a small, firm lump in the breast, not well defined or movable, which may be discovered only by careful examination. As the tumor increases in size, it attaches itself to the chest wall or to the skin above. A dimpling of the skin may be present, the nipple may be retracted or inverted, and a discharge from the nipple may occur. In some cases skin may become reddened and, if the tumor is large, the contour of the breast may change. Without treatment the axillary

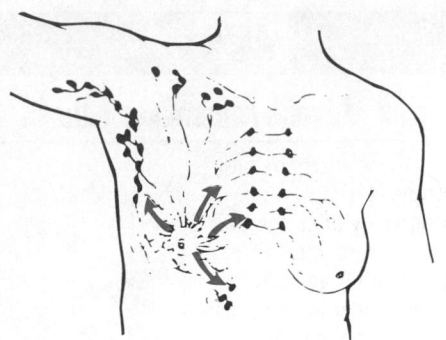

**Figure 43-13** Mode of dissemination of breast cancer. (From Bouchard R, Owens NF: *Nursing care of the patient*, ed 4, St Louis, 1981, Mosby.)

lymph nodes become involved, ulceration may develop, and metastasis to the lungs, bones, liver, and brain may occur. A gradual state of ill health occurs, with weight loss and poor appetite later in the illness.

Carcinoma of the breast usually occurs in a single area in one breast. Almost half of these tumors occur in the upper outer quadrant and another fourth in the central or inner half of the breast. Tumors in the upper outer quadrant tend to metastasize first to the axillary lymph nodes, whereas those from the central portion metastasize to the internal mammary chain lymph nodes (Figure 43-13).

Assessment should include exploration of the patient's feelings about treatment choices, which may include breast conservation surgery, modified mastectomy, and reconstructive surgery. Reconstruction can be more successful when tissue is conserved at the time of surgery. Methods of and indications for breast reconstruction are covered later in this chapter.

## Breast Conservation Surgery (Lumpectomy)

Early-stage breast carcinoma can be treated by breast conservation surgery (lumpectomy) combined with partial axillary node dissection and radiation or a modified mastectomy and lymph node dissection. When the malignancy is less than 1½ inches in diameter, the physician commonly offers breast conservation surgery as an alternative to mastectomy. Informed patients who refuse a mastectomy are seen as a major force in advancing research on conservative management of breast cancer. Several studies performed over the last 20 years have shown that rates of survival, distant metastasis, and local recurrence are similar in patients treated with lumpectomy plus radiation and mastectomy plus radiation (Knobf, 1994). If the likelihood of "cure" is considered equal, one can consider

the cosmetic advantage of removing only the malignant tumor and a small amount (¼ to ½ inch) of surrounding breast tissue. In breast conservation surgery the surgeon removes a minimum amount of skin and the breast tissues are approximated to preserve the appearance of the breast where the tumor has been removed. The incision is made to follow the contour of the breast. A separate incision is made in the axilla to dissect the axillary nodes for biopsy. At least five nodes lying lateral to (level I) and under (level II) the pectoralis minor muscles should be removed for review. If the nodes are removed from the lower two thirds of the axilla, the patient has better function and tolerance and less postoperative edema. If the nodes are negative, the axilla need not receive radiation therapy. Radiation treatments are given to the tumor site and the whole breast up to five times weekly for 6 to 7 weeks.

## Mastectomy

**Mastectomy,** the surgical removal of the breast for treatment of malignancy can be simple, modified radical, or radical. In a *simple mastectomy* the skin and tissue of the breast are removed, the edges of the remaining skin are sutured together, and the lymph nodes are left in place. Some surgeons think that preserving the lymph nodes is important in controlling the spread of malignant cells.

A *modified radical mastectomy* involves removal of all breast tissue and an axillary node dissection, but the pectoralis major and minor muscles are left in place. Preserving these muscles prevents the formation of a hollow depression below the clavicle, reducing disfigurement. Hand and arm swelling is uncommon, and arm and shoulder motion is rarely affected. For more advanced cancer, irradiation may precede or follow a surgical procedure but sufficient time must be allowed before or after surgery to avoid interference with healing.

A radical mastectomy involves removal of the breast and the underlying tissues, including the muscles, axillary lymph nodes, vessels, and perhaps the entire mammary lymph node chain and supraclavicular nodes. The extent of surgery depends on the spread of the neoplasm. However, radical mastectomy is rarely performed today. When the malignant tumor is localized and examination of the lymph nodes is negative, most surgeons believe that a modified radical mastectomy should be performed.

## Breast Reconstruction after Mastectomy

Although mastectomy is a curative treatment, the amputation of a breast is usually viewed as a tragic event, accompanied by loss of body image. Advances in the techniques of reconstructive mammoplasty hold the promise of restoring the contour and consistency of breast tissue to many mastectomy patients. Early detection and treatment make the patient a good candidate for less extensive surgery. Most women experience some dissatisfaction with any type of external prosthesis, whether it be difficulty in wearing clothing or lack of normalcy in sexual relationships. Replacement of the missing breast with an internal prosthesis or an implant of the patient's own tissues is becoming more common. Consultation with a plastic surgeon before mastectomy provides the opportunity to explore the possibilities for reconstruction and to perform the surgical procedure in a manner more likely to result in success.

The patient considering reconstruction can choose between an artificial implant or a procedure that uses her own tissues (autogenous implant). The artificial implant usually involves insertion of a temporary expander that is gradually filled with saline to stretch the breast tissue before insertion of the permanent implant. Some patients can receive the implant immediately without stretching the skin. The autogenous implant uses tissue and muscle from the back or the abdomen to create a new breast. Either procedure can be performed immediately after mastectomy or can be elected at a later date. The options for breast reconstruction must be considered carefully, and some patients are not ready to make the decision at the time of mastectomy.

## Skin Expansion with Implant

A saline implant is inserted immediately or sometime after the breast tissue is removed in a modified radical mastectomy (Figure 43-14). Saline is added gradually to inflate the implant and stretch the breast tissue. The tissue does stretch, just as abdominal tissue stretches during pregnancy. The permanent implant is then inserted in a second surgical procedure. After the incision has healed, the nipple and areola are reconstructed during an outpatient procedure. The nipple is created from a flap of skin, and the areola can be created either by injecting dark color, as done with a tattoo, or by using darker tissue from the inner thigh. The permanent implant is filled with saline and has a texture surface intended to reduce the amount of scar tissue that forms around it. If scar tissue does form, it may create a firm capsule that needs to be broken up manually or surgically. Silicone gel implants used previously are not often used because of continued controversy. There is conflicting evidence about the dangers of silicone leaking into the system. While there is any question, sur-

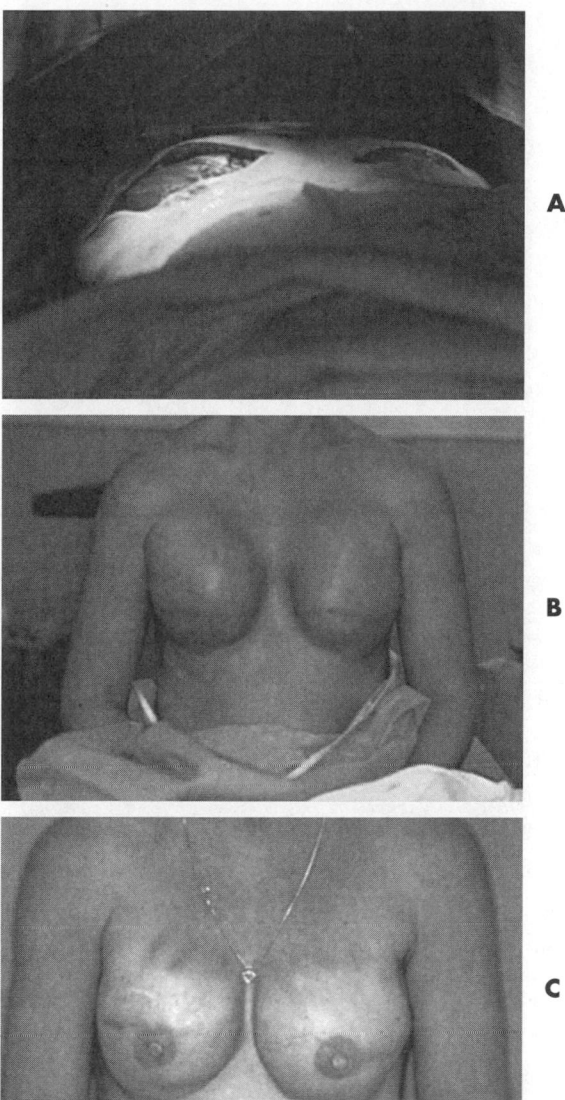

**Figure 43-14**    Breast reconstruction. Immediate reconstruction by means of tissue expansion, eventual insertion of saline-filled breast implants, and nipple and areola reconstructions. **A,** Removal of bilateral breasts. **B,** Hyperexpansion phase using temporary, saline-filled implants. **C,** Final results after insertion of permanent implants and nipple and areola reconstruction. (Courtesy Michael A. Epstein, MD, Elk Grove Village, Ill.)

geons and patients are hesitant to use silicone implants.

## Flap Reconstruction

An autogenous implant involves the use of the patient's own tissue taken from another part of her body (Figure 43-15). The latissimus dorsi muscle from the back was the first donor site. Now the tissue of the

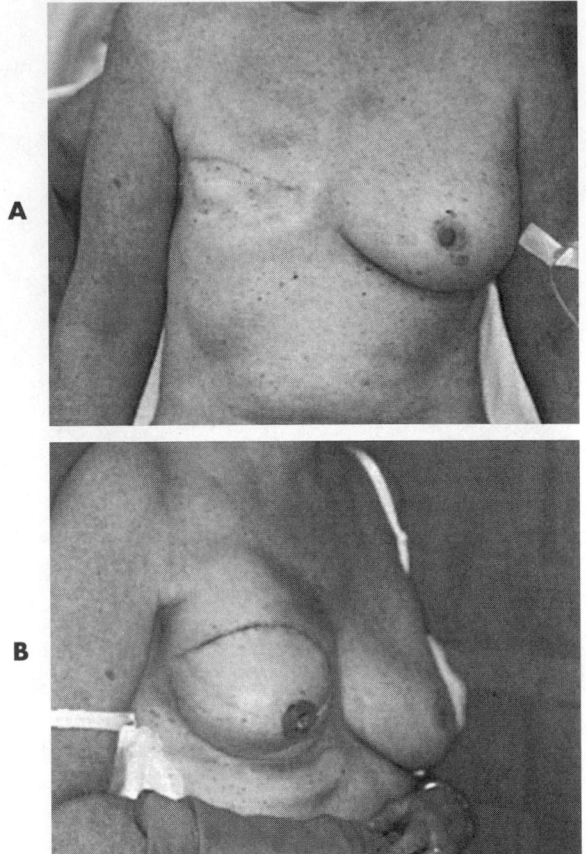

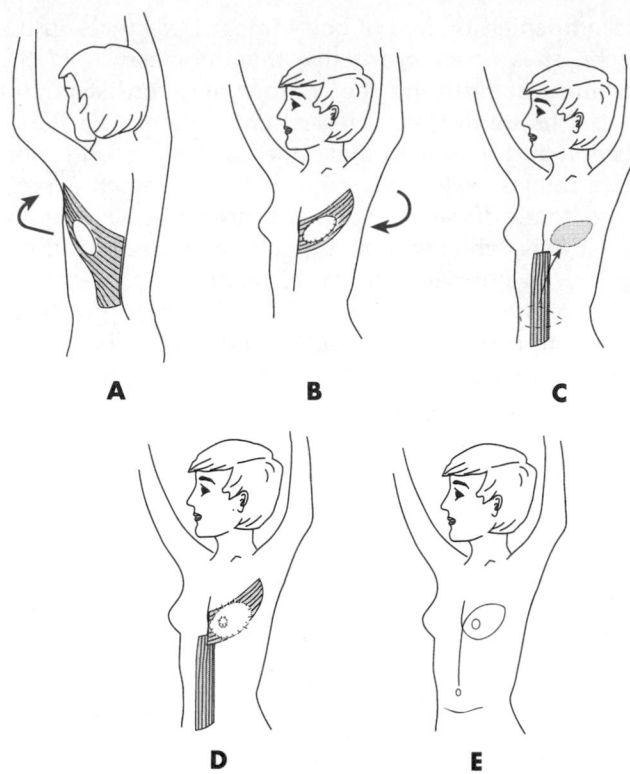

**Figure 43-16**   Flap surgery, breast reconstruction.

**Figure 43-15**   Reconstruction 2 years after mastectomy using TRAM procedure. **A,** Two years after mastectomy. **B,** After reconstruction with autogenous implant (TRAM) and nipple and areola reconstruction. (Courtesy Michael A. Epstein, MD, Elk Grove Village, Ill.)

abdomen over the rectus muscle is more commonly used. The flap of skin and muscle may remain attached to the blood supply and be tunneled under the skin to the breast site, or it may be completely dissected and the blood supply reestablished through microsurgery (Figure 43-16). The abdominal area is reconstructed to restore abdominal strength and prevent hernia. The nipple and areola are reconstructed in the same manner as with a saline implant. The reconstructed breast can be close in form and appearance to a natural breast. However, normal sensation cannot be restored with breast reconstruction.

**Preoperative intervention.** The emotional preparation of the patient may be more important than the physical preparation. When a biopsy is positive, the patient and the physician together decide on the best course of action. The possibility of reconstructive surgery can be discussed at this time (Table 43-5). Although reconstruction improves the patient's ability to accept the

diagnosis and loss, it remains an enormous psychologic trauma. The patient's partner may be unable to provide the understanding that she needs and should be given the opportunity to express feelings and concerns. It is important to discuss the patient's fears openly, and this is best done by a nurse who has established a therapeutic relationship with the patient and family. The relationship must begin on the day of admission. The nurse should demonstrate an awareness of the patient's concerns and help her to express them. Identifying and labeling fears make them more manageable. The nurse should respond to all questions in a way that keeps the patient talking. The "Reach to Recovery" program, sponsored by local chapters of the American Cancer Society, sends volunteers who have had breast surgery and reconstructive surgery to speak to patients at their request. Providing an opportunity to discuss the effects of a mastectomy with someone who has had one often gives needed reassurance to the patient facing or recuperating from such surgery. Unfortunately, these services are not available in all communities.

The physical preparation of the patient requires that a wide area of skin be shaved, including the axilla. If the patient's condition permits, a pint of blood is taken

**TABLE 43-5**

## Breast Cancer Treatment Options, Side Effects, Complications, and Patient Issues

| PROCEDURE | DESCRIPTION OF PROCEDURE | HOSPITALIZATION | SIDE EFFECTS | POTENTIAL COMPLICATIONS | | PATIENT ISSUES |
|---|---|---|---|---|---|---|
| | | | | SHORT-TERM | LONG-TERM | |
| Modified radical mastectomy | Removal of breast; preservation of pectoralis muscle; axillary dissection | Hospital stay 1–4 days | Chest wall tightness; phantom breast sensations; arm swelling; sensory changes | Skin flap necrosis; seroma; hematoma; infection | Muscle atrophy; muscle weakness; lymphedema | Loss of breast; incision; body image; need for prosthesis; impaired arm mobility |
| Breast conservation surgery with radiation therapy | Wide excision of tumor; axillary dissection; radiation therapy | Hospital stay 1–3 days; radiation 6–7 weeks | Breast soreness; breast edema; skin reactions; arm swelling; sensory changes (surgery—arm); sensory changes (breast—XRT); fatigue | Moist desquamation; hematoma; seroma; infection | Fibrosis; rib fractures; lymphedema; myositis; pneumonitis | Prolonged treatment; impaired arm mobility; change in texture and sensitivity of breast |
| Immediate reconstruction—implant | Implantation of prosthesis under musculofascial layer of chest wall | Hospital stay 1–4 days | Discomfort (greater than mastectomy alone because of elevation and stretching of muscles) | Skin flap necrosis; wound separation; seroma, hematoma; infection; delayed wound healing; cellulitis | Capsular contractions; loss of implant; questionable risks of sil cone implants | Body image; prolonged physician visits (expander implants); opposite breast (desire for additional procedures); prolonged postoperative recovery |
| Immediate reconstruction—flap procedures | Musculocutaneous flap (muscle, skin, blood supply) transposed to chest wall area | Hospital stay 5–7 days | Pain related to two surgical sites and extensiveness of the surgery | | | |

From Knobf MT: *Med Surg Nurs* 3(4):249, 1994.

preoperatively for administration at the time of surgery, if needed, to avoid a chance of reaction to donated blood. Other preparation is the same as for other types of major surgery.

**Postoperative intervention.** Postoperative nursing care should include checking vital signs and observing for symptoms of shock or hemorrhage because many large blood vessels are involved in the procedure. Jackson-Pratt drains, attached to low suction, may be placed in the axilla to facilitate drainage. Dressings are usually applied rather tightly and may cause pain and discomfort. When the vital signs are stable, the patient is placed in a 45-degree Fowler's position to promote drainage. The position should be changed often, and deep-breathing exercises should be encouraged. The patient may have some pain and should be given pain-relieving medication. The arm is elevated on a pillow with the hand and wrist higher than the elbow and the elbow higher than the shoulder joint. This facilitates the flow of fluids by the lymph and venous routes and prevents lymphedema. The arm should be observed for signs of circulatory disturbance such as coldness, lack of radial pulse, cyanosis, or blanching. The arm should also be observed for edema, numbness, or inability to move the fingers, which should be reported immediately. Fluids are permitted as soon as nausea ceases, and diet is usually ordered as tolerated. The patient may need help in cutting meat and arranging food conveniently because use of the arm on the affected side may be difficult. When drawing blood, administering intravenous fluids, or taking blood pressure, the nurse should use the unaffected arm. The patient is discharged 1 to 2 days postoperatively (Box 43-6).

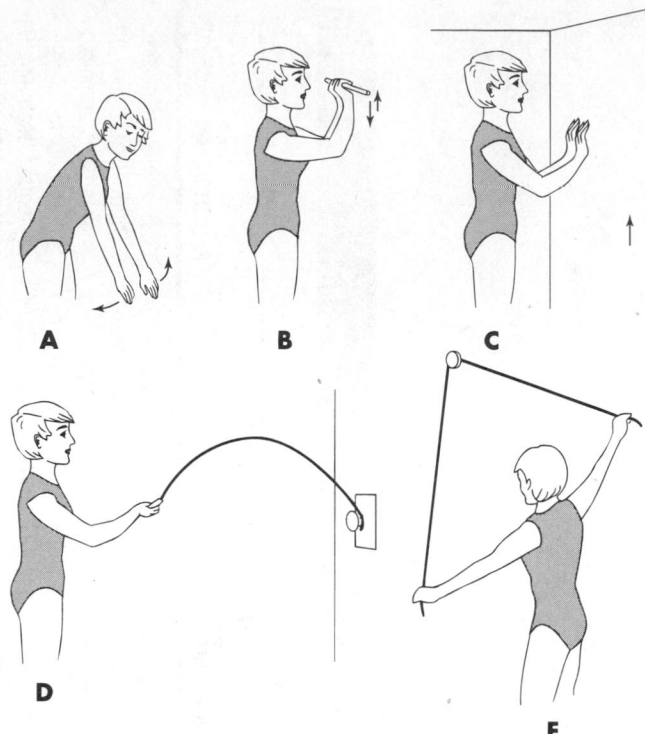

**Figure 43-17**    Arm exercises after mastectomy. **A,** Pendulum swinging with arms relaxed and swinging free. **B,** Arm raising over head. **C,** Wall climbing by standing with face to wall and climbing wall with hands, with fingers reaching as far as possible. **D,** Rope swinging with length of rope tied to doorknob and swinging with shoulder motion. **E,** Rope sliding by placing length of rope over pulley and sliding rope up and down.

> ### NURSE ALERT
>
> Swelling and discomfort in the arm may occur after mastectomy. The nurse should check for coolness, cyanosis, and lack of a radial pulse. The arm can be elevated with pillows to aid drainage.

## Rehabilitation

A primary aim of rehabilitation is to restore the use of the affected arm as soon as possible to prevent contracture. The physician determines the time at which exercises may be started. Some exercises that help the patient regain use of the arm are shown in Figure 43-17. A small handbook titled "Help Yourself to Recovery" is available from the American Cancer Society for use by the nurse in teaching patients. If a "Reach to Recovery" visitor is requested, she brings a kit containing this manual along with a small pillow to aid in positioning, a length of rope and ball to use in exercising, and a temporary prosthesis made of washable cotton. The kit also contains information about permanent prostheses. The visitor demonstrates and helps the patient with the exercises if indicated by the physician. Conversation centers on clothing, prostheses, and return to day-to-day routines. When the patient is discharged, the home health nurse may visit the patient to encourage and reassure her and to supervise exercises. Another important area for patient teaching is monthly self-examination of the chest wall and remaining breast if she has had a mastectomy or of both breasts if she has had breast conservation surgery. Evaluation of the patient's ability to perform breast self-examination and her understanding of its importance is essential. A discussion of nursing diag-

| BOX 43-6 | NURSING PROCESS |
|---|---|

## MASTECTOMY

### ASSESSMENT

- Vital signs (often)
- Dressings and drain (often)
- Lymphedema of the affected arm
- Intake and output
- Elimination patterns
- Lung and bowel sounds
- Level of comfort
- Self-esteem/self-concept

### NURSING DIAGNOSES

- Anxiety related to uncertainty of prognosis or decisions about treatment
- Pain related to incision in skin and muscles of chest wall
- Ineffective breathing pattern related to incision in chest wall
- Risk for injury to lymphatic system related to obstruction of lymph drainage
- Risk for infection related to interrupted skin integrity and presence of drainage
- Ineffective individual or family coping related to loss of breast and perceived loss of attractiveness
- Disturbance in self concept (body image or self-esteem) related to loss of breast
- Knowledge deficit related to prosthesis or reconstruction, activity restrictions, rehabilitation exercises, and support groups

### NURSING INTERVENTIONS

- Maintain in bed in semi-Fowler's position to promote drainage.
- Elevate affected arm with pillows above level of heart.
- Use *unaffected* arm only for blood pressures, venipunctures, and injections.
- Encourage early movement of affected arm, and exercise as soon as medically permitted.
- Check dressings for signs of hemorrhage; reinforce as necessary.

- Maintain patency and suction of drain, if present.
- Maintain intravenous fluids as ordered; do not infuse in arm on affected side.
- Encourage deep breathing, coughing, and turning every 2 hours.
- Encourage active range of motion exercises of the legs.
- Encourage expression of grief related to loss of breast and possible change in self-image.
- Discuss sexuality if indicated.
- Discuss the "Reach to Recovery" program and encourage participation.
- Encourage early use of temporary breast forms and well-fitting brassiere as soon as permitted by physician.
- Provide information on available community resources (Visiting Nurse Association, American Cancer Society, prosthetic suppliers).

### EVALUATION OF EXPECTED OUTCOMES

- Meets discharge criteria for the postsurgical patient (see Box 20-10)
- No edema in arm of affected side
- Demonstrates exercises as ordered by physician
- Verbalizes fears, concerns, and feelings related to loss of breast and change in body image
- Donor site of graft (if present) is dry and healing, with granulation tissue present
- States plans for use of appropriate temporary prosthesis and identifies need to postpone fitting of permanent prosthesis until physician permits
- Demonstrates procedure for breast self-examination and verbalizes understanding of need to perform it monthly on remaining breast or breast tissue
- Maintains self-esteem, evidenced by attention to personal hygiene and appearance
- Discusses fears and concerns with significant other

---

noses and interventions for the patient after breast cancer surgery appears earlier in this chapter.

## Choosing a Prosthesis

The patient should not be fitted for a prosthesis until at least 6 weeks after surgery to allow adequate healing.

A list of recommended fitters in the patient's geographic area assists the patient in her selection. Information about types of prostheses available is also helpful. The "Reach to Recovery" visitor usually has this information. The public health nurse may be of help to the patient in following up on suggestions concerning a prosthesis.

Breast prostheses are available in a variety of types, sizes, weights, and prices. They may be filled with rubber, air, fluid, or a gelatinlike substance. The ideal weight of the prosthesis to provide proper balance and the type of brassiere to offer comfortable support must be considered. A properly fitting prosthesis is essential to allow normal posture and provide a natural appearance under clothing. A natural appearance is important because it can help the patient regain a positive self-image.

## Inoperable Conditions

When patients have delayed medical care and surgery so that the cancer has become invasive and therefore inoperable, radiation, chemotherapy, or both may be used to retard the damaging effects of the malignant growth. The goal is to improve the quality of the patient's life while increasing the duration of survival with the fewest untoward effects for the patient. The patient cannot be cured, but, if she responds to treatment, she can live a longer and less painful life than if not treated. Radiation, chemotherapy, and hormonal therapy can be used. Treatment decisions should be considered individually and center on the woman's age, health status, tumor staging and type, axillary node status, and hormone receptor status of the tumor. A woman needs assistance from her health care team in choosing treatment options.

# CONDITIONS OF PREGNANCY

Care of the obstetric patient is beyond the scope of this book, but several common problems of pregnancy are discussed because they fall within the scope of medical-surgical nursing.

## Abortion

The term abortion means the termination of pregnancy at any time before the fetus has attained the stage of viability, which is approximately 20 to 24 weeks. There are two main types of abortion: *spontaneous* and *induced*. The layperson often uses the word "miscarriage" to denote a spontaneous abortion. An estimated 15% of pregnancies end in spontaneous abortion. At least half of these are the result of a defective fetoplacental unit, genetic defects, or implantation abnormalities.

The weight of the fetus is the customary criterion for defining abortion. Many authorities maintain that the fetus must weigh less than 500 g and have a crown-rump length of less than 16.5 cm. In many states a birth certificate is prepared for any pregnancy terminating after the twentieth week of gestation or when the fetus weighs 500 g or more.

## Types of Spontaneous Abortions

**Habitual abortion.** A woman is said to undergo habitual abortion when three or more successive pregnancies are spontaneously interrupted. The situation commonly creates a severe emotional problem when a woman wants to have children.

**Threatened abortion.** Threatened abortion is indicated when vaginal bleeding or spotting occurs during the first 20 weeks of gestation. The cervix is not dilated, and with conservative treatment the pregnancy may continue uninterrupted. Treatment of threatened abortion includes limiting activity, and bed rest may be prescribed for 24 to 48 hours. If the bleeding stops, it usually does so within 48 hours. The woman should be encouraged to avoid stress and fatigue and may be instructed to avoid intercourse until the pregnancy seems stable.

**Inevitable abortion.** In inevitable abortion the vaginal bleeding may be only spotting or may be hemorrhage with passage of clots. The cervix is dilated, and mild pelvic cramping gradually increases until all or part of the uterine contents is expelled. There is no chance of saving the pregnancy.

**Incomplete abortion.** In incomplete abortion only a portion of the products of conception has been expelled; bleeding continues and may cause severe hemorrhage. The part retained is usually fragments of the placenta. Hospitalizing the patient and prescribing bed rest are necessary. Sedative drugs are administered, and blood transfusions are given if the hemorrhage has been severe. Oxytocin may be administered to stimulate contractions of the uterus. If the residue is not expelled and bleeding continues, the patient is prepared for surgery, taken to the operating room, and given a light anesthetic. Then a D&C is performed.

**Complete abortion.** In complete abortion all products of conception are expelled. Many complete abortions occur without major difficulty, but a physician should be seen to determine whether any of the products of conception remain and to administer Rho(D) immune globulin if necessary.

**Missed abortion.** In a missed abortion the fetus dies and is retained for 8 weeks or more before 20 weeks' gestation. The fibrinogen level in the blood is measured weekly. No attempt is made to empty the uterus unless the fibrinogen level begins to fall. Oxytocin may be administered to stimulate contractions and cause the fetus to be expelled.

**Septic abortion.** Evidence of septic abortion includes a temperature elevation to 40° C (104° F) or more, with threatened or incomplete loss of the products of conception. The presence or absence of any other focus of infection is ruled out before a diagnosis of septic abortion is established. The sepsis may be caused by any of several pathogenic organisms. If it is caused by *Clostridium perfringens,* a spore-forming organism, a powerful exotoxin is liberated. The patient is critically ill with an elevated temperature; the pulse is rapid; and headache, malaise, abdominal tenderness, and indications of pelvic peritonitis occur. The patient is isolated, and medical aseptic technique is carried out. Samples from the cervix and the uterus are taken for culture, and the appropriate antibiotics are administered. Intravenous fluids and blood transfusions may be given, and hydrocortisone and oxytocin (Pitocin) may be ordered. Septic abortion often results in serious complications, including acute renal failure, congestive heart failure, hemorrhage, and severe shock. The patient's condition is considered in the physician's decision to perform a D&C. However, opinions differ concerning the time when a D&C should be performed. In some cases a hysterectomy may be performed.

### NURSE ALERT

**Fever, severe abdominal pain, and bleeding heavier than a normal menses after an abortion may indicate a complication.**

**Induced abortion.** Legal abortion, the termination of a pregnancy at the request of the woman, is now available in all states as the result of a Supreme Court ruling. On January 22, 1973, the U.S. Supreme Court ruled that all antiabortion laws were unconstitutional. In general the court made the following ruling concerning abortion:

1. During the first 12 weeks the state could not bar a woman from obtaining an abortion by a licensed physician.
2. Between 12 and 24 weeks the state could regulate the performance of an abortion in ways reasonable to the woman's health.
3. During the third trimester the state could regulate and prohibit abortion except those deemed necessary to protect the woman's health or life (Hatcher et al, 1994).

In 1976 the U.S. Congress passed the Hyde Amendment, which forbids the use of federal funds for abortions except for situations in which the woman's life is threatened. As a result women with personal funds or private insurance are able to have abortions, whereas poor women who use federal funds for health care are denied the same opportunity. Legal abortion has

nonetheless become the most commonly performed surgical procedure in the United States, with 1.4 million abortions performed annually (Hatcher et al, 1994). On June 29, 1992, the Supreme Court ruled that states might impose restrictions such as waiting periods, parental notification, hospitalization requirements, and specific informed consent requirements. Thus the provision of abortion may vary considerably from state to state.

## Intervention

Interventions are planned according to the type of abortion, prognosis, and nursing diagnosis. All pregnant women should be taught to report any signs of vaginal bleeding or spotting to their health care provider. Women experiencing bleeding or spotting must be observed for hemorrhage. An exact pad count must be kept, and the pads may be weighed to determine the amount of blood loss. All clots and tissue must be saved for inspection and possible laboratory testing. The nurse must be aware of hospital policy concerning the disposal of the products of conception. The nurse should also understand and encourage the woman's religious beliefs and practices that might be appropriate at this time.

In preparing the woman for a D&C, the nurse uses the same procedures as those for a nonpregnant woman. Administration of medication, intravenous fluids, or blood transfusions is carried out according to physician's orders. Informed consent must be obtained.

Postoperatively vital signs should be monitored routinely. The woman must be observed for vaginal bleeding and any signs of infection. She should be taught good hygiene practices and good nutrition. Because there has been blood loss, she should be instructed to eat foods high in iron, folic acid, vitamin C, and protein. The nurse should listen to her speak about the meaning of the loss of the pregnancy. The nurse should recognize that abortion may precipitate grief and that the grieving process takes time before it is resolved. The woman may need advice about birth control before discharge. She may need to have a method of birth control prescribed by her physician, so she should be encouraged to consult with the physician before discharge.

## Abortion Counseling

Most women approach the decision to terminate a pregnancy with ambivalence, fear, and doubt. They worry about making the right decision for themselves, their families, and the unborn child. Sometimes the pregnancy is desired, but the woman may choose to abort after learning of fetal abnormalities in the second trimester. Under these circumstances the decision to abort may be particularly difficult and accompanied by regret and grief. More often the pregnancy is unplanned and not desired. On learning that she is pregnant, a woman may experience feelings of shock, disbelief, and anger. Before she can make a decision, she must cope with feelings generated by the confirmation of her pregnancy. The nurse must allow time to process her feelings. All options for continuing the pregnancy and support systems for the pregnancy should be addressed. If the woman is considering abortion, she will need information about the procedure, its safety, and its cost to make her decision. She may feel overwhelmed by such a decision and may need help assessing both her feelings about the pregnancy and her life plans. The nurse should try to remain empathetic and objective. Active listening on the part of the nurse, such as paraphrasing and clarifying what the patient tries to communicate, may help the woman to identify concerns and conflicts. A woman's decision may be complicated by an abusive partner, lack of financial resources, fear of parental involvement, and unfamiliarity with making important life decisions. Whether she maintains or terminates the pregnancy, the decision is ultimately hers to make.

Whatever the feelings of the individual nurse, the patient who enters the hospital seeking an abortion should never face hostility or discrimination. The decision to seek an abortion may be a difficult one, and these patients have problems and worries similar to those of any other hospitalized patient. Nurses who believe that they cannot morally assist with an abortion should not work in a setting in which they are performed.

## Types of Induced Abortions

**First-trimester abortion.** Five of every six abortions are performed before the 13th week of pregnancy (Hatcher et al, 1994). The most common method used in the first trimester is vacuum aspiration. The procedure is relatively simple and safe. Local anesthesia in the form of a paracervical block is typically provided. Although general anesthesia may be used, doing so adds to the risk of the procedure and to the cost. To perform suction curettage, the physician completes a bimanual examination to determine gestational size and uterine position. An injection of a local anesthetic such as lidocaine may be used before the cervix is dilated. Alternatively, laminaria (dried seaweed) may be used to dilate the cervix gently up to 1 day before the procedure. After the cervix is dilated, the vacuum cannula is introduced into the uterus and negative pressure is applied, which evacuates the contents of the uterus. Curettage is performed to complete evacuation of the uterus. The products of conception are examined briefly, weighed to confirm complete evacuation, and sent to a pathologist for closer scrutiny. The vacuum aspiration procedure may be performed on an outpatient basis up to the 14th week of gestation. The nurse may be responsible for sterilizing the equipment and assisting the physician during the procedure. The nurse may also play a central role in preparing the patient and offering emotional support during the surgery. The patient remains in recovery under the observation of a nurse for 1 to 3 hours after the procedure. The nurse checks vital signs and provides emotional support. The patient should be instructed to check and report the amount of vaginal bleeding to the nurse before leaving the recovery area. At discharge the patient should be instructed to immediately report bleeding heavier than normal menses, severe or increasing abdominal pain, or fever greater than 37.8° C (100° F) (Table 43-6). If future contraception needs have not been addressed, they should be discussed at this point. Birth control pills or DMPA may be started on the day of the procedure. Rho(D) immune globulin should be given to women with Rh-negative blood to avoid the

| TABLE 43-6 | | |
|---|---|---|
| **Patient Teaching—What to Expect After an Abortion** | | |
| | **EXPECTED EFFECT** | **WARNING SIGNS** |
| Vaginal bleeding | Bleeding lasting up to 2 weeks | Bleeding heavier than menses |
| | Spotting up to 4 weeks | Bleeding more than 2 weeks |
| | No bleeding | Foul odor |
| Cramps | Menstrual like | Severe, persistent, noncramplike abdominal pain |
| | Mild to moderate, relieved by mild analgesia | |
| Temperature (oral) | Less than 100° F | 100° F or higher |
| Menses | Resume within 4 weeks or after first package | No menses within 8 weeks |
| | of oral contraceptives completed | Continued symptoms of pregnancy |
| Other | Fatigue | Appearance of rash or hives if antibiotics were given |

From Lichtman R, Papera S: *Gynecology well-woman care*, Norwalk, Conn, 1990, Appleton & Lange.

risk of sensitization and problems in future pregnancies. Some physicians prescribe a short course of antibiotics or oxytocic drugs, such as methylergonovine (Methergine), to contract the uterus. The woman should be instructed not to put anything into her vagina for 2 weeks after the abortion. That is, she should not douche, use tampons, or engage in sexual intercourse. Bleeding and cramping may vary, but discomfort is usually relieved with mild analgesics. The patient should return for a checkup 2 weeks after the procedure. She can expect her next period 4 to 6 weeks after the procedure. She should contact her health care provider if she does not have her period as expected because this could indicate a continued pregnancy or adhesions of the uterus (Asherman's syndrome).

**Medical abortion.** Mifepristone (RU-486) is a synthetic steroid that can be used together with prostaglandins in the first trimester to induce abortion without the need for surgery. Combining RU-486 with an oral prostaglandin such as misoprostol (Cytotec) has been shown to have a 95% to 99% success rate as an abortifacient in the first 8 weeks of pregnancy (Mackenzie, Yeo, 1997). Mifepristone has recently been approved by the Food and Drug Administration for use in the early termination of pregnancy. This method of abortion allows greater privacy because the administration of RU-486 is a medical treatment rather than a surgical procedure and so does not require the services of an abortion clinic.

**Second-trimester abortion.** Second-trimester abortions account for less than 10% of abortions performed in the United States (Hatcher et al, 1994). The most common surgical procedure used is dilation and evacuation, which may be performed up to 20 weeks but typically takes place between 13 to 16 weeks' gestation. An ultrasound is usually obtained to confirm gestational age. Because the products of conception are greater in amount in the second trimester, the cervix requires greater dilation and osmotic agents such as laminaria are often used to achieve this. The uterine contents are evacuated by vacuum cannula as with first-trimester abortion. Less frequently agents such as hypertonic saline, hypertonic urea, and prostaglandin E$_2$ are used to induce abortion late in the second trimester. In these instances the usual procedure involves removing amniotic fluid by amniocentesis and instilling one of the above agents in its place. A local anesthetic is used, and most clinicians use laminaria to dilate the cervix. Oxytocin accelerates the uterine contractions and hastens expulsion of the fetus.

## Ectopic Pregnancy

Ectopic pregnancy is gestation anywhere outside the uterus. An ectopic pregnancy rarely occurs in the abdomen or the ovary. The most common site for an ectopic pregnancy is in the fallopian tube. When the ovum becomes implanted in the fallopian tube, it is referred to as *tubal pregnancy*. Infrequently a tubal pregnancy may be palpated during bimanual examination in the area near the uterus, but the first indication of tubal pregnancy often occurs when the tube ruptures. The incidence of ectopic pregnancies increased sharply to 108,800 ectopic pregnancies (1 in 50 reported pregnancies) in 1992 (Powell, Spellman, 1996). Tubal pregnancy results from some condition within the tube that slows or prevents passage of the ovum through the tube to the endometrium of the uterus. Conditions such as inflammation from disease, narrowing of the tube, and an elongated or immature tube create a situation conducive to tubal pregnancy. Thus a medical history of PID, tubal ligation, or previous ectopic pregnancy increases a woman's risk for this problem.

As the embryo increases in size, the tube stretches until it can no longer remain intact. The tube may rupture, releasing the entire products of conception into the abdominal cavity (*ectopic abortion*). The rupture may be small, with the embryo remaining within the tube, but severe bleeding may occur as a result of damage to the blood vessels. The length of time the tube remains intact with the developing fetus varies but averages 7 to 8 weeks from the last menstrual period.

**Assessment.** With an ectopic pregnancy, often the patient has missed one period and has noted slight spotting, but she may not know that she is pregnant. In the majority of patients rupture results in sudden acute abdominal pain. The pain may extend to the shoulder and the rectal area. The patient becomes faint and pale and may be in shock. Hemorrhage may be severe, and acute secondary anemia results. In other cases the clinician may consider the diagnosis based on nonspecific symptoms such as bleeding and a uterine size that does not correlate with the last menstrual period. In a nonemergency situation a patient may be evaluated by serial measurement of HCG levels and pelvic ultrasound. Ultrasound should be able to detect an intrauterine gestational sac by 5 to 6 weeks' gestation.

> ### NURSE ALERT
> Abdominal pain, nausea, and pain referred to the shoulder in early pregnancy may indicate an ectopic pregnancy.

**Intervention.** A ruptured tubal pregnancy is always an emergency and requires immediate surgery. There may be little time for preoperative preparation. The patient is treated immediately for shock with blood transfusions or intravenous infusion of lactated Ringer's solution. When an ectopic pregnancy has not yet ruptured, more choices are available for treatment. These include laparoscopic surgery and treatment with methotrexate or etoposide, which induces dissolution of the fetal tissue, coupled with close observation when the pregnancy is early and HCG level low and declining (Hatcher et al, 1994). In cases of this last sort, spontaneous abortion

and reabsorption of tissue may occur without surgical intervention.

Postoperative care of the patient is the same as in other abdominal surgery. Transfusions with whole blood may be necessary to combat anemia. Uterine bleeding occurs for several days, and the patient must be observed for any unusual bleeding from the abdominal incision or the vagina.

## KEY CONCEPTS

➤ Teaching a patient about menstruation must begin with an assessment of her knowledge and feelings about menstruation, then proceed to clarify misconceptions and provide additional information appropriate for her age and developmental level, using positive terms.

➤ Contraceptive methods vary in effectiveness, and the patient must be guided and assisted in reviewing choices and selecting the most appropriate method.

➤ Infertility can be a life crisis and emotionally devastating for a couple. Causes are multiple, and systematic evaluation is required.

➤ Supplementary estrogen therapy in menopausal women is most effective in relieving hot flashes and night sweats and is generally accepted as important in preventing osteoporosis and heart disease. Treatment must be individualized.

➤ If a patient's condition or treatment raises concerns about limitations of sexual ability, the nurse should provide an opportunity for discussion. This is best done after the nurse-patient relationship is established. It also requires privacy and an attitude of nonjudgmental concern and caring.

➤ Vesicovaginal and rectovaginal fistulas require increased vitamin C and protein intake and careful hygiene to promote healing and comfort. Sitz baths, deodorizing douches, perineal pads, and "baby wipes" should be used to cleanse the perineum after elimination.

➤ Colporrhaphy is the surgical procedure used to repair cystocele (bulging of the bladder against the vaginal wall) and rectocele (bulging of the rectum against the vaginal wall). The primary goal of postoperative care is prevention of strain on the suture lines.

➤ Endometriosis is an inflammatory condition of endometrial cells located outside the uterus. The inflammation causes pain during menstruation, fatigue, pressure in the pelvic organs, and general discomfort.

➤ Vague lower abdominal discomfort and mild digestive complaints are early symptoms of ovarian cancer in some women.

➤ Pelvic inflammatory disease (PID) may demonstrate symptoms so mild that they are ignored and untreated. Chronic PID then results. PID can cause infertility and predispose a woman to ectopic pregnancy.

➤ Postoperative care of the patient with a hysterectomy is concerned with prevention of urinary retention, intestinal distention, and venous thrombosis. The surgery should not usually affect capacity for sexual stimulation.

➤ The American Cancer Society recommends that women 40 to 49 years of age should have a mammogram every 1 or 2 years, and those 50 and over and those with a family history in first-degree relatives should be scheduled annually.

➤ With 10% to 14% of breast cancers found during physical examinations and missed by mammography, breast self-examination should be taught and encouraged.

➤ The patient must understand treatment choices available for breast cancer: breast conservation surgery (lumpectomy), modified mastectomy, and reconstructive surgery.

➤ The emotional preparation of the patient for breast surgery is as important as the physical preparation. The patient's selection of course of action must be facilitated, and the patient must be able to openly express fears, feelings, and concerns.

➤ Legal abortion has become the most commonly performed surgical procedure in the United States, with 1.4 million performed annually. Federal funds may not be used for abortion except for situations in which the woman's life is threatened.

## KEY CONCEPTS—cont'd

➤ Women considering a termination of pregnancy should have counseling to cope with and process feelings and to explore options; support systems for continuing the pregnancy; and information

about abortion procedures, safety, and cost. Active listening is essential.

➤ Abdominal pain, nausea, and referred pain to the shoulder in early pregnancy may indicate an ectopic pregnancy.

## CRITICAL THINKING EXERCISES

1. Consider your approaches in taking sexual histories from an adolescent and a postmenopausal woman.
2. Contrast oral contraceptive pills and Norplant with regard to risks and benefits.
3. What are the risks and benefits of hormonal replacement therapy for postmenopausal women?
4. Contrast the pros and cons of lumpectomy and modified radical mastectomy as treatments for breast cancer.
5. Explain a colposcopy to your 45-year-old patient.

### REFERENCES AND ADDITIONAL READINGS

American Cancer Society: *Cancer facts and figures—1997*, Atlanta, 1997, American Cancer Society.

Baird SB, editor: *A cancer source book for nurses*, Atlanta, 1991, American Cancer Society Professional Education Publication.

Bilodeau BA: Information needs, sources of information, and decisional roles in women with breast cancer, *Oncol Nurs Forum* 23(4):691-696, 1996.

Bostwick J: Breast reconstruction following mastectomy, *Ca Cancer J Clin* 45(5):289-304, 1995.

Boyle DM: Gynecologic nursing in the next millenium: projections and opportunities, *Gynecol Oncol Nurs* 6(4):8-16, 1996.

Brucks JA: Ovarian cancer, *Nurs Clin North Am* 27(4):835-845, 1992.

Buyske J et al: Breast cancer in the nineties, *AORN J* 64(1):64-72, 1996.

Colbry SL: A review of toxic shock syndrome: the need for education still exists, *Nurs Pract* 17(9):39-43, 1992.

Dest VM, Fisher SM: Breast cancer: dreaded diagnosis, complicated care, *RN* 57(6):49-54, 1994.

Edwards S: Women who have undergone a tubal sterilization have a reduced risk of contracting ovarian cancer, *Fam Plan Perspect* 26(2):90-91, 1994.

Garner C: Endometriosis: what you need to know, *RN* 60(1):27-31, 1997.

Harbin RE: Female adolescent contraception, *Pediatr Nurs* 21(3):221-226, 1995.

Hatcher RA et al: *Contraceptive technology*, ed 16, New York, 1994, Irvington.

Hinkle LT: Education and counseling for Norplant users, *J Obstet Gynecol Neonatal Nurs* 23(5):387-391, 1994.

Holm K, Penckofer S, Chandler P: Deciding on hormone replacement therapy, *Am J Nurs* 95(8):57-60, 1995.

Ivey CL, Gordon SI: Breast reconstruction: new image, new hope, *RN* 57(7):49-53, 1994.

Johnson JR: Caring for the woman who's had a mastectomy, *Am J Nurs* 94(5):25-31, 1994.

Kaunitz AM: Oral contraceptives and gynecologic cancer: an update for the 1990s, *Am J Obstet Gynecol* 167(4, pt2):1171-1176, 1992.

Kjerulff KH: Chronic gynecological conditions reported by US women: findings from the National Health Interview Survey, 1984 to 1992, *Am J Public Health* 86(2):195-199, 1996.

Klemm PR: Cervical cancer: a developmental perspective, *J Obstet Gynecol Neonatal Nurs* 25(7):629-634, 1996.

Knobf MT: Treatment options for early stage breast cancer, *Med Surg Nurs* 3(4):249-259, 1994.

Mackenzie SJ, Yeo S: Pregnancy interruption using mifepristone (RU-486), *J Nurse-Midwifery* 42(2):86-90, 1997.

Maiolatesi CR, Peddicord K: Methotrexate for nonsurgical treatment of ectopic pregnancy: nursing implications, *J Obstet Gynecol Neonatal Nurs* 25(3):205-208, 1996.

McCance KL, Huether SE: *Pathophysiology: the biologic basis for disease in adults and children*, St Louis, 1990, Mosby.

McMullin M: Holistic care of the patient with cervical cancer, *Nurs Clin North Am* 27(4):847-857, 1992.

Moore AA, Noonan MD: A nurse's guide to hormone replacement therapy, *J Obstet Gynecol Neonatal Nurs* 25(1):24-31, 1996.

Nishimoto PW: Sex and sexuality in the cancer patient, *Nurse Pract Forum* 6(4):221-227, 1995.

Phippen ML, Wells MP: *Perioperative nursing handbook,* Philadelphia, 1995, Saunders.

Powell MP, Spellman JR: Medical management of the patient with an ectopic pregnancy, *J Perinatol Neonatal Nurs* 9(4): 31-43, 1996.

Robinson BJH: The perioperative nurse's role in assisted fertility procedures, *AORN J* 65(1):87-89, 92-93, 1997.

Salazar MK: Hispanic women's beliefs about breast cancer and mammography, *Cancer Nurs* 19(6):437-446, 1996.

Segal S: Nursing rounds, postoperative TAH/BSO . . . total abdominal hysterectomy/bilateral salpingo-oophorectomy, *Am J Nurs* 96(1):45, 57, 1996.

Thomas DJ: Benefits and risks of hormone/estrogen replacement, *Nurs Clin North Am* 31(4):815-825, 1996.

Thompson DS, Szukiewicz-Nugent JM, Walczak JR: A woman's cancer: when ovarian cancer strikes, *Nursing* 26(10): 33-38, 44-45, 1996.

Trad PV: Teenage pregnancy: seeking patterns that promote family harmony, *Am J Fam Ther* 22(1):42-55, 1994.

Wyeth-Ayerst Laboratories: *Norplant system levonorgestrel implants product monograph,* St Davids, Penn, 1991, Wyeth-Ayerst Laboratories.

# APPENDIX A

## Abbreviations and Symbols for Units of Measurement

| | | | |
|---|---|---|---|
| $<$ | Less than | mm³ | Cubic millimeter |
| $\leq$ | Less than or equal to | mM | Millimole |
| $>$ | Greater than | mm Hg | Millimeter of mercury |
| $\geq$ | Greater than or equal to | mm H₂O | Millimeter of water |
| C | Celsius | mol | Mole |
| cc | Cubic centimeter | mmol | Millimole |
| cg | Centigram | mOsm | Milliosmole |
| cm | Centimeter | mμ | Millimicron |
| cm H₂O | Centimeter of water | mU | Milliunit |
| cu | Cubic | mV | Millivolt |
| dl | Deciliter (100 ml) | ng | Nanogram |
| g | Gram | nmol | Nanomole |
| IU | International unit | Pa | Pascal |
| ImU | International milliunit | pg | Picogram (or micromicrogram) |
| IμU | International microunit | pl | Picoliter |
| K | Kilo | pm | Picomole |
| kg | Kilogram | S | Second (SI) |
| L | Liter | sec | Second |
| m | Meter | SI units | International System of Units |
| m² | Square meter | μ | Micron |
| m³ | Cubic meter | μ³ | Cubic micron |
| mEq | Milliequivalent | μg | Microgram |
| mEq/L | Milliequivalent per liter | μIU | Microinternational unit |
| mg | Milligram | μmol | Micromole |
| min | Minute | μU | Microunit |
| ml | Milliliter | U | Unit |
| mm | Millimeter | yr | Year |

From Pagana KD, Pagana TJ: *Diagnostic testing and nursing implications: a case study approach,* ed 5, St Louis, 1998, Mosby.

# APPENDIX B

## 1997–1998 NANDA—Approved Nursing Diagnoses

Activity intolerance
Activity intolerance, risk for
Adaptive capacity, decreased: intracranial
Adjustment, impaired
Airway clearance, ineffective
Anxiety
Aspiration, risk for
Body image disturbance
Body temperature, altered, risk for
Bowel incontinence
Breastfeeding, effective
Breastfeeding, ineffective
Breastfeeding, interrupted
Breathing pattern, ineffective
Cardiac output, decreased
Caregiver role strain
Caregiver role strain, risk for
Communication, impaired verbal
Community coping, potential for enhanced
Community coping, ineffective
Confusion, acute
Confusion, chronic
Constipation
Constipation, colonic
Constipation, perceived
Coping, defensive
Coping, family: potential for growth
Coping, ineffective family: compromised
Coping, ineffective family: disabling
Coping, ineffective individual
Decisional conflict (specify)
Denial, ineffective
Diarrhea
Disuse syndrome, risk for
Diversional activity deficit
Dysreflexia
Energy field disturbance
Environmental interpretation syndrome, impaired
Family processes, altered
Family processes, altered: alcoholism
Fatigue
Fear
Fluid volume deficit
Fluid volume deficit, risk for
Fluid volume excess
Gas exchange, impaired
Grieving, anticipatory

Grieving, dysfunctional
Growth and development, altered
Health maintenance, altered
Health-seeking behaviors (specify)
Home maintenance management, impaired
Hopelessness
Hyperthermia
Hypothermia
Incontinence, functional
Incontinence, reflex
Incontinence, stress
Incontinence, total
Incontinence, urge
Infant behavior, disorganized
Infant behavior, disorganized: risk for
Infant behavior, organized: potential for enhanced
Infant feeding pattern, ineffective
Infection, risk for
Injury, perioperative positioning: risk for
Injury, risk for
Knowledge deficit (specify)
Loneliness, risk for
Management of therapeutic regimen, community: ineffective
Management of therapeutic regimen, families: ineffective
Management of therapeutic regimen, individual: effective
Management of therapeutic regimen, individual: ineffective
Memory, impaired
Mobility, impaired physical
Noncompliance (specify)
Nutrition, altered: less than body requirements
Nutrition, altered: more than body requirements
Nutrition, altered: risk for more than body requirements
Oral mucous membrane, altered
Pain
Pain, chronic
Parent/infant/child attachment, altered: risk for
Parental role conflict
Parenting, altered
Parenting, altered, risk for
Peripheral neurovascular dysfunction, risk for
Personal identity disturbance
Poisoning, risk for
Post-trauma response
Powerlessness
Protection, altered
Rape-trauma syndrome
Rape-trauma syndrome: compound reaction

*Continued*

## 1997–1998 NANDA—Approved Nursing Diagnoses—cont'd

Rape-trauma syndrome: silent reaction
Relocation stress syndrome
Role performance, altered
Self-care deficit, bathing/hygiene
Self-care deficit, dressing/grooming
Self-care deficit, feeding
Self-care deficit, toileting
Self-esteem disturbance
Self-esteem, chronic low
Self-esteem, situational low
Self-mutilation, risk for
Sensory/perceptual alterations (specify) (visual, auditory, kinesthetic, gustatory, tactile, olfactory)
Sexual dysfunction
Sexuality patterns, altered
Skin integrity, impaired
Skin integrity, impaired, risk for
Sleep pattern disturbance
Social interaction, impaired

Social isolation
Spiritual distress (distress of the human spirit)
Spiritual well-being, potential for enhanced
Suffocation, risk for
Swallowing, impaired
Thermoregulation, ineffective
Thought processes, altered
Tissue integrity, impaired
Tissue perfusion, altered (specify type) (renal, cerebral, cardiopulmonary, gastrointestinal, peripheral)
Trauma, risk for
Unilateral neglect
Urinary elimination, altered
Urinary retention
Ventilation, inability to sustain spontaneous
Ventilatory weaning response, dysfunction (DVWR)
Violence, risk for: directed at others
Violence, risk for: self-directed

# APPENDIX C

## Normal Reference Laboratory Values
### Blood, plasma, or serum values

| DETERMINATION | REFERENCE RANGE | |
|---|---|---|
| | CONVENTIONAL | SI |
| Acetoacetate plus acetone | 0.3-2.0 mg/100 ml | 3-20 mg/L |
| Aldolase | 1.3-8.2 mU/ml | 12-75 nmol · s$^{-1}$/L |
| Alpha-aminonitrogen | 3.0-5.5 mg/100 ml | 2.1-3.9 mmol/L |
| Ammonia | 80-110 $\mu$g/100 ml | 47-65 $\mu$mol/L |
| Ascorbic acid | 0.4-1.5 mg/100 ml | 23-85 $\mu$mol/L |
| Barbiturate | 0 | 0 $\mu$mol/L |
| | Coma level: phenobarbital, approximately 10 mg/100 ml; most other drugs, 1-3 mg/100 ml | |
| Bicarbonate | 24-32 mEq/L | |
| Bilirubin (van den Bergh test) | 1 min: 0.4 mg/100 ml | Up to 7 $\mu$mol/L |
| | Direct: 0.4 mg/100 ml | |
| | Total: 1.0 mg/100 ml | |
| | Indirect is total minus direct | Up to 17 $\mu$mol/L |
| Blood volume | 8.5%-9.0% of body weight in kg | 80-85 ml/kg |
| Bromide | 0 | 0 mmol/L |
| | Toxic level: 17 mEq/L | |
| Bromsulphalein | Less than 5% retention 45 min after 5 mg/kg IV | <0.051 |
| Calcium | 8.5-10.5 mg/100 ml (slightly higher in children) | 2.1-2.6 mmol/L |
| Carbon dioxide content | 24-30 mEq/L | 24-30 mmol/L |
| | 20-26 mEq/L in infants (as HCO$_3^-$) | |
| Carbon monoxide | Symptoms with over 20% saturation | 0(1) |
| Carotenoids | 0.8-4.0 $\mu$g/ml | 1.5-7.4 $\mu$mol/L |
| Ceruloplasmin | 27-37 mg/100 ml | 1.8-2.5 $\mu$mol/L |
| Chloride | 100-106 mEq/L | 100-106 mmol/L |
| Cholinesterase (pseudocholinesterase) | 0.5 pH U or more/h | 0.5 or more arb. unit |
| | 0.7 pH U or more/h for packed cells | |
| Copper | Total: 100-200 $\mu$g/100 ml | 16-31 $\mu$mol/L |
| Creatine phosphokinase | Female: 5-35 mU/ml | 0.08-0.58 mmol · s$^{-1}$/L |
| | Male: 5-55 mU/ml | |
| Creatinine | 0.6-1.5 mg/100 ml | 60-130 $\mu$mol/L |
| Ethanol | 0.3%-0.4%, marked intoxication; 0.4%-0.5%, alcoholic stupor; 0.5% or over, alcoholic coma | 65-87 mmol/L |
| | | 87-109 mmol/L |
| | | >109 mmol/L |
| Glucose | Fasting: 70-110 mg/100 ml | 3.9-5.6 mmol/L |
| Iron | 50-150 $\mu$g/100 ml (higher in males) | 9.0-26.9 $\mu$mol/L |
| Iron-binding capacity | 250-410 $\mu$g/100 ml | 44.8-73.4 $\mu$mol/L |
| Lactic acid | 0.6-118 mEq/L | 0.6-1.8 mmol/L |
| Lactic dehydrogenase | 60-120 U/ml | 1.00-2.00 $\mu$mol · s$^{-1}$/L |

From Potter PA, Perry AG: *Basic nursing: theory and practice*, ed 3, St Louis, 1994, Mosby.
Modified from Kaye DA and Rose LF: *Fundamentals of internal medicine*, St Louis, 1983, Mosby. Adapted from the New England Journal of Medicine, Vol 302, pages 37-48, 1980.
*SI*, Système international d/Unités (The SI for the Health Professions. World Health Organization, Office of Publications, Geneva, Switzerland, 1977); *arb.*, arbitrary; *L*, liter; *h*, hour; *s*, second; *d*, 24 hours, *P*, plasma; *S*, serum; *B*, blood; *U*, urine *ACTH*, adrenocorticotropin.

*Continued*

## Normal Reference Laboratory Values—cont'd
*Blood, plasma, or serum values—cont'd*

| | REFERENCE RANGE | |
|---|---|---|
| **DETERMINATION** | **CONVENTIONAL** | **SI** |
| Lead | 50 $\mu$g/100 ml or less | Up to 2.4 $\mu$mol/L |
| Lipase | 2 U/ml or less | Up to 2 arb, unit |
| Lipids | | |
|   Cholesterol | 120-220 mg/100 ml | 3.10-5.69 mmol/L |
|   Cholesterol esters | 60%-75% of cholesterol | |
|   Phospholipids | 9-16 mg/100 ml as lipid phosphorus | 2.9-5.2 mmol/L |
|   Total fatty acids | 190-420 mg/100 ml | 1.9-4.2 g/L |
|   Total lipids | 450-1000 mg/100 ml | 4.5-10.0 g/L |
|   Triglycerides | 40-150 mg/100 ml | 0.4-1.5 g/L |
| Lithium | Toxic level 2 mEq/L | 2 mmol/L |
| Magnesium | 1.5-2.0 mEq/L | 0.8-1.3 mmol/L |
| 5' Nucleotidase | 0.3-3.2 Bodansky U | 30-290 nmol $\cdot$ s$^{-1}$/L |
| Osmolality | 285-295 mOsm/kg water | 285-295 mmol kg |
| Oxygen saturation (arterial) | 96%-100% | 0.96-1.00 L |
| P$co_2$ | 35-43 mm Hg | 4.7-6.0 kPa |
| pH | 7.35-7.45 | Same |
| P$o_2$ | 75-100 mm Hg (dependent on age) while breathing room air | |
| | Above 500 mm Hg while on 100% $O_2$ | 10.0-13.3 kPa |
| Phenylalanine | 0-2 mg/100 ml | 0.120 $\mu$mol/L |
| Phenytoin (Dilantin) | Therapeutic level, 5-20 $\mu$g/ml | 19.8-79.5 $\mu$mol/L |
| Phosphorus (inorganic) | 3.0-4.5 mg/100 ml (infants in first yr up to 6.0 mg/100 ml) | 1.0-1.5 mmol/L |
| Potassium | 3.5-5.0 mEq/L | 3.5-5.0 mmol/L |
| Primidone (Mysoline) | Therapeutic level 4-12 mg/ml | 18-55 $\mu$mol/L |
| Protein: Total | 6.0-8.4 g/100 ml | 60-84 g/L |
|   Albumin | 3.5-5.0 g/100 ml | 35-50 g/L |
|   Globulin | 2.3-3.5 g/100 ml | 23.35 g/L |
|   Electrophoresis | *% of total protein* | *% of total protein* |
|     Albumin | 52-68 | 0.52-0.68 |
|     Globulin | | |
|       Alpha$_1$ | 4.2-7.2 | 0.042-0.072 |
|       Alpha$_2$ | 6.8-12 | 0.068-0.12 |
|       Beta | 9.3-15 | 0.093-0.15 |
|       Gamma | 13-23 | 0.13-0.23 |
| Pyruvic acid | 0-0.11 mEq/L | 0.0.11 mmol/L |
| Quinidine | Therapeutic: 1.5-3 mm/ml | 4.6-9.2 $\mu$mol/L |
| Salicylate | | |
|   Therapeutic | 20-25 mg/100 ml; 25-30 mg/100 ml to age 10 yr, 3 h post dose | 1.4-1.8 mmol/L |
| | | 1.8-2.2 mmol/L |
|   Toxic | Over 30 mg/100 ml | Over 2.2 mmol/L |
| | Over 20 mg/100 ml after age 60 | Over 1.4 mmol/L |
| Sodium | 135-145 mEq/L | 135-145 mmol/L |
| Sulfate | 0.5-1.5 mg/100 ml | 0.05-1.2 mmol/L |
| Sulfonamide | 0 mg/100 ml | 0 mmol/L |
| | Therapeutic: 5-15 mg/100 ml | |
| Transaminase (aspartate aminotransferase) | 10-40 U/ml | 0.08-0.32 $\mu$mol $\cdot$ s$^{-1}$/L |
| Urea nitrogen | 8.25 mg/100 ml | 2.9-8.9 mmol/L |
| Uric acid | 3.0-7.0 mg/100 ml | 0.18-0.42 mmol/L |
| Vitamin A | 0.15-0.6 $\mu$g/ml | 0.5-2.1 $\mu$mol/L |
| Vitamin A tolerance test | Rise to twice fasting level in 3 to 5 h | |

## *Urine values*

| DETERMINATION | REFERENCE RANGE | |
|---|---|---|
| | CONVENTIONAL | SI |
| Acetone plus acetoacetate (quantitative) | 0 | 0 mg/L |
| Alpha amino nitrogen | 64-199 mg/d not over 1.5% of total nitrogen | 4.6-14.2 mmol/d |
| Amylase | 24-76 U/ml | 24-76 arb. unit |
| Calcium | 150 mg/d or less | 3.8 or less mmol/d |
| Catecholamines | Epinephrine: under 20 $\mu$g/d | <55 nmol/d |
| Copper | Norepinephrine: under 100 $\mu$g/d | <590 nmol/d |
| Coproporphyrin | 0-100 $\mu$g/d | 0-1.6 $\mu$mol/d |
| Creatine | 50-250 $\mu$g/d | 80-380 nmol/d |
| | Children under 80 lb 0-75 $\mu$g/d | 0-115 nmol/d |
| | Under 100 mg/d or less than 6% of creatinine; in pregnancy: up to 12%; in children under 1 yr: may equal creatinine; in older children: up to 30% of creatinine | <0.75 mmol/d |
| Crystine or cysteine | 0 | 0 |
| Follicle-stimulating hormone | | |
|     Follicular phase | 5-20 IU/d | Same |
|     Midcycle | 15-60 IU/d | |
|     Luteal phase | 5-15 IU/d | |
|     Menopausal | 50-100 IU/d | |
|     Men | 5-25 IU/d | |
| Hemoglobin and myoglobin | 0 | |
| 5-Hydroxyindole acetic acid | 2-9 mg/d (women lower than men) | 10-45 $\mu$mol/d |
| Lead | 0.08 $\mu$g/ml or 120 mg or less/d | 0.39 $\mu$mol/L or less |
| Phenolsulfonphthalein | At least 25% excreted by 15 min; 40% by 30 min; 60% by 120 min | 0.25 L |
| Phosphorus (inorganic) | Varies with intake; average 1 g/d | 32 mmol/d |
| Porphobilinogen | 0 | 0 |
| Protein | | |
|     Quantitative | <150 mg/d | <0.15 g/d |
| Steroids | | |

### 17-Ketosteroids (per day)

| Age (64) | Male (mg) | Female (mg) | Male ($\mu$mol/d) | Female ($\mu$mol/d) |
|---|---|---|---|---|
| 10 | 1-4 | 1-4 | 3-14 | 3-14 |
| 20 | 6-21 | 4-16 | 21-73 | 14-56 |
| 30 | 8-26 | 4-14 | 28-90 | 14-49 |
| 50 | 5-18 | 3-9 | 17-62 | 10-31 |
| 70 | 2-10 | 1-7 | 7-35 | 3-24 |

| DETERMINATION | CONVENTIONAL | SI |
|---|---|---|
|     17-Hydroxysteroids | 3-8 mg/d (women lower than men) | 8-22 $\mu$mol/d as hydrocortisone |
| Sugar | | |
|     Quantitative glucose | 0 | 0 mmol/L |
|     Identification of reducing substances | | |
|     Fructose | 0 | 0 mmol/L |
|     Pentose | 0 | 0 mmol/L |
| Titratable acidity | 24-40 mEq/d | 20-40 mmol/d |
| Urobilinogen | Up to 1.0 Ehrlich U | To 1.0 arb. unit |
| Uroporphyrin | 0 | 0 nmol/d |
| Vanillylmandelic acid | Up to 9 mg/d | Up to 45 $\mu$mol/d |

*Continued*

*Special endocrine tests*

| DETERMINATION | REFERENCE RANGE | |
|---|---|---|
| | CONVENTIONAL | SI |
| **Steroid Hormones** | | |
| Aldosterone | Excretion: 5-19 $\mu$g/d | 14-53 nmol/d |
| Fasting, at rest, 210 mEq sodium diet | Supine: 48 $\pm$ 29 pg/ml | 180 $\pm$ 64 pmol/L |
| | Upright: (2 h) 65 $\pm$ 23 pg/ml | |
| Fasting, at rest, 110 mEq sodium diet | Supine: 107 $\pm$ 45 pg/ml | 279 $\pm$ 125 pmol/L |
| | Upright: (2 h) 239 $\pm$ 123 pg/ml | 663 $\pm$ 341 pmol/L |
| Fasting, at rest, 10 mEq sodium diet | Supine: 175 $\pm$ 75 pg/ml | 485 $\pm$ 108 pmol/L |
| | Upright: (2 h) 523 $\pm$ 228 pg/ml | 1476 $\pm$ 632 pmol/L |
| Cortisol | | |
| Fasting | 8 AM: 5-25 $\mu$g/100 ml | 0.14-0.69 $\mu$mol/L |
| At rest | 8 PM: below 10 $\mu$g/100 ml | 0-0.28 $\mu$mol/L |
| 20 U ACTH | 4 h ACTH test: 30-45 $\mu$g/100 ml | 0.83-1.24 $\mu$mol/L |
| Dexamethasone at midnight | Overnight suppression test: Below 5 $\mu$g/100 ml | <0.14 nmol/L |
| | Excretion: 20-70 $\mu$g/d | $\geq$0.22 nmol/L |
| 11-Deoxycortisol | Responsive; over 7.5 $\mu$g/100 ml (after metyrapone) | 10.4-38.1 nmol/L |
| | | >3.5 nmol/L |
| Testosterone | Adult male: 300-1100 ng/100 ml | 0.87-3.12 nmol/L |
| | Adolescent male: over 100 ng/100 ml | 106-832 pmol/L |
| | Female: 25-90 ng/100 ml | 3.1-44.4 pmol/L |
| Unbound testosterone | Adult male: 3.06-24.0 ng/100 ml | |
| | Adult female: 0.09-1.28 ng/100 ml | |
| **Polypeptide Hormones** | | |
| ACTH | 15-70 pg/ml | 3.3-15.4 pmol/L |
| Calcitonin | Undetectable in normals | 0 |
| | >100 pg/ml in medullary carcinoma | >29.3 pmol/L |
| Growth hormone | | |
| Fasting, at rest | Below 5 ng/ml | <233 pmol/L |
| After exercise | Child: over 10 ng/ml | >465 pmol/L |
| | Male: below 5 ng/ml | <233 pmol/L |
| | Female: up to 309 ng/ml | 0-1395 pmol/L |
| After glucose | Male: below 5 ng/ml | <233 pmol/L |
| | Female: below 10 ng/ml | 0-465 pmol/L |
| Insulin | | |
| Fasting | 6-26 $\mu$U/ml | 43-187 pmol/L |
| During hypoglycemia | Below 20 $\mu$U/ml | <144 pmol/L |
| After glucose | Up to 150 $\mu$U/ml | 0-1078 pmol/L |
| Leuteinizing hormone | Male: 6-18 mU/ml | 6-18 $\mu$/L |
| Preovulatory or postovulatory | Female: 5-22 mU/ml | 5-22 $\mu$/L |
| Midcycle peak | 30-250 mU/ml | 30-250 $\mu$/L |
| Parathyroid hormone | <10 $\mu$L equiv/ml | <10 ml equiv/L |
| Prolactin | 2-15 ng/ml | 0.08-6.0 nmol/L |
| Renin activity | | |
| Normal diet | Supine: 1.1 $\pm$ 0.8 ng/ml/h | 0.9 $\pm$ 0.6 (nmol/Dh) |
| | Upright: 1.9 $\pm$ 17 ng/ml/h | 1.5 $\pm$ 1.3 (nmol/Dh) |
| Low-sodium diet | Supine: 2.7 $\pm$ 118 ng/ml/h | 2.1 $\pm$ 1.4 (nmol/Dh) |
| | Upright: 6.6 $\pm$ 2.5 ng/ml/h | 5.1 $\pm$ 1.9 (nmol/Dh) |
| Low-sodium diet | Diuretics: 10.0 $\pm$ 3.7 ng/ml/h | 7.7 $\pm$ 2.9 (nmol/Dh) |

*Special endocrine tests*

| DETERMINATION | REFERENCE RANGE | |
| --- | --- | --- |
| | CONVENTIONAL | SI |
| **Thyroid Hormones** | | |
| Thyroid-stimulating hormone | 0.5-3.5 $\mu$U/ml | 0.5-3.5 mU/L |
| Thyroxine-binding globulin capacity | 15-25 $\mu$g $T_4$/100 ml | 193-322 nmol/L |
| Total triiodothyronine by radioimmunoassay ($T_3$) | | |
| Total thyroxine by RIA ($T_4$) | 4-12 $\mu$g/100 ml | 52-154 nmol/L |
| $T_3$ resin uptake | 25%-35% | 0.25-0.35 |
| Free thyroxine index ($FT_4I$) | 1-4 ng/100 ml | 12.8-51.2 pmol/L |

*Cerebrospinal fluid values*

| DETERMINATION | REFERENCE RANGE | | DETERMINATION | REFERENCE RANGE | |
| --- | --- | --- | --- | --- | --- |
| | CONVENTIONAL | SI | | CONVENTIONAL | SI |
| Bilirubin | 0 | 0 $\mu$mol/L | Glucose | 50-75 mg/100 ml | 2.8-4.2 mmol/L |
| Chloride | 120-130 mEq/l (20 mEq/l higher than serum) | | | (30%-50% less than blood) | |
| | | | Pressure (initial) | 70-180 mm of water | 70-80 arb. units |
| Albumin | Mean: 29.5 mg/100 ml ±2 SD: 11-48 mg/100 ml | 0.295 g/L ±2 SD: 0.11-48 | Protein: | | |
| IgG | Mean: 4.3 mg/100 ml ±2 SD: 0-8.6 mg/100 ml | 0.043 g/L ±2 SD: 0-0.086 | Lumbar | 15-45 mg/100 ml | 0.15-0.45 g/L |
| | | | Cisternal | 15-25 mg/100 ml | 0.15-0.25 g/L |
| | | | Ventricular | 5-15 mg/100 ml | 0.05-0.15 g/L |

*Hematologic values*

| DETERMINATION | REFERENCE RANGE | |
| --- | --- | --- |
| | CONVENTIONAL | SI |
| Coagulation factors: | | |
| Factor I (fibrinogen) | 0.15-0.35 g/100 ml | 4.0-10.0 μmol/l |
| Factor II (prothrombin) | 60%-140% | 0.60-1.40 |
| Factor V (accelerator globulin) | 60%-140% | 0.60-1.40 |
| Factor VII-X (proconvertin-Stuart) | 70%-130% | 0.70-1.30 |
| Factor X (Stuart factor) | 70%-130% | 0.70-1.30 |
| Factor VIII (antihemophilic globulin) | 50%-200% | 0.50-2.0 |
| Factor IX (plasma thromboplastic cofactor) | 60%-140% | 0.60-1.40 |
| Factor XI (plasma thromboplastic antecedent) | 60%-140% | 0.60-1.40 |
| Factor XII (Hageman factor) | 60%-140% | 0.60-1.40 |
| Coagulation screening tests: | | |
| Bleeding time (Simplate) | 3-9 min | 18-540 s |
| Prothrombin time | Less than 2-s deviation from control | Less than 2-s deviation from control |
| Partial thromboplastin time (activated) | 25-37 s | 25-37 s |
| Whole-blood clot lysis | No clot lysis in 24 h | 0/d |
| Fibrinolytic studies: | | |
| Euglobin lysis | No lysis in 2 h | 0 (in 2 h) |
| Fibrinogen split products | Negative reaction at greater than 1:4 dilution | 0 (at >1:4 dilution) |
| Thrombin time | Control ± 5 s | Control ± 5 s |
| Complete blood count: | | |
| Hematocrit | Male: 45%-52% | Male: 0.42-0.52 |
| | Female: 37%-52% | Female: 0.37-0.48 |
| Hemoglobin | Male: 13-18 g/100 ml | Male: 8.1-11.2 mmol/L |
| | Female: 12-16 g/100 ml | Female: 7.4-9.9 mmol/L |
| Leukocyte count | 4300-10,800/mm³ | $4.3\text{-}10.8 \times 10^9$/L |
| Erythrocyte count | 4.2-5.9 million/mm³ | $4.2\text{-}5.9 \times 10^{12}$/L |
| Mean corpuscular volume | 80-94 mm³ | 80-94 fl |
| Mean corpuscular hemoglobin | 27-32 pg | 1.7-2.0 fmol |
| Mean corpuscular hemoglobin | 32%-36% | 19-22.8 mmol/L |
| Mean corpuscular hemoglobin concentration | | |
| Erythrocyte sedimentation rate (Westergren method) | Male: 1-13 mm/h | Male: 1-13 mm/h |
| | Female: 1-20 mm/h | Female: 1-20 mm/h |
| Erythrocyte enzymes | | |
| Glucose-6-phosphate dehydrogenase | 5-15 U/gHb | 5-15 U/g |
| Pyruvate kinase | 13-17 U/gHb | 13-17 U/g |
| Ferritin (serum) | | |
| Iron deficiency | 0.20 ng/ml | 0-20 μg/L |
| Iron excess | Greater than 400 ng/L | >400 μg/L |
| Folic acid | | |
| Normal | Greater than 1.9 ng/ml | >4.3 mmol/L |
| Borderline | 1.0-1.9 ng/ml | 2.3-4.3 mmol/L |
| Haptoglobin | 100-300 mg/100 ml | 1.0-3.0 g/L |
| Hemoglobin studies | | |
| Electrophoresis for A₂ hemoglobin | 1.5%-3.5% | 0.015-0.035 |
| Hemoglobin F (fetal hemoglobin) | Less than 2% | <0.02 |
| Hemoglobin, met- and sulf- | 0 | 0 |
| Serum hemoglobin | 2-3 mg/100 ml | 1.2-1.9 μmol/L |
| Thermolabile hemoglobin | 0 | 0 |
| Lupus erythematosus preparation | | |
| Heparin as anticoagulant | 0 | 0 |
| Defibrinated blood | 0 | 0 |

## *Hematologic values—cont'd*

| DETERMINATION | CONVENTIONAL | SI |
|---|---|---|
| | REFERENCE RANGE | |
| Leukocyte alkaline phosphatase: | | |
| Quantitative method | 1-40 mg of phosphorus liberated/h/$10^{10}$ cells | 15-40 mg/h |
| Qualitative method | Males: 33-188 U | 33-188 U |
| | Females (off contraceptive pill): 30-160 U | 30-160 U |
| Muramidase | Serum, 4-13 $\mu$g/ml | 4-12 $\mu$g/ml |
| | Urine, 0-2 $\cong$ $\mu$g/ml | 0-2 $\mu$g/L |
| Osmotic fragility of erythrocytes | Increased if hemolysis occurs in over 0.5% NaCl; decreased if hemolysis is incomplete in 0.3% of NaCl | |
| Peroxide hemolysis | Less than 10% | <0.10 |
| Platelet count | 150,000-350,000/mm³ | 150-350 $\times$ $10^9$/L |
| Platelet function tests | | |
| Clot retraction | 50%-100%/2 h | 0.50-1.00/2 h |
| Platelet aggregation | Full response to ADP, epinephrine, and collagen | 1.0 |
| Platelet factor 3 | 33-57 s | 33-57 s |
| Prothrombin time | Less than 2 sec deviation from control | |
| Reticulocyte count | 0.5%-1.5% red cells | 0.005-0.015 |
| Vitamin B$_{12}$ | 90-280 pg/ml (borderline: 70-90) | 66-207 pmol/L (borderline: 52-66) |

## *Miscellaneous values*

| DETERMINATION | CONVENTIONAL | SI |
|---|---|---|
| | REFERENCE RANGE | |
| Autoantibodies in serum | | |
| Thyroid collaid and microsomal antigens | Absent | |
| Stomach parietal cells | Absent | |
| Smooth muscle | Absent | |
| Kidney mitochondria | Absent | |
| Rabbit renal collecting ducts | Absent | |
| Cytoplasm of ova, theca cells, testicular interstitial cells | Absent | |
| Skeletal muscle | Absent | |
| Adrenal gland | Absent | |
| Carcinoembryonic antigen in blood | 0-2.5 ng/ml, 97% healthy nonsmokers | 0-2.5 $\mu$g/L, 97% healthy nonsmokers |
| Cryoprecipitable proteins in blood | 0 | 0 arb. unit |
| Digitoxin in serum | 17 $\pm$ 6 ng/ml | 22 $\pm$ 7.8 nmol/L |
| Digoxin in serum | | |
| 0.25 mg/d | 1.2 $\pm$ 0.4 ng/ml | 1.54 $\pm$ 0.5 nmol/L |
| 0.5 mg/d | 1.5 $\pm$ 0.4 ng/ml | 1.92 $\pm$ 0.5 nmol/L |
| Duodenal drainage | | |
| pH | 5.5-7.5 | 5.5-7.5 |
| Amylase | Over 1200 U/total sample | >1.2 arb. unit |
| Trypsin | Values from 35% to 160% "normal" | 0.35-1.60 |
| Viscosity | 3 min or less | 180 s or less |

*Continued*

*Miscellaneous values—cont'd*

| DETERMINATION | REFERENCE RANGE | |
|---|---|---|
| | CONVENTIONAL | SI |
| Gastric analysis | Basal: | |
| | Females: 2.0 ± 1.8 mEq/h | 0.6 ± 0.5 |
| | Males: 3.0 ± 2.0 mEq/h | 0.8 ± 0.6 µmol/s |
| | Maximal: (after histalog or gastrin) | |
| | Females: 16 ± 5 mEq/h | 6.4 ± 1.4 µmol/s |
| | Males: 23 ± 5 mEq/h | 0-95 pmol/L |
| Gastrin-I in blood | 0-200 pg/ml | |
| Alpha-fetoglobulin | Abnormal if present | |
| Alpha 1-antitrypsin | 200-400 mg/100 ml | 2.0-4.0 g/L |
| Antinuclear antibodies | Positive if detected with serum diluted 1:10 | |
| Anti-DNA antibodies | Less than 15 units/ml | |
| Complement, total hemolytic | 150-250 U/ml | |
| C3 | Range 55-120 mg/100 ml | 0.55-1.2 g/L |
| C4 | Range 20-50 mg/100 ml | 0.2-0.5 g/L |
| Immunoglobulins in blood | | |
| IgG | 1140 mg/100 ml | 11.4 g/L |
| | Range 540-1663 | 5.5-16.6 g/L |
| IgA | 214 mg/100 ml | 2.14 g/L |
| | Range 66-344 | 0.66-3.44 g/L |
| IgM | 168 mg/100 ml | 1.68 g/L |
| | Range 39-290 | 0.39-2.9 g/L |
| Viscosity | 1.4-1.8 expressed as relative viscosity of serum compared with water | |
| Iontophoresis | Children: 0-40 mEq/L sodium | 0-40 mmol/L |
| | Adults: 0-60 mEq/L sodium | 0-60 mmol/L |
| Propranolol (includes bioactive 4-OH metabolite) in serum 4 h after last dose | | |
| Stool fat | Less than 5 g in 24 h or less than 4% of measured fat intake in 3-d period | <5 g/d |
| Stool nitrogen | Less than 2 g/d or 10% of urinary nitrogen | <2 g/d |
| Synovial fluid: | | |
| Glucose | Not less than 20 mg/100 ml lower than simultaneously drawn blood sugar | See blood glucose mmol/L |
| Mucin | Type 1 or 2 | 1-2 arb. unit |
| | Grades as | |
| | Type 1-tight clump | |
| | Type 2-soft clump | |
| | Type 3-soft clump that breaks up | |
| | Type 4-cloudy, no clump | |
| | 5-8 g/5 h in urine | |
| D-Xylose absorption | 40 mg/100 ml in blood 2 h after ingestion of 25 g of D-xylose | 33-53 mmol 2.7 mmol/L |

# GLOSSARY

**abduction**  Movement of the extremity away from the midline of the body.

**abortion**  The termination of pregnancy before the fetus is viable.

**abscess**  A localized infection with an accumulation of pus.

**abuse**  To use wrongly or excessively.

**acceptance**  Approval or the willingness to accept.

**accountability**  Being answerable for an action.

**acetone**  A by-product of fat metabolism.

**acetylcholine**  The neurotransmitter that is released at synapses of parasympathetic nerves and at neuromuscular junctions.

**acidosis**  Increase in hydrogen ion concentration as a result of accumulation of acid products or depletion of bicarbonate reserves.

**acquired immunodeficiency syndrome**  See AIDS.

**acromegaly**  A chronic disease caused by an oversecretion of the growth hormone of the pituitary gland. In the adult it may be caused by a tumor.

**active immunity**  Immunity acquired during a person's lifetime as a result of exposure to infectious organisms.

**activities of daily living (ADL)**  Bathing, grooming, dressing, feeding, walking, and toileting.

**acute care**  Those services that treat the acute phase of illness or disability, the purpose of which is the restoration of normal life processes and functions.

**acute pain**  Discomfort of relatively short duration; useful in that it provides information relating to injury or pathology.

**acute renal failure**  Temporary loss of renal function; usually has a sudden onset.

**adaptation**  Modification to meet a new or changed situation.

**addiction**  Psychologic dependence on a drug; a behavioral pattern of compulsive drug use characterized by overwhelming involvement with getting and using the drug. Withdrawal symptoms specific to the drug occur after cessation of intake.

**addictive disorders**  Physiologic dependence on a chemical or organic substance that results in withdrawal symptoms after cessation of intake.

**adduction**  Movement of the extremity toward the midline of the body.

**adhesion**  Joining of two parts by an abnormal fibrous band.

**adjustment disorders**  An inability of the individual to adapt to new situations or changes in life, or an inability to modify behavior, which overwhelms the person's coping skills and defense mechanisms.

**adrenergic receptors**  Sympathetic nervous system receptors classified as alpha and beta that are located in the heart, vascular system, respiratory tract, and central nervous system.

**advance directives**  A written document that indicates choices regarding medical treatments and designation of a health care agent.

**adventitious sounds**  Abnormal breath sounds such as crackles, wheezes, or pleural friction rubs.

**aerobic**  Describes a pathogen that requires free oxygen to live.

**affective disorders**  One of a group of disorders that has a primary disturbance of emotions or mood as a major feature. It can be chronic or episodic.

**against medical advice (AMA)**  A patient's decision to leave the hospital despite the increased risk for having their condition worsen; discharge not sanctioned by a physician.

**agent**  A factor, such as a microorganism, where presence or relative absence is essential for the occurrence of a disease.

**aging**  A nonpathologic process that gradually results in loss of cells and physiologic reserves.

**agitation**  A state of anxiety accompanied by motor restlessness.

**agnosia**  Disorder of the brain where there is an inability to interpret sensations correctly.

**AIDS (acquired immunodeficiency syndrome)**  A manifestation of infection with the human immunodeficiency virus (HIV); characterized by the presence of one or more diseases as defined by the Centers for Disease Control and Prevention (CDC). These diseases occur following a depression of an individual's immune system function. The affected person becomes susceptible to unusual infections and malignancies.

**AIDS-related complex**  See ARC.

**airborne precautions**  Special air-handling and ventilation procedures implemented in addition to standard precautions to reduce the risk of airborne transmission.

**airborne transmission**  Dissemination of either airborne droplet nuclei that remain suspended in the air for long periods or in dust particles containing the infectious agent.

**airway**  A metal, plastic, or rubber device used to keep the tongue from obstructing the trachea.

**aldosterone**  A steroid hormone produced by the adrenal cortex to regulate sodium and potassium in the blood.

**alkalosis**  A condition in which the alkalinity of the body is increased.

**alkylating agent**  A drug used in the treatment of cancer; examples include nitrogen mustard and cyclophosphamide (cytoxan).

**allergen**  Any substance to which some individuals react abnormally.

**allergist**  A physician trained in the diagnosis and treatment of allergic diseases and disorders.

**alveoli** Blind-ended air sacs of lung tissue, microscopic in size, where the exchange of oxygen and carbon dioxide occurs.

**Alzheimer's disease** A chronic brain disorder that involves a progressive destruction of brain tissue. This disease can begin when a patient is in his or her forties and results in slurred speech, growing memory lapses, involuntary muscle movements, and gradual intellectual deterioration.

**amblyopia** Decrease in visual acuity without underlying cause; not correctable with lenses.

**ambulation** Not confined to bed; walking.

**ambulatory care** All health services provided on an outpatient basis to those who visit a hospital or other health care facility and depart after treatment on the same day.

**amenorrhea** Absence of menses; normal before puberty and during pregnancy.

**Americans with Disabilities Act** (Public Law 101-336) Passed in July 1990, this legislation establishes equal opportunity for persons with disabilities regarding employment, public accommodation, transportation, state and local government services, and telecommunications.

**amputation** Removal of a limb or other part of the body.

**amputee** A person who has lost one or more of his or her extremities.

**anabolism** A constructive process by which food is converted into living cells.

**anaerobic** Describes a pathogen that cannot live in the presence of oxygen.

**analgesic** A drug that relieves pain.

**analysis** Second step in the nursing process, sometimes combined with or implied as part of the first step (assessment). Involves the evaluation of data for the purpose of determining the patient's needs and problems and developing a nursing diagnosis.

**anaphylaxis** An immediate reaction that results from sensitivity to a foreign protein.

**anastomosis** Surgical connection between two normally distinct structures or segments of a structure (arteriovenous anastomosis); connection of an artery to a vein (intestinal anastomosis); connection of two previously distant parts of the intestine. Can also occur pathologically.

**androgens** Steroid hormones, including testosterone and androsterone, that stimulate the development of male sex organs and male secondary characteristics.

**anemia** A blood disorder caused by a reduction of erythrocytes and hemoglobin.

**anesthesia** Administration of a substance that causes loss of bodily sensations.

**aneurysm** Dilation of blood vessels into a saclike bulge.

**anger** An expression of anxiety resulting from real or perceived threats.

**angina pectoris** Paroxysms of pain caused by decreased blood supply to the myocardium.

**angioplasty** Percutaneous transfusional coronary angioplasty dilates the coronary vessel wall through mechanical compression.

**angiotensin II** Peptide derived from renin, an enzyme synthesized and secreted by the kidney. It is a potent vasoconstrictor that influences the regulation of blood pressure.

**anhidrosis** Lack of sweating.

**anion** A negatively charged ion.

**ankylosis** Stiffening of a joint caused by infection or irritation and the development of fibrous tissue in the joint.

**anorexia** Loss of appetite.

**antibody** An immune substance produced within the body in response to a specific antigen.

**anticipatory grief** Expectation of loss of someone or something highly valued.

**anticoagulant** A drug that lengthens the prothrombin time and helps to prevent thrombosis and embolism.

**antigen** A substance that stimulates the immune process.

**antihistamine** A drug used in the treatment of allergic disorders and motion sickness.

**antimetabolite** An agent that is used primarily in treating leukemia in children.

**antiretroviral therapy** Treatment with medications that interfere with the viral life cycle and reproductive process.

**antiseptic** An agent that is used on the skin to inhibit or destroy microorganisms.

**antispasmodic** A drug used to relieve spasms of smooth muscles.

**antitoxin** A serum that is used to combat the toxin produced by a microorganism.

**anuria** Failure of the kidneys to secrete urine.

**anxiety** Feeling of uneasiness or apprehension in which the source is often unknown.

**anxiety disorders** Disorders that have anxiety as the most outstanding symptom. These disorders include posttraumatic stress disorder, phobic disorder, panic disorder, and obsessive-compulsive disorder.

**aphasia** Loss of the ability to speak.

**apnea** A temporary absence of breathing.

**apoplexy** Cerebrovascular accident.

**appendicitis** Acute inflammation of the appendix.

**apraxia** Disorder of the cerebral cortex, where there is an inability to organize movements.

**ARC (AIDS-related complex)** The syndrome of general systemic infections (e.g., fever, diarrhea) that occur in an individual before the development of the opportunistic infections or malignancies of AIDS.

**ARDS** Adult respiratory distress syndrome.

**arrhythmia** Any deviation from the normal heartbeat rhythm.

**arterial blood pressure** The force that blood exerts on the wall of an arterial blood vessel.

**arterial occlusive disease** Chronic occlusion of the arteries linked to atherosclerosis.

**arteries** Blood vessel that carries blood away from the heart.

**arteriosclerosis** Hardening of the arteries caused by the formation of fibrous plaques and loss of elasticity.

**arthritis** Inflammation of one or more joints.

**arthrodesis** Surgical fusion of a joint in a functional position.

**arthroplasty** Plastic surgery on a diseased joint to increase mobility.

**arthroscopy** Process of inserting an instrument into the cavity of a joint to inspect the tissue.

**arthrotomy** Incision of a joint.

**articulation** Point at which two bones are joined together, such as in a joint.

**ascites** Accumulation of fluid in the peritoneal cavity.

**asepsis** A condition of relative freedom from pathogenic organisms.

**asphyxia** Suffocation caused by a decrease of oxygen and an increase of carbon dioxide.

**assessment** The first step in the nursing process. It demands the collection and recording of data related to the patient and the family for the purpose of identifying patient problems. It includes the physical and emotional signs and symptoms presented by the patient, as well as information obtained from other sources (e.g., the patient's chart, laboratory report, and family visitors).

**asthma** A chronic bronchial disease that is caused by spasm of the bronchial tubes and is accompanied by edema.

**astigmatism** A defect in the curvature of the cornea or the lens of the eye.

**ataxia** A lack of coordination of motor movements.

**atelectasis** Collapse of the lung; may be total or partial.

**atherosclerosis** A degenerative process of the blood vessels that is characterized by fatlike deposits along the walls of the vessels.

**atopic** Pertaining to a state of hypersensitivity that is influenced by heredity.

**atrial fibrillation** An arrhythmia of the atria consisting of rapid, irregular, and ineffective contractions.

**atrophic** Wasting away of an organ or part of the body.

**atrophy** To waste away or decrease in size.

**atropine** An alkaloid of belladonna; may be administered with a narcotic as preoperative medication.

**audiologist** A person trained in the detection of hearing problems and the administration of hearing tests; a person who is trained in the use of hearing aids.

**audiometry** Hearing test using an audiometer, which is an instrument that produces tones of varying pitch and intensity; the tones are heard through earphones that are attached to the audiometer.

**auditory canal** Passage from the auricle or pinna of the external ear to the tympanic membrane.

**aura** A visual sensation experienced by a person with epilepsy before having a seizure.

**auricle** The visible portion of the external ear; also called the pinna.

**auricular fibrillation** An arrhythmia of the atria that is characterized by a rapid, irregular rate of contraction.

**auscultation** Use of a stethoscope to amplify sounds.

**authority** The right and power to act.

**autoclave** An apparatus that uses steam and pressure to sterilize.

**autogenous** Made from within the body. A vaccine made from organisms that are taken from a person is an autogenous vaccine.

**autograft** Tissue taken from the same donor as the recipient.

**autoimmunity** A condition in which antibodies are produced by one's own body, which causes immunization against the body's own proteins.

**autologous blood transfusion** Transfusion of blood that has either been donated by the patient in advance of surgery or collected from the surgical site during the procedure. Use of the patient's own blood rather than blood from a donor prevents possible exposure to the AIDS virus.

**automatism** Repetitive behavior that may be associated with convulsive disorders.

**autonomic hyperreflexia** Exaggerated and uncontrolled response of the sympathetic nervous system to external stimulation. Emergency condition occurring in patients with cervical or high thoracic injury.

**autonomic nervous system (ANS)** Part of the nervous system that is responsible for control of unconscious bodily functions, such as beating of the heart, gastrointestinal motility, and perspiration among others.

**autonomy** The ability or tendency to function independently.

**BAC** See Blood Alcohol Concentration.

**bacteremia** Presence of bacteria in the bloodstream.

**bacterial endocarditis** Infection that affects the valves and the lining of the heart.

**bactericidal** Describes an agent that kills bacteria.

**bacteriophage** A virus that attacks bacteria.

**bacteriostatic** Describes an agent that prevents multiplication of bacteria.

**bargaining** A mutual agreement.

**barium** A silver-white chemical agent used as a contrast medium in x-ray examination of the gastrointestinal tract.

**baroreceptors** Pressure-sensitive nerve cells located in the walls of the large arteries and in the arch of the aorta.

**Battle's sign** Bruising behind the ear with otorrhea.

**beliefs** Rules that guide human behavior.

**bends** Abdominal cramps caused by a rapid change from increased atmospheric pressure to normal atmospheric pressure.

**beneficence** Principle of ethics to do good.

**benign** Describes a nonmalignant growth or tumor.

**benign hypertension** Uncomplicated elevation of blood pressure.

**benign prostatic hypertrophy** Enlargement of the prostate gland.

**bereavement** Deprivation, such as in loss by death.

**bilateral** On both sides.

**biliary** Relating to the gallbladder, liver, and their ducts.

**biliary colic** Acute pain caused by obstruction of the cystic duct, usually as a result of a stone.

**bioethics** The application of normative ethics to issues in biology and medicine; sometimes referred to as healthcare ethics.

**biologic response modifiers** Natural products produced in large quantities by genetic engineering techniques. Proteins that stimulate and improve the cancer patient's biologic response against tumor cells.

**biopsychosocial** The interrelationship of physical, emotional, and social factors.

**biotherapy** Treatment of cancer using biologic response modifiers.

**blackout** Period of amnesia that occurs while a person seems to be functioning normally; seen in someone who is or has been drinking heavily.

**bleb** An irregular elevation of the epidermis that is filled with serous fluid.

**Blood Alcohol Concentration (BAC)** The test is expressed in a blood alcohol concentration percentage. All states consider a level of 0.10 as legally intoxicated. Some mental and physical impairment is noticed.

**blood dyscrasias**   Diseases of the blood and the blood-forming organs.

**blood urea nitrogen (BUN)**   An end product of protein metabolism found in the blood.

**bloodstream infection**   A pathogen found in the circulatory system.

**body image**   The way in which a person views own body; may mean acceptance in the care of a deformity.

**boil**   Cutaneous superficial infection of short duration.

**bone marrow transplantation**   Replacement of bone marrow after chemotherapy and/or radiotherapy.

**braces**   Mechanical device used for support, usually of an extremity.

**bradycardia**   A cardiac arrhythmia that is marked by an unusually slow heartbeat.

**bradykinesia**   Symptom of parkinsonism; difficulty in initiating movement, slowness in movement, and difficulty maintaining posture.

**brain stem**   Subdivision of the brain; located above the spinal cord and contains the midbrain, pons, and medulla.

**bronchiectasis**   A chronic disease of the lungs in which there is a dilation of the bronchi; may affect both lungs or only a portion of one lung.

**bronchitis**   An inflammatory condition of the bronchial tubes.

**bronchography**   X-ray examination of the bronchi using a radiopaque substance.

**bronchoscopy**   Examination of the bronchi and a portion of the lungs with a lighted instrument.

**bruit**   Swishing sound that indicates turbulent blood flow.

**Buerger's disease**   Acute inflammation of the arteries and veins of the upper or lower extremities.

**bulla**   A vesicle greater than 1 cm in diameter.

**burnout**   A manifestation of physical and/or psychologic symptoms (e.g., hopelessness, helplessness, fatigue) that may occur in nurses who care for persons with AIDS or a terminal illness. It is an ongoing process in which nurses may have negative feelings toward life, careers, and other people. Stresslike symptoms are common.

**bursa**   Small sac of fibrous tissue that is lined with synovial membrane and contains synovial fluid.

**bursitis**   Acute or chronic inflammation of a bursa caused by injury, disease, or an unknown factor.

**calculus**   Many stones.

**calibrated**   Marked or graduated to provide for accurate measurement.

**callus**   (1) Thickening of skin from continuous irritation; (2) fibrous tissue formed at the site of a fracture.

**candidiasis**   An infection with a fungus of the *Candida* family, generally *C. albicans*, that most commonly involves the skin (dermatocandidiasis), oral mucosa (thrush), respiratory tract (bronchocandidiasis), and vagina (vaginitis). Candidiasis of the esophagus, trachea, bronchi, or lungs is an indicator of AIDS.

**cannulation**   Procedure of placing a cannula into the body, as into a vein.

**capillaries**   Blood vessels, one cell in thickness, that enable exchange of fluid and electrolytes in body tissues.

**capillary refill**   A palpation technique for assessment of the vascular system of the extremities. Following elevation of the extremity above the heart, pressure is put on the nail bed or tip of the toe to cause blanching. The area should return to the preblanching color in less than 3 seconds.

**capsule**   Mucilaginous envelope that surrounds some forms of bacteria.

**carbonaceous sputum**   Sooty sputum.

**carbuncle**   A boil with an infiltration into adjacent tissues that finally opens in several places on the skin.

**carcinogenic**   Anything capable of producing cancer.

**carcinogens**   Environmental agents, such as viruses, chemicals, physical agents, hormones, and dietary factors, that contribute to malignant changes in cells.

**carcinoma**   A malignant tumor arising from epithelial cells. Tends to infiltrate or metastasize to other tissues.

**cardiac output**   Volume of blood pumped out by the left ventricle with each heart beat (stroke volume) multiplied by the heart rate for 1 minute.

**cardiogenic shock**   Interference with pumping action of the heart, which causes insufficient vascular circulation.

**cardiogram**   A tracing of the electric activity of the heart.

**cardiopulmonary**   Pertaining to the heart and lungs.

**cardiopulmonary resuscitation (CPR)**   Process of externally supporting the circulation and ventilation of a person who has had a cardiac arrest; course offered by the American Red Cross.

**cardiospasm**   A spasm of the cardiac valve between the esophagus and the stomach; generally a functional disorder.

**cardioversion**   External electric stimulation of the heart.

**Care Map**   A prewritten and adopted statement of specific activities to be achieved at each phase of the illness. It is broader in scope than nursing care plans; care maps include all activities, not just nursing activities.

**carrier**   One who harbors germs of a disease and transmits the disease to others while having no symptoms of the disease.

**case management**   Coordination and supervision of all aspects of healthcare for an individual patient, including delivery of care and evaluation of effectiveness.

**catabolism**   Destructive process by which complex substances are broken down into simpler ones; opposite of anabolism.

**cataract**   An opacity of the lens of the eye.

**catecholamines**   Hormones that tend to increase and prolong the effects of the sympathetic nervous system.

**cation**   A positively charged ion.

**CD4 Cell Count (T4 count)**   The most characterized of all the surrogate markers of immunodeficiency; the number of CD4 (T4 helper) cells. As an HIV-infected individual's CD4 cells decline, the risk of developing opportunistic infections increases. The trend of several consecutive CD4 counts is more important than any one measurement.

**CD4 lymphocyte**   Helper T cell; T4 cell; see CD4 cell count (T4 count).

**cell body**   The enlarged portion of a nerve cell that contains the nucleus.

**cell-mediated immunity**   Acquired immunity characterized by the dominant role of small T-cell lymphocytes.

**cellular immunity**   Acquired immunity that results in sensitization of whole lymphocytes to the invading agent.

**central nervous system (CNS)**   The brain and the spinal cord.

**central venous pressure**  A measurement to determine the ability of the right side of the heart to receive and pump blood.

**cerebellum**  Part of the hindbrain; functions to coordinate movements.

**cerebral edema**  Increased fluid accumulation in the interstitial areas of the cerebrum.

**cerebral palsy**  A chronic neuromuscular disorder that affects motor coordination.

**cerebral perfusion pressure (CPP)**  Blood pressure gradient across the brain. Calculated by subtracting the intracranial pressure from the mean arterial pressure to estimate the adequacy of cerebral circulation.

**cerebrospinal fluid**  Fluid surrounding the brain and spinal cord.

**cerebrum**  Main portion of the brain in the upper half of the cranium; forms the largest part of the central nervous system.

**cerumen**  Earwax; a yellowish or brownish waxy secretion in the external ear canal.

**chain of custody**  Tracing who handled evidence from the time it was obtained.

**chancre**  Lesion of primary syphilis occurring at the point of inoculation.

**chemical restraints**  Sedative and antipsychotic drugs that are inappropriately used as a means of controlling wandering, anxiety, fidgeting, nervousness, agitation, and anxiety.

**chemoreceptors**  Nerve cells, located in close proximity to the baroreceptors in the aortic arch and carotid sinus, that transmit impulses to the vasomotor center when there is a decrease in the oxygen or hydrogen ion content or a decrease in the carbon dioxide content of the blood.

**chemotherapy**  Treatment of disease with drugs or medications. Most commonly refers to the treatment of cancer with antineoplastic drugs.

**Cheyne-Stokes respiration**  Respiration in which the rhythm and depth vary with periods of apnea.

**child abuse/maltreatment**  Any threat to a child's health or welfare.

**cholangiography**  X-ray examination of the biliary tree after injection of a radiopaque dye.

**cholecystectomy**  Surgical removal of the gallbladder.

**cholecystitis**  Inflammation of the gallbladder.

**cholecystography**  X-ray examination of the gallbladder.

**cholelithiasis**  A condition in which calculi are present in the gallbladder or one of its ducts.

**cholesterol**  A substance present in all body tissues and fluids. It may be increased or is thought to be a factor in the development of atherosclerosis.

**cholinergic**  Nerve fibers that liberate acetylcholine when an impulse passes through the nerve; a drug that resembles the action of acetylcholine.

**cholinergic crisis**  Generalized weakness caused by overmedication of anticholinesterase drugs.

**chordotomy**  Surgical division of the anterolateral tracts of the spinal cord to relieve pain.

**choreiform**  Resembling chorea.

**chronic disease**  A disease involving structure or function or both; may be expected to continue over an extended period.

**chronic pain**  Pain lasting more than several months.

**chronic renal failure**  Loss of renal function; usually has a prolonged onset.

**Chvostek's sign**  Muscle spasm that occurs when the face is tapped below the temple.

**cilia**  Hairlike structures of some epithelial cells; characteristic of respiratory epithelial cells whose continual movement serves to remove inhaled particles.

**CircOlectric bed**  A type of electrically operated bed that permits easy turning and moving of the patient.

**circumcision**  A surgical procedure in which the prepuce of the penis is excised.

**circumferential**  Covering all sides, especially of an extremity.

**circumvent**  To go around or to prevent.

**cirrhosis**  Disease characterized by death of liver cells and their replacement by scar tissue.

**client**  Recipient of service.

**client problem**  Nursing diagnosis.

**climacteric**  Synonymous with menopause.

**clinical ethics**  The application of bioethics in the identification, analysis, and resolution of moral problems that arise in the care of a particular patient.

**clinical latency**  A period following the acute events of primary infection when there may be no clinical signs or symptoms of infection.

**CMV (cytomegalovirus)**  A member of the herpes virus family that can cause fever, fatigue, enlarged lymph glands, aching, and a mild sore throat. In persons with AIDS, CMV infections can produce hepatitis, pneumonia, retinitis, and colitis. CMV infection may lead to blindness, chronic diarrhea, or death.

**coalesce**  To run together, such as in measles.

**coccidioidomycosis**  A disease of the lungs caused by inhaling spores of fungi from the soil.

**cochlea**  Part of the inner ear. A snail-shaped tube containing the organ of Corti (the receptor end organ of hearing).

**colectomy**  Surgical removal of part or all of the colon.

**collagenase (ABC) ointment**  Ointment found to be effective in the treatment of decubitus ulcers.

**colonization**  Presence of an infective agent in the body. Similar to infection.

**colostomy**  Surgical procedure in which a part of the colon is brought through the abdominal wall and opened so that the colon may be drained.

**colporrhaphy**  A surgical procedure used to remove redundant vaginal tissue when prolapse of the anterior or posterior vaginal wall has occurred.

**colposcopy**  Examination of the cervix and vagina by means of a lighted instrument with a magnifying lens, which is called a colposcope and is inserted into the vagina.

**coma**  State of unconsciousness where the person cannot be aroused even when stimulated.

**comedones**  Blackheads.

**communicable disease**  An infectious disease or infestation that is transmitted from one person or animal to another, directly or indirectly.

**community-acquired infections**  Public exposure to an infectious agent resulting in infectious disease.

**community-focused nursing practice**   Synthesis of nursing and public health principles that incorporate a comprehensive, culturally sensitive, and holistic approach to health care and services that range from health promotion and disease prevention to sickness care for individuals, families, groups, and communities.

**compartment syndrome**   The progressive development of arterial blood vessel compression and circulatory compromise (reduced blood supply). Can rapidly result in permanent contracture deformity of the hand or foot, which is called Volkmann's contracture; can occur with injury to forearm and lower leg, with or without fracture.

**compromised host**   A person with deficient defense mechanisms and who is therefore at an increased risk for infection.

**computerized tomography**   A computer-aided x-ray examination that visualizes soft tissues better than conventional x-ray examinations.

**concurrent disinfection**   Daily handling and disposal of contaminated material or equipment.

**concussion**   A violent jarring of the brain against the skull.

**condom**   A sheath used to cover the penis during sexual intercourse to prevent conception and sexually transmitted diseases. Correct use of a rubber (latex) condom during every act of intercourse greatly reduces, but does not eliminate, the risk of infection with HIV. Lambskin's or "natural" condoms do not offer protection because they are too porous.

**confusion**   Altered orientation to time, person, or place.

**congenital**   Existing at birth.

**congestive heart failure**   Condition occurring when cardiac output can no longer meet the needs of the body.

**conization**   A surgical procedure in which a cone-shaped piece of tissue is removed from the cervix.

**conjunctivitis**   Inflammation of the conjunctiva of the eye.

**conscious**   The part of the mind that is one's awareness.

**consciousness**   Normal continuum from state of being fully awake to sleep.

**Consolidated Omnibus Reconciliation Act (COBRA)**   Legislation passed by Congress in 1986. Considered the "anti-dumping" law. Requires all hospitals that receive Medicare dollars to perform a medical examination on all patients to determine if a medical emergency exists. This law sets standards for transferring patients.

**contact precautions**   Procedures used in addition to standard precautions for patients known or suspected to be infected or colonized with microorganisms that can be transmitted by touch.

**contact transmission**   Dissemination of microorganisms from one person to another through direct touch, indirect touch, or droplet contact.

**contamination**   Soiling with any infectious material.

**continuity**   Uninterrupted connection, succession, or union.

**contracture**   A shortening or tension of a muscle, which affects extension.

**contrecoup injury**   Injury of a part of the body resulting from a blow to the opposite point of impact.

**control**   Restricting the spread of infectious processes.

**contusion**   Bruise; black-and-blue spot that is caused by rupture of small blood vessels.

**convulsion**   Involuntary contraction of voluntary muscles.

**coronary care unit**   Specially designed hospital unit providing continuous monitoring of the patient's cardiopulmonary status.

**cor pulmonale**   Hypertrophy of the right ventricle secondary to a respiratory disorder.

**corpus callosum**   Broad band of nervous tissue that connects the two cerebral hemispheres.

**corpuscle**   Blood cell; any small mass in the body.

**corticosteroids**   Hormones or synthetic hormones that suppress the inflammatory and immune response.

**coryza**   An acute upper respiratory infection; a common cold.

**cotton-wool spots/patches**   Fluffy-looking white deposits on the retina that represent small areas that have lost their blood supply as a result of blockage of local vessels.

**countertraction**   An opposing force or pulling in the opposite direction.

**coup injury**   Area of injury that occurs directly below the point of contact.

**Cowper's gland**   Either of two round, pea-sized glands embedded in the male urethral sphincter. Also called the bulbourethral gland.

**crackles**   Fine rustling or cracking sounds in the lung resulting from air passing through moisture.

**craniotomy**   A surgical opening of the cranium for exploration or removal of a tumor or blood clot.

**creatinine**   Nonprotein substance in the blood; synthesized from three amino acids. Normally excreted by the kidney.

**crepitus**   Grating sensation caused by the rubbing action of abnormal synovial surfaces in a joint.

**cretinism**   A condition resulting from complete absence of the thyroid gland or its secretions at birth.

**cricothyroidotomy**   Incision made into the cricothyroid membrane to establish an emergency airway.

**critical pathways**   Interdisciplinary plan of care and method of documentation that indicate specific results and behaviors expected for a patient with a given diagnoses (see Care Maps).

**critical thinking**   A process used to make sound, accurate, and reasonable decisions on the basis of thorough data collection and analysis.

**cross-infection**   Transmission of an infection from one patient to another who is already ill with another disease.

**cross-tolerance**   Development of a tolerance for substances in the same or similar category.

**crust**   A dry exudate; commonly called a scab.

**cryoprecipitate**   A fraction of fresh blood plasma; used to control bleeding in a person with hemophilia.

**cryosurgery**   Surgical techniques that use an instrument to apply extreme cold either to destroy tissue or to cause tissues to adhere to one another. Used in retinal surgery.

**cryptorchidism**   A condition of an undescended testicle.

**culdoscopy**   Procedure whereby a tubular, lighted instrument is used for direct observation of the uterus, ovaries, and fallopian tubes.

**cultural blindness**   Occurs when the differences of the individual are not acknowledged.

**cultural conflict**   Discord occurring between people who have different values, beliefs, and customs.

**cultural imposition**   An expectation that individuals will conform to the cultural norms of the caregiver.

**cultural relativity**   Attitude of openness to the characteristics of culture and the wide variety of beliefs and practices that result from being reared in different environments with different societal needs.

**culture**   Values, beliefs, attitudes, and customs shared by a group of people and passed from one generation to the next.

**curettage**   A surgical procedure in which a cavity is scraped with an instrument called a curet.

**customs**   Habitual practices, or the usual way of acting under certain circumstances.

**cutdown**   Incision through the skin for the purpose of placing a needle or catheter into a vein.

**cyanosis**   A bluish color of the skin; caused by inadequate oxygenation of the blood.

**cyst**   Saclike, nonmalignant tumor; may contain fluid or cheeselike material.

**cystectomy**   Removal of the urinary bladder.

**cystitis**   Inflammation of the urinary bladder.

**cystocele**   Protrusion of the bladder into the vagina.

**cystography**   X-ray examination of the urinary bladder after injection of a radiopaque substance.

**cystoscope**   Lighted instrument for examination of the inside of the urinary bladder.

**cystostomy**   A surgical opening of the urinary bladder through an abdominal incision and drainage by a catheter through the abdominal wound.

**cytomegalovirus**   See CMV.

**deafness**   Hearing at 85-90 decibels below normal.

**debridement**   Removal of infected or necrotic tissue from a wound.

**decibel**   A ratio that compares the relationship between two sound intensities; used to measure hearing.

**decomposition**   Dissolution into simpler chemical forms.

**decompression**   Reduction of pressure.

**decubitus ulcer**   Necrotic ulcer caused by pressure over bones, where there is little fat and subcutaneous tissue.

**deep venous thrombosis (DVT)**   Blood clots in a deep vein.

**defense mechanisms**   Unconscious processes used to alleviate anxiety; physical structures or processes that protect against stresses from the environment.

**defibrillation**   Application of a current countershock to the chest wall to stop ventricular fibrillation.

**degeneration**   Gradual deterioration of the normal cells and body functions.

**dehiscence**   Separation of a surgical incision.

**delegatee**   The person who performs a selected act upon direction from another.

**delegation**   Transferring a selected task to someone else who takes accountability for the action.

**delegator**   The person who is doing the actual delegating.

**delirium**   A global cognitive impairment of memory and organization of thought.

**delirium tremens**   A form of alcoholic psychosis.

**delusion**   False belief that contradicts the individual's knowledge or experience.

**dementia**   A global cognitive dysfunction characterized by impairment in short-term and long-term memory, orienta-

tion, abstract thinking, and judgment, as well as by personality changes. Also referred to as organic brain syndrome.

**demineralization**   A decrease of mineral or inorganic salts; occurs in some diseases.

**denial**   Refusal to accept a situation.

**depolarization**   The reduction of a membrane potential to a less negative value.

**depression**   Feeling of inadequacy or sadness.

**dermatologist**   A physician trained in the diagnosis and treatment of skin diseases and disorders.

**dermatomycosis**   Superficial mycotic infections of the skin, hair, and nails.

**dermis**   True skin just below the epidermis.

**desensitization**   Injection of extracts of antigenic substances; causes immunization against specific antigens.

**desired objective**   Preferred outcome.

**desquamation**   A scaling or flaking of the skin following certain infectious diseases, in psoriasis, or in reaction to radiation therapy.

**diabetes mellitus**   Disorder of carbohydrate metabolism; sugars in the body are not oxidized to produce energy because of lack of the pancreatic enzyme, insulin.

**diabetic**   A person with diabetes, which is caused by a deficiency of insulin secretin from the islets of Langerhans.

**diagnosis-related group**   See DRG.

**dialyzer**   A machine used to separate or remove certain substances from the blood when the kidneys fail to perform their normal function.

**diastolic blood pressure**   The pressure in the blood vessels during ventricular relaxation; primarily affected by peripheral vascular resistance.

**diffusion**   Movement of molecules from an area of higher concentration to an area of lower concentration.

**digitalization**   Administration of digitalis in doses sufficient to achieve the maximum physiologic effect without toxic symptoms.

**dignity**   Feeling of worth.

**dilation**   Increasing the diameter of an opening either by normal physiologic processes, drugs, or mechanical means.

**dilation and curettage (D&C)**   Surgical procedure in which the cervix of the uterus is dilated and the lining of the uterus is lightly scraped with a curette.

**dilemma**   A situation that demands a choice between two or more equally undesirable actions.

**diplopia**   A condition of the eye in which a person sees double.

**direct contact**   Touching of two individuals or organisms; done in association with a carrier in an infective state.

**disability**   Alteration in performing social roles and activities such as work, family life, or independent living.

**disease**   Any condition in which either the physiologic or psychologic functions of the body deviate from what is considered to be normal.

**disinfectant**   A chemical that destroys microorganisms when applied to inanimate objects.

**disinfection**   The elimination of many pathogenic organisms, with the exception of bacterial spores.

**diskectomy**   Surgical procedure to remove herniated intervertebral disk material.

**dislocation** Separation of a bone in a joint from its normal position.

**disseminated intravascular coagulation (DIC)** An acute bleeding disorder that results in a hypercoagulable state.

**dissociative disorders** Disorders that involve the mental defense of splitting off some part of consciousness, identity, or particular behavior on a temporary basis.

**distraction techniques** Procedures that prevent or lessen the perception of pain sensations by focusing attention on sensations unrelated to pain.

**distributive care** The pattern of healthcare that concerns itself with environment, heredity, living conditions, lifestyle, and early detection; usually directed toward continuous care of persons who are not confined to healthcare institutions.

**diuresis** Increase in urinary output.

**diuretic** A drug used to increase urinary output.

**diverticula** Outpouching of weakened intestinal musculature.

**diverticulitis** Inflammation of a sac or pouch that has formed at weak points in the walls of the gastrointestinal tract.

**DNR (do not resuscitate)** Orders that cardiopulmonary resuscitation or other heroic measures will not be started if a patient's heartbeat or respirations stop.

**documentation** The act of recording patient assessments and nursing interventions in the patient's chart. The chart is a permanent record, is considered a legal document, and is also audited to evaluate charges and quality of care.

**domestic violence** An abuse of power within an intimate relationship. Occurs when efforts are made to gain or maintain control over another person through intimidation.

**donor** A person who gives or furnishes blood, skin, or body organs for use by another person.

**dopamine** Neurotransmitter that acts on specific receptors throughout the body; stimulates the release of noradrenaline from nerve endings. Can be used as a drug to stimulate contraction of the heart.

**doppler** Transcutaneous ultrasound devices that can detect blood flow at various levels; method of listening to arterial blood flow.

**dorsiflexion** A bending backward from a neutral position.

**DRG (diagnosis-related group)** A designation in a system that classifies patients by age, sex, diagnosis, treatment procedure, and discharge status to predict the use of hospital resources and length of stay. Currently used as the basis for a system of prospective payment under Medicare.

**droplet precautions** Procedures used in addition to standard precautions for patients known or suspected to be infected with a microorganism transmitted by droplets (larger than 5 mm).

**droplet transmission** A type of contact transmission occurring when an infectious agent briefly passes through air; considered contact rather than airborne because droplets usually travel no more than 3 feet.

**drug dependency** Addiction to a drug.

**drug interactions** Reactions between food or medications that may affect the action of a drug.

**dry drunk** A person who abstains from alcohol completely but still exhibits the attitudes, impaired thinking, and behaviors of an active alcoholic.

**dwarfism** Abnormal smallness of body; caused by undersecretion of the growth hormone from the anterior pituitary gland.

**dysarthria** A speech disorder where pronunciation is unclear although the linguistic content and meaning are normal; slurred speech.

**dyscrasias** Diseases of the blood.

**dysmenorrhea** Painful menstruation.

**dysphagia** Difficulty in swallowing.

**dyspnea** Shortness of breath; difficult, labored breathing.

**dysrhythmia** Any disturbance or abnormality in a normal rhythmic pattern; specifically irregularity in the brain waves or cadence of speech.

**ecchymosis** Large amount of bleeding into the tissues.

**ECF (extracellular fluid)** Fluid surrounding cells.

**eclampsia** A condition that can occur during pregnancy and is characterized by convulsions, hypertension, and edema.

**edema** Swelling caused by accumulation of fluid in tissues.

**effusion** Collection of fluid in a body space.

**ego** In Freudian theory, the part of the personality structure that contains the instinctive drives and urges.

**electrocardiogram** Graphic recording of brain waves within the deep structures of the skull.

**electrolytes** Ions that play an important role in regulating body processes. Ions are substances that break apart into electrically charged particles when placed in a solution.

**ELISA (Enzyme-linked immunosorbent assay)** The most common assay for HIV antibodies. Used for screening donated blood, it is usually the first clinical screening test used to detect HIV infection. A positive ELISA or EIA test result should be confirmed with a Western Blot or an immunofluorescent assay test to conclusively diagnose HIV infection.

**embolectomy** Surgical removal of a blood clot from a vein.

**embolism** Foreign substance in the bloodstream; may be a fragment from a blood clot or an air bubble.

**embolus** Material such as a blood clot, air, fat, or foreign body that is carried by the blood from one part of the circulatory system to another.

**embryonic** Pertaining to the embryo.

**emergent** Arising or becoming known. First stage and initial care of a burn injury.

**emmetropia** Absence of refractive error; "normal" vision.

**emphysema** Overinflation and other destructive changes in alveolar walls; results in loss of lung elasticity and decreased gas exchange.

**empyema** Presence of pus in the pleural cavity.

**endemic** Describes the continuous presence of a few cases of a disease in a community.

**endogenous** From within.

**endogenous depression** A depression that has no recognizable loss, stressor, or other identifiable cause; is seen as arising from intrapsychic sources.

**endolymph** Fluid in the inner ear (within the utricle, saccule, and a portion of the cochlea). Protects the cochlea and the semicircular canals.

**endometriosis** A disease caused by groups of cells growing in the pelvic cavity. The cells are similar to those of the uterine mucous membrane.

**endorphins** Substances produced by the brain that mimic the effects of opiates such as morphine.

**endotoxin** A toxin that is released when a cell disintegrates.

**enteric fistula** An abnormal communication between portions or loops of the bowel.

**enteritis** Inflammation of the intestines.

**enucleation** Surgical removal of the eyeball.

**enuresis** Involuntary voiding of urine; bedwetting.

**environment** All factors that influence the life and survival of a person.

**enzyme-linked immunosorbent assay** See ELISA.

**eosinophils** Granular leukocytes. Number is increased during an allergic reaction.

**epidemic** Occurrence of a large number of cases of a disease in a specific area at a given time.

**epidemiology** Study of factors related to epidemics of disease, their control, and their methods of spread.

**epidermis** The superficial layers of the skin; made up of an outer, dead portion and a deeper living, cellular portion.

**epididymis** One of a pair of long tightly coiled ducts that carry sperm from the semiinferous tubules of the testes to the vas deferens.

**epididymitis** Inflammation of the epididymis.

**epidural analgesia** The process of achieving regional anesthesia of the pelvic, abdominal, genital, or other area by the injection of a local anesthetic into the epidural space of the spinal column.

**epinephrine** A hormone secreted by the adrenal medulla; prepared commercially as Adrenalin.

**epiphora** Abnormal tearing; often associated with lacrimal system disorders, congenital glaucoma, or lid misalignment.

**episodic care** Care provided by the nurse to the medical or surgical patient who is hospitalized in an acute care or extended-care facility with a goal of cure or improvement in a specific illness or crisis.

**epistaxis** Nosebleed.

**equilibrium** A state of balance.

**erythema** A redness of the skin.

**erythroblastosis** A congenital blood disease of the newborn in which there is a reaction of the Rh-negative antibodies of the mother with the Rh-positive antibodies of the infant.

**erythrocytes** Red blood cells.

**erythropoiesis** Production of erythrocytes.

**erythropoietin** A hormone secreted by specialized kidney cells in response to a reduction in the amount of oxygen in the tissues.

**eschar** Slough of tissue resulting from a burn.

**escharotomy** Cutting through burned skin layers to relieve edema.

**Escherichia coli** A species of organism found in the intestinal tract of humans and animals.

**esophageal varices** Fragile, collateral vessels that develop in the esophagus as a result of portal hypertension.

**esophagogastroduodenoscopy** Visualization of the upper gastrointestinal tract (esophagus, stomach, duodenum) by the use of an endoscope.

**esophagoscopy** Examination of the esophagus by the use of the endoscope.

**estrogen** A hormone excreted by the ovaries.

**ethical dilemma** A situation in which a choice must be made among two or more undesirable alternatives and in which the reasons for the alternatives are valid and important; no choice is obviously right or wrong. It occurs in a context in which the facts, as known, do not make it clear which is the right choice.

**ethics** A branch of philosophy that studies two facets of human existence: how people should act and what type of character they should have. Normative ethics involves principles and rules.

**ethnocentric** Attitude that one's own culture is the best one.

**ethylene oxide** A gas used in sterilization of surgical supplies and equipment.

**etiology/etiologic** Describes the causes of diseases and disorders.

**eustachian tube** Tube connecting the middle ear with the pharynx.

**euthanasia** The intentional death of a person who has been suffering from an incurable disease; mercy death.

**evaluation** The final stage of the nursing process. Patient progress is compared to previously identified expected outcomes of each nursing action prescribed for a problem. Evaluation requires the continued assessment of the patient.

**evisceration** Opening of a surgical incision, which permits the viscera to protrude to the outside.

**excoriation** An abrasion or a denuded area of the skin.

**exfoliate** Flaking off of the upper layers of the skin.

**exfoliative cytology** Microscopic study of the cell; used for diagnostic purposes.

**exogenous** From outside the body.

**exotoxin** A toxin or poison secreted by an organism.

**expected outcomes** Statements that describe specific, desired patient behaviors or results.

**expertise** Skill and knowledge of a person by reason of special training.

**extended-care facility** Institution devoted to providing medical, nursing, or custodial care for an individual over a prolonged period of time. Includes intermediate- and skilled-care facilities.

**external rotation** Turning away of a limb from the midline of the body.

**extracorporeal** Outside the body; used to describe a method of bypassing a patient's heart and lungs by using the heart-lung machine; used in open heart surgery.

**extrasystole** A form of cardiac arrhythmia in which heartbeats occur sooner than expected.

**extrinsic asthma** Hypersensitivity of the bronchial tissue to substances (antigens) outside of the body; results in narrow and inflamed bronchi.

**exudate** Pus containing dead cells, phagocytes, bacteria, and tissue fluids.

**faces rating scale** A series of faces ranging from very happy ones with smiles to very sad ones with tears; person points to the face that best describes how he or she feels at this time.

**factitious disorders** Symptoms or disorders voluntarily produced by a patient for unconscious reasons.

**family** Two or more persons who are related by blood, marriage, or adoption and who live together over a period of time.

**fibrillation** Tremor or rapid contraction of the heart.

**fidelity** Being faithful to one's duty, commitments, and promises.

**filter** A device for separating one substance from another.

**filtration** Movement of fluid and electrolytes by the pressure or force that is exerted as a result of the weight of the solution.

**fimbriated** Demonstrating fingerlike projections at the end of the fallopian tubes.

**fissure** A crack or slit in the skin.

**flaccid** Limp; cannot be controlled.

**flagella** Hairlike projections extending from some bacterial cells, which makes the cells capable of movement.

**flashbacks** An experience of the original sensations that occur during substance abuse even when no drug has been taken.

**flotation therapy** Semiweightlessness produced by various types of equipment; used in prevention and treatment of decubitus ulcers.

**fluid resuscitation** Replacement of fluids in the burned patient.

**fomite** Any object or material that may hold or transmit pathogenic organisms.

**fremitus** Palpation of the vibrations of the thoracic wall that are produced by the normal spoken word. Increased with secretions or consolidation in the lung; decreased with bronchial obstruction or presence of air or fluid in the pleural space.

**frostbite** Freezing caused by exposure to extreme cold; seen as white patches on skin that do not redden on pressure or as deeper lesions that involve subcutaneous tissue.

**full-thickness skin graft** Skin graft that includes the epidermis and all of the dermis; used for reconstruction.

**functional assessment** Admission examination of patient's functional abilities.

**functional limitation** Alterations in activities such as walking and dressing.

**functional nursing** An approach to nursing service that uses auxiliary health workers who are trained in a variety of skills. Each person is assigned specific duties or functions that are carried out for all patients on a given unit. Assignments are made in relationship to the skill levels of the worker. This type of nursing follows the "assembly line" approach.

**functional psychosis** Major emotional disorder characterized by derangement of the personality and loss of the ability to function in reality; not directly related to physical processes.

**fungi** Microbes from the plant kingdom, of which there are many different types. Some are harmless and some cause disease.

**ganglia** Structures containing a collection of nerve cell bodies and synapses.

**gangrene** Necrosis of tissue caused by cutting off the blood supply.

**gastrectomy** Partial or complete surgical removal of the stomach.

**gastritis** Inflammation of the stomach; generally caused by ingestion of contaminated food.

**gastroscopy** A direct visualization of the stomach with a gastroscope.

**gate control theory** Proposes that pain impulses that are transmitted from nerve receptors, through the spinal cord, and to the brain can be altered or blocked in the spinal cord or brain.

**genetic** Pertaining to origin; inherited.

**genitalia** The reproductive organs.

**geriatrics** A medical specialty that deals with problems of aging and the aged.

**germicide** An agent that destroys bacteria.

**gerontology** The scientific study of the process of aging and of the problems of the aged. The science of gerontology is interdisciplinary and includes the social, biologic, and psychologic aspects of aging.

**giantism** Abnormal growth resulting in excessive height; usually caused by oversecretion of growth hormone by the pituitary gland in childhood.

**glans penis** The conical tip of the penis; the urethral opening is usually located at the center of the distal tip of the glans penis.

**Glasgow Coma Scale** Numeric scale used to estimate a patient's level of consciousness.

**glaucoma** An eye disease characterized by increased intraocular pressure; leads to visual field loss, optic atrophy, and eventually blindness if untreated.

**glomerular capillaries** Cluster of blood vessels surrounded by Bowman's capsule.

**glomerulonephritis** A type of nephritis that involves the glomerulus of the kidney.

**glucagon** A hormone that is produced by the alpha cells in the islets of Langerhans and that stimulates the conversion of glycogen to glucose in the liver.

**glucocorticoids** A primary group of corticosteroids, including hydrocortisone (cortisol), that are essential for the metabolism of carbohydrates, fats, and proteins by the body and for a normal response to stress.

**glycohemoglobin** A type of hemoglobin that has a sugar attached (glycosylated) and that is increased in poorly controlled diabetes. It is an indicator of glucose levels over several weeks.

**glycosuria** Presence of sugar in the urine.

**goiter** Any abnormal enlargement of the thyroid gland.

**goitrogens** Some foods and drugs that inhibit synthesis of thyroid hormones.

**gonads** Sex glands; testes in the male and ovaries in the female.

**gram-negative** Term used in identifying bacteria after staining with a dye. Color can be removed with a solvent.

**gram-positive** Term used in identifying bacteria after staining with a dye. Color cannot be removed with a solvent.

**granulocytes** Leukocytes identified by the shape of the nuclei and the coloring of their cytoplasm.

**grief** A severe emotional reaction to loss.

**gumma** A tumorlike lesion that is similar in appearance to an abscess.

**gynecology** A medical specialty concerned with diseases and disorders of the female reproductive system.

**habitat** The natural environment in which a plant or animal (including humans), resides.

**habituation** An acquired tolerance that results from repeated exposure to a particular substance.

**hallucination** A mental aberration that is based on seeing or hearing things that do not exist in reality.

**hallucinogenic** Describes an agent that causes hallucinations or changes in personality.

**hashish** A resinous mixture contained in the flowering tops of the *Cannabis sativa* plant.

**health** Defined by the World Health Organization as "a state of complete physical, mental, and social well-being and not merely the absence of disease."

**health care delivery system** The regulation, structure, and organization for distribution of health care services.

**health maintenance organization (HMO)** Created by the Social Security Amendments of 1972 to provide comprehensive services to enrollees on the basis of a predetermined fixed cost or rate and without regard to the extent or frequency of services. These services may be given directly by the HMO or through arrangements with others and include the services of primary care, specialty physicians, and institutional services.

**Healthy People 2000** U.S. national health objectives to be completed by the year 2000.

**heat stroke** Disturbance in the body heat-regulating mechanism; results in elevated body temperature and hot, dry skin; may be damaging to brain cells.

**hematemesis** Vomiting of blood.

**hematocrit** A measure of the volume of red blood cells and the plasma.

**hematogenic shock** A shock state caused by an internal or external loss of blood or plasma.

**hematuria** Blood in the urine.

**hemianopia** Defective vision or blindness in half the visual field.

**hemiparesis** Hemiplegia; paralysis of one side of the body.

**hemiplegia** Paralysis affecting one side of the body.

**hemodialysis** Artificial method of removing urea and nitrogenous wastes from the blood when the kidneys fail to function normally.

**hemoglobin electrophoresis** A test used to identify various abnormal hemoglobins in the blood; may indicate genetic disorders such as sickle cell anemia.

**hemophilia** A group of hereditary bleeding disorders.

**hemoptysis** Hemorrhage that may be from the lungs, trachea, or larynx.

**hemorrhage** Escape of blood from a broken vessel.

**hemorrhagic stroke** A cerebral accident caused by a bleeding blood vessel in the brain.

**hemorrhoids** Varicosities of the anal canal; may be internal or external.

**hemotympanum** Bulging of the tympanic membrane (ear drum) caused by blood.

**hepatic coma** Comatose condition caused by liver failure; believed to result from the accumulation of nitrogenous substances in the blood, especially ammonia.

**hepatitis** Inflammation of the cells of the liver; two types-hepatitis A and hepatitis B.

**hernia** A projection of a loop of an organ, tissue, or structure through a congenital or acquired defect.

**herniation** Process of protrusion of an organ or tissue out of the body cavity in which it normally lies.

**herniorrhaphy** Surgical repair of a hernia.

**herpes simplex** Cold sore or fever blister.

**herpes zoster** Shingles; caused by a virus that affects the nerve roots of the posterior ganglia; same virus that causes chickenpox.

**heterograft** Tissue taken from an animal or a species other than a human donor.

**hiatus hernia** Protrusion of a structure through the diaphragm around the esophageal opening.

**High Efficiency Particulate Air Respiratory (HEPA)** Special mask that filters out dust that is one micron in size; is to be worn when caring for patients with tuberculosis. Presently the mask has not been tested for the TB bacillus.

**high risk** Applied to groups of persons considered to be more susceptible to infections or diseases than other individuals.

**hirsutism** Condition characterized by the excessive growth of hair or the presence of hair in unusual places.

**histoplasmosis** A benign disease of the lungs; caused by a fungus.

**HIV (human immunodeficiency virus)** The organism isolated and recognized as the etiologic agent of AIDS. HIV is classified as a lentivirus in a subgroup of the retroviruses. It infects and destroys a class of lymphocytes, CD4 cells, thereby causing progressive damage to the immune system. This family of retroviruses has RNA as its genetic material and makes an enzyme, reverse transcriptase, that converts viral RNA into viral DNA. The viral DNA is then incorporated into the host cell's DNA and is replicated along with it. There are two known types of HIV:HIV-1 is the most common in the United States; HIV-2 causes a milder immune suppression and is found primarily in West Africa.

**HIV antibody (HIV-Ab)** The antibody to HIV; usually appears within 6 weeks after infection. Antibody testing early in the infection process may not produce accurate results because recently infected people may have not yet begun producing antibodies and therefore test negative even though they are infected. Therefore a single negative antibody test result is not a guarantee that a person is free from infection. The change from HIV-negative to HIV-positive status is called seroconversion.

**HIV infections** A clinical spectrum of symptoms of an underlying immunodeficiency that predisposes an individual infected with the HIV virus.

**Hodgkin's disease** A malignant disease affecting the lymph nodes; was once considered highly fatal but can now be cured.

**holistic care** Care of the total or whole person, including physiologic, psychologic, and sociologic needs.

**home health care** Health services provided in the client's place of residence for the purpose of promoting, maintaining, or restoring health or minimizing the effects of illness and disability.

**homemaker service** A service to provide assistance in the home for elderly or sick persons; federal program under the Older Americans Act.

**homeostasis** A relative constancy in the internal environment of the body; naturally maintained by adaptive responses that promote health survival.

**homograft** A graft taken from a person other than the recipient.

**hormone** A chemical substance secreted by an endocrine gland; some are prepared commercially.

**hospice** An approach to providing support for the terminally ill patient and significant others; addresses physical, emotional, and spiritual needs.

**host** An organism, which may be a human, from which another obtains its nourishment.

**HPV (human papillomavirus)** Organism causing oral as well as anogenital warts; cauliflowerlike surface or slightly raised and smooth.

**human immunodeficiency virus** See HIV.

**human needs** Those needs basic to every individual; identified by Maslow as physiologic, safety and comfort, love and belonging, esteem, and self-actualization.

**humoral immunity** Acquired immunity that results in lymphocytes forming antibodies that are specific to the invading agent.

**Huntington's chorea** A rare abnormal hereditary condition that is characterized by chronic, progressive chorea and mental deterioration that terminates in dementia.

**hydrocele** A collection of fluid in the testicle.

**hydrolysis** Splitting of a compound into parts by adding water. In digestion, enzymes reduce large molecules into small particles so that they may be absorbed.

**hydronephrosis** Distention of the kidney pelvis with urine; caused by an obstruction along the urinary route.

**hydrotherapy** Immersing a burn victim in a tub to cleanse and debride the wound.

**hypaxial** Beneath the axis of the vertebral column.

**hyperalimentation** A method of providing complete nutritional requirements by the intravenous route.

**hypercalcemia** Excess of calcium in the extracellular fluid.

**hypercapnia** Excess of carbon dioxide in the blood.

**hyperchloremia** Excess of chloride in the blood.

**hyperglycemia** Excess of glucose in the blood.

**hyperglycemic, hyperosmolar nonketotic coma** A diabetic coma in which the level of ketone bodies is normal; caused by hyperosmolarity of extracellular fluid.

**hyperkalemia** Excess of potassium in the extracellular fluid.

**hypernatremia** Excess of sodium in the extracellular fluid.

**hyperopia** Farsightedness.

**hyperphosphatemia** Abnormally high amounts of phosphate in the blood.

**hyperplasia** Increased number of cells, which causes a part to be enlarged.

**hyperreflexia** Exaggeration of reflexes.

**hypersensitivity** An abnormal sensitivity to certain substances.

**hypertension** A consistent elevation of blood pressure above normal.

**hypertensive crisis** An acute rise in blood pressure accompanied by severe symptoms and potential target organ complications; a life-threatening emergency.

**hyperthermia** Abnormally high body temperature.

**hypertonic (hyperosmolar)** A solution with a greater osmotic pressure than another solution.

**hypertrophy** Enlargement of an organ that may or may not be caused by disease; increase in the size of the cells that comprise an organ.

**hypervolemia** Increase in the amount of extracellular fluid.

**hypocalcemia** Deficit of calcium in the extracellular fluid.

**hypochloremia** A decrease in the chloride level in the blood serum.

**hypochromia** Below normal color, as in a low index of the color of hemoglobin.

**hypoglycemia** A condition in which the glucose in the blood is abnormally low.

**hypokalemia** Abnormally low amounts of potassium in the blood.

**hypomagnesemia** Abnormally low amounts of magnesium in the blood.

**hyponatremia** Deficit of sodium in the extracellular fluid.

**hypophosphatemia** Abnormally low amounts of phosphate in the blood.

**hypospadias** Congenital malformation of the male urethra.

**hypostatic pneumonia** Pneumonia caused by a patient remaining in the same position for long periods.

**hypothermia** A low body temperature as produced by exposure to cold weather or as an adjunct to anethesia.

**hypotonic** A solution having an osmotic pressure lower than the one with which it is being compared.

**hypovolemia** Decrease in the amount of extracellular fluid.

**hypovolemic shock** A state of physical collapse and prostration; caused by massive blood loss and inadequate tissue perfusion.

**hypoxia** Deficiency of oxygen in the tissues.

**hysterectomy** Surgical removal of the uterus; may be abdominal or vaginal, total or partial.

**iatrogenic** A disorder produced inadvertently by a physician as a result of treatment for another disorder.

**icterus index** A test to measure the amount of yellowness in the blood serum.

**id** In Freudian theory, the part of the personality structure that contains the instinctive drives and urges.

**idiopathic** Disease or condition that arises spontaneously or has an unknown cause.

**IFA (immunofluorescence antibody)** A serologic assay using an antibody tagged by a fluorescent molecule. There is an HIV-specific IFA assay available to confirm the results of a positive HIV ELISA test.

**ileal conduit** Method of urinary diversion. Ureters are implanted into a section of dissected ileum, which is then sewed to an opening in the abdomen.

**ileostomy** A surgical procedure in which an artificial passage from the ileum to the outside of the abdomen is constructed.

**ileus** Failure of peristalsis, which leads to intestinal constructed.

**immunity** Resistance to a specific disease.

**immunization** Process of becoming immune to certain diseases; usually refers to injections that are given to develop active acquired immunity.

**immunofluorescence antibody** See IFA.

**immunogenicity** Ability of an agent to produce specific immunity within the host.

**immunoglobulins (Ig)** Serum proteins that include several groups of globulins; formerly called gamma globulins.

**immunologist** A person trained in the science of immunity.

**immunotherapy** A special treatment of allergic responses; administers increasingly large doses of the offending allergens to gradually develop immunity.

**impairment**   Physiologic alteration.

**impetigo**   Contagious skin disease.

**implementation**   Category of nursing behavior. One of five steps in the nursing process in which the actions necessary for accomplishing the healthcare plan are initiated and completed. Includes performance of or assistance in the performance of activities of daily living, counseling and teaching, caregiving, supervising, and evaluating staff members, and recording and exchanging information relevant to the client's continued health care.

**incontinence**   Inability to retain urine in the bladder.

**incubation period**   The interval between initial infection and the appearance of the first symptom or sign of disease.

**incus**   One of three small bones in the middle ear; shaped like an anvil and lies between the malleus and the stapes.

**independence**   Capable of performing activities of daily living without assistance.

**indirect contact**   Touching an object contaminated with an infective organism.

**induration**   An abnormal hardening of tissue.

**infection**   Entry and multiplication of an infective agent in the body of man or animal. May or may not cause infectious disease.

**infectious disease**   A disease that may be transmitted from person to person, either by direct or indirect contact.

**infectivity**   Ability of an agent to invade the host and replicate; varies with the route of entry, source of the agent, and host susceptibility.

**infestation**   Arthropods on the surface of the body; considered a communicable disease.

**infiltration**   Passing of fluid through, as when intravenous fluid passes into the tissues; usually caused by a needle being displaced from the vein.

**inflammation**   A sequential response to cell injury that includes vascular response, cellular response, production of exudate, and healing.

**inhalation injury**   A direct insult at the alveolar level secondary to the inhalation of chemical fumes or smoke.

**inner child**   Refers to the child ego state as described by the Redecision Theory, which states that it is found in any person, regardless of chronologic age.

**inotropes**   Drugs that affect contraction of heart muscle.

**inspection**   Directly observing an area of the body to assess its condition.

**insulin reaction**   Syndrome caused by too much circulating insulin.

**interdisciplinary team**   Group of health care professionals that, together with the patient, develops and evaluates a plan of care.

**intermediate-care facility**   A facility that provides care for chronically ill or disabled individuals; room and board are provided, but skilled nursing care is not.

**intermittent claudication**   A cramping pain that is induced through exercise, improves with rest, and is caused by inadequate blood flow to muscles.

**internal rotation**   Turning of the limb toward the midline of the body.

**interstitial fluid**   Fluid found between body cells and in the lymphatic system.

**intervention**   One step in the nursing process. The actual implementation of the most suitable actions chosen for a given situation. In substance abuse, the action by the patient's significant others and a professional taken to break through denial and obtain treatment.

**intracranial pressure**   Pressure within the cranium.

**intracellular fluid (ICF)**   Fluid found within the body cells; comprises $3/4$ of the total body fluid.

**intrathecal analgesia**   Injection into the subarachnoid space of the spinal cord; a lumbar puncture must be performed.

**intravascular fluid**   Fluid found within the vascular system.

**intravenous therapy**   Administration of fluids, drugs, or both into the general circulation through a venipuncture.

**intrinsic asthma**   Narrow and edematous small bronchi occurring from chronic recurrent respiratory tract infection.

**intussusception**   Telescoping of the intestine; may involve any part of the small or large intestine.

**iodophor**   An antiseptic or disinfectant agent that combines iodine with another agent (usually a detergent).

**ion**   An atom or group of atoms that carry an electric charge.

**ionizing radiation**   Rays of energy that break atoms into smaller, electrically charged particles called ions.

**iridectomy**   Surgical procedure in which a small hole is made in the iris to provide drainage of aqueous humour when acute, narrow-angle glaucoma has caused the angle to narrow and obstruct drainage.

**ischemia**   A temporary interruption of the blood supply to any area.

**ischemic heart disease**   Pathology of the heart resulting from lack of oxygen.

**ischemic stroke**   A cerebrovascular accident caused by obstruction of a blood vessel in the brain.

**isoenzyme**   An enzyme that may appear in multiple forms with slightly different chemical or other characteristics; can be produced in different organs, although each enzyme performs essentially the same function.

**isolation**   Use of barriers to interrupt the transmission of infectious organisms.

**isometric exercise**   Exercise done by a patient in which he or she contracts and relaxes a muscle.

**isotonic**   Solution that is compatible with the normal tissue by having the same osmotic pressure.

**isotope**   A chemical element that has been made radioactive.

**jaundice**   A condition in which a yellow color affects the skin and the sclera of the eyes; caused by an accumulation of bile pigments in the blood.

**justice**   Principle of ethics concerned with distribution of social benefits and burdens.

**Kaposi's sarcoma**   A painless tumor of the wall of blood vessels or of the lymphatic system; usually appears on the skin as pink-to-purple spots. It may also occur internally, independent of skin lesions.

**keloid**   A benign overgrowth of fibrous tissue.

**keratisis**   Inflammation of the cornea of the eye with formation of ulcers.

**keratoplasty**   Corneal transplant. Can be full thickness or partial thickness graft.

**ketoacidosis**   Acidosis resulting from the body's inability to neutralize keto acids from abnormal fat metabolism.

**ketone** Organic compounds produced during the metabolism of fats in the body.

**ketonuria** Presence in the urine of excessive amounts of ketone bodies.

**ketosis** The abnormal accumulation of ketones in the body as a result of a deficiency or inadequate use of carbohydrates.

***Klebsiella*** A genus of bacteria that lives in the intestinal tract and may cause serious infections.

**Koplik's spots** White spots on a reddened base; found in the throat in measles.

**labyrinthitis** Inflammation of the labyrinth of the inner ear.

**lacrimal fluid** Tears secreted by the lacrimal glands.

**lacrimation** Increased secretion from the lacrimal glands.

**laminectomy** Surgical procedure for a ruptured intervertebral disk or for fusion.

**laparoscopic surgery** An operation performed through a laparoscope.

**laparoscopy** Examination of the interior of the abdomen with a laparoscope.

**laparotomy** Any surgical procedure in which the abdomen is opened.

**laryngectomy** Surgical procedure for the removal of the larynx.

**laser surgery** Procedures that use an instrument to create a narrow, highly focused beam of light that can cut, coagulate, or vaporize tissue.

**leukapheresis** Selective removal of leukocytes from blood that has been withdrawn from and reinfused into the patient.

**leukemia** Neoplastic disorder resulting in widespread proliferation of white blood cells and their precursors throughout the body.

**leukocyte** White blood cell.

**leukocytopenia** A reduction in the number of leukocytes.

**leukocytosis** Great increase in leukocytes; occurs in many types of infections.

**leukopenia** An abnormal decrease in the number of white blood cells to fewer than 5000 cells per cubic millimeter.

**leukoplakia** White spots formed on the mucous membrane of the mouth; may become malignant.

**leukorrhea** White or yellow vaginal discharge.

**lichenification** Thickening of the epidermis of the skin that exaggerates normal creases.

**life-island** A plastic bubble enclosing a bed; used to provide a germ-free environment.

**life span** The longest period of time for which a typical individual can be expected to live.

**ligature** Suture used in surgery to tie or ligate a blood vessel.

**lipodystrophy** Atrophy of subcutaneous fat at the site of injection of insulin.

**lipoproteins** Proteins combined with fats found in blood plasma and lymph.

**lithiasis** Formation of stones of calculi.

**living will** A written agreement between a patient and his or her physician to withhold heroic measures if the patient's condition is irreversible.

**lobectomy** Surgical removal of a lobe of a lung.

**long-term care** Those services designed to provide symptomatic treatment, maintenance, and rehabilitative services for patients of all age groups in a variety of health care settings.

**lumen** Passageway within a tube, such as the lumen of blood vessels.

**lymph nodes** Small structures of lymphatic tissue containing lymphocytes, the function of which is filtration and phagocytosis.

**lymphangitis** Inflammation of one or more lymph vessels.

**lymphedema** Accumulation of lymph in the tissues that causes swelling; often affects the legs.

**lymphocytes** A lymph cell or white blood cell; develops in the bone marrow.

**lymphoma** A malignant tumor involving abnormal lymphocyte production.

**lysergic acid diethylamide (LSD)** A hallucinogenic agent that causes changes in mood and personality.

**lysis** A gradual decrease of symptoms of a disease; also a laboratory procedure to indicate decomposing of an agent by another agent.

**MAC (mycobacterium avium-intracellular complex)** An acid-fast microorganism that causes lung and other organ system infections in individuals whose immune systems are severely damaged. Evidence of MAC has been found in approximately 50 percent of adult AIDS patients at autopsy.

**macrophage** Large phagocyte cell that wanders.

**macule** A discolored spot on the skin that may be of various colors and shapes. It is neither raised nor depressed.

**magnetic resonance imaging** An imaging method that provides superior visualization of soft tissue. Uses harmless low-energy radio waves to create a magnetic field. When introduced into the hydrogen nuclei of soft tissues, a complex series of events occurs and is assembled as a tomogram.

**malaria** A disease caused by a protozoan and transmitted by the *Anopheles* mosquito.

**malignant** Describes a disease that is a threat to life; usually applied to cancer.

**malignant hypertension** Accelerated hypertension; rapidly progressive elevation of blood pressure associated with acute end-organ damage.

**malleus** Hammer-shaped bone in the middle ear; attached to the tympanic membrane and the incus; transmits sound vibrations.

**mammary gland** Synonymous with the female breast.

**mammography** X-ray examination of the breast.

**marijuana *(Cannabis sativa)*** Same plant as hashish but contains less resin and is less psychoactive.

**mastectomy** Surgical removal of the breast. A simple mastectomy removes only breast tissue. A modified radical mastectomy removes the breast and axillary lymph nodes.

**mastitis** Inflammation of the breast.

**mastoiditis** Inflammation of the cells of the mastoid process.

**Meals on Wheels** Program designed to prepare food and take hot meals to elderly or physically handicapped persons.

**mediastinum** Space between the lungs that contains the heart.

**Medicaid** Federal- and state-supported program to provide hospital and medical care for certain eligible persons.

**medical-surgical nursing** The nursing care of patients whose conditions or disorders are treated pharmacologically or surgically.

**Medicare**  Federal program to provide hospital and medical care for persons 65 years of age or older.

**menarche**  First menstruation; occurs at puberty.

**Meniere's syndrome**  A condition involving an increase in pressure following an increase in the endolymph in the inner ear; produces the symptoms of vertigo, nausea and vomiting, and ringing in the ears.

**meninges**  Membrane enclosing the brain and spinal cord.

**meningitis**  Infection and inflammation of the meninges.

**menopause**  Climacteric or the cessation of menses; represents the end of the reproductive period.

**menorrhagia**  Excessive menstrual flow either in quantity or duration.

**mental health**  A state of being in which a person has a reasonably satisfactory balance of personality structure.

**mental illness**  Any psychiatric illness that has been identified by various recognized authorities. A condition in which the person experiences enough psychic pain to cause interference with successful life functioning.

**mental retardation**  A condition in which there is an absence of normal mental growth and development.

**mental status assessment**  The degree of competence shown by a person in intellectual, emotional, psychologic, and personality functioning (as measured by psychologic testing) with reference to a statistic norm.

**mescaline**  Derivation of peyote cactus; classified as a halucinogenic agent.

**metabolism**  Sum of all processes within the body, including the breaking-down and wearing-out processes and the regeneration and building-up processes.

**metastasis**  Spreading of cancer cells by the bloodstream or lymph from one part of the body to another.

**methadone**  Synthetic narcotic analgesic agent used to replace heroin; considered addictive.

**metrorrhagia**  Bleeding between regular menstrual periods.

**mineralocorticoids**  A primary group of corticosteroids, including aldosterone, that regulates salt and water balance in the body.

**mini-mental status examination (MMSE)**  Assessment of orientation, short-term memory, ability to attend to tasks, calculation, recall, and language.

**minimizing**  Denying, making less of.

**minimum data set (MDS)**  Holistic assessment completed upon admission.

**miotic**  A drug that causes constriction of the pupil of the eye.

**molecule**  Smallest particle of an element or compound.

**monochronic time**  Linear form of time perception; prioritizing according to time.

**monocyte**  A large mononuclear leukocyte.

**mononucleosis**  An infectious disease characterized by swelling of the lymph nodes, especially the cervical nodes.

**mood disorders**  Affective disorders.

**morals**  The set of values or principles to which a person is committed, often used interchangeably with ethics.

**motivation**  Providing an incentive to cause a person to move or to act in a particular way.

**MTB (mycobacterium tuberculosis)**  The microorganism that causes tuberculosis.

**multiple myeloma**  Malignant disease of the bone marrow.

**multisystem**  A corporation that manages a group of hospitals. Hospitals may or may not be owned by the managing system.

**muscle spasm**  A severe muscular contraction.

**myasthenic crisis**  Acute episode of muscular weakness.

**mycobacterium avium-intracellular complex**  See MAC.

**mycobacterium tuberculosis**  See MTB.

**mycotic**  Pertaining to a disease caused by a fungus.

**mydriatic**  A drug that dilates the pupils of the eyes.

**myelin**  Fatlike substance forming a sheath around certain nerve fibers.

**myelography**  X-ray examination of the spinal column after injection of a radiopaque substance.

**myelosuppression**  Inhibition of the function of the bone marrow.

**myocardial infarction**  Disorder caused by obstruction or thrombus of a coronary artery or its branches; deprives the myocardium of its blood supply and causes death of the affected tissue.

**myopia**  Nearsightedness.

**myringotomy**  A surgical incision of a portion of the tympanic membrane.

**myxedema**  Condition resulting from hypofunction of the thyroid gland; characterized by large tongue, slow speech, puffiness of hands and face, coarse and thickened skin, mental apathy, and sensitivity to cold.

**narcotic**  A drug that may be an opium derivative or synthetic, narcoticlike agent used to relieve pain and produce sleep. All narcotic drugs are habit forming and under government control.

**natural immunity**  Immunity acquired by an infant as a result of maternal antibodies crossing the placental barrier and entering fetal circulation.

**nebulization**  A method of spraying a drug into the respiratory passages; may be used with or without oxygen to carry the drug to the lungs.

**necrosis**  Death of tissue.

**necrotic tissue**  Dead tissue or small groups of cells.

**neglect**  Perceptual problems occurring with right hemisphere damage from a cerebrovascular accident; the hemiplegic part may not be recognized and may therefore be ignored by the patient.

**neobladder**  Urinary diversion resulting from transplantation of the ureters into a constructed segment of the sigmoid colon.

**neoplasm**  Abnormal tumor growth; may be benign or malignant.

**nephrectomy**  Surgical removal of a kidney.

**nephritis**  Inflammation of the kidney; may be acute or chronic.

**nephron**  Basic unit of kidney excretion.

**nephrosclerosis**  Sclerosis of the blood vessels of the kidney, usually associated with hypertension.

**nephrosis (nephrotic syndrome)**  Degeneration of renal tissue with inflammation; may occur with glomerulonephritis.

**nephrostomy**  Surgical wound on the flank and placement of a catheter into the kidney pelvis for the purpose of drainage.

**nephrotoxin**  A substance that is destructive to the kidney; nephrotoxic.

**neurectomy** Surgical division of the sensory portion of a peripheral or spinal nerve to relieve pain.

**neurogenic shock** Shock resulting from peripheral vascular dilation as a result of neurologic injury.

**neuron** Nerve cell; the basic functional unit of the nervous system.

**neurotransmitters** The chemicals responsible for message transmission across the synapse. Examples include dopamine, substance P, endorphins, and enkephalins.

**nodule** Small, solid node that can be detected by touch.

**nonmaleficence** Principle of ethics to do no harm.

**nonproprietary** Not-for-profit operation.

**normal flora** Microscopic cells normally present on skin and mucosal surfaces that may include *Staphylococcus* organisms, *Streptococcus* organisms, and other bacteria.

**normovolemic shock** Shock resulting from a disproportion between the normal volume of blood and the size of the vascular bed.

**nosocomial** Hospital-acquired infection.

**nuccal rigidity** Severely rigid, stiff neck; symptom of meningitis.

**nucleus pulposus** Soft, gelantinous substance that comprises the center of an intervertebral disk.

**nursing care plan** The proposed plan of care for each patient, preferably written; intended to communicate, prevent complications, ensure continuity of care, identify and ensure patient teaching, and provide for discharge planning. It must include statements that identify the patient's problems and proposed nursing interventions, as well as measurable expected outcomes.

**nursing diagnosis** A concise statement describing a combination of signs and symptoms that indicate an acute or potential health problem that nurses are licensed to treat and are capable of treating.

**nursing history** The documented findings of a thorough patient assessment, including the physical and emotional signs and symptoms presented by the patient, as well as information obtained from other sources.

**nursing home** A long-term or extended-care facility that provides nursing, medical, and rehabilitative care, as well as furnishes residential and personal services.

**nursing process** A dynamic interpersonal problem-solving process that facilitates a person's potential for health. The steps in the process include assessment, planning, intervention, and evaluation.

**nystagmus** A continuous movement of the eyeball; may be associated with labyrinthitis.

**objective data** Data obtained directly through measurement, inspection, palpation, percussion, or auscultation.

**occlusion** Blockage of a passageway.

**occult blood** A minute or hidden quantity of blood that can be detected only by means of a chemical test or by microscopic or spectroscopic examination. Often present in stools of patients with gastrointestinal lesions.

**occupational exposure** Transmission of an infectious agent to an employee in the workplace.

**Omaha system** A research-based assessment care plan that incorporates a comprehensive vocabulary intended to help users describe and measure their practice.

**oncogenes** Certain genes in the cell that can somehow be activated and cause cells to become malignant.

**oncology** Branch of medicine dealing with tumors.

**oophorectomy** Surgical removal of an ovary.

**opacity** Omitting light, or opaque to light rays.

**ophthalmia neonatorum** Infection of the eyes of the newborn with the gonococcus organism.

**ophthalmologist** A medical doctor who has completed 4 years of residency and, in some instances, 1 to 3 years of additional training in a subspecialty. Ophthalmologists diagnose and treat patients with eye diseases and vision problems. They perform surgery and prescribe medications, glasses, and contact lenses.

**opiate, opiod** Drug derived from opium.

**opisthotonos** Arching of the body caused by rigidity of the spine.

**opportunistic infections** Illnesses caused by organisms that do not usually cause disease in a person with a healthy immune system. When an individual's immune system is compromised, such organisms may cause serious, even life-threatening illness.

**opportunistic pathogen** A microbe that produces illness only in the compromised host.

**optician** A person who can test people for glasses and can dispense glasses.

**optometrist** Has a degree in optometry after attending optometry school for 4 years postbaccalaureate degree. Optometrists examine eyes, prescribe glasses and contact lenses, check intraocullar-pressure, and prescribe exercises for various eye muscle problems. They provide low-vision examinations, visual devices, and adaptive training for patients with limited vision.

**orchitis** Inflammatory condition of the testes caused by infection, injury, or malignancy.

**organic brain syndrome** Mental illness resulting from pathophysiologic changes in the brain.

**organic psychosis** Major emotional disorder characterized by derangement of the personality and loss of the ability to function in reality; caused by an underlying physical process, resulting in damage to the brain.

**orthopedic** Describes disorders of the musculoskeletal system.

**orthopnea** Inability to breathe except in a sitting position.

**orthostatic** Upright position of the body.

**oscilloscope** An instrument that records a visual wave on a screen.

**osmolality** Measures the total milliosmoles of solute per unit weight of solvent.

**osmolarity** Measures the total milliosmoles of solute per unit of total volume of solution.

**osmole** Unit of osmotic pressure equal to the molecular weight of a solution in grams divided by the number of ions or other particles that occur following dissociation in a solution.

**osmosis** Diffusion of water through a semipermeable membrane.

**osmotic pressure** Pressure of a fluid that determines its ability to pass through a semipermeable membrane.

**osseous** Pertaining to bone.

**osteoarthritis** A degenerative type of arthritis affecting the joints; characteristic of the aging process.

**osteomyelitis**   Infection and inflammation of a bone.

**osteoporosis**   A decrease in total bone mass that results in weak and brittle bones.

**osteotomy**   Cutting of bone to correct joint or bone deformities.

**otitis media**   Infection of the middle ear.

**otologist**   A physician trained in the diagnosis and treatment of diseases and disorders of the ear.

**otorrhea**   Discharge from the ear.

**otosclerosis**   A disease of the middle ear in which new growth of bone forms in the stapes and prevents transmission of sound to the inner ear.

**otoscopy**   Direct visualization of the external auditory canal and the tympanic membrane using an otoscope.

**outcomes**   The desired specific behaviors or results.

**ovulation**   Discharge of a mature ovum from the ovarian follicle.

**oxygenation**   The process of combining or treating with oxygen.

**pacemaker**   A mechanical device used to provide electric stimulation in heart block; may be temporary or permanent.

**pain**   Whatever the patient experiencing it says it is, existing whenever he or she says it exists.

**pain management**   Control of discomfort that is appropriate for the patient's condition.

**pain threshold**   The point at which a sensation is perceived as pain.

**pain tolerance**   The point at which a pain sensation is no longer voluntarily endured.

**palliative**   Therapy designed to relieve or reduce discomfort of symptoms but not produce a cure.

**pallor**   Lacking color.

**palpation**   Examination of a body area through the sense of touch.

**pancreatitis**   Inflammation of the pancreas.

**pandemic**   A disease that is widespread in a geographic area or throughout the world.

**panhysterectomy**   Surgical removal of the uterus and the cervix.

**Papanicolaou's (Pap) smear**   A cytologic test for the detection of cancer cells. Best known as the cervical Pap smear.

**papilledema**   Swelling of the optic disc or optic papilla, the first part of the optic nerve.

**papule**   A small, solid elevation on the skin that varies in size from a pinhead to a pea.

**paralytic ileus**   A decrease or absence of intestinal peristalsis.

**paraplegia**   Paralysis of the lower part of the body below a point of injury to the spinal cord.

**paresthesia**   Numbness, tingling, "pins and needles."

**parietal pleura**   Membrane covering the inner surface of the chest wall.

**paroxysm**   Spasmodic attacks that recur at intervals.

**paroxysmal atrial tachycardia**   Very rapid heartbeat that begins suddenly and ends abruptly.

**passive immunity**   Immunity acquired by injecting into the body a serum that produces an immediate but temporary immune response.

**pathogen**   An organism capable of causing disease.

**pathogenic**   The ability of an organism to produce disease.

**pathogenicity**   Ability of an agent to produce an infectious disease in a susceptible host.

**pathophysiology**   Changes in the physiologic function as a result of pathologic disease.

**patient**   The individual who initiates, plans, and actively participates in his or her healthcare.

**patient-controlled analgesia**   Self-administration of pain medications by means of a mechanical device.

**PCP (*Pneumocystis carinii* pneumonia)**   Form of pneumonia seen in persons with an impaired immune system, such as those who are HIV infected. PCP is the leading cause of death in patients with AIDS. It is caused by the opportunistic pathogen *P. carinii* (unclear whether fungal or protozoan), which can infect the eyes, skin, spleen, liver, and heart, as well as the lungs.

**pelvic exenteration**   Removal of all reproductive organs and adjacent tissues.

**penicillinase**   An enzymelike substance that is produced by some bacteria and that affects the antimicrobial properties of penicillin.

**peptic ulcer**   An ulcer occurring in the wall of the stomach or the duodenum.

**percussion**   Observing for the differences in sound and resonance through striking a part of the body with the fingers that indicates presence of fluid, air, or masses.

**percutaneous transluminal angioplasty (PTA)**   Insertion of a balloon-tipped catheter into an artery that is guided into an area of narrowing or occlusion. The balloon is then inflated, flattening the atherosclerotic plaque against the arterial wall.

**perfusion**   Procedure of introducing a chemical drug to an isolated part of the body by way of the bloodstream.

**perilymph**   Inner ear fluid contained within the space between the bony and membranous labyrinths, as well as in a portion of the cochlea.

**periosteum**   Specialized connective tissue covering all bones.

**peripheral nervous system**   Components of the nervous system that lie outside the brain and spinal cord.

**peripheral vascular resistance**   Sum of all the resistive forces that oppose the movement of blood flow in the circulatory system.

**peristalsis**   Involuntary wavelike contraction of muscles of the gastrointestinal tract.

**peritoneal dialysis**   A method of removal of waste products from the blood by way of the peritoneal membrane.

**periungual**   Around the fingernails or toenails.

**personality**   The unique combination of behavior patterns, attitudes, and traits of an individual.

**personality disorders**   A group of mental disorders in which there are maladaptive patterns of behavior, often identifiable by adolescence or earlier.

**pertussis**   Whooping cough.

**pessary**   A device used to support the uterus in a normal position.

**petechiae**   Small, pinpoint hemorrhagic spots on the skin.

**Peyer's patches**   Areas of lymphoid tissue on the mucous membrane of the small intestine that become elevated and inflamed in typhoid fever; may become ulcerated and rupture, causing hemorrhage.

**phacoemulsification** Technique of extracapsular cataract extraction in which the lens nucleus is broken into pieces ultrasonically and then aspirated through a small incision.

**phagocyte** Cell that engulfs and ingests bacteria or other material.

**phagocytosis** Ingestion and digestion of bacteria at the scene of an infection.

**phantom pain** Painful sensations in an amputated body part, such as a leg or breast.

**phenylketonuria** Hereditary disease in which there is a faulty utilization of the amino acid phenylalanine.

**phimosis** A narrowing of the prepuce opening so that the foreskin of the penis cannot be retracted.

**phlebotomy** Incision of a vein for the purpose of removing blood.

**phobia** Abnormal fear.

**photophobia** Abnormal sensitivity to light; often found in congenital glaucoma, corneal abrasions, and conjunctivitis.

**physical dependence** The altered state produced by the repeated administration of a drug. When the drug is stopped, withdrawal symptoms occur.

**physical restraints** Any manual method or physical device that the patient cannot remove, that restricts physical activity, and that is not a usual and customary part of a medical, diagnostic, or treatment procedure.

**pica** A craving to eat substances that are not foods, such as dirt, clay, chalk, glue, or hair.

**pinna** Auricle of the ear, or the cartilaginous external ear.

**pinworm** Small parasitic worm that matures in the large intestine and crawls to the outside of the rectum to deposit its eggs.

**placebo** Any substance or procedure that is used as a supposedly effective treatment and that produces an effect in the patient because of its intent and not because of its specific physical or chemical properties. It is used to satisfy a patient's need for therapy or as a means of control in research studies.

**planning** That stage of the nursing process that involves the development of an orderly mental or written design of action on the basis of needs and the real or potential problems that have been identified in the patient. It is this stage in which nursing actions or interventions are proposed and goals or expected outcomes are identified.

**plaques** Atherosclerotic fatty deposits found in the intima of blood vessels; often the coronary arteries are affected.

**plasmapheresis** Process of separating the plasma and the red blood cells.

**Platyhelminthes** Flatworms.

**pleural friction rub** Grating, squeeking sound caused by inflamed and roughened pleura surfaces rubbing together.

**pleurisy** Inflammation of the pleura.

*Pneumocystis carinii* **pneumonia** See PCP.

**pneumonectomy** Surgical removal of a lung.

**pneumonia** An acute inflammation of the lungs; often caused by inhaled pneumococci.

**pneumothorax** A collection of air or gas in the pleural space, which causes the lung to collapse.

**poikilothermy** Variations in body temperature in relation to the environment as a result of a loss of sympathetic nerve activity.

**pollinosis** An allergic condition; same as hay fever.

**polychronic time** Perception that time is not linear, placing a higher value on people rather than on a specific time schedule.

**polycythemia** An abnormal increase in the number of erythrocytes in the blood.

**polyendocrine deficiency syndrome** More than one endocrine deficiency; usually associated with hypofunction of the adrenal cortex (Addison's disease).

**polyp** A small, tumorlike growth that projects from a mucous membrane.

**polyuria** Increased urinary output.

**populations** Aggregation of individuals, often with specific characteristics in common.

**porcine graft** Temporary biologic heterograft taken from the skin of a pig.

**Post Anesthesia Care Unit (PACU)** Specifically equipped unit where a patient recovers from anesthesia; airway reflexes return and breathing is satisfactory.

**posttraumatic stress disorder** An anxiety disorder that originates with a traumatic event and is characterized by nightmares, flashbacks, physiologic symptoms, and acute anxiety attacks. This disorder can occur soon after the traumatic event or can occur years later.

**power of attorney for health care** A document establishing a health care agent to make a health care decision for you if you are not capable of making them for yourself.

**preferred provider organization (PPO)** An organization of physicians, hospitals, and pharmacists whose members discount their healthcare services to subscriber patients.

**prepuce** A fold of skin that forms a retractable cover as the foreskin of the penis.

**presbycusis** Impairment of hearing as a result of degenerative changes; a common cause of sensorineural loss associated with aging.

**pressure ulcer** Bedsore, decubitus ulcer; an ulcerated area of the skin caused by continuous irritation and pressure on part of the body.

**primary care** The first contact in a given episode of illness that leads to a decision of what must be done to help resolve the problem. It is provided by the individual who is responsible for the continuum of care and includes maintenance of health, evaluation and management of symptoms, and appropriate referral. Primary care is usually provided by a physician; however, some primary care functions are now handled by nurses with advanced education and experience.

**primary hypertension** Elevated blood pressure with no identifiable cause that accounts for approximately 90% to 95% of all cases.

**primary infection** Intense, uncontrolled viral replication with a burst of virus in the blood occurring within the first few weeks after infection.

**primary nursing** An approach to nursing service that closely resembles the original case method. The primary nurse assumes complete responsibility for the total care of the patient from a mission to discharge. When off duty, the primary nurse is assisted by other nurses, who follow the directives of the plan of care established. Each primary nurse is assigned a group of patients, preferably no more than five.

**primary prevention** Involves activities that promote general well-being, as well as specific protection for selected diseases, such as immunizations for diphtheria, measles, and tetanus.

**prioritization** Process of determining order of importance.

**priority** Order of importance.

**problem-oriented medical record (POMR)** A system of record-keeping that involves the identification and numbering of patient problems. All progress notes and orders are directly related to patient problems, and each entry must consist of four parts designated by the acronym SOAP—subjective data, objective data, assessment, and plan.

**problem-oriented record (POR)** See problem-oriented medical record.

**proctoscopy** Examination of the rectum with an endoscope that is passed through the anus (proctoscope).

**proctosigmoidoscopy** Visualization of the sigmoid colon and rectum.

**prognosis** Expected outcome of a disease.

**progression** Advancing; developing steadily or in stages.

**prophylaxis** Treatment for preventative purposes occurring before or after exposure.

**proprietary** Operated for profit.

**proprioception** The brain's ability to know the spatial relation of the body's parts.

**prospective payment** Third party reimbursement on the basis of predetermined cost rather than actual costs incurred.

**prostate gland** A chestnut-sized gland in men that surrounds the neck of the bladder and the urethra. The ejaculatory ducts pass through the prostate to the urethra.

**prostatitis** Inflammation of the prostate gland.

**prosthesis** Any artificial device used to replace a missing part of the body.

**prosthetist** A person skilled in making and fitting prostheses.

*Proteus morganii* A species of bacteria that may cause infectious diarrhea in infants.

*Proteus vulgaris* A species of bacteria found in feces, water, and soil; a frequent cause of urinary tract infection.

**Protozoa** A phylum of unicellular organisms.

**pruritus** Itching of the skin.

*Pseudomonas* Microorganism found on the skin or in the intestinal tract of humans; may be the cause of hospital-acquired infections. It is resistant to most antibiotics.

**pseudophakia** The condition of the eye after the lens is removed and an artificial lens has been implanted (IOL—intraocular lens implant).

**psilocybin** Active agent of the *Psilocybe mexicana* mushroom; classified as a hallucinogenic agent.

**psoriasis** A chronic skin disease characterized by scaly patches and desquamation.

**psychoneurosis** An emotional maladaptation in which the chief characteristic is anxiety.

**psychophysiologic reactions** Physical disorders resulting from an inward bodily channeling of anxiety and stress.

**psychoses** A major organic or emotional disorder resulting in an inability to function effectively in life; there may be loss of contact with reality.

**psychosomatic** Refers to disorders for which no pathologic condition can be found.

**ptosis** A dropping from the normal position, such as ptosis of the eyelid in facial paralysis.

**puberty** Period at which the ability to reproduce begins.

**pulmonary edema** A condition in which left ventricular heart failure occurs, which causes a slowing of the systemic circulation and backup of returning blood; a serious condition.

**pulmonary embolism** A condition that is usually caused by a blood clot that breaks away from its place of origin and travels by the bloodstream to the lungs, where it lodges in a small vessel.

**pulmonary emphysema** A chronic obstructive disease of the lungs in which there is an overdistention of the alveoli.

**pulse deficit** Difference between the radial pulse rate and apical pulse rate.

**Purkinje's fibers** Continuation of the bundle of His that extends into the muscle walls of the ventricles.

**purpura** Bleeding into the skin.

**purulent** Describes a discharge that contains pus.

**pustule** An elevated skin lesion that contains pus.

**pyelitis** Inflammatory condition of the kidney pelvis.

**pyelography** X-ray examination of the kidney pelvis; may include the ureters after injection of a radiopaque medium.

**pyelonephritis** An inflammatory condition that involves the kidney pelvis and extends into kidney tissue.

**pyloric spasm** Severe and painful spasm of the pyloric valve.

**pyurla** Pus in the urine.

**quadriplegia** Paralysis of all four extremities.

**quality assurance/quality improvement** Planned, systematic process for monitoring and evaluating the appropriateness of care, evaluating quality of service, and resolving existing problems.

**quality of life** Expression used in speaking of issues relating to normalizing the life of a chronically ill individual. In defining quality of life, healthcare providers must consider not only the physical responses to medical therapy but also the psychologic implications of illness for both the patient and family. The overriding goal of care should be to relieve suffering and increase patient well-being. This concept varies among individuals but may include autonomy, security, and freedom in interpersonal relationships.

**quarantine** Isolation for a given time that prohibits person-to-person contact; used in infectious diseases.

**Queckenstedt's test** A test used in diagnosing an obstruction of the spinal cord.

**radiation therapy** Treatment of neoplastic disease by use of gamma ray or x-rays.

**radioactive substance** Any substance that is capable of giving off rays as a result of disintegration, such as radium.

**radioisotope** A chemical element that has been made radioactive and that emits rays of energy.

**radiopaque** A substance that cannot be penetrated by any form of radiation; used in x-ray examination of internal structures.

**range of joint motion (ROJM)** Motion of the limbs of the body to stretch the muscles, ligaments, and tendons that surround and support each joint.

**Raynaud's phenomenon** Vasospasm of cold hands resulting in pallor, numbness, and pain of unknown cause; arteriospastic disease.

**reaginic antibody** IgE immunoglobulin that is elevated in hypersensitive individuals.

**reality orientation** A small group activity in which the group leader emphasizes such concepts as time, day, month, and weather.

**receptors** Membrane proteins that enable neurotransmitters to exert their effects.

**recovery room** A postanesthesia care unit.

**referred pain** Pain felt at a site other than its origin.

**reflex** An involuntary act.

**refraction** Bending of light rays entering the eye; also used to describe the technique of selecting lenses to correct optical defects of the eye (e.g., myopia, hyperopia).

**regression** Going backward.

**regurgitation** Usually applied to the return of food or fluids from the stomach.

**rehabilitation** Process of assisting an individual after a disabling event has occurred.

**rehabilitation nursing** Specialty practice area focusing on diagnosis and treatment of human responses of individuals and groups to actual or potential health problems stemming from altered functional ability and altered life-style.

**reimbursement** Repayment for an expense or loan.

**relapse** Falling back into a previous or worse condition; in substance abuse, the return to drinking or use of any mind-altering drug.

**relaxation techniques** Procedures that help the patient achieve freedom from mental and physical tension or stress.

**reminiscing** Recalling past events or experiences.

**remission** Relief from or temporary improvement of symptoms; opposite of exacerbation.

**remodeling** Reorganization or renovation of a preexisting structure, such as a bone or joint.

**remotivation** The use of special techniques that stimulate patients to become motivated to learn and interact.

**renal threshold** The maximum amount of a substance that can be reabsorbed by the renal tubules, at which point the excess is excreted into the urine.

**reservoir** Location where an infectious agent is usually found; where it lives and reproduces under normal circumstances.

**residual** Refers to the part remaining, such as urine remaining in the bladder after catheterization.

**respite** Period of relief from responsibilities for the care of a patient.

**responsibility** Condition of accepting important duties or obligations.

**resuscitation** The restoration of life or consciousness of one apparently dead.

**reticular activating system** Nerve pathways in the brain concerned with level of consciousness; integrates information and determines overall activity of the brain and autonomic nervous system.

**reticular formation** Network of nerve pathways connecting sensory and motor nerves to the spinal cord, cerebellum, cerebrum, and cranial nerves.

**reticulocyte** Immature red blood cell.

**retinopathy** Noninflammatory condition resulting in small vessel changes in the eyes.

**retirement** Period in one's life when one leaves a job and enters another phase of life.

**retrospective payment** Reimbursement payment to agencies after service has been provided.

**rheumatoid arthritis** Autoimmune disease that causes chronic inflammation of connective tissue primarily in the joints.

**rhinitis** Inflammation of the nasal mucosa.

**rhinorrhea** Watery mucus discharge from the nose.

**rhizotomy** A neurosurgical procedure in which the anterior or posterior root of a spinal nerve is resected either by surgery or radiofrequency electrodes to relieve pain.

**rickettsiae** Small bodies that occupy an intermediate position between bacteria and viruses.

**rigidity** Inflexibility.

**ringworm** A skin disorder caused by a fungus.

**risk factors** A factor that causes a person or a group of people to be particularly vulnerable to an unwanted, unpleasant, or unhealthy event.

**roentgen** Unit for measuring radiation, such as in x-rays.

**roles and responsibilities** The characteristics of a job and the duties or obligations that it requires.

**rose spots** Small rose-colored spots on the abdomen; occur in typhoid fever.

**Ryan White Act (Comprehensive AIDS Resources Emergency) Act** Passed in 1990 to provide services for persons with HIV infection, this act seeks "to improve the quality and availability of care for individuals and families with HIV disease." It directs financial assistance for emergency services to metropolitan areas that have the largest numbers of reported cases of AIDS and to all states for improved care, support, and early intervention services.

**saccule** One of two small sacs that separate the semicircular canals from the cochlea. Serve as vestibular receptors.

**sarcoma** A type of malignant tumor that arises from connective tissue such as bone, muscle, and cartilage.

**scale** A small, thin flake of dry epidermis.

**scar** A mark left on the skin after repair of tissue.

**Schick's test** A subcutaneous skin test to determine immunity to diphtheria.

**schizophrenia** Psychotic behavior in which there are a variety of subgroups; consists of alterations in association, affect, ambivalence, autism, and attention.

**scintillator** A device used to measure the amount of radioactive material in a part of the body.

**scolex** Segment of the tapeworm that forms the head with hooks or suckers.

**scrotum** The pouch of skin containing the testes and spermatic cords.

**sebaceous gland** Gland in the skin that opens into hair follicles and secretes an oily substance called sebum.

**seborrhea** An increased secretion of sebum from the sebaceous glands.

**sebum** Secretion from the sebaceous glands.

**secondary hypertension** Hypertension that is associated with problems within the renal or endocrine system; often reversible when the underlying problem is controlled.

**secondary prevention** The level of prevention of illness that focuses on making early diagnoses and implementing measures to stop the progression of disease processes or handicapping disabilities.

**sedimentation rate**   Rate at which red blood cells settle when blood is placed in a test tube.

**seizure**   A sudden loss of consciousness, such as in epilepsy.

**self-actualization**   The fundamental tendency toward the maximum realization and fulfillment of one's human potential. Highest need in Maslow's hierarchy of human needs.

**semen**   Thick, whitish secretion of male reproductive organs; discharged from the urethra during ejaculation.

**semicircular canals**   Part of the inner ear. Contain fluid and hair cells; help to maintain a sense of balance.

**seminal vesicles**   Male accessory sex glands that open into the vas deferens before it joins the urethera.

**senescence**   Process of becoming old, or old age.

**sensitized**   Describes tissues that have been made susceptible to antigenic substances.

**sepsis**   Destruction of tissue by infectious organisms or their toxins.

**septicemia**   A bloodstream infection resulting from invasion of the blood by bacteria or their toxins.

**sequential compression device (SCD)**   Devices used to increase venous return after surgery.

**sexual assault**   Any sexual act done without permission.

**sexuality**   A person's need for comfort, touch, companionship, and love that may or may not be expressed through sexual activity.

**shear**   Clip or cut off.

**shearing force**   Causing two contracting parts to slide on one another.

**shearlings**   Sheepskins used on the bed to help prevent decubitus ulcers.

**sickle-cell anemia**   Congenital disease marked by sickle-shaped red blood cells; occurs most commonly in blacks.

**sigmoidoscopy**   Examination of the sigmoid colon with a sigmoidoscope.

**sinoatrial node**   Cells located in the right atrial wall that contract to set the rate of the heartbeat; initiated electric conduction system of the heart; called the pacemaker.

**sinus bradycardia**   A slowing of the heart action to 60 or fewer beats per minute.

**sinus tachycardia**   Rapid beating of the heart in excess of 100 beats per minute.

**situational depression**   A depression that occurs as a result of a specific, identifiable event or events in which feelings of sadness and loss do not resolve within a normal period of time.

**skilled-nursing facility (SNF)**   A nursing home that provides 24-hour nursing services, regular medical supervision, and rehabilitation therapy.

**SOAP**   The acronym that designates the four parts of each entry in a problem-oriented record—subjective data, objective data, assessment, and plan.

**socioeconomic**   Interaction of social and economic factors.

**sordes**   A foul accumulation of secretions and crusts around the teeth and gums; caused by lack of oral care.

**source**   Location from which the infectious agent is immediately transmitted to the host.

**spastic**   Describes involuntary muscular contractions that result in rigidity.

**spasticity**   Resistance to passive movement of a limb that is greatest at the initiation of movement and gives way as increased pressure is applied; symptom of damage to the corticospinal tracts in the brain or spinal cord.

**spermatogenesis**   The process of development of spermatozoa.

**spermatozoa**   Mature male sex cell.

**sphincter**   Muscles that are circular in shape and that constrict an anatomic opening, such as the anal spincter.

**spinal shock**   Syndrome directly following acute spinal cord injury.

**spirometer**   Mechanical device to measure vital capacity.

**splenectomy**   Surgical removal of the spleen.

**splenomegaly**   Enlargement of the spleen.

**split-thickness skin graft**   Skin graft that leaves some dermis at the donor site, allowing that site to heal.

**spores**   Bacilli that are capable of changing into resistant forms and that can exist at high temperatures and in the presence of ordinary disinfectants.

**stabilization**   The creation of a stable state.

**standard precautions**   Procedures designed to reduce the risk of transmission of microorganisms from both known and unknown sources of infection; a synthesis of the major features of universal precautions and body substance isolation.

**standardized care plan**   A prewritten plan of care that includes outcomes, interventions, and evaluation that can be adapted or tailored to fit a particular patient situation.

**standards**   An evaluation that serves as a basis for comparison when evaluating similar phenomena or substances; also serves as a standard for the practice of a profession.

**stapedectomy**   Surgical procedure to correct otosclerosis, a disorder that prevents sound from reaching the inner ear.

**stapes**   One of three small bones in the middle ear—attached to the incus bone on one side and to the oval window on the other to transmit sound vibrations.

**Staphylococcus**   Species of bacteria that are often responsible for hospital-acquired infections.

**stasis**   Slowing or stopping the normal flow.

**stenosis**   Narrowing or constriction of a passageway, such as in the valves of the heart—mitral stenosis.

**stereotyping**   Considering a person to be representative of a particular group in all ways.

**sterilization**   Process of destroying all pathogenic microorganisms.

**stigma**   A mark of disgrace.

**stimulus**   Any action or agent that causes changes or action in an organ or part.

**stoma**   An opening onto the skin that is created by an artificial passageway; may also apply to the normal opening of a pore.

**stomatitis**   Inflammation of the mucous membranes of the mouth.

**strabismus**   Condition in which the muscles of the eyes are not aligned properly for three-dimensional vision. Eyes can turn inward, outward, upward, or downward.

**strawberry tongue**   Strawberrylike appearance of the tongue in scarlet fever.

**Streptococcus**   Species of bacteria that probably causes the most illness in man.

**stump**   Distal portion of an extremity after amputation.

**stuporous** Describes deep sleep with a diminished sense of feeling and responsiveness.

**subconscious** Partial responsiveness of the mind to impressions made by the senses.

**subculture** An ethnic, regional, economic, or social group with characteristic patterns of behavior that distinguish it from the larger culture or society.

**subjective data** Information obtained from the patient or family, either spontaneously or in response to direct questioning.

**substance abuse** Pathologic use of a mind-altering chemical that is accompanied by a loss of control over how much and how often the chemical is used.

**substance dependence** Addiction; the total psychophysical state of one who must receive an increasing amount of the chemical to prevent the onset of withdrawal symptoms.

**substance P** A chemical secreted by pain nerves; a neurotransmitter.

**suicide** Self-destruction.

**sunstroke** Disorder caused by overexposure to the sun.

**superego** In Freudian theory, that part of the personality structure that contains society's mores. It may often be self-critical.

**supervision/supervisory** The process of directing the work or actions of others; includes the assessment of the appropriateness of delegation.

**surfactant** Liquid secreted by alveolar cells that enhances lung inflation and keeps alveoli dry.

**surgical asepsis** The complete absence of organisms (germs).

**surgical procedure** Operation; commonly classified as emergency, scheduled, or elective.

**surveillance** Supervising or watching a person or a condition.

**sync time** Type of time perception involving rhythmic interactions.

**synovectomy** Excision of the synovial membrane of a joint.

**synovial membrane** Sac that encloses a freely moving joint; secretes synovial fluid that lubricates the joint.

**systolic blood pressure** Peak pressure within the vessels immediately following ventricular contraction; primarily affected by cardiac output.

**systemic infection** Infection spread throughout the body.

**tachycardia** A cardiac arrhythmia that results in a very rapid heartbeat.

**tangential** A change in direction although somewhat related to the original subject.

**team** A decentralized system in which the care of a patient is distributed among the members of a team of various professionals and/or family and friends.

**team nursing** A nursing service approach that uses the skills of a variety of nursing personnel in providing comprehensive care for the patient. The leader, a registered nurse, is assisted in the care of a group of patients by other nurses, LVN/LPNs, nursing assistants, and orderlies. The leader assigns and directs patient care on the basis of input from team members.

**telangiectasia** A localized group of distended capillaries in the skin.

**tenacious** Describes secretions that are sticky and stringy and tend to hold together.

**tentorium** Sheet of dura mater that separates the cerebellum from the occipital lobes of the cerebral hemispheres.

**terminal disinfection** Cleaning of equipment and airing of room after the release of a person who has had an infectious disease.

**tertiary prevention** The level of prevention of illness that deals with rehabilitation of a disabled person to return the person to a level of maximum usefulness.

**testes** Male sex organs that produce spermatozoa and secrete androgen.

**testosterone** The primary male sex hormone; a type of androgen.

**tetany** A condition characterized by cramps, convulsions, muscle twitching, and sharp flexion of the wrist and ankle joints (carpopedal spasm).

**thanatology** Study of death and dying.

**therapist** A person skilled in various therapeutic techniques.

**thermography** Technique of determining surface temperature of the body through photography.

**third spacing** The accumulation of fluid in areas that normally have no fluid or a minimal amount of fluid, as seen in ascites or in the edema associated with burns.

**thoracic cage** Part of the body between the neck and the diaphragm that is enclosed by the sternum, costal cartilage, ribs, and thoracic vertebrae of the spine; encloses the heart, lungs, esophagus, and related structures.

**thoracotomy** A surgical opening into the thoracic cavity.

**thrombocytes** Platelets; disc-shaped cell structures circulating in the blood that assist in coagulation of blood.

**thrombocytopenia** Decreased number of platelets in the circulating blood.

**thrombophlebitis** Inflammation of a vein; caused by a thrombus.

**thrombosis** Presence of a blood clot.

**thrush** An infection of the mouth and throat; caused by a fungus and usually occurs in infants.

**tinea** Ringworm; disease is further differentiated by the area of body affected. Tinea capitis—scalp; tinea barbae—beard and mustache; tinea corporis—body; tinea cruris—groin (jock itch); tinea manus—hand; tinea pedis—foot (athlete's foot).

**tinnitus** Ringing in the ears.

**tissue macrophage** Any phagocytic cell of the reticuloendothelial system, including cells in the liver, spleen, and connective tissue.

**tolerance** State in which increasingly larger doses of a drug are needed to provide the same effect as was produced by the original dose.

**tonic** Refers to tension of contraction.

**tonometry** Measurement of intraocular pressure.

**tonsillectomy** Surgical removal of tonsils.

**tophus, tophi** deposit of urates in tissues around joints; seen in gout.

**total body surface area (TBSA)** Measurement used to determine fluid and nutritional needs of the burn patient.

**total parenteral nutrition** An intravenous technique to provide for nutritional needs.

**total quality management** A type of quality assurance program.

**toxemia**   Presence of toxins or poisons in the blood.

**toxicity**   State of being poisonous.

**toxoid**   Toxins produced by microorganisms that have been treated with chemicals or heat to decrease their toxic effect and retain their ability to stimulate the immune system.

**trabeculae**   Portion of the eye in front of Schlemm's canal and within the angle created by the iris and the cornea.

**trabeculectomy**   Surgical removal of a section of corneoscleral tissue, usually including Schlemm's canal and the trabecular meshwork. Increases outflow of aqueous humor in patients with chronic side-angle glaucoma.

**trabeculoplasty**   Use of the laser to apply burns in the trabecular meshwork to improve aqueous humour outflow in chronic, open-angle glaucoma.

**tracheostomy**   Permanent opening into the trachea after a tracheotomy.

**tracheotomy**   An incision is made into the trachea through the neck and below the larynx to gain access to the airway below the blockage that has been caused by a foreign body, tumor, or edema of the glottis.

**traction**   Exerting a force that pulls or draws on a muscle or organ.

**transcultural nursing**   Area of nursing that focuses on study of the health-illness caring practices, beliefs, and values of different cultures and subcultures.

**transcutaneous electrical neural stimulation (TENS)**   Alteration of pain sensations by stimulating peripheral nerves with electric current that is applied to the skin.

**transected**   Cut across or severed.

**transient ischemic attack (TIA)**   Temporary disruption of the circulation to a portion of the brain caused by emboli, thrombi, or spasm of cerebral blood vessels.

**transplantation**   Surgical transfer of an organ from a donor to a recipient.

**tremor**   Involuntary trembling of the body or the extremities.

**triage**   System of assigning priorities in treating patients in a disaster or emergency situation.

**trichinosis**   Infection with trichina, a worm found in pork.

**trichomoniasis**   Infection with the *Trichomonas* parasite.

**Trousseau's phenomenon**   Carpopedal spasm following interruption of arterial circulation by a blood pressure cuff for 3 minutes.

**tuning fork**   A metal, two-pronged fork that vibrates to test hearing.

**turgor**   The elasticity of the skin.

**tympanic membrane (eardrum)**   A thin, semitransparent membrane in the middle ear that transmits sound vibrations to the inner ear by means of the auditory vessicles.

**tympanoplasty**   A group of surgical procedures to restore hearing; involves the eardrum or the bones of the middle ear.

**type I diabetes**   Insulin-dependent diabetes mellitus.

**type II diabetes**   Noninsulin-dependent diabetes mellitus.

**ulcer**   An open lesion on the skin with loss of deep tissue.

**ultrasonogram**   An instrument that measures and records the reflection of pulsed or continuous high-frequency sound waves to detect abnormalities.

**unconscious**   The part of the mind that is only rarely in one's awareness. It contains experiences or data that may be too painful to recall.

**unfinished business**   Concerns of the dying patient that require resolution before death can be accepted; range from financial factors to interpersonal relationships.

**universal precautions**   CDC-recommended "universal blood and body fluid precautions." Includes preventing injury from needles and sharp objects; wearing protective devices during resuscitation; avoiding patient and equipment contact if a draining lesion exists in healthcare worker.

**unlicensed worker**   A worker whose role and responsibilities are not governed by law.

**urea**   Chief end-product of protein metabolism; excreted by the kidney.

**uremia**   Accumulation of urinary constituents in the blood; causes a general toxic condition.

**ureter**   One of two tubes that conduct urine from the pelvis of the kidneys to the bladder.

**ureterotomy**   Incision into a ureter.

**urinalysis**   Analysis of components of urine.

**urine osmolality**   Measurement of the concentration of urine.

**urticaria**   Hives; an allergic reaction characterized by the appearance of wheals on the skin.

**uveitis**   Inflammation of one or more parts of the uveal tract, which includes the ciliary body, iris, and cornea.

**vaccine**   A pathogen whose virulence has been reduced and which is used as prophylaxis against a disease.

**vaginitis**   Inflammation of the vagina.

**values**   Used subjectively to identify what a person considers worthwhile; used objectively to identify the intrinsic quality (good) of a thing.

**varicocele**   A varicosity or dilation of veins in the spermatic cord.

**varicosities**   Dilated, tortous vericosed veins.

**vasogenic shock**   Shock resulting from peripheral vascular dilation; caused by factors (toxins) that directly affect blood vessels.

**vector**   An insect, rodent, or arthropod that carries disease and transmits it to humans.

**vectorborne transmission**   Occurs when insects or other animals serve as intermediate hosts for an infectious agent and then transmit it to humans through a sting or bite.

**vegetative bacteria**   Bacteria that do not form spores.

**vehicle**   Mode of transmission of an infective agent from its source to a susceptible host.

**vehicle transmission**   Occurs when contaminated items such as blood, blood products, food, water, or drugs serve as the source of transmission.

**veins**   Blood vessels that carry blood to the heart.

**venous access device**   An intravenous pump that patients use to give themselves limited doses of fast-acting analgesics at the onset of pain.

**venous stasis**   Obstruction and pooling of blood in the veins.

**ventilation**   The movement of air into and out of the lungs.

**ventricles**   Small cavities, such as in the heart or brain.

**ventricular fibrillation**   Disorganization of the heartbeat; may cause cardiac arrest without prompt treatment.

**ventricular tachycardia**   Rapid contraction of the ventricle with reduced cardiac output.

**ventriculogram**   A diagnostic procedure in which air is injected into the cerebral ventricles and x-ray films are taken.

**veracity** Telling the truth habitually.

**vertigo** A sensation characterized by the movement of objects or of self-movement; an extreme form of dizziness.

**vesicant** A drug that induces blistering. Vesicant chemotherapeutic agents cause tissue damage if they leak out of the vein during administration.

**vesicle** A blisterlike elevation on the skin that contains serous fluid.

**vesiculation** Formation of vesicles.

**vestibule** A cavity in the inner ear that contains two small sacs, the utricle and saccule.

**viral load** The amount of virus in the body.

**viral resistance** Ability of a virus to become unaffected by drug therapy.

**virology** Study of viruses.

**virulence** Strength of an organism to produce disease.

**viruses** Infective agents that cause several diseases.

**visceral pleura** Membrane covering the surface of the lungs.

**viscosity** Thickness of a fluid that causes it to resist flow.

**visual analog scale** A rating scale that uses a line to represent a continuum; the ends are marked for the two extremes of pain.

**vital capacity** Amount of air that can be retained in the lungs after a full inspiration.

**vitrectomy** Removal of blood, opacities, or disease from the posterior segment of the eye; vitreous gel is replaced with an isotonic solution.

**vulvovaginitis** Inflammation of the vagina, the vulva, and usually the vulvovaginal glands.

**Wangensteen suction** A suction-siphonage method to remove secretions from the stomach.

**wen** A cyst that often occurs on the back of the scalp.

**Western Blot** A test for the presence of antibodies to multiple antigens of HIV; used to confirm HIV infection following a positive ELISA test. The Western Blot displays antibodies to specific HIV viral proteins in a separate, well-defined band. A positive result shows stripes at the locations for two or more viral proteins. A negative result is blank at these locations.

**wheal** An elevated type of rash on the skin, such as in urticaria.

**wheezes** Musical, continuous, adventitious sounds caused by airway narrowing or bronchoconstriction.

**withdrawal syndrome** A syndrome of serious symptoms that occurs when the use of a drug is discontinued.

**wound healing** Repair of a break in the skin.

**wound infection** Invasion of a wound by pathogenic microorganisms that reproduce and multiply, causing injury.

# Index

Page numbers in italics indicate illustrations; *t* indicates tables.

Urostomy, continent, procedure for, 1159-1160
Urticaria
  symptoms and treatment, *1287*, 1287-1288
  testing for, 131
US TOO, 269
Uterine cancer
  checkup guidelines for people without symptoms, 245*t*
  risk factors for, 244
  symptoms and treatment, 1366
Uterine prolapse
  in elderly, 176
  pathophysiology, assessment, interventions, 1363
Uterus
  cross-section of, *1333*
  fibroid tumors of, 1366
  positions of, 1333, *1334*
  structure and function of, 1332-1333
Utilitarianism, 65
Uveal tract, structure and function of, 1173-1174
Uveitis, symptoms and interventions, 1197-1198
Uvula, assessment of, 50

**V**

Vaccines; *see also* Immunizations
  types of, 296
Vagina
  after menopause, 1342
  structure and function of, 1332
Vaginal cancer, treatment of, 1365
Vaginitis
  in elderly, 176
  pathophysiology, assessment, intervention, 1362
Vagotomy for peptic ulcer disease, 1078
Vagus nerve, function of, 919*t*
Validation therapy, 178
Valium; *see* Diazepam
Valproic acid for neurologic problems, 937*t*
Valsalva, sinus of, 628
Values
  in death/dying, 276
  defined, 64, 145
  examples, 145
Valves, cardiac, 627, *627*
Varicella; *see also* Chickenpox
  complications of, 1281
  immunizations against, 297*t*
  symptoms of, 1277-1278
Varicella-zoster virus
  in chickenpox, 312
  in symptomatic HIV disease, 361-362
Varices, esophageal, causes of, 1108
Varicocele, symptoms and treatment, 1314
Varicosed veins, 718, *752*, 752-756
  assessment of, 724-725, 753
  causes of, 753
  exacerbating factors, 753
  medical and nursing interventions, 753-756
    conservative, 754-755
    invasive, 755-756
  risk factors for, 721*t*, 722
  types of, 752-753
Vasa recta capillaries, 1123
Vascular purpuras, pathophysiology, assessment, interventions, 817
Vasectomy, 1315-1316, *1316*, 1354

Vasodilators
  in antihypertensive therapy, 780
  for congestive heart failure, 703-704
Vasogenic shock, causes and treatment, 862-863
Vasopressin; *see* Antidiuretic hormone
Vasotec; *see* Enalapril
Vector-borne transmission
  characteristics of, 296
  of nosocomial infections, 331
Vecuronium, perioperative applications, 494*t*
Vehicle transmission
  characteristics of, 296
  of nosocomial infections, 330-331
Vein(s), *717*
  coronary, *628*, 628-629
  peripheral, assessment of, 635
  structure and function of, 718, *718*
  varicosed; *see* Varicosed veins
Vein stripping for varicosed veins, 755
Velban; *see* Vinblastine
Vena cava(e), 630
Venereal warts with symptomatic HIV infection, 368
Venous circulation, impairment of, 995
Venous problems, 752-761; *see also* specific conditions
  anxiety associated with, 762
  characteristics of, 722*t*
  deep vein thrombosis, 758-760
  superficial venous thrombophlebitis, 757
  varicosed veins, 752-756
  venous stasis ulcers, 761
  venous thrombosis, 756-757
Venous stasis
  causes of, 723
  defined, 718
Venous stasis ulcers, assessment and interventions, 761
Venous thrombophlebitis; *see* Thrombophlebitis
Venous thrombosis, 756-757; *see also* Deep vein thrombosis
  characteristics of, 722*t*
  during pregnancy, 720
  unilateral edema in, 724
  Virchow's triad in, 756
Ventilation
  diseases interfering with, 596
  mechanical, indications and procedures, 582
  process of, 560
Ventricles, cardiac, 626
Ventricular aneurysm as complication of MI, 679*t*
Ventricular arrhythmias, 655-657
  asystole, 656-657, *658*
  premature ventricular contractions, 655, *655*
  ventricular fibrillation, 656, *657*
  ventricular tachycardia, 656, *656*
Ventricular fibrillation, 656, *657*
Ventricular rate, ECG evaluation of, 646-647
Ventricular standstill, 656-657, *658*
Ventricular tachycardia, 656, *656*
Venturi mask, 579, *579*
  oxygen concentration for, 580*t*
Venules, structure and function of, 718
VePesid; *see* Etoposide
Verapamil
  in antihypertensive therapy, 777*t*
  for cardiac problems, 674*t*
Vermiform appendix, 1042

Versed; *see* Midazolam
Vertigo
  ambulation and, 1237
  assessing, 1226
  defined, 1223
Vesicles
  characteristics and examples, *1248*
  defined, 1249
Vesicovaginal fistula, causes, symptoms, treatment, 1362-1363
Vestibule, 1222
Veterans Administration, rehabilitative services of, 412
Vibramycin; *see* Doxycycline
Vibration
  contraindications to, 576
  during postural drainage, 576
*Vibrio parahaemolyticus*, food poisoning due to, characteristics and transmission, 307*t*
Vicodin; *see* Hydrocodone
Vidarabine for vision problems, 1189*t*
Videx; *see* Didanosine
Vinblastine for cancer, 261*t*
Vincent de Paul, St., 466
Vincristine for cancer, 261*t*
Violence, 538-543
  in emergency departments, 538-539
  as epidemic health problem, 538
  family; *see* Family violence
  patients prone to, 539
  prevention of, 538
Vira-A Ophthalmic; *see* Vidarabine
Viracept; *see* Nelfinavir
Viral hepatitis; *see also* Hepatitis
  cause, findings, treatment, 314-315
  immunizations against, 299
Viral infections, 310-315
  chickenpox, 312
  complications of, 1281
  hepatitis, 314-315
  herpes zoster, 312
  infectious mononucleosis, 313
  influenza, 313-314
  measles, 310-311
  mumps, 312-313
  nursing process for, 1279
  rubella, 311-312
  of skin, 1276-1279
  in symptomatic HIV infection, gastrointestinal, 362-363
Viral load
  defined, 355
  guide for test results, 386
  measures of, 385-386
  testing for, 385-386
Virchow's triad, 756
Viridans streptococci, 109-110
Viroptic Ophthalmic Solution; *see* Trifluridine
Virtue ethics, 65
Virulence, defined, 118, 294
Virus(es)
  cancer-inducing, 242
  characteristics and infections, 110
  classification of, 110, 111*t*
  disinfection of, 340
  structure of, mutations in, 388
Visceral pleura, 559
Vision, 1173-1220; *see also* Eye(s); Eye problems; specific conditions
  aging and, 60*t*, 167-168, 451
  light refraction in, 1175-1176